ANESTHESIOLOGY & CRITICAL CARE DRUG HANDBOOK

Including Select Disease States & Perioperative Management

Also includes an International Brand Name Index

Andrew J. Donnelly, PharmD, MBA
Verna L. Baughman, MD
Jeffrey P. Gonzales, PharmD, BCPS
Julie Golembiewski, PharmD
Elizabeth A. Tomsik, PharmD, BCPS

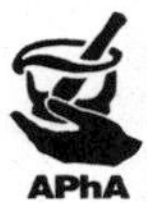

Lexi-Comp is the official drug reference for the American Pharmacists Association

7th Edition

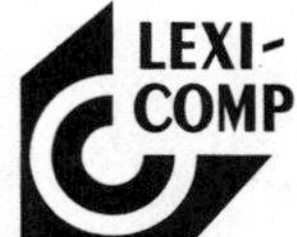

ANESTHESIOLOGY & CRITICAL CARE DRUG HANDBOOK

Including Select Disease States & Perioperative Management

Also includes an International Brand Name Index

Andrew J. Donnelly, PharmD, MBA
Director of Pharmacy
University of Illinois Hospital
Clinical Professor
Department of Pharmacy Practice
University of Illinois at Chicago College of Pharmacy
Chicago, Illinois

Verna L. Baughman, MD
Professor, Anesthesiology and Neurosurgery
University of Illinois
Chicago, Illinois

Jeffrey P. Gonzales, PharmD, BCPS
Critical Care Clinical Pharmacy Specialist
University of Maryland Medical Center
Baltimore, Maryland

Julie Golembiewski, PharmD
Clinical Pharmacist, Anesthesia/Pain
Clinical Associate Professor
Departments of Pharmacy Practice and Anesthesiology
University of Illinois at Chicago College of Pharmacy and Medicine
Chicago, Illinois

Elizabeth A. Tomsik, PharmD, BCPS
Pharmacotherapy Specialist
Medical Science Division
Lexi-Comp, Inc.
Hudson, Ohio

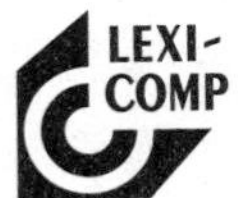

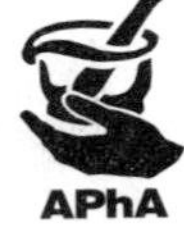

This data is intended to serve the user as a handy reference and not as a complete drug information resource. It does not include information on every therapeutic agent available. The publication covers 546 commonly used drugs and is specifically designed to present important aspects of drug data in a more concise format than is typically found in medical literature or product material supplied by manufacturers.

The nature of drug information is that it is constantly evolving because of ongoing research and clinical experience and is often subject to interpretation. While great care has been taken to ensure the accuracy of the information presented, the reader is advised that the authors, editors, reviewers, contributors, and publishers cannot be responsible for the continued currency of the information or for any errors, omissions, or the application of this information, or for any consequences arising therefrom. Therefore, the author(s) and/or the publisher shall have no liability to any person or entity with regard to claims, loss, or damage caused, or alleged to be caused, directly or indirectly, by the use of information contained herein. Because of the dynamic nature of drug information, readers are advised that decisions regarding drug therapy must be based on the independent judgment of the clinician, changing information about a drug (eg, as reflected in the literature and manufacturer's most current product information), and changing medical practices. Therefore, this data is designed to be used in conjunction with other necessary information and is not designed to be solely relied upon by any user. The user of this data hereby and forever releases the authors of this data for any and all liability of any kind that might arise out of the use of this data. The editors are not responsible for any inaccuracy of quotation or for any false or misleading implication that may arise due to the text or formulas as used or due to the quotation of revisions no longer official.

The authors, editors, and contributors have written this book in their private capacities. No official support or endorsement by any federal or state agency or pharmaceutical company is intended or inferred.

The publishers have made every effort to trace the copyright holders for borrowed material. If they have inadvertently overlooked any, they will be pleased to make the necessary arrangements at the first opportunity.

If you have any suggestions or questions regarding any information presented in this data, please contact our drug information pharmacists at (330) 650-6506.

This manual was produced using the FormuLex™ Program —
a complete publishing service of Lexi-Comp Inc.

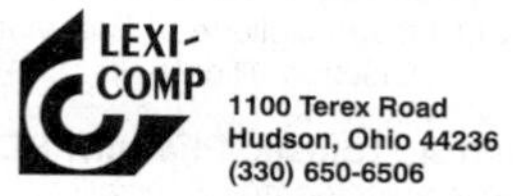

1100 Terex Road
Hudson, Ohio 44236
(330) 650-6506

ISBN 1-59195-144-5

TABLE OF CONTENTS

TABLE OF CONTENTS *(Continued)*

ABOUT THE AUTHORS

Andrew J. Donnelly, PharmD, MBA

Dr Donnelly received his Doctor of Pharmacy and Masters of Business Administration degrees from the University of Illinois. He has over 20 years of active pharmacy experience, with the majority concentrated in the areas of operating room pharmacy and anesthesiology. Dr Donnelly is currently Director of Pharmacy at the University of Illinois Hospital at Chicago. In addition, he holds the appointment of Clinical Professor in the Department of Pharmacy Practice at the University of Illinois at Chicago College of Pharmacy.

Throughout his years of operating room/anesthesiology pharmacy practice, Dr Donnelly has strived to expand the pharmacist's role in ensuring optimal patient outcome by developing methods to improve drug selection and use in the operating room setting. In recognition of this work, he was named a Fellow of the American Society of Health-System Pharmacists (FASHP). Dr Donnelly has published extensively in the areas of anesthesiology and operating room pharmacy and is frequently invited to speak at professional meetings on topics related to these areas.

Dr Donnelly is Associate Editor-in-Chief of *Anesthesia Today* and he serves on the editorial board of the *OR Pharmacy Services Bulletin*. He is an active member of the American Society of Health-System Pharmacists (ASHP); American Pharmacists Association (APhA); Society of Critical Care Medicine (SCCM); Operating Room Pharmacy Services Association; as well as various state and local pharmacy organizations.

Verna L. Baughman, MD

Dr Baughman is Professor of Anesthesiology and Neurosurgery at the University of Illinois at Chicago. She received her BA in 1968 from DePauw University, Greencastle, Indiana, with a major in both French and Biology. She then worked as a research editor/writer for the Encyclopaedia Britannica and as a hospital administrator. She attended Stritch School of Medicine at Loyola University, Chicago, receiving her medical degree in 1981. Following an internship and residency in Anesthesiology at Michael Reese Medical Center in Chicago, she spent a year as a Neuroanesthesia Research Fellow. Her interest in neuroanesthesia has dominated her laboratory research program, with a focus on stroke and the effects of various drug therapies in ameliorating neuronal damage from ischemia. She is also interested in the effects of estrogen and menopause in relation to cerebral ischemia.

Dr Baughman has to her credit over 100 publications including original research papers, textbook chapters, and editorials. She has been an active member of the editorial board for the Journal of Neurosurgical Anesthesia and Critical Care for sixteen years. She currently reviews papers for *Anesthesiology, Anesthesia & Analgesia, Journal of Clinical Anesthesia, Stroke* and *American Journal of Physiology.* She has been a visiting professor at many universities and a frequent lecturer at national meetings. Dr Baughman was cited in "Best Doctors in America" in 1995 and again in 1996.

Dr Baughman's interest in education is evidenced by consistently being voted by the resident staff as one of the best departmental teachers. She was selected to receive the 2001-2002 Excellence in Teaching Award, which recognizes quality teachers at the University of Illinois. In 2003 Dr Baughman was honored as the first Distinguished Teacher of the Year by the Society of Neurosurgical Anesthesia and Critical Care. She is also a consultant to the pharmaceutical industry, evaluating new drugs and equipment. Dr Baughman is an active member of the American Society of Anesthesiologists, Society of Neurosurgical Anesthesia and Critical Care, International Anesthesia Research Society, and Stroke Council of the American Heart Association.

ABOUT THE AUTHORS *(Continued)*

Jeffrey P. Gonzales, PharmD, BCPS

Dr Gonzales is currently the Critical Care Clinical Pharmacy Specialist at the University of Maryland Medical Center and holds a clinical practice in a 29-bed, state-of-the-art, Medical Intensive Care Unit. Dr Gonzales received his Doctor of Pharmacy degree at Idaho State University in Pocatello, Idaho. He completed a Pharmacy Practice Residency at the University of Nebraska Medical Center, then went on for specialized training with a Critical Care Residency at Detroit Receiving Hospital-Detroit Medical Center. Following his residency training, Dr Gonzales completed a Postdoctoral Fellowship in Critical Care at The University of Michigan College of Pharmacy, where he was the recipient of the 1999 American College of Clinical Pharmacy-Bayer Critical Care Fellowship Award.

After completion of his postgraduate training, he was the Critical Care Clinical Specialist at The Cleveland Clinic Foundation and practiced in the Medical Intensive Care Unit for 6 years. During that time, he was awarded the Ohio College of Clinical Pharmacy Bayer Board Certification Award and became a Board-Certified Pharmacotherapy Specialist (BCPS). At the Cleveland Clinic, he was involved with medical and pharmacy resident/student education, precepted numerous research projects, and created the Critical Care Pharmacy Residency. He was a member of the Pharmacology Curriculum Committee, Cleveland Clinic Lerner College of Medicine at Case Western Reserve University. He also received the 2004 Cleveland Clinic Foundation Department of Pharmacy Research and Education Award, as well as the 2005 Ohio College of Clinical Pharmacy-Pfizer Research Award. His areas of interests and research are sedation, sepsis, ARDS, pulmonary hypertension, and alterations in absorption in the critically ill.

Dr Gonzales is an active member of the Society of Critical Care Medicine (SCCM), the American College of Clinical Pharmacy (ACCP), and the American Society of Health-Systems Pharmacists (ASHP).

Julie Golembiewski, PharmD

Dr Golembiewski received her bachelor's degree in pharmacy and Doctor of Pharmacy degree from the University of Illinois at Chicago. She has over 20 years of active pharmacy experience, with the majority concentrated in the areas of operating room pharmacy and anesthesiology. She worked in the operating room pharmacy at the University of Illinois Medical Center at Chicago, then went on to manage an operating room pharmacy at Bergan Mercy Medical Center in Omaha, NE and The University of Michigan Health System in Ann Arbor, MI where she also held a faculty appointment of Clinical Associate Professor in the Clinical Sciences Department at the University of Michigan College of Pharmacy and Adjunct Assistant Professor of Anesthesiology at the University of Michigan Medical School.

Currently, Dr Golembiewski is a clinical pharmacist in anesthesia/pain at the University of Illinois Medical Center at Chicago (UIMCC) with a shared appointment in the Departments of Pharmacy Services and Anesthesiology. In addition, she holds the appointments of Clinical Associate Professor in the Departments of Pharmacy Practice and Anesthesiology at the University of Illinois at Chicago (UIC) College of Pharmacy and Medicine. At the UIMCC, Dr Golembiewski is a member of several committees including the Surgical Infection Prevention Team, the Pharmacy Resident Research Committee, the Medical Staff Committee on the Operating Room, and the Graduate Medical Education Committee for the Department of Anesthesiology. She is co-coordinator for the UIC Department of Anesthesiology for the Midwest Anesthesia Residents Conference, as well as co-chair of the Perioperative Beta-Blocker Quality Improvement Team. Dr Golembiewski teaches second and third year pharmacy students at the UIC College of Pharmacy and serves as a clerkship preceptor for fourth-year pharmacy students and pharmacy residents.

Dr Golembiewski has published extensively in the areas of anesthesiology and operating room pharmacy and is often invited to speak at professional meetings on topics related to these areas. She is on the editorial advisory board of *Anesthesia Today* and Pharmacy Practice News, and writes a regular column for the *Journal of PeriAnesthesia Nursing*. Dr Golembiewski is an active member of the Illinois Society of Health-System Pharmacists, the American Society of Health-System Pharmacists, and the American Pharmacists Association.

Elizabeth A. Tomsik, Pharm.D, BCPS

Dr Tomsik received her bachelor's degree in pharmacy from the Albany College of Pharmacy and her Doctor of Pharmacy degree from the University of Sciences in Philadelphia. She completed a one-year residency at Truman Medical Center in Kansas City and went on to work at Hahnemann University Hospital for 2 years in the field of nutrition. She continued her work at Louis Stokes Veterans Affairs Medical Center in Cleveland for 12 years. Her areas of practice included intensive care, coronary care, nutrition support, and anticoagulation. She was actively involved in residency training and was in charge of the pharmacy residency program for many years. She held faculty appointments from Case Western Reserve University, College of Medicine and The University of Toledo, College of Pharmacy. She has been a Board Certified Pharmacotherapy Specialist since 1999.

Dr Tomsik has been with Lexi-Comp, Inc since 1999. She is actively involved in developing and maintaining the patient education series (LEXI-PALS™ and PEDI-PALS™), enhancing the database with particular focus on the areas of critical care and coronary care, and working as an active participant in the Medical Science Division at Lexi-Comp, Inc.

Dr Tomsik is a member of the Ohio College of Clinical Pharmacy and the American College of Clinical Pharmacy, and the Society of Critical Care Medicine.

EDITORIAL ADVISORY PANEL

Larisa H. Cavallari, PharmD, BCPS
Assistant Professor, Section of Cardiology
University of Illinois
Chicago, Illinois

Harold L. Crossley, DDS, PhD
Associate Professor of Pharmacology
Baltimore College of Dental Surgery
Dental School
University of Maryland Baltimore
Baltimore, Maryland

Wayne R. DeMott, MD
Consultant in Pathology and Laboratory Medicine
Shawnee Mission, Kansas

Samir Desai, MD
Assistant Professor of Medicine
Department of Medicine
Baylor College of Medicine
Houston, Texas
Staff Physician
Veterans Affairs Medical Center
Houston, Texas

Andrew J. Donnelly, PharmD, MBA
Director of Pharmacy
and
Clinical Professor of Pharmacy Practice
University of Illinois Medical Center at Chicago
Chicago, Illinois

Thom C. Dumsha, DDS
Associate Professor and Chair
Dental School
University of Maryland Baltimore
Baltimore, Maryland

Michael S. Edwards, PharmD, MBA
Assistant Director, Weinberg Pharmacy
Johns Hopkins Hospital
Baltimore, Maryland

Vicki L. Ellingrod, PharmD, BCPP
Associate Professor
University of Iowa
Iowa City, Iowa

Kelley K. Engle, BSPharm
Pharmacotherapy Specialist
Lexi-Comp, Inc
Hudson, Ohio

Margaret A. Fitzgerald, MS, APRN, BC, NP-C, FAANP
President
Fitzgerald Health Education Associates, Inc.
North Andover, Massachusetts
Family Nurse Practitioner
Greater Lawrence Family Health Center
Lawrence, Massachusetts

EDITORIAL ADVISORY PANEL *(Continued)*

Martin D. Higbee, PharmD
Associate Professor
Department of Pharmacy Practice and Science
The University of Arizona
Tucson, Arizona

Jane Hurlburt Hodding, PharmD
Director, Pharmacy
Miller Children's Hospital
Long Beach, California

Collin A. Hovinga, PharmD
Neuropharmacologist
Miami Children's Hospital
Miami, Florida

Darrell T. Hulisz, PharmD
Department of Family Medicine
Case Western Reserve University
Cleveland, Ohio

David S. Jacobs, MD
President, Pathologists Chartered
Consultant in Pathology and Laboratory Medicine
Overland Park, Kansas

Polly E. Kintzel, PharmD, BCPS, BCOP
Clinical Pharmacy Specialist-Oncology
Spectrum Health
Grand Rapids, Michigan

Jill M. Kolesar, PharmD, FCCP, BCPS
Associate Professor of Pharmacy
University of Wisconsin
Madison, Wisconsin

Donna M. Kraus, PharmD, FAPhA
Associate Professor of Pharmacy Practice
Departments of Pharmacy Practice and Pediatrics
Pediatric Clinical Pharmacist
University of Illinois
Chicago, Illinois

Daniel L. Krinsky, RPh, MS
Director, Pharmacotherapy Sales and Marketing
Lexi-Comp, Inc
Hudson, Ohio

Kay Kyllonen, PharmD
Clinical Specialist
The Cleveland Clinic Children's Hospital
Cleveland, Ohio

Charles Lacy, RPh, PharmD, FCSHP
Vice President, Information Technologies
Professor, Pharmacy Practice
Professor, Business Leadership
University of Southern Nevada
Las Vegas, Nevada

Brenda R. Lance, RN, MSN
Program Development Director
Northcoast HealthCare Management Company
Northcoast Infusion Therapies
Oakwood Village, Ohio

EDITORIAL ADVISORY PANEL *(Continued)*

Franklin A. Michota, Jr, MD
Head, Section of Hospital and Preoperative Medicine
Department of General Internal Medicine
The Cleveland Clinic Foundation
Cleveland, Ohio

Michael A. Militello, PharmD, BCPS
Clinical Cardiology Specialist
Department of Pharmacy
The Cleveland Clinic Foundation
Cleveland, Ohio

J. Robert Newland, DDS, MS
Professor
Department of Diagnostic Sciences
University of Texas Health Science Center
Houston, Texas

Cecelia O'Keefe, PharmD
Pharmacotherapy Specialist
Lexi-Comp, Inc.
Hudson, Ohio

Dwight K. Oxley, MD
Consultant in Pathology and Laboratory Medicine
Wichita, Kansas

Frank P. Paloucek, PharmD, DABAT
Clinical Associate Professor in Pharmacy Practice
Director, Residency Programs
University of Illinois
Chicago, Illinois

Christopher J. Papasian, PhD
Director of Diagnostic Microbiology and Immunology Laboratories
Truman Medical Center
Kansas City, Missouri

Alpa Patel, PharmD
Clinical Specialist, Infectious Diseases
Johns Hopkins Hospital
Baltimore, Maryland

Luis F. Ramirez, MD
Adjunct Associate Professor of Psychiatry
Case Western Reserve University
Cleveland, Ohio

A.J. (Fred) Remillard, PharmD
Assistant Dean, Research and Graduate Affairs
College of Pharmacy and Nutrition
University of Saskatchewan
Saskatoon, Saskatchewan

Martha Sajatovic, MD
Associate Professor of Psychiatry
Case Western Reserve University
Cleveland, Ohio

EDITORIAL ADVISORY PANEL *(Continued)*

Todd P. Semla, PharmD, BCPS, FCCP
Clinical Pharmacy Specialist
Department of Veterans Affairs
Pharmacy Benefits Management
Associate Professor of Clinical Psychiatry
Feinberg School of Medicine
Northwestern University
Chicago, Illinois

Francis G. Serio, DMD, MS
Professor & Chairman
Department of Periodontics
University of Mississippi
Jackson, Mississippi

Dominic A. Solimando, Jr, MA, FAPhA, FASHP, BCOP
Oncology Pharmacist
President, Oncology Pharmacy Services, Inc
Arlington, VA

Joni Lombardi Stahura, BS, PharmD, RPh
Pharmacotherapy Specialist
Lexi-Comp, Inc
Hudson, Ohio

Carol K. Taketomo, PharmD
Pharmacy Manager
Children's Hospital Los Angeles
Los Angeles, California

Mary Temple, PharmD
Pediatric Clinical Research Specialist
Hillcrest Hospital
Mayfield Heights, Ohio

Elizabeth A. Tomsik, PharmD, BCPS
Pharmacotherapy Specialist
Lexi-Comp, Inc
Hudson, Ohio

Beatrice B. Turkoski, RN, PhD
Associate Professor, Graduate Faculty
Advanced Pharmacology
College of Nursing
Kent State University
Kent, Ohio

David M. Weinstein, PhD
Pharmacotherapy Specialist
Lexi-Comp, Inc.
Hudson, Ohio

Anne Marie Whelan, PharmD
College of Pharmacy
Dalhouise University
Halifax, Nova Scotia

Richard L. Wynn, PhD
Professor of Pharmacology
Baltimore College of Dental Surgery
Dental School
University of Maryland Baltimore
Baltimore, Maryland

PREFACE

Drug therapy in the perioperative and critical care settings continues to evolve as new medications are introduced into clinical practice and additional uses for existing medications are developed. Since patients undergoing surgery or admitted to an intensive care unit (ICU) are not confined to the operating room or ICU for the duration of their hospital stay, it is critical for all healthcare practitioners and students responsible for patient care to have a basic understanding of the medications used in these patient populations. The *Anesthesiology and Critical Care Drug Handbook* is designed to provide this information in a practical and convenient manner.

As in previous editions, special emphasis continues to be placed on medications used during the perioperative period (eg, neuromuscular blocking agents, antiemetic agents, volatile inhalation agents) and in critical care patients (eg, sedative agents, vasopressors, antiarrhythmics), with comparative tables provided for the key drug classes. Monographs for other commonly prescribed medications in these patient populations are also contained in the handbook, which increases its usefulness as a drug reference. All of the monographs follow a standard format, with frequently used information (eg, use, mechanism of action, pharmacodynamics/kinetics, dosage, monitoring parameters, anesthesia and critical care concerns). In each of the monographs, special consideration has been given to including anesthetic drug interactions when applicable.

The Special Topics/Issues section of the handbook contains clear, concise summaries of frequently encountered patient conditions (eg, latex allergy), select uses of anesthesia-related medications (eg, conscious sedation), critical care issues (eg, stress replacement of corticosteroids) and the management of various patient types (eg, cardiac patients undergoing noncardiac surgery). This handbook presents recent literature related to specific treatments. The information will provide the practitioner with a quick overview of the most salient facts to consider for the particular condition or therapy being discussed.

The appendix contains information valuable to the anesthesia/critical care practitioner such as summaries of the various anesthesia discharge scoring systems, airway classification, stress replacement of glucocorticoids, treatment of malignant hyperthermia, and ACLS guidelines. Many useful comparative medication tables can also be found in the appendix. The "Commonly Used Herbal Medicines" table should see frequent use based on the widespread use of alternative therapies by patients.

We know you will find this handbook to be a valuable and practical source of clinical drug information. We welcome comments to further enhance future editions.

ACKNOWLEDGMENTS

This handbook exists in its present form as the result of the concerted efforts of the following individuals: Robert D. Kerscher, publisher and chief executive officer of Lexi-Comp, Inc; Steven Kerscher, president and chief operating officer; Mark Bonfiglio, BS, PharmD, RPh, chief content officer; Stacy S. Robinson, editorial manager; Dawn M. Conover, project manager; David C. Marcus, chief information officer; Tracey J. Henterly, senior graphic designer; Alexandra Hart, composition specialist; Leslie Jo Hoppes, pharmacology database manager; Matthew C. Kerscher, business unit manager.

Special acknowledgment to all Lexi-Comp staff for their contributions to this handbook.

Much of the material contained in this book was a result of pharmacy contributors throughout the United States and Canada. Lexi-Comp has assisted many medical institutions to develop hospital-specific formulary manuals that contain clinical drug information as well as dosing. Working with clinical pharmacists, hospital pharmacy and therapeutics committees, and hospital drug information centers, Lexi-Comp has developed an evolutionary drug database that reflects the practice of pharmacy in these major institutions.

In addition, the authors wish to thank their families, friends, and colleagues who supported them in their efforts to complete this handbook.

Dr Donnelly would like to especially thank Jan Engle, PharmD, for her ongoing professional and personal support.

DESCRIPTION OF SECTIONS AND FIELDS

The *Anesthesiology & Critical Care Drug Handbook* is divided into five sections.

The first section is a compilation of introductory text pertinent to the use of this book.

The drug information section of the handbook, in which all drugs are listed alphabetically, details information pertinent to each drug. Extensive cross-referencing is provided by brand names and synonyms.

The third section is comprised of several text chapters dealing with various subjects and issues pertinent to perianesthetic patient management.

The fourth section is an invaluable appendix with charts, tables, nomograms, algorithms, management guidelines, and conversion information which can be helpful for patient care.

The last section of this handbook incorporates two indices, a pharmacologic category index and an international brand name index.

Alphabetical Listing of Drugs

Drug information is presented in a consistent format and provides the following:

Generic Name	U.S. adopted name
Pronunciation	Phonetic pronunciation guide
Medication Safety Issues	In an effort to promote the safe use of medications, this field is intended to highlight possible sources of medication errors such as look-alike/sound-alike drugs or highly concentrated formulations which require vigilance on the part of healthcare professionals. In addition, medications which have been associated with severe consequences in the event of a medication error are also identified in this field.
Related Information	Cross-reference to other pertinent drug information found elsewhere in this handbook
U.S. Brand Names	Trade names (manufacturer-specific) found in the United States. The symbol [DSC] appears after trade names that have been recently discontinued.
Canadian Brand Names	Trade names found in Canada
Synonyms	Other names or accepted abbreviations of the generic drug
Pharmacologic Category	Unique systematic classification of medications
Restrictions	The controlled substance classification from the Drug Enforcement Agency (DEA). U.S. schedules are I-V. Schedules vary by country and sometimes state (ie, Massachusetts uses I-VI)
Generic Available	Informs user if a generic product is available by a "yes" or "no"
Use	Information pertaining to appropriate FDA approved indications of the drug.
Unlabeled/ Investigational Use	Information pertaining to non-FDA approved and investigational indications of the drug
Mechanism of Action	How the drug works in the body to elicit a response
Pharmacodynamics/ Kinetics	The magnitude of a drug's effect depends on the drug concentration at the site of action. The pharmacodynamics are expressed in terms of onset of action and duration of action. Pharmacokinetics are expressed in terms of absorption, distribution (including appearance in breast milk and crossing of the placenta), protein binding, metabolism, bioavailability, half-life, time to peak serum concentration, and elimination.

DESCRIPTION OF SECTIONS AND FIELDS *(Continued)*

Dosage	The amount of the drug to be typically given or taken during therapy for children and adults; also includes any dosing adjustment/comments for renal impairment or hepatic impairment and other suggested dosing adjustments (eg, hematological toxicity)
Stability	Information regarding storage of product or steps for reconstitution. Provides the time and conditions for which a solution or mixture will maintain full potency. For example, some solutions may require refrigeration after reconstitution while stored at room temperature prior to preparation. Also includes compatibility information. **Note:** Professional judgment of the individual pharmacist in application of this information is imperative. While drug products may exhibit stability over longer durations of time, it may not be appropriate to utilize the drug product due to concerns in sterility.
Administration	Information regarding the recommended final concentrations, rates of administration for parenteral drugs, or other guidelines when giving the medication
Monitoring Parameters	Laboratory tests and patient physical parameters that should be monitored for safety and efficacy of drug therapy
Reference Range	Therapeutic and toxic serum concentrations listed including peak and trough levels
Anesthesia and Critical Care Concerns/Other Considerations	This field provides a focused summary of some of the important issues concerning anesthesia and critical care applications relevant to the drug; other additional information may be included
Pregnancy Risk Factor	Five categories established by the FDA to indicate the potential of a systemically absorbed drug for causing birth defects
Contraindications	Information pertaining to inappropriate use of the drug
Warnings/Precautions	Hazardous conditions related to use of the drug and disease states or patient populations in which the drug should be cautiously used
Adverse Reactions	Side effects are grouped by percentage of incidence and body system
Overdosage/ Toxicology	Comments and/or considerations are offered when appropriate and include signs/symptoms of excess drug and suggested management of the patient
Drug Interactions	If a drug has demonstrated involvement with cytochrome P450 enzymes, the initial line of this field will identify the drug as an inhibitor, inducer, or substrate of specific isoenzymes (eg, CYP1A2). A summary of this information can also be found in a tabular format within the appendix section of this handbook. The remainder of the field presents a description of the interactions between the drug listed in the monograph and other drugs or drug classes. May include possible mechanisms and effect of combined therapy. May also include a strategy to manage the patient on combined therapy.
Ethanol/Nutrition/Herb Interactions	Information regarding potential interactions with food, nutritionals (including herbal products or vitamins), or ethanol.
Test Interactions	Information regarding effect or implications of laboratory tests while taking the medication
Dietary Considerations	Includes information on how the medication should be taken relative to meals or food.
Dosage Forms	Information regarding form, strength, and availability of the drug
References	Sources and literature used in the writing of the monograph

FDA PREGNANCY CATEGORIES

Throughout this book there is a field labeled Pregnancy Risk Factor (PRF) and the letter A, B, C, D, or X immediately following which signifies a category. The FDA has established these five categories to indicate the potential of a systemically absorbed drug for causing birth defects. The key differentiation among the categories rests upon the reliability of documentation and the risk:benefit ratio. Pregnancy Category X is particularly notable in that if any data exists that may implicate a drug as a teratogen and the risk:benefit ratio is clearly negative, the drug is contraindicated during pregnancy.

These categories are summarized as follows:

A Controlled studies in pregnant women fail to demonstrate a risk to the fetus in the first trimester with no evidence of risk in later trimesters. The possibility of fetal harm appears remote.

B Either animal-reproduction studies have not demonstrated a fetal risk but there are no controlled studies in pregnant women, or animal-reproduction studies have shown an adverse effect (other than a decrease in fertility) that was not confirmed in controlled studies in women in the first trimester and there is no evidence of a risk in later trimesters.

C Either studies in animals have revealed adverse effects on the fetus (teratogenic or embryocidal effects or other) and there are no controlled studies in women, or studies in women and animals are not available. Drugs should be given only if the potential benefits justify the potential risk to the fetus.

D There is positive evidence of human fetal risk, but the benefits from use in pregnant women may be acceptable despite the risk (eg, if the drug is needed in a life-threatening situation or for a serious disease for which safer drugs cannot be used or are ineffective).

X Studies in animals or human beings have demonstrated fetal abnormalities or there is evidence of fetal risk based on human experience, or both, and the risk of the use of the drug in pregnant women clearly outweighs any possible benefit. The drug is contraindicated in women who are or may become pregnant.

FDA NAME DIFFERENTIATION PROJECT THE USE OF TALL-MAN LETTERS

Confusion between similar drug names is an important cause of medication errors. For years, The Institute For Safe Medication Practices (ISMP), has urged generic manufacturers to use a combination of large and small letters as well as bolding (ie, chlorpro**MAZINE** and chlorpro**PAMIDE**) to help distinguish drugs with look-alike names, especially when they share similar strengths. Recently the FDA's Division of Generic Drugs began to issue recommendation letters to manufacturers suggesting this novel way to label their products to help reduce this drug name confusion. Although this project has had marginal success, the method has successfully eliminated problems with products such as diphenhydr**AMINE** and dimenhy**DRINATE**. Hospitals should also follow suit by making similar changes in their own labels, preprinted order forms, computer screens and printouts, and drug storage location labels.

Lexi-Comp Medical Publishing will use "Tall-Man" letters for the drugs suggested by the FDA.

The following is a list of product names and recommended FDA revisions.

Drug Product	Recommended Revision
acetazolamide	aceta**ZOLAMIDE**
acetohexamide	aceto**HEXAMIDE**
bupropion	bu**PROP**ion
buspirone	bus**PIR**one
chlorpromazine	chlorpro**MAZINE**
chlorpropamide	chlorpro**PAMIDE**
clomiphene	clomi**PHENE**
clomipramine	clomi**PRAMINE**
cycloserine	cyclo**SERINE**
cyclosporine	cyclo**SPORINE**
daunorubicin	**DAUNO**rubicin
dimenhydrinate	dimenhy**DRINATE**
diphenhydramine	diphenhydr**AMINE**
dobutamine	**DOBUT**amine
dopamine	**DOP**amine
doxorubicin	**DOXO**rubicin
glipizide	glipi**ZIDE**
glyburide	gly**BURIDE**
hydralazine	hydr**ALAZINE**
hydroxyzine	hydr**OXY**zine
medroxyprogesterone	medroxy**PROGESTER**one
methylprednisolone	methyl**PREDNIS**olone
methyltestosterone	methyl**TESTOSTER**one
nicardipine	ni**CAR**dipine
nifedipine	**NIFE**dipine
prednisolone	predniso**LONE**
prednisone	predni**SONE**
sulfadiazine	sulfa**DIAZINE**
sulfisoxazole	sulfi**SOXAZOLE**
tolazamide	**TOLAZ**amide
tolbutamide	**TOLBUT**amide
vinblastine	vin**BLAS**tine
vincristine	vin**CRIS**tine

Institute for Safe Medication Practices. "New Tall-Man Lettering Will Reduce Mix-Ups Due to Generic Drug Name Confusion," *ISMP Medication Safety Alert*, September 19, 2001. Available at: http://www.ismp.org.

Institute for Safe Medication Practices. "Prescription Mapping, Can Improve Efficiency While Minimizing Errors With Look-Alike Products," *ISMP Medication Safety Alert*, October 6, 1999. Available at: http://www.ismp.org.

U.S. Pharmacopeia, "USP Quality Review: Use Caution-Avoid Confusion," March 2001, No. 76. Available at: http://www.usp.org.

SAFE WRITING PRACTICES

Health professionals and their support personnel frequently produce handwritten copies of information they see in print; therefore, such information is subjected to even greater possibilities for error or misinterpretation on the part of others. Thus, particular care must be given to how drug names and strengths are expressed when creating written healthcare documents.

The following are a few examples of safe writing rules suggested by the Institute for Safe Medication Practices, Inc.[1]

1. There should be a space between a number and its units as it is easier to read. There should be no periods after the abbreviations mg or mL.

Correct	Incorrect
10 mg	10mg
100 mg	100mg

2. Never place a decimal and a zero after a whole number (2 mg is correct and 2.0 mg is **incorrect**). If the decimal point is not seen because it falls on a line or because individuals are working from copies where the decimal point is not seen, this causes a tenfold overdose.
3. Just the opposite is true for numbers less than one. Always place a zero before a naked decimal (0.5 mL is correct, .5 mL is **incorrect**).
4. Never abbreviate the word unit. The handwritten U or u, looks like a 0 (zero), and may cause a tenfold overdose error to be made.
5. IU is not a safe abbreviation for international units. The handwritten IU looks like IV. Write out international units or use int. units.
6. Q.D. is not a safe abbreviation for once daily, as when the Q is followed by a sloppy dot, it looks like QID which means four times daily.
7. O.D. is not a safe abbreviation for once daily, as it is properly interpreted as meaning "right eye" and has caused liquid medications such as saturated solution of potassium iodide and Lugol's solution to be administered incorrectly. There is no safe abbreviation for once daily. It must be written out in full.
8. Do not use chemical names such as 6-mercaptopurine or 6-thioguanine, as sixfold overdoses have been given when these were not recognized as chemical names. The proper names of these drugs are mercaptopurine or thioguanine.
9. Do not abbreviate drug names (5FC, 6MP, 5-ASA, MTX, HCTZ, CPZ, PBZ, etc) as they are misinterpreted and cause error.
10. Do not use the apothecary system or symbols.
11. Do not abbreviate microgram as µg; instead use mcg as there is less likelihood of misinterpretation.
12. When writing an outpatient prescription, write a complete prescription. A complete prescription can prevent the prescriber, the pharmacist, and/or the patient from making a mistake and can eliminate the need for further clarification. The legible prescriptions should contain:
    a. patient's full name
    b. for pediatric or geriatric patients: their age (or weight where applicable)
    c. drug name, dosage form and strength; if a drug is new or rarely prescribed, print this information
    d. number or amount to be dispensed
    e. complete instructions for the patient, including the purpose of the medication
    f. when there are recognized contraindications for a prescribed drug, indicate to the pharmacist that you are aware of this fact (ie, when prescribing a potassium salt for a patient receiving an ACE inhibitor, write "K serum leveling being monitored")

[1]From "Safe Writing" by Davis NM, PharmD and Cohen MR, MS, Lecturers and Consultants for Safe Medication Practices, 1143 Wright Drive, Huntington Valley, PA 19006. Phone: (215) 947-7566.

ALPHABETICAL LISTING OF DRUGS

Abacavir (a BAK a veer)

U.S. Brand Names Ziagen®

Canadian Brand Names Ziagen®

Synonyms Abacavir Sulfate; ABC

Pharmacologic Category Antiretroviral Agent, Reverse Transcriptase Inhibitor (Nucleoside)

Restrictions An FDA-approved medication guide is available at http://www.fda.gov/cder/Offices/ODS/labeling.htm; distribute to each patient to whom this medication is dispensed.

Generic Available No

Use Treatment of HIV infections in combination with other antiretroviral agents

Mechanism of Action Nucleoside reverse transcriptase inhibitor. Abacavir is a guanosine analogue which is phosphorylated to carbovir triphosphate which interferes with HIV viral RNA-dependent DNA polymerase resulting in inhibition of viral replication.

Pharmacodynamics/Kinetics

Absorption: Rapid and extensive absorption

Distribution: V_d: 0.86 L/kg

Protein binding: 50%

Metabolism: Hepatic via alcohol dehydrogenase and glucuronyl transferase to inactive carboxylate and glucuronide metabolites

Bioavailability: 83%

Half-life elimination: 1.5 hours

Time to peak: 0.7-1.7 hours

Excretion: Primarily urine (as metabolites, 1.2% as unchanged drug); feces (16% total dose)

Dosage Oral:

Children: 3 months to 16 years: 8 mg/kg body weight twice daily (maximum: 300 mg twice daily) in combination with other antiretroviral agents

Adults: 300 mg twice daily or 600 mg once daily in combination with other antiretroviral agents

Dosage adjustment in hepatic impairment:

Mild dysfunction (Child-Pugh score 5-6): 200 mg twice daily (oral solution is recommended)

Moderate-to-severe dysfunction: Use is contraindicated by the manufacturer

Stability Store oral solution and tablets at controlled room temperature of 20°C to 25°C (68°F to 77°F). Oral solution may be refrigerated; do not freeze.

Administration May be administered with or without food.

Pregnancy Risk Factor C

Contraindications Hypersensitivity to abacavir (or carbovir) or any component of the formulation (do not rechallenge patients who have experienced hypersensitivity to abacavir); moderate-to-severe hepatic impairment

Warnings/Precautions Abacavir should always be used as a component of a multidrug regimen. **[U.S. Boxed Warning]: Serious and sometimes fatal hypersensitivity reactions have occurred.** Patients exhibiting symptoms from two or more of the following: Fever, skin rash, constitutional symptoms (malaise, fatigue, aches), respiratory symptoms (eg, pharyngitis, dyspnea, cough), and GI symptoms (eg, abdominal pain, diarrhea, nausea, vomiting) should discontinue therapy immediately and call for medical attention. Abacavir should be permanently discontinued if hypersensitivity cannot be ruled out, even when other diagnoses are possible. Abacavir SHOULD NOT be restarted because more severe symptoms may occur within hours, including LIFE-THREATENING HYPOTENSION AND DEATH. Fatal hypersensitivity reactions have occurred following the reintroduction of abacavir in patients whose therapy was interrupted (ie, interruption in drug supply, temporary discontinuation while treating other conditions). Reactions occurred within hours. In some cases, signs of hypersensitivity may have been previously present, but attributed to other medical conditions (eg, acute onset respiratory diseases, gastroenteritis, reactions to other medications). If abacavir is restarted following an interruption in therapy, evaluate the patient for previously unsuspected symptoms of hypersensitivity. Do not restart if hypersensitivity is suspected or if hypersensitivity cannot be ruled out. To report these events on abacavir hypersensitivity, a registry has been established (1-800-270-0425). Use with caution in patients with mild hepatic dysfunction (contraindicated in moderate-to-severe dysfunction). **[U.S. Boxed Warning]: Lactic acidosis and severe hepatomegaly with steatosis (sometimes fatal)**

have occurred with antiretroviral nucleoside analogues. Female gender, obesity, and prolonged treatment may increase the risk of hepatotoxicity.

Adverse Reactions Hypersensitivity reactions (which may be fatal) occur in ~5% of patients (see Warnings/Precautions). Symptoms may include anaphylaxis, fever, rash (including erythema multiforme), fatigue, diarrhea, abdominal pain; respiratory symptoms (eg, pharyngitis, dyspnea, cough, adult respiratory distress syndrome, or respiratory failure); headache, malaise, lethargy, myalgia, myolysis, arthralgia, edema, paresthesia, nausea and vomiting, mouth ulcerations, conjunctivitis, lymphadenopathy, hepatic failure, and renal failure.

Note: Rates of adverse reactions were defined during combination therapy with other antiretrovirals (lamivudine and efavirenz **or** lamivudine and zidovudine). Only reactions which occurred at a higher frequency than in the comparator group are noted. Adverse reaction rates attributable to abacavir alone are not available.

>10%:
- Central nervous system: Headache (7% to 13%), fatigue and malaise (7% to 12%)
- Gastrointestinal: Nausea (7% to 19%, children 9%)

1% to 10%:
- Central nervous system: Depression (6%), dizziness (6%), fever (6%, children 9%), anxiety (5%), abnormal dreams (10%)
- Dermatologic: Rash (5% to 6%, children 7%)
- Gastrointestinal: Diarrhea (7%), vomiting (2% to 10%, children 9%), abdominal pain (6%)
- Hematologic: Thrombocytopenia (1%)
- Hepatic: AST increased (6%)
- Neuromuscular and skeletal: Musculoskeletal pain (5% to 6%)
- Respiratory: Bronchitis (4%), respiratory viral infection (5%)
- Miscellaneous: Hypersensitivity reactions (9%; may include reactions to other components of antiretroviral regimen), infection (EENT 5%)

<1% (Limited to important or life-threatening): Erythema multiforme, hepatotoxicity, lactic acidosis, pancreatitis, Stevens-Johnson syndrome, toxic epidermal necrolysis

Drug Interactions

Amprenavir: Abacavir increases the AUC of amprenavir.

Methadone: Abacavir may decrease the serum concentration of methadone (clearance increased 22%); in a minority of patients, methadone dosage increase may be required.

Ribavirin: Concomitant use of ribavirin and nucleoside analogues may increase the risk of developing lactic acidosis (includes adefovir, didanosine, lamivudine, stavudine, zalcitabine, zidovudine).

Ethanol/Nutrition/Herb Interactions Ethanol: Ethanol may increase the risk of toxicity.

Dietary Considerations May be taken with or without food.

Dosage Forms

Solution, oral: 20 mg/mL (240 mL) [strawberry-banana flavor]

Tablet: 300 mg

- ♦ **Abacavir Sulfate** *see* Abacavir *on page 22*
- ♦ **Abbokinase® [DSC]** *see* Urokinase *on page 1323*
- ♦ **ABC** *see* Abacavir *on page 22*
- ♦ **ABCD** *see* Amphotericin B Cholesteryl Sulfate Complex *on page 93*

Abciximab (ab SIK si mab)

U.S. Brand Names ReoPro®

Canadian Brand Names Reopro®

Synonyms C7E3; 7E3

Pharmacologic Category Antiplatelet Agent, Glycoprotein IIb/IIIa Inhibitor

Generic Available No

Use Prevention of acute cardiac ischemic complications in patients at high risk for abrupt closure of the treated coronary vessel and patients at risk of restenosis; an adjunct with heparin to prevent cardiac ischemic complications in patients with unstable angina not responding to conventional therapy when a percutaneous coronary intervention (PCI) is scheduled within 24 hours

Unlabeled/Investigational Use Acute MI — combination regimen of abciximab (full dose), tenecteplase (half dose), and heparin (unlabeled dose)

(Continued)

Abciximab *(Continued)*

Mechanism of Action Fab antibody fragment of the chimeric human-murine monoclonal antibody 7E3; this agent binds to platelet IIb/IIIa receptors, resulting in steric hindrance, thus inhibiting platelet aggregation

Pharmacodynamics/Kinetics Half-life elimination: ~30 minutes

Dosage

Acute coronary syndromes: PCI: I.V.: 0.25 mg/kg bolus administered 10-60 minutes before the start of intervention followed by an infusion of 0.125 mcg/kg/minute (maximum: 10 mcg/minute) for 12 hours

Patients with unstable angina not responding to conventional medical therapy and who are planning to undergo percutaneous coronary intervention within 24 hours may be treated with abciximab 0.25 mg/kg intravenous bolus followed by an 18- to 24-hour intravenous infusion of 10 mcg/minute, concluding 1 hour after the percutaneous coronary intervention.

Acute MI combination regimen (unlabeled): Half-dose tenecteplase (15-25 mg based on weight), abciximab 0.25 mg/kg bolus then 0.125 mcg/kg/minute (maximum: 10 mcg/minute) for 12 hours and heparin dosing as follows: Concurrent bolus of 40 units/kg (maximum: 3000 units), then 7 units/kg/hour (maximum: 800 units/hour) as continuous infusion. Adjust to aPTT target of 50-70 seconds.

Stability Vials should be stored at 2°C to 8°C; do not freeze or shake. After admixture, the prepared solution is stable for 12 hours. Abciximab should be administered in a separate intravenous line. No incompatibilities have been observed with glass bottles or PVC bags.

Administration Abciximab is intended for coadministration with aspirin postangioplasty and heparin infused and weight adjusted to maintain a therapeutic bleeding time (eg, ACT 300-500 seconds). Solution must be filtered prior to administration. Do not shake the vial.

Bolus dose: Aseptically withdraw the necessary amount of abciximab for the bolus dose into a syringe using a 0.2 or 5 micron low protein-binding syringe filter (or equivalent); the bolus should be administered 10-60 minutes before the procedure.

Continuous infusion: Aseptically withdraw 4.5 mL (9 mg) of abciximab for the infusion through a 0.2 or 5 micron low protein-binding syringe filter into a syringe; inject this into 250 mL of NS or D_5W to make a solution with a final concentration of 35 mcg/mL. Infuse at a rate of 17 mL/hour (10 mcg/minute) for 12 hours via pump. If a syringe filter was not used when preparing the infusion, administer using an in-line 0.02 or 0.22 low protein-binding filter.

Monitoring Parameters Prothrombin time, activated partial thromboplastin time (aPTT), hemoglobin, hematocrit, platelet count, fibrinogen, fibrin split products, transfusion requirements, signs of hypersensitivity reactions, guaiac stools, Hemastix® urine. Platelet count should be monitored at baseline, 2-4 hours following bolus infusion, and at 24 hours (or prior to discharge, if before 24 hours).

To minimize risk of bleeding:

- Abciximab initiated 18-24 hours prior to PCI: Maintain aPTT between 60-85 seconds during the heparin/abciximab infusion period
- During PCI: Maintain ACT between 200-300 seconds
- Following PCI (if anticoagulation is maintained): Maintain aPTT between 50-75 seconds

Sheath removal should not occur until aPTT is ≤50 seconds or ACT ≤175 seconds.

Maintain bleeding precautions, avoid unnecessary arterial and venous punctures, use saline or heparin lock for blood drawing, assess sheath insertion site and distal pulses of affected leg every 15 minutes for the first hour and then every 1 hour for the next 6 hours. Arterial access site care is important to prevent bleeding. Care should be taken when attempting vascular access that only the anterior wall of the femoral artery is punctured, avoiding a Seldinger (through and through) technique for obtaining sheath access. Femoral vein sheath placement should be avoided unless needed. While the vascular sheath is in place, patients should be maintained on complete bedrest with the head of the bed at a 30° angle and the affected limb restrained in a straight position.

Observe patient for mental status changes, hemorrhage; assess nose and mouth mucous membranes, puncture sites for oozing, ecchymosis, and hematoma formation; and examine urine, stool, and emesis for presence of occult or frank blood; gentle care should be provided when removing dressings.

Anesthesia and Critical Care Concerns/Other Considerations Platelet Effects: Abciximab has a long duration of action and platelet effects reverse slowly. It can take 24-48 hours for platelet function to return to normal after discontinuation of infusion making it difficult to use in patients likely to need CABG. Antiplatelet effects can be reversed with platelet transfusions. Platelet count monitoring is recommended 2-4 hours after initiation, and at 24 hours or prior to discharge, whichever is first. Acute profound thrombocytopenia with abciximab occurs within 24 hours of administration and may be treated by discontinuing the infusion (if still running) and administering platelets. Platelet counts should recover rapidly after discontinuation.

Pregnancy Risk Factor C

Contraindications Hypersensitivity to abciximab, to murine proteins, or any component of the formulation; active internal hemorrhage or recent (within 6 weeks) clinically-significant GI or GU bleeding; history of cerebrovascular accident within 2 years or cerebrovascular accident with significant neurological deficit; clotting abnormalities or administration of oral anticoagulants within 7 days unless prothrombin time (PT) is ≤1.2 times control PT value; thrombocytopenia (<100,000 cells/μL); recent (within 6 weeks) major surgery or trauma; intracranial tumor, arteriovenous malformation, or aneurysm; severe uncontrolled hypertension; history of vasculitis; use of dextran before PTCA or intent to use dextran during PTCA; concomitant use of another parenteral GP IIb/IIIa inhibitor

Warnings/Precautions Administration of abciximab is associated with increased frequency of major bleeding complications, including retroperitoneal bleeding, pulmonary bleeding, spontaneous GI or GU bleeding, and bleeding at the arterial access. Risk may be increased with patients weighing <75 kilograms, elderly patients (>65 years of age), history of previous GI disease, and recent thrombolytic therapy. Avoid the creation of venous access at noncompressible sites.

The risk of major bleeds may increase with concurrent use of thrombolytics. Anticoagulation, such as with heparin, may contribute to the risk of bleeding. In serious, uncontrolled bleeding, abciximab and heparin should be stopped. Increased risk of hemorrhage during or following angioplasty is associated with unsuccessful PTCA, PTCA procedure >70 minutes duration, or PTCA performed within 12 hours of symptom onset for acute myocardial infarction.

Administration of abciximab may result in human antichimeric antibody formation that can cause hypersensitivity reactions (including anaphylaxis), thrombocytopenia, or diminished efficacy. Readministration of abciximab within 30 days or in patients with human antichimeric antibodies (HACA) increases the incidence and severity of thrombocytopenia.

Adverse Reactions As with all drugs which may affect hemostasis, bleeding is associated with abciximab. Hemorrhage may occur at virtually any site. Risk is dependent on multiple variables, including the concurrent use of multiple agents which alter hemostasis and patient susceptibility.

>10%:
- Cardiovascular: Hypotension (14.4%), chest pain (11.4%)
- Gastrointestinal: Nausea (13.6%)
- Hematologic: Minor bleeding (4.0% to 16.8%)
- Neuromuscular & skeletal: Back pain (17.6%)

1% to 10%:
- Cardiovascular: Bradycardia (4.5%), peripheral edema (1.6%)
- Central nervous system: Headache (6.45)
- Gastrointestinal: Vomiting (7.3%), abdominal pain (3.1%)
- Hematologic: Major bleeding (1.1% to 14%), thrombocytopenia: <100,000 cells/mm^3 (2.5% to 5.6%); <50,000 cells/mm^3 (0.4% to 1.7%)
- Local: Injection site pain (3.6%)

<1% (Limited to important or life-threatening): Abnormal thinking, allergic reactions/anaphylaxis (possible), AV block, bronchospasm, bullous eruption, coma, confusion, diabetes mellitus, embolism, hyperkalemia, ileus, inflammation, intracranial hemorrhage, myalgia, nodal arrhythmia, pleural effusion, pulmonary embolism, prostatitis, pruritus, stroke, urinary retention, ventricular tachycardia, xerostomia

Overdosage/Toxicology Since abciximab is a platelet antiaggregate, patients who bleed following administration may be best treated with platelet infusions.

Drug Interactions

Heparin and aspirin: Use with aspirin and heparin may increase bleeding over aspirin and heparin alone. However, aspirin and heparin were used concurrently in the majority of patients in the major clinical studies of abciximab.

(Continued)

Abciximab *(Continued)*

Monoclonal antibodies: Allergic reactions may be increased in patients who have received diagnostic or therapeutic monoclonal antibodies due to the presence of HACA antibodies.

Thrombolytic agents theoretically may increase the risk of bleeding; use with caution.

Warfarin and oral anticoagulants: Risk of bleeding may be increased during concurrent therapy.

Other IIb/IIIa antagonists: Avoid concomitant use of other glycoprotein IIb/IIIa antagonists (see Contraindications).

Dosage Forms Injection, solution: 2 mg/mL (5 mL)

- **Abelcet®** *see* Amphotericin B (Lipid Complex) *on page 99*
- **Abenol® (Can)** *see* Acetaminophen *on page 26*
- **ABLC** *see* Amphotericin B (Lipid Complex) *on page 99*
- **Absorbable Cotton** *see* Cellulose (Oxidized Regenerated) *on page 258*
- **AccuNeb®** *see* Albuterol *on page 50*
- **Accupril®** *see* Quinapril *on page 1091*
- **ACE** *see* Captopril *on page 221*
- **Aceon®** *see* Perindopril Erbumine *on page 1002*
- **Acephen™ [OTC]** *see* Acetaminophen *on page 26*
- **Acetadote®** *see* Acetylcysteine *on page 35*

Acetaminophen (a seet a MIN oh fen)

Medication Safety Issues

Sound-alike/look-alike issues:

Acephen® may be confused with AcipHex®

FeverALL® may be confused with Fiberall®

Tylenol® may be confused with atenolol, timolol, Tuinal®, Tylox®

Related Information

Acetaminophen and NSAIDS, Dosing Data *on page 1543*

Acute Postoperative Pain *on page 1388*

Chronic Pain Management *on page 1430*

U.S. Brand Names Acephen™ [OTC]; Apra Children's [OTC]; Aspirin Free Anacin® Maximum Strength [OTC]; Cetafen® [OTC]; Cetafen Extra® [OTC]; Comtrex® Sore Throat Maximum Strength [OTC]; ElixSure™ Fever/Pain [OTC] [DSC]; FeverALL® [OTC]; Genapap™ [OTC]; Genapap™ Children [OTC]; Genapap™ Extra Strength [OTC]; Genapap™ Infant [OTC]; Genebs [OTC]; Genebs Extra Strength [OTC]; Infantaire [OTC]; Mapap [OTC]; Mapap Children's [OTC]; Mapap Extra Strength [OTC]; Mapap Infants [OTC]; Nortemp Children's [OTC]; Pain Eze [OTC]; Silapap® Children's [OTC]; Silapap® Infants [OTC]; Tycolene [OTC]; Tycolene Maximum Strength [OTC]; Tylenol® [OTC]; Tylenol® 8 Hour [OTC]; Tylenol® Arthritis Pain [OTC]; Tylenol® Children's [OTC]; Tylenol® Children's with Flavor Creator [OTC]; Tylenol® Extra Strength [OTC]; Tylenol® Infants [OTC]; Tylenol® Junior [OTC]; Valorin [OTC]; Valorin Extra [OTC]

Canadian Brand Names Abenol®; Apo-Acetaminophen®; Atasol®; Novo-Gesic; Pediatrix; Tempra®; Tylenol®

Synonyms APAP; N-Acetyl-P-Aminophenol; Paracetamol

Pharmacologic Category Analgesic, Miscellaneous

Generic Available Yes: Excludes extended release products

Use Treatment of mild-to-moderate pain and fever (antipyretic/analgesic); does not have antirheumatic or anti-inflammatory effects

Mechanism of Action Inhibits the synthesis of prostaglandins in the central nervous system and peripherally blocks pain impulse generation; produces antipyresis from inhibition of hypothalamic heat-regulating center

Pharmacodynamics/Kinetics

Onset of action: <1 hour

Duration: 4-6 hours

Absorption: Incomplete; varies by dosage form

Protein binding: 8% to 43% at toxic doses

Metabolism: At normal therapeutic dosages, hepatic to sulfate and glucuronide metabolites, while a small amount is metabolized by CYP to a highly reactive intermediate (acetylimidoquinone) which is conjugated with glutathione and inactivated; at toxic doses (as little as 4 g daily) glutathione conjugation becomes insufficient to meet the metabolic demand causing an increase in acetylimidoquinone concentration, which may cause hepatic cell necrosis

Half-life elimination: Prolonged following toxic doses

Neonates: 2-5 hours

Adults: 1-3 hours (may be increased in elderly; however, this should not affect dosing)

Time to peak, serum: Oral: 10-60 minutes; may be delayed in acute overdoses

Excretion: Urine (2% to 5% unchanged; 55% as glucuronide metabolites; 30% as sulphate metabolites)

Dosage Oral, rectal:

Children <12 years: 10-15 mg/kg/dose every 4-6 hours as needed; do **not** exceed 5 doses (2.6 g) in 24 hours; alternatively, the following age-based doses may be used; see table.

Acetaminophen Dosing

Age	Dosage (mg)	Age	Dosage (mg)
0-3 mo	40	4-5 y	240
4-11 mo	80	6-8 y	320
1-2 y	120	9-10 y	400
2-3 y	160	11 y	480

Note: Higher rectal doses have been studied for use in preoperative pain control in children. However, specific guidelines are not available and dosing may be product dependent. The safety and efficacy of alternating acetaminophen and ibuprofen dosing has not been established.

Adults: 325-650 mg every 4-6 hours or 1000 mg 3-4 times/day; do **not** exceed 4 g/day

Dosing interval in renal impairment:

Cl_{cr} 10-50 mL/minute: Administer every 6 hours

Cl_{cr} <10 mL/minute: Administer every 8 hours (metabolites accumulate)

Hemodialysis: Moderately dialyzable (20% to 50%)

Dosing adjustment/comments in hepatic impairment: Use with caution. Limited, low-dose therapy is usually well tolerated in hepatic disease/cirrhosis. However, cases of hepatotoxicity at daily acetaminophen dosages <4 g/day have been reported. Avoid chronic use in hepatic impairment.

Stability Do not freeze suppositories.

Administration

Suppositories: Do not freeze.

Suspension, oral: Shake well before pouring a dose.

Monitoring Parameters Relief of pain or fever

Reference Range

Therapeutic concentration (analgesic/antipyretic): 10-30 mcg/mL

Toxic concentration (acute ingestion) with probable hepatotoxicity: >200 mcg/mL at 4 hours or 50 mcg/mL at 12 hours after ingestion

Anesthesia and Critical Care Concerns/Other Considerations Avoid excessive doses of acetaminophen particularly in patients with a significant alcohol history or poor nutritional habits. The 2002 ACCM/SCCM guidelines for analgesia (critically-ill adult) recommend prescribing <2 g/day for patients with a significant alcohol history or those with malnutrition. Other patients may be limited to <4 g/day. Susceptibility to acetaminophen hepatotoxicity may be due to induction of hepatic enzymes caused by chronic alcohol ingestion, depletion of glutathione, malnutrition, and impaired glucuronidation caused by fasting.

Pregnancy Risk Factor B

Contraindications Hypersensitivity to acetaminophen or any component of the formulation

Warnings/Precautions Limit dose to <4 g/day. May cause severe hepatic toxicity on acute overdose; in addition, chronic daily dosing in adults has resulted in liver damage in some patients. Use with caution in patients with alcoholic liver disease; consuming ≥3 alcoholic drinks/day may increase the risk of liver damage. Use caution in patients with known G6PD deficiency.

OTC labeling: When used for self-medication, patients should be instructed to contact healthcare provider if used for fever lasting >3 days or for pain lasting >10 days in adults or >5 days in children.

Adverse Reactions Frequency not defined.

Dermatologic: Rash

(Continued)

Acetaminophen *(Continued)*

Endocrine & metabolic: May increase chloride, uric acid, glucose; may decrease sodium, bicarbonate, calcium
Hematologic: Anemia, blood dyscrasias (neutropenia, pancytopenia, leukopenia)
Hepatic: Bilirubin increased, alkaline phosphatase increased
Renal: Ammonia increased, nephrotoxicity with chronic overdose, analgesic nephropathy
Miscellaneous: Hypersensitivity reactions (rare)

Overdosage/Toxicology Symptoms of overdose include hepatic necrosis, transient azotemia, renal tubular necrosis with acute toxicity, anemia, and GI disturbances with chronic toxicity. Treatment consists of acetylcysteine 140 mg/kg orally (loading) followed by 70 mg/kg every 4 hours for 17 doses; therapy should be initiated based upon laboratory analysis suggesting a high probability of hepatotoxic potential. Activated charcoal is very effective at binding acetaminophen. Intravenous acetylcysteine should be reserved for patients unable to take oral forms.

Drug Interactions **Substrate** (minor) of CYP1A2, 2A6, 2C9, 2D6, 2E1, 3A4; **Inhibits** CYP3A4 (weak)

Decreased effect: Barbiturates, carbamazepine, hydantoins, rifampin, sulfinpyrazone may decrease the analgesic effect of acetaminophen. Cholestyramine may decrease acetaminophen absorption (separate dosing by at least 1 hour).
Increased toxicity: Barbiturates, carbamazepine, hydantoins, isoniazid, rifampin, sulfinpyrazone may increase the hepatotoxic potential of acetaminophen. Chronic ethanol abuse increases risk for acetaminophen toxicity; effect of warfarin may be enhanced.

Ethanol/Nutrition/Herb Interactions

Ethanol: Excessive intake of ethanol may increase the risk of acetaminophen-induced hepatotoxicity. Avoid ethanol or limit to <3 drinks/day.
Food: Rate of absorption may be decreased when given with food.
Herb/Nutraceutical: St John's wort may decrease acetaminophen levels.

Test Interactions Increased chloride, bilirubin, uric acid, glucose, ammonia (B), chloride (S), uric acid (S), alkaline phosphatase (S), chloride (S); decreased sodium, bicarbonate, calcium (S)

Dietary Considerations Chewable tablets may contain phenylalanine (amount varies, ranges between 3-12 mg/tablet); consult individual product labeling.

Dosage Forms [DSC] = Discontinued product

Caplet: 500 mg
  Cetafen Extra® Strength, Genapap™ Extra Strength, Genebs Extra Strength, Mapap Extra Strength, Tycolene Maximum Strength, Tylenol® Extra Strength: 500 mg
Caplet, extended release:
  Tylenol® 8 Hour, Tylenol® Arthritis Pain: 650 mg
Capsule: 500 mg
Elixir: 160 mg/5 mL (120 mL, 480 mL, 3780 mL)
  Apra Children's: 160 mg/5 mL (120 mL, 480 mL, 3780 mL) [alcohol free; contains benzoic acid; cherry and grape flavors]
  Mapap Children's: 160 mg/5 mL (120 mL) [alcohol free; contains benzoic acid and sodium benzoate; cherry flavor]
Gelcap:
  Mapap Extra Strength, Tylenol® Extra Strength: 500 mg
Geltab:
  Tylenol® Extra Strength: 500 mg
Geltab, extended release:
  Tylenol® 8 Hour: 650 mg
Liquid, oral: 500 mg/15 mL (240 mL)
  Comtrex® Sore Throat Maximum Strength: 500 mg/15 mL (240 mL) [contains sodium benzoate; honey lemon flavor]
  Genapap™ Children: 160 mg/5 mL (120 mL) [contains sodium benzoate; cherry and grape flavors]
  Silapap®: 160 mg/5 mL (120 mL, 240 mL, 480 mL) [sugar free; contains sodium benzoate; cherry flavor]
  Tylenol® Extra Strength: 500 mg/15 mL (240 mL) [contains sodium benzoate; cherry flavor]
Solution, oral: 160 mg/5 mL (120 mL, 480 mL)
Solution, oral drops: 80 mg/0.8 mL (15 mL) [droppers are marked at 0.4 mL (40 mg) and at 0.8 mL (80 mg)]

Genapap™ Infant: 80 mg/0.8 mL (15 mL) [fruit flavor]
Infantaire: 80 mg/0.8mL (15 mL, 30 mL)
Silapap® Infant's: 80 mg/0.8 mL (15 mL, 30 mL) [contains sodium benzoate; cherry flavor]
Suppository, rectal: 120 mg, 325 mg, 650 mg
Acephen™: 120 mg, 325 mg, 650 mg
FeverALL®: 80 mg, 120 mg, 325 mg, 650 mg
Mapap: 125 mg, 650 mg
Suspension, oral:
Mapap Children's: 160 mg/5 mL (120 mL) [contains sodium benzoate; cherry flavor]
Nortemp Children's: 160 mg/5 mL (120 mL) [alcohol free; contains sodium benzoate; cotton candy flavor]
Tylenol® Children's: 160 mg/5 mL (120 mL, 240 mL) [contains sodium benzoate; bubble gum yum, cherry blast, dye free cherry, grape splash, and very berry strawberry flavors]
Tylenol® Children's with Flavor Creator: 160 mg/5 mL (120 mL) [contains sodium 2 mg/5 mL and sodium benzoate; cherry blast flavor; packaged with apple (4), bubblegum (8), chocolate (4), & strawberry (4) sugar free flavor packets]
Suspension, oral drops:
Mapap Infants: 80 mg/0.8 mL (15 mL, 30 mL) [contains sodium benzoate; cherry flavor]
Tylenol® Infants: 80 mg/0.8 mL (15 mL, 30 mL) [contains sodium benzoate; cherry, dye free cherry, and grape flavors]
Syrup, oral:
ElixSure™ Fever/Pain: 160 mg/5 mL (120 mL) [bubble gum, cherry, and grape flavors] [DSC]
Tablet: 325 mg, 500 mg
Aspirin Free Anacin® Extra Strength, Genapap™ Extra Strength, Genebs Extra Strength, Mapap Extra Strength, Pain Eze, Tylenol® Extra Strength, Valorin Extra: 500 mg
Cetafen®, Genapap™, Genebs, Mapap, Tycolene, Tylenol®, Valorin: 325 mg
Tablet, chewable: 80 mg
Genapap™ Children: 80 mg [contains phenylalanine 6 mg/tablet; fruit and grape flavors]
Mapap Children's: 80 mg [contains phenylalanine 3 mg/tablet; bubble gum, fruit, and grape flavors]
Mapap Junior Strength: 160 mg [contains phenylalanine 12 mg/tablet; grape flavor]
Tylenol® Children's: 80 mg [fruit and grape flavors contain phenylalanine 3 mg/tablet; bubble gum flavor contains phenylalanine 6 mg/tablet] [DSC]
Tylenol® Junior: 160 mg [contains phenylalanine 6 mg/tablet; fruit and grape flavors] [DSC]
Tablet, orally disintegrating: 80 mg, 160 mg
Tylenol® Children's Meltaways: 80 mg [bubble gum, grape, and watermelon flavors]
Tylenol® Junior Meltaways: 160 mg [bubble gum and grape flavors]

Acetaminophen and Codeine (a seet a MIN oh fen & KOE deen)

Medication Safety Issues
Sound-alike/look-alike issues:
Capital® may be confused with Capitrol®
Tylenol® may be confused with atenolol, timolol, Tuinal®, Tylox®

T3 is an error-prone abbreviation (mistaken as liothyronine)

U.S. Brand Names Capital® and Codeine; Tylenol® With Codeine

Canadian Brand Names ratio-Emtec; ratio-Lenoltec; Triatec-8; Triatec-8 Strong; Triatec-30; Tylenol Elixir with Codeine; Tylenol No. 1; Tylenol No. 1 Forte; Tylenol No. 2 with Codeine; Tylenol No. 3 with Codeine; Tylenol No. 4 with Codeine

Synonyms Codeine and Acetaminophen

Pharmacologic Category Analgesic, Narcotic

Restrictions C-III; C-V

Note: In countries outside of the U.S., some formulations of Tylenol® with Codeine (eg, Tylenol® No. 3) include caffeine.

Generic Available Yes

(Continued)

Acetaminophen and Codeine *(Continued)*

Use Relief of mild-to-moderate pain

Mechanism of Action Inhibits the synthesis of prostaglandins in the central nervous system and peripherally blocks pain impulse generation; produces antipyresis from inhibition of hypothalamic heat-regulating center; binds to opiate receptors in the CNS, causing inhibition of ascending pain pathways, altering the perception of and response to pain; causes cough supression by direct central action in the medulla; produces generalized CNS depression. Caffeine (contained in some non-U.S. formulations) is a CNS stimulant; use with acetaminophen and codeine increases the level of analgesia provided by each agent.

Pharmacodynamics/Kinetics See individual agents.

Dosage Doses should be adjusted according to severity of pain and response of the patient. Adult doses ≥60 mg codeine fail to give commensurate relief of pain but merely prolong analgesia and are associated with an appreciably increased incidence of side effects. Oral:

Children: Analgesic:
- Codeine: 0.5-1 mg codeine/kg/dose every 4-6 hours
- Acetaminophen: 10-15 mg/kg/dose every 4 hours up to a maximum of 2.6 g/24 hours for children <12 years; **alternatively, the following can be used:**
  - 3-6 years: 5 mL 3-4 times/day as needed of elixir
  - 7-12 years: 10 mL 3-4 times/day as needed of elixir
  - >12 years: 15 mL every 4 hours as needed of elixir

Adults:
- Antitussive: Based on codeine (15-30 mg/dose) every 4-6 hours (maximum: 360 mg/24 hours based on codeine component)
- Analgesic: Based on codeine (30-60 mg/dose) every 4-6 hours (maximum: 4000 mg/24 hours based on acetaminophen component)

Dosing adjustment in renal impairment: See individual agents.

Dosing adjustment in hepatic impairment: Use with caution. Limited, low-dose therapy is usually well tolerated in hepatic disease/cirrhosis; however, cases of hepatotoxicity at daily acetaminophen dosages <4 g/day have been reported. Avoid chronic use in hepatic impairment.

Monitoring Parameters Relief of pain, respiratory and mental status, blood pressure, bowel function

Pregnancy Risk Factor C

Contraindications Hypersensitivity to acetaminophen, codeine, or any component of the formulation; significant respiratory depression (in unmonitored settings); acute or severe bronchial asthma; hypercapnia; paralytic ileus

Warnings/Precautions Use with caution in patients with hypersensitivity reactions to other phenanthrene derivative opioid agonists (morphine, hydrocodone, hydromorphone, levorphanol, oxycodone, oxymorphone); tablets contain metabisulfite which may cause allergic reactions. Tolerance or drug dependence may result from extended use.

Limit total acetaminophen dose to <4 g/day. May cause severe hepatic toxicity on acute overdose; in addition, chronic daily dosing in adults has resulted in liver damage in some patients. Use with caution in patients with alcoholic liver disease; consuming 3 alcoholic drinks/day may increase the risk of liver damage. Use caution in patients with known G6PD deficiency.

This combination should be used with caution in elderly or debilitated patients, hypotension, adrenocortical insufficiency, thyroid disorders, prostatic hyperplasia, urethral stricture, seizure disorder, CNS depression, head injury or increased intracranial pressure. Causes sedation; caution must be used in performing tasks which require alertness (eg, operating machinery or driving). Safety and efficacy in pediatric patients have not been established.

Note: Some non-U.S. formulations (including most Canadian formulations) may contain caffeine as an additional ingredient. Caffeine may cause CNS and cardiovascular stimulation, as well as GI irritation in high doses. Use with caution in patients with a history of peptic ulcer or GERD; avoid in patients with symptomatic cardiac arrhythmias.

Adverse Reactions

>10%:
- Central nervous system: Lightheadedness, dizziness, sedation
- Gastrointestinal: Nausea, vomiting
- Respiratory: Dyspnea

1% to 10%:
- Central nervous system: Euphoria, dysphoria
- Dermatologic: Pruritus
- Gastrointestinal: Constipation, abdominal pain
- Miscellaneous: Histamine release

<1% (Limited to important or life-threatening): Antidiuretic hormone release, biliary tract spasm, bradycardia, hypotension, intracranial pressure increased, physical and psychological dependence, respiratory depression, urinary retention

Overdosage/Toxicology Symptoms of overdose include hepatic necrosis, blood dyscrasias, respiratory depression.

Acetylcysteine 140 mg/kg orally (loading) followed by 70 mg/kg every 4 hours for 17 doses; therapy should be initiated based upon laboratory analysis suggesting high probability of hepatotoxic potential.

Naloxone 2 mg I.V. (0.01 mg/kg for children) with repeat administration as necessary up to a total of 10 mg; can also be used to reverse the toxic effects of the opiate.

Activated charcoal is effective at binding certain chemicals, and this is especially true for acetaminophen (use within 2 hours of ingestion).

Drug Interactions Acetaminophen: **Substrate** (minor) of CYP1A2, 2A6, 2C9, 2D6, 2E1, 3A4; **Inhibits** CYP3A4 (weak)

Increased toxicity: CNS depressants, phenothiazines, tricyclic antidepressants, guanabenz, MAO inhibitors (may also decrease blood pressure); effect of warfarin may be enhanced.

Ethanol/Nutrition/Herb Interactions Ethanol: Excessive intake of ethanol may increase the risk of acetaminophen-induced hepatotoxicity. Avoid ethanol or limit to <3 drinks/day.

Dietary Considerations May be taken with food.

Dosage Forms [DSC] = Discontinued product; [CAN] = Canadian brand name

Caplet:
- ratio-Lenoltec No. 1 [CAN], Tylenol No. 1 [CAN]: Acetaminophen 300 mg, codeine phosphate 8 mg, and caffeine 15 mg [not available in the U.S.]
- Tylenol No. 1 Forte [CAN]: Acetaminophen 500 mg, codeine phosphate 8 mg, and caffeine 15 mg [not available in the U.S.]

Elixir, oral [C-V]: Acetaminophen 120 mg and codeine phosphate 12 mg per 5 mL (5 mL, 10 mL, 12.5 mL, 15 mL, 120 mL, 480 mL) [contains alcohol 7%]
- Tylenol® with Codeine [DSC]: Acetaminophen 120 mg and codeine phosphate 12 mg per 5 mL (480 mL) [contains alcohol 7%; cherry flavor]
- Tylenol Elixir with Codeine [CAN]: Acetaminophen 160 mg and codeine phosphate 8 mg per 5 mL (500 mL) [contains alcohol 7%, sucrose 31%; cherry flavor; not available in the U.S.]

Suspension, oral [C-V] (Capital® and Codeine): Acetaminophen 120 mg and codeine phosphate 12 mg per 5 mL (480 mL) [alcohol free; fruit punch flavor]

Tablet [C-III]: Acetaminophen 300 mg and codeine phosphate 15 mg; acetaminophen 300 mg and codeine phosphate 30 mg; acetaminophen 300 mg and codeine phosphate 60 mg
- ratio-Emtec [CAN], Triatec-30 [CAN]: Acetaminophen 300 mg and codeine phosphate 30 mg [not available in the U.S.]
- ratio-Lenoltec No. 1 [CAN]: Acetaminophen 300 mg, codeine phosphate 8 mg, and caffeine 15 mg [not available in the U.S.]
- ratio-Lenoltec No. 2 [CAN], Tylenol No. 2 with Codeine [CAN]: Acetaminophen 300 mg, codeine phosphate 15 mg, and caffeine 15 mg [not available in the U.S.]
- ratio-Lenoltec No. 3 [CAN], Tylenol No. 3 with Codeine [CAN]: Acetaminophen 300 mg, codeine phosphate 30 mg, and caffeine 15 mg [not available in the U.S.]
- ratio-Lenoltec No. 4 [CAN], Tylenol No. 4 with Codeine [CAN]: Acetaminophen 300 mg and codeine phosphate 60 mg [not available in the U.S.]
- Triatec-8 [CAN]: Acetaminophen 325 mg, codeine phosphate 8 mg, and caffeine 30 mg [not available in the U.S.]
- Triatec-8 Strong [CAN]: Acetaminophen 500 mg, codeine phosphate 8 mg, and caffeine 30 mg [not available in the U.S.]
- Tylenol® with Codeine No. 3: Acetaminophen 300 mg and codeine phosphate 30 mg [contains sodium metabisulfite]
- Tylenol® with Codeine No. 4: Acetaminophen 300 mg and codeine phosphate 60 mg [contains sodium metabisulfite]

- **Acetaminophen and Hydrocodone** *see* Hydrocodone and Acetaminophen *on page 636*
- **Acetaminophen and Oxycodone** *see* Oxycodone and Acetaminophen *on page 969*
- **Acetaminophen and Propoxyphene** *see* Propoxyphene and Acetaminophen *on page 1076*
- **Acetaminophen, Caffeine, Codeine, and Butalbital** *see* Butalbital, Acetaminophen, Caffeine, and Codeine *on page 207*

AcetaZOLAMIDE (a set a ZOLE a mide)

Medication Safety Issues

Sound-alike/look-alike issues:

AcetaZOLAMIDE may be confused with acetoHEXAMIDE

Diamox® Sequels® may be confused with Dobutrex®, Trimox®

U.S. Brand Names Diamox® Sequels®

Canadian Brand Names Apo-Acetazolamide®; Diamox®

Pharmacologic Category Anticonvulsant, Miscellaneous; Carbonic Anhydrase Inhibitor; Diuretic, Carbonic Anhydrase Inhibitor; Ophthalmic Agent, Antiglaucoma

Generic Available Yes: Injection, tablet

Use Treatment of glaucoma (chronic simple open-angle, secondary glaucoma, preoperatively in acute angle-closure); drug-induced edema or edema due to congestive heart failure (adjunctive therapy); centrencephalic epilepsies (immediate release dosage form); prevention or amelioration of symptoms associated with acute mountain sickness

Unlabeled/Investigational Use Urine alkalinization; respiratory stimulant in COPD; metabolic alkalosis

Mechanism of Action Reversible inhibition of the enzyme carbonic anhydrase resulting in reduction of hydrogen ion secretion at renal tubule and an increased renal excretion of sodium, potassium, bicarbonate, and water to decrease production of aqueous humor; also inhibits carbonic anhydrase in central nervous system to retard abnormal and excessive discharge from CNS neurons

Pharmacodynamics/Kinetics

Onset of action: Capsule, extended release: 2 hours; I.V.: 2 minutes

Peak effect: Capsule, extended release: 8-12 hours; I.V.: 15 minutes; Tablet: 2-4 hours

Duration: Inhibition of aqueous humor secretion: Capsule, extended release: 18-24 hours; I.V.: 4-5 hours; Tablet: 8-12 hours

Distribution: Erythrocytes, kidneys; blood-brain barrier and placenta; distributes into milk (~30% of plasma concentrations)

Excretion: Urine (70% to 100% as unchanged drug)

Dosage Note: I.M. administration is not recommended because of pain secondary to the alkaline pH

Children:

Glaucoma:

Oral: 8-30 mg/kg/day or 300-900 mg/m^2/day divided every 8 hours

I.V.: 20-40 mg/kg/24 hours divided every 6 hours, not to exceed 1 g/day

Edema: Oral, I.V.: 5 mg/kg or 150 mg/m^2 once every day

Epilepsy: Oral: 8-30 mg/kg/day in 1-4 divided doses, not to exceed 1 g/day; extended release capsule is not recommended for treatment of epilepsy

Adults:

Glaucoma:

Chronic simple (open-angle): Oral: 250 mg 1-4 times/day or 500 mg extended release capsule twice daily

Secondary, acute (closed-angle): I.V.: 250-500 mg, may repeat in 2-4 hours to a maximum of 1 g/day

Edema: Oral, I.V.: 250-375 mg once daily

Epilepsy: Oral: 8-30 mg/kg/day in 1-4 divided doses; **extended release capsule is not recommended for treatment of epilepsy**

Metabolic alkalosis (unlabeled use): I.V. 250 mg every 6 hours for 4 doses or 500 mg single dose; reassess need based upon acid-base status

Mountain sickness: Oral: 250 mg every 8-12 hours (or 500 mg extended release capsules every 12-24 hours)

Therapy should begin 24-48 hours before and continue during ascent and for at least 48 hours after arrival at the high altitude

Note: In situations of rapid ascent (such as rescue or military operations), 1000 mg/day is recommended.

Urine alkalinization (unlabeled use): Oral: 5 mg/kg/dose repeated 2-3 times over 24 hours

Respiratory stimulant in COPD (unlabeled use): Oral, I.V.: 250 mg twice daily

Elderly: Oral: Initial: 250 mg twice daily; use lowest effective dose

Dosing adjustment in renal impairment:

Cl_{cr} 10-50 mL/minute: Administer every 12 hours

Cl_{cr} <10 mL/minute: Avoid use (ineffective)

Hemodialysis: Moderately dialyzable (20% to 50%)

Peritoneal dialysis: Supplemental dose is not necessary

Stability

Capsules, tablets: Store at controlled room temperature.

Injection: Store vial for injection (prior to reconstitution) at controlled room temperature. Reconstitute with at least 5 mL sterile water to provide a solution containing not more than 100 mg/mL. Reconstituted solution may be refrigerated (2°C to 8°C) for 1 week, however, use within 12 hours is recommended. Further dilute in D_5W or NS for I.V. infusion. Stability of IVPB solution is 5 days at room temperature (25°C) and 44 days at refrigeration (5°C).

Administration

Oral: May cause an alteration in taste, especially carbonated beverages. Short-acting tablets may be crushed and suspended in cherry or chocolate syrup to disguise the bitter taste of the drug; do not use fruit juices. Alternatively, submerge tablet in 10 mL of hot water and add 10 mL honey or syrup.

I.M.: I.M. administration is painful because of the alkaline pH of the drug; use by this route is not recommended.

Monitoring Parameters Intraocular pressure, potassium, serum bicarbonate; serum electrolytes, periodic CBC with differential; monitor growth in pediatric patients

Pregnancy Risk Factor C

Contraindications Hypersensitivity to acetazolamide, sulfonamides, or any component of the formulation; hepatic disease or insufficiency; decreased sodium and/or potassium levels; adrenocortical insufficiency, cirrhosis; hyperchloremic acidosis, severe renal disease or dysfunction; severe pulmonary obstruction; long-term use in noncongestive angle-closure glaucoma

Warnings/Precautions Use in impaired hepatic function may result in coma. Use with caution in patients with respiratory acidosis and diabetes mellitus. Impairment of mental alertness and/or physical coordination may occur. Chemical similarities are present among sulfonamides, sulfonylureas, carbonic anhydrase inhibitors, thiazides, and loop diuretics (except ethacrynic acid). Use in patients with sulfonamide allergy is specifically contraindicated in product labeling, however, a risk of cross-reaction exists in patients with allergy to any of these compounds; avoid use when previous reaction has been severe. Discontinue if signs of hypersensitivity are noted.

I.M. administration is painful because of the alkaline pH of the drug; use by this route is not recommended.

Drug may cause substantial increase in blood glucose in some diabetic patients; malaise and complaints of tiredness and myalgia are signs of excessive dosing and acidosis in the elderly.

Adverse Reactions Frequency not defined.

Cardiovascular: Flushing

Central nervous system: Ataxia, confusion, convulsions, depression, dizziness, drowsiness, excitement, fatigue, fever, headache, malaise

Dermatologic: Allergic skin reactions, photosensitivity, Stevens-Johnson syndrome, toxic epidermal necrolysis, urticaria

Endocrine & metabolic: Electrolyte imbalance, growth retardation (children), hyperglycemia, hypoglycemia, hypokalemia, hyponatremia, metabolic acidosis

Gastrointestinal: Appetite decreased, diarrhea, melena, nausea, taste alteration, vomiting

Genitourinary: Crystalluria, glycosuria, hematuria, polyuria, renal failure

Hematologic: Agranulocytosis, aplastic anemia, leukopenia, thrombocytopenia, thrombocytopenic purpura

Hepatic: Cholestatic jaundice, fulminant hepatic necrosis, hepatic insufficiency, liver function tests abnormal

Local: Pain at injection site

Neuromuscular & skeletal: Flaccid paralysis, paresthesia

(Continued)

AcetaZOLAMIDE *(Continued)*

Ocular: Myopia
Otic: Hearing disturbance, tinnitus
Miscellaneous: Anaphylaxis

Overdosage/Toxicology Symptoms of overdose include low blood sugar, tingling of lips and tongue, nausea, yawning, confusion, agitation, tachycardia, sweating, convulsions, stupor, and coma. Hypoglycemia should be managed with 50 mL I.V. dextrose 50% followed immediately with a continuous infusion of 10% dextrose in water (administer at a rate sufficient enough to approach a serum glucose level of 100 mg/dL). The use of corticosteroids to treat hypoglycemia is controversial, however, adding 100 mg of hydrocortisone to the dextrose infusion may prove helpful. In certain instances, hemodialysis may be helpful.

Drug Interactions Inhibits CYP3A4 (weak)

Amphetamines: Urinary excretion of amphetamine may be decreased; magnitude and duration of effects may be enhanced.

Carbamazepine: May increase serum concentrations of carbamazepine.

Cyclosporine trough concentrations may be increased resulting in possible nephrotoxicity and neurotoxicity.

Flecainide: May decrease excretion of flecainide.

Lithium: Serum concentrations may be decreased by acetazolamide; monitor.

Memantine: May decrease excretion of memantine.

Methenamine: Urinary antiseptic effect may be prevented by acetazolamide.

Phenytoin: Serum concentrations of phenytoin may be increased; incidence of osteomalacia may be enhanced or increased in patients on chronic phenytoin therapy.

Primidone serum concentrations may be decreased; carbonic anhydrase inhibitors may enhance the adverse/toxic effects of primidone.

Quinidine: Urinary excretion of quinidine may be decreased and effects may be enhanced.

Salicylate use (high dose) may result in carbonic anhydrase inhibitor accumulation and toxicity including CNS depression and metabolic acidosis. Salicylate toxicity might also be enhanced.

Test Interactions May cause false-positive results for urinary protein with Albustix®, Labstix®, Albutest®, Bumintest®; interferes with HPLC theophylline assay and serum uric acid levels

Dietary Considerations May be taken with food to decrease GI upset. May have additive effects with other folic acid antagonists. Sodium content of 500 mg injection: 47.2 mg (2.05 mEq).

Dosage Forms

Capsule, extended release:
  Diamox® Sequels®: 500 mg
Injection, powder for reconstitution: 500 mg
Tablet: 125 mg, 250 mg

Acetylcholine (a se teel KOE leen)

Medication Safety Issues

Sound-alike/look-alike issues:
  Acetylcholine may be confused with acetylcysteine

U.S. Brand Names Miochol-E®

Canadian Brand Names Miochol-E®

Synonyms Acetylcholine Chloride

Pharmacologic Category Cholinergic Agonist; Ophthalmic Agent, Miotic

Generic Available No

Use Produces complete miosis in cataract surgery, keratoplasty, iridectomy, and other anterior segment surgery where rapid miosis is required

Mechanism of Action Causes contraction of the sphincter muscles of the iris, resulting in miosis and contraction of the ciliary muscle, leading to accommodation spasm

Pharmacodynamics/Kinetics

Onset of action: Rapid
Duration: ~10 minutes

Dosage Adults: Intraocular: 0.5-2 mL of 1% injection (5-20 mg) instilled into anterior chamber before or after securing one or more sutures

Stability Prepare solution immediately before use and discard unused portion. Acetylcholine solutions are unstable; reconstitute immediately before use.

Administration Open under aseptic conditions only.

Anesthesia and Critical Care Concerns/Other Considerations Systemic effects are rare after intraocular administration, but can occur. Caution should be used in patients with cardiovascular disease.

Pregnancy Risk Factor C

Contraindications Hypersensitivity to acetylcholine chloride or any component of the formulation; acute iritis and acute inflammatory disease of the anterior chamber

Warnings/Precautions Systemic effects rarely occur but can cause problems for patients with acute cardiac failure, bronchial asthma, peptic ulcer, hyperthyroidism, GI spasm, urinary tract obstruction, and Parkinson's disease; open under aseptic conditions only.

Adverse Reactions Frequency not defined.

Cardiovascular: Bradycardia, hypotension, flushing

Central nervous system: Headache

Ocular: Distance vision altered, night vision decreased, transient lenticular opacities

Respiratory: Dyspnea

Miscellaneous: Diaphoresis

Overdosage/Toxicology Treatment includes flushing eyes with water or normal saline and supportive measures. If accidentally ingested, induce emesis or perform gastric lavage.

Drug Interactions

Decreased effect possible with flurbiprofen and suprofen, ophthalmic.

Increased effect may be prolonged or enhanced in patients receiving tacrine.

Dosage Forms Powder for intraocular solution, as chloride: 1:100 [10 mg/mL] (2 mL)

♦ **Acetylcholine Chloride** *see* Acetylcholine *on page 34*

Acetylcysteine (a se teel SIS teen)

Medication Safety Issues

Sound-alike/look-alike issues:

- Acetylcysteine may be confused with acetylcholine
- Mucomyst® may be confused with Mucinex®

U.S. Brand Names Acetadote®

Canadian Brand Names Acetylcysteine Solution; Mucomyst®; Parvolex®

Synonyms Acetylcysteine Sodium; Mercapturic Acid; Mucomyst; NAC; *N*-Acetylcysteine; *N*-Acetyl-L-cysteine

Pharmacologic Category Antidote; Mucolytic Agent

Generic Available Yes: Solution for inhalation

Use Adjunctive mucolytic therapy in patients with abnormal or viscid mucous secretions in acute and chronic bronchopulmonary diseases; pulmonary complications of surgery and cystic fibrosis; diagnostic bronchial studies; antidote for acute acetaminophen toxicity

Unlabeled/Investigational Use Prevention of radiocontrast-induced renal dysfunction (oral, I.V.); distal intestinal obstruction syndrome (DIOS, previously referred to as meconium ileus equivalent)

Mechanism of Action Exerts mucolytic action through its free sulfhydryl group which opens up the disulfide bonds in the mucoproteins thus lowering mucous viscosity. The exact mechanism of action in acetaminophen toxicity is unknown; thought to act by providing substrate for conjugation with the toxic metabolite.

Pharmacodynamics/Kinetics

Onset of action: Inhalation: 5-10 minutes

Duration: Inhalation: >1 hour

Distribution: 0.47 L/kg

Protein binding, plasma: 83%

Half-life elimination:

- Reduced acetylcysteine: 2 hours
- Total acetylcysteine: Adults: 5.5 hours; Newborns: 11 hours

Time to peak, plasma: Oral: 1-2 hours

Excretion: Urine

(Continued)

Acetylcysteine *(Continued)*

Dosage

Acetaminophen poisoning: Children and Adults:

Oral: 140 mg/kg; followed by 17 doses of 70 mg/kg every 4 hours; repeat dose if emesis occurs within 1 hour of administration; therapy should continue until acetaminophen levels are undetectable and there is no evidence of hepatotoxicity.

I.V. (Acetadote®): Loading dose: 150 mg/kg over 60 minutes. Loading dose is followed by 2 additional infusions: Initial maintenance dose of 50 mg/kg infused over 4 hours, followed by a second maintenance dose of 100 mg/kg infused over 16 hours. To avoid fluid overload in patients <40 kg and those requiring fluid restriction, decrease volume of D_5W proportionally. Total dosage: 300 mg/kg administered over 21 hours.

Note: If commercial I.V. form is unavailable, the following dose has been reported using solution for oral inhalation (unlabeled): Loading dose: 140 mg/kg, followed by 70 mg/kg every 4 hours, for a total of 13 doses (loading dose and 48 hours of treatment); infuse each dose over 1 hour through a 0.2 micron Millipore filter (in-line).

Experts suggest that the duration of acetylcysteine administration may vary depending upon serial acetaminophen levels and liver function tests obtained during treatment. In general, patients without measurable acetaminophen levels and without significant LFT elevations (>3 times the ULN) can safely stop acetylcysteine after ≤24 hours of treatment. The patients who still have detectable levels of acetaminophen, and/or LFT elevations (>1000 units/L) continue to benefit from additional acetylcysteine administration

Adjuvant therapy in respiratory conditions: **Note:** Patients should receive an aerosolized bronchodilator 10-15 minutes prior to acetylcysteine.

Inhalation, nebulization (face mask, mouth piece, tracheostomy): Acetylcysteine 10% and 20% solution (dilute 20% solution with sodium chloride or sterile water for inhalation); 10% solution may be used undiluted

Infants: 1-2 mL of 20% solution or 2-4 mL of 10% solution until nebulized given 3-4 times/day

Children and Adults: 3-5 mL of 20% solution or 6-10 mL of 10% solution until nebulized given 3-4 times/day; dosing range: 1-10 mL of 20% solution or 2-20 mL of 10% solution every 2-6 hours

Inhalation, nebulization (tent, croupette): Children and Adults: Dose must be individualized; may require up to 300 mL solution/treatment

Direct instillation: Adults:

Into tracheostomy: 1-2 mL of 10% to 20% solution every 1-4 hours

Through percutaneous intratracheal catheter: 1-2 mL of 20% or 2-4 mL of 10% solution every 1-4 hours via syringe attached to catheter

Diagnostic bronchogram: Nebulization or intratracheal: Adults: 1-2 mL of 20% solution or 2-4 mL of 10% solution administered 2-3 times prior to procedure

Prevention of radiocontrast-induced renal dysfunction (unlabeled use): Adults: Oral: 600 mg twice daily for 2 days (beginning the day before the procedure); may be given as powder in capsules, some centers use solution (diluted in cola beverage or juice). Hydrate patient with saline concurrently.

Stability

Solution for injection (Acetadote®): Store vials at room temperature, 20°C to 25°C (68°F to 77°F). Following reconstitution with D_5W, solution is stable for 24 hours at room temperature.

Note: To avoid fluid overload in patients <40 kg and those requiring fluid restriction, decrease volume of D_5W proportionally. Discard unused portion.

Loading dose: Dilute 150 mg/kg in D_5W 200 mL

Initial maintenance dose: Dilute 50 mg/kg in D_5W 500 mL

Second maintenance dose: Dilute 100 mg/kg in D_5W 1000 mL

Solution for inhalation (Mucomyst®): Store unopened vials at room temperature; once opened, store under refrigeration and use within 96 hours. The 20% solution may be diluted with sodium chloride or sterile water; the 10% solution may be used undiluted. A color change may occur in opened vials (light purple) and does not affect the safety or efficacy.

Intravenous administration of solution for inhalation (unlabeled route): Using D_5W, dilute acetylcysteine 20% oral solution to a 3% solution.

Administration

Inhalation: Acetylcysteine is incompatible with tetracyclines, erythromycin, amphotericin B, iodized oil, chymotrypsin, trypsin, and hydrogen peroxide. Administer separately. Intermittent aerosol treatments are commonly given when patient arises, before meals, and just before retiring at bedtime.

Oral: For treatment of acetaminophen overdosage, administer orally as a 5% solution. Dilute the 20% solution 1:3 with a cola, orange juice, or other soft drink. Use within 1 hour of preparation. Unpleasant odor becomes less noticeable as treatment progresses. If patient vomits within 1 hour of dose, readminister.

I.V. :

Intravenous formulation (Acetadote®): Administer loading dose of 150 mg/kg over 60 minutes, followed by two separate maintenance infusions: 50 mg/kg over 4 hours followed by 100 mg/kg over 16 hours.

If not using commercially available I.V. formulation, use a 0.2-μ millipore filter (in-line).

Monitoring Parameters Acetaminophen overdose: AST, ALT, bilirubin, PT, serum creatinine, BUN, serum glucose, and electrolytes. Acetaminophen levels at ~4 hours postingestion (every 4-6 hours if extended release acetaminophen; plot on the nomogram) and every 4-6 hours to assess serum levels, and LFTs for possible hepatotoxicity. Assess patient for nausea, vomiting, and skin rash following oral administration for treatment of acetaminophen poisoning. If administered I.V., monitor for anaphylaxis/anaphylactoid reactions.

Reference Range Determine acetaminophen level as soon as possible, but no sooner than 4 hours after ingestion (to ensure peak levels have been obtained); administer for acetaminophen level >150 mcg/mL at 4 hours following ingestion; toxic concentration with probable hepatotoxicity: >200 mcg/mL at 4 hours or 50 mcg at 12 hours

Anesthesia and Critical Care Concerns/Other Considerations Intravenous acetylcysteine may be indicated over oral formulation in treatment of acetaminophen overdose for a restricted number of indications (oral cannot be tolerated; coingested toxin requires ongoing gastrointestinal decontamination; gastrointestinal tract nonfunctional; late presentation of acetaminophen overdose; neonatal toxicity from maternal overdose) (Yip, 1998). A commercially manufactured intravenous product is now available in the United States. If this formulation is unavailable, the product normally administered by inhalation can be administered intravenously. The inhalation preparation is sterile, but not labeled "pyrogen free." In Yip's retrospective case series, adverse reactions occurred in 4 (~5%) cases. Flushing, pruritus, and phlebitis were reported; one was labeled as an "anaphylactic reaction."

Bailey and McGuigan reviewed a retrospective case series of patients who received intravenous acetylcysteine and the literature to develop management guideline for anaphylactoid reactions (Bailey, 1998). Their recommendations for treatment of nonlife-threatening allergic reactions include reassessing the need for intravenous acetylcysteine, and administering diphenhydramine (1 mg/kg I.V.; maximum dose: 50 mg). If the acetylcysteine infusion was stopped initially and symptoms resolved, consider restarting infusion 1 hour after diphenhydramine's administration. Anaphylactoid reactions have also been reported with the commercial I.V. formulation. Monitor closely for allergic reactions. Be prepared to handle anaphylactoid reaction if it occurs.

Pregnancy Risk Factor B

Contraindications Hypersensitivity to acetylcysteine or any component of the formulation

Warnings/Precautions

Inhalation: Since increased bronchial secretions may develop after inhalation, percussion, postural drainage, and suctioning should follow. If bronchospasm occurs, administer a bronchodilator; discontinue acetylcysteine if bronchospasm progresses.

Intravenous: Acute flushing and erythema have been reported; usually occurs within 30-60 minutes and may resolve spontaneously. Serious anaphylactoid reactions have also been reported. Acetylcysteine infusion may be interrupted until treatment of allergic symptoms is initiated; the infusion can then be carefully restarted. Treatment for anaphylactic reactions should be immediately available. Use caution with asthma or history of bronchospasm.

Acetaminophen overdose: The modified Rumack-Matthew nomogram allows for stratification of patients into risk categories based on the relationship between

(Continued)

Acetylcysteine *(Continued)*

the serum acetaminophen level and time after ingestion. There are several situations where the nomogram is of limited use. Serum acetaminophen levels obtained prior to 4-hour postingestion are not interpretable; patients presenting late may have undetectable serum concentrations, but have received a lethal dose. The nomogram is less predictive in a chronic ingestion or in an overdose with an extended release product. Acetylcysteine should be administered for any signs of hepatotoxicity even if acetaminophen serum level is low or undetectable. The nomogram also does not take into account patients at higher risk of acetaminophen toxicity (eg, alcoholics, malnourished patients).

Adverse Reactions

Inhalation: Frequency not defined.

Central nervous system: Drowsiness, chills, fever

Gastrointestinal: Vomiting, nausea, stomatitis

Local: Irritation, stickiness on face following nebulization

Respiratory: Bronchospasm, rhinorrhea, hemoptysis

Miscellaneous: Acquired sensitization (rare), clamminess, unpleasant odor during administration

Intravenous:

>10%: Miscellaneous: Anaphylactoid reaction (~17%; reported as severe in 1% or moderate in 10% of patients within 15 minutes of first infusion; severe in 1% or mild to moderate in 6% to 7% of patients after 60-minute infusion)

1% to 10%:

Cardiovascular: Angioedema (2% to 8%), vasodilation (1% to 6%), hypotension (1% to 4%), tachycardia (1% to 4%), syncope (1% to 3%), chest tightness (1%), flushing (1%)

Central nervous system: Dysphoria (<1% to 2%)

Dermatologic: Urticaria (2% to 7%), rash (1% to 5%), facial erythema (≤1%), palmar erythema (≤1%), pruritus (≤1% to 3%), pruritus with rash and vasodilation (2% to 9%)

Gastrointestinal: Vomiting (<1% to 10%), nausea (1% to 10%), dyspepsia (≤1%)

Neuromuscular & skeletal: Gait disturbance (<1% to 2%)

Ocular: Eye pain (<1% to 3%)

Otic: Ear pain (1%)

Respiratory: Bronchospasm (1% to 6%), cough (1% to 4%), dyspnea (<1% to 3%), pharyngitis (1%), rhinorrhea (1%), rhonchi (1%), throat tightness (1%)

Miscellaneous: Diaphoresis (≤1%)

Overdosage/Toxicology Treatment of acetylcysteine toxicity is usually aimed at reversing anaphylactoid symptoms or controlling nausea and vomiting. The use of epinephrine, antihistamines, and steroids may be beneficial.

Drug Interactions Adsorbed by activated charcoal; clinical significance is minimal, though, once a pure acetaminophen ingestion requiring N-acetylcysteine is established; further charcoal dosing is unnecessary once the appropriate initial charcoal dose is achieved (5-10 g:g acetaminophen)

Dosage Forms

Injection, solution:

Acetadote®: 20% [200 mg/mL] (30 mL) [contains disodium edetate]

Solution, inhalation/oral: 10% [100 mg/mL] (4 mL, 10 mL, 30 mL); 20% [200 mg/mL] (4 mL, 10 mL, 30 mL)

References

Allaqaband S, Tumuluri R, Malik AM, et al, "Prospective Randomized Study of N-Acetylcysteine, Fenoldopam, and Saline for Prevention of Radiocontrast-Induced Nephropathy," *Catheter Cardiovasc Interv*, 2002, 57(3):279-83.

Appelboam AV, Dargan PI, and Knighton J, "Fatal Anaphylactoid Reaction to N-Acetylcysteine: Caution in Patients With Asthma," *Emerg Med J*, 2002, 19(6):594-5.

Bailey B and McGuigan MA, "Management of Anaphylactoid Reactions to Intravenous N-Acetylcysteine," *Ann Emerg Med*, 1998, 31(6):710-5.

Curhan GC, "Prevention of Contrast Nephropathy," *JAMA*, 2003, 289(5):606-8.

Falk JL, "Oral N-Acetylcysteine Given Intravenously for Acetaminophen Overdose: We Shouldn't Have To, But We Must," *Crit Care Med*, 1998, 26(1):7.

Mokhlesi B, Leikin JB, Murray P, et al, "Adult Toxicology in Critical Care: Part II: Specific Poisonings," *Chest*, 2003, 123(3):897-922.

Prescott LF, Donovan JW, Jarvie DR, et al, "The Disposition and Kinetics of Intravenous N-acetylcysteine in Patients With Paracetamol Overdosage," *Eur J Clin Pharmacol*, 1989, 37(5):501-6.

Prescott LF, Illingworth RN, Critchley JA, et al, "Intravenous N-Acetylcysteine: The Treatment of Choice for Paracetamol Poisoning," *Br Med J*, 1979, 2(6198):1097-100.

Smilkstein MJ, Bronstein AC, Linden C, et al, "Acetaminophen Overdose: A 48-Hour Intravenous N-Acetylcysteine Treatment Protocol," *Ann Emerg Med*, 1991, 20(10):1058-63.

Tepel M, van der Giet M, Schwarzfeld C, et al, "Prevention of Radiographic-Contrast-Agent-Induced Reductions in Renal Function by Acetylcysteine," *N Engl J Med*, 2000, 343(3):180-4.

Yankaskas JR, Marshall BC, Sufian B, et al, "Cystic Fibrosis Adult Care: Consensus Conference Report," *Chest*, 2004, 125(1 Suppl):1-39.

Yip L, Dart RC, and Hurlbut KM, "Intravenous Administration of Oral N-Acetylcysteine," *Crit Care Med*, 1998, 26(1):40-3.

- ♦ **Acetylcysteine Sodium** *see* Acetylcysteine *on page 35*
- ♦ **Acetylcysteine Solution (Can)** *see* Acetylcysteine *on page 35*
- ♦ **Acetylsalicylic Acid** *see* Aspirin *on page 129*
- ♦ **Aciclovir** *see* Acyclovir *on page 39*
- ♦ **Acilac (Can)** *see* Lactulose *on page 724*
- ♦ **AcipHex®** *see* Rabeprazole *on page 1099*
- ♦ **Aclasta® (Can)** *see* Zoledronic Acid *on page 1377*
- ♦ **Actidose-Aqua® [OTC]** *see* Charcoal *on page 259*
- ♦ **Actidose® with Sorbitol [OTC]** *see* Charcoal *on page 259*
- ♦ **Actiq®** *see* Fentanyl *on page 514*
- ♦ **Activase®** *see* Alteplase *on page 72*
- ♦ **Activase® rt-PA (Can)** *see* Alteplase *on page 72*
- ♦ **Activated Carbon** *see* Charcoal *on page 259*
- ♦ **Activated Charcoal** *see* Charcoal *on page 259*
- ♦ **Activated Protein C, Human, Recombinant** *see* Drotrecogin Alfa *on page 434*
- ♦ **Acular®** *see* Ketorolac *on page 717*
- ♦ **Acular LS™** *see* Ketorolac *on page 717*
- ♦ **Acular® PF** *see* Ketorolac *on page 717*
- ♦ **ACV** *see* Acyclovir *on page 39*
- ♦ **Acycloguanosine** *see* Acyclovir *on page 39*

Acyclovir (ay SYE kloe veer)

Medication Safety Issues
Sound-alike/look-alike issues:
Zovirax® may be confused with Zostrix®, Zyvox™

U.S. Brand Names Zovirax®

Canadian Brand Names Apo-Acyclovir®; Gen-Acyclovir; Nu-Acyclovir; ratio-Acyclovir; Zovirax®

Synonyms Aciclovir; ACV; Acycloguanosine

Pharmacologic Category Antiviral Agent

Generic Available Yes: Excludes cream, ointment

Use Treatment of genital herpes simplex virus (HSV), herpes labialis (cold sores), herpes zoster (shingles), HSV encephalitis, neonatal HSV, mucocutaneous HSV in immunocompromised patients, varicella-zoster (chickenpox)

Unlabeled/Investigational Use Prevention of HSV reactivation in HIV-positive patients; prevention of HSV reactivation in hematopoietic stem-cell transplant (HSCT); prevention of HSV reactivation during periods of neutropenia in patients with acute leukemia

Mechanism of Action Acyclovir is converted to acyclovir monophosphate by virus-specific thymidine kinase then further converted to acyclovir triphosphate by other cellular enzymes. Acyclovir triphosphate inhibits DNA synthesis and viral replication by competing with deoxyguanosine triphosphate for viral DNA polymerase and being incorporated into viral DNA.

Pharmacodynamics/Kinetics
Absorption: Oral: 15% to 30%
Distribution: V_d: 0.8 L/kg (63.6 L): Widely (eg, brain, kidney, lungs, liver, spleen, muscle, uterus, vagina, CSF)
Protein binding: 9% to 33%
Metabolism: Converted by viral enzymes to acyclovir monophosphate, and further converted to diphosphate then triphosphate (active form) by cellular enzymes
Bioavailability: Oral: 10% to 20% with normal renal function (bioavailability decreases with increased dose)
Half-life elimination: Terminal: Neonates: 4 hours; Children 1-12 years: 2-3 hours; Adults: 3 hours
Time to peak, serum: Oral: Within 1.5-2 hours
(Continued)

Acyclovir *(Continued)*

Excretion: Urine (62% to 90% as unchanged drug and metabolite)

Dosage Note: Obese patients should be dosed using ideal body weight

Genital HSV:

I.V.: Children ≥12 years and Adults (immunocompetent): Initial episode, severe: 5 mg/kg every 8 hours for 5-7 days

Oral:

Children:

Initial episode (unlabeled use): 40-80 mg/kg/day divided into 3-4 doses for 5-10 days (maximum: 1 g/day)

Chronic suppression (unlabeled use; limited data): 80 mg/kg/day in 3 divided doses (maximum: 1 g/day), re-evaluate after 12 months of treatment

Adults:

Initial episode: 200 mg every 4 hours while awake (5 times/day) for 10 days (per manufacturer's labeling); 400 mg 3 times/day for 5-10 days has also been reported

Recurrence: 200 mg every 4 hours while awake (5 times/day) for 5 days (per manufacturer's labeling; begin at earliest signs of disease); 400 mg 3 times/day for 5 days has also been reported

Chronic suppression: 400 mg twice daily or 200 mg 3-5 times/day, for up to 12 months followed by re-evaluation (per manufacturer's labeling); 400-1200 mg/day in 2-3 divided doses has also been reported

Topical: Adults (immunocompromised): Ointment: Initial episode: ½" ribbon of ointment for a 4" square surface area every 3 hours (6 times/day) for 7 days

Herpes labialis (cold sores): Topical: Children ≥12 years and Adults: Cream: Apply 5 times/day for 4 days

Herpes zoster (shingles):

Oral: Adults (immunocompetent): 800 mg every 4 hours (5 times/day) for 7-10 days

I.V.:

Children <12 years (immunocompromised): 20 mg/kg/dose every 8 hours for 7 days

Children ≥12 years and Adults (immunocompromised): 10 mg/kg/dose or 500 mg/m^2/dose every 8 hours for 7 days

HSV encephalitis: I.V.:

Children 3 months to 12 years: 20 mg/kg/dose every 8 hours for 10 days (per manufacturer's labeling); dosing for 14-21 days also reported

Children ≥12 years and Adults: 10 mg/kg/dose every 8 hours for 10 days (per manufacturer's labeling); 10-15 mg/kg/dose every 8 hours for 14-21 days also reported

Mucocutaneous HSV:

I.V.:

Children <12 years (immunocompromised): 10 mg/kg/dose every 8 hours for 7 days

Children ≥12 years and Adults (immunocompromised): 5 mg/kg/dose every 8 hours for 7 days (per manufacturer's labeling); dosing for up to 14 days also reported

Oral: Adults (immunocompromised, unlabeled use): 400 mg 5 times a day for 7-14 days

Topical: Ointment: Adults (nonlife-threatening, immunocompromised): ½" ribbon of ointment for a 4" square surface area every 3 hours (6 times/day) for 7 days

Neonatal HSV: I.V.: Neonate: Birth to 3 months: 10 mg/kg/dose every 8 hours for 10 days (manufacturer's labeling); 15 mg/kg/dose or 20 mg/kg/dose every 8 hours for 14-21 days has also been reported

Varicella-zoster (chickenpox): Begin treatment within the first 24 hours of rash onset:

Oral:

Children ≥2 years and ≤40 kg (immunocompetent): 20 mg/kg/dose (up to 800 mg/dose) 4 times/day for 5 days

Children >40 kg and Adults (immunocompetent): 800 mg/dose 4 times a day for 5 days

I.V.:

Children <1 year (immunocompromised, unlabeled use): 10 mg/kg/dose every 8 hours for 7-10 days

Children ≥1 year and Adults (immunocompromised, unlabeled use): 1500 mg/m^2/day divided every 8 hours or 10 mg/kg/dose every 8 hours for 7-10 days

Prevention of HSV reactivation in HIV-positive patients, for use only when recurrences are frequent or severe (unlabeled use): Oral:

Children: 80 mg/kg/day in 3-4 divided doses

Adults: 200 mg 3 times/day or 400 mg 2 times/day

Prevention of HSV reactivation in HSCT (unlabeled use): Note: Start at the beginning of conditioning therapy and continue until engraftment or until mucositis resolves (~30 days)

Oral: Adults: 200 mg 3 times/day

I.V.:

Children: 250 mg/m^2/dose every 8 hours or 125 mg/m^2/dose every 6 hours

Adults: 250 mg/m^2/dose every 12 hours

Bone marrow transplant recipients (unlabeled use): I.V.: Children and Adults: Allogeneic patients who are HSV and CMV seropositive: 500 mg/m^2/dose (10 mg/kg) every 8 hours; for clinically-symptomatic CMV infection, consider replacing acyclovir with ganciclovir

Dosing adjustment in renal impairment:

Oral:

Cl_{cr} 10-25 mL/minute/1.73 m^2: Normal dosing regimen 800 mg every 4 hours: Administer 800 mg every 8 hours

Cl_{cr} <10 mL/minute/1.73 m^2:

Normal dosing regimen 200 mg every 4 hours, 200 mg every 8 hours, or 400 mg every 12 hours: Administer 200 mg every 12 hours

Normal dosing regimen 800 mg every 4 hours: Administer 800 mg every 12 hours

I.V.:

Cl_{cr} 25-50 mL/minute/1.73 m^2: Administer recommended dose every 12 hours

Cl_{cr} 10-25 mL/minute/1.73 m^2: Administer recommended dose every 24 hours

Cl_{cr} <10 mL/minute/1.73 m^2: Administer 50% of recommended dose every 24 hours

Hemodialysis: Administer dose after dialysis

Peritoneal dialysis: No supplemental dose needed

CAVH: 3.5 mg/kg/day

CVVHD/CVVH: Adjust dose based upon Cl_{cr} 30 mL/minute

Stability

Capsule, tablet: Store at controlled room temperature of 15°C to 25°C (59°F to 77°F); protect from moisture.

Cream, suspension: Store at controlled room temperature of 15°C to 25°C (59°F to 77°F).

Ointment: Store at controlled room temperature of 15°C to 25°C (59°F to 77°F) in a dry place.

Injection: Store powder at controlled room temperature of 15°C to 25°C (59°F to 77°F). Reconstitute acyclovir 500 mg with SWFI 10 mL; do not use bacteriostatic water containing benzyl alcohol or parabens. For intravenous infusion, dilute to a final concentration ≤7 mg/mL. Concentrations >10 mg/mL increase the risk of phlebitis. Reconstituted solutions remain stable for 12 hours at room temperature. Do not refrigerate reconstituted solutions as they may precipitate. Once diluted for infusion, use within 24 hours.

Administration

Oral: May be administered with or without food.

I.V.: Avoid rapid infusion; infuse over 1 hour to prevent renal damage; maintain adequate hydration of patient; check for phlebitis and rotate infusion sites

Topical: Not for use in the eye. Apply using a finger cot or rubber glove to avoid transmission to other parts of the body or to other persons.

Monitoring Parameters Urinalysis, BUN, serum creatinine, liver enzymes, CBC

Pregnancy Risk Factor B

Contraindications Hypersensitivity to acyclovir, valacyclovir, or any component of the formulation

Warnings/Precautions Use with caution in immunocompromised patients; thrombocytopenic purpura/hemolytic uremic syndrome (TTP/HUS) has been reported. Use caution in the elderly, pre-existing renal disease, or in those receiving other nephrotoxic drugs. Maintain adequate hydration during oral or intravenous therapy. Use I.V. preparation with caution in patients with underlying

(Continued)

Acyclovir *(Continued)*

neurologic abnormalities, serious hepatic or electrolyte abnormalities, or substantial hypoxia.

Safety and efficacy of oral formulations have not been established in pediatric patients <2 years of age.

Chickenpox: Treatment should begin within 24 hours of appearance of rash; oral route not recommended for routine use in otherwise healthy children with varicella, but may be effective in patients at increased risk of moderate to severe infection (>12 years of age, chronic cutaneous or pulmonary disorders, long-term salicylate therapy, corticosteroid therapy).

Genital herpes: Physical contact should be avoided when lesions are present; transmission may also occur in the absence of symptoms. Treatment should begin with the first signs or symptoms.

Herpes labialis: For external use only to the lips and face; do not apply to eye or inside the mouth or nose. Treatment should begin with the first signs or symptoms.

Herpes zoster: Acyclovir should be started within 72 hours of appearance of rash to be effective.

Adverse Reactions

Systemic: Oral:

>10%: Central nervous system: Malaise (12%)

1% to 10%:

Central nervous system: Headache (2%)

Gastrointestinal: Nausea (2% to 5%), vomiting (3%), diarrhea (2% to 3%)

Systemic: Parenteral:

1% to 10%:

Dermatologic: Hives (2%), itching (2%), rash (2%)

Gastrointestinal: Nausea/vomiting (7%)

Hepatic: Liver function tests increased (1% to 2%)

Local: Inflammation at injection site or phlebitis (9%)

Renal: BUN increased (5% to 10%), creatinine increased (5% to 10%), acute renal failure

Topical:

>10%: Dermatologic: Mild pain, burning, or stinging (ointment 30%)

1% to 10%: Dermatologic: Pruritus (ointment 4%), itching

All forms: <1% (Limited to important or life-threatening): Abdominal pain, aggression, agitation, alopecia, anaphylaxis, anemia, angioedema, anorexia, ataxia, coma, confusion, consciousness decreased, delirium, desquamation, diarrhea, disseminated intravascular coagulopathy, dizziness, dry lips, dysarthria, encephalopathy, erythema multiforme, fatigue, fever, gastrointestinal distress, hallucinations, hematuria, hemolysis, hepatitis, hyperbilirubinemia, hypotension, insomnia, jaundice, leukocytoclastic vasculitis, leukocytosis, leukopenia, local tissue necrosis (following extravasation), lymphadenopathy, mental depression, myalgia, neutrophilia, paresthesia, peripheral edema, photosensitization, pruritus, psychosis, renal failure, seizure, somnolence, sore throat, Stevens-Johnson syndrome, thrombocytopenia, thrombocytopenic purpura/hemolytic uremic syndrome (TTP/HUS), thrombocytosis, toxic epidermal necrolysis, tremor, urticaria, visual disturbances

Overdosage/Toxicology Overdoses of up to 20 g have been reported. Symptoms of overdose include agitation, seizures, somnolence, confusion, elevated serum creatinine, and renal failure. In the event of overdose, sufficient urine flow must be maintained to avoid drug precipitation within renal tubules. Hemodialysis has resulted in up to 60% reduction in serum acyclovir levels.

Ethanol/Nutrition/Herb Interactions Food: Does not affect absorption of oral acyclovir.

Dietary Considerations May be taken with or without food. Acyclovir 500 mg injection contains sodium ~50 mg (~2 mEq).

Dosage Forms [DSC] = Discontinued product

Capsule: 200 mg

Zovirax®: 200 mg

Cream, topical:

Zovirax®: 5% (2 g)

Injection, powder for reconstitution, as sodium: 500 mg, 1000 mg

Zovirax®: 500 mg [DSC]

Injection, solution, as sodium [preservative free]: 25 mg/mL (20 mL, 40 mL); 50 mg/mL (10 mL, 20 mL)
Ointment, topical:
Zovirax®: 5% (15 g)
Suspension, oral: 200 mg/5 mL (480 mL)
Zovirax®: 200 mg/5 mL (480 mL) [banana flavor]
Tablet: 400 mg, 800 mg
Zovirax®: 400 mg, 800 mg

- **Adalat® XL® (Can)** *see* NIFEdipine *on page 920*
- **Adalat® CC** *see* NIFEdipine *on page 920*
- **Adamantanamine Hydrochloride** *see* Amantadine *on page 77*

Adefovir (a DEF o veer)

U.S. Brand Names Hepsera™
Synonyms Adefovir Dipivoxil
Pharmacologic Category Antiretroviral Agent, Reverse Transcriptase Inhibitor (Nucleoside)
Generic Available No
Use Treatment of chronic hepatitis B with evidence of active viral replication (based on persistent elevation of ALT/AST or histologic evidence), including patients with lamivudine-resistant hepatitis B
Mechanism of Action Acyclic nucleotide reverse transcriptase inhibitor (adenosine analog) which interferes with HBV viral RNA-dependent DNA polymerase resulting in inhibition of viral replication.
Pharmacodynamics/Kinetics
Distribution: 0.35-0.39 L/kg
Protein binding: ≤4%
Metabolism: Prodrug; rapidly converted to adefovir (active metabolite) in intestine
Bioavailability: 59%
Half-life elimination: 7.5 hours; prolonged in renal impairment
Time to peak: 1.75 hours
Excretion: Urine (45% as active metabolite within 24 hours)
Dosage Oral: Adults: 10 mg once daily
Dosage adjustment in renal impairment:
Cl_{cr} 20-49 mL/minute: 10 mg every 48 hours
Cl_{cr} 10-19 mL/minute: 10 mg every 72 hours
Hemodialysis: 10 mg every 7 days (following dialysis)
Dosage adjustment in hepatic impairment: No adjustment necessary
Stability Store at 25°C (77 °F); excursions permitted to 15°C to 30°C (59°F to 86°F).
Administration May be administered without regard to food.
Monitoring Parameters HIV status (prior to initiation of therapy); serum creatinine (prior to initiation and during therapy); viral load; LFTs for several months following discontinuation of adefovir
Pregnancy Risk Factor C
Contraindications Hypersensitivity to adefovir or any component of the formulation
Warnings/Precautions [U.S. Boxed Warning]: Use with caution in patients with renal dysfunction or in patients at risk of renal toxicity (including concurrent nephrotoxic agents or NSAIDs). Chronic administration may result in nephrotoxicity. Dosage adjustment is required in patients with renal dysfunction or in patients who develop renal dysfunction during therapy. **[U.S. Boxed Warnings]: May cause the development of resistance in patients with unrecognized or untreated HIV infection. Lactic acidosis and severe hepatomegaly with steatosis (sometimes fatal) have occurred with antiretroviral nucleoside analogues.** Female gender, obesity, and prolonged treatment may increase the risk of hepatotoxicity. Treatment should be discontinued in patients with lactic acidosis or signs/symptoms of hepatotoxicity (which may occur without marked transaminase elevations). **[U.S. Boxed Warning]: Acute exacerbations of hepatitis may occur (in up to 25% of patients) when antihepatitis therapy is discontinued.** Exacerbations typically occur within 12 weeks and may be self-limited or resolve upon resuming treatment; monitor patients following discontinuation of therapy. Safety and efficacy in pediatric patients have not been established.
(Continued)

Adefovir *(Continued)*

Adverse Reactions For a majority of adverse reactions, the incidence in adefovir-receiving patients was similar to or less than that observed with placebo treatment.

>10%:

Hepatic: ALT increased (20% grade ≥3)

Renal: Hematuria (11% grade ≥3)

1% to 10%:

Central nervous system: Headache (9%)

Dermatologic: Rash, pruritus

Endocrine & metabolic: Hypophosphatemia (1% to 2%)

Gastrointestinal: Abdominal pain (9%), nausea (5%), amylase increased (4% grade ≥3), flatulence (4%), dyspepsia (3%), vomiting, diarrhea

Hepatic: AST increased (8% grade ≥3), abnormal liver function, hepatic failure

Neuromuscular & skeletal: Weakness (13%)

Renal: Serum creatinine increased (2% to 10%; 7% grade ≥3), glycosuria (1% grade ≥3), renal failure, renal insufficiency

Note: In liver transplant patients with baseline renal dysfunction, frequency of increased serum creatinine has been observed to be as high as 32% to 53%; considering the concomitant use of other potentially nephrotoxic medications, baseline renal insufficiency, and predisposing comorbidities, the role of adefovir in these changes could not be established.

Respiratory: Cough increased, sinusitis, pharyngitis

Postmarketing and/or case reports: Hepatitis, hepatomegaly with steatosis, lactic acidosis, nephrotoxicity

Overdosage/Toxicology Limited experience in acute overdose. Chronic overdose may be associated with renal toxicity and gastrointestinal adverse effects. Hemodialysis may be effective in the removal of adefovir (35% of a 10 mg dose removed in 4 hours).

Drug Interactions

Aminoglycosides: May increase the risk of renal toxicity with adefovir.

Ganciclovir, valganciclovir: May increase the adverse effects/toxicity of reverse transcriptase inhibitors; monitor.

Ibuprofen: Increases the bioavailability of adefovir.

Immunosuppressants (cyclosporine, tacrolimus): May increase the risk of renal toxicity with adefovir.

Nephrotoxic agents: May increase the risk of renal toxicity with adefovir.

NSAIDs: May increase the risk of renal toxicity with adefovir (also see Ibuprofen above).

Ribavirin: May increase the adverse effects (eg, lactic acidosis) of reverse transcriptase inhibitors; monitor.

Vancomycin: May increase the risk of renal toxicity with adefovir.

Ethanol/Nutrition/Herb Interactions

Ethanol: Should be avoided in hepatitis B infection due to potential hepatic toxicity.

Food: Does not have a significant effect on adefovir absorption.

Dietary Considerations May be taken without regard to food.

Dosage Forms Tablet, as dipivoxil: 10 mg

◆ **Adefovir Dipivoxil** *see* Adefovir *on page 43*

◆ **Adenocard®** *see* Adenosine *on page 44*

◆ **Adenoscan®** *see* Adenosine *on page 44*

Adenosine (a DEN oh seen)

Related Information

Management of Postoperative Arrhythmias *on page 1451*

U.S. Brand Names Adenocard®; Adenoscan®

Canadian Brand Names Adenocard®; Adenoscan®; Adenosine Injection, USP

Synonyms 9-Beta-D-Ribofuranosyladenine

Pharmacologic Category Antiarrhythmic Agent, Class IV; Diagnostic Agent

Generic Available Yes

Use

Adenocard®: Treatment of paroxysmal supraventricular tachycardia (PSVT) including that associated with accessory bypass tracts (Wolff-Parkinson-White syndrome); when clinically advisable, appropriate vagal maneuvers should be attempted prior to adenosine administration; **not effective in atrial flutter, atrial fibrillation, or ventricular tachycardia**

Adenoscan®: Pharmacologic stress agent used in myocardial perfusion thallium-201 scintigraphy

Unlabeled/Investigational Use

Adenoscan®: Acute vasodilator testing in pulmonary artery hypertension

Mechanism of Action Slows conduction time through the AV node, interrupting the re-entry pathways through the AV node, restoring normal sinus rhythm

Pharmacodynamics/Kinetics

Onset of action: Rapid

Duration: Very brief

Metabolism: Blood and tissue to inosine then to adenosine monophosphate (AMP) and hypoxanthine

Half-life elimination: <10 seconds

Dosage

Adenocard®: **Rapid I.V. push (over 1-2 seconds) via peripheral line:**

Infants and Children:

Manufacturer's recommendation:

<50 kg: 0.05-0.1 mg/kg. If conversion of PSVT does not occur within 1-2 minutes, may increase dose by 0.05-0.1 mg/kg. May repeat until sinus rhythm is established or to a maximum single dose of 0.3 mg/kg or 12 mg. Follow each dose with normal saline flush.

≥50 kg: Refer to Adult dosing

Pediatric advanced life support (PALS): Treatment of SVT: I.V., I.O.: 0.1 mg/kg; if not effective, administer 0.2 mg/kg of PSVT; medium dose required: 0.15 mg/kg; maximum single dose: 12 mg. Follow each dose with normal saline flush.

Adults: 6 mg; if not effective within 1-2 minutes, 12 mg may be given; may repeat 12 mg bolus if needed

Maximum single dose: 12 mg

Follow each I.V. bolus of adenosine with normal saline flush

Note: Preliminary results in adults suggest adenosine may be administered via a central line at lower doses (ie, initial adult dose: 3 mg).

Adenoscan®:

Stress testing: Continuous I.V. infusion via peripheral line: 140 mcg/kg/minute for 6 minutes using syringe or columetric infusion pump; total dose: 0.84 mg/kg. Thallium-201 is injected at midpoint (3 minutes) of infusion.

Acute vasodilator testing (unlabeled use): I.V.: Initial: 50 mcg/kg/minute increased by 50 mcg/kg/minute every 2 minutes to a maximum dose of 500 mcg/kg/minute; acutely assess vasodilator response

Hemodialysis: Significant drug removal is unlikely based on physiochemical characteristics.

Peritoneal dialysis: Significant drug removal is unlikely based on physiochemical characteristics.

Note: Higher doses may be needed for administration via peripheral versus central vein.

Stability Store at controlled room temperature of 15°C to 30°C (59°F to 86°F). Do **not** refrigerate; precipitation may occur (may dissolve by warming to room temperature).

Administration For rapid bolus I.V. use only; administer I.V. push over 1-2 seconds at a peripheral I.V. site as proximal as possible to trunk (not in lower arm, hand, lower leg, or foot); follow each bolus with normal saline flush. **Note:** Preliminary results in adults suggest adenosine may be administered via central line at lower doses (eg, adults initial dose: 3 mg)

Monitoring Parameters ECG monitoring, heart rate, blood pressure

Anesthesia and Critical Care Concerns/Other Considerations Short action is an advantage; has prolonged effects in patients taking dipyridamole or carbamazepine and in denervated transplanted hearts; adjust doses or choose alternative agent accordingly.

Adenosine acts via interruption of AV-nodal conduction and, when used for this purpose, requires administration as rapid intravenous push in increasing doses. Because of more direct access when administered through a central line, lower doses of adenosine may be tried in these situations. It is not uncommon to see heart block and sinus pause soon after adenosine administration. May aid in the

(Continued)

Adenosine *(Continued)*

identification of the arrhythmia by making the atrial fibrillation or flutter electrocardiographic morphology more apparent.

Pregnancy Risk Factor C

Contraindications Hypersensitivity to adenosine or any component of the formulation; second- or third-degree AV block or sick sinus syndrome (except in patients with a functioning artificial pacemaker), atrial flutter, atrial fibrillation, and ventricular tachycardia (this drug is not effective in converting these arrhythmias to sinus rhythm). The manufacturer states that Adenoscan® should be avoided in patients with known or suspected bronchoconstrictive or bronchospastic lung disease.

Warnings/Precautions Adenosine decreases conduction through the AV node and may produce first-, second-, or third-degree heart block. Patients with pre-existing S-A nodal dysfunction may experience prolonged sinus pauses after adenosine; use caution in patients with first-degree AV block or bundle branch block; avoid use of adenosine for pharmacologic stress testing in patients with high-grade AV block or sinus node dysfunction (unless a functional pacemaker is in place). There have been reports of atrial fibrillation/flutter in patients with PSVT associated with accessory conduction pathways after adenosine. Rare, prolonged episodes of asystole have been reported, with fatal outcomes in some cases. Use caution in patients receiving other drugs which slow AV conduction (eg, digoxin, verapamil). Drugs which affect adenosine (theophylline, caffeine) should be withheld for five half-lives prior to adenosine use. Avoid dietary caffeine for 12-24 hours prior to pharmacologic stress testing.

Adenosine may also produce profound vasodilation with subsequent hypotension. When used as a bolus dose (PSVT), effects are generally self-limiting (due to the short half-life of adenosine). However, when used as a continuous infusion (pharmacologic stress testing), effects may be more pronounced and persistent, corresponding to continued exposure. Adenosine infusions should be used with caution in patients with autonomic dysfunction, stenotic valvular heart disease, pericarditis, pleural effusion, carotid stenosis (with cerebrovascular insufficiency), or uncorrected hypovolemia. Use caution in elderly patients; may be at increased risk of hemodynamic effects, bradycardia, and/or AV block.

A limited number of patients with asthma have received adenosine and have not experienced exacerbation of their asthma. Adenosine may cause bronchoconstriction in patients with asthma, and should be used cautiously in patients with obstructive lung disease not associated with bronchoconstriction (eg, emphysema, bronchitis).

Adenocard®: Transient AV block is expected. When used in PSVT, at the time of conversion to normal sinus rhythm, a variety of new rhythms may appear on the ECG. Administer as a rapid bolus, either directly into a vein or (if administered into an I.V. line), as close to the patient as possible (followed by saline flush).

Adverse Reactions Note: Frequency varies based on use; higher frequency of infusion-related effects, such as flushing and lightheadedness, were reported with continuous infusion (Adenoscan®).

>10%:
- Cardiovascular: Facial flushing (18% to 44%)
- Central nervous system: Headache (2% to 18%), lightheadedness (2% to 12%)
- Neuromuscular & skeletal: Discomfort of neck, throat, jaw (<1% to 15%)
- Respiratory: Dyspnea (12% to 28%), chest pressure/discomfort (7% to 40%)

1% to 10%:
- Cardiovascular: Hypotension (<1% to 2%), AV block (infusion 6%; third degree <1%), ST segment depression (3%), palpitation, chest pain
- Central nervous system: Dizziness, nervousness (2%), apprehension
- Gastrointestinal: Nausea (3%)
- Neuromuscular & skeletal: Upper extremity discomfort (up to 4%), numbness (up to 2%), paresthesia (up to 2%)
- Respiratory: Hyperventilation
- Miscellaneous: Diaphoresis

<1% (Limited to important or life-threatening): Asystole (prolonged), atrial fibrillation, back discomfort, bradycardia, bronchospasm, blurred vision, burning sensation, hypertension (transient), injection site reaction, intracranial pressure increased, metallic taste, pressure in groin, respiratory arrest, seizure, torsade de pointes, ventricular fibrillation, ventricular tachycardia

Overdosage/Toxicology Since adenosine half-life is <10 seconds, adverse effects are rapidly self-limiting. Treatment of prolonged effects requires individualization. To reverse the effects of Adenoscan®, administer theophylline 50-125 mg slow I.V. push.

Drug Interactions

Carbamazepine may increase heart block.

Dipyridamole potentiates effects of adenosine; reduce dose of adenosine.

Theophylline and caffeine (methylxanthines) antagonize adenosine's effects; may require increased dose of adenosine.

Ethanol/Nutrition/Herb Interactions Food: Avoid food or drugs with caffeine. Adenosine's therapeutic effect may be decreased if used concurrently with caffeine. Avoid dietary caffeine for 12-24 hours prior to pharmacologic stress testing.

Dietary Considerations Avoid dietary caffeine for 12-24 hours prior to pharmacologic stress testing.

Dosage Forms

Injection, solution [preservative free]: 3 mg/mL (2 mL)

Adenocard®: 3 mg/mL (2 mL, 4 mL)

Adenoscan®: 3 mg/mL (20 mL, 30 mL)

- **Adenosine Injection, USP (Can)** *see* Adenosine *on page 44*
- **ADH** *see* Vasopressin *on page 1342*
- **Adoxa™** *see* Doxycycline *on page 426*
- **Adrenalin®** *see* Epinephrine *on page 457*
- **Adrenaline** *see* Epinephrine *on page 457*
- **Adsorbent Charcoal** *see* Charcoal *on page 259*
- **Advate** *see* Antihemophilic Factor (Recombinant) *on page 113*
- **Advil® [OTC]** *see* Ibuprofen *on page 651*
- **Advil® Children's [OTC]** *see* Ibuprofen *on page 651*
- **Advil® Infants' [OTC]** *see* Ibuprofen *on page 651*
- **Advil® Junior [OTC]** *see* Ibuprofen *on page 651*
- **Advil® Migraine [OTC]** *see* Ibuprofen *on page 651*
- **AeroBid®** *see* Flunisolide *on page 537*
- **AeroBid®-M** *see* Flunisolide *on page 537*
- **Aerospan™** *see* Flunisolide *on page 537*
- **Afeditab™ CR** *see* NIFEdipine *on page 920*
- **Afrin® Extra Moisturizing [OTC]** *see* Oxymetazoline *on page 973*
- **Afrin® Original [OTC]** *see* Oxymetazoline *on page 973*
- **Afrin® Severe Congestion [OTC]** *see* Oxymetazoline *on page 973*
- **Afrin® Sinus [OTC]** *see* Oxymetazoline *on page 973*
- **Agenerase®** *see* Amprenavir *on page 109*
- **Aggrastat®** *see* Tirofiban *on page 1275*
- **Aggrenox®** *see* Aspirin and Dipyridamole *on page 133*
- **$AgNO_3$** *see* Silver Nitrate *on page 1172*
- **AH-chew® D [OTC] [DSC]** *see* Phenylephrine *on page 1015*
- **AHF (Recombinant)** *see* Antihemophilic Factor (Recombinant) *on page 113*
- **A-hydroCort** *see* Hydrocortisone *on page 639*
- **Airomir (Can)** *see* Albuterol *on page 50*
- **AK-Dilate®** *see* Phenylephrine *on page 1015*
- **Akne-Mycin®** *see* Erythromycin *on page 476*
- **AK-Pred®** *see* PrednisoLONE *on page 1046*
- **AKTob®** *see* Tobramycin *on page 1278*
- **AK-Tracin® [DSC]** *see* Bacitracin *on page 155*
- **Alamag [OTC]** *see* Aluminum Hydroxide and Magnesium Hydroxide *on page 76*
- **Alatrofloxacin Mesylate** *see* Trovafloxacin *on page 1320*
- **Albert® Glyburide (Can)** *see* GlyBURIDE *on page 598*
- **Albumarc®** *see* Albumin *on page 48*

Albumin (al BYOO min)

Medication Safety Issues

Sound-alike/look-alike issues:

Albutein® may be confused with albuterol

Buminate® may be confused with bumetanide

U.S. Brand Names Albumarc®; Albuminar®; Albutein®; Buminate®; Flexbumin; Plasbumin®

Canadian Brand Names Plasbumin®-5; Plasbumin®-25

Synonyms Albumin (Human); Normal Human Serum Albumin; Normal Serum Albumin (Human); Salt Poor Albumin; SPA

Pharmacologic Category Blood Product Derivative; Plasma Volume Expander, Colloid

Generic Available Yes

Use Plasma volume expansion and maintenance of cardiac output in the treatment of certain types of shock or impending shock; may be useful for burn patients, ARDS, and cardiopulmonary bypass; other uses considered by some investigators (but not proven) are retroperitoneal surgery, peritonitis, and ascites; unless the condition responsible for hypoproteinemia can be corrected, albumin can provide only symptomatic relief or supportive treatment

Unlabeled/Investigational Use In cirrhotics, administered with diuretics to help facilitate diuresis; large volume paracentesis; volume expansion in dehydrated, mildly-hypotensive cirrhotics

Mechanism of Action Provides increase in intravascular oncotic pressure and causes mobilization of fluids from interstitial into intravascular space

Dosage I.V.:

5% should be used in hypovolemic patients or intravascularly-depleted patients

25% should be used in patients in whom fluid and sodium intake must be minimized

Dose depends on condition of patient:

Children: Hypovolemia: 0.5-1 g/kg/dose (10-20 mL/kg/dose of albumin 5%); maximum dose: 6 g/kg/day

Adults: Usual dose: 25 g; initial dose may be repeated in 15-30 minutes if response is inadequate; no more than 250 g should be administered within 48 hours

Hypoproteinemia: 0.5-1 g/kg/dose; repeat every 1-2 days as calculated to replace ongoing losses

Hypovolemia: 5% albumin: 0.5-1 g/kg/dose; repeat as needed. **Note:** May be considered after inadequate response to crystalloid therapy and when nonprotein colloids are contraindicated. The volume administered and the speed of infusion should be adapted to individual response.

Stability Store at a temperature ≤30°C (86°F); do not freeze. Do not use solution if it is turbid or contains a deposit; use within 4 hours after opening vial; discard unused portion.

If 5% human albumin is unavailable, it may be prepared by diluting 25% human albumin with 0.9% sodium chloride or 5% dextrose in water. Do not use sterile water to dilute albumin solutions, as this has been associated with hypotonic-associated hemolysis.

Administration For I.V. administration only. Use within 4 hours after opening vial; discard unused portion. In emergencies, may administer as rapidly as necessary to improve clinical condition. After initial volume replacement:

5%: Do not exceed 2-4 mL/minute in patients with normal plasma volume; 5-10 mL/minute in patients with hypoproteinemia

25%: Do not exceed 1 mL/minute in patients with normal plasma volume; 2-3 mL/minute in patients with hypoproteinemia

Do not dilute 5% solution. Rapid infusion may cause vascular overload. Albumin 25% may be given undiluted or diluted in normal saline. May give in combination or through the same administration set as saline or carbohydrates. Do not use with ethanol or protein hydrolysates, precipitation may form.

Monitoring Parameters Blood pressure, pulmonary edema, hematocrit

Anesthesia and Critical Care Concerns/Other Considerations An Australian/New Zealand group recently published results from their evaluation of resuscitation fluid (4% albumin versus normal saline) in a heterogeneous intensive care population (Finfer, 2004). They conducted this multicenter, randomized, double-blind trial to compare the effects of resuscitation fluid on mortality from any cause during the 28-day period after randomization. Patients were eligible for inclusion if the treating clinician judged that fluid resuscitation was required for intravascular fluid depletion as supported by one of the following criteria:

Heart rate >90 bpm,
Systolic BP <100 mm Hg,
Mean arterial BP <75 mm Hg,
Decrease of 40 mm Hg in systolic or mean arterial BP (as compared with baseline),
CVP <10 mm Hg,
PCWP <12 mm Hg,
Respiratory variation in systolic or mean BP >5 mm Hg,
Capillary refill time >1 second, or
Urine output <0.5 mL/kg for 1 hour

Patients were excluded for a variety of reasons, including ICU transfer following cardiac or liver transplantation surgery, or burn treatment. Almost 7000 patients were randomized; 3497 to albumin and 3500 to saline. Baseline characteristics were similar between the groups, except CVP pressure was slightly higher in the albumin group (9.0 in albumin versus 8.6 in saline). There was no significant mortality difference between groups (726 deaths in albumin group; 729 deaths in saline group). There were no significant differences in secondary endpoints (length of stay in the ICU or hospital, days of mechanical ventilation, and days of renal replacement therapy). Similar outcomes resulted from use of either fluid for resuscitation in this patient population.

Pregnancy Risk Factor C

Contraindications Hypersensitivity to albumin or any component of the formulation; patients with severe anemia or cardiac failure

Warnings/Precautions Use with caution in patients with hepatic or renal failure because of added protein load; rapid infusion of albumin solutions may cause vascular overload. All patients should be observed for signs of hypervolemia such as pulmonary edema. Use with caution in those patients for whom sodium restriction is necessary. Avoid 25% concentration in preterm infants due to risk of intraventricular hemorrhage. Nutritional supplementation is not an appropriate indication for albumin.

Adverse Reactions Frequency not defined.

Cardiovascular: CHF precipitation, edema, hyper-/hypotension, hypervolemia, tachycardia
Central nervous system: Chills, fever, headache
Dermatologic: Pruritus, rash, urticaria
Gastrointestinal: Nausea, vomiting
Respiratory: Bronchospasm, pulmonary edema
Miscellaneous: Anaphylaxis

Overdosage/Toxicology Symptoms of overdose include hypervolemia, congestive heart failure, and pulmonary edema.

Drug Interactions ACE inhibitors: May have increased risk of atypical reactions; withhold ACEIs for at least 24 hours prior to plasma exchanges using large volumes of albumin

Dietary Considerations

Albumarc®, Albuminar®, Albutein®, Buminate®, Flexbumin: 5% [50 mg/mL] and 25% [250 mg/mL] contain sodium 130-160 mEq/L
Plasbumin®: 5% [50 mg/mL] and 25% [250 mg/mL] contain sodium ~145 mEq/L

Dosage Forms

Injection, solution, human [preservative free]: 5% [50 mg/mL] (50 mL, 250 mL, 500 mL) [contains sodium 130-160 mEq/L]; 25% [250 mg/mL] (50 mL, 100 mL) [contains sodium 130-160 mEq/L]

Albumarc®: 5% [50 mg/mL] (250 mL, 500 mL) [contains sodium 130-160 mEq/L]; 25% [250 mg/mL] (50 mL, 100 mL) [contains sodium 130-160 mEq/L]

Albuminar®: 5% [50 mg/mL] (50 mL, 250 mL, 500 mL, 1000 mL) [contains sodium 130-160 mEq/L]; 25% [250 mg/mL] (20 mL, 50 mL, 100 mL) [contains sodium 130-160 mEq/L]

Albutein®, Buminate®: 5% [50 mg/mL] (250 mL, 500 mL) [contains sodium 130-160 mEq/L]; 25% [250 mg/mL] (20 mL, 50 mL, 100 mL) [contains sodium 130-160 mEq/L]

Flexbumin: 25% [250 mg/mL] (50 mL, 100 mL) [contains sodium 130-160 mEq/L]

(Continued)

Albumin *(Continued)*

Plasbumin®: 5% [50 mg/mL] (50 mL, 250 mL, 500 mL) [contains sodium ~145 mEq/L]; 25% [250 mg/mL] (20 mL, 50 mL, 100 mL) [contains sodium ~145 mEq/L]

References

American Thoracic Society, "Evidence-Based Colloid Use in the Critically Ill: American Thoracic Society Consensus Statement," *Am J Respir Crit Care Med*, 2004, 170(11):1247-59.

Finfer S, Bellomo R, Boyce N, et al, "A Comparison of Albumin and Saline for Fluid Resuscitation in the Intensive Care Unit, SAFE Study Investigators," *N Engl J Med*, 2004, 350(22):2247-56.

♦ **Albuminar®** *see* Albumin *on page 48*

♦ **Albumin (Human)** *see* Albumin *on page 48*

♦ **Albutein®** *see* Albumin *on page 48*

Albuterol (al BYOO ter ole)

Medication Safety Issues

Sound-alike/look-alike issues:

Albuterol may be confused with Albutein®, atenolol
Proventil® may be confused with Bentyl®, Prilosec® Prinivil®
Salbutamol may be confused with salmeterol
Ventolin® may be confused with phentolamine, Benylin®, Vantin®
Volmax® may be confused with Flomax®

Related Information

Allergic Reactions *on page 1395*

U.S. Brand Names AccuNeb®; Proventil®; Proventil® HFA; Ventolin® HFA; VoSpire ER®

Canadian Brand Names Airomir; Alti-Salbutamol; Apo-Salvent®; Gen-Salbutamol; PMS-Salbutamol; ratio-Inspra-Sal; ratio-Salbutamol; Rhoxal-salbutamol; Salbu-2; Salbu-4; Ventolin®; Ventolin® Diskus; Ventolin® HFA; Ventrodisk

Synonyms Albuterol Sulfate; Salbutamol

Pharmacologic Category Beta$_2$-Adrenergic Agonist

Generic Available Yes: Excludes extended release

Use Bronchodilator in reversible airway obstruction due to asthma or COPD; prevention of exercise-induced bronchospasm

Mechanism of Action Relaxes bronchial smooth muscle by action on beta$_2$-receptors with little effect on heart rate

Pharmacodynamics/Kinetics

Onset of action: Peak effect:
- Nebulization/oral inhalation: 0.5-2 hours
  - CFC-propelled albuterol: 10 minutes
  - Ventolin® HFA: 25 minutes
- Oral: 2-3 hours

Duration: Nebulization/oral inhalation: 3-4 hours; Oral: 4-6 hours
Metabolism: Hepatic to an inactive sulfate
Half-life elimination: Inhalation: 3.8 hours; Oral: 3.7-5 hours
Excretion: Urine (30% as unchanged drug)

Dosage

Oral:
- Children: Bronchospasm (treatment):
  - 2-6 years: 0.1-0.2 mg/kg/dose 3 times/day; maximum dose not to exceed 12 mg/day (divided doses)
  - 6-12 years: 2 mg/dose 3-4 times/day; maximum dose not to exceed 24 mg/day (divided doses)
    - Extended release: 4 mg every 12 hours; maximum dose not to exceed 24 mg/day (divided doses)
- Children >12 years and Adults: Bronchospasm (treatment): 2-4 mg/dose 3-4 times/day; maximum dose not to exceed 32 mg/day (divided doses)
  - Extended release: 8 mg every 12 hours; maximum dose not to exceed 32 mg/day (divided doses). A 4 mg dose every 12 hours may be sufficient in some patients, such as adults of low body weight.
- Elderly: Bronchospasm (treatment): 2 mg 3-4 times/day; maximum: 8 mg 4 times/day

Inhalation: MDI 90 mcg/puff:

Children ≤12 years:

Bronchospasm (acute): 4-8 puffs every 20 minutes for 3 doses, then every 1-4 hours; spacer/holding-chamber device should be used

Exercise-induced bronchospasm (prophylaxis): 1-2 puffs 5 minutes prior to exercise

Children >12 years and Adults:

Bronchospasm (acute): 4-8 puffs every 20 minutes for up to 4 hours, then every 1-4 hours as needed

Exercise-induced bronchospasm (prophylaxis): 2 puffs 5-30 minutes prior to exercise

Children ≥4 years and Adults: Bronchospasm (chronic treatment): 1-2 inhalations every 4-6 hours; maximum: 12 inhalations/day

NIH guidelines: 2 puffs 3-4 times a day as needed; may double dose for mild exacerbations

Nebulization:

Children ≤12 years:

Bronchospasm (treatment): 0.05 mg/kg every 4-6 hours; minimum dose: 1.25 mg, maximum dose: 2.5 mg

2-12 years: AccuNeb®: 0.63 mg or 1.25 mg 3-4 times/day, as needed, delivered over 5-15 minutes

Children >40 kg, patients with more severe asthma, or children 11-12 years: May respond better with a 1.25 mg dose

Bronchospasm (acute): Solution 0.5%: 0.15 mg/kg (minimum dose: 2.5 mg) every 20 minutes for 3 doses, then 0.15-0.3 mg/kg (up to 10 mg) every 1-4 hours as needed; may also use 0.5 mg/kg/hour by continuous infusion. Continuous nebulized albuterol at 0.3 mg/kg/hour has been used safely in the treatment of severe status asthmaticus in children; continuous nebulized doses of 3 mg/kg/hour ± 2.2 mg/kg/hour in children whose mean age was 20.7 months resulted in no cardiac toxicity; the optimal dosage for continuous nebulization remains to be determined.

Note: Use of the 0.5% solution should be used for bronchospasm (acute or treatment) in children <15 kg. AccuNeb® has not been studied for the treatment of acute bronchospasm; use of the 0.5% concentrated solution may be more appropriate.

Children >12 years and Adults:

Bronchospasm (treatment): 2.5 mg, diluted to a total of 3 mL, 3-4 times/day over 5-15 minutes

NIH guidelines: 1.25-5 mg every 4-8 hours

Bronchospasm (acute) in intensive care patients: 2.5-5 mg every 20 minutes for 3 doses, then 2.5-10 mg every 1-4 hours as needed, **or** 10-15 mg/hour continuously

Hemodialysis: Not removed

Peritoneal dialysis: Significant drug removal is unlikely based on physiochemical characteristics

Stability

HFA aerosols: Store at 15°C to 25°C (59°F to 77°F)

Ventolin® HFA: Discard after using 200 actuations or 3 months after removal from protective pouch, whichever comes first. Store with mouthpiece down.

Inhalation solution: AccuNeb®: Store at 2°C to 25°C (36°F to 77°F). Do not use if solution changes color or becomes cloudy. Use within 1 week of opening foil pouch.

Nebulization 0.5% solution: Store at 2°C to 30°C (36°F to 86°F). To prepare a 2.5 mg dose, dilute 0.5 mL of solution to a total of 3 mL with normal saline; also compatible with cromolyn or ipratropium nebulizer solutions

Syrup: Store at 2°C to 30°C (36°F to 86°F)

Administration

Inhalation: MDI: Shake well before use; prime prior to first use, and whenever inhaler has not been used for >2 weeks or when it has been dropped, by releasing 4 test sprays into the air (away from face)

Oral: Do not crush or chew extended release tablets.

Monitoring Parameters FEV_1, peak flow, and/or other pulmonary function tests; blood pressure, heart rate; CNS stimulation; serum glucose, serum potassium; asthma symptoms; arterial or capillary blood gases (if patients condition warrants)

Anesthesia and Critical Care Concerns/Other Considerations Frequent use of inhaled beta agonists when used in patients with atrial fibrillation may

(Continued)

Albuterol *(Continued)*

counteract pharmacologic interventions directed at rate control. Inhaled beta agonists may be used to treat acute hyperkalemia in patients with renal failure.

Wait at least 1 minute between first and second puff of MDI. Because of its minimal effect on $beta_1$ receptors and its relatively long duration of action, albuterol is a rational choice in the elderly when a beta agonist is indicated. All patients should utilize a spacer device when using a metered-dose inhaler.

Pregnancy Risk Factor C

Contraindications Hypersensitivity to albuterol, adrenergic amines, or any component of the formulation

Warnings/Precautions Optimize anti-inflammatory treatment before initiating maintenance treatment with albuterol. Do not use as a component of chronic therapy without an anti-inflammatory agent. Only the mildest forms of asthma (Step 1 and/or exercise-induced) would not require concurrent use based upon asthma guidelines. Patient must be instructed to seek medical attention in cases where acute symptoms are not relieved or a previous level of response is diminished. The need to increase frequency of use may indicate deterioration of asthma, and treatment must not be delayed.

Use caution in patients with cardiovascular disease (arrhythmia or hypertension or CHF), convulsive disorders, diabetes, glaucoma, hyperthyroidism, or hypokalemia. Beta agonists may cause elevation in blood pressure, heart rate, and result in CNS stimulation/excitation. $Beta_2$ agonists may increase risk of arrhythmia, increase serum glucose, or decrease serum potassium.

Do not exceed recommended dose; serious adverse events, including fatalities, have been associated with excessive use of inhaled sympathomimetics. Rarely, paradoxical bronchospasm may occur with use of inhaled bronchodilating agents; this should be distinguished from inadequate response. All patients should utilize a spacer device when using a metered-dose inhaler; in addition, face masks should be used in children <4 years of age.

Because of its minimal effect on $beta_1$-receptors and its relatively long duration of action, albuterol is a rational choice in the elderly when an inhaled beta agonist is indicated. Oral use should be avoided in the elderly due to adverse effects. Patient response may vary between inhalers that contain chlorofluorocarbons and those which are chlorofluorocarbon-free.

Adverse Reactions Incidence of adverse effects is dependent upon age of patient, dose, and route of administration.

Cardiovascular: Angina, atrial fibrillation, chest discomfort, extrasystoles, flushing, hypertension, palpitation, tachycardia

Central nervous system: CNS stimulation, dizziness, drowsiness, headache, insomnia, irritability, lightheadedness, migraine, nervousness, nightmares, restlessness, sleeplessness, tremor

Dermatologic: Angioedema, erythema multiforme, rash, Stevens-Johnson syndrome, urticaria

Endocrine & metabolic: Hypokalemia, serum glucose increased, serum potassium decreased

Gastrointestinal: Diarrhea, dry mouth, gastroenteritis, nausea, unusual taste, vomiting, tooth discoloration

Genitourinary: Micturition difficulty

Neuromuscular & skeletal: Muscle cramps, weakness

Otic: Otitis media, vertigo

Respiratory: Asthma exacerbation, bronchospasm, cough, epistaxis, laryngitis, oropharyngeal drying/irritation, oropharyngeal edema

Miscellaneous: Allergic reaction, lymphadenopathy

Overdosage/Toxicology Symptoms of overdose include tachycardia, tremor, hypertension, angina, and seizures. Hypokalemia also may occur. Cardiac arrest and death may be associated with abuse of beta-agonist bronchodilators. Treatment includes immediate discontinuation and symptomatic and supportive therapies. Cautious use of beta-adrenergic blocking agents may be considered in severe cases.

Drug Interactions **Substrate** of CYP3A4 (major)

Beta-adrenergic blockers (eg, propranolol) antagonize albuterol's effects; avoid concurrent use.

CYP3A4 inducers: CYP3A4 inducers may decrease the levels/effects of albuterol. Example inducers include aminoglutethimide, carbamazepine, nafcillin, nevirapine, phenobarbital, phenytoin, and rifamycins.

Halothane may increase risk of malignant arrhythmias; avoid concurrent use.

Inhaled ipratropium may increase duration of bronchodilation.

MAO inhibitors may increase side effects; monitor heart rate and blood pressure.

TCAs may increase side effects; monitor heart rate and blood pressure.

Sympathomimetics may increase side effects; monitor heart rate and blood pressure.

Ethanol/Nutrition/Herb Interactions

Food: Avoid or limit caffeine (may cause CNS stimulation).

Herb/Nutraceutical: Avoid ephedra, yohimbe (may cause CNS stimulation).

Test Interactions Increased renin (S), increased aldosterone (S)

Dietary Considerations Oral forms should be administered with water 1 hour before or 2 hours after meals.

Dosage Forms

Aerosol, for oral inhalation: 90 mcg/metered inhalation (17 g) [200 metered inhalations; contains chlorofluorocarbons]

Proventil®: 90 mcg/metered inhalation (17 g) [200 metered inhalations; contains chlorofluorocarbons]

Aerosol, for oral inhalation: 90 mcg/metered inhalation (8.5 g) [200 metered inhalations; chlorofluorocarbon free]

Proventil® HFA: 90 mcg/metered inhalation (6.7 g) [200 metered inhalations; chlorofluorocarbon free]

Ventolin® HFA: 90 mcg/metered inhalation (18 g) [200 metered inhalations; chlorofluorocarbon free]

Solution for nebulization: 0.042% (3 mL); 0.083% (3 mL); 0.5% (0.5 mL, 20 mL)

AccuNeb® [preservative free]: 0.63 mg/3 mL (3 mL) [0.021%]; 1.25 mg/3 mL (3 mL) [0.042%]

Proventil®: 0.083% (3 mL) [preservative free]; 0.5% (20 mL) [contains benzalkonium chloride]

Syrup, as sulfate: 2 mg/5 mL (480 mL)

Tablet: 2 mg, 4 mg

Tablet, extended release:

VoSpire ER®: 4 mg, 8 mg

References

Katz RW, Kelly HW, Crowley MR, et al, "Safety of Continuous Nebulized Albuterol for Bronchospasm in Infants and Children," *Pediatrics*, 1993, 92(5):666-9.

Leikin JB, Linowiecki KA, Soglin DF, et al, "Hypokalemia After Pediatric Albuterol Overdose: A Case Series," *Am J Emerg Med*, 1994, 12(1):64-6.

Manthous CA, Chatila W, Schmidt GA, et al, "Treatment of Bronchospasm by Metered-Dose Inhaler Albuterol in Mechanically Ventilated Patients," *Chest*, 1995, 107(1):210-3.

Marik P, Hogan J, and Krikorian J, "A Comparison of Bronchodilator Therapy Delivered by Nebulization and Metered-Dose Inhaler in Mechanically Ventilated Patients," *Chest*, 1999, 115(6):1653-7.

National Asthma Education and Prevention Program, "Expert Panel Report 2: Guidelines for the Diagnosis and Management of Asthma," Bethesda, MD, National Institutes of Health, 1997. NIH publication 97-4051.

National Asthma Education and Prevention Program, "Expert Panel Report: Guidelines for the Diagnosis and Management of Asthma Update on Selected Topics - 2002," *J Allergy Clin Immunol*, 2002, 110(5 Suppl):141-219. Available at: www.nhlbi.nih.gov/guidelines/asthma/index.

Papo MC, Frank J, and Thompson AE, "A Prospective, Randomized Study of Continuous Versus Intermittent Nebulized Albuterol for Severe Status Asthmaticus in Children," *Crit Care Med*, 1993, 21(10):1479-86.

Schuh S, Parkin P, Rajan A, et al, "Bronchodilator Therapy With Metered Dose Inhaler Versus Nebulizer in Mechanically Ventilated Patients," *Respiratory Care*, (July) 2000, 817.

Schuh S, Parkin P, Rajan A, et al, "High- Versus Low-Dose, Frequently Administered, Nebulized Albuterol in Children With Severe, Acute Asthma," *Pediatrics*, 1989, 83(4):513-8.

Udezue E, D'Souza L, and Mahajan M, "Hypokalemia After Normal Doses of Nebulized Albuterol (Salbutamol)," *Am J Emerg Med*, 1995, 13(2):168-71.

♦ **Albuterol Sulfate** *see* Albuterol *on page 50*

♦ **Alcohol, Absolute** *see* Alcohol (Ethyl) *on page 53*

♦ **Alcohol, Dehydrated** *see* Alcohol (Ethyl) *on page 53*

Alcohol (Ethyl) (AL koe hol, ETH il)

Medication Safety Issues

Sound-alike/look-alike issues:

Ethanol may be confused with Ethyol®, Ethamolin®

(Continued)

Alcohol (Ethyl) *(Continued)*

U.S. Brand Names Lavacol® [OTC]

Canadian Brand Names Biobase™; Biobase-G™

Synonyms Alcohol, Absolute; Alcohol, Dehydrated; Ethanol; Ethyl Alcohol; EtOH

Pharmacologic Category Antidote; Pharmaceutical Aid

Generic Available Yes

Use Topical anti-infective; pharmaceutical aid; therapeutic neurolysis (nerve or ganglion block); replenishment of fluid and carbohydrate calories

Unlabeled/Investigational Use Antidote for ethylene glycol overdose; antidote for methanol overdose; treatment of fat occlusion of central venous catheters

Mechanism of Action When used to treat ethylene glycol or methanol toxicity, ethyl alcohol competitively inhibits their metabolism and decreases the formation of toxic metabolites.

Pharmacodynamics/Kinetics

Absorption: Oral: Rapid

Distribution: V_d: 0.6-0.7 L/kg; decreased in women

Metabolism: Hepatic (90% to 98%) to acetaldehyde or acetate

Half-life elimination: Rate: 15-20 mg/dL/hour (range: 10-34 mg/dL/hour); increased in alcoholics

Excretion: Kidneys and lungs (~2% unchanged)

Dosage

Treatment of methanol or ethylene glycol ingestion (unlabeled use): Children and Adults: Absolute ethanol (86 proof = 34 g EtOH/dL)/ethyl alcohol: **Note:** Continue until methanol or ethylene glycol are no longer detected **or** <20 mg/dL and metabolic acidosis is corrected:

- Oral: **Note:** Oral dosing is not recommended outside of a hospital setting: Initial: 600 mg/kg [equivalent to 1.8 mL/kg using a 43% solution]
  - Maintenance dose:
    - Nondrinker: 66 mg/kg/hour [equivalent to 0.2 mL/kg/hour using a 43% solution]
    - Chronic drinker: 154 mg/kg/hour [equivalent to 0.46 mL/kg/hour using a 43% solution]
  - **Dosage adjustment for hemodialysis:** Maintenance dose:
    - Nondrinker: 169 mg/kg/hour [equivalent to 0.5 mL/kg/hour using a 43% solution]
    - Chronic drinker: 257 mg/kg/hour [equivalent to 0.77 mL/kg/hour using a 43% solution]
- I.V.: Initial: 600 mg/kg [equivalent to 7.6 mL/kg using a 10% solution]
  - Maintenance dose:
    - Nondrinker: 66 mg/kg/hour [equivalent to 0.83 mL/kg/hour using a 10% solution]
    - Chronic drinker: 154 mg/kg/hour [equivalent to 1.96 mL/kg/hour using a 10% solution]
  - **Dosage adjustment for hemodialysis:** Maintenance dose:
    - Nondrinker: 169 mg/kg/hour [equivalent to 2.13 mL/kg/hour using a 10% solution]
    - Chronic drinker: 257 mg/kg/hour [equivalent to 3.26 mL/kg/hour using a 10% solution]

Treatment of fat occlusion of central venous catheters (unlabeled use): Children and Adults: Dehydrated alcohol injection: I.V. (see institutional-based protocol for catheter clearance assessment, the following assessment is a general methodology): Up to 3 mL of ethanol 70% (maximum: 0.55 mL/kg); the volume to instill is equal to the internal volume of the catheter

Antiseptic: Children and Adults: Liquid denatured alcohol: Topical: Apply 1-3 times/day as needed

Therapeutic neurolysis (nerve or ganglion block): Adults: Dehydrated alcohol injection: Intraneural: Dosage variable depending upon the site of injection (eg, trigeminal neuralgia: 0.05-0.5 mL as a single injection per interspace vs subarachnoid injection: 0.5-1 mL as a single injection per interspace); single doses >1.5 mL are seldom required

Replenishment of fluid and carbohydrate calories: Adults: Dehydrated alcohol infusion: Alcohol 5% and dextrose 5%: 1-2 L/day by slow infusion

Administration

Oral: Ethylene glycol or methanol poisoning: Dilute ethyl alcohol to 20% solution and administer hourly via NG tube. Oral treatment is not recommended outside of a hospital setting.

I.V.: Ethylene glycol or methanol poisoning: Administer as a 10% solution in D_5W. Initial dose should be administered over 1 hour.

Treatment of occluded central venous catheter: Instill a 70% solution with a volume equal to the internal volume of the catheter. Assess patency at 30-60 minutes (or per institutional protocol).

Intraneural: Separate needles should be used for each of multiple injections or sites to prevent residual alcohol deposition at sites not intended for tissue destruction. Inject slowly after determining proper placement of needle. Since dehydrated alcohol is hypobaric when compared with spinal fluid, proper positioning of the patient is essential to control localization of injections into the subarachnoid space.

Monitoring Parameters Antidotal therapy: Blood ethanol levels every 1-2 hours until steady state, then every 2-4 hours; blood glucose, electrolytes (including serum magnesium), arterial pH, blood gases, methanol or ethylene glycol blood levels; heart rate, blood pressure

Reference Range Antidote for methanol/ethylene glycol: Blood ethanol level: Goal range: 100-150 mg/dL

Anesthesia and Critical Care Concerns/Other Considerations

Neurolytic block: Pain will occur after initial injection for a short period of time and will subside when neurolysis occurs. This agent will destroy nerve and should be administered when pain is from malignant origin only; administer carefully.

Methanol/ethylene glycol poisoning: Treatment involves inhibiting the formation of toxic metabolites by inhibiting alcohol dehydrogenase and/or urgent dialytic removal of these alcohols and their metabolites. Fomepizole and ethanol are both inhibitors of alcohol dehydrogenase and have been used to prevent toxicity. Currently, fomepizole is the drug of choice because of its ease of use and lack of CNS toxicity. When ethanol is used, a target serum level of 100-200 mg/dL is maintained during treatment. Patients are treated until serum levels of the poison (ethylene glycol/methanol) are <20 mg/dL.

Pregnancy Risk Factor C (D per expert opinion)/X (prolonged use or high doses at term)

Contraindications Hypersensitivity to ethyl alcohol or any component of the formulation; seizure disorder and diabetic coma; subarachnoid injection of dehydrated alcohol in patients receiving anticoagulants; pregnancy

Warnings/Precautions Ethyl alcohol is a flammable liquid and should be kept cool and away from any heat source. Proper positioning of the patient for neurolytic administration is essential to control localization of the injection of dehydrated alcohol (which is hypobaric) into the subarachnoid space; avoid extravasation. Not for SubQ administration. Do not administer simultaneously with blood due to the possibility of pseudoagglutination or hemolysis; may potentiate severe hypoprothrombic bleeding. Clinical evaluation and periodic lab determinations, including serum ethanol levels, are necessary to monitor effectiveness, changes in electrolyte concentrations, and acid-base balance (when used as an antidote).

Use with caution in patients with diabetes (ethyl alcohol decreases blood sugar), hepatic impairment, patients with gout, shock, following cranial surgery, and in anticipated postpartum hemorrhage. Monitor blood glucose closely, particularly in children as treatment of ingestions is associated with hypoglycemia. Avoid extravasation during I.V. administration. Ethyl alcohol passes freely into breast milk at a level approximately equivalent to maternal serum level; minimize dermal exposure of ethyl alcohol in infants as significant systemic absorption and toxicity can occur.

Adverse Reactions Frequency not defined.

Central nervous system: Disorientation, encephalopathy, flushing, sedation, seizures (rare), vertigo

Endocrine & metabolic: Hypoglycemia

Genitourinary: Urinary retention

Local: Nerve and tissue destruction

Miscellaneous: Intoxication

Dosage Forms

Infusion [in D_5W, dehydrated]: Alcohol 5% (1000 mL); alcohol 10% (1000 mL)

Injection, solution [dehydrated]: 98% (1 mL, 5 mL)

Liquid, topical [denatured] (Lavacol®): 70% (473 mL)

References

Mokhlesi B, Leikin JB, Murray P, et al, "Adult Toxicology in Critical Care. Part 11:Specific Poisonings," *Chest*, 2003, 123(3):897-922.

♦ **Alcomicin® (Can)** *see* Gentamicin *on page 589*

♦ **Aldactone®** *see* Spironolactone *on page 1203*
♦ **Aldomet** *see* Methyldopa *on page 826*
♦ **Aler-Cap [OTC]** *see* DiphenhydrAMINE *on page 399*
♦ **Aler-Dryl [OTC]** *see* DiphenhydrAMINE *on page 399*
♦ **Aler-Tab [OTC]** *see* DiphenhydrAMINE *on page 399*
♦ **Aleve® [OTC]** *see* Naproxen *on page 899*
♦ **Alfenta®** *see* Alfentanil *on page 56*

Alfentanil (al FEN ta nil)

Medication Safety Issues

Sound-alike/look-alike issues:

Alfentanil may be confused with Anafranil®, fentanyl, remifentanil, sufentanil
Alfenta® may be confused with Sufenta®

Related Information

Anesthesia Considerations for Neurosurgery *on page 1401*
Anesthesia for Patients With Liver Disease *on page 1421*
Chronic Pain Management *on page 1430*
Chronic Renal Failure *on page 1437*
Narcotic / Opioid Analgesics *on page 1568*
Opioids *on page 1535*
Substance Abuse and Anesthesia *on page 1496*

U.S. Brand Names Alfenta®

Canadian Brand Names Alfenta®; Alfentanil Injection, USP

Synonyms Alfentanil Hydrochloride

Pharmacologic Category Analgesic, Narcotic

Restrictions C-II

Generic Available Yes

Use Analgesic adjunct given by continuous infusion or in incremental doses in maintenance of anesthesia with barbiturate or N_2O or a primary anesthetic agent for the induction of anesthesia in patients undergoing general surgery in which endotracheal intubation and mechanical ventilation are required

Mechanism of Action Binds with stereospecific receptors at many sites within the CNS, increases pain threshold, alters pain perception, inhibits ascending pain pathways; is an ultra short-acting narcotic

Alfentanil

Indication	Approx Duration of Anesthesia (min)	Induction Period (Initial Dose) (mcg/kg)	Maintenance Period (Increments/ Infusion)	Total Dose (mcg/kg)	Effects
Incremental injection	≤30	8-20	3-5 mcg/kg or 0.5-1 mcg/kg/ min	8-40	Spontaneously breathing or assisted ventilation when required.
	30-60	20-50	5-15 mcg/kg	Up to 75	Assisted or controlled ventilation required. Attenuation of response to laryngoscopy and intubation.
Continuous infusion	>45	50-75	0.5-3 mcg/kg/ min average infusion rate 1-1.5 mcg/kg/ min	Dependent on duration of procedure	Assisted or controlled ventilation required. Some attenuation of response to intubation and incision, with intraoperative stability.
Anesthetic induction	>45	130-245	0.5-1.5 mcg/ kg/min or general anesthetic	Dependent on duration of procedure	Assisted or controlled ventilation required. Administer slowly (over 3 minutes). Concentration of inhalation agents reduced by 30% to 50% for initial hour.

Pharmacodynamics/Kinetics

Onset of action: Rapid
Duration (dose dependent): 30-60 minutes

Distribution: V_d: Newborns, premature: 1 L/kg; Children: 0.163-0.48 L/kg; Adults: 0.46 L/kg

Half-life elimination: Newborns, premature: 5.33-8.75 hours; Children: 40-60 minutes; Adults: 83-97 minutes

Dosage Doses should be titrated to appropriate effects; wide range of doses is dependent upon desired degree of analgesia/anesthesia

Children <12 years: Dose not established

Adults: Dose should be based on ideal body weight as follows (see table on previous page)

Stability Dilute in D_5W, NS, or LR

Administration Administer I.V. slowly over 3-5 minutes or by I.V. continuous infusion.

Monitoring Parameters Respiratory rate, blood pressure, heart rate

Reference Range 100-340 ng/mL (depending upon procedure)

Anesthesia and Critical Care Concerns/Other Considerations Alfentanil may produce more muscle rigidity compared to fentanyl, therefore, be sure to administer slowly.

Pregnancy Risk Factor C

Contraindications Hypersensitivity to alfentanil hydrochloride, to narcotics, or any component of the formulation; increased intracranial pressure, severe respiratory depression

Warnings/Precautions Use with caution in patients with drug dependence, head injury, acute asthma and respiratory conditions; hypotension has occurred in neonates with respiratory distress syndrome; use caution when administering to patients with bradyarrhythmias; rapid I.V. infusion may result in skeletal muscle and chest wall rigidity, impaired ventilation, or respiratory distress/arrest; inject slowly over 3-5 minutes; nondepolarizing skeletal muscle relaxant may be required. Alfentanil may produce more hypotension compared to fentanyl, therefore, be sure to administer slowly and ensure patient has adequate hydration.

Adverse Reactions

>10%:

- Cardiovascular: Bradycardia, peripheral vasodilation
- Central nervous system: Drowsiness, sedation, intracranial pressure increased
- Endocrine & metabolic: Antidiuretic hormone release
- Gastrointestinal: Nausea, vomiting, constipation
- Ocular: Miosis

1% to 10%:

- Cardiovascular: Cardiac arrhythmia, orthostatic hypotension
- Central nervous system: Confusion, CNS depression
- Ocular: Blurred vision

<1% (Limited to important or life-threatening): Convulsions, mental depression, paradoxical CNS excitation or delirium, dizziness, dysesthesia, rash, urticaria, itching, biliary tract spasm, urinary tract spasm, respiratory depression, bronchospasm, laryngospasm, physical and psychological dependence with prolonged use; cold, clammy skin

Overdosage/Toxicology Symptoms of overdose include miosis, respiratory depression, seizures, and CNS depression. Naloxone 2 mg I.V. (0.01 mg/kg for children) with repeat administration as necessary up to a total of 10 mg; may precipitate withdrawal.

Drug Interactions Substrate of CYP3A4 (major)

Dextroamphetamine: May enhance the analgesic effect of morphine and other opiate agonists.

Increased toxicity with CNS depressants (eg, benzodiazepines, barbiturates, tricyclic antidepressants), erythromycin, reserpine, beta-blockers.

CYP3A4 inhibitors: May increase the levels/effects of alfentanil. Example inhibitors include azole antifungals, clarithromycin, diclofenac, doxycycline, erythromycin, imatinib, isoniazid, nefazodone, nicardipine, propofol, protease inhibitors, quinidine, telithromycin, and verapamil.

Dosage Forms

Injection, solution [preservative free]: 500 mcg/mL (2 mL, 5 mL, 10 mL)

Alfenta®: 500 mcg/mL (2 mL, 5 mL, 10 mL, 20 mL)

References

Bartkowski RR and McDonnell TE, "Prolonged Alfentanil Effect Following Erythromycin Administration," *Anesthesiology*, 1990, 73(3):566-8.

Bartkowski RR, Goldberg ME, Larijani GE, et al, "Inhibition of Alfentanil Metabolism by Erythromycin," *Clin Pharmacol Ther*, 1989, 46(1):99-102.

Bodenham A and Park GR, "Alfentanil Infusions in Patients Requiring Intensive Care," *Clin Pharmacokinet*, 1988, 15(4):216-26.

(Continued)

Alfentanil *(Continued)*

Davis PJ, Killian A, Stiller RL, et al, "Pharmacokinetics of Alfentanil in Newborn Premature Infants and Older Children," *Dev Pharmacol Ther*, 1989, 13(1):21-7.

Kirkham SR and Pugh R, "Opioid Analgesia in Uraemic Patients," *Lancet*, 1995, 345(8958):1185.

Marlow N, Weindling AM, Van Peer A, et al, "Alfentanil Pharmacokinetics in Preterm Infants," *Arch Dis Child*, 1990, 65(4 Spec No):349-51.

Meistelman C, Saint-Maurice C, Lepaul M, et al, "A Comparison of Alfentanil Pharmacokinetics in Children and Adults," *Anesthesiology*, 1987, 66(1):13-6.

Mokhlesi B, Leikin JB, Murray P, et al, "Adult Toxicology in Critical Care. Part 11: Specific Poisonings," *Chest*, 2003, 123(3):897-922.

Pokela ML, Ryhanen PT, Koivisto ME, et al, "Alfentanil-Induced Rigidity in Newborn Infants," *Anesth Analg*, 1992, 75(2):252-7.

Scholz J, Steinfath M, and Schulz M, "Clinical Pharmacokinetics of Alfentanil, Fentanyl, and Sufentanil. An Update," *Clin Pharmacokinet*, 1996, 31(4):275-92.

♦ **Alfentanil Hydrochloride** *see* Alfentanil *on page 56*

♦ **Alfentanil Injection, USP (Can)** *see* Alfentanil *on page 56*

Alfuzosin (al FYOO zoe sin)

U.S. Brand Names Uroxatral®

Canadian Brand Names Xatral

Synonyms Alfuzosin Hydrochloride

Pharmacologic Category $Alpha_1$ Blocker

Generic Available No

Use Treatment of the functional symptoms of benign prostatic hyperplasia (BPH)

Mechanism of Action An antagonist of $alpha_1$ adrenoreceptors in the lower urinary tract. Smooth muscle tone is mediated by the sympathetic nervous stimulation of $alpha_1$ adrenoreceptors, which are abundant in the prostate, prostatic capsule, prostatic urethra, and bladder neck. Blockade of these adrenoreceptors can cause smooth muscles in the bladder neck and prostate to relax, resulting in an improvement in urine flow rate and a reduction in symptoms of BPH.

Pharmacodynamics/Kinetics

Absorption: Decreased 50% under fasting conditions

Distribution: V_d: 3.2 L/kg

Protein binding: 82% to 90%

Metabolism: Hepatic, primarily via CYP3A4; metabolism includes oxidation, O-demethylation, and N-dealkylation; forms metabolites (inactive)

Bioavailability: 49% following a meal

Half-life elimination: 10 hours

Time to peak, plasma: 8 hours following a meal

Excretion: Feces (69%); urine (24%)

Dosage Oral: Adults: 10 mg once daily

Dosage adjustment in renal impairment: Bioavailability and maximum serum concentrations are increased by ~50% with mild, moderate, or severe renal impairment

Note: Safety has not been evaluated in patients with creatinine clearances <30 mL/minute.

Dosage adjustment in hepatic impairment:

Mild hepatic impairment: Use has not been studied

Moderate or severe hepatic impairment (Child-Pugh class B and C): Clearance is decreased $^1/_3$ to $^1/_4$ and serum concentration is increased three- to fourfold; use is contraindicated

Stability Store at controlled room temperature of 15°C to 30°C (59°F to 86°F). Protect from light and moisture.

Administration Tablet should be swallowed whole; do not crush or chew. Administer once daily (with a meal); should be taken at the same time each day.

Monitoring Parameters Urine flow; blood pressure

Pregnancy Risk Factor B

Contraindications Hypersensitivity to alfuzosin or any component of the formulation; moderate or severe hepatic insufficiency (Child-Pugh class B and C); potent CYP3A4 inhibitors (eg, itraconazole, ketoconazole, ritonavir)

Warnings/Precautions Not intended for use as an antihypertensive drug. May cause orthostasis, syncope, or dizziness. Patients should avoid situations where injury may occur as a result of syncope. Discontinue if symptoms of angina occur or worsen. Use caution with history of QT prolongation or use with medications which may prolong the QT interval. Rule out prostatic carcinoma before beginning therapy. Use caution with renal or mild hepatic impairment. Intraoperative floppy iris syndrome has been observed in cataract surgery patients who were on or were previously treated with $alpha_1$ blockers. Causality has not been established and there appears to be no benefit in discontinuing alpha blocker therapy prior to surgery. Safety and efficacy in children have not been established.

Adverse Reactions

1% to 10%:

Central nervous system: Dizziness (6%), fatigue (3%), headache (3%), pain (1% to 2%)

Gastrointestinal: Abdominal pain (1% to 2%), constipation (1% to 2%), dyspepsia (1% to 2%), nausea (1% to 2%)

Genitourinary: Impotence (1% to 2%)

Respiratory: Upper respiratory tract infection (3%), bronchitis (1% to 2%), pharyngitis (1% to 2%), sinusitis (1% to 2%)

<1% (Limited to important or life-threatening): Chest pain, hypotension, intraoperative floppy iris syndrome (with cataract surgery), postural hypotension, priapism, rash, syncope, tachycardia

Overdosage/Toxicology Hypotension would be expected in case of overdose. Treatment is symptom-directed and supportive. Dialysis not likely to benefit.

Drug Interactions Substrate of CYP3A4 (major)

CYP3A4 inducers: CYP3A4 inducers may decrease the levels/effects of alfuzosin. Example inducers include aminoglutethimide, carbamazepine, nafcillin, nevirapine, phenobarbital, phenytoin, and rifamycins.

CYP3A4 inhibitors: May increase the levels/effects of alfuzosin. Example inhibitors include azole antifungals, clarithromycin, diclofenac, doxycycline, erythromycin, imatinib, isoniazid, nefazodone, nicardipine, propofol, protease inhibitors, quinidine, telithromycin, and verapamil. Concurrent use of itraconazole, ketoconazole, or ritonavir is contraindicated.

Ethanol/Nutrition/Herb Interactions Food: Food increases the extent of absorption.

Dietary Considerations Take following a meal at the same time each day.

Dosage Forms Tablet, extended release, as hydrochloride: 10 mg

◆ **Alfuzosin Hydrochloride** *see* Alfuzosin *on page 58*
◆ **Allerdryl® (Can)** *see* DiphenhydrAMINE *on page 399*
◆ **AllerMax® [OTC]** *see* DiphenhydrAMINE *on page 399*
◆ **Allernix (Can)** *see* DiphenhydrAMINE *on page 399*
◆ **Alloprin® (Can)** *see* Allopurinol *on page 59*

Allopurinol (al oh PURE i nole)

Medication Safety Issues

Sound-alike/look-alike issues:

Allopurinol may be confused with Apresoline

Zyloprim® may be confused with Xylo-Pfan®, ZORprin®

Related Information

Chronic Renal Failure *on page 1437*

U.S. Brand Names Aloprim™; Zyloprim®

Canadian Brand Names Alloprin®; Apo-Allopurinol®; Novo-Purol; Zyloprim®

Synonyms Allopurinol Sodium

Pharmacologic Category Xanthine Oxidase Inhibitor

Generic Available Yes

Use

Oral: Prevention of attack of gouty arthritis and nephropathy; treatment of secondary hyperuricemia which may occur during treatment of tumors or leukemia; prevention of recurrent calcium oxalate calculi

I.V.: Treatment of elevated serum and urinary uric acid levels when oral therapy is not tolerated in patients with leukemia, lymphoma, and solid tumor malignancies who are receiving cancer chemotherapy

Mechanism of Action Allopurinol inhibits xanthine oxidase, the enzyme responsible for the conversion of hypoxanthine to xanthine to uric acid. Allopurinol is metabolized to oxypurinol which is also an inhibitor of xanthine oxidase; allopurinol acts on purine catabolism, reducing the production of uric acid without disrupting the biosynthesis of vital purines.

Pharmacodynamics/Kinetics

Onset of action: Peak effect: 1-2 weeks

Absorption: Oral: ~80%; Rectal: Poor and erratic

(Continued)

Allopurinol *(Continued)*

Distribution: V_d: ~1.6 L/kg; V_{ss}: 0.84-0.87 L/kg; enters breast milk
Protein binding: <1%
Metabolism: ~75% to active metabolites, chiefly oxypurinol
Bioavailability: 49% to 53%
Half-life elimination:
Normal renal function: Parent drug: 1-3 hours; Oxypurinol: 18-30 hours
End-stage renal disease: Prolonged
Time to peak, plasma: Oral: 30-120 minutes
Excretion: Urine (76% as oxypurinol, 12% as unchanged drug)
Allopurinol and oxypurinol are dialyzable

Dosage

Oral: Doses >300 mg should be given in divided doses.

Children ≤10 years: Secondary hyperuricemia associated with chemotherapy: 10 mg/kg/day in 2-3 divided doses **or** 200-300 mg/m²/day in 2-4 divided doses, maximum: 800 mg/24 hours

Alternative (manufacturer labeling): <6 years: 150 mg/day in 3 divided doses; 6-10 years: 300 mg/day in 2-3 divided doses

Children >10 years and Adults:

Secondary hyperuricemia associated with chemotherapy: 600-800 mg/day in 2-3 divided doses for prevention of acute uric acid nephropathy for 2-3 days starting 1-2 days before chemotherapy

Gout: Mild: 200-300 mg/day; Severe: 400-600 mg/day; to reduce the possibility of acute gouty attacks, initiate dose at 100 mg/day and increase weekly to recommended dosage.

Recurrent calcium oxalate stones: 200-300 mg/day in single or divided doses

Elderly: Initial: 100 mg/day, increase until desired uric acid level is obtained

I.V.: Hyperuricemia secondary to chemotherapy: Intravenous daily dose can be given as a single infusion or in equally divided doses at 6-, 8-, or 12-hour intervals. A fluid intake sufficient to yield a daily urinary output of at least 2 L in adults and the maintenance of a neutral or, preferably, slightly alkaline urine are desirable.

Children ≤10 years: Starting dose: 200 mg/m²/day

Children >10 years and Adults: 200-400 mg/m²/day (maximum: 600 mg/day)

Dosing adjustment in renal impairment: Must be adjusted due to accumulation of allopurinol and metabolites:

Oral: Removed by hemodialysis; adult maintenance doses of allopurinol (mg) based on creatinine clearance (mL/minute): See table.

Adult Maintenance Doses of Allopurinol[1]

Creatinine Clearance (mL/min)	Maintenance Dose of Allopurinol (mg)
140	400 daily
120	350 daily
100	300 daily
80	250 daily
60	200 daily
40	150 daily
20	100 daily
10	100 every 2 days
0	100 every 3 days

[1]This table is based on a standard maintenance dose of 300 mg of allopurinol per day for a patient with a creatinine clearance of 100 mL/min.

Hemodialysis: Administer dose posthemodialysis or administer 50% supplemental dose

I.V.:

Cl_{cr} 10-20 mL/minute: 200 mg/day
Cl_{cr} 3-10 mL/minute: 100 mg/day
Cl_{cr} <3 mL/minute: 100 mg/day at extended intervals

Stability

Powder for injection: Store at controlled room temperature of 15°C to 30°C (59°F to 86°F). Further dilution with NS or D_5W (50-100 mL) to ≤6 mg/mL is recommended. Following reconstitution, intravenous solutions should be stored at

20°C to 25°C (68°F to 77°F). Do not refrigerate reconstituted and/or diluted product. Must be administered within 10 hours of solution preparation.

Tablet: Store at controlled room temperature of 15°C to 25°C (59°F to 77°F).

Administration

Oral: Should administer oral forms after meals with plenty of fluid.

I.V.: Infuse over 15-60 minutes. The rate of infusion depends on the volume of the infusion. Whenever possible, therapy should be initiated at 24-48 hours before the start of chemotherapy known to cause tumor lysis (including adrenocorticosteroids). I.V. daily dose can be administered as a single infusion or in equally divided doses at 6-, 8-, or 12-hour interval.

Monitoring Parameters CBC, serum uric acid levels, I & O, hepatic and renal function, especially at start of therapy

Reference Range Uric acid, serum: An increase occurs during childhood

Adults:

Male: 3.4-7 mg/dL or slightly more

Female: 2.4-6 mg/dL or slightly more

Values >7 mg/dL are sometimes arbitrarily regarded as hyperuricemia, but there is no sharp line between normals on the one hand, and the serum uric acid of those with clinical gout. Normal ranges cannot be adjusted for purine ingestion, but high purine diet increases uric acid. Uric acid may be increased with body size, exercise, and stress.

Pregnancy Risk Factor C

Contraindications Hypersensitivity to allopurinol or any component of the formulation

Warnings/Precautions Do not use to treat asymptomatic hyperuricemia. Discontinue at first signs of rash. Caution in renal impairment, dosage adjustments needed. Use with caution in patients taking diuretics concurrently. Risk of skin rash may be increased in patients receiving amoxicillin or ampicillin. The risk of hypersensitivity may be increased in patients receiving thiazides, and possibly ACE inhibitors. Use caution with mercaptopurine or azathioprine.

Adverse Reactions

>1%:

Dermatologic: Rash (increased with ampicillin or amoxicillin use, 1.5% per manufacturer, >10% in some reports)

Gastrointestinal: Nausea (1.3%), vomiting (1.2%)

Renal: Renal failure/impairment (1.2%)

<1% (Limited to important or life-threatening): Acute tubular necrosis, agranulocytosis, angioedema, aplastic anemia, bronchospasm, cataracts, exfoliative dermatitis, granuloma annulare, granulomatous hepatitis, hypersensitivity syndrome, interstitial nephritis, macular retinitis, nephrolithiasis, neuritis, pancreatitis, paresthesia, peripheral neuropathy, Stevens-Johnson syndrome, toxic epidermal necrolysis, toxic pustuloderma, vasculitis

Overdosage/Toxicology If significant amounts of allopurinol have been absorbed, it is theoretically possible that oxypurinol stones could form, but no record of such occurrence exists. Alkalinization of urine and forced diuresis can help prevent potential xanthine stone formation.

Drug Interactions

Ampicillin, amoxicillin: Incidence of rash may be increased.

Anticoagulants: Allopurinol may prolong the half-life of anticoagulants, effect seen with dicumarol; monitor.

ACE inhibitors: Captopril may increase risk of hypersensitivity.

Azathioprine: Metabolism inhibited by allopurinol; reduce azathioprine dose by $^1/_3$ or $^1/_4$.

Chlorpropamide: Half-life of chlorpropamide may be increased.

Cyclosporine: Allopurinol may increase cyclosporine serum levels.

Mercaptopurine: Metabolism inhibited by allopurinol; reduce mercaptopurine dose by $^1/_3$ or $^1/_4$.

Thiazide diuretics: Toxicity and risk of hypersensitivity may be increased.

Theophylline: Half-life of theophylline may be increased.

Vidarabine: Neurotoxicity may be enhanced.

Ethanol/Nutrition/Herb Interactions

Ethanol: May decrease effectiveness.

Iron supplements: Hepatic iron uptake may be increased.

Vitamin C: Large amounts of vitamin C may acidify urine and increase kidney stone formation.

(Continued)

Allopurinol *(Continued)*

Dietary Considerations Should administer oral forms after meals with plenty of fluid. Fluid intake should be administered to yield neutral or slightly alkaline urine and an output of ~2 L (in adults).

Dosage Forms

Injection, powder for reconstitution, as sodium (Aloprim™): 500 mg
Tablet (Zyloprim®): 100 mg, 300 mg

♦ **Allopurinol Sodium** *see* Allopurinol *on page 59*

Almotriptan (al moh TRIP tan)

Medication Safety Issues

Sound-alike/look-alike issues:
Axert™ may be confused with Antivert®

U.S. Brand Names Axert™

Canadian Brand Names Axert™

Synonyms Almotriptan Malate

Pharmacologic Category Serotonin 5-HT_{1D} Receptor Agonist

Generic Available No

Use Acute treatment of migraine with or without aura

Mechanism of Action Selective agonist for serotonin (5-HT_{1B}, 5-HT_{1D}, 5-HT_{1F} receptors) in cranial arteries; causes vasoconstriction and reduce sterile inflammation associated with antidromic neuronal transmission correlating with relief of migraine

Pharmacodynamics/Kinetics

Absorption: Well absorbed
Distribution: V_d: 180-200 L
Protein binding: ~35%
Metabolism: MAO type A oxidative deamination (~27% of dose); via CYP3A4 and 2D6 (~12% of dose) to inactive metabolites
Bioavailability: 70%
Half-life elimination: 3-4 hours
Time to peak: 1-3 hours
Excretion: Urine (40% as unchanged drug); feces (13% unchanged and metabolized)

Dosage Oral: Adults: Migraine: Initial: 6.25-12.5 mg in a single dose; if the headache returns, repeat the dose after 2 hours; no more than 2 doses in 24-hour period

Note: If the first dose is ineffective, diagnosis needs to be re-evaluated. Safety of treating more than 4 migraines/month has not been established.

Dosage adjustment in renal impairment: Initial: 6.25 mg in a single dose; maximum daily dose: ≤12.5 mg

Dosage adjustment in hepatic impairment: Initial: 6.25 mg in a single dose; maximum daily dose: ≤12.5 mg

Stability Store at 15°C to 30°C (59°F to 86°F).

Anesthesia and Critical Care Concerns/Other Considerations Almotriptan should not be used in patients with a history of vasospastic disease, Prinzmetal's angina, or any critical vascular disease.

Pregnancy Risk Factor C

Contraindications Hypersensitivity to almotriptan or any component of the formulation; use as prophylactic therapy for migraine; hemiplegic or basilar migraine; cluster headache; known or suspected ischemic heart disease (angina pectoris, MI, documented silent ischemia, coronary artery vasospasm, Prinzmetal's variant angina); peripheral vascular syndromes (including ischemic bowel disease); uncontrolled hypertension; use within 24 hours of another 5-HT_1 agonist; use within 24 hours of ergotamine derivative; concurrent administration or within 2 weeks of discontinuing an MAO inhibitor (specifically MAO type A inhibitors)

Warnings/Precautions Almotriptan is indicated only in patients ≥18 years of age with a clear diagnosis of migraine headache. If a patient does not respond to the first dose, the diagnosis of migraine should be reconsidered. Do not give to patients with risk factors for CAD until a cardiovascular evaluation has been performed; if evaluation is satisfactory, the healthcare provider should administer the first dose and cardiovascular status should be periodically evaluated. Cardiac events (coronary artery vasospasm, transient ischemia, myocardial infarction, ventricular tachycardia/fibrillation, cardiac arrest, and death), cerebral/subarachnoid hemorrhage, stroke, peripheral vascular ischemia, and colonic ischemia have been reported with 5-HT_1 agonist administration. Significant elevation in blood pressure, including hypertensive crisis, has also been reported on rare occasions in patients with and without a history of hypertension. Use with caution in liver or renal dysfunction. Safety and efficacy in pediatric patients have not been established.

Adverse Reactions

1% to 10%:

Central nervous system: Headache (>1%), dizziness (>1%), somnolence (>1%)
Gastrointestinal: Nausea (1% to 2%), xerostomia (1%)
Neuromuscular & skeletal: Paresthesia (1%)

<1% (Limited to important or life-threatening): Colitis, coronary artery vasospasm, hypertension, myocardial ischemia, MI, neuropathy, rash, syncope, tachycardia, ventricular fibrillation, ventricular tachycardia, vertigo

Overdosage/Toxicology Hypertension or more serious cardiovascular symptoms may occur. Clinical and electrocardiographic monitoring needed for at least 20 hours even if patient is asymptomatic. Treatment is symptom-directed and supportive.

Drug Interactions **Substrate** (minor) of CYP2D6, 3A4

Ergot-containing drugs: Prolong vasospastic reactions; do not use almotriptan or ergot-containing drugs within 24 hours of each other.

Ketoconazole: Increases almotriptan serum concentration. Monitor for increased almotriptan response.

MAO inhibitors (moclobemide [MAO type A inhibitor]): Almotriptan clearance decreased by 27%; C_{max} increased by 6%. Avoid concurrent administration of MAO inhibitors or within 2 weeks of discontinuing an MAO inhibitor, specifically MAO type A inhibitors.

Selegiline: Selegiline is a selective MAO type B inhibitor; while not specifically contraindicated, combination has not been studied.

Verapamil: Increased almotriptan serum concentration by 24%. Dose adjustment not necessary.

SSRIs: Concurrent use may lead to symptoms of hyper-reflexia, weakness, and lack of coordination; monitor.

Dietary Considerations May be taken without regard to meals

Dosage Forms Tablet, as malate: 6.25 mg, 12.5 mg

♦ **Almotriptan Malate** *see* Almotriptan *on page 62*

♦ **Aloprim™** *see* Allopurinol *on page 59*

Alosetron (a LOE se tron)

Medication Safety Issues

Sound-alike/look-alike issues:

Lotronex® may be confused with Lovenox®, Protonix®

U.S. Brand Names Lotronex®

Pharmacologic Category Selective 5-HT_3 Receptor Antagonist

Restrictions Only physicians enrolled in GlaxoSmithKline's Prescribing Program for Lotronex® may prescribe this medication. Program stickers must be affixed to all prescriptions; no phone, fax, or computerized prescriptions are permitted with this program. n FDA-approved medication guide is available at www.fda.gov/cder/Offices/ODS/labeling.htm; distribute to each patient to whom this medication is dispensed

Generic Available No

Use Treatment of women with severe diarrhea-predominant irritable bowel syndrome (IBS) who have failed to respond to conventional therapy

Mechanism of Action Alosetron is a potent and selective antagonist of a subtype of the serotonin 5-HT_3 receptor. 5-HT_3 receptors are ligand-gated ion channels extensively distributed on enteric neurons in the human gastrointestinal tract, as well as other peripheral and central locations. Activation of these channels affect the regulation of visceral pain, colonic transit, and gastrointestinal secretions. In patients with irritable bowel syndrome, blockade of these channels may reduce pain, abdominal discomfort, urgency, and diarrhea.

Pharmacodynamics/Kinetics

Distribution: V_d: 65-95 L

Protein binding: 82%

(Continued)

Alosetron *(Continued)*

Metabolism: Extensive hepatic metabolism. Alosetron is metabolized by CYP2C9, 3A4, and 1A2. Thirteen metabolites have been detected in the urine. Biological activity of these metabolites in unknown.

Bioavailability: Mean: 50% to 60% (range: 30% to >90%); decreased with food (25%)

Half-life elimination: 1.5 hours for alosetron

Time to peak: 1 hour after oral administration

Excretion: Urine (73%) and feces (24%); 7% as unchanged drug (1% feces, 6% urine)

Dosage Oral:

Children: Safety and efficacy have not been established.

Adults: Female: Initial: 0.5 mg twice daily for 4 weeks, with or without food; if tolerated, but response is inadequate, may be increased after 4 weeks to 1 mg twice daily. If response is inadequate after 4 weeks of 1 mg twice-daily dosing, discontinue treatment.

Note: Discontinue immediately if constipation or signs/symptoms of ischemic colitis occur. Do not reinitiate in patients who develop ischemic colitis.

Elderly: Dosage adjustment is not required; however, postmarketing experience suggests that elderly patients may be at greater risk for complications of constipation.

Dosage adjustment in renal impairment: The need for dosage adjustment has not been defined (due to limited information on activity of metabolites).

Dosage adjustment in hepatic impairment: In mild-to-moderate dysfunction (Child-Pugh score ≤9), use caution. Avoid use in severe hepatic dysfunction (Child-Pugh score >9).

Stability Store at 15°C to 30°C (59°F to 86°F).

Administration May be administered with or with food; however, absorption may be reduced by approximately 25%.

Anesthesia and Critical Care Concerns/Other Considerations Alosetron has been linked to reports of ischemic colitis, which prompted a call for withdrawal by a prominent U.S. consumer group. The manufacturer initially withdrew this drug voluntarily in response to this concern. It has been reintroduced with restrictions on prescribing.

Pregnancy Risk Factor B

Contraindications Do not start treatment in patients who are constipated. Hypersensitivity to alosetron or any component of the formulation; history of severe or chronic constipation; history of ischemic colitis, intestinal obstruction, stricture, toxic megacolon, gastrointestinal perforation and/or adhesions; active diverticulitis, current or history of Crohn's disease, severe hepatic dysfunction, or ulcerative colitis; history of impaired intestinal circulation, thrombophlebitis, or hypercoagulable state; patients unable to understand or comply with "Patient-Physician" agreement; concomitant administration with fluvoxamine

Warnings/Precautions [U.S. Boxed Warning]: Patients must read and sign a "Patient-Physician" agreement before receiving the initial prescription. Constipation is a frequent, dose-related side effect. Serious complications of constipation have been infrequently reported (obstruction, perforation, impaction, toxic megacolon, secondary ischemia); risk may be increased in elderly, debilitated patients, or with concurrent use of other medications which decrease GI motility. **[U.S. Boxed Warning]: Discontinue immediately in patients with constipation.** Nonsevere constipation may be managed by temporarily interrupting therapy. **[U.S. Boxed Warning]: Acute ischemic colitis has been reported during alosetron treatment.** Discontinue immediately in patients who experience rectal bleeding or a sudden worsening of abdominal pain, and do not restart therapy if ischemic colitis is diagnosed. Use caution in mild-to-moderate hepatic impairment (Child-Pugh score ≤9) or renal impairment. Safety and efficacy have not been established in pediatric or male patients.

Adverse Reactions

>10%: Gastrointestinal: Constipation (dose related) (29%)

1% to 10%: Gastrointestinal: Abdominal discomfort and pain (7%), nausea (6%), gastrointestinal discomfort and pain (6%), abdominal distention (2%), hemorrhoids (2%), regurgitation and reflux (2%)

<1% (Limited to important or life-threatening): Allergic skin reactions, anxiety, bilirubin level changes, bladder inflammation, bone pain, breathing disorder, cholecystitis, cognitive function disorders, confusion, cramps, colitis, depression, diaphoresis, diverticulitis, dyspepsia symptoms, fatigue, gastroenteritis, GI

lesions, GI motility decreased, GI obstructions, GI spasms, headache, hemorrhage, hepatitis, hyperacidity, hyper-/hypoglycemia, hypertension, hypnagogic effects, hypoesthesia, hypothalamus/pituitary dysfunction, ileus, impaction, ischemic colitis, memory effects, muscle pain/stiffness, obstruction, occult stools, pain, perforation, rash, RBC/hemoglobin defects, sedation, sexual dysfunction, skeletal pain, small bowel mesenteric ischemia, tachyarrhythmia, temperature regulation impairment, tremor, ulceration, ulcerative colitis, urinary frequency, urticaria

Overdosage/Toxicology There is not a specific antidote for overdose; manage with appropriate supportive therapy.

Drug Interactions Substrate of CYP1A2 (major), 2C9 (minor), 3A4 (minor); **Inhibits** CYP1A2 (weak), 2E1 (weak)

CYP1A2 inhibitors: May increase the levels/effects of alosetron. Example inhibitors include ciprofloxacin, fluvoxamine, ketoconazole, norfloxacin, ofloxacin, and rofecoxib.

Fluvoxamine: Concomitant use is contraindicated.

Ethanol/Nutrition/Herb Interactions Food: When administered with food, absorption may be reduced by ~25%.

Dietary Considerations May be taken with or without food.

Dosage Forms Tablet: 0.5 mg, 1 mg

- **Aloxi®** *see* Palonosetron *on page 977*
- **AlphaNine® SD** *see* Factor IX *on page 502*

Alprazolam (al PRAY zoe lam)

Medication Safety Issues

Sound-alike/look-alike issues:

Alprazolam may be confused with alprostadil, lorazepam, triazolam

Xanax® may be confused with Lanoxin®, Tenex®, Tylox®, Xopenex®, Zantac®, Zyrtec®

Related Information

Anesthesia Considerations for Neurosurgery *on page 1401*

Benzodiazepines *on page 1555*

U.S. Brand Names Alprazolam Intensol®; Niravam™; Xanax®; Xanax XR®

Canadian Brand Names Alti-Alprazolam; Apo-Alpraz®; Gen-Alprazolam; Novo-Alprazol; Nu-Alprax; Xanax®; Xanax TS™

Pharmacologic Category Benzodiazepine

Restrictions C-IV

Generic Available Yes: Extended release tablet, immediate release tablet

Use Treatment of anxiety disorder (GAD); panic disorder, with or without agoraphobia; anxiety associated with depression

Unlabeled/Investigational Use Anxiety in children

Mechanism of Action Binds to stereospecific benzodiazepine receptors on the postsynaptic GABA neuron at several sites within the central nervous system, including the limbic system, reticular formation. Enhancement of the inhibitory effect of GABA on neuronal excitability results by increased neuronal membrane permeability to chloride ions. This shift in chloride ions results in hyperpolarization (a less excitable state) and stabilization.

Pharmacodynamics/Kinetics

Distribution: V_d: 0.9-1.2 L/kg; enters breast milk

Protein binding: 80%

Metabolism: Hepatic via CYP3A4; forms two active metabolites (4-hydroxyalprazolam and α-hydroxyalprazolam)

Bioavailability: 90%

Half-life elimination:

Adults: 11.2 hours (range: 6.3-26.9)

Elderly: 16.3 hours (range: 9-26.9 hours)

Alcoholic liver disease: 19.7 hours (range: 5.8-65.3 hours)

Obesity: 21.8 hours (range: 9.9-40.4 hours)

Time to peak, serum: 1-2 hours

Excretion: Urine (as unchanged drug and metabolites)

Dosage Oral: **Note:** Treatment >4 months should be re-evaluated to determine the patient's continued need for the drug

(Continued)

Alprazolam *(Continued)*

Children: Anxiety (unlabeled use): Immediate release: Initial: 0.005 mg/kg/dose or 0.125 mg/dose 3 times/day; increase in increments of 0.125-0.25 mg, up to a maximum of 0.02 mg/kg/dose or 0.06 mg/kg/day (0.375-3 mg/day)

Adults:

Anxiety: Immediate release: Effective doses are 0.5-4 mg/day in divided doses; the manufacturer recommends starting at 0.25-0.5 mg 3 times/day; titrate dose upward; usual maximum: 4 mg/day. Patients requiring doses >4 mg/day should be increased cautiously. Periodic reassessment and consideration of dosage reduction is recommended.

Anxiety associated with depression: Immediate release: Average dose required: 2.5-3 mg/day in divided doses

Ethanol withdrawal (unlabeled use): Immediate release: Usual dose: 2-2.5 mg/day in divided doses

Panic disorder:

Immediate release: Initial: 0.5 mg 3 times/day; dose may be increased every 3-4 days in increments ≤1 mg/day. Mean effective dosage: 5-6 mg/day; many patients obtain relief at 2 mg/day, as much as 10 mg/day may be required

Extended release: 0.5-1 mg once daily; may increase dose every 3-4 days in increments ≤1 mg/day (range: 3-6 mg/day)

Switching from immediate release to extended release: Patients may be switched to extended release tablets by taking the total daily dose of the immediate release tablets and giving it once daily using the extended release preparation.

Preoperative sedation: 0.5 mg in evening at bedtime and 0.5 mg 1 hour before procedure

Dose reduction: Abrupt discontinuation should be avoided. Daily dose may be decreased by 0.5 mg every 3 days, however, some patients may require a slower reduction. If withdrawal symptoms occur, resume previous dose and discontinue on a less rapid schedule.

Elderly: Initial: 0.125-0.25 mg twice daily; increase by 0.125 mg/day as needed. The smallest effective dose should be used. **Note:** Elderly patients may be more sensitive to the effects of alprazolam including ataxia and oversedation. The elderly may also have impaired renal function leading to decreased clearance. Titrate gradually, if needed.

Immediate release: Initial: 0.25 mg 2-3 times/day

Extended release: Initial: 0.5 mg once daily

Dosing adjustment in renal impairment: No guidelines for adjustment; use caution

Dosing adjustment in hepatic impairment: Reduce dose by 50% to 60% or avoid in cirrhosis

Stability Orally-disintegrating tablet: Store at room temperature of 20°C to 25°C (68°F to 77°F). Protect from moisture. Seal bottle tightly and discard any cotton packaged inside bottle.

Administration

Immediate release preparations: Can be administered sublingually with comparable onset and completeness of absorption.

Extended release tablet: Should be taken once daily in the morning; do not crush, break, or chew.

Orally-disintegrating tablets: Using dry hands, place tablet on top of tongue. If using one-half of tablet, immediately discard remaining half (may not remain stable). Administration with water is not necessary.

Monitoring Parameters Respiratory and cardiovascular status

Anesthesia and Critical Care Concerns/Other Considerations Chronic use of this agent may increase the perioperative benzodiazepine dose needed to achieve desired effect; not intended for management of anxieties and minor distresses associated with everyday life. Treatment >4 months should be re-evaluated to determine the patient's need for the drug. Patients who become physically dependent on alprazolam tend to have a difficult time discontinuing it; withdrawal symptoms may be severe. To minimize withdrawal symptoms, taper dosage slowly; do not discontinue abruptly. Abrupt discontinuation after sustained use (generally >10 days) may cause withdrawal symptoms.

Pregnancy Risk Factor D

Contraindications Hypersensitivity to alprazolam or any component of the formulation (cross-sensitivity with other benzodiazepines may exist);

narrow-angle glaucoma; concurrent use with ketoconazole or itraconazole; pregnancy

Warnings/Precautions Rebound or withdrawal symptoms, including seizures, may occur 18 hours to 3 days following abrupt discontinuation or large decreases in dose (more common in patients receiving >4 mg/day or prolonged treatment). Dose reductions or tapering must be approached with extreme caution. Breakthrough anxiety may occur at the end of dosing interval. Use with caution in patients receiving concurrent CYP3A4 inhibitors, particularly when these agents are added to therapy. Has weak uricosuric properties, use with caution in renal impairment or predisposition to urate nephropathy. Use with caution in elderly or debilitated patients, patients with hepatic disease (including alcoholics), renal impairment, or obese patients.

Causes CNS depression (dose related) resulting in sedation, dizziness, confusion, or ataxia which may impair physical and mental capabilities. Patients must be cautioned about performing tasks which require mental alertness (eg, operating machinery or driving). Use with caution in patients receiving other CNS depressants or psychoactive agents. Effects with other sedative drugs or ethanol may be potentiated. Benzodiazepines have been associated with falls and traumatic injury and should be used with extreme caution in patients who are at risk of these events (especially the elderly). Use with caution in patients with respiratory disease or impaired gag reflex.

Use caution in patients with depression, particularly if suicidal risk may be present. Episodes of mania or hypomania have occurred in depressed patients treated with alprazolam. May cause physical or psychological dependence - use with caution in patients with a history of drug dependence. Acute withdrawal, including seizures, may be precipitated in patients after administration of flumazenil to patients receiving long-term benzodiazepine therapy.

Benzodiazepines have been associated with anterograde amnesia. Paradoxical reactions, including hyperactive or aggressive behavior, have been reported with benzodiazepines, particularly in adolescent/pediatric or psychiatric patients. Does not have analgesic, antidepressant, or antipsychotic properties.

Benzodiazepines have the potential to cause harm to the fetus, particularly when administered during the first trimester. In addition, withdrawal symptoms may occur in the neonate following *in utero* exposure. Use of alprazolam during pregnancy should be avoided. In addition, symptoms of withdrawal, lethargy, and loss of body weight have been reported in infants exposed to alprazolam and/or benzodiazepines while nursing; use during breast-feeding is not recommended.

Adverse Reactions

>10%:

Central nervous system: Abnormal coordination, cognitive disorder, depression, drowsiness, fatigue, irritability, lightheadedness, memory impairment, sedation, somnolence

Gastrointestinal: Appetite increased/decreased, constipation, salivation decreased, weight gain/loss, xerostomia

Genitourinary: Micturition difficulty

Neuromuscular & skeletal: Dysarthria

1% to 10%:

Cardiovascular: Hypotension

Central nervous system: Agitation, attention disturbance, confusion, depersonalization, derealization, disorientation, disinhibition, dizziness, dream abnormalities, fear, hallucinations, hypersomnia, nightmares, seizure, talkativeness

Dermatologic: Dermatitis, pruritus, rash

Endocrine & metabolic: Libido decreased/increased, menstrual disorders

Gastrointestinal: Salivation increased

Genitourinary: Incontinence

Hepatic: Bilirubin increased, jaundice, liver enzymes increased

Neuromuscular & skeletal: Arthralgia, ataxia, myalgia, paresthesia

Ocular: Diplopia

Respiratory: Allergic rhinitis, dyspnea

<1% (Limited to important or life-threatening): Amnesia, falls, galactorrhea, gynecomastia, hepatic failure, hepatitis, hyperprolactinemia, Stevens-Johnson syndrome

Overdosage/Toxicology Symptoms of overdose include somnolence, confusion, coma, and diminished reflexes. Treatment for benzodiazepine overdose is

(Continued)

Alprazolam *(Continued)*

supportive. Flumazenil has been shown to selectively block the binding of benzodiazepines to CNS receptors, resulting in a reversal of benzodiazepine-induced sedation; however, its use may not reverse respiratory depression.

Drug Interactions Substrate of CYP3A4 (major)

CNS depressants: Sedative effects and/or respiratory depression may be additive with CNS depressants. Includes ethanol, barbiturates, narcotic analgesics, and other sedative agents; monitor for increased effect.

CYP3A4 inducers: CYP3A4 inducers may decrease the levels/effects of alprazolam. Example inducers include aminoglutethimide, carbamazepine, nafcillin, nevirapine, phenobarbital, phenytoin, and rifamycins.

CYP3A4 inhibitors: May increase the levels/effects of alprazolam. Example inhibitors include azole antifungals, clarithromycin, diclofenac, doxycycline, erythromycin, imatinib, isoniazid, nefazodone, nicardipine, propofol, protease inhibitors, quinidine, telithromycin, and verapamil. Contraindicated with itraconazole and ketoconazole.

Fluoxetine: May increase plasma concentrations/effects of alprazolam.

Oral contraceptives: May increase serum levels/effects of alprazolam.

Theophylline: May partially antagonize some of the effects of benzodiazepines; monitor for decreased response; may require higher doses for sedation.

Tricyclic antidepressants: Plasma concentrations of imipramine and desipramine have been reported to be increased 31% and 20%, respectively, by concomitant administration; monitor.

Ethanol/Nutrition/Herb Interactions

Cigarette smoking: May decrease alprazolam concentrations up to 50%.

Ethanol: Avoid ethanol (may increase CNS depression).

Food: Alprazolam serum concentration is unlikely to be increased by grapefruit juice because of alprazolam's high oral bioavailability. The C_{max} of the extended release formulation is increased by 25% when a high-fat meal is given 2 hours before dosing. T_{max} is decreased 30% when food is given immediately prior to dose. T_{max} is increased by 30% when food is given ≥1 hour after dose.

Herb/Nutraceutical: St John's wort may decrease alprazolam levels. Avoid valerian, St John's wort, kava kava, gotu kola (may increase CNS depression).

Dosage Forms

Solution, oral [concentrate]:
- Alprazolam Intensol®: 1 mg/mL (30 mL)

Tablet: 0.25 mg, 0.5 mg, 1 mg, 2 mg
- Xanax®: 0.25 mg, 0.5 mg, 1 mg, 2 mg

Tablet, extended release: 0.5 mg, 1 mg, 2 mg, 3 mg
- Xanax XR®: 0.5 mg, 1 mg, 2 mg, 3 mg

Tablet, orally disintegrating [scored]:
- Niravam™: 0.25 mg, 0.5 mg, 1 mg, 2 mg [orange flavor]

♦ **Alprazolam Intensol®** *see* Alprazolam *on page 65*

Alprostadil (al PROS ta dill)

Medication Safety Issues

Sound-alike/look-alike issues:
- Alprostadil may be confused with alprazolam

U.S. Brand Names Caverject®; Caverject Impulse®; Edex®; Muse®; Prostin VR Pediatric®

Canadian Brand Names Caverject®; Muse® Pellet; Prostin® VR

Synonyms PGE_1; Prostaglandin E_1

Pharmacologic Category Prostaglandin

Generic Available Yes: Solution for injection

Use

Prostin VR Pediatric®: Temporary maintenance of patency of ductus arteriosus in neonates with ductal-dependent congenital heart disease until surgery can be performed. These defects include cyanotic (eg, pulmonary atresia, pulmonary stenosis, tricuspid atresia, Fallot's tetralogy, transposition of the great vessels) and acyanotic (eg, interruption of aortic arch, coarctation of aorta, hypoplastic left ventricle) heart disease.

Caverject®: Treatment of erectile dysfunction of vasculogenic, psychogenic, or neurogenic etiology; adjunct in the diagnosis of erectile dysfunction

Edex®, Muse®: Treatment of erectile dysfunction of vasculogenic, psychogenic, or neurogenic etiology

Unlabeled/Investigational Use Investigational: Treatment of pulmonary hypertension in infants and children with congenital heart defects with left-to-right shunts

Mechanism of Action Causes vasodilation by means of direct effect on vascular and ductus arteriosus smooth muscle; relaxes trabecular smooth muscle by dilation of cavernosal arteries when injected along the penile shaft, allowing blood flow to and entrapment in the lacunar spaces of the penis (ie, corporeal veno-occlusive mechanism)

Pharmacodynamics/Kinetics

Onset of action: Rapid

Duration: <1 hour

Distribution: Insignificant following penile injection

Protein binding, plasma: 81% to albumin

Metabolism: ~75% by oxidation in one pass via lungs

Half-life elimination: 5-10 minutes

Excretion: Urine (90% as metabolites) within 24 hours

Dosage

Patent ductus arteriosus (Prostin VR Pediatric®):

I.V. continuous infusion into a large vein, or alternatively through an umbilical artery catheter placed at the ductal opening: 0.05-0.1 mcg/kg/minute with therapeutic response, rate is reduced to lowest effective dosage; with unsatisfactory response, rate is increased gradually; maintenance: 0.01-0.4 mcg/kg/minute

PGE_1 is usually given at an infusion rate of 0.1 mcg/kg/minute, but it is often possible to reduce the dosage to $^1/_2$ or even $^1/_{10}$ without losing the therapeutic effect. The mixing schedule is as follows. Infusion rates deliver 0.1 mcg/kg/minute: See table.

Alprostadil

Add 1 Ampul (500 mcg) to:	Concentration (mcg/mL)	Infusion Rate	
		mL/min/kg Needed to Infuse 0.1 mcg/kg/min	mL/kg/24 h
250 mL	2	0.05	72
100 mL	5	0.02	28.8
50 mL	10	0.01	14.4
25 mL	20	0.005	7.2

Therapeutic response is indicated by increased pH in those with acidosis or by an increase in oxygenation (PO_2) usually evident within 30 minutes

Erectile dysfunction:

Caverject®, Edex®: Intracavernous: Individualize dose by careful titration; doses >40 mcg (Edex®) or >60 mcg (Caverject®) are not recommended: Initial dose must be titrated in physician's office. Patient must stay in the physician's office until complete detumescence occurs; if there is no response, then the next higher dose may be given within 1 hour; if there is still no response, a 1-day interval before giving the next dose is recommended; increasing the dose or concentration in the treatment of impotence results in increasing pain and discomfort

Vasculogenic, psychogenic, or mixed etiology: Initiate dosage titration at 2.5 mcg, increasing by 2.5 mcg to a dose of 5 mcg and then in increments of 5-10 mcg depending on the erectile response until the dose produces an erection suitable for intercourse, not lasting >1 hour; if there is absolutely no response to initial 2.5 mcg dose, the second dose may be increased to 7.5 mcg, followed by increments of 5-10 mcg

Neurogenic etiology (eg, spinal cord injury): Initiate dosage titration at 1.25 mcg, increasing to a dose of 2.5 mcg and then 5 mcg; increase further in increments 5 mcg until the dose is reached that produces an erection suitable for intercourse, not lasting >1 hour

Maintenance: Once appropriate dose has been determined, patient may self-administer injections at a frequency of no more than 3 times/week with at least 24 hours between doses

(Continued)

Alprostadil *(Continued)*

Muse® Pellet: Intraurethral:

Initial: 125-250 mcg

Maintenance: Administer as needed to achieve an erection; duration of action is about 30-60 minutes; use only two systems per 24-hour period

Elderly: Elderly patients may have a greater frequency of renal dysfunction; lowest effective dose should be used. In clinical studies with Edex®, higher minimally effective doses and a higher rate of lack of effect were noted.

Stability

Caverject® Impulse™: Store at controlled room temperature of 15°C to 30°C (59°F to 86°F). Provided as a dual-chamber syringe with diluent in one chamber. To mix, hold syringe with needle pointing upward and turn plunger clockwise; turn upside down several times to mix. Device can be set to deliver specified dose, each device can be set at various increments. Following reconstitution, use within 24 hours and discard any unused solution.

Caverject® powder: The 5 mcg, 10 mcg, and 20 mcg vials should be stored at or below 25°C (77°F). The 40 mcg vial should be stored at 2°C to 8°C until dispensed. After dispensing, stable for up to 3 months at or below 25°C. Use only the supplied diluent for reconstitution (ie, bacteriostatic/sterile water with benzyl alcohol 0.945%). Following reconstitution, all strengths should be stored at or below 25°C (77°F); do not refrigerate or freeze; use within 24 hours.

Caverject® solution: Prior to dispensing, store frozen at -20°C to -10°C (-4°F to -14°F); once dispensed, may be stored frozen for up to 3 months, or under refrigeration at 2°C to 8°C (36°F to 46°F) for up to 7 days. Do not refreeze. Once removed from foil wrap, solution may be allowed to warm to room temperature prior to use. If not used immediately, solution should be discarded. Shake well prior to use.

Edex®: Store at controlled room temperature of 15°C to 30°C (59°F to 86°F); following reconstitution with NS, use immediately and discard any unused solution.

Muse®: Refrigerate at 2°C to 8°C (36°F to 46°F); may be stored at room temperature for up to 14 days.

Prostin VR Pediatric®: Refrigerate at 2°C to 8°C (36°F to 46°F); prior to infusion, dilute with D_5W or NS; use within 24 hours.

Administration Erectile dysfunction: Use a ½ inch, 27- to 30-gauge needle. Inject into the dorsolateral aspect of the proximal third of the penis, avoiding visible veins; alternate side of the penis for injections.

Monitoring Parameters Arterial pressure, respiratory rate, heart rate, temperature, degree of penile pain, length of erection, signs of infection

Pregnancy Risk Factor X/C (Muse®)

Contraindications Hypersensitivity to alprostadil or any component of the formulation; hyaline membrane disease or persistent fetal circulation and when a dominant left-to-right shunt is present; respiratory distress syndrome; conditions predisposing patients to priapism (sickle cell anemia, multiple myeloma, leukemia); patients with anatomical deformation of the penis, penile implants; use in men for whom sexual activity is inadvisable or contraindicated; pregnancy

Warnings/Precautions Use cautiously in neonates with bleeding tendencies. **[U.S. Boxed Warning]: Apnea may occur in 10% to 12% of neonates with congenital heart defects, especially in those weighing <2 kg at birth.** Apnea usually appears during the first hour of drug infusion.

When used in erectile dysfunction, priapism may occur; patient must be instructed to report to physician or seek immediate medical assistance if an erection persists for longer than 4 hours. Treat immediately to avoid penile tissue damage and permanent loss of potency; discontinue therapy if signs of penile fibrosis develop (penile angulation, cavernosal fibrosis, or Peyronie's disease). When used in erectile dysfunction (Muse®), syncope occurring within 1 hour of administration has been reported. The potential for drug-drug interactions may occur when Muse® is prescribed concomitantly with antihypertensives. Some lowering of blood pressure may occur without symptoms, and swelling of leg veins, leg pain, perineal pain, and rapid pulse have been reported in <2% of patients during in-clinic titration and home treatment.

Adverse Reactions

Intraurethral:

>10%: Genitourinary: Penile pain, urethral burning

2% to 10%:

Central nervous system: Headache, dizziness, pain

Genitourinary: Vaginal itching (female partner), testicular pain, urethral bleeding (minor)

<2% (Limited to important or life-threatening): Tachycardia, perineal pain, leg pain

Intracavernosal injection:

>10%: Genitourinary: Penile pain

1% to 10%:

Cardiovascular: Hypertension

Central nervous system: Headache, dizziness

Genitourinary: Prolonged erection (>4 hours, 4%), penile fibrosis, penis disorder, penile rash, penile edema

Local: Injection site hematoma and/or bruising

<1% (Limited to important or life-threatening): Balanitis, injection site hemorrhage, priapism (0.4%)

Intravenous:

>10%:

Cardiovascular: Flushing

Central nervous system: Fever

Respiratory: Apnea

1% to 10%:

Cardiovascular: Bradycardia, hyper-/hypotension, tachycardia, cardiac arrest, edema

Central nervous system: Seizures, headache, dizziness

Endocrine & metabolic: Hypokalemia

Gastrointestinal: Diarrhea

Hematologic: Disseminated intravascular coagulation

Neuromuscular & skeletal: Back pain

Respiratory: Upper respiratory infection, flu syndrome, sinusitis, nasal congestion, cough

Miscellaneous: Sepsis, localized pain in structures other than the injection site

<1% (Limited to important or life-threatening): Anemia, anuria, bleeding, bradypnea, bronchial wheezing, cerebral bleeding, CHF, gastric regurgitation, hematuria, hyperbilirubinemia, hyperemia, hyperextension of neck, hyperirritability, hyperkalemia, hypoglycemia, hypothermia, jitteriness, lethargy, peritonitis, second degree heart block, shock, stiffness, supraventricular tachycardia, thrombocytopenia, ventricular fibrillation

Overdosage/Toxicology Symptoms of overdose when treating patent ductus arteriosus include apnea, bradycardia, hypotension, and flushing. If hypotension or pyrexia occurs, the infusion rate should be reduced until symptoms subside. Apnea or bradycardia requires drug discontinuation. If intracavernous overdose occurs, supervise until systemic effects have resolved or until penile detumescence has occurred.

Drug Interactions Risk of hypotension and syncope may be increased with antihypertensives.

Ethanol/Nutrition/Herb Interactions Ethanol: Avoid concurrent use (vasodilating effect).

Dosage Forms

Injection, powder for reconstitution:

Caverject®: 20 mcg, 40 mcg [contains lactose; diluent contains benzyl alcohol]

Caverject Impulse®: 10 mcg, 20 mcg [prefilled injection system; contains lactose; diluent contains benzyl alcohol]

Edex®: 10 mcg, 20 mcg, 40 mcg [contains lactose; packaged in kits containing diluent, syringe, and alcohol swab]

Injection, solution: 500 mcg/mL (1 mL)

Prostin VR Pediatric®: 500 mcg/mL (1 mL) [contains dehydrated alcohol]

Pellet, urethral (Muse®): 125 mcg (6s), 250 mcg (6s), 500 mcg (6s), 1000 mcg (6s)

- **Alrex®** *see* Loteprednol *on page 781*
- **Altace®** *see* Ramipril *on page 1103*
- **Altachlore [OTC]** *see* Sodium Chloride *on page 1183*
- **Altafrin** *see* Phenylephrine *on page 1015*
- **Altamist [OTC]** *see* Sodium Chloride *on page 1183*
- **Altaryl [OTC]** *see* DiphenhydrAMINE *on page 399*

Alteplase (AL te plase)

Medication Safety Issues

Sound-alike/look-alike issues:

Alteplase may be confused with Altace®

"tPA" abbreviation should not be used when writing orders for this medication; has been misread as TNKase (tenecteplase)

High alert medication: The Institute for Safe Medication Practices (ISMP) includes this medication (I.V.) among its list of drugs which have a heightened risk of causing significant patient harm when used in error.

U.S. Brand Names Activase®; Cathflo® Activase®

Canadian Brand Names Activase® rt-PA; Cathflo® Activase®

Synonyms Alteplase, Recombinant; Alteplase, Tissue Plasminogen Activator, Recombinant; tPA

Pharmacologic Category Thrombolytic Agent

Generic Available No

Use Management of acute myocardial infarction for the lysis of thrombi in coronary arteries; management of acute massive pulmonary embolism (PE) in adults

Acute myocardial infarction (AMI): Chest pain ≥20 minutes, ≤12-24 hours; S-T elevation ≥0.1 mV in at least two ECG leads

Acute pulmonary embolism (APE): Age ≤75 years: Documented massive pulmonary embolism by pulmonary angiography or echocardiography or high probability lung scan with clinical shock

Cathflo® Activase®: Restoration of central venous catheter function

Unlabeled/Investigational Use Acute peripheral arterial occlusive disease

Mechanism of Action Initiates local fibrinolysis by binding to fibrin in a thrombus (clot) and converts entrapped plasminogen to plasmin

Pharmacodynamics/Kinetics

Duration: >50% present in plasma cleared ~5 minutes after infusion terminated, ~80% cleared within 10 minutes

Excretion: Clearance: Rapidly from circulating plasma (550-650 mL/minute), primarily hepatic; >50% present in plasma is cleared within 5 minutes after the infusion is terminated, ~80% cleared within 10 minutes

Dosage

I.V.:

Coronary artery thrombi: Front loading dose (weight-based):

Patients >67 kg: Total dose: 100 mg over 1.5 hours; infuse 15 mg over 1-2 minutes. Infuse 50 mg over 30 minutes. See "Note."

Patients ≤67 kg: Total dose: 1.25 mg/kg; infuse 15 mg I.V. bolus over 1-2 minutes, then infuse 0.75 mg/kg (not to exceed 50 mg) over next 30 minutes, followed by 0.5 mg/kg over next 60 minutes (not to exceed 35 mg). See "Note."

Note: Concurrently, begin heparin 60 units/kg bolus (maximum: 4000 units) followed by continuous infusion of 12 units/kg/hour (maximum: 1000 units/hour) and adjust to aPTT target of 1.5-2 times the upper limit of control. Infuse remaining 35 mg of alteplase over the next hour.

Acute pulmonary embolism: 100 mg over 2 hours.

Acute ischemic stroke: Doses should be given within the first 3 hours of the onset of symptoms; recommended total dose: 0.9 mg/kg (maximum dose should not exceed 90 mg) infused over 60 minutes.

Load with 0.09 mg/kg (10% of the 0.9 mg/kg dose) as an I.V. bolus over 1 minute, followed by 0.81 mg/kg (90% of the 0.9 mg/kg dose) as a continuous infusion over 60 minutes. Heparin should not be started for 24 hours or more after starting alteplase for stroke.

Intracatheter: Central venous catheter clearance: Cathflo® Activase® 1 mg/mL:

Patients <30 kg: 110% of the internal lumen volume of the catheter, not to exceed 2 mg/2 mL; retain in catheter for 0.5-2 hours; may instill a second dose if catheter remains occluded

Patients ≥30 kg: 2 mg (2 mL); retain in catheter for 0.5-2 hours; may instill a second dose if catheter remains occluded

Intra-arterial: Acute peripheral arterial occlusive disease (unlabeled use): 0.02-0.1 mg/kg/hour for up to 36 hours

Advisory Panel to the Society for Cardiovascular and Interventional Radiology on Thrombolytic Therapy recommendation: ≤2 mg/hour and subtherapeutic heparin (aPTT <1.5 times baseline)

Stability

Activase®: The lyophilized product may be stored at room temperature (not to exceed 30°C/86°F), or under refrigeration; once reconstituted it should be used within 8 hours. Reconstitution:

50 mg vial: Use accompanying diluent (50 mL sterile water for injection); do not shake; final concentration: 1 mg/mL

100 mg vial: Use transfer set with accompanying diluent (100 mL vial of sterile water for injection); no vacuum is present in 100 mg vial; final concentration: 1 mg/mL

Cathflo® Activase®: Store lyophilized product under refrigeration. Reconstitution: Add 2.2 mL SWFI to vial; do not shake. Final concentration: 1 mg/mL. Once reconstituted, store at 2°C to 30°C (36°F to 86°F) and use within 8 hours. Do not mix other medications into infusion solution.

Administration

Activase®: Acute MI: Accelerated infusion:

Bolus dose may be prepared by one of three methods:

1) removal of 15 mL reconstituted (1 mg/mL) solution from vial
2) removal of 15 mL from a port on the infusion line after priming
3) programming an infusion pump to deliver a 15 mL bolus at the initiation of infusion

Remaining dose may be administered as follows:

50 mg vial: Either PVC bag or glass vial and infusion set

100 mg vial: Insert spike end of the infusion set through the same puncture site created by transfer device and infuse from vial

If further dilution is desired, may be diluted in equal volume of 0.9% sodium chloride or D_5W to yield a final concentration of 0.5 mg/mL AD

Cathflo® Activase®: Intracatheter: Instill dose into occluded catheter. Do not force solution into catheter. After a 30-minute dwell time, assess catheter function by attempting to aspirate blood. If catheter is functional, aspirate 4-5 mL of blood in patients ≥10 kg or 3 mL in patients <10 kg to remove Cathflo® Activase® and residual clots. Gently irrigate the catheter with NS. If catheter remains nonfunctional, let Cathflo® Activase® dwell for another 90 minutes (total dwell time: 120 minutes) and reassess function. If catheter function is not restored, a second dose may be instilled.

Monitoring Parameters

When using for central venous catheter clearance: Assess catheter function by attempting to aspirate blood.

When using for management of acute myocardial infarction: Assess for evidence of cardiac reperfusion through resolution of chest pain, resolution of baseline ECG changes, preserved left ventricular function, cardiac enzyme washout phenomenon, and/or the appearance of reperfusion arrhythmias; assess for bleeding potential through clinical evidence of GI bleeding, hematuria, gingival bleeding, fibrinogen levels, fibrinogen degradation products, prothrombin times, and partial thromboplastin times.

Reference Range

Not routinely measured; literature supports therapeutic levels of 0.52-1.8 mcg/mL

Fibrinogen: 200-400 mg/dL

Activated partial thromboplastin time (aPTT): 22.5-38.7 seconds

Prothrombin time (PT): 10.9-12.2 seconds

Anesthesia and Critical Care Concerns/Other Considerations The Surgery Versus Thrombolysis for Ischemia of the Lower Extremity (STILE) trial (Ann Surg, 1994) compared surgery to intra-arterial thrombolytic therapy with either urokinase (250,000 units bolus, followed by 4000 units/minute for 4 hours, followed by 2000 units/minute for ≤36 hours) or alteplase (0.05 mg/kg/hour for ≤12 hours) in patients with acute (<14 days) or chronic peripheral arterial occlusive disease (PAOD). Patients with acute PAOD who received either fibrinolytic treatment had a shorter hospital stay and an improved amputation-free survival rate. There was no difference between alteplase or urokinase with regard to efficacy or bleeding events. A group from Stanford University recently did a retrospective comparison evaluating efficacy, safety, and cost of low-dose alteplase (<2 mg/hour) and subtherapeutic heparin to urokinase and therapeutic heparin for the treatment of PAOD or DVT (Sugimoto K, 2003). Efficacy was similar for both groups. The average dose of alteplase was 0.86 mg/hour and the dose of urokinase was 2250 units/minute. Alteplase infusions were shorter and less expensive than urokinase.

Pregnancy Risk Factor C

(Continued)

Alteplase *(Continued)*

Contraindications Hypersensitivity to alteplase or any component of the formulation

Treatment of acute MI or PE: Active internal bleeding; history of CVA; recent intracranial or intraspinal surgery or trauma; intracranial neoplasm; arteriovenous malformation or aneurysm; known bleeding diathesis; severe uncontrolled hypertension

Treatment of acute ischemic stroke: Evidence of intracranial hemorrhage or suspicion of subarachnoid hemorrhage on pretreatment evaluation; recent (within 3 months) intracranial or intraspinal surgery; prolonged external cardiac massage; suspected aortic dissection; serious head trauma or previous stroke; history of intracranial hemorrhage; uncontrolled hypertension at time of treatment (eg, >185 mm Hg systolic or >110 mm Hg diastolic); seizure at the onset of stroke; active internal bleeding; intracranial neoplasm; arteriovenous malformation or aneurysm; known bleeding diathesis including but not limited to: current use of anticoagulants or an INR >1.7, administration of heparin within 48 hours preceding the onset of stroke and an elevated aPTT at presentation, platelet count <100,000/mm^3.

Other exclusion criteria (NINDS recombinant tPA study): Stroke or serious head injury within 3 months, major surgery or serious trauma within 2 weeks, GI or urinary tract hemorrhage within 3 weeks, aggressive treatment required to lower blood pressure, glucose level <50 mg/dL or >400 mg/dL, arterial puncture at a noncompressible site or lumbar puncture within 1 week, clinical presentation suggesting post-MI pericarditis, pregnancy, breast-feeding.

Warnings/Precautions Concurrent heparin anticoagulation may contribute to bleeding. Monitor all potential bleeding sites. Doses >150 mg are associated with increased risk of intracranial hemorrhage. Intramuscular injections and nonessential handling of the patient should be avoided. Venipunctures should be performed carefully and only when necessary. If arterial puncture is necessary, use an upper extremity vessel that can be manually compressed. If serious bleeding occurs, the infusion of alteplase and heparin should be stopped.

For the following conditions, the risk of bleeding is higher with use of thrombolytics and should be weighed against the benefits of therapy: Recent major surgery (eg, CABG, obstetrical delivery, organ biopsy, previous puncture of noncompressible vessels), cerebrovascular disease, recent gastrointestinal or genitourinary bleeding, recent trauma, hypertension (systolic BP >175 mm Hg and/or diastolic BP >110 mm Hg), high likelihood of left heart thrombus (eg, mitral stenosis with atrial fibrillation), acute pericarditis, subacute bacterial endocarditis, hemostatic defects including ones caused by severe renal or hepatic dysfunction, significant hepatic dysfunction, pregnancy, diabetic hemorrhagic retinopathy or other hemorrhagic ophthalmic conditions, septic thrombophlebitis or occluded AV cannula at seriously infected site, advanced age (eg, >75 years), patients receiving oral anticoagulants, any other condition in which bleeding constitutes a significant hazard or would be particularly difficult to manage because of location.

Coronary thrombolysis may result in reperfusion arrhythmias. Treatment of patients with acute ischemic stroke more than 3 hours after symptom onset is not recommended Treatment of patients with minor neurological deficit or with rapidly improving symptoms is not recommended.

Cathflo® Activase®: When used to restore catheter function, use Cathflo® cautiously in those patients with known or suspected catheter infections. Evaluate catheter for other causes of dysfunction before use. Avoid excessive pressure when instilling into catheter.

Adverse Reactions As with all drugs which may affect hemostasis, bleeding is the major adverse effect associated with alteplase. Hemorrhage may occur at virtually any site. Risk is dependent on multiple variables, including the dosage administered, concurrent use of multiple agents which alter hemostasis, and patient predisposition. Rapid lysis of coronary artery thrombi by thrombolytic agents may be associated with reperfusion-related atrial and/or ventricular arrhythmia. **Note:** Lowest rate of bleeding complications expected with dose used to restore catheter function.

1% to 10%:
- Cardiovascular: Hypotension
- Central nervous system: Fever
- Dermatologic: Bruising (1%)

Gastrointestinal: GI hemorrhage (5%), nausea, vomiting
Genitourinary: GU hemorrhage (4%)
Hematologic: Bleeding (0.5% major, 7% minor: GUSTO trial)
Local: Bleeding at catheter puncture site (15.3%, accelerated administration)

<1% (Limited to important or life-threatening): Allergic reactions: Anaphylaxis, anaphylactoid reactions, laryngeal edema, rash, and urticaria (<0.02%); epistaxis; gingival hemorrhage; intracranial hemorrhage (0.4% to 0.87% when dose is ≤100 mg); pericardial hemorrhage; retroperitoneal hemorrhage

Additional cardiovascular events associated **with use in MI:** AV block, cardiogenic shock, heart failure, cardiac arrest, recurrent ischemia/infarction, myocardial rupture, electromechanical dissociation, pericardial effusion, pericarditis, mitral regurgitation, cardiac tamponade, thromboembolism, pulmonary edema, asystole, ventricular tachycardia, bradycardia, ruptured intracranial AV malformation, seizure, hemorrhagic bursitis, cholesterol crystal embolization

Additional events associated **with use in pulmonary embolism:** Pulmonary re-embolization, pulmonary edema, pleural effusion, thromboembolism

Additional events associated **with use in stroke:** Cerebral edema, cerebral herniation, seizure, new ischemic stroke

Overdosage/Toxicology Symptoms of overdose include increased incidence of intracranial bleeding.

Drug Interactions

Aminocaproic acid (antifibrinolytic agent) may decrease effectiveness.

Drugs which affect platelet function (eg, NSAIDs, dipyridamole, ticlopidine, clopidogrel, IIb/IIIa antagonists) may potentiate the risk of hemorrhage; use with caution.

Heparin and aspirin: Use with aspirin and heparin may increase the risk of bleeding. However, aspirin and heparin were used concomitantly with alteplase in many patients in myocardial infarction or pulmonary embolism trials. This combination was prohibited in the NINDS tPA stroke trial.

Nitroglycerin may increase the hepatic clearance of alteplase, potentially reducing lytic activity (limited clinical information).

Warfarin or oral anticoagulants: Risk of bleeding may be increased during concurrent therapy.

Ethanol/Nutrition/Herb Interactions Herb/Nutraceutical: Avoid cat's claw, dong quai, evening primrose, feverfew, red clover, horse chestnut, garlic, green tea, ginseng, ginkgo (all have additional antiplatelet activity).

Test Interactions Altered results of coagulation and fibrinolytic agents

Dosage Forms

Injection, powder for reconstitution, recombinant:

Activase®: 50 mg [29 million int. units; contains polysorbate 80; packaged with diluent]; 100 mg [58 million int. units; contains polysorbate 80; packaged with diluent and transfer device]

Cathflo® Activase®: 2 mg [contains polysorbate 80]

References

Albers GW, Bates VE, Clark WM, et al, "Intravenous Tissue-Type Plasminogen Activator for Treatment of Acute Stroke: The Standard Treatment With Alteplase to Reverse Stroke (STARS) Study," *JAMA*, 2000, 283(9):1145-50.

"NINDS tPA Stroke Study Group. Generalized Efficacy for Acute Stroke: Subgroup Analysis of the NINDS tPA Stroke Study Group," *Stroke*, 1997, 28(11):2119-25.

Ouriel K, "Current Status of Thrombolysis for Peripheral Arterial Occlusive Disease," *Ann Vasc Surg*, 2002, 16(6):797-804.

Ponec D, Irwin D, Haire WD, et al, "Recombinant Tissue Plasminogen Activator (Alteplase) for Restoration of Flow in Occluded Central Venous Access Devices: A Double-Blind Placebo-Controlled Trial - The Cardiovascular Thrombolytic to Open Occluded Lines (COOL) Efficacy Trial," *J Vasc Interv Radiol*, 2001, 12(8):951-5.

Semba CP, Murphy TP, Bakal CW, et al, "Thrombolytic Therapy With Use of Alteplase (rtPA) in Peripheral Arterial Occlusive Disease: Review of the Clinical Literature. The Advisory Panel," *J Vasc Interv Radiol*, 2000, 11(2 Pt 1):149-61.

Sugimoto K, Hofmann LV, Razavi MK, et al, "The Safety, Efficacy, and Pharmacoeconomics of Low-Dose Alteplase Compared With Urokinase for Catheter-Directed Thrombolysis of Arterial and Venous Occlusions," *J Vasc Surg*, 2003, 37(3):512-7.

"The Seventh ACCP Conference on Antithrombotic and Thrombolytic Therapy: Evidence-Based Guidelines," *Chest*, 2004, 126(3 Suppl):163-703.

The Surgery Versus Thrombolysis for Ischemia of the Lower Extremity Investigators, "Results of a Prospective, Randomised Trial Evaluating Surgery Versus Thrombolysis for Ischemia of the Lower Extremity. The STILE Trial," *Ann Surg*, 1994, 220(3):251-68.

Valji K, "Evolving Strategies for Thrombolytic Therapy of Peripheral Vascular Occlusion," *J Vasc Interv Radiol*, 2000, 11(4):411-20.

Zacharias JM, Weatherston CP, Spewak CR, et al, "Alteplase Versus Urokinase for Occluded Hemodialysis Catheters," *Ann Pharmacother*, 2003, 37(1):27-33.

♦ **Alteplase, Recombinant** *see* Alteplase *on page 72*

- ♦ **Alteplase, Tissue Plasminogen Activator, Recombinant** *see* Alteplase *on page 72*
- ♦ **Alti-Alprazolam (Can)** *see* Alprazolam *on page 65*
- ♦ **Alti-Amiodarone (Can)** *see* Amiodarone *on page 83*
- ♦ **Alti-Azathioprine (Can)** *see* Azathioprine *on page 148*
- ♦ **Alti-Captopril (Can)** *see* Captopril *on page 221*
- ♦ **Alti-Clindamycin (Can)** *see* Clindamycin *on page 304*
- ♦ **Alti-Clonazepam (Can)** *see* Clonazepam *on page 313*
- ♦ **Alti-Desipramine (Can)** *see* Desipramine *on page 359*
- ♦ **Alti-Diltiazem CD (Can)** *see* Diltiazem *on page 394*
- ♦ **Alti-Divalproex (Can)** *see* Valproic Acid and Derivatives *on page 1329*
- ♦ **Alti-Doxazosin (Can)** *see* Doxazosin *on page 420*
- ♦ **Alti-Flunisolide (Can)** *see* Flunisolide *on page 537*
- ♦ **Alti-Fluoxetine (Can)** *see* Fluoxetine *on page 539*
- ♦ **Alti-Flurbiprofen (Can)** *see* Flurbiprofen *on page 550*
- ♦ **Alti-Ipratropium (Can)** *see* Ipratropium *on page 698*
- ♦ **Alti-Metformin (Can)** *see* Metformin *on page 810*
- ♦ **Alti-Minocycline (Can)** *see* Minocycline *on page 854*
- ♦ **Alti-Nadolol (Can)** *see* Nadolol *on page 886*
- ♦ **Alti-Nortriptyline (Can)** *see* Nortriptyline *on page 938*
- ♦ **Alti-Ranitidine (Can)** *see* Ranitidine *on page 1105*
- ♦ **Alti-Salbutamol (Can)** *see* Albuterol *on page 50*
- ♦ **Alti-Sotalol (Can)** *see* Sotalol *on page 1198*
- ♦ **Alti-Terazosin (Can)** *see* Terazosin *on page 1243*
- ♦ **Alti-Ticlopidine (Can)** *see* Ticlopidine *on page 1266*
- ♦ **Alti-Timolol (Can)** *see* Timolol *on page 1268*
- ♦ **Alti-Trazodone (Can)** *see* Trazodone *on page 1306*
- ♦ **Alti-Verapamil (Can)** *see* Verapamil *on page 1352*
- ♦ **Altoprev™** *see* Lovastatin *on page 782*

Aluminum Hydroxide and Magnesium Hydroxide

(a LOO mi num hye DROKS ide & mag NEE zhum hye DROK side)

Medication Safety Issues

Sound-alike/look-alike issues:

Maalox® may be confused with Maox®, Monodox®

U.S. Brand Names Alamag [OTC]; Rulox [OTC]; Rulox No. 1 [DSC]

Canadian Brand Names Diovol®; Diovol® Ex; Gelusil® Extra Strength; Mylanta™

Synonyms Magnesium Hydroxide and Aluminum Hydroxide

Pharmacologic Category Antacid

Generic Available Yes

Use Antacid, hyperphosphatemia in renal failure

Dosage Oral: 5-10 mL 4-6 times/day, between meals and at bedtime; may be used every hour for severe symptoms

Pregnancy Risk Factor C

Adverse Reactions

>10%: Gastrointestinal: Constipation, chalky taste, stomach cramps, fecal impaction

1% to 10%: Gastrointestinal: Nausea, vomiting, discoloration of feces (white speckles)

<1% (Limited to important or life-threatening): Hypomagnesemia, hypophosphatemia

Drug Interactions Decreased effect: Tetracyclines, digoxin, indomethacin, iron salts, isoniazid, allopurinol, benzodiazepines, corticosteroids, penicillamine, phenothiazines, ranitidine, ketoconazole, itraconazole

Dietary Considerations Should be taken 1-3 hours after meals.

Dosage Forms [DSC] = Discontinued product

Suspension: Aluminum hydroxide 225 mg and magnesium hydroxide 200 mg per 5 mL (360 mL)

Alamag, Rulox: Aluminum hydroxide 225 mg and magnesium hydroxide 200 mg per 5 mL (360 mL)

Tablet, chewable:

Alamag: Aluminum hydroxide 300 mg and magnesium hydroxide 150 mg

Rulox No. 1: Aluminum hydroxide 200 mg and magnesium hydroxide 200 mg [DSC]

- **Aluminum Sucrose Sulfate, Basic** *see* Sucralfate *on page 1212*
- **Alupent®** *see* Metaproterenol *on page 808*

Amantadine (a MAN ta deen)

Medication Safety Issues
Sound-alike/look-alike issues:
Amantadine may be confused with ranitidine, rimantadine
Symmetrel® may be confused with Synthroid®

U.S. Brand Names Symmetrel®

Canadian Brand Names Endantadine®; PMS-Amantadine; Symmetrel®

Synonyms Adamantanamine Hydrochloride; Amantadine Hydrochloride

Pharmacologic Category Anti-Parkinson's Agent, Dopamine Agonist; Antiviral Agent, Adamantane

Generic Available Yes

Use Prophylaxis and treatment of influenza A viral infection; treatment of parkinsonism; treatment of drug-induced extrapyramidal symptoms

Mechanism of Action As an antiviral, blocks the uncoating of influenza A virus preventing penetration of virus into host; antiparkinsonian activity may be due to its blocking the reuptake of dopamine into presynaptic neurons or by increasing dopamine release from presynaptic fibers

Pharmacodynamics/Kinetics
Onset of action: Antidyskinetic: Within 48 hours
Absorption: Well absorbed
Distribution: V_d: Normal: 1.5-6.1 L/kg; Renal failure: 5.1 ± 0.2 L/kg; in saliva, tear film, and nasal secretions; in animals, tissue (especially lung) concentrations higher than serum concentrations; crosses blood-brain barrier
Protein binding: Normal renal function: ~67%; Hemodialysis: ~59%
Metabolism: Not appreciable; small amounts of an acetyl metabolite identified
Bioavailability: 86% to 90%
Half-life elimination: Normal renal function: 16 ± 6 hours (9-31 hours); End-stage renal disease: 7-10 days
Excretion: Urine (80% to 90% unchanged) by glomerular filtration and tubular secretion
Total clearance: 2.5-10.5 L/hour

Dosage Oral:
Children:
Influenza A treatment:
1-9 years: 5 mg/kg/day in 2 divided doses (manufacturers range: 4.4-8.8 mg/kg/day); maximum dose: 150 mg/day
≥10 years and <40 kg: 5 mg/kg/day; maximum dose: 150 mg/day
≥10 years and ≥40 kg: 100 mg twice daily
Note: Initiate within 24-48 hours after onset of symptoms; discontinue as soon as possible based on clinical response (generally within 3-5 days or within 24-48 hours after symptoms disappear)
Influenza A prophylaxis: Refer to "Influenza A treatment" dosing
Note: Continue treatment throughout the peak influenza activity in the community or throughout the entire influenza season in patients who cannot be vaccinated. Development of immunity following vaccination takes ~2 weeks; amantadine therapy should be considered for high-risk patients from the time of vaccination until immunity has developed. For children <9 years receiving influenza vaccine for the first time, amantadine prophylaxis should continue for 6 weeks (4 weeks after the first dose and 2 weeks after the second dose).
Adults:
Drug-induced extrapyramidal symptoms: 100 mg twice daily; may increase to 300-400 mg/day, if needed
Parkinson's disease or Creutzfeldt-Jakob disease (unlabeled use): 100 mg twice daily as sole therapy; may increase to 400 mg/day if needed with close monitoring; initial dose: 100 mg/day if with other serious illness or with high doses of other anti-Parkinson drugs
Influenza A viral infection: 100 mg twice daily; initiate within 24-48 hours after onset of symptoms; discontinue as soon as possible based on clinical

(Continued)

Amantadine *(Continued)*

response (generally within 3-5 days or within 24-48 hours after symptoms disappear)

Influenza A prophylaxis: 100 mg twice daily

Note: Continue treatment throughout the peak influenza activity in the community or throughout the entire influenza season in patients who cannot be vaccinated. Development of immunity following vaccination takes ~2 weeks; amantadine therapy should be considered for high-risk patients from the time of vaccination until immunity has developed.

Elderly: Adjust dose based on renal function; some patients tolerate the drug better when it is given in 2 divided daily doses (to avoid adverse neurologic reactions).

Influenza A prophylaxis or treatment: ≤100 mg/day in patients ≥65 years

Dosing interval in renal impairment:

Cl_{cr} 30-50 mL/minute: Administer 200 mg on day 1, then 100 mg/day

Cl_{cr} 15-29 mL/minute: Administer 200 mg on day 1, then 100 mg on alternate days

Cl_{cr} <15 mL/minute: Administer 200 mg every 7 days

Hemodialysis: Administer 200 mg every 7 days

Peritoneal dialysis: No supplemental dose is needed

Continuous arteriovenous or venous-venous hemofiltration: No supplemental dose is needed

Stability Store at 15°C to 30°C (59°F to 86°F); protect from freezing.

Monitoring Parameters Renal function, Parkinson's symptoms, mental status, influenza symptoms, blood pressure

Pregnancy Risk Factor C

Contraindications Hypersensitivity to amantadine, rimantadine, or any component of the formulation

Warnings/Precautions Use with caution in patients with liver disease, history of recurrent and eczematoid dermatitis, uncontrolled psychosis or severe psychoneurosis, seizures, and in those receiving CNS stimulant drugs; reduce dose in renal disease. When treating Parkinson's disease, do not discontinue abruptly. In many patients, the therapeutic benefits of amantadine are limited to a few months. Elderly patients may be more susceptible to CNS effects (using 2 divided daily doses may minimize this effect). Has been associated with neuroleptic malignant syndrome (associated with dose reduction or abrupt discontinuation). Has not been shown to prevent bacterial infection or complications when used as prophylaxis or treatment of influenza A. Use with caution in patients with CHF, peripheral edema, or orthostatic hypotension. Avoid in angle closure glaucoma.

Adverse Reactions

1% to 10%:

Cardiovascular: Orthostatic hypotension, peripheral edema

Central nervous system: Insomnia, depression, anxiety, irritability, dizziness, hallucinations, ataxia, headache, somnolence, nervousness, dream abnormality, agitation, fatigue, confusion

Dermatologic: Livedo reticularis

Gastrointestinal: Nausea, anorexia, constipation, diarrhea, xerostomia

Respiratory: Dry nose

<1% (Limited to important or life-threatening): Amnesia, CHF, convulsions, dyspnea, eczematoid dermatitis, euphoria, hyperkinesis, hypertension, leukopenia, libido decreased, neutropenia, oculogyric episodes, photosensitivity, psychosis, rash, slurred speech, urinary retention, visual disturbances, vomiting, weakness; withdrawal reactions may include delirium, hallucinations, and psychosis

Overdosage/Toxicology Symptoms of overdose include nausea, vomiting, slurred speech, blurred vision, lethargy, hallucinations, seizures, and myoclonic jerking. Acute toxicity may be primarily due to anticholinergic effects. The minimum lethal dose may be as low as 1 g. Treatment should be directed at reducing CNS stimulation, controlling seizures, and maintaining cardiovascular function.

Drug Interactions

Anticholinergics may potentiate CNS side effects of amantadine; monitor for altered response. Includes benztropine and trihexyphenidyl, as well as agents with anticholinergic activity such as quinidine, tricyclics, and antihistamines.

Thiazide diuretics: Hydrochlorothiazide has been reported to increase the potential for toxicity with amantadine (limited documentation); monitor response.

Triamterene: Has been reported to increase the potential for toxicity with amantadine (limited documentation); monitor response.
Trimethoprim: Has been reported to increase the potential for toxicity with amantadine (limited documentation); monitor for acute confusion.

Ethanol/Nutrition/Herb Interactions Ethanol: Avoid ethanol (may increase CNS adverse effects).

Dosage Forms [DSC] = Discontinued product
Capsule, as hydrochloride: 100 mg
Syrup, as hydrochloride: 50 mg/5 mL (480 mL)
Symmetrel®: 50 mg/5 mL (480 mL) [raspberry flavor] [DSC]
Tablet, as hydrochloride (Symmetrel®): 100 mg

- **Amantadine Hydrochloride** *see* Amantadine *on page 77*
- **Ambien®** *see* Zolpidem *on page 1382*
- **Ambien CR™** *see* Zolpidem *on page 1382*
- **AmBisome®** *see* Amphotericin B (Liposomal) *on page 100*
- **Amerge®** *see* Naratriptan *on page 903*
- **A-Methapred** *see* MethylPREDNISolone *on page 830*
- **Amethocaine Hydrochloride** *see* Tetracaine *on page 1248*
- **Amethopterin** *see* Methotrexate *on page 821*
- **Ametop™ (Can)** *see* Tetracaine *on page 1248*
- **Amicar®** *see* Aminocaproic Acid *on page 81*
- **Amidate®** *see* Etomidate *on page 500*
- **Amigesic®** *see* Salsalate *on page 1147*

Amikacin (am i KAY sin)

Medication Safety Issues
Sound-alike/look-alike issues:
Amikacin may be confused with Amicar®, anakinra
Amikin® may be confused with Amicar®

U.S. Brand Names Amikin®

Canadian Brand Names Amikacin Sulfate Injection, USP; Amikin®

Synonyms Amikacin Sulfate

Pharmacologic Category Antibiotic, Aminoglycoside

Generic Available Yes

Use Treatment of serious infections due to organisms resistant to gentamicin and tobramycin, including *Pseudomonas*, *Proteus*, *Serratia*, and other gram-negative bacilli (bone infections, respiratory tract infections, endocarditis, and septicemia); documented infection of mycobacterial organisms susceptible to amikacin

Mechanism of Action Inhibits protein synthesis in susceptible bacteria by binding to 30S ribosomal subunits

Pharmacodynamics/Kinetics
Absorption:
I.M.: Rapid
Oral: Poorly absorbed
Distribution: Primarily into extracellular fluid (highly hydrophilic); penetrates blood-brain barrier when meninges inflamed; crosses placenta
Relative diffusion of antimicrobial agents from blood into CSF: Good only with inflammation (exceeds usual MICs)
CSF:blood level ratio: Normal meninges: 10% to 20%; Inflamed meninges: 15% to 24%
Half-life elimination (renal function and age dependent):
Infants: Low birth weight (1-3 days): 7-9 hours; Full-term >7 days: 4-5 hours
Children: 1.6-2.5 hours
Adults: Normal renal function: 1.4-2.3 hours; Anuria/end-stage renal disease: 28-86 hours
Time to peak, serum: I.M.: 45-120 minutes
Excretion: Urine (94% to 98%)

Dosage Note: Individualization is critical because of the low therapeutic index
Use of ideal body weight (IBW) for determining the mg/kg/dose appears to be more accurate than dosing on the basis of total body weight (TBW)
In morbid obesity, dosage requirement may best be estimated using a dosing weight of IBW + 0.4 (TBW - IBW)
(Continued)

Amikacin *(Continued)*

Initial and periodic peak and trough plasma drug levels should be determined, particularly in critically-ill patients with serious infections or in disease states known to significantly alter aminoglycoside pharmacokinetics (eg, cystic fibrosis, burns, or major surgery)

Usual dosage range:

Infants and Children: I.M., I.V.: 5-7.5 mg/kg/dose every 8 hours

Adults: I.M., I.V.: 5-7.5 mg/kg/dose every 8 hours

Note: Some clinicians suggest a daily dose of 15-20 mg/kg for all patients with normal renal function. This dose is at least as efficacious with similar, if not less, toxicity than conventional dosing.

Indication-specific dosing:

Adults: I.V.:

Hospital-acquired pneumonia (HAP): 20 mg/kg/day with antipseudomonal beta-lactam or carbapenem (American Thoracic Society/ATS guidelines)

Meningitis *(Pseudomonas aeruginosa):* 5 mg/kg every 8 hours (administered with another bacteriocidal drug)

Mycobacterium fortuitum, M. chelonae, or M. abscessus: 10-15 mg/kg twice daily for at least 2 weeks with high dose cefoxitin

Dosing interval in renal impairment: Some patients may require larger or more frequent doses if serum levels document the need (ie, cystic fibrosis or febrile granulocytopenic patients)

Cl_{cr} ≥60 mL/minute: Administer every 8 hours

Cl_{cr} 40-60 mL/minute: Administer every 12 hours

Cl_{cr} 20-40 mL/minute: Administer every 24 hours

Cl_{cr} <20 mL/minute: Loading dose, then monitor levels

Hemodialysis: Dialyzable (50% to 100%); administer dose postdialysis or administer ²/₃ normal dose as a supplemental dose postdialysis and follow levels

Peritoneal dialysis: Dose as Cl_{cr} <20 mL/minute: Follow levels

Continuous arteriovenous or venovenous hemodiafiltration effects: Dose as for Cl_{cr} 10-40 mL/minute and follow levels

Stability Stable for 24 hours at room temperature and 2 days at refrigeration when mixed in D_5W, $D_5\frac{1}{4}NS$, $D_5\frac{1}{2}NS$, NS, LR

Administration Administer around-the-clock to promote less variation in peak and trough serum levels. Do not mix with other drugs, administer separately.

I.M.: Administer I.M. injection in large muscle mass.

I.V.: Infuse over 30-60 minutes.

Some penicillins (eg, carbenicillin, ticarcillin, and piperacillin) have been shown to inactivate *in vitro.* This has been observed to a greater extent with tobramycin and gentamicin, while amikacin has shown greater stability against inactivation. Concurrent use of these agents may pose a risk of reduced antibacterial efficacy *in vivo*, particularly in the setting of profound renal impairment. However, definitive clinical evidence is lacking. If combination penicillin/aminoglycoside therapy is desired in a patient with renal dysfunction, separation of doses (if feasible), and routine monitoring of aminoglycoside levels, CBC, and clinical response should be considered.

Monitoring Parameters Urinalysis, BUN, serum creatinine, appropriately timed peak and trough concentrations, vital signs, temperature, weight, I & O, hearing parameters

Some penicillin derivatives may accelerate the degradation of aminoglycosides*in vitro.* This may be clinically-significant for certain penicillin (ticarcillin, piperacillin, carbenicillin) and aminoglycoside (gentamicin, tobramycin) combination therapy in patients with significant renal impairment. Close monitoring of aminoglycoside levels is warranted.

Reference Range

Sample size: 0.5-2 mL blood (red top tube) or 0.1-1 mL serum (separated)

Therapeutic levels:

Peak:

Life-threatening infections: 25-30 mcg/mL

Serious infections: 20-25 mcg/mL

Urinary tract infections: 15-20 mcg/mL

Trough:

Serious infections: 1-4 mcg/mL

Life-threatening infections: 4-8 mcg/mL

The American Thoracic Society (ATS) recommends trough levels of <4-5 mcg/mL for patients with hospital-acquired pneumonia.

Toxic concentration: Peak: >35 mcg/mL; Trough: >10 mcg/mL

Timing of serum samples: Draw peak 30 minutes after completion of 30-minute infusion or at 1 hour following initiation of infusion or I.M. injection; draw trough within 30 minutes prior to next dose

Pregnancy Risk Factor D

Contraindications Hypersensitivity to amikacin sulfate or any component of the formulation; cross-sensitivity may exist with other aminoglycosides

Warnings/Precautions **[U.S. Boxed Warning]: Amikacin may cause neurotoxicity, nephrotoxicity, and/or neuromuscular blockade and respiratory paralysis;** usual risk factors include prexisiting renal impairment, concomitant neuro-/nephrotoxic medications, advanced age and dehydration. Dose and/or frequency of administration must be monitored and modified in patients with renal impairment. Drug should be discontinued if signs of ototoxicity, nephrotoxicity, or hypersensitivity occur. Ototoxicity is proportional to the amount of drug given and the duration of treatment. Tinnitus or vertigo may be indications of vestibular injury and impending bilateral irreversible damage. Renal damage is usually reversible.

Adverse Reactions

1% to 10%:

- Central nervous system: Neurotoxicity
- Otic: Ototoxicity (auditory), ototoxicity (vestibular)
- Renal: Nephrotoxicity

<1% (Limited to important or life-threatening): Allergic reaction, dyspnea, eosinophilia

Overdosage/Toxicology Symptoms of overdose include ototoxicity, nephrotoxicity, and neuromuscular toxicity. Treatment of choice, following a single acute overdose, appears to be maintenance of urine output of at least 3 mL/kg/hour during the acute treatment phase. Dialysis is of questionable value in enhancing aminoglycoside elimination. If required, hemodialysis is preferred over peritoneal dialysis in patients with normal renal function.

Drug Interactions

Decreased effect of aminoglycoside: High concentrations of penicillins and/or cephalosporins (*in vitro* data)

Increased toxicity of aminoglycoside: Indomethacin I.V., amphotericin, loop diuretics, vancomycin, enflurane, methoxyflurane; increased effect of neuromuscular-blocking agents and polypeptide antibiotics with administration of aminoglycosides

Test Interactions Some penicillin derivatives may accelerate the degradation of aminoglycosides *in vitro*, leading to a potential underestimation of aminoglycoside serum concentration.

Dietary Considerations Sodium content of 1 g: 29.9 mg (1.3 mEq)

Dosage Forms [DSC] = Discontinued product

Injection, solution, as sulfate: 50 mg/mL (2 mL, 4 mL); 62.5 mg/mL (8 mL) [DSC]; 250 mg/mL (2 mL, 4 mL)

Amikin®: 50 mg/mL (2 mL); 250 mg/mL (2 mL, 4 mL) [contains metabisulfite]

References

American Thoracic Society and Infectious Diseases Society of America, "Guidelines for the Management of Adults With Hospital-Acquired, Ventilator-Associated, and Healthcare-Associated Pneumonia," *Am J Respir Crit Care Med*, 2005, 171(4):388-416.

Tunkel AR, Hartman BJ, Kaplan SL, et al, "Practice Guidelines for the Management of Bacterial Meningitis," *Clin Infect Dis*, 2004, 39(9):1267-84.

♦ **Amikacin Sulfate** *see* Amikacin *on page 79*

♦ **Amikacin Sulfate Injection, USP (Can)** *see* Amikacin *on page 79*

♦ **Amikin®** *see* Amikacin *on page 79*

♦ **Aminobenzylpenicillin** *see* Ampicillin *on page 104*

Aminocaproic Acid (a mee noe ka PROE ik AS id)

Medication Safety Issues

Sound-alike/look-alike issues:

Amicar® may be confused with amikacin, Amikin®, Omacor®

(Continued)

Aminocaproic Acid *(Continued)*

U.S. Brand Names Amicar®

Synonyms Epsilon Aminocaproic Acid

Pharmacologic Category Hemostatic Agent

Generic Available Yes

Use Treatment of excessive bleeding from fibrinolysis

Unlabeled/Investigational Use Treatment of traumatic hyphema; control bleeding in thrombocytopenia; control oral bleeding in congenital and acquired coagulation disorders

Mechanism of Action Competitively inhibits activation of plasminogen to plasmin, also, a lesser antiplasmin effect

Pharmacodynamics/Kinetics

Onset of action: ~1-72 hours

Distribution: Widely through intravascular and extravascular compartments

V_d: Oral: 23 L, I.V.: 30 L

Metabolism: Minimally hepatic

Half-life elimination: 2 hours

Time to peak: Oral: Within 2 hours

Excretion: Urine (65% as unchanged drug, 11% as metabolite)

Dosage

Acute bleeding syndrome:

Children (unlabeled use): Oral, I.V.: 100-200 mg/kg during the first hour, followed by continuous infusion at 33.3 mg/kg/hour or 100 mg/kg (oral or I.V.) every 6 hours

Adults: Oral, I.V.: 4-5 g during the first hour, followed by 1 g/hour for 8 hours or until bleeding controlled (maximum daily dose: 30 g)

Control bleeding in thrombocytopenia (unlabeled use): Adults:

Initial: I.V.: 0.1 g/kg over 30-60 minutes

Maintenance: Oral: 1-3 g every 6 hours

Control oral bleeding in congenital and acquired coagulation disorder (unlabeled use): Adults: Oral: 50-60 mg/kg every 4 hours

Traumatic hyphema (unlabeled use): Children and Adults: Oral: 100 mg/kg/dose every 4 hours (maximum daily dose: 30 g)

Dosing adjustment in renal impairment: May accumulate in patients with decreased renal function.

Stability Store at 15°C to 30°C (59°F to 86°F). Dilute I.V. solution (1 g/50 mL of diluent) with D_5W, 0.9% sodium chloride, or lactated Ringer's.

Administration I.V.: May be administered over 30-60 minutes or by continuous infusion; rapid I.V. injection (IVP) should be avoided due to possible hypotension, bradycardia, and arrhythmia.

Monitoring Parameters Fibrinogen, fibrin split products, creatine phosphokinase (with long-term therapy)

Reference Range Therapeutic concentration: >130 mcg/mL (concentration necessary for inhibition of fibrinolysis)

Pregnancy Risk Factor C

Contraindications Hypersensitivity to aminocaproic acid or any component of the formulation; disseminated intravascular coagulation (without heparin); evidence of an intravascular clotting process

Warnings/Precautions Avoid rapid I.V. administration; may induce hypotension, bradycardia, or arrhythmia. Aminocaproic acid may accumulate in patients with decreased renal function. Intrarenal obstruction may occur secondary to glomerular capillary thrombosis or clots in the renal pelvis and ureters. Do not use in hematuria of upper urinary tract origin unless possible benefits outweigh risks. Use with caution in patients with cardiac, renal, or hepatic disease. Do not administer without a definite diagnosis of laboratory findings indicative of hyperfibrinolysis. Inhibition of fibrinolysis may promote clotting or thrombosis; more likely due to the presence of DIC. Subsequently, use with great caution in patients with, or at risk for, veno-occlusive disease of the liver. Benzyl alcohol is used as a preservative in the injection, therefore, these products should not be used in the neonate. Do not administer with factor IX complex concentrates or anti-inhibitor coagulant complexes.

Adverse Reactions Frequency not defined.

Cardiovascular: Arrhythmia, bradycardia, hypotension, peripheral ischemia, syncope, thrombosis

Central nervous system: Confusion, delirium, dizziness, fatigue, hallucinations, headache, intracranial hypertension, malaise, seizure, stroke
Dermatologic: Rash, pruritus
Gastrointestinal: Abdominal pain, anorexia, cramps, diarrhea, GI irritation, nausea
Genitourinary: Dry ejaculation
Hematologic: Agranulocytosis, bleeding time increased, leukopenia, thrombocytopenia
Neuromuscular & skeletal: CPK increased, myalgia, myositis, myopathy, rhabdomyolysis (rare), weakness
Ophthalmic: Watery eyes, vision decreased
Otic: Tinnitus
Renal: Failure (rare), myoglobinuria (rare)
Respiratory: Dyspnea, nasal congestion, pulmonary embolism

Overdosage/Toxicology Symptoms of overdose include acute renal failure, delirium, diarrhea, hepatic necrosis, nausea, seizures, transient hypotension, and thromboembolism. Aminocaproic acid may be removed by hemodialysis.

Drug Interactions Increased toxic effect with oral contraceptives, estrogens.

Test Interactions Increased potassium, creatine phosphokinase [CPK] (S)

Dosage Forms
Injection, solution: 250 mg/mL (20 mL)
Amicar®: 250 mg/mL (20 mL) [contains benzyl alcohol]
Solution, oral: 1.25 g/5 mL (240 mL, 480 mL)
Syrup:
Amicar®: 1.25 g/5 mL (480 mL) [raspberry flavor]
Tablet [scored]: 500 mg, 1000 mg
Amicar®: 500 mg, 1000 mg

♦ **Aminoxin® [OTC]** *see* Pyridoxine *on page 1090*

Amiodarone (a MEE oh da rone)

Medication Safety Issues
Sound-alike/look-alike issues:
Amiodarone may be confused with amiloride, amrinone
Cordarone® may be confused with Cardura®, Cordran®

High alert medication: The Institute for Safe Medication Practices (ISMP) includes this medication among its list of drugs which have a heightened risk of causing significant patient harm when used in error.

Related Information
Antiarrhythmic Drugs *on page 1548*
Management of Postoperative Arrhythmias *on page 1451*

U.S. Brand Names Cordarone®; Pacerone®

Canadian Brand Names Alti-Amiodarone; Amiodarone Hydrochloride for Injection®; Apo-Amiodarone®; Cordarone®; Gen-Amiodarone; Novo-Amiodarone; Rhoxal-amiodarone; Sandoz-Amiodarone

Synonyms Amiodarone Hydrochloride

Pharmacologic Category Antiarrhythmic Agent, Class III

Restrictions An FDA-approved medication guide is available at www.fda.gov/cder/Offices/ODS/labeling.htm; distribute to each patient to whom this medication is dispensed.

Generic Available Yes

Use Management of life-threatening recurrent ventricular fibrillation (VF) or hemodynamically-unstable ventricular tachycardia (VT) refractory to other antiarrhythmic agents or in patients intolerant of other agents used for these conditions

Unlabeled/Investigational Use
Conversion of atrial fibrillation to normal sinus rhythm; maintenance of normal sinus rhythm
Prevention of postoperative atrial fibrillation during cardiothoracic surgery
Paroxysmal supraventricular tachycardia (SVT)
Control of rapid ventricular rate due to accessory pathway conduction in pre-excited atrial arrhythmias [ACLS guidelines]
Cardiac arrest with persistent ventricular tachycardia (VT) or ventricular fibrillation (VF) if defibrillation, CPR, and vasopressor administration have failed [ACLS/PALS guidelines]
Control of hemodynamically-stable VT, polymorphic VT with a normal QT interval, or wide-complex tachycardia of uncertain origin [ACLS/PALS guidelines]
(Continued)

Amiodarone *(Continued)*

Mechanism of Action Class III antiarrhythmic agent which inhibits adrenergic stimulation (alpha- and beta-blocking properties), affects sodium, potassium, and calcium channels, prolongs the action potential and refractory period in myocardial tissue; decreases AV conduction and sinus node function

Pharmacodynamics/Kinetics

Onset of action: Oral: 2 days to 3 weeks; I.V.: May be more rapid

Peak effect: 1 week to 5 months

Duration after discontinuing therapy: 7-50 days

Note: Mean onset of effect and duration after discontinuation may be shorter in children than adults

Distribution: V_d: 66 L/kg (range: 18-148 L/kg); crosses placenta; enters breast milk in concentrations higher than maternal plasma concentrations

Protein binding: 96%

Metabolism: Hepatic via CYP2C8 and 3A4 to active N-desethylamiodarone metabolite; possible enterohepatic recirculation

Bioavailability: Oral: ~50%

Half-life elimination: Terminal: 40-55 days (range: 26-107 days); shorter in children than adults

Excretion: Feces; urine (<1% as unchanged drug)

Dosage Note: Lower loading and maintenance doses are preferable in women and all patients with low body weight.

Oral:

Children: Arrhythmias (unlabeled use):

Loading dose: 10-20 mg/kg/day in 1-2 doses for 4-14 days or until adequate control of arrhythmia or prominent adverse effects occur; alternative loading dose in children <1 year: 600-800 mg/1.73 m^2/day in 1-2 divided doses/day

Maintenance dose: Dose may be reduced to 5 mg/kg/day for several weeks (or 200-400 mg/1.73 m^2/day given once daily); if no recurrence of arrhythmia, dose may be further reduced to 2.5 mg/kg/day; maintenance doses may be given 5-7 days/week

Adults:

Ventricular arrhythmias: 800-1600 mg/day in 1-2 doses for 1-3 weeks, then when adequate arrhythmia control is achieved, decrease to 600-800 mg/day in 1-2 doses for 1 month; maintenance: 400 mg/day. Lower doses are recommended for supraventricular arrhythmias.

Prophylaxis of atrial fibrillation following open heart surgery (unlabeled use): 400 mg twice daily (starting in postop recovery) for up to 7 days. An alternative regimen of amiodarone 600 mg/day for 7 days prior to surgery, followed by 200 mg/day until hospital discharge, has also been shown to decrease the risk of postoperative atrial fibrillation. **Note:** A variety of regimens have been used in clinical trials.

Recurrent atrial fibrillation (unlabeled use): No standard regimen defined; examples of regimens include: Initial: 10 mg/kg/day for 14 days; followed by 300 mg/day for 4 weeks, followed by maintenance dosage of 100-200 mg/day. Other regimens have been described and are used clinically (ie, 400 mg 3 times/day for 5-7 days, then 400 mg/day for 1 month, then 200 mg/day).

I.V.:

Children:

Arrhythmias (unlabeled use, dosing based on limited data): Loading dose: 5 mg/kg over 30 minutes; may repeat up to 3 times if no response. Maintenance dose: 2-20 mg/kg/day (5-15 mcg/kg/minute) by continuous infusion

Note: I.V. administration at low flow rates (potentially associated with use in pediatrics) may result in leaching of plasticizers (DEHP) from intravenous tubing. DEHP may adversely affect male reproductive tract development. Alternative means of dosing and administration (1 mg/kg aliquots) may need to be considered.

Pulseless VF or VT (PALS dosing): 5 mg/kg rapid I.V. bolus or I.O.; repeat up to a maximum dose of 15 mg/kg (300 mg)

Perfusing tachycardias (PALS dosing): Loading dose: 5 mg/kg I.V. over 20-60 minutes or I.O.; may repeat up to maximum dose of 15 mg/kg/day

Adults:

Breakthrough VF or VT: 150 mg supplemental doses in 100 mL D_5W over 10 minutes

Pulseless VF or VT: I.V. push: Initial: 300 mg in 20-30 mL NS or D_5W; if VF or VT recurs, supplemental dose of 150 mg followed by infusion of 1 mg/minute for 6 hours, then 0.5 mg/minute (maximum daily dose: 2.1 g)

Prophylaxis of atrial fibrillation following open heart surgery (unlabeled use): 1000 mg infused over 24 hours (starting at postop recovery) for 2 days has been shown to reduce the risk of postoperative atrial fibrillation. **Note:** A variety of regimens have been used in clinical trials.

Stable VT or SVT (unlabeled use): First 24 hours: 1050 mg according to following regimen

Step 1: 150 mg (100 mL) over first 10 minutes (mix 3 mL in 100 mL D_5W)

Step 2: 360 mg (200 mL) over next 6 hours (mix 18 mL in 500 mL D_5W): 1 mg/minute

Step 3: 540 mg (300 mL) over next 18 hours: 0.5 mg/minute

Note: After the first 24 hours: 0.5 mg/minute utilizing concentration of 1-6 mg/mL

Note: When switching from I.V. to oral therapy, use the following as a guide:

<1-week I.V. infusion: 800-1600 mg/day

1- to 3-week I.V. infusion: 600-800 mg/day

>3-week I.V. infusion: 400 mg/day

Recommendations for conversion to intravenous amiodarone after oral administration: During long-term amiodarone therapy (ie, ≥4 months), the mean plasma-elimination half-life of the active metabolite of amiodarone is 61 days. Replacement therapy may not be necessary in such patients if oral therapy is discontinued for a period <2 weeks, since any changes in serum amiodarone concentrations during this period may **not** be clinically significant.

Elderly: No specific guidelines available. Dose selection should be cautious, at low end of dosage range, and titration should be slower to evaluate response.

Hemodialysis: Not dialyzable (0% to 5%); supplemental dose is not necessary.

Peritoneal dialysis effects: Not dialyzable (0% to 5%); supplemental dose is not necessary.

Dosing adjustment in hepatic impairment: Probably necessary in substantial hepatic impairment. No specific guidelines available.

Stability Store at room temperature; protect from light. When admixed in D_5W to a final concentration of 1-6 mg/mL, the solution is stable at room temperature for 24 hours in polyolefin or glass, or for 2 hours in PVC. Infusions >2 hours must be administered in glass or polyolefin bottles.

Administration

Oral: Administer consistently with regard to meals. Take in divided doses with meals if high daily dose or if GI upset occurs. If GI intolerance occurs with single-dose therapy, use twice daily dosing.

I.V.: Adjust administration rate to urgency (give more slowly when perfusing arrhythmia present). Give I.V. therapy using an infusion pump at a concentration <2 mg/mL. Slow the infusion rate if hypotension or bradycardia develops. Infusions >2 hours must be administered in glass or polyolefin bottles. **Note:** I.V. administration at lower flow rates (potentially associated with use in pediatrics) and higher concentrations than recommended may result in leaching of plasticizers (DEHP) from intravenous tubing. DEHP may adversely affect male reproductive tract development. Alternative means of dosing and administration (1 mg/kg aliquots) may need to be considered. Use only volumetric infusion pump; use of drop counting may lead to under-dosing. Administer through I.V. line with in-line filter.

Monitoring Parameters Blood pressure, heart rate (ECG) and rhythm throughout therapy; assess patient for signs of lethargy, edema of the hands or feet, weight loss, and pulmonary toxicity (baseline pulmonary function tests); liver function tests; monitor serum electrolytes, especially potassium and magnesium. Assess for thyroid dysfunction (thyroid function tests): Amiodarone partially inhibits the peripheral conversion of thyroxine (T_4) to triiodothyronine (T_3); serum T_4 and reverse triiodothyronine (rT_3) concentrations may be increased and serum T_3 may be decreased; most patients remain clinically euthyroid, however, clinical hypothyroidism or hyperthyroidism may occur.

Reference Range Therapeutic: 0.5-2.5 mg/L (SI: 1-4 μmol/L) (parent); desethyl metabolite is active and is present in equal concentration to parent drug

Anesthesia and Critical Care Concerns/Other Considerations

Cardiac Arrest: The ARREST trial was a randomized, placebo-controlled trial evaluating amiodarone's efficacy in patients who had an out-of-hospital cardiac arrest with pulseless ventricular tachycardia or ventricular fibrillation. The primary

(Continued)

Amiodarone *(Continued)*

endpoint was admission to the hospital with a spontaneous perfusing rhythm. Patients were randomized to receive 300 mg of intravenous amiodarone or placebo after being shocked >3 times, intubated, and receiving 1 mg of epinephrine. Ventricular fibrillation was the most common initial arrhythmia (88%). More patients in the amiodarone group were successfully resuscitated (44% amiodarone; 34% placebo; P=0.03) and admitted to the hospital, but mortality was similar in both groups (possibly due to sample size). More recently, the ALIVE trial compared amiodarone to lidocaine in out-of-hospital cardiac arrest victims whose ventricular fibrillation was resistant to three defibrillation attempts in addition to epinephrine and a fourth defibrillation attempt (Dorian, 2002). This was a randomized, double-blind comparison. Other inclusion criteria included ventricular fibrillation unrelated to trauma (or with other arrhythmias that converted to ventricular fibrillation) and recurrent ventricular fibrillation after successful initial defibrillation. The primary endpoint was the number of patients who were admitted to the hospital intensive care unit alive. Three hundred and forty-seven patients were enrolled. The initial amiodarone dose was 5 mg/kg and the lidocaine dose was 1.5 mg/kg. If ventricular fibrillation persisted after another shock, then the study drug could be administered again (amiodarone 2.5 mg/kg, lidocaine 1.5 mg/kg). Significantly more amiodarone patients (~23%) were admitted to the hospital alive than lidocaine patients (12%). The majority (>90%) of patients in the ALIVE trial had ventricular fibrillation as the initial arrhythmia. The authors concluded that intravenous amiodarone is superior to lidocaine in the treatment of shock-resistant, out-of-hospital ventricular fibrillation.

Arrhythmias: In patients with severe left ventricular dysfunction, amiodarone is preferable over other antiarrhythmics.

Adverse Events: Although adverse events are less common with 200 mg/day, amiodarone-induced pulmonary toxicity can occur and the patient must be monitored. Patients may present with very mild, nonspecific signs such as dyspnea on exertion or cough.

Pregnancy Risk Factor D

Contraindications Hypersensitivity to amiodarone, iodine, or any component of the formulation; severe sinus-node dysfunction; second- and third-degree heart block (except in patients with a functioning artificial pacemaker); bradycardia causing syncope (except in patients with a functioning artificial pacemaker); pregnancy

Warnings/Precautions Monitor for pulmonary toxicity, liver toxicity, or exacerbation of the arrhythmia (including torsade de pointes). Use very cautiously and with close monitoring in patients with thyroid or liver disease. May cause hyper- or hypothyroidism. Hyperthyroidism may aggravate or cause breakthrough arrhythmias. Significant heart block or sinus bradycardia can occur. Patients should be hospitalized when amiodarone is initiated. Amiodarone is a potent inhibitor of CYP enzymes and transport proteins (including p-glycoprotein), which may lead to increased serum concentrations/toxicity of a number of medications. Particular caution must be used when a drug with QT_c-prolonging potential relies on metabolism via these enzymes, since the effect of elevated concentrations may be additive with the effect of amiodarone. Carefully assess risk:benefit of coadministration of other drugs which may prolong QT_c interval. Correct electrolyte disturbances, especially hypokalemia or hypomagnesemia, prior to use and throughout therapy.

Pre-existing pulmonary disease does not increase risk of developing pulmonary toxicity, but if pulmonary toxicity develops then the prognosis is worse. Due to complex pharmacokinetics, it is difficult to predict when an arrhythmia or interaction with a subsequent treatment will occur following discontinuation of amiodarone. May cause optic neuropathy and/or optic neuritis, usually resulting in visual impairment. Corneal microdeposits occur in a majority of patients, and may cause visual disturbances in some patients (blurred vision, halos); these are not generally considered a reason to discontinue treatment.

May cause hypotension and bradycardia (infusion-rate related). Caution in surgical patients; may enhance hemodynamic effect of anesthetics; associated with increased risk of adult respiratory distress syndrome (ARDS) postoperatively. Injection contains benzyl alcohol, which has been associated with "gasping syndrome" in neonates. Safety and efficacy of amiodarone in children has not been fully established.

Adverse Reactions In a recent meta-analysis, patients taking lower doses of amiodarone (152-330 mg daily for at least 12 months) were more likely to develop thyroid, neurologic, skin, ocular, and bradycardic abnormalities than those taking placebo. Pulmonary toxicity was similar in both the low dose amiodarone group and in the placebo group but there was a trend towards increased toxicity in the amiodarone group. Gastrointestinal and hepatic events were seen to a similar extent in both the low dose amiodarone group and placebo group. As the frequency of adverse events varies considerably across studies as a function of route and dose, a consolidation of adverse event rates is provided by Goldschlager, 2000.

Cardiovascular: Hypotension (I.V. 16%, refractory in rare cases)

Central nervous system (3% to 40%): Abnormal gait/ataxia, dizziness, fatigue, headache, malaise, impaired memory, involuntary movement, insomnia, poor coordination, peripheral neuropathy, sleep disturbances, tremor

Dermatologic: Photosensitivity (10% to 75%)

Endocrine & Metabolic: Hypothyroidism (1% to 22%)

Gastrointestinal: Nausea, vomiting, anorexia, and constipation (10% to 33%); AST or ALT level >2x normal (15% to 50%)

Ocular: Corneal microdeposits (>90%; causes visual disturbance in <10%)

1% to 10%:

Cardiovascular: CHF (3%), bradycardia (3% to 5%), AV block (5%), conduction abnormalities, SA node dysfunction (1% to 3%), cardiac arrhythmia, flushing, edema. Additional effects associated with I.V. administration include asystole, cardiac arrest, electromechanical dissociation, ventricular tachycardia, and cardiogenic shock.

Dermatologic: Slate blue skin discoloration (<10%)

Endocrine & metabolic: Hyperthyroidism (<3%), libido decreased

Gastrointestinal: Abdominal pain, abnormal salivation, abnormal taste (oral)

Hematologic: Coagulation abnormalities

Hepatic: Hepatitis and cirrhosis (<3%)

Local: Phlebitis (I.V., with concentrations >3 mg/mL)

Ocular: Visual disturbances (2% to 9%), halo vision (<5% occurring especially at night), optic neuritis (1%)

Respiratory: Pulmonary toxicity has been estimated to occur at a frequency between 2% and 7% of patients (some reports indicate a frequency as high as 17%). Toxicity may present as hypersensitivity pneumonitis; pulmonary fibrosis (cough, fever, malaise); pulmonary inflammation; interstitial pneumonitis; or alveolar pneumonitis. ARDS has been reported in up to 2% of patients receiving amiodarone, and postoperatively in patients receiving oral amiodarone.

Miscellaneous: Abnormal smell (oral)

<1% (Limited to important or life-threatening): Acute intracranial hypertension (I.V.), acute renal failure, agranulocytosis, alopecia, anaphylactic shock, angioedema, aplastic anemia, bone marrow granuloma, bronchiolitis obliterans organizing pneumonia (BOOP), bronchospasm, confusion, disorientation, dyspnea, encephalopathy, epididymitis (noninfectious), erectile dysfunction, erythema multiforme, exfoliative dermatitis, hallucination, hemolytic anemia, hemoptysis, hyperglycemia, hypertriglyceridemia, hypotension (oral), hypoxia, impotence, injection site reactions, leukocytoclastic vasculitis, muscle weakness, myopathy, neutropenia, optic neuropathy, pancreatitis, pancytopenia, parkinsonian symptoms, photophobia, pleuritis, proarrhythmia, pruritus, pseudotumor cerebri, pulmonary edema, QT interval increased, rash, renal impairment, renal insufficiency, SIADH, sinus arrest, spontaneous ecchymosis, Stevens-Johnson syndrome, thrombocytopenia, toxic epidermal necrolysis, vasculitis, ventricular fibrillation, wheezing

Overdosage/Toxicology Symptoms of overdose include extension of pharmacologic effects, sinus bradycardia and/or heart block, hypotension, and QT prolongation. Patients should be monitored for several days following ingestion. Intoxication with amiodarone necessitates ECG monitoring. Bradycardia may be atropine resistant. Injectable isoproterenol or a temporary pacemaker may be required. Dialysis is not beneficial.

Drug Interactions Substrate of CYP1A2 (minor), 2C8 (major at low concentrations), 2C19 (minor), 2D6 (minor), 3A4 (major); **Inhibits** CYP1A2 (weak), 2A6 (moderate), 2B6 (weak), 2C9 (moderate), 2C19 (weak), 2D6 (moderate), 3A4 (moderate)

(Continued)

Amiodarone *(Continued)*

Anesthetics (halogenated, inhaled): Amiodarone enhances the myocardial depressant and conduction effects of inhalation anesthetics; monitor.

Azole antifungals: May prolong QT_c, potentially leading to malignant arrhythmias; use caution.

Beta-blockers may cause excessive AV block; monitor response.

Calcium channel blockers (diltiazem, verapamil): May cause excessive AV block; monitor.

Cimetidine: May increase amiodarone blood levels.

Cholestyramine: May decrease amiodarone blood levels.

Cisapride: May prolong QT_c interval potentially leading to malignant arrhythmias.

Clonazepam effects may be increased by amiodarone.

Cyclosporine: Serum levels may be increased by amiodarone; monitor.

CYP2A6 substrates: Amiodarone may increase the levels/effects of CYP2A6 substrates. Example substrates include dexmedetomidine and ifosfamide.

CYP2C8 inducers: May decrease the levels/effects of amiodarone. Example inducers include carbamazepine, phenobarbital, phenytoin, rifampin, rifapentine, and secobarbital.

CYP2C8 inhibitors: May increase the levels/effects of amiodarone. Example inhibitors include atazanavir, gemfibrozil, and ritonavir.

CYP2C9 substrates: Amiodarone may increase the levels/effects of CYP2C9 substrates. Example substrates include bosentan, dapsone, fluoxetine, glimepiride, glipizide, losartan, montelukast, nateglinide, paclitaxel, phenytoin, warfarin, and zafirlukast.

CYP2D6 substrates: Amiodarone may increase the levels/effects of CYP2D6 substrates. Example substrates include amphetamines, selected beta-blockers, dextromethorphan, fluoxetine, lidocaine, mirtazapine, nefazodone, paroxetine, risperidone, ritonavir, thioridazine, tricyclic antidepressants, and venlafaxine.

CYP2D6 prodrug substrates: Amiodarone may decrease the levels/effects of CYP2D6 prodrug substrates. Example prodrug substrates include codeine, hydrocodone, oxycodone, and tramadol.

CYP3A4 inducers: CYP3A4 inducers may decrease the levels/effects of amiodarone. Example inducers include aminoglutethimide, carbamazepine, nafcillin, nevirapine, phenobarbital, phenytoin, and rifamycins.

CYP3A4 inhibitors: May increase the levels/effects of amiodarone. Example inhibitors include azole antifungals, clarithromycin, diclofenac, doxycycline, erythromycin, imatinib, isoniazid, nefazodone, nicardipine, propofol, protease inhibitors, quinidine, telithromycin, and verapamil.

CYP3A4 substrates: Amiodarone may increase the levels/effects of CYP3A4 substrates. Example substrates include benzodiazepines, calcium channel blockers, ergot derivatives, mirtazapine, nateglinide, nefazodone, tacrolimus, and venlafaxine.

Digoxin levels may be increased by amiodarone; consider reducing digoxin dose by 50% and monitor digoxin blood levels closely.

Fentanyl: Concurrent use may lead to bradycardia, sinus arrest, and hypotension.

Flecainide blood levels may be increased; consider reducing flecainide dose by 25% to 33% with concurrent use.

Fluoroquinolones (sparfloxacin, gatifloxacin, moxifloxacin): May result in additional prolongation of the QT interval; concurrent use of sparfloxacin is contraindicated.

HMG-CoA reductase inhibitors (lovastatin, simvastatin, and others dependent on CYP3A4 metabolism): Amiodarone inhibits metabolism of lovastatin and/or simvastatin and may increase the risk of myopathy and rhabdomyolysis. Concurrent use of lovastatin or simvastatin is not recommended, but if unavoidable, dose of lovastatin should not exceed 40 mg/day. The dose of simvastatin should not exceed 20 mg/day; consider alternative HMG-CoA reductase inhibitor.

Lidocaine: Amiodarone may increase serum levels/toxicity of lidocaine. Sinus bradycardia may occur with concurrent use.

Macrolide antibiotics: May prolong QT_c, potentially leading to malignant arrhythmias. Use caution and evaluate risk:benefit.

Metoprolol blood levels may be increased; monitor response.

Phenytoin blood levels may be increased by amiodarone; amiodarone blood levels may be decreased by phenytoin.

Procainamide and NAPA plasma levels may be increased; consider reducing procainamide dosage by 25% with concurrent use.

Propranolol blood levels may be increased.

Protease inhibitors (amprenavir, indinavir, ritonavir): May increase amiodarone blood levels and toxicity; concurrent use is contraindicated.

QT_c interval prolonging agents (including but may not be limited to amitriptyline, bepridil, disopyramide, erythromycin, haloperidol, imipramine, quinidine, pimozide, procainamide, sotalol, and thioridazine): Effect/toxicity increased; use with caution.

Quinidine blood levels may be increased; monitor quinidine trough concentration.

Rifampin may decrease amiodarone blood levels.

Theophylline blood levels may be increased.

Thyroid supplements: Amiodarone may alter thyroid function; monitor closely.

Warfarin: Hypoprothrombinemic response increased. Monitor INR closely when amiodarone is initiated or discontinued. Reduce warfarin's dose by $^1/_3$ to $^1/_2$ when amiodarone is started.

Ethanol/Nutrition/Herb Interactions

Food: Increases the rate and extent of absorption of amiodarone. Grapefruit juice increases bioavailability of oral amiodarone by 50% and decreases the conversion of amiodarone to N-DEA (active metabolite); altered effects are possible; use should be avoided during therapy.

Herb/Nutraceutical: St John's wort may decrease amiodarone levels or enhance photosensitization. Avoid ephedra (may worsen arrhythmia). Avoid dong quai.

Dietary Considerations Administer consistently with regard to meals. Amiodarone contains iodine 37.3% by weight. Grapefruit juice is not recommended.

Dosage Forms [DSC] = Discontinued product

Injection, solution, as hydrochloride: 50 mg/mL (3 mL, 9 mL, 18 mL) [contains benzyl alcohol and polysorbate (Tween®) 80]

Cordarone®: 50 mg/mL (3 mL) [contains benzyl alcohol and polysorbate (Tween®) 80]

Tablet, as hydrochloride [scored]: 200 mg, 400 mg

Cordarone®: 200 mg

Pacerone®: 100 mg [not scored], 200 mg, 300 mg [DSC], 400 mg

References

"2005 American Heart Association Guidelines for Cardiopulmonary Resuscitation and Emergency Cardiovascular Care," *Circulation*, 2005, 112(24 Suppl): 1-211.

Daoud EG, Strickberger SA, Man KC, et al, "Preoperative Amiodarone as Prophylaxis Against Atrial Fibrillation After Heart Surgery," *N Engl J Med*, 1997, 337(25):1785-91.

Dorian P, Cass D, Schwartz B, et al, "Amiodarone as Compared With Lidocaine for Shock-Resistant Ventricular Fibrillation," *N Engl J Med*, 2002, 346(12):884-90.

Goldschlager N, Epstein AE, Naccarelli G, et al, "Practical Guidelines for Clinicians Who Treat Patients With Amiodarone. Practice Guidelines Subcommittee, North American Society of Pacing and Electrophysiology," *Arch Intern Med*, 2000, 160(12):1741-8.

Guarnieri T, Nolan S, Gottlieb SO, et al, "Intravenous Amiodarone for the Prevention of Atrial Fibrillation After Open Heart Surgery: The Amiodarone Reduction in Coronary Heart (ARCH) Trial," *J Am Coll Cardiol*, 1999, 34(2):343-7.

Kudenchuk PJ, Cobb LA, Copass MK, et al, "Amiodarone for Resuscitation After Out-of-Hospital Cardiac Arrest Due to Ventricular Fibrillation," *N Engl J Med*, 1999, 341(12):871-8.

Ott MC, Khoor A, Leventhal JP, et al, "Pulmonary Toxicity in Patients Receiving Low-Dose Amiodarone," *Chest*, 2003, 123:646-54.

Perry JC, Fenrich AL, Hulse JE, et al, "Pediatric Use of Intravenous Amiodarone: Efficacy and Safety in Critically Ill Patients From a Multicenter Protocol," *J Am Coll Cardiol*, 1996, 27(5):1246-50.

Stamou SC, Hill PC, Sample GA, et al, "Prevention of Atrial Fibrillation After Cardiac Surgery: The Significance of Postoperative Oral Amiodarone," *Chest*, 2001, 120(6):1936-41.

- ♦ **Amiodarone Hydrochloride** *see* Amiodarone *on page 83*
- ♦ **Amiodarone Hydrochloride for Injection® (Can)** *see* Amiodarone *on page 83*

Amitriptyline (a mee TRIP ti leen)

Medication Safety Issues

Sound-alike/look-alike issues:

Amitriptyline may be confused with aminophylline, imipramine, nortriptyline

Elavil® may be confused with Aldoril®, Eldepryl®, enalapril, Equanil®, Mellaril®, Oruvail®, Plavix®

Related Information

Antidepressant Agents *on page 1551*

Chronic Pain Management *on page 1430*

Canadian Brand Names Apo-Amitriptyline®; Levate®; Novo-Triptyn; PMS-Amitriptyline

(Continued)

Amitriptyline *(Continued)*

Synonyms Amitriptyline Hydrochloride; Elavil

Pharmacologic Category Antidepressant, Tricyclic (Tertiary Amine)

Restrictions A medication guide concerning the use of antidepressants in children and teenagers can be found on the FDA website at www.fda.gov/cder/Offices/ODS/labeling.htm. It should be dispensed to parents or guardians of children and teenagers receiving this medication.

Generic Available Yes

Use Relief of symptoms of depression

Unlabeled/Investigational Use Analgesic for certain chronic and neuropathic pain; prophylaxis against migraine headaches; treatment of depressive disorders in children

Mechanism of Action Increases the synaptic concentration of serotonin and/or norepinephrine in the central nervous system by inhibition of their reuptake by the presynaptic neuronal membrane

Pharmacodynamics/Kinetics

Onset of action: Migraine prophylaxis: 6 weeks, higher dosage may be required in heavy smokers because of increased metabolism; Depression: 4-6 weeks, reduce dosage to lowest effective level

Distribution: Crosses placenta; enters breast milk

Metabolism: Hepatic to nortriptyline (active), hydroxy and conjugated derivatives; may be impaired in the elderly

Half-life elimination: Adults: 9-27 hours (average: 15 hours)

Time to peak, serum: ~4 hours

Excretion: Urine (18% as unchanged drug); feces (small amounts)

Dosage

Children:

Chronic pain management (unlabeled use): Oral: Initial: 0.1 mg/kg at bedtime, may advance as tolerated over 2-3 weeks to 0.5-2 mg/kg at bedtime

Depressive disorders (unlabeled use): Oral: Initial doses of 1 mg/kg/day given in 3 divided doses with increases to 1.5 mg/kg/day have been reported in a small number of children (n=9) 9-12 years of age; clinically, doses up to 3 mg/kg/day (5 mg/kg/day if monitored closely) have been proposed

Migraine prophylaxis (unlabeled use): Oral: Initial: 0.25 mg/kg/day, given at bedtime; increase dose by 0.25 mg/kg/day to maximum 1 mg/kg/day. Reported dosing ranges: 0.1-2 mg/kg/day; maximum suggested dose: 10 mg.

Adolescents: Depressive disorders: Oral: Initial: 25-50 mg/day; may administer in divided doses; increase gradually to 100 mg/day in divided doses

Adults:

Depression:

Oral: 50-150 mg/day single dose at bedtime or in divided doses; dose may be gradually increased up to 300 mg/day

Migraine prophylaxis (unlabeled use): Oral: Initial: 10-25 mg at bedtime; usual dose: 150 mg; reported dosing ranges: 10-400 mg/day

Pain management (unlabeled use): Oral: Initial: 25 mg at bedtime; may increase as tolerated to 100 mg/day

Elderly: Depression: Oral: Initial: 10-25 mg at bedtime; dose should be increased in 10-25 mg increments every week if tolerated; dose range: 25-150 mg/day

Dosing interval in hepatic impairment: Use with caution and monitor plasma levels and patient response

Hemodialysis: Nondialyzable

Stability Protect injection and Elavil® 10 mg tablets from light.

Monitoring Parameters Monitor blood pressure and pulse rate prior to and during initial therapy; evaluate mental status; monitor weight; ECG in older adults and patients with cardiac disease

Reference Range Therapeutic: Amitriptyline and nortriptyline 100-250 ng/mL (SI: 360-900 nmol/L); nortriptyline 50-150 ng/mL (SI: 190-570 nmol/L); Toxic: >0.5 mcg/mL; plasma levels do not always correlate with clinical effectiveness

Anesthesia and Critical Care Concerns/Other Considerations Plasma levels do not always correlate with clinical effectiveness. Desired therapeutic effect (for analgesia) may take as long as 1-3 weeks. When used for migraine headache prophylaxis, therapeutic effect may take as long as 6 weeks.

Tricyclic antidepressants affect conduction and have anticholinergic effects and, therefore, should be used with caution in patients with underlying cardiovascular disease. Therapy is relatively contraindicated in patients with conduction abnormalities or in patients with symptomatic hypotension. Heart block may be precipitated in patients with pre-existing conduction system disease. Cardiovascular signs of toxicity may include tachycardia, ventricular arrhythmia, impaired conduction, and shock.

Pregnancy Risk Factor C

Contraindications Hypersensitivity to amitriptyline or any component of the formulation (cross-sensitivity with other tricyclics may occur); use of MAO inhibitors within past 14 days; acute recovery phase following myocardial infarction; concurrent use of cisapride

Warnings/Precautions **[U.S. Boxed Warning]: Antidepressants increase the risk of suicidal thinking and behavior in children and adolescents with major depressive disorder (MDD) and other depressive disorders;** consider risk prior to prescribing. Closely monitor for clinical worsening, suicidality, or unusual changes in behavior; the child's family or caregiver should be instructed to closely observe the patient and communicate condition with healthcare provider. Such observation would generally include at least weekly face-to-face contact with patients or their family members or caregivers during the first 4 weeks of treatment, then every other week visits for the next 4 weeks, then at 12 weeks, and as clinically indicated beyond 12 weeks. Additional contact by telephone may be appropriate between face-to-face visits. Adults treated with antidepressants should be observed similarly for clinical worsening and suicidality, especially during the initial few months of a course of drug therapy, or at times of dose changes, either increases or decreases. A medication guide should be dispensed with each prescription. **Amitriptyline is not FDA-approved for use in children <12 years of age.**

The possibility of a suicide attempt is inherent in major depression and may persist until remission occurs. Monitor for worsening of depression or suicidality, especially during initiation of therapy or with dose increases or decreases. Worsening depression and severe abrupt suicidality that are not part of the presenting symptoms may require discontinuation or modification of drug therapy. Use caution in high-risk patients during initiation of therapy. Prescriptions should be written for the smallest quantity consistent with good patient care. The patient's family or caregiver should be alerted to monitor patients for the emergence of suicidality and associated behaviors such as anxiety, agitation, panic attacks, insomnia, irritability, hostility, impulsivity, akathisia, hypomania, and mania; patients should be instructed to notify their healthcare provider if any of these symptoms or worsening depression occur.

May worsen psychosis in some patients or precipitate a shift to mania or hypomania in patients with bipolar disorder. Monotherapy in patients with bipolar disorder should be avoided. Patients presenting with depressive symptoms should be screened for bipolar disorder. **Amitriptyline is not FDA approved for the treatment of bipolar depression.**

Often causes drowsiness/sedation, resulting in impaired performance of tasks requiring alertness (eg, operating machinery or driving). Sedative effects may be additive with other CNS depressants and/or ethanol. The degree of sedation is very high relative to other antidepressants. May cause hyponatremia/SIADH. May increase the risks associated with electroconvulsive therapy. Consider discontinuing, when possible, prior to elective surgery. Therapy should not be abruptly discontinued in patients receiving high doses for prolonged periods.

May cause orthostatic hypotension; the risk of this problem is very high relative to other antidepressants. Use with caution in patients at risk of hypotension or in patients where transient hypotensive episodes would be poorly tolerated (cardiovascular disease or cerebrovascular disease). The degree of anticholinergic blockade produced by this agent is very high relative to other cyclic antidepressants; use with caution in patients with urinary retention, benign prostatic hyperplasia, narrow-angle glaucoma, xerostomia, visual problems, constipation, or a history of bowel obstruction. May alter glucose control - use with caution in patients with diabetes.

Use with caution in patients with a history of cardiovascular disease (including previous MI, stroke, tachycardia, or conduction abnormalities). The risk of conduction abnormalities with this agent is high relative to other antidepressants. May lower seizure threshold - use caution in patients with a previous seizure disorder or condition predisposing to seizures such as brain damage, alcoholism, or concurrent therapy with other drugs which lower the seizure threshold. Use

(Continued)

Amitriptyline *(Continued)*

with caution in hyperthyroid patients or those receiving thyroid supplementation. Use with caution in patients with hepatic or renal dysfunction and in elderly patients.

Adverse Reactions Anticholinergic effects may be pronounced; moderate to marked sedation can occur (tolerance to these effects usually occurs).

Frequency not defined.

Cardiovascular: Orthostatic hypotension, tachycardia, ECG changes (nonspecific), AV conduction changes, cardiomyopathy (rare), MI, stroke, heart block, arrhythmia, syncope, hypertension, palpitation

Central nervous system: Restlessness, dizziness, insomnia, sedation, fatigue, anxiety, cognitive function impaired, seizure, extrapyramidal symptoms, coma, hallucinations, confusion, disorientation, coordination impaired, ataxia, headache, nightmares, hyperpyrexia

Dermatologic: Allergic rash, urticaria, photosensitivity, alopecia

Endocrine & metabolic: Syndrome of inappropriate ADH secretion

Gastrointestinal: Weight gain, xerostomia, constipation, paralytic ileus, nausea, vomiting, anorexia, stomatitis, peculiar taste, diarrhea, black tongue

Genitourinary: Urinary retention

Hematologic: Bone marrow depression, purpura, eosinophilia

Neuromuscular & skeletal: Numbness, paresthesia, peripheral neuropathy, tremor, weakness

Ocular: Blurred vision, mydriasis, ocular pressure increased

Otic: Tinnitus

Miscellaneous: Diaphoresis, withdrawal reactions (nausea, headache, malaise)

Postmarketing and/or case reports: Neuroleptic malignant syndrome (rare), serotonin syndrome (rare)

Overdosage/Toxicology Symptoms of overdose include agitation, confusion, hallucinations, urinary retention, hypothermia, hypotension, ventricular tachycardia, and seizures. Treatment is symptomatic and supportive. Alkalinization by sodium bicarbonate and/or hyperventilation may limit cardiac toxicity.

Drug Interactions Substrate of CYP1A2 (minor), 2B6 (minor), 2C9 (minor), 2C19 (minor), 2D6 (major), 3A4 (minor); **Inhibits** CYP1A2 (weak), 2C9 (weak), 2C19 (weak), 2D6 (weak), 2E1 (weak)

Altretamine: Concurrent use may cause orthostatic hypertension.

Amphetamines: TCAs may enhance the effect of amphetamines; monitor for adverse CV effects.

Anticholinergics: Combined use with TCAs may produce additive anticholinergic effects.

Antihypertensives: Amitriptyline inhibits the antihypertensive response to bethanidine, clonidine, debrisoquin, guanadrel, guanethidine, guanabenz, guanfacine; monitor BP; consider alternate antihypertensive agent.

Beta-agonists: When combined with TCAs may predispose patients to cardiac arrhythmias.

Bupropion: May increase the levels of tricyclic antidepressants; based on limited information, monitor response.

Carbamazepine: Tricyclic antidepressants may increase carbamazepine levels; monitor.

Cholestyramine and colestipol: May bind TCAs and reduce their absorption; monitor for altered response.

Cisapride: May increase the risk of QT_c prolongation and/or arrhythmia; concurrent use is contraindicated.

Clonidine: Abrupt discontinuation of clonidine may cause hypertensive crisis; amitriptyline may enhance the response (also see note on antihypertensives).

CNS depressants: Sedative effects may be additive with TCAs; monitor for increased effect; includes benzodiazepines, barbiturates, antipsychotics, ethanol, and other sedative medications.

CYP2D6 inhibitors: May increase the levels/effects of amitriptyline; example inhibitors include chlorpromazine, delavirdine, fluoxetine, miconazole, paroxetine, pergolide, quinidine, quinine, ritonavir, and ropinirole.

Epinephrine (and other direct alpha-agonists): Pressor response to I.V. epinephrine, norepinephrine, and phenylephrine may be enhanced in patients receiving TCAs. (**Note:** Effect is unlikely with epinephrine or levonordefrin dosages typically administered as infiltration in combination with local anesthetics.)

Fenfluramine: May increase tricyclic antidepressant levels/effects.

Hypoglycemic agents (including insulin): TCAs may enhance the hypoglycemic effects of tolazamide, chlorpropamide, or insulin; monitor for changes in blood glucose levels; reported with chlorpropamide, tolazamide, and insulin.

Levodopa: Tricyclic antidepressants may decrease the absorption (bioavailability) of levodopa; rare hypertensive episodes have also been attributed to this combination.

Linezolid: Hyperpyrexia, hypertension, tachycardia, confusion, seizures, and **deaths have been reported** with agents which inhibit MAO (serotonin syndrome); this combination should be avoided.

Lithium: Concurrent use with a TCA may increase the risk for neurotoxicity.

MAO inhibitors: Hyperpyrexia, hypertension, tachycardia, confusion, seizures, and **deaths have been reported** (serotonin syndrome); this combination should be avoided.

Methylphenidate: Metabolism of amitriptyline may be decreased.

Phenothiazines: Serum concentrations of some TCAs may be increased; in addition, TCAs may increase concentration of phenothiazines; monitor for altered clinical response.

QT_c prolonging agents: Concurrent use of tricyclic agents with other drugs which may prolong QT_c interval may increase the risk of potentially fatal arrhythmias; includes type Ia and type III antiarrhythmics agents, selected quinolones (sparfloxacin, gatifloxacin, moxifloxacin, grepafloxacin), cisapride, and other agents.

Ritonavir: Combined use of high-dose tricyclic antidepressants with ritonavir may cause serotonin syndrome in HIV-positive patients; monitor.

Sucralfate: Absorption of tricyclic antidepressants may be reduced with coadministration.

Sympathomimetics, indirect-acting: Tricyclic antidepressants may result in a decreased sensitivity to indirect-acting sympathomimetics; includes dopamine and ephedrine; also see interaction with epinephrine (and direct-acting sympathomimetics).

Tramadol: Tramadol's risk of seizures may be increased with TCAs.

Valproic acid: May increase serum concentrations/adverse effects of some tricyclic antidepressants.

Warfarin (and other oral anticoagulants): Amitriptyline may increase the anticoagulant effect in patients stabilized on warfarin; monitor INR.

Ethanol/Nutrition/Herb Interactions

Ethanol: Avoid ethanol (may increase CNS depression).

Food: Grapefruit juice may inhibit the metabolism of some TCAs and clinical toxicity may result.

Herb/Nutraceutical: St John's wort may decrease amitriptyline levels. Avoid valerian, St John's wort, kava kava, gotu kola (may increase CNS depression).

Test Interactions May cause false-positive reaction to EMIT immunoassay for imipramine

Dosage Forms

Tablet, as hydrochloride: 10 mg, 25 mg, 50 mg, 75 mg, 100 mg, 150 mg

References

Mokhlesi B, Leikin JB, Murray P, et al, "Adult Toxicology in Critical Care. Part 11: Specific Poisonings," *Chest*, 2003, 123(3):897-922.

♦ **Amitriptyline Hydrochloride** *see* Amitriptyline *on page 89*

♦ **Amphadase**™ *see* Hyaluronidase *on page 631*

♦ **Amphocin**® *see* Amphotericin B (Conventional) *on page 96*

♦ **Amphotec**® *see* Amphotericin B Cholesteryl Sulfate Complex *on page 93*

Amphotericin B Cholesteryl Sulfate Complex

(am foe TER i sin bee kole LES te ril SUL fate KOM plecks)

Medication Safety Issues

Safety issues:

Lipid-based amphotericin formulations (Amphotec®) may be confused with conventional formulations (Amphocin®, Fungizone®)

Large overdoses have occurred when conventional formulations were dispensed inadvertently for lipid-based products. Single daily doses of conventional amphotericin formulation never exceed 1.5 mg/kg.

Related Information

Antifungal Agents *on page 1554*

(Continued)

Amphotericin B Cholesteryl Sulfate Complex (Continued)

U.S. Brand Names Amphotec®

Canadian Brand Names Amphotec®

Synonyms ABCD; Amphotericin B Colloidal Dispersion

Pharmacologic Category Antifungal Agent, Parenteral

Generic Available No

Use Treatment of invasive aspergillosis in patients who have failed amphotericin B deoxycholate treatment, or who have renal impairment or experience unacceptable toxicity which precludes treatment with amphotericin B deoxycholate in effective doses.

Unlabeled/Investigational Use Effective in patients with serious *Candida* species infections

Mechanism of Action Binds to ergosterol altering cell membrane permeability in susceptible fungi and causing leakage of cell components with subsequent cell death. Proposed mechanism suggests that amphotericin causes an oxidation-dependent stimulation of macrophages.

Pharmacodynamics/Kinetics

Distribution: V_d: Total volume increases with higher doses, reflects increasing uptake by tissues (with 4 mg/kg/day = 4 L/kg); predominantly distributed in the liver; concentrations in kidneys and other tissues are lower than observed with conventional amphotericin B

Half-life elimination: 28-29 hours; prolonged with higher doses

Dosage Children and Adults: I.V.:

Premedication: For patients who experience chills, fever, hypotension, nausea, or other nonanaphylactic infusion-related immediate reactions, premedicate with the following drugs 30-60 minutes prior to drug administration: A nonsteroidal (eg, ibuprofen, choline magnesium trisalicylate) with or without diphenhydramine **or** acetaminophen with diphenhydramine **or** hydrocortisone 50-100 mg. If the patient experiences rigors during the infusion, meperidine may be administered.

Range: 3-4 mg/kg/day (infusion of 1 mg/kg/hour); maximum: 7.5 mg/kg/day

Stability

Store intact vials under refrigeration.

Reconstitute 50 mg and 100 mg vials with 10 mL and 20 mL of SWI, respectively. The reconstituted vials contain 5 mg/mL of amphotericin B. Shake the vial gently by hand until all solid particles have dissolved. After reconstitution, the solution should be refrigerated at 2°C to 8°C (36°F to 46°F) and used within 24 hours.

Further dilute amphotericin B colloidal dispersion with dextrose 5% in water. Concentrations of 0.1-2 mg/mL in dextrose 5% in water are stable for 14 days at 4°C and 23°C if protected from light, however, due to the occasional formation of subvisual particles, solutions should be used within 48 hours.

Administration Avoid injection faster than 1 mg/kg/hour. For a patient who experiences chills, fever, hypotension, nausea, or other nonanaphylactic infusion-related reactions, premedicate with the following drugs 30-60 minutes prior to drug administration: A nonsteroidal (eg, ibuprofen, choline magnesium trisalicylate) with or without diphenhydramine **or** acetaminophen with diphenhydramine **or** hydrocortisone 50-100 mg. If the patient experiences rigors during the infusion, meperidine may be administered. If severe respiratory distress occurs, the infusion should be immediately discontinued.

Monitoring Parameters Liver function tests, electrolytes, BUN, Cr, temperature, CBC, I/O, signs of hypokalemia (muscle weakness, cramping, drowsiness, ECG changes)

Anesthesia and Critical Care Concerns/Other Considerations Patients may be premedicated with acetaminophen and diphenhydramine 30 minutes prior to infusion. Meperidine (Demerol®) may help reduce rigors.

Controlled trials which compare the original formulation of amphotericin B to the newer liposomal formulations (ie, Amphotec®) are lacking. Thus, comparative data discussing differences among the formulations should be interpreted cautiously. Although the risk of nephrotoxicity and infusion-related adverse effects may be less with Amphotec®, the efficacy profiles of Amphotec® and the original amphotericin formulation are comparable. Consequently, Amphotec® should be restricted to those patients who cannot tolerate or who fail a standard amphotericin B formulation. This product is significantly more expensive than conventional amphotericin B; Infectious Disease consult is recommended.

Pregnancy Risk Factor B

Contraindications Hypersensitivity to amphotericin B or any component of the formulation

Warnings/Precautions Anaphylaxis has been reported with other amphotericin B-containing drugs. Facilities for cardiopulmonary resuscitation should be available during administration due to the possibility of anaphylactic reaction. If severe respiratory distress occurs, the infusion should be immediately discontinued. During the initial dosing, the drug should be administered under close clinical observation. Infusion reactions, sometimes severe, usually subside with continued therapy - manage with decreased rate of infusion and pretreatment with antihistamines/corticosteroids. Pulmonary reactions may occur in neutropenic patients receiving leukocyte transfusions; separation of the infusions as much as possible is advised.

Adverse Reactions

>10%: Central nervous system: Chills, fever

1% to 10%:

Cardiovascular: Hypotension, tachycardia

Central nervous system: Headache

Dermatologic: Rash

Endocrine & metabolic: Hypokalemia, hypomagnesemia

Gastrointestinal: Nausea, diarrhea, abdominal pain

Hematologic: Thrombocytopenia

Hepatic: LFT change

Neuromuscular & skeletal: Rigors

Renal: Creatinine increased

Respiratory: Dyspnea

Note: Amphotericin B colloidal dispersion has an improved therapeutic index compared to conventional amphotericin B, and has been used safely in patients with amphotericin B-related nephrotoxicity; however, continued decline of renal function has occurred in some patients.

Overdosage/Toxicology Symptoms of overdose include renal dysfunction, anemia, thrombocytopenia, granulocytopenia, fever, nausea, and vomiting. Treatment is supportive.

Drug Interactions

Increased nephrotoxicity: Aminoglycosides, cyclosporine, other nephrotoxic drugs.

Potentiation of hypokalemia: Corticosteroids, corticotropin.

Increased digitalis and neuromuscular-blocking agent toxicity due to hypokalemia.

Decreased effect: Pharmacologic antagonism may occur with azole antifungal agents (eg, miconazole, ketoconazole).

Pulmonary toxicity has occurred with concomitant administration of amphotericin B and leukocyte transfusions.

Dosage Forms Injection, powder for reconstitution: 50 mg, 100 mg

References

Lister J, "Amphotericin B Lipid Complex (Abelcet®) in the Treatment of Invasive Mycoses: The North American Experience," *Eur J Haematol Suppl*, 1996, 57:18-23.

Mora-Duarte J, Betts R, Rotstein C, et al, "Comparison of Caspofungin and Amphotericin B for Invasive Candidiasis," *N Engl J Med*, 2002, 347(25):2020-9.

Prentice HG, Hann IM, Herbrecht R, et al, "A Randomized Comparison of Liposomal Versus Conventional Amphotericin B for the Treatment of Pyrexia of Unknown Origin in Neutropenic Patients," *Br J Haematol*, 1997, 98(3):711-8.

Rex JH, Walsh TJ, Sobel JD, et al, "Practice Guidelines for the Treatment of Candidiasis. Infectious Diseases Society of America," *Clin Infect Dis*, 2000, 30(4):662-78.

Slain D, "Lipid-Based Amphotericin B for the Treatment of Fungal Infections," *Pharmacotherapy*, 1999, 19(3):306-23.

♦ **Amphotericin B Colloidal Dispersion** *see* Amphotericin B Cholesteryl Sulfate Complex *on page 93*

Amphotericin B (Conventional)

(am foe TER i sin bee con VEN sha nal)

Medication Safety Issues

Safety issues:

Conventional amphotericin formulations (Amphocin®, Fungizone®) may be confused with lipid-based formulations (AmBisome®, Abelcet®, Amphotec®).

Large overdoses have occurred when conventional formulations were dispensed inadvertently for lipid-based products. Single daily doses of conventional amphotericin formulation never exceed 1.5 mg/kg.

Related Information

Antifungal Agents *on page 1554*

U.S. Brand Names Amphocin®

Canadian Brand Names Fungizone®

Synonyms Amphotericin B Desoxycholate

Pharmacologic Category Antifungal Agent, Parenteral

Generic Available Yes

Use Treatment of severe systemic and central nervous system infections caused by susceptible fungi such as *Candida* species, *Histoplasma capsulatum, Cryptococcus neoformans, Aspergillus* species, *Blastomyces dermatitidis, Torulopsis glabrata*, and *Coccidioides immitis*; fungal peritonitis; irrigant for bladder fungal infections; used in fungal infection in patients with bone marrow transplantation, amebic meningoencephalitis, ocular aspergillosis (intraocular injection), candidal cystitis (bladder irrigation), chemoprophylaxis (low-dose I.V.), immunocompromised patients at risk of aspergillosis (intranasal/nebulized), refractory meningitis (intrathecal), coccidioidal arthritis (intra-articular/I.M.).

Low-dose amphotericin B has been administered after bone marrow transplantation to reduce the risk of invasive fungal disease.

Mechanism of Action Binds to ergosterol altering cell membrane permeability in susceptible fungi and causing leakage of cell components with subsequent cell death. Proposed mechanism suggests that amphotericin causes an oxidation-dependent stimulation of macrophages.

Pharmacodynamics/Kinetics

Distribution: Minimal amounts enter the aqueous humor, bile, CSF (inflamed or noninflamed meninges), amniotic fluid, pericardial fluid, pleural fluid, and synovial fluid

Protein binding, plasma: 90%

Half-life elimination: Biphasic: Initial: 15-48 hours; Terminal: 15 days

Time to peak: Within 1 hour following a 4- to 6-hour dose

Excretion: Urine (2% to 5% as biologically active form); ~40% eliminated over a 7-day period and may be detected in urine for at least 7 weeks after discontinued use

Dosage

Premedication: For patients who experience infusion-related immediate reactions, premedicate with the following drugs 30-60 minutes prior to drug administration: NSAID (with or without diphenhydramine) **or** acetaminophen with diphenhydramine **or** hydrocortisone 50-100 mg. If the patient experiences rigors during the infusion, meperidine may be administered.

Infants and Children: I.V.:

Test dose: 0.1 mg/kg/dose to a maximum of 1 mg; infuse over 30-60 minutes. Many clinicians believe a test dose is unnecessary.

Maintenance dose: 0.25-1 mg/kg/day given once daily; infuse over 2-6 hours. Once therapy has been established, amphotericin B can be administered on an every-other-day basis at 1-1.5 mg/kg/dose; cumulative dose: 1.5-2 g over 6-10 weeks.

Adults: I.V.:

Test dose: 1 mg infused over 20-30 minutes. Many clinicians believe a test dose is unnecessary.

Maintenance dose: Usual: 0.25-1.5 mg/kg/day; 1-1.5 mg/kg over 4-6 hours every other day may be given once therapy is established; aspergillosis, mucormycosis, rhinocerebral phycomycosis often require 1-1.5 mg/kg/day; do not exceed 1.5 mg/kg/day

Duration of therapy varies with nature of infection: Usual duration is 4-12 weeks or cumulative dose of 1-4 g

Meningitis, coccidioidal or cryptococcal: I.T.:

Children.: 25-100 mcg every 48-72 hours; increase to 500 mcg as tolerated

Adults: Initial: 25-300 mcg every 48-72 hours; increase to 500 mcg to 1 mg as tolerated; maximum total dose: 15 mg has been suggested

Bone marrow transplantation (prophylaxis): Adults: I.V.: Low-dose amphotericin B 0.1-0.25 mg/kg/day has been administered after bone marrow transplantation to reduce the risk of invasive fungal disease.

Bladder irrigation: Candidal cystitis: Irrigate with 50 mcg/mL solution instilled periodically or continuously for 5-10 days or until cultures are clear

Note: Alternative routes of administration and extemporaneous preparations have been used when standard antifungal therapy is not available (eg, inhalation, intraocular injection, subconjunctival application, intracavitary administration into various joints and the pleural space).

Dosing adjustment in renal impairment: If renal dysfunction is due to the drug, the daily total can be decreased by 50% or the dose can be given every other day; I.V. therapy may take several months

Dialysis: Poorly dialyzed; no supplemental dosage necessary when using hemo- or peritoneal dialysis or continuous arteriovenous or venovenous hemodiafiltration effects

Administration in dialysate: Children and Adults: 1-2 mg/L of peritoneal dialysis fluid either with or without low-dose I.V. amphotericin B (a total dose of 2-10 mg/kg given over 7-14 days). Precipitate may form in ionic dialysate solutions.

Stability Store intact vials under refrigeration; protect from light. Add 10 mL of SWFI (without a bacteriostatic agent) to each vial of amphotericin B. Further dilute with 250-500 mL D_5W; final concentration should not exceed 0.1 mg/mL (peripheral infusion) or 0.25 mg/mL (central infusion).

Reconstituted vials are stable, protected from light, for 24 hours at room temperature and 1 week when refrigerated. Parenteral admixtures are stable, protected from light, for 24 hours at room temperature and 2 days under refrigeration. Short-term exposure (<24 hours) to light during I.V. infusion does **not** appreciably affect potency.

Administration May be infused over 4-6 hours. For a patient who experiences chills, fever, hypotension, nausea, or other nonanaphylactic infusion-related reactions, premedicate with the following drugs 30-60 minutes prior to drug administration: A nonsteroidal (eg, ibuprofen, choline magnesium trisalicylate) with or without diphenhydramine **or** acetaminophen with diphenhydramine **or** hydrocortisone 50-100 mg. If the patient experiences rigors during the infusion, meperidine may be administered. Bolus infusion of normal saline immediately preceding, or immediately preceding and following amphotericin B may reduce drug-induced nephrotoxicity. Risk of nephrotoxicity increases with amphotericin B doses >1 mg/kg/day. Infusion of admixtures more concentrated than 0.25 mg/mL should be limited to patients absolutely requiring volume contraction.

Monitoring Parameters Renal function (monitor frequently during therapy), electrolytes (especially potassium and magnesium), liver function tests, temperature, PT/PTT, CBC; monitor input and output; monitor for signs of hypokalemia (muscle weakness, cramping, drowsiness, ECG changes, etc)

Reference Range Therapeutic: 1-2 mcg/mL (SI: 1-2.2 μmol/L)

Anesthesia and Critical Care Concerns/Other Considerations Patients may be premedicated with acetaminophen and diphenhydramine 30 minutes prior to the amphotericin infusion. Meperidine (Demerol®) may help to reduce rigors. Avoid rapid injection (usually 4- to 6-hour infusion required). Dosage adjustments are not necessary with renal impairment. If decreased renal function is due to amphotericin, the daily dose can be decreased by 50% or the dose can be given every other day.

Hydrocortisone may be used in patients with severe or refractory infusion-related reactions. Bolus infusion of normal saline immediately preceding, or immediately preceding and following amphotericin B may reduce drug-induced nephrotoxicity. Risk of nephrotoxicity increases with amphotericin B doses >1 mg/kg/day. Infusion of admixtures more concentrated than 0.25 mg/mL should be limited to patients absolutely requiring volume restriction. Amphotericin B does not have a bacteriostatic constituent, subsequently admixture expiration is determined by sterility more than chemical stability.

Pregnancy Risk Factor B

Contraindications Hypersensitivity to amphotericin or any component of the formulation

(Continued)

Amphotericin B (Conventional) *(Continued)*

Warnings/Precautions Anaphylaxis has been reported with other amphotericin B-containing drugs. During the initial dosing, the drug should be administered under close clinical observation. Avoid use with other nephrotoxic drugs; drug-induced renal toxicity usually improves with interrupting therapy, decreasing dosage, or increasing dosing interval. Infusion reactions are most common 1-3 hours after starting the infusion and diminish with continued therapy. Use amphotericin B with caution in patients with decreased renal function. Pulmonary reactions may occur in neutropenic patients receiving leukocyte transfusions; separation of the infusions as much as possible is advised.

Adverse Reactions

Systemic:

>10%:

Cardiovascular: Hypotension, tachypnea

Central nervous system: Fever, chills, headache (less frequent with I.T.), malaise

Endocrine & metabolic: Hypokalemia, hypomagnesemia

Gastrointestinal: Anorexia, nausea (less frequent with I.T.), vomiting (less frequent with I.T.), diarrhea, heartburn, cramping epigastric pain

Hematologic: Normochromic-normocytic anemia

Local: Pain at injection site with or without phlebitis or thrombophlebitis (incidence may increase with peripheral infusion of admixtures)

Neuromuscular & skeletal: Generalized pain, including muscle and joint pains (less frequent with I.T.)

Renal: Decreased renal function and renal function abnormalities including azotemia, renal tubular acidosis, nephrocalcinosis (>0.1 mg/mL)

1% to 10%:

Cardiovascular: Hypertension, flushing

Central nervous system: Delirium, arachnoiditis, pain along lumbar nerves (especially I.T. therapy)

Genitourinary: Urinary retention

Hematologic: Leukocytosis

Neuromuscular & skeletal: Paresthesia (especially with I.T. therapy)

<1% (Limited to important or life-threatening): Acute liver failure, agranulocytosis, anuria, bone marrow suppression, cardiac arrest, coagulation defects, convulsions, dyspnea, hearing loss, leukopenia, maculopapular rash, renal failure, renal tubular acidosis, thrombocytopenia, vision changes

Overdosage/Toxicology Symptoms of overdose include renal dysfunction, cardiac arrest, anemia, thrombocytopenia, granulocytopenia, fever, nausea, and vomiting. Treatment is supportive.

Drug Interactions

Increased nephrotoxicity: Aminoglycosides, cyclosporine, other nephrotoxic drugs.

Potentiation of hypokalemia: Corticosteroids, corticotropin.

Increased digitalis and neuromuscular-blocking agent toxicity due to hypokalemia.

Decreased effect: Pharmacologic antagonism may occur with azole antifungal agents (eg, miconazole, ketoconazole).

Pulmonary toxicity has occurred with concomitant administration of amphotericin B and leukocyte transfusions.

Test Interactions Increased BUN (S), serum creatinine, alkaline phosphate, bilirubin; decreased magnesium, potassium (S)

Dosage Forms Injection, powder for reconstitution, as desoxycholate: 50 mg

References

Branch RA, "Prevention of Amphotericin B-Induced Renal Impairment. A Review on the Use of Sodium Supplementation," *Arch Intern Med*, 1988, 148(11):2389-94.

Mora-Duarte J, Betts R, Rotstein C, et al, "Comparison of Caspofungin and Amphotericin B for Invasive Candidiasis," *N Engl J Med*, 2002, 347(25):2020-9.

Rex JH, Walsh TJ, Sobel JD, et al, "Practice Guidelines for the Treatment of Candidiasis. Infectious Diseases Society of America," *Clin Infect Dis*, 2000, 30(4):662-78.

♦ **Amphotericin B Desoxycholate** *see* Amphotericin B (Conventional) *on page 96*

Amphotericin B (Lipid Complex)

(am foe TER i sin bee LIP id KOM pleks)

Medication Safety Issues

Safety issues:

Lipid-based amphotericin formulations (Abelcet®) may be confused with conventional formulations (Amphocin®, Fungizone®)

Large overdoses have occurred when conventional formulations were dispensed inadvertently for lipid-based products. Single daily doses of conventional amphotericin formulation never exceed 1.5 mg/kg.

Related Information

Antifungal Agents *on page 1554*

U.S. Brand Names Abelcet®

Canadian Brand Names Abelcet®; Amphotec®

Synonyms ABLC

Pharmacologic Category Antifungal Agent, Parenteral

Generic Available No

Use Treatment of aspergillosis or any type of progressive fungal infection in patients who are refractory to or intolerant of conventional amphotericin B therapy

Unlabeled/Investigational Use Effective in patients with serious *Candida* species infections

Mechanism of Action Binds to ergosterol altering cell membrane permeability in susceptible fungi and causing leakage of cell components with subsequent cell death. Proposed mechanism suggests that amphotericin causes an oxidation-dependent stimulation of macrophages.

Pharmacodynamics/Kinetics

Distribution: V_d: Increases with higher doses; reflects increased uptake by tissues (131 L/kg with 5 mg/kg/day)

Half-life elimination: ~24 hours

Excretion: Clearance: Increases with higher doses (5 mg/kg/day): 400 mL/hour/kg

Dosage Children and Adults: I.V.:

Premedication: For patients who experience infusion-related immediate reactions, premedicate with the following drugs 30-60 minutes prior to drug administration: A nonsteroidal anti-inflammatory agent ± diphenhydramine **or** acetaminophen with diphenhydramine **or** hydrocortisone 50-100 mg. If the patient experiences rigors during the infusion, meperidine may be administered.

Range: 2.5-5 mg/kg/day as a single infusion

Dosing adjustment in renal impairment: None necessary; effects of renal impairment are not currently known

Hemodialysis: No supplemental dosage necessary

Peritoneal dialysis: No supplemental dosage necessary

Continuous arteriovenous or venovenous hemofiltration: No supplemental dosage necessary

Stability Intact vials should be stored at 2°C to 8°C (35°F to 46°F) and protected from exposure to light; do not freeze intact vials. Solutions for infusion are stable for 48 hours under refrigeration and for 6 hours at room temperature. Shake the vial gently until there is no evidence of any yellow sediment at the bottom. Dilute with D_5W to 1-2 mg/mL. Protect from light.

Do not dilute with saline solutions or mix with other drugs or electrolytes - compatibility has not been established

Do not use an in-line filter during administration.

Administration For patients who experience nonanaphylactic infusion-related reactions, premedicate 30-60 minutes prior to drug administration with a nonsteroidal anti-inflammatory agent ± diphenhydramine **or** acetaminophen with diphenhydramine **or** hydrocortisone 50-100 mg. If the patient experiences rigors during the infusion, meperidine may be administered.

Invert infusion container several times prior to administration and every 2 hours during infusion.

Monitoring Parameters Renal function (monitor frequently during therapy), electrolytes (especially potassium and magnesium), liver function tests, temperature, PT/PTT, CBC; monitor input and output; monitor for signs of hypokalemia (muscle weakness, cramping, drowsiness, ECG changes, etc)

Anesthesia and Critical Care Concerns/Other Considerations This product is significantly more expensive than conventional amphotericin B. The incidence of nephrotoxicity with ABLC appears to be less when compared to

(Continued)

Amphotericin B (Lipid Complex) *(Continued)*

conventional amphotericin B. The incidence of infusion-related reactions does not appear to be decreased with ABLC, but tolerance usually develops. Premedication may be considered to prevent/attenuate infusion-related adverse events. To prevent aggregation of the lipid products, it is important to shake the bag before hanging and once every 2 hours. *In vitro* experiments confirm that liposomal amphotericin B is at least as active as amphotericin B against clinical isolates of *Candida*, *Cryptococcus*, *Blastomyces*, and *Aspergillus*. Their activities also have appeared to be equal against *Fusarium*. Abelcet® may be restricted to patients who cannot tolerate or fail a standard amphotericin B formulation.

Pregnancy Risk Factor B

Contraindications Hypersensitivity to amphotericin or any component of the formulation

Warnings/Precautions Anaphylaxis has been reported with other amphotericin B-containing drugs. Facilities for cardiopulmonary resuscitation should be available during administration due to the possibility of anaphylactic reaction. If severe respiratory distress occurs, the infusion should be immediately discontinued. During the initial dosing, the drug should be administered under close clinical observation. Acute reactions (including fever and chills) may occur 1-2 hours after starting an intravenous infusion. These reactions are usually more common with the first few doses and generally diminish with subsequent doses. Pulmonary reactions may occur in neutropenic patients receiving leukocyte transfusions; separation of the infusions as much as possible is advised.

Adverse Reactions Nephrotoxicity and infusion-related hyperpyrexia, rigor, and chilling are reduced relative to amphotericin deoxycholate.

>10%:
- Central nervous system: Chills, fever
- Renal: Serum creatinine increased
- Miscellaneous: Multiple organ failure

1% to 10%:
- Cardiovascular: Hypotension, cardiac arrest
- Central nervous system: Headache, pain
- Dermatologic: Rash
- Endocrine & metabolic: Bilirubinemia, hypokalemia, acidosis
- Gastrointestinal: Nausea, vomiting, diarrhea, gastrointestinal hemorrhage, abdominal pain
- Renal: Renal failure
- Respiratory: Respiratory failure, dyspnea, pneumonia

Drug Interactions

Increased nephrotoxicity: Aminoglycosides, cyclosporine, other nephrotoxic drugs.

Potentiation of hypokalemia: Corticosteroids, corticotropin.

Increased digitalis and neuromuscular-blocking agent toxicity due to hypokalemia.

Decreased effect: Pharmacologic antagonism may occur with azole antifungal agents (eg, miconazole, ketoconazole).

Pulmonary toxicity has occurred with concomitant administration of amphotericin B and leukocyte transfusions.

Test Interactions Increased BUN (S), serum creatinine, alkaline phosphate, bilirubin; decreased magnesium, potassium (S)

Dosage Forms Injection, suspension [preservative free]: 5 mg/mL (20 mL)

References

Mora-Duarte J, Betts R, Rotstein C, et al, "Comparison of Caspofungin and Amphotericin B for Invasive Candidiasis," *N Engl J Med*, 2002, 347(25):2020-9.

Rex JH, Walsh TJ, Sobel JD, et al, "Practice Guidelines for the Treatment of Candidiasis. Infectious Diseases Society of America," *Clin Infect Dis*, 2000, 30(4):662-78.

Slain D, "Lipid-Based Amphotericin B for the Treatment of Fungal Infections," *Pharmacotherapy*, 1999, 19(3):306-23.

Amphotericin B (Liposomal) (am foe TER i sin bee lye po SO mal)

Medication Safety Issues

Safety issues:

Lipid-based amphotericin formulations (AmBisome®) may be confused with conventional formulations (Amphocin®, Fungizone®)

Large overdoses have occurred when conventional formulations were dispensed inadvertently for lipid-based products. Single daily doses of conventional amphotericin formulation never exceed 1.5 mg/kg.

Related Information

Antifungal Agents *on page 1554*

U.S. Brand Names AmBisome®

Canadian Brand Names AmBisome®

Synonyms L-AmB

Pharmacologic Category Antifungal Agent, Parenteral

Generic Available No

Use Empirical therapy for presumed fungal infection in febrile, neutropenic patients; treatment of patients with *Aspergillus* species, *Candida* species, and/or *Cryptococcus* species infections refractory to amphotericin B desoxycholate, or in patients where renal impairment or unacceptable toxicity precludes the use of amphotericin B desoxycholate; treatment of cryptococcal meningitis in HIV-infected patients; treatment of visceral leishmaniasis

Unlabeled/Investigational Use Effective in patients with serious *Candida* species infections

Mechanism of Action Binds to ergosterol altering cell membrane permeability in susceptible fungi and causing leakage of cell components with subsequent cell death. Proposed mechanism suggests that amphotericin causes an oxidation-dependent stimulation of macrophages.

Pharmacodynamics/Kinetics

Distribution: V_d: 131 L/kg

Half-life elimination: Terminal: 174 hours

Dosage

Usual dosage range:

Children: I.V.: 3-5 mg/kg/day

Adults: I.V.: 2-6 mg/kg/day; **Note:** Higher doses (15 mg/kg/day) have been used clinically.

Note: Premedication: For patients who experience nonanaphylactic infusion-related immediate reactions, premedicate with the following drugs 30-60 minutes prior to drug administration: A nonsteroidal anti-inflammatory agent ± diphenhydramine; **or** acetaminophen with diphenhydramine; **or** hydrocortisone 50-100 mg. If the patient experiences rigors during the infusion, meperidine may be administered.

Indication-specific dosing:

Children: I.V.:

Candidal infection:

Endocarditis: 3-6 mg/kg/day with flucytosine 25-37.5 mg/kg 4 times daily

Meningitis: 5 mg/kg/day with flucytosine 100 mg/kg/day

Cryptococcal meningitis (HIV-positive): 6 mg/kg/day

Note: IDSA guidelines (April, 2000) report doses of 3-6 mg/kg/day, noting that 4 mg/kg/day was effective in a small, open-label trial. The manufacturer's labeled dose of 6 mg/kg/day was approved in June, 2000.

Empiric therapy: 3 mg/kg/day

Systemic fungal infections *(Aspergillus, Candida, Cryptococcus)*: 3-5 mg/kg/day

Visceral leishmaniasis:

Immunocompetent: 3 mg/kg/day on days 1-5, and 3 mg/kg/day on days 14 and 21; a repeat course may be given in patients who do not achieve parasitic clearance

Note: Alternate regimen of 10 mg/kg/day for 2 days has been reportedly effective.

Immunocompromised: 4 mg/kg/day on days 1-5, and 4 mg/kg/day on days 10, 17, 24, 31, and 38

Adults: I.V.:

Candidal infection:

Endocarditis: 3-6 mg/kg/day with flucytosine 25-37.5 mg/kg 4 times daily

Meningitis: 5 mg/kg/day with flucytosine 100 mg/kg/day

Cryptococcal meningitis (HIV-positive): 6 mg/kg/day

Note: IDSA guidelines (April, 2000) report doses of 3-6 mg/kg/day, noting that 4 mg/kg/day was effective in a small, open-label trial. The manufacturer's labeled dose of 6 mg/kg/day was approved in June, 2000.

Empiric therapy: 3 mg/kg/day

Fungal sinusitis: 5-7.5 mg/kg/day

(Continued)

Amphotericin B (Liposomal) *(Continued)*

Note: Use azole antifungal if causative organism is *Pseudallescheria boydii* (*Scedosporium* sp).

Systemic fungal infections *(Aspergillus, Candida, Cryptococcus)*: 3-5 mg/kg/day

Visceral leishmaniasis:

Immunocompetent: 3 mg/kg/day on days 1-5, and 3 mg/kg/day on days 14 and 21; a repeat course may be given in patients who do not achieve parasitic clearance

Note: Alternate regimen of 2 mg/kg/day for 5 days has been reportedly effective.

Immunocompromised: 4 mg/kg/day on days 1-5, and 4 mg/kg/day on days 10, 17, 24, 31, and 38

Dosing adjustment in renal impairment: None necessary; effects of renal impairment are not currently known

Hemodialysis: No supplemental dosage necessary

Peritoneal dialysis effects: No supplemental dosage necessary

Continuous arteriovenous or venovenous hemofiltration: No supplemental dosage necessary

Stability Unopened vials should be refrigerated at 2°C to 8°C (36°F to 46°F). Vials reconstituted with SWFI are stable for 24 hours under refrigeration. Infusion should begin with 6 hours of dilution with D_5W.

Reconstitution: Add 12 mL SWFI to vial. The use of any solution other than those recommended, or the presence of a bacteriostatic agent in the solution, may cause precipitation. **Shake the vial vigorously** for 30 seconds.

Filtration and dilution: The 5-micron filter should be on the syringe used to remove the reconstituted AmBisome®. Dilute to a final concentration of 1-2 mg/mL (0.2-0.5 mg/mL for infants and small children).

Administration Administer via intravenous infusion, over a period of approximately 2 hours. Infusion time may be reduced to approximately 1 hour in patients in whom the treatment is well-tolerated. If the patient experiences discomfort during infusion, the duration of infusion may be increased. Administer at a rate of 2.5 mg/kg/hour. Existing intravenous line should be flushed with D_5W prior to infusion (if not feasible, administer through a separate line). An in-line membrane filter (not less than 1 micron) may be used.

Monitoring Parameters Renal function (monitor frequently during therapy), electrolytes (especially potassium and magnesium), liver function tests, temperature, PT/PTT, CBC; monitor input and output; monitor for signs of hypokalemia (muscle weakness, cramping, drowsiness, ECG changes, etc)

Anesthesia and Critical Care Concerns/Other Considerations This product is significantly more expensive than conventional amphotericin B; Infectious Disease consult is recommended. AmBisome® is a true single bilayer liposomal drug delivery system. Liposomes are closed, spherical vesicles created by mixing specific proportions of amphophilic substances such as phospholipids and cholesterol so that they arrange themselves into multiple concentric bilayer membranes when hydrated in aqueous solutions. Single bilayer liposomes are then formed by microemulsification of multilamellar vesicles using a homogenizer. AmBisome® consists of these unilamellar bilayer liposomes with amphotericin B intercalated within the membrane. Due to the nature and quantity of amphophilic substances used, and the lipophilic moiety in the amphotericin B molecule, the drug is an integral part of the overall structure of the AmBisome® liposomes. AmBisome® contains true liposomes that are <100 nm in diameter.

Pregnancy Risk Factor B

Contraindications Hypersensitivity to amphotericin B or any component of the formulation

Warnings/Precautions Although amphotericin B (liposomal) has been shown to be significantly less toxic than amphotericin B desoxycholate, adverse events may still occur. Patients should be under close clinical observation during initial dosing. As with other amphotericin B-containing products, anaphylaxis has been reported. Facilities for cardiopulmonary resuscitation should be available during administration. Acute reactions (including fever and chills) may occur 1-2 hours after starting infusions; reactions are more common with the first few doses and generally diminish with subsequent doses. Immediately discontinue infusion if severe respiratory distress occurs; the patient should not receive further infusions. Safety and efficacy have not been established in patients <1 year of age.

Adverse Reactions Percentage of adverse reactions is dependent upon population studied and may vary with respect to premedications and underlying illness. Incidence of decreased renal function and infusion-related events are lower than rates observed with amphotericin B deoxycholate.

>10%:

Cardiovascular: Peripheral edema (15%), edema (12% to 14%), tachycardia (9% to 18%), hypotension (7% to 14%), hypertension (8% to 20%), chest pain (8% to 12%), hypervolemia (8% to 12%)

Central nervous system: Chills (29% to 48%), insomnia (17% to 22%), headache (9% to 20%), anxiety (7% to 14%), pain (14%), confusion (9% to 13%)

Dermatologic: Rash (5% to 25%), pruritus (11%)

Endocrine & metabolic: Hypokalemia (31% to 51%), hypomagnesemia (15% to 50%), hyperglycemia (8% to 23%), hypocalcemia (5% to 18%), hyponatremia (8% to 12%)

Gastrointestinal: Nausea (16% to 40%), vomiting (10% to 32%), diarrhea (11% to 30%), abdominal pain (7% to 20%), constipation (15%), anorexia (10% to 14%)

Hematologic: Anemia (27% to 48%), blood transfusion reaction (9% to 18%), leukopenia (15% to 17%), thrombocytopenia (6% to 13%)

Hepatic: Alkaline phosphatase increased (7% to 22%), BUN increased (7% to 21%), bilirubinemia (9% to 18%), ALT increased (15%), AST increased (13%), liver function tests abnormal (not specified) (4% to 13%)

Local: Phlebitis (9% to 11%)

Neuromuscular & skeletal: Weakness (6% to 13%), back pain (12%)

Renal: Creatinine increased (18% to 40%), hematuria (14%)

Respiratory: Dyspnea (18% to 23%), lung disorder (14% to 18%), cough increased (2% to 18%), epistaxis (8% to 15%), pleural effusion (12%), rhinitis (11%)

Miscellaneous: Sepsis (7% to 14%), infection (11% to 12%)

2% to 10% (Limited to important or life-threatening):

Cardiovascular: Arrhythmia, atrial fibrillation, bradycardia, cardiac arrest, cardiomegaly, postural hypotension

Central nervous system: Agitation, coma, convulsion, depression, dizziness (7% to 8%), hallucinations, malaise, somnolence

Dermatologic: Alopecia, rash, petechia, purpura, skin discoloration, urticaria

Endocrine & metabolic: Acidosis, hypernatremia (4%), hyperchloremia, hyperkalemia, hypermagnesemia, hyperphosphatemia, hypophosphatemia

Gastrointestinal: Gastrointestinal hemorrhage (10%), hematemesis, gum/oral hemorrhage, ileus, ulcerative stomatitis

Genitourinary: Vaginal hemorrhage

Hematologic: Coagulation disorder, hemorrhage, prothrombin decreased, thrombocytopenia

Hepatic: Hepatocellular damage, veno-occlusive liver disease

Local: Injection site inflammation

Neuromuscular & skeletal: Arthralgia, bone pain, dystonia, paresthesia, rigors, tremor

Ocular: Conjunctivitis, eye hemorrhage

Renal: Acute kidney failure, toxic nephropathy

Respiratory: Asthma, atelectasis, hemoptysis, pulmonary edema, respiratory alkalosis, respiratory failure, hypoxia (6% to 8%)

Miscellaneous: Allergic reaction, cell-mediated immunological reaction, flu-like syndrome, procedural complication (8% to 10%), diaphoresis (7%)

<1% (Limited to important or life-threatening): Agranulocytosis, angioedema, cyanosis/hypoventilation, erythema, hemorrhagic cystitis, pulmonary edema, urticaria

Overdosage/Toxicology The toxicity due to overdose has not been defined. Repeated daily doses up to 7.5 mg/kg have been administered in clinical trials with no reported dose-related toxicity. If overdosage should occur, cease administration immediately. Symptomatic supportive measures should be instituted. Particular attention should be given to monitoring renal function.

Drug Interactions

Increased nephrotoxicity: Aminoglycosides, cyclosporine, other nephrotoxic drugs.

Potentiation of hypokalemia: Corticosteroids, corticotropin.

Increased digitalis and neuromuscular-blocking agent toxicity due to hypokalemia.

(Continued)

Amphotericin B (Liposomal) *(Continued)*

Decreased effect: Pharmacologic antagonism may occur with azole antifungal agents (eg, miconazole, ketoconazole).

Pulmonary toxicity has occurred with concomitant administration of amphotericin B and leukocyte transfusions.

Dosage Forms

Injection, powder for reconstitution:

AmBisome®: 50 mg [contains soy and sucrose]

References

Mora-Duarte J, Betts R, Rotstein C, et al, "Comparison of Caspofungin and Amphotericin B for Invasive Candidiasis," *N Engl J Med*, 2002, 347(25):2020-9.

Rex JH, Walsh TJ, Sobel JD, et al, "Practice Guidelines for the Treatment of Candidiasis. Infectious Diseases Society of America," *Clin Infect Dis*, 2000, 30(4):662-78.

Slain D, "Lipid-Based Amphotericin B for the Treatment of Fungal Infections," *Pharmacotherapy*, 1999, 19(3):306-23.

Ampicillin (am pi SIL in)

Medication Safety Issues

Sound-alike/look-alike issues:

Ampicillin may be confused with aminophylline

Related Information

Anesthesia for Patients With Liver Disease *on page 1421*

Prevention of Bacterial Endocarditis *on page 1583*

U.S. Brand Names Principen®

Canadian Brand Names Apo-Ampi®; Novo-Ampicillin; Nu-Ampi

Synonyms Aminobenzylpenicillin; Ampicillin Sodium; Ampicillin Trihydrate

Pharmacologic Category Antibiotic, Penicillin

Generic Available Yes

Use Treatment of susceptible bacterial infections (nonbeta-lactamase-producing organisms); susceptible bacterial infections caused by streptococci, pneumococci, nonpenicillinase-producing staphylococci, *Listeria*, meningococci; some strains of *H. influenzae*, *Salmonella*, *Shigella*, *E. coli*, *Enterobacter*, and *Klebsiella*

Mechanism of Action Inhibits bacterial cell wall synthesis by binding to one or more of the penicillin-binding proteins (PBPs) which in turn inhibits the final transpeptidation step of peptidoglycan synthesis in bacterial cell walls, thus inhibiting cell wall biosynthesis. Bacteria eventually lyse due to ongoing activity of cell wall autolytic enzymes (autolysins and murein hydrolases) while cell wall assembly is arrested.

Pharmacodynamics/Kinetics

Absorption: Oral: 50%

Distribution: Bile, blister, and tissue fluids; penetration into CSF occurs with inflamed meninges only, good only with inflammation (exceeds usual MICs)

Normal meninges: Nil; Inflamed meninges: 5% to 10%

Protein binding: 15% to 25%

Half-life elimination:

Children and Adults: 1-1.8 hours

Anuria/end-stage renal disease: 7-20 hours

Time to peak: Oral: Within 1-2 hours

Excretion: Urine (~90% as unchanged drug) within 24 hours

Dosage

Usual dosage range:

Infants and Children:

Oral: 50-100 mg/kg/day in doses divided every 6 hours (maximum: 2-4 g/day)

I.M., I.V.: 100-400 mg/kg/day in divided doses every 6 hours (maximum: 12 g/day)

Adults: Oral, I.M., I.V.: 250-500 mg every 6 hours

Indication-specific dosing:

Infants and Children:

Endocarditis prophylaxis:

Dental, oral, respiratory tract, or esophageal procedures: I.M., I.V.: 50 mg/kg within 30 minutes prior to procedure in patients unable to take oral amoxicillin

Genitourinary and gastrointestinal tract (except esophageal) procedures:
I.M., I.V.:
High-risk patients: 50 mg/kg (maximum: 2 g) within 30 minutes prior to procedure, followed by ampicillin 25 mg/kg (or amoxicillin 25 mg/kg orally) 6 hours later; must be used in combination with gentamicin.
Moderate-risk patients: 50 mg/kg within 30 minutes prior to procedure

Mild-to-moderate infections:
Oral: 50-100 mg/kg/day in doses divided every 6 hours (maximum: 2-4 g/day)
I.M., I.V.: 100-150 mg/kg/day in divided doses every 6 hours (maximum: 2-4 g/day)

Severe infections, meningitis: I.M., I.V.: 200-400 mg/kg/day in divided doses every 6 hours (maximum: 6-12 g/day)

Adults:
Actinomycosis: I.V.: 50 mg/kg/day for 4-6 weeks then oral amoxicillin
Cholangitis (acute): I.V.: 2 g every 4 hours with gentamicin
Diverticulitis: I.M., I.V.: 2 g every 6 hours with metronidazole
Endocarditis:
Infective: I.V.: 12 g/day via continuous infusion or divided every 4 hours
Prophylaxis: Dental, oral, respiratory tract, or esophageal procedures: I.M., I.V.: 2 g within 30 minutes prior to procedure in patients unable to take oral amoxicillin
Genitourinary and gastrointestinal tract (except esophageal) procedures:
High-risk patients: I.M., I.V.: 2 g within 30 minutes prior to procedure, followed by ampicillin 1 g (or amoxicillin 1g orally) 6 hours later; must be used in combination with gentamicin.
Moderate-risk patients: I.M., I.V.: 2 g within 30 minutes prior to procedure

Group B strep prophylaxis (intrapartum): I.V.: 2 g initial dose, then 1 g every 4 hours until delivery
***Listeria* infections:** I.V.: 200 mg/kg/day divided every 6 hours
Sepsis/meningitis: I.M., I.V.: 150-250 mg/kg/day divided every 3-4 hours (range: 6-12 g/day)
Urinary tract infections (enterococcus suspected): I.V.: 1-2 g every 6 hours with gentamicin

Dosing interval in renal impairment:
Cl_{cr} >50 mL/minute: Administer every 6 hours
Cl_{cr} 10-50 mL/minute: Administer every 6-12 hours
Cl_{cr} <10 mL/minute: Administer every 12-24 hours

Hemodialysis: Moderately dialyzable (20% to 50%); administer dose after dialysis
Peritoneal dialysis: Moderately dialyzable (20% to 50%)
Administer 250 mg every 12 hours
Continuous arteriovenous or venovenous hemofiltration effects: Dose as for Cl_{cr} 10-50 mL/minute; ~50 mg of ampicillin per liter of filtrate is removed

Stability
Oral: Oral suspension is stable for 7 days at room temperature or for 14 days under refrigeration.
I.V.:
Solutions for I.M. or direct I.V. should be used within 1 hour. Solutions for I.V. infusion will be inactivated by dextrose at room temperature. If dextrose-containing solutions are to be used, the resultant solution will only be stable for 2 hours versus 8 hours in the 0.9% sodium chloride injection. D_5W has limited stability.
Stability of parenteral admixture in NS at room temperature (25°C) is 8 hours.
Stability of parenteral admixture in NS at refrigeration temperature (4°C) is 2 days.
Standard diluent: 500 mg/50 mL NS; 1 g/50 mL NS; 2 g/100 mL NS

Administration Administer around-the-clock to promote less variation in peak and trough serum levels.
Oral: Administer on an empty stomach (ie, 1 hour prior to, or 2 hours after meals) to increase total absorption.
I.V.: Administer over 3-5 minutes (125-500 mg) or over 10-15 minutes (1-2 g). More rapid infusion may cause seizures. Ampicillin and gentamicin should not be mixed in the same I.V. tubing.
Some penicillins (eg, carbenicillin, ticarcillin, and piperacillin) have been shown to inactivate aminoglycosides *in vitro*. This has been observed to a greater extent with tobramycin and gentamicin, while amikacin has shown greater stability against inactivation. Concurrent use of these agents may pose a risk of reduced

(Continued)

Ampicillin *(Continued)*

antibacterial efficacy *in vivo*, particularly in the setting of profound renal impairment. However, definitive clinical evidence is lacking. If combination penicillin/aminoglycoside therapy is desired in a patient with renal dysfunction, separation of doses (if feasible), and routine monitoring of aminoglycoside levels, CBC, and clinical response should be considered.

Monitoring Parameters With prolonged therapy, monitor renal, hepatic, and hematologic function periodically; observe signs and symptoms of anaphylaxis during first dose

Pregnancy Risk Factor B

Contraindications Hypersensitivity to ampicillin, any component of the formulation, or other penicillins

Warnings/Precautions Dosage adjustment may be necessary in patients with renal impairment. A low incidence of cross-allergy with other beta-lactams exists. High percentage of patients with infectious mononucleosis have developed rash during therapy with ampicillin. Appearance of a rash should be carefully evaluated to differentiate a nonallergic ampicillin rash from a hypersensitivity reaction. Ampicillin rash occurs in 5% to 10% of children receiving ampicillin and is a generalized dull red, maculopapular rash, generally appearing 3-14 days after the start of therapy. It normally begins on the trunk and spreads over most of the body. It may be most intense at pressure areas, elbows, and knees.

Adverse Reactions Frequency not defined.

Central nervous system: Fever, penicillin encephalopathy, seizure

Dermatologic: Erythema multiforme, exfoliative dermatitis, rash, urticaria

Note: Appearance of a rash should be carefully evaluated to differentiate (if possible) nonallergic ampicillin rash from hypersensitivity reaction. Incidence is higher in patients with viral infection, *Salmonella* infection, lymphocytic leukemia, or patients that have hyperuricemia.

Gastrointestinal: Black hairy tongue, diarrhea, enterocolitis, glossitis, nausea, pseudomembranous colitis, sore mouth or tongue, stomatitis, vomiting

Hematologic: Agranulocytosis, anemia, hemolytic anemia, eosinophilia, leukopenia, thrombocytopenia purpura

Hepatic: AST increased

Renal: Interstitial nephritis (rare)

Respiratory: Laryngeal stridor

Miscellaneous: Anaphylaxis, serum sickness-like reaction

Overdosage/Toxicology Symptoms of penicillin overdose include neuromuscular hypersensitivity (eg, agitation, hallucinations, asterixis, encephalopathy, confusion, and seizures). Electrolyte imbalance may occur if the preparation contains potassium or sodium salts, especially in renal failure. Hemodialysis may be helpful to aid in removal of the drug from blood; otherwise, treatment is supportive or symptom-directed.

Drug Interactions

Allopurinol: Theoretically has an additive potential for ampicillin/amoxicillin rash.

Aminoglycosides: May be synergistic against selected organisms.

Methotrexate: Penicillins may increase the exposure to methotrexate during concurrent therapy; monitor.

Oral contraceptives: Anecdotal reports suggesting decreased contraceptive efficacy with penicillins have been refuted by more rigorous scientific and clinical data.

Probenecid, disulfiram: May increase levels of penicillins (ampicillin).

Warfarin: Effects of warfarin may be increased.

Ethanol/Nutrition/Herb Interactions Food: Food decreases ampicillin absorption rate; may decrease ampicillin serum concentration.

Test Interactions May interfere with urinary glucose tests using cupric sulfate (Benedict's solution, Clinitest®)

Some penicillin derivatives may accelerate the degradation of aminoglycosides *in vitro*, leading to a potential underestimation of aminoglycoside serum concentration.

Dietary Considerations Take on an empty stomach 1 hour before or 2 hours after meals.

Sodium content of 5 mL suspension (250 mg/5 mL): 10 mg (0.4 mEq)

Sodium content of 1 g: 66.7 mg (3 mEq)

Dosage Forms

Capsule (Principen®): 250 mg, 500 mg

Injection, powder for reconstitution, as sodium: 125 mg, 250 mg, 500 mg, 1 g, 2 g, 10 g
Powder for oral suspension (Principen®): 125 mg/5 mL (100 mL, 200 mL); 250 mg/5 mL (100 mL, 200 mL)

Ampicillin and Sulbactam (am pi SIL in & SUL bak tam)

U.S. Brand Names Unasyn®
Canadian Brand Names Unasyn®
Synonyms Sulbactam and Ampicillin
Pharmacologic Category Antibiotic, Penicillin
Generic Available Yes
Use Treatment of susceptible bacterial infections involved with skin and skin structure, intra-abdominal infections, gynecological infections; spectrum is that of ampicillin plus organisms producing beta-lactamases such as *S. aureus*, *H. influenzae*, *E. coli*, *Klebsiella*, *Acinetobacter*, *Enterobacter*, and anaerobes
Mechanism of Action The addition of sulbactam, a beta-lactamase inhibitor, to ampicillin extends the spectrum of ampicillin to include some beta-lactamase-producing organisms; inhibits bacterial cell wall synthesis by binding to one or more of the penicillin-binding proteins (PBPs) which in turn inhibits the final transpeptidation step of peptidoglycan synthesis in bacterial cell walls, thus inhibiting cell wall biosynthesis. Bacteria eventually lyse due to ongoing activity of cell wall autolytic enzymes (autolysins and murein hydrolases) while cell wall assembly is arrested.

Pharmacodynamics/Kinetics
Ampicillin: See Ampicillin.
Sulbactam:
Distribution: Bile, blister, and tissue fluids
Protein binding: 38%
Half-life elimination: Normal renal function: 1-1.3 hours
Excretion: Urine (~75% to 85% as unchanged drug) within 8 hours

Dosage Note: Unasyn® (ampicillin/sulbactam) is a combination product. Dosage recommendations for Unasyn® are based on the ampicillin component.
Usual dosage range:
Children ≥1 year: I.V.: 100-400 mg ampicillin/kg/day divided every 6 hours (maximum: 8 g ampicillin/day, 12 g Unasyn®). **Note:** The American Academy of Pediatrics recommends a dose of up to 300 mg/kg/day for severe infection in infants >1 month of age.
Adults: I.M., I.V.: 1-2 g ampicillin (1.5-3 g Unasyn®) every 6 hours (maximum: 8 g ampicillin/day, 12 g Unasyn®)
Indication-specific dosing:
Children:
Epiglottitis: I.V.: 100-200 mg ampicillin/kg/day divided in 4 doses
Mild-to-moderate infections: I.M., I.V.: 100-200 mg ampicillin/kg/day (150-300 mg Unasyn®) divided every 6 hours (maximum: 8 g ampicillin/day, 12 g Unasyn®)
Peritonsillar and retropharyngeal abscess: I.V.: 50 mg ampicillin/kg/dose every 6 hours
Severe infections: I.M., I.V.: 200-400 mg ampicillin/kg/day divided every 6 hours (maximum: 8 g ampicillin/day, 12 g Unasyn®)
Adults: Doses expressed as ampicillin/sulbactam combination:
Amnionitis, cholangitis, diverticulitis, endometritis, endophthalmitis, epididymitis/orchitis, liver abscess, osteomyelitis (diabetic foot), peritonitis: I.V.: 3 g every 6 hours
Endocarditis: I.V.: 3 g every 6 hours with gentamicin or vancomycin for 4-6 weeks
Orbital cellulitis: I.V.: 1.5 g every 6 hours
Parapharyngeal space infections: I.V.: 3 g every 6 hours
***Pasteurella multocida* (human, canine/feline bites):** I.V.: 1.5-3 g every 6 hours
Pelvic inflammatory disease: I.V.: 3 g every 6 hours with doxycycline
Peritonitis (CAPD): Intraperitoneal:
Anuric, intermittent: 3 g every 12 hours
Anuric, continuous: Loading dose: 1.5 g; maintenance dose: 150 mg
Pneumonia:
Aspiration, community-acquired: I.V.: 1.5-3 g every 6 hours

(Continued)

Ampicillin and Sulbactam *(Continued)*

Hospital-acquired: I.V.: 3 g every 6 hours

Urinary tract infections, pyelonephritis: I.V.: 3 g every 6 hours for 14 days

Dosing interval in renal impairment:

Cl_{cr} 15-29 mL/minute: Administer every 12 hours

Cl_{cr} 5-14 mL/minute: Administer every 24 hours

Stability Prior to reconstitution, store at ≤30°C (86°F).

I.M. and direct I.V. administration: Use within 1 hour after preparation. Reconstitute with sterile water for injection or 0.5% or 2% lidocaine hydrochloride injection (I.M.). Sodium chloride 0.9% (NS) is the diluent of choice for I.V. piggyback use. Solutions made in NS are stable up to 72 hours when refrigerated whereas dextrose solutions (same concentration) are stable for only 4 hours

Administration Administer around-the-clock to promote less variation in peak and trough serum levels. Administer by slow injection over 10-15 minutes or I.V. over 15-30 minutes. Ampicillin and gentamicin should not be mixed in the same I.V. tubing.

Some penicillins (eg, carbenicillin, ticarcillin, and piperacillin) have been shown to inactivate aminoglycosides *in vitro*. This has been observed to a greater extent with tobramycin and gentamicin, while amikacin has shown greater stability against inactivation. Concurrent use of these agents may pose a risk of reduced antibacterial efficacy *in vivo*, particularly in the setting of profound renal impairment. However, definitive clinical evidence is lacking. If combination penicillin/aminoglycoside therapy is desired in a patient with renal dysfunction, separation of doses (if feasible), and routine monitoring of aminoglycoside levels, CBC, and clinical response should be considered.

Monitoring Parameters With prolonged therapy, monitor hematologic, renal, and hepatic function; monitor for signs of anaphylaxis during first dose

Pregnancy Risk Factor B

Contraindications Hypersensitivity to ampicillin, sulbactam, penicillins, or any component of the formulations

Warnings/Precautions Dosage adjustment may be necessary in patients with renal impairment. A low incidence of cross-allergy with other beta-lactams exists. High percentage of patients with infectious mononucleosis have developed rash during therapy with ampicillin. Appearance of a rash should be carefully evaluated to differentiate a nonallergic ampicillin rash from a hypersensitivity reaction. Ampicillin rash occurs in 5% to 10% of children receiving ampicillin and is a generalized dull red, maculopapular rash, generally appearing 3-14 days after the start of therapy. It normally begins on the trunk and spreads over most of the body. It may be most intense at pressure areas, elbows, and knees.

Adverse Reactions Also see Ampicillin.

>10%: Local: Pain at injection site (I.M.)

1% to 10%:

Dermatologic: Rash

Gastrointestinal: Diarrhea

Local: Pain at injection site (I.V.), thrombophlebitis

Miscellaneous: Allergic reaction (may include serum sickness, urticaria, bronchospasm, hypotension, etc)

<1% (Limited to important or life-threatening): Abdominal distension, candidiasis, chest pain, chills, dysuria, edema, epistaxis, erythema, facial swelling, fatigue, flatulence, glossitis, hairy tongue, headache, interstitial nephritis, itching, liver enzymes increased, malaise, mucosal bleeding, nausea, pseudomembranous colitis, seizure, substernal pain, throat tightness, thrombocytopenia, urine retention, vomiting

Overdosage/Toxicology Symptoms of penicillin overdose include neuromuscular hypersensitivity (eg, agitation, hallucinations, asterixis, encephalopathy, confusion, and seizures). Electrolyte imbalance may occur if the preparation contains potassium or sodium salts, especially in renal failure. Hemodialysis may be helpful to aid in removal of the drug from blood; otherwise, treatment is supportive or symptom-directed.

Drug Interactions

Allopurinol: Theoretically has an additive potential for ampicillin/amoxicillin rash.

Aminoglycosides: May be synergistic against selected organisms.

Methotrexate: Penicillins may increase the exposure to methotrexate during concurrent therapy; monitor.

Oral contraceptives: Anecdotal reports suggesting decreased contraceptive efficacy with penicillins have been refuted by more rigorous scientific and clinical data.

Probenecid, disulfiram: May increase levels of penicillins (ampicillin).

Warfarin: Effects of warfarin may be increased.

Test Interactions May interfere with urinary glucose tests using cupric sulfate (Benedict's solution, Clinitest®).

Some penicillin derivatives may accelerate the degradation of aminoglycosides. *in vitro*, leading to a potential underestimation of aminoglycoside serum concentration.

Dietary Considerations Sodium content of 1.5 g injection: 115 mg (5 mEq)

Dosage Forms Injection, powder for reconstitution (Unasyn®): 1.5 g [ampicillin sodium 1 g and sulbactam sodium 0.5 g]; 3 g [ampicillin sodium 2 g and sulbactam sodium 1 g]; 15 g [ampicillin sodium 10 g and sulbactam sodium 5 g] [bulk package]

◆ **Ampicillin Sodium** *see* Ampicillin *on page 104*

◆ **Ampicillin Trihydrate** *see* Ampicillin *on page 104*

Amprenavir (am PREN a veer)

U.S. Brand Names Agenerase®

Canadian Brand Names Agenerase®

Pharmacologic Category Antiretroviral Agent, Protease Inhibitor

Generic Available No

Use Treatment of HIV infections in combination with at least two other antiretroviral agents; oral solution should only be used when capsules or other protease inhibitors are not therapeutic options

Mechanism of Action Binds to the protease activity site and inhibits the activity of the enzyme. HIV protease is required for the cleavage of viral polyprotein precursors into individual functional proteins found in infectious HIV. Inhibition prevents cleavage of these polyproteins, resulting in the formation of immature, noninfectious viral particles.

Pharmacodynamics/Kinetics

Absorption: 63%

Distribution: 430 L

Protein binding: 90%

Metabolism: Hepatic via CYP (primarily CYP3A4)

Bioavailability: Not established; increased sixfold with high-fat meal; oral solution: 86% relative to capsule formulation (14% less bioavailable than capsule)

Half-life elimination: 7.1-10.6 hours

Time to peak: 1-2 hours

Excretion: Feces (75%, ~68% as metabolites); urine (14% as metabolites)

Dosage Oral: **Note:** Capsule and oral solution are **not** interchangeable on a mg-per-mg basis.

Capsule:

Children 4-12 years **or** 13-16 years (<50 kg): 20 mg/kg twice daily or 15 mg/kg 3 times daily; maximum: 2400 mg/day

Children >13 years (≥50 kg) and Adults: 1200 mg twice daily

Note: Dosage adjustments for amprenavir when administered in combination therapy:

Efavirenz: Adjustments necessary for both agents:

Amprenavir 1200 mg 3 times/day (single protease inhibitor) **or**

Amprenavir 1200 mg twice daily plus ritonavir 200 mg twice daily

Ritonavir: Adjustments necessary for both agents:

Amprenavir 1200 mg plus ritonavir 200 mg once daily **or**

Amprenavir 600 mg plus ritonavir 100 mg twice daily

Note: Oral solution of ritonavir and amprenavir should not be coadministered.

Solution:

Children 4-12 years **or** 13-16 years (<50 kg): 22.5 mg/kg twice daily or 17 mg/kg 3 times daily; maximum: 2800 mg/day

Children >13 years (≥50 kg) and Adults: 1400 mg twice daily

Dosage adjustment in renal impairment: Oral solution is contraindicated in renal failure.

(Continued)

Amprenavir *(Continued)*

Dosage adjustment in hepatic impairment:

Child-Pugh score between 5-8:

Capsule: 450 mg twice daily

Solution: 513 mg twice daily; contraindicated in hepatic failure

Child-Pugh score between 9-12:

Capsule: 300 mg twice daily

Solution: 342 mg twice daily; contraindicated in hepatic failure

Anesthesia and Critical Care Concerns/Other Considerations Propylene glycol is included in the oral solution; a dose of 22.5 mg/kg twice daily corresponds to an intake of 1650 mg/kg of propylene glycol. Capsule and oral solution are not interchangeable on a mg-per-mg basis.

Pregnancy Risk Factor C

Contraindications Hypersensitivity to amprenavir or any component of the formulation; concurrent therapy with cisapride, ergot derivatives, midazolam, pimozide, and triazolam; severe previous allergic reaction to sulfonamides; oral solution is contraindicated in infants or children <4 years of age, pregnant women, patients with renal or hepatic failure, and patients receiving concurrent metronidazole or disulfiram

Warnings/Precautions Because of hepatic metabolism and effect on cytochrome P450 enzymes, amprenavir should be used with caution in combination with other agents metabolized by this system (see Contraindications and Drug Interactions). Avoid use of lovastatin or simvastatin (risk of rhabdomyolysis may be increased). Avoid concurrent use of hormonal contraceptives, rifampin, and/or St John's wort (may lead to loss of virologic response and/or resistance). New onset or worsening diabetes mellitus and hyperglycemia have been reported, including cases of diabetic ketoacidosis; use with caution in patients with impaired glucose control. Use with caution in patients with sulfonamide allergy, hepatic impairment, or hemophilia. Redistribution of fat may occur (eg, buffalo hump, peripheral wasting, cushingoid appearance). Immune reconstitution syndrome may develop resulting in the occurrence of an inflammatory response to an indolent or residual opportunistic infection; further evaluation and treatment may be required.

Amprenavir formulations contain vitamin E; additional vitamin E supplements should be avoided. **[U.S. Boxed Warning]: Certain ethnic populations (Asians, Eskimos, Native Americans) may be at increased risk of propylene glycol-associated adverse effects; use of the oral solution of amprenavir should be avoided.** Use oral solution only when capsules or other protease inhibitors are not options. Dosage adjustment is required for combination therapy with amprenavir and ritonavir; in addition, the risk of hyperlipidemia may be increased during concurrent therapy. Safety and efficacy in children <4 years of age have not been established.

Adverse Reactions

>10%:

Central nervous system: Depression/mood disorder (9% to 16%), paresthesia (peripheral 10% to 14%)

Dermatologic: Rash (20% to 27%)

Endocrine & metabolic: Hyperglycemia (>160 mg/dL: 37% to 41%), hypertriglyceridemia (>399 mg/dL: 36% to 47%; >750 mg/dL: 8% to 13%)

Gastrointestinal: Nausea (43% to 74%), vomiting (24% to 34%), diarrhea (39% to 60%), abdominal symptoms

Miscellaneous: Perioral tingling/numbness (26% to 31%)

1% to 10%:

Central nervous system: Headache, fatigue

Dermatologic: Stevens-Johnson syndrome (1% of total, 4% of patients who develop a rash)

Endocrine & metabolic: Hypercholesterolemia (>260 mg/dL: 4% to 9%), hyperglycemia (>251 mg/dL: 2% to 3%), fat redistribution

Gastrointestinal: Taste disorders (2% to 10%), amylase increased (3% to 4%)

Hepatic: AST increased (3% to 5%), ALT increased (4%)

<1% (Limited to important or life-threatening): New-onset diabetes

Overdosage/Toxicology Monitor for signs and symptoms of propylene glycol toxicity if the oral solution is administered.

Drug Interactions **Substrate** of CYP2C9 (minor), 3A4 (major); **Inhibits** CYP2C19 (weak), 3A4 (strong)

Antacids, didanosine (buffered formulation): May decrease serum concentrations of amprenavir. Administer amprenavir 1 hour before or after didanosine.
Antiarrhythmics: Amprenavir may increase serum concentrations/toxicity of several antiarrhythmic agents. Use extreme caution with amiodarone, bepridil, lidocaine, and quinidine.
Anticonvulsants (phenytoin, phenobarbital, carbamazepine): May decrease serum concentrations of amprenavir.
Benzodiazepines (alprazolam, clorazepate, diazepam, flurazepam, midazolam, triazolam) toxicity may be increased; concurrent use of midazolam and triazolam is specifically contraindicated.
Calcium channel blockers: Amprenavir may increase serum concentrations/effects.
Cisapride: Amprenavir may increase serum concentrations of cisapride, increasing the risk of malignant arrhythmias; use is contraindicated.
Clarithromycin: May increase serum concentrations of amprenavir.
CYP3A4 inducers: CYP3A4 inducers may decrease the levels/effects of amprenavir. Example inducers include aminoglutethimide, carbamazepine, nafcillin, nevirapine, phenobarbital, phenytoin, and rifamycins.
CYP3A4 substrates: Amprenavir may increase the levels/effects of CYP3A4 substrates. Example substrates include benzodiazepines, calcium channel blockers, mirtazapine, nateglinide, nefazodone, tacrolimus, and venlafaxine. Selected benzodiazepines (midazolam and triazolam), cisapride, ergot alkaloids, selected HMG-CoA reductase inhibitors (lovastatin and simvastatin), and pimozide are generally contraindicated with strong CYP3A4 inhibitors.
Delavirdine: Amprenavir decreases the serum concentrations of delavirdine; may lead to loss of virologic response and possible resistance to delavirdine. Concomitant use is not recommended.
Disulfiram: Concurrent use with amprenavir oral solution is contraindicated due to risk of propylene glycol toxicity.
Efavirenz: May decrease serum concentrations of amprenavir.
Ergot alkaloids (dihydroergotamine, ergotamine, ergonovine, methylergonovine): Toxicity (peripheral ischemia, vasospasm) is increased by amprenavir; concurrent use is contraindicated.
HMG-CoA reductase inhibitors (atorvastatin, cerivastatin, lovastatin, simvastatin) serum concentrations may be increased by amprenavir, increasing the risk of myopathy/rhabdomyolysis. Lovastatin and simvastatin are not recommended. Use lowest possible dose of atorvastatin. Fluvastatin and pravastatin may be safer alternatives.
Immunosuppressants (cyclosporine, tacrolimus): Amprenavir may increase serum concentrations of immunosuppressive agents.
Inhaled corticosteroids (eg, fluticasone, budesonide): Amprenavir may increase the levels/effects of inhaled corticosteroids; monitor for adrenal suppression, Cushing's syndrome; concomitant use of fluticasone with amprenavir/ritonavir is not recommended.
Methadone: Effect of amprenavir may be diminished (consider alternative antiretroviral). In addition, the effect of methadone may be reduced (dosage increase may be required).
Metronidazole: Concurrent use with amprenavir oral solution is contraindicated due to risk of propylene glycol toxicity.
Nelfinavir: May increase serum concentrations of amprenavir.
Nevirapine: May decrease serum concentrations of amprenavir.
Oral contraceptives: Concurrent use of ethinyl estradiol/norethindrone may lead to decreased effect of amprenavir; avoid use. Nonhormonal contraception is recommended.
Pimozide: Toxicity is significantly increased by amprenavir; concurrent use is contraindicated.
Rifampin/rifabutin: May decrease serum concentrations of amprenavir. Concurrent use of rifampin is not recommended. Serum concentrations of rifabutin may be increased by amprenavir; dosage adjustment required.
Ritonavir: The serum concentrations of amprenavir may be increased by ritonavir. In addition, the risk of cholesterol/triglyceride elevations may be increased, specific dosing has been recommended for both agents. Concurrent use of amprenavir oral solution with ritonavir oral solution is not recommended (due to competition for metabolic elimination between propylene glycol and ethanol in these formulations).
Sildenafil, tadalafil, vardenafil: Serum concentrations may be increased by amprenavir. When used concurrently with sildenafil, do not exceed a maximum

(Continued)

Amprenavir *(Continued)*

sildenafil dose of 25 mg in a 48-hour period. When used concurrently with tadalafil, do not exceed a maximum tadalafil dose of 10 mg in a 72-hour period. When used concurrently with vardenafil, do not exceed vardenafil dose of 2.5 mg in a 24-hour period (2.5 mg in a 72-hour period if used with ritonavir).

St John's wort: May decrease serum concentrations of amprenavir.

Trazodone: Amprenavir may increase the levels/effects of trazodone; monitor for signs of hypotension/syncope. Use with caution and reduce dose of trazodone.

Tricyclic antidepressants: Amprenavir may increase serum concentrations/toxicity, potentially leading to serious arrhythmias.

Ethanol/Nutrition/Herb Interactions

Ethanol: Avoid ethanol with amprenavir oral solution.

Food: Levels increased sixfold with high-fat meals.

Herb/Nutraceutical: Amprenavir serum concentration may be decreased by St John's wort; avoid concurrent use. Formulations contain vitamin E; avoid additional supplements.

Dietary Considerations May be taken with or without food; do not take with high-fat meal. The 50 mg capsules contain 36.3 int. units of vitamin E per capsule; oral solution contains 46 int. units of vitamin E per mL; avoid additional vitamin E-containing supplements.

Dosage Forms

Capsule: 50 mg [contains vitamin E 36.3 int. units (as TPGS)]

Solution, oral [use only when there are no other options]: 15 mg/mL (240 mL) [contains propylene glycol 550 mg/mL and vitamin E 46 int. units/mL; grape-bubble gum-peppermint flavor]

♦ **Amrinone Lactate** *see* Inamrinone *on page 670*

Amyl Nitrite (AM il NYE trite)

Synonyms Isoamyl Nitrite

Pharmacologic Category Antidote; Vasodilator

Generic Available Yes

Use Coronary vasodilator in angina pectoris; adjunct in treatment of cyanide poisoning; produce changes in the intensity of heart murmurs

Mechanism of Action Relaxes vascular smooth muscle; decreased venous ratios and arterial blood pressure; reduces left ventricular work; decreases myocardial O_2 consumption; in cyanide poisoning, amyl nitrite converts hemoglobin to methemoglobin that binds with cyanide to form cyanate hemoglobin

Pharmacodynamics/Kinetics

Onset of action: Angina: Within 30 seconds

Duration: 3-15 minutes

Dosage Nasal inhalation:

Cyanide poisoning: Children and Adults: Inhale the vapor from a 0.3 mL crushed ampul every minute for 15-30 seconds until I.V. sodium nitrite infusion is available

Angina: Adults: 1-6 inhalations from 1 crushed ampul; may repeat in 3-5 minutes

Stability Store in cool place; protect from light

Administration Administer nasally. Patient should not be sitting. Crush ampul in woven covering between fingers and then hold under patient's nostrils.

Monitoring Parameters Monitor blood pressure during therapy

Anesthesia and Critical Care Concerns/Other Considerations Highly flammable - do not use where it might be ignited. Amyl nitrate is also used as a recreational drug during intercourse. However, when used in combination with phosphodiesterase-5 enzyme inhibitors, significant and profound hypotension may result.

Pregnancy Risk Factor X

Contraindications Hypersensitivity to nitrates; severe anemia; head injury; angle-closure glaucoma; postural hypotension; head trauma or cerebral hemorrhage; pregnancy

Warnings/Precautions Use with caution in patients with increased intracranial pressure, low systolic blood pressure, and coronary artery disease.

Adverse Reactions

1% to 10%:

Cardiovascular: Postural hypotension; cutaneous flushing of head, neck, and clavicular area; tachycardia

Central nervous system: Headache, restlessness

Gastrointestinal: Nausea, vomiting

<1% (Limited to important or life-threatening): Hemolytic anemia

Overdosage/Toxicology Symptoms of overdose include hypotension. Treatment includes general supportive measures.

Drug Interactions

Ethanol taken with amyl nitrite may have additive side effects.

Sildenafil: Avoid concurrent use of sildenafil; severe reactions may result.

Dosage Forms Vapor for inhalation [crushable covered glass capsules]: Amyl nitrite USP (0.3 mL)

References

Dudley MJ and Solomon T, "A Case of Methaemoglobinaemia," *Arch Emerg Med*, 1993, 10(2):117-9.

Laaban JP, Bodenan P, and Rochemaure J, "Amyl Nitrate Poppers and Methemoglobinemia," *Ann Intern Med*, 1985, 103(5):804-5.

Mokhlesi B, Leikin JB, Murray P, et al, "Adult Toxicology in Critical Care. Part 11: Specific Poisonings," *Chest*, 2003, 123(3):897-922.

Osterloh J and Olson K, "Toxicities of Alkyl Nitrites," *Ann Intern Med*, 1986, 104(5):727.

Schwartz RH, "When to Suspect Inhalant Abuse," *Patient Care*, 1989, 23:39-64.

♦ **AN100226** *see* Natalizumab *on page 904*

♦ **Anafranil®** *see* ClomiPRAMINE *on page 309*

♦ **Anaprox®** *see* Naproxen *on page 899*

♦ **Anaprox® DS** *see* Naproxen *on page 899*

♦ **Ancef®** *see* Cefazolin *on page 236*

♦ **Anestacon®** *see* Lidocaine *on page 755*

♦ **Anexate® (Can)** *see* Flumazenil *on page 534*

♦ **Anexsia®** *see* Hydrocodone and Acetaminophen *on page 636*

♦ **Angiomax®** *see* Bivalirudin *on page 178*

♦ **Ansaid® [DSC]** *see* Flurbiprofen *on page 550*

♦ **Anti-4 Alpha Integrin** *see* Natalizumab *on page 904*

♦ **Antidigoxin Fab Fragments, Ovine** *see* Digoxin Immune Fab *on page 392*

♦ **Antidiuretic Hormone** *see* Vasopressin *on page 1342*

Antihemophilic Factor (Recombinant)

(an tee hee moe FIL ik FAK tor ree KOM be nant)

U.S. Brand Names Advate; Helixate® FS; Kogenate® FS; Recombinate; ReFacto®

Canadian Brand Names Helixate® FS; Kogenate®; Kogenate® FS; Recombinate; ReFacto®

Synonyms AHF (Recombinant); Factor VIII (Recombinant); rAHF

Pharmacologic Category Antihemophilic Agent

Generic Available No

Use Prevention and treatment of hemorrhagic episodes in patients with hemophilia A (classic hemophilia); perioperative management of hemophilia A; can be of significant therapeutic value in patients with acquired factor VIII inhibitors ≤10 Bethesda units/mL

Mechanism of Action Factor VIII replacement, necessary for clot formation and maintenance of hemostasis. It activates factor X in conjunction with activated factor IX; activated factor X converts prothrombin to thrombin, which converts fibrinogen to fibrin, and with factor XIII forms a stable clot.

Pharmacodynamics/Kinetics Half-life elimination: Mean: 9-19 hours

Dosage Children and Adults: I.V.: Individualize dosage based on coagulation studies performed prior to treatment and at regular intervals during treatment. In general, administration of factor VIII 1 int. unit/kg will increase circulating factor VIII levels by ~2 int. units/dL. (General guidelines presented; consult individual product labeling for specific dosing recommendations.)

Dosage based on desired factor VIII increase (%):

To calculate dosage needed based on desired factor VIII increase (%):

[Body weight (kg) x desired factor VIII increase (%)] divided by 2%/int. units/kg = int. units factor VIII required

For example:

50 kg x 30 (% increase) divided by 2%/int. units/kg = 750 int. units factor VIII

(Continued)

Antihemophilic Factor (Recombinant) *(Continued)*

Dosage based on expected factor VIII increase (%):

It is also possible to calculate the **expected** % factor VIII increase:

(# int. units administered x 2%/int. units/kg) divided by body weight (kg) = expected % factor VIII increase

For example:

(1400 int. units x 2%/int. units/kg) divided by 70 kg = 40%

General guidelines:

Minor hemorrhage: 10-20 int. units/kg as a single dose to achieve FVIII plasma level ~20% to 40% of normal. Mild superficial or early hemorrhages may respond to a single dose; may repeat dose every 12-24 hours for 1-3 days until bleeding is resolved or healing achieved.

Moderate hemorrhage/minor surgery: 15-30 int. units/kg to achieve FVIII plasma level 30% to 60% of normal. May repeat 1 dose at 12-24 hours if needed. Some products suggest continuing for ≥3 days until pain and disability are resolved

Major to life-threatening hemorrhage: Initial dose 40-50 int. units/kg followed by a maintenance dose of 20-25 int. units/kg every 8-12 hours until threat is resolved, to achieve FVIII plasma level 80% to 100% of normal.

Major surgery: 50 int. units/kg given preoperatively to raise factor VIII level to 100% before surgery begins. May repeat as necessary after 6-12 hours initially and for a total of 10-14 days until healing is complete. Intensity of therapy may depend on type of surgery and postoperative regimen.

Bleeding prophylaxis: May be administered on a regular basis for bleeding prophylaxis. Doses of 24-40 int. units/kg 3 times/week have been reported in patients with severe hemophilia to prevent joint bleeding.

If bleeding is not controlled with adequate dose, test for presence of inhibitor. It may not be possible or practical to control bleeding if inhibitor titers >10 Bethesda units/mL.

Elderly: Response in the elderly is not expected to differ from that of younger patients; dosage should be individualized

Stability Store under refrigeration, 2°C to 8°C (36°F to 46°F); avoid freezing. Use within 3 hours of reconstitution. Gently agitate or rotate vial after adding diluent, do not shake vigorously. Do not refrigerate after reconstitution, a precipitation may occur.

Advate: May also be stored at room temperature for up to 6 months.

Helixate® FS, Kogenate® FS, ReFacto®: May also be stored at room temperature for up to 3 months; avoid prolonged exposure to light during storage.

Recombinate: May also be stored at room temperature, not to exceed 30°C (86°F).

If refrigerated, the dried concentrate and diluent should be warmed to room temperature before reconstitution. Gently swirl or rotate vial after adding diluent, do not shake vigorously.

Administration I.V. infusion over 5-10 minutes (maximum: 10 mL/minute).

Advate: Infuse over ≤5 minutes (maximum: 10 mL/minute).

Monitoring Parameters Heart rate and blood pressure (before and during I.V. administration); AHF levels prior to and during treatment; development of factor VIII inhibitors; bleeding

Reference Range Classification of hemophilia; normal is defined as 1 int. unit/mL of factor VIII

Severe: Factor level <1% of normal

Moderate: Factor level 1% to 5% of normal

Mild: Factor level >5% to <40% of normal

Pregnancy Risk Factor C

Contraindications Hypersensitivity to any component of the formulation

Warnings/Precautions Monitor for signs of formation of antibodies to factor VIII; may occur at anytime but more common in young children with severe hemophilia. The dosage requirement will vary in patients with factor VIII inhibitors; optimal treatment should be determined by clinical response. Monitor for allergic hypersensitivity reactions. Products vary by preparation method. Recombinate is stabilized using human albumin. Helixate® FS and Kogenate® FS are stabilized with sucrose. Advate, Helixate® FS, Kogenate® FS and ReFacto® may contain trace amounts of mouse or hamster protein. Recombinate and may contain mouse, hamster or bovine protein. Products may contain vonWillebrand factor for stabilization; however, efficacy has not been established for the treatment of von Willebrand's disease.

Adverse Reactions Actual frequency may vary by product.

$>1\%$:

Central nervous system: Chills, dizziness, fever, headache, pain
Dermatologic: Pruritus
Gastrointestinal: Nausea, taste perversion
Hematologic: Hemorrhage
Local: Injection-site pain
Neuromuscular & skeletal: Arthralgia, weakness
Respiratory: Dyspnea, nasopharyngitis, pharyngolaryngeal pain
Miscellaneous: Catheter thrombosis, factor VIII inhibitor formation

$\leq 1\%$ (Limited to important or life-threatening): Abdominal pain, adenopathy, allergic reactions, anaphylaxis, anemia, anorexia, arthralgia, chest discomfort, constipation, depersonalization, diaphoresis, diarrhea, edema, epistaxis, facial flushing, factor VIII decreased, fatigue, fever, GI hemorrhage, hot flashes, hyper-/hypotension (slight), infection, injection-site reactions, joint swelling, lethargy, otitis media, pallor, rash, rhinitis, rigors, SGOT increased, somnolence, urinary tract infection, urticaria, vasodilation, venous catheter access complications, vomiting

Overdosage/Toxicology Massive doses of antihemophilic factor (human) have been reported to cause acute hemolytic anemia, increased bleeding tendency, or hyperfibrinogenemia. Occurrence is rare.

Dietary Considerations Advate contains sodium 108 mEq/L; Helixate® FS and Kogenate® FS contain sodium 27-36 mEq/L; Recombinate contains sodium 180 mEq/L

Dosage Forms

Injection, powder for reconstitution, recombinant [preservative free]:

Advate: 250 int. units, 500 int. units, 1000 int. units, 1500 int. units, 2000 int. units [plasma/albumin free; contains sodium 108 mEq/L, mannitol; derived from hamster or mouse proteins]

Helixate® FS, Kogenate® FS: 250 int. units, 500 int. units, 1000 int. units [albumin free; contains sucrose 28 mg/vial, sodium 27-36 mEq/L; derived from hamster or mouse protein]

Recombinate: 250 int. units, 500 units, 1000 int. units [contains human albumin, sodium 180 mEq/L; derived from bovine, hamster or mouse proteins; packaging contains natural rubber latex]

ReFacto®: 250 int. units, 500 units, 1000 int. units, 2000 int. units [contains sucrose; derived from hamster or mouse proteins]

Antithrombin III (an tee THROM bin three)

U.S. Brand Names Thrombate III®

Canadian Brand Names Thrombate III®

Synonyms AT-III; Heparin Cofactor I

Pharmacologic Category Anticoagulant; Blood Product Derivative

Generic Available No

Use Treatment of hereditary antithrombin III deficiency in connection with surgical procedures, obstetrical procedures, or thromboembolism

Unlabeled/Investigational Use Acquired antithrombin III deficiencies related to disseminated intravascular coagulation (DIC)

Mechanism of Action Antithrombin III is the primary physiologic inhibitor of *in vivo* coagulation. It is an alpha$_2$-globulin. Its principal actions are the inactivation of thrombin, plasmin, and other active serine proteases of coagulation, including factors IXa, Xa, XIa, and XIIa. The inactivation of proteases is a major step in the normal clotting process. The strong activation of clotting enzymes at the site of every bleeding injury facilitates fibrin formation and maintains normal hemostasis. Thrombosis in the circulation would be caused by active serine proteases if they were not inhibited by antithrombin III after the localized clotting process.

Pharmacodynamics/Kinetics Half-life elimination: Biologic: 2.5 days (immunologic assay); 3.8 days (functional AT-III assay). Half-life may be decreased following surgery, with hemorrhage, acute thrombosis, and/or during heparin administration.

Dosage Adults:

Initial dose: Dosing is individualized based on pretherapy AT-III levels. The initial dose should raise antithrombin III levels (AT-III) to 120% and may be calculated based on the following formula:

[desired AT-III level % — baseline AT-III level %] x body weight (kg) divided by 1.4%/int. units/kg

(Continued)

Antithrombin III *(Continued)*

For example, if a 70 kg adult patient had a baseline AT-III level of 57%, the initial dose would be

[(120% — 57%) x 70] divided by 1.4 = 3150 int. units

Maintenance dose: Subsequent dosing should be targeted to keep levels between 80% to 120% which may be achieved by administering 60% of the initial dose every 24 hours. Adjustments may be made by adjusting dose or interval. Maintain level within normal range for 2-8 days depending on type of procedure.

Stability Store vials under refrigeration at 2°C to 8°C (36°F to 46°F); avoid freezing. Bring drug and diluent to room temperature prior to reconstitution. Reconstitute with sterile water for injection. Do not shake; swirl to mix to avoid foaming. Filter through sterile filter needle provided prior to administration. Administer within 3 hours of mixing.

Administration I.V.: Infuse over 10-20 minutes.

Monitoring Parameters Monitor antithrombin III peak and trough levels (preinfusion and 20 minutes postinfusion) for each dose and monitor levels 12 hours after initial loading dose; liver function tests; monitor antithrombin III levels in neonates of parents with hereditary antithrombin III deficiency immediately after birth

Reference Range Maintain antithrombin III level in plasma >80%; plasma AT-III levels are ~60% lower near term infants than levels observed in adults; premature infants may have levels lower than other neonates.

Pregnancy Risk Factor B

Contraindications Hypersensitivity to any component of the formulation

Warnings/Precautions Product of human plasma; may potentially contain infectious agents which could transmit disease; screening of donors, as well as testing and/or inactivation or removal of certain viruses, reduces this risk. Infections thought to be transmitted by this product should be reported to Talecris Biotherapeutics at 1-800-520-2807. Safety and efficacy in children have not been established.

Adverse Reactions

1% to 10%: Central nervous system: Dizziness (2%)

<1% (Limited to important or life-threatening): Bowel fullness, chest pain, chest tightness, chills, cramps, dyspnea, fever, film over eye, foul taste, hematoma, hives, lightheadedness, nausea

Drug Interactions

Drotrecogin alfa: Concurrent use may increase risk of bleeding.

Drugs which affect platelet function (eg, aspirin, NSAIDs, dipyridamole, ticlopidine, clopidogrel) may potentiate the risk of hemorrhage.

Heparin: Anticoagulant effects of heparin are potentiated by antithrombin III (ATIII); reduced doses of heparin are recommended. May require more frequent administration of ATIII; monitor.

Thrombolytic agents increase the risk of hemorrhage.

Treprostinil: Concurrent use may increase risk of bleeding.

Warfarin (and other oral anticoagulants) may increase the risk of bleeding with antithrombin III.

Ethanol/Nutrition/Herb Interactions Herb/Nutraceutical: Recent use/intake of herbs with anticoagulant or antiplatelet activity (including cat's claw, dong quai, evening primrose, garlic, ginkgo and ginseng) may increase the risk of bleeding.

Dietary Considerations Contains sodium 110-210 mEq/L

Dosage Forms Injection, powder for reconstitution [preservative free]: 500 int. units, 1000 int. units [contains heparin, sodium chloride 110-210 mEq/L; packaged with diluent]

- ♦ **Antizol®** *see* Fomepizole *on page 555*
- ♦ **Anucort-HC®** *see* Hydrocortisone *on page 639*
- ♦ **Anu-Med [OTC]** *see* Phenylephrine *on page 1015*
- ♦ **Anusol-HC®** *see* Hydrocortisone *on page 639*
- ♦ **Anusol® HC-1 [OTC]** *see* Hydrocortisone *on page 639*
- ♦ **Anzemet®** *see* Dolasetron *on page 412*
- ♦ **APAP** *see* Acetaminophen *on page 26*
- ♦ **Apidra®** *see* Insulin Glulisine *on page 685*
- ♦ **Aplonidine** *see* Apraclonidine *on page 119*

- ♦ **Apo-Acetaminophen® (Can)** *see* Acetaminophen *on page 26*
- ♦ **Apo-Acetazolamide® (Can)** *see* AcetaZOLAMIDE *on page 32*
- ♦ **Apo-Acyclovir® (Can)** *see* Acyclovir *on page 39*
- ♦ **Apo-Allopurinol® (Can)** *see* Allopurinol *on page 59*
- ♦ **Apo-Alpraz® (Can)** *see* Alprazolam *on page 65*
- ♦ **Apo-Amiodarone® (Can)** *see* Amiodarone *on page 83*
- ♦ **Apo-Amitriptyline® (Can)** *see* Amitriptyline *on page 89*
- ♦ **Apo-Ampi® (Can)** *see* Ampicillin *on page 104*
- ♦ **Apo-Atenol® (Can)** *see* Atenolol *on page 136*
- ♦ **Apo-Azathioprine® (Can)** *see* Azathioprine *on page 148*
- ♦ **Apo-Azithromycin® (Can)** *see* Azithromycin *on page 149*
- ♦ **Apo-Baclofen® (Can)** *see* Baclofen *on page 156*
- ♦ **Apo-Beclomethasone® (Can)** *see* Beclomethasone *on page 161*
- ♦ **Apo-Benazepril® (Can)** *see* Benazepril *on page 163*
- ♦ **Apo-Benztropine® (Can)** *see* Benztropine *on page 166*
- ♦ **Apo-Benzydamine® (Can)** *see* Benzydamine *on page 167*
- ♦ **Apo-Bromocriptine® (Can)** *see* Bromocriptine *on page 191*
- ♦ **Apo-Buspirone® (Can)** *see* BusPIRone *on page 205*
- ♦ **Apo-Butorphanol® (Can)** *see* Butorphanol *on page 208*
- ♦ **Apo-Capto® (Can)** *see* Captopril *on page 221*
- ♦ **Apo-Carbamazepine® (Can)** *see* Carbamazepine *on page 225*
- ♦ **Apo-Carvedilol® (Can)** *see* Carvedilol *on page 231*
- ♦ **Apo-Cefuroxime® (Can)** *see* Cefuroxime *on page 253*
- ♦ **Apo-Chlordiazepoxide® (Can)** *see* Chlordiazepoxide *on page 264*
- ♦ **Apo-Chlorhexadine® (Can)** *see* Chlorhexidine Gluconate *on page 267*
- ♦ **Apo-Chlorpromazine® (Can)** *see* ChlorproMAZINE *on page 273*
- ♦ **Apo-Cimetidine® (Can)** *see* Cimetidine *on page 281*
- ♦ **Apo-Ciproflox® (Can)** *see* Ciprofloxacin *on page 285*
- ♦ **Apo-Citalopram® (Can)** *see* Citalopram *on page 297*
- ♦ **Apo-Clindamycin® (Can)** *see* Clindamycin *on page 304*
- ♦ **Apo-Clomipramine® (Can)** *see* ClomiPRAMINE *on page 309*
- ♦ **Apo-Clonazepam® (Can)** *see* Clonazepam *on page 313*
- ♦ **Apo-Clonidine® (Can)** *see* Clonidine *on page 316*
- ♦ **Apo-Clorazepate® (Can)** *see* Clorazepate *on page 321*
- ♦ **Apo-Cyclosporine® (Can)** *see* CycloSPORINE *on page 337*
- ♦ **Apo-Desipramine® (Can)** *see* Desipramine *on page 359*
- ♦ **Apo-Desmopressin® (Can)** *see* Desmopressin *on page 363*
- ♦ **Apo-Dexamethasone® (Can)** *see* Dexamethasone *on page 366*
- ♦ **Apo-Diazepam® (Can)** *see* Diazepam *on page 374*
- ♦ **Apo-Diclo® (Can)** *see* Diclofenac *on page 378*
- ♦ **Apo-Diclo Rapide® (Can)** *see* Diclofenac *on page 378*
- ♦ **Apo-Diclo SR® (Can)** *see* Diclofenac *on page 378*
- ♦ **Apo-Diflunisal® (Can)** *see* Diflunisal *on page 385*
- ♦ **Apo-Diltiaz® (Can)** *see* Diltiazem *on page 394*
- ♦ **Apo-Diltiaz CD® (Can)** *see* Diltiazem *on page 394*
- ♦ **Apo-Diltiaz SR® (Can)** *see* Diltiazem *on page 394*
- ♦ **Apo-Dipyridamole FC® (Can)** *see* Dipyridamole *on page 402*
- ♦ **Apo-Divalproex® (Can)** *see* Valproic Acid and Derivatives *on page 1329*
- ♦ **Apo-Doxazosin® (Can)** *see* Doxazosin *on page 420*
- ♦ **Apo-Doxepin® (Can)** *see* Doxepin *on page 422*
- ♦ **Apo-Doxy® (Can)** *see* Doxycycline *on page 426*
- ♦ **Apo-Doxy Tabs® (Can)** *see* Doxycycline *on page 426*
- ♦ **Apo-Erythro Base® (Can)** *see* Erythromycin *on page 476*
- ♦ **Apo-Erythro E-C® (Can)** *see* Erythromycin *on page 476*
- ♦ **Apo-Erythro-ES® (Can)** *see* Erythromycin *on page 476*
- ♦ **Apo-Erythro-S® (Can)** *see* Erythromycin *on page 476*
- ♦ **Apo-Etidronate® (Can)** *see* Etidronate Disodium *on page 495*
- ♦ **Apo-Etodolac® (Can)** *see* Etodolac *on page 496*
- ♦ **Apo-Famotidine® (Can)** *see* Famotidine *on page 506*

- ♦ **Apo-Flecainide® (Can)** *see* Flecainide *on page 527*
- ♦ **Apo-Fluconazole® (Can)** *see* Fluconazole *on page 530*
- ♦ **Apo-Flunisolide® (Can)** *see* Flunisolide *on page 537*
- ♦ **Apo-Fluoxetine® (Can)** *see* Fluoxetine *on page 539*
- ♦ **Apo-Fluphenazine® (Can)** *see* Fluphenazine *on page 545*
- ♦ **Apo-Fluphenazine Decanoate® (Can)** *see* Fluphenazine *on page 545*
- ♦ **Apo-Flurazepam® (Can)** *see* Flurazepam *on page 548*
- ♦ **Apo-Flurbiprofen® (Can)** *see* Flurbiprofen *on page 550*
- ♦ **Apo-Fosinopril® (Can)** *see* Fosinopril *on page 562*
- ♦ **Apo-Furosemide® (Can)** *see* Furosemide *on page 572*
- ♦ **Apo-Gabapentin® (Can)** *see* Gabapentin *on page 577*
- ♦ **Apo-Gain® (Can)** *see* Minoxidil *on page 856*
- ♦ **Apo-Glyburide® (Can)** *see* GlyBURIDE *on page 598*
- ♦ **Apo-Haloperidol® (Can)** *see* Haloperidol *on page 604*
- ♦ **Apo-Haloperidol LA® (Can)** *see* Haloperidol *on page 604*
- ♦ **Apo-Hydralazine® (Can)** *see* HydrALAZINE *on page 632*
- ♦ **Apo-Hydro® (Can)** *see* Hydrochlorothiazide *on page 634*
- ♦ **Apo-Hydroxyurea® (Can)** *see* Hydroxyurea *on page 648*
- ♦ **Apo-Ibuprofen® (Can)** *see* Ibuprofen *on page 651*
- ♦ **Apo-Imipramine® (Can)** *see* Imipramine *on page 663*
- ♦ **Apo-Indomethacin® (Can)** *see* Indomethacin *on page 674*
- ♦ **Apo-Ipravent® (Can)** *see* Ipratropium *on page 698*
- ♦ **Apo-Keto® (Can)** *see* Ketoprofen *on page 714*
- ♦ **Apo-Ketoconazole® (Can)** *see* Ketoconazole *on page 711*
- ♦ **Apo-Keto-E® (Can)** *see* Ketoprofen *on page 714*
- ♦ **Apo-Ketorolac® (Can)** *see* Ketorolac *on page 717*
- ♦ **Apo-Ketorolac Injectable® (Can)** *see* Ketorolac *on page 717*
- ♦ **Apo-Keto SR® (Can)** *see* Ketoprofen *on page 714*
- ♦ **Apo-Labetalol® (Can)** *see* Labetalol *on page 721*
- ♦ **Apo-Lactulose® (Can)** *see* Lactulose *on page 724*
- ♦ **Apo-Lamotrigine® (Can)** *see* Lamotrigine *on page 727*
- ♦ **Apo-Levocarb® (Can)** *see* Levodopa and Carbidopa *on page 743*
- ♦ **Apo-Levocarb® CR (Can)** *see* Levodopa and Carbidopa *on page 743*
- ♦ **Apo-Lisinopril® (Can)** *see* Lisinopril *on page 767*
- ♦ **Apo-Lithium® (Can)** *see* Lithium *on page 770*
- ♦ **Apo-Lithium® Carbonate SR (Can)** *see* Lithium *on page 770*
- ♦ **Apo-Lorazepam® (Can)** *see* Lorazepam *on page 773*
- ♦ **Apo-Lovastatin® (Can)** *see* Lovastatin *on page 782*
- ♦ **Apo-Mefenamic® (Can)** *see* Mefenamic Acid *on page 795*
- ♦ **Apo-Meloxicam® (Can)** *see* Meloxicam *on page 798*
- ♦ **Apo-Metformin® (Can)** *see* Metformin *on page 810*
- ♦ **Apo-Methotrexate® (Can)** *see* Methotrexate *on page 821*
- ♦ **Apo-Methyldopa® (Can)** *see* Methyldopa *on page 826*
- ♦ **Apo-Metoclop® (Can)** *see* Metoclopramide *on page 834*
- ♦ **Apo-Metoprolol® (Can)** *see* Metoprolol *on page 839*
- ♦ **Apo-Metronidazole® (Can)** *see* Metronidazole *on page 842*
- ♦ **Apo-Midazolam® (Can)** *see* Midazolam *on page 847*
- ♦ **Apo-Minocycline® (Can)** *see* Minocycline *on page 854*
- ♦ **Apo-Misoprostol® (Can)** *see* Misoprostol *on page 857*
- ♦ **Apo-Nabumetone® (Can)** *see* Nabumetone *on page 883*
- ♦ **Apo-Nadol® (Can)** *see* Nadolol *on page 886*
- ♦ **Apo-Napro-Na® (Can)** *see* Naproxen *on page 899*
- ♦ **Apo-Napro-Na DS® (Can)** *see* Naproxen *on page 899*
- ♦ **Apo-Naproxen® (Can)** *see* Naproxen *on page 899*
- ♦ **Apo-Naproxen SR® (Can)** *see* Naproxen *on page 899*
- ♦ **Apo-Nifed® (Can)** *see* NIFEdipine *on page 920*
- ♦ **Apo-Nifed PA® (Can)** *see* NIFEdipine *on page 920*
- ♦ **Apo-Nitrofurantoin® (Can)** *see* Nitrofurantoin *on page 927*
- ♦ **Apo-Nizatidine® (Can)** *see* Nizatidine *on page 935*

- ♦ **Apo-Nortriptyline® (Can)** *see* Nortriptyline *on page 938*
- ♦ **Apo-Oflox® (Can)** *see* Ofloxacin *on page 950*
- ♦ **Apo-Ofloxacin® (Can)** *see* Ofloxacin *on page 950*
- ♦ **Apo-Omeprazole® (Can)** *see* Omeprazole *on page 957*
- ♦ **Apo-Oxaprozin® (Can)** *see* Oxaprozin *on page 964*
- ♦ **Apo-Paroxetine® (Can)** *see* Paroxetine *on page 988*
- ♦ **Apo-Piroxicam® (Can)** *see* Piroxicam *on page 1032*
- ♦ **Apo-Pravastatin® (Can)** *see* Pravastatin *on page 1042*
- ♦ **Apo-Prazo® (Can)** *see* Prazosin *on page 1044*
- ♦ **Apo-Prednisone® (Can)** *see* PredniSONE *on page 1050*
- ♦ **Apo-Procainamide® (Can)** *see* Procainamide *on page 1056*
- ♦ **Apo-Prochlorperazine® (Can)** *see* Prochlorperazine *on page 1061*
- ♦ **Apo-Propafenone® (Can)** *see* Propafenone *on page 1067*
- ♦ **Apo-Propranolol® (Can)** *see* Propranolol *on page 1077*
- ♦ **Apo-Quin-G® (Can)** *see* Quinidine *on page 1094*
- ♦ **Apo-Quinidine® (Can)** *see* Quinidine *on page 1094*
- ♦ **Apo-Ranitidine® (Can)** *see* Ranitidine *on page 1105*
- ♦ **Apo-Salvent® (Can)** *see* Albuterol *on page 50*
- ♦ **Apo-Selegiline® (Can)** *see* Selegiline *on page 1157*
- ♦ **Apo-Sertraline® (Can)** *see* Sertraline *on page 1161*
- ♦ **Apo-Simvastatin® (Can)** *see* Simvastatin *on page 1174*
- ♦ **Apo-Sotalol® (Can)** *see* Sotalol *on page 1198*
- ♦ **Apo-Sucralate® (Can)** *see* Sucralfate *on page 1212*
- ♦ **Apo-Sulfatrim® (Can)** *see* Sulfamethoxazole and Trimethoprim *on page 1215*
- ♦ **Apo-Sulin® (Can)** *see* Sulindac *on page 1219*
- ♦ **Apo-Sumatriptan® (Can)** *see* Sumatriptan *on page 1222*
- ♦ **Apo-Temazepam® (Can)** *see* Temazepam *on page 1239*
- ♦ **Apo-Terazosin® (Can)** *see* Terazosin *on page 1243*
- ♦ **Apo-Theo LA® (Can)** *see* Theophylline *on page 1253*
- ♦ **Apo-Thioridazine® (Can)** *see* Thioridazine *on page 1259*
- ♦ **Apo-Ticlopidine® (Can)** *see* Ticlopidine *on page 1266*
- ♦ **Apo-Timol® (Can)** *see* Timolol *on page 1268*
- ♦ **Apo-Timop® (Can)** *see* Timolol *on page 1268*
- ♦ **Apo-Tobramycin® (Can)** *see* Tobramycin *on page 1278*
- ♦ **Apo-Trazodone® (Can)** *see* Trazodone *on page 1306*
- ♦ **Apo-Trazodone D® (Can)** *see* Trazodone *on page 1306*
- ♦ **Apo-Triazo® (Can)** *see* Triazolam *on page 1316*
- ♦ **Apo-Verap® (Can)** *see* Verapamil *on page 1352*
- ♦ **Apo-Warfarin® (Can)** *see* Warfarin *on page 1362*
- ♦ **Apra Children's [OTC]** *see* Acetaminophen *on page 26*

Apraclonidine (a pra KLOE ni deen)

Medication Safety Issues

Sound-alike/look-alike issues:

Iopidine® may be confused with indapamide, iodine, Lodine®

U.S. Brand Names Iopidine®

Canadian Brand Names Iopidine®

Synonyms Aplonidine; Apraclonidine Hydrochloride; p-Aminoclonidine

Pharmacologic Category $Alpha_2$ Agonist, Ophthalmic

Generic Available No

Use Prevention and treatment of postsurgical intraocular pressure (IOP) elevation; short-term, adjunctive therapy in patients who require additional reduction of IOP

Mechanism of Action Apraclonidine is a potent alpha-adrenergic agent similar to clonidine; relatively selective for $alpha_2$-receptors but does retain some binding to $alpha_1$-receptors; appears to result in reduction of aqueous humor formation; its penetration through the blood-brain barrier is more polar than clonidine which reduces its penetration through the blood-brain barrier and suggests that its pharmacological profile is characterized by peripheral rather than central effects.

Pharmacodynamics/Kinetics

Onset of action: 1 hour

(Continued)

Apraclonidine *(Continued)*

Peak effect: Decreased intraocular pressure: 3-5 hours
Absorption: Ocular: Systemically absorbed
Half-life elimination, systemic: 8 hours

Dosage Adults: Ophthalmic:

0.5%: Instill 1-2 drops in the affected eye(s) 3 times/day

1%: Instill 1 drop in operative eye 1 hour prior to anterior segment laser surgery, second drop in eye immediately upon completion of procedure

Dosing adjustment in renal impairment: Although the topical use of apraclonidine has not been studied in renal failure patients, structurally-related clonidine undergoes a significant increase in half-life in patients with severe renal impairment; close monitoring of cardiovascular parameters in patients with impaired renal function is advised.

Dosing adjustment in hepatic impairment: Close monitoring of cardiovascular parameters in patients with impaired liver function is advised because the systemic dosage form of clonidine is partially metabolized in the liver.

Stability Store between 2°C to 27°C (36°F to 80°F); protect from freezing and light.

Administration Wait 5 minutes between instillation of other ophthalmic agents to avoid washout of previous dose. After topical instillation, finger pressure should be applied to lacrimal sac to decrease drainage into the nose and throat and minimize possible systemic absorption.

Monitoring Parameters Closely monitor patients who develop exaggerated reductions in intraocular pressure

Pregnancy Risk Factor C

Contraindications Hypersensitivity to apraclonidine, clonidine, or any component of the formulation; use with or within 14 days of MAO inhibitors

Warnings/Precautions IOP-lowering efficacy decreases over time in some patients. Most patients will experience decreased benefit from therapy lasting longer than 1 month. Closely monitor patients who develop exaggerated reductions in intraocular pressure. Use with caution in patients with cardiovascular disease, coronary insufficiency, recent myocardial infarction, cerebrovascular disease, history of vasovagal reactions, Raynaud's disease, thromboangiitis obliterans, depression, chronic renal failure, or severe renal or hepatic impairment.

Adverse Reactions

Ocular:

5% to 15%: Discomfort, hyperemia, pruritus

1% to 5%: Blanching, blurred vision, conjunctivitis, discharge, dry eye, foreign body sensation, lid edema, tearing

<1% (Limited to important or life-threatening): Abnormal vision, blepharitis, blepharoconjunctivitis, conjunctival edema, conjunctival follicles, corneal erosion, corneal infiltrate, corneal staining, edema, irritation, keratitis, keratopathy, lid disorder, lid erythema, lid margin crusting, lid retraction, lid scales, pain, photophobia

Other body systems:

1% to 10%: Gastrointestinal: Dry mouth (10%)

<3%:

Cardiovascular: Arrhythmia, chest pain, facial edema, peripheral edema

Central nervous system: Depression, dizziness, headache, insomnia, malaise, nervousness, somnolence

Dermatologic: Contact dermatitis, dermatitis

Gastrointestinal: Constipation, nausea, taste perversion

Neuromuscular & skeletal: Abnormal coordination, myalgia, paresthesia, weakness

Respiratory: Asthma, dry nose, dyspnea, parosmia, pharyngitis, rhinitis

Postmarketing and/or case reports: Allergic reactions, bradycardia

Overdosage/Toxicology Bradycardia, drowsiness, and hypothermia have been reported following ingestion of the ophthalmic solution.

Drug Interactions

Antihypertensive agents: Apraclonidine may reduce pulse and blood pressure, use systemic agents with caution.

Beta-blockers: Ophthalmic agents may have additive effect on IOP; apraclonidine may reduce pulse and blood pressure, use systemic agents with caution.

CNS depressants: May have additive CNS depression.

MAO inhibitors: Concomitant use is contraindicated.

Pilocarpine: Ophthalmic use may have additive effect on IOP.

Dosage Forms Solution, ophthalmic, as hydrochloride: 0.5% (5 mL, 10 mL); 1% (0.1 mL) [contains benzalkonium chloride]

♦ **Apraclonidine Hydrochloride** *see* Apraclonidine *on page 119*

Aprepitant (ap RE pi tant)

U.S. Brand Names Emend®

Synonyms L 754030; MK 869

Pharmacologic Category Antiemetic; Substance P/Neurokinin 1 Receptor Antagonist

Generic Available No

Use Prevention of acute and delayed nausea and vomiting associated with moderately- and highly -emetogenic chemotherapy in combination with a corticosteroid and 5-HT_3 receptor antagonist

Mechanism of Action Prevents acute and delayed vomiting by selectively inhibiting the substance P/neurokinin 1 (NK_1) receptor.

Pharmacodynamics/Kinetics

Distribution: V_d: 70 L; crosses the blood brain barrier

Protein binding: >95%

Metabolism: Extensively hepatic via CYP3A4 (major); CYP1A2 and CYP2C19 (minor); forms seven metabolites (weakly active)

Bioavailability: 60% to 65%

Half-life elimination: Terminal: 9-13 hours

Time to peak, plasma: 4 hours

Dosage Oral: Adults: 125 mg on day 1, followed by 80 mg on days 2 and 3 in combination with a corticosteroid and 5-HT_3 receptor antagonist

In clinical trials, the following regimens were used:

For highly-emetogenic chemotherapy:

Aprepitant: Oral: 125 mg on day 1, followed by 80 mg on days 2 and 3

Dexamethasone: Oral: 12 mg on day 1, followed 8 mg on days 2, 3, and 4

Ondansetron: I.V.: 32 mg on day 1

For moderately-emetogenic chemotherapy:

Aprepitant: Oral: 125 mg on day 1, followed by 80 mg on days 2 and 3

Dexamethasone: Oral: 12 mg on day 1 only

Ondansetron: Oral: Two 8 mg doses on day 1 only

Dosage adjustment in renal impairment: No dose adjustment necessary in patients with renal disease or end-stage renal disease maintained on hemodialysis.

Dosage adjustment in hepatic impairment:

Mild-to-moderate impairment (Child-Pugh score 5-9): No adjustment necessary

Severe impairment (Child-Pugh score >9): No data available

Stability Store at controlled room temperature of 20°C to 25°C (68°F to 77°F).

Administration Administer with or without food. First dose should be given 1 hour prior to antineoplastic therapy; subsequent doses should be given in the morning.

Pregnancy Risk Factor B

Contraindications Hypersensitivity to aprepitant or any component of the formulation; use with cisapride or pimozide

Warnings/Precautions Use caution with agents primarily metabolized via CYP3A4. Use caution with hepatic impairment. Not intended for treatment of nausea and vomiting or for chronic continuous therapy. Safety and efficacy in pediatric patients have not been established.

Adverse Reactions Note: Adverse reactions reported as part of a combination chemotherapy regimen.

>10%:

Central nervous system: Fatigue (18% to 22%)

Dermatologic: Alopecia (24%; placebo 22%)

Gastrointestinal: Nausea (7% to 13%), constipation (10% to 12%)

Neuromuscular & skeletal: Weakness (3% to 18%)

Miscellaneous: Hiccups (11%)

1% to 10%:

Central nervous system: Dizziness (3% to 7%)

Endocrine & metabolic: Dehydration (6%), hot flushing (3%)

Gastrointestinal: Diarrhea (6% to 10%), dyspepsia (8%), abdominal pain (5%), stomatitis (5%), epigastric discomfort (4%), gastritis (4%), mucous membrane disorder (3%), throat pain (3%)

(Continued)

Aprepitant *(Continued)*

Hematologic: Neutropenia (3% to 9%), leukopenia (9%), hemoglobin decreased (2% to 5%)

Hepatic: ALT increased (6%), AST increased (3%)

Renal: BUN increased (5%), proteinuria (7%), serum creatinine increased (4%)

>0.5% (Limited to important or life-threatening): Acid reflux, acne, alkaline phosphatase increased, anemia, angioedema, anxiety, appetite decreased, back pain, bradycardia, candidiasis, confusion, conjunctivitis, cough, deglutition disorder, disorientation, depression, diabetes mellitus, diaphoresis, dry mouth, duodenal ulcer (perforating), DVT, dysgeusia, dysphagia, dyspnea, dysuria, edema, enterocolitis, eructation, erythrocyturia, febrile neutropenia, flatulence, flushing, hyperglycemia, hyper-/hypotension, hypoesthesia, hypokalemia, hyponatremia, leukocytes increased, leukocyturia, malaise, MI, muscular weakness, musculoskeletal pain, myalgia, nasal secretion, neutropenic sepsis, obstipation, pelvic pain, peripheral neuropathy, pharyngitis, pneumonia, pneumonitis, pulmonary embolism, rash, renal insufficiency, respiratory infection, respiratory insufficiency, rigors, salivation, sensory neuropathy, septic shock, sinus tachycardia, Stevens-Johnson syndrome, tachycardia, taste disturbance, thrombocytopenia, tremor, urinary tract infection, urticaria, vocal disturbance, weight loss

Overdosage/Toxicology Single doses up to 600 mg and daily doses of 375 mg for up to 42 days were well-tolerated in healthy subjects; drowsiness and headache were noted at a dose of 1440 mg. In cancer patients, a single dose of 375 mg followed by 250 mg on days 2 to 5 was well tolerated. In case of overdose, treatment should be symptom-directed and supportive. Not removed by hemodialysis.

Drug Interactions **Substrate** of CYP1A2 (minor), 2C19 (minor), 3A4 (major); **Inhibits** CYP2C9 (weak), 2C19 (weak), 3A4 (moderate); **Induces** CYP2C9 (weak), 3A4 (weak)

CYP3A4 inducers: CYP3A4 inducers may decrease the levels/effects of aprepitant. Example inducers include aminoglutethimide, carbamazepine, nafcillin, nevirapine, phenobarbital, phenytoin, and rifamycins.

CYP3A4 inhibitors: May increase the levels/effects of aprepitant. Example inhibitors include azole antifungals, clarithromycin, diclofenac, doxycycline, erythromycin, imatinib, isoniazid, nefazodone, nicardipine, propofol, protease inhibitors, quinidine, telithromycin, and verapamil.

CYP3A4 substrates: Aprepitant may increase the levels/effects of CYP3A4 substrates. Example substrates include benzodiazepines, calcium channel blockers, ergot derivatives, mirtazapine, nateglinide, nefazodone, tacrolimus, and venlafaxine.

Corticosteroids: Bioavailability of corticosteroids may be increased. Dexamethasone doses should be decreased by 50% (oral) when compared to dose given without aprepitant. Methylprednisolone doses should be decreased by 25% (I.V.) or 50% (oral) when compared to dose given without aprepitant. Doses used in clinical studies reflect this reduction.

Diltiazem: May increase plasma levels of aprepitant.

Ketoconazole: May increase plasma levels of aprepitant; use with caution.

Rifampin: May significantly decrease the bioavailability of aprepitant.

Oral contraceptives: Aprepitant may decrease the plasma levels of ethinyl estradiol. Contraceptive efficacy may be reduced; a nonhormonal form of contraception is recommended by the manufacturer during treatment and for 1 month following the last dose.

Warfarin: Aprepitant may increase warfarin metabolism and the INR may be decreased; monitoring recommended in the 2-week period (particularly days 7-10) following start of each cycle.

Ethanol/Nutrition/Herb Interactions

Food: Aprepitant serum concentration may be increased when taken with grapefruit juice; avoid concurrent use.

Herb/Nutraceutical: St John's wort may decrease aprepitant levels.

Dietary Considerations May be taken with or without food.

Dosage Forms

Capsule: 80 mg, 125 mg

Combination package: Capsule 80 mg (2s), capsule 125 mg (1s)

♦ **Apresoline® (Can)** *see* HydrALAZINE *on page 632*

Aprotinin (a proe TYE nin)

U.S. Brand Names Trasylol®

Canadian Brand Names Trasylol®

Pharmacologic Category Blood Product Derivative; Hemostatic Agent

Generic Available No

Use Reduction of blood loss in patients undergoing cardiopulmonary bypass in coronary artery bypass graft surgery

Mechanism of Action Bleeding from CABG surgery is thought to result from a systemic inflammatory response induced by the procedure. Contact of blood cells with the cardiopulmonary bypass (CPB) equipment leads to deregulated activation of the coagulation and fibrinolysis systems, with concurrent upregulation of proinflammatory cytokines. Aprotinin is a broad spectrum serine protease inhibitor that attenuates the coagulation, fibrinolytic and inflammatory pathways by interfering with the chemical mediators (thrombin, plasmin, kallikrein). Additionally, it protects platelet-expressed glycoproteins from mechanical shear forces. This preserves normal hemostatic activity through protease receptor-independent mechanisms (eg, via ADP, IIb/IIIa), while blocking CPB-induced thrombin-mediated aggregation.

Pharmacodynamics/Kinetics

Distribution: Extracellular space; renal phagolysomes

Metabolism: Aprotinin is slowly degraded by lysosomal enzymes.

Half-life elimination: 2.5 hours (plasma); terminal: 10 hours

Excretion: Urine (25% to 40%; <10% as unchanged drug)

Dosage Adults:

Test dose: **All** patients should receive a 1 mL (1.4 mg) I.V. test dose at least 10 minutes prior to the loading dose to assess the potential for allergic reactions. **Note:** To avoid physical incompatibility with heparin when adding to pump-prime solution, each agent should be added during recirculation to assure adequate dilution.

Regimen A (standard dose):
- 2 million KIU (280 mg; 200 mL) loading dose I.V. over 20-30 minutes
- 2 million KIU (280 mg; 200 mL) into pump prime volume
- 500,000 KIU/hour (70 mg/hour; 50 mL/hour) I.V. during operation

Regimen B (low dose):
- 1 million KIU (140 mg; 100 mL) loading dose I.V. over 20-30 minutes
- 1 million KIU (140 mg; 100 mL) into pump prime volume
- 250,000 KIU/hour (35 mg/hour; 25 mL/hour) I.V. during operation

Dosage adjustment in renal impairment: No adjustment required

Dosage adjustment in hepatic impairment: No information available

Stability Store at 2°C to 25°C (36°F to 77°F); protect from freezing.

Administration Administer through a central line. Infuse loading dose over 20-30 minutes, then continuous infusion at 50 mL/hour (regimen A) or 25 mL/hour (regimen B). Rapid infusion (<20 minutes) can cause transient blood pressure decrease; to avoid incompatibility with heparin, add while recirculating the prime fluid of the cardiac bypass circuit.

Monitoring Parameters Bleeding times, prothrombin time, activated clotting time, platelet count, red blood cell counts, hematocrit, hemoglobin and fibrinogen degradation products; for toxicity also include renal function tests and blood pressure

Because aPPT and ACT are difficult to interpret with aprotinin use, the manufacturer recommends two different ways to administer heparin:

1). Fixed heparin dosing where a standard loading dose of heparin plus the quantity of heparin added to the prime volume of the CPB circuit should total at least 350 units/kg. Additional heparin should be administered based on patient's weight and duration of CPB.

2). Heparin dosing based upon a protamine titration method. A heparin dose response, assessed by protamine titration, should be performed prior to administration of aprotinin to determine the heparin loading dose.

Reference Range Antiplasmin effects occur when plasma aprotinin concentrations are 125 KIU/mL and antikallikrein effects occur when plasma levels are 250-500 KIU/mL; it remains unknown if these plasma concentrations are required for clinical benefits to occur during cardiopulmonary bypass; **Note:** KIU = Kallikrein inhibitor unit

(Continued)

Aprotinin *(Continued)*

While institutional protocols may vary, a minimal celite ACT of 750 seconds or kaolin-ACT of 480 seconds is recommended in the presence of aprotinin. Consult the manufacturer's information on specific ACT test interpretation in the presence of aprotinin.

Anesthesia and Critical Care Concerns/Other Considerations An observational, international study evaluating the safety of three agents (aprotinin, aminocaproic acid, tranexamic acid) versus no agent in the treatment of 4374 patients undergoing cardiac revascularization (primary or complex) was recently published (Mangano, 2006). Three thousand patients from 64 centers received an antifibrinolytic (1295 aprotinin, 883 aminocaproic acid, 822 tranexamic acid) and 1374 patients were in the control group (no antifibrinolytic agent). Patients received aprotinin (low dose >2 million kallikrein-inhibitor units or high dose >4 million), aminocaproic acid (>10 g), or tranexamic acid (>1 g). Overall, the use of aprotinin was associated with an increased risk of renal, cardiovascular, and cerebrovascular events when compared with the aminocaproic acid, tranexamic acid, or no treatment therapies. Aminocaproic acid and tranexamic acid were not associated with increased risk.

BayerHealthcare, the manufacturer of Trasylol® (aprotinin), has studied aprotinin in a series of prospective, randomized, double-blind, placebo-controlled clinical trials involving almost 6500 open-heart surgery patients (aprotinin 3817, placebo 2682). In these trials, Bayer did not observe the increased risk of renal, cardiovascular, or cerebrovascular adverse events that was reported in the Mangano observational study. Bayer is in the process of contacting the study authors to discuss the details of their study. The Food and Drug Administration (FDA) has not issued any comments or mandated any changes to package labeling at this point.

Aprotinin is the only agent that has an FDA-approved indication (since 1993) to reduce perioperative blood loss and the need for blood transfusion in patients undergoing cardiopulmonary bypass in the course of coronary artery bypass graft surgery.

Pregnancy Risk Factor B

Contraindications Hypersensitivity to aprotinin or any component of the formulation

Warnings/Precautions [U.S. Boxed Warning]: Anaphylactic reactions are possible. Hypersensitivity reactions are more common with repeated use, especially when re-exposure is within 6 months. All patients should receive a test dose at least 10 minutes before loading dose. Patients with a history of allergic reactions to drugs or other agents may be more likely to develop a reaction. Epinephrine, steroids, and facilities for cardiopulmonary resuscitation should be available in case such a reaction occurs. Patients with a previous exposure to aprotinin (particularly when re-exposure is within 6 months) are at an increased risk for hypersensitivity reactions including anaphylactic or anaphylactoid reactions; pretreatment with an antihistamine and H_2 blocker before administration of the loading dose is recommended in these patients; delay the addition of aprotinin into the pump prime solution until the loading dose has been safely administered. Safety and efficacy in children have not been established.

Adverse Reactions

>10%:

Central nervous system: Fever (15%)

Gastrointestinal: Nausea (11%)

1% to 10%:

Cardiovascular: Atrial flutter (6%), MI (6%; not statistically different from placebo), ventricular extrasystoles (6%), ventricular tachycardia (1% to 5%), heart failure (1% to 5%), arrhythmia (4%), supraventricular arrhythmia (4%), bradycardia (1% to 2%), bundle branch block (1% to 2%), heart block (1% to 2%), hemorrhage (1% to 2%), myocardial ischemia (1% to 2%), pericardia effusion (1% to 2%), shock (<1% to 2%), ventricular fibrillation (1% to 2%), thrombosis (1% to 2%)

Central nervous system: Agitation (1% to 2%), anxiety (1% to 2%), dizziness (1% to 2%), seizure (1% to 2%)

Endocrine & metabolic: Creatinine phosphokinase increase (2%), acidosis (1% to 2%), hyperglycemia (1% to 2%), hypervolemia (1% to 2%), hypokalemia

Gastrointestinal: Diarrhea (3%), dyspepsia (1% to 2%), gastrointestinal hemorrhage (1% to 2%)

Hematologic: Disseminated intravascular coagulation (DIC), leukocytosis (1% to 2%), prothrombin decreased (1% to 2%), thrombocytopenia (1% to 2%)

Hepatic: Liver function tests increased (3%), jaundice (1% to 2%), hepatic failure (1% to 2%)

Neuromuscular & skeletal: Arthralgia (1% to 2%)

Renal: Kidney function abnormality (3%), oliguria (1% to 2%), kidney failure (1%)

Respiratory: Hypoxia (2%), pulmonary hypertension (1% to 2%), pneumonia (1% to 2%), apnea (1% to 2%), cough increased (1% to 2%), lung edema (1% to 2%)

Miscellaneous: Sepsis (1% to 2%), multisystem organ failure (1% to 2%)

<1% (Limited to important or life-threatening): Anaphylactic reaction/hypersensitivity (re-exposure within 6 months 5%; re-exposure >6 months <1%), hemoperitoneum, skin discoloration, tubular necrosis

Note: In controlled trials, thrombosis has **not** been reported more frequently in the aprotinin versus placebo group. However, thrombosis has been reported in uncontrolled trials, compassionate use trials, and spontaneous postmarketing reports.

Overdosage/Toxicology The maximum amount of aprotinin that can safely be given has not yet been determined. Doses as high as 17.5 million KIU/24 hours have been tolerated. However, one case report of aprotinin overdose (>15 million KIU/24 hours) was associated with the development of hepatic and renal failure and eventually death. Autopsy demonstrated severe hepatic necrosis and extensive renal tubular and glomerular necrosis. The patient had pre-existing hepatic dysfunction.

Drug Interactions

Captopril (and other ACE inhibitors): Antihypertensive effects may be blocked; monitor.

Fibrinolytic drugs may have poorer activity. Aprotinin blocks this fibrinolytic activity; monitor.

Test Interactions Aprotinin significantly increases aPTT and celite Activated Clotting Time (ACT) which may not reflect the actual degree of anticoagulation by heparin. Kaolin-based ACTs are not affected by aprotinin to the same degree as celite ACTs.

Dosage Forms Injection, solution: 1.4 mg/mL [10,000 KIU/mL] (100 mL, 200 mL) [bovine derived]

References

Bidstrup BP, Royston D, Sapsford RN, et al, "Reduction in Blood Loss and Blood Use After Cardiovascular Bypass With High Dose Aprotinin," *J Thorac Cardiovasc Surg*, 1989, 97(3):364-72.

Boldt J, "Endothelial-Related Coagulation in Pediatric Surgery," *Ann Thorac Surg*, 1998, 65(6 Suppl):56-9.

Carrel TP, Schwanda M, Vogt P, et al, "Aprotinin in Pediatric Cardiac Operations: A Benefit in Complex Malformations and With High-Dose Regimen Only," *Ann Thorac Surg*, 1998, 66(1):153-8.

Cosgrove DM 3d, Heric B, Lytle BW, et al, "Aprotinin Therapy for Reoperative Myocardial Revascularization: A Placebo-Controlled Study," *Ann Thorac Surg*, 1992, 54(6):1031-6.

Huang H, Ding W, Su Z, et al, "Mechanism of the Preserving Effect of Aprotinin on Platelet Function and Its Use in Cardiac Surgery," *J Thorac Cardiovasc Surg*. 1993, 106(1):11-8.

Mangano DT, Tudor IC, Dietzel C, et al, "The Risk Associated With Aprotinin in Cardiac Surgery," *N Engl J Med*, 2006, 354(4):353-65.

Miller BE, Tosone SR, Tam VK, et al, "Hematologic and Economic Impact of Aprotinin in Reoperative Pediatric Cardiac Operations," *Ann Thorac Surg*, 1998, 66(2):535-41.

Penkoske P, Entwistle LM, Marchak BE, et al, "Aprotinin in Children Undergoing Repair of Congenital Heart Defects," *Ann Thorac Surg*, 1995, 60(6 Suppl):529-32.

Schulze K, Graeter T, Schaps D, et al, "Severe Anaphylactic Shock Due to Repeated Application of Aprotinin in Patients Following Intrathoracic Aortic Replacement," *Eur J Cardiothorac Surg*, 1993, 7(9):495-6.

Spray TL, "Use of Aprotinin in Pediatric Organ Transplantation," *Ann Thorac Surg*, 1998, 65(6 Suppl):71-3.

Woodman RC and Harker LA, "Bleeding Complications Associated With Cardiopulmonary Bypass," *Blood*, 1990, 76(9):1680-97.

♦ **Aquachloral® Supprettes®** *see* Chloral Hydrate *on page 261*

♦ **Aquacort® (Can)** *see* Hydrocortisone *on page 639*

♦ **AquaMEPHYTON® (Can)** *see* Phytonadione *on page 1027*

♦ **Aquanil™ HC [OTC]** *see* Hydrocortisone *on page 639*

♦ **Aranesp®** *see* Darbepoetin Alfa *on page 353*

♦ **Aredia®** *see* Pamidronate *on page 978*

Argatroban (ar GA troh ban)

Medication Safety Issues

Sound-alike/look-alike issues:

Argatroban may be confused with Aggrastat®

Related Information

Continuous Renal Replacement Therapy *on page 1447*

Pharmacologic Category Anticoagulant, Thrombin Inhibitor

Generic Available No

Use Prophylaxis or treatment of thrombosis in adults with heparin-induced thrombocytopenia; adjunct to percutaneous coronary intervention (PCI) in patients who have or are at risk of thrombosis associated with heparin-induced thrombocytopenia

Mechanism of Action A direct, highly-selective thrombin inhibitor. Reversibly binds to the active thrombin site of free and clot-associated thrombin. Inhibits fibrin formation; activation of coagulation factors V, VIII, and XIII; protein C; and platelet aggregation.

Pharmacodynamics/Kinetics

Onset of action: Immediate

Distribution: 174 mL/kg

Protein binding: Albumin: 20%; α_1-acid glycoprotein: 35%

Metabolism: Hepatic via hydroxylation and aromatization. Metabolism via CYP3A4/5 to four known metabolites plays a minor role. Unchanged argatroban is the major plasma component. Plasma concentration of metabolite M1 is 0% to 20% of the parent drug and is three- to fivefold weaker.

Half-life elimination: 39-51 minutes; Hepatic impairment: ≤181 minutes

Time to peak: Steady-state: 1-3 hours

Excretion: Feces (65%); urine (22%); low quantities of metabolites M2-4 in urine

Dosage I.V.: Adults:

Heparin-induced thrombocytopenia:

Initial dose: 2 mcg/kg/minute

Maintenance dose: Measure aPTT after 2 hours, adjust dose until the steady-state aPTT is 1.5-3.0 times the initial baseline value, not exceeding 100 seconds; dosage should not exceed 10 mcg/kg/minute

Conversion to oral anticoagulant: Because there may be a combined effect on the INR when argatroban is combined with warfarin, loading doses of warfarin should not be used. Warfarin therapy should be started at the expected daily dose.

Patients receiving ≤2 mcg/kg/minute of argatroban: Argatroban therapy can be stopped when the combined INR on warfarin and argatroban is >4; repeat INR measurement in 4-6 hours; if INR is below therapeutic level, argatroban therapy may be restarted. Repeat procedure daily until desired INR on warfarin alone is obtained.

Patients receiving >2 mcg/kg/minute of argatroban: Reduce dose of argatroban to 2 mcg/kg/minute; measure INR for argatroban and warfarin 4-6 hours after dose reduction; argatroban therapy can be stopped when the combined INR on warfarin and argatroban is >4. Repeat INR measurement in 4-6 hours; if INR is below therapeutic level, argatroban therapy may be restarted. Repeat procedure daily until desired INR on warfarin alone is obtained.

Note: Critically-ill patients with normal hepatic function became excessively anticoagulated with FDA-approved or lower starting doses of argatroban (Reichert MG, 2003). Doses between 0.15-1.3 mcg/kg/minute were required to maintain aPTTs in the target range. Another report of a cardiac patient with anasarca secondary to acute renal failure had a reduction in argatroban clearance similar to patients with hepatic dysfunction (de Denus S, 2003). Reduced clearance may have been attributed to reduced perfusion to the liver. Consider reducing starting dose to 0.5-1 mcg/kg/minute in critically-ill patients who may have impaired hepatic perfusion (eg, patients requiring vasopressors, having decreased cardiac output, having fluid overload). In a retrospective review of critical care patients, patients with three organ system failure required 0.5 mcg/kg/minute. The mean argatroban dose of ICU patients was 0.9 mcg/kg/minute.

Percutaneous coronary intervention (PCI):

Initial: Begin infusion of 25 mcg/kg/minute and administer bolus dose of 350 mcg/kg (over 3-5 minutes). ACT should be checked 5-10 minutes after bolus infusion; proceed with procedure if ACT >300 seconds. Following initial bolus:

ACT <300 seconds: Give an additional 150 mcg/kg bolus, and increase infusion rate to 30 mcg/kg/minute (recheck ACT in 5-10 minutes)

ACT >450 seconds: Decrease infusion rate to 15 mcg/kg/minute (recheck ACT in 5-10 minutes)

Once a therapeutic ACT (300-450 seconds) is achieved, infusion should be continued at this dose for the duration of the procedure.

If dissection, impending abrupt closure, thrombus formation during PCI, or inability to achieve ACT >300 seconds: An additional bolus of 150 mcg/kg, followed by an increase in infusion rate to 40 mcg/kg/minute may be administered.

Note: Post-PCI anticoagulation, if required, may be achieved by continuing infusion at a reduced dose of 2-10 mcg/kg/minute, with close monitoring of aPTT.

Dosage adjustment in renal impairment: Removal during hemodialysis and continuous venovenous hemofiltration is clinically insignificant. No dosage adjustment required.

Dosage adjustment in hepatic impairment: Decreased clearance and increased elimination half-life are seen with hepatic impairment; dose should be reduced. Initial dose for moderate hepatic impairment is 0.5 mcg/kg/minute. **Note:** During PCI, avoid use in patients with elevations of ALT/AST (>3 times ULN); the use of argatroban in these patients has not been evaluated.

Elderly: No adjustment is necessary for patients with normal liver function

Stability Prior to use, store at 15°C to 30°C (59°F to 86°F). Protect from light. The prepared solution is stable for 24 hours at 15°C to 30°C (59°F to 86°F) in ambient indoor light. Do not expose to direct sunlight. May be mixed with 0.9% sodium chloride injection, 5% dextrose injection, or lactated Ringer's injection. Do not mix with other medications.

To prepare solution for I.V. administration, dilute each 250 mg vial with 250 mL of diluent. Mix by repeated inversion for 1 minute. Once mixed, final concentration should be 1 mg/mL. A slight but brief haziness may occur prior to mixing. Prepared solutions that are protected from light and kept at controlled room temperature of 20°C to 25°C (68°F to 77°F) or under refrigeration at 2°C to 8°C (36°F to 46°F) are stable for up to 96 hours.

Administration Solution **must be diluted to 1 mg/mL** prior to administration.

Monitoring Parameters Obtain baseline aPTT prior to start of therapy. Check aPTT 2 hours after start of therapy to adjust dose, keeping the steady-state aPTT 1.5-3 times the initial baseline value (not exceeding 100 seconds). Monitor hemoglobin, hematocrit, signs and symptoms of bleeding.

PCI: Monitor ACT before dosing, 5-10 minutes after bolus dosing, and after any change in infusion rate and at the end of the procedure. Additional ACT assessments should be made every 20-30 minutes during extended PCI procedures.

Anesthesia and Critical Care Concerns/Other Considerations Argatroban achieves steady state rapidly (4-5 hours after initiating therapy) when administered I.V., with a predictable dose-response effect. PTTs generally remain stable at a given dose. Argatroban does not induce formation of antibodies that can alter its clearance, as is seen with lepirudin. Reduce dose in critically-ill patients, particularly those who may have impaired hepatic perfusion.

Pregnancy Risk Factor B

Contraindications Hypersensitivity to argatroban or any component of the formulation; overt major bleeding

Warnings/Precautions Hemorrhage can occur at any site in the body. Extreme caution should be used when there is an increased danger of hemorrhage, such as severe hypertension, immediately following lumbar puncture, spinal anesthesia, major surgery (including brain, spinal cord, or eye surgery), congenital or acquired bleeding disorders, and gastrointestinal ulcers. Use caution in critically-ill patients; reduced clearance may require dosage reduction. Use caution with hepatic dysfunction. Concomitant use with warfarin will cause increased prolongation of the PT and INR greater than that of warfarin alone; alternative guidelines for monitoring therapy should be followed. Safety and efficacy for use with other thrombolytic agents has not been established. Discontinue all parenteral anticoagulants prior to starting therapy. Allow reversal of heparin's effects before initiation. Patients with hepatic dysfunction may require >4 hours to achieve full reversal of argatroban's anticoagulant effect following treatment. Avoid use during PCI in patients with elevations of ALT/AST (>3 times ULN); the

(Continued)

Argatroban *(Continued)*

use of argatroban in these patients has not been evaluated. Safety and efficacy in children <18 years of age have not been established.

Adverse Reactions As with all anticoagulants, bleeding is the major adverse effect of argatroban. Hemorrhage may occur at virtually any site. Risk is dependent on multiple variables, including the intensity of anticoagulation and patient susceptibility.

>10%:
- Cardiovascular: Chest pain (<1% to 15%), hypotension (7% to 11%)
- Gastrointestinal: Gastrointestinal bleed (minor, 3% to 14%)
- Genitourinary: Genitourinary bleed and hematuria (minor, 2% to 12%)

1% to 10%:
- Cardiovascular: Cardiac arrest (6%), ventricular tachycardia (5%), bradycardia (5%), myocardial infarction (PCI: 4%), atrial fibrillation (3%), angina (2%), CABG-related bleeding (minor, 2%), myocardial ischemia (2%), cerebrovascular disorder (<1% to 2%), thrombosis (<1% to 2%)
- Central nervous system: Fever (<1% to 7%), headache (5%), pain (5%), intracranial bleeding (1% to 4%)
- Gastrointestinal: Nausea (5% to 7%), diarrhea (6%), vomiting (4% to 6%), abdominal pain (3% to 4%), bleeding (major, <1% to 2%)
- Genitourinary: Urinary tract infection (5%)
- Hematologic: Hemoglobin (<2 g/dL) and hematocrit (minor, 2% to 10%) decreased
- Local: Bleeding at injection or access site (minor, 2% to 5%)
- Neuromuscular & skeletal: Back pain (8%)
- Renal: Abnormal renal function (3%)
- Respiratory: Dyspnea (8% to 10%), cough (3% to 10%), hemoptysis (minor, <1% to 3%), pneumonia (3%)
- Miscellaneous: Sepsis (6%), infection (4%)

<1% (Limited to important or life-threatening): Aortic stenosis, genitourinary bleeding and hematuria (major), GERD, hemoglobin/hematocrit decreased (major), limb and below-the-knee stump bleed, pulmonary edema, multisystem hemorrhage and DIC, retroperitoneal bleeding, vascular disorder

Overdosage/Toxicology No specific antidote is available. Treatment should be symptomatic and supportive. Discontinue or decrease infusion to control excessive anticoagulation with or without bleeding. Reversal of anticoagulant effects may be longer than 4 hours in patients with hepatic impairment. Hemodialysis may remove up to 20% of the drug; however, this is considered clinically insignificant.

Drug Interactions Substrate of CYP3A4 (minor)
- Drugs which affect platelet function (eg, aspirin, NSAIDs, dipyridamole, ticlopidine, clopidogrel): May potentiate the risk of hemorrhage.
- Erythromycin: Concurrent therapy failed to demonstrate a significant effect on argatroban pharmacokinetics, indicating CYP3A4/5 is not a major route of argatroban metabolism.
- Glycoprotein IIb/IIIa antagonists: Concurrent therapy has not been evaluated. An increased risk of bleeding would be expected.
- Heparin: Sufficient time must pass after heparin therapy is discontinued; allow heparin's effect on the aPTT to decrease.
- Thrombolytics: Safety and efficacy for concomitant use have not been established. May increase risk of bleeding. Intracranial bleeding has been reported.
- Warfarin: Concomitant use with argatroban increases PT and INR greater than that of warfarin alone. Argatroban is commonly continued during the initiation of warfarin therapy to assure anticoagulation and to protect against possible transient hypercoagulability.

Dosage Forms Injection, solution: 100 mg/mL (2.5 mL) [contains dehydrated alcohol 1000 mg/mL]

References

Dager WE and White RH, "Pharmacotherapy of Heparin-Induced Thrombocytopenia," *Expert Opin Pharmacother*, 2003, 4(6):919-40.

de Denus S and Spinler SA, "Decreased Argatrogan Clearance Unaffected by Hemodialysis in Anasarca," *Ann Pharmacother*, 2003, 37(9):1237-40.

Lewis BE, Wallis DE, Berkowitz SD, et al, "Argatroban Anticoagulant Therapy in Patients With Heparin-Induced Thrombocytopenia," *Circulation*, 2001, 103(14):1838-43.

Reichert MG, "Excessive Argatroban Anticoagulation for Heparin-Induced Thrombocytopenia," *Ann Pharmacother*, 2003, 37(5):652-4.

♦ **8-Arginine Vasopressin** *see* Vasopressin *on page 1342*

- **Aristocort®** *see* Triamcinolone *on page 1311*
- **Aristocort® A** *see* Triamcinolone *on page 1311*
- **Aristospan®** *see* Triamcinolone *on page 1311*
- **Arixtra®** *see* Fondaparinux *on page 557*
- **ASA** *see* Aspirin *on page 129*
- **Asaphen (Can)** *see* Aspirin *on page 129*
- **Asaphen E.C. (Can)** *see* Aspirin *on page 129*
- **Ascriptin® [OTC]** *see* Aspirin *on page 129*
- **Ascriptin® Extra Strength [OTC]** *see* Aspirin *on page 129*
- **Aspart Insulin** *see* Insulin Aspart *on page 681*
- **Aspercin [OTC]** *see* Aspirin *on page 129*
- **Aspercin Extra [OTC]** *see* Aspirin *on page 129*
- **Aspergum® [OTC]** *see* Aspirin *on page 129*

Aspirin (AS pir in)

Medication Safety Issues

Sound-alike/look-alike issues:

Aspirin may be confused with Afrin®, Asendin®

Ascriptin® may be confused with Aricept®

Ecotrin® may be confused with Akineton®, Edecrin®, Epogen®

Halfprin® may be confused with Halfan®, Haltran®

ZORprin® may be confused with Zyloprim®

Related Information

Acetaminophen and NSAIDS, Dosing Data *on page 1543*

Chronic Pain Management *on page 1430*

U.S. Brand Names Ascriptin® [OTC]; Ascriptin® Extra Strength [OTC]; Aspercin [OTC]; Aspercin Extra [OTC]; Aspergum® [OTC]; Bayer® Aspirin [OTC]; Bayer® Aspirin Extra Strength [OTC]; Bayer® Aspirin Regimen Adult Low Strength [OTC]; Bayer® Aspirin Regimen Children's [OTC]; Bayer® Aspirin Regimen Regular Strength [OTC]; Bayer® Extra Strength Arthritis Pain Regimen [OTC]; Bayer® Plus Extra Strength [OTC]; Bayer® Women's Aspirin Plus Calcium [OTC]; Bufferin® [OTC]; Bufferin® Extra Strength [OTC]; Buffinol [OTC]; Buffinol Extra [OTC]; Easprin®; Ecotrin® [OTC]; Ecotrin® Low Strength [OTC]; Ecotrin® Maximum Strength [OTC]; Halfprin® [OTC]; St. Joseph® Adult Aspirin [OTC]; Sureprin 81™ [OTC]; ZORprin®

Canadian Brand Names Asaphen; Asaphen E.C.; Entrophen®; Novasen

Synonyms Acetylsalicylic Acid; ASA

Pharmacologic Category Salicylate

Generic Available Yes: Excludes gum

Use Treatment of mild-to-moderate pain, inflammation, and fever; may be used as prophylaxis of myocardial infarction; prophylaxis of stroke and/or transient ischemic episodes; management of rheumatoid arthritis, rheumatic fever, osteoarthritis, and gout (high dose); adjunctive therapy in revascularization procedures (coronary artery bypass graft [CABG], percutaneous transluminal coronary angioplasty [PTCA], carotid endarterectomy), stent implantation

Unlabeled/Investigational Use Low doses have been used in the prevention of pre-eclampsia, complications associated with autoimmune disorders such as lupus or antiphospholipid syndrome

Mechanism of Action Inhibits prostaglandin synthesis, acts on the hypothalamus heat-regulating center to reduce fever, blocks prostaglandin synthetase action which prevents formation of the platelet-aggregating substance thromboxane A_2

Pharmacodynamics/Kinetics

Duration: 4-6 hours

Absorption: Rapid

Distribution: V_d: 10 L; readily into most body fluids and tissues

Metabolism: Hydrolyzed to salicylate (active) by esterases in GI mucosa, red blood cells, synovial fluid, and blood; metabolism of salicylate occurs primarily by hepatic conjugation; metabolic pathways are saturable

Bioavailability: 50% to 75% reaches systemic circulation

Half-life elimination: Parent drug: 15-20 minutes; Salicylates (dose dependent): 3 hours at lower doses (300-600 mg), 5-6 hours (after 1 g), 10 hours with higher doses

Time to peak, serum: ~1-2 hours

(Continued)

Aspirin *(Continued)*

Excretion: Urine (75% as salicyluric acid, 10% as salicylic acid)

Serum Salicylate: Clinical Correlations

Serum Salicylate Concentration (mcg/mL)	Desired Effects	Adverse Effects / Intoxication
~100	Antiplatelet Antipyresis Analgesia	GI intolerance and bleeding, hypersensitivity, hemostatic defects
150-300	Anti-inflammatory	Mild salicylism
250-400	Treatment of rheumatic fever	Nausea/vomiting, hyperventilation, salicylism, flushing, sweating, thirst, headache, diarrhea, and tachycardia
>400-500		Respiratory alkalosis, hemorrhage, excitement, confusion, asterixis, pulmonary edema, convulsions, tetany, metabolic acidosis, fever, coma, cardiovascular collapse, renal and respiratory failure

Dosage

Children:

Analgesic and antipyretic: Oral, rectal: 10-15 mg/kg/dose every 4-6 hours, up to a total of 4 g/day

Anti-inflammatory: Oral: Initial: 60-90 mg/kg/day in divided doses; usual maintenance: 80-100 mg/kg/day divided every 6-8 hours; monitor serum concentrations

Antiplatelet effects: Adequate pediatric studies have not been performed; pediatric dosage is derived from adult studies and clinical experience and is not well established; suggested doses have ranged from 3-5 mg/kg/day to 5-10 mg/kg/day given as a single daily dose. Doses are rounded to a convenient amount (eg, 1/2 of 80 mg tablet).

Mechanical prosthetic heart valves: 6-20 mg/kg/day given as a single daily dose (used in combination with an oral anticoagulant in children who have systemic embolism despite adequate oral anticoagulation therapy (INR 2.5-3.5) and used in combination with low-dose anticoagulation (INR 2-3) and dipyridamole when full-dose oral anticoagulation is contraindicated)

Blalock-Taussig shunts: 3-5 mg/kg/day given as a single daily dose

Kawasaki disease: Oral: 80-100 mg/kg/day divided every 6 hours; monitor serum concentrations; after fever resolves: 3-5 mg/kg/day once daily; in patients without coronary artery abnormalities, give lower dose for at least 6-8 weeks or until ESR and platelet count are normal; in patients with coronary artery abnormalities, low-dose aspirin should be continued indefinitely

Antirheumatic: Oral: 60-100 mg/kg/day in divided doses every 4 hours

Adults:

Analgesic and antipyretic: Oral, rectal: 325-650 mg every 4-6 hours up to 4 g/day

Anti-inflammatory: Oral: Initial: 2.4-3.6 g/day in divided doses; usual maintenance: 3.6-5.4 g/day; monitor serum concentrations

Myocardial infarction prophylaxis: 75-325 mg/day; use of a lower aspirin dosage has been recommended in patients receiving ACE inhibitors

Acute myocardial infarction: 160-325 mg/day (have patient chew tablet if not taking aspirin before presentation)

CABG: 75-325 mg/day starting 6 hours following procedure; if bleeding prevents administration at 6 hours after CABG, initiate as soon as possible

PTCA: Initial: 80-325 mg/day starting 2 hours before procedure; longer pretreatment durations (up to 24 hours) should be considered if lower dosages (80-100 mg) are used

Stent implantation: Oral: 325 mg 2 hours prior to implantation and 160-325 mg daily thereafter

Carotid endarterectomy: 81-325 mg/day preoperatively and daily thereafter

Acute stroke: 160-325 mg/day, initiated within 48 hours (in patients who are not candidates for thrombolytics and are not receiving systemic anticoagulation)

Stroke prevention/TIA: 30-325 mg/day (dosages up to 1300 mg/day in 2-4 divided doses have been used in clinical trials)

Pre-eclampsia prevention (unlabeled use): 60-80 mg/day during gestational weeks 13-26 (patient selection criteria not established)

Dosing adjustment in renal impairment: Cl_{cr} <10 mL/minute: Avoid use.

Hemodialysis: Dialyzable (50% to 100%)

Dosing adjustment in hepatic disease: Avoid use in severe liver disease.

Stability Keep suppositories in refrigerator; do not freeze. Hydrolysis of aspirin occurs upon exposure to water or moist air, resulting in salicylate and acetate, which possess a vinegar-like odor. Do not use if a strong odor is present.

Administration Do not crush sustained release or enteric coated tablet. Administer with food or a full glass of water to minimize GI distress. For acute myocardial infarction, have patient chew tablet.

Reference Range Timing of serum samples: Peak levels usually occur 2 hours after ingestion. Salicylate serum concentrations correlate with the pharmacological actions and adverse effects observed. The serum salicylate concentration (mcg/mL) and the corresponding clinical correlations are as follows: See table on previous page.

Anesthesia and Critical Care Concerns/Other Considerations

Primary Prevention: The U.S. Preventive Services Task Force strongly recommends that clinicians discuss aspirin therapy for primary prevention of heart disease with adults who are at increased risk. The balance of benefits and harm is most favorable in patients at high risk for coronary heart disease (those with a 5-year risk ≥3%). Risk can be calculated at www.med-decisions.com. Adequate blood pressure control is necessary in hypertensive patients who are candidates for aspirin.

Secondary Prevention: In unstable angina, aspirin reduces the rate of refractory angina, nonfatal MI, and death. Aspirin reduces the rate of recurrent ischemia and infarction, stroke, and death following MI. In patients who have acute coronary syndrome (ACS) but are not already receiving aspirin, the first dose may be chewed to rapidly establish a high blood level.

Pregnancy Risk Factor C/D (full-dose aspirin in 3rd trimester - expert analysis)

Contraindications Hypersensitivity to salicylates, other NSAIDs, or any component of the formulation; asthma; rhinitis; nasal polyps; inherited or acquired bleeding disorders (including factor VII and factor IX deficiency); do not use in children (<16 years of age) for viral infections (chickenpox or flu symptoms), with or without fever, due to a potential association with Reye's syndrome; pregnancy (3rd trimester especially)

Warnings/Precautions Use with caution in patients with platelet and bleeding disorders, renal dysfunction, dehydration, erosive gastritis, or peptic ulcer disease. Heavy ethanol use (>3 drinks/day) can increase bleeding risks. Avoid use in severe renal failure or in severe hepatic failure. Discontinue use if tinnitus or impaired hearing occurs. Caution in mild-to-moderate renal failure (only at high dosages). Patients with sensitivity to tartrazine dyes, nasal polyps, and asthma may have an increased risk of salicylate sensitivity. Surgical patients should avoid ASA if possible, for 1-2 weeks prior to surgery, to reduce the risk of excessive bleeding.

When used for self-medication (OTC labeling): Children and teenagers who have or are recovering from chickenpox or flu-like symptoms should not use this product. Changes in behavior (along with nausea and vomiting) may be an early sign of Reye's syndrome; patients should be instructed to contact their healthcare provider if these occur.

Adverse Reactions As with all drugs which may affect hemostasis, bleeding is associated with aspirin. Hemorrhage may occur at virtually any site. Risk is dependent on multiple variables including dosage, concurrent use of multiple agents which alter hemostasis, and patient susceptibility. Many adverse effects of aspirin are dose related, and are extremely rare at low dosages. Other serious reactions are idiosyncratic, related to allergy or individual sensitivity. Accurate estimation of frequencies is not possible.

Cardiovascular: Hypotension, tachycardia, dysrhythmias, edema

Central nervous system: Fatigue, insomnia, nervousness, agitation, confusion, dizziness, headache, lethargy, cerebral edema, hyperthermia, coma

Dermatologic: Rash, angioedema, urticaria

Endocrine & metabolic: Acidosis, hyperkalemia, dehydration, hypoglycemia (children), hyperglycemia, hypernatremia (buffered forms)

(Continued)

Aspirin *(Continued)*

Gastrointestinal: Nausea, vomiting, dyspepsia, epigastric discomfort, heartburn, stomach pain, gastrointestinal ulceration (6% to 31%), gastric erosions, gastric erythema, duodenal ulcers

Hematologic: Anemia, disseminated intravascular coagulation, prothrombin times prolonged, coagulopathy, thrombocytopenia, hemolytic anemia, bleeding, iron-deficiency anemia

Hepatic: Hepatotoxicity, transaminases increased, hepatitis (reversible)

Neuromuscular & skeletal: Rhabdomyolysis, weakness, acetabular bone destruction (OA)

Otic: Hearing loss, tinnitus

Renal: Interstitial nephritis, papillary necrosis, proteinuria, renal failure (including cases caused by rhabdomyolysis), BUN increased, serum creatinine increased

Respiratory: Asthma, bronchospasm, dyspnea, laryngeal edema, hyperpnea, tachypnea, respiratory alkalosis, noncardiogenic pulmonary edema

Miscellaneous: Anaphylaxis, prolonged pregnancy and labor, stillbirths, low birth weight, peripartum bleeding, Reye's syndrome

Postmarketing and/or case reports: Colonic ulceration, esophageal stricture, esophagitis with esophageal ulcer, esophageal hematoma, oral mucosal ulcers (aspirin-containing chewing gum), coronary artery spasm, conduction defect and atrial fibrillation (toxicity), delirium, ischemic brain infarction, colitis, rectal stenosis (suppository), cholestatic jaundice, periorbital edema, rhinosinusitis

Overdosage/Toxicology Symptoms of overdose include tinnitus, headache, dizziness, confusion, metabolic acidosis, hyperpyrexia, hypoglycemia, and coma. Treatment should be based upon symptomatology.

Drug Interactions Substrate of CYP2C9 (minor)

ACE inhibitors: The effects of ACE inhibitors may be blunted by aspirin administration, particularly at higher dosages.

Buspirone increases aspirin's free % *in vitro.*

Carbonic anhydrase inhibitors and corticosteroids have been associated with alteration in salicylate serum concentrations.

Heparin and low molecular weight heparins: Concurrent use may increase the risk of bleeding.

Methotrexate serum levels may be increased; consider discontinuing aspirin 2-3 days before high-dose methotrexate treatment or avoid concurrent use.

NSAIDs may increase the risk of gastrointestinal adverse effects and bleeding. Serum concentrations of some NSAIDs may be decreased by aspirin. Ibuprofen, and possibly other COX-1 inhibitors, may reduce the cardioprotective effects of aspirin. Avoid giving prior to aspirin therapy or on a regular basis in patients with CAD.

Platelet inhibitors (IIb/IIIa antagonists): Risk of bleeding may be increased.

Probenecid effects may be antagonized by aspirin.

Sulfonylureas: The effects of older sulfonylurea agents (tolazamide, tolbutamide) may be potentiated due to displacement from plasma proteins. This effect does not appear to be clinically significant for newer sulfonylurea agents (glyburide, glipizide, glimepiride).

Valproic acid may be displaced from its binding sites which can result in toxicity.

Verapamil may potentiate the prolongation of bleeding time associated with aspirin.

Warfarin and oral anticoagulants may increase the risk of bleeding.

Ethanol/Nutrition/Herb Interactions

Ethanol: Avoid ethanol (may enhance gastric mucosal damage).

Food: Food may decrease the rate but not the extent of oral absorption.

- Folic acid: Hyperexcretion of folate; folic acid deficiency may result, leading to macrocytic anemia.
- Iron: With chronic aspirin use and at doses of 3-4 g/day, iron-deficiency anemia may result.
- Sodium: Hypernatremia resulting from buffered aspirin solutions or sodium salicylate containing high sodium content. Avoid or use with caution in CHF or any condition where hypernatremia would be detrimental.
- Benedictine liqueur, prunes, raisins, tea, and gherkins: Potential salicylate accumulation.
- Fresh fruits containing vitamin C: Displace drug from binding sites, resulting in increased urinary excretion of aspirin.

Herb/Nutraceutical: Avoid cat's claw, dong quai, evening primrose, feverfew, garlic, ginger, ginkgo, red clover, horse chestnut, green tea, ginseng (all have additional antiplatelet activity). Limit curry powder, paprika, licorice; may cause salicylate accumulation. These foods contain 6 mg salicylate/100 g. An ordinarily American diet contains 10-200 mg/day of salicylate.

Test Interactions False-negative results for glucose oxidase urinary glucose tests (Clinistix®); false-positives using the cupric sulfate method (Clinitest®); also, interferes with Gerhardt test, VMA determination; 5-HIAA, xylose tolerance test and T_3 and T_4

Dietary Considerations Take with food or large volume of water or milk to minimize GI upset.

Dosage Forms

Caplet:
- Bayer® Aspirin: 325 mg
- Bayer® Aspirin Extra Strength: 500 mg
- Bayer® Extra Strength Arthritis Pain Regimen: 500 mg [enteric coated]
- Bayer® Women's Aspirin Plus Calcium: 81 mg [contains elemental calcium 300 mg]

Caplet, buffered (Ascriptin® Extra Strength): 500 mg [contains aluminum hydroxide, calcium carbonate, and magnesium hydroxide]

Gelcap (Bayer® Aspirin Extra Strength): 500 mg

Gum (Aspergum®): 227 mg [cherry or orange flavor]

Suppository, rectal: 300 mg, 600 mg

Tablet: 325 mg
- Aspercin: 325 mg
- Aspercin Extra: 500 mg
- Bayer® Aspirin: 325 mg [film coated]

Tablet, buffered: 325 mg
- Ascriptin®: 325 mg [contains aluminum hydroxide, calcium carbonate, and magnesium hydroxide]
- Bayer® Plus Extra Strength: 500 mg [contains calcium carbonate]
- Bufferin®: 325 mg [contains citric acid]
- Bufferin® Extra Strength: 500 mg [contains citric acid]
- Buffinol: 325 mg [contains magnesium oxide]
- Buffinol Extra: 500 mg [contains magnesium oxide]

Tablet, chewable: 81 mg
- Bayer® Aspirin Regimen Children's Chewable: 81 mg [cherry, mint or orange flavor]
- St. Joseph® Adult Aspirin: 81 mg [orange flavor]

Tablet, controlled release (ZORprin®): 800 mg

Tablet, enteric coated: 81 mg, 325 mg, 500 mg, 650 mg
- Bayer® Aspirin Regimen Adult Low Strength, Ecotrin® Low Strength, St. Joseph Adult Aspirin: 81 mg
- Bayer® Aspirin Regimen Regular Strength, Ecotrin®: 325 mg
- Easprin®: 975 mg
- Ecotrin® Maximum Strength: 500 mg
- Halfprin®: 81 mg, 162 mg
- Sureprin 81™: 81 mg

Aspirin and Dipyridamole (AS pir in & dye peer ID a mole)

Medication Safety Issues

Sound-alike/look-alike issues:
- Aggrenox® may be confused with Aggrastat®

U.S. Brand Names Aggrenox®

Canadian Brand Names Aggrenox®

Synonyms Aspirin and Extended-Release Dipyridamole; Dipyridamole and Aspirin

Pharmacologic Category Antiplatelet Agent

Generic Available No

Use Reduction in the risk of stroke in patients who have had transient ischemia of the brain or completed ischemic stroke due to thrombosis

Mechanism of Action The antithrombotic action results from additive antiplatelet effects. Dipyridamole inhibits the uptake of adenosine into platelets, endothelial cells, and erythrocytes. Aspirin inhibits platelet aggregation by irreversible inhibition of platelet cyclooxygenase and thus inhibits the generation of thromboxane A_2.

Pharmacodynamics/Kinetics See individual agents.

(Continued)

Aspirin and Dipyridamole *(Continued)*

Dosage Adults: Oral: 1 capsule (dipyridamole 200 mg, aspirin 25 mg) twice daily

Dosage adjustment in renal impairment: Avoid use in patients with severe renal dysfunction (Cl_{cr} <10 mL/minute). Studies have not been done in patients with renal impairment.

Dosage adjustment in hepatic impairment: Avoid use in patients with severe hepatic impairment. Studies have not been done in patients with varying degrees of hepatic impairment.

Elderly: Plasma concentrations were 40% higher, but specific dosage adjustments have not been recommended.

Stability Store at 25°C (77°F); excursions permitted to 15°C to 30°C (59°F to 86°F). Protect from excessive moisture.

Administration Capsule should be swallowed whole; do not crush or chew. May be given with or without food.

Monitoring Parameters Hemoglobin, hematocrit, signs or symptoms of bleeding, signs or symptoms of stroke or transient ischemic attack

Pregnancy Risk Factor D

Contraindications Hypersensitivity to dipyridamole, aspirin, or any component of the formulation; allergy to NSAIDs; patients with asthma, rhinitis, and nasal polyps; bleeding disorders (factor VII or IX deficiencies); children <16 years of age with viral infections; pregnancy (aspirin)

Warnings/Precautions Patients who consume ≥3 alcoholic drinks per day are at risk of bleeding. Cautious use in patients with inherited or acquired bleeding disorders including those of liver disease or vitamin K deficiency. Watch for signs and symptoms of GI ulcers and bleeding. Avoid use in patients with active peptic ulcer disease. Discontinue use if dizziness, tinnitus, or impaired hearing occurs. Discontinue 1-2 weeks before elective surgical procedures to avoid bleeding. Use caution in the elderly who are at high risk for adverse events. Cautious use in patients with hypotension, patients with unstable angina, recent MI, and hepatic dysfunction. Avoid in patients with severe renal failure. Dose of aspirin in this combination is inadequate to prevent MI. Safety and efficacy in children have not been established.

Adverse Reactions

>10%:

- Central nervous system: Headache (38%)
- Gastrointestinal: Dyspepsia, abdominal pain (18%), nausea (16%), diarrhea (13%)

1% to 10%:

- Cardiovascular: Cardiac failure (2%), syncope (1%)
- Central nervous system: Pain (6%), seizure (2%), fatigue (6%), malaise (2%), amnesia (2%), confusion (1%), somnolence (1%)
- Dermatologic: Purpura (1%)
- Gastrointestinal: Vomiting (8%), bleeding (4%), rectal bleeding (2%), hemorrhoids (1%), hemorrhage (1%), anorexia (1%)
- Hematologic: Anemia (2%)
- Neuromuscular & skeletal: Back pain (5%), weakness (2%), arthralgia (6%), arthritis (2%), arthrosis (1%), myalgia (1%)
- Respiratory: Cough (2%), upper respiratory tract infection (1%), epistaxis (2%)

<1% (Limited to important or life-threatening): Allergic reaction, allergic vasculitis, alopecia, anaphylaxis, anemia (aplastic), angina pectoris, angioedema, antepartum and postpartum bleeding, arrhythmia, bronchospasm, cerebral edema, cerebral hemorrhage, cholelithiasis, coma, deafness, disseminated intravascular coagulation, dyspnea, hematemesis, hemoptysis, hepatic failure, hepatitis, interstitial nephritis, intracranial hemorrhage (0.6%), jaundice, lower weight infants, pancreatitis, pancytopenia, papillary necrosis, paresthesia, PT time prolonged, pruritus, pulmonary edema, rash, renal failure, Reye's syndrome, rhabdomyolysis, Stevens-Johnson syndrome, stillbirths, subarachnoid hemorrhage, tachypnea, thrombocytopenia, ulceration, urticaria, uterine hemorrhage

Overdosage/Toxicology Symptoms of dipyridamole overdose might predominate. Symptoms may include hypotension and peripheral vasodilation.

Drug Interactions Aspirin: **Substrate** of CYP2C9 (minor)

Increased effects: Plasma levels and cardiovascular effects of adenosine are increased; decrease adenosine dose. Use of aspirin-dipyridamole with anticoagulants (heparin, low molecular weight heparins, warfarin) or antiplatelet agents (NSAIDs, IIb/IIIa antagonists) may increase the risk of bleeding. Serum concentrations and toxicity of methotrexate may be increased when used concurrently with aspirin; avoid concurrent use. Serum concentrations of acetazolamide, phenytoin, or valproic acid may be increased with aspirin. Concurrent use of verapamil may prolong bleeding times.

Decreased effect: ACE inhibitors may have diminished pharmacologic effect with aspirin (at higher dosages). The effect of cholinesterase inhibitors may be reduced with concurrent aspirin-dipyridamole therapy; avoid concurrent use. Aspirin may diminish the effect of diuretics, probenecid, and sulfinpyrazone.

Ethanol/Nutrition/Herb Interactions Ethanol: Avoid ethanol (due to GI irritation).

Dietary Considerations May be taken with or without food.

Dosage Forms Capsule: Dipyridamole (extended release) 200 mg and aspirin 25 mg [contains lactose]

- **Aspirin and Extended-Release Dipyridamole** *see* Aspirin and Dipyridamole *on page 133*
- **Aspirin and Oxycodone** *see* Oxycodone and Aspirin *on page 971*

Aspirin and Pravastatin (AS pir in & PRA va stat in)

U.S. Brand Names Pravigard™ PAC [DSC]

Canadian Brand Names PravASA

Synonyms Buffered Aspirin and Pravastatin Sodium; Pravastatin and Aspirin

Pharmacologic Category Antilipemic Agent, HMG-CoA Reductase Inhibitor; Salicylate

Generic Available No

Use Combination therapy in patients who need treatment with aspirin and pravastatin to reduce the incidence of cardiovascular events, including myocardial infarction, stroke, and death

Mechanism of Action

Aspirin: Inhibits prostaglandin synthesis, acts on the hypothalamus heat-regulating center to reduce fever, blocks prostaglandin synthetase action which prevents formation of the platelet-aggregating substance thromboxane A_2

Pravastatin: Competitive inhibitor of 3-hydroxy-3-methylglutaryl coenzyme A (HMG-CoA) reductase, which is the rate-limiting enzyme involved in *de novo* cholesterol synthesis.

Pharmacodynamics/Kinetics See individual agents.

Dosage Oral: Adults:

Initial: Pravastatin 40 mg with aspirin (either 81 mg or 325 mg); both medications taken once daily. If pravastatin 40 mg does not achieve the desired cholesterol result, dosage may be increased to 80 mg once daily with aspirin (either 81 mg or 325 mg) once daily. Some patients may achieve/maintain goal cholesterol levels at a pravastatin dosage of 20 mg.

See Pravastatin for dosing in renal or hepatic impairment, as well as, dosing with concurrent immunosuppressant therapy.

Stability Store at 20°C to 25°C (68°F to 77°F).

Monitoring Parameters Pravastatin: Obtain baseline LFTs and total cholesterol profile; creatine phosphokinase. Repeat LFTs prior to elevation of dose. May be measured when clinically indicated and/or periodically thereafter.

Pregnancy Risk Factor X

Contraindications Hypersensitivity to pravastatin, aspirin, salicylates, or other NSAIDs, or any component of the formulation; syndrome of asthma, rhinitis, and nasal polyps; inherited or acquired bleeding disorders (including factor VII and factor IX deficiency); active liver disease; unexplained persistent elevations of serum transaminases; pregnancy; breast-feeding

Warnings/Precautions

Aspirin: Use with caution in patients with platelet and bleeding disorders, renal dysfunction, dehydration, erosive gastritis, or peptic ulcer disease. Heavy ethanol use (>3 drinks/day) can increase bleeding risks. Avoid use in severe renal failure or in severe hepatic failure. Discontinue use if tinnitus or impaired hearing occurs. Patients with sensitivity to tartrazine dyes, nasal polyps, and asthma may have an increased risk of salicylate sensitivity. Surgical patients should avoid ASA if possible, for 1-2 weeks prior to surgery, to reduce the risk of excessive bleeding.

Pravastatin: Secondary causes of hyperlipidemia should be ruled out prior to therapy. Liver function must be monitored by periodic laboratory assessment. Rhabdomyolysis with acute renal failure has occurred. Risk may be increased

(Continued)

Aspirin and Pravastatin *(Continued)*

with concurrent use of other drugs which may cause rhabdomyolysis (including gemfibrozil, fibric acid derivatives, or niacin at doses ≥1 g/day). Temporarily discontinue in any patient experiencing an acute or serious condition predisposing to renal failure secondary to rhabdomyolysis. Use caution in patients with previous liver disease or heavy ethanol use.

Combination product is not appropriate for use in pediatric patients.

Adverse Reactions Clinical studies of this combination product have not been conducted. See individual agents.

Overdosage/Toxicology See individual agents.

Drug Interactions

Aspirin: **Substrate** of CYP2C9 (minor)

Pravastatin: **Substrate** of CYP3A4 (minor); **Inhibits** CYP2C9 (weak), 2D6 (weak), 3A4 (weak)

Also see individual agents.

Ethanol/Nutrition/Herb Interactions See individual agents.

Dietary Considerations May be taken with or without food. Red yeast rice contains an estimated 2.4 mg lovastatin per 600 mg rice.

Dosage Forms [DSC] = Discontinued product

Combination package (Pravigard™ PAC) [each administration card contains] [DSC]:

81/20:

Tablet: Aspirin, buffered 81 mg (5/card) [contains calcium carbonate, and magnesium oxide, and magnesium carbonate]

Tablet (Pravachol®): Pravastatin sodium 20 mg (5/card) [contains lactose]

81/40:

Tablet: Aspirin, buffered 81 mg (5/card) [contains calcium carbonate, and magnesium oxide, and magnesium carbonate]

Tablet (Pravachol®): Pravastatin sodium 40 mg (5/card) [contains lactose]

81/80:

Tablet: Aspirin, buffered 81 mg (5/card) [contains calcium carbonate, and magnesium oxide, and magnesium carbonate]

Tablet (Pravachol®): Pravastatin sodium 80 mg (5/card) [contains lactose]

325/20:

Tablet: Aspirin, buffered 325 mg (5/card) [contains calcium carbonate, and magnesium oxide, and magnesium carbonate]

Tablet (Pravachol®): Pravastatin sodium 20 mg (5/card) [contains lactose]

325/40:

Tablet: Aspirin, buffered 325 mg (5/card) [contains calcium carbonate, and magnesium oxide, and magnesium carbonate]

Tablet (Pravachol®): Pravastatin sodium 40 mg (5/card) [contains lactose]

325/80:

Tablet: Aspirin, buffered 325 mg (5/card) [contains calcium carbonate, and magnesium oxide, and magnesium carbonate]

Tablet (Pravachol®): Pravastatin sodium 80 mg (5/card) [contains lactose]

- **Aspirin Free Anacin® Maximum Strength [OTC]** *see* Acetaminophen *on page 26*
- **Astramorph/PF™** *see* Morphine Sulfate *on page 867*
- **AT-III** *see* Antithrombin III *on page 115*
- **Atacand®** *see* Candesartan *on page 219*
- **Atasol® (Can)** *see* Acetaminophen *on page 26*

Atenolol (a TEN oh lole)

Medication Safety Issues

Sound-alike/look-alike issues:

Atenolol may be confused with albuterol, Altenol®, timolol, Tylenol®

Tenormin® may be confused with Imuran®, Norpramin®, thiamine, Trovan®

Related Information

Anesthesia for Patients With Liver Disease *on page 1421*

Antiarrhythmic Drugs *on page 1548*

Beta-Blockers *on page 1557*

Preoperative Evaluation of the Cardiac Patient for Noncardiac Surgery *on page 1485*

U.S. Brand Names Tenormin®

Canadian Brand Names Apo-Atenol®; Gen-Atenolol; Novo-Atenol; Nu-Atenol; PMS-Atenolol; Rhoxal-atenolol; Riva-Atenolol; Sandoz-Atenolol; Tenolin; Tenormin®

Pharmacologic Category Beta Blocker, $Beta_1$ Selective

Generic Available Yes: Tablet

Use Treatment of hypertension, alone or in combination with other agents; management of angina pectoris, postmyocardial infarction patients

Unlabeled/Investigational Use Acute ethanol withdrawal, supraventricular and ventricular arrhythmias, and migraine headache prophylaxis

Mechanism of Action Competitively blocks response to beta-adrenergic stimulation, selectively blocks $beta_1$-receptors with little or no effect on $beta_2$-receptors except at high doses

Pharmacodynamics/Kinetics

Onset of action: Peak effect: Oral: 2-4 hours

Duration: Normal renal function: 12-24 hours

Absorption: Incomplete

Distribution: Low lipophilicity; does not cross blood-brain barrier

Protein binding: 3% to 15%

Metabolism: Limited hepatic

Half-life elimination: Beta:

Neonates: ≤35 hours; Mean: 16 hours

Children: 4.6 hours; children >10 years may have longer half-life (>5 hours) compared to children 5-10 years (<5 hours)

Adults: Normal renal function: 6-9 hours, prolonged with renal impairment; End-stage renal disease: 15-35 hours

Excretion: Feces (50%); urine (40% as unchanged drug)

Dosage

Oral:

Children: 0.8-1 mg/kg/dose given daily; range of 0.8-1.5 mg/kg/day; maximum dose: 2 mg/kg/day

Adults:

Hypertension: 25-50 mg once daily, may increase to 100 mg/day. Doses >100 mg are unlikely to produce any further benefit.

Angina pectoris: 50 mg once daily, may increase to 100 mg/day. Some patients may require 200 mg/day.

Postmyocardial infarction: Follow I.V. dose with 100 mg/day or 50 mg twice daily for 6-9 days postmyocardial infarction.

I.V.:

Hypertension: Dosages of 1.25-5 mg every 6-12 hours have been used in short-term management of patients unable to take oral enteral beta-blockers

Postmyocardial infarction: Early treatment: 5 mg slow I.V. over 5 minutes; may repeat in 10 minutes. If both doses are tolerated, may start oral atenolol 50 mg every 12 hours or 100 mg/day for 6-9 days postmyocardial infarction.

Dosing interval for oral atenolol in renal impairment:

Cl_{cr} 15-35 mL/minute: Administer 50 mg/day maximum.

Cl_{cr} <15 mL/minute: Administer 50 mg every other day maximum.

Hemodialysis: Moderately dialyzable (20% to 50%) via hemodialysis; administer dose postdialysis or administer 25-50 mg supplemental dose.

Peritoneal dialysis: Elimination is not enhanced; supplemental dose is not necessary.

Stability Protect from light.

Administration When administered acutely for cardiac treatment, monitor ECG and blood pressure. The injection can be administered undiluted or diluted with a compatible I.V. solution. May administer by rapid infusion (I.V. push) at a rate of 1 mg/minute or by slow infusion over ~30 minutes. Necessary monitoring for surgical patients who are unable to take oral beta-blockers (prolonged ileus) has not been defined. Some institutions require monitoring of baseline and postinfusion heart rate and blood pressure when a patient's response to beta-blockade has not been characterized (ie, the patient's initial dose or following a change in dose). Consult individual institutional policies and procedures.

Monitoring Parameters Acute cardiac treatment: Monitor ECG and blood pressure with I.V. administration; heart rate and blood pressure with oral administration

(Continued)

Atenolol *(Continued)*

Anesthesia and Critical Care Concerns/Other Considerations Atenolol may mask signs and symptoms of hypoglycemia; may potentiate hypoglycemia in a diabetic patient.

Myocardial Infarction: Beta-blockers, in general without intrinsic sympathomimetic activity (ISA), have been shown to decrease morbidity and mortality when initiated in the acute treatment of myocardial infarction and continued long-term. In this setting, therapy should be avoided in patients with hypotension, cardiogenic shock, or heart block.

Surgery: Atenolol has also been shown to improve cardiovascular outcomes when used in the perioperative period in patients with underlying cardiovascular disease who are undergoing noncardiac surgery. Bisoprolol in high-risk patients undergoing vascular surgery reduced the perioperative incidence of death from cardiac causes and nonfatal myocardial infarction.

Withdrawal: Beta-blocker therapy should not be withdrawn abruptly, but gradually tapered to avoid acute tachycardia and hypertension.

Pregnancy Risk Factor D

Contraindications Hypersensitivity to atenolol or any component of the formulation; sinus bradycardia; sinus node dysfunction; heart block greater than first-degree (except in patients with a functioning artificial pacemaker); cardiogenic shock; uncompensated cardiac failure; pulmonary edema; pregnancy

Warnings/Precautions Safety and efficacy in children have not been established. Administer cautiously in compensated heart failure and monitor for a worsening of the condition (efficacy of atenolol in heart failure has not been established). **[U.S. Boxed Warning]: Beta-blocker therapy should not be withdrawn abruptly (particularly in patients with CAD), but gradually tapered to avoid acute tachycardia, hypertension, and/or ischemia.** Use caution with concurrent use of beta-blockers and either verapamil or diltiazem; bradycardia or heart block can occur. Avoid concurrent I.V. use of both agents. Beta-blockers should be avoided in patients with bronchospastic disease (asthma). Atenolol, with B1 selectivity, has been used cautiously in bronchospastic disease with close monitoring. Use cautiously in peripheral arterial disease, especially if severe disease is present. Use cautiously in patients with diabetes - may mask hypoglycemic symptoms. May mask signs of thyrotoxicosis. May cause fetal harm when administered in pregnancy. Use cautiously in the renally impaired (dosage adjustment required). Use care with anesthetic agents which decrease myocardial function. Caution in myasthenia gravis.

Adverse Reactions

1% to 10%:

- Cardiovascular: Persistent bradycardia, hypotension, chest pain, edema, heart failure, second- or third-degree AV block, Raynaud's phenomenon
- Central nervous system: Dizziness, fatigue, insomnia, lethargy, confusion, mental impairment, depression, headache, nightmares
- Gastrointestinal: Constipation, diarrhea, nausea
- Genitourinary: Impotence
- Miscellaneous: Cold extremities

<1% (Limited to important or life-threatening): Alopecia, dyspnea (especially with large doses), hallucinations, impotence, liver enzymes increased, lupus syndrome, Peyronie's disease, positive ANA, psoriaform rash, psychosis, thrombocytopenia, wheezing

Overdosage/Toxicology Symptoms of toxicity include lethargy, respiratory drive disorder, wheezing, sinus pause, and bradycardia. Additional effects associated with any beta-blocker are congestive heart failure, hypotension, bronchospasm, and hypoglycemia. Treatment includes removal of unabsorbed drug by induced emesis, gastric lavage, or administration of activated charcoal and symptomatic treatment of toxic responses. Atenolol can be removed by hemodialysis.

Drug Interactions

Alpha-blockers (prazosin, terazosin): Concurrent use of beta-blockers may increase risk of orthostasis.

Ampicillin, in single doses of 1 gram, decreases atenolol's pharmacologic actions.

Antacids (magnesium-aluminum, calcium antacids or salts) may reduce the bioavailability of atenolol.

Clonidine: Hypertensive crisis after or during withdrawal of either agent.

Drugs which slow AV conduction (digoxin): Effects may be additive with beta-blockers.

Glucagon: Atenolol may blunt the hyperglycemic action of glucagon.

Insulin and oral hypoglycemics: Atenolol masks the tachycardia that usually accompanies hypoglycemia.

NSAIDs (ibuprofen, indomethacin, naproxen, piroxicam) may reduce the antihypertensive effects of beta-blockers.

Salicylates may reduce the antihypertensive effects of beta-blockers.

Sulfonylureas: Beta-blockers may alter response to hypoglycemic agents.

Verapamil or diltiazem may have synergistic or additive pharmacological effects when taken concurrently with beta-blockers.

Ethanol/Nutrition/Herb Interactions

Food: Atenolol serum concentrations may be decreased if taken with food.

Herb/Nutraceutical: Avoid dong quai if using for hypertension (has estrogenic activity). Avoid ephedra, yohimbe, ginseng (may worsen hypertension). Avoid garlic (may have increased antihypertensive effect).

Test Interactions Increased glucose; decreased HDL

Dietary Considerations May be taken without regard to meals.

Dosage Forms

Injection, solution: 0.5 mg/mL (10 mL)

Tablet: 25 mg, 50 mg, 100 mg

References

Radack K and Deck C, "Beta-Adrenergic Blocker Therapy Does Not Worsen Intermittent Claudication in Subjects With Peripheral Arterial Disease. A Meta-Analysis of Randomized Controlled Trials," *Arch Intern Med*, 1991, 151(9):1769-76.

♦ **Ativan®** *see* Lorazepam *on page 773*

Atorvastatin (a TORE va sta tin)

Medication Safety Issues

Sound-alike/look-alike issues:

Lipitor® may be confused with Levatol®

Related Information

Hyperlipidemia Management *on page 1614*

U.S. Brand Names Lipitor®

Canadian Brand Names Lipitor®

Pharmacologic Category Antilipemic Agent, HMG-CoA Reductase Inhibitor

Generic Available No

Use Treatment of dyslipidemias or primary prevention of cardiovascular disease (atherosclerotic) as detailed below:

Primary prevention of cardiovascular disease (high-risk for CVD): To reduce the risk of MI or stroke in patients without evidence of heart disease who have multiple CVD risk factors or type 2 diabetes. Treatment reduces the risk for angina or revascularization procedures in patients with multiple risk factors.

Treatment of dyslipidemias: To reduce elevations in total cholesterol, LDL-C, apolipoprotein B, and triglycerides in patients with elevations of one or more components, and/or to increase HDL-C as present in Fredrickson type IIa, IIb, III, and IV hyperlipidemias; treatment of primary dysbetalipoproteinemia, homozygous familial hypercholesterolemia

Treatment of heterozygous familial hypercholesterolemia (HeFH) in adolescent patients (10-17 years of age, females >1 year postmenarche) having LDL-C ≥190 mg/dL or LDL-C ≥160 mg/dL with positive family history of premature cardiovascular disease (CVD) or with two or more CVD risk factors.

Mechanism of Action Inhibitor of 3-hydroxy-3-methylglutaryl coenzyme A (HMG-CoA) reductase, the rate-limiting enzyme in cholesterol synthesis (reduces the production of mevalonic acid from HMG-CoA); this then results in a compensatory increase in the expression of LDL receptors on hepatocyte membranes and a stimulation of LDL catabolism

Pharmacodynamics/Kinetics

Onset of action: Initial changes: 3-5 days; Maximal reduction in plasma cholesterol and triglycerides: 2 weeks

Absorption: Rapid

Distribution: V_d: 318 L

Protein binding: ≥98%

Metabolism: Hepatic; forms active ortho- and parahydroxylated derivates and an inactive beta-oxidation product

Half-life elimination: Parent drug: 14 hours

Time to peak, serum: 1-2 hours

(Continued)

Atorvastatin *(Continued)*

Excretion: Bile; urine (2% as unchanged drug)

Dosage Oral: **Note:** Doses should be individualized according to the baseline LDL-cholesterol levels, the recommended goal of therapy, and patient response; adjustments should be made at intervals of 2-4 weeks

Children 10-17 years (females >1 year postmenarche): HeFH: 10 mg once daily (maximum: 20 mg/day)

Adults:

Hyperlipidemias: Initial: 10-20 mg once daily; patients requiring >45% reduction in LDL-C may be started at 40 mg once daily; range: 10-80 mg once daily

Primary prevention of CVD: 10 mg once daily

Dosing adjustment in renal impairment: No dosage adjustment is necessary.

Dosing adjustment in hepatic impairment: Do not use in active liver disease.

Administration May be administered with food if desired; may take without regard to time of day.

Monitoring Parameters Lipid levels after 2-4 weeks; LFTs, CPK

It is recommended that liver function tests (LFTs) be performed prior to and at 12 weeks following both the initiation of therapy and any elevation in dose, and periodically (eg, semiannually) thereafter

Anesthesia and Critical Care Concerns/Other Considerations **Myopathy:** Currently-marketed HMG-CoA reductase inhibitors appear to have a similar potential for causing myopathy. Incidence of severe myopathy is about 0.08% to 0.09%. The factors that increase risk include advanced age (especially >80 years), gender (occurs in women more frequently than men), small body frame, frailty, multisystem disease (eg, chronic renal insufficiency especially due to diabetes), multiple medications, **perioperative periods (higher risk when continued during hospitalization for major surgery)**, and drug interactions (use with caution or avoid).

Pregnancy Risk Factor X

Contraindications Hypersensitivity to atorvastatin or any component of the formulation; active liver disease; unexplained persistent elevations of serum transaminases; pregnancy

Warnings/Precautions Secondary causes of hyperlipidemia should be ruled out prior to therapy. May cause hepatic dysfunction. Use with caution in patients who consume large amounts of ethanol or have a history of liver disease. Monitoring is recommended. Rhabdomyolysis with acute renal failure has occurred. Risk is dose related and is increased with concurrent use of lipid-lowering agents which may cause rhabdomyolysis (gemfibrozil, fibric acid derivatives, or niacin at doses ≥1 g/day) or during concurrent use with potent CYP3A4 inhibitors (including amiodarone, clarithromycin, cyclosporine, erythromycin, itraconazole, ketoconazole, nefazodone, grapefruit juice in large quantities, verapamil, or protease inhibitors such as indinavir, nelfinavir, or ritonavir). Weigh the risk versus benefit when combining any of these drugs with atorvastatin. Discontinue in any patient experiencing an acute or serious condition predisposing to renal failure secondary to rhabdomyolysis. Safety and efficacy have not been established in patients <10 years of age or in premenarcheal girls.

Adverse Reactions

>10%: Central nervous system: Headache (3% to 17%)

2% to 10%:

Cardiovascular: Chest pain, peripheral edema

Central nervous system: Insomnia, dizziness

Dermatologic: Rash (1% to 4%)

Gastrointestinal: Abdominal pain (up to 4%), constipation (up to 3%), diarrhea (up to 4%), dyspepsia (1% to 3%), flatulence (1% to 3%), nausea

Genitourinary: Urinary tract infection

Hepatic: Transaminases increased (2% to 3% with 80 mg/day dosing)

Neuromuscular & skeletal: Arthralgia (up to 5%), arthritis, back pain (up to 4%), myalgia (up to 6%), weakness (up to 4%)

Respiratory: Sinusitis (up to 6%), pharyngitis (up to 3%), bronchitis, rhinitis

Miscellaneous: Infection (3% to 10%), flu-like syndrome (up to 3%), allergic reaction (up to 3%)

<2% (Limited to important or life-threatening): Alopecia, anaphylaxis, angina, angioneurotic edema, arrhythmia, bullous rash, cholestatic jaundice, deafness, dyspnea, erythema multiforme, esophagitis, facial paralysis, fatigue, glaucoma, gout, hepatitis, hyperkinesias, impotence, migraine, myasthenia, myopathy, myositis, nephritis, pancreatitis, paresthesia, peripheral neuropathy, petechiae,

photosensitivity, postural hypotension, pruritus, rectal hemorrhage, rhabdomyolysis, somnolence, Stevens-Johnson syndrome, syncope, tendinous contracture, thrombocytopenia, tinnitus, torticollis, toxic epidermal necrolysis, urticaria, vaginal hemorrhage, vomiting

Overdosage/Toxicology Treatment is supportive.

Drug Interactions Substrate of CYP3A4 (major); **Inhibits** CYP3A4 (weak)

Antacids: Plasma concentrations may be decreased when given with magnesium-aluminum hydroxide containing antacids (reported with atorvastatin and pravastatin). Clinical efficacy is not altered, no dosage adjustment is necessary.

Bile acid sequestrants (cholestyramine and colestipol): Reduce absorption of several HMG-CoA reductase inhibitors; separate administration times by at least 4 hours. Cholesterol-lowering effects are additive.

Cyclosporine: May increase serum concentrations of atorvastatin, increasing the risk of myopathy; monitor.

CYP3A4 inhibitors: May increase the levels/effects of atorvastatin. Example inhibitors include azole antifungals, clarithromycin, diclofenac, doxycycline, erythromycin, imatinib, isoniazid, nefazodone, nicardipine, propofol, protease inhibitors, quinidine, telithromycin, and verapamil.

Digoxin: Plasma concentrations of digoxin may be increased by ~20%; monitor.

Fibric acid derivatives (clofibrate and fenofibrate): May increase the risk of myopathy and rhabdomyolysis.

Grapefruit juice: May inhibit metabolism of atorvastatin via CYP3A4; more likely to occur with lovastatin or simvastatin; avoid high dietary intake of grapefruit juice.

Niacin: May increase the risk of myopathy and rhabdomyolysis.

Ethanol/Nutrition/Herb Interactions

Ethanol: Avoid excessive ethanol consumption (due to potential hepatic effects).

Food: Atorvastatin serum concentrations may be increased by grapefruit juice; avoid concurrent intake of large quantities (>1 quart/day). Red yeast rice contains an estimated 2.4 mg lovastatin per 600 mg rice.

Herb/Nutraceutical: St John's wort may decrease atorvastatin levels.

Dietary Considerations May take with food if desired; may take without regard to time of day. Before initiation of therapy, patients should be placed on a standard cholesterol-lowering diet for 3-6 months and the diet should be continued during drug therapy. Red yeast rice contains an estimated 2.4 mg lovastatin per 600 mg rice.

Dosage Forms Tablet: 10 mg, 20 mg, 40 mg, 80 mg

Atracurium (a tra KYOO ree um)

Medication Safety Issues

High alert medication: The Institute for Safe Medication Practices (ISMP) includes this medication among its list of drugs which have a heightened risk of causing significant patient harm when used in error.

Related Information

Anesthesia for Patients With Liver Disease *on page 1421*
Chronic Renal Failure *on page 1437*
Neuromuscular Blocking Agents *on page 1572*

U.S. Brand Names Tracrium®

Canadian Brand Names Atracurium Besylate Injection

Synonyms Atracurium Besylate

Pharmacologic Category Neuromuscular Blocker Agent, Nondepolarizing

Generic Available Yes

Use Adjunct to general anesthesia to facilitate endotracheal intubation and to relax skeletal muscles during surgery; to facilitate mechanical ventilation in ICU patients; does not relieve pain or produce sedation

Mechanism of Action Blocks neural transmission at the myoneural junction by binding with cholinergic receptor sites

Pharmacodynamics/Kinetics

Onset of action (dose dependent): 2-3 minutes

Duration: Recovery begins in 20-35 minutes following initial dose of 0.4-0.5 mg/kg under balanced anesthesia; recovery to 95% of control takes 60-70 minutes

Metabolism: Undergoes ester hydrolysis and Hofmann elimination (nonbiologic process independent of renal, hepatic, or enzymatic function); metabolites have no neuromuscular blocking properties; laudanosine, a product of Hofmann elimination, is a CNS stimulant and can accumulate with prolonged use. Laudanosine is hepatically metabolized.

(Continued)

Atracurium *(Continued)*

Half-life elimination: Biphasic: Adults: Initial (distribution): 2 minutes; Terminal: 20 minutes

Excretion: Urine (<5%)

Dosage I.V. (not to be used I.M.): Dose to effect; doses must be individualized due to interpatient variability; use ideal body weight for obese patients

Children 1 month to 2 years: Initial: 0.3-0.4 mg/kg followed by maintenance doses as needed to maintain neuromuscular blockade

Children >2 years to Adults: 0.4-0.5 mg/kg, then 0.08-0.1 mg/kg 20-45 minutes after initial dose to maintain neuromuscular block, followed by repeat doses of 0.08-0.1 mg/kg at 15- to 25-minute intervals

Initial dose after succinylcholine for intubation (balanced anesthesia): Adults: 0.2-0.4 mg/kg

Pretreatment/priming: 10% of intubating dose given 3-5 minutes before initial dose

Continuous infusion:

Surgery: Initial: 9-10 mcg/kg/minute at initial signs of recovery from bolus dose; block usually maintained by a rate of 5-9 mcg/kg/minute under balanced anesthesia

ICU: Block usually maintained by rate of 11-13 mcg/kg/minute (rates for pediatric patients may be higher)

See table.

Atracurium Besylate Infusion Chart

Drug Delivery Rate (mcg/kg/min)	Infusion Rate (mL/kg/min) 0.2 mg/mL (20 mg/100 mL)	Infusion Rate (mL/kg/min) 0.5 mg/mL (50 mg/100 mL)
5	0.025	0.01
6	0.03	0.012
7	0.035	0.014
8	0.04	0.016
9	0.045	0.018
10	0.05	0.02

Dosage adjustment for hepatic or renal impairment is not necessary

Stability Refrigerate; unstable in alkaline solutions; **compatible** with D_5W, D_5NS, and NS; do not dilute in LR

Administration May be given undiluted as a bolus injection; not for I.M. injection due to tissue irritation; administration via infusion requires the use of an infusion pump; use infusion solutions within 24 hours of preparation

Monitoring Parameters Vital signs (heart rate, blood pressure, respiratory rate); degree of muscle relaxation (via peripheral nerve stimulator and presence of spontaneous movement); renal function (serum creatinine, BUN) and liver function when in ICU

In the ICU setting, prolonged paralysis and generalized myopathy, following discontinuation of agent, may be minimized by appropriately monitoring degree of blockade.

Anesthesia and Critical Care Concerns/Other Considerations Atracurium is classified as an intermediate duration neuromuscular-blocking agent; does not appear to have a cumulative effect on the duration of blockade.

Critically-Ill Adult Patients:

The 2004 Surviving Sepsis Campaign guidelines recommend avoiding use of neuromuscular blockers if at all possible in the septic patient due to the risk of prolonged neuromuscular blockade following discontinuation. If one is required, monitor carefully and observe the following recommendations.

The 2002 ACCM/SCCM/ASHP clinical practice guidelines for sustained neuromuscular blockade in the adult critically-ill patient recommend:

Optimize sedatives and analgesics prior to initiation, and monitor and adjust accordingly during course. Neuromuscular blockers do not relieve pain or produce sedation.

Protect patient's eyes from development of keratitis and corneal abrasion by administering ophthalmic ointment and taping eyelids closed or using eye patches. Reposition patient routinely to protect pressure points from breakdown. Address DVT prophylaxis.

Concurrent use of a neuromuscular blocker and corticosteroids appear to increase the risk of certain ICU myopathies; avoid or administer the corticosteroid at the lowest dose possible. Reassess need for neuromuscular blocker daily.

Using daily drug holidays (stopping neuromuscular-blocking agent until patient requires it again) may decrease the incidence of acute quadriplegic myopathy syndrome.

Tachyphylaxis can develop; switch to another neuromuscular blocker (taking into consideration the patient's organ function) if paralysis is still necessary.

Acidosis and severe hypothermia may delay the elimination of atracurium and cisatracurium.

Atracurium or cisatracurium is recommended for patients with significant hepatic or renal disease due to organ-independent Hofmann elimination.

Monitor patients clinically and via "Train of Four" (TOF) testing with a goal of adjusting the degree of blockade to 1-2 twitches or based upon the patient's clinical condition.

Pregnancy Risk Factor C

Contraindications Hypersensitivity to atracurium besylate or any component of the formulation

Warnings/Precautions Reduce initial dosage and inject slowly (over 1-2 minutes) in patients in whom substantial histamine release would be potentially hazardous (eg, patients with clinically-important cardiovascular disease). Maintenance of an adequate airway and respiratory support is critical. Certain clinical conditions may result in potentiation or antagonism of neuromuscular blockade:

Potentiation: Electrolyte abnormalities, severe hyponatremia, severe hypocalcemia, severe hypokalemia, hypermagnesemia, neuromuscular diseases, acidosis, acute intermittent porphyria, renal failure, hepatic failure

Antagonism: Alkalosis, hypercalcemia, demyelinating lesions, peripheral neuropathies, diabetes mellitus

Increased sensitivity in patients with myasthenia gravis, Eaton-Lambert syndrome; resistance in burn patients (>30% of body) for period of 5-70 days postinjury; resistance in patients with muscle trauma, denervation, immobilization, infection, chronic treatment with atracurium. Cross-sensitivity with other neuromuscular-blocking agents may occur; use extreme caution in patients with previous anaphylactic reactions. Bradycardia may be more common with atracurium than with other neuromuscular-blocking agents since it has no clinically-significant effects on heart rate to counteract the bradycardia produced by anesthetics.

Adverse Reactions Mild, rare, and generally suggestive of histamine release

1% to 10%: Cardiovascular: Flushing

<1%: Bronchial secretions, erythema, hives, itching, wheezing

Postmarketing and/or case reports: Allergic reaction, bradycardia, bronchospasm, dyspnea, hypotension, injection site reaction, seizure, acute quadriplegic myopathy syndrome (prolonged use), laryngospasm, myositis ossificans (prolonged use), tachycardia, urticaria

Causes of prolonged neuromuscular blockade: Excessive drug administration; cumulative drug effect, metabolism/excretion decreased (hepatic and/or renal impairment); accumulation of active metabolites; electrolyte imbalance (hypokalemia, hypocalcemia, hypermagnesemia, hypernatremia); hypothermia

Overdosage/Toxicology Symptoms of overdose include respiratory depression and cardiovascular collapse.

Neostigmine 1-3 mg slow I.V. push in adults (0.5 mg in children) antagonizes the neuromuscular blockade and should be administered with or immediately after atropine 1-1.5 mg I.V. push (adults). This may be especially useful in the presence of bradycardia.

Drug Interactions

Prolonged neuromuscular blockade: Local anesthetics, calcium channel blockers, corticosteroids, antiarrhythmics (eg, quinidine or procainamide), antibiotics (eg, aminoglycosides, tetracyclines, vancomycin, clindamycin), immunosuppressants (eg, cyclosporine).

Increased sensitivity to muscle relaxants (eg, neuromuscular disorders such as myasthenia gravis or polymyositis).

Dosage Forms

Injection, as besylate: 10 mg/mL (10 mL) [contains benzyl alcohol]

(Continued)

Atracurium *(Continued)*

Injection, as besylate [preservative free]: 10 mg/mL (5 mL)

References

Dellinger RP, Carlet JM, Masur H, et al, "Surviving Sepsis Campaign Guidelines for Management of Severe Sepsis and Septic Shock," *Crit Care Med*, 2004, 32(3):858-73.

Peat SJ, Potter DR, and Hunter JM, "The Prolonged Use of Atracurium in a Patient With Tetanus," *Anaesthesia*, 1988, 43(11):962-3.

Yate PM, Flynn PJ, Arnold RW, et al, "Clinical Experience and Plasma Laudanosine Concentrations During the Infusion of Atracurium in the Intensive Therapy Unit," *Br J Anaesth*, 1987, 59(2):211-7.

♦ **Atracurium Besylate** *see* Atracurium *on page 141*

♦ **Atracurium Besylate Injection (Can)** *see* Atracurium *on page 141*

♦ **AtroPen®** *see* Atropine *on page 144*

Atropine (A troe peen)

Related Information

Cycloplegic Mydriatics *on page 1564*

Management of Postoperative Arrhythmias *on page 1451*

U.S. Brand Names AtroPen®; Atropine-Care®; Isopto® Atropine; Sal-Tropine™

Canadian Brand Names Dioptic's Atropine Solution; Isopto® Atropine

Synonyms Atropine Sulfate

Pharmacologic Category Anticholinergic Agent; Anticholinergic Agent, Ophthalmic; Antidote; Antispasmodic Agent, Gastrointestinal; Ophthalmic Agent, Mydriatic

Restrictions The AtroPen® formulation is available for use primarily by the Department of Defense.

Generic Available Yes: Excludes tablet

Use

Injection: Preoperative medication to inhibit salivation and secretions; treatment of symptomatic sinus bradycardia; AV block (nodal level); ventricular asystole; antidote for organophosphate pesticide poisoning

Ophthalmic: Produce mydriasis and cycloplegia for examination of the retina and optic disc and accurate measurement of refractive errors; uveitis

Oral: Inhibit salivation and secretions

Unlabeled/Investigational Use Pulseless electric activity, asystole, neuromuscular blockade reversal; treatment of nerve agent toxicity (chemical warfare) in combination with pralidoxime

Mechanism of Action Blocks the action of acetylcholine at parasympathetic sites in smooth muscle, secretory glands, and the CNS; increases cardiac output, dries secretions, antagonizes histamine and serotonin

Pharmacodynamics/Kinetics

Onset of action: I.V.: Rapid

Absorption: Complete

Distribution: Widely throughout the body; crosses placenta; trace amounts enter breast milk; crosses blood-brain barrier

Metabolism: Hepatic

Half-life elimination: 2-3 hours

Excretion: Urine (30% to 50% as unchanged drug and metabolites)

Dosage

Neonates, Infants, and Children: Doses <0.1 mg have been associated with paradoxical bradycardia.

Inhibit salivation and secretions (preanesthesia): Oral, I.M., I.V., SubQ:

<5 kg: 0.02 mg/kg/dose 30-60 minutes preop then every 4-6 hours as needed. Use of a minimum dosage of 0.1 mg in neonates <5 kg will result in dosages >0.02 mg/kg. There is no documented minimum dosage in this age group.

>5 kg: 0.01-0.02 mg/kg/dose to a maximum 0.4 mg/dose 30-60 minutes preop; minimum dose: 0.1 mg

Alternate dosing:

3-7 kg (7-16 lb): 0.1 mg

8-11 kg (17-24 lb): 0.15 mg

11-18 kg (24-40 lb): 0.2 mg

18-29 kg (40-65 lb): 0.3 mg

>30 kg (>65 lb): 0.4 mg

Bradycardia: I.V., intratracheal: 0.02 mg/kg, minimum dose 0.1 mg, maximum single dose: 0.5 mg in children and 1 mg in adolescents; may repeat in

5-minute intervals to a maximum total dose of 1 mg in children or 2 mg in adolescents. (**Note:** For intratracheal administration, the dosage must be diluted with normal saline to a total volume of 1-5 mL). When treating bradycardia in neonates, reserve use for those patients unresponsive to improved oxygenation and epinephrine.

Infants and Children: Nerve agent toxicity management (unlabeled use): See **Note** under adult dosing.

Prehospital ("in the field"): I.M.:

Birth to <2 years: Mild-to-moderate symptoms: 0.05 mg/kg; severe symptoms: 0.1 mg/kg

2-10 years: Mild-to-moderate symptoms: 1 mg; severe symptoms: 2 mg

>10 years: Mild-to-moderate symptoms: 2 mg; severe symptoms: 4 mg

Hospital/emergency department: I.M.:

Birth to <2 years: Mild-to-moderate symptoms: 0.05 mg/kg I.M. **or** 0.02 mg/kg I.V.; severe symptoms: 0.1 mg/kg I.M. **or** 0.02 mg/kg I.V.

2-10 years: Mild-to-moderate symptoms: 1 mg; severe symptoms: 2 mg

>10 years: Mild-to-moderate symptoms: 2 mg; severe symptoms: 4 mg

Note: Pralidoxime is a component of the management of nerve agent toxicity; consult Pralidoxime for specific route and dose. For prehospital ("in the field") management, repeat atropine I.M. (children: 0.05-0.1 mg/kg) at 5-10 minute intervals until secretions have diminished and breathing is comfortable or airway resistance has returned to near normal. For hospital management, repeat atropine I.M. (infants 1 mg; all others: 2 mg) at 5-10 minute intervals until secretions have diminished and breathing is comfortable or airway resistance has returned to near normal.

Children: Organophosphate or carbamate poisoning:

I.V.: 0.03-0.05 mg/kg every 10-20 minutes until atropine effect, then every 1-4 hours for at least 24 hours

I.M. (AtroPen®): Mild symptoms: Administer dose listed below as soon as exposure is known or suspected. If severe symptoms develop after first dose, 2 additional doses should be repeated in 10 minutes; do not administer more than 3 doses. Severe symptoms: Immediately administer 3 doses as follows:

<6.8 kg (15 lb): Use of **AtroPen® formulation not recommended;** administer atropine 0.05 mg/kg

6.8-18 kg (15-40 lb): 0.5 mg/dose

18-41 kg (40-90 lb): 1 mg/dose

>41 kg (>90 lb): 2 mg/dose

Adults (doses <0.5 mg have been associated with paradoxical bradycardia):

Asystole or pulseless electrical activity:

I.V.: 1 mg; repeat in 3-5 minutes if asystole persists; total dose of 0.04 mg/kg.

Intratracheal: Administer 2-2.5 times the recommended I.V. dose; dilute in 10 mL NS or distilled water. **Note:** Absorption is greater with distilled water, but causes more adverse effects on PaO_2.

Inhibit salivation and secretions (preanesthesia):

I.M., I.V., SubQ: 0.4-0.6 mg 30-60 minutes preop and repeat every 4-6 hours as needed

Oral: 0.4 mg; may repeat in 4 hours if necessary

Bradycardia: I.V.: 0.5-1 mg every 5 minutes, not to exceed a total of 3 mg or 0.04 mg/kg; may give intratracheally in 10 mL NS (intratracheal dose should be 2-2.5 times the I.V. dose)

Neuromuscular blockade reversal: I.V.: 25-30 mcg/kg 30-60 seconds before neostigmine or 7-10 mcg/kg 30-60 seconds before edrophonium

Organophosphate or carbamate poisoning:

I.V.: 2 mg, followed by 2 mg every 5-60 minutes until adequate atropinization has occurred; initial doses of up to 6 mg may be used in life-threatening cases

I.M. (AtroPen®): Mild symptoms: Administer 2 mg as soon as exposure is known or suspected. If severe symptoms develop after first dose, 2 additional doses should be repeated in 10 minutes; do not administer more than 3 doses. Severe symptoms: Immediately administer three 2 mg doses.

Nerve agent toxicity management (unlabeled use): I.M.: See **Note**. Prehospital ("in the field") or hospital/emergency department: Mild-to-moderate symptoms: 2-4 mg; severe symptoms: 6 mg

Note: Pralidoxime is a component of the management of nerve agent toxicity; consult Pralidoxime for specific route and dose. For prehospital ("in the field") management, repeat atropine I.M. (2 mg) at 5-10 minute intervals until secretions have diminished and breathing is comfortable or airway

(Continued)

Atropine *(Continued)*

resistance has returned to near normal. For hospital management, repeat atropine I.M. (2 mg) at 5-10 minute intervals until secretions have diminished and breathing is comfortable or airway resistance has returned to near normal.

Mydriasis, cycloplegia (preprocedure): Ophthalmic (1% solution): Instill 1-2 drops 1 hour before procedure.

Uveitis: Ophthalmic:

1% solution: Instill 1-2 drops 4 times/day

Ointment: Apply a small amount in the conjunctival sac up to 3 times/day; compress the lacrimal sac by digital pressure for 1-3 minutes after instillation

Elderly, frail patients: Nerve agent toxicity management (unlabeled use): I.M.: See **Note** under adult dosing.

Prehospital ("in the field"): Mild-to-moderate symptoms: 1 mg; severe symptoms: 2-4 mg

Hospital/emergency department: Mild-to-moderate symptoms: 1 mg; severe symptoms: 2 mg

Stability Store injection at controlled room temperature of 15°C to 30°C (59°F to 86°F); avoid freezing. In addition, AtroPen® should be protected from light.

Administration

I.M.: AtroPen®: Administer to outer thigh. May be given through clothing as long as pockets at the injection site are empty. Hold autoinjector in place for 10 seconds following injection; massage the injection site.

I.V.: Administer undiluted by rapid I.V. injection; slow injection may result in paradoxical bradycardia.

Intratracheal: Dilute in NS or distilled water. Absorption is greater with distilled water, but causes more adverse effects on PaO_2. Pass catheter beyond tip of tracheal tube, stop compressions, spray drug quickly down tube. Follow immediately with several quick insufflations and continue chest compressions.

Monitoring Parameters Heart rate, blood pressure, pulse, mental status; intravenous administration requires a cardiac monitor

Anesthesia and Critical Care Concerns/Other Considerations Atropine, at usual recommended cardiovascular doses, causes blockade of muscarinic receptors at the cardiac SA-node and is parasympatholytic (ie, blocks vagal activity increasing heart rate). A dose 0.5-1 mg is recommended for the treatment of bradyarrhythmias. In administering atropine, it is important to recognize that lower doses (<0.5 mg) may have vagalmimetic effects (ie, increase vagal tone causing paradoxical bradycardia). A total dose of 3 mg (0.04 mg/kg) results in full vagal blockade in humans. In the absence of vascular access, atropine can be administered intratracheally.

Pregnancy Risk Factor C

Contraindications Hypersensitivity to atropine or any component of the formulation; narrow-angle glaucoma; adhesions between the iris and lens; tachycardia; obstructive GI disease; paralytic ileus; intestinal atony of the elderly or debilitated patient; severe ulcerative colitis; toxic megacolon complicating ulcerative colitis; hepatic disease; obstructive uropathy; renal disease; myasthenia gravis (unless used to treat side effects of acetylcholinesterase inhibitor); asthma; thyrotoxicosis; Mobitz type II block

Warnings/Precautions Heat prostration can occur in the presence of a high environmental temperature. Psychosis can occur in sensitive individuals. The elderly may be sensitive to side effects. Use caution in patients with myocardial ischemia. Use caution in hyperthyroidism, autonomic neuropathy, BPH, CHF, tachyarrhythmias, hypertension, and hiatal hernia associated with reflux esophagitis. Use with caution in children with spastic paralysis.

AtroPen®: There are no absolute contraindications for the use of atropine in organophosphate poisonings, however, use caution in those patients where the use of atropine would be otherwise contraindicated. Formulation for use by trained personnel only.

Adverse Reactions Severity and frequency of adverse reactions are dose related and vary greatly; listed reactions are limited to significant and/or life-threatening.

Cardiovascular: Arrhythmia, flushing, hypotension, palpitation, tachycardia

Central nervous system: Ataxia, coma, delirium, disorientation, dizziness, drowsiness, excitement, fever, hallucinations, headache, insomnia, nervousness

Dermatologic: Anhidrosis, urticaria, rash, scarlatiniform rash

Gastrointestinal: Bloating, constipation, delayed gastric emptying, loss of taste, nausea, paralytic ileus, vomiting, xerostomia

Genitourinary: Urinary hesitancy, urinary retention

Neuromuscular & skeletal: Weakness

Ocular: Angle-closure glaucoma, blurred vision, cycloplegia, dry eyes, mydriasis, ocular tension increased

Respiratory: Dyspnea, laryngospasm, pulmonary edema

Miscellaneous: Anaphylaxis

Overdosage/Toxicology Symptoms of overdose include dilated, unreactive pupils; blurred vision; hot, dry flushed skin; dryness of mucous membranes; difficulty swallowing; foul breath; diminished or absent bowel sounds; urinary retention; tachycardia; hyperthermia; hypertension; and increased respiratory rate. For anticholinergic overdose with severe life-threatening symptoms, physostigmine 1-2 mg SubQ or I.V. slowly, may be given to reverse these effects.

Drug Interactions

Drugs with anticholinergic activity (including phenothiazines and TCAs) may increase anticholinergic effects when used concurrently.

Sympathomimetic amines may cause tachyarrhythmias; avoid concurrent use.

Dosage Forms

Injection, solution, as sulfate: 0.05 mg/mL (5 mL); 0.1 mg/mL (5 mL, 10 mL); 0.4 mg/mL (0.5 mL, 1 mL, 20 mL); 0.5 mg/mL (1 mL); 1 mg/mL (1 mL)

AtroPen® [prefilled autoinjector]: 0.5 mg/0.7 mL (0.7 mL); 1 mg/0.7 mL (0.7 mL); 2 mg/0.7 mL (0.7 mL)

Ointment, ophthalmic, as sulfate: 1% (3.5 g)

Solution, ophthalmic, as sulfate: 1% (5 mL, 15 mL)

Atropine-Care®: 1% (2 mL)

Isopto® Atropine: 1% (5 mL, 15 mL)

Tablet, as sulfate (Sal-Tropine™): 0.4 mg

References

American Heart Association and the International Liaison Committee on Resuscitation (ILCOR), "Guidelines 2000 Conference for Cardiopulmonary Resuscitation and Emergency Cardiovascular Care: International Consensus on Science," *Circulation*, 2000, 102(8):I1-252.

Eisenberg MS and Mengert TJ, "Cardiac Resuscitation," *N Engl J Med*, 2001, 344(17):1304-13.

"Medical Management Guidelines (MMGs) for Nerve Agents: Tabun (GA); Sarin (GB); Soman (GD); and VX". Available at: www.atsdr.cdc.gov/MHMI/mmg166.html.

Mokhlesi B, Leikin JB, Murray P, et al, "Adult Toxicology in Critical Care. Part 11:Specific Poisonings," *Chest*, 2003, 123(3):897-922.

♦ **Atropine-Care®** *see* Atropine *on page 144*

♦ **Atropine Sulfate** *see* Atropine *on page 144*

♦ **Atrovent®** *see* Ipratropium *on page 698*

♦ **Atrovent® HFA** *see* Ipratropium *on page 698*

♦ **A/T/S®** *see* Erythromycin *on page 476*

♦ **Avagard™ [OTC]** *see* Chlorhexidine Gluconate *on page 267*

♦ **Avapro®** *see* Irbesartan *on page 700*

♦ **Avaxim® (Can)** *see* Hepatitis A Vaccine *on page 616*

♦ **Avaxim®-Pediatric (Can)** *see* Hepatitis A Vaccine *on page 616*

♦ **Avelox®** *see* Moxifloxacin *on page 873*

♦ **Avelox® I.V.** *see* Moxifloxacin *on page 873*

♦ **Aventyl® (Can)** *see* Nortriptyline *on page 938*

♦ **Avinza®** *see* Morphine Sulfate *on page 867*

♦ **Avodart™** *see* Dutasteride *on page 437*

♦ **Axert™** *see* Almotriptan *on page 62*

♦ **Axid®** *see* Nizatidine *on page 935*

♦ **Axid® AR [OTC]** *see* Nizatidine *on page 935*

♦ **Ayr® Baby Saline [OTC]** *see* Sodium Chloride *on page 1183*

♦ **Ayr® Saline [OTC]** *see* Sodium Chloride *on page 1183*

♦ **Ayr® Saline No-Drip [OTC]** *see* Sodium Chloride *on page 1183*

♦ **Azactam®** *see* Aztreonam *on page 153*

♦ **Azasan®** *see* Azathioprine *on page 148*

Azathioprine (ay za THYE oh preen)

Medication Safety Issues

Sound-alike/look-alike issues:

Azathioprine may be confused with azatadine, azidothymidine, Azulfidine®

Imuran® may be confused with Elmiron®, Enduron®, Imdur®, Inderal®, Tenormin®

U.S. Brand Names Azasan®; Imuran®

Canadian Brand Names Alti-Azathioprine; Apo-Azathioprine®; Gen-Azathioprine; Imuran®; Novo-Azathioprine

Synonyms Azathioprine Sodium

Pharmacologic Category Immunosuppressant Agent

Generic Available Yes

Use Adjunctive therapy in prevention of rejection of kidney transplants; active rheumatoid arthritis

Unlabeled/Investigational Use Adjunct in prevention of rejection of solid organ (nonrenal) transplants; maintenance of remission in Crohn's disease

Mechanism of Action Azathioprine is an imidazolyl derivative of mercaptopurine; antagonizes purine metabolism and may inhibit synthesis of DNA, RNA, and proteins; may also interfere with cellular metabolism and inhibit mitosis. The 6-thioguanine nucleotides appear to mediate the majority of azathioprine's immunosuppressive and toxic effects.

Pharmacodynamics/Kinetics

Distribution: Crosses placenta

Protein binding: ~30%

Metabolism: Hepatic, to 6-mercaptopurine (6-MP), possibly by glutathione S-transferase (GST). Further metabolism of 6-MP (in the liver and GI tract), via three major pathways: Hypoxanthine guanine phosphoribosyltransferase (to 6-thioguanine-nucleotides, or 6-TGN), xanthine oxidase (to 6-thiouric acid), and thiopurine methyltransferase (TPMT), which forms 6-methylmercapotpurine (6-MMP).

Half-life elimination: Parent drug: 12 minutes; mercaptopurine: 0.7-3 hours; End-stage renal disease: Slightly prolonged

Time to peak, plasma: 1-2 hours (including metabolites)

Excretion: Urine (primarily as metabolites)

Dosage I.V. dose is equivalent to oral dose (dosing should be based on ideal body weight):

Children (unlabeled) and Adults:

Renal transplantation: Oral, I.V.: Initial: 3-5 mg/kg/day usually given as a single daily dose, then 1-3 mg/kg/day maintenance

Rheumatoid arthritis: Oral:

Initial: 1 mg/kg/day given once daily or divided twice daily for 6-8 weeks; increase by 0.5 mg/kg every 4 weeks until response or up to 2.5 mg/kg/day; an adequate trial should be a minimum of 12 weeks

Maintenance dose: Reduce dose by 0.5 mg/kg every 4 weeks until lowest effective dose is reached; optimum duration of therapy not specified; may be discontinued abruptly

Adults: Oral: Adjunctive management of severe recurrent aphthous stomatitis (unlabeled use): 50 mg once daily in conjunction with prednisone

Dosing adjustment in renal impairment:

Cl_{cr} 10-50 mL/minute: Administer 75% of normal dose daily

Cl_{cr} <10 mL/minute: Administer 50% of normal dose daily

Hemodialysis: Dialyzable (~45% removed in 8 hours)

Administer dose posthemodialysis: CAPD effects: Unknown; CAVH effects: Unknown

Stability

Tablet: Store at room temperature of 15°C to 25°C (59°F to 77°F); protect from light.

Powder for injection: Store at room temperature of 15°C to 25°C (59°F to 77°F) and protect from light. Parenteral admixture is stable at room temperature (25°C) for 24 hours, and stable under refrigeration (4°C) for 16 days.

Administration

I.V.: Azathioprine can be administered IVP over 5 minutes at a concentration not to exceed 10 mg/mL **or** azathioprine can be further diluted with normal saline or D_5W and administered by intermittent infusion usually over 30-60 minutes; may be extended up to 8 hours.

Oral: Administering tablets after meals or in divided doses may decrease adverse GI events.

Monitoring Parameters CBC, platelet counts, total bilirubin, liver function tests, TPMT genotyping or phenotyping

Pregnancy Risk Factor D

Contraindications Hypersensitivity to azathioprine or any component of the formulation; pregnancy

Warnings/Precautions [U.S. Boxed Warning]: Chronic immunosuppression increases the risk of neoplasia and serious infections. Azathioprine has mutagenic potential to both men and women and with possible hematologic toxicities; hematologic toxicities are dose related and may be more severe with renal transplants undergoing rejection. Gastrointestinal toxicity may occur within the first several weeks of therapy and is reversible. Symptoms may include severe nausea, vomiting, diarrhea, rash, fever, malaise, myalgia, hypotension, and liver enzyme abnormalities. Use with caution in patients with liver disease, renal impairment; monitor hematologic function closely. Patients with genetic deficiency of thiopurine methyltransferase (TPMT) or concurrent therapy with drugs which may inhibit TPMT may be sensitive to myelosuppressive effects.

Adverse Reactions Frequency not defined; dependent upon dose, duration, and concomitant therapy.

Central nervous system: Fever, malaise
Dermatologic: Alopecia, rash
Gastrointestinal: Diarrhea, nausea, pancreatitis, vomiting
Hematologic: Bleeding, leukopenia, macrocytic anemia, pancytopenia, thrombocytopenia
Hepatic: Hepatotoxicity, hepatic veno-occlusive disease, steatorrhea
Neuromuscular & skeletal: Arthralgia, myalgia
Respiratory: Interstitial pneumonitis
Miscellaneous: Hypersensitivity reactions (rare), infection secondary to immunosuppression, neoplasia

Overdosage/Toxicology Symptoms of overdose include nausea, vomiting, diarrhea, and hematologic toxicity. Following initiation of essential overdose management, symptomatic and supportive treatment should be instituted. Dialysis has been reported to remove significant amounts of the drug and its metabolites, and should be considered as a treatment option in those patients who deteriorate despite established forms of therapy.

Drug Interactions

ACE inhibitors: Concomitant therapy may induce anemia and severe leukopenia.
Allopurinol: May increase serum levels of azathioprine's active metabolite (mercaptopurine). Decrease azathioprine dose to 1/3 to 1/4 of normal dose.
Aminosalicylates (olsalazine, mesalamine, sulfasalazine): May inhibit TPMT, increasing toxicity/myelosuppression of azathioprine. Use caution.
Warfarin: Effect may be decreased by azathioprine.

Ethanol/Nutrition/Herb Interactions Herb/Nutraceutical: Avoid cat's claw, echinacea (have immunostimulant properties).

Dietary Considerations May be taken with food.

Dosage Forms

Injection, powder for reconstitution: 100 mg
Tablet [scored]: 50 mg
  Azasan®: 75 mg, 100 mg
  Imuran®: 50 mg

♦ **Azathioprine Sodium** *see* Azathioprine *on page 148*
♦ **Azidothymidine** *see* Zidovudine *on page 1371*

Azithromycin (az ith roe MYE sin)

Medication Safety Issues

Sound-alike/look-alike issues:
  Azithromycin may be confused with erythromycin
  Zithromax® may be confused with Zinacef®

U.S. Brand Names Zithromax®; Zmax™

Canadian Brand Names Apo-Azithromycin®; CO Azithromycin; GMD-Azithromycin; Novo-Azithromycin; PMS-Azithromycin; ratio-Azithromycin; Sandoz-Azithromycin; Zithromax®

(Continued)

Azithromycin *(Continued)*

Synonyms Azithromycin Dihydrate; Zithromax® TRI-PAK™; Zithromax® Z-PAK®

Pharmacologic Category Antibiotic, Macrolide

Generic Available Yes: Tablet

Use Treatment of acute otitis media due to *H. influenzae, M. catarrhalis,* or *S. pneumoniae*; pharyngitis/tonsillitis due to *S. pyogenes*; treatment of mild-to-moderate upper and lower respiratory tract infections, infections of the skin and skin structure, community-acquired pneumonia, pelvic inflammatory disease (PID), sexually-transmitted diseases (urethritis/cervicitis), pharyngitis/tonsillitis (alternative to first-line therapy), and genital ulcer disease (chancroid) due to susceptible strains of *C. trachomatis, M. catarrhalis, H. influenzae, S. aureus, S. pneumoniae, Mycoplasma pneumoniae,* and *C. psittaci*; acute bacterial exacerbations of chronic obstructive pulmonary disease (COPD) due to *H. influenzae, M. catarrhalis,* or *S. pneumoniae*; acute bacterial sinusitis

Unlabeled/Investigational Use Prevention of (or to delay onset of) or treatment of MAC in patients with advanced HIV infection; prophylaxis of bacterial endocarditis in patients who are allergic to penicillin and undergoing surgical or dental procedures; pertussis

Mechanism of Action Inhibits RNA-dependent protein synthesis at the chain elongation step; binds to the 50S ribosomal subunit resulting in blockage of transpeptidation

Pharmacodynamics/Kinetics

Absorption: Rapid

Distribution: Extensive tissue; distributes well into skin, lungs, sputum, tonsils, and cervix; penetration into CSF is poor; I.V.: 33.3 L/kg; Oral: 31.1 L/kg

Protein binding (concentration dependent): 7% to 51%

Metabolism: Hepatic

Bioavailability: 38%, decreased by 17% with extended release suspension; variable effect with food (increased with immediate or delayed release oral suspension, unchanged with tablet)

Half-life elimination: Terminal: Immediate release: 68-72 hours; Extended release: 59 hours

Time to peak, serum: Immediate release: 2-3 hours; Extended release: 5 hours

Excretion: Biliary (major route); urine (6%)

Dosage Note: Extended release suspension (Zmax™) is not interchangeable with immediate release formulations. Use should be limited to approved indications. All doses are expressed as immediate release azithromycin unless otherwise specified.

Usual dosage range:

Children ≥6 months: Oral: 5-12 mg/kg given once daily (maximum: 500 mg/day) **or** 30 mg/kg as a single dose (maximum: 1500 mg)

Adolescents ≥16 years and Adults:

Oral: 250-600 mg once daily **or** 1-2 g as a single dose

I.V.: 250-500 mg once daily

Indication-specific dosing:

Children: Oral:

Bacterial sinusitis: 10 mg/kg once daily for 3 days (maximum: 500 mg/day)

Cat scratch disease (unlabeled use): <45.5 kg: 10 mg/kg as a single dose, then 5 mg/kg once daily for 4 days

Community-acquired pneumonia: 10 mg/kg on day 1 (maximum: 500 mg/day) followed by 5 mg/kg/day once daily on days 2-5 (maximum: 250 mg/day)

Disseminated *M. avium* (unlabeled use):

HIV-infected patients: 5 mg/kg/day once daily (maximum: 250 mg/day) or 20 mg/kg (maximum: 1200 mg) once weekly given alone or in combination with rifabutin

Treatment and secondary prevention in HIV-negative patients: 5 mg/kg/day once daily (maximum: 250 mg/day) in combination with ethambutol, with or without rifabutin

Endocarditis, prophylaxis (unlabeled use): 15 mg/kg 1 hour before procedure (maximum: 500 mg)

Otitis media:

1-day regimen: 30 mg/kg as a single dose (maximum: 1500 mg)

3-day regimen: 10 mg/kg once daily for 3 days (maximum: 500 mg/day)

5-day regimen: 10 mg/kg on day 1 (maximum: 500 mg/day) followed by 5 mg/kg/day once daily on days 2-5 (maximum: 250 mg/day)

Pharyngitis, tonsillitis: Children ≥2 years: 12 mg/kg/day once daily for 5 days (maximum: 500 mg/day)

Pertussis (CDC guidelines):

Children <6 months: 10 mg/kg/day for 5 days

Children ≥6 months: 10 mg/kg on day 1 (maximum: 500 mg/day) followed by 5 mg/kg/day once daily on days 2-5 (maximum: 250 mg/day)

Uncomplicated chlamydial urethritis or cervicitis (unlabeled use): Children ≥45 kg: 1 g as a single dose

Adolescents ≥16 years and Adults:

Bacterial sinusitis: Oral: 500 mg/day for a total of 3 days

Extended release suspension (Zmax™): 2 g as a single dose

Cat scratch disease (unlabeled use): >45.5 kg: 500 mg as a single dose, then 250 mg once daily for 4 days

Chancroid due to *H. ducreyi*: 1 g as a single dose

Community-acquired pneumonia:

Oral (Zmax™): 2 g as a single dose

I.V.: 500 mg as a single dose for at least 2 days, follow I.V. therapy by the oral route with a single daily dose of 500 mg to complete a 7- to 10-day course of therapy.

Disseminated *M. avium* complex disease in patients with advanced HIV infection (unlabeled use): Oral:

Prophylaxis: 1200 mg once weekly (may be combined with rifabutin)

Treatment: 600 mg daily (in combination with ethambutol 15 mg/kg)

Endocarditis, prophylaxis (unlabeled use): Oral: 500 mg 1 hour prior to the procedure

Mild-to-moderate respiratory tract, skin, and soft tissue infections: Oral: 500 mg in a single loading dose on day 1 followed by 250 mg/day as a single dose on days 2-5

Alternative regimen: Bacterial exacerbation of COPD: 500 mg/day for a total of 3 days

Pelvic inflammatory disease (PID): I.V.: 500 mg as a single dose for 1-2 days, follow I.V. therapy by the oral route with a single daily dose of 250 mg to complete a 7-day course of therapy

Pertussis (CDC guidelines): Oral: 500 mg on day 1 followed by 250 mg/day on days 2-5 (maximum: 500 mg/day)

Urethritis/cervicitis: Oral:

Due to C. trachomatis: 1 g as a single dose

Due to N. gonorrhoeae: 2 g as a single dose

Dosage adjustment in renal impairment: Use caution in patients with Cl_{cr} <10 mL/minute

Dosage adjustment in hepatic impairment: Use with caution due to potential for hepatotoxicity (rare). Specific guidelines for dosing in hepatic impairment have not been established.

Stability

Injection: Store intact vials of injection at room temperature. Reconstitute the 500 mg vial with 4.8 mL of sterile water for injection and shake until all of the drug is dissolved. Each mL contains 100 mg azithromycin. Reconstituted solution is stable for 24 hours when stored below 30°C (86°F). Use of a standard syringe is recommended due to the vacuum in the vial (which may draw additional solution through an automated syringe).

The initial solution should be further diluted to a concentration of 1 mg/mL (500 mL) to 2 mg/mL (250 mL) in 0.9% sodium chloride, 5% dextrose in water, or lactated Ringer's. The diluted solution is stable for 24 hours at or below room temperature (30°C or 86°F) and for 7 days if stored under refrigeration (5°C or 41°F).

Other medications should not be infused simultaneously through the same I.V. line.

Suspension, immediate release: Store dry powder below 30°C (86°F). Following reconstitution, store at 5°C to 30°C (41°F to 86°F).

Suspension, extended release: Store dry powder below 30°C (86°F). Following reconstitution, store at 15°C to 30°C (59°F to 86°F); do not freeze. Should be consumed within 12 hours following reconstitution.

Tablets: Store between 15°C to 30°C (59°F to 86°F).

(Continued)

Azithromycin *(Continued)*

Administration

I.V.: Infusate concentration and rate of infusion for azithromycin for injection should be either 1 mg/mL over 3 hours or 2 mg/mL over 1 hour. Other medications should not be infused simultaneously through the same I.V. line.

Oral: Immediate release suspension and tablet may be taken without regard to food; extended release suspension should be taken on an empty stomach (at least 1 hour before or 2 hours following a meal), within 12 hours of reconstitution.

Monitoring Parameters Liver function tests, CBC with differential

Pregnancy Risk Factor B

Contraindications Hypersensitivity to azithromycin, other macrolide antibiotics, or any component of the formulation

Warnings/Precautions Use with caution in patients with hepatic dysfunction; hepatic impairment with or without jaundice has occurred chiefly in older children and adults. It may be accompanied by malaise, nausea, vomiting, abdominal colic, and fever; discontinue use if these occur. May mask or delay symptoms of incubating gonorrhea or syphilis, so appropriate culture and susceptibility tests should be performed prior to initiating azithromycin. Pseudomembranous colitis has been reported with use of macrolide antibiotics; use caution with renal dysfunction. Prolongation of the QT_c interval has been reported with macrolide antibiotics; use caution in patients at risk of prolonged cardiac repolarization. Safety and efficacy have not been established in children <6 months of age with acute otitis media, acute bacterial sinusitis, or community-acquired pneumonia, or in children <2 years of age with pharyngitis/tonsillitis. Suspensions (immediate release and extended release) are not interchangeable.

Adverse Reactions

>10%: Gastrointestinal: Diarrhea (4% to 11%)

1% to 10%:

Central nervous system: Headache

Gastrointestinal: Nausea, abdominal pain, cramping, vomiting (especially with high single-dose regimens)

<1% (Limited to important or life-threatening): Acute renal failure, allergic reaction, aggressive behavior, anaphylaxis, angioedema, arrhythmia (including ventricular tachycardia), cholestatic jaundice, constipation, convulsion, deafness, dehydration, enteritis, erythema multiforme (rare), hearing loss, hepatic necrosis (rare), hepatitis, hypertrophic pyloric stenosis, hypotension, interstitial nephritis, leukopenia, LFTs increased, neutropenia, oral candidiasis, oral moniliasis, palpitations, pancreatitis, paresthesia, pruritus, pseudomembranous colitis, QT_c prolongation (rare), seizure, somnolence, Stevens-Johnson syndrome (rare), syncope, taste perversion, thrombocytopenia, tinnitus, tongue discoloration (rare), torsade de pointes (rare), urticaria, vertigo

Overdosage/Toxicology Symptoms of overdose include nausea, vomiting, diarrhea, and prostration. Treatment is supportive and symptomatic.

Drug Interactions **Substrate** of CYP3A4 (minor); **Inhibits** CYP3A4 (weak)

Cardiac glycosides: Macrolides may increase the serum concentrations of cardiac glycosides; monitor.

Colchicine: Macrolides may increase the adverse/toxic effects of colchicine.

Nelfinavir: May increase azithromycin serum levels; monitor for adverse effects.

Warfarin: Azithromycin and other macrolides may decrease metabolism, via CYP isoenzymes, of warfarin. Monitor for increased effects.

Ethanol/Nutrition/Herb Interactions Food: Rate and extent of GI absorption may be altered depending upon the formulation. Azithromycin suspension, not tablet form, has significantly increased absorption (46%) with food.

Dietary Considerations

Oral suspension, immediate release, may be administered with or without food.

Oral suspension, extended release, should be taken on an empty stomach (at least 1 hour before or 2 hours following a meal).

Tablet may be administered with food to decrease GI effects.

Sodium content:

Injection: 114 mg (4.96 mEq) per vial

Oral suspension, immediate release: 3.7 mg per 100 mg/5 mL of constituted suspension; 7.4 mg per 200 mg/5 mL of constituted suspension; 37 mg per 1 g single-dose packet

Oral suspension, extended release: 148 mg per 2 g constituted suspension

Tablet: 0.9 mg/250 mg tablet; 1.8 mg/500 mg tablet; 2.1 mg/600 mg tablet

Dosage Forms Note: Strength expressed as base

Injection, powder for reconstitution, as dihydrate (Zithromax®): 500 mg [contains sodium 114 mg (4.96 mEq) per vial]

Microspheres for oral suspension, extended release, as dihydrate (Zmax™): 2 g [single-dose bottle; contains sodium 148 mg per bottle; cherry and banana flavor]

Powder for oral suspension, immediate release, as dihydrate (Zithromax®): 100 mg/5 mL (15 mL) [contains sodium 3.7 mg/ 5 mL; cherry creme de vanilla and banana flavor]; 200 mg/5 mL (15 mL, 22.5 mL, 30 mL) [contains sodium 7.4 mg/ 5 mL; cherry creme de vanilla and banana flavor]; 1 g [single-dose packet; contains sodium 37 mg per packet; cherry creme de vanilla and banana flavor]

Tablet, as dihydrate:

Zithromax®: 250 mg [contains sodium 0.9 mg per tablet]; 500 mg [contains sodium 1.8 mg per tablet]; 600 mg [contains sodium 2.1 mg per tablet]

Zithromax® TRI-PAK™ [unit-dose pack]: 500 mg (3s)

Zithromax® Z-PAK® [unit-dose pack]: 250 mg (6s)

Tablet, as monohydrate: 250 mg, 500 mg, 600 mg

- **Azithromycin Dihydrate** *see* Azithromycin *on page 149*
- **Azmacort®** *see* Triamcinolone *on page 1311*
- **AZT™ (Can)** *see* Zidovudine *on page 1371*
- **AZT (error-prone abbreviation)** *see* Zidovudine *on page 1371*
- **Azthreonam** *see* Aztreonam *on page 153*

Aztreonam (AZ tree oh nam)

Medication Safety Issues

Sound-alike/look-alike issues:

Aztreonam may be confused with azidothymidine

U.S. Brand Names Azactam®

Canadian Brand Names Azactam®

Synonyms Azthreonam

Pharmacologic Category Antibiotic, Miscellaneous

Generic Available No

Use Treatment of patients with urinary tract infections, lower respiratory tract infections, septicemia, skin/skin structure infections, intra-abdominal infections, and gynecological infections caused by susceptible gram-negative bacilli

Mechanism of Action Inhibits bacterial cell wall synthesis by binding to one or more of the penicillin binding proteins (PBPs) which in turn inhibits the final transpeptidation step of peptidoglycan synthesis in bacterial cell walls, thus inhibiting cell wall biosynthesis. Bacteria eventually lyse due to ongoing activity of cell wall autolytic enzymes (autolysins and murein hydrolases) while cell wall assembly is arrested. Monobactam structure makes cross-allergenicity with beta-lactams unlikely.

Pharmacodynamics/Kinetics

Absorption: I.M.: Well absorbed; I.M. and I.V. doses produce comparable serum concentrations

Distribution: Widely to most body fluids and tissues; crosses placenta; enters breast milk

V_d: Children: 0.2-0.29 L/kg; Adults: 0.2 L/kg

Relative diffusion of antimicrobial agents from blood into CSF: Good only with inflammation (exceeds usual MICs)

CSF:blood level ratio: Meninges: Inflamed: 8% to 40%; Normal: ~1%

Protein binding: 56%

Metabolism: Hepatic (minor %)

Half-life elimination:

Children 2 months to 12 years: 1.7 hours

Adults: Normal renal function: 1.7-2.9 hours

End-stage renal disease: 6-8 hours

Time to peak: I.M., I.V. push: Within 60 minutes; I.V. infusion: 1.5 hours

Excretion: Urine (60% to 70% as unchanged drug); feces (~13% to 15%)

Dosage

Children >1 month: I.M., I.V.:

Mild-to-moderate infections: I.M., I.V.: 30 mg/kg every 8 hours

Moderate-to-severe infections: I.M., I.V.: 30 mg/kg every 6-8 hours; maximum: 120 mg/kg/day (8 g/day)

(Continued)

Aztreonam *(Continued)*

Cystic fibrosis: I.V.: 50 mg/kg/dose every 6-8 hours (ie, up to 200 mg/kg/day); maximum: 8 g/day

Adults:

Urinary tract infection: I.M., I.V.: 500 mg to 1 g every 8-12 hours

Moderately-severe systemic infections: 1 g I.V. or I.M. or 2 g I.V. every 8-12 hours

Severe systemic or life-threatening infections (especially caused by *Pseudomonas aeruginosa*): I.V.: 2 g every 6-8 hours; maximum: 8 g/day

Meningitis (gram-negative): I.V.: 2 g every 6-8 hours

Dosing adjustment in renal impairment: Adults: Following initial dose, maintenance doses should be given as follows:

Cl_{cr} 10-30 mL/minute: 50% of usual dose at the usual interval

Cl_{cr} <10 mL/minute: 25% of usual dosage at the usual interval

Hemodialysis: Moderately dialyzable (20% to 50%); $^1/_8$ of initial dose after each hemodialysis session (given in addition to the maintenance doses)

Peritoneal dialysis: Administer as for Cl_{cr} <10 mL/minute

Continuous arteriovenous or venovenous hemofiltration: Dose as for Cl_{cr} 10-30 mL/minute

Stability Prior to reconstitution, store at room temperature; avoid excessive heat. Reconstituted solutions are colorless to light yellow straw and may turn pink upon standing without affecting potency. Use reconstituted solutions and I.V. solutions (in NS and D_5W) within 48 hours if kept at room temperature (25°C) or 7 days under refrigeration (4°C).

I.M.: Reconstitute with at least 3 mL SWFI, sterile bacteriostatic water for injection, NS, or bacteriostatic sodium chloride.

I.V.:

Bolus injection: Reconstitute with 6-10 mL SWFI.

Infusion: Reconstitute to a final concentration ≤2%; the final concentration should not exceed 20 mg/mL. Solution for infusion may be frozen at less than -2°C (less than -4°F) for up to 3 months. Thawed solution should be used within 24 hours if thawed at room temperature or within 72 hours if thawed under refrigeration. **Do not refreeze.**

Administration Doses >1 g should be administered I.V.

I.M.: Administer by deep injection into large muscle mass, such as upper outer quadrant of gluteus maximus or the lateral part of the thigh

I.V.: Administer by slow I.V. push over 3-5 minutes or by intermittent infusion over 20-60 minutes.

Monitoring Parameters Periodic liver function test; monitor for signs of anaphylaxis during first dose

Anesthesia and Critical Care Concerns/Other Considerations Although marketed as an agent similar to aminoglycosides, aztreonam is a monobactam antimicrobial with almost pure gram-negative aerobic activity. It cannot be used for gram-positive infections, whereas aminoglycosides are often used for synergy in gram-positive infections.

Pregnancy Risk Factor B

Contraindications Hypersensitivity to aztreonam or any component of the formulation

Warnings/Precautions Rare cross-allergenicity to penicillins and cephalosporins has been reported. Use caution in renal impairment; dosing adjustment required.

Adverse Reactions As reported in adults:

1% to 10%:

Dermatologic: Rash

Gastrointestinal: Diarrhea, nausea, vomiting

Local: Thrombophlebitis, pain at injection site

<1% (Limited to important or life-threatening): Abdominal cramps, abnormal taste, anaphylaxis, anemia, angioedema, aphthous ulcer, breast tenderness, bronchospasm, *C. difficile*-associated diarrhea, chest pain, confusion, diaphoresis, diplopia, dizziness, dyspnea, eosinophilia, erythema multiforme, exfoliative dermatitis, fever, flushing, halitosis, headache, hepatitis, hypotension, insomnia, jaundice, leukopenia, liver enzymes increased, muscular aches myalgia, neutropenia, numb tongue, pancytopenia, paresthesia, petechiae, pruritus, pseudomembranous colitis, purpura, seizure, sneezing, thrombocytopenia, tinnitus, toxic epidermal necrolysis, urticaria, vaginitis, vertigo, weakness, wheezing

Overdosage/Toxicology Symptoms of overdose include seizures. Treatment is supportive. If necessary, dialysis can reduce the drug concentration in the blood.

Drug Interactions Avoid antibiotics that induce beta-lactamase production (cefoxitin, imipenem).

Test Interactions May interfere with urine glucose tests containing cupric sulfate (Benedict's solution, Clinitest®); positive Coombs' test

Dosage Forms

Infusion [premixed]: 1 g (50 mL); 2 g (50 mL)

Injection, powder for reconstitution: 500 mg, 1 g, 2 g

References

Tunkel AR, Hartman BJ, Kaplan SL, et al, "Practice Guidelines for the Management of Bacterial Meningitis," *Clin Infect Dis*, 2004, 39(9):1267-84.

- ♦ **BabyBIG®** *see* Botulism Immune Globulin (Intravenous-Human) *on page 190*
- ♦ **Baciguent® [OTC]** *see* Bacitracin *on page 155*
- ♦ **BaciiM®** *see* Bacitracin *on page 155*
- ♦ **Baciject® (Can)** *see* Bacitracin *on page 155*

Bacitracin (bas i TRAY sin)

Medication Safety Issues

Sound-alike/look-alike issues:

Bacitracin may be confused with Bactrim®, Bactroban®

U.S. Brand Names AK-Tracin® [DSC]; Baciguent® [OTC]; BaciiM®

Canadian Brand Names Baciguent®; Baciject®

Pharmacologic Category Antibiotic, Miscellaneous; Antibiotic, Ophthalmic; Antibiotic, Topical

Generic Available Yes

Use Treatment of susceptible bacterial infections mainly; has activity against gram-positive bacilli; due to toxicity risks, systemic and irrigant uses of bacitracin should be limited to situations where less toxic alternatives would not be effective

Unlabeled/Investigational Use Oral administration: Successful in antibiotic-associated colitis; has been used for enteric eradication of vancomycin-resistant enterococci (VRE)

Mechanism of Action Inhibits bacterial cell wall synthesis by preventing transfer of mucopeptides into the growing cell wall

Pharmacodynamics/Kinetics

Duration: 6-8 hours

Absorption: Poor from mucous membranes and intact or denuded skin; rapidly following I.M. administration; not absorbed by bladder irrigation, but absorption can occur from peritoneal or mediastinal lavage

Distribution: CSF: Nil even with inflammation

Protein binding, plasma: Minimal

Time to peak, serum: I.M.: 1-2 hours

Excretion: Urine (10% to 40%) within 24 hours

Dosage Do not administer I.V.:

Infants: I.M.:

≤2.5 kg: 900 units/kg/day in 2-3 divided doses

>2.5 kg: 1000 units/kg/day in 2-3 divided doses

Children: I.M.: 800-1200 units/kg/day divided every 8 hours

Adults: Oral:

Antibiotic-associated colitis: 25,000 units 4 times/day for 7-10 days

VRE eradication (unlabeled use): 25,000 units 4 times/day for 7-10 days

Children and Adults:

Topical: Apply 1-5 times/day

Ophthalmic, ointment: Instill 1/4" to 1/2" ribbon every 3-4 hours into conjunctival sac for acute infections, or 2-3 times/day for mild-to-moderate infections for 7-10 days

Irrigation, solution: 50-100 units/mL in normal saline, lactated Ringer's, or sterile water for irrigation; soak sponges in solution for topical compresses 1-5 times/day or as needed during surgical procedures

Stability For I.M. use. Bacitracin sterile powder should be dissolved in 0.9% sodium chloride injection containing 2% procaine hydrochloride. Once reconstituted, bacitracin is stable for 1 week under refrigeration (2°C to 8°C). Sterile powder should be stored in the refrigerator. Do not use diluents containing parabens.

(Continued)

Bacitracin *(Continued)*

Administration For I.M. administration only, **do not administer I.V.** Confirm any orders for parenteral use. pH of urine should be kept >6 by using sodium bicarbonate. Bacitracin sterile powder should be dissolved in 0.9% sodium chloride injection containing 2% procaine hydrochloride. Do not use diluents containing parabens.

Monitoring Parameters I.M.: Urinalysis, renal function tests

Pregnancy Risk Factor C

Contraindications Hypersensitivity to bacitracin or any component of the formulation; I.M. use is contraindicated in patients with renal impairment

Warnings/Precautions [U.S. Boxed Warning]: I.M. use may cause renal failure due to tubular and glomerular necrosis; monitor renal function daily. Prolonged use may result in overgrowth of nonsusceptible organisms. Do not administer intravenously because severe thrombophlebitis occurs.

Adverse Reactions 1% to 10%:

Cardiovascular: Hypotension, edema of the face/lips, chest tightness
Central nervous system: Pain
Dermatologic: Rash, itching
Gastrointestinal: Anorexia, nausea, vomiting, diarrhea, rectal itching
Hematologic: Blood dyscrasias
Miscellaneous: Diaphoresis

Overdosage/Toxicology Symptoms of overdose include nephrotoxicity (parenteral), nausea, and vomiting (oral). Treatment is symptomatic and supportive.

Drug Interactions Increased toxicity: Nephrotoxic drugs, neuromuscular blocking agents, and anesthetics (increases neuromuscular blockade).

Dosage Forms [DSC] = Discontinued product

Injection, powder for reconstitution (BaciiM®): 50,000 units
Ointment, ophthalmic (AK-Tracin® [DSC]): 500 units/g (3.5 g)
Ointment, topical: 500 units/g (0.9 g, 15 g, 30 g, 120 g, 454 g)
  Baciguent®: 500 units/g (15 g, 30 g)

Baclofen (BAK loe fen)

Medication Safety Issues

Sound-alike/look-alike issues:
  Baclofen may be confused with Bactroban®
  Lioresal® may be confused with lisinopril, Loniten®, Lotensin®

Related Information

Chronic Pain Management *on page 1430*

U.S. Brand Names Lioresal®

Canadian Brand Names Apo-Baclofen®; Gen-Baclofen; Lioresal®; Liotec; Nu-Baclo; PMS-Baclofen

Pharmacologic Category Skeletal Muscle Relaxant

Generic Available Yes: Tablets only

Use Treatment of reversible spasticity associated with multiple sclerosis or spinal cord lesions

Orphan drug: Intrathecal: Treatment of intractable spasticity caused by spinal cord injury, multiple sclerosis, and other spinal disease (spinal ischemia or tumor, transverse myelitis, cervical spondylosis, degenerative myelopathy)

Unlabeled/Investigational Use Intractable hiccups, intractable pain relief, bladder spasticity, trigeminal neuralgia, cerebral palsy, Huntington's chorea

Mechanism of Action Inhibits the transmission of both monosynaptic and polysynaptic reflexes at the spinal cord level, possibly by hyperpolarization of primary afferent fiber terminals, with resultant relief of muscle spasticity

Pharmacodynamics/Kinetics

Onset of action: 3-4 days
  Peak effect: 5-10 days
Absorption (dose dependent): Oral: Rapid
Protein binding: 30%
Metabolism: Hepatic (15% of dose)
Half-life elimination: 3.5 hours
Time to peak, serum: Oral: Within 2-3 hours
Excretion: Urine and feces (85% as unchanged drug)

Dosage

Oral (avoid abrupt withdrawal of drug):

Children:

2-7 years: Initial: 10-15 mg/24 hours divided every 8 hours; titrate dose every 3 days in increments of 5-15 mg/day to a maximum of 40 mg/day

≥8 years: Maximum: 60 mg/day in 3 divided doses

Adults: 5 mg 3 times/day, may increase 5 mg/dose every 3 days to a maximum of 80 mg/day

Hiccups: Adults: Usual effective dose: 10-20 mg 2-3 times/day

Intrathecal: Children and Adults:

Test dose: 50-100 mcg, doses >50 mcg should be given in 25 mcg increments, separated by 24 hours. A screening dose of 25 mcg may be considered in very small patients. Patients not responding to screening dose of 100 mcg should not be considered for chronic infusion/implanted pump.

Maintenance: After positive response to test dose, a maintenance intrathecal infusion can be administered via an implanted intrathecal pump. Initial dose via pump: Infusion at a 24-hour rate dosed at twice the test dose. Avoid abrupt discontinuation.

Elderly: Oral (the lowest effective dose is recommended): Initial: 5 mg 2-3 times/day, increasing gradually as needed; if benefits are not seen, withdraw the drug slowly.

Dosing adjustment in renal impairment: May be necessary to reduce dosage in renal impairment, but there are no specific guidelines available

Hemodialysis: Poor water solubility allows for accumulation during chronic hemodialysis. Low-dose therapy is recommended. There have been several case reports of accumulation of baclofen resulting in toxicity symptoms (organic brain syndrome, myoclonia, deceleration and steep potentials in EEG) in patients with renal failure who have received normal doses of baclofen.

Administration Intrathecal: For screening dosages, dilute with preservative-free sodium chloride to a final concentration of 50 mcg/mL for bolus injection into the subarachnoid space. For maintenance infusions, concentrations of 500-2000 mcg/mL may be used.

Anesthesia and Critical Care Concerns/Other Considerations Avoid abrupt withdrawal of the drug; abrupt withdrawal of intrathecal baclofen has resulted in severe sequelae (hyperpyrexia, obtundation, rebound/exaggerated spasticity, muscle rigidity, and rhabdomyolysis), leading to organ failure and some fatalities. Risk may be higher in patients with injuries at T-6 or above, history of baclofen withdrawal, or limited ability to communicate. Elderly are more sensitive to the effects of baclofen and are more likely to experience adverse CNS effects at higher doses.

Pregnancy Risk Factor C

Contraindications Hypersensitivity to baclofen or any component of the formulation

Warnings/Precautions Use with caution in patients with seizure disorder or impaired renal function. **[U.S. Boxed Warning]: Avoid abrupt withdrawal of the drug; abrupt withdrawal of intrathecal baclofen has resulted in severe sequelae (hyperpyrexia, obtundation, rebound/exaggerated spasticity, muscle rigidity, and rhabdomyolysis), leading to organ failure and some fatalities.** Risk may be higher in patients with injuries at T-6 or above, history of baclofen withdrawal, or limited ability to communicate. Elderly are more sensitive to the effects of baclofen and are more likely to experience adverse CNS effects at higher doses.

Adverse Reactions

>10%:

Central nervous system: Drowsiness, vertigo, dizziness, psychiatric disturbances, insomnia, slurred speech, ataxia, hypotonia

Neuromuscular & skeletal: Weakness

1% to 10%:

Cardiovascular: Hypotension

Central nervous system: Fatigue, confusion, headache

Dermatologic: Rash

Gastrointestinal: Nausea, constipation

Genitourinary: Polyuria

<1% (Limited to important or life-threatening): Chest pain, dyspnea, dysuria, enuresis, hematuria, impotence, inability to ejaculate, nocturia, palpitation, syncope, urinary retention; withdrawal reactions have occurred with abrupt discontinuation (particularly severe with intrathecal use).

(Continued)

Baclofen *(Continued)*

Overdosage/Toxicology Symptoms of overdose include vomiting, muscle hypotonia, salivation, drowsiness, coma, seizures, and respiratory depression. Atropine has been used to improve ventilation, heart rate, blood pressure, and core body temperature. Treatment is symptom-directed and supportive.

For toxicity following intrathecal administration: For adults, administer physostigmine 2 mg I.M. or I.V. (not to exceed 1 mg/minute). For pediatric patients, administer physostigmine 0.02 mg/kg I.M. or I.V. (not to exceed 0.5 mg/minute). Consider withdrawal of 30-40 mL of CSF to reduce baclofen concentration. Abrupt withdrawal of intrathecal baclofen has resulted in severe sequelae (hyperpyrexia, obtundation, muscle rigidity, and rhabdomyolysis).

Drug Interactions

Increased effect: Opiate analgesics, benzodiazepines, hypertensive agents

Increased toxicity: CNS depressants and ethanol (sedation), tricyclic antidepressants (short-term memory loss), clindamycin (neuromuscular blockade), guanabenz (sedation), MAO inhibitors (decrease blood pressure, CNS, and respiratory effects)

Ethanol/Nutrition/Herb Interactions

Ethanol: Avoid ethanol (may increase CNS depression).

Herb/Nutraceutical: Avoid valerian, St John's wort, kava kava, gotu kola.

Test Interactions Increased alkaline phosphatase, AST, glucose, ammonia (B); decreased bilirubin (S)

Dosage Forms

Injection, solution, intrathecal [preservative free] (Lioresal®): 50 mcg/mL (1 mL); 500 mcg/mL (20 mL); 2000 mcg/mL (5 mL)

Tablet: 10 mg, 20 mg

- **BactoShield® CHG [OTC]** *see* Chlorhexidine Gluconate *on page 267*
- **Bactrim™** *see* Sulfamethoxazole and Trimethoprim *on page 1215*
- **Bactrim™ DS** *see* Sulfamethoxazole and Trimethoprim *on page 1215*
- **Bactroban®** *see* Mupirocin *on page 876*
- **Bactroban® Nasal** *see* Mupirocin *on page 876*
- **Baking Soda** *see* Sodium Bicarbonate *on page 1181*
- **Balacet 325™** *see* Propoxyphene and Acetaminophen *on page 1076*
- **Balminil Decongestant (Can)** *see* Pseudoephedrine *on page 1085*
- **Bancap HC®** *see* Hydrocodone and Acetaminophen *on page 636*
- **Band-Aid® Hurt-Free™ Antiseptic Wash [OTC]** *see* Lidocaine *on page 755*
- **Banophen® [OTC]** *see* DiphenhydrAMINE *on page 399*
- **Banophen® Anti-Itch [OTC]** *see* DiphenhydrAMINE *on page 399*

Basiliximab (ba si LIK si mab)

U.S. Brand Names Simulect®

Canadian Brand Names Simulect®

Pharmacologic Category Monoclonal Antibody

Generic Available No

Use Prophylaxis of acute organ rejection in renal transplantation

Mechanism of Action Chimeric (murine/human) monoclonal antibody which blocks the alpha-chain of the interleukin-2 (IL-2) receptor complex; this receptor is expressed on activated T lymphocytes and is a critical pathway for activating cell-mediated allograft rejection

Pharmacodynamics/Kinetics

Duration: Mean: 36 days (determined by IL-2R alpha saturation)

Distribution: Mean: V_d: Children 1-11 years: 4.8 ± 2.1 L; Adolescents 12-16 years: 7.8 ± 5.1 L; Adults: 8.6 ± 4.1 L

Half-life elimination: Children 1-11 years: 9.5 days; Adolescents 12-16 years: 9.1 days; Adults: Mean: 7.2 days

Excretion: Clearance: Children 1-11 years: 17 mL/hour; Adolescents 12-16 years: 31 mL/hour; Adults: Mean: 41 mL/hour

Dosage Note: Patients previously administered basiliximab should only be re-exposed to a subsequent course of therapy with extreme caution.

I.V.:

Children <35 kg: Renal transplantation: 10 mg within 2 hours prior to transplant surgery, followed by a second 10 mg dose 4 days after transplantation; the second dose should be withheld if complications occur (including severe hypersensitivity reactions or graft loss)

Children ≥35 kg and Adults: Renal transplantation: 20 mg within 2 hours prior to transplant surgery, followed by a second 20 mg dose 4 days after transplantation; the second dose should be withheld if complications occur (including severe hypersensitivity reactions or graft loss)

Dosing adjustment/comments in renal or hepatic impairment: No specific dosing adjustment recommended

Stability Store intact vials under refrigeration 2°C to 8°C (36°F to 46°F). Reconstitute vials with sterile water for injection, USP. Shake the vial gently to dissolve. It is recommended that after reconstitution, the solution should be used immediately. If not used immediately, it can be stored at 2°C to 8°C for up to 24 hours or at room temperature for up to 4 hours. Discard the reconstituted solution within 24 hours. Further dilute reconstituted solution with 25-50 mL 0.9% sodium chloride or dextrose 5% in water. When mixing the solution, gently invert the bag to avoid foaming. Do not shake.

Administration For intravenous administration only. Infuse as a bolus or I.V. infusion over 20-30 minutes. (Bolus dosing is associated with nausea, vomiting, and local pain at the injection site.)

Monitoring Parameters Signs and symptoms of acute rejection

Pregnancy Risk Factor B (manufacturer)

Contraindications Hypersensitivity to basiliximab, murine proteins, or any component of the formulation

Warnings/Precautions To be used as a component of immunosuppressive regimen which includes cyclosporine and corticosteroids. The incidence of lymphoproliferative disorders and/or opportunistic infections may be increased by immunosuppressive therapy. Severe hypersensitivity reactions, occurring within 24 hours, have been reported. Reactions, including anaphylaxis, have occurred both with the initial exposure and/or following re-exposure after several months. Use caution during re-exposure to a subsequent course of therapy in a patient who has previously received basiliximab. Discontinue the drug permanently if a reaction occurs. Medications for the treatment of hypersensitivity reactions should be available for immediate use. Treatment may result in the development of human antimurine antibodies (HAMA); however, limited evidence suggesting the use of muromonab-CD3 or other murine products is not precluded. **[U.S. Boxed Warning]: Should be administered under the supervision of a physician experienced in immunosuppression therapy.**

Adverse Reactions Administration of basiliximab did not appear to increase the incidence or severity of adverse effects in clinical trials. Adverse events were reported in 96% of both the placebo and basiliximab groups.

>10%:

- Cardiovascular: Hypertension, peripheral edema
- Central nervous system: Fever, headache, insomnia, pain
- Dermatologic: Acne, wound complications
- Endocrine & metabolic: Hypercholesterolemia, hyperglycemia, hyper-/hypokalemia, hyperuricemia, hypophosphatemia
- Gastrointestinal: Abdominal pain, constipation, diarrhea, dyspepsia, nausea, vomiting
- Genitourinary: Urinary tract infection
- Hematologic: Anemia
- Neuromuscular & skeletal: Tremor
- Respiratory: Dyspnea, infection (upper respiratory)
- Miscellaneous: Viral infection

3% to 10%:

- Cardiovascular: Abnormal heart sounds, angina pectoris, arrhythmia, atrial fibrillation, cardiac failure, chest pain, generalized edema, hypotension, tachycardia
- Central nervous system: Agitation, anxiety, depression, dizziness, fatigue, hypoesthesia, malaise, neuropathy, rigors
- Dermatologic: Cyst, hypertrichosis, pruritus, rash, skin disorder, skin ulceration
- Endocrine & metabolic: Acidosis, dehydration, diabetes mellitus, fluid overload, hyper-/hypocalcemia, hyperlipidemia, hypertriglyceridemia, hypoglycemia, hypomagnesemia, hyponatremia
- Gastrointestinal: Abdomen enlarged, esophagitis, flatulence, gastroenteritis, GI hemorrhage, gingival hyperplasia, melena, moniliasis, stomatitis (including ulcerative), weight gain

(Continued)

Basiliximab *(Continued)*

Genitourinary: Albuminuria, bladder disorder, dysuria, genital edema, hematuria, impotence, oliguria, renal function abnormal, renal tubular necrosis, ureteral disorder, urinary frequency, urinary retention

Hematologic: Hematoma, hemorrhage, leukopenia, polycythemia, purpura, thrombocytopenia, thrombosis

Neuromuscular & skeletal: Arthralgia, arthropathy, back pain, cramps, fracture, hernia, leg pain, myalgia, paresthesia, weakness

Ocular: Abnormal vision, cataract, conjunctivitis

Respiratory: Bronchitis, bronchospasm, cough, pharyngitis, pneumonia, pulmonary edema, sinusitis, rhinitis

Miscellaneous: Accidental trauma, facial edema, glucocorticoids increased, herpes infection, sepsis

Postmarketing and/or case reports: Capillary leak syndrome, cytokine release syndrome; severe hypersensitivity reactions, including anaphylaxis, have been reported (symptoms may include hypotension, tachycardia, cardiac failure, dyspnea, bronchospasm, pulmonary edema, urticaria, rash, pruritus, sneezing, and respiratory failure)

Overdosage/Toxicology The maximum tolerated dose has not been determined. Single doses up to 60 mg and divided doses up to 120 mg were administered without adverse event in clinical trials; a pediatric patient received a single 20 mg dose without adverse event. Treatment is symptom-directed and supportive.

Drug Interactions

Monoclonal antibodies: Allergic reactions may be increased in patients who have received diagnostic or therapeutic monoclonal antibodies due to the presence of human antichimeric antibody (HACA).

Vaccine (dead organism): Basiliximab may decrease the effect of vaccines (dead organisms).

Vaccine (live organism): Basiliximab may increase the risk of vaccinial infection.

Ethanol/Nutrition/Herb Interactions Herb/Nutraceutical: Echinacea may diminish the therapeutic effect of basiliximab. Avoid hypoglycemic herbs, including alfalfa, bilberry, bitter melon, burdock, celery, damiana, fenugreek, garcinia, garlic, ginger, ginseng, gymnema, marshmallow, and stinging nettle (may enhance the hypoglycemic effect of basiliximab).

Dosage Forms

Injection, powder for reconstitution:

Simulect®: 10 mg, 20 mg

- **Bayer® Aspirin [OTC]** *see* Aspirin *on page 129*
- **Bayer® Aspirin Extra Strength [OTC]** *see* Aspirin *on page 129*
- **Bayer® Aspirin Regimen Adult Low Strength [OTC]** *see* Aspirin *on page 129*
- **Bayer® Aspirin Regimen Children's [OTC]** *see* Aspirin *on page 129*
- **Bayer® Aspirin Regimen Regular Strength [OTC]** *see* Aspirin *on page 129*
- **Bayer® Extra Strength Arthritis Pain Regimen [OTC]** *see* Aspirin *on page 129*
- **Bayer® Plus Extra Strength [OTC]** *see* Aspirin *on page 129*
- **Bayer® Women's Aspirin Plus Calcium [OTC]** *see* Aspirin *on page 129*
- **BayHep B®** *see* Hepatitis B Immune Globulin *on page 618*
- **BayRab®** *see* Rabies Immune Globulin (Human) *on page 1100*
- **BayTet™** *see* Tetanus Immune Globulin (Human) *on page 1246*
- **BCI-Fluoxetine (Can)** *see* Fluoxetine *on page 539*
- **BCI-Gabapentin (Can)** *see* Gabapentin *on page 577*
- **BCI-Metformin (Can)** *see* Metformin *on page 810*
- **BCI-Ranitidine (Can)** *see* Ranitidine *on page 1105*
- **BCI-Simvastatin (Can)** *see* Simvastatin *on page 1174*
- **Bebulin® VH** *see* Factor IX Complex (Human) *on page 504*

Becaplermin (be KAP ler min)

Medication Safety Issues

Sound-alike/look-alike issues:

Regranex® may be confused with Granulex®, Repronex®

U.S. Brand Names Regranex®

Canadian Brand Names Regranex®

Synonyms Recombinant Human Platelet-Derived Growth Factor B; rPDGF-BB

Pharmacologic Category Growth Factor, Platelet-Derived; Topical Skin Product

Generic Available No

Use Debridement adjunct for the treatment of diabetic ulcers that occur on the lower limbs and feet

Mechanism of Action Recombinant B-isoform homodimer of human platelet-derived growth factor (rPDGF-BB) which enhances formation of new granulation tissue, induces fibroblast proliferation and differentiation to promote wound healing

Pharmacodynamics/Kinetics

Onset of action: Complete healing: 15% of patients within 8 weeks, 25% at 10 weeks

Absorption: Minimal

Distribution: Binds to PDGF-beta receptors in normal skin and granulation tissue

Dosage Topical: Adults:

Diabetic ulcers: Apply appropriate amount of gel once daily with a cotton swab or similar tool, as a coating over the ulcer

The amount of becaplermin to be applied will vary depending on the size of the ulcer area. To calculate the length of gel applied to the ulcer, measure the greatest length of the ulcer by the greatest width of the ulcer in inches. Tube size will determine the formula used in the calculation. For a 15 or 7.5 g tube, multiply length x width x 0.6. For a 2 g tube, multiply length x width x 1.3.

Note: If the ulcer does not decrease in size by ~30% after 10 weeks of treatment or complete healing has not occurred in 20 weeks, continued treatment with becaplermin gel should be reassessed.

Stability Refrigerate at 2°C to 8°C (36°F to 46°F); do not freeze.

Monitoring Parameters Ulcer volume (pressure ulcers); wound area; evidence of closure; drainage (diabetic ulcers); signs/symptoms of toxicity (erythema, local infections)

Pregnancy Risk Factor C

Contraindications Hypersensitivity to becaplermin or any component of the formulation; known neoplasm(s) at the site(s) of application; active infection at ulcer site

Warnings/Precautions Concurrent use of corticosteroids, cancer chemotherapy, or other immunosuppressive agents; ulcer wounds related to arterial or venous insufficiency. Thermal, electrical, or radiation burns at wound site. Malignancy (potential for tumor proliferation, although unproven; topical absorption is minimal). Should not be used in wounds that close by primary intention. For external use only.

Adverse Reactions <1%: Erythema with purulent discharge, exuberant granulation tissue, local pain, skin ulceration, tunneling of ulcer, ulcer infection

Dosage Forms Gel, topical: 0.01% (15 g)

Beclomethasone (be kloe METH a sone)

Medication Safety Issues

Sound-alike/look-alike issues:

Vanceril® may be confused with Vancenase®

Related Information

Asthma *on page 1594*

U.S. Brand Names Beconase® AQ; QVAR®

Canadian Brand Names Apo-Beclomethasone® ; Gen-Beclo; Nu-Beclomethasone; Propaderm®; QVAR®; Rivanase AQ; Vanceril® AEM

Synonyms Beclomethasone Dipropionate

Pharmacologic Category Corticosteroid, Inhalant (Oral); Corticosteroid, Nasal

Generic Available No

Use

Oral inhalation: Maintenance and prophylactic treatment of asthma; includes those who require corticosteroids and those who may benefit from a dose reduction/elimination of systemically-administered corticosteroids. Not for relief of acute bronchospasm.

(Continued)

Beclomethasone *(Continued)*

Nasal aerosol: Symptomatic treatment of seasonal or perennial rhinitis; prevent recurrence of nasal polyps following surgery.

Mechanism of Action Controls the rate of protein synthesis; depresses the migration of polymorphonuclear leukocytes, fibroblasts; reverses capillary permeability and lysosomal stabilization at the cellular level to prevent or control inflammation

Pharmacodynamics/Kinetics

Onset of action: Therapeutic effect: 1-4 weeks

Absorption: Readily; quickly hydrolyzed by pulmonary esterases prior to absorption

Distribution: Beclomethasone: 20 L; active metabolite: 424 L

Protein binding: 87%

Metabolism: Hepatic via CYP3A4 to active metabolites

Bioavailability: Of active metabolite, 44% following nasal inhalation (43% from swallowed portion)

Half-life elimination: Initial: 3 hours

Excretion: Feces (60%); urine (12%)

Dosage Nasal inhalation and oral inhalation dosage forms are not to be used interchangeably

Inhalation, nasal: Rhinitis, nasal polyps (Beconase® AQ): Children ≥6 years and Adults: 1-2 inhalations each nostril twice daily; total dose 168-336 mcg/day

Inhalation, oral: Asthma (doses should be titrated to the lowest effective dose once asthma is controlled) (QVAR®):

Children 5-11 years: Initial: 40 mcg twice daily; maximum dose: 80 mcg twice daily

Children ≥12 years and Adults:

Patients previously on bronchodilators only: Initial dose 40-80 mcg twice daily; maximum dose: 320 mcg twice day

Patients previously on inhaled corticosteroids: Initial dose 40-160 mcg twice daily; maximum dose: 320 mcg twice daily

NIH Asthma Guidelines (NAEPP, 2002; NIH, 1997): HFA formulation (eg, QVAR®): Administer in divided doses:

Children ≤12 years:

"Low" dose: 80-160 mcg/day

"Medium" dose: 160-320 mcg/day

"High" dose: >320 mcg/day

Children >12 years and Adults:

"Low" dose: 80-240 mcg/day

"Medium" dose: 240-480 mcg/day

"High" dose: >480 mcg/day

Stability Do not store near heat or open flame. Do not puncture canisters. Store at room temperature. Rest QVAR® on concave end of canister with actuator on top.

Administration

Beconase AQ®: Shake well before use. Nasal applicator and dust cap may be washed in warm water and dry thoroughly.

QVAR®: Rinse mouth and throat after use to prevent *Candida* infection. Do not wash or put inhaler in water; mouth piece may be cleaned with a dry tissue or cloth. Prime canister before using.

Pregnancy Risk Factor C

Contraindications Hypersensitivity to beclomethasone or any component of the formulation; status asthmaticus

Warnings/Precautions Not to be used in status asthmaticus or for the relief of acute bronchospasm. Safety and efficacy in children <5 years of age have not been established. May cause suppression of hypothalamic-pituitary-adrenal (HPA) axis, particularly in younger children or in patients receiving high doses for prolonged periods. Particular care is required when patients are transferred from systemic corticosteroids to inhaled products due to possible adrenal insufficiency or withdrawal from steroids, including an increase in allergic symptoms. Patients receiving 20 mg per day of prednisone (or equivalent) may be most susceptible. Fatalities have occurred due to adrenal insufficiency in asthmatic patients during and after transfer from systemic corticosteroids to aerosol steroids; aerosol steroids do **not** provide the systemic steroid needed to treat steroid-dependent patients having trauma, surgery, or infections. Withdrawal and discontinuation of the corticosteroid should be done slowly and carefully.

Controlled clinical studies have shown that orally-inhaled and intranasal corticosteroids may cause a reduction in growth velocity in pediatric patients. (In studies of orally-inhaled corticosteroids, the mean reduction in growth velocity was approximately 1 centimeter per year [range 0.3-1.8 cm per year] and appears to be related to dose and duration of exposure.) The growth of pediatric patients receiving inhaled corticosteroids should be monitored routinely (eg, via stadiometry). To minimize the systemic effects of orally-inhaled and intranasal corticosteroids, each patient should be titrated to the lowest effective dose.

May suppress the immune system, patients may be more susceptible to infection. Use with caution in patients with systemic infections or ocular herpes simplex. Avoid exposure to chickenpox and measles. Corticosteroids should be used with caution in patients with diabetes, hypertension, osteoporosis, peptic ulcer, glaucoma, cataracts, or tuberculosis. Use caution in hepatic impairment.

Adverse Reactions Frequency not defined.

Central nervous system: Agitation, depression, dizziness, dysphonia, headache, lightheadedness, mental disturbances

Dermatologic: Acneiform lesions, angioedema, atrophy, bruising, pruritus, purpura, striae, rash, urticaria

Endocrine & metabolic: Cushingoid features, growth velocity reduction in children and adolescents, HPA function suppression

Gastrointestinal: Dry/irritated nose, throat and mouth, hoarseness, localized *Candida* or *Aspergillus* infection, loss of smell, loss of taste, nausea, unpleasant smell, unpleasant taste, vomiting, weight gain

Local: Nasal spray: Burning, epistaxis, localized *Candida* infection, nasal septum perforation (rare), nasal stuffiness, nosebleeds, rhinorrhea, sneezing, transient irritation, ulceration of nasal mucosa (rare)

Ocular: Cataracts, glaucoma, intraocular pressure increased

Respiratory: Cough, paradoxical bronchospasm, pharyngitis, sinusitis, wheezing

Miscellaneous: Anaphylactic/anaphylactoid reactions, death (due to adrenal insufficiency, reported during and after transfer from systemic corticosteroids to aerosol in asthmatic patients), immediate and delayed hypersensitivity reactions

Overdosage/Toxicology Symptoms of overdose include irritation and burning of the nasal mucosa, sneezing, intranasal and pharyngeal *Candida* infections, nasal ulceration, epistaxis, rhinorrhea, nasal stuffiness, and headache. When consumed in high doses over prolonged periods, systemic hypercorticism and adrenal suppression may occur. In those cases, discontinuation of the corticosteroid should be done judiciously.

Drug Interactions Salmeterol: The addition of salmeterol has been demonstrated to improve response to inhaled corticosteroids (as compared to increasing steroid dosage).

Dosage Forms

Aerosol for oral inhalation, as dipropionate (QVAR®): 40 mcg/inhalation [100 metered doses] (7.3 g); 80 mcg/inhalation [100 metered doses] (7.3 g)

Suspension, intranasal, aqueous, as dipropionate [spray] (Beconase® AQ): 42 mcg/inhalation [180 metered doses] (25 g)

- **Beclomethasone Dipropionate** *see* Beclomethasone *on page 161*
- **Beconase® AQ** *see* Beclomethasone *on page 161*
- **Benadryl® (Can)** *see* DiphenhydrAMINE *on page 399*
- **Benadryl® Allergy [OTC]** *see* DiphenhydrAMINE *on page 399*
- **Benadryl® Children's Allergy [OTC]** *see* DiphenhydrAMINE *on page 399*
- **Benadryl® Children's Allergy Fastmelt® [OTC]** *see* DiphenhydrAMINE *on page 399*
- **Benadryl® Dye-Free Allergy [OTC]** *see* DiphenhydrAMINE *on page 399*
- **Benadryl® Injection** *see* DiphenhydrAMINE *on page 399*
- **Benadryl® Itch Stopping [OTC]** *see* DiphenhydrAMINE *on page 399*
- **Benadryl® Itch Stopping Extra Strength [OTC]** *see* DiphenhydrAMINE *on page 399*

Benazepril (ben AY ze pril)

Medication Safety Issues

Sound-alike/look-alike issues:

Benazepril may be confused with Benadryl®

Lotensin® may be confused with Lioresal®, Loniten®, lovastatin

(Continued)

Benazepril *(Continued)*

Related Information

Angiotensin Agents *on page 1544*

Preoperative Evaluation of the Cardiac Patient for Noncardiac Surgery *on page 1485*

U.S. Brand Names Lotensin®

Canadian Brand Names Apo-Benazepril®; Lotensin®

Synonyms Benazepril Hydrochloride

Pharmacologic Category Angiotensin-Converting Enzyme (ACE) Inhibitor

Generic Available Yes

Use Treatment of hypertension, either alone or in combination with other antihypertensive agents

Mechanism of Action Competitive inhibition of angiotensin I being converted to angiotensin II, a potent vasoconstrictor, through the angiotensin I-converting enzyme (ACE) activity, with resultant lower levels of angiotensin II which causes an increase in plasma renin activity and a reduction in aldosterone secretion

Pharmacodynamics/Kinetics

Reduction in plasma angiotensin-converting enzyme (ACE) activity:

Onset of action: Peak effect: 1-2 hours after 2-20 mg dose

Duration: >90% inhibition for 24 hours after 5-20 mg dose

Reduction in blood pressure:

Peak effect: Single dose: 2-4 hours; Continuous therapy: 2 weeks

Absorption: Rapid (37%); food does not alter significantly; metabolite (benazeprilat) itself unsuitable for oral administration due to poor absorption

Distribution: V_d: ~8.7 L

Metabolism: Rapidly and extensively hepatic to its active metabolite, benazeprilat, via enzymatic hydrolysis; extensive first-pass effect

Half-life elimination: Benazeprilat: Effective: 10-11 hours; Terminal: Children: 5 hours, Adults: 22 hours

Time to peak: Parent drug: 0.5-1 hour

Excretion: Clearance: Nonrenal clearance (ie, biliary, metabolic) appears to contribute to the elimination of benazeprilat (11% to 12%), particularly patients with severe renal impairment; hepatic clearance is the main elimination route of unchanged benazepril

Dialysis: ~6% of metabolite removed within 4 hours of dialysis following 10 mg of benazepril administered 2 hours prior to procedure; parent compound not found in dialysate

Dosage Oral: Hypertension:

Children ≥6 years: Initial: 0.2 mg/kg/day as monotherapy; dosing range: 0.1-0.6 mg/kg/day (maximum dose: 40 mg/day)

Adults: Initial: 10 mg/day in patients not receiving a diuretic; 20-40 mg/day as a single dose or 2 divided doses; the need for twice-daily dosing should be assessed by monitoring peak (2-6 hours after dosing) and trough responses.

Note: Patients taking diuretics should have them discontinued 2-3 days prior to starting benazepril. If they cannot be discontinued, then initial dose should be 5 mg; restart after blood pressure is stabilized if needed.

Elderly: Oral: Initial: 5-10 mg/day in single or divided doses; usual range: 20-40 mg/day; adjust for renal function; also see **Note** in adult dosing.

Dosing interval in renal impairment: Cl_{cr} <30 mL/minute:

Children: Use is not recommended.

Adults: Administer 5 mg/day initially; maximum daily dose: 40 mg.

Hemodialysis: Moderately dialyzable (20% to 50%); administer dose postdialysis or administer 25% to 35% supplemental dose.

Peritoneal dialysis: Supplemental dose is not necessary.

Monitoring Parameters CBC, renal function tests, electrolytes

Anesthesia and Critical Care Concerns/Other Considerations Aging patients with a decrease in glomerular filtration (also creatinine clearance), severe congestive heart failure, and renal failure may experience an exaggerated response with administration of ACE inhibitors. Diabetic proteinuria is reduced and insulin sensitivity is enhanced. In general, the side effect profile is favorable in elderly and causes little or no CNS confusion.

ACE inhibitors decrease morbidity and mortality in patients with asymptomatic and symptomatic left ventricular dysfunction. In this situation, they decrease hospitalizations for, and retard progression to, congestive heart failure. ACE inhibitors are also indicated in patients postmyocardial infarction in whom left ventricular ejection fraction is <40%. When used in patients with heart failure, the target dose or maximum tolerated dose, should be achieved, if possible. Lower daily doses of ACE inhibitors have not demonstrated the same cardioprotective effects. ACE inhibitors have renal protective effects in patients with proteinuria and possibly cardioprotective effects in high-risk patients.

ACE inhibitor therapy may elicit rapid increases in potassium and creatinine, especially when used in patients with bilateral renal artery stenosis. When ACE inhibition is introduced in patients with pre-existing diuretic therapy who are hypovolemic, the ACE inhibitor may induce acute hypotension. In those patients experiencing cough on an ACE inhibitor, the ACE inhibitor may be discontinued and, if necessary, angiotensin-receptor blocker therapy instituted. Concomitant NSAID therapy may attenuate blood pressure control; use of NSAIDs should be avoided or limited, with monitoring of blood pressure control. In the setting of heart failure, NSAID use may be associated with an increased risk for fluid accumulation and edema. Because of the potent teratogenic effects of ACE inhibitors, these drugs should be avoided, if possible, when treating women of childbearing potential not on effective birth control measures.

Pregnancy Risk Factor C (1st trimester)/D (2nd and 3rd trimesters)

Contraindications Hypersensitivity to benazepril or any component of the formulation; angioedema or serious hypersensitivity related to previous treatment with an ACE inhibitor; bilateral renal artery stenosis; patients with idiopathic or hereditary angioedema; pregnancy (2nd and 3rd trimesters)

Warnings/Precautions Anaphylactic reactions can occur. Angioedema can occur at any time during treatment (especially following first dose). Angioedema can occur at any time during treatment (especially following first dose). It may involve head and neck (potentially affecting the airway) or the intestine (presenting with abdominal pain). Prolonged monitoring may be required especially if tongue, glottis, or larynx are involved as they are associated with airway obstruction. Those with a history of airway surgery in this situation have a higher risk. Careful blood pressure monitoring with first dose (hypotension can occur especially in volume-depleted patients). **[U.S. Boxed Warning]: Based on human data, ACEIs can cause injury and death to the developing fetus when used in the second and third trimesters. ACEIs should be discontinued as soon as possible once pregnancy is detected.** Dosage adjustment needed in renal impairment. Use with caution in hypovolemia; collagen vascular diseases; valvular stenosis (particularly aortic stenosis); hyperkalemia; or before, during, or immediately after anesthesia. Avoid rapid dosage escalation which may lead to renal insufficiency. Rare toxicities associated with ACE inhibitors include cholestatic jaundice (which may progress to hepatic necrosis) and neutropenia/agranulocytosis with myeloid hyperplasia. Hypersensitivity reactions may be seen during hemodialysis with high-flux dialysis membranes (eg, AN69). Deterioration in renal function can occur with initiation. Use with caution in unilateral renal artery stenosis and pre-existing renal insufficiency.

Adverse Reactions

1% to 10%:

Cardiovascular: Postural dizziness (1.5%)

Central nervous system: Headache (6.2%), dizziness (3.6%), fatigue (2.4%), somnolence (1.6%)

Endocrine & metabolic: Hyperkalemia (1%), uric acid increased

Gastrointestinal: Nausea (1.3%)

Renal: Serum creatinine increased (2%), worsening of renal function may occur in patients with bilateral renal artery stenosis or hypovolemia

Respiratory: Cough (1.2% to 10%)

<1% (Limited to important or life-threatening): Alopecia, angina, angioedema, asthma, dermatitis, dyspnea, hemolytic anemia, hypersensitivity, hypotension, impotence, insomnia, pancreatitis, paresthesia, photosensitivity, postural hypotension (0.3%), rash, shock, Stevens-Johnson syndrome, syncope, thrombocytopenia, vomiting

Eosinophilic pneumonitis, neutropenia, anaphylaxis, renal insufficiency, and renal failure have been reported with other ACE inhibitors. In addition, a syndrome including fever, myalgia, arthralgia, interstitial nephritis, vasculitis, rash, eosinophilia, and elevated ESR has been reported to be associated with ACE inhibitors.

Overdosage/Toxicology Mild hypotension has been the primary toxic effect seen with acute overdose. Bradycardia may also occur. Hyperkalemia occurs

(Continued)

Benazepril *(Continued)*

even with therapeutic doses, especially in patients with renal insufficiency and those taking NSAIDs. Treatment is symptom-directed and supportive.

Drug Interactions

Alpha$_1$ blockers: Hypotensive effect increased.

Aspirin: The effects of ACE inhibitors may be blunted by aspirin administration, particularly at higher dosages, and/or increase adverse renal effects.

Diuretics: Hypovolemia due to diuretics may precipitate acute hypotensive events or acute renal failure.

Insulin: Risk of hypoglycemia may be increased.

Lithium: Risk of lithium toxicity may be increased; monitor lithium levels.

NSAIDs: May attenuate hypertensive efficacy; effect has been seen with captopril and may occur with other ACE inhibitors; monitor blood pressure. May increase adverse renal effects.

Potassium-sparing diuretics or potassium supplements (amiloride, potassium, spironolactone, triamterene): Increased risk of hyperkalemia.

Trimethoprim (high dose) may increase the risk of hyperkalemia.

Ethanol/Nutrition/Herb Interactions Herb/Nutraceutical: Avoid dong quai if using for hypertension (has estrogenic activity). Avoid ephedra, yohimbe, ginseng (may worsen hypertension). Avoid garlic (may have increased antihypertensive effect).

Dosage Forms Tablet, as hydrochloride: 5 mg, 10 mg, 20 mg, 40 mg

- ♦ **Benazepril Hydrochloride** *see* Benazepril *on page 163*
- ♦ **BeneFix®** *see* Factor IX *on page 502*
- ♦ **Benemid [DSC]** *see* Probenecid *on page 1055*
- ♦ **Benicar®** *see* Olmesartan *on page 953*
- ♦ **Benuryl™ (Can)** *see* Probenecid *on page 1055*
- ♦ **Benylin® D for Infants (Can)** *see* Pseudoephedrine *on page 1085*

Benztropine (BENZ troe peen)

Medication Safety Issues

Sound-alike/look-alike issues:

Benztropine may be confused with bromocriptine

U.S. Brand Names Cogentin®

Canadian Brand Names Apo-Benztropine®

Synonyms Benztropine Mesylate

Pharmacologic Category Anti-Parkinson's Agent, Anticholinergic; Anticholinergic Agent

Generic Available Yes: Tablet

Use Adjunctive treatment of Parkinson's disease; treatment of drug-induced extrapyramidal symptoms (except tardive dyskinesia)

Mechanism of Action Possesses both anticholinergic and antihistaminic effects. *In vitro* anticholinergic activity approximates that of atropine; *in vivo* it is only about half as active as atropine. Animal data suggest its antihistaminic activity and duration of action approach that of pyrilamine maleate. May also inhibit the reuptake and storage of dopamine and thereby, prolong the action of dopamine.

Pharmacodynamics/Kinetics

Onset of action: Oral: Within 1 hour; Parenteral: Within 15 minutes

Duration: 6-48 hours

Metabolism: Hepatic (N-oxidation, N-dealkylation, and ring hydroxylation)

Bioavailability: 29%

Dosage Use in children ≤3 years of age should be reserved for life-threatening emergencies

Drug-induced extrapyramidal symptom: Oral, I.M., I.V.:

Children >3 years: 0.02-0.05 mg/kg/dose 1-2 times/day

Adults: 1-4 mg/dose 1-2 times/day

Acute dystonia: Adults: I.M., I.V.: 1-2 mg

Parkinsonism: Oral:

Adults: 0.5-6 mg/day in 1-2 divided doses; if one dose is greater, administer at bedtime; titrate dose in 0.5 mg increments at 5- to 6-day intervals

Elderly: Initial: 0.5 mg once or twice daily; increase by 0.5 mg as needed at 5-6 days; maximum: 4 mg/day

Monitoring Parameters Symptoms of EPS or Parkinson's, pulse, anticholinergic effects

Pregnancy Risk Factor C

Contraindications Hypersensitivity to benztropine or any component of the formulation; pyloric or duodenal obstruction, stenosing peptic ulcers; bladder neck obstructions; achalasia; myasthenia gravis; children <3 years of age

Warnings/Precautions Use with caution in older children (dose has not been established). Use with caution in hot weather or during exercise. May cause anhidrosis and hyperthermia, which may be severe. The risk is increased in hot environments, particularly in the elderly, alcoholics, patients with CNS disease, and those with prolonged outdoor exposure.

Elderly patients frequently develop increased sensitivity and require strict dosage regulation - side effects may be more severe in elderly patients with atherosclerotic changes. Use with caution in patients with tachycardia, cardiac arrhythmias, hypertension, hypotension, prostatic hyperplasia (especially in the elderly), any tendency toward urinary retention, liver or kidney disorders, and obstructive disease of the GI or GU tract. When given in large doses or to susceptible patients, may cause weakness and inability to move particular muscle groups.

May be associated with confusion or hallucinations (generally at higher dosages). Intensification of symptoms or toxic psychosis may occur in patients with mental disorders. Benztropine does not relieve symptoms of tardive dyskinesia.

Adverse Reactions Frequency not defined.

Cardiovascular: Tachycardia

Central nervous system: Confusion, disorientation, memory impairment, toxic psychosis, visual hallucinations

Dermatologic: Rash

Endocrine & metabolic: Heat stroke, hyperthermia

Gastrointestinal: Xerostomia, nausea, vomiting, constipation, ileus

Genitourinary: Urinary retention, dysuria

Ocular: Blurred vision, mydriasis

Miscellaneous: Fever

Overdosage/Toxicology Symptoms of overdose include CNS depression, confusion, nervousness, hallucinations, dizziness, blurred vision, nausea, vomiting, and hyperthermia. For anticholinergic overdose with severe life-threatening symptoms, physostigmine 1-2 mg SubQ or I.V. slowly, may be given to reverse these effects.

Drug Interactions Substrate of CYP2D6 (minor)

Amantadine, rimantadine: Central and/or peripheral anticholinergic syndrome can occur when administered with amantadine or rimantadine.

Anticholinergic agents: Central and/or peripheral anticholinergic syndrome can occur when administered with narcotic analgesics, phenothiazines and other antipsychotics (especially with high anticholinergic activity), tricyclic antidepressants, quinidine and some other antiarrhythmics, and antihistamines.

Atenolol: Anticholinergics may increase the bioavailability of atenolol (and possibly other beta-blockers); monitor for increased effect.

Cholinergic agents: Anticholinergics may antagonize the therapeutic effect of cholinergic agents; includes tacrine and donepezil.

Digoxin: Anticholinergics may decrease gastric degradation and increase the amount of digoxin absorbed by delaying gastric emptying.

Levodopa: Anticholinergics may increase gastric degradation and decrease the amount of levodopa absorbed by delaying gastric emptying.

Neuroleptics: Anticholinergics may antagonize the therapeutic effects of neuroleptics.

Ethanol/Nutrition/Herb Interactions Ethanol: Avoid ethanol (may increase CNS depression).

Dosage Forms

Injection, solution, as mesylate (Cogentin®): 1 mg/mL (2 mL)

Tablet, as mesylate: 0.5 mg, 1 mg, 2 mg

♦ **Benztropine Mesylate** *see* Benztropine *on page 166*

Benzydamine (ben ZID a meen)

Canadian Brand Names Apo-Benzydamine®; Dom-Benzydamine; Novo-Benzydamine; PMS-Benzydamine; ratio-Benzydamine; Sun-Benz®; Tantum®

(Continued)

Benzydamine *(Continued)*

Synonyms Benzydamine Hydrochloride

Pharmacologic Category Local Anesthetic, Oral

Restrictions Not available in U.S.

Generic Available Yes

Use Symptomatic treatment of pain associated with acute pharyngitis; treatment of pain associated with radiation-induced oropharyngeal mucositis

Mechanism of Action Local anesthetic and anti-inflammatory, reduces local pain and inflammation. Does not interfere with arachidonic acid metabolism.

Pharmacodynamics/Kinetics

Absorption: Oral rinse may be absorbed, at least in part, through the oral mucosa

Excretion: Urine (primarily as unchanged drug)

Dosage Oral rinse: Adults:

Acute pharyngitis: Gargle with 15 mL of undiluted solution every 1½-3 hours until symptoms resolve. Patient should expel solution from mouth following use; solution should not be swallowed.

Mucositis: 15 mL of undiluted solution as a gargle or rinse 3-4 times/day; contact should be maintained for at least 30 seconds, followed by expulsion from the mouth. Clinical studies maintained contact for ~2 minutes, up to 8 times/day. Patient should not swallow the liquid. Begin treatment 1day prior to initiation of radiation therapy and continue daily during treatment. Continue oral rinse treatments after the completion of radiation therapy until desired result/healing is achieved.

Dosage adjustment in renal impairment: No adjustment required.

Stability Store at 15°C to 30°C; protect from freezing

Contraindications Hypersensitivity to benzydamine or any component of the formulation

Warnings/Precautions May cause local irritation and/or burning sensation in patients with altered mucosal integrity. Dilution (1:1 in warm water) may attenuate this effect. Use caution in renal impairment. Safety and efficacy have not been established in children ≤5 years of age.

Adverse Reactions

Central nervous system: Drowsiness, headache

Gastrointestinal: Nausea and/or vomiting (2%), dry mouth

Local: Numbness (10%), burning/stinging sensation (8%)

Respiratory: Pharyngeal irritation, cough

Drug Interactions **Substrate** (minor) of CYP1A2, 2C19, 2D6, 3A4

No drug interactions established.

Dosage Forms

Oral rinse: 0.15% (100 mL, 250 mL) [not available in the U.S.]

- **Benzydamine Hydrochloride** *see* Benzydamine *on page 167*
- **Benzylpenicillin Potassium** *see* Penicillin G (Parenteral/Aqueous) *on page 994*
- **Benzylpenicillin Sodium** *see* Penicillin G (Parenteral/Aqueous) *on page 994*

Beractant (ber AKT ant)

Medication Safety Issues

Sound-alike/look-alike issues:

Survanta® may be confused with Sufenta®

U.S. Brand Names Survanta®

Canadian Brand Names Survanta®

Synonyms Bovine Lung Surfactant; Natural Lung Surfactant

Pharmacologic Category Lung Surfactant

Generic Available No

Use Prevention and treatment of respiratory distress syndrome (RDS) in premature infants

Prophylactic therapy: Body weight <1250 g in infants at risk for developing, or with evidence of, surfactant deficiency (administer within 15 minutes of birth)

Rescue therapy: Treatment of infants with RDS confirmed by x-ray and requiring mechanical ventilation (administer as soon as possible - within 8 hours of age)

Mechanism of Action Replaces deficient or ineffective endogenous lung surfactant in neonates with respiratory distress syndrome (RDS) or in neonates at risk

... as the
... more frequently than every

... protect from light. Prior to administration, warm by standing at room temperature for 20 minutes or held in hand for 8 minutes. **Artificial warming methods should not be used.** Unused, unopened vials warmed to room temperature may be returned to the refrigerator within 8 hours of warming only once.

Administration

For intratracheal administration only

Suction infant prior to administration. Inspect solution to verify complete mixing of the suspension.

Administer intratracheally by instillation through a 5-French end-hole catheter inserted into the infant's endotracheal tube.

Administer the dose in four 1 mL/kg aliquots. Each quarter-dose is instilled over 2-3 seconds; each quarter-dose is administered with the infant in a different position. Slightly downward inclination with head turned to the right, then repeat with head turned to the left; then slightly upward inclination with head turned to the right, then repeat with head turned to the left.

Monitoring Parameters Continuous ECG and transcutaneous O_2 saturation should be monitored during administration; frequent arterial blood gases are necessary to prevent postdosing hyperoxia and hypocarbia

Warnings/Precautions Rapidly affects oxygenation and lung compliance and should be restricted to a highly-supervised use in a clinical setting with immediate availability of clinicians experienced with intubation and ventilatory management of premature infants. If transient episodes of bradycardia and decreased oxygen saturation occur, discontinue the dosing procedure and initiate measures to alleviate the condition. Produces rapid improvements in lung oxygenation and compliance that may require immediate reductions in ventilator settings and FiO_2.

Adverse Reactions During the dosing procedure:

>10%: Cardiovascular: Transient bradycardia

1% to 10%: Respiratory: Oxygen desaturation

<1% (Limited to important or life-threatening): Apnea, endotracheal tube blockage, hypercarbia, hyper-/hypotension, post-treatment nosocomial sepsis probability increased, pulmonary air leaks, pulmonary interstitial emphysema, vasoconstriction

Drug Interactions No data reported

Dosage Forms Suspension for inhalation: 25 mg/mL (4 mL, 8 mL)

- ♦ **9-Beta-D-Ribofuranosyladenine** *see* Adenosine *on page 44*
- ♦ **Betacaine® (Can)** *see* Lidocaine *on page 755*
- ♦ **Betaderm (Can)** *see* Betamethasone *on page 169*
- ♦ **Betadine® [OTC]** *see* Povidone-Iodine *on page 1039*
- ♦ **Betadine® Ophthalmic** *see* Povidone-Iodine *on page 1039*
- ♦ **Beta-HC®** *see* Hydrocortisone *on page 639*
- ♦ **Betaject™ (Can)** *see* Betamethasone *on page 169*
- ♦ **Betaloc® (Can)** *see* Metoprolol *on page 839*
- ♦ **Betaloc® Durules® (Can)** *see* Metoprolol *on page 839*

Betamethasone (bay ta METH a sone)

Medication Safety Issues

Sound-alike/look-alike issues:

Luxiq® may be confused with Lasix®

Related Information

Corticosteroids *on page 1561*

(Continued)

Exc...

Dosage Base...

Children: Use lowest ...

(physiologic replacement)

I.M.: 0.0175-0.125 mg base/kg/day divi... g base/m^2/day divided every 6-12 hours

Oral: 0.0175-0.25 mg/kg/day divided every 6-8 hours **or** ... ay divided every 6-8 hours

Topical:

≤12 years: Use is not recommended.

≥13 years: Use minimal amount for shortest period of time to avoid HPA axis suppression

Gel, augmented formulation: Apply once or twice daily; rub in gently. **Note:** Do not exceed 2 weeks of treatment or 50 g/week.

Lotion: Apply a few drops twice daily

Augmented formulation: Apply a few drops once or twice daily; rub in gently. **Note:** Do not exceed 2 weeks of treatment or 50 mL/week.

Cream/ointment: Apply once or twice daily.

Augmented formulation: Apply once or twice daily. **Note:** Do not exceed 2 weeks of treatment or 45 g/week.

Adolescents and Adults:

Oral: 2.4-4.8 mg/day in 2-4 doses; range: 0.6-7.2 mg/day

I.M.: Betamethasone sodium phosphate and betamethasone acetate: 0.6-9 mg/day (generally, 1/3 to 1/2 of oral dose) divided every 12-24 hours

Adults:

Intrabursal, intra-articular, intradermal: 0.25-2 mL

Intralesional: Rheumatoid arthritis/osteoarthritis:

Very large joints: 1-2 mL

Large joints: 1 mL

Medium joints: 0.5-1 mL

Small joints: 0.25-0.5 mL

Topical:

Foam: Apply to the scalp twice daily, once in the morning and once at night

Gel, augmented formulation: Apply once or twice daily; rub in gently. **Note:** Do not exceed 2 weeks of treatment or 50 g/week.

Lotion: Apply a few drops twice daily

Augmented formulation: Apply a few drops once or twice daily; rub in gently. **Note:** Do not exceed 2 weeks of treatment or 50 mL/week.

Cream/ointment: Apply once or twice daily

Augmented formulation: Apply once or twice daily. **Note:** Do not exceed 2 weeks of treatment or 45 g/week.

Dosing adjustment in hepatic impairment: Adjustments may be necessary in patients with liver failure because betamethasone is extensively metabolized in the liver

Administration

Oral: Not for alternate day therapy; once daily doses should be given in the morning.

I.M.: Do **not** give injectable sodium phosphate/acetate suspension I.V.

Topical: Apply topical sparingly to areas. Not for use on broken skin or in areas of infection. Do not apply to wet skin unless directed; do not cover with occlusive dressing. Do not apply very high potency agents to face, groin, axillae, or diaper area.

Foam: Invert can and dispense a small amount onto a saucer or other cool surface. Do not dispense directly into hands. Pick up small amounts of foam and gently massage into affected areas until foam disappears. Repeat until entire affected scalp area is treated.

Anesthesia and Critical Care Concerns/Other Considerations

Neuromuscular Effects: ICU-acquired paresis was recently studied in five ICUs (three medical and two surgical) at four French hospitals. All ICU patients without pre-existing neuromuscular disease admitted from March 1999 through June 2000 were evaluated (De Jonghe, 2002). Each patient had to be mechanically ventilated for ≥7 days and was screened daily for awakening. The first day the patient was considered awake was Study Day 1. Patients with severe muscle weakness on Study Day 7 were considered to have ICU-acquired paresis. Among the 95 patients who were evaluable, about 25% developed ICU-acquired paresis. Independent predictors included female gender, the number of days with two or more organ dysfunctions, and administration of corticosteroids. Further studies may be required to verify and characterize the association between the development of ICU-acquired paresis and use of corticosteroids. Concurrent use of a corticosteroid and muscle relaxant appear to increase the risk of certain ICU myopathies; avoid or administer the corticosteroid at the lowest dose possible.

Adrenal Insufficiency: Patients will often have steroid-induced adverse effects on glucose tolerance and lipid profiles. When discontinuing steroid therapy in patients on long-term steroid supplementation, it is important that the steroid therapy be discontinued gradually. Abrupt withdrawal may result in adrenal insufficiency with hypotension and hyperkalemia. Patients on long-term steroid supplementation will require higher corticosteroid doses when subject to stress (ie, trauma, surgery, severe infection). Guidelines for glucocorticoid replacement during various surgical procedures has been published (Salem, 1994; Coursin, 2002).

Septic Shock: A recent randomized, double-blind, placebo-controlled trial assessed whether low-dose corticosteroid administration could improve 28-day survival in patients with septic shock and relative adrenal insufficiency. Relative adrenal insufficiency was defined as an inappropriate response to corticotropin administration (increase of serum cortisol ≤9 mcg/dL from baseline). Cortisol levels were drawn immediately before corticotropin administration and 30-60 minutes afterwards. Three hundred adult septic shock patients requiring mechanical ventilation and vasopressor support were randomized to either hydrocortisone (50 mg IVP every 6 hours) and fludrocortisone (50 mcg tablet daily via nasogastric tube) or matching placebos for 7 days. In patients who did not appropriately respond to corticotropin (nonresponders), there were significantly fewer deaths in the active treatment group. Vasopressor therapy was withdrawn more frequently in this subset of the active treatment group. Adverse events were similar in both groups. Patients who lack adrenal reserve and thus have relative adrenal insufficiency during the stress of septic shock may benefit from physiologic steroid replacement. However, there was a trend for increased mortality in patients who responded to the corticotropin test (increase of serum cortisol >9 mcg/dL from baseline). These patients may not benefit from physiologic steroid replacement. Further study is required to better characterize the patient populations who may benefit.

Pregnancy Risk Factor C

Contraindications Hypersensitivity to betamethasone, other corticosteroids, or any component of the formulation; systemic fungal infections

Warnings/Precautions Topical use in patients ≤12 years of age is not recommended. May cause suppression of hypothalamic-pituitary-adrenal (HPA) axis, particularly in younger children or in patients receiving high doses for prolonged periods.

(Continued)

Betamethasone *(Continued)*

Very high potency topical products are not for treatment of rosacea, perioral dermatitis; not for use on face, groin, or axillae; not for use in a diapered area. Avoid concurrent use of other corticosteroids.

May suppress the immune system; patients may be more susceptible to infection. Use with caution in patients with systemic infections or ocular herpes simplex. Avoid exposure to chickenpox and measles.

Use with caution in patients with hypothyroidism, cirrhosis, ulcerative colitis; do not use occlusive dressings on weeping or exudative lesions and general caution with occlusive dressings should be observed; adverse effects may be increased. Discontinue if skin irritation or contact dermatitis should occur; do not use in patients with decreased skin circulation.

Adverse Reactions

Systemic:

Cardiovascular: Congestive heart failure, edema, hyper-/hypotension

Central nervous system: Dizziness, headache, insomnia, intracranial pressure increased, lightheadedness, nervousness, pseudotumor cerebri, seizure, vertigo

Dermatologic: Ecchymoses, facial erythema, fragile skin, hirsutism, hyper-/hypopigmentation, perioral dermatitis (oral), petechiae, striae, wound healing impaired

Endocrine & metabolic: Amenorrhea, Cushing's syndrome, diabetes mellitus, growth suppression, hyperglycemia, hypokalemia, menstrual irregularities, pituitary-adrenal axis suppression, protein catabolism, sodium retention, water retention

Gastrointestinal: Abdominal distention, appetite increased, hiccups, indigestion, peptic ulcer, pancreatitis, ulcerative esophagitis

Local: Injection site reactions (intra-articular use), sterile abscess

Neuromuscular & skeletal: Arthralgia, muscle atrophy, fractures, muscle weakness, myopathy, osteoporosis, necrosis (femoral and humeral heads)

Ocular: Cataracts, glaucoma, intraocular pressure increased

Miscellaneous: Anaphylactoid reaction, diaphoresis, hypersensitivity, secondary infection

Topical:

Dermatologic: Acneiform eruptions, allergic dermatitis, burning, dry skin, erythema, folliculitis, hypertrichosis, irritation, miliaria, pruritus, skin atrophy, striae, vesiculation

Endocrine and metabolic effects have occasionally been reported with topical use.

Overdosage/Toxicology When consumed in high doses for prolonged periods, systemic hypercorticism and adrenal suppression may occur. In those cases, discontinuation of the corticosteroid should be done judiciously.

Drug Interactions Inhibits CYP3A4 (weak)

Phenytoin, phenobarbital, rifampin increase clearance of betamethasone.

Potassium-depleting diuretics increase potassium loss.

Skin test antigens, immunizations: Betamethasone may decrease response and increase potential infections.

Insulin or oral hypoglycemics: Betamethasone may increase blood glucose.

Ethanol/Nutrition/Herb Interactions

Ethanol: Avoid ethanol (may enhance gastric mucosal irritation).

Food: Betamethasone interferes with calcium absorption.

Herb/Nutraceutical: Avoid cat's claw, echinacea (have immunostimulant properties).

Dietary Considerations May be taken with food to decrease GI distress.

Dosage Forms Note: Potency expressed as betamethasone base.

Cream, topical, as dipropionate: 0.05% (15 g, 45 g)

Maxivate®: 0.05% (45 g)

Cream, topical, as dipropionate augmented (Diprolene® AF): 0.05% (15 g, 50 g)

Cream, topical, as valerate (Beta-Val®): 0.1% (15 g, 45 g)

Foam, topical, as valerate (Luxiq®): 0.12% (50 g, 100 g, 150 g) [contains alcohol 60.4%]

Gel, topical, as dipropionate augmented: 0.05% (15 g, 50 g)

Injection, suspension (Celestone® Soluspan®): Betamethasone sodium phosphate 3 mg/mL and betamethasone acetate 3 mg/mL [6 mg/mL] (5 mL)

Lotion, topical, as dipropionate (Maxivate®): 0.05% (60 mL)
Lotion, topical, as dipropionate augmented (Diprolene®): 0.05% (30 mL, 60 mL)
Lotion, topical, as valerate (Beta-Val®): 0.1% (60 mL)
Ointment, topical, as dipropionate: 0.05% (15 g, 45 g)
Maxivate®: 0.05% (45 g)
Ointment, topical, as dipropionate augmented (Diprolene®): 0.05% (15 g, 50 g)
Ointment, topical, as valerate: 0.1% (15 g, 45 g)
Syrup, as base (Celestone®): 0.6 mg/5 mL (118 mL)

References

Abraham E and Evans T, "Corticosteroids and Septic Shock (editorial)," *JAMA*, 2002, 288(7):886-7.
Annane D, Sebille V, Charpentier C, et al, "Effect of Treatment With Low Doses of Hydrocortisone and Fludrocortisone on Mortality in Patients With Septic Shock," *JAMA*, 2002, 288(7):862-71.
Cooper MS and Stewart PM, "Corticosteroid Insufficiency in Acutely Ill Patients," *N Engl J Med*, 2003, 348(8):727-34.
Coursin DB and Wood KE, "Corticosteroid Supplementation for Adrenal Insufficiency," *JAMA*, 2002, 287(2):236-40.
De Jonghe B, Sharshar T, Lefaucheur JP, et al, "Paresis Acquired in the Intensive Care Unit. A Prospective Multicenter Study," *JAMA*, 2002, 288(22):2859-67.
Gamsu HR, Mullinger BM, Donnai P, et al, "Antenatal Administration of Betamethasone to Prevent Respiratory Distress Syndrome in Preterm Infants: Report of a UK Multicentre Trial," *Br J Obstet Gynaecol*, 1989, 96(4):401-10.
Hotchkiss RS and Karl IE, "The Pathophysiology and Treatment of Sepsis," *N Engl J Med*, 2003, 348(2):138-50.
Liggins GC and Howie RN, "A Controlled Trial of Antepartum Glucocorticoid Treatment of Respiratory Distress Syndrome in Premature Infants," *Pediatrics*, 1972, 50(4):515-25.
Salem M, Tainsh RE, Jr, Bromberg J, et al, "Perioperative Glucocorticoid Coverage: A Reassessment 42 Years After Emergence of a Problem," *Ann Surg*, 1994, 219(4):416-25.

♦ **Betamethasone Dipropionate** *see* Betamethasone *on page 169*
♦ **Betamethasone Dipropionate, Augmented** *see* Betamethasone *on page 169*
♦ **Betamethasone Sodium Phosphate** *see* Betamethasone *on page 169*
♦ **Betamethasone Valerate** *see* Betamethasone *on page 169*
♦ **Betapace®** *see* Sotalol *on page 1198*
♦ **Betapace AF®** *see* Sotalol *on page 1198*
♦ **Betasept® [OTC]** *see* Chlorhexidine Gluconate *on page 267*
♦ **Beta-Val®** *see* Betamethasone *on page 169*

Betaxolol (be TAKS oh lol)

Medication Safety Issues
Sound-alike/look-alike issues:
Betaxolol may be confused with bethanechol, labetalol

Related Information
Antiarrhythmic Drugs *on page 1548*
Beta-Blockers *on page 1557*
Preoperative Evaluation of the Cardiac Patient for Noncardiac Surgery *on page 1485*

U.S. Brand Names Betoptic® S; Kerlone®

Canadian Brand Names Betoptic® S; Sandoz-Betaxolol

Synonyms Betaxolol Hydrochloride

Pharmacologic Category Beta Blocker, Beta$_1$ Selective

Generic Available Yes: Solution, tablet

Use Treatment of chronic open-angle glaucoma and ocular hypertension; management of hypertension

Mechanism of Action Competitively blocks beta$_1$-receptors, with little or no effect on beta$_2$-receptors; ophthalmic reduces intraocular pressure by reducing the production of aqueous humor

Pharmacodynamics/Kinetics
Onset of action: Ophthalmic: 30 minutes; Oral: 1-1.5 hours
Duration: Ophthalmic: ≥12 hours
Absorption: Ophthalmic: Some systemic; Oral: ~100%
Metabolism: Hepatic to multiple metabolites
Protein binding: Oral: 50%
Bioavailability: Oral: 89%
Half-life elimination: Oral: 12-22 hours
Time to peak: Ophthalmic: ~2 hours; Oral: 1.5-6 hours
Excretion: Urine

Dosage Adults:
Ophthalmic: Instill 1-2 drops twice daily.
(Continued)

Betaxolol *(Continued)*

Oral: 5-10 mg/day; may increase dose to 20 mg/day after 7-14 days if desired response is not achieved. Initial dose in elderly: 5 mg/day.

Dosage adjustment in renal impairment: Administer 5 mg/day. Can increase every 2 weeks up to a maximum of 20 mg/day.

Cl_{cr} <10 mL/minute: Administer 50% of usual dose.

Stability Avoid freezing. Store ophthalmic drops at room temperature.

Administration Ophthalmic: Shake suspension well before using. Tilt head back and instill in eye. Keep eye open and do not blink for 30 seconds. Apply gentle pressure to lacrimal sac for 1 minute. Wipe away excess from skin. Do not touch applicator to eye and do not contaminate tip of applicator.

Monitoring Parameters Ophthalmic: Intraocular pressure. Systemic: Blood pressure, pulse.

Anesthesia and Critical Care Concerns/Other Considerations Due to alterations in the autonomic nervous system, beta-blockade may result in less hemodynamic response in the elderly. Studies indicate that despite decreased sensitivity to the chronotropic effects of beta-blockade with age, there appears to be an increased myocardial sensitivity to the negative inotropic effect.

Myocardial Infarction: Beta-blockers, in general without intrinsic sympathomimetic activity (ISA), have been shown to decrease morbidity and mortality when initiated in the acute treatment of myocardial infarction and continued long-term. In this setting, therapy should be avoided in patients with hypotension, cardiogenic shock, or heart block.

Surgery: Atenolol has also been shown to improve cardiovascular outcomes when used in the perioperative period in patients with underlying cardiovascular disease who are undergoing noncardiac surgery. Bisoprolol in high-risk patients undergoing vascular surgery reduced the perioperative incidence of death from cardiac causes and nonfatal myocardial infarction.

Atrial Fibrillation: Beta-blocker therapy provides effective rate control in patients with atrial fibrillation.

Withdrawal: Beta-blocker therapy should not be withdrawn abruptly, but gradually tapered to avoid acute tachycardia and hypertension.

Pregnancy Risk Factor C (manufacturer); D (2nd and 3rd trimesters - expert analysis)

Contraindications Hypersensitivity to betaxolol or any component of the formulation; sinus bradycardia; heart block greater than first-degree (except in patients with a functioning artificial pacemaker); cardiogenic shock; uncompensated cardiac failure; pulmonary edema; pregnancy (2nd and 3rd trimester)

Warnings/Precautions Administer cautiously in compensated heart failure and monitor for a worsening of the condition. Beta-blocker therapy should not be withdrawn abruptly (particularly in patients with CAD), but gradually tapered to avoid acute tachycardia, hypertension, and/or ischemia. Use caution with concurrent use of beta-blockers and either verapamil or diltiazem; bradycardia or heart block can occur. Use caution in patients with PVD (can aggravate arterial insufficiency). In general, beta-blockers should be avoided in patients with bronchospastic disease. Betaxolol, with $beta_1$ selectivity, should be used cautiously in bronchospastic disease with close monitoring. Use cautiously in diabetics because it can mask prominent hypoglycemic symptoms. Can mask signs of thyrotoxicosis. Dosage adjustment required in severe renal impairment and in patients on dialysis. Use care with anesthetic agents which decrease myocardial function. Safety and efficacy in pediatric patients have not been established.

Adverse Reactions

Ophthalmic:

>10%: Ocular: Short-term discomfort (25%)

<1% (Limited to important or life-threatening): Alopecia, asthma, bradycardia, bronchospasm, depression, dizziness, dyspnea, glossitis, heart block, heart failure, headache, hives, insomnia, myasthenia gravis exacerbation, respiratory failure, toxic epidermal necrolysis, vertigo

Frequency not defined: Ocular: Anisocoria, blurred vision, corneal sensitivity decreased, corneal staining, crusty lashes, discharge, dry eyes, edema, erythema, foreign body sensation, inflammation, itching sensation, keratitis, photophobia, tearing, visual acuity decreased

Systemic:

>10%:

Central nervous system: Drowsiness, insomnia

Endocrine & metabolic: Sexual ability decreased

1% to 10%:

Cardiovascular: Bradycardia, palpitation, edema, CHF, peripheral circulation reduced

Central nervous system: Mental depression

Gastrointestinal: Diarrhea or constipation, nausea, vomiting, stomach discomfort

Respiratory: Bronchospasm

Miscellaneous: Cold extremities

<1% (Limited to important or life-threatening): Chest pain, thrombocytopenia

Overdosage/Toxicology Symptoms of significant overdose include bradycardia, hypotension, AV block, CHF, bronchospasm, hypoglycemia. Treat initially with fluids. Sympathomimetics (eg, epinephrine or dopamine), glucagon, or a pacemaker can be used to treat toxic bradycardia, asystole, and/or hypotension.

Drug Interactions Substrate (major) of CYP1A2, 2D6; **Inhibits** CYP2D6 (weak)

Acetylcholinesterase inhibitors: May enhance the bradycardic effect of beta-blockers.

Alpha-/beta-agonists (direct-acting): Beta-blockers may enhance the vasopressor effect of alpha-/beta-agonists (direct-acting).

Alpha$_1$-blockers: Beta-blockers may enhance the orthostatic effect of alpha$_1$-blockers. The risk associated with ophthalmic products is probably less than systemic products.

Alpha$_2$-agonists: Beta-blockers may enhance the rebound hypertensive effect of alpha$_2$-agonists. This effect can occur when the alpha$_2$-agonist is abruptly withdrawn.

Aminoquinolines (antimalarial): May decrease the metabolism, via cyp isoenzymes, of beta-blockers.

Amiodarone: May enhance the bradycardic effect of beta-blockers.

Antipsychotic agents (phenothiazines): May enhance the hypotensive effect of beta-blockers. Either group may decrease the metabolism of the other.

Barbiturates: May increase the metabolism, via cyp isoenzymes, of beta-blockers.

Beta$_2$-agonists: May diminish the bradycardic effect of beta-blockers (beta$_1$ selective).

Calcium channel blockers (nondihydropyridine): May enhance the hypotensive effect of beta-blockers; may also decrease the metabolism of beta-blockers.

Cardiac glycosides: Beta-blockers may enhance the bradycardic effect of cardiac glycosides.

CYP1A2 inducers: May decrease the levels/effects of betaxolol. Example inducers include aminoglutethimide, carbamazepine, phenobarbital, and rifampin.

CYP1A2 inhibitors: May increase the levels/effects of betaxolol. Example inhibitors include ciprofloxacin, fluvoxamine, ketoconazole, norfloxacin, ofloxacin, and rofecoxib.

CYP2D6 inhibitors: May increase the levels/effects of betaxolol. Example inhibitors include chlorpromazine, delavirdine, fluoxetine, miconazole, paroxetine, pergolide, quinidine, quinine, ritonavir, and ropinirole.

Dipyridamole: May enhance the bradycardic effect of beta-blockers.

Disopyramide: May enhance the bradycardic effect of beta-blockers.

Insulin: Beta-blockers may enhance the hypoglycemic effect of insulin.

Lidocaine: Beta-blockers may decrease the metabolism of lidocaine.

Nonsteroidal anti-inflammatory agents (NSAIDs): May diminish the antihypertensive effect of beta-blockers.

Propafenone: May decrease the metabolism, via cyp isoenzymes, of beta-blockers. Propafenone possesses some independent beta-blocking activity.

Propoxyphene: May decrease the metabolism, via cyp isoenzymes, of beta-blockers.

Quinidine: May decrease the metabolism, via cyp isoenzymes, of beta-blockers.

Rifamycin derivatives: May increase the metabolism, via cyp isoenzymes, of beta-blockers.

Selective serotonin reuptake inhibitors (SSRIs): May enhance the bradycardic effect of beta-blockers.

(Continued)

Betaxolol *(Continued)*

Sulfonylureas: Beta-blockers may enhance the hypoglycemic effect of sulfonylureas; beta-blockers appear to mask tachycardia as an initial symptom of hypoglycemia. Ophthalmic beta-blockers are probably associated with lower risk than systemic agents.

Theophylline derivatives: Beta-blockers (beta$_1$ selective) may diminish the bronchodilatory effect of theophylline derivatives. this is true at higher beta-blockers doses where cardioselectivity is lost.

Ethanol/Nutrition/Herb Interactions Herb/Nutraceutical: Avoid bayberry; blue cohosh, cayenne, ephedra, ginger, ginseng (American), kola, and licorice (may worsen hypertension). Avoid black cohosh, California poppy, coleus, golden seal, hawthorn, mistletoe, periwinkle, quinine, shepherd's purse (may have increased antihypertensive effects).

Dosage Forms

Solution, ophthalmic, as hydrochloride: 0.5% (5 mL, 10 mL, 15 mL) [contains benzalkonium chloride]

Suspension, ophthalmic, as hydrochloride (Betoptic® S): 0.25% (2.5 mL, 5 mL, 10 mL, 15 mL) [contains benzalkonium chloride]

Tablet, as hydrochloride (Kerlone®): 10 mg, 20 mg

- ♦ **Betaxolol Hydrochloride** *see* Betaxolol *on page 173*
- ♦ **Betimol®** *see* Timolol *on page 1268*
- ♦ **Betnesol® (Can)** *see* Betamethasone *on page 169*
- ♦ **Betnovate® (Can)** *see* Betamethasone *on page 169*
- ♦ **Betoptic® S** *see* Betaxolol *on page 173*
- ♦ **Bextra®** ***[Withdrawn from Market]*** *see* Valdecoxib *on page 1325*
- ♦ **Biaxin®** *see* Clarithromycin *on page 300*
- ♦ **Biaxin® XL** *see* Clarithromycin *on page 300*
- ♦ **BIG-IV** *see* Botulism Immune Globulin (Intravenous-Human) *on page 190*
- ♦ **Biobase™ (Can)** *see* Alcohol (Ethyl) *on page 53*
- ♦ **Biobase-G™ (Can)** *see* Alcohol (Ethyl) *on page 53*
- ♦ **Biofed [OTC]** *see* Pseudoephedrine *on page 1085*
- ♦ **BioQuin® Durules™ (Can)** *see* Quinidine *on page 1094*
- ♦ **Bio-Statin®** *see* Nystatin *on page 945*

Bisoprolol (bis OH proe lol)

Medication Safety Issues

Sound-alike/look-alike issues:

Zebeta® may be confused with DiaBeta®

Related Information

Antiarrhythmic Drugs *on page 1548*

Beta-Blockers *on page 1557*

Heart Failure (Systolic) *on page 1607*

Preoperative Evaluation of the Cardiac Patient for Noncardiac Surgery *on page 1485*

U.S. Brand Names Zebeta®

Canadian Brand Names Monocor®; Novo-Bisoprolol; Sandoz-Bisoprolol; Zebeta®

Synonyms Bisoprolol Fumarate

Pharmacologic Category Beta Blocker, Beta$_1$ Selective

Generic Available Yes

Use Treatment of hypertension, alone or in combination with other agents

Unlabeled/Investigational Use Angina pectoris, supraventricular arrhythmias, PVCs, CHF

Mechanism of Action Selective inhibitor of beta$_1$-adrenergic receptors; competitively blocks beta$_1$-receptors, with little or no effect on beta$_2$-receptors at doses <10 mg

Pharmacodynamics/Kinetics

Onset of action: 1-2 hours

Absorption: Rapid and almost complete

Distribution: Widely; highest concentrations in heart, liver, lungs, and saliva; crosses blood-brain barrier; enters breast milk

Protein binding: 26% to 33%

Metabolism: Extensively hepatic; significant first-pass effect
Half-life elimination: 9-12 hours
Time to peak: 1.7-3 hours
Excretion: Urine (3% to 10% as unchanged drug); feces (<2%)

Dosage Oral:

Adults: 2.5-5 mg once daily; may be increased to 10 mg and then up to 20 mg once daily, if necessary

Hypertension (JNC 7): 2.5-10 mg once daily

CHF (unlabeled use): Initial: 1.25 mg once daily; maximum recommended dose: 10 mg once daily

Elderly: Initial dose: 2.5 mg/day; may be increased by 2.5-5 mg/day; maximum recommended dose: 20 mg/day

Dosing adjustment in renal/hepatic impairment: Cl_{cr} <40 mL/minute: Initial: 2.5 mg/day; increase cautiously.

Hemodialysis: Not dialyzable

Monitoring Parameters Blood pressure, ECG, neurologic status

Anesthesia and Critical Care Concerns/Other Considerations Bisoprolol may mask signs and symptoms of hypoglycemia; may potentiate hypoglycemia in a diabetic patient.

Surgery: Atenolol has also been shown to improve cardiovascular outcomes when used in the perioperative period in patients with underlying cardiovascular disease who are undergoing noncardiac surgery. Bisoprolol in high-risk patients undergoing vascular surgery reduced the perioperative incidence of death from cardiac causes and nonfatal myocardial infarction.

Withdrawal: Beta-blocker therapy should not be withdrawn abruptly, but gradually tapered to avoid acute tachycardia and hypertension.

Pregnancy Risk Factor C (manufacturer); D (2nd and 3rd trimesters - expert analysis)

Contraindications Hypersensitivity to bisoprolol or any component of the formulation; sinus bradycardia; heart block greater than first-degree (except in patients with a functioning artificial pacemaker); cardiogenic shock; uncompensated cardiac failure; pulmonary edema; pregnancy (2nd and 3rd trimesters)

Warnings/Precautions Administer cautiously in compensated heart failure and monitor for a worsening of the condition. Beta-blocker therapy should not be withdrawn abruptly (particularly in patients with CAD), but gradually tapered to avoid acute tachycardia, hypertension, and/or ischemia. Use caution in patients with PVD (can aggravate arterial insufficiency). Use caution with concurrent use of beta-blockers and either verapamil or diltiazem; bradycardia or heart block can occur. In general, beta-blockers should be avoided in patients with bronchospastic disease. Bisoprolol, with B1 selectivity, should be used cautiously in bronchospastic disease with close monitoring. Use cautiously in diabetics because it can mask prominent hypoglycemic symptoms. Can mask signs of thyrotoxicosis. Can cause fetal harm when administered in pregnancy. Dosage adjustment is required in patients with significant hepatic or renal dysfunction. Use care with anesthetic agents which decrease myocardial function.

Adverse Reactions

>10%:

Central nervous system: Drowsiness, insomnia
Endocrine & metabolic: Sexual ability decreased

1% to 10%:

Cardiovascular: Bradycardia, palpitation, edema, CHF, peripheral circulation reduced
Central nervous system: Mental depression
Gastrointestinal: Diarrhea, constipation, nausea, vomiting, stomach discomfort
Ocular: Mild ocular stinging and discomfort, tearing, photophobia, corneal sensitivity decreased, keratitis
Respiratory: Bronchospasm
Miscellaneous: Cold extremities

<1% (Limited to important or life-threatening): Angioedema, arrhythmia, bronchospasm, confusion (especially in the elderly), depression, dyspnea, exfoliative dermatitis, hallucinations, leukopenia, orthostatic hypotension, Peyronie's disease, psoriasiform eruption, syncope, thrombocytopenia, vasculitis

Overdosage/Toxicology Symptoms of overdose include severe hypotension, bradycardia, heart failure, bronchospasm, and hypoglycemia. Treat initially with I.V. fluids. Sympathomimetics (eg, epinephrine or dopamine), glucagon, or a pacemaker can be used to treat toxic bradycardia, asystole, and/or hypotension.

(Continued)

Bisoprolol *(Continued)*

Bisoprolol may be removed by hemodialysis. Other treatment is symptomatic and supportive.

Drug Interactions Substrate of CYP2D6 (minor), 3A4 (major)

Alpha-blockers (prazosin, terazosin): Concurrent use of beta-blockers may increase risk of orthostasis.

AV conduction-slowing agents (digoxin): Effects may be additive with beta-blockers.

Clonidine: Hypertensive crisis after or during withdrawal of either agent.

CYP3A4 inducers: CYP3A4 inducers may decrease the levels/effects of bisoprolol. Example inducers include aminoglutethimide, carbamazepine, nafcillin, nevirapine, phenobarbital, phenytoin, and rifamycins.

CYP3A4 inhibitors: May increase the levels/effects of bisoprolol. Example inhibitors include azole antifungals, clarithromycin, diclofenac, doxycycline, erythromycin, imatinib, isoniazid, nefazodone, nicardipine, propofol, protease inhibitors, quinidine, telithromycin, and verapamil.

Glucagon: Bisoprolol may blunt the hyperglycemic action of glucagon.

Insulin: Bisoprolol may mask tachycardia from hypoglycemia.

NSAIDs (ibuprofen, indomethacin, naproxen, piroxicam) may reduce the antihypertensive effects of beta-blockers.

Salicylates may reduce the antihypertensive effects of beta-blockers.

Sulfonylureas: Beta-blockers may alter response to hypoglycemic agents.

Ethanol/Nutrition/Herb Interactions Herb/Nutraceutical: Avoid dong quai if using for hypertension (has estrogenic activity). Avoid ephedra, yohimbe, ginseng (may worsen hypertension). Avoid garlic (may have increased antihypertensive effect).

Test Interactions Increased thyroxine (S), cholesterol (S), glucose, triglycerides, uric acid; decreased HDL

Dietary Considerations May be taken without regard to meals.

Dosage Forms Tablet, as fumarate: 5 mg, 10 mg

♦ **Bisoprolol Fumarate** *see* Bisoprolol *on page 176*
♦ **Bistropamide** *see* Tropicamide *on page 1320*

Bivalirudin (bye VAL i roo din)

U.S. Brand Names Angiomax®

Canadian Brand Names Angiomax®

Synonyms Hirulog

Pharmacologic Category Anticoagulant, Thrombin Inhibitor

Generic Available No

Use Anticoagulant used in conjunction with aspirin for patients with unstable angina undergoing percutaneous transluminal coronary angioplasty (PTCA) or percutaneous coronary intervention (PCI) with provisional glycoprotein IIb/IIIa inhibitor; anticoagulant used in patients undergoing PCI with (or at risk of) heparin-induced thrombocytopenia (HIT) / thrombosis syndrome (HITTS)

Mechanism of Action Bivalirudin acts as a specific and reversible direct thrombin inhibitor; it binds to the catalytic and anionic exosite of both circulating and clot-bound thrombin. Catalytic binding site occupation functionally inhibits coagulant effects by preventing thrombin-mediated cleavage of fibrinogen to fibrin monomers, and activation of factors V, VIII, and XIII. Shows linear dose- and concentration-dependent prolongation of ACT, aPTT, PT, and TT.

Pharmacodynamics/Kinetics

Onset of action: Immediate

Duration: Coagulation times return to baseline ~1 hour following discontinuation of infusion

Distribution: 0.2 L/kg

Protein binding, plasma: Does not bind other than thrombin

Half-life elimination: Normal renal function: 25 minutes; Cl_{cr} 10-29 mL/minute: 57 minutes

Excretion: Urine, proteolytic cleavage

Dosage I.V.: Adults: Anticoagulant in patients undergoing PTCA/PCI or PCI with HITS/HITTS (treatment should be started just prior to procedure): Initial: Bolus: 0.75 mg/kg, followed by continuous infusion: 1.75 mg/kg/hour for the duration of procedure and up to 4 hours postprocedure if needed; determine ACT 5 minutes after bolus dose; may administer additional bolus of 0.3 mg/kg if necessary.

A glycoprotein IIb/IIIa inhibitor may be administered concomitantly during the procedure.

If needed, infusion may be continued beyond initial 4 hours at 0.2 mg/kg/hour for up to 20 hours.

Dosage adjustment in renal impairment: Infusion dose should be reduced based on degree of renal impairment; initial bolus dose remains unchanged; monitor activated coagulation time (ACT)

Cl_{cr} ≥30 mL/minute: No adjustment required

Cl_{cr} 10-29 mL/minute: Decrease infusion rate to 1 mg/kg/hour

Dialysis-dependent patients (off dialysis): Decrease infusion rate to 0.25 mg/kg/hour

Clearance of bivalirudin remains 1.8-fold greater than the glomerular filtration rate, regardless of the degree in renal impairment.

Dosage adjustment in hepatic impairment: No dosage adjustment is needed

Elderly: No dosage adjustment is needed in elderly patients with normal renal function. Puncture site hemorrhage and catheterization site hemorrhage were seen in more patients ≥65 years of age than in patients <65 years of age

Stability Store unopened vials at 15°C to 30°C. Reconstitute each 250 mg with 5 mL SWFI. Gently swirl to dissolve. Further dilution in D_5W or NS (50 mL to make 5 mg/mL solution **or** 500 mL to make 0.5 mg/mL solution) is required prior to infusion. Do not administer in same line with other medications. Following reconstitution, vials should be stored at 2°C to 8°C. Do not freeze. Final dilutions of 0.5 mg/mL or 5 mg/mL are stable at room temperature for up to 24 hours.

Administration For I.V. administration only.

Monitoring Parameters ACT; depending upon indication for use of bivalirudin: aPTT, PT

Anesthesia and Critical Care Concerns/Other Considerations

Percutaneous Coronary Intervention (PCI): Compared with heparin, bivalirudin reduced the composite endpoint of death, myocardial infarction, or revascularization in patients undergoing PCI. Bleeding complications were significantly decreased as well.

Heparin-induced thrombocytopenia (HIT): Because bivalirudin has no structural similarity to heparin, it may be safely administered to patients with HIT or heparin-induced thrombotic thrombocytopenia syndrome (HITTS) or a history of HIT or HITTS.

Pregnancy Risk Factor B

Contraindications Hypersensitivity to bivalirudin or any component of the formulation; active major bleeding

Warnings/Precautions Not for intramuscular use. Safety and efficacy have not been established in patients with unstable angina or acute coronary syndromes who are not undergoing PTCA or PCI. Increased risk of thrombus formation (some fatal) has been reported with bivalirudin use in gamma brachytherapy. As with all anticoagulants, bleeding may occur at any site and should be considered following an unexplained fall in blood pressure or hematocrit, or any unexplained symptom. Use with caution in patients with disease states associated with increased risk of bleeding. Safety and efficacy in pediatric patients have not been established.

Adverse Reactions As with all anticoagulants, bleeding is the major adverse effect of bivalirudin. Hemorrhage may occur at virtually any site. Risk is dependent on multiple variables, including the intensity of anticoagulation and patient susceptibility. Additional adverse effects are often related to idiosyncratic reactions, and the frequency is difficult to estimate.

Adverse reactions reported were generally less than those seen with heparin.

>10%:
- Cardiovascular: Hypotension (3% to 12%)
- Central nervous system: Pain (15%), headache (3% to 12%)
- Gastrointestinal: Nausea (3% to 15%)
- Neuromuscular & skeletal: Back pain (9% to 42%)

1% to 10%:
- Cardiovascular: Hypertension (6%), bradycardia (5%), angina (up to 5%)
- Central nervous system: Insomnia (7%), anxiety (6%), fever (5%), nervousness (5%)
- Gastrointestinal: Vomiting (6%), dyspepsia (5%), abdominal pain (5%)
- Genitourinary: Urinary retention (4%)

(Continued)

Bivalirudin *(Continued)*

Hematologic: Major hemorrhage (2% to 4%, compared to 4% to 9% with heparin); transfusion required (1% to 2%, compared to 2% to 6% with heparin), thrombocytopenia (<1% to 4%)

Local: Injection site pain (3% to 8%)

Neuromuscular & skeletal: Pelvic pain (6%)

<1% (Limited to important or life-threatening): Allergic reaction (including anaphylaxis), cerebral ischemia, confusion, facial paralysis, fatal bleeding, intracranial bleeding, kidney failure, pulmonary edema, retroperitoneal bleeding, syncope, thrombus formation (during PCI, including intracoronary brachytherapy), ventricular fibrillation

Overdosage/Toxicology Single bolus doses of up to 7.5 mg/kg have been reported without bleeding complications or other adverse events. Discontinue bivalirudin and monitor patients for signs of bleeding. Bivalirudin is hemodialyzable (~25% removed).

Drug Interactions

Aspirin: May increase anticoagulant effect; all clinical trials included coadministration of aspirin

Other anticoagulants: May increase the risk of bleeding complications; monitor.

Treprostinil: May enhance the adverse/toxic effect of anticoagulants. Bleeding may occur.

Dosage Forms Injection, powder for reconstitution: 250 mg

♦ **Blenoxane®** *see* Bleomycin *on page 180*

♦ **Bleo** *see* Bleomycin *on page 180*

Bleomycin (blee oh MYE sin)

Medication Safety Issues

Sound-alike/look-alike issues:

Bleomycin may be confused with Cleocin®

U.S. Brand Names Blenoxane®

Canadian Brand Names Blenoxane®; Bleomycin Injection, USP

Synonyms Bleo; Bleomycin Sulfate; BLM; NSC-125066

Pharmacologic Category Antineoplastic Agent, Antibiotic

Generic Available Yes

Use Treatment of squamous cell carcinomas, melanomas, sarcomas, testicular carcinoma, Hodgkin's lymphoma, and non-Hodgkin's lymphoma; sclerosing agent for malignant pleural effusion

Mechanism of Action Inhibits synthesis of DNA; binds to DNA leading to single- and double-strand breaks

Pharmacodynamics/Kinetics

Absorption: I.M. and intrapleural administration: 30% to 50% of I.V. serum concentrations; intraperitoneal and SubQ routes produce serum concentrations equal to those of I.V.

Distribution: V_d: 22 L/m^2; highest concentrations in skin, kidney, lung, heart tissues; lowest in testes and GI tract; does not cross blood-brain barrier

Protein binding: 1%

Metabolism: Via several tissues including hepatic, GI tract, skin, pulmonary, renal, and serum

Half-life elimination: Biphasic (renal function dependent):

Normal renal function: Initial: 1.3 hours; Terminal: 9 hours

End-stage renal disease: Initial: 2 hours; Terminal: 30 hours

Time to peak, serum: I.M.: Within 30 minutes

Excretion: Urine (50% to 70% as active drug)

Dosage Maximum cumulative lifetime dose: 400 units; refer to individual protocols; 1 unit = 1 mg

May be administered I.M., I.V., SubQ, or intracavitary

Children and Adults:

Test dose for lymphoma patients: I.M., I.V., SubQ: Because of the possibility of an anaphylactoid reaction, ≤2 units of bleomycin for the first 2 doses; monitor vital signs every 15 minutes; wait a minimum of 1 hour before administering remainder of dose; if no acute reaction occurs, then the regular dosage schedule may be followed. **Note:** Test doses may produce false-negative results.

Single-agent therapy:

I.M./I.V./SubQ: Squamous cell carcinoma, lymphoma, testicular carcinoma: 0.25-0.5 units/kg (10-20 units/m^2) 1-2 times/week

CIV: 15 units/m^2 over 24 hours daily for 4 days

Pleural sclerosing: Intrapleural: 60 units as a single instillation (some recommend limiting the dose in the elderly to 40 units/m^2; usual maximum: 60 units). Dose may be repeated at intervals of several days if fluid continues to accumulate (mix in 50-100 mL of NS); may add lidocaine 100-200 mg to reduce local discomfort.

Dosing adjustment in renal impairment:

Cl_{cr} 10-50 mL/minute: Administer 75% of normal dose

Cl_{cr} <10 mL/minute: Administer 50% of normal dose

Stability

Refrigerate intact vials of powder; intact vials are stable for up to one month at 45°C. Solutions for infusion are stable for 96 hours at room temperature and 14 days under refrigeration.

Reconstitute powder with 1-5 mL BWFI or BNS which is stable at room temperature or under refrigeration for 28 days.

Standard I.V. dilution: Dose/50-1000 mL NS

Administration

I.V. doses should be administered slowly (manufacturer recommends giving over a period of 10 minutes)

I.M. or SubQ: May cause pain at injection site

Intrapleural: 60 units in 50-100 mL NS; use of topical anesthetics or narcotic analgesia is usually not necessary

Monitoring Parameters Pulmonary function tests (total lung volume, forced vital capacity, carbon monoxide diffusion), renal function, liver function, chest x-ray, temperature initially; check body weight at regular intervals

Anesthesia and Critical Care Concerns/Other Considerations The use of oxygen concentrations (>30%) in animals previously treated with bleomycin has been reported to promote pulmonary toxicity. Although this is still controversial, supplemental oxygen should be used judiciously in patients who have received bleomycin.

Pregnancy Risk Factor D

Contraindications Hypersensitivity to bleomycin or any component of the formulation; severe pulmonary disease; pregnancy

Warnings/Precautions Hazardous agent — use appropriate precautions for handling and disposal. **[U.S. Boxed Warnings]: Occurrence of pulmonary fibrosis (commonly presenting as pneumonitis) is higher in elderly patients, patients receiving >400 units total lifetime dose or single doses >30 units, smokers, and patients with prior radiation therapy or receiving concurrent oxygen. A severe idiosyncratic reaction consisting of hypotension, mental confusion, fever, chills, and wheezing (similar to anaphylaxis) has been reported in 1% of lymphoma patients treated with bleomycin.** Since these reactions usually occur after the first or second dose, careful monitoring is essential after these doses. Follow manufacturer recommendations for administering O_2 during surgery to patients who have received bleomycin. Use caution with renal impairment, may require dose adjustment. May cause renal or hepatic toxicity. **[U.S. Boxed Warning]: Should be administered under the supervision of an experienced cancer chemotherapy physician.** Safety and efficacy in children have not been established.

Adverse Reactions

>10%:

Dermatologic: Pain at the tumor site, phlebitis. About 50% of patients develop erythema, rash, striae, induration, hyperkeratosis, vesiculation, and peeling of the skin, particularly on the palmar and plantar surfaces of the hands and feet. Hyperpigmentation (50%), alopecia, nailbed changes may also occur. These effects appear dose related and reversible with discontinuation.

Gastrointestinal: Stomatitis and mucositis (30%), anorexia, weight loss

Respiratory: Tachypnea, rales, acute or chronic interstitial pneumonitis, and pulmonary fibrosis (5% to 10%); hypoxia and death (1%). Symptoms include cough, dyspnea, and bilateral pulmonary infiltrates. The pathogenesis is not certain, but may be due to damage of pulmonary, vascular, or connective tissue. Response to steroid therapy is variable and somewhat controversial.

Miscellaneous: Acute febrile reactions (25% to 50%)

(Continued)

Bleomycin *(Continued)*

1% to 10%:

Dermatologic: Skin thickening, diffuse scleroderma, onycholysis, pruritus

Miscellaneous: Anaphylactoid-like reactions (characterized by hypotension, confusion, fever, chills, and wheezing; onset may be immediate or delayed for several hours); idiosyncratic reactions (1% in lymphoma patients)

<1% (Limited to important or life-threatening): Angioedema, cerebrovascular accident, cerebral arteritis, hepatotoxicity, malaise, MI, nausea, Raynaud's phenomenon, renal toxicity, scleroderma-like skin changes, thrombotic microangiopathy, vomiting; Myelosuppression (rare); Onset: 7 days, Nadir: 14 days, Recovery: 21 days

Overdosage/Toxicology Symptoms of overdose include chills, fever, pulmonary fibrosis, and hyperpigmentation. Treatment is symptom-directed and supportive.

Drug Interactions

Cisplatin: May decrease bleomycin elimination.

Digitalis glycosides: Bleomycin may decrease plasma levels of digoxin.

Phenytoin: Results in decreased phenytoin levels.

Dosage Forms Injection, powder for reconstitution, as sulfate: 15 units, 30 units

- **Bleomycin Injection, USP (Can)** *see* Bleomycin *on page 180*
- **Bleomycin Sulfate** *see* Bleomycin *on page 180*
- **BLM** *see* Bleomycin *on page 180*
- **Blocadren®** *see* Timolol *on page 1268*
- **Bonefos® (Can)** *see* Clodronate *on page 308*

Bosentan (boe SEN tan)

U.S. Brand Names Tracleer®

Canadian Brand Names Tracleer®

Pharmacologic Category Endothelin Antagonist

Restrictions Bosentan (Tracleer®) is available only through a limited distribution program directly from the manufacturer (Actelion Pharmaceuticals 1-866-228-3546). It will not be available through wholesalers or individual pharmacies. An FDA-approved medication guide is available at www.fda.gov/cder/Offices/ODS/labeling.htm; distribute to each patient to whom this medication is dispensed.

Generic Available No

Use Treatment of pulmonary artery hypertension (PAH) (WHO Group I) in patients with World Health Organization (WHO) Class III or IV symptoms to improve exercise capacity and decrease the rate of clinical deterioration

Unlabeled/Investigational Use Investigational: Congestive heart failure

Mechanism of Action Blocks endothelin receptors on vascular endothelium and smooth muscle. Stimulation of these receptors is associated with vasoconstriction. Although bosentan blocks both ET_A and ET_B receptors, the affinity is higher for the A subtype. Improvement in symptoms of pulmonary artery hypertension and a decrease in the rate of clinical deterioration have been demonstrated in clinical trials.

Pharmacodynamics/Kinetics

Distribution: V_d: 18 L

Protein binding, plasma: >98% primarily to albumin

Metabolism: Hepatic via CYP2C9 and 3A4 to three primary metabolites (one contributing ~10% to 20% pharmacologic activity)

Bioavailability: 50%

Half-life elimination: 5 hours; prolonged with heart failure, possibly in PAH

Time to peak, plasma: 3-5 hours

Excretion: Feces (as metabolites); urine (<3% as unchanged drug)

Dosage Oral:

Children ≤12 years (unlabeled use):

10-20 kg: Initial: 31.25 mg once daily for 4 weeks; increase to maintenance dose of 31.25 mg twice daily

>20"40 kg: Initial: 31.25 mg twice daily for 4 weeks; increase to maintenance dose of 62.5 mg twice daily

>40 kg: Initial: 62.5 mg twice daily for 4 weeks; increase to maintenance dose of 125 mg twice daily

Adolescents >12 years and ≥40 kg and Adults: Initial: 62.5 mg twice daily for 4 weeks; increase to maintenance dose of 125 mg twice daily; patients <40 kg should be maintained at 62.5 mg twice daily. Doses >125 mg twice daily do not appear to confer additional clinical benefit but may increase risk of liver toxicity.

Note: When discontinuing treatment, consider a reduction in dosage to 62.5 mg twice daily for 3-7 days (to avoid clinical deterioration).

Dosage adjustment in renal impairment: No dosage adjustment required.

Dosage adjustment in hepatic impairment: Avoid use in patients with **pretreatment** moderate to severe hepatic insufficiency.

Modification based on transaminase elevation:

If any elevation, regardless of degree, is accompanied by clinical symptoms of hepatic injury (unusual fatigue, nausea, vomiting, abdominal pain, fever, or jaundice) or a serum bilirubin ≥2 times the upper limit of normal, treatment should be stopped.

AST/ALT >3 times but ≤5 times upper limit of normal: Confirm with additional test; if confirmed, reduce dose or interrupt treatment. Monitor transaminase levels at least every 2 weeks. May continue or reintroduce treatment, as appropriate, following return to pretreatment values. Begin with initial dose (above) and recheck transaminases within 3 days

AST/ALT >5 times but ≤8 times upper limit of normal: Confirm with additional test; if confirmed, stop treatment. Monitor transaminase levels at least every 2 weeks. May reintroduce treatment, as appropriate, at starting dose, following return to pretreatment values. Recheck within 3 days and thereafter following reinitiation.

AST/ALT >8 times upper limit of normal: Stop treatment. No experience with reintroduction.

Stability Store at 20°C to 25°C (68°F to 77°F).

Administration May be administered with or without food, once in the morning and once in the evening. Women of childbearing potential should avoid excessive handling broken tablets.

Monitoring Parameters Serum transaminase (AST and ALT) and bilirubin should be determined prior to the initiation of therapy and at monthly intervals thereafter. A woman of childbearing potential must have a negative pregnancy test prior to the initiation of therapy and monthly thereafter (prior to shipment of monthly refill). Hemoglobin and hematocrit should be measured at baseline, at 1 month and 3 months of treatment, and every 3 months thereafter. Monitor for clinical signs and symptoms of liver injury.

Pregnancy Risk Factor X

Contraindications Hypersensitivity to bosentan or any component of the formulation; concurrent use of cyclosporine or glyburide; pregnancy

Warnings/Precautions **[U.S. Boxed Warning]: Avoid use in moderate-to-severe hepatic impairment.** Has been associated with a high incidence (11%) of significant transaminase elevations, and rare cases of unexplained hepatic cirrhosis have occurred, including after long-term therapy. Transaminase elevations are dose dependent, generally asymptomatic, occur both early and late in therapy, progress slowly, and are usually reversible. Avoid use in patients with elevated serum transaminases (>3 times upper limit of normal) at baseline. Monitor hepatic function closely (at least monthly) for the duration of treatment. Treatment should be stopped in patients who develop elevated transaminases (ALT or AST) in combination with symptoms of hepatic injury (unusual fatigue, jaundice, nausea, vomiting, abdominal pain, and/or fever) or elevated serum bilirubin ≥2 times upper limit of normal.

[U.S. Boxed Warning]: Use in pregnancy is contraindicated; exclude pregnancy prior to initiation of therapy. Pregnancy must be excluded prior to shipment of each monthly refill. Efficacy of hormonal contraceptive may be decreased, and should not be the sole contraceptive method in patients receiving bosentan. Women of childbearing potential should avoid excessive handling broken tablets. Use caution in patients with low hemoglobin levels or ischemic cardiovascular disease. May cause dose-related decreases in hemoglobin and hematocrit (monitoring of hemoglobin is recommended). May cause fluid retention evidenced by signs and symptoms of CHF, weight gain, and leg edema. Bosentan should be discontinued in any patient with signs of pulmonary edema due to the possibility of pulmonary veno-occlusive disease (PVOD). Safety and efficacy in pediatric patients ≤12 years of age have not been established.

Adverse Reactions

>10%:

Central nervous system: Headache (16% to 22%)

(Continued)

Bosentan *(Continued)*

Hematologic: Hemoglobin decreased (≥1 g/dL in up to 57%; typically in first 6 weeks of therapy)

Hepatic: Transaminases increased (>3 times upper limit of normal; up to 11%)

Respiratory: Nasopharyngitis (11%)

1% to 10%:

Cardiovascular: Flushing (7% to 9%), edema (lower limb, 8%; generalized 4%), hypotension (7%), palpitation (5%)

Central nervous system: Fatigue (4%)

Dermatologic: Pruritus (4%)

Gastrointestinal: Dyspepsia (4%)

Hematologic: Anemia (3%)

Hepatic: Abnormal hepatic function (6% to 8%)

<1% (Limited to important or life-threatening): Angioneurotic edema, CHF (exacerbation), cirrhosis (prolonged therapy), hypersensitivity, leukocytoclastic vasculitis, liver failure (rare), peripheral edema, rash, weight gain

Overdosage/Toxicology No specific experience in overdose. Single doses of 2400 mg or 2000 mg/day for 2 months have been tolerated. Symptoms may include headache, nausea, vomiting, and hypotension. Treatment is symptom-directed and supportive.

Drug Interactions Substrate (major) of CYP2C9, 3A4; **Induces** CYP2C9 (strong), 3A4 (strong)

Cyclosporine: Bosentan may enhance the metabolism of cyclosporine, decreasing its serum concentrations by ~50%; effect on sirolimus and/or tacrolimus has not been specifically evaluated, but may be similar. Cyclosporine increases serum concentrations of bosentan (approximately 3-4 times baseline). Concurrent use of cyclosporine is contraindicated.

CYP2C9 inducers: May decrease the levels/effects of bosentan. Example inducers include carbamazepine, phenobarbital, phenytoin, rifampin, rifapentine, and secobarbital.

CYP2C9 inhibitors: May increase the levels/effects of bosentan. Example inhibitors include delavirdine, fluconazole, gemfibrozil, ketoconazole, nicardipine, NSAIDs, pioglitazone, and sulfonamides.

CYP2C9 substrates: Bosentan may decrease the levels/effects of CYP2C9 substrates. Example substrates include celecoxib, dapsone, fluoxetine, glimepiride, glipizide, losartan, montelukast, nateglinide, paclitaxel, phenytoin, sulfonamides, trimethoprim, warfarin, zafirlukast

CYP3A4 inducers: CYP3A4 inducers may decrease the levels/effects of bosentan. Example inducers include aminoglutethimide, carbamazepine, nafcillin, nevirapine, phenobarbital, phenytoin, and rifamycins.

CYP3A4 inhibitors: May increase the levels/effects of bosentan. Example inhibitors include azole antifungals, clarithromycin, diclofenac, doxycycline, erythromycin, imatinib, isoniazid, nefazodone, nicardipine, propofol, protease inhibitors, quinidine, telithromycin, and verapamil.

CYP3A4 substrates: Bosentan may decrease the levels/effects of CYP3A4 substrates. Example substrates include benzodiazepines, calcium channel blockers, ergot derivatives, mirtazapine, nateglinide, nefazodone, tacrolimus, and venlafaxine.

Glyburide: An increased risk of serum transaminase elevations was observed during concurrent therapy with bosentan. Concurrent use is contraindicated.

HMG-CoA reductase inhibitors: Agents metabolized via CYP3A4 may be decreased by bosentan; includes atorvastatin, lovastatin, and simvastatin.

Hormonal contraceptives: Bosentan may decrease levels of hormonal contraceptives; additional methods of contraception are recommended.

Ketoconazole: May increase the serum concentrations of bosentan; concentrations are increased approximately twofold; monitor for increased effects.

Sildenafil: Bosentan may increase the metabolism, via CYP isoenzymes, of sildenafil. Sildenafil may increase the serum concentration of bosentan.

Warfarin: Bosentan may increase the metabolism of oral anticoagulants; monitor for changes in INR.

Ethanol/Nutrition/Herb Interactions

Food: Bioavailability of bosentan is not affected by food.

Herb/Nutraceutical: Avoid St John's wort (may decrease serum concentrations of bosentan).

Dietary Considerations May be taken with or without food.

Dosage Forms

Tablet:

Tracleer®: 62.5 mg, 125 mg

♦ **Botox®** *see* Botulinum Toxin Type A *on page 185*
♦ **Botox® Cosmetic** *see* Botulinum Toxin Type A *on page 185*

Botulinum Toxin Type A (BOT yoo lin num TOKS in type aye)

U.S. Brand Names Botox®; Botox® Cosmetic

Canadian Brand Names Botox®; Botox® Cosmetic

Synonyms BTX-A

Pharmacologic Category Neuromuscular Blocker Agent, Toxin; Ophthalmic Agent, Toxin

Generic Available No

Use Treatment of strabismus and blepharospasm associated with dystonia (including benign essential blepharospasm or VII nerve disorders in patients ≥12 years of age); cervical dystonia (spasmodic torticollis) in patients ≥16 years of age; temporary improvement in the appearance of lines/wrinkles of the face (moderate to severe glabellar lines associated with corrugator and/or procerus muscle activity) in adult patients ≤65 years of age; treatment of severe primary axillary hyperhidrosis in adults not adequately controlled with topical treatments

Orphan drug: Treatment of dynamic muscle contracture in pediatric cerebral palsy patients

Unlabeled/Investigational Use Treatment of oromandibular dystonia, spasmodic dysphonia (laryngeal dystonia) and other dystonias (ie, writer's cramp, focal task-specific dystonias); migraine treatment and prophylaxis

Mechanism of Action Botulinum A toxin is a neurotoxin produced by *Clostridium botulinum*, spore-forming anaerobic bacillus, which appears to affect only the presynaptic membrane of the neuromuscular junction in humans, where it prevents calcium-dependent release of acetylcholine and produces a state of denervation. Muscle inactivation persists until new fibrils grow from the nerve and form junction plates on new areas of the muscle-cell walls.

Pharmacodynamics/Kinetics

Onset of action (improvement):

- Blepharospasm: ~3 days
- Cervical dystonia: ~2 weeks
- Strabismus: ~1-2 days
- Reduction of glabellar lines (Botox® Cosmetic): 1-2 days, increasing in intensity during first week

Duration:

- Blepharospasm: ~3 months
- Cervical dystonia: <3 months
- Strabismus: ~2-6 weeks
- Primary axillary hyperhydrosis: 201 days (mean)
- Reduction of glabellar lines (Botox® Cosmetic): Up to 3 months

Absorption: Not expected to be present in peripheral blood at recommended doses

Time to peak:

- Blepharospasm: 1-2 weeks
- Cervical dystonia: ~6 weeks
- Strabismus: Within first week

Dosage

Cervical dystonia: Children ≥16 years and Adults: I.M.: For dosing guidance, the mean dose is 236 units (25th to 75th percentile range 198-300 units) divided among the affected muscles in patients previously treated with botulinum toxin. Initial dose in previously untreated patients should be lower. Sequential dosing should be based on the patient's head and neck position, localization of pain, muscle hypertrophy, patient response, and previous adverse reactions. The total dose injected into the sternocleidomastoid muscles should be ≤100 units to decrease the occurrence of dysphagia.

Blepharospasm: Children ≥12 years and Adults: I.M.: Initial dose: 1.25-2.5 units injected into the medial and lateral pretarsal orbicularis oculi of the upper and lower lid; dose may be increased up to twice the previous dose if the response from the initial dose lasted ≤2 months; maximum dose per site: 5 units; cumulative dose in a 30-day period: ≤200 units. Tolerance may occur if treatments are given more often than every 3 months, but the effect is not usually permanent.

(Continued)

Botulinum Toxin Type A *(Continued)*

Strabismus: Children ≥12 years and Adults: I.M.:

Initial dose:

Vertical muscles and for horizontal strabismus <20 prism diopters: 1.25-2.5 units in any one muscle

Horizontal strabismus of 20-50 prism diopters: 2.5-5 units in any one muscle

Persistent VI nerve palsy >1 month: 1.5-2.5 units in the medial rectus muscle

Re-examine patients 7-14 days after each injection to assess the effect of that dose. Subsequent doses for patients experiencing incomplete paralysis of the target may be increased up to twice the previous administered dose. The maximum recommended dose as a single injection for any one muscle is 25 units. Do not administer subsequent injections until the effects of the previous dose are gone.

Primary axillary hyperhidrosis: Adults ≥18 years: Intradermal: 50 units/axilla. Injection area should be defined by standard staining techniques. Injections should be evenly distributed into multiple sites (10-15), administered in 0.1-0.2 mL aliquots, ~1-2 cm apart.

Reduction of glabellar lines: Adults ≤65 years: I.M.: An effective dose is determined by gross observation of the patient's ability to activate the superficial muscles injected. The location, size and use of muscles may vary markedly among individuals. Inject 0.1 mL dose into each of five sites, two in each corrugator muscle and one in the procerus muscle (total dose 0.5 mL).

Elderly: No specific adjustment recommended

Dosage adjustment in renal impairment: No specific adjustment recommended

Dosage adjustment in hepatic impairment: No specific adjustment recommended

Stability Store undiluted vials under refrigeration at 2°C to 8°C for up to 24 months. Administer within 4 hours after the vial is reconstituted. Reconstitute with sterile normal saline without a preservative. Mix gently. After reconstitution, store in refrigerator (2°C to 8°C) and use within 4 hours (does not contain preservative). Do not freeze.

Botox®: Reconstitute vials with 1 mL of diluent to get 10 units per 0.1 mL; 2 mL of diluent to get 5 units per 0.1 mL; 4 mL of diluent to get 2.5 units per 0.1 mL; 8 mL of diluent to get 1.25 units per 0.1 mL.

Botox® Cosmetic: Reconstitute vials with 2.5 mL of diluent to get 0.4 units per 0.1 mL (20 units per 0.5 mL).

Administration

Cervical dystonia: Use 25-, 27-, or 30-gauge needle for superficial muscles and a longer 22-gauge needle for deeper musculature; electromyography may help localize the involved muscles.

Blepharospasm: Use a 27- or 30-gauge needle without electromyography guidance. Avoid injecting near the levator palpebrae superioris (may decrease ptosis); avoid medial lower lid injections (may decrease diplopia). Apply pressure at the injection site to prevent ecchymosis in the soft eyelid tissues.

Strabismus injections: Must use surgical exposure or electromyographic guidance; use the electrical activity recorded from the tip of the injections needle as a guide to placement within the target muscle. Local anesthetic and ocular decongestant should be given before injection. The volume of injection should be 0.05-0.15 mL per muscle. Many patients will require additional doses because of inadequate response to initial dose.

Primary axillary hyperhidrosis: Inject each dose intradermally to a depth of ~2 mm and at a 45° angle. Do not inject directly into areas marked in ink (to avoid permanent tattoo effect). Prior to administration, injection area should be defined by standard staining techniques such as Minor's Iodine-Starch Test.

Instructions for Minor's Iodine-Starch Test: Patient should shave underarms and refrain from using deodorants or antiperspirants for 24 hours prior to test. At 30 minutes prior to test, patient should be at rest, no exercise, and not consume hot beverages. Underarm area should be dried and immediately painted with iodine solution. After area dries, lightly sprinkle with starch powder. Gently blow off excess powder. A deep blue-black color will develop over the hyperhidrotic area in ~10 minutes.

Reduction of glabellar lines (Botox® Cosmetic): Use a 30-gauge needle. Ensure injected volume/dose is accurate and where feasible keep to a minimum. Avoid injection near the levator palpebrae superioris. Medial corrugator injections should be at least 1 cm above the bony supraorbital ridge. Do not inject toxin closer than 1 cm above the central eyebrow.

Pregnancy Risk Factor C (manufacturer)

Contraindications Hypersensitivity to albumin, botulinum toxin, or any component of the formulation; infection at the proposed injection site(s); pregnancy. Relative contraindications include diseases of neuromuscular transmission; coagulopathy including therapeutic anticoagulation; uncooperative patient.

Warnings/Precautions Higher doses or more frequent administration may result in neutralizing antibody formation and loss of efficacy. Product contains albumin and may carry a remote risk of virus transmission. Use caution if there is inflammation, excessive weakness, or atrophy at the proposed injection site(s). Have appropriate support in case of anaphylactic reaction. Use with caution in patients with neuromuscular diseases (such as myasthenia gravis), neuropathic disorders (such as amyotrophic lateral sclerosis), or patients taking aminoglycosides or other drugs that interfere with neuromuscular transmission. Ensure adequate contraception in women of childbearing years. Long-term effects of chronic therapy unknown.

Cervical dystonia: Dysphagia is common. It may be severe requiring alternative feeding methods. Risk factors include smaller neck muscle mass, bilateral injections into the sternocleidomastoid muscle, or injections into the levator scapulae. Dysphasia may be associated with increased risk of upper respiratory infection.

Blepharospasm: Reduced blinking from injection of the orbicularis muscle can lead to corneal exposure and ulceration.

Strabismus: Retrobulbar hemorrhages may occur from needle penetration into orbit. Spatial disorientation, double vision, or past pointing may occur if one or more extraocular muscles are paralyzed. Covering the affected eye may help. Careful testing of corneal sensation, avoidance of lower lid injections, and treatment of epithelial defects are necessary.

Primary axillary hyperhidrosis: Evaluate for secondary causes prior to treatment (eg, hyperthyroidism). Safety and efficacy for treatment of hyperhidrosis in other areas of the body have not been established.

Temporary reduction in glabellar lines: Do not use more frequently than every 3 months. Patients with marked facial asymmetry, ptosis, excessive dermatochalasis, deep dermal scarring, thick sebaceous skin, or the inability to substantially lessen glabellar lines by physically spreading them apart were excluded from clinical trials. Reduced blinking from injection of the orbicularis muscle can lead to corneal exposure and ulceration. Spatial disorientation, double vision, or past pointing may occur if one or more extraocular muscles are paralyzed.

Adverse Reactions Adverse effects usually occur in 1 week and may last up to several months

>10%:

- Central nervous system: Headache (cervical dystonia up to 11%, reduction of glabellar lines up to 13%; can occur with other uses)
- Gastrointestinal: Dysphagia (cervical dystonia 19%)
- Neuromuscular & skeletal: Neck pain (cervical dystonia 11%)
- Ocular: Ptosis (blepharospasm 10% to 40%, strabismus 1% to 38%, reduction of glabellar lines 1% to 5%), vertical deviation (strabismus 17%)
- Respiratory: Upper respiratory infection (cervical dystonia 12%)

2% to 10%:

- Central nervous system: Anxiety (primary axillary hyperhydrosis), dizziness (cervical dystonia, reduction of glabellar lines), drowsiness (cervical dystonia), fever (cervical dystonia, primary axillary hyperhydrosis), speech disorder (cervical dystonia)
- Dermatologic: Nonaxillary sweating (primary axillary hyperhydrosis), pruritus (primary axillary hyperhydrosis)
- Gastrointestinal: Xerostomia (cervical dystonia), nausea (cervical dystonia, reduction of glabellar lines)
- Local: Injection site reaction
- Neuromuscular & skeletal: Back pain (cervical dystonia), facial pain (reduction of glabellar lines), hypertonia (cervical dystonia), weakness (cervical dystonia, reduction of glabellar lines)
- Ocular: Dry eyes (blepharospasm 6%), superficial punctate keratitis (blepharospasm 6%)

(Continued)

Botulinum Toxin Type A *(Continued)*

Respiratory: Cough (cervical dystonia), infection (reduction of glabellar lines, primary axillary hyperhydrosis), pharyngitis (primary axillary hyperhydrosis), rhinitis (cervical dystonia)

Miscellaneous: Flu syndrome (cervical dystonia, reduction of glabellar lines, primary axillary hyperhydrosis)

<2%: Stiffness, diplopia (cervical dystonia, blepharospasm), ptosis (cervical dystonia), dyspnea (cervical dystonia), numbness (cervical dystonia), ectropion (blepharospasm), lagophthalmos (blepharospasm), facial weakness (blepharospasm), ecchymoses (blepharospasm), eyelid edema (blepharospasm), tearing (blepharospasm), photophobia (blepharospasm), entropion (blepharospasm)

Postmarketing and/or case reports: Allergic reactions, arrhythmia, erythema multiforme, MI, pruritus, psoriasiform eruption, skin rash, urticaria

Reported following treatment of cervical dystonia: Brachial plexopathy, dysphonia, aspiration

Reported following treatment of blepharospasm: Reduced blinking leading to corneal ulceration, corneal perforation, acute angle-closure glaucoma, focal facial paralysis, exacerbation of myasthenia gravis, syncope, vitreous hemorrhage

Reported following treatment of strabismus: Retrobulbar hemorrhage, ciliary ganglion damage, anterior segment eye ischemia

Reported following reduction of glabellar lines: Exacerbation of myasthenia gravis, retinal vein occlusion, abnormal hearing/hearing loss, glaucoma, vertigo with nystagmus

Overdosage/Toxicology Systemic weakness or muscle paralysis could occur for up to several weeks after overdose. Signs and symptoms of overdose are not apparent immediately. An antitoxin is available if there is immediate knowledge of an overdose or misinjection. Contact Allergan for additional information at (800) 433-8871 or (714) 246-5954. The antitoxin will not reverse toxin-induced muscle weakness already present.

Drug Interactions

Aminoglycosides: May increase neuromuscular blockade.

Neuromuscular-blocking agents: May increase neuromuscular blockade.

Other agents which may have neuromuscular-blocking activity: Calcium channel blockers, catecholamines, chloroquine, clindamycin, colistin, corticosteroids, digitalis glycosides, diuretics, inhalation anesthetics, lidocaine, lincomycin, magnesium salts, opioids, phenytoin, phenelzine, polymixin B, procainamide, propranolol, quinidine, and tetracyclines.

Dosage Forms Injection, powder for reconstitution [preservative free]: *Clostridium botulinum* toxin type A 100 units [contains human albumin]

Botulinum Toxin Type B (BOT yoo lin num TOKS in type bee)

U.S. Brand Names Myobloc®

Pharmacologic Category Neuromuscular Blocker Agent, Toxin

Generic Available No

Use Treatment of cervical dystonia (spasmodic torticollis)

Unlabeled/Investigational Use Treatment of cervical dystonia in patients who have developed resistance to botulinum toxin type A

Mechanism of Action Botulinum B toxin is a neurotoxin produced by *Clostridium botulinum*, spore-forming anaerobic bacillus. It cleaves synaptic Vesicle Association Membrane Protein (VAMP; synaptobrevin) which is a component of the protein complex responsible for docking and fusion of the synaptic vesicle to the presynaptic membrane. By blocking neurotransmitter release, botulinum B toxin paralyzes the muscle.

Pharmacodynamics/Kinetics

Duration: 12-16 weeks

Absorption: Not expected to be present in peripheral blood at recommended doses

Dosage

Children: Not established in pediatric patients

Adults: Cervical dystonia: I.M.: Initial: 2500-5000 units divided among the affected muscles in patients **previously treated** with botulinum toxin; initial dose in **previously untreated** patients should be lower. Subsequent dosing should be optimized according to patient's response.

Elderly: No dosage adjustments required, but limited experience in patients ≥75 years old

Dosage adjustment in renal impairment: No specific adjustment recommended

Dosage adjustment in hepatic impairment: No specific adjustment recommended

Stability Store vials under refrigeration at 2°C to 8°C (36°F to 46°F) for up to 21 months. May be diluted with normal saline; once diluted, use within 4 hours. Does not contain preservative. Single-use vial. Do not shake; do not freeze. Do not mix with any other medicines.

Anesthesia and Critical Care Concerns/Other Considerations Units of biological activity of Myobloc® cannot be compared with units of any other botulinum toxin.

Pregnancy Risk Factor C (manufacturer)

Contraindications Hypersensitivity to albumin, botulinum toxin, or any component of the formulation; infection at the injection site(s); pregnancy; coadministration of agents known to potentiate neuromuscular blockade. Relative contraindications include diseases of neuromuscular transmission; coagulopathy, including therapeutic anticoagulation; inability of patient to cooperate.

Warnings/Precautions Higher doses or more frequent administration may result in neutralizing antibody formation and loss of efficacy. Product contains albumin and may carry a remote risk of virus transmission. Use caution if there is inflammation, excessive weakness, or atrophy at the proposed injection site(s). Concurrent use of botulinum toxin type A or within <4 months of type B is not recommended. Have appropriate support in case of anaphylactic reaction. Use with caution in patients taking aminoglycosides or other drugs that interfere with neuromuscular transmission. Ensure adequate contraception in women of childbearing years. Long-term effects of chronic therapy unknown. Increased risk of dysphagia and respiratory complications. Safety and efficacy in children have not been established.

Adverse Reactions

>10%:

Central nervous system: Headache (10% to 16%), pain (6% to 13%; placebo 10%)

Gastrointestinal: Dysphagia (10% to 25%), xerostomia (3% to 34%)

Local: Injection site pain (12% to 16%)

Neuromuscular & skeletal: Neck pain (up to 17%; placebo: 16%)

Miscellaneous: Infection (13% to 19%; placebo: 15%)

1% to 10%:

Cardiovascular: Chest pain, vasodilation, peripheral edema

Central nervous system: Dizziness (3% to 6%), fever, malaise, migraine, anxiety, tremor, hyperesthesia, somnolence, confusion, vertigo

Dermatologic: Pruritus, bruising

Gastrointestinal: Nausea (3% to 10%; placebo: 5%), dyspepsia (up to 10%; placebo: 5%), vomiting, stomatitis, taste perversion

Genitourinary: Urinary tract infection, cystitis, vaginal moniliasis

Hematologic: Serum neutralizing activity

Neuromuscular & skeletal: Torticollis (up to 8%; placebo: 7%), arthralgia (up to 7%; placebo: 5%), back pain (3% to 7%; placebo: 3%), myasthenia (3% to 6%; placebo: 3%), weakness (up to 6%; placebo: 4%), arthritis

Ocular: Amblyopia, abnormal vision

Otic: Otitis media, tinnitus

Respiratory: Cough (3% to 7%; placebo: 3%), rhinitis (1% to 5%; placebo: 6%), dyspnea, pneumonia

Miscellaneous: Flu-syndrome (6% to 9%), allergic reaction, viral infection, abscess, cyst

Overdosage/Toxicology Systemic weakness or muscle paralysis could occur for up to several weeks after overdose. Signs and symptoms of overdose are not apparent immediately. An antitoxin is available if there is immediate knowledge of an overdose or misinjection. Contact Elan Pharmaceuticals for additional information at (888) 638-7605 and your State Health Department to process a request for antitoxin through the CDC. The antitoxin will not reverse toxin-induced muscle weakness already present.

Drug Interactions

Aminoglycosides: May increase neuromuscular blockade.

Botulinum toxin type A: Potentiation of paralysis with concurrent or overlapping use; separate by ≥4 months.

Neuromuscular-blocking agents: May increase neuromuscular blockade.

(Continued)

Botulinum Toxin Type B *(Continued)*

Other agents which may have neuromuscular-blocking activity: Inhalation anesthetics, calcium channel blockers, catecholamines, chloroquine, clarithromycin, clindamycin, colistin, corticosteroids, digitalis glycosides, diuretics, erythromycin, inhalation anesthetics, lidocaine, lincomycin, magnesium salts, opioids, phenytoin, phenelzine, polymixin B, procainamide, propranolol, quinidine, tetracyclines, and vancomycin.

Dosage Forms Injection, solution [single-dose vial]: 5000 units/mL (0.5 mL, 1 mL, 2 mL) [contains albumin 0.05%]

Botulism Immune Globulin (Intravenous-Human)

(BOT yoo lism i MYUN GLOB you lin, in tra VEE nus, YU man)

U.S. Brand Names BabyBIG®

Synonyms BIG-IV

Pharmacologic Category Immune Globulin

Restrictions Available from the California Department of Health

Generic Available No

Use Treatment of infant botulism caused by toxin type A or B

Mechanism of Action BIG-IV is purified immunoglobulin derived from the plasma of adults immunized with botulinum toxoid types A and B. BIG-IV provides antibodies to neutralize circulating toxins.

Pharmacodynamics/Kinetics

Duration: Protective neutralizing antibody levels: 6 months

Half-life elimination: 28 days

Dosage I.V.: Children <1 year: Infant botulism: 1 mL/kg (50 mg/kg) as a single dose; infuse at 0.5 mL/kg/hour (25 mg/kg/hour) for the first 15 minutes; if well tolerated, may increase to 1 mL/kg/hour (50 mg/kg/hour)

Stability Prior to reconstitution, store between 2°C to 8°C (35.6°F to 46.4°F). Infusion should begin within 2 hours of reconstitution and be completed within 4 hours of reconstitution. Reconstitute with SWFI 2 mL; swirl gently to wet powder, do not shake. Powder should dissolve in ~30 minutes.

Administration For I.V. infusion only. Do not administer if solution is turbid. Epinephrine should be available for the treatment of acute allergic reaction. Administer using low volume tubing and infusion pump with an in-line or syringe tip 18 μm filter. Infuse at 0.5 mL/kg/hour (25 mg/kg/hour) for the first 15 minutes; if well tolerated, may increase to 1 mL/kg/hour (50 mg/kg/hour). Infusion should take ~67.5 minutes. Infusion should be slowed or temporarily interrupted for minor side effects; discontinue in case of hypotension or anaphylaxis.

Monitoring Parameters Renal function (BUN, serum creatinine, urinary output); vital signs (continuously during infusion); aseptic meningitis syndrome (may occur hours to days following IGIV therapy); signs of relapse (may occur up to 1 month following recovery)

Contraindications Hypersensitivity to human immune globulin preparations or any component of the formulation; selective immunoglobulin A deficiency

Warnings/Precautions Use caution with renal dysfunction or those at increased risk for renal disease, including concomitant nephrotoxic drugs, diabetes mellitus, paraproteinemia, sepsis, or volume depletion. Patients should not be volume depleted prior to therapy. For I.V. infusion only; do not exceed recommended rate of administration. Not indicated for use in adults or children; safety and efficacy established for infants <1 year of age.

Adverse Reactions Percentages reported in open-label study except where otherwise noted; may reflect pathophysiology of infant botulism.

>10%:

Cardiovascular: Blood pressure increased (transient, 75%), pallor (28%), edema (18%); blood pressure decreased (transient, 16%), cardiac murmur (15%)

Central nervous system: Irritability (41%), pyrexia (17%), body temperature decreased (16%)

Dermatologic: Contact dermatitis (24%), erythematous rash (22%, reported as 14% vs 8% in placebo-controlled study)

Gastrointestinal: Dysphagia (65%), loose stools (25%), vomiting (20%), abdominal distension (11%)

Otic: Otitis media (11%, reported in placebo-controlled study)

Respiratory: Atelectasis (39%), rhonchi (34%), nasal congestion (18%), oxygen saturation decreased (17%), cough (13%), rales (13%)

1% to 10%:

Cardiovascular: Tachycardia (7%), peripheral coldness (7%)

Central nervous system: Agitation (10%)

Endocrine & metabolic: Dehydration (10%), hyponatremia (6%), metabolic acidosis (5%)

Hematologic: Hemoglobin decreased (9%), anemia (5%)

Local: Injection site reaction (7%), injection site erythema (5%)

Renal: Neurogenic bladder

Respiratory: Breath sounds decreased (10%), stridor (9%), lower respiratory tract infection (8%), dyspnea (6%), tachypnea (5%)

Miscellaneous: Oral candidiasis (8%), intubation (5%), infusion rate reactions (<5%, includes chills, back pain, fever, muscle cramps, nausea, vomiting, wheezing)

Overdosage/Toxicology Limited data; adverse reactions related to volume overload may be expected

Drug Interactions

Vaccines: Immune globulins may interfere with live virus vaccines; defer vaccination for ~5 months following therapy. Revaccinations may be needed if given shortly before or after BIG-IV administration.

Dosage Forms Injection, powder for reconstitution [preservative free]: ~100 mg [contains albumin 1% and sucrose 5%; packaged with SWFI]

- **Bovine Lung Surfactant** *see* Beractant *on page 168*
- **Breathe Right® Saline [OTC]** *see* Sodium Chloride *on page 1183*
- **Brethaire [DSC]** *see* Terbutaline *on page 1244*
- **Brethine®** *see* Terbutaline *on page 1244*
- **Brevibloc®** *see* Esmolol *on page 481*
- **Brevital® (Can)** *see* Methohexital *on page 819*
- **Brevital® Sodium** *see* Methohexital *on page 819*
- **Bricanyl® (Can)** *see* Terbutaline *on page 1244*
- **Brioschi® [OTC]** *see* Sodium Bicarbonate *on page 1181*
- **BRL 43694** *see* Granisetron *on page 602*

Bromocriptine (broe moe KRIP teen)

Medication Safety Issues

Sound-alike/look-alike issues:

Bromocriptine may be confused with benztropine, brimonidine

Parlodel® may be confused with pindolol, Provera®

U.S. Brand Names Parlodel®

Canadian Brand Names Apo-Bromocriptine®; Parlodel®; PMS-Bromocriptine

Synonyms Bromocriptine Mesylate

Pharmacologic Category Anti-Parkinson's Agent, Dopamine Agonist; Ergot Derivative

Generic Available Yes

Use Treatment of hyperprolactinemia associated with amenorrhea with or without galactorrhea, infertility, or hypogonadism; treatment of prolactin-secreting adenomas; treatment of acromegaly; treatment of Parkinson's disease

Unlabeled/Investigational Use Neuroleptic malignant syndrome

Mechanism of Action Semisynthetic ergot alkaloid derivative and a dopamine receptor agonist which activates postsynaptic dopamine receptors in the tuberoinfundibular (inhibiting pituitary prolactin secretion) and nigrostriatal pathways (enhancing coordinated motor control).

Pharmacodynamics/Kinetics

Bioavailability: 28%

Protein binding: 90% to 96%

Metabolism: Primarily hepatic

Half-life elimination: Biphasic: Initial: 6-8 hours; Terminal: 50 hours

Time to peak, serum: 1-2 hours

Excretion: Feces; urine (2% to 6% as unchanged drug)

(Continued)

Bromocriptine *(Continued)*

Dosage Oral:

Children: Hyperprolactinemia:

11-15 years (based on limited information): Initial: 1.25-2.5 mg daily; dosage may be increased as tolerated to achieve a therapeutic response (range: 2.5-10 mg daily).

≥16 years: Refer to adult dosing

Adults:

Parkinsonism: 1.25 mg twice daily, increased by 2.5 mg/day in 2- to 4-week intervals (usual dose range is 30-90 mg/day in 3 divided doses), though elderly patients can usually be managed on lower doses

Neuroleptic malignant syndrome (unlabeled use): 2.5-5 mg 3 times/day

Acromegaly: Initial: 1.25-2.5 mg daily increasing by 1.25-2.5 mg daily as necessary every 3-7 days; usual dose: 20-30 mg/day (maximum: 100 mg/day)

Hyperprolactinemia: Initial: 1.25-2.5 mg/day; may be increased by 2.5 mg/day as tolerated every 2-7 days until optimal response (range: 2.5-15 mg/day)

Dosing adjustment in hepatic impairment: No guidelines are available, however, may be necessary

Monitoring Parameters Monitor blood pressure closely as well as hepatic, hematopoietic, and cardiovascular function; visual field monitoring is recommended (prolactinoma); pregnancy test during amenorrheic peroid; growth hormone and prolactin levels.

Pregnancy Risk Factor B

Contraindications Hypersensitivity to bromocriptine, ergot alkaloids, or any component of the formulation; ergot alkaloids are contraindicated with potent inhibitors of CYP3A4 (includes protease inhibitors, azole antifungals, and some macrolide antibiotics); uncontrolled hypertension; severe ischemic heart disease or peripheral vascular disorders; pregnancy (risk to benefit evaluation must be performed in women who become pregnant during treatment for acromegaly, prolactinoma, or Parkinson's disease - hypertension during treatment should generally result in efforts to withdraw)

Warnings/Precautions Complete evaluation of pituitary function should be completed prior to initiation of treatment. Use caution in patients with impaired renal or hepatic function, a history of peptic ulcer disease, dementia, psychosis, or cardiovascular disease (myocardial infarction, arrhythmia). Symptomatic hypotension may occur in a significant number of patients. In addition, hypertension, seizures, MI, and stroke have been rarely associated with bromocriptine therapy. Severe headache or visual changes may precede events. The onset of reactions may be immediate or delayed (often may occur in the second week of therapy).

Concurrent antihypertensives or drugs which may alter blood pressure should be used with caution. Concurrent use with levodopa has been associated with an increased risk of hallucinations. Consider dosage reduction and/or discontinuation in patients with hallucinations. Hallucinations may require weeks to months before resolution.

In the treatment of acromegaly, discontinuation is recommended if tumor expansion occurs during therapy. Digital vasospasm (cold sensitive) may occur in some patients with acromegaly; may require dosage reduction. Patients who receive bromocriptine during and immediately following pregnancy as a continuation of previous therapy (eg, acromegaly) should be closely monitored for cardiovascular effects. Should not be used post-partum in women with coronary artery disease or other cardiovascular disease. Use of bromocriptine to control or prevent lactation or in patients with uncontrolled hypertension is not recommended.

Monitoring and careful evaluation of visual changes during the treatment of hyperprolactinemia is recommended to differentiate between tumor shrinkage and traction on the optic chiasm; rapidly progressing visual field loss requires neurosurgical consultation. Discontinuation of bromocriptine in patients with macroadenomas has been associated with rapid regrowth of tumor and increased prolactin serum levels. Pleural and retroperitoneal fibrosis have been reported with prolonged daily use. Cardiac valvular fibrosis has also been associated with ergot alkaloids. Safety and effectiveness in patients <15 years of age (for pituitary adenoma) have not been established.

Adverse Reactions Note: Frequency of adverse effects may vary by dose and/or indication.

>10%:

Cardiovascular: Hypotension (up to 30%)

Central nervous system: Headache, dizziness
Gastrointestinal: Nausea, constipation

1% to 10%:
Cardiovascular: Orthostasis, vasospasm (cold-sensitive), Raynaud's syndrome, syncope
Central nervous system: Fatigue, lightheadedness, drowsiness
Gastrointestinal: Anorexia, vomiting, abdominal cramps, diarrhea, dyspepsia, GI bleeding, xerostomia
Respiratory: Nasal congestion

<1%(Limited to important or life-threatening): Arrhythmias, erythromelalgia, ethanol potentiation, hallucinations (visual), hypertension, MI, paranoia, paresthesia, psychosis, pulmonary infiltrates, pleural effusion, peritoneal fibrosis, rash, retroperitoneal fibrosis, skin mottling, status epilepticus, vasovagal reaction, vertigo, visual changes

Withdrawal reactions: Abrupt discontinuation has resulted in rare cases of a withdrawal reaction with symptoms similar to neuroleptic malignant syndrome.

Overdosage/Toxicology Symptoms of overdose include nausea, vomiting, and hypotension. Treatment is symptomatic and supportive.

Drug Interactions Substrate of CYP3A4 (major); **Inhibits** CYP1A2 (weak), 3A4 (weak)

Alpha agonists/sympathomimetics: May enhance the adverse/toxic effect of bromocriptine, including increased blood pressure, ventricular arrhythmias, and seizures. Monitor. **Note:** The use of epinephrine in combination local anethetics should pose no clinical concern.

Antihypertensives: Concurrent use with bromocriptine may increase the risk of hypotension and/or orthostasis. Use caution.

Antifungals, azole derivatives (itraconazole, ketoconazole) increase levels of ergot alkaloids by inhibiting CYP3A4 metabolism, resulting in toxicity; concomitant use is contraindicated.

Antipsychotics: May diminish the effects of bromocriptine (due to dopamine antagonism); these combinations should generally be avoided.

CYP3A4 inhibitors: May increase the levels/effects of bromocriptine. Example inhibitors include azole antifungals, clarithromycin, diclofenac, doxycycline, erythromycin, imatinib, isoniazid, nefazodone, nicardipine, propofol, protease inhibitors, quinidine, telithromycin, and verapamil.

Levodopa: Concurrent use may increase the risk of hallucinations. Dosage reduction may be required.

Macrolide antibiotics: Erythromycin, clarithromycin, and troleandomycin may increase levels of ergot alkaloids by inhibiting CYP3A4 metabolism, resulting in toxicity (ischemia, vasospasm); concomitant use is contraindicated.

MAO inhibitors: The serotonergic effects of ergot derivatives may be increased by MAO inhibitors. Monitor for signs and symptoms of serotonin syndrome.

Metoclopramide: May diminish the effects of bromocriptine (due to dopamine antagonism); concurrent therapy should generally be avoided.

Protease inhibitors (ritonavir, amprenavir, indinavir, nelfinavir, and saquinavir) increase blood levels of ergot alkaloids by inhibiting CYP3A4 metabolism, acute ergot toxicity has been reported; concomitant use is contraindicated.

Serotonin agonists: Concurrent use with bromocriptine may increase the risk of serotonin syndrome (includes buspirone, SSRIs, TCAs, nefazodone, sumatriptan, and trazodone).

Sibutramine: May cause serotonin syndrome; concurrent use with ergot alkaloids is contraindicated.

Telithromycin: May increase levels of ergot alkaloids by inhibiting CYP3A4 metabolism, resulting in toxicity (ischemia, vasospasm); concomitant use is contraindicated.

Ethanol/Nutrition/Herb Interactions

Ethanol: Avoid ethanol (may increase GI side effects or ethanol intolerance).
Herb/Nutraceutical: St John's wort may decrease bromocriptine levels.

Dietary Considerations May be taken with food to decrease GI distress.

Dosage Forms

Capsule, as mesylate: 5 mg
Parlodel®: 5 mg
Tablet, as mesylate: 2.5 mg
Parlodel®: 2.5 mg

♦ **Bromocriptine Mesylate** *see* Bromocriptine *on page 191*
♦ **Broncho Saline® [OTC]** *see* Sodium Chloride *on page 1183*

- **BTX-A** *see* Botulinum Toxin Type A *on page 185*
- **B-type Natriuretic Peptide (Human)** *see* Nesiritide *on page 913*
- **Bubbli-Pred™ [DSC]** *see* PrednisoLONE *on page 1046*
- **Budeprion™ SR** *see* BuPROPion *on page 201*
- **Buffered Aspirin and Pravastatin Sodium** *see* Aspirin and Pravastatin *on page 135*
- **Bufferin® [OTC]** *see* Aspirin *on page 129*
- **Bufferin® Extra Strength [OTC]** *see* Aspirin *on page 129*
- **Buffinol [OTC]** *see* Aspirin *on page 129*
- **Buffinol Extra [OTC]** *see* Aspirin *on page 129*

Bumetanide (byoo MET a nide)

Medication Safety Issues

Sound-alike/look-alike issues:

Bumetanide may be confused with Buminate®

Bumex® may be confused with Brevibloc®, Buprenex®, Permax®

Related Information

Diuretics, Loop *on page 1565*

Heart Failure (Systolic) *on page 1607*

U.S. Brand Names Bumex®

Canadian Brand Names Bumex®; Burinex®

Pharmacologic Category Diuretic, Loop

Generic Available Yes

Use Management of edema secondary to congestive heart failure or hepatic or renal disease including nephrotic syndrome; may be used alone or in combination with antihypertensives in the treatment of hypertension; can be used in furosemide-allergic patients

Mechanism of Action Inhibits reabsorption of sodium and chloride in the ascending loop of Henle and proximal renal tubule, interfering with the chloride-binding cotransport system, thus causing increased excretion of water, sodium, chloride, magnesium, phosphate, and calcium; it does not appear to act on the distal tubule

Pharmacodynamics/Kinetics

Onset of action: Oral, I.M.: 0.5-1 hour; I.V.: 2-3 minutes

Duration: 4-6 hours

Distribution: V_d: 13-25 L/kg

Protein binding: 95%

Metabolism: Partially hepatic

Half-life elimination: Neonates: ~6 hours; Infants (1 month): ~2.4 hours; Adults: 1-1.5 hours

Excretion: Primarily urine (as unchanged drug and metabolites)

Dosage

Oral, I.M., I.V.:

Neonates (see Warnings/Precautions): 0.01-0.05 mg/kg/dose every 24-48 hours

Infants and Children: 0.015-0.1 mg/kg/dose every 6-24 hours (maximum dose: 10 mg/day)

Adults:

Edema:

Oral: 0.5-2 mg/dose (maximum dose: 10 mg/day) 1-2 times/day

I.M., I.V.: 0.5-1 mg/dose; may repeat in 2-3 hours for up to 2 doses if needed (maximum dose: 10 mg/day)

Continuous I.V. infusion: Initial: 1 mg I.V. load then 0.5-2 mg/hour (ACC/AHA 2005 practice guidelines for chronic heart failure)

Hypertension: Oral: 0.5 mg daily (maximum dose: 5 mg/day); usual dosage range (JNC 7): 0.5-2 mg/day in 2 divided doses

Stability

I.V.: Store vials at 15°C to 30°C (59°F to 86°F). Infusion solutions should be used within 24 hours after preparation. Light sensitive; discoloration may occur when exposed to light.

Tablet: Store at 15°C to 30°C (59°F to 86°F).

Administration Administer I.V. slowly, over 1-2 minutes. An alternate-day schedule or a 3-4 daily dosing regimen with rest periods of 1-2 days in between may be the most tolerable and effective regimen for the continued control of edema. Reserve I.V. administration for those unable to take oral medications.

Monitoring Parameters Blood pressure, serum electrolytes, renal function

Anesthesia and Critical Care Concerns/Other Considerations If given the morning of surgery, it may render the patient volume depleted and blood pressure may be labile during general anesthesia.

Patients with impaired hepatic function must be monitored carefully, often requiring reduced doses. Larger doses may be necessary in patients with impaired renal function to obtain the same therapeutic response.

It is important that patients be closely followed for hypokalemia, hypomagnesemia, and volume depletion because of significant diuresis.

Pregnancy Risk Factor C (manufacturer); D (expert analysis)

Contraindications Hypersensitivity to bumetanide, any component of the formulation, or sulfonylureas; anuria; patients with hepatic coma or in states of severe electrolyte depletion until the condition improves or is corrected; pregnancy (based on expert analysis)

Warnings/Precautions Adjust dose to avoid dehydration. In cirrhosis, avoid electrolyte and acid/base imbalances that might lead to hepatic encephalopathy. Ototoxicity is associated with I.V. rapid administration, renal impairment, excessive doses, and concurrent use of other ototoxins. Hypersensitivity reactions can rarely occur. Monitor fluid status and renal function in an attempt to prevent oliguria, azotemia, and reversible increases in BUN and creatinine. Close medical supervision of aggressive diuresis required. Watch for and correct electrolyte disturbances. Coadministration of antihypertensives may increase the risk of hypotension.

Chemical similarities are present among sulfonamides, sulfonylureas, carbonic anhydrase inhibitors, thiazides, and loop diuretics (except ethacrynic acid). Use in patients with sulfonylurea allergy is specifically contraindicated in product labeling, however, a risk of cross-reaction exists in patients with allergy to any of these compounds; avoid use when previous reaction has been severe.

[U.S. Boxed Warning]: Loop diuretics are potent diuretics; excess amounts can lead to profound diuresis with fluid and electrolyte loss; close medical supervision and dose evaluation are required. *In vitro* studies using pooled sera from critically-ill neonates have shown bumetanide to be a potent displacer of bilirubin; avoid use in neonates at risk for kernicterus.

Adverse Reactions

>10%:

- Endocrine & metabolic: Hyperuricemia (18%), hypochloremia (15%), hypokalemia (15%)
- Renal: Azotemia (11%)

1% to 10%:

- Central nervous system: Dizziness (1%)
- Endocrine & metabolic: Hyponatremia (9%); hyperglycemia (7%); variations in phosphorus (5%), CO_2 content (4%), bicarbonate (3%), and calcium (2%)
- Neuromuscular & skeletal: Muscle cramps (1%)
- Otic: Ototoxicity (1%)
- Renal: Serum creatinine increased (7%)

<1% (Limited to important or life-threatening): Asterixis, dehydration, encephalopathy, hearing impaired, hypernatremia, hypotension, orthostatic hypotension, pruritus, rash, renal failure, vertigo, vomiting

Overdosage/Toxicology Symptoms of overdose include electrolyte and volume depletion. Treatment is symptomatic and supportive.

Drug Interactions

ACE inhibitors: Hypotensive effects and/or renal effects are potentiated by hypovolemia.

Antidiabetic agents: Glucose tolerance may be decreased.

Antihypertensive agents: Hypotensive effects may be enhanced.

Cholestyramine or colestipol may reduce bioavailability of bumetanide.

Digoxin: Bumetanide-induced hypokalemia may predispose to digoxin toxicity; monitor potassium.

Indomethacin (and other NSAIDs) may reduce natriuretic and hypotensive effects of diuretics.

Lithium: Renal clearance may be reduced. Isolated reports of lithium toxicity have occurred; monitor lithium levels.

(Continued)

Bumetanide *(Continued)*

NSAIDs: Risk of renal impairment may increase when used in conjunction with diuretics.

Ototoxic drugs (aminoglycosides, cis-platinum): Concomitant use of bumetanide may increase risk of ototoxicity, especially in patients with renal dysfunction.

Peripheral adrenergic-blocking drugs or ganglionic blockers: Effects may be increased.

Salicylates (high dose) with diuretics may predispose patients to salicylate toxicity due to reduced renal excretion or alter renal function.

Thiazides: Synergistic diuretic effects occur.

Ethanol/Nutrition/Herb Interactions Herb/Nutraceutical: Avoid ephedra, yohimbe, ginseng (may worsen hypertension). Avoid dong quai if using for hypertension (has estrogenic activity). Avoid garlic (may have increased antihypertensive effect).

Dietary Considerations May require increased intake of potassium-rich foods.

Dosage Forms

Injection, solution: 0.25 mg/mL (2 mL, 4 mL, 10 mL) [contains benzyl alcohol]

Tablet (Bumex®): 0.5 mg, 1 mg, 2 mg

♦ **Bumex®** *see* Bumetanide *on page 194*

♦ **Buminate®** *see* Albumin *on page 48*

Bupivacaine (byoo PIV a kane)

Medication Safety Issues

Sound-alike/look-alike issues:

Bupivacaine may be confused with mepivacaine, ropivacaine

Marcaine® may be confused with Narcan®

Related Information

Acute Postoperative Pain *on page 1388*

Local Anesthetics *on page 1532*

U.S. Brand Names Marcaine®; Marcaine® Spinal; Sensorcaine®; Sensorcaine®-MPF

Canadian Brand Names Marcaine®; Sensorcaine®

Synonyms Bupivacaine Hydrochloride

Pharmacologic Category Local Anesthetic

Generic Available Yes

Use Local anesthetic (injectable) for peripheral nerve block, infiltration, sympathetic block, caudal or epidural block, retrobulbar block

Mechanism of Action Blocks both the initiation and conduction of nerve impulses by decreasing the neuronal membrane's permeability to sodium ions, which results in inhibition of depolarization with resultant blockade of conduction

Pharmacodynamics/Kinetics

Onset of action: Anesthesia (route and dose dependent): 1-17 minutes

Duration (route and dose dependent): 2-9 hours

Protein binding: ~95%

Metabolism: Hepatic; forms metabolite (PPX)

Half-life elimination (age dependent): Neonates: 8.1 hours; Adults: 1.5-5.5 hours

Excretion: Urine (~6% unchanged)

Dosage Dose varies with procedure, depth of anesthesia, vascularity of tissues, duration of anesthesia, and condition of patient. Do not use solutions containing preservatives for caudal or epidural block.

Children >12 years and Adults:

Local anesthesia: Infiltration: 0.25% infiltrated locally; maximum: 175 mg

Caudal block (preservative free): 15-30 mL of 0.25% or 0.5%

Epidural block (other than caudal block; preservative free): Administer in 3-5 mL increments, allowing sufficient time to detect toxic manifestations of inadvertent I.V. or I.T. administration: 10-20 mL of 0.25% or 0.5%

Surgical procedures requiring a high degree of muscle relaxation and prolonged effects **only**: 10-20 mL of 0.75% (**Note:** Not to be used in obstetrical cases)

Peripheral nerve block: 5 mL of 0.25 or 0.5%; maximum: 400 mg/day

Sympathetic nerve block: 20-50 mL of 0.25%

Retrobulbar anesthesia: 2-4 mL of 0.75%

Adults: Spinal anesthesia: Preservative free solution of 0.75% bupivacaine in 8.25% dextrose:
- Lower extremity and perineal procedures: 1 mL
- Lower abdominal procedures: 1.6 mL
- Normal vaginal delivery: 0.8 mL (higher doses may be required in some patients)
- Cesarean section: 1-1.4 mL

Stability Store at controlled room temperature of 15°C to 30°C (59°F to 86°F).

Administration Solutions containing preservatives should not be used for epidural or caudal blocks.

Monitoring Parameters Vital signs, state of consciousness; signs of CNS toxicity; fetal heart rate during paracervical anesthesia

Pregnancy Risk Factor C

Contraindications Hypersensitivity to bupivacaine hydrochloride, amide-type local anesthetics, or any component of the formulation; obstetrical paracervical block anesthesia

Warnings/Precautions Use with caution in patients with hepatic impairment. Not recommended for use in children <12 years of age. The solution for spinal anesthesia should not be used in children <18 years of age. **Do not use solutions containing preservatives for caudal or epidural block**. Local anesthetics have been associated with rare occurrences of sudden respiratory arrest; convulsions due to systemic toxicity leading to cardiac arrest have also been reported, presumably following unintentional intravascular injection. **[U.S. Boxed Warning]: The 0.75% is not recommended for obstetrical anesthesia.** A test dose is recommended prior to epidural administration (prior to initial dose) and all reinforcing doses with continuous catheter technique. Use caution with cardiovascular dysfunction. Use caution in debilitated, elderly, or acutely ill patients; dose reduction may be required.

Adverse Reactions Note: Incidence of adverse reactions is difficult to define. Most effects are dose related, and are often due to accelerated absorption from the injection site, unintentional intravascular injection, or slow metabolic degradation. The development of any central nervous system symptoms may be an early indication of more significant toxicity (seizure).

- Cardiovascular: Hypotension, bradycardia, palpitation, heart block, ventricular arrhythmia, cardiac arrest
- Central nervous system: Restlessness, anxiety, dizziness, seizure (0.1%); rare symptoms (usually associated with unintentional subarachnoid injection during high spinal anesthesia) include persistent anesthesia, paresthesia, paralysis, headache, septic meningitis, and cranial nerve palsies
- Gastrointestinal: Nausea, vomiting; rare symptoms (usually associated with unintentional subarachnoid injection during high spinal anesthesia) include fecal incontinence and loss of sphincter control
- Genitourinary: Rare symptoms (usually associated with unintentional subarachnoid injection during high spinal anesthesia) include urinary incontinence, loss of perineal sensation, and loss of sexual function
- Neuromuscular & skeletal: Weakness
- Ocular: Blurred vision, pupillary constriction
- Otic: Tinnitus
- Respiratory: Apnea, hypoventilation (usually associated with unintentional subarachnoid injection during high spinal anesthesia)
- Miscellaneous: Allergic reactions (urticaria, pruritus, angioedema), anaphylactoid reactions

Overdosage/Toxicology Treatment is symptomatic and supportive. Termination of anesthesia by pneumatic tourniquet inflation should be attempted when bupivacaine is administered by infiltration or regional injection. Treatment is symptomatic and supportive. Methemoglobinemia should be treated with methylene blue 1-2 mg/kg in a 1% sterile aqueous solution by I.V. push over 4-6 minutes, repeated up to a total dose of 7 mg/kg.

Drug Interactions Substrate (minor) of CYP1A2, 2C19, 2D6, 3A4

Dosage Forms

Injection, solution, as hydrochloride [preservative free]: 0.25% [2.5 mg/mL] (10 mL, 20 mL, 30 mL, 50 mL); 0.5% [5 mg/mL] (10 mL, 20 mL, 30 mL); 0.75% [7.5 mg/mL] (10 mL, 20 mL, 30 mL)
- Marcaine®: 0.25% [2.5 mg/mL] (10 mL, 30 mL); 0.5% [5 mg/mL] (10 mL, 30 mL); 0.75% [7.5 mg/mL] (10 mL, 30 mL)
- Marcaine® Spinal: 0.75% [7.5 mg/mL] (2 mL) [in dextrose 8.25%]

(Continued)

Bupivacaine *(Continued)*

Sensorcaine®-MPF: 0.25% [2.5 mg/mL] (10 mL, 30 mL); 0.5% [5 mg/mL] (10 mL, 30 mL); 0.75% [7.5 mg/mL] (10 mL, 30 mL)

Injection, solution, as hydrochloride (Marcaine®, Sensorcaine®): 0.25% [2.5 mg/mL] (50 mL); 0.5% [5 mg/mL] (50 mL) [contains methylparaben]

References

Lehmann LJ and Pallares VS, "Subdural Injection of a Local Anesthetic With Steroids: Complication of Epidural Anesthesia," *South Med J*, 1995, 88(4):467-9.

Long WB, Rosenblum S, and Grady IP, "Successful Resuscitation of Bupivacaine-Induced Cardiac Arrest Using Cardiopulmonary Bypass," *Anesth Analg*, 1989, 69(3):403-6.

Scott DB, Lee A, Fagan D, et al, "Acute Toxicity of Ropivacaine Compared With That of Bupivacaine," *Anesth Analg*, 1989, 69(5):563-9.

Sun KO, "Convulsion Following Spinal Anaesthesia," *Anaesth Intensive Care*, 1995, 23(4):520-1.

Tuominen MK, Pere P, and Rosenberg PH, "Unintentional Arterial Catheterization and Bupivacaine Toxicity Associated With Continuous Interscalene Brachial Plexus Block," *Anesthesiology*, 1991, 75(2):356-8.

- ♦ **Bupivacaine and Lidocaine** *see* Lidocaine and Bupivacaine *on page 761*
- ♦ **Bupivacaine Hydrochloride** *see* Bupivacaine *on page 196*
- ♦ **Buprenex®** *see* Buprenorphine *on page 198*

Buprenorphine (byoo pre NOR feen)

Medication Safety Issues

Sound-alike/look-alike issues:

Buprenex® may be confused with Brevibloc®, Bumex®

Related Information

Anesthesia Considerations for Neurosurgery *on page 1401*
Chronic Pain Management *on page 1430*
Narcotic / Opioid Analgesics *on page 1568*
Opioids *on page 1535*

U.S. Brand Names Buprenex®; Subutex®

Canadian Brand Names Buprenex®; Subutex®

Synonyms Buprenorphine Hydrochloride

Pharmacologic Category Analgesic, Narcotic

Restrictions Injection: C-V; Tablet: C-III

Prescribing of tablets for opioid dependence is limited to physicians who have met the qualification criteria and have received a DEA number specific to prescribing this product. Tablets will be available through pharmacies and wholesalers which normally provide controlled substances.

Generic Available Yes: Injection

Use

Injection: Management of moderate to severe pain

Tablet: Treatment of opioid dependence

Unlabeled/Investigational Use Injection: Heroin and opioid withdrawal

Mechanism of Action Buprenorphine exerts its analgesic effect via high affinity binding to μ opiate receptors in the CNS; displays both agonist and antagonist activity

Pharmacodynamics/Kinetics

Onset of action: Analgesic: 10-30 minutes

Duration: 6-8 hours

Absorption: I.M., SubQ: 30% to 40%

Distribution: V_d: 97-187 L/kg

Protein binding: High

Metabolism: Primarily hepatic; extensive first-pass effect

Half-life elimination: 2.2-3 hours

Excretion: Feces (70%); urine (20% as unchanged drug)

Dosage Long-term use is not recommended

Note: These are guidelines and do not represent the maximum doses that may be required in all patients. Doses should be titrated to pain relief/prevention. In high-risk patients (eg, elderly, debilitated, presence of respiratory disease) and/or concurrent CNS depressant use, reduce dose by one-half. Buprenorphine has an analgesic ceiling.

Acute pain (moderate to severe):

Children 2-12 years: I.M., slow I.V.: 2-6 mcg/kg every 4-6 hours

Children ≥13 years and Adults:

I.M.: Initial: Opiate-naive: 0.3 mg every 6-8 hours as needed; initial dose (up to 0.3 mg) may be repeated once in 30-60 minutes after the initial dose if needed; usual dosage range: 0.15-0.6 mg every 4-8 hours as needed

Slow I.V.: Initial: Opiate-naive: 0.3 mg every 6-8 hours as needed; initial dose (up to 0.3 mg) may be repeated once in 30-60 minutes after the initial dose if needed

Elderly: I.M., slow I.V.: 0.15 mg every 6 hours; elderly patients are more likely to suffer from confusion and drowsiness compared to younger patients

Heroin or opiate withdrawal (unlabeled use): Children ≥13 years and Adults: I.M., slow I.V.: Variable; 0.1-0.4 mg every 6 hours

Sublingual: Children ≥16 years and Adults: Opioid dependence:

Induction: Range: 12-16 mg/day (doses during an induction study used 8 mg on day 1, followed by 16 mg on day 2; induction continued over 3-4 days). Treatment should begin at least 4 hours after last use of heroin or short-acting opioid, preferably when first signs of withdrawal appear. Titrating dose to clinical effectiveness should be done as rapidly as possible to prevent undue withdrawal symptoms and patient drop-out during the induction period.

Maintenance: Target dose: 16 mg/day; range: 4-24 mg/day; patients should be switched to the buprenorphine/naloxone combination product for maintenance and unsupervised therapy

Stability

Tablet: Store at room temperature of 25°C (77°F).

Injection: Protect from excessive heat >40°C (>104°F) and light.

Administration

I.V.: Administer slowly, over at least 2 minutes.

Sublingual: Tablet should be placed under the tongue until dissolved; should not be swallowed. If two or more tablets are needed per dose, all may be placed under the tongue at once, or two at a time. To ensure consistent bioavailability, subsequent doses should always be taken the same way.

Monitoring Parameters Pain relief, respiratory and mental status, CNS depression, blood pressure; LFTs

Anesthesia and Critical Care Concerns/Other Considerations Buprenorphine has a longer duration of action than either morphine or meperidine. It may precipitate withdrawal in narcotic-dependent patients. Buprenorphine is not readily reversed by naloxone. Avoid in labor.

Equivalent dosing: Buprenorphine 0.3 mg = morphine 10 mg or meperidine 75 mg I.M.

Pregnancy Risk Factor C

Contraindications Hypersensitivity to buprenorphine or any component of the formulation

Warnings/Precautions An opioid-containing analgesic regimen should be tailored to each patient's needs and based upon the type of pain being treated (acute versus chronic), the route of administration, degree of tolerance for opioids (naive versus chronic user), age, weight, and medical condition. The optimal analgesic dose varies widely among patients. Doses should be titrated to pain relief/prevention.

May cause respiratory depression - use caution in patients with respiratory disease or pre-existing respiratory depression. Potential for drug dependency exists, abrupt cessation may precipitate withdrawal. Use caution in elderly, debilitated, or pediatric patients. Use with caution in patients with depression or suicidal tendencies, or in patients with a history of drug abuse. Tolerance, psychological and physical dependence may occur with prolonged use. Use with caution in patients with hepatic, pulmonary, or renal function impairment. May cause CNS depression, which may impair physical or mental abilities. Patients must be cautioned about performing tasks which require mental alertness (eg, operating machinery or driving). Effects with other sedative drugs or ethanol may be potentiated. Elderly may be more sensitive to CNS depressant and constipating effects. Use with caution in patients with head injury or increased ICP, biliary tract dysfunction, pancreatitis, patients with history of ileus or bowel obstruction, glaucoma, hyperthyroidism, adrenal insufficiency, prostatic hyperplasia, urinary stricture, CNS depression, toxic psychosis, alcoholism, delirium tremens, or kyphoscoliosis. Partial antagonist activity may precipitate acute narcotic withdrawal in opioid-dependent individuals. Tablets, which are used for induction treatment of opioid dependence, should not be started until effects of withdrawal are evident.

(Continued)

Buprenorphine *(Continued)*

Adverse Reactions

Injection:

>10%: Central nervous system: Sedation

1% to 10%:

Cardiovascular: Hypotension

Central nervous system: Respiratory depression, dizziness, headache

Gastrointestinal: Vomiting, nausea

Ocular: Miosis

Otic: Vertigo

Miscellaneous: Diaphoresis

<1% (Limited to important or life-threatening): Agitation, allergic reaction, apnea, appetite decreased, blurred vision, bradycardia, confusion, constipation, convulsion, coma, cyanosis, depersonalization, depression, diplopia, dyspnea, dysphoria, euphoria, fatigue, flatulence, flushing, hallucinations, hypertension, injection site reaction, malaise, nervousness, pallor, paresthesia, pruritus, psychosis, rash, slurred speech, tachycardia, tinnitus, tremor, urinary retention, urticaria, weakness, Wenckebach block, xerostomia

Tablet:

>10%:

Central nervous system: Headache (30%), pain (24%), insomnia (21% to 25%), anxiety (12%), depression (11%)

Gastrointestinal: Nausea (10% to 14%), abdominal pain (12%), constipation (8% to 11%)

Neuromuscular & skeletal: Back pain (14%), weakness (14%)

Respiratory: Rhinitis (11%)

Miscellaneous: Withdrawal syndrome (19%; placebo 37%), infection (12% to 20%), diaphoresis (12% to 13%)

1% to 10%:

Central nervous system: Chills (6%), nervousness (6%), somnolence (5%), dizziness (4%), fever (3%)

Gastrointestinal: Vomiting (5% to 8%), diarrhea (5%), dyspepsia (3%)

Ocular: Lacrimation (5%)

Respiratory: Cough (4%), pharyngitis (4%)

Miscellaneous: Flu-like syndrome (6%)

Overdosage/Toxicology Symptoms of overdose include CNS depression, pinpoint pupils, hypotension, and bradycardia. Treatment is supportive. Naloxone may have limited effects in reversing respiratory depression; doxapram has also been used to stimulate respirations.

Drug Interactions **Substrate** of CYP3A4 (major); **Inhibits** CYP1A2 (weak), 2A6 (weak), 2C19 (weak), 2D6 (weak)

Cimetidine: May increase sedation from narcotic analgesics; however, histamine blockers may attenuate the cardiovascular response from histamine release associated with narcotic analgesics.

CNS depressants: May produce additive respiratory and CNS depression; includes benzodiazepines, barbiturates, ethanol, and other sedatives. Respiratory and CV collapse was reported in a patient who received diazepam and buprenorphine.

CYP3A4 inducers: CYP3A4 inducers may decrease the levels/effects of buprenorphine. Example inducers include aminoglutethimide, carbamazepine, nafcillin, nevirapine, phenobarbital, phenytoin, and rifamycins.

CYP3A4 inhibitors: May increase the levels/effects of buprenorphine. Example inhibitors include azole antifungals, clarithromycin, diclofenac, doxycycline, erythromycin, imatinib, isoniazid, nefazodone, nicardipine, propofol, protease inhibitors, quinidine, and verapamil.

Naltrexone: May antagonize the effect of narcotic analgesics; concurrent use or use within 7-10 days of injection for pain relief is contraindicated.

Ethanol/Nutrition/Herb Interactions

Ethanol: Avoid ethanol (may increase CNS depression).

Herb/Nutraceutical: Avoid valerian, St John's wort, kava kava, gotu kola (may increase CNS depression).

Dosage Forms

Injection, solution (Buprenex®): 0.3 mg/mL (1 mL)

Tablet, sublingual (Subutex®): 2 mg, 8 mg

Additional dosage strength available in Canada: 0.4 mg

References

Carr DB, Jacox AK, Chapman RC, et al, "Acute Pain Management," Guideline Technical Report, No. 1. Rockville, MD: U.S. Department of Health and Human Services, Public Health Service, Agency for Health Care Policy and Research. AHCPR Publication No. 95-0034. February 1995.

"Drugs for Pain," *Treat Guidel Med Lett*, 2004, 2(23):47-54.

Gal TJ, "Naloxone Reversal of Buprenorphine-Induced Respiratory Depression," *Clin Pharmacol Ther*, 1989, 45(1):66-71.

Harcus AH, Ward AE, and Smith DW, "Buprenorphine: Experience in an Elderly Population of 975 Patients During a Year's Monitored Release," *Br J Clin Pract*, 1980, 34(5):144-6.

Jain PN and Shah SC, "Respiratory Depression Following Combination of Epidural Buprenorphine and Intramuscular Ketorolac," *Anaesthesia*, 1993, 48(10):898-9.

MacEvilly M and O'Carroll C, "Hallucinations After Epidural Buprenorphine," *Br Med J*, 1989, 298(6678):928-9.

Mokhlesi B, Leikin JB, Murray P, et al, "Adult Toxicology in Critical Care. Part 11: Specific Poisonings," *Chest*, 2003, 123(3):897-922.

"Principles of Analgesic Use in the Treatment of Acute Pain and Chronic Cancer Pain," 5th ed, Glenview, IL: American Pain Society, 2003.

- **Buprenorphine Hydrochloride** *see* Buprenorphine *on page 198*
- **Buproban™** *see* BuPROPion *on page 201*

BuPROPion (byoo PROE pee on)

Medication Safety Issues

Sound-alike/look-alike issues:

BuPROPion may be confused with busPIRone
Wellbutrin SR® may be confused with Wellbutrin XL™
Wellbutrin XL™ may be confused with Wellbutrin SR®
Zyban® may be confused with Zagam®

Related Information

Antidepressant Agents *on page 1551*
Chronic Pain Management *on page 1430*

U.S. Brand Names Budeprion™ SR; Buproban™; Wellbutrin®; Wellbutrin SR®; Wellbutrin XL™; Zyban®

Canadian Brand Names Novo-Bupropion SR; Wellbutrin®; Wellbutrin XL™; Zyban®

Pharmacologic Category Antidepressant, Dopamine-Reuptake Inhibitor; Smoking Cessation Aid

Restrictions A medication guide concerning the use of antidepressants in children and teenagers can be found on the FDA website at http://www.fda.gov/cder/Offices/ODS/labeling.htm. It should be dispensed to parents or guardians of children and teenagers receiving this medication.

Generic Available Yes: Excludes Wellbutrin XL™

Use Treatment of depression; adjunct in smoking cessation

Unlabeled/Investigational Use Attention-deficit/hyperactivity disorder (ADHD)

Mechanism of Action Aminoketone antidepressant structurally different from all other marketed antidepressants; like other antidepressants the mechanism of bupropion's activity is not fully understood. Bupropion is a relatively weak inhibitor of the neuronal uptake of serotonin, norepinephrine, and dopamine, and does not inhibit monoamine oxidase. Metabolite inhibits the reuptake of norepinephrine. The primary mechanism of action is thought to be dopaminergic and/or noradrenergic.

Pharmacodynamics/Kinetics

Absorption: Rapid
Distribution: V_d: 19-21 L/kg
Protein binding: 82% to 88%
Metabolism: Extensively hepatic to 3 active metabolites: Hydroxybupropion, erythrohydrobupropion, threohydrobupropion (metabolite activity ranges from $^1/_5$ to $^1/_2$ potency of bupropion)
Bioavailability: 5% to 20% in animals
Half-life:
Distribution: 3-4 hours
Elimination: 21 $\pm$ 9 hours; Metabolites: Hydroxybupropion: 20 $\pm$ 5 hours; Erythrohydrobupropion: 33 $\pm$ 10 hours; Threohydrobupropion: 37 $\pm$ 13 hours
Time to peak, serum: Bupropion: ~3 hours; bupropion extended release: ~5 hours
Metabolites: Hydroxybupropion, erythrohydrobupropion, threohydrobupropion: 6 hours
Excretion: Urine (87%); feces (10%)
(Continued)

BuPROPion *(Continued)*

Dosage Oral:

Children and Adolescents: ADHD (unlabeled use): 1.4-6 mg/kg/day

Adults:

Depression:

Immediate release: 100 mg 3 times/day; begin at 100 mg twice daily; may increase to a maximum dose of 450 mg/day

Sustained release: Initial: 150 mg/day in the morning; may increase to 150 mg twice daily by day 4 if tolerated; target dose: 300 mg/day given as 150 mg twice daily; maximum dose: 400 mg/day given as 200 mg twice daily

Extended release: Initial: 150 mg/day in the morning; may increase as early as day 4 of dosing to 300 mg/day; maximum dose: 450 mg/day

Smoking cessation (Zyban®): Initiate with 150 mg once daily for 3 days; increase to 150 mg twice daily; treatment should continue for 7-12 weeks

Elderly: Depression: 50-100 mg/day, increase by 50-100 mg every 3-4 days as tolerated; there is evidence that the elderly respond at 150 mg/day in divided doses, but some may require a higher dose

Dosing adjustment/comments in renal impairment: Effect of renal disease on bupropion's pharmacokinetics has not been studied; elimination of the major metabolites of bupropion may be affected by reduced renal function. Patients with renal failure should receive a reduced dosage initially and be closely monitored.

Dosing adjustment in hepatic impairment:

Note: The mean AUC increased by ~1.5-fold for hydroxybupropion and ~2.5-fold for erythro/threohydrobupropion; median T_{max} was observed 19 hours later for hydroxybupropion, 31 hours later for erythro/threohydrobupropion; mean half-life for hydroxybupropion increased fivefold, and increased twofold for erythro/threohydrobupropion in patients with severe hepatic cirrhosis compared to healthy volunteers.

Mild-to-moderate hepatic impairment: Use with caution and/or reduced dose/frequency

Severe hepatic cirrhosis: Use with extreme caution; maximum dose:

Wellbutrin®: 75 mg/day

Wellbutrin SR®: 100 mg/day or 150 mg every other day

Wellbutrin XL™: 150 mg every other day

Zyban®: 150 mg every other day

Stability Store at controlled of 20°C to 25°C (68°F to 77°F).

Administration May be taken without regard to meals. Zyban® and extended release tablets should be swallowed whole; do not crush, chew, or divide. The insoluble shell of the extended-release tablet may remain intact during GI transit and is eliminated in the feces. Wellbutrin® SR may be divided, but not crushed or chewed.

Monitoring Parameters Body weight; mental status for depression, suicidal ideation (especially at the beginning of therapy or when doses are increased or decreased), anxiety, social functioning, mania, panic attacks

Reference Range Therapeutic levels (trough, 12 hours after last dose): 50-100 ng/mL

Anesthesia and Critical Care Concerns/Other Considerations There are relatively few cardiovascular side effects compared to tricyclic antidepressants. However, several case reports include cardiovascular complications, including hypotension and MI. Use with caution in patients with recent MI or unstable angina. Recent information suggests that hypertension, in some cases severe and requiring acute treatment, has been reported in patients receiving bupropion alone, and especially when bupropion is used in conjunction with nicotine replacement therapy. Monitoring of blood pressure is recommended in patients receiving the combination of bupropion and nicotine replacement, particularly in those with hypertension and/or significant coronary artery disease.

Pregnancy Risk Factor B

Contraindications Hypersensitivity to bupropion or any component of the formulation; seizure disorder; anorexia/bulimia; use of MAO inhibitors within 14 days; patients undergoing abrupt discontinuation of ethanol or sedatives (including benzodiazepines); patients receiving other dosage forms of bupropion

Warnings/Precautions [U.S. Boxed Warning]: Antidepressants increase the risk of suicidal thinking and behavior in children and adolescents with major depressive disorder (MDD) and other depressive disorders; consider risk prior to prescribing. Closely monitor for clinical worsening, suicidality, or unusual changes in behavior; the child's family or caregiver should be instructed to closely observe the patient and communicate condition with healthcare provider. Such observation would generally include at least weekly face-to-face contact with patients or their family members or caregivers during the first 4 weeks of treatment, then every other week visits for the next 4 weeks, then at 12 weeks, and as clinically indicated beyond 12 weeks. Additional contact by telephone may be appropriate between face-to-face visits. Adults treated with antidepressants should be observed similarly for clinical worsening and suicidality, especially during the initial few months of a course of drug therapy, or at times of dose changes, either increases or decreases. A medication guide should be dispensed with each prescription. **Bupropion is not FDA approved for use in children.**

The possibility of a suicide attempt is inherent in major depression and may persist until remission occurs. Monitor for worsening of depression or suicidality, especially during initiation of therapy or with dose increases or decreases. Worsening depression and severe abrupt suicidality that are not part of the presenting symptoms may require discontinuation or modification of drug therapy. Use caution in high-risk patients during initiation of therapy. Prescriptions should be written for the smallest quantity consistent with good patient care. The patient's family or caregiver should be alerted to monitor patients for the emergence of suicidality and associated behaviors such as anxiety, agitation, panic attacks, insomnia, irritability, hostility, impulsivity, akathisia, hypomania, and mania; patients should be instructed to notify their healthcare provider if any of these symptoms or worsening depression occur.

May worsen psychosis in some patients or precipitate a shift to mania or hypomania in patients with bipolar disorder. Monotherapy in patients with bipolar disorder should be avoided. Patients presenting with depressive symptoms should be screened for bipolar disorder. **Bupropion is not FDA approved for bipolar depression.**

When using immediate release tablets, seizure risk is increased at total daily dosage >450 mg, individual dosages >150 mg, or by sudden, large increments in dose. Data for the immediate-release formulation of bupropion revealed a seizure incidence of 0.4% in patients treated at doses in the 300-450 mg/day range. The estimated seizure incidence increases almost 10-fold between 450 mg and 600 mg per day. Data for the sustained release dosage form revealed a seizure incidence of 0.1% in patients treated at a dosage range of 100-300 mg/day, and increases to ~0.4% at the maximum recommended dose of 400 mg/day. The risk of seizures is increased in patients with a history of seizures, anorexia/bulimia, head trauma, CNS tumor, severe hepatic cirrhosis, abrupt discontinuation of sedative-hypnotics or ethanol, medications which lower seizure threshold (antipsychotics, antidepressants, theophyllines, systemic steroids), stimulants, or hypoglycemic agents. Discontinue and do not restart in patients experiencing a seizure. May cause CNS stimulation (restlessness, anxiety, insomnia) or anorexia. May increase the risks associated with electroconvulsive therapy. Consider discontinuing, when possible, prior to elective surgery. May cause weight loss; use caution in patients where weight loss is not desirable. The incidence of sexual dysfunction with bupropion is generally lower than with SSRIs.

Use caution in patients with cardiovascular disease, history of hypertension, or coronary artery disease; treatment-emergent hypertension (including some severe cases) has been reported, both with bupropion alone and in combination with nicotine transdermal systems. Use with caution in patients with hepatic or renal dysfunction and in elderly patients. Elderly patients may be at greater risk of accumulation during chronic dosing. May cause motor or cognitive impairment in some patients; use with caution if tasks requiring alertness such as operating machinery or driving are undertaken. Arthralgia, myalgia, and fever with rash and other symptoms suggestive of delayed hypersensitivity resembling serum sickness reported.

Adverse Reactions Frequencies, when reported, reflect highest incidence reported with sustained release product.

>10%:

Central nervous system: Dizziness (11%), headache (25%), insomnia (16%)

Gastrointestinal: Nausea (18%), xerostomia (24%)

Respiratory: Pharyngitis (11%)

(Continued)

BuPROPion *(Continued)*

1% to 10%:

Cardiovascular: Arrhythmias, chest pain (4%), flushing, hypertension (may be severe), hypotension, palpitation (5%), syncope, tachycardia

Central nervous system: Agitation (9%), anxiety (6%), confusion, depression, euphoria, hostility, irritability (2%), memory decreased (3%), migraine, nervousness (3%), sleep disturbance, somnolence (3%)

Dermatologic: Pruritus (4%), rash (4%), sweating increased (5%), urticaria (1%)

Endocrine & metabolic: Hot flashes, libido decreased, menstrual complaints

Gastrointestinal: Abdominal pain, anorexia (3%), appetite increased, constipation (5%), diarrhea (7%), dyspepsia, dysphagia (2%), taste perversion (4%), vomiting (2%)

Genitourinary: Urinary frequency (5%)

Neuromuscular & skeletal: Arthralgia (4%), arthritis (2%), myalgia (6%), neck pain, paresthesia (2%), tremor (3%), twitching (2%)

Ocular: Amblyopia (2%), blurred vision

Otic: Auditory disturbance, tinnitus (6%)

Respiratory: Cough increased (2%), sinusitis (1%)

Miscellaneous: Allergic reaction (including anaphylaxis, pruritus, urticaria), infection

Postmarketing and/or case reports (limited to important or life-threatening): Akinesia, amnesia, angioedema, aphasia, ataxia, atrioventricular block, bronchospasm, delirium, depersonalization, dysarthria, dyskinesia, dyspareunia, dystonia, edema, EEG abnormality, ejaculation abnormality, exfoliative dermatitis, extrapyramidal syndrome, gynecomastia, hallucinations, hepatitis, hostility, hyperkinesia, hypoglycemia, impotence, jaundice, leukopenia, maculopapular rash, manic reaction, myoclonus, neuralgia, neuropathy, nocturia, painful erection, pancreatitis, pancytopenia, paranoia, paresthesia, photosensitivity, postural hypotension, seizure, SIADH, suicidal ideation, tardive dyskinesia, thrombocytopenia, tongue edema, urinary incontinence, vaginitis, vertigo

Overdosage/Toxicology Symptoms of overdose include labored breathing, salivation, ataxia, and convulsions. Dialysis may be of limited value after drug absorption because of slow tissue-to-plasma diffusion. Treatment is symptomatic and supportive.

Drug Interactions Substrate of CYP1A2 (minor), 2A6 (minor), 2B6 (major), 2C9 (minor), 2D6 (minor), 2E1 (minor), 3A4 (minor); **Inhibits** CYP2D6 (weak)

Note: Seizure threshold-lowering agents: Use with caution in individuals receiving other agents that may lower seizure threshold (antipsychotics, antidepressants, fluoroquinolones, theophylline, abrupt discontinuation of benzodiazepines, systemic steroids)

Amantadine: Concurrent use appears to result in a higher incidence of adverse effects; use caution.

Cimetidine: May increase effect of bupropion (due to effect on bupropion metabolites).

CYP2B6 inducers: May decrease the levels/effects of bupropion. Example inducers include carbamazepine, nevirapine, phenobarbital, phenytoin, and rifampin.

CYP2B6 inhibitors: May increase the levels/effects of bupropion. Example inhibitors include desipramine, paroxetine, and sertraline.

Levodopa: Toxicity of bupropion is enhanced by levodopa.

MAO inhibitors: Toxicity of bupropion is enhanced by MAO inhibitors (phenelzine); concurrent use is contraindicated.

Nicotine: Treatment-emergent hypertension may occur; monitor BP in patients treated with bupropion and nicotine patch.

Selegiline: When used in low doses (<10 mg/day), risk of interaction is theoretically lower than with nonselective MAO inhibitors.

Tricyclic antidepressants: Serum levels may be increased by bupropion; in addition, these agents lower seizure threshold (see Note).

Warfarin: Coadministration has resulted in altered PT/INR and thrombotic or hemorrhagic events. Monitor INR.

Ethanol/Nutrition/Herb Interactions

Ethanol: Ethanol (may increase CNS depression).

Herb/Nutraceutical: Avoid valerian, St John's wort, SAMe, gotu kola, kava kava (may increase CNS depression).

Dosage Forms

Tablet, as hydrochloride (Wellbutrin®): 75 mg, 100 mg

Tablet, extended release, as hydrochloride:

Budeprion™ SR: 100 mg [contains tartrazine; equivalent to Wellbutrin® SR], 150 mg [equivalent to Wellbutrin® SR]

Buproban™: 150 mg [equivalent to Zyban®]

Wellbutrin XL™: 150 mg, 300 mg

Tablet, sustained release, as hydrochloride: 100 mg, 150 mg [equivalent to Wellbutrin® SR], 150 mg [equivalent to Zyban®]

Wellbutrin® SR: 100 mg, 150 mg, 200 mg

Zyban®: 150 mg

- ♦ **Burinex® (Can)** *see* Bumetanide *on page 194*
- ♦ **Burnamycin [OTC]** *see* Lidocaine *on page 755*
- ♦ **Burn Jel [OTC]** *see* Lidocaine *on page 755*
- ♦ **Burn-O-Jel [OTC]** *see* Lidocaine *on page 755*
- ♦ **Buscopan® (Can)** *see* Scopolamine *on page 1152*
- ♦ **BuSpar®** *see* BusPIRone *on page 205*
- ♦ **Buspirex (Can)** *see* BusPIRone *on page 205*

BusPIRone (byoo SPYE rone)

Medication Safety Issues

Sound-alike/look-alike issues:

BusPIRone may be confused with buPROPion

U.S. Brand Names BuSpar®

Canadian Brand Names Apo-Buspirone®; BuSpar®; Buspirex; Bustab®; Gen-Buspirone; Lin-Buspirone; Novo-Buspirone; Nu-Buspirone; PMS-Buspirone

Synonyms Buspirone Hydrochloride

Pharmacologic Category Antianxiety Agent, Miscellaneous

Generic Available Yes

Use Management of generalized anxiety disorder (GAD)

Unlabeled/Investigational Use Management of aggression in mental retardation and secondary mental disorders; major depression; potential augmenting agent for antidepressants; premenstrual syndrome

Mechanism of Action The mechanism of action of buspirone is unknown. Buspirone has a high affinity for serotonin 5-HT_{1A} and 5-HT_2 receptors, without affecting benzodiazepine-GABA receptors. Buspirone has moderate affinity for dopamine D_2 receptors.

Pharmacodynamics/Kinetics

Absorption: Oral: ~100%

Distribution: V_d: 5.3 L/kg

Protein binding: 95%

Metabolism: Hepatic via oxidation; extensive first-pass effect

Bioavailability: ~4%

Half-life elimination: Mean: 2.4 hours (range: 2-11 hours)

Time to peak, serum: Within 0.7-1.5 hours

Excretion: Urine: 65%; feces: 35%; ~1% dose excreted unchanged

Dosage Oral:

Generalized anxiety disorder:

Children and Adolescents: Initial: 5 mg daily; increase in increments of 5 mg/day at weekly intervals as needed, to a maximum dose of 60 mg/day divided into 2-3 doses

Adults: 15 mg/day (7.5 mg twice daily); may increase in increments of 5 mg/day every 2-4 days to a maximum of 60 mg/day; target dose for most people is 30 mg/day (15 mg twice daily)

Elderly: Initial: 5 mg twice daily, increase by 5 mg/day every 2-3 days as needed up to 20-30 mg/day; maximum daily dose: 60 mg/day.

Dosing adjustment in renal or hepatic impairment: Buspirone is metabolized by the liver and excreted by the kidneys. Patients with impaired hepatic or renal function demonstrated increased plasma levels and a prolonged half-life of buspirone. Therefore, use in patients with severe hepatic or renal impairment cannot be recommended.

Monitoring Parameters Mental status, symptoms of anxiety

Anesthesia and Critical Care Concerns/Other Considerations Takes 2-3 weeks for full effect. Because of slow onset, not appropriate for "as needed" (prn)

(Continued)

BusPIRone *(Continued)*

use or for brief, situational anxiety; not effective for severe anxiety; does not show cross-tolerance with benzodiazepines or other sedatives; less sedating than other anxiolytics; has shown little potential for abuse; needs continuous use; ineffective for benzodiazepine or ethanol withdrawal

Pregnancy Risk Factor B

Contraindications Hypersensitivity to buspirone or any component of the formulation

Warnings/Precautions Use in hepatic or renal impairment is not recommended; does not prevent or treat withdrawal from benzodiazepines. Low potential for cognitive or motor impairment. Use with MAO inhibitors may result in hypertensive reactions.

Adverse Reactions

>10%: Central nervous system: Dizziness

1% to 10%:

Central nervous system: Drowsiness, EPS, serotonin syndrome, confusion, nervousness, lightheadedness, excitement, anger, hostility, headache

Dermatologic: Rash

Gastrointestinal: Diarrhea, nausea

Neuromuscular & skeletal: Muscle weakness, numbness, paresthesia, incoordination, tremor

Ocular: Blurred vision, tunnel vision

Miscellaneous: Diaphoresis, allergic reactions

Overdosage/Toxicology Symptoms of overdose include dizziness, drowsiness, pinpoint pupils, nausea, and vomiting. There is no known antidote for buspirone. Treatment is supportive.

Drug Interactions Substrate of CYP2D6 (minor), 3A4 (major)

Calcium channel blockers: Diltiazem and verapamil may increase serum concentrations of buspirone; consider a dihydropyridine calcium channel blocker.

CYP3A4 inducers: CYP3A4 inducers may decrease the levels/effects of buspirone. Example inducers include aminoglutethimide, carbamazepine, nafcillin, nevirapine, phenobarbital, phenytoin, and rifamycins.

CYP3A4 inhibitors: May increase the levels/effects of buspirone. Example inhibitors include azole antifungals, clarithromycin, diclofenac, doxycycline, erythromycin, imatinib, isoniazid, nefazodone, nicardipine, propofol, protease inhibitors, quinidine, telithromycin, and verapamil.

MAO inhibitors: Buspirone should not be used concurrently with an MAO inhibitor due to reports of increased blood pressure; includes classic MAO inhibitors and linezolid (due to ability to inhibit MAO).

Nefazodone: Concurrent use may increase risk of CNS adverse events. Limit buspirone initial dose (eg, 2.5 mg/day).

Selegiline: Theoretically, risk of interaction with selective MAO type B inhibitor would be less than with nonselective inhibitors; however, this combination is generally best avoided.

SSRIs: Concurrent use of buspirone with SSRIs may cause serotonin syndrome. Some SSRIs may increase buspirone serum concentrations (see CYP3A4 inhibitors). Buspirone may increase the efficacy of fluoxetine in some patients; however, the anxiolytic activity of buspirone may be lost when combined with SSRIs (fluoxetine).

Trazodone: Concurrent use of buspirone with trazodone may cause serotonin syndrome.

Ethanol/Nutrition/Herb Interactions

Ethanol: Ethanol (may increase CNS depression).

Food: Food may decrease the absorption of buspirone, but it may also decrease the first-pass metabolism, thereby increasing the bioavailability of buspirone. Grapefruit juice may cause increased buspirone concentrations; avoid concurrent use.

Herb/Nutraceutical: St John's wort may decrease buspirone levels or increase CNS depression. Avoid valerian, gotu kola, kava kava (may increase CNS depression).

Test Interactions Increased AST, ALT, growth hormone(s), prolactin (S)

Dosage Forms

Tablet, as hydrochloride: 5 mg, 7.5 mg, 10 mg, 15 mg, 30 mg

BuSpar®: 5 mg, 10 mg, 15 mg, 30 mg

♦ **Buspirone Hydrochloride** *see* BusPIRone *on page 205*

♦ **Bustab® (Can)** *see* BusPIRone *on page 205*

Butalbital, Acetaminophen, Caffeine, and Codeine

(byoo TAL bi tal, a seet a MIN oh fen, KAF een, & KOE deen)

Medication Safety Issues

Sound-alike/look-alike issues:

Fioricet® may be confused with Fiorinal®, Lorcet®

U.S. Brand Names Fioricet® with Codeine

Synonyms Acetaminophen, Caffeine, Codeine, and Butalbital; Caffeine, Acetaminophen, Butalbital, and Codeine; Codeine, Acetaminophen, Butalbital, and Caffeine

Pharmacologic Category Analgesic Combination (Narcotic); Barbiturate

Restrictions C-III

Generic Available Yes

Use Relief of symptoms of complex tension (muscle contraction) headache

Mechanism of Action Combination product for the treatment of tension headache. Contains codeine (narcotic analgesic), butalbital (barbiturate), caffeine (CNS stimulant), and acetaminophen (nonopiate, nonsalicylate analgesic).

Dosage Oral: Adults: 1-2 capsules every 4 hours. Total daily dosage should not exceed 6 capsules.

Dosing adjustment/comments in hepatic impairment: Use with caution. Limited, low-dose therapy usually well tolerated in hepatic disease/cirrhosis. However, cases of hepatotoxicity at daily acetaminophen dosages <4 g/day have been reported. Avoid chronic use in hepatic impairment.

Stability Store below 30°C (86°F).

Pregnancy Risk Factor C (per manufacturer); D (prolonged use or high doses at term)

Contraindications Hypersensitivity to butalbital, codeine, caffeine, acetaminophen, or any component of the formulation; porphyria; known G6PD deficiency; pregnancy (prolonged use or high doses at term)

Warnings/Precautions Limit acetaminophen to <4 g/day. May cause severe hepatic toxicity in acute overdose. In addition, chronic daily dosing in adults has resulted in liver damage in some patients. Use with caution in patients with hypersensitivity reactions to other phenanthrene derivative opioid agonists (eg, morphine, hydrocodone, oxycodone). Use caution with Addison's disease, severe renal or hepatic impairment. Use caution in patients with head injury or other intracranial lesions, acute abdominal conditions, urethral stricture of BPH, or in patients with respiratory diseases. Elderly (not recommended for use) and/or debilitated patients may be more susceptible to CNS depressants, as well as constipating effects of narcotics. Tolerance or drug dependence may result from extended use. Safety and efficacy in pediatric patients have not been established.

Adverse Reactions Frequency not defined.

Cardiovascular: Tachycardia, palpitation, hypotension, edema, syncope

Central nervous system: Drowsiness, fatigue, mental confusion, disorientation, nervousness, hallucination, euphoria, depression, seizure, headache, agitation, fainting, excitement, fever

Dermatologic: Rash, erythema, pruritus, urticaria, erythema multiforme, exfoliative dermatitis, toxic epidermal necrolysis

Gastrointestinal: Nausea, xerostomia, constipation, gastrointestinal spasm, heartburn, flatulence

Genitourinary: Urinary retention, diuresis

Neuromuscular & skeletal: Leg pain, weakness, numbness

Otic: Tinnitus

Miscellaneous: Allergic reaction, anaphylaxis

Note: Potential reactions associated with components of Fioricet® with Codeine include agranulocytosis, irritability, nausea, thrombocytopenia, tremor, vomiting

Overdosage/Toxicology Symptoms of opiate overdose include unsteady gait, slurred speech, confusion, respiratory depression, hypotension, and coma. Opioid symptoms may be reversed by naloxone, 2 mg I.V., with repeated doses as necessary up to a total of 10 mg. Barbiturate treatment is symptomatic and supportive.

Symptoms of acetaminophen overdose include hepatic necrosis, transient azotemia, renal tubular necrosis with acute toxicity, anemia, and GI disturbances with chronic toxicity. Treatment consists of acetylcysteine 140 mg/kg orally (loading) followed by 70 mg/kg every 4 hours for 17 doses; therapy should be

(Continued)

Butalbital, Acetaminophen, Caffeine, and Codeine *(Continued)*

initiated based upon laboratory analysis suggesting a high probability of hepatotoxic potential. Activated charcoal is very effective at binding acetaminophen. Intravenous acetylcysteine should be reserved for patients unable to take oral forms.

Drug Interactions

Acetaminophen: **Substrate** of (minor) CYP1A2, 2A6, 2C9, 2D6, 2E1, 3A4; **Inhibits** CYP3A4 (weak)

Caffeine: **Substrate** of CYP1A2 (major), 2C9 (minor), 2D6 (minor), 2E1 (minor), 3A4 (minor); **Inhibits** CYP1A2 (weak), 3A4 (moderate)

Butalbital: Refer to Phenobarbital.

See also Acetaminophen, Caffeine, and Codeine.

Ethanol/Nutrition/Herb Interactions Ethanol: Avoid ethanol (may increase CNS depression).

Test Interactions Acetaminophen may produce false-positive tests for urinary 5-hydroxyindoleacetic acid.

Dosage Forms Capsule: Butalbital 50 mg, caffeine 40 mg, acetaminophen 325 mg, and codeine phosphate 30 mg

Butorphanol (byoo TOR fa nole)

Medication Safety Issues

Sound-alike/look-alike issues:

Stadol® may be confused with Haldol®, sotalol

Related Information

Chronic Pain Management *on page 1430*

Narcotic / Opioid Analgesics *on page 1568*

Opioids *on page 1535*

U.S. Brand Names Stadol®

Canadian Brand Names Apo-Butorphanol®; PMS-Butorphanol

Synonyms Butorphanol Tartrate

Pharmacologic Category Analgesic, Narcotic

Restrictions C-IV

Generic Available Yes

Use

Parenteral: Management of moderate-to-severe pain; preoperative medication; supplement to balanced anesthesia; management of pain during labor

Nasal spray: Management of moderate-to-severe pain, including migraine headache pain

Mechanism of Action Mixed narcotic agonist-antagonist with central analgesic actions; binds to opiate receptors in the CNS, causing inhibition of ascending pain pathways, altering the perception of and response to pain; produces generalized CNS depression

Pharmacodynamics/Kinetics

Onset of action: I.M.: 5-10 minutes; I.V.: <10 minutes; Nasal: Within 15 minutes

Peak effect: I.M.: 0.5-1 hour; I.V.: 4-5 minutes

Duration: I.M., I.V.: 3-4 hours; Nasal: 4-5 hours

Absorption: Rapid and well absorbed

Protein binding: 80%

Metabolism: Hepatic

Bioavailability: Nasal: 60% to 70%

Half-life elimination: 2.5-4 hours

Excretion: Primarily urine

Dosage Note: These are guidelines and do not represent the maximum doses that may be required in all patients. Doses should be titrated to pain relief/prevention. Butorphanol has an analgesic ceiling.

Adults:

Parenteral:

Acute pain (moderate to severe):

I.M.: Initial: 2 mg, may repeat every 3-4 hours as needed; usual range: 1-4 mg every 3-4 hours as needed

I.V.: Initial: 1 mg, may repeat every 3-4 hours as needed; usual range: 0.5-2 mg every 3-4 hours as needed

Preoperative medication: I.M.: 2 mg 60-90 minutes before surgery

Supplement to balanced anesthesia: I.V.: 2 mg shortly before induction and/or an incremental dose of 0.5-1 mg (up to 0.06 mg/kg), depending on previously administered sedative, analgesic, and hypnotic medications

Pain during labor (fetus >37 weeks gestation and no signs of fetal distress): I.M., I.V.: 1-2 mg; may repeat in 4 hours

Note: Alternative analgesia should be used for pain associated with delivery or if delivery is anticipated within 4 hours

Nasal spray:

Moderate to severe pain (including migraine headache pain): Initial: 1 spray (~1 mg per spray) in 1 nostril; if adequate pain relief is not achieved within 60-90 minutes, an additional 1 spray in 1 nostril may be given; may repeat initial dose sequence in 3-4 hours after the last dose as needed

Alternatively, an initial dose of 2 mg (1 spray in each nostril) may be used in patients who will be able to remain recumbent (in the event drowsiness or dizziness occurs); additional 2 mg doses should not be given for 3-4 hours

Note: In some clinical trials, an initial dose of 2 mg (as 2 doses 1 hour apart or 2 mg initially - 1 spray in each nostril) has been used, followed by 1 mg in 1 hour; side effects were greater at these dosages

Elderly:

I.M., I.V.: Initial dosage should generally be ½ of the recommended dose; repeated dosing must be based on initial response rather than fixed intervals, but generally should be at least 6 hours apart

Nasal spray: Initial dose should not exceed 1 mg; a second dose may be given after 90-120 minutes

Dosage adjustment in renal impairment:

I.M., I.V.: Initial dosage should generally be ½ of the recommended dose; repeated dosing must be based on initial response rather than fixed intervals, but generally should be at least 6 hours apart

Nasal spray: Initial dose should not exceed 1 mg; a second dose may be given after 90-120 minutes

Dosage adjustment in hepatic impairment:

I.M., I.V.: Initial dosage should generally be ½ of the recommended dose; repeated dosing must be based on initial response rather than fixed intervals, but generally should be at least 6 hours apart

Nasal spray: Initial dose should not exceed 1 mg; a second dose may be given after 90-120 minutes

Stability Store at room temperature. Protect from freezing.

Administration Intranasal: Consider avoiding simultaneous intranasal migraine sprays; may want to separate by at least 30 minutes

Monitoring Parameters Pain relief, respiratory and mental status, blood pressure

Reference Range 0.7-1.5 ng/mL

Anesthesia and Critical Care Concerns/Other Considerations Butorphanol is a mixed agonist-antagonist opiate; may precipitate withdrawal in narcotic-dependent patients. Abrupt discontinuation after sustained use (generally >10 days) may cause withdrawal symptoms. This agent can potentially cause hallucinations.

Pregnancy Risk Factor C/D (prolonged use or high doses at term)

Contraindications Hypersensitivity to butorphanol or any component of the formulation; avoid use in opiate-dependent patients who have not been detoxified, may precipitate opiate withdrawal; pregnancy (prolonged use or high doses at term)

Warnings/Precautions An opioid-containing analgesic regimen should be tailored to each patient's needs and based upon the type of pain being treated (acute versus chronic), the route of administration, degree of tolerance for opioids (naive versus chronic user), age, weight, and medical condition. The optimal analgesic dose varies widely among patients. Doses should be titrated to pain relief/prevention. May cause CNS depression, which may impair physical or mental abilities. Effects with other sedative drugs or ethanol may be potentiated. Use with caution in patients with hepatic/renal dysfunction. Tolerance or drug dependence may result from extended use. Concurrent use of sumatriptan nasal spray and butorphanol nasal spray may increase risk of transient high blood pressure.

(Continued)

Butorphanol *(Continued)*

Adverse Reactions

>10%:

Central nervous system: Drowsiness (43%), dizziness (19%), insomnia (Stadol® NS)

Gastrointestinal: Nausea/vomiting (13%)

Respiratory: Nasal congestion (Stadol® NS)

1% to 10%:

Cardiovascular: Vasodilation, palpitation

Central nervous system: Lightheadedness, headache, lethargy, anxiety, confusion, euphoria, somnolence

Dermatologic: Pruritus

Gastrointestinal: Anorexia, constipation, xerostomia, stomach pain, unpleasant aftertaste

Neuromuscular & skeletal: Tremor, paresthesia, weakness

Ocular: Blurred vision

Otic: Ear pain, tinnitus

Respiratory: Bronchitis, cough, dyspnea, epistaxis, nasal irritation, pharyngitis, rhinitis, sinus congestion, sinusitis, upper respiratory infection

Miscellaneous: Diaphoresis increased

<1% (Limited to important or life-threatening): Dependence (with prolonged use), depression, difficulty speaking (transient), dyspnea, hallucinations, hypertension, nightmares, paradoxical CNS stimulation, rash, respiratory depression, syncope, tinnitus, vertigo, withdrawal symptoms

Stadol® NS: Apnea, chest pain, convulsions, delusions, depressions, edema, hypertension, shallow breathing, tachycardia

Overdosage/Toxicology Symptoms of overdose include respiratory depression, cardiac and CNS depression. Treatment is supportive. Naloxone, 2 mg I.V. with repeat administration as necessary up to a total of 10 mg, can also be used to reverse toxic effects of the opiate.

Drug Interactions Increased toxicity: CNS depressants, phenothiazines, barbiturates, skeletal muscle relaxants, alfentanil, guanabenz, and MAO inhibitors.

Ethanol/Nutrition/Herb Interactions

Ethanol: Avoid or limit ethanol (may increase CNS depression). Watch for sedation.

Herb/Nutraceutical: Avoid valerian, St John's wort, kava kava, gotu kola (may increase CNS depression).

Dosage Forms

Injection, solution, as tartrate [preservative free] (Stadol®): 1 mg/mL (1 mL); 2 mg/mL (1 mL, 2 mL)

Injection, solution, as tartrate [with preservative] (Stadol®): 2 mg/mL (10 mL)

Solution, intranasal, as tartrate [spray]: 10 mg/mL (2.5 mL) [14-15 doses]

References

Bennie RE, Boehringer LA, Dierdorf SF, et al, "Transnasal Butorphanol Is Effective for Postoperative Pain Relief in Children Undergoing Myringotomy," *Anesthesiology*, 1998, 89(2):385-90.

Carr DB, Jacox AK, Chapman RC, et al, "Acute Pain Management," Guideline Technical Report, No. 1. Rockville, MD: U.S. Department of Health and Human Services, Public Health Service, Agency for Health Care Policy and Research. AHCPR Publication No. 95-0034. February 1995.

"Drugs for Pain," *Treat Guidel Med Lett*, 2004, 2(23):47-54.

Melanson SW, Morse JW, Pronchik DJ, et al, "Transnasal Butorphanol in the Emergency Department Management of Migraine Headache," *Am J Emerg Med*, 1997, 15(1):57-61.

Mokhlesi B, Leikin JB, Murray P, et al, "Adult Toxicology in Critical Care. Part 11: Specific Poisonings," *Chest*, 2003, 123(3):897-922.

"Principles of Analgesic Use in the Treatment of Acute Pain and Chronic Cancer Pain," 5th ed, Glenview, IL: American Pain Society, 2003.

Shyu WC, Morgenthien EA, and Barbhaiya RH, "Pharmacokinetics of Butorphanol Nasal Spray in Patients With Renal Impairment," *Br J Clin Pharmacol*, 1996, 41(5):397-402.

◆ **Butorphanol Tartrate** *see* Butorphanol *on page 208*

◆ **BW-430C** *see* Lamotrigine *on page 727*

◆ **BW524W91** *see* Emtricitabine *on page 445*

◆ **C7E3** *see* Abciximab *on page 23*

◆ **311C90** *see* Zolmitriptan *on page 1380*

◆ **Cafcit®** *see* Caffeine *on page 211*

◆ **Caffedrine® [OTC]** *see* Caffeine *on page 211*

Caffeine (KAF een)

U.S. Brand Names Cafcit®; Caffedrine® [OTC]; Enerjets [OTC]; Lucidex [OTC]; No Doz® Maximum Strength [OTC]; Vivarin® [OTC]

Synonyms Caffeine and Sodium Benzoate; Caffeine Citrate; Sodium Benzoate and Caffeine

Pharmacologic Category Stimulant

Generic Available Yes: Caffeine and sodium benzoate injection

Use

Caffeine citrate: Treatment of idiopathic apnea of prematurity

Caffeine and sodium benzoate: Treatment of acute respiratory depression (not a preferred agent)

Caffeine [OTC labeling]: Restore mental alertness or wakefulness when experiencing fatigue

Unlabeled/Investigational Use Caffeine and sodium benzoate: Treatment of spinal puncture headache; CNS stimulant; diuretic

Mechanism of Action Increases levels of 3'5' cyclic AMP by inhibiting phosphodiesterase; CNS stimulant which increases medullary respiratory center sensitivity to carbon dioxide, stimulates central inspiratory drive, and improves skeletal muscle contraction (diaphragmatic contractility); prevention of apnea may occur by competitive inhibition of adenosine

Pharmacodynamics/Kinetics

Distribution: V_d:

Neonates: 0.8-0.9 L/kg

Children >9 months to Adults: 0.6 L/kg

Protein binding: 17% (children) to 36% (adults)

Metabolism: Hepatic, via demethylation by CYP1A2. **Note:** In neonates, interconversion between caffeine and theophylline has been reported (caffeine levels are ~25% of measured theophylline after theophylline administration and ~3% to 8% of caffeine would be expected to be converted to theophylline)

Half-life elimination:

Neonates: 72-96 hours (range: 40-230 hours)

Children >9 months and Adults: 5 hours

Time to peak, serum: Oral: Within 30 minutes to 2 hours

Excretion:

Neonates ≤1 month: 86% excreted unchanged in urine

Infants >1 month and Adults: In urine, as metabolites

Dosage

Note: Caffeine citrate should not be interchanged with the caffeine sodium benzoate formulation.

Caffeine citrate: Neonates: Apnea of prematurity: Oral, I.V.:

Loading dose: 10-20 mg/kg as caffeine citrate (5-10 mg/kg as caffeine base). If theophylline has been administered to the patient within the previous 3 days, a full or modified loading dose (50% to 75% of a loading dose) may be given.

Maintenance dose: 5 mg/kg/day as caffeine citrate (2.5 mg/kg/day as caffeine base) once daily starting 24 hours after the loading dose. Maintenance dose is adjusted based on patient's response and serum caffeine concentrations.

Caffeine and sodium benzoate:

Children: Stimulant: I.M., I.V., SubQ: 8 mg/kg every 4 hours as needed

Children ≥12 years and Adults: OTC labeling (stimulant): Oral: 100-200 mg every 3-4 hours as needed

Adults:

Respiratory depression: I.M., I.V.: 250 mg as a single dose; may repeat as needed. Maximum single dose should be limited to 500 mg; maximum amount in any 24-hour period should generally be limited to 2500 mg.

Spinal puncture headache (unlabeled use):

I.V.: 500 mg in 1000 mL NS infused over 1 hour, followed by 1000 mL NS infused over 1 hour; a second course of caffeine can be given for unrelieved headache pain in 4 hours.

Oral: 300 mg as a single dose

Stimulant/diuretic (unlabeled use): I.M., I.V.: 500 mg, maximum single dose: 1 g

Dosage adjustment in renal impairment: No dosage adjustment required.

Stability Store at 20°C to 25°C (68°F to 77°F).

Caffeine citrate: Injection and oral solution contain no preservatives; injection is chemically stable for at least 24 hours at room temperature when diluted to

(Continued)

Caffeine *(Continued)*

10 mg/mL (as caffeine citrate) with D_5W, $D_{50}W$, Intralipid® 20%, and Aminosyn® 8.5%; also compatible with dopamine (600 mcg/mL), calcium gluconate 10%, heparin (1 unit/mL), and fentanyl (10 mcg/mL) at room temperature for 24 hours.

Administration

Oral: May be administered without regard to feedings or meals. May administer injectable formulation (caffeine citrate) orally.

Parenteral:

Caffeine citrate: Infuse loading dose over at least 30 minutes; maintenance dose may be infused over at least 10 minutes. May administer without dilution or diluted with D_5W to 10 mg caffeine citrate/mL.

Caffeine and sodium benzoate: I.V. as slow direct injection. For spinal headaches, dilute in 1000 mL NS and infuse over 1 hour. Follow with 1000 mL NS; infuse over 1 hour. May administer I.M. undiluted.

Reference Range

Therapeutic: Apnea of prematurity: 8-20 mcg/mL

Potentially toxic: >20 mcg/mL

Toxic: >50 mcg/mL

Anesthesia and Critical Care Concerns/Other Considerations Caffeine has 40% of the bronchodilatory activity of theophylline. Lithium blood levels may increase during caffeine withdrawal. Analgesia from transcutaneous electrical nerve stimulation may be lessened with concomitant caffeine use.

Pregnancy Risk Factor C

Contraindications Hypersensitivity to caffeine or any component of the formulation; sodium benzoate is not for use in neonates

Warnings/Precautions Use with caution in patients with a history of peptic ulcer, gastroesophageal reflux, impaired renal or hepatic function, seizure disorders, or cardiovascular disease. Avoid use in patients with symptomatic cardiac arrhythmias, agitation, anxiety, or tremor. Over-the-counter [OTC] products contain an amount of caffeine similar to one cup of coffee; limit the use of other caffeine-containing beverages or foods.

Caffeine citrate should not be interchanged with caffeine and sodium benzoate. Avoid use of products containing sodium benzoate in neonates; has been associated with a potentially fatal toxicity ("gasping syndrome") in neonates, including metabolic acidosis, respiratory distress, gasping respirations, seizures, intracranial hemorrhage, hypotension, and cardiovascular collapse. *In vitro* and animal studies have shown that benzoate also displaces bilirubin from protein-binding sites. Neonates receiving caffeine citrate should be closely monitored for the development of necrotizing enterocolitis. Caffeine serum levels should be closely monitored to optimize therapy and prevent serious toxicity.

Adverse Reactions Frequency not specified; primarily serum-concentration related.

Cardiovascular: Angina, arrhythmia (ventricular), chest pain, flushing, palpitation, sinus tachycardia, tachycardia (supraventricular), vasodilation

Central nervous system: Agitation, delirium, dizziness, hallucinations, headache, insomnia, irritability, psychosis, restlessness

Dermatologic: Urticaria

Gastrointestinal: Esophageal sphincter tone decreased, gastritis

Neuromuscular & skeletal: Fasciculations

Ocular: Intraocular pressure increased (>180 mg caffeine), miosis

Renal: Diuresis

Overdosage/Toxicology Symptoms of overdose may include CNS stimulation, tachyarrhythmias, and tremor. Treatment is symptomatic and supportive.

Drug Interactions Substrate of CYP1A2 (major), 2C9 (minor), 2D6 (minor), 2E1 (minor), 3A4 (minor); **Inhibits** CYP1A2 (weak), 3A4 (moderate)

Benzodiazepines: Caffeine may diminish the sedative or anxiolytic effects of benzodiazepines.

CYP1A2 inducers: May decrease the levels/effects of caffeine. Example inducers include aminoglutethimide, carbamazepine, phenobarbital, and rifampin.

CYP1A2 inhibitors: May increase the levels/effects of caffeine. Example inhibitors include fluvoxamine, ketoconazole, and rofecoxib.

Quinolone antibiotics (specifically ciprofloxacin, norfloxacin, ofloxacin): May increase the levels/effects of caffeine.

Dosage Forms

Caplet (Caffedrine®, Vivarin®): 200 mg [OTC]

Injection, solution, as citrate [preservative free] (Cafcit®): 20 mg/mL (3 mL) [equivalent to 10 mg/mL caffeine base]

Injection, solution [with sodium benzoate]: Caffeine 125 mg/mL and sodium benzoate 125 mg/mL (2 mL); caffeine 121 mg/mL and sodium benzoate 129 mg/mL (2 mL)

Lozenge (Enerjets): 75 mg [OTC; Hazelnut coffee or mochamint flavor]

Solution, oral, as citrate (Cafcit®): 20 mg/mL (3 mL) [equivalent to 10 mg/mL caffeine base]

Tablet:

Lucidex: 100 mg [OTC]

NoDoz® Maximum Strength, Vivarin®: 200 mg [OTC]

- **Caffeine, Acetaminophen, Butalbital, and Codeine** *see* Butalbital, Acetaminophen, Caffeine, and Codeine *on page 207*
- **Caffeine and Sodium Benzoate** *see* Caffeine *on page 211*
- **Caffeine Citrate** *see* Caffeine *on page 211*
- **Calan®** *see* Verapamil *on page 1352*
- **Calan® SR** *see* Verapamil *on page 1352*

Calcium Chloride (KAL see um KLOR ide)

Pharmacologic Category Calcium Salt; Electrolyte Supplement, Parenteral

Generic Available Yes

Use Cardiac resuscitation when epinephrine fails to improve myocardial contractions, cardiac disturbances of hyperkalemia, hypocalcemia; emergent treatment of hypocalcemic tetany; treatment of hypermagnesemia

Unlabeled/Investigational Use

Calcium channel blocker overdose

Mechanism of Action Moderates nerve and muscle performance via action potential excitation threshold regulation

Pharmacodynamics/Kinetics

Distribution: Crosses placenta; enters breast milk

Excretion: Primarily feces (as unabsorbed calcium); urine (20%)

Dosage Note: Calcium chloride has 3 times more elemental calcium than calcium gluconate. Calcium chloride is 27% elemental calcium; calcium gluconate is 9% elemental calcium. One gram of calcium chloride is equal to 270 mg of elemental calcium; one gram of calcium gluconate is equal to 90 mg of elemental calcium. Dosages are expressed in terms of the calcium chloride salt based on a solution concentration of 100 mg/mL (10%) containing 1.4 mEq (27.3 mg)/mL elemental calcium.

Cardiac arrest in the presence of hyperkalemia or hypocalcemia, magnesium toxicity: I.V.:

Infants and Children: 20 mg/kg; may repeat in 10 minutes if necessary

Adolescents and Adults: 2-4 mg/kg, repeated every 10 minutes if necessary

Calcium channel blocker overdose (unlabeled use): Adults:

I.V.: 1 g every 15-20 minutes (total of 4 doses) **or** 1 g every 2-3 minutes until clinical effect is achieved

I.V. infusion: 0.2-0.4 mL/kg/hour

Hypocalcemia: I.V.:

Children (manufacturer's recommendation): 2.7-5 mg/kg/dose every 4-6 hours

Alternative pediatric dosing: Infants and Children: 10-20 mg/kg/dose, repeat every 4-6 hours if needed

Adults: 500 mg to 1 g/dose repeated every 4-6 hours if needed

Hypocalcemic tetany: I.V.:

Neonates: Divided doses totaling approximately 170 mg/kg/24 hours

Infants and Children: 10 mg/kg over 5-10 minutes; may repeat after 6-8 hours or follow with an infusion with a maximum dose of 200 mg/kg/day; alternatively, higher doses of 35-50 mg/kg/dose repeated every 6-8 hours have been used

Adults: 1 g over 10-30 minutes; may repeat after 6 hours

Hypocalcemia secondary to citrated blood transfusion: I.V.: **Note:** Routine administration of calcium, in the absence of signs/symptoms of hypocalcemia, is generally not recommended. A number of recommendations have been published seeking to address potential hypocalcemia during massive transfusion of citrated blood; however, many practitioners recommend replacement

(Continued)

Calcium Chloride *(Continued)*

only as guided by clinical evidence of hypocalcemia and/or serial monitoring of ionized calcium.

Neonates, Infants, and Children: Give 32 mg (0.45 mEq elemental calcium) for each 100 mL citrated blood infused

Adults: 200-500 mg per 500 mL of citrated blood (infused into another vein)

Dosing adjustment in renal impairment: Cl_{cr} <25 mL/minute: Dosage adjustments may be necessary depending on the serum calcium levels

Stability

Do not refrigerate solutions; IVPB solutions/I.V. infusion solutions are stable for 24 hours at room temperature.

Maximum concentration in parenteral nutrition solutions: 15 mEq/L of calcium and 30 mmol/L of phosphate.

Administration For I.V. administration only; avoid extravasation. Administer slowly (0.7-1.8 mEq per minute or between 0.5 mL and 1.5 mL per minute of calcium chloride 10%); for I.V. infusion, dilute to a maximum concentration of 20 mg/mL and infuse over 1 hour or no greater than 45-90 mg/kg/hour (0.6-1.2 mEq/kg/hour); administration via a central or deep vein is preferred; do not use scalp, small hand or foot veins for I.V. administration since severe necrosis and sloughing may occur. Monitor ECG if calcium is infused faster than 2.5 mEq/minute; **stop the infusion if the patient complains of pain or discomfort.** Warm to body temperature. If used as intraventricular injection, inject into ventricular cavity - not myocardium; **do not infuse calcium chloride in the same I.V. line as phosphate-containing solutions**.

Monitoring Parameters Serum calcium, albumin, ionized calcium

Reference Range

Serum calcium: 8.4-10.2 mg/dL

Due to a poor correlation between the serum ionized calcium (free) and total serum calcium, particularly in states of low albumin or acid/base imbalances, direct measurement of ionized calcium is recommended.

In low albumin states, the corrected **total** serum calcium may be estimated by the following equation (assuming a normal albumin of 4 g/dL).

Corrected total calcium = total serum calcium + 0.8 (4.0 - measured serum albumin)

or

Corrected calcium = measured calcium - measured albumin + 4.0

Serum/plasma chloride: 95-108 mEq/L

Anesthesia and Critical Care Concerns/Other Considerations

Hypercalcemia is evident on ECG by shortening of the QT interval and possibly lengthening of the PR interval. Hypocalcemia causes prolongation of the QT interval. This prolongation is due to lengthening of the ST segment; the T waves remain unchanged. However, in severe hypocalcemia, T waves may be inverted. Note that only hypocalcemia and hypothermia lengthen the ST segment without altering T-wave duration. Hypocalcemia may also present clinically with skeletal muscle spasm.

Calcium salts may enhance the arrhythmogenic effects of digoxin. Part of the inotropic action of digoxin appears to be associated with increased intracellular calcium availability. Chronotropic effects are also calcium mediated. The administration of exogenous calcium (especially by parenteral routes) can lead to cardiac arrhythmias.

Pregnancy Risk Factor C

Contraindications In ventricular fibrillation during cardiac resuscitation, hypercalcemia, and in patients with risk of digitalis toxicity, renal or cardiac disease; not recommended in treatment of asystole and electromechanical dissociation; patients with suspected digoxin toxicity

Warnings/Precautions Avoid too rapid I.V. administration (<1 mL/minute) and extravasation. Use with caution in digitalized patients, respiratory failure, or acidosis. Hypercalcemia may occur in patients with renal failure, and frequent determination of serum calcium is necessary. Avoid metabolic acidosis (ie, administer only 2-3 days then change to another calcium salt).

Adverse Reactions <1% (Limited to important or life-threatening): Bradycardia, cardiac arrhythmia, coma, serum magnesium decreased, serum amylase increased, erythema, hypercalcemia, hypercalciuria, hypotension, lethargy, mania, muscle weakness, syncope, tissue necrosis, vasodilation, ventricular fibrillation

Overdosage/Toxicology

Symptoms of overdose include lethargy, nausea, vomiting, coma

Following withdrawal of the drug, treatment consists of bedrest, liberal intake of fluids, reduced calcium intake, and cathartic administration. Severe hypercalcemia requires I.V. hydration and forced diuresis. Urine output should be monitored and maintained at >3 mL/kg/hour. I.V. saline and natriuretic agents (eg, furosemide) can quickly and significantly increase excretion of calcium.

Drug Interactions

Calcium channel blockers (eg, verapamil) effects may be diminished; monitor response.

Levothyroxine: Calcium carbonate (and possibly other calcium salts) may decrease T_4 absorption; separate dose from levothyroxine by at least 4 hours.

Thiazide diuretics can cause hypercalcemia; monitor response.

May potentiate digoxin toxicity. High doses of calcium with thiazide diuretics may result in milk-alkali syndrome and hypercalcemia.

Test Interactions Increased calcium (S); decreased magnesium

Dosage Forms Injection, solution [preservative free]: 10% [100 mg/mL] (10 mL) [equivalent to elemental calcium 27.2 mg/mL, calcium 1.36 mEq/mL]

References

DeRoos F, "Calcium Channel Blockers," Goldfrank LG, et al, ed,*Goldfrank's Toxicologic Emergencies*, 7th ed, New York, (NY):McGraw-Hill Medical Publishing, 2002, 762-74.

Howarth DM, Dawson AH, Smith AJ, et al, "Calcium Channel Blocking Drug Overdose: An Australian Series," *Hum Exp Toxicol*, 1994, 13(3):161-6.

Isbister GK, "Continuous Calcium Chloride Infusion for Massive Nifedipine Overdose," *Emerg Med J*, 2002, 19(4):355-7.

Lam YM, Tse HF, and Lau CP, "Delayed Asystolic Cardiac Arrest After Diltiazem Overdose: Resuscitation With High Dose Intravenous Calcium," *Chest*, 2001, 119(4):1280-2.

Luscher TF, Noll G, and Sturmer T, "Calcium Gluconate in Severe Verapamil Intoxication," *N Engl J Med*, 1994, 330(10):718-20.

Mokhlesi B, Leikin JB, Murray P, et al, "Adult Toxicology in Critical Care: Part II: Specific Poisonings," *Chest*, 2003, 123(3):897-922.

Salhanick SD and Shannon MW, "Management of Calcium Channel Antagonist Overdose," *Drug Saf*, 2003, 26(2):65-79.

Calcium Gluconate (KAL see um GLOO koe nate)

Medication Safety Issues

Sound-alike/look-alike issues:

Calcium gluconate may be confused with calcium glubionate

Pharmacologic Category Calcium Salt; Electrolyte Supplement, Oral; Electrolyte Supplement, Parenteral

Generic Available Yes

Use Treatment and prevention of hypocalcemia; treatment of tetany, cardiac disturbances of hyperkalemia, cardiac resuscitation when epinephrine fails to improve myocardial contractions, hypocalcemia; calcium supplementation

Unlabeled/Investigational Use Hydrofluoric acid (HF) burns; calcium channel blocker overdose

Mechanism of Action As dietary supplement, used to prevent or treat negative calcium balance; in osteoporosis, it helps to prevent or decrease the rate of bone loss. The calcium in calcium salts moderates nerve and muscle performance and allows normal cardiac function.

Pharmacodynamics/Kinetics

Absorption: Requires vitamin D; calcium is absorbed in soluble, ionized form; solubility of calcium is increased in an acid environment

Distribution: Primarily in bones and teeth; crosses placenta; enters breast milk

Protein binding: Primarily albumin

Excretion: Primarily feces (as unabsorbed calcium); urine (20%)

Dosage

Adequate Intake (as elemental calcium):

0-6 months: 210 mg/day

7-12 months: 270 mg/day

1-3 years: 500 mg/day

4-8 years: 800 mg/day

9-18 years: 1300 mg/day

Adults, Male/Female:

19-50 years: 1000 mg/day

≥51 years: 1200 mg/day

(Continued)

Calcium Gluconate *(Continued)*

Female: Pregnancy: Same as for Adults, Male/Female

Female: Lactating: Same as for Adults, Male/Female

Dosage note: Calcium chloride has 3 times more elemental calcium than calcium gluconate. Calcium chloride is 27% elemental calcium; calcium gluconate is 9% elemental calcium. One gram of calcium chloride is equal to 270 mg of elemental calcium; 1 gram of calcium gluconate is equal to 90 mg of elemental calcium. The following dosages are expressed in terms of the calcium gluconate salt based on a solution concentration of 100 mg/mL (10%) containing 0.465 mEq (9.3 mg)/mL elemental calcium:

Hypocalcemia: I.V.:

Neonates: 200-800 mg/kg/day as a continuous infusion or in 4 divided doses (maximum: 1 g/dose)

Infants and Children: 200-500 mg/kg/day as a continuous infusion or in 4 divided doses (maximum: 2-3 g/dose)

Adults: 2-15 g/24 hours as a continuous infusion or in divided doses

Hypocalcemia: Oral:

Children: 200-500 mg/kg/day divided every 6 hours

Adults: 500 mg to 2 g 2-4 times/day

Hypocalcemia secondary to citrated blood infusion: I.V.: **Note:** Routine administration of calcium, in the absence of signs/symptoms of hypocalcemia, is generally not recommended. A number of recommendations have been published seeking to address potential hypocalcemia during massive transfusion of citrated blood; however, many practitioners recommend replacement only as guided by clinical evidence of hypocalcemia and/or serial monitoring of ionized calcium.

Neonates, Infants, and Children: Give 98 mg (0.45 mEq **elemental** calcium) for each 100 mL citrated blood infused

Adults: 500 mg to 1 g per 500 mL of citrated blood (infused into another vein). Single doses up to 2 g have also been recommended.

Hypocalcemic tetany: I.V.:

Neonates, Infants, and Children: 100-200 mg/kg/dose over 5-10 minutes; may repeat every 6-8 hours **or** follow with an infusion of 500 mg/kg/day

Adults: 1-3 g may be administered until therapeutic response occurs

Magnesium intoxication, cardiac arrest in the presence of hyperkalemia or hypocalcemia: I.V.:

Infants and Children: 60-100 mg/kg/dose (maximum: 3 g/dose)

Adults: 500-800 mg/dose (maximum: 3 g/dose)

Maintenance electrolyte requirements for total parenteral nutrition: I.V.: Daily requirements: Adults: 1.7-3.4 g/1000 kcal/24 hours

Calcium channel blocker overdose (unlabeled use): Adults: I.V. infusion: 10% solution: 0.6-1.2 mL/kg/hour or I.V. 0.2-0.5 ml/kg every 15-20 minutes for 4 doses (maximum: 2-3 g/dose). In life-threatening situations, 1 g has been given every 1-10 minutes until clinical effect is achieved (case reports of resistant hypotension reported use of 12-18 g total).

Dosing adjustment in renal impairment: Cl_{cr} <25 mL/minute: Dosage adjustments may be necessary depending on the serum calcium levels

Stability

Do not refrigerate solutions. IVPB solutions/I.V. infusion solutions are stable for 24 hours at room temperature.

Standard diluent: 1 g/100 mL D_5W or NS; 2 g/100 mL D_5W or NS

Maximum concentration in parenteral nutrition solutions is variable depending upon concentration and solubility (consult detailed reference).

Administration Not for I.M. or SubQ administration. For I.V. administration only; administer slowly (~1.5 mL calcium gluconate 10% per minute) through a small needle into a large vein in order to avoid too rapid increased in serum calcium and extravasation.

Extravasation treatment example: Hyaluronidase: Add 1 mL NS to 150 unit vial to make 150 units/mL of concentration; mix 0.1 mL of above with 0.9 mL NS in 1 mL syringe to make final concentration = 15 units/mL

Reference Range

Serum calcium: 8.4-10.2 mg/dL: Monitor plasma calcium levels if using calcium salts as electrolyte supplements for deficiency

Due to a poor correlation between the serum ionized calcium (free) and total serum calcium, particularly in states of low albumin or acid/base imbalances, direct measurement of ionized calcium is recommended

In low albumin states, the corrected **total** serum calcium may be estimated by: Corrected total calcium = total serum calcium + 0.8 (4.0 - measured serum albumin)

Pregnancy Risk Factor C

Contraindications Ventricular fibrillation during cardiac resuscitation; digitalis toxicity or suspected digoxin toxicity; hypercalcemia

Warnings/Precautions Injection solution is for I.V. use only; do not inject SubQ or I.M. Avoid too rapid I.V. administration and avoid extravasation. Use with caution in digitalized patients, severe hyperphosphatemia, respiratory failure, or acidosis. May produce cardiac arrest. Hypercalcemia may occur in patients with renal failure; frequent determination of serum calcium is necessary. Use caution with renal disease. Solutions may contain aluminum; toxic levels may occur following prolonged administration in premature neonates or patients with renal dysfunction.

Adverse Reactions Frequency not defined.

I.V.:

Cardiovascular: Arrhythmia, bradycardia, cardiac arrest, hypotension, vasodilation, and syncope may occur following rapid I.V. injection

Central nervous system: Sense of oppression

Gastrointestinal: Chalky taste

Local: Abscess and necrosis following I.M. administration

Neuromuscular & skeletal: Tingling sensation

Miscellaneous: Heat waves

Postmarketing and/or case reports: Calcinosis cutis

Oral: Gastrointestinal: Constipation

Overdosage/Toxicology

Acute single oral ingestions of calcium salts may produce mild gastrointestinal distress, but hypercalcemia or other toxic manifestations are extremely unlikely. Symptoms of hypercalcemia include lethargy, nausea, vomiting, and coma.

Treatment is supportive. Severe hypercalcemia following parenteral overdose requires I.V. hydration. Urine output should be monitored and maintained at >3 mL/kg/hour. I.V. saline and natriuretic agents (eg, furosemide) can quickly and significantly increase excretion of calcium into urine.

Drug Interactions

Bisphosphonate derivatives: Absorption may be decreased by calcium salts.

Calcium channel blockers (eg, verapamil) effects may be diminished; monitor response.

Digoxin: May potentiate digoxin toxicity.

Dobutamine: Calcium salts may diminish the therapeutic effect of dobutamine.

Levothyroxine: Calcium carbonate (and possibly other calcium salts) may decrease T_4 absorption; separate dose from levothyroxine by at least 4 hours.

Phosphate supplements: Calcium salts may decrease the absorption of phosphate supplements.

Quinolone antibiotics: Calcium salts may decrease the absorption of quinolone antibiotics with oral administration of both agents.

Thiazide diuretics: Thiazide diuretics may decrease the excretion of calcium salts. Continued concomitant use can also result in metabolic alkalosis.

Test Interactions Increased calcium (S); decreased magnesium

Dosage Forms

Injection, solution [preservative free]: 10% [100 mg/mL] (10 mL, 50 mL, 100 mL, 200 mL) [equivalent to elemental calcium 9 mg/mL; calcium 0.46 mEq/mL]

Powder: 347 mg/tablespoonful (480 g)

Tablet: 500 mg [equivalent to elemental calcium 45 mg]; 650 mg [equivalent to elemental calcium 58.5 mg]; 975 mg [equivalent to elemental calcium 87.75 mg]

References

DeRoos F, "Calcium Channel Blockers," Goldfrank LG, et al, ed, *Goldfrank's Toxicologic Emergencies*, 7th ed, New York, (NY):McGraw-Hill Medical Publishing, 2002, 762-74.

Howarth DM, Dawson AH, Smith AJ, et al, "Calcium Channel Blocking Drug Overdose: An Australian Series," *Hum Exp Toxicol*, 1994, 13(3):161-6.

Isbister GK, "Continuous Calcium Chloride Infusion for Massive Nifedipine Overdose," *Emerg Med J*, 2002, 19(4):355-7.

Lam YM, Tse HF, and Lau CP, "Delayed Asystolic Cardiac Arrest After Diltiazem Overdose: Resuscitation With High Dose Intravenous Calcium," *Chest*, 2001, 119(4):1280-2.

Luscher TF, Noll G, and Sturmer T, "Calcium Gluconate in Severe Verapamil Intoxication," *N Engl J Med*, 1994, 330(10):718-20.

(Continued)

Calcium Gluconate *(Continued)*

Mokhlesi B, Leikin JB, Murray P, et al, "Adult Toxicology in Critical Care: Part II: Specific Poisonings," *Chest*, 2003, 123(3):897-922.

Salhanick SD and Shannon MW, "Management of Calcium Channel Antagonist Overdose," *Drug Saf*, 2003, 26(2):65-79.

♦ **Calcium Leucovorin** *see* Leucovorin *on page 738*

♦ **Caldecort® [OTC]** *see* Hydrocortisone *on page 639*

Calfactant (kaf AKT ant)

U.S. Brand Names Infasurf®

Pharmacologic Category Lung Surfactant

Generic Available No

Use Prevention of respiratory distress syndrome (RDS) in premature infants at high risk for RDS and for the treatment ("rescue") of premature infants who develop RDS

Prophylaxis: Therapy at birth with calfactant is indicated for premature infants <29 weeks of gestational age at significant risk for RDS. Should be administered as soon as possible, preferably within 30 minutes after birth.

Treatment: For infants ≤72 hours of age with RDS (confirmed by clinical and radiologic findings) and requiring endotracheal intubation.

Mechanism of Action Endogenous lung surfactant is essential for effective ventilation because it modifies alveolar surface tension, thereby stabilizing the alveoli. Lung surfactant deficiency is the cause of respiratory distress syndrome (RDS) in premature infants and lung surfactant restores surface activity to the lungs of these infants.

Pharmacodynamics/Kinetics No human studies of absorption, biotransformation, or excretion have been performed

Dosage Intratracheal administration **only**: Each dose is 3 mL/kg body weight at birth; should be administered every 12 hours for a total of up to 3 doses

Stability Gentle swirling or agitation of the vial of suspension is often necessary for redispersion. **Do not shake**. Visible flecks of the suspension and foaming under the surface are normal. Calfactant should be stored at refrigeration (2°C to 8°C/ 36°F to 46°F). Warming before administration is not necessary. Unopened and unused vials of calfactant that have been warmed to room temperature can be returned to the refrigeration storage within 24 hours for future use. Repeated warming to room temperature should be avoided. Each single-use vial should be entered only once and the vial with any unused material should be discarded after the initial entry.

Administration Gentle swirling or agitation of the vial is often necessary for redispersion as suspension settles during storage; do **not** shake; visible flecks in the suspension and foaming at the surface are normal; does not require reconstitution; do not dilute or sonicate.

Should be administered intratracheally through an endotracheal tube. Dose is drawn into a syringe from the single-use vial using a 20-gauge or larger needle with care taken to avoid excessive foaming. Should be administered in two aliquots of 1.5 mL/kg each. After each aliquot is instilled, the infant should be positioned with either the right or the left side dependent. Administration is made while ventilation is continued over 20-30 breaths for each aliquot, with small bursts timed only during the inspiratory cycles. A pause followed by evaluation of the respiratory status and repositioning should separate the two aliquots.

Monitoring Parameters Following administration, patients should be carefully monitored so that oxygen therapy and ventilatory support can be modified in response to changes in respiratory status.

Warnings/Precautions For intratracheal administration only; the administration of exogenous surfactants often rapidly improves oxygenation and lung compliance. Transient episodes of cyanosis, bradycardia, reflux of surfactant into the endotracheal tube, and airway obstruction were observed more frequently among infants treated with calfactant in clinical trials.

Adverse Reactions

Cardiovascular: Bradycardia (34%), cyanosis (65%)

Respiratory: Airway obstruction (39%), reflux (21%), requirement for manual ventilation (16%), reintubation (1% to 10%)

Overdosage/Toxicology There have been no known reports of overdosage. While there are no known reports of excess lung surfactant, overdoses would result in overloading the lungs with an isotonic solution. Ventilation should be supported until clearance of the liquid is accomplished.

Dosage Forms Suspension, intratracheal [preservative free]: 35 mg/mL (6 mL)

- **Camphorated Tincture of Opium (error-prone synonym)** *see* Paregoric *on page 987*
- **Cancidas®** *see* Caspofungin *on page 234*

Candesartan (kan de SAR tan)

Related Information

Angiotensin Agents *on page 1544*

U.S. Brand Names Atacand®

Canadian Brand Names Atacand®

Synonyms Candesartan Cilexetil

Pharmacologic Category Angiotensin II Receptor Blocker

Generic Available No

Use Alone or in combination with other antihypertensive agents in treating essential hypertension; treatment of heart failure (NYHA class II-IV)

Mechanism of Action Candesartan is an angiotensin receptor antagonist. Angiotensin II acts as a vasoconstrictor. In addition to causing direct vasoconstriction, angiotensin II also stimulates the release of aldosterone. Once aldosterone is released, sodium as well as water are reabsorbed. The end result is an elevation in blood pressure. Candesartan binds to the AT1 angiotensin II receptor. This binding prevents angiotensin II from binding to the receptor thereby blocking the vasoconstriction and the aldosterone secreting effects of angiotensin II.

Pharmacodynamics/Kinetics

Onset of action: 2-3 hours

Peak effect: 6-8 hours

Duration: >24 hours

Distribution: V_d: 0.13 L/kg

Protein binding: 99%

Metabolism: To candesartan by the intestinal wall cells

Bioavailability: 15%

Half-life elimination (dose dependent): 5-9 hours

Time to peak: 3-4 hours

Excretion: Urine (26%)

Clearance: Total body: 0.37 mL/kg/minute; Renal: 0.19 mL/kg/minute

Dosage Adults: Oral:

Hypertension: Usual dose is 4-32 mg once daily; dosage must be individualized. Blood pressure response is dose related over the range of 2-32 mg. The usual recommended starting dose of 16 mg once daily when it is used as monotherapy in patients who are not volume depleted. It can be administered once or twice daily with total daily doses ranging from 8-32 mg. Larger doses do not appear to have a greater effect and there is relatively little experience with such doses.

Congestive heart failure: Initial: 4 mg once daily; double the dose at 2-week intervals, as tolerated; target dose: 32 mg

Note: In selected cases, concurrent therapy with an ACE inhibitor may provide additional benefit.

Elderly: No initial dosage adjustment is necessary for elderly patients (although higher concentrations (C_{max}) and AUC were observed in these populations), for patients with mildly impaired renal function, or for patients with mildly impaired hepatic function.

Dosage adjustment in hepatic impairment: No initial dosage adjustment required in mild hepatic impairment. Consider initiation at lower dosages in moderate hepatic impairment (AUC increased by 145%). No data available concerning dosing in severe hepatic impairment.

Monitoring Parameters Supine blood pressure, electrolytes, serum creatinine, BUN, urinalysis, symptomatic hypotension, and tachycardia; in CHF, serum potassium during dose escalation and periodically thereafter

Anesthesia and Critical Care Concerns/Other Considerations The angiotensin II receptor antagonists appear to have similar indications as the ACE inhibitors. In heart failure, the angiotensin II antagonists are especially useful in providing an alternative therapy in those patients who have intractable cough in response to ACE inhibitor therapy. Candesartan has been studied as an alternative therapy in chronic heart failure patients who cannot tolerate an ACE-I

(Continued)

Candesartan *(Continued)*

(CHARM-Alternative) and as an added therapy in heart failure patients who are maintained on an ACE-I (CHARM-Added). In both studies the combined endpoint of cardiovascular death or heart failure hospitalizations was significantly improved over the placebo treated group. Similar to ACE inhibitors, pre-existing volume depletion caused by diuretic therapy may potentiate hypotension in response to angiotensin II antagonists. Concomitant NSAID therapy may attenuate blood pressure control; use of NSAIDs should be avoided or limited, with monitoring of blood pressure control. In the setting of heart failure, NSAID use may be associated with an increased risk for fluid accumulation and edema.

Pregnancy Risk Factor C/D (2nd and 3rd trimesters)

Contraindications Hypersensitivity to candesartan or any component of the formulation; hypersensitivity to other A-II receptor antagonists; bilateral renal artery stenosis; pregnancy (2nd and 3rd trimesters)

Warnings/Precautions [U.S. Boxed Warning]: Based on human data, drugs that act on the angiotensin system can cause injury and death to the developing fetus when used in the second and third trimesters. Angiotensin receptor blockers should be discontinued as soon as possible once pregnancy is detected. Avoid use or use a smaller dose in patients who are volume depleted; correct depletion first. May be associated with deterioration of renal function and/or increases in serum creatinine, particularly in patients dependent on renin-angiotensin-aldosterone system; deterioration may result in oliguria, acute renal failure, and progressive azotemia. Small increases in serum creatinine may occur following initiation; consider discontinuation only in patients with progressive and/or significant deterioration in renal function. Use with caution in unilateral renal artery stenosis, hepatic dysfunction, pre-existing renal insufficiency, or significant aortic/mitral stenosis. Use caution when initiating in heart failure; may need to adjust dose, and/or concurrent diuretic therapy, because of candesartan-induced hypotension. Although some properties may be shared between these agents, concurrent therapy with ACE inhibitor may be rational in selected patients.

Adverse Reactions

Cardiovascular: Angina, hypotension (CHF 19%), MI, palpitation, tachycardia

Central nervous system: Dizziness, lightheadedness, drowsiness, headache, vertigo, anxiety, depression, somnolence, fever

Dermatologic: Angioedema, rash

Endocrine & metabolic: Hyperglycemia, hyperkalemia (CHF <1% to 6%), hypertriglyceridemia, hyperuricemia

Gastrointestinal: Dyspepsia, gastroenteritis

Genitourinary: Hematuria

Neuromuscular & skeletal: Back pain, CPK increased, myalgia, paresthesia, weakness

Renal: Serum creatinine increased (up to 13% in patients with CHF with drug discontinuation required in 6%)

Respiratory: Dyspnea, epistaxis, pharyngitis, rhinitis, upper respiratory tract infection

Miscellaneous: Diaphoresis increased

<1%, postmarketing, and/or case reports: Abnormal hepatic function, agranulocytosis, anemia, hepatitis, hyponatremia, leukopenia, neutropenia, pruritus, renal failure, renal impairment, rhinitis, sinusitis, thrombocytopenia, urticaria; rhabdomyolysis has been reported (rarely) with angiotensin-receptor antagonists

Overdosage/Toxicology Symptoms of overdose include hypotension and tachycardia. Treatment is supportive.

Drug Interactions Substrate of CYP2C9 (minor); **Inhibits** CYP2C8 (weak), 2C9 (weak)

Lithium: Risk of toxicity may be increased by candesartan; monitor lithium levels.

NSAIDs: May decrease angiotensin II antagonist efficacy; effect has been seen with losartan, but may occur with other medications in this class; monitor blood pressure.

Potassium-sparing diuretics (amiloride, spironolactone, triamterene): May increase risk of hyperkalemia.

Potassium supplements: May increase the risk of hyperkalemia.

Trimethoprim (high dose): May increase the risk of hyperkalemia.

Ethanol/Nutrition/Herb Interactions

Food: Food reduces the time to maximal concentration and increases the C_{max}.

Herb/Nutraceutical: Avoid dong quai if using for hypertension (has estrogenic activity). Avoid ephedra, yohimbe, ginseng (may worsen hypertension). Avoid garlic (may have increased antihypertensive effect).

Dosage Forms Tablet, as cilexetil: 4 mg, 8 mg, 16 mg, 32 mg

- **Candesartan Cilexetil** *see* Candesartan *on page 219*
- **Candistatin® (Can)** *see* Nystatin *on page 945*
- **Capital® and Codeine** *see* Acetaminophen and Codeine *on page 29*
- **Capoten®** *see* Captopril *on page 221*

Captopril (KAP toe pril)

Medication Safety Issues

Sound-alike/look-alike issues:

Captopril may be confused with Capitrol®, carvedilol

Related Information

Angiotensin Agents *on page 1544*
Heart Failure (Systolic) *on page 1607*
Hypertension *on page 1620*
Preoperative Evaluation of the Cardiac Patient for Noncardiac Surgery *on page 1485*

U.S. Brand Names Capoten®

Canadian Brand Names Alti-Captopril; Apo-Capto®; Capoten™; Gen-Captopril; Novo-Captopril; Nu-Capto; PMS-Captopril

Synonyms ACE

Pharmacologic Category Angiotensin-Converting Enzyme (ACE) Inhibitor

Generic Available Yes

Use Management of hypertension; treatment of congestive heart failure, left ventricular dysfunction after myocardial infarction, diabetic nephropathy

Unlabeled/Investigational Use Treatment of hypertensive crisis, rheumatoid arthritis; diagnosis of anatomic renal artery stenosis, hypertension secondary to scleroderma renal crisis; diagnosis of aldosteronism, idiopathic edema, Bartter's syndrome, postmyocardial infarction for prevention of ventricular failure; increase circulation in Raynaud's phenomenon, hypertension secondary to Takayasu's disease

Mechanism of Action Competitive inhibitor of angiotensin-converting enzyme (ACE); prevents conversion of angiotensin I to angiotensin II, a potent vasoconstrictor; results in lower levels of angiotensin II which causes an increase in plasma renin activity and a reduction in aldosterone secretion

Pharmacodynamics/Kinetics

Onset of action: Peak effect: Blood pressure reduction: 1-1.5 hours after dose

Duration: Dose related, may require several weeks of therapy before full hypotensive effect

Absorption: 60% to 75%; reduced 30% to 40% by food

Protein binding: 25% to 30%

Metabolism: 50%

Half-life elimination (renal and cardiac function dependent):

Adults, healthy volunteers: 1.9 hours; Congestive heart failure: 2.06 hours; Anuria: 20-40 hours

Excretion: Urine (95%) within 24 hours

Dosage Note: Dosage must be titrated according to patient's response; use lowest effective dose. Oral:

Infants: Initial: 0.15-0.3 mg/kg/dose; titrate dose upward to maximum of 6 mg/kg/day in 1-4 divided doses; usual required dose: 2.5-6 mg/kg/day

Children: Initial: 0.5 mg/kg/dose; titrate upward to maximum of 6 mg/kg/day in 2-4 divided doses

Older Children: Initial: 6.25-12.5 mg/dose every 12-24 hours; titrate upward to maximum of 6 mg/kg/day

Adolescents: Initial: 12.5-25 mg/dose given every 8-12 hours; increase by 25 mg/dose to maximum of 450 mg/day

Adults:

Acute hypertension (urgency/emergency): 12.5-25 mg, may repeat as needed (may be given sublingually, but no therapeutic advantage demonstrated)

(Continued)

Captopril *(Continued)*

Hypertension:

Initial dose: 12.5-25 mg 2-3 times/day; may increase by 12.5-25 mg/dose at 1- to 2-week intervals up to 50 mg 3 times/day; maximum dose: 150 mg 3 times/day; add diuretic before further dosage increases

Usual dose range (JNC 7): 25-100 mg/day in 2 divided doses

Congestive heart failure:

Initial dose: 6.25-12.5 mg 3 times/day in conjunction with cardiac glycoside and diuretic therapy; initial dose depends upon patient's fluid/electrolyte status

Target dose: 50 mg 3 times/day

LVD after MI: Initial dose: 6.25 mg followed by 12.5 mg 3 times/day; then increase to 25 mg 3 times/day during next several days and then over next several weeks to target dose of 50 mg 3 times/day

Diabetic nephropathy: 25 mg 3 times/day; other antihypertensives often given concurrently

Dosing adjustment in renal impairment:

Cl_{cr} 10-50 mL/minute: Administer at 75% of normal dose.

Cl_{cr} <10 mL/minute: Administer at 50% of normal dose.

Note: Smaller dosages given every 8-12 hours are indicated in patients with renal dysfunction; renal function and leukocyte count should be carefully monitored during therapy.

Hemodialysis: Moderately dialyzable (20% to 50%); administer dose postdialysis or administer 25% to 35% supplemental dose.

Peritoneal dialysis: Supplemental dose is not necessary.

Administration Unstable in aqueous solutions; to prepare solution for oral administration, mix prior to administration and use within 10 minutes.

Monitoring Parameters BUN, serum creatinine, urine dipstick for protein, complete leukocyte count, and blood pressure

Anesthesia and Critical Care Concerns/Other Considerations Severe hypotension may occur in patients who are sodium and/or volume depleted.

ACE inhibitors are indicated in patients postmyocardial infarction in whom left ventricular ejection fraction is <40%. When used in patients with heart failure, the target dose of 50 mg 3 times/day should be achieved, if possible. Lower daily doses of ACE inhibitors have not demonstrated the same cardioprotective effects.

ACE inhibitor therapy may elicit rapid increases in potassium and creatinine, especially when used in patients with bilateral renal artery stenosis. When ACE inhibition is introduced in patients with pre-existing diuretic therapy who are hypovolemic, the ACE inhibitor may induce acute hypotension. Because of the potent teratogenic effects of ACE inhibitors, these drugs should be avoided, if possible, when treating women of childbearing potential not on effective birth control measures.

Pregnancy Risk Factor C (1st trimester)/D (2nd and 3rd trimesters)

Contraindications Hypersensitivity to captopril or any component of the formulation; angioedema related to previous treatment with an ACE inhibitor; idiopathic or hereditary angioedema; bilateral renal artery stenosis; pregnancy (2nd or 3rd trimester)

Warnings/Precautions Anaphylactic reactions can occur. Angioedema can occur at any time during treatment (especially following first dose). It may involve head and neck (potentially affecting the airway) or the intestine (presenting with abdominal pain). Prolonged monitoring may be required especially if tongue, glottis, or larynx are involved as they are associated with airway obstruction. Those with a history of airway surgery in this situation have a higher risk. Careful blood pressure monitoring with first dose (hypotension can occur especially in volume-depleted patients). **[U.S. Boxed Warning]: Based on human data, ACEIs can cause injury and death to the developing fetus when used in the second and third trimesters. ACEIs should be discontinued as soon as possible once pregnancy is detected.** Dosage adjustment needed in renal impairment. Use with caution in hypovolemia; collagen vascular diseases; valvular stenosis (particularly aortic stenosis); hyperkalemia; or before, during, or immediately after anesthesia. Avoid rapid dosage escalation which may lead to renal insufficiency. Rare toxicities associated with ACE inhibitors include cholestatic jaundice (which may progress to hepatic necrosis) and neutropenia/agranulocytosis with myeloid hyperplasia. If patient has renal impairment, then a baseline WBC with differential and serum creatinine should be evaluated and monitored closely during the first 3 months of therapy. Hypersensitivity reactions may be seen during hemodialysis with high-flux dialysis membranes (eg, AN69). Deterioration in renal function can occur with initiation. Use with caution in unilateral renal artery stenosis and pre-existing renal insufficiency.

Adverse Reactions

1% to 10%:

Cardiovascular: Hypotension (1% to 2.5%), tachycardia (1%), chest pain (1%), palpitation (1%)

Dermatologic: Rash (maculopapular or urticarial) (4% to 7%), pruritus (2%); in patients with rash, a positive ANA and/or eosinophilia has been noted in 7% to 10%.

Endocrine & metabolic: Hyperkalemia (1% to 11%)

Hematologic: Neutropenia may occur in up to 3.7% of patients with renal insufficiency or collagen-vascular disease.

Renal: Proteinuria (1%), serum creatinine increased, worsening of renal function (may occur in patients with bilateral renal artery stenosis or hypovolemia)

Respiratory: Cough (0.5% to 2%)

Miscellaneous: Hypersensitivity reactions (rash, pruritus, fever, arthralgia, and eosinophilia) have occurred in 4% to 7% of patients (depending on dose and renal function); dysgeusia - loss of taste or diminished perception (2% to 4%)

Frequency not defined:

Cardiovascular: Angioedema, cardiac arrest, cerebrovascular insufficiency, rhythm disturbances, orthostatic hypotension, syncope, flushing, pallor, angina, MI, Raynaud's syndrome, CHF

Central nervous system: Ataxia, confusion, depression, nervousness, somnolence

Dermatologic: Bullous pemphigus, erythema multiforme, Stevens-Johnson syndrome, exfoliative dermatitis

Endocrine & metabolic: Alkaline phosphatase increased, bilirubin increased, gynecomastia

Gastrointestinal: Pancreatitis, glossitis, dyspepsia

Genitourinary: Urinary frequency, impotence

Hematologic: Anemia, thrombocytopenia, pancytopenia, agranulocytosis

Hepatic: Jaundice, hepatitis, hepatic necrosis (rare), cholestasis, hyponatremia (symptomatic), transaminases increased

Neuromuscular & skeletal: Asthenia, myalgia, myasthenia

Ocular: Blurred vision

Renal: Renal insufficiency, renal failure, nephrotic syndrome, polyuria, oliguria

Respiratory: Bronchospasm, eosinophilic pneumonitis, rhinitis

Miscellaneous: Anaphylactoid reactions

Postmarketing and/or case reports: Alopecia, aplastic anemia, exacerbations of Huntington's disease, Guillain-Barré syndrome, hemolytic anemia, Kaposi's sarcoma, pericarditis, seizure (in premature infants), systemic lupus erythematosus. A syndrome which may include fever, myalgia, arthralgia, interstitial nephritis, vasculitis, rash, eosinophilia, and elevated ESR has been reported for captopril and other ACE inhibitors.

Overdosage/Toxicology Mild hypotension has been the primary toxic effect seen with acute overdose. Bradycardia may also occur. Hyperkalemia occurs even with therapeutic doses, especially in patients with renal insufficiency and those taking NSAIDs. Treatment is symptom-directed and supportive.

Drug Interactions Substrate of CYP2D6 (major)

Allopurinol: Case reports (rare) indicate a possible increased risk of Stevens-Johnson syndrome when combined with captopril.

$Alpha_1$ blockers: Hypotensive effect increased.

Aspirin: The effects of ACE inhibitors may be blunted by aspirin administration, particularly at higher dosages and/or increase adverse renal effects.

CYP2D6 inhibitors: May increase the levels/effects of captopril. Example inhibitors include chlorpromazine, delavirdine, fluoxetine, miconazole, paroxetine, pergolide, quinidine, quinine, ritonavir, and ropinirole.

Diuretics: Hypovolemia due to diuretics may precipitate acute hypotensive events or acute renal failure.

Insulin: Risk of hypoglycemia may be increased.

Lithium: Risk of lithium toxicity may be increased; monitor lithium levels, especially the first 4 weeks of therapy.

Mercaptopurine: Risk of neutropenia may be increased.

(Continued)

Captopril *(Continued)*

NSAIDs: May attenuate hypertensive efficacy; effect has been seen with captopril and may occur with other ACE inhibitors; monitor blood pressure. May increase adverse renal effects.

Potassium-sparing diuretics (amiloride, potassium, spironolactone, triamterene): Increased risk of hyperkalemia.

Potassium supplements may increase the risk of hyperkalemia.

Trimethoprim (high dose) may increase the risk of hyperkalemia.

Ethanol/Nutrition/Herb Interactions

Food: Captopril serum concentrations may be decreased if taken with food. Long-term use of captopril may result in a zinc deficiency which can result in a decrease in taste perception.

Herb/Nutraceutical: Avoid dong quai if using for hypertension (has estrogenic activity). Avoid ephedra, yohimbe, ginseng (may worsen hypertension). Avoid garlic (may have increased antihypertensive effect).

Test Interactions Increased BUN, creatinine, potassium, positive Coombs' [direct]; decreased cholesterol (S); may cause false-positive results in urine acetone determinations using sodium nitroprusside reagent

Dietary Considerations Should be taken at least 1 hour before or 2 hours after eating.

Dosage Forms Tablet: 12.5 mg, 25 mg, 50 mg, 100 mg

- **Carafate®** *see* Sucralfate *on page 1212*
- **Carapres® (Can)** *see* Clonidine *on page 316*

Carbachol (KAR ba kole)

Medication Safety Issues

Sound-alike/look-alike issues:

Isopto® Carbachol may be confused with Isopto® Carpine

U.S. Brand Names Carbastat® [DSC]; Isopto® Carbachol; Miostat®

Canadian Brand Names Isopto® Carbachol; Miostat®

Synonyms Carbacholine; Carbamylcholine Chloride

Pharmacologic Category Cholinergic Agonist; Ophthalmic Agent, Antiglaucoma; Ophthalmic Agent, Miotic

Generic Available No

Use Lowers intraocular pressure in the treatment of glaucoma; cause miosis during surgery

Mechanism of Action Synthetic direct-acting cholinergic agent that causes miosis by stimulating muscarinic receptors in the eye

Pharmacodynamics/Kinetics

Ophthalmic instillation:

Onset of action: Miosis: 10-20 minutes

Duration: Reduction in intraocular pressure: 4-8 hours

Intraocular administration:

Onset of action: Miosis: 2-5 minutes

Duration: 24 hours

Dosage Adults:

Ophthalmic: Instill 1-2 drops up to 3 times/day

Intraocular: 0.5 mL instilled into anterior chamber before or after securing sutures

Stability

Intraocular: Store at room temperature of 15°C to 30°C (59°F to 86°F).

Topical: Store at 8°C to 27°C (46°F to 80°F).

Administration

Ophthalmic: Finger pressure should be applied on the lacrimal sac for 1-2 minutes following topical instillation; remove excess around the eye with a tissue.

Intraocular: Instillation for miosis prior to eye surgery should be gentle and parallel to the iris face and tangential to the pupil border; discard unused portion. Do not inject >0.5 mL into the anterior chamber. Instillation may occur before or after securing sutures. Sterile technique must be used.

Pregnancy Risk Factor C

Contraindications Hypersensitivity to carbachol or any component of the formulation; acute iritis, acute inflammatory disease of the anterior chamber

Warnings/Precautions Use with caution in patients undergoing general anesthesia and in presence of corneal abrasion. Use caution with acute cardiac failure, asthma, peptic ulcer, hyperthyroidism, gastrointestinal spasm, urinary tract obstruction, and Parkinson's disease.

Adverse Reactions Frequency not defined.

Cardiovascular: Arrhythmia, flushing, hypotension, syncope

Central nervous system: Headache

Gastrointestinal: Abdominal cramps, diarrhea, epigastric distress, salivation, vomiting

Genitourinary: Urinary bladder tightness

Ocular: Bullous keratopathy, burning (transient), ciliary spasm, conjunctival injection, corneal clouding, irritation, postoperative iritis (following cataract extraction), retinal detachment, stinging (transient)

Respiratory: Asthma

Miscellaneous: Diaphoresis

Overdosage/Toxicology Symptoms of overdose include miosis, flushing, vomiting, bradycardia, bronchospasm, involuntary urination Atropine is the treatment of choice for intoxications manifesting with significant muscarinic symptoms. Atropine I.V. 1-2 mg every 5-60 minutes (or 0.04-0.08 mg/kg I.V. every 5-60 minutes if needed for children) should be repeated to control symptoms and then continued as needed for 1-2 days following the acute ingestion. Epinephrine 0.1-1 mg SubQ may be useful in reversing severe cardiovascular or pulmonary sequelae.

Drug Interactions Decreased effect of carbachol possible with topical NSAIDs

Dosage Forms [DSC] = Discontinued product

Solution, intraocular (Carbastat® [DSC], Miostat®): 0.01% (1.5 mL)

Solution, ophthalmic (Isopto® Carbachol): 1.5% (15 mL); 3% (30 mL) [contains benzalkonium chloride]

♦ **Carbacholine** *see* Carbachol *on page 224*

Carbamazepine (kar ba MAZ e peen)

Medication Safety Issues

Sound-alike/look-alike issues:

Carbatrol® may be confused with Cartrol®

Epitol® may be confused with Epinal®

Tegretol®, Tegretol®-XR may be confused with Mebaral®, Tegrin®, Toprol-XL®, Toradol®, Trental®

Related Information

Chronic Pain Management *on page 1430*

Epilepsy *on page 1604*

Perioperative Management of Patients on Antiseizure Medication *on page 1458*

U.S. Brand Names Carbatrol®; Epitol®; Equetro™; Tegretol®; Tegretol®-XR

Canadian Brand Names Apo-Carbamazepine®; Gen-Carbamazepine CR; Mapezine®; Novo-Carbamaz; Nu-Carbamazepine; PMS-Carbamazepine; Taro-Carbamazepine Chewable; Tegretol®

Synonyms CBZ; SPD417

Pharmacologic Category Anticonvulsant, Miscellaneous

Generic Available Yes: Excludes capsule (extended release), tablet (extended release)

Use

Carbatrol®, Tegretol®, Tegretol®-XR: Partial seizures with complex symptomatology (psychomotor, temporal lobe), generalized tonic-clonic seizures (grand mal), mixed seizure patterns, trigeminal neuralgia

Equetro™: Acute manic and mixed episodes associated with bipolar 1 disorder

Unlabeled/Investigational Use Treatment of resistant schizophrenia, ethanol withdrawal, restless leg syndrome, psychotic behavior associated with dementia, post-traumatic stress disorders

Mechanism of Action In addition to anticonvulsant effects, carbamazepine has anticholinergic, antineuralgic, antidiuretic, muscle relaxant, antimanic, antidepressive, and antiarrhythmic properties; may depress activity in the nucleus ventralis of the thalamus or decrease synaptic transmission or decrease summation of temporal stimulation leading to neural discharge by limiting influx of sodium ions across cell membrane or other unknown mechanisms; stimulates the release of ADH and potentiates its action in promoting reabsorption of water; chemically related to tricyclic antidepressants

(Continued)

Carbamazepine *(Continued)*

Pharmacodynamics/Kinetics

Absorption: Slow

Distribution: V_d: Neonates: 1.5 L/kg; Children: 1.9 L/kg; Adults: 0.59-2 L/kg

Protein binding: Carbamazepine: 75% to 90%, may be decreased in newborns; Epoxide metabolite: 50%

Metabolism: Hepatic via CYP3A4 to active epoxide metabolite; induces hepatic enzymes to increase metabolism

Bioavailability: 85%

Half-life elimination:

Carbamazepine: Initial: 18-55 hours; Multiple doses: Children: 8-14 hours; Adults: 12-17 hours

Epoxide metabolite: Initial: 25-43 hours

Time to peak, serum: Unpredictable:

Immediate release: Suspension: 1.5 hour; tablet: 4-5 hours

Extended release: Carbatrol®, Equetro™: 12-26 hours (single dose), 4-8 hours (multiple doses); Tegretol®-XR: 3-12 hours

Excretion: Urine 72% (1% to 3% as unchanged drug); feces (28%)

Dosage Dosage must be adjusted according to patient's response and serum concentrations. Administer tablets (chewable or conventional) in 2-3 divided doses daily and suspension in 4 divided doses daily.

Oral:

Epilepsy:

Children:

<6 years: Initial: 10-20 mg/kg/day divided twice or 3 times daily as tablets or 4 times/day as suspension; increase dose every week until optimal response and therapeutic levels are achieved

Maintenance dose: Divide into 3-4 doses daily (tablets or suspension); maximum recommended dose: 35 mg/kg/day

6-12 years: Initial: 100 mg twice daily (tablets or extended release tablets) or 50 mg of suspension 4 times/day (200 mg/day); increase by up to 100 mg/day at weekly intervals using a twice daily regimen of extended release tablets or 3-4 times daily regimen of other formulations until optimal response and therapeutic levels are achieved

Maintenance: Usual: 400-800 mg/day; maximum recommended dose: 1000 mg/day

Note: Children <12 years who receive ≥400 mg/day of carbamazepine may be converted to extended release capsules (Carbatrol®) using the same total daily dosage divided twice daily

Children >12 years and Adults: Initial: 200 mg twice daily (tablets, extended release tablets, or extended release capsules) or 100 mg of suspension 4 times/day (400 mg daily); increase by up to 200 mg/day at weekly intervals using a twice daily regimen of extended release tablets or capsules, or a 3-4 times/day regimen of other formulations until optimal response and therapeutic levels are achieved; usual dose: 800-1200 mg/day

Maximum recommended doses:

Children 12-15 years: 1000 mg/day

Children >15 years: 1200 mg/day

Adults: 1600 mg/day; however, some patients have required up to 1.6-2.4 g/day

Trigeminal or glossopharyngeal neuralgia: Adults: Initial: 100 mg twice daily with food, gradually increasing in increments of 100 mg twice daily as needed

Maintenance: Usual: 400-800 mg daily in 2 divided doses; maximum dose: 1200 mg/day

Elderly: 100 mg 1-2 times daily, increase in increments of 100 mg/day at weekly intervals until therapeutic level is achieved; usual dose: 400-1000 mg/day

Bipolar disorder (Equetro™): Adults: Initial: 400 mg/day in divided doses, twice daily; may adjust by 200 mg daily increments; maximum dose: 1600 mg/day

Administration

Suspension: Must be given on a 3-4 times/day schedule versus tablets which can be given 2-4 times/day. When carbamazepine suspension has been combined with chlorpromazine or thioridazine solutions, a precipitate forms which may result in loss of effect. Therefore, it is recommended that the carbamazepine suspension dosage form not be administered at the same time with other liquid medicinal agents or diluents. Since a given dose of suspension will produce higher peak levels than the same dose given as the tablet form, patients given the suspension should be started on lower doses and increased slowly to avoid unwanted side effects. Should be administered with meals.

Extended release capsule (Carbatrol®, Equetro™): Consists of three different types of beads: Immediate release, extended-release, and enteric release. The bead types are combined in a ratio to allow twice daily dosing. May be opened and contents sprinkled over food such as a teaspoon of applesauce; may be administered with or without food; do not crush or chew.

Extended release tablet: Should be inspected for damage. Damaged extended release tablets (without release portal) should not be administered. Should be administered with meals; swallow whole, do not crush or chew.

Monitoring Parameters CBC with platelet count, reticulocytes, serum iron, lipid panel, liver function tests, urinalysis, BUN, serum carbamazepine levels, thyroid function tests, serum sodium; ophthalmic exams (pupillary reflexes); observe patient for excessive sedation, especially when instituting or increasing therapy

Reference Range

Timing of serum samples: Absorption is slow, peak levels occur 6-8 hours after ingestion of the first dose; the half-life ranges from 8-60 hours, therefore, steady-state is achieved in 2-5 days

Therapeutic levels: 4-12 mcg/mL (SI: 17-51 μmol/L)

Toxic concentration: >15 mcg/mL; patients who require higher levels of 8-12 mcg/mL (SI: 34-51 μmol/L) should be watched closely. Side effects including CNS effects occur commonly at higher dosage levels. If other anticonvulsants are given therapeutic range is 4-8 mcg/mL.

Anesthesia and Critical Care Concerns/Other Considerations Carbamazepine is not effective in absence, myoclonic, or akinetic seizures; exacerbation of certain seizure types has been seen after initiation of carbamazepine therapy in children with mixed seizure disorders. Elderly may have increase risk of SIADH-like syndrome and psychosis. Simultaneous administration of carbamazepine suspension with other liquids can precipitate the drug.

Pregnancy Risk Factor D

Contraindications Hypersensitivity to carbamazepine, tricyclic antidepressants, or any component of the formulation; bone marrow depression; with or within 14 days of MAO inhibitor use; pregnancy

Warnings/Precautions Administer carbamazepine with caution to patients with history of cardiac damage, hepatic or renal disease. **[U.S. Boxed Warning]: Potentially fatal blood cell abnormalities have been reported following treatment.** Patients with a previous history of adverse hematologic reaction to any drug may be at increased risk. Early detection of hematologic change is important; advise patients of early signs and symptoms including fever, sore throat, mouth ulcers, infections, easy bruising, petechial or purpuric hemorrhage. Prescriptions should be written for the smallest quantity consistent with good patient care. The smallest effective dose is suggested for use in bipolar disorder to reduce the risk for overdose; high-risk patients should be monitored. Actuation of latent psychosis is possible.

Carbamazepine is not effective in absence, myoclonic, or akinetic seizures; exacerbation of certain seizure types have been seen after initiation of carbamazepine therapy in children with mixed seizure disorders. Abrupt discontinuation is not recommended in patients being treated for seizures. Dizziness or drowsiness may occur; caution should be used when performing tasks which require alertness (operating machinery or driving) until the effects are known. Coadministration of carbamazepine and delavirdine may lead to loss of virologic response and possible resistance. Elderly may have increased risk of SIADH-like syndrome. Carbamazepine has mild anticholinergic activity; use with caution in patients with increased intraocular pressure (monitor closely), or sensitivity to anticholinergic effects (urinary retention, constipation). Severe dermatologic reactions, including Lyell and Stevens-Johnson syndromes, although rarely reported, have resulted in fatalities. Drug should be discontinued if there are any signs of hypersensitivity.

Adverse Reactions Frequency not defined, unless otherwise specified.

Cardiovascular: Arrhythmias, AV block, bradycardia, chest pain (bipolar use), CHF, edema, hyper-/hypotension, lymphadenopathy, syncope, thromboembolism, thrombophlebitis

Central nervous system: Amnesia (bipolar use), anxiety (bipolar use), aseptic meningitis (case report), ataxia (bipolar use 15%), confusion, depression (bipolar use), dizziness (bipolar use 44%), fatigue, headache (bipolar use 22%), sedation, slurred speech, somnolence (bipolar use 32%)

(Continued)

Carbamazepine *(Continued)*

Dermatologic: Alopecia, alterations in skin pigmentation, erythema multiforme, exfoliative dermatitis, photosensitivity reaction, pruritus (bipolar use 8%), purpura, rash, Stevens-Johnson syndrome, toxic epidermal necrolysis, urticaria

Endocrine & metabolic: Chills, fever, hyponatremia, syndrome of inappropriate ADH secretion (SIADH)

Gastrointestinal: Abdominal pain, anorexia, constipation, diarrhea, dyspepsia (bipolar use), gastric distress, nausea (bipolar use 29%), pancreatitis, vomiting (bipolar use 18%), xerostomia (bipolar use)

Genitourinary: Azotemia, impotence, renal failure, urinary frequency, urinary retention

Hematologic: Acute intermittent porphyria, agranulocytosis, aplastic anemia, bone marrow suppression, eosinophilia, leukocytosis, leukopenia, pancytopenia, thrombocytopenia

Hepatic: Abnormal liver function tests, hepatic failure, hepatitis, jaundice

Neuromuscular & skeletal: Back pain, pain (bipolar use 12%), peripheral neuritis, weakness

Ocular: Blurred vision, conjunctivitis, lens opacities, nystagmus

Otic: Hyperacusis, tinnitus

Miscellaneous: Diaphoresis, hypersensitivity (including multiorgan reactions, may include disorders mimicking lymphoma, eosinophilia, hepatosplenomegaly, vasculitis); infection (bipolar use 12%)

Overdosage/Toxicology Symptoms of overdose include dizziness ataxia, drowsiness, nausea, vomiting, tremor, agitation, nystagmus, urinary retention, dysrhythmias, coma, seizures, twitches, respiratory depression, and neuromuscular disturbances. Severe cardiac complications occur with very high doses. Activated charcoal is effective at binding carbamazepine. Other treatment is supportive and symptomatic.

Drug Interactions Substrate of CYP2C8 (minor), 3A4 (major); **Induces** CYP1A2 (strong), 2B6 (strong), 2C8 (strong), 2C9 (strong), 2C19 (strong), 3A4 (strong)

Acetaminophen: Carbamazepine may enhance hepatotoxic potential of acetaminophen; risk is greater in acetaminophen overdose.

Antimalarial drugs (chloroquine, mefloquine): Concomitant use with carbamazepine may reduce seizure control by lowering plasma levels; monitor.

Antipsychotics: Carbamazepine may enhance the metabolism (decrease the efficacy) of antipsychotics; monitor for altered response; dose adjustment may be needed.

Barbiturates: May reduce serum concentrations of carbamazepine; monitor.

Benzodiazepines: Serum concentrations and effect of benzodiazepines may be reduced by carbamazepine; monitor for decreased effect.

Calcium channel blockers: Diltiazem and verapamil may increase carbamazepine levels, due to enzyme inhibition (see below); other calcium channel blockers (felodipine) may be decreased by carbamazepine due to enzyme induction.

Chlorpromazine: **Note:** Carbamazepine suspension is incompatible with chlorpromazine solution. Schedule carbamazepine suspension at least 1-2 hours apart from other liquid medicinals.

Corticosteroids: Metabolism may be increased by carbamazepine.

Cyclosporine (and other immunosuppressants): Carbamazepine may enhance the metabolism of immunosuppressants, decreasing its clinical effect; includes both cyclosporine and tacrolimus.

CYP1A2 substrates: Carbamazepine may decrease the levels/effects of CYP1A2 substrates. Example substrates include aminophylline, estrogens, fluvoxamine, mirtazapine, ropinirole, and theophylline.

CYP2B6 substrates: Carbamazepine may decrease the levels/effects of CYP2B6 substrates. Example substrates include bupropion, efavirenz, promethazine, selegiline, and sertraline.

CYP2C8 Substrates: Carbamazepine may decrease the levels/effects of CYP2C8 substrates. Example substrates include amiodarone, paclitaxel, pioglitazone, repaglinide, and rosiglitazone.

CYP2C9 Substrates: Carbamazepine may decrease the levels/effects of CYP2C9 substrates. Example substrates include bosentan, celecoxib, dapsone, fluoxetine, glimepiride, glipizide, losartan, montelukast, nateglinide, paclitaxel, phenytoin, sulfonamides, trimethoprim, warfarin, and zafirlukast.

CYP2C19 substrates: Carbamazepine may decrease the levels/effects of CYP2C19 substrates. Example substrates include citalopram, diazepam, methsuximide, phenytoin, propranolol, proton pump inhibitors, sertraline, and voriconazole.

CYP3A4 inducers: CYP3A4 inducers may decrease the levels/effects of carbamazepine. Example inducers include aminoglutethimide, nafcillin, nevirapine, phenobarbital, phenytoin, and rifamycins. Carbamazepine may induce its own metabolism.

CYP3A4 inhibitors: May increase the levels/effects of carbamazepine. Example inhibitors include azole antifungals, clarithromycin, diclofenac, doxycycline, erythromycin, imatinib, isoniazid, nefazodone, nicardipine, propofol, protease inhibitors, quinidine, telithromycin, and verapamil.

CYP3A4 substrates: Carbamazepine may decrease the levels/effects of CYP3A4 substrates. Example substrates include benzodiazepines, calcium channel blockers, clarithromycin, cyclosporine, erythromycin, estrogens, mirtazapine, nateglinide, nefazodone, nevirapine, protease inhibitors, tacrolimus, and venlafaxine.

Danazol: May increase serum concentrations of carbamazepine; monitor.

Delavirdine: May lead to loss of virologic response and possible resistance.

Doxycycline: Carbamazepine may enhance the metabolism of doxycycline, decreasing its clinical effect.

Ethosuximide: Serum levels may be reduced by carbamazepine.

Felbamate: May increase carbamazepine levels and toxicity (increased epoxide metabolite concentrations); carbamazepine may decrease felbamate levels due to enzyme induction.

Immunosuppressants: Carbamazepine may enhance the metabolism of immunosuppressants, decreasing its clinical effect; includes both cyclosporine and tacrolimus.

Isoniazid: May increase the serum concentrations and toxicity of carbamazepine; in addition, carbamazepine may increase the hepatic toxicity of isoniazid (INH).

Isotretinoin: May decrease the effect of carbamazepine.

Lamotrigine: Increases the epoxide metabolite of carbamazepine resulting in toxicity; carbamazepine increases the metabolism of lamotrigine.

Lithium: Neurotoxicity may result in patients receiving concurrent carbamazepine.

Loxapine: May increase concentrations of epoxide metabolite and toxicity of carbamazepine.

Methadone: Carbamazepine may enhance the metabolism of methadone resulting in methadone withdrawal.

Methylphenidate: concurrent use of carbamazepine may reduce the therapeutic effect of methylphenidate; limited documentation; monitor for decreased effect.

Neuromuscular blocking agents, nondepolarizing: Effects may be of shorter duration when administered to patients receiving carbamazepine.

Oral contraceptives: Metabolism may be increased by carbamazepine, resulting in a loss of efficacy.

Phenytoin: Carbamazepine levels may be decreased by phenytoin. Metabolism of phenytoin may be altered by carbamazepine; phenytoin levels may be increased or decreased.

SSRIs: Metabolism may be increased by carbamazepine (due to enzyme induction).

Theophylline: Serum levels may be reduced by carbamazepine.

Thioridazine: **Note:** Carbamazepine suspension is incompatible with thioridazine liquid. Schedule carbamazepine suspension at least 1-2 hours apart from other liquid medicinals.

Thyroid: Serum levels may be reduced by carbamazepine.

Tramadol: Tramadol's risk of seizures may be increased with TCAs (carbamazepine may be associated with similar risk due to chemical similarity to TCAs).

Tricyclic antidepressants: May increase serum concentrations of carbamazepine; carbamazepine may decrease concentrations of tricyclics due to enzyme induction.

Valproic acid: Serum levels may be reduced by carbamazepine; carbamazepine levels may also be altered by valproic acid.

Warfarin: Carbamazepine may inhibit the hypoprothrombinemic effects of oral anticoagulants via increased metabolism; this combination should generally be avoided.

Ethanol/Nutrition/Herb Interactions

Ethanol: Avoid ethanol (may increase CNS depression).

(Continued)

Carbamazepine *(Continued)*

Food: Carbamazepine serum levels may be increased if taken with food. Carbamazepine serum concentration may be increased if taken with grapefruit juice; avoid concurrent use.

Herb/Nutraceutical: Avoid evening primrose (seizure threshold decreased). Avoid valerian, St John's wort, kava kava, gotu kola (may increase CNS depression).

Test Interactions May interact with some pregnancy tests; increased BUN, AST, ALT, bilirubin, alkaline phosphatase (S); decreased calcium, T_3, T_4, sodium (S)

Dietary Considerations Drug may cause GI upset, take with large amount of water or food to decrease GI upset. May need to split doses to avoid GI upset.

Dosage Forms

Capsule, extended release (Carbatrol®, Equetro™): 100 mg, 200 mg, 300 mg
Suspension, oral: 100 mg/5 mL (10 mL, 450 mL)
  Tegretol®: 100 mg/5 mL (450 mL) [citrus vanilla flavor]
Tablet (Epitol®, Tegretol®): 200 mg
Tablet, chewable (Tegretol®): 100 mg
Tablet, extended release (Tegretol®-XR): 100 mg, 200 mg, 400 mg

- **Carbamylcholine Chloride** *see* Carbachol *on page 224*
- **Carbastat® [DSC]** *see* Carbachol *on page 224*
- **Carbatrol®** *see* Carbamazepine *on page 225*
- **Carbidopa and Levodopa** *see* Levodopa and Carbidopa *on page 743*
- **Carbocaine®** *see* Mepivacaine *on page 804*
- **Carbolic Acid** *see* Phenol *on page 1012*
- **Carbolith™ (Can)** *see* Lithium *on page 770*
- **Carbose D** *see* Carboxymethylcellulose *on page 230*

Carboxymethylcellulose (kar boks ee meth il SEL yoo lose)

U.S. Brand Names Refresh Liquigel™ [OTC]; Refresh Plus® [OTC]; Refresh Tears® [OTC]; Tears Again® Gel Drops™ [OTC]; Tears Again® Night and Day™ [OTC]; Theratears®

Canadian Brand Names Celluvisc™; Refresh Plus®; Refresh Tears®

Synonyms Carbose D; Carboxymethylcellulose Sodium

Pharmacologic Category Ophthalmic Agent, Miscellaneous

Generic Available Yes

Use Artificial tear substitute

Dosage Ophthalmic: Adults: Instill 1-2 drops into eye(s) 3-4 times/day

Dosage Forms

Gel, ophthalmic, as sodium (Tears Again® Night and Day™): 1.5% (3.5 g)
Solution ophthalmic, as sodium:
  Refresh Liquigel™: 1% (15 mL) [liquid gel formulation]
  Refresh Plus® preservative free: 0.5% (0.4 mL) [available in packages of 30 or 50]
  Refresh Tears®: 0.5% (15 mL)
  Tears Again® Gel Drops™: 0.7% (15 mL)
  Theratears®: 0.25% (0.6 mL [preservative free], 15 mL)

- **Carboxymethylcellulose Sodium** *see* Carboxymethylcellulose *on page 230*
- **Cardene®** *see* NiCARdipine *on page 918*
- **Cardene® I.V.** *see* NiCARdipine *on page 918*
- **Cardene® SR** *see* NiCARdipine *on page 918*
- **Cardizem®** *see* Diltiazem *on page 394*
- **Cardizem® CD** *see* Diltiazem *on page 394*
- **Cardizem® LA** *see* Diltiazem *on page 394*
- **Cardizem® SR [DSC]** *see* Diltiazem *on page 394*
- **Cardura®** *see* Doxazosin *on page 420*
- **Cardura-1™ (Can)** *see* Doxazosin *on page 420*
- **Cardura-2™ (Can)** *see* Doxazosin *on page 420*
- **Cardura-4™ (Can)** *see* Doxazosin *on page 420*
- **Cardura® XL** *see* Doxazosin *on page 420*
- **Carimune™ NF** *see* Immune Globulin (Intravenous) *on page 666*
- **Cartia XT™** *see* Diltiazem *on page 394*

Carvedilol (KAR ve dil ole)

Medication Safety Issues

Sound-alike/look-alike issues:

Carvedilol may be confused with captopril, carteolol

Related Information

Antiarrhythmic Drugs *on page 1548*
Beta-Blockers *on page 1557*
Heart Failure (Systolic) *on page 1607*
Preoperative Evaluation of the Cardiac Patient for Noncardiac Surgery *on page 1485*

U.S. Brand Names Coreg®

Canadian Brand Names Apo-Carvedilol®; Coreg®; Novo-Carvedilol; PMS-Carvedilol; RAN™-Carvedilol; ratio-Carvedilol

Pharmacologic Category Beta Blocker With Alpha-Blocking Activity

Generic Available No

Use Mild-to-severe heart failure of ischemic or cardiomyopathic origin (usually in addition to standardized therapy); left ventricular dysfunction following myocardial infarction (MI); management of hypertension

Unlabeled/Investigational Use Angina pectoris

Mechanism of Action As a racemic mixture, carvedilol has nonselective beta-adrenoreceptor and alpha-adrenergic blocking activity. No intrinsic sympathomimetic activity has been documented. Associated effects in hypertensive patients include reduction of cardiac output, exercise- or beta agonist-induced tachycardia, reduction of reflex orthostatic tachycardia, vasodilation, decreased peripheral vascular resistance (especially in standing position), decreased renal vascular resistance, reduced plasma renin activity, and increased levels of atrial natriuretic peptide. In CHF, associated effects include decreased pulmonary capillary wedge pressure, decreased pulmonary artery pressure, decreased heart rate, decreased systemic vascular resistance, increased stroke volume index, and decreased right arterial pressure (RAP).

Pharmacodynamics/Kinetics

Onset of action: 1-2 hours

Peak antihypertensive effect: ~1-2 hours

Absorption: Rapid; food decreases rate but not extent of absorption; administration with food minimizes risks of orthostatic hypotension

Distribution: V_d: 115 L

Protein binding: >98%, primarily to albumin

Metabolism: Extensively hepatic, via **CYP2C9, 2D6,** 3A4, and 2C19 (2% excreted unchanged); three active metabolites (4-hydroxyphenyl metabolite is 13 times more potent than parent drug for beta-blockade); first-pass effect; plasma concentrations in the elderly and those with cirrhotic liver disease are 50% and 4-7 times higher, respectively

Bioavailability: 25% to 35%

Half-life elimination: 7-10 hours

Excretion: Primarily feces

Dosage Oral: Adults: Reduce dosage if heart rate drops to <55 beats/minute.

Hypertension: 6.25 mg twice daily; if tolerated, dose should be maintained for 1-2 weeks, then increased to 12.5 mg twice daily. Dosage may be increased to a maximum of 25 mg twice daily after 1-2 weeks. Maximum dose: 50 mg/day.

Congestive heart failure: 3.125 mg twice daily for 2 weeks; if this dose is tolerated, may increase to 6.25 mg twice daily. Double the dose every 2 weeks to the highest dose tolerated by patient. (Prior to initiating therapy, other heart failure medications should be stabilized and fluid retention minimized.)

Maximum recommended dose:

Mild-to-moderate heart failure:

<85 kg: 25 mg twice daily

>85 kg: 50 mg twice daily

Severe heart failure: 25 mg twice daily

Left ventricular dysfunction following MI: Initial 3.125-6.25 mg twice daily; increase dosage incrementally (ie, from 6.25-12.5 mg twice daily) at intervals of 3-10 days, based on tolerance, to a target dose of 25 mg twice daily. **Note**: Should be initiated only after patient is hemodynamically stable and fluid retention has been minimized.

Angina pectoris (unlabeled use): 25-50 mg twice daily

Dosing adjustment in renal impairment: None necessary

(Continued)

Carvedilol *(Continued)*

Dosing adjustment in hepatic impairment: Use is contraindicated in severe liver dysfunction.

Stability Store at 30°C (86°F).

Administration Administer with food.

Monitoring Parameters Heart rate, blood pressure (base need for dosage increase on trough blood pressure measurements and for tolerance on standing systolic pressure 1 hour after dosing); renal studies, BUN, liver function; in patient with increase risk for developing renal dysfunction, monitor during dosage titration.

Anesthesia and Critical Care Concerns/Other Considerations

Withdrawal: Beta-blocker therapy should not be withdrawn abruptly, but gradually tapered to avoid acute tachycardia and hypertension.

Heart Failure: Carvedilol is a nonselective beta-blocker with alpha-blocking and antioxidant properties.

Pregnancy Risk Factor C (manufacturer); D (2nd and 3rd trimesters - expert analysis)

Contraindications Hypersensitivity to carvedilol or any component of the formulation; patients with decompensated cardiac failure requiring intravenous inotropic therapy; bronchial asthma or related bronchospastic conditions; second- or third-degree AV block, sick sinus syndrome, and severe bradycardia (except in patients with a functioning artificial pacemaker); cardiogenic shock; severe hepatic impairment; pregnancy (2nd and 3rd trimesters)

Warnings/Precautions Initiate cautiously and monitor for possible deterioration in patient status (including symptoms of CHF). Adjustment of other medications (ACE inhibitors and/or diuretics) may be required. In severe chronic heart failure, trial patients were excluded if they had cardiac-related rales, ascites, or a serum creatinine >2.8 mg/dL. Congestive heart failure patients may experience a worsening of renal function; risks include ischemic disease, diffuse vascular disease, underlying renal dysfunction; systolic BP <100 mm Hg. Patients should be advised to avoid driving or other hazardous tasks during initiation of therapy due to the risk of syncope. Avoid abrupt discontinuation (may exacerbate underlying condition), particularly in patients with coronary artery disease; dose should be tapered over 1-2 weeks with close monitoring.

Manufacturer recommends discontinuation of therapy if liver injury occurs (confirmed by laboratory testing). Use caution in patients with PVD (can aggravate arterial insufficiency). Use caution with concurrent use of verapamil or diltiazem; bradycardia or heart block can occur. Use caution in patients with bronchospastic disease. Use cautiously in diabetics because it can mask prominent hypoglycemic symptoms. May mask signs of thyrotoxicosis. Use care with anesthetic agents that decrease myocardial function. Safety and efficacy in children <18 years of age have not been established.

Adverse Reactions Note: Frequency ranges include data from hypertension and heart failure trials. Higher rates of adverse reactions have generally been noted in patients with CHF. However, the frequency of adverse effects associated with placebo is also increased in this population. Events occurring at a frequency > placebo in clinical trials.

>10%:

- Cardiovascular: Hypotension (9% to 20%)
- Central nervous system: Dizziness (6% to 32%), fatigue (4% to 24%)
- Endocrine & metabolic: Hyperglycemia (5% to 12%), weight gain (10% to 12%)
- Gastrointestinal: Diarrhea (2% to 12%)
- Neuromuscular & skeletal: Weakness (11%)

1% to 10%:

- Cardiovascular: Bradycardia (2% to 10%), hypertension (3%), AV block (3%), angina (2% to 6%), postural hypotension (2%), syncope (3% to 8%), dependent edema (4%), palpitation, peripheral edema (1% to 7%), generalized edema (5% to 6%)
- Central nervous system: Headache (5% to 8%), fever (3%), paresthesia (2%), somnolence (2%), insomnia (2%), malaise, hypoesthesia, vertigo
- Endocrine & metabolic: Alkaline phosphatase increased, gout (6%), hypercholesterolemia (4%), dehydration (2%), hyperkalemia (3%), hypervolemia (2%), hypertriglyceridemia (1%), hyperuricemia, hypoglycemia, hyponatremia
- Gastrointestinal: Nausea (4% to 9%), vomiting (6%), melena, periodontitis

Genitourinary: Hematuria (3%), impotence
Hematologic: Thrombocytopenia (1% to 2%), prothrombin decreased, purpura
Hepatic: Transaminases increased
Neuromuscular & skeletal: Back pain (2% to 7%), arthralgia (6%), myalgia (3%), muscle cramps
Ocular: Blurred vision (3% to 5%), lacrimation
Renal: BUN increased (6%), renal function abnormal, albuminuria, glycosuria, creatinine increased (3%), kidney failure
Respiratory: Rhinitis (2%), cough increased (5%)
Miscellaneous: Injury (3% to 6%), allergy, sudden death

<1% (Limited to important or life-threatening): Aggravated depression, anaphylactoid reaction, anemia, aplastic anemia (rare, all events occurred in patients receiving other medications capable of causing this effect); asthma, AV block (complete), bronchospasm, bundle branch block, cholestatic jaundice, convulsion, diabetes mellitus, erythema multiforme, exfoliative dermatitis, GI hemorrhage, interstitial pneumonitis, leukopenia, migraine, myocardial ischemia, neuralgia, pancytopenia, peripheral ischemia, pulmonary edema, Stevens-Johnson syndrome, toxic epidermal necrolysis, urinary incontinence

Overdosage/Toxicology Symptoms of intoxication include cardiac disturbances, CNS toxicity, bronchospasm, hypoglycemia, and hyperkalemia. The most common cardiac symptoms include hypotension and bradycardia. Atrioventricular block, intraventricular conduction disturbances, cardiogenic shock, and asystole may occur with severe overdose, especially with membrane-depressant drugs (eg, propranolol). CNS effects include convulsions, coma, and respiratory arrest (commonly seen with propranolol and other membrane-depressant and lipid-soluble drugs). Treatment is symptom-directed and supportive. Carvedilol does not appear to be significantly cleared by hemodialysis.

Drug Interactions Substrate of CYP1A2 (minor), 2C9 (major), 2D6 (major), 2E1 (minor), 3A4 (minor)

Alpha-blockers (prazosin, terazosin): Concurrent use of beta-blockers may increase risk of orthostasis.
Beta-agonists: Beta-blockers may counteract desired effects of beta-agonists.
Calcium channel blockers (nondihydropyridine): May enhance hypotensive effects of beta-blockers.
Cimetidine: May increase carvedilol serum levels.
CYP2C9 inducers: May decrease the levels/effects of carvedilol. Example inducers include carbamazepine, phenobarbital, phenytoin, rifampin, rifapentine, and secobarbital.
CYP2C9 Inhibitors may increase the levels/effects of carvedilol. Example inhibitors include delavirdine, fluconazole, gemfibrozil, ketoconazole, nicardipine, NSAIDs, sulfonamides and tolbutamide.
CYP2D6 inhibitors: May increase the levels/effects of carvedilol. Example inhibitors include chlorpromazine, delavirdine, fluoxetine, miconazole, paroxetine, pergolide, quinidine, quinine, ritonavir, and ropinirole.
Digoxin: Carvedilol may increase the serum levels of digoxin.
Disopyramide: May exacerbate heart failure or enhance bradycardic effect of beta-blockers.
Drugs which slow AV conduction (digoxin): Effects may be additive with beta-blockers.
Insulin and oral hypoglycemics: Carvedilol may mask symptoms of hypoglycemia.
NSAIDs (ibuprofen, indomethacin, naproxen, piroxicam) may reduce the antihypertensive effects of beta-blockers.
Rifampin: May increase the metabolism of carvedilol.
Salicylates: May reduce the antihypertensive effects of beta-blockers.
SSRIs: May decrease the metabolism of carvedilol.
Sulfonylureas: Beta-blockers may alter response to hypoglycemic agents.
Verapamil, diltiazem: May have synergistic or additive pharmacological effects when taken concurrently with beta-blockers.

Ethanol/Nutrition/Herb Interactions Herb/Nutraceutical: Avoid dong quai if using for hypertension (has estrogenic activity). Avoid ephedra, yohimbe, ginseng (may worsen hypertension). Avoid garlic (may have increased antihypertensive effect).

Test Interactions Increased hepatic enzymes, BUN, NPN, alkaline phosphatase; decreased HDL

Dietary Considerations Should be taken with food to minimize the risk of orthostatic hypotension.

Dosage Forms Tablet: 3.125 mg, 6.25 mg, 12.5 mg, 25 mg

Caspofungin (kas poe FUN jin)

U.S. Brand Names Cancidas®
Canadian Brand Names Cancidas®
Synonyms Caspofungin Acetate
Pharmacologic Category Antifungal Agent, Parenteral; Echinocandin
Generic Available No

Use Treatment of invasive *Aspergillus* infections in patients who are refractory or intolerant of other therapy; treatment of candidemia and other *Candida* infections (intra-abdominal abscesses, esophageal, peritonitis, pleural space); empirical treatment for presumed fungal infections in febrile neutropenic patient

Mechanism of Action Inhibits synthesis of β(1,3)-D-glucan, an essential component of the cell wall of susceptible fungi. Highest activity in regions of active cell growth. Mammalian cells do not require β(1,3)-D-glucan, limiting potential toxicity.

Pharmacodynamics/Kinetics

Protein binding: 97% to albumin

Metabolism: Slowly, via hydrolysis and *N*-acetylation as well as by spontaneous degradation, with subsequent metabolism to component amino acids. Overall metabolism is extensive.

Half-life elimination: Beta (distribution): 9-11 hours; Terminal: 40-50 hours

Excretion: Urine (41% as metabolites, 1% to 9% unchanged) and feces (35% as metabolites)

Dosage I.V.:

Children: Safety and efficacy in pediatric patients have not been established

Adults: **Note:** Duration of caspofungin treatment should be determined by patient status and clinical response. Empiric therapy should be given until neutropenia resolves. In patients with positive cultures, treatment should continue until 14 days after last positive culture. In neutropenic patients, treatment should be given at least 7 days after both signs and symptoms of infection **and** neutropenia resolve.

Empiric therapy: Initial dose: 70 mg on day 1; subsequent dosing: 50 mg/day; may increase up to 70 mg/day if tolerated, but clinical response is inadequate

Invasive *Aspergillus*, candidiasis: Initial dose: 70 mg on day 1; subsequent dosing: 50 mg/day

Esophageal candidiasis: 50 mg/day; **Note:** The majority of patients studied for this indication also had oropharyngeal involvement.

Concomitant use of an enzyme inducer:

Patients receiving rifampin: 70 mg caspofungin daily

Patients receiving carbamazepine, dexamethasone, efavirenz, nevirapine, **or** phenytoin (and possibly other enzyme inducers) may require an increased daily dose of caspofungin (70 mg/day).

Elderly: The number of patients >65 years of age in clinical studies was not sufficient to establish whether a difference in response may be anticipated.

Dosage adjustment in renal impairment: No specific dosage adjustment is required; supplemental dose is not required following dialysis

Dosage adjustment in hepatic impairment:

Mild hepatic insufficiency (Child-Pugh score 5-6): No adjustment necessary

Moderate hepatic insufficiency (Child-Pugh score 7-9): 35 mg/day; initial 70 mg loading dose should still be administered in treatment of invasive infections

Severe hepatic insufficiency (Child-Pugh score >9): No clinical experience

Stability Store vials at 2°C to 8°C (36°F to 46°F). Reconstituted solution may be stored at less than 25°C (77°F) for 1 hour prior to preparation of infusion solution. Infusion solutions may be stored at less than 25°C (77°F) and should be used within 24 hours; up to 48 hours if stored at 2°C to 8°C (36°F to 46°F).

Bring refrigerated vial to room temperature. Reconstitute vials using 0.9% sodium chloride for injection, SWFI, or bacteriostatic water for injection. Mix gently until clear solution is formed; do not use if cloudy or contains particles. Solution should be further diluted with 0.9%, 0.45%, or 0.225% sodium chloride or LR. Do not mix with dextrose-containing solutions. Do not coadminister with other medications.

Administration Infuse slowly, over 1 hour; monitor during infusion. Isolated cases of possible histamine-related reactions have occurred during clinical trials (rash, flushing, pruritus, facial edema).

Pregnancy Risk Factor C

Contraindications Hypersensitivity to caspofungin or any component of the formulation

Warnings/Precautions Concurrent use of cyclosporine should be limited to patients for whom benefit outweighs risk, due to a high frequency of hepatic transaminase elevations observed during concurrent use. Limited data are available concerning treatment durations longer than 4 weeks; however, treatment appears to be well tolerated. Use caution in hepatic impairment; dosage reduction required in moderate impairment. Safety and efficacy in pediatric patients have not been established.

Adverse Reactions

>10%:

Central nervous system: Headache (up to 11%), fever (3% to 26%), chills (up to 14%)

Endocrine & metabolic: Hypokalemia (4% to 11%)

Hematologic: Hemoglobin decreased (1% to 12%)

Hepatic: Serum alkaline phosphatase increased (3% to 11%), transaminases increased (up to 13%)

Local: Infusion site reactions (2% to 12%), phlebitis/thrombophlebitis (up to 16%)

1% to 10%:

Cardiovascular: Flushing (2% to 3%), facial edema (up to 3%), hypertension (1% to 2%), tachycardia (1% to 2%), hypotension (1%)

Central nervous system: Dizziness (2%), pain (1% to 5%), insomnia (1%)

Dermatologic: Rash (<1% to 6%), pruritus (1% to 3%), erythema (1% to 2%)

Gastrointestinal: Nausea (2% to 6%), vomiting (1% to 4%), abdominal pain (1% to 4%), diarrhea (1% to 4%), anorexia (1%)

Hematologic: Eosinophils increased (3%), neutrophils decreased (2% to 3%), WBC decreased (5% to 6%), anemia (up to 4%), platelet count decreased (2% to 3%)

Hepatic: Bilirubin increased (3%)

Local: Induration (up to 3%)

Neuromuscular & skeletal: Myalgia (up to 3%), paresthesia (1% to 3%), tremor (≤2%)

Renal: Nephrotoxicity (8%)*, proteinuria (5%), hematuria (2%), serum creatinine increased (<1% to 4%), urinary WBCs increased (up to 8%), urinary RBCs increased (1% to 4%), blood urea nitrogen increased (1%)

*Nephrotoxicity defined as serum creatinine ≥2x baseline value or ≥1 mg/dL in patients with serum creatinine above ULN range (patients with Cl_{cr} <30 mL/minute were excluded)

Miscellaneous: Flu-like syndrome (3%), diaphoresis (up to 3%)

<1% (Limited to important or life-threatening): Adult respiratory distress syndrome (ARDS), anaphylaxis, hepatic dysfunction, pulmonary edema, renal insufficiency; histamine-mediated reaction (including facial swelling, bronchospasm, sensation of warmth) have been reported

Overdosage/Toxicology No experience with overdosage has been reported. Caspofungin is not dialyzable. Treatment is symptomatic and supportive.

Drug Interactions

Cyclosporine: Concurrent administration may increase caspofungin concentrations. Serum hepatic transaminases may be increased. Limit use to patients for whom benefit outweighs risk.

Rifampin: May decrease caspofungin concentrations. Caspofungin dose should be 70 mg daily during concomitant therapy.

Tacrolimus: Caspofungin may decrease blood concentrations of tacrolimus; monitor.

Dosage Forms Injection, powder for reconstitution, as acetate: 50 mg [contains sucrose 39 mg], 70 mg [contains sucrose 54 mg]

References

Mora-Duarte J, Betts R, Rotstein C, et al, "Comparison of Caspofungin and Amphotericin B for Invasive Candidiasis," *N Engl J Med*, 2002, 347(25):2020-9.

- **Caspofungin Acetate** *see* Caspofungin *on page 234*
- **Castellani Paint Modified [OTC]** *see* Phenol *on page 1012*
- **Cataflam®** *see* Diclofenac *on page 378*
- **Catapres®** *see* Clonidine *on page 316*
- **Catapres-TTS®** *see* Clonidine *on page 316*
- **Cathflo® Activase®** *see* Alteplase *on page 72*
- **Caverject®** *see* Alprostadil *on page 68*
- **Caverject Impulse®** *see* Alprostadil *on page 68*
- **CBZ** *see* Carbamazepine *on page 225*

♦ **CEE** *see* Estrogens (Conjugated/Equine) *on page 488*

Cefazolin (sef A zoe lin)

Medication Safety Issues

Sound-alike/look-alike issues:

Cefazolin may be confused with cefprozil, cephalexin, cephalothin

Kefzol® may be confused with Cefzil®

Related Information

Anesthesia for Patients With Liver Disease *on page 1421*
Prevention of Bacterial Endocarditis *on page 1583*
Prevention of Wound Infection and Sepsis in Surgical Patients *on page 1588*

U.S. Brand Names Ancef®

Synonyms Cefazolin Sodium

Pharmacologic Category Antibiotic, Cephalosporin (First Generation)

Generic Available Yes

Use Treatment of respiratory tract, skin and skin structure, genital, urinary tract, biliary tract, bone and joint infections, and septicemia due to susceptible gram-positive cocci (except enterococcus); some gram-negative bacilli including *E. coli*, *Proteus*, and *Klebsiella* may be susceptible; perioperative prophylaxis

Unlabeled/Investigational Use Prophylaxis against bacterial endocarditis

Mechanism of Action Inhibits bacterial cell wall synthesis by binding to one or more of the penicillin-binding proteins (PBPs) which in turn inhibits the final transpeptidation step of peptidoglycan synthesis in bacterial cell walls, thus inhibiting cell wall biosynthesis. Bacteria eventually lyse due to ongoing activity of cell wall autolytic enzymes (autolysins and murein hydrolases) while cell wall assembly is arrested.

Pharmacodynamics/Kinetics

Distribution: Widely into most body tissues and fluids including gallbladder, liver, kidneys, bone, sputum, bile, pleural, and synovial; CSF penetration is poor; crosses placenta; enters breast milk

Protein binding: 74% to 86%

Metabolism: Minimally hepatic

Half-life elimination: 90-150 minutes; prolonged with renal impairment

Time to peak, serum: I.M.: 0.5-2 hours

Excretion: Urine (80% to 100% as unchanged drug)

Dosage

Usual dosage range: I.M., I.V.:

Children >1 month: 25-100 mg/kg/day divided every 6-8 hours; maximum: 6 g/day

Adults: 250 mg to 2 g every 6-12 (usually 8) hours, depending on severity of infection; maximum dose: 12 g/day

Indication-specific dosing:

Prophylaxis against bacterial endocarditis (unlabeled use):

Infants and Children: 25 mg/kg 30 minutes before procedure; maximum dose: 1 g

Adults: 1 g 30 minutes before procedure

Mild-to-moderate infections: Adults: 500 mg to 1 g every 6-8 hours

Mild infection with gram-positive cocci: Adults: 250-500 mg every 8 hours

Perioperative prophylaxis: Adults: 1 g given 30 minutes prior to surgery (repeat with 500 mg to 1 g during prolonged surgery); followed by 500 mg to 1 g every 6-9 hours for 24 hours postop

Pneumococcal pneumonia: Adults: 500 mg every 12 hours

Severe infection: Adults: 1-2 g every 6 hours

Prophylaxis against bacterial endocarditis (unlabeled use): Adults: 1 g 30 minutes before procedure

UTI (uncomplicated): Adults: 1 g every 12 hours

Dosing adjustment in renal impairment:

Cl_{cr} 10-30 mL/minute: Administer every 12 hours

Cl_{cr} <10 mL/minute: Administer every 24 hours

Hemodialysis: Moderately dialyzable (20% to 50%); administer dose postdialysis or administer supplemental dose of 0.5-1 g after dialysis

Peritoneal dialysis: Administer 0.5 g every 12 hours

Continuous arteriovenous or venovenous hemofiltration: Dose as for Cl_{cr} 10-30 mL/minute; removes 30 mg of cefazolin per liter of filtrate per day

Stability Store intact vials at room temperature and protect from temperatures exceeding 40°C. Dilute large vial with 2.5 mL SWFI; 10 g vial may be diluted with 45 mL to yield 1 g/5 mL or 96 mL to yield 1 g/10 mL. May be injected or further dilution for I.V. administration in 50-100 mL compatible solution. Standard diluent is 1 g/50 mL D_5W or 2 g/50 mL D_5W.

Reconstituted solutions of cefazolin are light yellow to yellow. Protection from light is recommended for the powder and for the reconstituted solutions. Reconstituted solutions are stable for 24 hours at room temperature and for 10 days under refrigeration. Stability of parenteral admixture at room temperature (25°C) is 48 hours. Stability of parenteral admixture at refrigeration temperature (4°C) is 14 days.

DUPLEX™: Store at 20°C to 25°C (68°F to 77°F); excursions permitted to 15°C to 30°C (59°F to 86°F) prior to activation. Following activation, stable for 24 hours at room temperature and for 7 days under refrigeration.

Administration

I.M.: Inject deep I.M. into large muscle mass.

I.V.: Inject direct I.V. over 5 minutes. Infuse intermittent infusion over 30-60 minutes.

Some penicillins (eg, carbenicillin, ticarcillin and piperacillin) have been shown to inactivate aminoglycosides *in vitro*. This has been observed to a greater extent with tobramycin and gentamicin, while amikacin has shown greater stability against inactivation. Concurrent use of these agents may pose a risk of reduced antibacterial efficacy *in vivo*, particularly in the setting of profound renal impairment. However, definitive clinical evidence is lacking. If combination penicillin/aminoglycoside therapy is desired in a patient with renal dysfunction, separation of doses (if feasible), and routine monitoring of aminoglycoside levels, CBC, and clinical response should be considered.

Monitoring Parameters Renal function periodically when used in combination with other nephrotoxic drugs, hepatic function tests, CBC; monitor for signs of anaphylaxis during first dose

Pregnancy Risk Factor B

Contraindications Hypersensitivity to cefazolin sodium, any component of the formulation, or other cephalosporins

Warnings/Precautions Modify dosage in patients with severe renal impairment. Prolonged use may result in superinfection. Use with caution in patients with a history of penicillin allergy, especially IgE-mediated reactions (eg, anaphylaxis, angioedema, urticaria). May cause antibiotic-associated colitis or colitis secondary to *C. difficile*.

Adverse Reactions Frequency not defined.

Central nervous system: Fever, seizure

Dermatologic: Rash, pruritus, Stevens-Johnson syndrome

Gastrointestinal: Diarrhea, nausea, vomiting, abdominal cramps, anorexia, pseudomembranous colitis, oral candidiasis

Genitourinary: Vaginitis

Hepatic: Transaminases increased, hepatitis

Hematologic: Eosinophilia, neutropenia, leukopenia, thrombocytopenia, thrombocytosis

Local: Pain at injection site, phlebitis

Renal: BUN increased, serum creatinine increased, renal failure

Miscellaneous: Anaphylaxis

Reactions reported with other cephalosporins: Toxic epidermal necrolysis, abdominal pain, cholestasis, superinfection, toxic nephropathy, aplastic anemia, hemolytic anemia, hemorrhage, prothrombin time prolonged, pancytopenia

Overdosage/Toxicology Symptoms of overdose include neuromuscular hypersensitivity and convulsions. Many beta-lactam containing antibiotics have the potential to cause neuromuscular hyperirritability or convulsive seizures. Hemodialysis may be helpful to aid in the removal of drug from blood; otherwise, treatment is supportive or symptom-directed.

Drug Interactions

Aminoglycosides: Aminoglycosides increase nephrotoxic potential.

Probenecid: High-dose probenecid decreases clearance.

Warfarin: Cefazolin may increase the hypothrombinemic response to warfarin (due to alteration of GI microbial flora).

(Continued)

Cefazolin *(Continued)*

Test Interactions Positive direct Coombs', false-positive urinary glucose test using cupric sulfate (Benedict's solution, Clinitest®, Fehling's solution), false-positive serum or urine creatinine with Jaffé reaction.

Some penicillin derivatives may accelerate the degradation of aminoglycosides *in vitro*, leading to a potential underestimation of aminoglycoside serum concentration.

Dietary Considerations Sodium content of 1 g: 48 mg (2 mEq)

Dosage Forms [DSC] = Discontinued product

Infusion [premixed in D_5W]: 500 mg (50 mL); 1 g (50 mL)

Injection, powder for reconstitution: 500 mg, 1 g, 10 g, 20 g

Ancef®: 1 g; 10 g [DSC]

References

"Antimicrobial Prophylaxis for Surgery," *Treat Guidel Med Lett*, 2004, 2(20):27-32.

Dajani AS, Taubert KA, Wilson WW, et al, "Prevention of Bacterial Endocarditis. Recommendations by the American Heart Association," *JAMA*, 1997, 277(22):1794-801.

Gentry LO, Zeluff BJ, and Cooley DA, "Antibiotic Prophylaxis in Open-Heart Surgery: A Comparison of Cefamandole, Cefuroxime, and Cefazolin," *Ann Thorac Surg*, 1988, 46(2):167-71.

♦ **Cefazolin Sodium** *see* Cefazolin *on page 236*

Cefepime (SEF e pim)

U.S. Brand Names Maxipime®

Canadian Brand Names Maxipime®

Synonyms Cefepime Hydrochloride

Pharmacologic Category Antibiotic, Cephalosporin (Fourth Generation)

Generic Available No

Use Treatment of uncomplicated and complicated urinary tract infections, including pyelonephritis caused by typical urinary tract pathogens; monotherapy for febrile neutropenia; uncomplicated skin and skin structure infections caused by *Streptococcus pyogenes*; moderate-to-severe pneumonia caused by pneumococcus, *Pseudomonas aeruginosa*, and other gram-negative organisms; complicated intra-abdominal infections (in combination with metronidazole). Also active against methicillin-susceptible staphylococci, *Enterobacter* sp, and many other gram-negative bacilli.

Children 2 months to 16 years: Empiric therapy of febrile neutropenia patients, uncomplicated skin/soft tissue infections, pneumonia, and uncomplicated/complicated urinary tract infections.

Mechanism of Action Inhibits bacterial cell wall synthesis by binding to one or more of the penicillin-binding proteins (PBPs) which in turn inhibits the final transpeptidation step of peptidoglycan synthesis in bacterial cell walls, thus inhibiting cell wall biosynthesis. Bacteria eventually lyse due to ongoing activity of cell wall autolytic enzymes (autolysis and murein hydrolases) while cell wall assembly is arrested.

Pharmacodynamics/Kinetics

Absorption: I.M.: Rapid and complete

Distribution: V_d: Adults: 14-20 L; penetrates into inflammatory fluid at concentrations ~80% of serum levels and into bronchial mucosa at levels ~60% of those reached in the plasma; crosses blood-brain barrier

Protein binding, plasma: 16% to 19%

Metabolism: Minimally hepatic

Half-life elimination: 2 hours

Time to peak: 0.5-1.5 hours

Excretion: Urine (85% as unchanged drug)

Dosage

Usual dosage range:

Children: I.V.: 50 mg/kg every 8-12 hours

Adults: I.V.: 1-2 g every 6-12 hours

Indication-specific dosing:

Children >2 months: I.V.:

Febrile neutropenia: 50 mg/kg every 8 hours for 7-10 days

Uncomplicated skin/soft tissue infections, pneumonia, complicated/uncomplicated UTI: 50 mg/kg twice daily

Adults:

Brain abscess *(Pseudomonas)*, meningitis (postsurgical): I.V.: 2 g every 8 hours

Hospital"acquired pneumonia (HAP): I.V.: 1-2 g every 8-12 hours (American Thoracic Society/ATS guidelines)

Monotherapy for febrile neutropenic patients: I.V: 2 g every 8 hours for 7 days or until the neutropenia resolves

Otitis externa (malignant), pneumonia: I.V.: 2 g every 12 hours

Peritonitis (spontaneous): I.V.: 2 g every 12 hours with metronidazole

Septic lateral/cavernous sinus thrombosis: I.V.: 2 g every 6 hours; with metronidazole for lateral

Urinary tract infections (mild to moderate) I.M., I.V.: 500-1000 mg every 12 hours

Dosing adjustment in renal impairment: Adults: Recommended maintenance schedule based on creatinine clearance (mL/minute), compared to normal dosing schedule: See table.

Cefepime Hydrochloride

Creatinine Clearance (mL/minute)	Recommended Maintenance Schedule			
>60 Normal recommended dosing schedule	500 mg every 12 hours	1 g every 12 hours	2 g every 12 hours	2 g every 8 hours
30-60	500 mg every 24 hours	1 g every 24 hours	2 g every 24 hours	2 g every 12 hours
11-29	500 mg every 24 hours	500 mg every 24 hours	1 g every 24 hours	2 g every 24 hours
<11	250 mg every 24 hours	250 mg every 24 hours	500 mg every 24 hours	1 g every 24 hours

Hemodialysis: Initial: 1 g (single dose) on day 1. Maintenance: 500 mg once daily (1 g once daily in febrile neutropenic patients). Dosage should be administered after dialysis on dialysis days.

Peritoneal dialysis: Removed to a lesser extent than hemodialysis; administer 250 mg every 48 hours

Continuous arteriovenous or venovenous hemofiltration: Dose as normal Cl_{cr} (eg, >30 mL/minute)

Stability Cefepime is **compatible** and stable with normal saline, D_5W, and a variety of other solutions for 24 hours at room temperature and 7 days refrigerated

Administration May be administered either I.M. or I.V.

Monitoring Parameters Obtain specimen for culture and sensitivity prior to the first dose. Monitor for signs of anaphylaxis during first dose.

Pregnancy Risk Factor B

Contraindications Hypersensitivity to cefepime, any component of the formulation, or other cephalosporins

Warnings/Precautions Modify dosage in patients with severe renal impairment; prolonged use may result in superinfection; use with caution in patients with a history of penicillin or cephalosporin allergy, especially IgE-mediated reactions (eg, anaphylaxis, urticaria). May cause antibiotic-associated colitis or colitis secondary to *C. difficile*.

Adverse Reactions

>10%: Hematologic: Positive Coombs' test without hemolysis

1% to 10%:

Central nervous system: Fever (1%), headache (1%)

Dermatologic: Rash, pruritus

Gastrointestinal: Diarrhea, nausea, vomiting

Local: Pain, erythema at injection site

<1% (Limited to important or life-threatening): Agranulocytosis, anaphylactic shock, anaphylaxis, coma, encephalopathy, hallucinations, leukopenia, myoclonus, neuromuscular excitability, neutropenia, seizure, thrombocytopenia

Reactions reported with other cephalosporins: Aplastic anemia, erythema multiforme, hemolytic anemia, hemorrhage, pancytopenia, PT prolonged, renal dysfunction, Stevens-Johnson syndrome, superinfection, toxic epidermal necrolysis, toxic nephropathy, vaginitis

Overdosage/Toxicology Symptoms of overdose include neuromuscular hypersensitivity and CNS toxicity (including hallucinations, confusion, seizures, and coma). Many beta-lactam containing antibiotics have the potential to cause

(Continued)

Cefepime *(Continued)*

neuromuscular hyperirritability or convulsive seizures. Hemodialysis may be helpful to aid in removal of the drug from blood; otherwise, treatment is supportive and symptom-directed.

Drug Interactions

Increased effect: High-dose probenecid decreases clearance

Increased toxicity: Aminoglycosides increase nephrotoxic potential

Test Interactions Positive direct Coombs', false-positive urinary glucose test using cupric sulfate (Benedict's solution, Clinitest®, Fehling's solution), false-positive serum or urine creatinine with Jaffé reaction, false-positive urinary proteins and steroids

Dosage Forms Injection, powder for reconstitution, as hydrochloride: 500 mg, 1 g, 2 g

References

American Thoracic Society and Infectious Diseases Society of America, "Guidelines for the Management of Adults With Hospital-Acquired, Ventilator-Associated, and Healthcare-Associated Pneumonia," *Am J Respir Crit Care Med*, 2005, 171(4):388-416.

Tunkel AR, Hartman BJ, Kaplan SL, et al, "Practice Guidelines for the Management of Bacterial Meningitis," *Clin Infect Dis*, 2004, 39(9):1267-84.

◆ **Cefepime Hydrochloride** *see* Cefepime *on page 238*

◆ **Cefizox®** *see* Ceftizoxime *on page 248*

◆ **Cefotan® [DSC]** *see* Cefotetan *on page 242*

Cefotaxime (sef oh TAKS eem)

Medication Safety Issues

Sound-alike/look-alike issues:

Cefotaxime may be confused with cefoxitin, ceftizoxime, cefuroxime

U.S. Brand Names Claforan®

Canadian Brand Names Claforan®

Synonyms Cefotaxime Sodium

Pharmacologic Category Antibiotic, Cephalosporin (Third Generation)

Generic Available Yes: Powder

Use Treatment of susceptible infection in respiratory tract, skin and skin structure, bone and joint, urinary tract, gynecologic as well as septicemia, and documented or suspected meningitis. Active against most gram-negative bacilli (not *Pseudomonas*) and gram-positive cocci (not enterococcus). Active against many penicillin-resistant pneumococci.

Mechanism of Action Inhibits bacterial cell wall synthesis by binding to one or more of the penicillin-binding proteins (PBPs) which in turn inhibits the final transpeptidation step of peptidoglycan synthesis in bacterial cell walls, thus inhibiting cell wall biosynthesis. Bacteria eventually lyse due to ongoing activity of cell wall autolytic enzymes (autolysins and murein hydrolases) while cell wall assembly is arrested.

Pharmacodynamics/Kinetics

Distribution: Widely to body tissues and fluids including aqueous humor, ascitic and prostatic fluids, bone; penetrates CSF best when meninges are inflamed; crosses placenta; enters breast milk

Metabolism: Partially hepatic to active metabolite, desacetylcefotaxime

Half-life elimination:

Cefotaxime: Premature neonates <1 week: 5-6 hours; Full-term neonates <1 week: 2-3.4 hours; Adults: 1-1.5 hours; prolonged with renal and/or hepatic impairment

Desacetylcefotaxime: 1.5-1.9 hours; prolonged with renal impairment

Time to peak, serum: I.M.: Within 30 minutes

Excretion: Urine (as unchanged drug and metabolites)

Dosage

Usual dosage range:

Infants and Children 1 month to 12 years <50 kg: I.M., I.V.: 50-200 mg/kg/day in divided doses every 4-6 hours

Children >12 years and Adults: I.M., I.V.: 1-2 g every 4-12 hours

Indication-specific dosing:

Infants and Children 1 month to 12 years:

Epiglottitis: I.M., I.V.: 150-200 mg/kg/day in 4 divided doses with clindamycin for 7-10 days

Meningitis: I.M., I.V.: 200 mg/kg/day in divided doses every 6 hours

Pneumonia: I.V.: 200 mg/kg/day divided every 8 hours
Sepsis: I.V.: 150 mg/kg/day divided every 8 hours
Typhoid fever: I.M., I.V.: 150-200 mg/kg/day in 3-4 divided doses (maximum: 12 g/day); fluoroquinolone resistant: 80 mg/kg/day in 3-4 divided doses (maximum: 12 g/day)

Children >12 years and Adults:
Arthritis (septic): I.V.: 1 g every 8 hours
Brain abscess, meningitis: I.V.: 2 g every 4-6 hours
Caesarean section: I.M., I.V.: 1 g as soon as the umbilical cord is clamped, then 1 g at 6- and 12-hour intervals
Epiglottitis: I.V.: 2 g every 4-8 hours
Gonorrhea: I.M.: 1 g as a single dose
Disseminated: I.V.: 1 g every 8 hours
Life-threatening infections: I.V.: 2 g every 4 hours
Liver abscess: I.V.: 1-2 g every 6 hours
Lyme disease:
Cardiac manifestations: I.V.: 2 g every 4 hours
CNS manifestations: I.V.: 2 g every 8 hours for 14-28 days
Moderate-to-severe infections: I.M., I.V.: 1-2 g every 8 hours
Orbital cellulitis: I.V.: 2 g every 4 hours
Peritonitis (spontaneous): I.V.: 2 g every 8 hours, unless life-threatening then 2 g every 4 hours
Septicemia: I.V.: 2 g every 6-8 hours
Skin and soft tissue:
Mixed, necrotizing: I.V.: 2 g every 6 hours, with metronidazole or clindamycin
Bite wounds (animal): I.V.: 2 g every 6 hours
Surgical prophylaxis: I.M., I.V.: 1 g 30-90 minutes before surgery
Uncomplicated infections: I.M., I.V.: 1 g every 12 hours

Dosing interval in renal impairment:
Cl_{cr} 10-50 mL/minute: Administer every 8-12 hours
Cl_{cr} <10 mL/minute: Administer every 24 hours
Hemodialysis: Moderately dialyzable

Dosing adjustment in hepatic impairment: Moderate dosage reduction is recommended in severe liver disease

Continuous arteriovenous or venovenous hemodiafiltration effects: Administer 1 g every 12 hour

Stability Reconstituted solution is stable for 12-24 hours at room temperature and 7-10 days when refrigerated and for 13 weeks when frozen. For I.V. infusion in NS or D_5W, solution is stable for 24 hours at room temperature, 5 days when refrigerated, or 13 weeks when frozen in Viaflex® plastic containers. Thawed solutions previously of frozen premixed bags are stable for 24 hours at room temperature or 10 days when refrigerated.

Administration Can be administered IVP over 3-5 minutes or I.V. intermittent infusion over 15-30 minutes.

Monitoring Parameters Observe for signs and symptoms of anaphylaxis during first dose; CBC with differential (especially with long courses)

Pregnancy Risk Factor B

Contraindications Hypersensitivity to cefotaxime, any component of the formulation, or other cephalosporins

Warnings/Precautions Modify dosage in patients with severe renal impairment. Prolonged use may result in superinfection. A potentially life-threatening arrhythmia has been reported in patients who received a rapid bolus injection via central line. Use caution in patients with colitis. Minimize tissue inflammation by changing infusion sites when needed. Use with caution in patients with a history of penicillin allergy, especially IgE-mediated reactions (eg, anaphylaxis, urticaria). May cause antibiotic-associated colitis or colitis secondary to *C. difficile*.

Adverse Reactions

1% to 10%:
Dermatologic: Rash, pruritus
Gastrointestinal: Diarrhea, nausea, vomiting, colitis
Local: Pain at injection site

<1% (Limited to important or life-threatening): Anaphylaxis, arrhythmia (after rapid I.V. injection via central catheter), BUN increased, candidiasis, creatinine increased, eosinophilia, erythema multiforme, fever, headache, interstitial nephritis, neutropenia, phlebitis, pseudomembranous colitis, Stevens-Johnson

(Continued)

Cefotaxime *(Continued)*

syndrome, thrombocytopenia, transaminases increased, toxic epidermal necrolysis, urticaria, vaginitis

Reactions reported with other cephalosporins: Agranulocytosis, aplastic anemia, cholestasis, hemolytic anemia, hemorrhage, pancytopenia, renal dysfunction, seizure, superinfection, toxic nephropathy.

Overdosage/Toxicology Symptoms of overdose include neuromuscular hypersensitivity and convulsions. Many beta-lactam containing antibiotics have the potential to cause neuromuscular hyperirritability or convulsive seizures. Hemodialysis may be helpful to aid in removal of the drug from blood; otherwise, treatment is supportive or symptom-directed.

Drug Interactions

Increased effect: Probenecid may decrease cephalosporin elimination

Increased toxicity: Furosemide, aminoglycosides may be a possible additive to nephrotoxicity

Test Interactions Positive direct Coombs', false-positive urinary glucose test using cupric sulfate (Benedict's solution, Clinitest®, Fehling's solution), false-positive serum or urine creatinine with Jaffé reaction

Dietary Considerations Sodium content of 1 g: 50.5 mg (2.2 mEq)

Dosage Forms

Infusion, as sodium [premixed in D_5W]: 1 g (50 mL); 2 g (50 mL)

Injection, powder for reconstitution, as sodium: 500 mg, 1 g, 2 g, 10 g, 20 g

Claforan®: 500 mg, 1 g, 2 g, 10 g [contains sodium 50.5 mg (2.2 mEq) per cefotaxime 1 g]

References

Tunkel AR, Hartman BJ, Kaplan SL, et al, "Practice Guidelines for the Management of Bacterial Meningitis," *Clin Infect Dis*, 2004, 39(9):1267-84.

♦ **Cefotaxime Sodium** *see* Cefotaxime *on page 240*

Cefotetan (SEF oh tee tan)

Medication Safety Issues

Sound-alike/look-alike issues:

Cefotetan may be confused with cefoxitin, Ceftin®

Cefotan® may be confused with Ceftin®

Related Information

Anesthesia for Patients With Liver Disease *on page 1421*

Prevention of Wound Infection and Sepsis in Surgical Patients *on page 1588*

U.S. Brand Names Cefotan® [DSC]

Canadian Brand Names Cefotan®

Synonyms Cefotetan Disodium

Pharmacologic Category Antibiotic, Cephalosporin (Second Generation)

Generic Available No

Use Surgical prophylaxis; intra-abdominal infections and other mixed infections; respiratory tract, skin and skin structure, bone and joint, urinary tract and gynecologic as well as septicemia; active against gram-negative enteric bacilli including *E. coli*, *Klebsiella*, and *Proteus*; less active against staphylococci and streptococci than first generation cephalosporins, but active against anaerobes including *Bacteroides fragilis*

Mechanism of Action Inhibits bacterial cell wall synthesis by binding to one or more of the penicillin-binding proteins (PBPs) which in turn inhibits the final transpeptidation step of peptidoglycan synthesis in bacterial cell walls, thus inhibiting cell wall biosynthesis. Bacteria eventually lyse due to ongoing activity of cell wall autolytic enzymes (autolysins and murein hydrolases) while cell wall assembly is arrested.

Pharmacodynamics/Kinetics

Distribution: Widely to body tissues and fluids including bile, sputum, prostatic, peritoneal; low concentrations enter CSF; crosses placenta; enters breast milk

Protein binding: 76% to 90%

Half-life elimination: 3-5 hours

Time to peak, serum: I.M.: 1.5-3 hours

Excretion: Primarily urine (as unchanged drug); feces (20%)

Dosage

Usual dosage range:

Children (unlabeled use): I.M., I.V.: 20-40 mg/kg/dose every 12 hours (maximum: 6 g/day)

Adults: I.M., I.V.: 1-6 g/day in divided doses every 12 hours

Indication-specific dosing:

Children (unlabeled use):

Preoperative prophylaxis: I.M., I.V.: 40 mg/kg 30-60 minutes prior to surgery

Adolescents and Adults:

Pelvic inflammatory disease: I.V.: 2 g every 12 hours; used in combination with doxycycline

Adults:

Orbital cellulitis, odontogenic infections: I.V.: 2 g every 12 hours

Preoperative prophylaxis: I.M., I.V.: 1-2 g 30-60 minutes prior to surgery; when used for cesarean section, dose should be given as soon as umbilical cord is clamped

Urinary tract infection: I.M., I.V.: 1-2 g may be given every 24 hours

Dosing interval in renal impairment:

Cl_{cr} 10-30 mL/minute: Administer every 24 hours

Cl_{cr} <10 mL/minute: Administer every 48 hours

Hemodialysis: Dialyzable (5% to 20%); administer 1/4 the usual dose every 24 hours on days between dialysis; administer 1/2 the usual dose on the day of dialysis.

Continuous arteriovenous or venovenous hemodiafiltration effects: Administer 750 mg every 12 hours

Stability Reconstituted solution is stable for 24 hours at room temperature and 96 hours when refrigerated. For I.V. infusion in NS or D_5W solution and after freezing, thawed solution is stable for 24 hours at room temperature or 96 hours when refrigerated. Frozen solution is stable for 12 weeks.

Administration

I.M.: Inject deep I.M. into large muscle mass.

I.V.: Inject direct I.V. over 3-5 minutes. Infuse intermittent infusion over 30 minutes.

Monitoring Parameters Observe for signs and symptoms of anaphylaxis during first dose; monitor for signs and symptoms of hemolytic anemia, including hematologic parameters where appropriate.

Pregnancy Risk Factor B

Contraindications Hypersensitivity to cefotetan, any component of the formulation, or other cephalosporins; previous cephalosporin-associated hemolytic anemia

Warnings/Precautions Modify dosage in patients with severe renal impairment. Prolonged use may result in superinfection. Although cefotetan contains the methyltetrazolethiol side chain, bleeding has not been a significant problem. Use with caution in patients with a history of penicillin allergy, especially IgE-mediated reactions (eg, anaphylaxis, urticaria). Cefotetan has been associated with a higher risk of hemolytic anemia relative to other cephalosporins (approximately threefold); monitor carefully during use and consider cephalosporin-associated immune anemia in patients who have received cefotetan within 2-3 weeks (either as treatment or prophylaxis). May cause antibiotic-associated colitis or colitis secondary to *C. difficile*.

Adverse Reactions

1% to 10%:

Gastrointestinal: Diarrhea (1%)

Hepatic: Transaminases increased (1%)

Miscellaneous: Hypersensitivity reactions (1%)

<1%: Anaphylaxis, urticaria, rash, pruritus, pseudomembranous colitis, nausea, vomiting, eosinophilia, thrombocytosis, agranulocytosis, hemolytic anemia, leukopenia, thrombocytopenia, prolonged PT, bleeding, BUN increased, creatinine increased, nephrotoxicity, phlebitis, fever

Reactions reported with other cephalosporins: Seizure, Stevens-Johnson syndrome, toxic epidermal necrolysis, renal dysfunction, toxic nephropathy, cholestasis, aplastic anemia, hemolytic anemia, hemorrhage, pancytopenia, agranulocytosis, colitis, superinfection

Overdosage/Toxicology Symptoms of overdose include neuromuscular hypersensitivity and convulsions. Many beta-lactam containing antibiotics have the

(Continued)

Cefotetan *(Continued)*

potential to cause neuromuscular hyperirritability or convulsive seizures. Hemodialysis may be helpful to aid in removal of the drug from blood; otherwise, treatment is supportive or symptom-directed.

Drug Interactions

Ethanol: Disulfiram-like reaction may occur if ethanol is consumed by a patient taking cefotetan.

Probenecid: May increase cefotetan plasma levels.

Warfarin: Cefotetan may increase risk of bleeding in patients receiving warfarin.

Ethanol/Nutrition/Herb Interactions Ethanol: Avoid ethanol (may cause a disulfiram-like reaction).

Test Interactions Positive direct Coombs', false-positive urinary glucose test using cupric sulfate (Benedict's solution, Clinitest®, Fehling's solution), false-positive serum or urine creatinine with Jaffé reaction

Dietary Considerations Contains sodium of 80 mg (3.5 mEq) per cefotetan 1 g

Dosage Forms [DSC] = Discontinued product

Infusion [premixed iso-osmotic solution]: 1 g (50 mL); 2 g (50 mL) [contains sodium 80 mg/g (3.5 mEq/g)] [DSC]

Injection, powder for reconstitution: 1 g, 2 g [contains sodium 80 mg/g (3.5 mEq/g)] [DSC]

References

"Antimicrobial Prophylaxis for Surgery," *Treat Guidel Med Lett*, 2004, 2(20):27-32.

Martin C, Thomachot L, and Albanese J, "Clinical Pharmacokinetics of Cefotetan," *Clin Pharmacokinet*, 1994, 26(4):248-58.

♦ **Cefotetan Disodium** *see* Cefotetan *on page 242*

Cefoxitin (se FOKS i tin)

Medication Safety Issues

Sound-alike/look-alike issues:

Cefoxitin may be confused with cefotaxime, cefotetan, Cytoxan®

Mefoxin® may be confused with Lanoxin®

Related Information

Anesthesia for Patients With Liver Disease *on page 1421*

Prevention of Wound Infection and Sepsis in Surgical Patients *on page 1588*

U.S. Brand Names Mefoxin®

Synonyms Cefoxitin Sodium

Pharmacologic Category Antibiotic, Cephalosporin (Second Generation)

Generic Available Yes: Powder for injection

Use Less active against staphylococci and streptococci than first generation cephalosporins, but active against anaerobes including *Bacteroides fragilis*; active against gram-negative enteric bacilli including *E. coli*, *Klebsiella*, and *Proteus*; used predominantly for respiratory tract, skin and skin structure, bone and joint, urinary tract and gynecologic as well as septicemia; surgical prophylaxis; intra-abdominal infections and other mixed infections; indicated for bacterial *Eikenella corrodens* infections

Mechanism of Action Inhibits bacterial cell wall synthesis by binding to one or more of the penicillin-binding proteins (PBPs) which in turn inhibits the final transpeptidation step of peptidoglycan synthesis in bacterial cell walls, thus inhibiting cell wall biosynthesis. Bacteria eventually lyse due to ongoing activity of cell wall autolytic enzymes (autolysins and murein hydrolases) while cell wall assembly is arrested.

Pharmacodynamics/Kinetics

Distribution: Widely to body tissues and fluids including pleural, synovial, ascitic, bile; poorly penetrates into CSF even with inflammation of the meninges; crosses placenta; small amounts enter breast milk

Protein binding: 65% to 79%

Half-life elimination: 45-60 minutes; significantly prolonged with renal impairment

Time to peak, serum: I.M.: 20-30 minutes

Excretion: Urine (85% as unchanged drug)

Dosage

Usual dosage range:

Infants >3 months and Children: I.M., I.V.: 80-160 mg/kg/day in divided doses every 4-6 hours (maximum dose: 12 g/day)

Adults: I.M., I.V.: 1-2 g every 6-8 hours (maximum dose: 12 g/day)

Note: I.M. injection is painful

Indication-specific dosing:

Infants >3 months and Children:

Mild-to-moderate infection: I.M., I.V.: 80-100 mg/kg/day in divided doses every 4-6 hours

Perioperative prophylaxis: I.V.: 30-40 mg/kg 30-60 minutes prior to surgery followed by 30-40 mg/kg/dose every 6 hours for no more than 24 hours after surgery depending on the procedure

Severe infection: I.M., I.V.: 100-160 mg/kg/day in divided doses every 4-6 hours

Adolescents and Adults:

Perioperative prophylaxis: I.M., I.V.: 1-2 g 30-60 minutes prior to surgery followed by 1-2 g every 6-8 hours for no more than 24 hours after surgery depending on the procedure

Adults:

Amnionitis, endomyometritis: I.M., I.V.: 2 g every 6-8 hours

Aspiration pneumonia, empyema, orbital cellulitis, parapharyngeal space, human bites: I.M., I.V.: 2 g every 8 hours

Liver abscess: I.V.: 1 g every 4 hours

Mycobacterium species, not MTB or MAI: I.V.: 12 g/day with amikacin

Pelvic inflammatory disease:

Inpatients: I.V.: 2 g every 6 hours **plus** doxycycline 100 mg I.V. or 100 mg orally every 12 hours until improved, followed by doxycycline 100 mg orally twice daily to complete 14 days

Outpatients: I.M.: 2 g **plus** probenecid 1 g orally as a single dose, followed by doxycycline 100 mg orally twice daily for 14 days

Dosing interval in renal impairment:

Cl_{cr} 30-50 mL/minute: Administer 1-2 g every 8-12 hours

Cl_{cr} 10-29 mL/minute: Administer 1-2 g every 12-24 hours

Cl_{cr} 5-9 mL/minute: Administer 0.5-1 g every 12-24 hours

Cl_{cr} <5 mL/minute: Administer 0.5-1 g every 24-48 hours

Hemodialysis: Moderately dialyzable (20% to 50%); administer a loading dose of 1-2 g after each hemodialysis; maintenance dose as noted above based on Cl_{cr}

Continuous arteriovenous or venovenous hemodiafiltration effects: Dose as for Cl_{cr} 10-50 mL/minute

Stability Reconstitute vials with SWFI, bacteriostatic water for injection, NS, or D_5W. For I.V. infusion, solutions may be further diluted in NS, $D_5{}^1/_4NS$, $D_5{}^1/_2NS$, D_5NS, D_5W, $D_{10}W$, LR, D_5LR, mannitol 10%, or sodium bicarbonate 5%. Reconstituted solution is stable for 6 hours at room temperature or 7 days when refrigerated; I.V. infusion in NS or D_5W solution is stable for 18 hours at room temperature or 48 hours when refrigerated. Premixed frozen solution, when thawed, is stable for 24 hours at room temperature or 21 days when refrigerated.

Administration

I.M.: Inject deep I.M. into large muscle mass.

I.V.: Can be administered IVP over 3-5 minutes at a maximum concentration of 100 mg/mL or I.V. intermittent infusion over 10-60 minutes at a final concentration for I.V. administration not to exceed 40 mg/mL

Monitoring Parameters Monitor renal function periodically when used in combination with other nephrotoxic drugs; observe for signs and symptoms of anaphylaxis during first dose

Pregnancy Risk Factor B

Contraindications Hypersensitivity to cefoxitin, any component of the formulation, or other cephalosporins

Warnings/Precautions Use with caution in patients with history of colitis. Cefoxitin may increase resistance of organisms by inducing beta-lactamase. Modify dosage in patients with severe renal impairment. Prolonged use may result in superinfection. Use with caution in patients with a history of penicillin allergy, especially IgE-mediated reactions (eg, anaphylaxis, urticaria). May cause antibiotic-associated colitis or colitis secondary to *C. difficile*.

Adverse Reactions

1% to 10%: Gastrointestinal: Diarrhea

<1% (Limited to important or life-threatening): Anaphylaxis, angioedema, bone marrow suppression, BUN increased, creatinine increased, dyspnea, eosinophilia, exacerbation of myasthenia gravis, exfoliative dermatitis, fever, hemolytic anemia, hypotension, interstitial nephritis, jaundice, leukopenia, nausea,

(Continued)

Cefoxitin *(Continued)*

nephrotoxicity (with aminoglycosides), phlebitis, prolonged PT, pruritus, pseudomembranous colitis, rash, thrombocytopenia, thrombophlebitis, toxic epidermal necrolysis, transaminases increased, urticaria, vomiting

Reactions reported with other cephalosporins: Agranulocytosis, aplastic anemia, cholestasis, colitis, erythema multiforme, hemolytic anemia, hemorrhage, pancytopenia, renal dysfunction, seizure, serum-sickness reactions, Stevens-Johnson syndrome, superinfection, toxic nephropathy, vaginitis

Overdosage/Toxicology Symptoms of overdose include neuromuscular hypersensitivity and convulsions. Many beta-lactam containing antibiotics have the potential to cause neuromuscular hyperirritability or convulsive seizures. Hemodialysis may be helpful to aid in removal of the drug from blood; otherwise, treatment is supportive or symptom-directed.

Drug Interactions

Increased effect: Probenecid may decrease cephalosporin elimination

Increased toxicity: Aminoglycosides and furosemide may increase nephrotoxic potential

Test Interactions Positive direct Coombs', false-positive urinary glucose test using cupric sulfate (Benedict's solution, Clinitest®, Fehling's solution), false-positive serum or urine creatinine with Jaffé reaction

Dietary Considerations Sodium content of 1 g: 53 mg (2.3 mEq)

Dosage Forms

Infusion, as sodium [premixed iso-osmotic solution]: 1 g (50 mL); 2 g (50 mL) [contains sodium 53.8 mg/g (2.3 mEq/g)]

Injection, powder for reconstitution, as sodium: 1 g, 2 g, 10 g [contains sodium 53.8 mg/g (2.3 mEq/g)]

References

"Antimicrobial Prophylaxis for Surgery," *Treat Guidel Med Lett*, 2004, 2(20):27-32.

Feldman WE, Moffitt S, and Sprow N, "Clinical and Pharmacokinetic Evaluation of Parenteral Cefoxitin in Infants and Children," *Antimicrob Agents Chemother*, 1980, 17(4):669-74.

Marshall WF and Blair JE, "The Cephalosporins," *Mayo Clin Proc*, 1999, 74(2):187-95.

Regazzi MB, Chirico G, Cristiani D, et al, "Cefoxitin in Newborn Infants. A Clinical and Pharmacokinetic Study," *Eur J Clin Pharmacol*, 1983, 25(4):507-9.

♦ **Cefoxitin Sodium** *see* Cefoxitin *on page 244*

Ceftazidime (SEF tay zi deem)

Medication Safety Issues

Sound-alike/look-alike issues:

Ceftazidime may be confused with ceftizoxime

Ceptaz® may be confused with Septra®

Tazicef® may be confused with Tazidime®

Tazidime® may be confused with Tazicef®

U.S. Brand Names Ceptaz® [DSC]; Fortaz®; Tazicef®

Canadian Brand Names Fortaz®

Pharmacologic Category Antibiotic, Cephalosporin (Third Generation)

Generic Available No

Use Treatment of documented susceptible *Pseudomonas aeruginosa* infection and infections due to other susceptible aerobic gram-negative organisms; empiric therapy of a febrile, granulocytopenic patient

Mechanism of Action Inhibits bacterial cell wall synthesis by binding to one or more of the penicillin-binding proteins (PBPs) which in turn inhibits the final transpeptidation step of peptidoglycan synthesis in bacterial cell walls, thus inhibiting cell wall biosynthesis. Bacteria eventually lyse due to ongoing activity of cell wall autolytic enzymes (autolysins and murein hydrolases) while cell wall assembly is arrested.

Pharmacodynamics/Kinetics

Distribution: Widely throughout the body including bone, bile, skin, CSF (higher concentrations achieved when meninges are inflamed), endometrium, heart, pleural and lymphatic fluids

Protein binding: 17%

Half-life elimination: 1-2 hours, prolonged with renal impairment; Neonates <23 days: 2.2-4.7 hours

Time to peak, serum: I.M.: ~1 hour

Excretion: Urine (80% to 90% as unchanged drug)

Dosage

Usual dosage range:

Infants and Children 1 month to 12 years: I.V.: 30-50 mg/kg/dose every 8 hours (maximum dose: 6 g/day)

Adults: I.M., I.V.: 500 mg to 2 g every 8-12 hours

Indication-specific dosing:

Bacterial arthritis (gram-negative bacilli): I.V.: 1-2 g every 8 hours

Cystic fibrosis: I.V.: 30-50 mg/kg every 8 hours (maximum: 6 g/day)

Melioidosis: I.V.: 40 mg/kg every 8 hours for 10 days, followed by oral therapy with doxycycline or TMP/SMX

Otitis externa: I.V.: 2 g every 8 hours

Peritonitis (CAPD):

Anuric, intermittent: 1000-1500 mg/day

Anuric, continuous (per liter exchange): Loading dose: 250 mg; maintenance dose: 125 mg

Severe infections, including meningitis, complicated pneumonia, endophthalmitis, CNS infection, osteomyelitis, intra-abdominal and gynecological, skin and soft tissue: I.V.: 2 g every 8 hours

Dosing interval in renal impairment:

Cl_{cr} 30-50 mL/minute: Administer every 12 hours

Cl_{cr} 10-30 mL/minute: Administer every 24 hours

Cl_{cr} <10 mL/minute: Administer every 48-72 hours

Hemodialysis: Dialyzable (50% to 100%)

Continuous arteriovenous or venovenous hemodiafiltration effects: Dose as for Cl_{cr} 30-50 mL/minute

Stability Reconstituted solution and I.V. infusion in NS or D_5W solution are stable for 24 hours at room temperature, 10 days when refrigerated, or 12 weeks when frozen. After freezing, thawed solution is stable for 24 hours at room temperature or 4 days when refrigerated; 96 hours under refrigeration, after mixing.

Administration Any carbon dioxide bubbles that may be present in the withdrawn solution should be expelled prior to injection. Administer around-the-clock to promote less variation in peak and trough serum levels. Ceftazidime can be administered deep I.M. into large mass muscle, IVP over 3-5 minutes, or I.V. intermittent infusion over 15-30 minutes. Do not admix with aminoglycosides in same bottle/bag. Final concentration for I.V. administration should not exceed 100 mg/mL.

Monitoring Parameters Observe for signs and symptoms of anaphylaxis during first dose

Pregnancy Risk Factor B

Contraindications Hypersensitivity to ceftazidime, any component of the formulation, or other cephalosporins

Warnings/Precautions Modify dosage in patients with severe renal impairment. Prolonged use may result in superinfection. Use with caution in patients with a history of penicillin allergy, especially IgE-mediated reactions (eg, anaphylaxis, urticaria). May cause antibiotic-associated colitis or colitis secondary to *C. difficile.*

Adverse Reactions

1% to 10%:

Gastrointestinal: Diarrhea (1%)

Local: Pain at injection site (1%)

Miscellaneous: Hypersensitivity reactions (2%)

<1% (Limited to important or life-threatening): Anaphylaxis, angioedema, asterixis, BUN increased, candidiasis, creatinine increased, dizziness, encephalopathy, eosinophilia, erythema multiforme, fever, headache, hemolytic anemia, hyperbilirubinemia, jaundice, leukopenia, myoclonus, nausea, neuromuscular excitability, paresthesia, phlebitis, pruritus, pseudomembranous colitis, rash, Stevens-Johnson syndrome, thrombocytosis, toxic epidermal necrolysis, transaminases increased, vaginitis, vomiting

Reactions reported with other cephalosporins: Agranulocytosis, aplastic anemia, cholestasis, colitis, hemolytic anemia, hemorrhage, interstitial nephritis, pancytopenia, prolonged PT, renal dysfunction, seizure, serum-sickness reactions, superinfection, toxic nephropathy, urticaria

Overdosage/Toxicology Symptoms of overdose include neuromuscular hypersensitivity and convulsions. Many beta-lactam containing antibiotics have the

(Continued)

Ceftazidime *(Continued)*

potential to cause neuromuscular hyperirritability or convulsive seizures. Hemodialysis may be helpful to aid in removal of the drug from blood; otherwise, treatment is supportive or symptom-directed.

Drug Interactions

Increased effect: Probenecid may decrease cephalosporin elimination; aminoglycosides: *in vitro* studies indicate additive or synergistic effect against some strains of Enterobacteriaceae and *Pseudomonas aeruginosa*

Increased toxicity: Aminoglycosides and furosemide may increase nephrotoxic potential

Test Interactions Positive direct Coombs', false-positive urinary glucose test using cupric sulfate (Benedict's solution, Clinitest®, Fehling's solution), false-positive serum or urine creatinine with Jaffé reaction

Dietary Considerations Sodium content of 1 g: 2.3 mEq

Dosage Forms [DSC] = Discontinued product

Infusion, as sodium [premixed iso-osmotic solution] (Fortaz®): 1 g (50 mL); 2 g (50 mL)

Injection, powder for reconstitution:

- Ceptaz® [DSC]: 10 g [L-arginine formulation]
- Fortaz®: 500 mg, 1 g, 2 g, 6 g [contains sodium carbonate]
- Tazicef®: 1 g, 2 g, 6 g [contains sodium carbonate]

References

American Thoracic Society and Infectious Diseases Society of America, "Guidelines for the Management of Adults With Hospital-Acquired, Ventilator-Associated, and Healthcare-Associated Pneumonia," *Am J Respir Crit Care Med*, 2005, 171(4):388-416.

Tunkel AR, Hartman BJ, Kaplan SL, et al, "Practice Guidelines for the Management of Bacterial Meningitis," *Clin Infect Dis*, 2004, 39(9):1267-84.

♦ **Ceftin®** *see* Cefuroxime *on page 253*

Ceftizoxime (sef ti ZOKS eem)

Medication Safety Issues

Sound-alike/look-alike issues:

Ceftizoxime may be confused with cefotaxime, ceftazidime, cefuroxime

U.S. Brand Names Cefizox®

Canadian Brand Names Cefizox®

Synonyms Ceftizoxime Sodium

Pharmacologic Category Antibiotic, Cephalosporin (Third Generation)

Generic Available No

Use Treatment of susceptible bacterial infections, mainly respiratory tract, skin and skin structure, bone and joint, urinary tract and gynecologic, as well as septicemia; active against many gram-negative bacilli (not *Pseudomonas*), some gram-positive cocci (not *Enterococcus*), and some anaerobes

Mechanism of Action Inhibits bacterial cell wall synthesis by binding to one or more of the penicillin-binding proteins (PBPs) which in turn inhibits the final transpeptidation step of peptidoglycan synthesis in bacterial cell walls, thus inhibiting cell wall biosynthesis. Bacteria eventually lyse due to ongoing activity of cell wall autolytic enzymes (autolysins and murein hydrolases) while cell wall assembly is arrested.

Pharmacodynamics/Kinetics

Distribution: V_d: 0.35-0.5 L/kg; widely into most body tissues and fluids including gallbladder, liver, kidneys, bone, sputum, bile, pleural and synovial fluids; has good CSF penetration; crosses placenta; small amounts enter breast milk

Protein binding: 30%

Half-life elimination: 1.6 hours; Cl_{cr} <10 mL/minute: 25 hours

Time to peak, serum: I.M.: 0.5-1 hour

Excretion: Urine (as unchanged drug)

Dosage

Usual dosage range:

Children ≥6 months: I.M., I.V.: 150-200 mg/kg/day divided every 6-8 hours (maximum: 12 g/24 hours)

Adults: I.M., I.V.: 1-4 g every 8-12 hours

Indication-specific dosing:

Adults:

Gonococcal:

Disseminated infection: I.M., I.V.: 1 g every 8 hours

Uncomplicated: I.M.: 1 g as single dose

Life-threatening infections: I.V.: 2 g every 4 hours or 4 g every 8 hours

Dosing adjustment in renal impairment: Adults:

Cl_{cr} 10-30 mL/minute: Administer 1 g every 12 hours

Cl_{cr} <10 mL/minute: Administer 1 g every 24 hours

Moderately dialyzable (20% to 50%)

Continuous arteriovenous or venovenous hemodiafiltration effects: Dose as for Cl_{cr} 10-50 mL/minute

Stability Reconstituted solution is stable for 24 hours at room temperature and 96 hours when refrigerated. For I.V. infusion in NS or D_5W solution is stable for 24 hours at room temperature, 96 hours when refrigerated, or 12 weeks when frozen. After freezing, thawed solution is stable for 24 hours at room temperature or 10 days when refrigerated.

Administration

I.M.: Inject deep I.M. into large muscle mass.

I.V.: Inject direct I.V. over 3-5 minutes. Infuse intermittent infusion over 30 minutes.

Monitoring Parameters Observe for signs and symptoms of anaphylaxis during first dose

Pregnancy Risk Factor B

Contraindications Hypersensitivity to ceftizoxime, any component of the formulation, or other cephalosporins

Warnings/Precautions Modify dosage in patients with severe renal impairment. Prolonged use may result in superinfection. Use with caution in patients with a history of penicillin allergy, especially IgE-mediated reactions (eg, anaphylaxis, urticaria). May cause antibiotic-associated colitis or colitis secondary to *C. difficile*.

Adverse Reactions

1% to 10%:

Central nervous system: Fever

Dermatologic: Rash, pruritus

Hematologic: Eosinophilia, thrombocytosis

Hepatic: Alkaline phosphatase increased, transaminases increased

Local: Pain, burning at injection site

<1% (Limited to important or life-threatening): Anaphylaxis, anemia, bilirubin increased, BUN increased, creatinine increased, diarrhea, injection site reactions, leukopenia, nausea, neutropenia, numbness, paresthesia, phlebitis, thrombocytopenia, vaginitis, vomiting

Reactions reported with other cephalosporins: Agranulocytosis, angioedema, aplastic anemia, asterixis, candidiasis, cholestasis, colitis, encephalopathy, erythema multiforme, hemolytic anemia, hemorrhage, interstitial nephritis, neuromuscular excitability, pancytopenia, prolonged PT, pseudomembranous colitis, renal dysfunction, seizure, serum-sickness reactions, Stevens-Johnson syndrome, superinfection, toxic epidermal necrolysis, toxic nephropathy

Overdosage/Toxicology Symptoms of overdose include neuromuscular hypersensitivity and convulsions. Many beta-lactam containing antibiotics have the potential to cause neuromuscular hyperirritability or convulsive seizures. Hemodialysis may be helpful to aid in removal of the drug from blood; otherwise, treatment is supportive or symptom-directed.

Drug Interactions

Increased effect: Probenecid may decrease cephalosporin elimination

Increased toxicity: Aminoglycosides and furosemide may increase nephrotoxic potential

Test Interactions Positive direct Coombs', false-positive urinary glucose test using cupric sulfate (Benedict's solution, Clinitest®, Fehling's solution), false-positive serum or urine creatinine with Jaffé reaction

Dietary Considerations Sodium content of 1 g: 60 mg (2.6 mEq)

Dosage Forms

Infusion [premixed iso-osmotic solution]: 1 g (50 mL); 2 g (50 mL)

Injection, powder for reconstitution: 1 g, 2 g, 10 g

♦ **Ceftizoxime Sodium** *see* Ceftizoxime *on page 248*

Ceftriaxone (sef trye AKS one)

Medication Safety Issues

Sound-alike/look-alike issues:

Rocephin® may be confused with Roferon®

U.S. Brand Names Rocephin®

Canadian Brand Names Rocephin®

Synonyms Ceftriaxone Sodium

Pharmacologic Category Antibiotic, Cephalosporin (Third Generation)

Generic Available Yes

Use Treatment of lower respiratory tract infections, acute bacterial otitis media, skin and skin structure infections, bone and joint infections, intra-abdominal and urinary tract infections, pelvic inflammatory disease (PID), uncomplicated gonorrhea, bacterial septicemia, and meningitis; used in surgical prophylaxis

Unlabeled/Investigational Use Treatment of chancroid, epididymitis, complicated gonococcal infections; sexually-transmitted diseases (STD); periorbital or buccal cellulitis; salmonellosis or shigellosis; atypical community-acquired pneumonia; Lyme disease; used in chemoprophylaxis for high-risk contacts and persons with invasive meningococcal disease; sexual assault

Mechanism of Action Inhibits bacterial cell wall synthesis by binding to one or more of the penicillin-binding proteins (PBPs) which in turn inhibits the final transpeptidation step of peptidoglycan synthesis in bacterial cell walls, thus inhibiting cell wall biosynthesis. Bacteria eventually lyse due to ongoing activity of cell wall autolytic enzymes (autolysins and murein hydrolases) while cell wall assembly is arrested.

Pharmacodynamics/Kinetics

Absorption: I.M.: Well absorbed

Distribution: Widely throughout the body including gallbladder, lungs, bone, bile, CSF (higher concentrations achieved when meninges are inflamed); crosses placenta; enters amniotic fluid and breast milk

Protein binding: 85% to 95%

Half-life elimination: Normal renal and hepatic function: 5-9 hours

Time to peak, serum: I.M.: 1-2 hours

Excretion: Urine (33% to 65% as unchanged drug); feces

Dosage

Usual dosage range:

Infants and Children: I.M., I.V.: 50-100 mg/kg/day in 1-2 divided doses (maximum: 4 g/day)

Adults: I.M., I.V.: 1-2 g every 12-24 hours

Indication-specific dosing:

Infants and Children:

Epiglottitis: I.M., I.V.: 50-100 mg/kg once daily for 7-10 days with clindamycin

Gonococcal infections:

Conjunctivitis, complicated (unlabeled use): I.M.:

<45 kg: 50 mg/kg in a single dose (maximum: 1 g)

>45 kg: 1 g in a single dose

Disseminated (unlabeled use): I.M., I.V.:

<45 kg: 25-50 mg/kg once daily (maximum: 1 g)

>45 kg: 1 g once daily for 7 days

Endocarditis (unlabeled use):

<45 kg: I.M., I.V.: 50 mg/kg/day every 12 hours (maximum: 2 g/day) for at least 28 days

>45 kg: I.V.: 1-2 g every 12 hours, for at least 28 days

Uncomplicated: I.M.: 125 mg in a single dose

Mild-to-moderate infections: I.M., I.V.: 50-75 mg/kg/day in 1-2 divided doses every 12-24 hours (maximum: 2 g/day); continue until at least 2 days after signs and symptoms of infection have resolved

Meningitis:

Gonococcal, complicated:

<45 kg: I.V.: 50 mg/kg/day given every 12 hours (maximum: 2 g/day); usual duration of treatment is 10-14 days

>45 kg: I.V.: 1-2 g every 12 hours; usual duration of treatment is 10-14 days

Uncomplicated: I.M., I.V.: Loading dose of 100 mg/kg (maximum: 4 g), followed by 100 mg/kg/day divided every 12-24 hours (maximum: 4 g/day); usual duration of treatment is 7-14 days

Otitis media:

Acute: I.M., I.V.: 50 mg/kg in a single dose (maximum: 1 g)

Persistent or relapsing (unlabeled use): I.M., I.V.: 50 mg/kg once daily for 3 days

Pneumonia: I.V.: 50-75 mg/kg once daily

Serious infections: I.V.: 80-100 mg/kg/day in 1-2 divided doses (maximum: 4 g/day)

STD, sexual assault (unlabeled use): I.M.: 125 mg in a single dose

Typhoid fever: I.V.: 100 mg/kg once daily (maximum 4 g)

Children >8 years (≥45 kg) and Adolescents:

Epididymitis, acute (unlabeled use): I.M.: 125 mg in a single dose

Children ≤15 years:

Chemoprophylaxis for high-risk contacts and persons with invasive meningococcal disease (unlabeled use): I.M.: 125 mg in a single dose. Children >15 years: Refer to adult dosing.

Adults:

Arthritis (septic): I.V.: 1-2 g once daily

Brain abscess and necrotizing fasciitis: I.V.: 2 g every 12 hours

Cavernous sinus thrombosis: I.V.: 1 g every 12 hours with vancomycin or linezolid

Chancroid (unlabeled use): I.M.: 250 mg as single dose

Chemoprophylaxis for high-risk contacts and persons with invasive meningococcal disease (unlabeled use): I.M.: 250 mg in a single dose

Endocarditis, acute native valve: I.V.: 2 g once daily for 2-4 weeks

Epididymitis, acute (unlabeled use) and prostatitis: I.M.: 250 mg in a single dose with doxycycline

Gonococcal infections:

Conjunctivitis, complicated (unlabeled use): I.M., I.V.: 1 g in a single dose

Disseminated (unlabeled use): I.M., I.V.: 1 g once daily for 7 days

Endocarditis (unlabeled use): I.M., I.V.: 1-2 g every 12 hours for at least 28 days

Uncomplicated: I.M.: 125-250 mg in a single dose

Lyme disease: I.V.: 2 g once daily for 14-28 days

Mastoiditis (hospitalized): I.V.: 2 g once daily; >60 years old: 1 g once daily

Meningitis: I.V.: 2 g every 12 hours for 7-14 days (longer courses may be necessary for selected organisms)

Orbital cellulitis (unlabeled use) and endophthalmitis: I.V.: 2 g once daily

Pelvic inflammatory disease: I.M.: 250 mg in a single dose

Pneumonia, community-acquired: I.V.: 2 g once daily; >65 years of age: 1 g once daily

Septic/toxic shock: I.V.: 2 g once daily; with clindamycin for toxic shock

Surgical prophylaxis: I.V.: 1 g 30 minutes to 2 hours before surgery

Syphilis: I.M., I.V.: 1 g once daily for 8-10 days

Typhoid fever: I.V.: 2-3 g once daily for 7-14 days

Dosage adjustment in renal/hepatic impairment: No adjustment necessary

Hemodialysis: Not dialyzable (0% to 5%); administer dose postdialysis

Peritoneal dialysis effects: Administer 750 mg every 12 hours

Continuous arteriovenous or venovenous hemofiltration: Removes 10 mg of ceftriaxone of liter of filtrate per day

Stability

Powder for injection: Prior to reconstitution, store at room temperature of 25°C (77°F); protect from light.

Premixed solution (manufacturer premixed): Store at -20°C; once thawed, solutions are stable for 3 days at room temperature of 25°C (77°F) or for 21 days refrigerated at 5°C (41°F). Do not refreeze.

Stability of reconstituted solutions:

10-40 mg/mL: Reconstituted in D_5W or NS: Stable for 2 days at room temperature of 25°C (77°F) or for 10 days when refrigerated at 5°C (41°F).

100 mg/mL:

Reconstituted in D_5W or NS: Stable for 2 days at room temperature of 25°C (77°F) or for 10 days when refrigerated at 5°C (41°F). Stable for 26 weeks when frozen at -20°C. Once thawed, solutions are stable for 2 days at room temperature of 25°C (77°F) or for 10 days when refrigerated at 5°C (41°F); does not apply to manufacturer's premixed bags. Do not refreeze.

(Continued)

Ceftriaxone *(Continued)*

Reconstituted in lidocaine 1% solution: Stable for 24 hours at room temperature of 25°C (77°F) or for 10 days when refrigerated at 5°C (41°F).

250-350 mg/mL: Reconstituted in D_5W, NS, lidocaine 1% solution, or SWFI: Stable for 24 hours at room temperature of 25°C (77°F) or for 3 days when refrigerated at 5°C (41°F).

Reconstitution:

I.M. injection: Vials should be reconstituted with appropriate volume of diluent (including D_5W, NS, or 1% lidocaine) to make a final concentration of 250 mg/mL or 350 mg/mL.

Volume to add to create a **250 mg/mL** solution:
250 mg vial: 0.9 mL
500 mg vial: 1.8 mL
1 g vial: 3.6 mL
2 g vial: 7.2 mL

Volume to add to create a **350 mg/mL** solution:
500 mg vial: 1.0 mL
1 g vial: 2.1 mL
2 g vial: 4.2 mL

I.V. infusion: Infusion is prepared in two stages: Initial reconstitution of powder, followed by dilution to final infusion solution.

Vials: Reconstitute powder with appropriate I.V. diluent (including SWFI, D_5W, NS) to create an initial solution of ~100 mg/mL. Recommended volume to add:
250 mg vial: 2.4 mL
500 mg vial: 4.8 mL
1 g vial: 9.6 mL
2 g vial: 19.2 mL

Note: After reconstitution of powder, further dilution into a volume of compatible solution (eg, 50-100 mL of D_5W or NS) is recommended.

Piggyback bottle: Reconstitute powder with appropriate I.V. diluent (D_5W or NS) to create a resulting solution of ~100 mg/mL. Recommended initial volume to add:
1 g bottle:10 mL
2 g bottle: 20 mL

Note: After reconstitution, to prepare the final infusion solution, further dilution to 50 mL or 100 mL volumes with the appropriate I.V. diluent (including D_5W or NS) is recommended.

Administration Do not admix with aminoglycosides in same bottle/bag.

I.M.: Inject deep I.M. into large muscle mass; a concentration of 250 mg/mL or 350 mg/mL is recommended for all vial sizes except the 250 mg size (250 mg/mL is suggested); can be diluted with 1:1 water and 1% lidocaine for I.M. administration

I.V.: Infuse intermittent infusion over 30 minutes

Monitoring Parameters Observe for signs and symptoms of anaphylaxis

Pregnancy Risk Factor B

Contraindications Hypersensitivity to ceftriaxone sodium, any component of the formulation, or other cephalosporins; **do not use in hyperbilirubinemic neonates**, particularly those who are premature since ceftriaxone is reported to displace bilirubin from albumin binding sites

Warnings/Precautions Modify dosage in patients with severe renal impairment, prolonged use may result in superinfection. Use with caution in patients with a history of penicillin allergy, especially IgE-mediated reactions (eg, anaphylaxis, urticaria). May cause antibiotic-associated colitis or colitis secondary to *C. difficile.* Discontinue in patients with signs and symptoms of gallbladder disease.

Adverse Reactions

1% to 10%:
Dermatologic: Rash (2%)
Gastrointestinal: Diarrhea (3%)
Hematologic: Eosinophilia (6%), thrombocytosis (5%), leukopenia (2%)
Hepatic: Transaminases increased (3.1% to 3.3%)
Local: Pain, induration at injection site (I.V. 1%); warmth, tightness, induration (5% to 17%) following I.M. injection
Renal: Increased BUN (1%)

<1% (Limited to important or life-threatening): Agranulocytosis, allergic pneumonitis, anaphylaxis, anemia, basophilia, bronchospasm, candidiasis, chills,

colitis, diaphoresis, dizziness, dysgeusia, flushing, gallstones, glycosuria, headache, hematuria, hemolytic anemia, jaundice, leukocytosis, lymphocytosis, lymphopenia, monocytosis, nausea, nephrolithiasis, neutropenia, phlebitis, prolonged or decreased PT, pruritus, pseudomembranous colitis, renal precipitations, renal stones, seizure, serum sickness, thrombocytopenia, urinary casts, vaginitis, vomiting; increased alkaline phosphatase, bilirubin, and creatinine

Reactions reported with other cephalosporins: Angioedema, aplastic anemia, asterixis, cholestasis, encephalopathy, erythema multiforme, hemorrhage, interstitial nephritis, neuromuscular excitability, pancytopenia, paresthesia, renal dysfunction, Stevens-Johnson syndrome, superinfection, toxic epidermal necrolysis, toxic nephropathy

Overdosage/Toxicology Symptoms of overdose include neuromuscular hypersensitivity and convulsions. Many beta-lactam containing antibiotics have the potential to cause neuromuscular hyperirritability or convulsive seizures. Hemodialysis may be helpful to aid in removal of the drug from blood; otherwise, treatment is supportive or symptom-directed.

Drug Interactions

Coumarin derivative (eg, dicumarol, warfarin): Cephalosporins may increase the anticoagulant effect of coumarin derivatives.

Uricosuric agents (eg, probenecid, sulfinpyrazone): Uricosuric agents may decrease the excretion of cephalosporin; monitor for toxic effects.

Test Interactions Positive direct Coombs', false-positive urinary glucose test using cupric sulfate (Benedict's solution, Clinitest®, Fehling's solution), false-positive serum or urine creatinine with Jaffé reaction

Dietary Considerations Sodium contents: 83 mg (3.6 mEq) per ceftriaxone 1 g

Dosage Forms Note: Contains sodium 83 mg (3.6 mEq) per ceftriaxone 1 g

Infusion [premixed in dextrose]: 1 g (50 mL); 2 g (50 mL)

Injection, powder for reconstitution: 250 mg, 500 mg, 1 g, 2 g, 10 g

References

Tunkel AR, Hartman BJ, Kaplan SL, et al, "Practice Guidelines for the Management of Bacterial Meningitis," *Clin Infect Dis*, 2004, 39(9):1267-84.

♦ **Ceftriaxone Sodium** *see* Ceftriaxone *on page 250*

Cefuroxime (se fyoor OKS eem)

Medication Safety Issues

Sound-alike/look-alike issues:

Cefuroxime may be confused with cefotaxime, cefprozil, ceftizoxime, deferoxamine

Ceftin® may be confused with Cefotan®, cefotetan, Cefzil®, Cipro®

Zinacef® may be confused with Zithromax®

Related Information

Prevention of Wound Infection and Sepsis in Surgical Patients *on page 1588*

U.S. Brand Names Ceftin®; Zinacef®

Canadian Brand Names Apo-Cefuroxime®; Ceftin®; ratio-Cefuroxime; Zinacef®

Synonyms Cefuroxime Axetil; Cefuroxime Sodium

Pharmacologic Category Antibiotic, Cephalosporin (Second Generation)

Generic Available Yes

Use Treatment of infections caused by staphylococci, group B streptococci, *H. influenzae* (type A and B), *E. coli*, *Enterobacter*, *Salmonella*, and *Klebsiella*; treatment of susceptible infections of the lower respiratory tract, otitis media, urinary tract, skin and soft tissue, bone and joint, sepsis and gonorrhea

Mechanism of Action Inhibits bacterial cell wall synthesis by binding to one or more of the penicillin-binding proteins (PBPs) which in turn inhibits the final transpeptidation step of peptidoglycan synthesis in bacterial cell walls, thus inhibiting cell wall biosynthesis. Bacteria eventually lyse due to ongoing activity of cell wall autolytic enzymes (autolysins and murein hydrolases) while cell wall assembly is arrested.

Pharmacodynamics/Kinetics

Absorption: Oral (cefuroxime axetil): Increases with food

Distribution: Widely to body tissues and fluids; crosses blood-brain barrier; therapeutic concentrations achieved in CSF even when meninges are not inflamed; crosses placenta; enters breast milk

Protein binding: 33% to 50%

Bioavailability: Tablet: Fasting: 37%; Following food: 52%

(Continued)

Cefuroxime *(Continued)*

Half-life elimination: Adults: 1-2 hours; prolonged with renal impairment
Time to peak, serum: I.M.: ~15-60 minutes; I.V.: 2-3 minutes
Excretion: Urine (66% to 100% as unchanged drug)

Dosage Note: Cefuroxime axetil film-coated tablets and oral suspension are not bioequivalent and are not substitutable on a mg/mg basis

Usual dosage range:
Neonates: I.M., I.V.: 50-100 mg/kg/day divided every 12 hours
Children <13 years:
Oral: 20-30 mg/kg/day in 2 divided doses
I.M., I.V.: 75-150 mg/kg/day divided every 8 hours (maximum dose: 6 g/day)
Children ≥13 years and Adults:
Oral: 250-500 mg twice daily
I.M., I.V.: 750 mg to 1.5 g every 6-8 hours or 100-150 mg/kg/day in divided doses every 6-8 hours (maximum: 6 g/day)

Indication-specific dosing:
Children ≥3 months to 12 years:
Acute bacterial maxillary sinusitis, acute otitis media, and impetigo:
Oral: Suspension: 30 mg/kg/day in 2 divided doses for 10 days (maximum dose: 1 g/day); tablet: 250 mg twice daily for 10 days
I.M., I.V.: 75-150 mg/kg/day divided every 8 hours (maximum dose: 6 g/day)
Epiglottitis: Oral: 150 mg/kg/day in 3 divided doses for 7-10 days
Pharyngitis/tonsillitis:
Oral: Suspension: 20 mg/kg/day (maximum: 500 mg/day) in 2 divided doses for 10 days; tablet: 125 mg every 12 hours for 10 days
I.M., I.V.: 75-150 mg/kg day divided every 8 hours (maximum: 6 g/day)
Children ≥13 years and Adults:
Bronchitis (acute and exacerbations of chronic bronchitis):
Oral: 250-500 mg every 12 hours for 10 days
I.V.: 500-750 mg every 8 hours (complete therapy with oral dosing)
Cellulitis:
Oral: 500 mg every 12 hours
Orbital: I.V.: 1.5 g every 8 hours
Gonorrhea:
Disseminated: I.M., I.V.: 750 mg every 8 hours
Uncomplicated:
Oral: 1 g as a single dose
I.M.: 1.5 g as single dose (administer in 2 different sites with probenecid)
Lyme disease (early): Oral: 500 mg twice daily for 20 days
Pharyngitis/tonsillitis and sinusitis: Oral: 250 mg twice daily for 10 days
Pneumonia (uncomplicated): I.V.: 750 mg every 8 hours
Severe or complicated infections: I.M., I.V.: 1.5 g every 8 hours (up to 1.5 g every 6 hours in life-threatening infections)
Skin/skin structure infection (uncomplicated):
Oral: 250-500 mg every 12 hours for 10 days
I.M., I.V.: 750 mg every 8 hours
Surgical prophylaxis:
I.V.: 1.5 g 30 minutes to 1 hour prior to procedure (if procedure is prolonged can give 750 mg every 8 hours I.M.)
Open heart: I.V.: 1.5 g every 12 hours to a total of 6 g
Urinary tract infection (uncomplicated):
Oral: 125-250 mg every 12 hours for 7-10 days
I.M., I.V.: 750 mg every 8 hours

Dosing adjustment in renal impairment:
Cl_{cr} 10-20 mL/minute: Administer every 12 hours
Cl_{cr} <10 mL/minute: Administer every 24 hours
Hemodialysis: Dialyzable (25%)
Continuous arteriovenous or venovenous hemodiafiltration effects: Dose as for Cl_{cr} 10-20 mL/minute

Stability Reconstituted solution is stable for 24 hours at room temperature and 48 hours when refrigerated; I.V. infusion in NS or D_5W solution is stable for 24 hours at room temperature, 7 days when refrigerated, or 26 weeks when frozen; after freezing, thawed solution is stable for 24 hours at room temperature or 21 days when refrigerated

Administration

Oral: Administer around-the-clock to promote less variation in peak and trough serum levels.

Oral suspension: Administer with food. Shake well before use.

I.M.: Inject deep I.M. into large muscle mass.

I.V.: Inject direct I.V. over 3-5 minutes. Infuse intermittent infusion over 15-30 minutes.

Monitoring Parameters Observe for signs and symptoms of anaphylaxis during first dose; with prolonged therapy, monitor renal, hepatic, and hematologic function periodically; monitor prothrombin time in patients at risk of prolongation during cephalosporin therapy (nutritionally-deficient, prolonged treatment, renal or hepatic disease)

Pregnancy Risk Factor B

Contraindications Hypersensitivity to cefuroxime, any component of the formulation, or other cephalosporins

Warnings/Precautions Modify dosage in patients with severe renal impairment, prolonged use may result in superinfection; use with caution in patients with a history of penicillin allergy, especially IgE-mediated reactions (eg, anaphylaxis, urticaria). May cause antibiotic-associated colitis or colitis secondary to *C. difficile*. May be associated with increased INR, especially in nutritionally-deficient patients, prolonged treatment, hepatic or renal disease. Tablets and oral suspension are not bioequivalent (do not substitute on a mg-per-mg basis).

Adverse Reactions

1% to 10%:

Hematologic: Eosinophilia (7%), decreased hemoglobin and hematocrit (10%)

Hepatic: Increased transaminases (4%), increased alkaline phosphatase (2%)

Local: Thrombophlebitis (1.7%)

<1% (Limited to important or life-threatening): Anaphylaxis, angioedema, BUN increased, cholestasis, colitis, creatinine increased, diarrhea, dizziness, erythema multiforme, fever, GI bleeding, hemolytic anemia, headache, hepatitis, interstitial nephritis, jaundice, leukopenia, nausea, neutropenia, pain at injection site, pancytopenia, prolonged PT/INR, pseudomembranous colitis, rash, seizure, Stevens-Johnson syndrome, stomach cramps, thrombocytopenia, toxic epidermal necrolysis, vaginitis, vomiting

Reactions reported with other cephalosporins: Agranulocytosis, aplastic anemia, asterixis, colitis, encephalopathy, hemorrhage, neuromuscular excitability, serum-sickness reactions, superinfection, toxic nephropathy

Overdosage/Toxicology Symptoms of overdose include neuromuscular hypersensitivity and convulsions. Many beta-lactam containing antibiotics have the potential to cause neuromuscular hyperirritability or convulsive seizures. Hemodialysis may be helpful to aid in removal of the drug from blood; otherwise, treatment is supportive or symptom-directed.

Drug Interactions

Increased effect: High-dose probenecid decreases clearance

Increased toxicity: Aminoglycosides increase nephrotoxic potential

Ethanol/Nutrition/Herb Interactions Food: Bioavailability is increased with food; cefuroxime serum levels may be increased if taken with food or dairy products.

Test Interactions Positive direct Coombs', false-positive urinary glucose test using cupric sulfate (Benedict's solution, Clinitest®, Fehling's solution), false-positive serum or urine creatinine with Jaffé reaction

Dietary Considerations May be taken with food.

Zinacef®: Sodium content: 4.8 mEq (111 mg) per 750 mg

Ceftin®: Powder for oral suspension 125 mg/5 mL contains phenylalanine 11.8 mg/5 mL; 250 mg/5 mL contains phenylalanine 25.2 mg/5 mL.

Dosage Forms

Infusion, as sodium [premixed] (Zinacef®): 750 mg (50 mL); 1.5 g (50 mL) [contains sodium 4.8 mEq (111 mg) per 750 mg]

Injection, powder for reconstitution, as sodium (Zinacef®): 750 mg, 1.5 g, 7.5 g [contains sodium 4.8 mEq (111 mg) per 750 mg]

Powder for oral suspension, as axetil (Ceftin®): 125 mg/5 mL (100 mL) [contains phenylalanine 11.8 mg/5 mL; tutti-frutti flavor]; 250 mg/5 mL (50 mL, 100 mL) [contains phenylalanine 25.2 mg/5 mL; tutti-frutti flavor]

Tablet, as axetil (Ceftin®): 250 mg, 500 mg

♦ **Cefuroxime Axetil** *see* Cefuroxime *on page 253*

♦ **Cefuroxime Sodium** *see* Cefuroxime *on page 253*

♦ **Celebrex®** *see* Celecoxib *on page 256*

Celecoxib (se le KOKS ib)

Medication Safety Issues

Sound-alike/look-alike issues:

Celebrex® may be confused with Celexa™, cerebra, Cerebyx®

Related Information

Acetaminophen and NSAIDS, Dosing Data *on page 1543*

U.S. Brand Names Celebrex®

Canadian Brand Names Celebrex®

Pharmacologic Category Nonsteroidal Anti-inflammatory Drug (NSAID), COX-2 Selective

Restrictions A medication guide should be dispensed with each prescription. A template for the required MedGuide can be found on the FDA website at http://www.fda.gov/medwatch/SAFETY/2005/safety05.htm#NSAID

Generic Available No

Use Relief of the signs and symptoms of osteoarthritis, ankylosing spondylitis, and rheumatoid arthritis; management of acute pain; treatment of primary dysmenorrhea; decreasing intestinal polyps in familial adenomatous polyposis (FAP). **Note:** The Notice of Compliance for the use of celecoxib in FAP has been suspended by Health Canada.

Mechanism of Action Inhibits prostaglandin synthesis by decreasing the activity of the enzyme, cyclooxygenase-2 (COX-2), which results in decreased formation of prostaglandin precursors. Celecoxib does not inhibit cyclooxygenase-1 (COX-1) at therapeutic concentrations.

Pharmacodynamics/Kinetics

Distribution: V_d (apparent): 400 L

Protein binding: 97% to albumin

Metabolism: Hepatic via CYP2C9; forms inactive metabolites

Bioavailability: Absolute: Unknown

Half-life elimination: 11 hours (fasted)

Time to peak: 3 hours

Excretion: Urine (27% as metabolites, <3% as unchanged drug); feces (57%)

Dosage Adults: Oral:

Acute pain or primary dysmenorrhea: Initial dose: 400 mg, followed by an additional 200 mg if needed on day 1; maintenance dose: 200 mg twice daily as needed

Ankylosing spondylitis: 200 mg/day as a single dose or in divided doses twice daily; if no effect after 6 weeks, may increase to 400 mg/day. If no response following 6 weeks of treatment with 400 mg/day, consider discontinuation and alternative treatment.

Familial adenomatous polyposis: 400 mg twice daily

Osteoarthritis: 200 mg/day as a single dose or in divided dose twice daily

Rheumatoid arthritis: 100-200 mg twice daily

Elderly: No specific adjustment is recommended. However, the AUC in elderly patients may be increased by 50% as compared to younger subjects. Use the lowest recommended dose in patients weighing <50 kg.

Dosing adjustment in renal impairment: No specific dosage adjustment is recommended; not recommended in patients with advanced renal disease

Dosing adjustment in hepatic impairment: Reduced dosage is recommended (AUC may be increased by 40% to 180%); decrease dose by 50% in patients with moderate hepatic impairment (Child-Pugh class B)

Stability Store at controlled room temperature of 25°C (77°F).

Monitoring Parameters Periodic LFTs; in patients treated for FAP, continue routine endoscopic exams

Anesthesia and Critical Care Concerns/Other Considerations Celecoxib does not inhibit platelets or prolong bleeding time.

Pregnancy Risk Factor C/D (3rd trimester)

Contraindications Hypersensitivity to celecoxib, sulfonamides, aspirin, other NSAIDs, or any component of the formulation; perioperative pain in the setting of coronary artery bypass surgery (CABG); pregnancy (3rd trimester)

Warnings/Precautions [U.S. Boxed Warning]: NSAIDs are associated with an increased risk of adverse cardiovascular events, including MI, and new onset or worsening of pre-existing hypertension. Risk may be increased with duration of use or pre-existing cardiovascular risk factors or disease. Carefully evaluate individual cardiovascular risk profiles prior to prescribing. Use caution with fluid retention, CHF, cerebrovascular disease, ischemic heart disease, or hypertension.

[U.S. Boxed Warning]: NSAIDs may increase risk of gastrointestinal irritation, ulceration, bleeding, and perforation. These events may occur at any time during therapy and without warning. Use caution with a history of GI disease (bleeding or ulcers), concurrent therapy with aspirin, anticoagulants and/or corticosteroids, smoking, use of alcohol, the elderly or debilitated patients. Use the lowest effective dose for the shortest duration of time, consistent with individual patient goals, to reduce risk of cardiovascular or GI adverse events. Alternate therapies should be considered for patients at high risk.

NSAIDs may cause serious skin adverse events including exfoliative dermatitis, Stevens-Johnson syndrome (SJS), and toxic epidermal necrolysis (TEN). Anaphylactoid reactions may occur, even without prior exposure; patients with "aspirin triad" (bronchial asthma, aspirin intolerance, rhinitis) may be at increased risk. Do not use in patients who experience bronchospasm, asthma, rhinitis, or urticaria with NSAID or aspirin therapy.

Use with caution in patients with dehydration, decreased renal or hepatic function. Use of NSAIDs can compromise existing renal function, especially when Cl_{cr} <30 mL/minute. Not recommended for use in severe renal or hepatic impairment.

Anaphylactoid reactions may occur, even with no prior exposure to celecoxib. Use caution in patients with known or suspected deficiency of cytochrome P450 isoenzyme 2C9. Safety and efficacy have not been established in patients <18 years of age. **[U.S. Boxed Warning]: Celecoxib is contraindicated for treatment of perioperative pain in the setting of coronary artery bypass surgery (CABG).**

Adverse Reactions

>10%: Central nervous system: Headache (15.8%)

2% to 10%:

- Cardiovascular: Peripheral edema (2.1%)
- Central nervous system: Insomnia (2.3%), dizziness (2%)
- Dermatologic: Skin rash (2.2%)
- Gastrointestinal: Dyspepsia (8.8%), diarrhea (5.6%), abdominal pain (4.1%), nausea (3.5%), flatulence (2.2%)
- Neuromuscular & skeletal: Back pain (2.8%)
- Respiratory: Upper respiratory tract infection (8.1%), sinusitis (5%), pharyngitis (2.3%), rhinitis (2%)
- Miscellaneous: Accidental injury (2.9%)

<2%, postmarketing, and/or case reports (limited to important or life-threatening): Acute renal failure, agranulocytosis, albuminuria, allergic reactions, alopecia, anaphylactoid reactions, angioedema, aplastic anemia, arthralgia, aseptic meningitis, ataxia, bronchospasm, cerebrovascular accident, CHF, colitis, conjunctivitis, cystitis, deafness, diabetes mellitus, dyspnea, dysuria, ecchymosis, erythema multiforme, esophageal perforation, esophagitis, exfoliative dermatitis, flu-like syndrome, gangrene, gastroenteritis, gastroesophageal reflux, gastrointestinal bleeding, glaucoma, hematuria, hepatic failure, hepatitis, hypertension, hypoglycemia, hypokalemia, hyponatremia, interstitial nephritis, intestinal perforation, intracranial hemorrhage (fatal in association with warfarin), jaundice, leukopenia, melena, migraine, myalgia, MI, neuralgia, neuropathy, pancreatitis, pancytopenia, paresthesia, photosensitivity, prostate disorder, pulmonary embolism, rash, renal calculi, sepsis, Stevens-Johnson syndrome, stomatitis, sudden death, syncope, thrombophlebitis, tinnitus, toxic epidermal necrolysis, urticaria, vaginal bleeding, vaginitis, vasculitis, ventricular fibrillation, vertigo, vomiting

Overdosage/Toxicology Doses up to 2400 mg/day for up to 10 days have been reported without serious toxicity. Symptoms of overdose may include epigastric pain, drowsiness, lethargy, nausea, and vomiting; gastrointestinal bleeding may occur. Rare manifestations include hypertension, respiratory depression, coma, and acute renal failure. Treatment is symptomatic and supportive. Forced diuresis, hemodialysis and/or urinary alkalinization may not be useful.

Drug Interactions **Substrate** of CYP2C9 (major), 3A4 (minor); **Inhibits** CYP2C8 (moderate), 2D6 (weak)

ACE inhibitors: Antihypertensive effect may be diminished by celecoxib.

Aminoglycosides: Celecoxib may decrease excretion; monitor levels.

(Continued)

Celecoxib *(Continued)*

Aspirin: Low-dose aspirin may be used with celecoxib, however, monitor for GI complications.
Beta-blockers: Antihypertensive effect may be diminished by celecoxib.
Bile acid sequestrants: May decrease absorption of NSAIDs.
CYP2C8 Substrates: Celecoxib may increase the levels/effects of CYP2C8 substrates. Example substrates include amiodarone, paclitaxel, pioglitazone, repaglinide, and rosiglitazone.
Cyclosporine: NSAIDs may increase levels/nephrotoxicity of cyclosporine.
Fluconazole: Fluconazole increases celecoxib concentrations twofold. Lowest dose of celecoxib should be used.
Hydralazine: Antihypertensive effect may be diminished by celecoxib.
Lithium: Plasma levels of lithium are increased by ~17% when used with celecoxib. Monitor lithium levels closely when treatment with celecoxib is started or withdrawn.
Loop diuretics (bumetanide, furosemide, torsemide): Natriuretic effect of furosemide and other loop diuretics may be decreased by celecoxib.
Methotrexate: Severe bone marrow suppression, aplastic anemia, and GI toxicity have been reported with concomitant NSAID therapy. Selective COX-2 inhibitors appear to have a lower risk of this toxicity, however, caution is warranted.
Thiazide diuretics: Natriuretic effects of thiazide diuretics may be decreased by celecoxib.
Vancomycin: Celecoxib may decrease excretion; monitor levels.
Warfarin: Bleeding events (including rare intracranial hemorrhage in association with increased prothrombin time) have been reported with concomitant use. Monitor closely, especially in the elderly.

Ethanol/Nutrition/Herb Interactions
Ethanol: Avoid ethanol (increased GI irritation).
Food: Peak concentrations are delayed and AUC is increased by 10% to 20% when taken with a high-fat meal.

Dietary Considerations Lower doses (200 mg twice daily) may be taken without regard to meals. Larger doses should be taken with food to improve absorption.

Dosage Forms Capsule: 100 mg, 200 mg, 400 mg

♦ **Celestone®** *see* Betamethasone *on page 169*
♦ **Celestone® Soluspan®** *see* Betamethasone *on page 169*
♦ **Celexa®** *see* Citalopram *on page 297*
♦ **CellCept®** *see* Mycophenolate *on page 877*

Cellulose (Oxidized Regenerated)

(SEL yoo lose, OKS i dyzed re JEN er aye ted)

Medication Safety Issues
Sound-alike/look-alike issues:
Surgicel® may be confused with Serentil®

U.S. Brand Names Surgicel®; Surgicel® Fibrillar; Surgicel® NuKnit

Synonyms Absorbable Cotton; Oxidized Regenerated Cellulose

Pharmacologic Category Hemostatic Agent

Generic Available No

Use Hemostatic; temporary packing for the control of capillary, venous, or small arterial hemorrhage

Mechanism of Action Cellulose, oxidized regenerated is saturated with blood at the bleeding site and swells into a brownish or black gelatinous mass which aids in the formation of a clot. When used in small amounts, it is absorbed from the sites of implantation with little or no tissue reaction. In addition to providing hemostasis, oxidized regenerated cellulose also has been shown *in vitro* to have bactericidal properties.

Pharmacodynamics/Kinetics Absorption: 7-14 days

Dosage Minimal amounts of the fabric strip are laid on the bleeding site or held firmly against the tissues until hemostasis occurs; remove excess material

Stability Store at controlled room temperature. Inactivated by autoclaving; do not resterilize. Do not use if package is damaged. Do not reuse after opening.

Pregnancy Risk Factor No data reported

Contraindications Hypersensitivity to any component of the formulation; implantation into bone defects; hemorrhage from large arteries; nonhemorrhagic oozing; use as an adhesion product

Warnings/Precautions Pain, numbness, or paralysis have been reported if used near a bony or neural space and left inside patient; use minimum amount necessary to achieve hemostasis. Remove as much of agent as possible after hemostasis is achieved. Do not leave in a contaminated or infected space. Always remove completely following hemostasis if applied in proximity to foramina in bone, areas of bony confine, the spinal cord or optic nerve and chasm; product may swell and exert unwanted pressure. The material should not be moistened before insertion since the hemostatic effect is greater when applied dry. The material should not be impregnated with anti-infective agents. Its hemostatic effect is not enhanced by the addition of thrombin.

Adverse Reactions Frequency not defined.

Central nervous system: Headache

Respiratory: Nasal burning or stinging, sneezing (rhinological procedures)

Miscellaneous: Encapsulation of fluid, foreign body reactions (with or without) infection

Postmarketing and/or case reports: Numbness, pain, paralysis

Drug Interactions No data reported

Dosage Forms

Fabric, fibrous (Surgicel® Fibrillar):

1" x 2" (10s)
2" x 4" (10s)
4" x 4" (10s)

Fabric, knitted (Surgicel® NuKnit):

1" x 1" (24s)
1" x 3½" (10s)
3" x 4" (24s)
6" x 9" (10s)

Fabric, sheer weave (Surgicel®):

½" x 2" (24s)
2" x 3" (24s)
2" x 14" (24s)
4" x 8" (24s)

- **Celluvisc™ (Can)** *see* Carboxymethylcellulose *on page 230*
- **Cenestin (Can)** *see* Estrogens (Conjugated/Equine) *on page 488*
- **Centany™** *see* Mupirocin *on page 876*
- **Cepastat® [OTC]** *see* Phenol *on page 1012*
- **Cepastat® Extra Strength [OTC]** *see* Phenol *on page 1012*
- **Ceptaz® [DSC]** *see* Ceftazidime *on page 246*
- **Cerebyx®** *see* Fosphenytoin *on page 564*
- **C.E.S.® (Can)** *see* Estrogens (Conjugated/Equine) *on page 488*
- **Cesamet™** *see* Nabilone *on page 882*
- **Cetacort®** *see* Hydrocortisone *on page 639*
- **Cetafen® [OTC]** *see* Acetaminophen *on page 26*
- **Cetafen Extra® [OTC]** *see* Acetaminophen *on page 26*
- **Ceta-Plus®** *see* Hydrocodone and Acetaminophen *on page 636*
- **CGP-42446** *see* Zoledronic Acid *on page 1377*
- **Charcadole® (Can)** *see* Charcoal *on page 259*
- **Charcadole®, Aqueous (Can)** *see* Charcoal *on page 259*
- **Charcadole® TFS (Can)** *see* Charcoal *on page 259*
- **Char-Caps [OTC]** *see* Charcoal *on page 259*
- **CharcoAid G® [OTC] [DSC]** *see* Charcoal *on page 259*

Charcoal (CHAR kole)

Medication Safety Issues

Sound-alike/look-alike issues:

Actidose® may be confused with Actos®

U.S. Brand Names Actidose-Aqua® [OTC]; Actidose® with Sorbitol [OTC]; Char-Caps [OTC]; CharcoAid G® [OTC] [DSC]; Charcoal Plus® DS [OTC]; Charcocaps® [OTC]; EZ-Char™ [OTC]; Kerr Insta-Char® [OTC]

Canadian Brand Names Charcadole®; Charcadole®, Aqueous; Charcadole® TFS

Synonyms Activated Carbon; Activated Charcoal; Adsorbent Charcoal; Liquid Antidote; Medicinal Carbon; Medicinal Charcoal

(Continued)

Charcoal *(Continued)*

Pharmacologic Category Antidote

Generic Available Yes

Use Emergency treatment in poisoning by drugs and chemicals; aids the elimination of certain drugs and improves decontamination of excessive ingestions of sustained-release products or in the presence of bezoars; repetitive doses have proven useful to enhance the elimination of certain drugs (eg, theophylline, phenobarbital, and aspirin); repetitive doses for gastric dialysis in uremia to adsorb various waste products; dietary supplement (digestive aid)

Mechanism of Action Adsorbs toxic substances or irritants, thus inhibiting GI absorption; adsorbs intestinal gas; the addition of sorbitol results in hyperosmotic laxative action causing catharsis

Pharmacodynamics/Kinetics Excretion: Feces (as charcoal)

Dosage Oral:

Acute poisoning: **Note:** ~10 g of activated charcoal for each 1 g of toxin is considered adequate; this may require multiple doses. If sorbitol is also used, sorbitol dose should not exceed 1.5 g/kg. When using multiple doses of charcoal, sorbitol should be given with every other dose (not to exceed 2 doses/day).

- Children: 1 g/kg as a single dose; if multiple doses are needed, additional doses can be given as 0.25 g/kg every hour or equivalent (ie, 0.5 g/kg every 2 hours) **or**
  - >1 year-12 years: 25-50 g as a single dose; smaller doses (10-25 g) may be used in children 1-5 years due to smaller gut lumen capacity
- Children >12 years and Adults: 25-100 g as a single dose; if multiple doses are needed, additional doses may be given as 12.5 g/hour or equivalent (ie, 25 g every 2 hours)

Dietary supplement: Adult: 500-520 mg after meals; may repeat in 2 hours if needed (maximum 10 g/day)

Stability Adsorbs gases from air, store in closed container. Dilute powder with at least 8 mL of water per 1 g of charcoal, or mix in a charcoal to water ratio of 1:4 to 1:8. Mix to form a slurry.

Administration Flavoring agents (eg, chocolate) and sorbitol can enhance charcoal's palatability. If treatment includes ipecac syrup, induce vomiting prior to administration of charcoal. Often given with a laxative or cathartic; check for presence of bowel sounds before administration.

Pregnancy Risk Factor C

Contraindications Intestinal obstruction; GI tract not anatomically intact; patients at risk of hemorrhage or GI perforation; if use would increase risk and severity of aspiration; not effective for cyanide, mineral acids, caustic alkalis, organic solvents, iron, ethanol, methanol poisoning, lithium; do not use charcoal with sorbitol in patients with fructose intolerance; charcoal with sorbitol not recommended in children <1 year of age

Warnings/Precautions When using ipecac with charcoal, induce vomiting with ipecac before administering activated charcoal since charcoal adsorbs ipecac syrup. Charcoal may cause vomiting which is hazardous in petroleum distillate and caustic ingestions. If charcoal in sorbitol is administered, doses should be limited to prevent excessive fluid and electrolyte losses. Use caution with decreased peristalsis. Most effective when administered within 1 hour of ingestion for most ingestions.

Adverse Reactions Frequency not defined.

Endocrine & metabolic: Hypernatremia, hypokalemia, and hypermagnesemia may occur with coadministration of cathartics

Gastrointestinal: Vomiting (incidence may increase with sorbitol), diarrhea (with sorbitol), constipation, swelling of abdomen, bowel obstruction

Miscellaneous: Fecal discoloration (black)

Drug Interactions Do not administer concomitantly with syrup of ipecac.

Ethanol/Nutrition/Herb Interactions Food: Do not mix with milk, ice cream, sherbet, or marmalade (may reduce charcoal's effectiveness).

Dosage Forms [DSC] = Discontinued product

Capsule, activated (Char-Caps, Charcocaps®): 260 mg

Granules, activated (CharcoAid G®): 15 g (120 mL) [DSC]

Liquid, activated:

- Actidose-Aqua®: 15 g (72 mL); 25 g (120 mL); 50 g (240 mL)
- Kerr Insta-Char®: 25 g (120 mL) [cherry flavor]; 50 g (240 mL) [unflavored or cherry flavor]

Liquid, activated [with sorbitol]:
  Actidose® with Sorbitol: 25 g (120 mL); 50 g (240 mL)
  Kerr Insta-Char®: 25 g (120 mL); 50 g (240 mL) [cherry flavor]
Pellets, activated (EZ-Char™): 25 g
Powder for suspension, activated: 30 g, 240 g
Tablets, activated (Charcoal Plus® DS): 250 mg

- **Charcoal Plus® DS [OTC]** *see* Charcoal *on page 259*
- **Charcocaps® [OTC]** *see* Charcoal *on page 259*
- **Cheracol® [OTC]** *see* Phenol *on page 1012*
- **CHG** *see* Chlorhexidine Gluconate *on page 267*
- **Chirocaine® [DSC]** *see* Levobupivacaine *on page 741*
- **Chloral** *see* Chloral Hydrate *on page 261*

Chloral Hydrate (KLOR al HYE drate)

Related Information
Moderate Sedation *on page 1442*

U.S. Brand Names Aquachloral® Supprettes®; Somnote™

Canadian Brand Names PMS-Chloral Hydrate

Synonyms Chloral; Hydrated Chloral; Trichloroacetaldehyde Monohydrate

Pharmacologic Category Hypnotic, Nonbenzodiazepine

Restrictions C-IV

Generic Available Yes: Syrup

Use Short-term sedative and hypnotic (<2 weeks); sedative/hypnotic for diagnostic procedures; sedative prior to EEG evaluations

Mechanism of Action Central nervous system depressant effects are due to its active metabolite trichloroethanol, mechanism unknown

Pharmacodynamics/Kinetics
Onset of action: Peak effect: 0.5-1 hour
Duration: 4-8 hours
Absorption: Oral, rectal: Well absorbed
Distribution: Crosses placenta; negligible amounts enter breast milk
Metabolism: Rapidly hepatic to trichloroethanol (active metabolite); variable amounts hepatically and renally to trichloroacetic acid (inactive)
Half-life elimination: Active metabolite: 8-11 hours
Excretion: Urine (as metabolites); feces (small amounts)

Dosage
Children:
  Sedation or anxiety: Oral, rectal: 5-15 mg/kg/dose every 8 hours (maximum: 500 mg/dose)
  Prior to EEG: Oral, rectal: 20-25 mg/kg/dose, 30-60 minutes prior to EEG; may repeat in 30 minutes to maximum of 100 mg/kg or 2 g total
  Hypnotic: Oral, rectal: 20-40 mg/kg/dose up to a maximum of 50 mg/kg/24 hours or 1 g/dose or 2 g/24 hours
  Conscious sedation: Oral: 50-75 mg/kg/dose 30-60 minutes prior to procedure; may repeat 30 minutes after initial dose if needed, to a total maximum dose of 120 mg/kg or 1 g total
Adults: Oral, rectal:
  Sedation, anxiety: 250 mg 3 times/day
  Hypnotic: 500-1000 mg at bedtime or 30 minutes prior to procedure, not to exceed 2 g/24 hours
Discontinuation: Withdraw gradually over 2 weeks if patient has been maintained on high doses for prolonged period of time. Do not stop drug abruptly; sudden withdrawal may result in delirium.

Dosing adjustment/comments in renal impairment: Cl_{cr} <50 mL/minute: Avoid use
Hemodialysis: Dialyzable (50% to 100%); supplemental dose is not necessary
Dosing adjustment/comments in hepatic impairment: Avoid use in patients with severe hepatic impairment

Stability Sensitive to light. Exposure to air causes volatilization. Store in light-resistant, airtight container.

Administration Chilling the syrup may help to mask unpleasant taste. Do not crush capsule (contains drug in liquid form). Gastric irritation may be minimized by diluting dose in water or other oral liquid.
(Continued)

Chloral Hydrate *(Continued)*

Monitoring Parameters Vital signs, O_2 saturation and blood pressure with doses used for conscious sedation

Pregnancy Risk Factor C

Contraindications Hypersensitivity to chloral hydrate or any component of the formulation; hepatic or renal impairment; gastritis or ulcers; severe cardiac disease

Warnings/Precautions Use with caution in patients with porphyria. Use with caution in neonates. Drug may accumulate with repeated use; prolonged use in neonates associated with hyperbilirubinemia. Tolerance to hypnotic effect develops, therefore, not recommended for use >2 weeks. Taper dosage to avoid withdrawal with prolonged use. Trichloroethanol (TCE), a metabolite of chloral hydrate, is a carcinogen in mice; there is no data in humans. Chloral hydrate is considered a second line hypnotic agent in the elderly. Recent interpretive guidelines from the Centers for Medicare and Medicaid Services (CMS) discourage the use of chloral hydrate in residents of long-term care facilities.

Adverse Reactions Frequency not defined.

Central nervous system: Ataxia, disorientation, sedation, excitement (paradoxical), dizziness, fever, headache, confusion, lightheadedness, nightmares, hallucinations, drowsiness, "hangover" effect

Dermatologic: Rash, urticaria

Gastrointestinal: Gastric irritation, nausea, vomiting, diarrhea, flatulence

Hematologic: Leukopenia, eosinophilia, acute intermittent porphyria

Miscellaneous: Physical and psychological dependence may occur with prolonged use of large doses

Overdosage/Toxicology Symptoms of overdose include hypotension, respiratory depression, coma, hypothermia, and cardiac arrhythmias. Treatment is supportive and symptomatic.

Drug Interactions

CNS depressants: Sedative effects and/or respiratory depression with chloral hydrate may be additive with other CNS depressants; monitor for increased effect; includes ethanol, sedatives, antidepressants, narcotic analgesics, and benzodiazepines.

Furosemide: Diaphoresis, flushing, and hypertension have occurred in patients who received I.V. furosemide within 24 hours after administration of chloral hydrate; consider using a benzodiazepine.

Phenytoin: Half-life may be decreased by chloral hydrate; limited documentation (small, single-dose study); monitor.

Warfarin: Effect of oral anticoagulants may be increased by chloral hydrate; monitor INR; warfarin dosage may require adjustment. Chloral hydrate's metabolite may displace warfarin from its protein binding sites resulting in an increase in the hypoprothrombinemic response to warfarin.

Ethanol/Nutrition/Herb Interactions

Ethanol: Avoid ethanol (may increase CNS depression).

Herb/Nutraceutical: Avoid valerian, St John's wort, kava kava, gotu kola (may increase CNS depression).

Test Interactions False-positive urine glucose using Clinitest® method; may interfere with fluorometric urine catecholamine and urinary 17-hydroxycorticosteroid tests

Dosage Forms

Capsule (Somnote™): 500 mg

Suppository, rectal (Aquachloral® Supprettes®): 325 mg [contains tartrazine], 650 mg

Syrup: 500 mg/5 mL (480 mL) [contains sodium benzoate]

Chloramphenicol (klor am FEN i kole)

Medication Safety Issues

Sound-alike/look-alike issues:

Chloromycetin® may be confused with chlorambucil, Chlor-Trimeton®

U.S. Brand Names Chloromycetin® Sodium Succinate

Canadian Brand Names Chloromycetin®; Chloromycetin® Succinate; Diochloram®; Pentamycetin®

Pharmacologic Category Antibiotic, Miscellaneous

Generic Available Yes

Use Treatment of serious infections due to organisms resistant to other less toxic antibiotics or when its penetrability into the site of infection is clinically superior to other antibiotics to which the organism is sensitive; useful in infections caused by *Bacteroides*, *H. influenzae*, *Neisseria meningitidis*, *Salmonella*, and *Rickettsia*; active against many vancomycin-resistant enterococci

Mechanism of Action Reversibly binds to 50S ribosomal subunits of susceptible organisms preventing amino acids from being transferred to growing peptide chains thus inhibiting protein synthesis

Pharmacodynamics/Kinetics

Distribution: To most tissues and body fluids; readily crosses placenta; enters breast milk

CSF:blood level ratio: Normal meninges: 66%; Inflamed meninges: >66%

Protein binding: 60%

Metabolism: Extensively hepatic (90%) to inactive metabolites, principally by glucuronidation; chloramphenicol sodium succinate is hydrolyzed by esterases to active base

Half-life elimination:

Normal renal function: 1.6-3.3 hours

End-stage renal disease: 3-7 hours

Cirrhosis: 10-12 hours

Excretion: Urine (5% to 15%)

Dosage

Meningitis: I.V.: Infants >30 days and Children: 50-100 mg/kg/day divided every 6 hours

Other infections: I.V.:

Infants >30 days and Children: 50-75 mg/kg/day divided every 6 hours; maximum daily dose: 4 g/day

Adults: 50-100 mg/kg/day in divided doses every 6 hours; maximum daily dose: 4 g/day

Dosing adjustment/comments in hepatic impairment: Avoid use in severe liver impairment as increased toxicity may occur

Hemodialysis: Slightly dialyzable (5% to 20%) via hemo- and peritoneal dialysis; no supplemental doses needed in dialysis or continuous arteriovenous or veno-venous hemofiltration

Stability Store at room temperature prior to reconstitution. Reconstituted solutions remain stable for 30 days. Use only clear solutions. Frozen solutions remain stable for 6 months.

Administration Do not administer I.M.; can be administered IVP over at least 1 minute at a concentration of 100 mg/mL, or I.V. intermittent infusion over 15-30 minutes at a final concentration for administration of ≤20 mg/mL.

Monitoring Parameters CBC with reticulocyte and platelet counts, periodic liver and renal function tests, serum drug concentration

Reference Range

Therapeutic levels:

Meningitis:

Peak: 15-25 mcg/mL; toxic concentration: >40 mcg/mL

Trough: 5-15 mcg/mL

Other infections:

Peak: 10-20 mcg/mL

Trough: 5-10 mcg/mL

Timing of serum samples: Draw levels 0.5-1.5 hours after completion of I.V. dose

Pregnancy Risk Factor C

Contraindications Hypersensitivity to chloramphenicol or any component of the formulation

Warnings/Precautions [U.S. Boxed Warning]: Serious and fatal blood dyscrasias have occurred after both short-term and prolonged therapy. Should not be used when less potentially toxic agents are effective. Prolonged use may result in superinfection. Use with caution in patients with impaired renal or hepatic function and in neonates. Reduce dose with impaired liver function. Use with care in patients with glucose 6-phosphate dehydrogenase deficiency.

Adverse Reactions

Three (3) major toxicities associated with chloramphenicol include:

Aplastic anemia, an idiosyncratic reaction which can occur with any route of administration; usually occurs 3 weeks to 12 months after initial exposure to chloramphenicol.

(Continued)

Chloramphenicol *(Continued)*

Bone marrow suppression is thought to be dose related with serum concentrations >25 mcg/mL and reversible once chloramphenicol is discontinued; anemia and neutropenia may occur during the first week of therapy.

Gray syndrome is characterized by circulatory collapse, cyanosis, acidosis, abdominal distention, myocardial depression, coma, and death. Reaction appears to be associated with serum levels ≥50 mcg/mL. May result from drug accumulation in patients with impaired hepatic or renal function.

Additional adverse reactions, frequency not defined:

Central nervous system: Confusion, delirium, depression, fever, headache

Dermatologic: Angioedema, rash, urticaria

Gastrointestinal: Diarrhea, enterocolitis, glossitis, nausea, stomatitis, vomiting

Hematologic: Granulocytopenia, hypoplastic anemia, pancytopenia, thrombocytopenia

Ocular: Optic neuritis

Miscellaneous: Anaphylaxis, hypersensitivity reactions

Overdosage/Toxicology Symptoms of overdose include anemia, metabolic acidosis, hypotension, and hypothermia. Treatment is supportive.

Drug Interactions Inhibits CYP2C9 (weak), 3A4 (weak)

Decreased effect: Phenobarbital and rifampin may decrease concentration of chloramphenicol.

Increased toxicity: Chloramphenicol inhibits the metabolism of chlorpropamide, phenytoin, oral anticoagulants.

Ethanol/Nutrition/Herb Interactions Food: May decrease intestinal absorption of vitamin B_{12} may have increased dietary need for riboflavin, pyridoxine, and vitamin B_{12}.

Test Interactions May cause false-positive results in urine glucose tests when using cupric sulfate (Benedict's solution, Clinitest®).

Dietary Considerations May have increased dietary need for riboflavin, pyridoxine, and vitamin B_{12}. Sodium content of 1 g injection: ~52 mg (2.25 mEq).

Dosage Forms Injection, powder for reconstitution: 1 g [contains sodium ~52 mg/g (2.25 mEq/g)]

- **ChloraPrep® [OTC]** *see* Chlorhexidine Gluconate *on page 267*
- **Chloraseptic® Gargle [OTC]** *see* Phenol *on page 1012*
- **Chloraseptic® Mouth Pain [OTC]** *see* Phenol *on page 1012*
- **Chloraseptic® Rinse [OTC]** *see* Phenol *on page 1012*
- **Chloraseptic® Spray [OTC]** *see* Phenol *on page 1012*
- **Chloraseptic® Spray for Kids [OTC]** *see* Phenol *on page 1012*

Chlordiazepoxide (klor dye az e POKS ide)

Medication Safety Issues

Sound-alike/look-alike issues:

Librium® may be confused with Librax®

Related Information

Anesthesia Considerations for Neurosurgery *on page 1401*

Benzodiazepines *on page 1555*

U.S. Brand Names Librium®

Canadian Brand Names Apo-Chlordiazepoxide®

Synonyms Methaminodiazepoxide Hydrochloride

Pharmacologic Category Benzodiazepine

Restrictions C-IV

Generic Available Yes: Capsule

Use Management of anxiety disorder or for the short-term relief of symptoms of anxiety; withdrawal symptoms of acute alcoholism; preoperative apprehension and anxiety

Mechanism of Action Binds to stereospecific benzodiazepine receptors on the postsynaptic GABA neuron at several sites within the central nervous system, including the limbic system, reticular formation. Enhancement of the inhibitory effect of GABA on neuronal excitability results by increased neuronal membrane permeability to chloride ions. This shift in chloride ions results in hyperpolarization (a less excitable state) and stabilization.

Pharmacodynamics/Kinetics

Distribution: V_d: 3.3 L/kg; crosses placenta; enters breast milk

Protein binding: 90% to 98%

Metabolism: Extensively hepatic to desmethyldiazepam (active and long-acting)

Half-life elimination: 6.6-25 hours; End-stage renal disease: 5-30 hours; Cirrhosis: 30-63 hours

Time to peak, serum: Oral: Within 2 hours; I.M.: Results in lower peak plasma levels than oral

Excretion: Urine (minimal as unchanged drug)

Dosage

Children:

<6 years: Not recommended

>6 years: Anxiety: Oral, I.M.: 0.5 mg/kg/24 hours divided every 6-8 hours

Adults:

Anxiety:

Oral: 15-100 mg divided 3-4 times/day

I.M., I.V.: Initial: 50-100 mg followed by 25-50 mg 3-4 times/day as needed

Preoperative anxiety: I.M.: 50-100 mg prior to surgery

Ethanol withdrawal symptoms: Oral, I.V.: 50-100 mg to start, dose may be repeated in 2-4 hours as necessary to a maximum of 300 mg/24 hours

Note: Up to 300 mg may be given I.M. or I.V. during a 6-hour period, but not more than this in any 24-hour period.

Dosing adjustment in renal impairment: Cl_{cr} <10 mL/minute: Administer 50% of dose

Hemodialysis: Not dialyzable (0% to 5%)

Dosing adjustment/comments in hepatic impairment: Avoid use

Stability Injection: Prior to reconstitution, store under refrigeration and protect from light. Solution should be used immediately following reconstitution.

I.M. use: Reconstitute by adding 2 mL of provided diluent; agitate gently until dissolved. Provided diluent is **not** for I.V. use.

I.V. use: Reconstitute by adding 5 mL NS or SWFI; agitate gently until dissolved; **do not administer this dilution I.M.**

Administration

I.M.: Administer by deep I.M. injection slowly into the upper outer quadrant of the gluteus muscle. Use only the diluent provided for I.M. use. Solutions made with SWFI or NS cause pain with I.M. administration.

I.V.: Administer slowly over at least 1 minute. Do not use the diluent provided for I.M. use. Air bubbles form during reconstitution.

Monitoring Parameters Respiratory and cardiovascular status, mental status, check for orthostasis

Reference Range Therapeutic: 0.1-3 mcg/mL (SI: 0-10 µmol/L); Toxic: >23 mcg/mL (SI: >77 µmol/L)

Anesthesia and Critical Care Concerns/Other Considerations Chronic use of this agent may increase the perioperative benzodiazepine dose needed to achieve desired effect. Abrupt discontinuation after sustained use (generally >10 days) may cause withdrawal symptoms.

Pregnancy Risk Factor D

Contraindications Hypersensitivity to chlordiazepoxide or any component of the formulation (cross-sensitivity with other benzodiazepines may also exist); narrow-angle glaucoma; pregnancy

Warnings/Precautions Active metabolites with extended half-lives may lead to delayed accumulation and adverse effects. Use with caution in elderly or debilitated patients, pediatric patients, patients with hepatic disease (including alcoholics) or renal impairment. Use with caution in patients with respiratory disease or impaired gag reflex. Use with caution in patients with porphyria.

Parenteral administration should be avoided in comatose patients or shock. Adequate resuscitative equipment/personnel should be available, and appropriate monitoring should be conducted at the time of injection and for several hours following administration. The parenteral formulation should be diluted for I.M. administration with the supplied diluent only. This diluent should not be used when preparing the drug for intravenous administration.

Causes CNS depression (dose related) resulting in sedation, dizziness, confusion, or ataxia which may impair physical and mental capabilities. Patients must be cautioned about performing tasks which require mental alertness (eg, operating machinery or driving). Use with caution in patients receiving other CNS depressants or psychoactive agents (lithium, phenothiazines). Effects with other

(Continued)

Chlordiazepoxide *(Continued)*

sedative drugs or ethanol may be potentiated. Benzodiazepines have been associated with falls and traumatic injury and should be used with extreme caution in patients who are at risk of these events (especially the elderly).

Use caution in patients with depression, particularly if suicidal risk may be present. Use with caution in patients with a history of drug dependence. Benzodiazepines have been associated with dependence and acute withdrawal symptoms on discontinuation or reduction in dose. Acute withdrawal, including seizures, may be precipitated in patients after administration of flumazenil to patients receiving long-term benzodiazepine therapy.

Benzodiazepines have been associated with anterograde amnesia. Paradoxical reactions, including hyperactive or aggressive behavior have been reported with benzodiazepines, particularly in adolescent/pediatric or psychiatric patients. Does not have analgesic, antidepressant, or antipsychotic properties.

Adverse Reactions

>10%:

Central nervous system: Drowsiness, fatigue, ataxia, lightheadedness, memory impairment, dysarthria, irritability

Dermatologic: Rash

Endocrine & metabolic: Libido decreased, menstrual disorders

Gastrointestinal: Xerostomia, salivation decreased, appetite increased or decreased, weight gain/loss

Genitourinary: Micturition difficulties

1% to 10%:

Cardiovascular: Hypotension

Central nervous system: Confusion, dizziness, disinhibition, akathisia

Dermatologic: Dermatitis

Endocrine & metabolic: Libido increased

Gastrointestinal: Salivation increased

Genitourinary: Sexual dysfunction, incontinence

Neuromuscular & skeletal: Rigidity, tremor, muscle cramps

Otic: Tinnitus

Respiratory: Nasal congestion

<1% (Limited to important or life-threatening): Photosensitivity

Overdosage/Toxicology Symptoms of overdose include hypotension, respiratory depression, coma, hypothermia, and cardiac arrhythmias. Treatment for benzodiazepine overdose is supportive. Flumazenil has been shown to selectively block the binding of benzodiazepines to CNS receptors, resulting in a reversal of benzodiazepine-induced CNS depression. Respiratory depression may not be reversed.

Drug Interactions Substrate of CYP3A4 (major)

CNS depressants: Sedative effects and/or respiratory depression may be additive with CNS depressants; includes ethanol, barbiturates, narcotic analgesics, and other sedative agents; monitor for increased effect.

CYP3A4 inducers: CYP3A4 inducers may decrease the levels/effects of chlordiazepoxide. Example inducers include aminoglutethimide, carbamazepine, nafcillin, nevirapine, phenobarbital, phenytoin, and rifamycins.

CYP3A4 inhibitors: May increase the levels/effects of chlordiazepoxide. Example inhibitors include azole antifungals, clarithromycin, diclofenac, doxycycline, erythromycin, imatinib, isoniazid, nefazodone, nicardipine, propofol, protease inhibitors, quinidine, telithromycin, and verapamil.

Levodopa: Therapeutic effects may be diminished in some patients following the addition of a benzodiazepine; limited/inconsistent data.

Oral contraceptives: May decrease the clearance of some benzodiazepines (those which undergo oxidative metabolism); monitor for increased benzodiazepine effect.

Theophylline: May partially antagonize some of the effects of benzodiazepines; monitor for decreased response; may require higher doses for sedation.

Ethanol/Nutrition/Herb Interactions

Ethanol: Avoid ethanol (may increase CNS depression).

Food: Serum concentrations/effects may be increased with grapefruit juice, but unlikely because of high oral bioavailability of chlordiazepoxide.

Herb/Nutraceutical: Avoid valerian, St John's wort, kava kava, gotu kola (may increase CNS depression).

Dosage Forms

Capsule, as hydrochloride: 5 mg, 10 mg, 25 mg

Injection, powder for reconstitution, as hydrochloride: 100 mg [diluent contains benzyl alcohol, polysorbate 80, and propylene glycol]

Chlorhexidine Gluconate (klor HEKS i deen GLOO koe nate)

Medication Safety Issues

Sound-alike/look-alike issues:

Peridex® may be confused with Precedex™

U.S. Brand Names Avagard™ [OTC]; BactoShield® CHG [OTC]; Betasept® [OTC]; ChloraPrep® [OTC]; Dyna-Hex® [OTC]; Hibiclens® [OTC]; Hibistat® [OTC]; Operand® Chlorhexidine Gluconate [OTC]; Peridex®; PerioChip®; PerioGard®

Canadian Brand Names Apo-Chlorhexadine®; Hibidil® 1:2000; ORO-Clense

Synonyms CHG; 3M™ Avagard™ [OTC]

Pharmacologic Category Antibiotic, Oral Rinse; Antibiotic, Topical

Generic Available Yes: Oral liquid

Use Skin cleanser for surgical scrub, cleanser for skin wounds, preoperative skin preparation, germicidal hand rinse, and as antibacterial dental rinse. Chlorhexidine is active against gram-positive and gram-negative organisms, facultative anaerobes, aerobes, and yeast.

Orphan drug: Peridex®: Oral mucositis with cytoreductive therapy when used for patients undergoing bone marrow transplant

Mechanism of Action The bactericidal effect of chlorhexidine is a result of the binding of this cationic molecule to negatively charged bacterial cell walls and extramicrobial complexes. At low concentrations, this causes an alteration of bacterial cell osmotic equilibrium and leakage of potassium and phosphorous resulting in a bacteriostatic effect. At high concentrations of chlorhexidine, the cytoplasmic contents of the bacterial cell precipitate and result in cell death.

Pharmacodynamics/Kinetics

Topical hand sanitizer (Avagard™): Duration of antimicrobial protection: 6 hours

Oral rinse (Peridex®, PerioGard®):

Absorption: ~30% retained in the oral cavity following rinsing and slowly released into oral fluids; poorly absorbed

Time to peak, plasma: Oral rinse: Detectable levels not present after 12 hours

Excretion: Feces (~90%); urine (<1%)

Dosage Adults:

Oral rinse (Peridex®, PerioGard®):

Floss and brush teeth, completely rinse toothpaste from mouth and swish 15 mL (one capful) undiluted oral rinse around in mouth for 30 seconds, then expectorate. Caution patient not to swallow the medicine and instruct not to eat for 2-3 hours after treatment. (Cap on bottle measures 15 mL.)

Treatment of gingivitis: Oral prophylaxis: Swish for 30 seconds with 15 mL chlorhexidine, then expectorate; repeat twice daily (morning and evening). Patient should have a re-evaluation followed by a dental prophylaxis every 6 months.

Periodontal chip: One chip is inserted into a periodontal pocket with a probing pocket depth ≥5 mm. Up to 8 chips may be inserted in a single visit. Treatment is recommended every 3 months in pockets with a remaining depth ≥5 mm. If dislodgment occurs 7 days or more after placement, the subject is considered to have had the full course of treatment. If dislodgment occurs within 48 hours, a new chip should be inserted. The chip biodegrades completely and does not need to be removed. Patients should avoid dental floss at the site of PerioChip® insertion for 10 days after placement because flossing might dislodge the chip.

Insertion of periodontal chip: Pocket should be isolated and surrounding area dried prior to chip insertion. The chip should be grasped using forceps with the rounded edges away from the forceps. The chip should be inserted into the periodontal pocket to its maximum depth. It may be maneuvered into position using the tips of the forceps or a flat instrument.

Cleanser:

Surgical scrub: Scrub 3 minutes and rinse thoroughly, wash for an additional 3 minutes

Hand sanitizer (Avagard™): Dispense 1 pumpful in palm of one hand; dip fingertips of opposite hand into solution and work it under nails. Spread remainder evenly over hand and just above elbow, covering all surfaces.

(Continued)

Chlorhexidine Gluconate *(Continued)*

Repeat on other hand. Dispense another pumpful in each hand and reapply to each hand up to the wrist. Allow to dry before gloving.

Hand wash: Wash for 15 seconds and rinse

Hand rinse: Rub 15 seconds and rinse

Stability Store at room temperature

Avagard™: Avoid excessive heat. Ethanol-containing products are flammable; keep away from flames or fire. Hand lotions and gel hand sanitizers are incompatible. The thickeners used in these products (eg, carbomer) react to form an insoluble salt and cause loss of antibacterial action.

Administration

Hand sanitizer (Avagard™): To facilitate drying, continue rubbing hand prep into hands until dry.

Periodontal chip insertion: Pocket should be isolated and surrounding area dried prior to chip insertion. The chip should be grasped using forceps with the rounded edges away from the forceps. The chip should be inserted into the periodontal pocket to its maximum depth. It may be maneuvered into position using the tips of the forceps or a flat instrument. The chip biodegrades completely and does not need to be removed. Patients should avoid dental floss at the site of PerioChip® insertion for 10 days after placement because flossing might dislodge the chip.

Topical: Keep out of eyes, ears, and mouth. Do not routinely apply to wounds which involve more than superficial layers of skin.

Pregnancy Risk Factor B

Contraindications Hypersensitivity to chlorhexidine gluconate or any component of the formulation

Warnings/Precautions

Oral: Staining of oral surfaces (mucosa, teeth, tooth restorations, dorsum of tongue) may occur; may be visible as soon as 1 week after therapy begins and is more pronounced when there is a heavy accumulation of unremoved plaque and when teeth fillings have rough surfaces. Stain does not have a clinically adverse effect, but because removal may not be possible, patient with frontal restoration should be advised of the potential permanency of the stain.

Topical: For topical use only. Keep out of eyes and ears. May stain fabric. There have been case reports of anaphylaxis following chlorhexidine disinfection. Not for preoperative preparation of face or head; avoid contact with meninges.

Adverse Reactions

Oral:

>10%: Increase of tartar on teeth, changes in taste. Staining of oral surfaces (mucosa, teeth, dorsum of tongue) may be visible as soon as 1 week after therapy begins and is more pronounced when there is a heavy accumulation of unremoved plaque and when teeth fillings have rough surfaces. Stain does not have a clinically adverse effect but because removal may not be possible, patient with frontal restoration should be advised of the potential permanency of the stain.

1% to 10%: Gastrointestinal: Tongue irritation, oral irritation

<1% (Limited to important or life-threatening): Dyspnea, facial edema, nasal congestion

Topical: Skin erythema and roughness, dryness, sensitization, allergic reactions

Overdosage/Toxicology Symptoms of oral overdose include gastric distress, nausea, or signs of ethanol intoxication

Drug Interactions No data reported

Dosage Forms

Chip, for periodontal pocket insertion (PerioChip®): 2.5 mg

Liquid, topical [surgical scrub]:

Avagard™: 1% (500 mL) [contains ethyl alcohol and moisturizers]

BactoShield® CHG: 2% (120 mL, 480 mL, 750 mL, 1000 mL, 3800 mL); 4% (120 mL, 480 mL, 750 mL, 1000 mL, 3800 mL) [contains isopropyl alcohol]

Betasept®: 4% (120 mL, 240 mL, 480 mL, 960 mL, 3840 mL) [contains isopropyl alcohol]

ChloraPrep®: 2% (0.67 mL, 1.5 mL, 3 mL, 10.5 mL) [contains isopropyl alcohol 70%; prefilled applicator]

Dyna-Hex®: 2% (120 mL, 960 mL, 3840 mL); 4% (120 mL, 960 mL, 3840 mL)

Hibiclens®: 4% (15 mL, 120 mL, 240 mL, 480 mL, 960 mL, 3840 mL) [contains isopropyl alcohol]

Operand® Chlorhexidine Gluconate: 2% (120 mL); 4% (120 mL, 240 mL, 480 mL, 960 mL, 3840 mL) [contains isopropyl alcohol]

Liquid, oral rinse: 0.12% (480 mL)

Peridex®: 0.12% (480 mL) [contains alcohol 11.6%]

PerioGard®: 0.12% (480 mL) [contains alcohol 11.6%; mint flavor]

Pad [prep pad] (Hibistat®): 0.5% (50s) [contains isopropyl alcohol]

Sponge/Brush (BactoShield® CHG): 4% per sponge/brush [contains isopropyl alcohol]

- ♦ **Chlormeprazine** *see* Prochlorperazine *on page 1061*
- ♦ **Chloromycetin® (Can)** *see* Chloramphenicol *on page 262*
- ♦ **Chloromycetin® Sodium Succinate** *see* Chloramphenicol *on page 262*
- ♦ **Chloromycetin® Succinate (Can)** *see* Chloramphenicol *on page 262*

Chloroprocaine (klor oh PROE kane)

Medication Safety Issues

Sound-alike/look-alike issues:

Nesacaine® may be confused with Neptazane®

Related Information

Local Anesthetics *on page 1532*

U.S. Brand Names Nesacaine®; Nesacaine®-MPF

Canadian Brand Names Nesacaine®-CE

Synonyms Chloroprocaine Hydrochloride

Pharmacologic Category Local Anesthetic

Generic Available Yes

Use Infiltration anesthesia and peripheral and epidural anesthesia

Mechanism of Action Chloroprocaine HCl is benzoic acid, 4-amino-2-chloro-2-(diethylamino) ethyl ester monohydrochloride. Chloroprocaine is an ester-type local anesthetic, which stabilizes the neuronal membranes and prevents initiation and transmission of nerve impulses thereby affecting local anesthetic actions. Local anesthetics including chloroprocaine, reversibly prevent generation and conduction of electrical impulses in neurons by decreasing the transient increase in permeability to sodium. The differential sensitivity generally depends on the size of the fiber; small fibers are more sensitive than larger fibers and require a longer period for recovery. Sensory pain fibers are usually blocked first, followed by fibers that transmit sensations of temperature, touch, and deep pressure. High concentrations block sympathetic somatic sensory and somatic motor fibers. The spread of anesthesia depends upon the distribution of the solution. This is primarily dependent on the volume of drug injected.

Pharmacodynamics/Kinetics

Onset of action: 6-12 minutes

Duration: 30-60 minutes

Distribution: V_d: Depends upon route of administration; high concentrations found in highly perfused organs such as liver, lungs, heart, and brain

Metabolism: Plasma cholinesterases

Excretion: Urine

Dosage Dosage varies with anesthetic procedure, the area to be anesthetized, the vascularity of the tissues, depth of anesthesia required, degree of muscle relaxation required, and duration of anesthesia; range.

Children >3 years (normally developed): Maximum dose (without epinephrine): 11 mg/kg; for infiltration, concentrations of 0.5% to 1% are recommended; for nerve block, concentrations of 1% to 1.5% are recommended

Adults:

Maximum single dose (without epinephrine): 11 mg/kg; maximum dose: 800 mg

Maximum single dose (with epinephrine): 14 mg/kg; maximum dose: 1000 mg

Infiltration and peripheral nerve block:

Mandibular: 2%: 2-3 mL; total dose 40-60 mg

Infraorbital: 2%: 0.5-1 mL; total dose 10-20 mg

Brachial plexus: 2%; 30-40 mL; total dose 600-800 mg

Digital (without epinephrine): 1%; 3-4 mL; total dose: 30-40 mg

Pudendal: 2%; 10 mL each side; total dose: 400 mg

Paracervical: 1%; 3 mL per each of four sites

Caudal block: Preservative-free: 2% or 3%: 15-25 mL; may repeat at 40-60 minute intervals

(Continued)

Chloroprocaine *(Continued)*

Lumbar epidural block: Preservative-free: 2% or 3%: 2-2.5 mL per segment; usual total volume: 15-25 mL; may repeat with doses that are 2-6 mL less than initial dose every 40-50 minutes.

Stability Store at 15°C to 30°C (59°F to 86°F); protect from light and freezing. Dilute with NS. To prepare 1:200,000 epinephrine-chloroprocaine HCl injection, add 0.1 mL of a 1:1000 epinephrine injection to 20 mL of preservative free chloroprocaine. Discard Nesacaine®-MPF following single use.

Administration Before injecting, withdraw syringe plunger to ensure injection is not into vein or artery.

Monitoring Parameters Cardiovascular and respiratory status; mental status

Anesthesia and Critical Care Concerns/Other Considerations Termination of anesthesia by pneumatic tourniquet inflation should be attempted when the agent is administered by infiltration or regional injection. Seizures commonly respond to diazepam, midazolam, or thiopental, while hypotension responds to I.V. fluids and Trendelenburg positioning. Bradyarrhythmias (when the heart rate is <60) can be treated with I.V., I.M., or SubQ atropine 15 mcg/kg. With the development of metabolic acidosis, I.V. sodium bicarbonate 0.5-2 mEq/kg and ventilatory assistance should be instituted.

Pregnancy Risk Factor C

Contraindications Hypersensitivity to chloroprocaine, other ester type anesthetics, or any component of the formulation; myasthenia gravis; do not use for subarachnoid administration

Warnings/Precautions Use with caution in patients with hepatic impairment. **Do not use solutions containing preservatives for caudal or epidural block.** Local anesthetics have been associated with rare occurrences of sudden respiratory arrest; seizures due to systemic toxicity leading to cardiac arrest have also been reported, presumably following unintentional intravascular injection. A test dose is recommended prior to epidural administration (prior to initial dose) and all reinforcing doses with continuous catheter technique.

Adverse Reactions

Frequency not defined.

Cardiovascular: Bradycardia, cardiac arrest, hypotension, ventricular arrhythmia

Central nervous system: Anxiety, dizziness, restlessness, tinnitus, unconsciousness

Dermatologic: Angioneurotic edema, erythema, pruritus, urticaria

Ocular: Blurred vision

Respiratory: Respiratory arrest

Miscellaneous: Allergic reactions, anaphylactoid reactions

<1% (Limited to important or life-threatening): Seizure (0.1%)

Overdosage/Toxicology Symptoms may include anxiety, blurred vision, bradyarrhythmias, CNS depression, dizziness, drowsiness, metabolic acidosis, methemoglobinemia, restlessness, seizures, and tremors. Treatment is symptomatic and supportive. Termination of anesthesia by pneumatic tourniquet inflation should be attempted when chloroprocaine is administered by infiltration or regional injection.

Drug Interactions

PABA (from ester-type anesthetics) may inhibit sulfonamides.

Dosage Forms

Injection, solution, as hydrochloride (Nesacaine®): 1% (30 mL); 2% (30 mL) [contains disodium EDTA and methylparaben]

Injection, solution, as hydrochloride [preservative free] (Nesacaine®-MPF): 2% (20 mL); 3% (20 mL)

References

Freeman DW and Arnold NI, "Paracervical Block With Low Doses of Chloroprocaine: Fetal and Maternal Effects," *JAMA*, 1975, 231(1):56-7.

Jankowsky EC, "Pharmacologic Aspects of Local Anesthetic Use," *Anesth Clin North Am*, 1990, 8:1-25.

♦ **Chloroprocaine Hydrochloride** *see* Chloroprocaine *on page 269*

Chlorothiazide (klor oh THYE a zide)

U.S. Brand Names Diuril®

Canadian Brand Names Diuril®

Pharmacologic Category Diuretic, Thiazide

Generic Available Yes: Tablet

Use Management of mild-to-moderate hypertension; adjunctive treatment of edema

Mechanism of Action Inhibits sodium reabsorption in the distal tubules causing increased excretion of sodium and water as well as potassium and hydrogen ions, magnesium, phosphate, calcium

Pharmacodynamics/Kinetics

Onset of action: Diuresis: Oral: 2 hours; I.V.: 15 minutes

Duration of diuretic action: Oral: 6-12 hours; I.V.: ~2 hours

Absorption: Oral: Poor

Half-life elimination: 1-2 hours

Time to peak, serum: Oral: ~4 hours; I.V.: 30 minutes

Excretion: Urine (as unchanged drug)

Dosage Note: The manufacturer states that I.V. and oral dosing are equivalent. Some clinicians may use lower I.V. doses, however, because of chlorothiazide's poor oral absorption. I.V. dosing in infants and children has not been well established.

Infants <6 months:

- Oral: 20-40 mg/kg/day in 2 divided doses (maximum dose: 375 mg/day)
- I.V. (unlabeled): 2-8 mg/kg/day in 2 divided doses; doses up to 20 mg/kg/day have been used (anecdotal reports)

Infants >6 months and Children:

- Oral: 10-20 mg/kg/day in 2 divided doses (maximum dose: 375 mg/day in children <2 years or 1 g/day in children 2-12 years)
- I.V. (unlabeled): 4 mg/kg/day in 1-2 divided doses; doses up to 20 mg/kg/day have been used (anecdotal reports)

Adults:

- Hypertension: Oral: 500-2000 mg/day divided in 1-2 doses (manufacturer labeling); doses of 125-500 mg/day have also been recommended
- Edema: Oral, I.V.: 250-1000 mg once or twice daily; intermittent treatment (eg, therapy on alternative days) may be appropriate for some patients. Maximum daily dose: 1000 mg (ACC/AHA 2005 Heart Failure Guidelines)

Elderly: Oral: 500 mg once daily **or** 1 g 3 times/week

Dosage adjustment in renal impairment: Cl_{cr} <10 mL/minute: Avoid use. Ineffective with low GFR

Note: ACC/AHA 2005 Heart Failure Guidelines suggest that thiazides lose their efficacy when Cl_{cr} <40 mL/minute

Stability

Powder for injection: Prior to reconstitution, store between 2°C to 25°C (36°F to 77°F). To reconstitute, add SWFI 18 mL to make 28 mg/mL. May be further diluted with dextrose or sodium chloride solutions. Reconstituted solution is stable for 24 hours at room temperature; precipitation will occur in <24 hours in pH <7.4. Single use only, discard any unused reconstituted solution.

Suspension, tablets: Store at room temperature 15°C to 30°C (59°F to 86°F); protect from freezing

Administration Do **not** administer injection via I.M. or SubQ route. Administer I.V. ≤0.5 g over 5 minutes.

Monitoring Parameters Serum electrolytes, renal function, blood pressure; assess weight, I & O reports daily to determine fluid loss

Anesthesia and Critical Care Concerns/Other Considerations Thiazide diuretics are effective first-line therapeutic agents in the management of hypertension and have proven to be of benefit in terms of cardiovascular outcome. If given the morning of surgery it may render the patient volume depleted and blood pressure may be labile during general anesthesia.

Pregnancy Risk Factor C (manufacturer); D (expert analysis)

Contraindications Hypersensitivity to chlorothiazide, any component of the formulation, thiazides, or sulfonamide-derived drugs; anuria; renal decompensation; pregnancy (see Pregnancy Implications)

Warnings/Precautions Use with caution in severe renal disease. Electrolyte disturbances (hypokalemia, hypochloremic alkalosis, hyponatremia) can occur. Use with caution in severe hepatic dysfunction; hepatic encephalopathy can be

(Continued)

Chlorothiazide *(Continued)*

caused by electrolyte disturbances. Gout can be precipitate in certain patients with a history of gout, a familial predisposition to gout, or chronic renal failure. Cautious use in diabetics; may see a change in glucose control. Can cause SLE exacerbation or activation. Use with caution in patients with moderate or high cholesterol concentrations. Photosensitization may occur. Correct hypokalemia before initiating therapy.

Chemical similarities are present among sulfonamides, sulfonylureas, carbonic anhydrase inhibitors, thiazides, and loop diuretics (except ethacrynic acid). Use in patients with thiazide or sulfonamide allergy is specifically contraindicated in product labeling. A risk of cross-reaction exists in patients with allergy to any of these compounds; avoid use when previous reaction has been severe.

Adverse Reactions Frequency not defined.

Cardiovascular: Hypotension, orthostatic hypotension, necrotizing angiitis
Central nervous system: Dizziness, headache, restlessness, vertigo
Dermatologic: Alopecia, erythema multiforme, exfoliative dermatitis, photosensitivity, Stevens-Johnson syndrome, toxic epidermal necrolysis
Endocrine & metabolic: Cholesterol increased, hypokalemia, hypomagnesemia, triglycerides increased
Gastrointestinal: Abdominal cramping, anorexia, constipation, diarrhea, gastric irritation, nausea, pancreatitis, sialadenitis, vomiting
Genitourinary: Impotence
Hematologic: Agranulocytosis, aplastic anemia, hemolytic anemia, leukopenia, thrombocytopenia
Hepatic: Jaundice
Neuromuscular & skeletal: Muscle spasm, paresthesia, weakness
Ocular: Blurred vision, xanthopsia
Renal: Azotemia, hematuria, interstitial nephritis, renal failure, renal dysfunction
Respiratory: Pneumonitis, pulmonary edema, respiratory distress
Miscellaneous: Anaphylactic reactions, systemic lupus erythematosus

Overdosage/Toxicology Symptoms of overdose include signs and symptoms of hypovolemia, hypermotility, diuresis, lethargy, confusion, muscle weakness, and coma. Treatment is supportive.

Drug Interactions

ACE inhibitors: Increased hypotension if aggressively diuresed with a thiazide diuretic
Antidiabetic agents (insulin, oral agents): Dosage adjustment of antidiabetic agent may be needed.
Beta-blockers increase hyperglycemic effects of thiazides in type 2 diabetes mellitus (noninsulin dependent, NIDDM)
Corticosteroids: May increase electrolyte-depletion effects of chlorothiazide.
Cyclosporine and thiazides can increase the risk of gout or renal toxicity; avoid concurrent use
Digoxin toxicity can be exacerbated if a thiazide induces hypokalemia or hypomagnesemia.
Lithium toxicity can occur by reducing renal excretion of lithium; monitor lithium concentration and adjust as needed
Neuromuscular-blocking agents can prolong blockade; monitor serum potassium and neuromuscular status
NSAIDs can decrease the efficacy of thiazides reducing the diuretic and antihypertensive effects

Ethanol/Nutrition/Herb Interactions

Ethanol: May increase risk of orthostatic hypotension.
Food: Chlorothiazide serum levels may be increased if taken with food.
Herb/Nutraceutical: Avoid dong quai if using for hypertension (has estrogenic activity). Avoid dong quai, St John's wort (may also cause photosensitization). Avoid ephedra, yohimbe, ginseng (may worsen hypertension). Avoid natural licorice (due to mineralocorticoid activity). Avoid garlic (may have increased antihypertensive effect).

Test Interactions Increased creatine phosphokinase [CPK] (S), ammonia (B), amylase (S), calcium (S), chloride (S), cholesterol (S), glucose, increased acid (S), decreased chloride (S), magnesium, potassium (S), sodium (S); may interfere with tests for parathyroid function

Dietary Considerations May need to decrease sodium and calcium, may need to increase potassium, zinc, magnesium, and riboflavin in diet. Sodium content of 500 mg injection: 57.5 mg (2 mEq).

Dosage Forms

Injection, powder for reconstitution, as sodium: 500 mg

Suspension, oral: 250 mg/5 mL (237 mL) [contains alcohol 0.5% and benzoic acid]

Tablet: 250 mg, 500 mg

ChlorproMAZINE (klor PROE ma zeen)

Medication Safety Issues

Sound-alike/look-alike issues:

ChlorproMAZINE may be confused with chlorproPAMIDE, clomiPRAMINE, prochlorperazine, promethazine

Thorazine® may be confused with thiamine, thioridazine

Canadian Brand Names Apo-Chlorpromazine®; Largactil®; Novo-Chlorpromazine

Synonyms Chlorpromazine Hydrochloride; CPZ

Pharmacologic Category Antipsychotic Agent, Typical, Phenothiazine

Generic Available Yes

Use Control of mania; treatment of schizophrenia; control of nausea and vomiting; relief of restlessness and apprehension before surgery; acute intermittent porphyria; adjunct in the treatment of tetanus; intractable hiccups; combativeness and/or explosive hyperexcitable behavior in children 1-12 years of age and in short-term treatment of hyperactive children

Unlabeled/Investigational Use Management of psychotic disorders

Mechanism of Action Chlorpromazine is an aliphatic phenothiazine antipsychotic which blocks postsynaptic mesolimbic dopaminergic receptors in the brain; exhibits a strong alpha-adrenergic blocking effect and depresses the release of hypothalamic and hypophyseal hormones; believed to depress the reticular activating system, thus affecting basal metabolism, body temperature, wakefulness, vasomotor tone, and emesis

Pharmacodynamics/Kinetics

Onset of action: I.M.: 15 minutes; Oral: 30-60 minutes

Absorption: Rapid

Distribution: V_d: 20 L/kg; crosses the placenta; enters breast milk

Protein binding: 92% to 97%

Metabolism: Extensively hepatic to active and inactive metabolites

Bioavailability: 20%

Half-life, biphasic: Initial: 2 hours; Terminal: 30 hours

Excretion: Urine (<1% as unchanged drug) within 24 hours

Dosage

Children ≥6 months:

Schizophrenia/psychoses:

Oral: 0.5-1 mg/kg/dose every 4-6 hours; older children may require 200 mg/day or higher

I.M., I.V.: 0.5-1 mg/kg/dose every 6-8 hours

<5 years (22.7 kg): Maximum: 40 mg/day

5-12 years (22.7-45.5 kg): Maximum: 75 mg/day

Nausea and vomiting:

Oral: 0.5-1 mg/kg/dose every 4-6 hours as needed

I.M., I.V.: 0.5-1 mg/kg/dose every 6-8 hours

<5 years (22.7 kg): Maximum: 40 mg/day

5-12 years (22.7-45.5 kg): Maximum: 75 mg/day

Adults:

Schizophrenia/psychoses:

Oral: Range: 30-2000 mg/day in 1-4 divided doses, initiate at lower doses and titrate as needed; usual dose: 400-600 mg/day; some patients may require 1-2 g/day

I.M., I.V.: Initial: 25 mg, may repeat (25-50 mg) in 1-4 hours, gradually increase to a maximum of 400 mg/dose every 4-6 hours until patient is controlled; usual dose: 300-800 mg/day

Intractable hiccups: Oral, I.M.: 25-50 mg 3-4 times/day

Nausea and vomiting:

Oral: 10-25 mg every 4-6 hours

I.M., I.V.: 25-50 mg every 4-6 hours

Elderly: Behavioral symptoms associated with dementia: Initial: 10-25 mg 1-2 times/day; increase at 4- to 7-day intervals by 10-25 mg/day. Increase dose

(Continued)

ChlorproMAZINE *(Continued)*

intervals (bid, tid, etc) as necessary to control behavior response or side effects; maximum daily dose: 800 mg; gradual increases (titration) may prevent some side effects or decrease their severity.

Dosing comments in renal impairment: Hemodialysis: Not dialyzable (0% to 5%)

Dosing adjustment/comments in hepatic impairment: Avoid use in severe hepatic dysfunction

Stability Injection: Protect from light; a slightly yellowed solution does not indicate potency loss, but a markedly discolored solution should be discarded; diluted injection (1 mg/mL) with NS and stored in 5 mL vials remains stable for 30 days

Administration Note: Avoid skin contact with oral solution or injection solution; may cause contact dermatitis.

I.V.: Direct or intermittent infusion: Infuse 1 mg or portion thereof over 1 minute.

Monitoring Parameters Vital signs; lipid profile, fasting blood glucose/Hgb A_{1c}; BMI; mental status; abnormal involuntary movement scale (AIMS); extrapyramidal symptoms (EPS)

Reference Range

Therapeutic: 50-300 ng/mL (SI: 157-942 nmol/L)

Toxic: >750 ng/mL (SI: >2355 nmol/L); serum concentrations poorly correlate with expected response

Pregnancy Risk Factor C

Contraindications Hypersensitivity to chlorpromazine or any component of the formulation (cross-reactivity between phenothiazines may occur); severe CNS depression; coma

Warnings/Precautions Highly sedating, use with caution in disorders where CNS depression is a feature. Use with caution in Parkinson's disease. Caution in patients with hemodynamic instability; bone marrow suppression; predisposition to seizures, subcortical brain damage, severe cardiac, hepatic, renal, or respiratory disease. Esophageal dysmotility and aspiration have been associated with antipsychotic use - use with caution in patients at risk of aspiration pneumonia (ie, Alzheimer's disease). Caution in breast cancer or other prolactin-dependent tumors (may elevate prolactin levels). May alter temperature regulation or mask toxicity of other drugs due to antiemetic effects. May alter cardiac conduction - life-threatening arrhythmias have occurred with therapeutic doses of neuroleptics. May cause orthostatic hypotension - use with caution in patients at risk of this effect or those who would tolerate transient hypotensive episodes (cerebrovascular disease, cardiovascular disease, or other medications which may predispose). Significant hypotension may occur, particularly with parenteral administration. Injection contains sulfites.

Phenothiazines may cause anticholinergic effects (confusion, agitation, constipation, xerostomia, blurred vision, urinary retention). Therefore, they should be used with caution in patients with decreased gastrointestinal motility, urinary retention, BPH, xerostomia, or visual problems. Conditions which also may be exacerbated by cholinergic blockade include narrow-angle glaucoma (screening is recommended) and worsening of myasthenia gravis. Relative to other neuroleptics, chlorpromazine has a moderate potency of cholinergic blockade.

May cause extrapyramidal symptoms, including pseudoparkinsonism, acute dystonic reactions, akathisia, and tardive dyskinesia (risk of these reactions is low-moderate relative to other neuroleptics). May be associated with neuroleptic malignant syndrome (NMS) or pigmentary retinopathy.

Adverse Reactions Frequency not defined.

Cardiovascular: Postural hypotension, tachycardia, dizziness, nonspecific QT changes

Central nervous system: Drowsiness, dystonias, akathisia, pseudoparkinsonism, tardive dyskinesia, neuroleptic malignant syndrome, seizure

Dermatologic: Photosensitivity, dermatitis, skin pigmentation (slate gray)

Endocrine & metabolic: Lactation, breast engorgement, false-positive pregnancy test, amenorrhea, gynecomastia, hyper- or hypoglycemia

Gastrointestinal: Xerostomia, constipation, nausea

Genitourinary: Urinary retention, ejaculatory disorder, impotence

Hematologic: Agranulocytosis, eosinophilia, leukopenia, hemolytic anemia, aplastic anemia, thrombocytopenic purpura

Hepatic: Jaundice

Ocular: Blurred vision, corneal and lenticular changes, epithelial keratopathy, pigmentary retinopathy

Overdosage/Toxicology Symptoms of overdose include deep sleep, coma, extrapyramidal symptoms, abnormal involuntary muscle movements, and hypotension. Following initiation of essential overdose management, toxic symptom treatment and supportive treatment should be initiated. Neuroleptics often cause extrapyramidal symptoms (eg, dystonic reactions) requiring management with anticholinergic agents such as benztropine mesylate 1-2 mg for adult patients (oral, I.M., I.V.) or diphenhydramine 25-50 mg (oral, I.M., I.V.) may be effective.

Drug Interactions **Substrate** of CYP1A2 (minor), 2D6 (major), 3A4 (minor); **Inhibits** CYP2D6 (strong), 2E1 (weak)

Acetylcholinesterase inhibitors (central): May increase the risk of antipsychotic-related extrapyramidal symptoms; monitor.

Aluminum salts: May decrease the absorption of phenothiazines; monitor

Amphetamines: Efficacy may be diminished by antipsychotics; in addition, amphetamines may increase psychotic symptoms; avoid concurrent use

Anticholinergics: May inhibit the therapeutic response to phenothiazines and excess anticholinergic effects may occur; includes benztropine, trihexyphenidyl, biperiden, and drugs with significant anticholinergic activity (TCAs, antihistamines, disopyramide)

Antihypertensives: Concurrent use of phenothiazines with an antihypertensive may produce additive hypotensive effects (particularly orthostasis)

Bromocriptine: Phenothiazines inhibit the ability of bromocriptine to lower serum prolactin concentrations

CNS depressants: Sedative effects may be additive with phenothiazines; monitor for increased effect; includes barbiturates, benzodiazepines, narcotic analgesics, ethanol and other sedative agents

CYP2D6 inhibitors: May increase the levels/effects of chlorpromazine. Example inhibitors include delavirdine, fluoxetine, miconazole, paroxetine, pergolide, quinidine, quinine, ritonavir, and ropinirole.

CYP2D6 substrates: Chlorpromazine may increase the levels/effects of CYP2D6 substrates. Example substrates include amphetamines, selected beta-blockers, dextromethorphan, fluoxetine, lidocaine, mirtazapine, nefazodone, paroxetine, risperidone, ritonavir, thioridazine, tricyclic antidepressants, and venlafaxine.

CYP2D6 prodrug substrates: Chlorpromazine may decrease the levels/effects of CYP2D6 prodrug substrates. Example prodrug substrates include codeine, hydrocodone, oxycodone, and tramadol.

Epinephrine: Chlorpromazine (and possibly other low potency antipsychotics) may diminish the pressor effects of epinephrine

Guanethidine and guanadrel: Antihypertensive effects may be inhibited by chlorpromazine

Levodopa: Chlorpromazine may inhibit the antiparkinsonian effect of levodopa; avoid this combination

Lithium: Chlorpromazine may produce neurotoxicity with lithium; this is a rare effect

Metoclopramide: May increase extrapyramidal symptoms (EPS) or risk.

Phenytoin: May reduce serum levels of phenothiazines; phenothiazines may increase phenytoin serum levels

Propranolol: Serum concentrations of phenothiazines may be increased; propranolol also increases phenothiazine concentrations

Polypeptide antibiotics: Rare cases of respiratory paralysis have been reported with concurrent use of phenothiazines

QT_c-prolonging agents: Effects on QT_c interval may be additive with phenothiazines, increasing the risk of malignant arrhythmias; includes type Ia antiarrhythmics, TCAs, and some quinolone antibiotics (sparfloxacin, moxifloxacin and gatifloxacin)

Sulfadoxine-pyrimethamine: May increase phenothiazine concentrations

Tricyclic antidepressants: Concurrent use may produce increased toxicity or altered therapeutic response

Trazodone: Phenothiazines and trazodone may produce additive hypotensive effects

Valproic acid: Serum levels may be increased by phenothiazines

Ethanol/Nutrition/Herb Interactions

Ethanol: Avoid ethanol (may increase CNS depression).

Herb/Nutraceutical: Avoid St John's wort (may decrease chlorpromazine levels, increase photosensitization, or enhance sedative effect). Avoid dong quai (may

(Continued)

ChlorproMAZINE *(Continued)*

enhance photosensitization). Avoid kava kava, gotu kola, valerian (may increase CNS depression).

Test Interactions False-positives for phenylketonuria, amylase, uroporphyrins, urobilinogen. May cause false-positive pregnancy test.

Dosage Forms

Injection, solution, as hydrochloride: 25 mg/mL (1 mL, 2 mL)

Tablet, as hydrochloride: 10 mg, 25 mg, 50 mg, 100 mg, 200 mg

♦ **Chlorpromazine Hydrochloride** *see* ChlorproMAZINE *on page 273*

Choline Magnesium Trisalicylate

(KOE leen mag NEE zhum trye sa LIS i late)

Related Information

Acetaminophen and NSAIDS, Dosing Data *on page 1543*

U.S. Brand Names Trilisate® [DSC]

Synonyms Tricosal

Pharmacologic Category Salicylate

Generic Available Yes

Use Management of osteoarthritis, rheumatoid arthritis, and other arthritis; acute painful shoulder

Mechanism of Action Inhibits prostaglandin synthesis; acts on the hypothalamus heat-regulating center to reduce fever; blocks the generation of pain impulses

Pharmacodynamics/Kinetics

Onset of action: Peak effect: ~2 hours

Absorption: Stomach and small intestines

Distribution: Readily into most body fluids and tissues; crosses placenta; enters breast milk

Half-life elimination (dose dependent): Low dose: 2-3 hours; High dose: 30 hours

Time to peak, serum: ~2 hours

Dosage Oral (based on total salicylate content):

Children <37 kg: 50 mg/kg/day given in 2 divided doses; 2250 mg/day for heavier children

Adults: 500 mg to 1.5 g 2-3 times/day **or** 3 g at bedtime; usual maintenance dose: 1-4.5 g/day

Elderly: 750 mg 3 times/day

Dosing adjustment/comments in renal impairment: Avoid use in severe renal impairment

Stability Store at controlled room temperature of 15°C to 30°C (59°F to 86°F).

Administration Liquid may be mixed with fruit juice just before drinking. Do not administer with antacids. Take with a full glass of water and remain in an upright position for 15-30 minutes after administration.

Monitoring Parameters Serum magnesium with high dose therapy or in patients with impaired renal function; serum salicylate levels, renal function, hearing changes or tinnitus, abnormal bruising, weight gain and response (ie, pain)

Reference Range Salicylate blood levels for anti-inflammatory effect: 150-300 mcg/mL; analgesia and antipyretic effect: 30-50 mcg/mL

Anesthesia and Critical Care Concerns/Other Considerations Salicylate salts do not inhibit platelet aggregation and, therefore, should not be substituted for aspirin in the prophylaxis of thrombosis.

Pregnancy Risk Factor C/D (3rd trimester)

Contraindications Hypersensitivity to salicylates, other nonacetylated salicylates, other NSAIDs, or any component of the formulation; bleeding disorders; pregnancy (3rd trimester)

Warnings/Precautions Salicylate salts may not inhibit platelet aggregation and, therefore, should not be substituted for aspirin in the prophylaxis of thrombosis. Use with caution in patients with impaired renal function, dehydration, erosive gastritis, asthma, or peptic ulcer. Discontinue use 1 week prior to surgical procedures. Children and teenagers who have or are recovering from chickenpox or flu-like symptoms should not use this product. Changes in behavior (along with nausea and vomiting) may be an early sign of Reye's syndrome; patients should be instructed to contact their healthcare provider if these occur.

Elderly are a high-risk population for adverse effects from NSAIDs. As many as 60% of elderly can develop peptic ulceration and/or hemorrhage asymptomatically. Use lowest effective dose for shortest period possible. Tinnitus or impaired hearing may indicate toxicity. Tinnitus may be a difficult and unreliable indication of toxicity due to age-related hearing loss or eighth cranial nerve damage. CNS adverse effects may be observed in the elderly at lower doses than younger adults.

Adverse Reactions

<20%:

Gastrointestinal: Nausea, vomiting, diarrhea, heartburn, dyspepsia, epigastric pain, constipation

Otic: Tinnitus

<2%:

Central nervous system: Headache, lightheadedness, dizziness, drowsiness, lethargy

Otic: Hearing impairment

<1%: Anorexia, asthma, BUN and creatinine increased, bruising, confusion, duodenal ulceration, dysgeusia, edema, epistaxis, erythema multiforme, esophagitis, hallucinations, hearing loss (irreversible), hepatic enzymes increased, gastric ulceration, occult bleeding, pruritus, rash, weight gain

Overdosage/Toxicology Symptoms of overdose include tinnitus, vomiting, acute renal failure, hyperthermia, irritability, seizures, coma, and metabolic acidosis. For acute ingestion, determine serum salicylate levels 6 hours after ingestion. Nomograms, such as the "Done" nomogram, may be helpful for estimating the severity of aspirin poisoning and directing treatment using serum salicylate levels. Treatment is based upon symptomatology.

Drug Interactions

ACE inhibitors: Effects of ACE inhibitors may be decreased by concurrent therapy with NSAIDs.

Antacids: Concomitant use may lead to decreased salicylate concentration.

Warfarin: Concomitant use may increase the hypoprothrombinemic effect of warfarin.

Ethanol/Nutrition/Herb Interactions

Ethanol: Avoid ethanol (may enhance gastric mucosal irritation).

Food: May decrease the rate but not the extent of oral absorption.

Herb/Nutraceutical: Avoid cat's claw, dong quai, evening primrose, feverfew, garlic, ginger, ginkgo, red clover, horse chestnut, green tea, ginseng (all have additional antiplatelet activity). Limit curry powder, paprika, licorice, Benedictine liqueur, prunes, raisins, tea, and gherkins; may cause salicylate accumulation. These foods contain 6 mg salicylate/100 g.

Test Interactions False-negative results for glucose oxidase urinary glucose tests (Clinistix®); false-positives using the cupric sulfate method (Clinitest®); also, interferes with Gerhardt test (urinary ketone analysis), VMA determination; 5-HIAA, xylose tolerance test, and T_3 and T_4; increased PBI

Dietary Considerations Take with food or large volume of water or milk to minimize GI upset. Liquid may be mixed with fruit juice just before drinking. Hypermagnesemia resulting from magnesium salicylate; avoid or use with caution in renal insufficiency.

Dosage Forms

Liquid: 500 mg/5 mL (240 mL) [choline salicylate 293 mg and magnesium salicylate 362 mg per 5 mL; cherry cordial flavor]

Tablet: 500 mg [choline salicylate 293 mg and magnesium salicylate 362 mg]; 750 mg [choline salicylate 440 mg and magnesium salicylate 544 mg]; 1000 mg [choline salicylate 587 mg and magnesium salicylate 725 mg]

- **Chromium** *see* Trace Metals *on page 1296*
- **Chronovera® (Can)** *see* Verapamil *on page 1352*
- **Cialis®** *see* Tadalafil *on page 1230*
- **Cidecin** *see* Daptomycin *on page 352*

Cilazapril (sye LAY za pril)

Related Information

Preoperative Evaluation of the Cardiac Patient for Noncardiac Surgery *on page 1485*

(Continued)

Cilazapril *(Continued)*

Canadian Brand Names Inhibace®; Novo-Cilazapril

Synonyms Cilazapril Monohydrate

Pharmacologic Category Angiotensin-Converting Enzyme (ACE) Inhibitor

Restrictions Not available in U.S.

Use Management of hypertension; treatment of congestive heart failure

Mechanism of Action Competitive inhibitor of angiotensin-converting enzyme (ACE); prevents conversion of angiotensin I to angiotensin II, a potent vasoconstrictor; results in lower levels of angiotensin II which causes an increase in plasma renin activity and a reduction in aldosterone secretion.

Pharmacodynamics/Kinetics

Onset of action: Antihypertensive: ~1 hour

Duration: Therapeutic effect: 24 hours

Absorption: Rapid

Metabolism: To active form (cilazaprilat)

Bioavailability: 57%

Half-life elimination: Cilazaprilat: Terminal: 36-49 hours

Time to peak: 3-7 hours

Excretion: In urine (91%)

Dosage Oral:

Hypertension: 2.5-5 mg once daily (maximum dose: 10 mg/day)

Congestive heart failure: Initial: 0.5 mg once daily; if tolerated, after 5 days increase to 1 mg/day (lowest maintenance dose); may increase to maximum of 2.5 mg once daily

Elderly: Initial: 1.25 mg once daily; titrate slowly as tolerated

Dosage adjustment in renal impairment:

Hypertension:

Cl_{cr} 10-40 mL/minute: Initial: 0.5 mg once daily (maximum dose: 2.5 mg once daily)

Cl_{cr} <10 mL/minute: 0.25-0.5 mg once or twice weekly

Congestive heart failure:

Cl_{cr} 10-40 mL/minute: Initial: 0.25-0.5 mg once daily (maximum dose: 2.5 mg once daily)

Cl_{cr} <10 mL/minute: 0.25-0.5 mg once or twice weekly

Dosage adjustment in hepatic impairment: Initial: ≤0.5 mg once daily (with caution)

Stability Store at 15°C to 30°C (59°F to 86°F).

Administration May be administered with or without food.

Pregnancy Risk Factor Not assigned; C/D (2nd and 3rd trimesters) based on other ACE inhibitors

Contraindications Hypersensitivity to cilazapril or any component of the formulation; angioedema related to previous treatment with an ACE inhibitor; idiopathic or hereditary angioedema; bilateral renal artery stenosis (unilateral if single kidney); ascites; pregnancy (2nd or 3rd trimester)

Warnings/Precautions Anaphylactic reactions can occur. Angioedema can occur at any time during treatment (especially following first dose). It may involve head and neck (potentially affecting the airway) or the intestine (presenting with abdominal pain). Prolonged monitoring may be required especially if tongue, glottis, or larynx are involved as they are associated with airway obstruction. Those with a history of airway surgery in this situation have a higher risk. Careful blood pressure monitoring with first dose (hypotension can occur especially in volume-depleted patients). Dosage adjustment needed in renal impairment. Use with caution in hypovolemia; collagen vascular diseases; valvular stenosis (particularly aortic stenosis); hyperkalemia; or before, during, or immediately after anesthesia. Avoid rapid dosage escalation which may lead to renal insufficiency.

Rare toxicities associated with ACE inhibitors include cholestatic jaundice (which may progress to hepatic necrosis) and neutropenia/agranulocytosis with myeloid hyperplasia. Patients with collagen vascular diseases or renal impairment may be at increased risk for hematologic toxicity. Consider baseline and periodic monitoring of WBC and serum creatinine. Hypersensitivity reactions may be seen during hemodialysis with high-flux dialysis membranes (eg, AN69). Deterioration in renal function can occur with initiation. Use with caution in unilateral renal artery stenosis and pre-existing renal insufficiency.

Adverse Reactions

1% to 10%

Cardiovascular: Palpitation (up to 1%), hypotension (symptomatic, up to 1% in CHF patients), orthostatic hypotension (2%)

Central nervous system: Headache (3% to 5%), dizziness (3% to 8%), fatigue (2% to 3%)

Gastrointestinal: Nausea (1% to 3%)

Neuromuscular & skeletal: Weakness (0.3% to 2%)

Renal: Serum creatinine increased

Respiratory: Cough (2% in hypertension, up to 7.5% in CHF patients)

<1% (Limited to important or life-threatening): Angina, angioedema, arrhythmia, atrial fibrillation, AV block, bronchospasm, cardiogenic shock, depression, dyspnea, gout, hemolytic anemia, hyperglycemia, hyperkalemia, MI, neutropenia, pancreatitis, paresthesia, rash, renal failure, Stevens-Johnson syndrome, stroke, syncope, thrombocytopenic purpura, vomiting

Overdosage/Toxicology Mild hypotension has been the primary toxic effect seen with acute overdose. Bradycardia may also occur. Hyperkalemia occurs even with therapeutic doses, especially in patients with renal insufficiency and those taking NSAIDs. Treatment is symptom-directed and supportive.

Drug Interactions

Allopurinol: Case reports (rare) indicate a possible increased risk of Stevens-Johnson syndrome when combined with captopril. Risk with other ACE inhibitors not established.

Alpha$_1$ blockers: Hypotensive effect increased.

Aspirin: The effects of ACE inhibitors may be blunted by aspirin administration, particularly at higher dosages and/or increase adverse renal effects.

Diuretics: Hypovolemia due to diuretics may precipitate acute hypotensive events or acute renal failure.

Insulin: Risk of hypoglycemia may be increased.

Lithium: Risk of lithium toxicity may be increased; monitor lithium levels, especially the first 4 weeks of therapy.

Mercaptopurine: Risk of neutropenia may be increased.

NSAIDs: May attenuate hypertensive efficacy; effect has been seen with captopril and may occur with other ACE inhibitors; monitor blood pressure. May increase adverse renal effects.

Potassium-sparing diuretics (amiloride, potassium, spironolactone, triamterene): Increased risk of hyperkalemia.

Potassium supplements: May increase the risk of hyperkalemia.

Trimethoprim (high dose): May increase the risk of hyperkalemia.

Ethanol/Nutrition/Herb Interactions

Food: Cilazapril serum concentrations may be decreased if taken with food (no apparent effect on activity). Long-term use of ACE inhibitors may result in a zinc deficiency which can result in a decrease in taste perception.

Herb/Nutraceutical: Avoid dong quai if using for hypertension (has estrogenic activity). Avoid ephedra, yohimbe, ginseng (may worsen hypertension). Avoid garlic (may have increased antihypertensive effect). Long-term use may result in zinc deficiency.

Dietary Considerations May be taken with or without food.

Dosage Forms [CAN] = Canadian brand name

Tablet:

Inhibace® [CAN], Novo-Cilazapril [CAN]: 1 mg, 2.5 mg, 5 mg [not available in the U.S.]

♦ **Cilazapril Monohydrate** *see* Cilazapril *on page 277*

Cilostazol (sil OH sta zol)

Medication Safety Issues

Sound-alike/look-alike issues:

Pletal® may be confused with Plendil®

U.S. Brand Names Pletal®

Canadian Brand Names Pletal®

Synonyms OPC-13013

Pharmacologic Category Antiplatelet Agent; Phosphodiesterase Enzyme Inhibitor

Generic Available Yes

(Continued)

Cilostazol *(Continued)*

Use Symptomatic management of peripheral vascular disease, primarily intermittent claudication

Unlabeled/Investigational Use Treatment of acute coronary syndromes and for graft patency improvement in percutaneous coronary interventions with or without stenting

Mechanism of Action Cilostazol and its metabolites are inhibitors of phosphodiesterase III. As a result, cyclic AMP is increased leading to reversible inhibition of platelet aggregation and vasodilation. Other effects of phosphodiesterase III inhibition include increased cardiac contractility, accelerated AV nodal conduction, increased ventricular automaticity, heart rate, and coronary blood flow.

Pharmacodynamics/Kinetics

Onset of action: 2-4 weeks; may require up to 12 weeks

Protein binding: 97% to 98%

Metabolism: Hepatic via CYP3A4 (primarily), 1A2, 2C19, and 2D6; at least one metabolite has significant activity

Half-life elimination: 11-13 hours

Excretion: Urine (74%) and feces (20%) as metabolites

Dosage Adults: Oral: 100 mg twice daily taken at least one-half hour before or 2 hours after breakfast and dinner; dosage should be reduced to 50 mg twice daily during concurrent therapy with inhibitors of CYP3A4 or CYP2C19 (see Drug Interactions)

Anesthesia and Critical Care Concerns/Other Considerations In some animal models, high-dose or long-term administration was associated with a variety of cardiovascular lesions, including endocardial hemorrhage, hemosiderin deposition and left ventricular fibrosis, coronary arteritis, and periarteritis.

Pregnancy Risk Factor C

Contraindications Hypersensitivity to cilostazol or any component of the formulation; heart failure (of any severity)

Warnings/Precautions Use with caution in patients receiving other platelet aggregation inhibitors or in patients with thrombocytopenia. Discontinue therapy if thrombocytopenia or leukopenia occur, progression to agranulocytosis (reversible) has been reported when cilostazol was not immediately stopped. When cilostazol and clopidogrel are used concurrently, manufacturer recommends checking bleeding times. Withhold for at least 4-6 half-lives prior to elective surgical procedures. Use with caution in patients receiving CYP3A4 inhibitors (eg, ketoconazole or erythromycin) or CYP2C19 inhibitors (eg, omeprazole). **[U.S. Boxed Warning]: Heart disease (of any severity);** use with caution in severe underlying heart disease. Use caution in moderate-to-severe hepatic impairment. Use cautiously in severe renal impairment (Cl_{cr} <25 mL/minute). Safety and efficacy in pediatric patients have not been established.

Adverse Reactions

>10%:

- Central nervous system: Headache (27% to 34%)
- Gastrointestinal: Abnormal stools (12% to 15%), diarrhea (12% to 19%)
- Respiratory: Rhinitis (7% to 12%)
- Miscellaneous: Infection (10% to 14%)

2% to 10%:

- Cardiovascular: Peripheral edema (7% to 9%), palpitation (5% to 10%), tachycardia (4%)
- Central nervous system: Dizziness (9% to 10%), vertigo (up to 3%)
- Gastrointestinal: Dyspepsia (6%), nausea (6% to 7%), abdominal pain (4% to 5%), flatulence (2% to 3%)
- Neuromuscular & skeletal: Back pain (6% to 7%), myalgia (2% to 3%)
- Respiratory: Pharyngitis (7% to 10%), cough (3% to 4%)

<2% (Limited to important or life-threatening): Agranulocytosis, anemia, asthma, atrial fibrillation, atrial flutter, blindness, bursitis, cardiac arrest, cerebral infarction/ischemia, cholelithiasis, colitis, CHF, cystitis, diabetes mellitus, duodenal ulcer, duodenitis, esophageal hemorrhage, esophagitis, extradural hematoma, gout, granulocytopenia, hemorrhage, hepatic dysfunction, hypotension, leukopenia, myocardial infarction/ischemia, neuralgia, nodal arrhythmia, periodontal abscess, peptic ulcer, pneumonia, polycythemia, postural hypotension, QT_c prolongation, rectal hemorrhage, retinal hemorrhage, retroperitoneal hemorrhage, Stevens-Johnson syndrome, subdural hematoma, supraventricular tachycardia, syncope, thrombocytopenia, thrombosis, torsade de pointes, ventricular tachycardia

Overdosage/Toxicology Experience with overdosage in humans is limited. Headache, diarrhea, hypotension, tachycardia, and/or cardiac arrhythmias may occur. Treatment is symptomatic and supportive. Hemodialysis is unlikely to be of value. In some animal models, high-dose or long-term administration was associated with a variety of cardiovascular lesions, including endocardial hemorrhage, hemosiderin deposition and left ventricular fibrosis, coronary arteritis, and periarteritis.

Drug Interactions **Substrate** of CYP1A2 (minor), 2C19 (major), 2D6 (minor), 3A4 (major)

Antifungal agents (imidazole): May decrease the metabolism, via CYP isoenzymes, of cilostazol. Manufacturer recommends a reduced dose of cilostazole during concurrent therapy.

CYP2C19 inhibitors may increase the levels/effects of cilostazol. Example inhibitors include delavirdine, fluconazole, fluvoxamine, gemfibrozil, isoniazid, omeprazole, and ticlopidine.

CYP3A4 inhibitors may increase the levels/effects of cilostazol. Example inhibitors include azole antifungals, clarithromycin, diclofenac, doxycycline, erythromycin, imatinib, isoniazid, nefazodone, nicardipine, propofol, protease inhibitors, quinidine, telithromycin, and verapamil.

Drotrecogin alfa: Antiplatelet agents may enhance the adverse/toxic effect of drotrecogin alfa. Bleeding may occur.

Macrolide antibiotics: May decrease the metabolism, via CYP isoenzymes, of cilostazol. Examples include clarithromycin, erythromycin, telithromycin. The manufacturer recommends considering a reduced dose (50 mg twice daily) during coadministration of these agents.

Nonsteroidal anti-inflammatory agents: May enhance the adverse/toxic effect of antiplatelet agents. An increased risk of bleeding may occur.

Omeprazole: May enhance the adverse/toxic effect of cilostazol. The manufacturer recommends considering a reduced dose (50 mg twice daily) during coadministration of omeprazole.

Salicylates: Antiplatelet agents such as cilostazol may enhance the adverse/toxic effect of salicylates. Increased risk of bleeding may result.

Treprostinil: May enhance the adverse/toxic effect of antiplatelet agents such as cilostazol. Bleeding may occur.

Ethanol/Nutrition/Herb Interactions Food: Taking cilostazol with a high-fat meal may increase peak concentration by 90%. Avoid concurrent ingestion of grapefruit juice due to the potential to inhibit CYP3A4.

Dietary Considerations It is best to take cilostazol 30 minutes before or 2 hours after meals.

Dosage Forms Tablet: 50 mg, 100 mg

♦ **Ciloxan®** *see* Ciprofloxacin *on page 285*

Cimetidine (sye MET i deen)

Medication Safety Issues

Sound-alike/look-alike issues:

Cimetidine may be confused with simethicone

Related Information

Anesthesia for Patients With Liver Disease *on page 1421*

Moderate Sedation *on page 1442*

U.S. Brand Names Tagamet®; Tagamet® HB 200 [OTC]

Canadian Brand Names Apo-Cimetidine®; Gen-Cimetidine; Novo-Cimetidine; Nu-Cimet; PMS-Cimetidine; Tagamet® HB

Pharmacologic Category Histamine H_2 Antagonist

Generic Available Yes

Use Short-term treatment of active duodenal ulcers and benign gastric ulcers; long-term prophylaxis of duodenal ulcer; gastric hypersecretory states; gastroesophageal reflux; prevention of upper GI bleeding in critically-ill patients; labeled for OTC use for prevention or relief of heartburn, acid indigestion, or sour stomach

Unlabeled/Investigational Use Part of a multidrug regimen for *H. pylori* eradication to reduce the risk of duodenal ulcer recurrence

Mechanism of Action Competitive inhibition of histamine at H_2 receptors of the gastric parietal cells resulting in reduced gastric acid secretion, gastric volume and hydrogen ion concentration reduced

(Continued)

Cimetidine *(Continued)*

Pharmacodynamics/Kinetics

Onset of action: 1 hour
Duration: 4-8 hours
Absorption: Rapid
Distribution: Crosses placenta; enters breast milk
Protein binding: 20%
Metabolism: Partially hepatic
Bioavailability: 60% to 70%
Half-life elimination: Neonates: 3.6 hours; Children: 1.4 hours; Adults: Normal renal function: 2 hours
Time to peak, serum: Oral: 1-2 hours
Excretion: Primarily urine (48% as unchanged drug); feces (some)

Dosage

Children: Oral, I.M., I.V.: 20-40 mg/kg/day in divided doses every 6 hours

Children ≥12 years and Adults: Oral: Heartburn, acid indigestion, sour stomach (OTC labeling): 200 mg up to twice daily; may take 30 minutes prior to eating foods or beverages expected to cause heartburn or indigestion

Adults:

Short-term treatment of active ulcers:

Oral: 300 mg 4 times/day or 800 mg at bedtime or 400 mg twice daily for up to 8 weeks

Note: Higher doses of 1600 mg at bedtime for 4 weeks may be beneficial for a subpopulation of patients with larger duodenal ulcers (>1 cm defined endoscopically) who are also heavy smokers (≥1 pack/day).

I.M., I.V.: 300 mg every 6 hours or 37.5 mg/hour by continuous infusion; I.V. dosage should be adjusted to maintain an intragastric pH ≥5

Prevention of upper GI bleed in critically-ill patients: 50 mg/hour by continuous infusion; I.V. dosage should be adjusted to maintain an intragastric pH ≥5

Note: Reduce dose by 50% if Cl_{cr} <30 mL/minute; treatment >7 days has not been evaluated.

Duodenal ulcer prophylaxis: Oral: 400 mg at bedtime

Gastric hypersecretory conditions: Oral, I.M., I.V.: 300-600 mg every 6 hours; dosage not to exceed 2.4 g/day

Gastroesophageal reflux disease: Oral: 400 mg 4 times/day or 800 mg twice daily for 12 weeks

Helicobacter pylori eradication (unlabeled use): 400 mg twice daily; requires combination therapy with antibiotics

Dosing adjustment/interval in renal impairment: Children and Adults:

Cl_{cr} 10-50 mL/minute: Administer 50% of normal dose

Cl_{cr} <10 mL/minute: Administer 25% of normal dose

Hemodialysis: Slightly dialyzable (5% to 20%); administer after dialysis

Dosing adjustment/comments in hepatic impairment: Usual dose is safe in mild liver disease but use with caution and in reduced dosage in severe liver disease; increased risk of CNS toxicity in cirrhosis suggested by enhanced penetration of CNS

Stability

Tablet: Store between 15°C and 30°C (59°F to 86°F); protect from light.

Solution for injection/infusion: Intact vials should be stored at room temperature, between 15°C and 30°C (59°F to 86°F); protect from light. May precipitate from solution upon exposure to cold, but can be redissolved by warming without degradation.

Stability at room temperature:

Prepared bags: 7 days

Premixed bags: Manufacturer expiration dating and out of overwrap stability: 15 days

Stable in parenteral nutrition solutions for up to 7 days when protected from light.

Physically incompatible with barbiturates, amphotericin B, and cephalosporins

Administration

Oral: Administer with meals so that the drug's peak effect occurs at the proper time (peak inhibition of gastric acid secretion occurs at 1 and 3 hours after dosing in fasting subjects and approximately 2 hours in nonfasting subjects; this correlates well with the time food is no longer in the stomach offering a buffering effect)

Injection: May be administered as a slow I.V. push or preferably as an I.V. intermittent or I.V. continuous infusion. Administer each 300 mg (or fraction thereof) over a minimum of 5 minutes when giving I.V. push. Give intermittent infusion over 15-30 minutes for each 300 mg dose. Intermittent infusions are administered over 15-30 minutes at a final concentration not to exceed 6 mg/mL; for patients with an active bleed, preferred method of administration is continuous infusion.

Monitoring Parameters CBC, gastric pH, occult blood with GI bleeding; monitor renal function to correct dose.

Anesthesia and Critical Care Concerns/Other Considerations Cimetidine has extensive drug interactions, particularly with antiarrhythmics (lidocaine, phenytoin, procainamide, quinidine) and may also increase the likelihood of theophylline and cyclosporine toxicity. Because of inhibition of warfarin metabolism, cimetidine may increase INR in patients on anticoagulation therapy.

Pregnancy Risk Factor B

Contraindications Hypersensitivity to cimetidine, any component of the formulation, or other H_2 antagonists

Warnings/Precautions Reversible confusional states, usually clearing within 3-4 days after discontinuation, have been linked to use. Increased age (>50 years) and renal or hepatic impairment are thought to be associated. Dosage should be adjusted in renal/hepatic impairment or in patients receiving drugs metabolized through the P450 system.

Over the counter (OTC) cimetidine should not be taken by individuals experiencing painful swallowing, vomiting with blood, or bloody or black stools; medical attention should be sought. A physician should be consulted prior to use when pain in the stomach, shoulder, arms or neck is present; if heartburn has occurred for >3 months; or if unexplained weight loss, or nausea and vomiting occur. Frequent wheezing, shortness of breath, lightheadedness, or sweating, especially with chest pain or heartburn, should also be reported. Consultation of a healthcare provider should occur by patients if also taking theophylline, phenytoin, or warfarin; if heartburn or stomach pain continues or worsens; or if use is required for >14 days. Pregnant or breast-feeding women should speak to a healthcare provider before use. OTC cimetidine is not approved for use in patients <12 years of age.

Adverse Reactions

1% to 10%:

Central nervous system: Headache (2% to 4%), dizziness (1%), somnolence (1%), agitation

Endocrine & metabolic: Gynecomastia (<1% to 4%)

Gastrointestinal: Diarrhea (1%), nausea, vomiting

<1% (Limited to important or life-threatening): Agranulocytosis, anaphylaxis, aplastic anemia, AST/ALT increased, bradycardia, confusion, creatinine increased, decreased sexual ability, hemolytic anemia (immune-based), hepatic fibrosis (case report), hypotension, interstitial nephritis, neutropenia, pancreatitis, pancytopenia, polymyositis, tachycardia, thrombocytopenia, vasculitis

Adverse reactions reported with H_2 antagonists: Alopecia, AV heart block, bradycardia, erythema multiforme, exfoliative dermatitis, Stevens-Johnson syndrome, toxic epidermal necrolysis

Overdosage/Toxicology Reported ingestions of up to 20 g have resulted in transient side effects seen with recommended doses. Reports of ingestions up to 40 g have documented severe CNS depression, including unresponsiveness. Treatment is symptom-directed and supportive. Animal data suggests that ventilation assistance and beta-blocker treatment may be effective in managing the possible respiratory depression and tachycardia, respectively.

Drug Interactions Inhibits CYP1A2 (moderate), 2C9 (weak), 2C19 (moderate), 2D6 (moderate), 2E1 (weak), 3A4 (moderate)

Note: There are many potential interactions. Listed are the most significant ones.

Alfentanil: Increased serum concentration; monitor for toxicity.

Amiodarone: Serum concentration of amiodarone is increased; avoid concurrent use.

Atazanavir: Absorption may be decreased by cimetidine; separate doses by 12 hours.

Benzodiazepines (except lorazepam, oxazepam, temazepam): Serum concentration of the benzodiazepine is increased; consider alternative H_2 antagonist or monitor for benzodiazepine toxicity.

(Continued)

Cimetidine *(Continued)*

Beta-blockers (except atenolol, betaxolol, bisoprolol, nadolol, penbutolol): Effects of the beta-blocker may be increased; use a renally-eliminated beta-blocker or alternative H_2 antagonist.

Calcium channel blockers (except amlodipine and nicardipine): Serum concentration of the CCB is increased; monitor for toxicity.

Carbamazepine: Plasma concentration of carbamazepine may increase transiently (1 week). Monitor for carbamazepine toxicity or use an alternative H_2 antagonist.

Carmustine: Myelotoxicity of carmustine is increased; avoid concurrent use.

Cefpodoxime, cefuroxime: Oral absorption of these agents may be reduced by increased pH; consider alternative antibiotic or separate dosing by at least 2 hours.

Cisapride: Bioavailability of cisapride is increased; avoid concurrent use.

Citalopram: Serum concentration of citalopram is increased; use an alternative H_2 antagonist or adjust citalopram dose.

Clozapine: Cimetidine may increase levels/effects; consider alternative H_2 antagonist

Cyclosporine: Serum concentration of cyclosporine may increase; monitor cyclosporine levels.

CYP1A2 substrates: Cimetidine may increase the levels/effects of CYP1A2 substrates. Example substrates include aminophylline, fluvoxamine, mexiletine, mirtazapine, ropinirole, theophylline, and trifluoperazine.

CYP2C19 substrates: Cimetidine may increase the levels/effects of CYP2C19 substrates. Example substrates include citalopram, diazepam, methsuximide, phenytoin, propranolol, and sertraline.

CYP2D6 substrates: Cimetidine may increase the levels/effects of CYP2D6 substrates. Example substrates include amphetamines, selected beta-blockers, dextromethorphan, fluoxetine, lidocaine, mirtazapine, nefazodone, paroxetine, risperidone, ritonavir, thioridazine, tricyclic antidepressants, and venlafaxine.

CYP2D6 prodrug substrates: Cimetidine may decrease the levels/effects of CYP2D6 prodrug substrates. Example prodrug substrates include codeine, hydrocodone, oxycodone, and tramadol.

CYP3A4 substrates: Cimetidine may increase the levels/effects of CYP3A4 substrates. Example substrates include benzodiazepines, calcium channel blockers, cyclosporine, mirtazapine, nateglinide, nefazodone, sildenafil (and other PDE-5 inhibitors), tacrolimus, and venlafaxine. Selected benzodiazepines (midazolam and triazolam), cisapride, ergot alkaloids, selected HMG-CoA reductase inhibitors (lovastatin and simvastatin), and pimozide are generally contraindicated with strong CYP3A4 inhibitors.

Delavirdine: Absorption of delavirdine is decreased; avoid concurrent use with H_2 antagonists.

Dofetilide: Cimetidine may increase the levels/effects of dofetilide; avoid concurrent use

Flecainide: Serum concentration of flecainide is increased, especially in patients with renal failure.

Ketoconazole, fluconazole, itraconazole (especially capsule): Decreased serum concentration; avoid concurrent use with H_2 antagonists.

Lidocaine: Serum concentration of lidocaine is increased; use alternative H_2 antagonist.

Metformin: Serum levels/effects may be increased by cimetidine; monitor for hypoglycemia.

Moricizine: Serum concentration of moricizine is increased; monitor for toxicity.

Phenytoin: Serum levels/effects may be increased by cimetidine; avoid concurrent use.

Procainamide: Cimetidine may increase levels/effects; monitor.

Propafenone: Serum concentration of propafenone is increased; monitor for toxicity.

Quinolones: Renal elimination of quinolone antibiotics may be decreased.

Selective serotonin reuptake inhibitors (eg, paroxetine, citalopram): Serum concentrations may be increased by cimetidine; monitor.

Sulfonylureas: Cimetidine may increase levels/effects; monitor for hypoglycemia

Tacrine: Plasma concentration of tacrine is increased; consider alternative H_2 antagonist.

TCAs: Serum concentration is increased; consider alternative H_2 antagonist or monitor for TCAs toxicity.

Theophylline: Serum concentration of theophylline is increased; consider alternative H_2 antagonist.

Thioridazine: Serum levels/effects may be increased by cimetidine; concurrent use contraindicated by manufacturer.

Warfarin: INR is increased; cimetidine's effect is dose related. Use an alternative H_2 antagonist if possible or monitor INR closely and adjust warfarin dose as needed.

Ethanol/Nutrition/Herb Interactions

Ethanol: Avoid ethanol (may enhance gastric mucosal irritation).

Food: Cimetidine may increase serum caffeine levels if taken with caffeine. Cimetidine peak serum levels may be decreased if taken with food.

Herb/Nutraceutical: St John's wort may decrease cimetidine levels.

Dosage Forms

Infusion, as hydrochloride [premixed in NS]: 300 mg (50 mL)

Injection, solution, as hydrochloride: 150 mg/mL (2 mL, 8 mL) [8 mL size contains benzyl alcohol]

Liquid, oral, as hydrochloride: 300 mg/5 mL (240 mL, 480 mL) [contains alcohol 2.8%; mint-peach flavor]

Tablet: 200 mg [OTC], 300 mg, 400 mg, 800 mg

Tagamet®: 300 mg, 400 mg

Tagamet® HB 200: 200 mg

◆ **Cipro®** *see* Ciprofloxacin *on page 285*

◆ **Cipro® XL (Can)** *see* Ciprofloxacin *on page 285*

Ciprofloxacin (sip roe FLOKS a sin)

Medication Safety Issues

Sound-alike/look-alike issues:

Ciprofloxacin may be confused with cephalexin

Ciloxan® may be confused with cinoxacin, Cytoxan®

Cipro® may be confused with Ceftin®

Related Information

Prevention of Wound Infection and Sepsis in Surgical Patients *on page 1588*

U.S. Brand Names Ciloxan®; Cipro®; Cipro® XR; Proquin® XR

Canadian Brand Names Apo-Ciproflox®; Ciloxan®; Cipro®; Cipro® XL; CO Ciprofloxacin; Gen-Ciprofloxacin; Novo-Ciprofloxacin; PMS-Ciprofloxacin; RAN™-Ciprofloxacin; ratio-Ciprofloxacin; Rhoxal-ciprofloxacin; Sandoz-Ciprofloxacin; Taro-Ciprofloxacin

Synonyms Ciprofloxacin Hydrochloride

Pharmacologic Category Antibiotic, Ophthalmic; Antibiotic, Quinolone

Generic Available Yes: Suspension, tablet

Use

Children: Complicated urinary tract infections and pyelonephritis due to *E. coli*. **Note:** Although effective, ciprofloxacin is not the drug of first choice in children.

Children and adults: To reduce incidence or progression of disease following exposure to aerolized *Bacillus anthracis*. Ophthalmologically, for superficial ocular infections (corneal ulcers, conjunctivitis) due to susceptible strains

Adults: Treatment of the following infections when caused by susceptible bacteria: Urinary tract infections; acute uncomplicated cystitis in females; chronic bacterial prostatitis; lower respiratory tract infections (including acute exacerbations of chronic bronchitis); acute sinusitis; skin and skin structure infections; bone and joint infections; complicated intra-abdominal infections (in combination with metronidazole); infectious diarrhea; typhoid fever due to *Salmonella typhi* (eradication of chronic typhoid carrier state has not been proven); uncomplicated cervical and urethra gonorrhea (due to *N. gonorrhoeae*); nosocomial pneumonia; empirical therapy for febrile neutropenic patients (in combination with piperacillin)

Unlabeled/Investigational Use Acute pulmonary exacerbations in cystic fibrosis (children); cutaneous/gastrointestinal/oropharyngeal anthrax (treatment, children and adults); disseminated gonococcal infection (adults); chancroid (adults); prophylaxis to *Neisseria meningitidis* following close contact with an infected person

Mechanism of Action Inhibits DNA-gyrase in susceptible organisms; inhibits relaxation of supercoiled DNA and promotes breakage of double-stranded DNA

Pharmacodynamics/Kinetics

Absorption: Oral: Immediate release tablet: Rapid (~50% to 85%)

(Continued)

Ciprofloxacin *(Continued)*

Distribution: V_d: 2.1-2.7 L/kg; tissue concentrations often exceed serum concentrations especially in kidneys, gallbladder, liver, lungs, gynecological tissue, and prostatic tissue; CSF concentrations: 10% of serum concentrations (noninflamed meninges), 14% to 37% (inflamed meninges); crosses placenta; enters breast milk

Protein binding: 20% to 40%

Metabolism: Partially hepatic; forms 4 metabolites (limited activity)

Half-life elimination: Children: 2.5 hours; Adults: Normal renal function: 3-5 hours

Time to peak: Oral:

Immediate release tablet: 0.5-2 hours

Extended release tablet: Cipro® XR: 1-2.5 hours, Proquin® XR: 3.5-8.7 hours

Excretion: Urine (30% to 50% as unchanged drug); feces (15% to 43%)

Dosage Note: Extended release tablets and immediate release formulations are not interchangeable. Unless otherwise specified, oral dosing reflects the use of immediate release formulations.

Usual dosage ranges:

Children (see Warnings/Precautions):

Oral: 20-30 mg/kg/day in 2 divided doses; maximum dose: 1.5 g/day

I.V.: 20-30 mg/kg/day divided every 12 hours; maximum dose: 800 mg/day

Adults:

Oral: 250-750 mg every 12 hours

I.V.: 200-400 mg every 12 hours

Indication-specific dosing:

Children:

Anthrax:

Inhalational (postexposure prophylaxis):

Oral: 15 mg/kg/dose every 12 hours for 60 days; maximum: 500 mg/dose

I.V.: 10 mg/kg/dose every 12 hours for 60 days; do **not** exceed 400 mg/dose (800 mg/day)

Cutaneous (treatment, CDC guidelines): Oral: 10-15 mg/kg every 12 hours for 60 days (maximum: 1 g/day); amoxicillin 80 mg/kg/day divided every 8 hours is an option for completion of treatment after clinical improvement. **Note:** In the presence of systemic involvement, extensive edema, lesions on head/neck, refer to I.V. dosing for treatment of inhalational/gastrointestinal/oropharyngeal anthrax.

Inhalational/gastrointestinal/oropharyngeal (treatment, CDC guidelines): I.V.: Initial: 10-15 mg/kg every 12 hours for 60 days (maximum: 500 mg/dose); switch to oral therapy when clinically appropriate; refer to adult dosing for notes on combined therapy and duration

Bacterial conjunctivitis: See adult dosing

Corneal ulcer: See adult dosing

Cystic fibrosis (unlabeled use):

Oral: 40 mg/kg/day divided every 12 hours administered following 1 week of I.V. therapy has been reported in a clinical trial; total duration of therapy: 10-21 days

I.V.: 30 mg/kg/day divided every 8 hours for 1 week, followed by oral therapy, has been reported in a clinical trial

Urinary tract infection (complicated) or pyelonephritis:

Oral: 20-30 mg/kg/day in 2 divided doses (every 12 hours) for 10-21 days; maximum: 1.5 g/day

I.V.: 6-10 mg/kg every 8 hours for 10-21 days (maximum: 400 mg/dose)

Adults:

Anthrax:

Inhalational (postexposure prophylaxis):

Oral: 500 mg every 12 hours for 60 days

I.V.: 400 mg every 12 hours for 60 days

Cutaneous (treatment, CDC guidelines): Oral: Immediate release formulation: 500 mg every 12 hours for 60 days. **Note:** In the presence of systemic involvement, extensive edema, lesions on head/neck, refer to I.V. dosing for treatment of inhalational/gastrointestinal/oropharyngeal anthrax

Inhalational/gastrointestinal/oropharyngeal (treatment, CDC guidelines): I.V.: 400 mg every 12 hours. **Note:** Initial treatment should include two or more agents predicted to be effective (per CDC recommendations). Agents suggested for use in conjunction with ciprofloxacin or doxycycline include rifampin, vancomycin, imipenem, penicillin, ampicillin, chloramphenicol, clindamycin, and clarithromycin. May switch to oral antimicrobial therapy when clinically appropriate. Continue combined therapy for 60 days.

Bacterial conjunctivitis:

Ophthalmic solution: Instill 1-2 drops in eye(s) every 2 hours while awake for 2 days and 1-2 drops every 4 hours while awake for the next 5 days

Ophthalmic ointment: Apply a ½" ribbon into the conjunctival sac 3 times/day for the first 2 days, followed by a ½" ribbon applied twice daily for the next 5 days

Bone/joint infections:

Oral: 500-750 mg twice daily for 4-6 weeks, depending on severity and susceptibility

I.V.: Mild to moderate: 400 mg every 12 hours for 4-6 weeks; Severe/complicated: 400 mg every 8 hours for 4-6 weeks

Chancroid (CDC guidelines): Oral: 500 mg twice daily for 3 days

Corneal ulcer: Ophthalmic solution: Instill 2 drops into affected eye every 15 minutes for the first 6 hours, then 2 drops into the affected eye every 30 minutes for the remainder of the first day. On day 2, instill 2 drops into the affected eye hourly. On days 3-14, instill 2 drops into affected eye every 4 hours. Treatment may continue after day 14 if re-epithelialization has not occurred.

Febrile neutropenia (with piperacillin): I.V.: 400 mg every 8 hours for 7-14 days

Gonococcal infections:

Urethral/cervical gonococcal infections: Oral: 250-500 mg as a single dose (CDC recommends concomitant doxycycline or azithromycin due to developing resistance; avoid use in Asian or Western Pacific travelers)

Disseminated gonococcal infection (CDC guidelines): Oral: 500 mg twice daily to complete 7 days of therapy (initial treatment with ceftriaxone 1 g I.M./I.V. daily for 24-48 hours after improvement begins)

Infectious diarrhea: Oral:

Salmonella: 500 mg twice daily for 5-7 days

Shigella: 500 mg twice daily for 3 days

Traveler's diarrhea: Mild: 750 mg for one dose; Severe: 500 mg twice daily for 3 days

Vibrio cholerae: 1 g for one dose

Intra-abdominal (in combination with metronidazole):

Oral: 500 mg every 12 hours for 7-14 days

I.V.: 400 mg every 12 hours for 7-14 days

Lower respiratory tract, skin/skin structure infections:

Oral: 500-750 mg twice daily for 7-14 days depending on severity and susceptibility

I.V.: Mild to moderate: 400 mg every 12 hours for 7-14 days; Severe/complicated: 400 mg every 8 hours for 7-14 days

Nosocomial pneumonia: I.V.: 400 mg every 8 hours for 10-14 days

Prostatitis (chronic, bacterial):

Oral: 500 mg every 12 hours for 28 days

I.V.: 400 mg every 12 hours for 28 days

Sinusitis (acute):

Oral: 500 mg every 12 hours for 10 days

I.V.: 400 mg every 12 hours for 10 days

Typhoid fever: Oral: 500 mg every 12 hours for 10 days

Urinary tract infection:

Acute uncomplicated: Oral: Immediate release formulation: 250 mg every 12 hours for 3 days; Extended release formulation (Cipro® XR, Proquin® XR): 500 mg every 24 hours for 3 days

Acute uncomplicated pyelonephritis: Oral: Extended release formulation (Cipro® XR): 1000 mg every 24 hours for 7-14 days

Mild to moderate:

Oral: Immediate release formulation: 250 mg every 12 hours for 7-14 days

I.V.: 200 mg every 12 hours for 7-14 days

Severe/complicated:

Oral:

Immediate release formulation: 500 mg every 12 hours for 7-14 days

(Continued)

Ciprofloxacin *(Continued)*

Extended release formulation (Cipro® XR): 1000 mg every 24 hours for 7-14 days

I.V.: 400 mg every 12 hours for 7-14 days

Elderly: No adjustment needed in patients with normal renal function

Dosing adjustment in renal impairment: Adults:

Cl_{cr} 30-50 mL/minute: Oral: 250-500 mg every 12 hours

Cl_{cr} <30 mL/minute: Acute uncomplicated pyelonephritis or complicated UTI: Oral: Extended release formulation: 500 mg every 24 hours

Cl_{cr} 5-29 mL/minute:

Oral: 250-500 mg every 18 hours

I.V.: 200-400 mg every 18-24 hours

Dialysis: Only small amounts of ciprofloxacin are removed by hemo- or peritoneal dialysis (<10%); usual dose: Oral: 250-500 mg every 24 hours following dialysis

Continuous arteriovenous or venovenous hemodiafiltration effects: Administer 200-400 mg I.V. every 12 hours

Stability

Injection:

Premixed infusion: Store between 5°C to 25°C (41°F to 77°F); avoid freezing. Protect from light.

Vial: Store between 5°C to 30°C (41°F to 86°F); avoid freezing. Protect from light. May be diluted with NS, D_5W, SWFI, $D_{10}W$, D_5¼NS, D_5½NS, LR. Diluted solutions of 0.5-2 mg/mL are stable for up to 14 days refrigerated or at room temperature.

Ophthalmic solution/ointment: Store at 36°F to 77°F (2°C to 25°C); protect from light.

Microcapsules for oral suspension: Prior to reconstitution, store below 25°C (77°F); protect from freezing. Following reconstitution, store below 30°C (86°F) for up to 14 days; protect from freezing.

Tablet:

Immediate release: Store below 30°C (86°F).

Extended release: Store at room temperature of 15°C to 30°C (59°F to 86°F).

Administration

Oral: May administer with food to minimize GI upset; avoid antacid use; maintain proper hydration and urine output. Administer immediate release ciprofloxacin and Cipro® XR at least 2 hours before or 6 hours after, and Proquin® XR at least 4 hours before or 6 hours after antacids or other products containing calcium, iron, or zinc (including dairy products or calcium-fortified juices). Separate oral administration from drugs which may impair absorption (see Drug Interactions).

Oral suspension: Should not be administered through feeding tubes (suspension is oil-based and adheres to the feeding tube). Patients should avoid chewing on the microcapsules.

Nasogastric/orogastric tube: Crush immediate-release tablet and mix with water. Flush feeding tube before and after administration. Hold tube feedings at least 1 hour before and 2 hours after administration.

Tablet, extended release: Do not crush, split, or chew. May be administered with meals containing dairy products (calcium content <800 mg), but not with dairy products alone. Proquin® XR should be administered with a main meal of the day; evening meal is preferred.

Parenteral: Administer by slow I.V. infusion over 60 minutes to reduce the risk of venous irritation (burning, pain, erythema, and swelling); final concentration for administration should not exceed 2 mg/mL.

Monitoring Parameters Patients receiving concurrent ciprofloxacin, theophylline, or cyclosporine should have serum levels monitored; CBC, renal and hepatic function during prolonged therapy

Reference Range Therapeutic: 2.6-3 mcg/mL; Toxic: >5 mcg/mL

Anesthesia and Critical Care Concerns/Other Considerations Ciprofloxacin may increase theophylline levels resulting in relevant cardiovascular side effects, including tachycardia.

Pregnancy Risk Factor C

Contraindications Hypersensitivity to ciprofloxacin, any component of the formulation, or other quinolones; concurrent administration of tizanidine

Warnings/Precautions CNS stimulation may occur (tremor, restlessness, confusion, and very rarely hallucinations or seizures). Use with caution in patients with known or suspected CNS disorder. Potential for seizures, although very rare, may be increased with concomitant NSAID therapy. Use with caution in individuals at risk of seizures. Prolonged use may result in superinfection. Tendon inflammation and/or rupture have been reported with ciprofloxacin and other quinolone antibiotics. Risk may be increased with concurrent corticosteroids, particularly in the elderly. Discontinue at first sign of tendon inflammation or pain. Adverse effects, including those related to joints and/or surrounding tissues, are increased in pediatric patients and therefore, ciprofloxacin should not be considered as drug of choice in children (exception is anthrax treatment). Rare cases of peripheral neuropathy may occur.

Severe hypersensitivity reactions, including anaphylaxis, have occurred with quinolone therapy. Quinolones may exacerbate myasthenia gravis, use with caution (rare, potentially life-threatening weakness of respiratory muscles may occur). Use caution in renal impairment. Avoid excessive sunlight; may cause moderate-to-severe phototoxicity reactions.

Ciprofloxacin is a potent inhibitor of CYP1A2. Coadministration of drugs which depend on this pathway may lead to substantial increases in serum concentrations and adverse effects.

Adverse Reactions

1% to 10%:

Central nervous system: Neurologic events (children 2%, includes dizziness, insomnia, nervousness, somnolence); fever (children 2%); headache (I.V. administration); restlessness (I.V. administration)

Dermatologic: Rash (children 2%, adults 1%)

Gastrointestinal: Nausea (children/adults 3%); diarrhea (children 5%, adults 2%); vomiting (children 5%, adults 1%); abdominal pain (children 3%, adults <1%); dyspepsia (children 3%)

Hepatic: ALT/AST increased (adults 1%)

Local: Injection site reactions (I.V. administration)

Respiratory: Rhinitis (children 3%)

<1% (Limited to important or life-threatening): Abnormal gait, acute renal failure, agitation, agranulocytosis, albuminuria, allergic reactions, anaphylactic shock, anaphylaxis, anemia, angina pectoris, angioedema, anorexia, anosmia, arthralgia, ataxia, atrial flutter, bone marrow depression (life-threatening), breast pain, bronchospasm, candidiasis, candiduria, cardiopulmonary arrest, cerebral thrombosis, chills, cholestatic jaundice, chromatopsia, confusion, constipation, crystalluria (particularly in alkaline urine), cylindruria, delirium, depersonalization, depression, dizziness, drowsiness, dyspepsia (adults), dysphagia, dyspnea, edema, eosinophilia, erythema multiforme, erythema nodosum, exfoliative dermatitis, fever (adults), fixed eruption, flatulence, gastrointestinal bleeding, hallucinations, headache (oral), hematuria, hemolytic anemia, hepatic failure, hepatic necrosis, hyperesthesia, hyperglycemia, hyperpigmentation, hyper-/hypotension, hypertonia, insomnia, interstitial nephritis, intestinal perforation, irritability, jaundice, joint pain, laryngeal edema, lightheadedness, lymphadenopathy, malaise, manic reaction, methemoglobinemia, MI, migraine, moniliasis, myalgia, myasthenia gravis, myoclonus, nephritis, nightmares, nystagmus, orthostatic hypotension, palpitation, pancreatitis, pancytopenia (life-threatening or fatal), paranoia, paresthesia, peripheral neuropathy, petechia, photosensitivity, prolongation of PT/INR, pseudomembranous colitis, psychosis, pulmonary edema, renal calculi, seizure; serum cholesterol, glucose, triglycerides increased; serum sickness-like reactions, Stevens-Johnson syndrome, syncope, tachycardia, taste loss, tendon rupture, tendonitis, thrombophlebitis, tinnitus, torsade de pointes, toxic epidermal necrolysis (Lyell's syndrome), tremor, twitching, urethral bleeding, vaginal candidiasis, vaginitis, vasculitis, ventricular ectopy, visual disturbance, weakness

Overdosage/Toxicology Symptoms of overdose include acute renal failure and seizures. Treatment is supportive and should include adequate hydration and renal function monitoring. Magnesium- or calcium-containing antacids may be given to decrease absorption of oral ciprofloxacin. Only a small amount of ciprofloxacin (<10%) is removed from the body after hemodialysis or peritoneal dialysis.

Drug Interactions **Inhibits** CYP1A2 (strong), 3A4 (weak)

Caffeine: Ciprofloxacin may decrease the metabolism of caffeine.

Corticosteroids: Concurrent use may increase the risk of tendon rupture, particularly in elderly patients (overall incidence rare).

(Continued)

Ciprofloxacin *(Continued)*

CYP1A2 substrates: Ciprofloxacin may increase the levels/effects of CYP1A2 substrates. Example substrates include aminophylline, fluvoxamine, mexiletine, mirtazapine, ropinirole, tizanidine, and trifluoperazine.

Foscarnet: Concomitant use with ciprofloxacin has been associated with an increased risk of seizures.

Glyburide: Quinolones may increase the effect of glyburide; monitor.

Metal cations (aluminum, calcium, iron, magnesium, and zinc) bind quinolones in the gastrointestinal tract and inhibit absorption. Concurrent administration of most antacids, oral electrolyte supplements, quinapril, sucralfate, some didanosine formulations (chewable/buffered tablets and pediatric powder for oral suspension), and other highly-buffered oral drugs, should be avoided. Ciprofloxacin should be administered 2 hours before or 6 hours after these agents.

Methotrexate: Ciprofloxacin may decrease renal secretion of methotrexate; monitor.

Pentoxifylline: Monitor for headache during concomitant therapy.

Phenytoin: Ciprofloxacin may decrease phenytoin levels; monitor.

Probenecid: May decrease renal secretion of quinolones.

Ropivacaine: Ciprofloxacin may decrease the metabolism of ropivacaine.

Sevelamer: May decrease absorption of oral ciprofloxacin.

Theophylline: Serum levels may be increased by ciprofloxacin; in addition, CNS stimulation/seizures may occur at lower theophylline serum levels due to additive CNS effects.

Tizanidine: Ciprofloxacin may increase serum levels of tizanidine. Concurrent administration is contraindicated.

Warfarin: The hypoprothrombinemic effect of warfarin may be enhanced by ciprofloxacin; monitor INR.

Ethanol/Nutrition/Herb Interactions

Food: Food decreases rate, but not extent, of absorption. Ciprofloxacin serum levels may be decreased if taken with dairy products or calcium-fortified juices. Ciprofloxacin may increase serum caffeine levels if taken with caffeine.

Enteral feedings may decrease plasma concentrations of ciprofloxacin probably by >30% inhibition of absorption. Ciprofloxacin should not be administered with enteral feedings. The feeding would need to be discontinued for 1-2 hours prior to and after ciprofloxacin administration. Nasogastric administration produces a greater loss of ciprofloxacin bioavailability than does nasoduodenal administration.

Herb/Nutraceutical: Avoid dong quai, St John's wort (may also cause photosensitization).

Test Interactions Some quinolones may produce a false-positive urine screening result for opiates using commercially-available immunoassay kits. This has been demonstrated most consistently for levofloxacin and ofloxacin, but other quinolones have shown cross-reactivity in certain assay kits. Confirmation of positive opiate screens by more specific methods should be considered.

Dietary Considerations

Food: Drug may cause GI upset; take without regard to meals (manufacturer prefers that immediate release tablet is taken 2 hours after meals). Extended release tablet may be taken with meals that contain dairy products (calcium content <800 mg), but not with dairy products alone.

Dairy products, calcium-fortified juices, oral multivitamins, and mineral supplements: Absorption of ciprofloxacin is decreased by divalent and trivalent cations. The manufacturer states that the usual dietary intake of calcium (including meals which include dairy products) has not been shown to interfere with ciprofloxacin absorption. Immediate release ciprofloxacin and Cipro® XR may be taken 2 hours before or 6 hours after, and Proquin® XR may be taken 4 hours before or 6 hours after, any of these products.

Caffeine: Patients consuming regular large quantities of caffeinated beverages may need to restrict caffeine intake if excessive cardiac or CNS stimulation occurs.

Dosage Forms [DSC] = Discontinued product

Infusion [premixed in D_5W] (Cipro®): 200 mg (100 mL); 400 mg (200 mL) [latex free]

Injection, solution (Cipro®): 10 mg/mL (20 mL, 40 mL, 120 mL [DSC])

Microcapsules for oral suspension (Cipro®): 250 mg/5 mL (100 mL); 500 mg/5 mL (100 mL) [strawberry flavor]

Ointment, ophthalmic, as hydrochloride (Ciloxan®): 3.33 mg/g [0.3% base] (3.5 g)

Solution, ophthalmic, as hydrochloride (Ciloxan®): 3.5 mg/mL [0.3% base] (2.5 mL, 5 mL, 10 mL) [contains benzalkonium chloride]

Tablet: 250 mg, 500 mg, 750 mg

Cipro®: 100 mg, 250 mg, 500 mg, 750 mg

Tablet, extended release:

Cipro® XR: 500 mg [equivalent to ciprofloxacin hydrochloride 287.5 mg and ciprofloxacin base 212.6 mg]; 1000 mg [equivalent to ciprofloxacin hydrochloride 574.9 mg and ciprofloxacin base 425.2 mg]

Proquin® XR: 500 mg

Tablet, extended release [dose pack]:

Proquin® XR: 500 mg (3s)

References

American Thoracic Society and Infectious Diseases Society of America, "Guidelines for the Management of Adults With Hospital-Acquired, Ventilator-Associated, and Healthcare-Associated Pneumonia," *Am J Respir Crit Care Med*, 2005, 171(4):388-416.

"Antimicrobial Prophylaxis for Surgery," *Treat Guidel Med Lett*, 2004, 2(20):27-32.

Centers for Disease Control and Prevention, "Update: Investigation of Bioterrorism-Related Anthrax and Interim Guidelines for Exposure Management and Antimicrobial Therapy, October 2001," *MMWR Morb Mortal Wkly Rep*, October 26, 2001, 50(42):909-19. Available at: http://www.cdc.gov/mmwr/preview/mmwrhtml/mm5042a1.htm.

Fish DN, Bainbridge JL, and Peloquin CA, "Variable Disposition of Ciprofloxacin in Critically Ill Patients Undergoing Continuous Arteriovenous Hemodiafiltration," *Pharmacotherapy*, 1995, 15(2):236-45.

Lomaestro BM and Bailie GR, "Quinolone-Cation Interactions: A Review," *DICP*, 1991, 25(11):1249-58.

Mackay AD and Mehta A, "Autoimmune Haemolytic Anemia Associated With Ciprofloxacin," *Clin Lab Haematol*, 1995, 17(1):97-8.

Schaad UB, abdus Salam M, Aujard Y, et al, "Use of Fluoroquinolones in Pediatrics: Consensus Report of an International Society of Chemotherapy Commission," *Pediatr Infect Dis J*, 1995, 14(1):1-9.

◆ **Ciprofloxacin Hydrochloride** *see* Ciprofloxacin *on page 285*

◆ **Cipro® XR** *see* Ciprofloxacin *on page 285*

Cisapride (SIS a pride)

Medication Safety Issues

Sound-alike/look-alike issues:

Propulsid® may be confused with propranolol

U.S. Brand Names Propulsid®

Pharmacologic Category Gastrointestinal Agent, Prokinetic

Restrictions In U.S., available via limited-access protocol only (1-800-JANSSEN).

Generic Available No

Use Treatment of nocturnal symptoms of gastroesophageal reflux disease (GERD); has demonstrated effectiveness for gastroparesis, refractory constipation, and nonulcer dyspepsia

Mechanism of Action Enhances the release of acetylcholine at the myenteric plexus. *In vitro* studies have shown cisapride to have serotonin-4 receptor agonistic properties which may increase gastrointestinal motility and cardiac rate; increases lower esophageal sphincter pressure and lower esophageal peristalsis; accelerates gastric emptying of both liquids and solids.

Pharmacodynamics/Kinetics

Onset of action: 0.5-1 hour

Protein binding: 97.5% to 98%

Metabolism: Extensively hepatic to norcisapride

Bioavailability: 35% to 40%

Half-life elimination: 6-12 hours

Excretion: Urine and feces (<10%)

Dosage Oral:

Children: 0.15-0.3 mg/kg/dose 3-4 times/day; maximum: 10 mg/dose

Adults: Initial: 10 mg 4 times/day at least 15 minutes before meals and at bedtime; in some patients the dosage will need to be increased to 20 mg to obtain a satisfactory result

Anesthesia and Critical Care Concerns/Other Considerations

IMPORTANT NOTE: On March 24, 2000, the FDA announced that the manufacturer of cisapride would voluntarily withdraw its product from the U.S. market on July 14, 2000. This decision was based on 341 reports of heart rhythm abnormalities including 80 reports of deaths. The company will continue to make the drug

(Continued)

Cisapride *(Continued)*

available to patients who meet specific clinical eligibility criteria for a limited-access protocol (contact 1-800-JANSSEN).

The potential for arrhythmogenic effects may also increase secondary to significant drug interactions (see Drug Interactions).

In the absence of a known disease or drug contraindication, all patients should have a 12-lead ECG and an electrolyte panel (potassium, calcium, and magnesium) completed prior to initiating cisapride therapy. Serum electrolytes and 12-lead ECG should be again evaluated within the first 48 hours of therapy and periodically thereafter. Patients on diuretic and cisapride therapies should be monitored more closely for the development of hypokalemia, hypocalcemia, and hypomagnesemia. Cisapride therapy should be stopped and the patient monitored closely in patients who develop hypokalemia, hypocalcemia, hypomagnesemia, or QT prolongation (QT_c >450 milliseconds).

Pregnancy Risk Factor C

Contraindications

Hypersensitivity to cisapride or any component of the formulations; GI hemorrhage, mechanical obstruction, GI perforation, or other situations when GI motility stimulation is dangerous

Serious cardiac arrhythmias including ventricular tachycardia, ventricular fibrillation, torsade de pointes, and QT prolongation have been reported in patients taking cisapride with other drugs that inhibit CYP3A4. Some of these events have been fatal. Concomitant oral or intravenous administration of the following drugs with cisapride may lead to elevated cisapride blood levels and is contraindicated:

Antibiotics: Oral or I.V. erythromycin, clarithromycin, troleandomycin

Antidepressants: Nefazodone

Antifungals: Oral or I.V. fluconazole, itraconazole, miconazole, oral ketoconazole

Protease inhibitors: Indinavir, ritonavir, amprenavir, atazanavir

Cisapride is also contraindicated for patients with a prolonged electrocardiographic QT intervals (QT_c >450 msec), a history of QT_c prolongation, or known family history of congenital long QT syndrome; clinically significant bradycardia, renal failure, history of ventricular arrhythmias, ischemic heart disease, and congestive heart failure; uncorrected electrolyte disorders (hypokalemia, hypomagnesemia); respiratory failure; and concomitant medications known to prolong the QT interval and increase the risk of arrhythmia, such as certain antiarrhythmics, certain antipsychotics, certain antidepressants, bepridil, sparfloxacin, and terodiline. The preceding lists of drugs are not comprehensive. Cisapride should not be used in patients with uncorrected hypokalemia or hypomagnesemia or who might experience rapid reduction of plasma potassium such as those administered potassium-wasting diuretics and/or insulin in acute settings.

Warnings/Precautions

On March 24, 2000, the FDA announced that the manufacturer of cisapride would voluntarily withdraw its product from the U.S. market on July 14, 2000. This decision was based on 341 reports of heart rhythm abnormalities including 80 reports of deaths. The company will continue to make the drug available to patients who meet specific clinical eligibility criteria for a limited-access protocol (contact 1-800-JANSSEN).

[U.S. Boxed Warning]: Serious cardiac arrhythmias including ventricular tachycardia, ventricular fibrillation, torsade de pointes, and QT prolongation have been reported in patients taking this drug. Many of these patients also took drugs expected to increase cisapride blood levels by inhibiting the cytochrome P450 3A4 enzymes that metabolize cisapride. These drugs include clarithromycin, erythromycin, troleandomycin, nefazodone, fluconazole, itraconazole, ketoconazole, indinavir and ritonavir. Some of these events have been fatal. Cisapride is contraindicated in patients taking any of these drugs. **QT prolongation, torsade de pointes (sometimes with syncope), cardiac arrest and sudden death have been reported in patients taking cisapride without the above-mentioned contraindicated drugs.** Most patients had disorders that may have predisposed them to arrhythmias with cisapride. Cisapride is contraindicated for those patients with: history of prolonged electrocardiographic QT intervals; renal failure; history of ventricular arrhythmias, ischemic heart disease, and CHF; uncorrected electrolyte disorders (hypokalemia, hypomagnesemia);

respiratory failure; and concomitant medications known to prolong the QT interval and increase the risk of arrhythmia, such as certain antiarrhythmics, including those of Class 1A (such as quinidine and procainamide) and Class III (such as sotalol); tricyclic antidepressants (such as amitriptyline); certain tetracyclic antidepressants (such as maprotiline); certain antipsychotic medications (such as certain phenothiazines and sertindole), protease inhibitors, bepridil, sparfloxacin and terodiline. (The preceding lists of drugs are not comprehensive.) Recommended doses of cisapride should not be exceeded.

Patients should have a baseline ECG and an electrolyte panel (magnesium, calcium, potassium) prior to initiating cisapride (see Contraindications). Potential benefits should be weighed against risks prior administration of cisapride to patients who have or may develop prolongation of cardiac conduction intervals, particularly QT_c. These include patients with conditions that could predispose them to the development of serious arrhythmias, such as multiple organ failure, COPD, apnea and advanced cancer. Cisapride should not be used in patients with uncorrected hypokalemia or hypomagnesemia, such as those with severe dehydration, vomiting or malnutrition, or those taking potassium-wasting diuretics. Cisapride should not be used in patients who might experience rapid reduction of plasma potassium, such as those administered potassium-wasting diuretics and/or insulin in acute settings. Safety and effectiveness in children have not been established.

Adverse Reactions

>10%:

- Central nervous system: Headache
- Gastrointestinal: Diarrhea (dose dependent)

1% to 10%:

- Cardiovascular: Tachycardia
- Central nervous system: Extrapyramidal effects, somnolence, fatigue, insomnia, anxiety
- Dermatologic: Rash
- Gastrointestinal: Abdominal cramping, constipation, nausea
- Respiratory: Sinusitis, rhinitis, cough, upper respiratory tract infection, increased incidence of viral infection

<1% (Limited to important or life-threatening): Apnea, bronchospasm, gynecomastia, hyperprolactinemia, methemoglobinemia, photosensitivity, psychiatric disturbances, seizure (have been reported only in patients with a history of seizure)

Drug Interactions Substrate of CYP1A2 (minor), 2A6 (minor), 2B6 (minor), 2C9 (minor), 2C19 (minor), 3A4 (major); **Inhibits** CYP2D6 (weak), 3A4 (weak)

Azole antifungals (fluconazole, itraconazole, ketoconazole, miconazole) increase cisapride's concentration. Pre-existing cardiovascular disease or electrolyte imbalances increase the risk of malignant arrhythmias; concurrent use is contraindicated.

Bepridil increases the risk of malignant arrhythmias; concurrent use is contraindicated

Cimetidine increases the bioavailability of cisapride; use an alternative H_2 antagonist

Class Ia (quinidine, procainamide) and Class III (amiodarone, sotalol) antiarrhythmics increase the risk of malignant arrhythmias; concurrent use is contraindicated

CYP3A4 inhibitors: May increase the levels/effects of cisapride. Example inhibitors include azole antifungals, clarithromycin, diclofenac, doxycycline, erythromycin, imatinib, isoniazid, nefazodone, nicardipine, propofol, protease inhibitors, quinidine, telithromycin, and verapamil. Concurrent use of azole antifungals, clarithromycin, erythromycin, nefazodone, and protease inhibitors is contraindicated.

Grapefruit juice may increase the bioavailability of cisapride; concomitant use should be avoided.

Macrolides (clarithromycin, erythromycin, troleandomycin) increase serum concentrations of cisapride. Risk of arrhythmias; concurrent use is contraindicated.

Nefazodone and maprotiline may increase the risk of malignant arrhythmias; concurrent use is contraindicated

Phenothiazines (prochlorperazine, promethazine) may increase the risk of malignant arrhythmias; concurrent use is contraindicated

Pimozide may prolong the QT interval; concurrent use is contraindicated.

(Continued)

Cisapride *(Continued)*

Protease inhibitors (amprenavir, atazanavir, indinavir, nelfinavir, ritonavir) increase cisapride's concentration. Increased risk of malignant arrhythmias; concurrent use is contraindicated.
Quinolone antibiotics: Sparfloxacin, gatifloxacin, moxifloxacin increase the risk of malignant arrhythmias; concurrent use is contraindicated
Sertindole may increase the risk of malignant arrhythmias; concurrent use is contraindicated
TCAs increase the risk of malignant arrhythmias; concurrent use is contraindicated
Warfarin: Isolated cases of increased INR; monitor closely

Ethanol/Nutrition/Herb Interactions
Ethanol: Avoid ethanol (may increase CNS depression).
Food: Coadministration of grapefruit juice with cisapride increases the bioavailability of cisapride and concomitant use should be avoided.
Herb/Nutraceutical: St John's wort may decrease cisapride levels.

Cisatracurium (sis a tra KYOO ree um)

Medication Safety Issues
Sound-alike/look-alike issues:
Nimbex® may be confused with Revex®

High alert medication: The Institute for Safe Medication Practices (ISMP) includes this medication among its list of drugs which have a heightened risk of causing significant patient harm when used in error.

Related Information
Chronic Renal Failure *on page 1437*
Neuromuscular Blocking Agents *on page 1572*

U.S. Brand Names Nimbex®
Canadian Brand Names Nimbex®
Synonyms Cisatracurium Besylate
Pharmacologic Category Neuromuscular Blocker Agent, Nondepolarizing
Generic Available No
Use Adjunct to general anesthesia to facilitate endotracheal intubation and to relax skeletal muscles during surgery; to facilitate mechanical ventilation in ICU patients; does not relieve pain or produce sedation
Mechanism of Action Blocks neural transmission at the myoneural junction by binding with cholinergic receptor sites

Pharmacodynamics/Kinetics
Onset of action: I.V.: 2-3 minutes
Peak effect: 3-5 minutes
Duration: Recovery begins in 20-35 minutes when anesthesia is balanced; recovery is attained in 90% of patients in 25-93 minutes
Metabolism: Undergoes rapid nonenzymatic degradation in the bloodstream (Hofmann elimination), additional metabolism occurs via ester hydrolysis; some active metabolites
Half-life elimination: 22-29 minutes

Dosage I.V. (not to be used I.M.):
Operating room administration:
Children 2-12 years: Intubating doses: 0.1 mg over 5-15 seconds during either halothane or opioid anesthesia. (**Note:** When given during stable opioid/nitrous oxide/oxygen anesthesia, 0.1 mg/kg produces maximum neuromuscular block in an average of 2.8 minutes and clinically effective block for 28 minutes.)
Adults: Intubating doses: 0.15-0.2 mg/kg as component of propofol/nitrous oxide/oxygen induction-intubation technique. (**Note:** May produce generally good or excellent conditions for tracheal intubation in 1.5-2 minutes with clinically effective duration of action during propofol anesthesia of 55-61 minutes.); initial dose after succinylcholine for intubation: 0.1 mg/kg; maintenance dose: 0.03 mg/kg 40-60 minutes after initial dose, then at ~20-minute intervals based on clinical criteria
Children ≥2 years and Adults: Continuous infusion: After an initial bolus, a diluted solution can be given by continuous infusion for maintenance of neuromuscular blockade during extended surgery; adjust the rate of administration according to the patient's response as determined by peripheral nerve

stimulation. An initial infusion rate of 3 mcg/kg/minute may be required to rapidly counteract the spontaneous recovery of neuromuscular function; thereafter, a rate of 1-2 mcg/kg/minute should be adequate to maintain continuous neuromuscular block in the 89% to 99% range in most pediatric and adult patients. Consider reduction of the infusion rate by 30% to 40% when administering during stable isoflurane, enflurane, sevoflurane, or desflurane anesthesia. Spontaneous recovery from neuromuscular blockade following discontinuation of infusion of cisatracurium may be expected to proceed at a rate comparable to that following single bolus administration.

Intensive care unit administration: Follow the principles for infusion in the operating room. At initial signs of recovery from bolus dose, begin the infusion at a dose of 3 mcg/kg/minute and adjust rates accordingly; dosage ranges of 0.5-10 mcg/kg/minute have been reported. If patient is allowed to recover from neuromuscular blockade, readministration of a bolus dose may be necessary to quickly re-establish neuromuscular block prior to reinstituting the infusion. See table.

Cisatracurium Besylate Infusion Chart

Drug Delivery Rate (mcg/kg/min)	Infusion Rate (mL/kg/min) 0.1 mg/mL (10 mg/100 mL)	Infusion Rate (mL/kg/min) 0.4 mg/mL (40 mg/100 mL)
1	0.01	0.0025
1.5	0.015	0.00375
2	0.02	0.005
3	0.03	0.0075
5	0.05	0.0125

Dosing adjustment in renal impairment: Because slower times to onset of complete neuromuscular block were observed in renal dysfunction patients, extending the interval between the administration of cisatracurium and intubation attempt may be required to achieve adequate intubation conditions.

Stability Refrigerate intact vials at 2°C to 8°C/36°F to 46°F; use vials within 21 days upon removal from the refrigerator to room temperature (25°C to 77°F). Dilutions of 0.1-0.2 mg/mL in 0.9% sodium chloride or dextrose 5% in water are stable for up to 24 hours at room temperature.

Administration Administer I.V. only; the use of a peripheral nerve stimulator will permit the most advantageous use of cisatracurium, minimize the possibility of overdosage or underdosage and assist in the evaluation of recovery

Give undiluted as a bolus injection; not for I.M. injection, too much tissue irritation; continuous administration requires the use of an infusion pump

Monitoring Parameters Vital signs (heart rate, blood pressure, respiratory rate)

Anesthesia and Critical Care Concerns/Other Considerations Cisatracurium is classified as an intermediate duration neuromuscular-blocking agent; does not appear to have a cumulative effect on the duration of blockade; neuromuscular-blocking potency is 3 times that of atracurium.

Critically-Ill Adult Patients:

The 2004 Surviving Sepsis Campaign guidelines recommend avoiding use of neuromuscular blockers if at all possible in the septic patient due to the risk of prolonged neuromuscular blockade following discontinuation. If one is required, monitor carefully and observe the following recommendations.

The 2002 ACCM/SCCM/ASHP clinical practice guidelines for sustained neuromuscular blockade in the adult critically-ill patient recommend:

Optimize sedatives and analgesics prior to initiation and monitor and adjust accordingly during course. Neuromuscular blockers do not relieve pain or produce sedation.

Protect patient's eyes from development of keratitis and corneal abrasion by administering ophthalmic ointment and taping eyelids closed or using eye patches. Reposition patient routinely to protect pressure points from breakdown. Address DVT prophylaxis.

Concurrent use of a neuromuscular blocker and corticosteroids appear to increase the risk of certain ICU myopathies; avoid or administer the corticosteroid at the lowest dose possible. Reassess need for neuromuscular blocker daily.

(Continued)

Cisatracurium *(Continued)*

Using daily drug holidays (stopping neuromuscular-blocking agent until patient requires it again) may decrease the incidence of acute quadriplegic myopathy syndrome.

Tachyphylaxis can develop; switch to another neuromuscular blocker (taking into consideration the patient's organ function) if paralysis is still necessary.

Acidosis and severe hypothermia may delay the elimination of atracurium and cisatracurium.

Atracurium or cisatracurium is recommended for patients with significant hepatic or renal disease, due to organ-independent Hofmann elimination.

Monitor patients clinically and via "Train of Four" (TOF) testing with a goal of adjusting the degree of blockade to 1-2 twitches or based upon the patient's clinical condition.

Pregnancy Risk Factor B

Contraindications Hypersensitivity to cisatracurium besylate or any component of the formulation

Warnings/Precautions Maintenance of an adequate airway and respiratory support is critical; certain clinical conditions may result in potentiation or antagonism of neuromuscular blockade:

Potentiation: Electrolyte abnormalities, severe hyponatremia, severe hypocalcemia, severe hypokalemia, hypermagnesemia, neuromuscular diseases, acidosis, acute intermittent porphyria, renal failure, hepatic failure

Antagonism: Alkalosis, hypercalcemia, demyelinating lesions, peripheral neuropathies, diabetes mellitus

Increased sensitivity in patients with myasthenia gravis, Eaton-Lambert syndrome; resistance in burn patients (>30% of body) for period of 5-70 days postinjury; resistance in patients with muscle trauma, denervation, immobilization, infection. Cross-sensitivity with other neuromuscular-blocking agents may occur; use extreme caution in patients with previous anaphylactic reactions. Bradycardia may be more common with cisatracurium than with other neuromuscular-blocking agents since it has no clinically significant effects on heart rate to counteract the bradycardia produced by anesthetics.

Adverse Reactions <1%: Effects are minimal and transient, bradycardia and hypotension, flushing, pruritus, rash, bronchospasm, acute quadriplegic myopathy syndrome (prolonged use), myositis ossificans (prolonged use)

Overdosage/Toxicology

Symptoms of overdose include respiratory depression and cardiovascular collapse.

Neostigmine 1-3 mg slow I.V. push in adults (0.5 mg in children) antagonizes the neuromuscular blockade, and should be administered with or immediately after atropine 1-1.5 mg I.V. push (adults). This may be especially useful in the presence of bradycardia.

Drug Interactions

Prolonged neuromuscular blockade:

- Inhaled anesthetics:
  - Halothane has only a marginal effect, enflurane and isoflurane increase the potency and prolong duration of neuromuscular blockade induced by cisatracurium
  - Dosage should be reduced by 30% to 40% in patients receiving isoflurane or enflurane
- Local anesthetics
- Lithium
- Magnesium salts
- Antiarrhythmics (eg, quinidine or procainamide)
- Antibiotics (eg, aminoglycosides, tetracyclines, vancomycin, clindamycin)

Resistance to neuromuscular blockade: Chronic phenytoin or carbamazepine

Dosage Forms

Injection, solution: 2 mg/mL (5 mL); 10 mg/mL (20 mL)

Injection, solution: 2 mg/mL (10 mL) [contains benzyl alcohol]

References

Belmont MR, Lien CA, Quessy S, et al, "The Clinical Neuromuscular Pharmacology of 51W89 in Patients Receiving Nitrous Oxide/Opioid/Barbiturate Anesthesia," *Anesthesiology*, 1995, 82(5):1139-45.

Dellinger RP, Carlet JM, Masur H, et al, "Surviving Sepsis Campaign Guidelines for Management of Severe Sepsis and Septic Shock," *Crit Care Med*, 2004, 32(3):858-73.

Konstadt SN, Reich DL, Stanley TE 3d, et al, "A Two Center Comparison of the Cardiovascular Effects of Cisatracurium (Nimbex®) and Vecuronium in Patients With Coronary Artery Disease," *Anesth Analg*, 1995, 81(5):1010-4.

Lien CA, Belmont MR, Abalos A, et al, "The Cardiovascular Effects and Histamine-Releasing Properties of 51W89 in Patients Receiving Nitrous Oxide/Opioid/Barbiturate Anesthesia," *Anesthesiology*, 1995, 82(5):1131-8.

Murray MJ, Cowen J, DeBlock H, et al, "Clinical Practice Guidelines for Sustained Neuromuscular Blockade in the Adult Critically Ill Patient. Task Force of the American College of Critical Care Medicine (ACCM) of the Society of Critical Care Medicine (SCCM), American Society of Health-System Pharmacists, American College of Chest Physicians," *Crit Care Med*, 2002, 30(1):142-56; viewable at http://www.sccm.org/pdf/NeuromuscularBlockade.pdf.

Prielipp RC, Coursin DB, Scuderi PE, et al, "Comparison of the Infusion Requirements and Recovery Profiles of Vecuronium and Cisatracurium 51W89 in Intensive Care Unit Patients," *Anesth Analg*, 1995, 81(1):3-12.

Sorooshian SS, Stafford MA, Eastwood NB, et al, "Pharmacokinetics and Pharmacodynamics of Cisatracurium in Young and Elderly Adult Patients," *Anesthesiology*, 1996, 84(5):1083-91.

♦ **Cisatracurium Besylate** *see* Cisatracurium *on page 294*

Citalopram (sye TAL oh pram)

Medication Safety Issues

Sound-alike/look-alike issues:

Celexa® may be confused with Celebrex®, Cerebra®, Cerebyx®, Zyprexa®

Related Information

Antidepressant Agents *on page 1551*

Chronic Pain Management *on page 1430*

U.S. Brand Names Celexa®

Canadian Brand Names Apo-Citalopram®; Celexa®; CO Citalopram; Dom-Citalopram; Gen-Citalopram; Novo-Citalopram; PHL-Citalopram; PMS-Citalopram; RAN™-Citalopram; ratio-Citalopram; Rhoxal-citalopram; Sandoz-Citalopram

Synonyms Citalopram Hydrobromide; Nitalapram

Pharmacologic Category Antidepressant, Selective Serotonin Reuptake Inhibitor

Restrictions A medication guide concerning the use of antidepressants in children and teenagers can be found on the FDA website at http://www.fda.gov/cder/Offices/ODS/labeling.htm. It should be dispensed to parents or guardians of children and teenagers receiving this medication.

Generic Available Yes

Use Treatment of depression

Unlabeled/Investigational Use Treatment of dementia, smoking cessation, ethanol abuse, obsessive-compulsive disorder (OCD) in children, diabetic neuropathy

Mechanism of Action A bicyclic phthalane derivative, citalopram selectively inhibits serotonin reuptake in the presynaptic neurons

Pharmacodynamics/Kinetics

Distribution: V_d: 12 L/kg

Protein binding, plasma: ~80%

Metabolism: Extensively hepatic, including CYP, to N-demethylated, N-oxide, and deaminated metabolites

Bioavailability: 80%

Half-life elimination: 24-48 hours; average 35 hours (doubled with hepatic impairment)

Time to peak, serum: 1-6 hours, average within 4 hours

Excretion: Urine (10% as unchanged drug)

Note: Clearance was decreased, while AUC and half-life were significantly increased in elderly patients and in patients with hepatic impairment. Mild-to-moderate renal impairment may reduce clearance (17%) and prolong half-life of citalopram. No pharmacokinetic information is available concerning patients with severe renal impairment.

Dosage Oral:

Children and Adolescents: OCD (unlabeled use): 10-40 mg/day

Adults: Depression: Initial: 20 mg/day, generally with an increase to 40 mg/day; doses of more than 40 mg are not usually necessary. Should a dose increase be necessary, it should occur in 20 mg increments at intervals of no less than 1 week. Maximum dose: 60 mg/day; reduce dosage in elderly or those with hepatic impairment.

Stability Store below 25°C.

(Continued)

Citalopram *(Continued)*

Monitoring Parameters Monitor patient periodically for symptom resolution; mental status for depression, suicidal ideation (especially at the beginning of therapy or when doses are increased or decreased), anxiety, social functioning, mania, panic attacks; akathisia

Pregnancy Risk Factor C

Contraindications Hypersensitivity to citalopram or any component of the formulation; hypersensitivity or other adverse sequelae during therapy with other SSRIs; concomitant use with MAO inhibitors or within 2 weeks of discontinuing MAO inhibitors

Warnings/Precautions

Major psychiatric warnings:

- **[U.S. Boxed Warning]: Antidepressants increase the risk of suicidal thinking and behavior in children and adolescents with major depressive disorder (MDD) and other depressive disorders;** consider risk prior to prescribing. Closely monitor for clinical worsening, suicidality, or unusual changes in behavior; the child's family or caregiver should be instructed to closely observe the patient and communicate condition with healthcare provider. A medication guide concerning the use of antidepressants in children and teenagers should be dispensed with each prescription. **Citalopram is not FDA approved for use in children.**
- The possibility of a suicide attempt is inherent in major depression and may persist until remission occurs. Patients treated with antidepressants should be observed for clinical worsening and suicidality, especially during the initial few months of a course of drug therapy, or at times of dose changes, either increases or decreases. Worsening depression and severe abrupt suicidality that are not part of the presenting symptoms may require discontinuation or modification of drug therapy. Use caution in high-risk patients during initiation of therapy.
- Prescriptions should be written for the smallest quantity consistent with good patient care. The patient's family or caregiver should be alerted to monitor patients for the emergence of suicidality and associated behaviors such as anxiety, agitation, panic attacks, insomnia, irritability, hostility, impulsivity, akathisia, hypomania, and mania; patients should be instructed to notify their healthcare provider if any of these symptoms or worsening depression or psychosis occur.
- May worsen psychosis in some patients or precipitate a shift to mania or hypomania in patients with bipolar disorder. Monotherapy in patients with bipolar disorder should be avoided. Patients presenting with depressive symptoms should be screened for bipolar disorder. **Citalopram is not FDA approved for the treatment of bipolar depression.**

Key adverse effects:

- Anticholinergic effects: Relatively devoid of these side effects.
- CNS depression: Has a low potential to impair cognitive or motor performance; caution operating hazardous machinery or driving.
- SIADH and hyponatremia: Has been associated with the development of SIADH; hyponatremia has been reported rarely, predominately in the elderly.

Concurrent disease:

- Hepatic impairment: Use caution; clearance is decreased and plasma concentrations are increased; a lower dosage may be needed.
- Platelet aggregation: May impair platelet aggregation, resulting in bleeding.
- Renal impairment: Use caution; clearance is decreased and plasma concentrations are increased; a lower dosage may be needed.
- Sexual dysfunction: May cause or exacerbate sexual dysfunction.

Concurrent drug therapy:

- Anticoagulants/Antiplatelets: Use caution with concomitant use of NSAIDs, ASA, or other drugs that affect coagulation; the risk of bleeding is potentiated.
- CNS depressants: Use caution with concomitant therapy.
- MAO inhibitors: Potential for severe reaction when used with MAO inhibitors; autonomic instability, coma, death, delirium, diaphoresis, hyperthermia, mental status changes/agitation, muscular rigidity, myoclonus, neuroleptic malignant syndrome features, and seizures may occur.

Special populations:

- Elderly: Use caution in elderly patients.
- Pregnancy: Use caution in pregnant patients; high doses of citalopram have been associated with teratogenicity in animals.

Special notes:

- Electroconvulsive therapy: May increase the risks associated with electroconvulsive therapy; consider discontinuing, when possible, prior to ECT treatment.
- Withdrawal syndrome: May cause dysphoric mood, irritability, agitation, dizziness, sensory disturbances, anxiety, confusion, headache, lethargy, emotional lability, insomnia, hypomania, tinnitus, and seizures. Upon discontinuation of citalopram therapy, gradually taper dose. If intolerable symptoms occur following a decrease in dosage or upon discontinuation of therapy, then resuming the previous dose with a more gradual taper should be considered.

Adverse Reactions

>10%:

Central nervous system: Somnolence, insomnia
Gastrointestinal: Nausea, xerostomia
Miscellaneous: Diaphoresis

<10%:

Central nervous system: Anxiety, anorexia, agitation, yawning
Dermatologic: Rash, pruritus
Endocrine & metabolic: Sexual dysfunction
Gastrointestinal: Diarrhea, dyspepsia, vomiting, abdominal pain, weight gain
Neuromuscular & skeletal: Tremor, arthralgia, myalgia
Respiratory: Cough, rhinitis, sinusitis

<1%, Postmarketing, and/or case reports (limited to important or life-threatening): Acute renal failure, anaphylaxis, angioedema, delirium, dyskinesia, epidermal necrolysis, erythema multiforme, hemolytic anemia, hepatic necrosis, neuroleptic malignant syndrome (NMS), pancreatitis, priapism, QT prolonged, rhabdomyolysis, serotonin syndrome, SIADH, ventricular arrhythmia, torsade de pointes, withdrawal syndrome

Overdosage/Toxicology Symptoms of overdose include dizziness, nausea, vomiting, sweating, tremor, somnolence, and sinus tachycardia. Rare symptoms have included amnesia, confusion, coma, seizures, hyperventilation, and ECG changes (including QT_c prolongation, ventricular arrhythmia, and torsade de pointes). Management is supportive and symptomatic.

Drug Interactions Substrate of CYP2C19 (major), 2D6 (minor), 3A4 (major); **Inhibits** CYP1A2 (weak), 2B6 (weak), 2C19 (weak), 2D6 (weak)

Aspirin: Concomitant use of citalopram and NSAIDs, aspirin, or other drugs affecting coagulation has been associated with an increased risk of bleeding; monitor.

Beta-blockers: Citalopram may increase levels of some beta-blockers (see Carvedilol and Metoprolol); monitor carefully.

Buspirone: Concurrent use of citalopram with buspirone may cause serotonin syndrome; avoid concurrent use.

Carbamazepine: May enhance the metabolism of citalopram.

Carvedilol: Serum concentrations may be increased; monitor carefully for increased carvedilol effect (hypotension and bradycardia).

Cimetidine: May inhibit the metabolism of citalopram.

CYP2C19 inducers: May decrease the levels/effects of citalopram. Example inducers include aminoglutethimide, carbamazepine, phenytoin, and rifampin.

CYP2C19 inhibitors: May increase the levels/effects of citalopram. Example inhibitors include delavirdine, fluconazole, fluvoxamine, gemfibrozil, isoniazid, omeprazole, and ticlopidine.

CYP3A4 inducers: CYP3A4 inducers may decrease the levels/effects of citalopram. Example inducers include aminoglutethimide, carbamazepine, nafcillin, nevirapine, phenobarbital, phenytoin, and rifamycins.

CYP3A4 inhibitors: May increase the levels/effects of citalopram. Example inhibitors include azole antifungals, clarithromycin, diclofenac, doxycycline, erythromycin, imatinib, isoniazid, nefazodone, nicardipine, propofol, protease inhibitors, quinidine, telithromycin, and verapamil.

Linezolid: Hyperpyrexia, hypertension, tachycardia, confusion, seizures, and **deaths have been reported** with agents which inhibit MAO (serotonin syndrome); this combination should be avoided.

MAO inhibitors: Hyperpyrexia, hypertension, tachycardia, confusion, seizures, and **deaths have been reported** with MAO inhibitors (serotonin syndrome); this combination should be avoided.

Meperidine: Combined use theoretically may increase the risk of serotonin syndrome.

(Continued)

Citalopram *(Continued)*

Metoprolol: Citalopram may increase plasma levels of metoprolol; monitor for increased effect.

Moclobemide: Concurrent use of citalopram with moclobemide may cause serotonin syndrome; avoid concurrent use.

Nefazodone: Concurrent use of citalopram with nefazodone may cause serotonin syndrome.

NSAIDs: Concomitant use of citalopram and NSAIDs, aspirin, or other drugs affecting coagulation has been associated with an increased risk of bleeding; monitor.

Ritonavir: Combined use of citalopram with ritonavir may cause serotonin syndrome in HIV-positive patients; monitor.

Selegiline: Concurrent use with citalopram has been reported to cause serotonin syndrome; as an MAO type B inhibitor, the risk of serotonin syndrome may be less than with nonselective MAO inhibitors, and reports indicate that this combination has been well tolerated in Parkinson's patients.

Serotonin reuptake inhibitors: Concurrent use with other reuptake inhibitors may increase the risk of serotonin syndrome.

Sibutramine: May increase the risk of serotonin syndrome with SSRIs.

Sumatriptan (and other serotonin agonists): Concurrent use may result in toxicity; weakness, hyper-reflexia, and incoordination have been observed with sumatriptan and SSRIs. In addition, concurrent use may theoretically increase the risk of serotonin syndrome; includes sumatriptan, naratriptan, rizatriptan, and zolmitriptan.

Tramadol: Concurrent use of citalopram with tramadol may cause serotonin syndrome; avoid concurrent use.

Trazodone: Concurrent use of citalopram with trazodone may cause serotonin syndrome.

Venlafaxine: Combined use with citalopram may increase the risk of serotonin syndrome.

Ethanol/Nutrition/Herb Interactions

Ethanol: Avoid ethanol (may increase CNS depression).

Herb/Nutraceutical: Avoid valerian, St John's wort, SAMe, kava kava, and gotu kola (may increase CNS depression).

Dietary Considerations May be taken without regard to food.

Dosage Forms

Solution, oral: 10 mg/5 mL (240 mL) [alcohol free, sugar free; peppermint flavor]

Tablet: 10 mg, 20 mg, 40 mg

- **Citalopram Hydrobromide** *see* Citalopram *on page 297*
- **Citanest® Plain** *see* Prilocaine *on page 1054*
- **Citrate of Magnesia** *see* Magnesium Citrate *on page 786*
- **Citro-Mag® (Can)** *see* Magnesium Citrate *on page 786*
- **Citrovorum Factor** *see* Leucovorin *on page 738*
- **Claforan®** *see* Cefotaxime *on page 240*

Clarithromycin (kla RITH roe mye sin)

Medication Safety Issues

Sound-alike/look-alike issues:

Clarithromycin may be confused with erythromycin

Related Information

Helicobacter pylori Treatment *on page 1613*

U.S. Brand Names Biaxin®; Biaxin® XL

Canadian Brand Names Biaxin®; Biaxin® XL; ratio-Clarithromycin

Pharmacologic Category Antibiotic, Macrolide

Generic Available Yes: Tablet

Use

Children:

Pharyngitis/tonsillitis, acute maxillary sinusitis, uncomplicated skin/skin structure infections, and mycobacterial infections

Acute otitis media (*H. influenzae*, *M. catarrhalis*, or *S. pneumoniae*)

Prevention of disseminated mycobacterial infections due to MAC disease in patients with advanced HIV infection

Adults:

Pharyngitis/tonsillitis due to susceptible *S. pyogenes*

Acute maxillary sinusitis and acute exacerbation of chronic bronchitis due to susceptible *H. influenzae, M. catarrhalis*, or *S. pneumoniae*

Community-acquired pneumonia due to susceptible *H. influenzae, H. parainfluenzae, Mycoplasma pneumoniae, S. pneumoniae*, or *Chlamydia pneumoniae* (TWAR)

Uncomplicated skin/skin structure infections due to susceptible *S. aureus, S. pyogenes*

Disseminated mycobacterial infections due to *M. avium* or *M. intracellulare*

Prevention of disseminated mycobacterial infections due to *M. avium* complex (MAC) disease (eg, patients with advanced HIV infection)

Duodenal ulcer disease due to *H. pylori* in regimens with other drugs including amoxicillin and lansoprazole or omeprazole, ranitidine bismuth citrate, bismuth subsalicylate, tetracycline, and/or an H_2 antagonist

Alternate antibiotic for prophylaxis of bacterial endocarditis in patients who are allergic to penicillin and undergoing surgical or dental procedures

Unlabeled/Investigational Use Pertussis

Mechanism of Action Exerts its antibacterial action by binding to 50S ribosomal subunit resulting in inhibition of protein synthesis. The 14-OH metabolite of clarithromycin is twice as active as the parent compound against certain organisms.

Pharmacodynamics/Kinetics

Absorption: Highly stable in presence of gastric acid (unlike erythromycin); food delays but does not affect extent of absorption

Distribution: Widely into most body tissues except CNS

Metabolism: Partially hepatic via CYP3A4; converted to 14-OH clarithromycin (active metabolite)

Bioavailability: 50%

Half-life elimination: Clarithromycin: 3-7 hours; 14-OH-clarithromycin: 5-9 hours

Time to peak: 2-4 hours

Excretion: Primarily urine

Clearance: Approximates normal GFR

Dosage

Usual dosage range:

Children ≥6 months: Oral: 7.5-15 mg/kg every 12 hours (maximum: 500 mg/dose)

Adults: Oral: 250-500 mg every 12 hours **or** 1000 mg (two 500 mg extended release tablets) once daily for 7-14 days

Indication-specific dosing:

Children: Oral:

Community-acquired pneumonia, sinusitis, bronchitis, skin infections: 15 mg/kg/day divided every 12 hours for 10 days

Endocarditis, prophylaxis: 15 mg/kg 1 hour before procedure (maximum: 500 mg)

Mycobacterial infection (prevention and treatment): 7.5 mg/kg (up to 500 mg) twice daily. **Note:** Safety of clarithromycin for MAC not studied in children <20 months.

Pertussis (CDC guidelines):

Children ≥1 months: 15 mg/kg/day divided every 12 hours for 7 days (maximum: 1 g/day)

Children ≥6 months: 15 mg/kg/day divided every 12 hours for 10 days

Adults: Oral:

Acute exacerbation of chronic bronchitis:

M. catarrhalis and *S. pneumoniae*: 250 mg every 12 hours for 7-14 days **or** 1000 mg (two 500 mg extended release tablets) once daily for 7 days

H. influenzae: 500 mg every 12 hours for 7-14 days or 1000 mg (two 500 mg extended release tablets) for 7 days

H. parainfluenzae: 500 mg every 12 hours for 7 days or 1000 mg (two 500 mg extended release tablets) for 7 days

Acute maxillary sinusitis: 500 mg every 12 hours **or** 1000 mg (two 500 mg extended release tablets) once daily for 14 days

Endocarditis, prophylaxis: 500 mg 1 hour prior to procedure

Mycobacterial infection (prevention and treatment): 500 mg twice daily (use with other antimycobacterial drugs, eg, ethambutol or rifampin)

Peptic ulcer disease: Eradication of *Helicobacter pylori*: Dual or triple combination regimen with bismuth subsalicylate, tetracycline, clarithromycin, and an H_2-receptor; or combination of omeprazole and clarithromycin; 500 mg every 8-12 hours for 10-14 days

(Continued)

Clarithromycin *(Continued)*

Pertussis (CDC guidelines): 500 mg twice daily for 7 days

Pharyngitis, tonsillitis: 250 mg every 12 hours for 10 days

Pneumonia:

C. pneumoniae, *M. pneumoniae*, and *S. pneumoniae*: 250 mg every 12 hours for 7-14 days **or** 1000 mg (two 500 mg extended release tablets) once daily for 7 days

H. influenzae: 250 mg every 12 hours for 7 days **or** 1000 mg (two 500 mg extended release tablets) once daily for 7 days

Skin and skin structure infection, uncomplicated: 250 mg every 12 hours for 7-14 days

Elderly: Pharmacokinetics are similar to those in younger adults; may have age-related reductions in renal function; monitor and adjust dose if necessary

Dosing adjustment in renal impairment:

Cl_{cr} <30 mL/minute: Half the normal dose or double the dosing interval

In combination with ritonavir:

Cl_{cr} 30-60 mL/minute: Decrease clarithromycin dose by 50%

Cl_{cr} <30 mL/minute: Decrease clarithromycin dose by 75%

Dosing adjustment in hepatic impairment: No dosing adjustment is needed as long as renal function is normal

Stability Store tablets and granules for oral suspension at controlled room temperature. Reconstituted oral suspension should not be refrigerated because it might gel; microencapsulated particles of clarithromycin in suspension is stable for 14 days when stored at room temperature

Administration Clarithromycin may be given with or without meals. Give every 12 hours rather than twice daily to avoid peak and trough variation.

Biaxin® XL: Should be given with food. Do not crush or chew extended release tablet.

Pregnancy Risk Factor C

Contraindications Hypersensitivity to clarithromycin, erythromycin, or any macrolide antibiotic; use with ergot derivatives, pimozide, cisapride; combination with ranitidine bismuth citrate should not be used in patients with history of acute porphyria or Cl_{cr} <25 mL/minute

Warnings/Precautions Dosage adjustment required with severe renal impairment, decreased dosage or prolonged dosing interval may be appropriate; antibiotic-associated colitis has been reported with use of clarithromycin. Macrolides (including clarithromycin) have been associated with rare QT prolongation and ventricular arrhythmias, including torsade de pointes. The extended release formulation consists of drug within a nondeformable matrix; following drug release/absorption, the matrix/shell is expelled in the stool. The use of nondeformable products in patients with known stricture/narrowing of the GI tract has been associated with symptoms of obstruction. Safety and efficacy in children <6 months of age have not been established.

Adverse Reactions

1% to 10%:

Central nervous system: Headache (adults and children 2%)

Dermatologic: Rash (children 3%)

Gastrointestinal: Abnormal taste (adults 3% to 7%), diarrhea (adults 3% to 6%; children 6%), vomiting (children 6%), nausea (adults 3%), heartburn (adults 2%), abdominal pain (adults 2%; children 3%), dyspepsia 2%

Hepatic: Prothrombin time increased (1%)

Renal: BUN increased (4%)

<1% (Limited to important or life-threatening): *Clostridium difficile* colitis, alkaline phosphatase increased, anaphylaxis, anorexia, anxiety, behavioral changes, bilirubin increased, confusion, disorientation, dizziness, dyspnea, glossitis, hallucinations, hearing loss (reversible), hepatic dysfunction, hepatic failure, hepatitis, hypoglycemia, insomnia, interstitial nephritis, jaundice, leukopenia, manic behavior, neuromuscular blockade (case reports), neutropenia, nightmares, oral moniliasis, pancreatitis, psychosis, QT prolongation, seizure, serum creatinine increased, smell alteration, Stevens-Johnson syndrome, stomatitis, thrombocytopenia, tinnitus, tongue discoloration, tooth discoloration, torsade de pointes, toxic epidermal necrolysis, transaminases increased, tremor, urticaria, ventricular tachycardia, ventricular arrhythmia, vertigo

Overdosage/Toxicology Symptoms of overdose include nausea, vomiting, diarrhea, prostration, reversible pancreatitis, hearing loss with or without tinnitus, or vertigo. Treatment includes symptomatic and supportive care. Dialysis not likely to benefit.

Drug Interactions Substrate of CYP3A4 (major); **Inhibits** CYP1A2 (weak), 3A4 (strong)

Alfentanil (and possibly other narcotic analgesics): Serum levels may be increased by clarithromycin; monitor for increased effect.

Benzodiazepines (those metabolized by CYP3A4, including alprazolam, midazolam, triazolam): Serum levels may be increased by clarithromycin; somnolence and confusion have been reported.

Bromocriptine: Serum levels may be increased by clarithromycin; monitor for increased effect.

Buspirone: Serum levels may be increased by clarithromycin; monitor.

Calcium channel blockers (felodipine, verapamil, and potentially others metabolized by CYP3A4): Serum levels may be increased by clarithromycin; monitor.

Carbamazepine: Serum levels may be increased by clarithromycin; monitor.

Cilostazol: Serum levels may be increased by clarithromycin; monitor.

Cisapride: Serum levels may be increased by clarithromycin; serious arrhythmias have occurred; concurrent use contraindicated.

Clopidogrel: Therapeutic effect may be decreased by clarithromycin; monitor.

Clozapine: Serum levels may be increased by clarithromycin; monitor.

Colchicine: Serum levels/toxicity may be increased by clarithromycin; monitor. Avoid use, if possible.

Cyclosporine: Serum levels may be increased by clarithromycin; monitor serum levels.

CYP3A4 inducers: CYP3A4 inducers may decrease the levels/effects of clarithromycin. Example inducers include aminoglutethimide, carbamazepine, nafcillin, nevirapine, phenobarbital, phenytoin, and rifamycins.

CYP3A4 inhibitors: May increase the levels/effects of clarithromycin. Example inhibitors include azole antifungals, diclofenac, doxycycline, erythromycin, imatinib, isoniazid, nefazodone, nicardipine, propofol, protease inhibitors, quinidine, telithromycin, and verapamil.

CYP3A4 substrates: Clarithromycin may increase the levels/effects of CYP3A4 substrates. Example substrates include benzodiazepines, calcium channel blockers, mirtazapine, nateglinide, nefazodone, tacrolimus, and venlafaxine. Selected benzodiazepines (midazolam and triazolam), cisapride, ergot alkaloids, selected HMG-CoA reductase inhibitors (lovastatin and simvastatin), and pimozide are generally contraindicated with strong CYP3A4 inhibitors.

Delavirdine: Serum levels may be increased by clarithromycin; monitor.

Digoxin: Serum levels may be increased by clarithromycin; digoxin toxicity and potentially fatal arrhythmias have been reported; monitor digoxin levels.

Disopyramide: Serum levels may be increased by clarithromycin; in addition, QT_c prolongation and risk of malignant arrhythmia may be increased; avoid combination.

Ergot alkaloids: Concurrent use may lead to acute ergot toxicity (severe peripheral vasospasm and dysesthesia).

Fluconazole: Increases clarithromycin levels and AUC by ~25%

HMG-CoA reductase inhibitors (atorvastatin, lovastatin, and simvastatin); Clarithromycin may increase serum levels of "statins" metabolized by CYP3A4, increasing the risk of myopathy/rhabdomyolysis (does not include fluvastatin and pravastatin). Switch to pravastatin/fluvastatin or suspend treatment during course of clarithromycin therapy.

Methylprednisolone: Serum levels may be increased by clarithromycin; monitor.

Phenytoin: Serum levels may be increased by clarithromycin; other evidence suggested phenytoin levels may be decreased in some patients; monitor.

Pimozide: Serum levels may be increased, leading to malignant arrhythmias; concomitant use is contraindicated.

Protease inhibitors (amprenavir, nelfinavir, and ritonavir): May increase serum levels of clarithromycin.

QT_c-prolonging agents: Concomitant use may increase the risk of malignant arrhythmias.

Quinidine: Serum levels may be increased by clarithromycin; in addition, the risk of QT_c prolongation and malignant arrhythmias may be increased during concurrent use.

Quinolone antibiotics (sparfloxacin, gatifloxacin, or moxifloxacin): Concurrent use may increase the risk of malignant arrhythmias.

Rifabutin: Serum levels may be increased by clarithromycin; monitor.

(Continued)

Clarithromycin *(Continued)*

Sildenafil, tadalafil, vardenafil: Serum levels may be increased by clarithromycin. Do not exceed single sildenafil doses of 25 mg in 48 hours, a single tadalafil dose of 10 mg in 72 hours, or a single vardenafil dose of 2.5 mg in 24 hours.
Tacrolimus: Serum levels may be increased by clarithromycin; monitor serum concentration.
Theophylline: Serum levels may be increased by clarithromycin; monitor.
Thioridazine: Risk of QT_c prolongation and malignant arrhythmias may be increased.
Valproic acid (and derivatives): Serum levels may be increased by clarithromycin; monitor.
Vinblastine (and vincristine): Serum levels may be increased by clarithromycin.
Warfarin: Effects may be potentiated; monitor INR closely and adjust warfarin dose as needed or choose another antibiotic
Zidovudine: Peak levels (but not AUC) of zidovudine may be increased; other studies suggest levels may be decreased.
Zopiclone: Serum levels may be increased by clarithromycin; monitor.

Ethanol/Nutrition/Herb Interactions
Food: Delays absorption; total absorption remains unchanged.
Herb/Nutraceutical: St John's wort may decrease clarithromycin levels.

Dietary Considerations May be taken with or without meals; may be taken with milk. Biaxin® XL should be taken with food.

Dosage Forms
Granules for oral suspension (Biaxin®): 125 mg/5 mL (50 mL, 100 mL); 250 mg/5 mL (50 mL, 100 mL) [fruit punch flavor]
Tablet (Biaxin®): 250 mg, 500 mg
Tablet, extended release (Biaxin® XL): 500 mg

♦ **Claritin® Allergic Decongestant (Can)** *see* Oxymetazoline *on page 973*
♦ **Clasteon® (Can)** *see* Clodronate *on page 308*
♦ **Cleocin®** *see* Clindamycin *on page 304*
♦ **Cleocin HCl®** *see* Clindamycin *on page 304*
♦ **Cleocin Pediatric®** *see* Clindamycin *on page 304*
♦ **Cleocin Phosphate®** *see* Clindamycin *on page 304*
♦ **Cleocin T®** *see* Clindamycin *on page 304*
♦ **Clindagel®** *see* Clindamycin *on page 304*
♦ **ClindaMax™** *see* Clindamycin *on page 304*

Clindamycin (klin da MYE sin)

Medication Safety Issues
Sound-alike/look-alike issues:
Cleocin® may be confused with bleomycin, Clinoril®, Lincocin®

Related Information
Anesthesia for Patients With Liver Disease *on page 1421*
Prevention of Bacterial Endocarditis *on page 1583*
Prevention of Wound Infection and Sepsis in Surgical Patients *on page 1588*

U.S. Brand Names Cleocin®; Cleocin HCl®; Cleocin Pediatric®; Cleocin Phosphate®; Cleocin T®; Clindagel®; ClindaMax™; Clindesse™; Clindets®; Evoclin™

Canadian Brand Names Alti-Clindamycin; Apo-Clindamycin®; Clindamycin Injection, USP; Clindoxyl®; Dalacin® C; Dalacin® T; Dalacin® Vaginal; Novo-Clindamycin; Taro-Clindamycin

Synonyms Clindamycin Hydrochloride; Clindamycin Palmitate; Clindamycin Phosphate

Pharmacologic Category Antibiotic, Lincosamide

Generic Available Yes: Excludes foam, vaginal suppositories, vaginal cream

Use Treatment against aerobic and anaerobic streptococci (except enterococci), most staphylococci, *Bacteroides* sp and *Actinomyces*; bacterial vaginosis (vaginal cream, vaginal suppository); pelvic inflammatory disease (I.V.); topically in treatment of severe acne; vaginally for *Gardnerella vaginalis*

Unlabeled/Investigational Use May be useful in PCP; alternate treatment for toxoplasmosis

Mechanism of Action Reversibly binds to 50S ribosomal subunits preventing peptide bond formation thus inhibiting bacterial protein synthesis; bacteriostatic or bactericidal depending on drug concentration, infection site, and organism

Pharmacodynamics/Kinetics

Absorption: Topical: ~10%; Oral: Rapid (90%)

Distribution: High concentrations in bone and urine; no significant levels in CSF, even with inflamed meninges; crosses placenta; enters breast milk

Metabolism: Hepatic

Bioavailability: Topical: <1%

Half-life elimination: Neonates: Premature: 8.7 hours; Full-term: 3.6 hours; Adults: 1.6-5.3 hours (average: 2-3 hours)

Time to peak, serum: Oral: Within 60 minutes; I.M.: 1-3 hours

Excretion: Urine (10%) and feces (~4%) as active drug and metabolites

Dosage

Usual dosage ranges:

Infants and Children:

Oral: 8-20 mg/kg/day as hydrochloride; 8-25 mg/kg/day as palmitate in 3-4 divided doses (minimum dose of palmitate: 37.5 mg 3 times/day)

I.M., I.V.:

<1 month: 15-20 mg/kg/day

>1 month: 20-40 mg/kg/day in 3-4 divided doses

Adults:

Oral: 150-450 mg/dose every 6-8 hours; maximum dose: 1.8 g/day

I.M., I.V.: 1.2-1.8 g/day in 2-4 divided doses; maximum dose: 4.8 g/day

Indication-specific dosing:

Children:

Anthrax: I.V.: 7.5 mg/kg every 6 hours

Babesiosis: Oral: 20-40 mg/kg/day divided every 8 hours for 7 days plus quinine

Orofacial infections: 8-25 mg/kg in 3-4 equally divided doses

Prevention of bacterial endocarditis (unlabeled use):

Oral: 20 mg/kg 1 hour before procedure with no follow-up dose needed

I.V.: 20 mg/kg within 30 minutes before procedure

Children ≥12 years and Adults:

Acne vulgaris: Topical:

Gel, pledget, lotion, solution: Apply a thin film twice daily

Foam (Evoclin™): Apply once daily

Adults:

Amnionitis: I.V.: 450-900 mg every 8 hours

Anthrax: I.V.: 900 mg every 8 hours with ciprofloxacin or doxycycline

Babesiosis:

Oral: 600 mg 3 times/day for 7 days with quinine

I.V.: 1.2 g twice daily

Bacterial vaginosis: Intravaginal:

Suppositories: Insert one ovule (100 mg clindamycin) daily into vagina at bedtime for 3 days

Cream:

Cleocin®: One full applicator inserted intravaginally once daily before bedtime for 3 or 7 consecutive days in nonpregnant patients or for 7 consecutive days in pregnant patients

Clindesse™: One full applicator inserted intravaginally as a single dose at anytime during the day in nonpregnant patients

Bite wounds (canine): Oral: 300 mg 4 times/day with a fluoroquinolone

Gangrenous myositis: I.V.: 900 mg every 8 hours with penicillin G

Group B streptococcus (neonatal prophylaxis): I.V.: 900 mg every 8 hours until delivery

Orofacial/parapharyngeal space infections:

Oral: 150-450 mg every 6 hours for 7 days, maximum 1.8 g/day

I.V.: 600-900 mg every 8 hours

Pelvic inflammatory disease: I.V.: 900 mg every 8 hours with gentamicin 2 mg/kg, then 1.5 mg/kg every 8 hours; continue after discharge with doxycycline 100 mg twice daily to complete 14 days of total therapy

***Pneumocystis jiroveci* pneumonia (unlabeled use):**

Oral: 300-450 mg 4 times/day with primaquine

I.M., I.V.: 1200-2400 mg/day with pyrimethamine or 600 mg 4 times/day with primaquine

Prevention of bacterial endocarditis (unlabeled use):

Oral: 600 mg 1 hour before procedure with no follow-up dose needed

I.V.: 600 mg within 30 minutes before procedure

(Continued)

Clindamycin *(Continued)*

Toxic shock syndrome: I.V.: 900 mg every 8 hours with penicillin G or ceftriaxone

Toxoplasmosis (unlabeled use): Oral, I.V.: 600 mg every 6 hours with pyrimethamine and folinic acid

Dosing adjustment in hepatic impairment: Adjustment recommended in patients with severe hepatic disease

Stability

Capsule: Store at room temperature of 20°C to 25°C (68°F to 77°F).

Cream: Store at room temperature.

Foam: Store at room temperature of 20°C to 25°C (68°F to 77°F); avoid fire, flame, or smoking during or following application.

Gel: Store at room temperature.

Clindagel®: Do not store in direct sunlight.

I.V.: Infusion solution in NS or D_5W solution is stable for 16 days at room temperature.

Lotion: Store at room temperature of 20°C to 25°C (68°F to 77°F).

Oral solution: Do not refrigerate reconstituted oral solution (it will thicken); following reconstitution, oral solution is stable for 2 weeks at room temperature of 20°C to 25°C (68°F to 77°F).

Ovule: Store at room temperature of 15°C to 30°C (68°F to 77°F).

Pledget: Store at room temperature.

Topical solution: Store at room temperature of 20°C to 25°C (68°F to 77°F).

Administration

I.M.: Deep I.M. sites, rotate sites; do not exceed 600 mg in a single injection.

Intravaginal:

Cream: Insertion should be as far as possible into the vagina without causing discomfort.

Ovule: The foil should be removed; if the applicator is used for insertion, it should be washed for additional use.

I.V.: **Never administer as bolus**; administer by I.V. intermittent infusion over at least 10-60 minutes, at a rate **not** to exceed 30 mg/minute (not exceed 1200 mg/hour); final concentration for administration should not exceed 18 mg/mL.

Oral: Administer with a full glass of water to minimize esophageal ulceration; give around-the-clock to promote less variation in peak and trough serum levels.

Topical foam: Dispense directly into cap or onto a cool surface; do not dispense directly into hands.

Monitoring Parameters Observe for changes in bowel frequency. Monitor for colitis and resolution of symptoms. During prolonged therapy monitor CBC, liver and renal function tests periodically.

Anesthesia and Critical Care Concerns/Other Considerations Clindamycin may increase the duration of neuromuscular blockade after anesthesia. In adults, clindamycin injection can usually be dosed effectively on an every-8-hour basis.

Pregnancy Risk Factor B

Contraindications Hypersensitivity to clindamycin or any component of the formulation; previous pseudomembranous colitis; regional enteritis, ulcerative colitis

Warnings/Precautions Dosage adjustment may be necessary in patients with severe hepatic dysfunction. **[U.S. Boxed Warning]: Can cause severe and possibly fatal colitis.** Discontinue drug if significant diarrhea, abdominal cramps, or passage of blood and mucus occurs. Vaginal products may weaken latex or rubber condoms, or contraceptive diaphragms. Barrier contraceptives are not recommended concurrently or for 3-5 days (depending on the product) following treatment. Some dosage forms contain benzyl alcohol or tartrazine. Use caution in atopic patients.

Adverse Reactions

Systemic:

>10%: Gastrointestinal: Diarrhea, abdominal pain

1% to 10%:

Cardiovascular: Hypotension

Dermatologic: Urticaria, rash, Stevens-Johnson syndrome

Gastrointestinal: Pseudomembranous colitis, nausea, vomiting

Local: Thrombophlebitis, sterile abscess at I.M. injection site

Miscellaneous: Fungal overgrowth, hypersensitivity

<1% (Limited to important or life-threatening): Granulocytopenia, neutropenia, polyarthritis, renal dysfunction (rare), thrombocytopenia

Topical:

>10%: Dermatologic: Dryness, burning, itching, scaliness, erythema, or peeling of skin (lotion, solution); oiliness (gel, lotion)

1% to 10%: Central nervous system: Headache

<1% (Limited to important or life-threatening): Pseudomembranous colitis, nausea, vomiting, diarrhea (severe), abdominal pain, folliculitis, hypersensitivity reactions

Vaginal:

>10%: Genitourinary: Fungal vaginosis, vaginitis or vulvovaginal pruritus (from *Candida albicans*)

1% to 10%:

Central nervous system: Back pain, headache
Gastrointestinal: Constipation, diarrhea
Genitourinary: Urinary tract infection
Respiratory: Nasopharyngitis
Miscellaneous: Fungal infection

<1% (Limited to important or life-threatening): Atrophic vaginitis, bladder infection, bladder spasm, cervical dysplasia, diarrhea, dizziness, epistaxis, erythema, fever, hypersensitivity, hyperthyroidism, local edema, menstrual disorder, nausea, pain, palpable lymph node, pruritus, pyelonephritis, pyrexia, rash, sciatica, stomach cramps, upper respiratory urticaria, uterine cervical disorder, uterine spasm, vaginal burning, vertigo, vomiting, vulvar erythema, vulvar laceration, wheezing

Overdosage/Toxicology Symptoms of overdose include diarrhea, nausea, and vomiting. Treatment is supportive.

Drug Interactions Increased duration of neuromuscular blockade from tubocurarine, pancuronium

Ethanol/Nutrition/Herb Interactions

Food: Peak concentrations may be delayed with food.

Herb/Nutraceutical: St John's wort may decrease clindamycin levels.

Dietary Considerations May be taken with food.

Dosage Forms Note: Strength is expressed as base

Capsule, as hydrochloride: 150 mg, 300 mg
  Cleocin HCl®: 75 mg [contains tartrazine], 150 mg [contains tartrazine], 300 mg
Cream, vaginal, as phosphate:
  Cleocin®: 2% (40 g) [contains benzyl alcohol and mineral oil; packaged with 7 disposable applicators]
  Clindesse™: 2% (5 g) [contains mineral oil; prefilled single disposable applicator]
Foam, topical, as phosphate (Evoclin™): 1% (50 g, 100 g) [contains ethanol 58%]
Gel, topical, as phosphate: 1% [10 mg/g] (30 g, 60 g)
  Cleocin T®: 1% [10 mg/g] (30 g, 60 g)
  Clindagel®: 1% [10 mg/g] (40 mL, 75 mL)
  ClindaMax™: 1% (30 g, 60 g)
Granules for oral solution, as palmitate (Cleocin Pediatric®): 75 mg/5 mL (100 mL) [cherry flavor]
Infusion, as phosphate [premixed in D_5W] (Cleocin Phosphate®): 300 mg (50 mL); 600 mg (50 mL); 900 mg (50 mL)
Injection, solution, as phosphate (Cleocin Phosphate®): 150 mg/mL (2 mL, 4 mL, 6 mL, 60 mL) [contains benzyl alcohol and disodium edetate 0.5 mg]
Lotion, as phosphate (Cleocin T®, ClindaMax™): 1% [10 mg/mL] (60 mL)
Pledgets, topical: 1% (60s) [contains alcohol]
  Cleocin T®: 1% (60s) [contains isopropyl alcohol 50%]
  Clindets®: 1% (69s) [contains isopropyl alcohol 52%]
Solution, topical, as phosphate (Cleocin T®): 1% [10 mg/mL] (30 mL, 60 mL) [contains isopropyl alcohol 50%]
Suppository (ovule), vaginal, as phosphate (Cleocin®): 100 mg (3s) [contains oleaginous base; single reusable applicator]

- **Clindamycin Hydrochloride** *see* Clindamycin *on page 304*
- **Clindamycin Injection, USP (Can)** *see* Clindamycin *on page 304*
- **Clindamycin Palmitate** *see* Clindamycin *on page 304*
- **Clindamycin Phosphate** *see* Clindamycin *on page 304*
- **Clindesse™** *see* Clindamycin *on page 304*
- **Clindets®** *see* Clindamycin *on page 304*

- **Clindoxyl® (Can)** *see* Clindamycin *on page 304*
- **Clinoril®** *see* Sulindac *on page 1219*

Clodronate (KLOE droh nate)

Canadian Brand Names Bonefos®; Clasteon®; Ostac®

Synonyms Clodronate Disodium

Pharmacologic Category Bisphosphonate Derivative

Restrictions Not available in U.S.

Use Management of hypercalcemia of malignancy

Mechanism of Action A bisphosphonate which inhibits bone resorption via actions on osteoclasts or on osteoclast precursors.

Pharmacodynamics/Kinetics

Onset of effect: 24-48 hours

Peak effect: 5-7 days

Duration: 2-3 weeks

Distribution: V_d: 20 L

Bioavailability: Oral: 1% to 3%

Half-life (terminal): 13 hours (serum); prolonged in bone tissue

Elimination: Urine (as unchanged drug)

Dosage

I.V.:

Multiple infusions: 300 mg/day; should not be prolonged beyond 10 days.

Single infusion: 1500 mg as a single dose

Oral: Recommended daily maintenance dose following I.V. therapy: Range: 1600 mg (4 capsules) to 2400 mg (6 capsules) given in single or 2 divided doses; maximum recommended daily dose: 3200 mg (8 capsules). Should be taken at least 1 hour before or after food, because food may decrease the amount of clodronate absorbed by the body.

Dosage adjustment in renal impairment:

Cl_{cr} >5 mg/dL: Use is contraindicated

Cl_{cr} ≥2.5-5 mg/dL: Dosage reduction is recommended; no specific guidelines available

Stability

Capsules: Store at room temperature of 15°C to 30°C.

Injection: Store undiluted ampuls at room temperature of 15°C to 30°C; must be diluted in 500 mL of NS or D_5W. Diluted solution should be infused within 12 hours of preparation.

Administration

Capsules: Administer with copious fluids (not milk).

Injection: Do not administer as bolus injection; infuse over 2-6 hours.

Monitoring Parameters Serum electrolytes, monitor for hypocalcemia for at least 2 weeks after therapy; serum calcium, phosphate, magnesium, potassium, serum creatinine, CBC with differential, hepatic function

Reference Range Calcium (total): Adults: 9.0-11.0 mg/dL (SI: 2.05-2.54 mmol/L), may slightly decrease with aging; Phosphorus: 2.5-4.5 mg/dL (SI: 0.81-1.45 mmol/L)

Pregnancy Risk Factor Not assigned; similar agents rated X

Contraindications Hypersensitivity to clodronate, bisphosphonates, or any component of the formulation; severe GI inflammation; renal impairment (serum creatinine >5 mg/dL, SI 440 μmol/L); pregnancy or breast-feeding

Warnings/Precautions Use caution in patients with renal impairment. May cause irritation to upper gastrointestinal mucosa. Esophagitis, esophageal ulcers, esophageal erosions, and esophageal stricture (rare) have been reported with bisphosphonates (oral). Use with caution in patients with dysphagia, esophageal disease, gastritis, duodenitis, or ulcers (may worsen underlying condition). Bisphosphonate therapy has been associated with osteonecrosis, primarily of the jaw; this has been observed mostly in cancer patients, but also in patients with postmenopausal osteoporosis and other diagnoses. Risk factors include a diagnosis of cancer, with concomitant chemotherapy, radiotherapy, or corticosteroids; anemia, coagulopathy, infection, or pre-existing dental disease. Symptoms included nonhealing extraction socket or an exposed jawbone. There are no data addressing whether discontinuation of therapy reduces the risk of developing osteonecrosis. However, as a precautionary measure, dental exams and preventative dentistry should be performed prior to placing patients with risk factors on chronic bisphosphonate therapy. Invasive dental procedures should be avoided during treatment. Safety and efficacy have not been established in pediatric patients.

For I.V. preparation: Dilute prior to use; adequate hydration should be ensured prior to infusion; avoid infiltration/extravasation. May cause venous irritation, hypocalcemia, or transient hypophosphatemia. Do not give as bolus injection.

Adverse Reactions

1% to 10%:

Endocrine & metabolic: Hypocalcemia (2%)

Gastrointestinal: Incidence highest with oral administration: Vomiting (4%), nausea (3%), diarrhea (2%), anorexia (1%)

Renal: Serum creatinine increased (1%), BUN increased

<1% (Limited to important or life-threatening): Bronchospasm, hypersensitivity reactions (angioedema, pruritus, rash, urticaria), oliguria, osteonecrosis, proteinuria, transaminases increased

Overdosage/Toxicology Symptoms of overdose include hypocalcemia, ECG changes, seizures, bleeding, paresthesia, carpopedal spasm, and fever. Treat with I.V. calcium gluconate, and general supportive care; fever and hypotension can be treated with corticosteroids.

Drug Interactions

Aminoglycosides: May lower serum calcium levels with prolonged administration. Concomitant use may have an additive hypocalcemic effect.

Antacids: May decrease the absorption of bisphosphonate derivatives; should be administered at a different time of the day. Antacids containing aluminum, calcium, or magnesium are of specific concern.

Calcium salts: May decrease the absorption of bisphosphonate derivatives. Separate oral dosing in order to minimize risk of interaction.

Iron salts: May decrease the absorption of bisphosphonate derivatives. Only oral iron salts and oral bisphosphonates are of concern.

Magnesium salts: May decrease the absorption of bisphosphonate derivatives. Only oral magnesium salts and oral bisphosphonates are of concern.

Nonsteroidal anti-inflammatory drugs (NSAIDs): May enhance the gastrointestinal adverse/toxic effects (increased incidence of GI ulcers) of bisphosphonate derivatives.

Phosphate supplements: Bisphosphonate derivatives may enhance the hypocalcemic effect of phosphate supplements.

Ethanol/Nutrition/Herb Interactions Food: All food and beverages may interfere with absorption. Coadministration with dairy products may decrease absorption. Beverages (especially orange juice and coffee), food, and medications (eg, antacids, calcium, iron, and multivalent cations) may reduce the absorption of bisphosphonates as much as 60%.

Test Interactions Bisphosphonates may interfere with diagnostic imaging agents such as technetium-99m-diphosphonate in bone scans.

Dosage Forms [CAN] = Canadian brand name

Injection:

Bonefos® [CAN], Ostac® [CAN]: 30 mg/mL (10 mL); 60 mg/mL (5 mL) [not available in the U.S.]

Capsule:

Bonefos® [CAN], Ostac® [CAN]: 400 mg [not available in the U.S.]

♦ **Clodronate Disodium** *see* Clodronate *on page 308*

ClomiPRAMINE (kloe MI pra meen)

Medication Safety Issues

Sound-alike/look-alike issues:

ClomiPRAMINE may be confused with chlorproMAZINE, clomiPHENE, desipramine, Norpramin®

Anafranil® may be confused with alfentanil, enalapril, nafarelin

Related Information

Antidepressant Agents *on page 1551*

U.S. Brand Names Anafranil®

Canadian Brand Names Anafranil®; Apo-Clomipramine®; CO Clomipramine; Gen-Clomipramine

(Continued)

ClomiPRAMINE *(Continued)*

Synonyms Clomipramine Hydrochloride

Pharmacologic Category Antidepressant, Tricyclic (Tertiary Amine)

Restrictions A medication guide concerning the use of antidepressants in children and teenagers can be found on the FDA website at http://www.fda.gov/cder/Offices/ODS/labeling.htm. It should be dispensed to parents or guardians of children and teenagers receiving this medication.

Generic Available Yes

Use Treatment of obsessive-compulsive disorder (OCD)

Unlabeled/Investigational Use Depression, panic attacks, chronic pain

Mechanism of Action Clomipramine appears to affect serotonin uptake while its active metabolite, desmethylclomipramine, affects norepinephrine uptake

Pharmacodynamics/Kinetics

Absorption: Rapid

Metabolism: Hepatic to desmethylclomipramine (active); extensive first-pass effect

Half-life elimination: 20-30 hours

Dosage Oral: Initial:

Children:

<10 years: Safety and efficacy have not been established.

≥10 years: OCD: 25 mg/day; gradually increase, as tolerated, to a maximum of 3 mg/kg/day or 200 mg/day (whichever is smaller)

Adults: OCD: 25 mg/day and gradually increase, as tolerated, to 100 mg/day the first 2 weeks, may then be increased to a total of 250 mg/day maximum

Monitoring Parameters Pulse rate and blood pressure prior to and during therapy; ECG/cardiac status in older adults and patients with cardiac disease

Pregnancy Risk Factor C

Contraindications Hypersensitivity to clomipramine, other tricyclic agents, or any component of the formulation; use of MAO inhibitors within 14 days; use in a patient during the acute recovery phase of MI

Warnings/Precautions [U.S. Boxed Warning]: Antidepressants increase the risk of suicidal thinking and behavior in children and adolescents with major depressive disorder (MDD) and other depressive disorders; consider risk prior to prescribing. Closely monitor for clinical worsening, suicidality, or unusual changes in behavior; the child's family or caregiver should be instructed to closely observe the patient and communicate condition with healthcare provider. Such observation would generally include at least weekly face-to-face contact with patients or their family members or caregivers during the first 4 weeks of treatment, then every other week visits for the next 4 weeks, then at 12 weeks, and as clinically indicated beyond 12 weeks. Additional contact by telephone may be appropriate between face-to-face visits. Adults treated with antidepressants should be observed similarly for clinical worsening and suicidality, especially during the initial few months of a course of drug therapy, or at times of dose changes, either increases or decreases. A medication guide should be dispensed with each prescription. **Clomipramine is FDA approved for the treatment of OCD in children ≥10 years of age.**

The possibility of a suicide attempt is inherent in major depression and may persist until remission occurs. Monitor for worsening of depression or suicidality, especially during initiation of therapy or with dose increases or decreases. Worsening depression and severe abrupt suicidality that are not part of the presenting symptoms may require discontinuation or modification of drug therapy. Use caution in high-risk patients during initiation of therapy. Prescriptions should be written for the smallest quantity consistent with good patient care. The patient's family or caregiver should be alerted to monitor patients for the emergence of suicidality and associated behaviors such as anxiety, agitation, panic attacks, insomnia, irritability, hostility, impulsivity, akathisia, hypomania, and mania; patients should be instructed to notify their healthcare provider if any of these symptoms or worsening depression occur.

May worsen psychosis in some patients or precipitate a shift to mania or hypomania in patients with bipolar disorder. Monotherapy in patients with bipolar disorder should be avoided. Patients presenting with depressive symptoms should be screened for bipolar disorder. **Clomipramine is not FDA approved for the treatment of bipolar depression.**

May cause seizures (relationship to dose and/or duration of therapy) - do not exceed maximum doses. Use caution in patients with a previous seizure disorder or condition predisposing to seizures such as brain damage, alcoholism, or concurrent therapy with other drugs which lower the seizure threshold. Has been associated with a high incidence of sexual dysfunction. Weight gain may occur. May cause sedation, resulting in impaired performance of tasks requiring alertness (eg, operating machinery or driving). Sedative effects may be additive with other CNS depressants and/or ethanol. The degree of sedation is very high relative to other antidepressants. May increase the risks associated with electroconvulsive therapy. Consider discontinuing, when possible, prior to elective surgery. Therapy should not be abruptly discontinued in patients receiving high doses for prolonged periods.

May cause orthostatic hypotension (risk is moderate to high relative to other antidepressants) - use with caution in patients at risk of hypotension or in patients where transient hypotensive episodes would be poorly tolerated (cardiovascular disease or cerebrovascular disease). The degree of anticholinergic blockade produced by this agent is very high relative to other cyclic antidepressants - use caution in patients with urinary retention, benign prostatic hyperplasia, narrow-angle glaucoma, xerostomia, visual problems, constipation, or history of bowel obstruction.

Use with caution in patients with a history of cardiovascular disease (including previous MI, stroke, tachycardia, or conduction abnormalities). The risk conduction abnormalities with this agent is high relative to other antidepressants. Use with caution in hyperthyroid patients or those receiving thyroid supplementation. Use with caution in patients with hepatic or renal dysfunction and in elderly patient.

Adverse Reactions

>10%:

Central nervous system: Dizziness, drowsiness, headache, insomnia, nervousness

Endocrine & metabolic: Libido changes

Gastrointestinal: Xerostomia, constipation, appetite increased, nausea, weight gain, dyspepsia, anorexia, abdominal pain

Neuromuscular & skeletal: Fatigue, tremor, myoclonus

Miscellaneous: Diaphoresis increased

1% to 10%:

Cardiovascular: Hypotension, palpitation, tachycardia

Central nervous system: Confusion, hypertonia, sleep disorder, yawning, speech disorder, abnormal dreaming, paresthesia, memory impairment, anxiety, twitching, coordination impaired, agitation, migraine, depersonalization, emotional lability, flushing, fever

Dermatologic: Rash, pruritus, dermatitis

Gastrointestinal: Diarrhea, vomiting

Genitourinary: Difficult urination

Ocular: Blurred vision, eye pain

<1% (Limited to important or life-threatening): Alopecia, galactorrhea, hyperacusis, marrow depression, photosensitivity, reflux, seizure, SIADH

Overdosage/Toxicology Symptoms of overdose include agitation, confusion, hallucinations, urinary retention, hypothermia, hypotension, tachycardia, ventricular tachycardia, seizures, and coma. Following initiation of essential overdose management, toxic symptoms should be treated.

Drug Interactions Substrate of CYP1A2 (major), 2C19 (major), 2D6 (major), 3A4 (minor); **Inhibits** CYP2D6 (moderate)

Altretamine: Concurrent use may cause orthostatic hypertension.

Amphetamines: TCAs may enhance the effect of amphetamines; monitor for adverse CV effects.

Anticholinergics: Combined use with TCAs may produce additive anticholinergic effects.

Antihypertensives: TCAs inhibit the antihypertensive response to bethanidine, clonidine, debrisoquin, guanadrel, guanethidine, guanabenz, guanfacine; monitor BP; consider alternate antihypertensive agent.

Beta-agonists: When combined with TCAs may predispose patients to cardiac arrhythmias.

Bupropion: May increase the levels of tricyclic antidepressants; based on limited information; monitor response.

(Continued)

ClomiPRAMINE *(Continued)*

Carbamazepine: Tricyclic antidepressants may increase carbamazepine levels; monitor.

Cholestyramine and colestipol: May bind TCAs and reduce their absorption; monitor for altered response.

Clonidine: Abrupt discontinuation of clonidine may cause hypertensive crisis, amitriptyline may enhance the response.

CNS depressants: Sedative effects may be additive with TCAs; monitor for increased effect; includes benzodiazepines, barbiturates, antipsychotics, ethanol, and other sedative medications.

CYP1A2 inducers: May decrease the levels/effects of clomipramine. Example inducers include aminoglutethimide, carbamazepine, phenobarbital, and rifampin.

CYP1A2 inhibitors: May increase the levels/effects of clomipramine. Example inhibitors include ciprofloxacin, fluvoxamine, ketoconazole, norfloxacin, ofloxacin, and rofecoxib.

CYP2C19 inducers: May decrease the levels/effects of clomipramine. Example inducers include aminoglutethimide, carbamazepine, phenytoin, and rifampin.

CYP2C19 inhibitors: May increase the levels/effects of clomipramine. Example inhibitors include delavirdine, fluconazole, fluvoxamine, gemfibrozil, isoniazid, omeprazole, and ticlopidine.

CYP2D6 inhibitors: May increase the levels/effects of clomipramine. Example inhibitors include chlorpromazine, delavirdine, fluoxetine, miconazole, paroxetine, pergolide, quinidine, quinine, ritonavir, and ropinirole.

CYP2D6 substrates: Clomipramine may increase the levels/effects of CYP2D6 substrates. Example substrates include amphetamines, selected beta-blockers, dextromethorphan, fluoxetine, lidocaine, mirtazapine, nefazodone, paroxetine, risperidone, ritonavir, thioridazine, tricyclic antidepressants, and venlafaxine.

CYP2D6 prodrug substrates: Clomipramine may decrease the levels/effects of CYP2D6 prodrug substrates. Example prodrug substrates include codeine, hydrocodone, oxycodone, and tramadol.

Epinephrine (and other direct alpha-agonists): Pressor response to I.V. epinephrine, norepinephrine, and phenylephrine may be enhanced in patients receiving TCAs. (**Note:** Effect is unlikely with epinephrine or levonordefrin dosages typically administered as infiltration in combination with local anesthetics.)

Fenfluramine: May increase tricyclic antidepressant levels/effects.

Hypoglycemic agents (including insulin): TCAs may enhance the hypoglycemic effects of tolazamide, chlorpropamide, or insulin; monitor for changes in blood glucose levels; reported with chlorpropamide, tolazamide, and insulin.

Levodopa: Tricyclic antidepressants may decrease the absorption (bioavailability) of levodopa; rare hypertensive episodes have also been attributed to this combination.

Linezolid: Hyperpyrexia, hypertension, tachycardia, confusion, seizures, and **deaths have been reported** with agents which inhibit MAO (serotonin syndrome); this combination should be avoided.

Lithium: Concurrent use with a TCA may increase the risk for neurotoxicity.

MAO inhibitors: Hyperpyrexia, hypertension, tachycardia, confusion, seizures, and **deaths have been reported** (serotonin syndrome); this combination should be avoided.

Methylphenidate: Metabolism of some TCAs may be decreased.

Olanzapine: When used in combination, clomipramine and olanzapine have been reported to be associated with the development of seizures; limited documentation (case report).

Phenothiazines: Serum concentrations of some TCAs may be increased; in addition, TCAs may increase concentration of phenothiazines; monitor for altered clinical response.

QT_c-prolonging agents: Concurrent use of tricyclic agents with other drugs which may prolong QT_c interval may increase the risk of potentially fatal arrhythmias; includes type Ia and type III antiarrhythmics agents, selected quinolones (sparfloxacin, gatifloxacin, moxifloxacin, grepafloxacin), cisapride, and other agents.

Ritonavir: Combined use of high-dose tricyclic antidepressants with ritonavir may cause serotonin syndrome in HIV-positive patients; monitor.

Sucralfate: Absorption of tricyclic antidepressants may be reduced with coadministration.

Sympathomimetics, indirect-acting: Tricyclic antidepressants may result in a decreased sensitivity to indirect-acting sympathomimetics; includes dopamine and ephedrine; also see interaction with epinephrine (and direct-acting sympathomimetics).

Tramadol: Tramadol's risk of seizures may be increased with TCAs.

Valproic acid: May increase serum concentrations/adverse effects of some tricyclic antidepressants.

Warfarin (and other oral anticoagulants): TCAs may increase the anticoagulant effect in patients stabilized on warfarin; monitor INR.

Ethanol/Nutrition/Herb Interactions

Ethanol: Avoid ethanol (may increase CNS depression).

Food: Serum concentrations/toxicity may be increased by grapefruit juice.

Herb/Nutraceutical: Avoid valerian, St John's wort, SAMe, kava kava.

Test Interactions Increased glucose

Dosage Forms Capsule, as hydrochloride: 25 mg, 50 mg, 75 mg

♦ **Clomipramine Hydrochloride** *see* ClomiPRAMINE *on page 309*

♦ **Clonapam (Can)** *see* Clonazepam *on page 313*

Clonazepam (kloe NA ze pam)

Medication Safety Issues

Sound-alike/look-alike issues:

Clonazepam may be confused with clofazimine, clonidine, clorazepate, clozapine, lorazepam

Klonopin® may be confused with clofazimine, clonidine, clorazepate, clozapine, lorazepam

Related Information

Anesthesia Considerations for Neurosurgery *on page 1401*

Benzodiazepines *on page 1555*

Chronic Pain Management *on page 1430*

Perioperative Management of Patients on Antiseizure Medication *on page 1458*

U.S. Brand Names Klonopin®

Canadian Brand Names Alti-Clonazepam; Apo-Clonazepam®; Clonapam; CO Clonazepam; Gen-Clonazepam; Klonopin®; Novo-Clonazepam; Nu-Clonazepam; PMS-Clonazepam; Rho®-Clonazepam; Rivotril®; Sandoz-Clonazepam

Pharmacologic Category Benzodiazepine

Restrictions C-IV

Generic Available Yes

Use Alone or as an adjunct in the treatment of petit mal variant (Lennox-Gastaut), akinetic, and myoclonic seizures; petit mal (absence) seizures unresponsive to succimides; panic disorder with or without agoraphobia

Unlabeled/Investigational Use Restless legs syndrome; neuralgia; multifocal tic disorder; parkinsonian dysarthria; bipolar disorder; adjunct therapy for schizophrenia

Mechanism of Action The exact mechanism is unknown, but believed to be related to its ability to enhance the activity of GABA; suppresses the spike-and-wave discharge in absence seizures by depressing nerve transmission in the motor cortex

Pharmacodynamics/Kinetics

Onset of action: 20-60 minutes

Duration: Infants and young children: 6-8 hours; Adults: ≤12 hours

Absorption: Well absorbed

Distribution: Adults: V_d: 1.5-4.4 L/kg

Protein binding: 85%

Metabolism: Extensively hepatic via glucuronide and sulfate conjugation

Half-life elimination: Children: 22-33 hours; Adults: 19-50 hours

Time to peak, serum: 1-3 hours; Steady-state: 5-7 days

Excretion: Urine (<2% as unchanged drug); metabolites excreted as glucuronide or sulfate conjugates

Dosage Oral:

Children <10 years or 30 kg: Seizure disorders:

Initial daily dose: 0.01-0.03 mg/kg/day (maximum: 0.05 mg/kg/day) given in 2-3 divided doses; increase by no more than 0.5 mg every third day until seizures are controlled or adverse effects seen

Usual maintenance dose: 0.1-0.2 mg/kg/day divided 3 times/day, not to exceed 0.2 mg/kg/day

(Continued)

Clonazepam *(Continued)*

Adults:

Burning mouth syndrome (dental use): 0.25-3 mg/day in 2 divided doses, in morning and evening

Seizure disorders:

Initial daily dose not to exceed 1.5 mg given in 3 divided doses; may increase by 0.5-1 mg every third day until seizures are controlled or adverse effects seen (maximum: 20 mg/day)

Usual maintenance dose: 0.05-0.2 mg/kg; do not exceed 20 mg/day

Panic disorder: 0.25 mg twice daily; increase in increments of 0.125-0.25 mg twice daily every 3 days; target dose: 1 mg/day (maximum: 4 mg/day)

Discontinuation of treatment: To discontinue, treatment should be withdrawn gradually. Decrease dose by 0.125 mg twice daily every 3 days until medication is completely withdrawn.

Elderly: Initiate with low doses and observe closely

Hemodialysis: Supplemental dose is not necessary

Administration Orally-disintegrating tablet: Open pouch and peel back foil on the blister; do not push tablet through foil. Use dry hands to remove tablet and place in mouth. May be swallowed with or without water. Use immediately after removing from package.

Monitoring Parameters CBC, liver function tests; observe patient for excess sedation, respiratory depression

Reference Range Relationship between serum concentration and seizure control is not well established

Timing of serum samples: Peak serum levels occur 1-3 hours after oral ingestion; the half-life is 20-40 hours; therefore, steady-state occurs in 5-7 days

Therapeutic levels: 20-80 ng/mL; Toxic concentration: >80 ng/mL

Anesthesia and Critical Care Concerns/Other Considerations Ethosuximide or valproic acid may be preferred for treatment of absence (petit mal) seizures. Flumazenil, a competitive benzodiazepine antagonist at the CNS receptor site, reverses benzodiazepine-induced CNS depression. Abrupt discontinuation after sustained use (generally >10 days) may cause withdrawal symptoms.

Pregnancy Risk Factor D

Contraindications Hypersensitivity to clonazepam or any component of the formulation (cross-sensitivity with other benzodiazepines may exist); significant liver disease; narrow-angle glaucoma; pregnancy

Warnings/Precautions Use with caution in elderly or debilitated patients, patients with hepatic disease (including alcoholics), or renal impairment. Use with caution in patients with respiratory disease or impaired gag reflex or ability to protect the airway from secretions (salivation may be increased). Worsening of seizures may occur when added to patients with multiple seizure types. Concurrent use with valproic acid may result in absence status. Monitoring of CBC and liver function tests has been recommended during prolonged therapy.

Causes CNS depression (dose related) resulting in sedation, dizziness, confusion, or ataxia which may impair physical and mental capabilities. Patients must be cautioned about performing tasks which require mental alertness (eg, operating machinery or driving). Use with caution in patients receiving other CNS depressants or psychoactive agents. Effects with other sedative drugs or ethanol may be potentiated. Benzodiazepines have been associated with falls and traumatic injury and should be used with extreme caution in patients who are at risk of these events (especially the elderly).

Use caution in patients with depression, particularly if suicidal risk may be present. Use with caution in patients with a history of drug dependence. Benzodiazepines have been associated with dependence and acute withdrawal symptoms, including seizures, on discontinuation or reduction in dose. Acute withdrawal, including seizures, may be precipitated in patients after administration of flumazenil to patients receiving long-term benzodiazepine therapy.

Benzodiazepines have been associated with anterograde amnesia. Paradoxical reactions, including hyperactive or aggressive behavior, have been reported with benzodiazepines, particularly in adolescent/pediatric or psychiatric patients. Does not have analgesic, antidepressant, or antipsychotic properties.

Adverse Reactions Reactions reported in patients with seizure and/or panic disorder. Frequency not defined.

Cardiovascular: Edema (ankle or facial), palpitation

Central nervous system: Amnesia, ataxia (seizure disorder ~30%; panic disorder 5%), behavior problems (seizure disorder ~25%), coma, confusion, depression, dizziness, drowsiness (seizure disorder ~50%), emotional lability, fatigue, fever, hallucinations, headache, hypotonia, hysteria, insomnia, intellectual ability reduced, memory disturbance, nervousness; paradoxical reactions (including aggressive behavior, agitation, anxiety, excitability, hostility, irritability, nervousness, nightmares, sleep disturbance, vivid dreams); psychosis, slurred speech, somnolence (panic disorder 37%), suicidal attempt, vertigo

Dermatologic: Hair loss, hirsutism, skin rash

Endocrine & metabolic: Dysmenorrhea, libido increased/decreased

Gastrointestinal: Abdominal pain, anorexia, appetite increased/decreased, coated tongue, constipation, dehydration, diarrhea, gastritis, gum soreness, nausea, weight changes (loss/gain), xerostomia

Genitourinary: Colpitis, dysuria, ejaculation delayed, enuresis, impotence, micturition frequency, nocturia, urinary retention, urinary tract infection

Hematologic: Anemia, eosinophilia, leukopenia, thrombocytopenia

Hepatic: Alkaline phosphatase increased (transient), hepatomegaly, transaminases increased (transient)

Neuromuscular & skeletal: Choreiform movements, coordination abnormal, dysarthria, muscle pain, muscle weakness, myalgia, tremor

Ocular: Blurred vision, eye movements abnormal, diplopia, nystagmus

Respiratory: Chest congestion, cough, bronchitis, hypersecretions, pharyngitis, respiratory depression, respiratory tract infection, rhinitis, rhinorrhea, shortness of breath, sinusitis

Miscellaneous: Allergic reaction, aphonia, dysdiadochokinesis, encopresis, "glassy-eyed" appearance, hemiparesis, lymphadenopathy

Overdosage/Toxicology May produce somnolence, confusion, ataxia, diminished reflexes, or coma. Treatment for benzodiazepine overdose is supportive. Flumazenil has been shown to selectively block the binding of benzodiazepines to CNS receptors, resulting in a reversal of benzodiazepine-induced CNS depression, but not respiratory depression.

Drug Interactions **Substrate** of CYP3A4 (major)

CNS depressants: Sedative effects and/or respiratory depression may be additive with CNS depressants; includes ethanol, barbiturates, narcotic analgesics, and other sedative agents; monitor for increased effect.

CYP3A4 inducers: CYP3A4 inducers may decrease the levels/effects of clonazepam. Example inducers include aminoglutethimide, carbamazepine, nafcillin, nevirapine, phenobarbital, phenytoin, and rifamycins.

CYP3A4 inhibitors: May increase the levels/effects of clonazepam. Example inhibitors include azole antifungals, clarithromycin, diclofenac, doxycycline, erythromycin, imatinib, isoniazid, nefazodone, nicardipine, propofol, protease inhibitors, quinidine, telithromycin, and verapamil.

Disulfiram: Disulfiram may inhibit the metabolism of clonazepam; monitor for increased benzodiazepine effect.

Levodopa: Therapeutic effects may be diminished in some patients following the addition of a benzodiazepine; limited/inconsistent data.

Oral contraceptives: May decrease the clearance of some benzodiazepines (those which undergo oxidative metabolism); monitor for increased benzodiazepine effect.

Theophylline: May partially antagonize some of the effects of benzodiazepines; monitor for decreased response; may require higher doses for sedation.

Valproic acid: The combined use of clonazepam and valproic acid has been associated with absence seizures.

Ethanol/Nutrition/Herb Interactions

Ethanol: Avoid ethanol (may increase CNS depression).

Food: Clonazepam serum concentration is unlikely to be increased by grapefruit juice because of clonazepam's high oral bioavailability.

Herb/Nutraceutical: St John's wort may decrease clonazepam levels. Avoid valerian, St John's wort, kava kava, gotu kola (may increase CNS depression).

Dosage Forms

Tablet: 0.5 mg, 1 mg, 2 mg

Tablet, orally disintegrating [wafer]: 0.125 mg, 0.25 mg, 0.5 mg, 1 mg, 2 mg

Clonidine (KLON i deen)

Medication Safety Issues

Sound-alike/look-alike issues:

Clonidine may be confused with Clomid®, clomiPHENE, clonazepam, clozapine, Klonopin™, Loniten®, quinidine

Catapres® may be confused with Cataflam®, Cetapred®, Combipres®

Transdermal patch may contain conducting metal (eg, aluminum); remove patch prior to MRI.

Related Information

Chronic Pain Management *on page 1430*
Hypertension *on page 1620*

U.S. Brand Names Catapres®; Catapres-TTS®; Duraclon™

Canadian Brand Names Apo-Clonidine®; Carapres®; Dixarit®; Novo-Clonidine; Nu-Clonidine

Synonyms Clonidine Hydrochloride

Pharmacologic Category $Alpha_2$-Adrenergic Agonist

Generic Available Yes: Tablet

Use Management of mild-to-moderate hypertension; either used alone or in combination with other antihypertensives

Orphan drug: Duraclon™: For continuous epidural administration as adjunctive therapy with intraspinal opiates for treatment of cancer pain in patients tolerant to or unresponsive to intraspinal opiates

Unlabeled/Investigational Use Heroin or nicotine withdrawal; severe pain; dysmenorrhea; vasomotor symptoms associated with menopause; ethanol dependence; prophylaxis of migraines; glaucoma; diabetes-associated diarrhea; impulse control disorder, attention-deficit/hyperactivity disorder (ADHD), clozapine-induced sialorrhea

Mechanism of Action Stimulates $alpha_2$-adrenoceptors in the brain stem, thus activating an inhibitory neuron, resulting in reduced sympathetic outflow from the CNS, producing a decrease in peripheral resistance, renal vascular resistance, heart rate, and blood pressure; epidural clonidine may produce pain relief at spinal presynaptic and postjunctional $alpha_2$-adrenoceptors by preventing pain signal transmission; pain relief occurs only for the body regions innervated by the spinal segments where analgesic concentrations of clonidine exist

Pharmacodynamics/Kinetics

Onset of action: Oral: 0.5-1 hour; Transdermal: Initial application: 2-3 days

Duration: 6-10 hours

Distribution: V_d: Adults: 2.1 L/kg; highly lipid soluble; distributes readily into extravascular sites

Protein binding: 20% to 40%

Metabolism: Extensively hepatic to inactive metabolites; undergoes enterohepatic recirculation

Bioavailability: 75% to 95%

Half-life elimination: Adults: Normal renal function: 6-20 hours; Renal impairment: 18-41 hours

Time to peak: 2-4 hours

Excretion: Urine (65%, 32% as unchanged drug); feces (22%)

Dosage

Children:

Oral:

Hypertension: Initial: 5-10 mcg/kg/day in divided doses every 8-12 hours; increase gradually at 5- to 7-day intervals to 25 mcg/kg/day in divided doses every 6 hours; maximum: 0.9 mg/day

Clonidine tolerance test (test of growth hormone release from pituitary): 0.15 mg/m^2 or 4 mcg/kg as single dose

ADHD (unlabeled use): Initial: 0.05 mg/day; increase every 3-7 days by 0.05 mg/day to 3-5 mcg/kg/day given in divided doses 3-4 times/day (maximum dose: 0.3-0.4 mg/day)

Epidural infusion: Pain management: Reserved for patients with severe intractable pain, unresponsive to other analgesics or epidural or spinal opiates: Initial: 0.5 mcg/kg/hour; adjust with caution, based on clinical effect

Adults:

Oral:

Acute hypertension (urgency): Initial 0.1-0.2 mg; may be followed by additional doses of 0.1 mg every hour, if necessary, to a maximum total dose of 0.6 mg.

Unlabeled route of administration: Sublingual clonidine 0.1-0.2 mg twice daily may be effective in patients unable to take oral medication

Hypertension: Initial dose: 0.1 mg twice daily (maximum recommended dose: 2.4 mg/day); usual dose range (JNC 7): 0.1-0.8 mg/day in 2 divided doses

Nicotine withdrawal symptoms: 0.1 mg twice daily to maximum of 0.4 mg/day for 3-4 weeks

Transdermal: Hypertension: Apply once every 7 days; for initial therapy start with 0.1 mg and increase by 0.1 mg at 1- to 2-week intervals (dosages >0.6 mg do not improve efficacy); usual dose range (JNC 7): 0.1-0.3 mg once weekly

Note: If transitioning from oral to transdermal therapy, overlap oral regimen for 1-2 days; transdermal route takes 2-3 days to achieve therapeutic effects.

Conversion from oral to transdermal:

Day 1: Place Catapres-TTS® 1; administer 100% of oral dose.

Day 2: Administer 50% of oral dose.

Day 3: Administer 25% of oral dose.

Day 4: Patch remains, no further oral supplement necessary.

Epidural infusion: Pain management: Starting dose: 30 mcg/hour; titrate as required for relief of pain or presence of side effects; minimal experience with doses >40 mcg/hour; should be considered an adjunct to intraspinal opiate therapy

Elderly: Initial: 0.1 mg once daily at bedtime, increase gradually as needed

Dosing adjustment in renal impairment: Cl_{cr} <10 mL/minute: Administer 50% to 75% of normal dose initially

Dialysis: Not dialyzable (0% to 5%) via hemo- or peritoneal dialysis; supplemental dose not necessary

Administration

Oral: Do not discontinue clonidine abruptly. if needed, gradually reduce dose over 2-4 days to avoid rebound hypertension

Transdermal patch: Patches should be applied weekly at bedtime to a clean, hairless area of the upper outer arm or chest. Rotate patch sites weekly. Redness under patch may be reduced if a topical corticosteroid spray is applied to the area before placement of the patch.

Monitoring Parameters Blood pressure, standing and sitting/supine, mental status, heart rate

Reference Range Therapeutic: 1-2 ng/mL (SI: 4.4-8.7 nmol/L)

Anesthesia and Critical Care Concerns/Other Considerations Abrupt withdrawal from clonidine therapy should be avoided. Clonidine patch has provided an important alternative to frequent daily dosing; may be used in patients unable to take oral medication. Transdermal therapy takes 2-3 days for therapeutic effects.

Pregnancy Risk Factor C

Contraindications Hypersensitivity to clonidine hydrochloride or any component of the formulation

Warnings/Precautions Gradual withdrawal is needed (over 1 week for oral, 2-4 days with epidural) if drug needs to be stopped. Patients should be instructed about abrupt discontinuation (causes rapid increase in BP and symptoms of sympathetic overactivity). In patients on both a beta-blocker and clonidine where withdrawal of clonidine is necessary, withdraw the beta-blocker first and several days before clonidine. Then slowly decrease clonidine.

Use with caution in patients with severe coronary insufficiency; conduction disturbances; recent MI, CVA, or chronic renal insufficiency. Caution in sinus node dysfunction. Discontinue within 4 hours of surgery then restart as soon as possible after. Clonidine injection should be administered via a continuous epidural infusion device. **[U.S. Boxed Warning]: Epidural clonidine is not recommended for perioperative, obstetrical, or postpartum pain.** It is not recommended for use in patients with severe cardiovascular disease or hemodynamic instability. In all cases, the epidural may lead to cardiovascular instability (hypotension, bradycardia). Transdermal patch may contain conducting metal (eg, aluminum); remove patch prior to MRI. Due to the potential for altered

(Continued)

Clonidine *(Continued)*

electrical conductivity, remove transdermal patch before cardioversion or defibrillation. Clonidine cause significant CNS depression and xerostomia. Caution in patients with pre-existing CNS disease or depression. Elderly may be at greater risk for CNS depressive effects, favoring other agents in this population.

Adverse Reactions Incidence of adverse events is not always reported.

>10%:

Central nervous system: Drowsiness (35% oral, 12% transdermal), dizziness (16% oral, 2% transdermal)

Dermatologic: Transient localized skin reactions characterized by pruritus, and erythema (15% to 50% transdermal)

Gastrointestinal: Dry mouth (40% oral, 25% transdermal)

Neuromuscular & skeletal: Weakness (10% transdermal)

1% to 10%:

Cardiovascular: Orthostatic hypotension (3% oral)

Central nervous system: Headache (1% oral, 5% transdermal), sedation (3% transdermal), fatigue (6% transdermal), lethargy (3% transdermal), insomnia (2% transdermal), nervousness (3% oral, 1% transdermal), mental depression (1% oral)

Dermatologic: Rash (1% oral), allergic contact sensitivity (5% transdermal), localized vesiculation (7%), hyperpigmentation (5% at application site), edema (3%), excoriation (3%), burning (3%), throbbing, blanching (1%), papules (1%), and generalized macular rash (1%) has occurred in patients receiving transdermal clonidine.

Endocrine & metabolic: Sodium and water retention, sexual dysfunction (3% oral, 2% transdermal), impotence (3% oral, 2% transdermal), weakness (10% transdermal)

Gastrointestinal: Nausea (5% oral, 1% transdermal), vomiting (5% oral), anorexia and malaise (1% oral), constipation (10% oral, 1% transdermal), dry throat (2% transdermal), taste disturbance (1% transdermal), weight gain (1% oral)

Genitourinary: Nocturia (1% oral)

Hepatic: Liver function test (mild abnormalities, 1% oral)

Miscellaneous: Withdrawal syndrome (1% oral)

<1% (Limited to important or life-threatening): Abdominal pain, agitation, alopecia, angioedema, AV block, behavioral changes, blurred vision, bradycardia, chest pain, CHF, contact dermatitis (transdermal), CVA, delirium, depression, dryness of eyes, ECG abnormalities, ethanol sensitivity increased, gynecomastia, hallucinations, hepatitis, localized hypo- or hyperpigmentation (transdermal), nightmares, orthostatic symptoms, pseudo-obstruction, rash, Raynaud's phenomenon, syncope, tachycardia, thrombocytopenia, urinary retention, urticaria, vomiting, withdrawal syndrome

Overdosage/Toxicology Symptoms of overdose include bradycardia, CNS depression, hypothermia, diarrhea, respiratory depression, and apnea. Treatment is supportive and symptomatic. Naloxone may be utilized in treating CNS depression and/or apnea and should be given I.V., 0.4-2 mg, with repeated doses as needed up to a total of 10 mg, or as an infusion.

Drug Interactions

Antipsychotics: Concurrent use with antipsychotics (especially low potency) or nitroprusside may produce additive hypotensive effects.

Beta-blockers: May potentiate bradycardia in patients receiving clonidine and may increase the rebound hypertension of withdrawal; discontinue beta-blocker several days before clonidine is tapered.

CNS depressants: Sedative effects may be additive; monitor for increased effect; includes barbiturates, benzodiazepines, narcotic analgesics, ethanol, and other sedative agents.

Cyclosporine: Clonidine may increase cyclosporine (and perhaps tacrolimus) serum concentrations; cyclosporine dosage adjustment may be needed.

Hypoglycemic agents: Clonidine may decrease the symptoms of hypoglycemia; monitor patients receiving antidiabetic agents.

Levodopa: Effects may be reduced by clonidine in some patients with Parkinson's disease (limited documentation); monitor.

Local anesthetics: Epidural clonidine may prolong the sensory and motor blockade of local anesthetics.

Mirtazapine: Antihypertensive effects of clonidine may be antagonized by mirtazapine (hypertensive urgency has been reported following addition of mirtazapine to clonidine). In addition, mirtazapine may potentially enhance the hypertensive response associated with abrupt clonidine withdrawal. Avoid this combination; consider an alternative agent.

Narcotic analgesics: May potentiate hypotensive effects of clonidine.

Tricyclic antidepressants: Antihypertensive effects of clonidine may be antagonized by tricyclic antidepressants. In addition, tricyclic antidepressants may enhance the hypertensive response associated with abrupt clonidine withdrawal; avoid this combination; consider an alternative agent.

Verapamil: Concurrent administration may be associated with hypotension and AV block in some patients (limited documentation); monitor.

Ethanol/Nutrition/Herb Interactions

Ethanol: Avoid ethanol (may increase CNS depression).

Herb/Nutraceutical: Avoid dong quai if using for hypertension (has estrogenic activity). Avoid ephedra, yohimbe, ginseng (may worsen hypertension). Avoid valerian, St John's wort, kava kava, gotu kola (may increase CNS depression).

Dietary Considerations Hypertensive patients may need to decrease sodium and calories in diet.

Dosage Forms

Injection, epidural solution, as hydrochloride [preservative free] (Duraclon™): 100 mcg/mL (10 mL); 500 mcg/mL (10 mL)

Patch, transdermal [once-weekly patch]:

Catapres-TTS®-1: 0.1 mg/24 hours (4s)

Catapres-TTS®-2: 0.2 mg/24 hours (4s)

Catapres-TTS®-3: 0.3 mg/24 hours (4s)

Tablet, as hydrochloride (Catapres®): 0.1 mg, 0.2 mg, 0.3 mg

♦ **Clonidine Hydrochloride** *see* Clonidine *on page 316*

Clopidogrel (kloh PID oh grel)

Medication Safety Issues

Sound-alike/look-alike issues:

Plavix® may be confused with Elavil®, Paxil®

U.S. Brand Names Plavix®

Canadian Brand Names Plavix®

Synonyms Clopidogrel Bisulfate

Pharmacologic Category Antiplatelet Agent

Generic Available No

Use Reduce atherosclerotic events (myocardial infarction, stroke, vascular deaths) in patients with atherosclerosis documented by recent myocardial infarction (MI), recent stroke, or established peripheral arterial disease; acute coronary syndrome (unstable angina or non-Q-wave MI) managed medically or through PCI (with or without stent)

Unlabeled/Investigational Use In aspirin-allergic patients, prevention of coronary artery bypass graft closure (saphenous vein)

Mechanism of Action Blocks the ADP receptors, which prevent fibrinogen binding at that site and thereby reduce the possibility of platelet adhesion and aggregation

Pharmacodynamics/Kinetics

Onset of action: Inhibition of platelet aggregation detected: 2 hours after 300 mg administered; after second day of treatment with 50-100 mg/day

Peak effect: 50-100 mg/day: Bleeding time: 5-6 days; Platelet function: 3-7 days

Absorption: Well absorbed

Metabolism: Extensively hepatic via hydrolysis; biotransformation primarily to carboxyl acid derivative (inactive). The active metabolite that inhibits platelet aggregation has not been isolated.

Half-life elimination: ~8 hours

Time to peak, serum: ~1 hour

Excretion: Urine

Dosage Oral: Adults:

Recent MI, recent stroke, or established arterial disease: 75 mg once daily

Acute coronary syndrome: Initial: 300 mg loading dose, followed by 75 mg once daily (in combination with aspirin 75-325 mg once daily). **Note:** A loading dose of 600 mg has been used in some investigations; limited research exists comparing the two doses.

(Continued)

Clopidogrel *(Continued)*

Prevention of coronary artery bypass graft closure (saphenous vein): Aspirin-allergic patients (unlabeled use): Loading dose: 300 mg 6 hours following procedure; maintenance: 50-100 mg/day

Dosing adjustment in renal impairment and elderly: None necessary

Stability Store at 25°C (77°F); excursions permitted to 15°C to 3°C (59°F to 86°F).

Monitoring Parameters Signs of bleeding; hemoglobin and hematocrit periodically

Anesthesia and Critical Care Concerns/Other Considerations Withhold clopidogrel for 5-7 days prior to elective CABG surgery.

Pregnancy Risk Factor B

Contraindications Hypersensitivity to clopidogrel or any component of the formulation; active pathological bleeding such as PUD or intracranial hemorrhage; coagulation disorders

Warnings/Precautions Use with caution in patients who may be at risk of increased bleeding, including patients with peptic ulcer disease, trauma, or surgery. Consider discontinuing 5 days before elective surgery. Use caution in concurrent treatment with other antiplatelet drugs; bleeding risk is increased. Use with caution in patients with severe liver disease (experience is limited). Cases of thrombotic thrombocytopenic purpura (usually occurring within the first 2 weeks of therapy) have been reported; urgent referral to a hematologist is required.

Adverse Reactions As with all drugs which may affect hemostasis, bleeding is associated with clopidogrel. Hemorrhage may occur at virtually any site. Risk is dependent on multiple variables, including the concurrent use of multiple agents which alter hemostasis and patient susceptibility.

>10%: Gastrointestinal: The overall incidence of gastrointestinal events (including abdominal pain, vomiting, dyspepsia, gastritis, and constipation) has been documented to be 27% compared to 30% in patients receiving aspirin.

3% to 10%:

- Cardiovascular: Chest pain (8%), edema (4%), hypertension (4%)
- Central nervous system: Headache (3% to 8%), dizziness (2% to 6%), depression (4%), fatigue (3%), general pain (6%)
- Dermatologic: Rash (4%), pruritus (3%)
- Endocrine & metabolic: Hypercholesterolemia (4%)
- Gastrointestinal: Abdominal pain (2% to 6%), dyspepsia (2% to 5%), diarrhea (2% to 5%), nausea (3%)
- Genitourinary: Urinary tract infection (3%)
- Hematologic: Bleeding (major 4%; minor 5%), purpura (5%), epistaxis (3%)
- Hepatic: Liver function test abnormalities (<3%; discontinued in 0.11%)
- Neuromuscular & skeletal: Arthralgia (6%), back pain (6%)
- Respiratory: Dyspnea (5%), rhinitis (4%), bronchitis (4%), cough (3%), upper respiratory infection (9%)
- Miscellaneous: Flu-like syndrome (8%)

1% to 3%:

- Cardiovascular: Atrial fibrillation, cardiac failure, palpitation, syncope
- Central nervous system: Fever, insomnia, vertigo, anxiety
- Dermatologic: Eczema
- Endocrine & metabolic: Gout, hyperuricemia
- Gastrointestinal: Constipation, GI hemorrhage, vomiting
- Genitourinary: Cystitis
- Hematologic: Hematoma, anemia
- Neuromuscular & skeletal: Arthritis, leg cramps, neuralgia, paresthesia, weakness
- Ocular: Cataract, conjunctivitis

<1% (Limited to important or life-threatening): Acute liver failure, agranulocytosis, allergic reaction, anaphylactoid reaction, angioedema, aplastic anemia, bilirubinemia, bronchospasm, bullous eruption, erythema multiforme, fatty liver, fever, granulocytopenia, hematuria, hemoptysis, hemothorax, hepatitis, hypersensitivity, hypochromic anemia, interstitial pneumonitis, intracranial hemorrhage (0.4%), ischemic necrosis, leukopenia, lichen planus, maculopapular rash, menorrhagia, neutropenia (0.05%), ocular hemorrhage, pancreatitis, pancytopenia, pulmonary hemorrhage, purpura, retroperitoneal bleeding, serum sickness, Stevens-Johnson syndrome, stomatitis, thrombocytopenia, thrombotic thrombocytopenic purpura (TTP), toxic epidermal necrolysis, urticaria, vasculitis

Overdosage/Toxicology

Symptoms of acute toxicity include vomiting, prostration, difficulty breathing, and gastrointestinal hemorrhage. Only one case of overdose with clopidogrel has been reported to date, no symptoms were reported with this case and no specific treatments were required.

Based on its pharmacology, platelet transfusions may be an appropriate treatment when attempting to reverse the effects of clopidogrel. After decontamination, treatment is symptomatic and supportive.

Drug Interactions Substrate (minor) of CYP1A2, 3A4; **Inhibits** CYP2C9 (weak)

Anticoagulants or other antiplatelet agents may increase the risk of bleeding. Use with heparin in acute coronary syndrome is clinically accepted.

Aspirin: Clopidogrel may increase the antiplatelet effect of aspirin; bleeding time is not prolonged relative to clopidogrel alone. Concurrent use is accepted in clinical practice (particularly in ACS treatment).

Atorvastatin: Atorvastatin may attenuate the effects of clopidogrel; monitor.

Drotrecogin alfa may increase the risk of bleeding.

Macrolide antibiotics: CYP3A4-inhibiting macrolides may attenuate the effects of clopidogrel. These include clarithromycin, erythromycin, and troleandomycin. Monitor.

NSAIDs: Concurrent use with clopidogrel may increase gastrointestinal effects, including GI blood loss. NSAID use was excluded in ACS trial (CURE).

Rifampin: Rifampin may increase the effects of clopidogrel; monitor.

Thrombolytics may increase the risk of bleeding.

Ethanol/Nutrition/Herb Interactions Herb/Nutraceutical: Avoid cat's claw, dong quai, evening primrose, feverfew, garlic, ginger, ginkgo, red clover, horse chestnut, green tea, ginseng (all have additional antiplatelet activity).

Dietary Considerations May be taken without regard to meals.

Dosage Forms Tablet: 75 mg

◆ **Clopidogrel Bisulfate** *see* Clopidogrel *on page 319*

Clorazepate (klor AZ e pate)

Medication Safety Issues

Sound-alike/look-alike issues:

Clorazepate may be confused with clofibrate, clonazepam

Related Information

Benzodiazepines *on page 1555*

U.S. Brand Names Tranxene® SD™; Tranxene® SD™-Half Strength; Tranxene® T-Tab®

Canadian Brand Names Apo-Clorazepate®; Novo-Clopate

Synonyms Clorazepate Dipotassium; Tranxene T-Tab®

Pharmacologic Category Benzodiazepine

Restrictions C-IV

Generic Available Yes

Use Treatment of generalized anxiety disorder; management of ethanol withdrawal; adjunct anticonvulsant in management of partial seizures

Mechanism of Action Binds to stereospecific benzodiazepine receptors on the postsynaptic GABA neuron at several sites within the central nervous system, including the limbic system, reticular formation. Enhancement of the inhibitory effect of GABA on neuronal excitability results by increased neuronal membrane permeability to chloride ions. This shift in chloride ions results in hyperpolarization (a less excitable state) and stabilization.

Pharmacodynamics/Kinetics

Onset of action: 1-2 hours

Duration: Variable, 8-24 hours

Distribution: Crosses placenta; appears in urine

Metabolism: Rapidly decarboxylated to desmethyldiazepam (active) in acidic stomach prior to absorption; hepatically to oxazepam (active)

Half-life elimination: Adults: Desmethyldiazepam: 48-96 hours; Oxazepam: 6-8 hours

Time to peak, serum: ~1 hour

Excretion: Primarily urine

Dosage Oral:

Children 9-12 years: Anticonvulsant: Initial: 3.75-7.5 mg/dose twice daily; increase dose by 3.75 mg at weekly intervals, not to exceed 60 mg/day in 2-3 divided doses

(Continued)

Clorazepate *(Continued)*

Children >12 years and Adults: Anticonvulsant: Initial: Up to 7.5 mg/dose 2-3 times/day; increase dose by 7.5 mg at weekly intervals, not to exceed 90 mg/day

Adults:

Anxiety:

Regular release tablets (Tranxene® T-Tab®): 7.5-15 mg 2-4 times/day

Sustained release (Tranxene® SD): 11.25 or 22.5 mg once daily at bedtime

Ethanol withdrawal: Initial: 30 mg, then 15 mg 2-4 times/day on first day; maximum daily dose: 90 mg; gradually decrease dose over subsequent days

Monitoring Parameters Respiratory and cardiovascular status, excess CNS depression

Reference Range Therapeutic: 0.12-1 mcg/mL (SI: 0.36-3.01 µmol/L)

Anesthesia and Critical Care Concerns/Other Considerations Abrupt discontinuation after sustained use (generally >10 days) may cause withdrawal symptoms.

Pregnancy Risk Factor D

Contraindications Hypersensitivity to clorazepate or any component of the formulation (cross-sensitivity with other benzodiazepines may exist); narrow-angle glaucoma; pregnancy

Warnings/Precautions Not recommended for use in patients <9 years of age or patients with depressive or psychotic disorders. Use with caution in elderly or debilitated patients, patients with hepatic disease (including alcoholics), or renal impairment. Active metabolites with extended half-lives may lead to delayed accumulation and adverse effects. Use with caution in patients with respiratory disease or impaired gag reflex. Avoid use in patients with sleep apnea.

Causes CNS depression (dose related) resulting in sedation, dizziness, confusion, or ataxia which may impair physical and mental capabilities. Patients must be cautioned about performing tasks which require mental alertness (eg, operating machinery or driving). Use with caution in patients receiving other CNS depressants or psychoactive agents. Effects with other sedative drugs or ethanol may be potentiated. Benzodiazepines have been associated with falls and traumatic injury and should be used with extreme caution in patients who are at risk of these events (especially the elderly).

Use caution in patients with depression, particularly if suicidal risk may be present. Use with caution in patients with a history of drug dependence. Benzodiazepines have been associated with dependence and acute withdrawal symptoms on discontinuation or reduction in dose. Acute withdrawal, including seizures, may be precipitated in patients after administration of flumazenil to patients receiving long-term benzodiazepine therapy.

Benzodiazepines have been associated with anterograde amnesia. Paradoxical reactions, including hyperactive or aggressive behavior, have been reported with benzodiazepines, particularly in adolescent/pediatric or psychiatric patients. Does not have analgesic, antidepressant, or antipsychotic properties.

Adverse Reactions Frequency not defined.

Cardiovascular: Hypotension

Central nervous system: Drowsiness, fatigue, ataxia, lightheadedness, memory impairment, insomnia, anxiety, headache, depression, slurred speech, confusion, nervousness, dizziness, irritability

Dermatologic: Rash

Endocrine & metabolic: Libido decreased

Gastrointestinal: Xerostomia, constipation, diarrhea, salivation decreased, nausea, vomiting, appetite increased or decreased

Neuromuscular & skeletal: Dysarthria, tremor

Ocular: Blurred vision, diplopia

Overdosage/Toxicology May produce somnolence, confusion, ataxia, diminished reflexes, and coma. Treatment for benzodiazepine overdose is supportive. Rarely is mechanical ventilation required. Flumazenil has been shown to selectively block the binding of benzodiazepines to CNS receptors, resulting in a reversal of benzodiazepine-induced CNS depression, but not respiratory depression.

Drug Interactions **Substrate** of CYP3A4 (major)

CNS depressants: Sedative effects and/or respiratory depression may be additive with CNS depressants; includes ethanol, barbiturates, narcotic analgesics, and other sedative agents; monitor for increased effect.

CYP3A4 inducers: CYP3A4 inducers may decrease the levels/effects of clorazepate. Example inducers include aminoglutethimide, carbamazepine, nafcillin, nevirapine, phenobarbital, phenytoin, and rifamycins.

CYP3A4 inhibitors: May increase the levels/effects of clorazepate. Example inhibitors include azole antifungals, clarithromycin, diclofenac, doxycycline, erythromycin, imatinib, isoniazid, nefazodone, nicardipine, propofol, protease inhibitors, quinidine, telithromycin, and verapamil.

Levodopa: Therapeutic effects may be diminished in some patients following the addition of a benzodiazepine; limited/inconsistent data.

Oral contraceptives: May decrease the clearance of some benzodiazepines (those which undergo oxidative metabolism); monitor for increased benzodiazepine effect.

Theophylline: May partially antagonize some of the effects of benzodiazepines; monitor for decreased response; may require higher doses for sedation.

Ethanol/Nutrition/Herb Interactions

Ethanol: Avoid ethanol (may increase CNS depression).

Food: Serum concentrations/toxicity may be increased by grapefruit juice.

Herb/Nutraceutical: Avoid valerian, St John's wort, kava kava, gotu kola (may increase CNS depression).

Dosage Forms

Tablet, as dipotassium: 3.75 mg, 7.5 mg, 15 mg

Tranxene® SD™: 22.5 mg [once daily]

Tranxene® SD™-Half Strength: 11.25 mg [once daily]

Tranxene® T-Tab®: 3.75 mg, 7.5 mg, 15 mg

♦ **Clorazepate Dipotassium** *see* Clorazepate *on page 321*

♦ **Coagulation Factor VIIa** *see* Factor VIIa (Recombinant) *on page 501*

♦ **CO Azithromycin (Can)** *see* Azithromycin *on page 149*

Cocaine (koe KANE)

Related Information

Anesthesia for Obstetric Patients in Nonobstetric Surgery *on page 1416*

Local Anesthetics *on page 1532*

Substance Abuse and Anesthesia *on page 1496*

Synonyms Cocaine Hydrochloride

Pharmacologic Category Local Anesthetic

Restrictions C-II

Generic Available Yes

Use Topical anesthesia for mucous membranes

Mechanism of Action Ester local anesthetic blocks both the initiation and conduction of nerve impulses by decreasing the neuronal membrane's permeability to sodium ions, which results in inhibition of depolarization with resultant blockade of conduction; interferes with the uptake of norepinephrine by adrenergic nerve terminals producing vasoconstriction

Pharmacodynamics/Kinetics Following topical administration to mucosa:

Onset of action: ~1 minute

Peak effect: ~5 minutes

Duration (dose dependent): ≥30 minutes; cocaine metabolites may appear in urine of neonates up to 5 days after birth due to maternal cocaine use shortly before birth

Absorption: Well absorbed through mucous membranes; limited by drug-induced vasoconstriction; enhanced by inflammation

Distribution: Enters breast milk

Metabolism: Hepatic; major metabolites are ecgonine methyl ester and benzoyl ecgonine

Half-life elimination: 75 minutes

Excretion: Primarily urine (<10% as unchanged drug and metabolites)

Dosage Topical application (ear, nose, throat, bronchoscopy): Dosage depends on the area to be anesthetized, tissue vascularity, technique of anesthesia, and individual patient tolerance; the lowest dose necessary to produce adequate anesthesia should be used; concentrations of 1% to 10% are used (not to exceed 1 mg/kg). Use reduced dosages for children, elderly, or debilitated patients.

Stability Store in well closed, light-resistant containers

Administration Topical: Use only on mucous membranes of the oral, laryngeal, and nasal cavities. Do not use on extensive areas of broken skin.

(Continued)

Cocaine *(Continued)*

Monitoring Parameters Vital signs

Reference Range Therapeutic: 100-500 ng/mL (SI: 330 nmol/L); Toxic: >1000 ng/mL (SI: >3300 nmol/L)

Anesthesia and Critical Care Concerns/Other Considerations Cocaine may also be associated with cerebral vascular accidents in young patients without any previous risk factors.

Pregnancy Risk Factor C/X (nonmedicinal use)

Contraindications Hypersensitivity to cocaine or any component of the topical solution; ophthalmologic anesthesia (causing sloughing of the corneal epithelium); pregnancy (nonmedicinal use)

Warnings/Precautions For topical use only. Limit to office and surgical procedures only. Resuscitative equipment and drugs should be immediately available when any local anesthetic is used. Debilitated, elderly patients, acutely ill patients, and children should be given reduced doses consistent with their age and physical status. Use caution in patients with severely traumatized mucosa and sepsis in the region of the proposed application. Use with caution in patients with cardiovascular disease or a history of cocaine abuse. In patients being treated for cardiovascular complication of cocaine abuse, avoid beta-blockers for treatment.

Adverse Reactions

>10%:

Central nervous system: CNS stimulation
Gastrointestinal: Loss of taste perception
Respiratory: Rhinitis, nasal congestion
Miscellaneous: Loss of smell

1% to 10%:

Cardiovascular: Heart rate (decreased) with low doses, tachycardia with moderate doses, hypertension, cardiomyopathy, cardiac arrhythmia, myocarditis, QRS prolongation, Raynaud's phenomenon, cerebral vasculitis, thrombosis, fibrillation (atrial), flutter (atrial), sinus bradycardia, CHF, pulmonary hypertension, sinus tachycardia, tachycardia (supraventricular), arrhythmia (ventricular), vasoconstriction

Central nervous system: Fever, nervousness, restlessness, euphoria, excitation, headache, psychosis, hallucinations, agitation, seizure, slurred speech, hyperthermia, dystonic reactions, cerebral vascular accident, vasculitis, clonic-tonic reactions, paranoia, sympathetic storm

Dermatologic: Skin infarction, pruritus, madarosis

Gastrointestinal: Nausea, anorexia, colonic ischemia, spontaneous bowel perforation

Genitourinary: Priapism, uterine rupture

Hematologic: Thrombocytopenia

Neuromuscular & skeletal: Chorea (extrapyramidal), paresthesia, tremor, fasciculations

Ocular: Mydriasis (peak effect at 45 minutes; may last up to 12 hours), sloughing of the corneal epithelium, ulceration of the cornea, iritis, chemosis

Renal: Myoglobinuria, necrotizing vasculitis

Respiratory: Tachypnea, nasal mucosa damage (when snorting), hyposmia, bronchiolitis obliterans organizing pneumonia

Miscellaneous: "Washed-out" syndrome

Overdosage/Toxicology Symptoms of overdose include anxiety, excitement, confusion, nausea, vomiting, headache, rapid pulse, irregular respiration, delirium, fever, seizures, respiratory arrest, hallucinations, dilated pupils, muscle spasms, sensory aberrations, and cardiac arrhythmias.

Fatal dose: Oral: 500 mg to 1.2 g; severe toxic effects have occurred with doses as low as 20 mg.

Since no specific antidote for cocaine exists, serious toxic effects are treated symptomatically.

Drug Interactions **Substrate** of CYP3A4 (major); **Inhibits** CYP2D6 (strong), 3A4 (weak)

Beta-blockers potentiate cocaine-induced coronary vasoconstriction (potentiate alpha-adrenergic effect of cocaine); avoid concurrent use.

CYP2D6 substrates: Cocaine may increase the levels/effects of CYP2D6 substrates. Example substrates include amphetamines, selected beta-blockers, dextromethorphan, fluoxetine, lidocaine, mirtazapine, nefazodone, paroxetine, risperidone, ritonavir, thioridazine, tricyclic antidepressants, and venlafaxine.

CYP2D6 prodrug substrates: Cocaine may decrease the levels/effects of CYP2D6 prodrug substrates. Example prodrug substrates include codeine, hydrocodone, oxycodone, and tramadol.

CYP3A4 inhibitors: May increase the levels/effects of cocaine. Example inhibitors include azole antifungals, clarithromycin, diclofenac, doxycycline, erythromycin, imatinib, isoniazid, nefazodone, nicardipine, propofol, protease inhibitors, quinidine, telithromycin, and verapamil.

Sympathomimetic amines may cause malignant arrhythmias; avoid concurrent use.

Dosage Forms

Powder, as hydrochloride: 1 g, 5 g, 25 g

Solution, topical, as hydrochloride: 4% [40 mg/mL] (4 mL, 10 mL); 10% [100 mg/mL] (4 mL, 10 mL)

References

Richards CF, Clark RF, Holbrook T, et al, "The Effect of Cocaine and Amphetamines on Vital Signs in Trauma Patients," *J Emerg Med*, 1995, 13(1):59-63.

- **Cocaine Hydrochloride** *see* Cocaine *on page 323*
- **CO Ciprofloxacin (Can)** *see* Ciprofloxacin *on page 285*
- **CO Citalopram (Can)** *see* Citalopram *on page 297*
- **CO Clomipramine (Can)** *see* ClomiPRAMINE *on page 309*
- **CO Clonazepam (Can)** *see* Clonazepam *on page 313*

Codeine (KOE deen)

Medication Safety Issues

Sound-alike/look-alike issues:

Codeine may be confused with Cardene®, Cophene®, Cordran®, iodine, Lodine®

Related Information

Acute Postoperative Pain *on page 1388*

Anesthesia Considerations for Neurosurgery *on page 1401*

Chronic Pain Management *on page 1430*

Narcotic / Opioid Analgesics *on page 1568*

Canadian Brand Names Codeine Contin®

Synonyms Codeine Phosphate; Codeine Sulfate; Methylmorphine

Pharmacologic Category Analgesic, Narcotic; Antitussive

Restrictions C-II

Generic Available Yes

Use Treatment of mild-to-moderate pain; antitussive in lower doses; dextromethorphan has equivalent antitussive activity but has much lower toxicity in accidental overdose

Mechanism of Action Binds to opiate receptors in the CNS, causing inhibition of ascending pain pathways, altering the perception of and response to pain; causes cough supression by direct central action in the medulla; produces generalized CNS depression

Pharmacodynamics/Kinetics

Onset of action: Oral: 0.5-1 hour; I.M.: 10-30 minutes

Peak effect: Oral: 1-1.5 hours; I.M.: 0.5-1 hour

Duration: 4-6 hours

Absorption: Oral: Adequate

Distribution: Crosses placenta; enters breast milk

Protein binding: 7%

Metabolism: Hepatic to morphine (active)

Half-life elimination: 2.5-3.5 hours

Excretion: Urine (3% to 16% as unchanged drug, norcodeine, and free and conjugated morphine)

Dosage Note: These are guidelines and do not represent the maximum doses that may be required in all patients. Doses should be titrated to pain relief/prevention. Doses >1.5 mg/kg body weight are not recommended.

Analgesic:

Children: Oral, I.M., SubQ: 0.5-1 mg/kg/dose every 4-6 hours as needed; maximum: 60 mg/dose

Adults:

Oral: 30 mg every 4-6 hours as needed; patients with prior opiate exposure may require higher initial doses. Usual range: 15-120 mg every 4-6 hours as needed

(Continued)

Codeine *(Continued)*

Oral, controlled release formulation (Codeine Contin®, not available in U.S.): 50-300 mg every 12 hours. **Note:** A patient's codeine requirement should be established using prompt release formulations; conversion to long acting products may be considered when chronic, continuous treatment is required. Higher dosages should be reserved for use only in opioid-tolerant patients.

I.M., SubQ: 30 mg every 4-6 hours as needed; patients with prior opiate exposure may require higher initial doses. Usual range: 15-120 mg every 4-6 hours as needed; more frequent dosing may be needed

Antitussive: Oral (for nonproductive cough):

Children: 1-1.5 mg/kg/day in divided doses every 4-6 hours as needed: Alternative dose according to age:

2-6 years: 2.5-5 mg every 4-6 hours as needed; maximum: 30 mg/day

6-12 years: 5-10 mg every 4-6 hours as needed; maximum: 60 mg/day

Adults: 10-20 mg/dose every 4-6 hours as needed; maximum: 120 mg/day

Dosing adjustment in renal impairment:

Cl_{cr} 10-50 mL/minute: Administer 75% of dose

Cl_{cr} <10 mL/minute: Administer 50% of dose

Dosing adjustment in hepatic impairment: Probably necessary in hepatic insufficiency

Stability Store injection between 15°C to 30°C, avoid freezing; do not use if injection is discolored or contains a precipitate; protect injection from light

Administration Not approved for I.V. administration (although this route has been used clinically). If given intravenously, must be given slowly and the patient should be lying down. Rapid intravenous administration of narcotics may increase the incidence of serious adverse effects, in part due to limited opportunity to assess response prior to administration of the full dose. Access to respiratory support should be immediately available.

Monitoring Parameters Pain relief, respiratory and mental status, blood pressure, heart rate

Reference Range Therapeutic: Not established; Toxic: >1.1 mcg/mL

Anesthesia and Critical Care Concerns/Other Considerations The 2002 ACCM/SCCM guidelines for analgesia (critically-ill adult) recommend against using codeine because of its lack of potency, histamine release (may cause hypotension), potential accumulation of active metabolites. The guidelines recommend fentanyl in patients who need immediate pain relief because of its rapid onset of action; fentanyl or hydromorphone is preferred in patients who are hypotensive or have renal dysfunction. Morphine or hydromorphone is recommended for intermittent, scheduled therapy. Both have a longer duration of action requiring less frequent administration.

Pregnancy Risk Factor C/D (prolonged use or high doses at term)

Contraindications Hypersensitivity to codeine or any component of the formulation; pregnancy (prolonged use or high doses at term)

Warnings/Precautions An opioid-containing analgesic regimen should be tailored to each patient's needs and based upon the type of pain being treated (acute versus chronic), the route of administration, degree of tolerance for opioids (naive versus chronic user), age, weight, and medical condition. The optimal analgesic dose varies widely among patients. Doses should be titrated to pain relief/prevention.

Use with caution in patients with hypersensitivity reactions to other phenanthrene derivative opioid agonists (morphine, hydrocodone, hydromorphone, levorphanol, oxycodone, oxymorphone); respiratory diseases including asthma, emphysema, COPD, or severe liver or renal insufficiency; some preparations contain sulfites which may cause allergic reactions; tolerance or drug dependence may result from extended use

Not recommended for use for cough control in patients with a productive cough; not recommended as an antitussive for children <2 years of age; the elderly may be particularly susceptible to the CNS depressant and confusion as well as constipating effects of narcotics

Not approved for I.V. administration (although this route has been used clinically). If given intravenously, must be given slowly and the patient should be lying down. Rapid intravenous administration of narcotics may increase the incidence of serious adverse effects, in part due to limited opportunity to assess response prior to administration of the full dose. Access to respiratory support should be immediately available

Adverse Reactions

>10%:

Central nervous system: Drowsiness

Gastrointestinal: Constipation

1% to 10%:

Cardiovascular: Tachycardia or bradycardia, hypotension

Central nervous system: Dizziness, lightheadedness, false feeling of well being, malaise, headache, restlessness, paradoxical CNS stimulation, confusion

Dermatologic: Rash, urticaria

Gastrointestinal: Dry mouth, anorexia, nausea, vomiting

Hepatic: Transaminases increased

Genitourinary: Decreased urination, ureteral spasm

Local: Burning at injection site

Neuromuscular & skeletal: Weakness

Ocular: Blurred vision

Respiratory: Dyspnea

Miscellaneous: Physical and psychological dependence, histamine release

<1% (Limited to important or life-threatening): Convulsions, hallucinations, insomnia, mental depression, nightmares

Overdosage/Toxicology Symptoms of overdose include CNS and respiratory depression, GI cramping, and constipation. Naloxone, 2 mg I.V. with repeat administration as necessary up to a total of 10 mg, can also be used to reverse toxic effects of the opiate.

Drug Interactions **Substrate** of CYP2D6 (major), 3A4 (minor); **Inhibits** CYP2D6 (weak)

CYP2D6 inhibitors: May decrease the effects of codeine. Example inhibitors include chlorpromazine, delavirdine, fluoxetine, miconazole, paroxetine, pergolide, quinidine, quinine, ritonavir, and ropinirole.

Decreased effect with cigarette smoking

Increased toxicity: CNS depressants, phenothiazines, TCAs, other narcotic analgesics, guanabenz, MAO inhibitors, neuromuscular blockers

Ethanol/Nutrition/Herb Interactions

Ethanol: Avoid or limit ethanol (may increase CNS depression).

Herb/Nutraceutical: St John's wort may decrease codeine levels. Avoid valerian, St John's wort, kava kava, gotu kola (may increase CNS depression).

Test Interactions

Some quinolones may produce a false-positive urine screening result for opiates using commercially-available immunoassay kits. This has been demonstrated most consistently for levofloxacin and ofloxacin, but other quinolones have shown cross-reactivity in certain assay kits. Confirmation of positive opiate screens by more specific methods should be considered.

Dosage Forms [CAN] = Canadian brand name

Injection, as phosphate: 15 mg/mL (2 mL); 30 mg/mL (2 mL) [contains sodium metabisulfite]

Solution, oral, as phosphate: 15 mg/5 mL (5 mL, 500 mL) [strawberry flavor]

Tablet, as phosphate: 30 mg, 60 mg

Tablet, as sulfate: 15 mg, 30 mg, 60 mg

Tablet, controlled release (Codeine Contin®) [CAN]: 50 mg, 100 mg, 150 mg, 200 mg [not available in U.S.]

- ♦ **Codeine, Acetaminophen, Butalbital, and Caffeine** *see* Butalbital, Acetaminophen, Caffeine, and Codeine *on page 207*
- ♦ **Codeine and Acetaminophen** *see* Acetaminophen and Codeine *on page 29*
- ♦ **Codeine Contin® (Can)** *see* Codeine *on page 325*
- ♦ **Codeine Phosphate** *see* Codeine *on page 325*
- ♦ **Codeine Sulfate** *see* Codeine *on page 325*
- ♦ **CO Fluoxetine (Can)** *see* Fluoxetine *on page 539*
- ♦ **Cogentin®** *see* Benztropine *on page 166*
- ♦ **Co-Gesic®** *see* Hydrocodone and Acetaminophen *on page 636*

Colchicine (KOL chi seen)

Medication Safety Issues

High alert medication: The Institute for Safe Medication Practices (ISMP) includes this medication among its list of drugs which have a heightened risk of causing significant patient harm when used in error.

Pharmacologic Category Colchicine

Generic Available Yes

Use Treatment of acute gouty arthritis attacks and prevention of recurrences of such attacks

Unlabeled/Investigational Use Primary biliary cirrhosis; management of familial Mediterranean fever; pericarditis

Mechanism of Action Decreases leukocyte motility, decreases phagocytosis in joints and lactic acid production, thereby reducing the deposition of urate crystals that perpetuates the inflammatory response

Pharmacodynamics/Kinetics

Onset of action: Oral: Pain relief: ~12 hours if adequately dosed

Distribution: Concentrates in leukocytes, kidney, spleen, and liver; does not distribute in heart, skeletal muscle, and brain

Protein binding: 10% to 31%

Metabolism: Partially hepatic via deacetylation

Half-life elimination: 12-30 minutes; End-stage renal disease: 45 minutes

Time to peak, serum: Oral: 0.5-2 hours, declining for the next 2 hours before increasing again due to enterohepatic recycling

Excretion: Primarily feces; urine (10% to 20%)

Dosage

Familial Mediterranean fever (unlabeled use): Prophylaxis: Oral:

Children:

≤5 years: 0.5 mg/day

>5 years: 1-1.5 mg/day in 2-3 divided doses

Adults: 1-2 mg daily in divided doses (occasionally reduced to 0.6 mg/day in patients with GI intolerance)

Gouty arthritis: Adults:

Prophylaxis of acute attacks: Oral: 0.6 mg twice daily; initial and/or subsequent dosage may be decreased (ie, 0.6 mg once daily) in patients at risk of toxicity or in those who are intolerant (including weakness, loose stools, or diarrhea); range: 0.6 mg every other day to 0.6 mg 3 times/day

Acute attacks:

Oral: Initial: 0.6-1.2 mg, followed by 0.6 every 1-2 hours; some clinicians recommend a maximum of 3 doses; more aggressive approaches have recommended a maximum dose of up to 6 mg. Wait at least 3 days before initiating another course of therapy

I.V.: Initial: 1-2 mg, then 0.5 mg every 6 hours until response, not to exceed total dose of 4 mg. If pain recurs, it may be necessary to administer additional daily doses. The amount of colchicine administered intravenously in an acute treatment period (generally ~1 week) should not exceed a total dose of 4 mg. Do not administer more colchicine by any route for at least 7 days after a full course of I.V. therapy.

Note: Many experts would avoid use because of potential for serious, life-threatening complications. Should not be administered to patients with renal insufficiency, hepatobiliary obstruction, patients >70 years of age, or recent oral colchicine use. Should be reserved for hospitalized patients who are under the care of a physician experienced in the use of intravenous colchicine.

Surgery: Gouty arthritis, prophylaxis of recurrent attacks: Adults: Oral: 0.6 mg/day or every other day; patients who are to undergo surgical procedures may receive 0.6 mg 3 times/day for 3 days before and 3 days after surgery

Primary biliary cirrhosis (unlabeled use): Adults: Oral: 0.6 mg twice daily

Pericarditis (unlabeled use): Adults: Oral: 0.6 mg twice daily

Elderly: Reduce maintenance/prophylactic dose by 50% in individuals >70 years

Dosing adjustment in renal impairment: Gouty arthritis, acute attacks: Oral: Specific dosing recommendations not available from the manufacturer:

Prophylaxis:

Cl_{cr} 35-49 mL/minute: 0.6 mg once daily

Cl_{cr} 10-34 mL/minute: 0.6 mg every 2-3 days

Cl_{cr} <10 mL/minute: Avoid chronic use of colchicine. Use in serious renal impairment is contraindicated by the manufacturer.

Treatment: Cl_{cr} <10 mL/minute: Use in serious renal impairment is contraindicated by the manufacturer. If a decision is made to use colchicine, decrease dose by 75%.

Peritoneal dialysis: Supplemental dose is not necessary

Dosage adjustment in hepatic impairment: Avoid in hepatobiliary dysfunction and in patients with hepatic disease.

Stability Protect tablets from light.

Administration

I.V.: Injection should be made over 2-5 minutes into tubing of free-flowing I.V. with compatible fluid. Do not administer I.M. or SubQ; severe local irritation can occur following SubQ or I.M. administration. Extravasation can cause tissue irritation.

Tablet: Administer orally with water and maintain adequate fluid intake.

Monitoring Parameters CBC and renal function test

Pregnancy Risk Factor C (oral); D (parenteral)

Contraindications Hypersensitivity to colchicine or any component of the formulation; severe renal, gastrointestinal, hepatic, or cardiac disorders; blood dyscrasias; pregnancy (parenteral)

Warnings/Precautions Use with caution in debilitated patients or elderly patients; use caution in patients with mild-to-moderate cardiac, GI, renal, or liver disease. Severe local irritation can occur following SubQ or I.M. administration. Dosage reduction is recommended in patients who develop weakness or gastrointestinal symptoms (anorexia, diarrhea, nausea, vomiting) related to drug therapy.

Intravenous: Use only with extreme caution; potential for serious, life-threatening complications. Should not be administered to patients with renal insufficiency, hepatobiliary obstruction, patients >70 years of age, or recent oral colchicine use. Should be reserved for hospitalized patients who are under the care of a physician experienced in the use of intravenous colchicine.

Adverse Reactions

>10%: Gastrointestinal: Nausea, vomiting, diarrhea, abdominal pain

1% to 10%:

Dermatologic: Alopecia

Gastrointestinal: Anorexia

<1% (Limited to important or life-threatening): Agranulocytosis, aplastic anemia, arrhythmia (with intravenous administration), bone marrow suppression, hepatotoxicity

Overdosage/Toxicology Symptoms of overdose include acute nausea, vomiting, abdominal pain, shock, kidney damage, muscle weakness, burning in throat, watery to bloody diarrhea, hypotension, anuria, cardiovascular collapse, delirium, convulsions, and respiratory paralysis. Treatment includes gastric lavage and measures to prevent shock, hemodialysis or peritoneal dialysis. Atropine and morphine may relieve abdominal pain.

Drug Interactions Substrate of CYP3A4 (major); **Induces** CYP2C8 (weak), 2C9 (weak), 2E1 (weak), 3A4 (weak)

Cyclosporine: Concurrent use with colchicine may increase toxicity of colchicine.

CYP3A4 inhibitors: May increase the levels/effects of colchicine. Example inhibitors include azole antifungals, diclofenac, doxycycline, imatinib, isoniazid, nefazodone, nicardipine, propofol, protease inhibitors, quinidine, telithromycin, and verapamil.

Macrolide antibiotics (clarithromycin, erythromycin, troleandomycin): May decrease the metabolism of colchicine resulting in severe colchicine toxicity. Avoid, if possible.

Telithromycin: May decrease the metabolism of colchicine resulting in colchicine toxicity. Avoid, if possible.

Verapamil: May increase colchicine toxicity (especially nephrotoxicity).

Ethanol/Nutrition/Herb Interactions

Ethanol: Avoid ethanol.

Food: Cyanocobalamin (vitamin B_{12}): Malabsorption of the substrate. May result in macrocytic anemia or neurologic dysfunction.

Herb/Nutraceutical: Vitamin B_{12} absorption may be decreased by colchicine.

Test Interactions May cause false-positive results in urine tests for erythrocytes or hemoglobin

Dietary Considerations May need to supplement with vitamin B_{12}.

(Continued)

Colchicine *(Continued)*

Dosage Forms
Injection, solution: 0.5 mg/mL (2 mL)
Tablet: 0.6 mg

Colistimethate (koe lis ti METH ate)

U.S. Brand Names Coly-Mycin® M
Canadian Brand Names Coly-Mycin® M
Synonyms Colistimethate Sodium
Pharmacologic Category Antibiotic, Miscellaneous
Generic Available Yes
Use Treatment of infections due to sensitive strains of certain gram-negative bacilli which are resistant to other antibacterials or in patients allergic to other antibacterials
Unlabeled/Investigational Use Used as inhalation in the prevention of *Pseudomonas aeruginosa* respiratory tract infections in immunocompromised patients, and used as inhalation adjunct agent for the treatment of *P. aeruginosa* infections in patients with cystic fibrosis and other seriously ill or chronically ill patients
Mechanism of Action Hydrolyzed to colistin, which acts as a cationic detergent which damages the bacterial cytoplasmic membrane causing leaking of intracellular substances and cell death
Pharmacodynamics/Kinetics
Distribution: Widely, except for CNS, synovial, pleural, and pericardial fluids
Half-life elimination: 1.5-8 hours; Anuria: ≤2-3 days
Time to peak: ~2 hours
Excretion: Primarily urine (as unchanged drug)
Dosage Children and Adults:
I.M., I.V.: 2.5-5 mg/kg/day in 2-4 divided doses
Inhalation: 50-75 mg in NS (3-4 mL total) via nebulizer 2-3 times/day
Dosing interval in renal impairment: Adults:
S_{cr} 0.7-1.2 mg/dL: 100-125 mg 2-4 times/day
S_{cr} 1.3-1.5 mg/dL: 75-115 mg twice daily
S_{cr} 1.6-2.5 mg/dL: 66-150 mg once or twice daily
S_{cr} 2.6-4 mg/dL: 100-150 mg every 36 hours
Stability Freshly prepare any infusion and use for no longer than 24 hours.
Administration
Parenteral: Reconstitute vial with 2 mL SWFI resulting in a concentration of 75 mg colistin/mL; swirl gently to avoid frothing. Administer by I.M., direct I.V. injection over 3-10 minutes, intermittent infusion over 30 minutes, or by continuous I.V. infusion. For continuous I.V. infusion, one-half of the total daily dose is administered by direct I.V. injection over 3-10 minutes followed 1-2 hours later by the remaining one-half of the total daily dose diluted in a compatible I.V. solution infused over 22-23 hours. The final concentration for administration should be based on the patient's fluid needs.
Inhalation: Further dilute dose to a total volume of 3-4 mL in NS and administer via nebulizer. If patient is on a ventilator, place medicine in a T-piece at the midinspiratory circuit of the ventilator.
Pregnancy Risk Factor C
Contraindications Hypersensitivity to colistimethate or any component of the formulation
Warnings/Precautions Use with caution in patients with pre-existing renal disease
Adverse Reactions 1% to 10%:
Central nervous system: Vertigo, slurring of speech
Dermatologic: Urticaria
Gastrointestinal: GI upset
Respiratory: Respiratory arrest
Renal: Nephrotoxicity
Drug Interactions Other nephrotoxic drugs, neuromuscular blocking agents
Dosage Forms Injection, powder for reconstitution: 150 mg

♦ **Colistimethate Sodium** *see* Colistimethate *on page 330*
♦ **Colocort**® *see* Hydrocortisone *on page 639*
♦ **CO Lovastatin (Can)** *see* Lovastatin *on page 782*

- **Coly-Mycin® M** *see* Colistimethate *on page 330*
- **CO Meloxicam (Can)** *see* Meloxicam *on page 798*
- **Compazine® (Can)** *see* Prochlorperazine *on page 1061*
- **Compound 347™** *see* Enflurane *on page 450*
- **Compound F** *see* Hydrocortisone *on page 639*
- **Compound S** *see* Zidovudine *on page 1371*
- **Compoz® Nighttime Sleep Aid [OTC]** *see* DiphenhydrAMINE *on page 399*
- **Compro™** *see* Prochlorperazine *on page 1061*
- **Comtrex® Sore Throat Maximum Strength [OTC]** *see* Acetaminophen *on page 26*

Conivaptan (koe NYE vap tan)

U.S. Brand Names Vaprisol®

Synonyms Conivaptan Hydrochloride; YM087

Pharmacologic Category Vasopressin Antagonist

Generic Available No

Use Treatment of euvolemic hyponatremia in hospitalized patients

Mechanism of Action Conivaptan is an arginine vasopressin (AVP) receptor antagonist with affinity for AVP receptor subtypes V_{1A} and V_2. The antidiuretic action of AVP is mediated through activation of the V_2 receptor, which functions to regulate water and electrolyte balance at the level of the collecting ducts in the kidney. Serum levels of AVP are commonly elevated in euvolemic or hypervolemic hyponatremia, which results in the dilution of serum sodium and the relative hyponatremic state. Antagonism of the V_2 receptor by conivaptan promotes the excretion of free water (without loss of serum electrolytes) resulting in net fluid loss, increased urine output, decreased urine osmolality, and subsequent restoration of normal serum sodium levels.

Pharmacodynamics/Kinetics

Protein binding: 99%

Metabolism: Hepatic via CYP3A4 to four minimally-active metabolites

Half-life elimination: 6.7-8.6 hours

Excretion: Feces (83%); urine (12%)

Dosage I.V.: Adults:

Loading dose: 20 mg infused over 30 minutes, followed by continuous infusion of 20 mg over 24 hours

Maintenance: 20 mg/day as continuous infusion over 24 hours; may titrate to maximum of 40 mg/day if serum sodium not rising sufficiently; total duration of therapy not to exceed 4 days

Stability Store ampuls in original cardboard container at 15°C to 30°C (59°F to 86°F); protect from light. Dilute loading dose of 20 mg in 100 mL D_5W and continuous infusion dose of 20-40 mg in 250 mL D_5W. After dilution, infusion bag (final concentration of 0.08-0.2 mg/mL) is stable at room temperature for 24 hours.

Administration For intravenous use only; do not administer undiluted; infuse into large veins and change infusion site every 24 hours to minimize vascular irritation

Monitoring Parameters Rate of serum sodium increase, urine output

Pregnancy Risk Factor C

Contraindications Hypersensitivity to conivaptan or any component of the formulation; use in hypovolemic hyponatremia; concurrent use with strong CYP3A4 inhibitors (eg, ketoconazole, itraconazole, ritonavir, indinavir, and clarithromycin)

Warnings/Precautions Monitor closely for rate of serum sodium increase and neurological status; overly rapid serum sodium correction (>12 mEq/L/24 hours) can lead to permanent neurological damage. Discontinue use if rate of serum sodium increase is undesirable; may reinitiate infusion (at reduced dose) if hyponatremia persists in the absence of neurological symptoms typically associated with rapid sodium rise. Use with caution in patients with hepatic and renal impairment. Safety and efficacy in pediatric patients, or patients with underlying heart failure, have not been established.

Adverse Reactions

>10%:

Central nervous system: Headache (12%)

Local: Injection site reactions including pain, erythema, phlebitis, swelling (53%)

(Continued)

Conivaptan *(Continued)*

1% to 10%:

Cardiovascular: Hypertension (6%), phlebitis (5%), atrial fibrillation (3%), hypotension (3%; orthostatic 6%)

Central nervous system: Fever (4%), confusion (4%), insomnia (3%), pain (2%)

Dermatologic: Erythema (3%)

Endocrine & metabolic: Hypokalemia (10%), hyper-/hypoglycemia (3%), hypomagnesemia (2%), hyponatremia (3%)

Gastrointestinal: Vomiting (7%), diarrhea (6%), constipation (5%), dry mouth (4%), nausea (4%), dehydration (2%), oral candidiasis (2%)

Genitourinary: Urinary tract infection (3%)

Hematologic: Anemia (4%)

Renal: Polyuria (5% to 6%), hematuria (2%)

Respiratory: Pneumonia (3%)

Miscellaneous: Thirst (10%)

Overdosage/Toxicology No specific overdose information available. Doses of up to 120 mg/day for 2 days have been evaluated, with no additional toxicity other than an expected increased incidence of hypotension and thirst. Treatment should be symptom-directed and supportive.

Drug Interactions Substrate of CYP3A4 (major); **Inhibits** CYP3A4 (strong)

CYP3A4 inducers may decrease the levels/effects of conivaptan. Example inducers include aminoglutethimide, carbamazepine, nafcillin, nevirapine, phenobarbital, phenytoin, and rifamycins.

CYP3A4 inhibitors may increase the levels/effects of conivaptan. Example inhibitors include azole antifungals, clarithromycin, diclofenac, doxycycline, erythromycin, imatinib, isoniazid, nefazodone, nicardipine, propofol, protease inhibitors, quinidine, telithromycin, and verapamil.

CYP3A4 substrates: Conivaptan may increase the levels/effects of CYP3A4 substrates. Example substrates include benzodiazepines, calcium channel blockers, cyclosporine, mirtazapine, nateglinide, nefazodone, sildenafil (and other PDE5 inhibitors), tacrolimus, and venlafaxine. Selected benzodiazepines (midazolam and triazolam), cisapride, ergot alkaloids, selected HMG-CoA reductase inhibitors (lovastatin and simvastatin), and pimozide are generally contraindicated with strong CYP3A4 inhibitors.

Digoxin: Conivaptan may increase the levels/toxicity of digoxin; monitor.

Ketoconazole: May increase the levels/effects of conivaptan; concomitant use is contraindicated.

Dosage Forms

Injection, solution:

Vaprisol®: 5 mg/mL (4 mL) [single-use ampul; contains propylene glycol and ethanol]

- **Conivaptan Hydrochloride** *see* Conivaptan *on page 331*
- **Constulose®** *see* Lactulose *on page 724*
- **Contac® Cold 12 Hour Relief Non Drowsy (Can)** *see* Pseudoephedrine *on page 1085*
- **Contact® Cold [OTC]** *see* Pseudoephedrine *on page 1085*
- **CO Paroxetine (Can)** *see* Paroxetine *on page 988*
- **Copegus®** *see* Ribavirin *on page 1116*
- **Copper** *see* Trace Metals *on page 1296*
- **CO Pravastatin (Can)** *see* Pravastatin *on page 1042*
- **CO Ranitidine (Can)** *see* Ranitidine *on page 1105*
- **Cordarone®** *see* Amiodarone *on page 83*
- **Coreg®** *see* Carvedilol *on page 231*
- **Corgard®** *see* Nadolol *on page 886*
- **Corlopam®** *see* Fenoldopam *on page 510*
- **Cortaid® Intensive Therapy [OTC]** *see* Hydrocortisone *on page 639*
- **Cortaid® Maximum Strength [OTC]** *see* Hydrocortisone *on page 639*
- **Cortaid® Sensitive Skin [OTC]** *see* Hydrocortisone *on page 639*
- **Cortamed® (Can)** *see* Hydrocortisone *on page 639*
- **Cortef®** *see* Hydrocortisone *on page 639*
- **Cortenema® (Can)** *see* Hydrocortisone *on page 639*
- **Corticool® [OTC]** *see* Hydrocortisone *on page 639*
- **Cortifoam®** *see* Hydrocortisone *on page 639*

- ♦ **Cortisol** *see* Hydrocortisone *on page 639*
- ♦ **Cortizone®-10 Maximum Strength [OTC]** *see* Hydrocortisone *on page 639*
- ♦ **Cortizone®-10 Plus Maximum Strength [OTC]** *see* Hydrocortisone *on page 639*
- ♦ **Cortizone®-10 Quick Shot [OTC]** *see* Hydrocortisone *on page 639*
- ♦ **Cortrosyn®** *see* Cosyntropin *on page 333*
- ♦ **Corvert®** *see* Ibutilide *on page 657*
- ♦ **CO Simvastatin (Can)** *see* Simvastatin *on page 1174*
- ♦ **CO Sotalol (Can)** *see* Sotalol *on page 1198*
- ♦ **CO Sumatriptan (Can)** *see* Sumatriptan *on page 1222*

Cosyntropin (koe sin TROE pin)

Medication Safety Issues

Sound-alike/look-alike issues:

Cortrosyn® may be confused with Cotazym®

U.S. Brand Names Cortrosyn®

Canadian Brand Names Cortrosyn®

Synonyms Synacthen; Tetracosactide

Pharmacologic Category Diagnostic Agent

Generic Available No

Use Diagnostic test to differentiate primary adrenal from secondary (pituitary) adrenocortical insufficiency

Mechanism of Action Stimulates the adrenal cortex to secrete adrenal steroids (including hydrocortisone, cortisone), androgenic substances, and a small amount of aldosterone

Pharmacodynamics/Kinetics Time to peak, serum: I.M., IVP: ~1 hour; plasma cortisol levels rise in healthy individuals within 5 minutes

Dosage

Adrenocortical insufficiency: I.M., I.V. (over 2 minutes): Peak plasma cortisol concentrations usually occur 45-60 minutes after cosyntropin administration

Children <2 years: 0.125 mg

Children >2 years and Adults: 0.25-0.75 mg

When greater cortisol stimulation is needed, an I.V. infusion may be used:

Children >2 years and Adults: 0.25 mg administered at 0.04 mg/hour over 6 hours

Stability Powder for injection: Store at controlled room temperature of 15°C to 30°C (59°F to 86°F).

I.M.: Reconstitute cosyntropin 0.25 mg with NS 1 mL

I.V. push: Reconstitute cosyntropin 0.25 mg with NS 2-5 mL

I.V. infusion: Mix in NS or D_5W; stable for 12 hours at room temperature; stable for 21 days under refrigeration

Administration Administer I.V. doses over 2 minutes

Reference Range Normal baseline cortisol; increase in serum cortisol after cosyntropin injection of >7 mcg/dL or peak response >18 mcg/dL; plasma cortisol concentrations should be measured immediately before and exactly 30 minutes after a dose

Anesthesia and Critical Care Concerns/Other Considerations

Septic Shock: A recent randomized, double-blind, placebo-controlled trial assessed whether low-dose corticosteroid administration could improve 28-day survival in patients with septic shock and relative adrenal insufficiency. Relative adrenal insufficiency was defined as an inappropriate response to corticotropin administration (increase of serum cortisol of ≤9 mcg/dL from baseline). Cortisol levels were drawn immediately before corticotropin administration and 30-60 minutes afterwards. Three hundred adult septic shock patients requiring mechanical ventilation and vasopressor support were randomized to either hydrocortisone (50 mg IVP every 6 hours) and fludrocortisone (50 mcg tablet daily via nasogastric tube) or matching placebos for 7 days. In patients who did not appropriately respond to corticotropin (nonresponders), there were significantly fewer deaths in the active treatment group. Vasopressor therapy was withdrawn more frequently in this subset of the active treatment group. Adverse events were similar in both groups. Patients who lack adrenal reserve and thus have relative adrenal insufficiency during the stress of septic shock may benefit from physiologic steroid replacement. However, there was a trend for increased mortality in patients who responded to the corticotropin test (increase serum cortisol >9 mcg/dL

(Continued)

Cosyntropin *(Continued)*

from baseline). These patients may not benefit from physiologic steroid replacement. Further study is required to better characterize the patient populations who may benefit.

Pregnancy Risk Factor C

Contraindications Hypersensitivity to cosyntropin or any component of the formulation

Warnings/Precautions Use with caution in patients with pre-existing allergic disease or a history of allergic reactions to corticotropin.

Adverse Reactions Frequency not defined.

Cardiovascular: Bradycardia, hypertension, peripheral edema, tachycardia
Dermatologic: Rash
Local: Whealing with redness at the injection site
Miscellaneous: Anaphylaxis, hypersensitivity reaction

Test Interactions Decreased effect: Spironolactone, hydrocortisone, cortisone, etomidate

Dosage Forms Injection, powder for reconstitution: 0.25 mg

References

Annane D, Sebille V, Charpentier C, et al, "Effect of Treatment With Low Doses of Hydrocortisone and Fludrocortisone on Mortality in Patients With Septic Shock," *JAMA*, 2002, 288(7):862-71.

♦ **CO Temazepam (Can)** *see* Temazepam *on page 1239*
♦ **Co-Trimoxazole** *see* Sulfamethoxazole and Trimethoprim *on page 1215*
♦ **Coumadin®** *see* Warfarin *on page 1362*
♦ **Covera® (Can)** *see* Verapamil *on page 1352*
♦ **Covera-HS®** *see* Verapamil *on page 1352*
♦ **Coversyl® (Can)** *see* Perindopril Erbumine *on page 1002*
♦ **Coviracil** *see* Emtricitabine *on page 445*
♦ **Cozaar®** *see* Losartan *on page 778*
♦ **CP-99,219-27** *see* Trovafloxacin *on page 1320*
♦ **CPM** *see* Cyclophosphamide *on page 334*
♦ **CPZ** *see* ChlorproMAZINE *on page 273*
♦ **Crestor®** *see* Rosuvastatin *on page 1142*
♦ **Crixivan®** *see* Indinavir *on page 671*
♦ **Crosseal™** *see* Fibrin Sealant Kit *on page 523*
♦ **Crystalline Penicillin** *see* Penicillin G (Parenteral/Aqueous) *on page 994*
♦ **CsA** *see* CycloSPORINE *on page 337*
♦ **CTX** *see* Cyclophosphamide *on page 334*
♦ **Cubicin®** *see* Daptomycin *on page 352*
♦ **Curosurf®** *see* Poractant Alfa *on page 1038*
♦ **CyA** *see* CycloSPORINE *on page 337*

Cyclophosphamide (sye kloe FOS fa mide)

Medication Safety Issues

Sound-alike/look-alike issues:

Cyclophosphamide may be confused with cycloSPORINE, ifosfamide
Cytoxan® may be confused with cefoxitin, Centoxin®, Ciloxan®, cytarabine, CytoGam®, Cytosar®, Cytosar-U®, Cytotec®

U.S. Brand Names Cytoxan®

Canadian Brand Names Cytoxan®; Procytox®

Synonyms CPM; CTX; CYT; NSC-26271

Pharmacologic Category Antineoplastic Agent, Alkylating Agent

Generic Available Yes: Tablet

Use

Oncologic: Treatment of Hodgkin's and non-Hodgkin's lymphoma, Burkitt's lymphoma, chronic lymphocytic leukemia (CLL), chronic myelocytic leukemia (CML), acute myelocytic leukemia (AML), acute lymphocytic leukemia (ALL), mycosis fungoides, multiple myeloma, neuroblastoma, retinoblastoma, rhabdomyosarcoma, Ewing's sarcoma; breast, testicular, endometrial, ovarian, and lung cancers, and in conditioning regimens for bone marrow transplantation

Nononcologic: Prophylaxis of rejection for kidney, heart, liver, and bone marrow transplants, severe rheumatoid disorders, nephrotic syndrome, Wegener's granulomatosis, idiopathic pulmonary hemosideroses, myasthenia gravis, multiple sclerosis, systemic lupus erythematosus, lupus nephritis, autoimmune hemolytic anemia, idiopathic thrombocytic purpura (ITP), macroglobulinemia, and antibody-induced pure red cell aplasia

Mechanism of Action Cyclophosphamide is an alkylating agent that prevents cell division by cross-linking DNA strands and decreasing DNA synthesis. It is a cell cycle phase nonspecific agent. Cyclophosphamide also possesses potent immunosuppressive activity. Cyclophosphamide is a prodrug that must be metabolized to active metabolites in the liver.

Pharmacodynamics/Kinetics

Absorption: Oral: Well absorbed

Distribution: V_d: 0.48-0.71 L/kg; crosses placenta; crosses into CSF (not in high enough concentrations to treat meningeal leukemia)

Protein binding: 10% to 56%

Metabolism: Hepatic to active metabolites acrolein, 4-aldophosphamide, 4-hydroperoxycyclophosphamide, and nor-nitrogen mustard

Bioavailability: >75%

Half-life elimination: 4-8 hours

Time to peak, serum: Oral: ~1 hour

Excretion: Urine (<30% as unchanged drug, 85% to 90% as metabolites)

Dosage Refer to individual protocols

Children:

SLE: I.V.: 500-750 mg/m^2 every month; maximum dose: 1 g/m^2

JRA/vasculitis: I.V.: 10 mg/kg every 2 weeks

Children and Adults:

Oral: 50-100 mg/m^2/day as continuous therapy or 400-1000 mg/m^2 in divided doses over 4-5 days as intermittent therapy

I.V.:

Single doses: 400-1800 mg/m^2 (30-50 mg/kg) per treatment course (1-5 days) which can be repeated at 2-4 week intervals

Continuous daily doses: 60-120 mg/m^2 (1-2.5 mg/kg) per day

Autologous BMT: IVPB: 50 mg/kg/dose x 4 days or 60 mg/kg/dose for 2 days; total dose is usually divided over 2-4 days

Nephrotic syndrome: Oral: 2-3 mg/kg/day every day for up to 12 weeks when corticosteroids are unsuccessful

Dosing adjustment in renal impairment: A large fraction of cyclophosphamide is eliminated by hepatic metabolism

Some authors recommend no dose adjustment unless severe renal insufficiency (Cl_{cr} <20 mL/minute)

Cl_{cr} >10 mL/minute: Administer 100% of normal dose

Cl_{cr} <10 mL/minute: Administer 75% of normal dose

Hemodialysis: Moderately dialyzable (20% to 50%); administer dose posthemodialysis

CAPD effects: Unknown

CAVH effects: Unknown

Dosing adjustment in hepatic impairment: The pharmacokinetics of cyclophosphamide are not significantly altered in the presence of hepatic insufficiency. No dosage adjustments are recommended.

Stability Store intact vials of powder at room temperature of 15°C to 30°C (59°F to 86°F). Reconstitute vials with sterile water, normal saline, or 5% dextrose to a concentration of 20 mg/mL. Reconstituted solutions are stable for 24 hours at room temperature and 6 days under refrigeration at 2°C to 8°C (36°F to 46°F). Further dilutions in D_5W or NS are stable for 24 hours at room temperature and 6 days at refrigeration.

Administration Administer I.P., intrapleurally, IVPB, or continuous I.V. infusion; may also be administered slow IVP in doses ≤1 g.

I.V. infusions may be administered over 1-24 hours

Doses >500 mg to approximately 2 g may be administered over 20-30 minutes

To minimize bladder toxicity, increase normal fluid intake during and for 1-2 days after cyclophosphamide dose. Most adult patients will require a fluid intake of at least 2 L/day. High-dose regimens should be accompanied by vigorous hydration with or without mesna therapy.

Oral: Tablets are not scored and should not be cut or crushed; should be administered during or after meals.

Monitoring Parameters CBC with differential and platelet count, BUN, UA, serum electrolytes, serum creatinine

Pregnancy Risk Factor D

(Continued)

Cyclophosphamide *(Continued)*

Contraindications Hypersensitivity to cyclophosphamide or any component of the formulation; pregnancy

Warnings/Precautions Hazardous agent - use appropriate precautions for handling and disposal. Dosage adjustment needed for renal or hepatic failure.

Adverse Reactions

>10%:

Dermatologic: Alopecia (40% to 60%) but hair will usually regrow although it may be a different color and/or texture. Hair loss usually begins 3-6 weeks after the start of therapy.

Endocrine & metabolic: Fertility: May cause sterility; interferes with oogenesis and spermatogenesis; may be irreversible in some patients; gonadal suppression (amenorrhea)

Gastrointestinal: Nausea and vomiting, usually beginning 6-10 hours after administration; anorexia, diarrhea, mucositis, and stomatitis are also seen

Genitourinary: Severe, potentially fatal acute hemorrhagic cystitis (7% to 40%)

Hematologic: Thrombocytopenia and anemia are less common than leukopenia

Onset: 7 days

Nadir: 10-14 days

Recovery: 21 days

1% to 10%:

Cardiovascular: Facial flushing

Central nervous system: Headache

Dermatologic: Skin rash

Renal: SIADH may occur, usually with doses >50 mg/kg (or 1 g/m^2); renal tubular necrosis, which usually resolves with discontinuation of the drug, is also reported

Respiratory: Nasal congestion occurs when I.V. doses are administered too rapidly; patients experience runny eyes, rhinorrhea, sinus congestion, and sneezing during or immediately after the infusion.

<1% (Limited to important or life-threatening): High-dose therapy may cause cardiac dysfunction manifested as CHF; cardiac necrosis or hemorrhagic myocarditis has occurred rarely, but may be fatal. Cyclophosphamide may also potentiate the cardiac toxicity of anthracyclines. Other adverse reactions include anaphylactic reactions, darkening of skin/fingernails, dizziness, hemorrhagic colitis, hemorrhagic ureteritis, hepatotoxicity, hyperuricemia, hypokalemia, jaundice, neutrophilic eccrine hidradenitis, radiation recall, renal tubular necrosis, secondary malignancy (eg, bladder carcinoma), Stevens-Johnson syndrome, toxic epidermal necrolysis; interstitial pneumonitis and pulmonary fibrosis are occasionally seen with high doses

BMT:

Cardiovascular: Heart failure, cardiac necrosis, pericardial tamponade

Endocrine & metabolic: Hyponatremia

Hematologic: Methemoglobinemia

Gastrointestinal: Severe nausea and vomiting

Miscellaneous: Hemorrhagic cystitis, secondary malignancy

Overdosage/Toxicology Symptoms of overdose include myelosuppression, alopecia, nausea, and vomiting. Treatment is supportive.

Drug Interactions **Substrate** of CYP2A6 (minor), 2B6 (major), 2C9 (minor), 2C19 (minor), 3A4 (major); **Inhibits** CYP3A4 (weak); **Induces** CYP2B6 (weak), 2C8 (weak), 2C9 (weak)

Allopurinol may cause increase in bone marrow depression and may result in significant elevations of cyclophosphamide cytotoxic metabolites.

Anesthetic agents: Cyclophosphamide reduces serum pseudocholinesterase concentrations and may prolong the neuromuscular blocking activity of succinylcholine; use with caution with halothane, nitrous oxide, and succinylcholine.

Chloramphenicol results in prolonged cyclophosphamide half-life to increase toxicity.

CYP2B6 inducers: May increase the levels/effects of acrolein (the active metabolite of cyclophosphamide). Example inducers include carbamazepine, nevirapine, phenobarbital, phenytoin, and rifampin.

CYP2B6 inhibitors: May decrease the levels/effects of acrolein (the active metabolite of cyclophosphamide). Example inhibitors include desipramine, paroxetine, and sertraline.

CYP3A4 inducers: CYP3A4 inducers may increase the levels/effects of acrolein (the active metabolite of cyclophosphamide). Example inducers include aminoglutethimide, carbamazepine, nafcillin, nevirapine, phenobarbital, phenytoin, and rifamycins.

CYP3A4 inhibitors: May decrease the levels/effects of acrolein (the active metabolite of cyclophosphamide). Example inhibitors include azole antifungals, ciprofloxacin, clarithromycin, diclofenac, doxycycline, erythromycin, imatinib, isoniazid, nefazodone, nicardipine, propofol, protease inhibitors, quinidine, and verapamil.

Digoxin: Cyclophosphamide may decrease digoxin serum levels.

Doxorubicin: Cyclophosphamide may enhance cardiac toxicity of anthracyclines.

Tetrahydrocannabinol results in enhanced immunosuppression in animal studies.

Thiazide diuretics: Leukopenia may be prolonged.

Ethanol/Nutrition/Herb Interactions Herb/Nutraceutical: Avoid black cohosh, dong quai in estrogen-dependent tumors.

Dietary Considerations Tablets should be administered during or after meals.

Dosage Forms

Injection, powder for reconstitution (Cytoxan®): 500 mg, 1 g, 2 g [contains mannitol 75 mg per cyclophosphamide 100 mg]

Tablet (Cytoxan®): 25 mg, 50 mg

♦ **Cyclosporin A** *see* CycloSPORINE *on page 337*

CycloSPORINE (SYE kloe spor een)

Medication Safety Issues

Sound-alike/look-alike issues:

CycloSPORINE may be confused with cyclophosphamide, Cyklokapron®, cycloSERINE

CycloSPORINE modified (Neoral®, Gengraf®) may be confused with cycloSPORINE non-modified (Sandimmne®)

Gengraf® may be confused with Prograf®

Neoral® may be confused with Neurontin®, Nizoral®

Sandimmune® may be confused with Sandostatin®

U.S. Brand Names Gengraf®; Neoral®; Restasis®; Sandimmune®

Canadian Brand Names Apo-Cyclosporine®; Neoral®; Rhoxal-cyclosporine; Sandimmune® I.V.; Sandoz-Cyclosporine

Synonyms CsA; CyA; Cyclosporin A

Pharmacologic Category Immunosuppressant Agent

Generic Available Yes

Use Prophylaxis of organ rejection in kidney, liver, and heart transplants, has been used with azathioprine and/or corticosteroids; severe, active rheumatoid arthritis (RA) not responsive to methotrexate alone; severe, recalcitrant plaque psoriasis in nonimmunocompromised adults unresponsive to or unable to tolerate other systemic therapy

Ophthalmic emulsion (Restasis®): Increase tear production when suppressed tear production is presumed to be due to keratoconjunctivitis sicca-associated ocular inflammation (in patients not already using topical anti-inflammatory drugs or punctal plugs)

Unlabeled/Investigational Use Short-term, high-dose cyclosporine as a modulator of multidrug resistance in cancer treatment; allogenic bone marrow transplants for prevention and treatment of graft-versus-host disease; also used in some cases of severe autoimmune disease (eg, SLE, myasthenia gravis) that are resistant to corticosteroids and other therapy; focal segmental glomerulosclerosis

Mechanism of Action Inhibition of production and release of interleukin II and inhibits interleukin II-induced activation of resting T-lymphocytes.

Pharmacodynamics/Kinetics

Absorption:

Ophthalmic emulsion: Serum concentrations not detectable.

Oral:

Cyclosporine (non-modified): Erratic and incomplete; dependent on presence of food, bile acids, and GI motility; larger oral doses are needed in pediatrics due to shorter bowel length and limited intestinal absorption

Cyclosporine (modified): Erratic and incomplete; increased absorption, up to 30% when compared to cyclosporine (non-modified); less dependent on

(Continued)

CycloSPORINE *(Continued)*

food, bile acids, or GI motility when compared to cyclosporine (non-modified)

Distribution: Widely in tissues and body fluids including the liver, pancreas, and lungs; crosses placenta; enters breast milk

V_{dss}: 4-6 L/kg in renal, liver, and marrow transplant recipients (slightly lower values in cardiac transplant patients; children <10 years have higher values)

Protein binding: 90% to 98% to lipoproteins

Metabolism: Extensively hepatic via CYP3A4; forms at least 25 metabolites; extensive first-pass effect following oral administration

Bioavailability: Oral:

Cyclosporine (non-modified): Dependent on patient population and transplant type (<10% in adult liver transplant patients and as high as 89% in renal transplant patients); bioavailability of Sandimmune® capsules and oral solution are equivalent; bioavailability of oral solution is ~30% of the I.V. solution

Children: 28% (range: 17% to 42%); gut dysfunction common in BMT patients and oral bioavailability is further reduced

Cyclosporine (modified): Bioavailability of Neoral® capsules and oral solution are equivalent:

Children: 43% (range: 30% to 68%)

Adults: 23% greater than with cyclosporine (non-modified) in renal transplant patients; 50% greater in liver transplant patients

Half-life elimination: Oral: May be prolonged in patients with hepatic impairment and shorter in pediatric patients due to the higher metabolism rate

Cyclosporine (non-modified): Biphasic: Alpha: 1.4 hours; Terminal: 19 hours (range: 10-27 hours)

Cyclosporine (modified): Biphasic: Terminal: 8.4 hours (range: 5-18 hours)

Time to peak, serum: Oral:

Cyclosporine (non-modified): 2-6 hours; some patients have a second peak at 5-6 hours

Cyclosporine (modified): Renal transplant: 1.5-2 hours

Excretion: Primarily feces; urine (6%, 0.1% as unchanged drug and metabolites)

Dosage Neoral®/Genraf® and Sandimmune® are not bioequivalent and cannot be used interchangeably.

Children: Transplant: Refer to adult dosing; children may require, and are able to tolerate, larger doses than adults.

Adults:

Newly-transplanted patients: Adjunct therapy with corticosteroids is recommended. Initial dose should be given 4-12 hours prior to transplant or may be given postoperatively; adjust initial dose to achieve desired plasma concentration

Oral: Dose is dependent upon type of transplant and formulation:

Cyclosporine (modified):

Renal: 9 ± 3 mg/kg/day, divided twice daily

Liver: 8 ± 4 mg/kg/day, divided twice daily

Heart: 7 ± 3 mg/kg/day, divided twice daily

Cyclosporine (non-modified): Initial dose: 15 mg/kg/day as a single dose (range 14-18 mg/kg); lower doses of 10-14 mg/kg/day have been used for renal transplants. Continue initial dose daily for 1-2 weeks; taper by 5% per week to a maintenance dose of 5-10 mg/kg/day; some renal transplant patients may be dosed as low as 3 mg/kg/day

Note: When using the non-modified formulation, cyclosporine levels may increase in liver transplant patients when the T-tube is closed; dose may need decreased

I.V.: Cyclosporine (non-modified): Manufacturer's labeling: Initial dose: 5-6 mg/kg/day as a single dose (1/3 the oral dose), infused over 2-6 hours; use should be limited to patients unable to take capsules or oral solution; patients should be switched to an oral dosage form as soon as possible

Note: Many transplant centers administer cyclosporine as "divided dose" infusions (in 2-3 doses/day) or as a continuous (24-hour) infusion; dosages range from 3-7.5 mg/kg/day. Specific institutional protocols should be consulted.

Conversion to cyclosporine (modified) from cyclosporine (non-modified): Start with daily dose previously used and adjust to obtain preconversion cyclosporine trough concentration. Plasma concentrations should be monitored every 4-7 days and dose adjusted as necessary, until desired trough level is obtained. When transferring patients with previously poor absorption of cyclosporine (non-modified), monitor trough levels at least twice weekly (especially if initial dose exceeds 10 mg/kg/day); high plasma levels are likely to occur.

Rheumatoid arthritis: Oral: Cyclosporine (modified): Initial dose: 2.5 mg/kg/day, divided twice daily; salicylates, NSAIDs, and oral glucocorticoids may be continued (refer to Drug Interactions); dose may be increased by 0.5-0.75 mg/kg/day if insufficient response is seen after 8 weeks of treatment; additional dosage increases may be made again at 12 weeks (maximum dose: 4 mg/kg/day). Discontinue if no benefit is seen by 16 weeks of therapy.

Note: Increase the frequency of blood pressure monitoring after each alteration in dosage of cyclosporine. Cyclosporine dosage should be decreased by 25% to 50% in patients with no history of hypertension who develop sustained hypertension during therapy and, if hypertension persists, treatment with cyclosporine should be discontinued.

Psoriasis: Oral: Cyclosporine (modified): Initial dose: 2.5 mg/kg/day, divided twice daily; dose may be increased by 0.5 mg/kg/day if insufficient response is seen after 4 weeks of treatment. Additional dosage increases may be made every 2 weeks if needed (maximum dose: 4 mg/kg/day). Discontinue if no benefit is seen by 6 weeks of therapy. Once patients are adequately controlled, the dose should be decreased to the lowest effective dose. Doses lower than 2.5 mg/kg/day may be effective. Treatment longer than 1 year is not recommended.

Note: Increase the frequency of blood pressure monitoring after each alteration in dosage of cyclosporine. Cyclosporine dosage should be decreased by 25% to 50% in patients with no history of hypertension who develop sustained hypertension during therapy and, if hypertension persists, treatment with cyclosporine should be discontinued.

Focal segmental glomerulosclerosis (unlabeled use): Initial: 3 mg/kg/day divided every 12 hours

Autoimmune diseases (unlabeled use): 1-3 mg/kg/day

Keratoconjunctivitis sicca: Ophthalmic: Children ≥16 years and Adults: Instill 1 drop in each eye every 12 hours

Dosage adjustment in renal impairment: For severe psoriasis:

Serum creatinine levels ≥25% above pretreatment levels: Take another sample within 2 weeks; if the level remains ≥25% above pretreatment levels, decrease dosage of cyclosporine (modified) by 25% to 50%. If two dosage adjustments do not reverse the increase in serum creatinine levels, treatment should be discontinued.

Serum creatinine levels ≥50% above pretreatment levels: Decrease cyclosporine dosage by 25% to 50%. If two dosage adjustments do not reverse the increase in serum creatinine levels, treatment should be discontinued.

Hemodialysis: Supplemental dose is not necessary.

Peritoneal dialysis: Supplemental dose is not necessary.

Dosage adjustment in hepatic impairment: Probably necessary; monitor levels closely

Stability

Capsule: Store at controlled room temperature

Injection: Store at controlled room temperature; do not refrigerate. Ampuls should be protected from light.

Ophthalmic emulsion: Store at 15°C to 25°C (59°F to 77°F). Vials are single-use; discard immediately following administration.

Oral solution: Store at controlled room temperature; do not refrigerate. Use within 2 months after opening; should be mixed in glass containers

Reconstitution:

Sandimmune® injection: Injection should be further diluted [1 mL (50 mg) of concentrate in 20-100 mL of D_5W or NS] for administration by intravenous infusion.

Stability of injection of parenteral admixture at room temperature (25°C) is 6 hours in PVC; 24 hours in Excel®, PAB® containers, or glass.

Compatibility:

Neoral® oral solution: Orange juice, apple juice; avoid changing diluents frequently; mix thoroughly and drink at once

Sandimmune® oral solution: Milk, chocolate milk, orange juice; avoid changing diluents frequently; mix thoroughly and drink at once

(Continued)

CycloSPORINE *(Continued)*

Administration

Oral solution: Do not administer liquid from plastic or styrofoam cup. May dilute Neoral® oral solution with orange juice or apple juice. May dilute Sandimmune® oral solution with milk, chocolate milk, or orange juice. Avoid changing diluents frequently. Mix thoroughly and drink at once. Use syringe provided to measure dose. Mix in a glass container and rinse container with more diluent to ensure total dose is taken. Do not rinse syringe before or after use (may cause dose variation).

I.V.: The manufacturer recommends that following dilution, intravenous admixture be administered over 2-6 hours. However, many transplant centers administer as divided doses (2-3 doses/day) or as a 24-hour continuous infusion. Discard solution after 24 hours. Anaphylaxis has been reported with I.V. use; reserve for patients who cannot take oral form. Patients should be under continuous observation for at least the first 30 minutes of the infusion, and should be monitored frequently thereafter. Maintain patent airway; other supportive measures and agents for treating anaphylaxis should be present when I.V. drug is given.

Ophthalmic emulsion: Prior to use, invert vial several times to obtain a uniform emulsion. Remove contact lenses prior to instillation of drops; may be reinserted 15 minutes after administration. May be used with artificial tears; allow 15 minute interval between products.

Monitoring Parameters Monitor blood pressure and serum creatinine after any cyclosporine dosage changes or addition, modification, or deletion of other medications. Monitor plasma concentrations periodically.

Transplant patients: Cyclosporine trough levels, serum electrolytes, renal function, hepatic function, blood pressure, lipid profile

Psoriasis therapy: Baseline blood pressure, serum creatinine (2 levels each), BUN, CBC, serum magnesium, potassium, uric acid, lipid profile. Biweekly monitoring of blood pressure, complete blood count, and levels of BUN, uric acid, potassium, lipids, and magnesium during the first 3 months of treatment for psoriasis. Monthly monitoring is recommended after this initial period. Also evaluate any atypical skin lesions prior to therapy. Increase the frequency of blood pressure monitoring after each alteration in dosage of cyclosporine. Cyclosporine dosage should be decreased by 25% to 50% in patients with no history of hypertension who develop sustained hypertension during therapy and, if hypertension persists, treatment with cyclosporine should be discontinued.

Rheumatoid arthritis: Baseline blood pressure, and serum creatinine (2 levels each); serum creatinine every 2 weeks for first 3 months, then monthly if patient is stable. Increase the frequency of blood pressure monitoring after each alteration in dosage of cyclosporine. Cyclosporine dosage should be decreased by 25% to 50% in patients with no history of hypertension who develop sustained hypertension during therapy and, if hypertension persists, treatment with cyclosporine should be discontinued.

Reference Range Reference ranges are method dependent and specimen dependent; use the same analytical method consistently

Method-dependent and specimen-dependent: Trough levels should be obtained:

Oral: 12-18 hours after dose (chronic usage)

I.V.: 12 hours after dose **or** immediately prior to next dose

Therapeutic range: Not absolutely defined, dependent on organ transplanted, time after transplant, organ function and CsA toxicity:

General range of 100-400 ng/mL

Toxic level: Not well defined, nephrotoxicity may occur at any level

Pregnancy Risk Factor C

Contraindications Hypersensitivity to cyclosporine or any component of the formulation. Rheumatoid arthritis and psoriasis: Abnormal renal function, uncontrolled hypertension, malignancies. Concomitant treatment with PUVA or UVB therapy, methotrexate, other immunosuppressive agents, coal tar, or radiation therapy are also contraindications for use in patients with psoriasis. Ophthalmic emulsion is contraindicated in patients with active ocular infections.

Warnings/Precautions [U.S. Boxed Warning]: Use caution with other potentially nephrotoxic drugs (eg, acyclovir, aminoglycoside antibiotics, amphotericin B, ciprofloxacin). **[U.S. Boxed Warning]: Increased risk of lymphomas, other malignancies, infection. [U.S. Boxed Warning]: May cause hypertension.**

Use caution when changing dosage forms; products are not equally interchangeable. Cyclosporine (modified) refers to the capsule dosage formulation of cyclosporine in an aqueous dispersion (previously referred to as "microemulsion"). **[U.S. Boxed Warning]: Cyclosporine (modified) has increased bioavailability as compared to cyclosporine (non-modified) and cannot be used interchangeably without close monitoring.** Monitor cyclosporine concentrations closely following the addition, modification, or deletion of other medications; live, attenuated vaccines may be less effective; use should be avoided.

Transplant patients: To be used initially with corticosteroids. May cause significant hyperkalemia and hyperuricemia. May cause seizures, particularly if used with high-dose corticosteroids. Encephalopathy has been reported, predisposing factors include hypertension, hypomagnesemia, hypocholesterolemia, high-dose corticosteroids, high cyclosporine serum concentration, and graft-versus-host disease; may be more common in patients with liver transplant. Make dose adjustments based on cyclosporine blood concentrations. **[U.S. Boxed Warning]: Adjustment of dose should only be made under the direct supervision of an experienced physician.** Anaphylaxis has been reported with I.V. use; reserve for patients who cannot take oral form.

Psoriasis: Patients should avoid excessive sun exposure; safety and efficacy in children <18 years of age have not been established. **[U.S. Boxed Warning]: Risk of skin cancer may be increased with a history of PUVA and possibly methotrexate or other immunosuppressants, UVB, coal tar, or radiation.**

Rheumatoid arthritis: Safety and efficacy for use in juvenile rheumatoid arthritis have not been established. If receiving other immunosuppressive agents, radiation or UV therapy, concurrent use of cyclosporine is not recommended.

Ophthalmic emulsion: Safety and efficacy have not been established in patients <16 years of age.

Products may contain corn oil, castor oil, ethanol, or propylene glycol; injection also contains Cremophor® EL (polyoxyethylated castor oil), which has been associated with rare anaphylactic reactions.

Adverse Reactions Adverse reactions reported with systemic use, including rheumatoid arthritis, psoriasis, and transplantation (kidney, liver, and heart). Percentages noted include the highest frequency regardless of indication/dosage. Frequencies may vary for specific conditions or formulation.

>10%:

Cardiovascular: Hypertension (8% to 53%), edema (5% to 14%)
Central nervous system: Headache (2% to 25%)
Dermatologic: Hirsutism (21% to 45%), hypertrichosis (5% to 19%)
Endocrine & metabolic: Triglycerides increased (15%), female reproductive disorder (9% to 11%)
Gastrointestinal: Nausea (23%), diarrhea (3% to 13%), gum hyperplasia (2% to 16%), abdominal discomfort (<1% to 15%), dyspepsia (2% to 12%)
Neuromuscular & skeletal: Tremor (7% to 55%), paresthesia (1% to 11%), leg cramps/muscle contractions (2% to 12%)
Renal: Renal dysfunction/nephropathy (10% to 38%), creatinine increased (16% to ≥50%)
Respiratory: Upper respiratory infection (1% to 14%)
Miscellaneous: Infection (3% to 25%)

1% to 10%:

Cardiovascular: Chest pain (4% to 6%), arrhythmia (2% to 5%), abnormal heart sounds, cardiac failure, flushes (<1% to 5%), MI, peripheral ischemia
Central nervous system: Dizziness (8%), pain (6%), convulsions (1% to 5%), insomnia (4%), psychiatric events (4% to 5%), pain (3% to 4%), depression (1% to 6%), migraine (2% to 3%), anxiety, confusion, fever, hypoesthesia, emotional lability, impaired concentration, insomnia, lethargy, malaise, nervousness, paranoia, somnolence, vertigo
Dermatologic: Hypertrichosis (5% to 7%), purpura (3% to 4%), acne (1% to 6%), brittle fingernails, hair breaking, abnormal pigmentation, angioedema, cellulitis, dermatitis, dry skin, eczema, folliculitis, keratosis, pruritus, rash, skin disorder, skin malignancies, urticaria
Endocrine & metabolic: Gynecomastia (<1% to 4%), menstrual disorder (1% to 3%), breast fibroadenosis, breast pain, hyper-/hypoglycemia, diabetes mellitus, goiter, hot flashes, hyperkalemia, hyperuricemia, libido increased/decreased

(Continued)

CycloSPORINE *(Continued)*

Gastrointestinal: Vomiting (2% to 10%), flatulence (5%), gingivitis (up to 4%), cramps (up to 4%), anorexia, constipation, dry mouth, dysphagia, enanthema, eructation, esophagitis, gastric ulcer, gastritis, gastroenteritis, gastrointestinal bleeding (upper), gingival bleeding, glossitis, mouth sores, peptic ulcer, pancreatitis, swallowing difficulty, salivary gland enlargement, taste perversion, tongue disorder, tooth disorder, weight loss/gain

Genitourinary: Leukorrhea (1%), abnormal urine, micturition increased, micturition urgency, nocturia, polyuria, pyelonephritis, urinary incontinence, uterine hemorrhage

Hematologic: Leukopenia (<1% to 6%), anemia, bleeding disorder, clotting disorder, platelet disorder, red blood cell disorder, thrombocytopenia

Hepatic: Hepatotoxicity (<1% to 7%), hyperbilirubinemia

Neuromuscular & skeletal: Arthralgia (1% to 6%), bone fracture, joint dislocation, joint pain, muscle pain, myalgia, neuropathy, stiffness, synovial cyst, tendon disorder, tingling, weakness

Ocular: Abnormal vision, cataract, conjunctivitis, eye pain, visual disturbance

Otic: Deafness, hearing loss, tinnitus, vestibular disorder

Renal: BUN increased, hematuria, renal abscess

Respiratory: Sinusitis (<1% to 7%), bronchospasm (up to 5%), cough (3% to 5%), pharyngitis (3% to 5%), dyspnea (1% to 5%), rhinitis (up to 5%), abnormal chest sounds, epistaxis, respiratory infection, pneumonia (up to 1%)

Miscellaneous: Flu-like symptoms (8% to 10%), lymphoma (<1% to 6% reported in transplant), abscess, allergic reactions, bacterial infection, carcinoma, diaphoresis increased, fungal infection, herpes simplex, herpes zoster, hiccups, lymphadenopathy, moniliasis, night sweats, tonsillitis, viral infection

Postmarketing and/or case reports (any indication): Anaphylaxis/anaphylactoid reaction (possibly associated with Cremophor® EL vehicle in injection formulation), benign intracranial hypertension, cholesterol increased, death (due to renal deterioration), encephalopathy, gout, hyperbilirubinemia, hyperkalemia, hypomagnesemia (mild), impaired consciousness, neurotoxicity, papilloedema, pulmonary edema (noncardiogenic), uric acid increased

Ophthalmic emulsion (Restasis®):

>10%: Ocular: Burning (17%)

1% to 10%: Ocular: Hyperemia (conjunctival 5%), eye pain, pruritus, stinging

Overdosage/Toxicology Symptoms of overdose include hepatotoxicity, nephrotoxicity, nausea, vomiting, tremor. CNS secondary to direct action of the drug may not be reflected in serum concentrations, may be more predictable by renal magnesium loss. Forced emesis may be beneficial if done within 2 hours of ingestion of oral cyclosporine. Treatment is symptom-directed and supportive. Cyclosporine is not dialyzable.

Drug Interactions **Substrate** of CYP3A4 (major); **Inhibits** CYP2C9 (weak), 3A4 (moderate)

ACE inhibitors: May enhance nephrotoxic effects of cyclosporine.

Allopurinol: Increases cyclosporine concentrations by inhibiting cyclosporine metabolism.

Amiodarone: May increase cyclosporine concentrations by inhibiting cyclosporine metabolism.

Antibiotics: Concomitant use may potentiate renal dysfunction (seen with ciprofloxacin, gentamicin, tobramycin, vancomycin, trimethoprim and sulfamethoxazole); increased cyclosporine concentrations by inhibiting cyclosporine metabolism (seen with azithromycin, clarithromycin, erythromycin, and norfloxacin, quinupristin/dalfopristin); may decrease cyclosporine concentrations by inducing cyclosporine metabolism (seen with nafcillin, and rifampin); may decrease immunosuppressant effects (seen with ciprofloxacin); CNS disturbances, seizures (seen with imipenem).

Anticonvulsants: May decrease cyclosporine concentrations by inducing cyclosporine metabolism (seen with carbamazepine, phenobarbital, and phenytoin)

Antineoplastics: Concomitant use may potentiate renal dysfunction (seen with melphalan)

Antifungals: Concomitant use may potentiate renal dysfunction (seen with amphotericin B, ketoconazole); increase cyclosporine concentrations by inhibiting cyclosporine metabolism (seen with fluconazole, itraconazole, and ketoconazole)

Bosentan: Cyclosporine may increase the serum concentration of bosentan. Bosentan may decrease the serum concentration of cyclosporine. Concurrent use is contraindicated..

Bromocriptine: Increases cyclosporine concentrations by inhibiting cyclosporine metabolism

Calcium channel blockers (diltiazem, nicardipine, verapamil): Increase cyclosporine concentrations by inhibiting cyclosporine metabolism. Nifedipine has been reported to increase the risk of gingival hyperplasia.

Colchicine: May potentiate renal dysfunction; colchicine may increase cyclosporine concentrations by inhibiting metabolism. Cyclosporine may decrease the clearance of colchicine.

Corticosteroids: Systemic corticosteroids may increase the serum concentration of cyclosporine (reported with methylprednisolone). Cyclosporine may increase the serum concentration of systemic corticosteroids. Convulsions have been reported with high-dose methylprednisolone.

CYP3A4 inducers: CYP3A4 inducers may decrease the levels/effects of cyclosporine. Example inducers include aminoglutethimide, carbamazepine, nafcillin, nevirapine, phenobarbital, phenytoin, and rifamycins.

CYP3A4 inhibitors: May increase the levels/effects of cyclosporine. Example inhibitors include azole antifungals, clarithromycin, diclofenac, doxycycline, erythromycin, imatinib, isoniazid, nefazodone, nicardipine, propofol, protease inhibitors, quinidine, telithromycin, and verapamil.

CYP3A4 substrates: Cyclosporine may increase the levels/effects of CYP3A4 substrates. Example substrates include benzodiazepines, calcium channel blockers, cyclosporine, mirtazapine, nateglinide, nefazodone, sildenafil (and other PDE-5 inhibitors), tacrolimus, and venlafaxine. Selected benzodiazepines (midazolam and triazolam), cisapride, ergot alkaloids, selected HMG-CoA reductase inhibitors (lovastatin and simvastatin), and pimozide are generally contraindicated with strong CYP3A4 inhibitors.

Danazol: Increases cyclosporine concentrations by inhibiting cyclosporine metabolism

Digoxin: Decreased clearance and decreased volume of distribution of digoxin; severe digitalis toxicity has been observed.

Fibric acid derivatives: May increase the risk of renal dysfunction and may alter cyclosporine concentrations; monitor.

H_2 blockers: Concomitant use may potentiate renal dysfunction (seen with cimetidine, ranitidine).

HMG-CoA reductase inhibitors: Cyclosporine may increase levels/effects of HMG-CoA reductase inhibitors, resulting in myalgias, rhabdomyolysis, acute renal failure; dosage adjustments of HMG-CoA reductase inhibitors are recommended.

Imatinib: May increase cyclosporine serum concentrations by inhibiting cyclosporine metabolism.

Immunosuppressives: Concomitant use may potentiate renal dysfunction (seen with tacrolimus, muromonab-CD3).

Metoclopramide: Increases cyclosporine concentrations by inhibiting cyclosporine metabolism.

Methotrexate: Cyclosporine increases plasma levels of methotrexate and decreases plasma levels of its metabolite; monitor closely for signs of toxicity.

Minoxidil: Concomitant use may lead to severe hypertrichosis.

NSAIDs: Concomitant use may potentiate renal dysfunction, especially in dehydrated patients (seen with diclofenac, naproxen, sulindac). In addition, diclofenac plasma levels are doubled when given with cyclosporine; the lowest possible dose of diclofenac should be used. Monitor serum creatinine.

Octreotide: May decrease cyclosporine concentrations by inducing cyclosporine metabolism.

Oral contraceptives (hormonal): May increase serum levels of cyclosporine; monitor for signs of toxicity.

Orlistat: May decrease absorption of cyclosporine; avoid concomitant use.

Protease inhibitors: Formal interaction studies have not been done; protease inhibitors are known to induce CYP3A4; use caution when using cyclosporine with indinavir, nelfinavir, ritonavir, or saquinavir.

Rifabutin: Formal interaction studies have not been done; rifabutin is known to increase the metabolism of medications via CYP3A4.

Sirolimus: Cyclosporine may increase serum levels/effects; monitor. Concurrent therapy may increase the risk of HUS/TTP/TMA. Administer sirolimus 4 hours after cyclosporine to minimize the increase in sirolimus blood levels.

(Continued)

CycloSPORINE *(Continued)*

Sulfinpyrazone: May decrease cyclosporine levels by inducing cyclosporine metabolism; monitor.

Ticlopidine: May decrease cyclosporine concentrations by inducing cyclosporine metabolism.

Vaccines: Vaccination may be less effective; avoid use of live vaccines during therapy.

Voriconazole: Cyclosporine serum concentrations may be increased; monitor serum concentrations and renal function. Decrease cyclosporine dosage by 50% when initiating voriconazole.

Ethanol/Nutrition/Herb Interactions

Food: Grapefruit juice increases absorption; unsupervised use should be avoided.

Herb/Nutraceutical: Avoid St John's wort; as an enzyme inducer, it may increase the metabolism of and decrease plasma levels of cyclosporine; organ rejection and graft loss have been reported. Avoid cat's claw, echinacea (have immunostimulant properties).

Test Interactions Specific whole blood, HPLC assay for cyclosporine may be falsely elevated if sample is drawn from the same line through which dose was administered (even if flush has been administered and/or dose was given hours before).

Dietary Considerations Administer this medication consistently with relation to time of day and meals. Avoid grapefruit juice.

Dosage Forms

Capsule, soft gel, modified: 25 mg, 100 mg [contains castor oil, ethanol]
- Gengraf®: 25 mg, 100 mg [contains ethanol, castor oil, propylene glycol]
- Neoral®: 25 mg, 100 mg [contains dehydrated ethanol, corn oil, castor oil, propylene glycol]

Capsule, soft gel, non-modified (Sandimmune®): 25 mg, 100 mg [contains dehydrated ethanol, corn oil]

Emulsion, ophthalmic [preservative free, single-use vial] (Restasis®): 0.05% (0.4 mL) [contains glycerin, castor oil, polysorbate 80, carbomer 1342; 32 vials/box]

Injection, solution, non-modified (Sandimmune®): 50 mg/mL (5 mL) [contains Cremophor® EL (polyoxyethylated castor oil), ethanol]

Solution, oral, modified:
- Gengraf®: 100 mg/mL (50 mL) [contains castor oil, propylene glycol]
- Neoral®: 100 mg/mL (50 mL) [contains dehydrated ethanol, corn oil, castor oil, propylene glycol]

Solution, oral, non-modified (Sandimmune®): 100 mg/mL (50 mL) [contains olive oil, ethanol]

Cyproheptadine (si proe HEP ta deen)

Medication Safety Issues

Sound-alike/look-alike issues:
- Cyproheptadine may be confused with cyclobenzaprine
- Periactin may be confused with Perative®, Percodan®, Persantine®

Synonyms Cyproheptadine Hydrochloride; Periactin

Pharmacologic Category Antihistamine

Generic Available Yes

Use Perennial and seasonal allergic rhinitis and other allergic symptoms including urticaria

Unlabeled/Investigational Use Appetite stimulation, blepharospasm, cluster headaches, migraine headaches, Nelson's syndrome, pruritus, schizophrenia, spinal cord damage associated spasticity, and tardive dyskinesia

Mechanism of Action A potent antihistamine and serotonin antagonist, competes with histamine for H_1-receptor sites on effector cells in the gastrointestinal tract, blood vessels, and respiratory tract

Pharmacodynamics/Kinetics

Absorption: Completely

Metabolism: Almost completely hepatic

Excretion: Urine (>50% primarily as metabolites); feces (~25%)

Dosage Oral:

Children:

Allergic conditions: 0.25 mg/kg/day or 8 mg/m²/day in 2-3 divided doses **or**

2-6 years: 2 mg every 8-12 hours (not to exceed 12 mg/day)
7-14 years: 4 mg every 8-12 hours (not to exceed 16 mg/day)
Migraine headaches: 4 mg 2-3 times/day
Children ≥12 years and Adults: Spasticity associated with spinal cord damage: 4 mg at bedtime; increase by a 4 mg dose every 3-4 days; average daily dose: 16 mg in divided doses; not to exceed 36 mg/day
Children >13 years and Adults: Appetite stimulation (anorexia nervosa): 2 mg 4 times/day; may be increased gradually over a 3-week period to 8 mg 4 times/day
Adults:
Allergic conditions: 4-20 mg/day divided every 8 hours (not to exceed 0.5 mg/kg/day)
Cluster headaches: 4 mg 4 times/day
Migraine headaches: 4-8 mg 3 times/day
Dosage adjustment in hepatic impairment: Reduce dosage in patients with significant hepatic dysfunction

Anesthesia and Critical Care Concerns/Other Considerations May stimulate appetite; in case reports, cyproheptadine has promoted weight gain in anorexic adults.

Pregnancy Risk Factor B

Contraindications Hypersensitivity to cyproheptadine or any component of the formulation; narrow-angle glaucoma; bladder neck obstruction; acute asthmatic attack; stenosing peptic ulcer; GI tract obstruction; concurrent use of MAO inhibitors; avoid use in premature and term newborns due to potential association with SIDS

Warnings/Precautions Do not use in neonates, safety and efficacy have not been established in children <2 years of age; symptomatic prostate hypertrophy; antihistamines are more likely to cause dizziness, excessive sedation, syncope, toxic confusion states, and hypotension in the elderly. In case reports, cyproheptadine has promoted weight gain in anorexic adults, though it has not been specifically studied in the elderly. All cases of weight loss or decreased appetite should be adequately assessed.

Adverse Reactions
>10%:
Central nervous system: Slight to moderate drowsiness
Respiratory: Thickening of bronchial secretions
1% to 10%:
Central nervous system: Headache, fatigue, nervousness, dizziness
Gastrointestinal: Appetite stimulation, nausea, diarrhea, abdominal pain, dry mouth
Neuromuscular & skeletal: Arthralgia
Respiratory: Pharyngitis
<1% (Limited to important or life-threatening): Bronchospasm, CNS stimulation, depression, epistaxis, hemolytic anemia, hepatitis, leukopenia, sedation, seizure, thrombocytopenia

Overdosage/Toxicology Symptoms of overdose include CNS depression or stimulation, dry mouth, flushed skin, fixed and dilated pupils, and apnea. There is no specific treatment for antihistamine overdose. Clinical toxicity is due to blockade of cholinergic receptors. For anticholinergic overdose with severe life-threatening symptoms, physostigmine 1-2 mg I.V. slowly, may be given to reverse these effects.

Drug Interactions
Cyproheptadine may potentiate the effect of CNS depressants.
MAO inhibitors may cause hallucinations when taken with cyproheptadine.

Ethanol/Nutrition/Herb Interactions Ethanol: Avoid ethanol (may increase CNS sedation).

Test Interactions Diagnostic antigen skin test results may be suppressed; false positive serum TCA screen

Dosage Forms
Syrup, as hydrochloride: 2 mg/5 mL (473 mL) [contains alcohol 5%; mint flavor]
Tablet, as hydrochloride: 4 mg

- **Cyproheptadine Hydrochloride** *see* Cyproheptadine *on page 344*
- **CYT** *see* Cyclophosphamide *on page 334*
- **Cytomel®** *see* Liothyronine *on page 765*
- **Cytotec®** *see* Misoprostol *on page 857*
- **Cytovene®** *see* Ganciclovir *on page 581*

◆ **Cytoxan®** *see* Cyclophosphamide *on page 334*

◆ **d4T** *see* Stavudine *on page 1205*

Daclizumab (dac KLYE zue mab)

U.S. Brand Names Zenapax®

Canadian Brand Names Zenapax®

Pharmacologic Category Immunosuppressant Agent

Generic Available No

Use Part of an immunosuppressive regimen (including cyclosporine and corticosteroids) for the prophylaxis of acute organ rejection in patients receiving renal transplant

Unlabeled/Investigational Use Graft-versus-host disease; prevention of organ rejection after heart transplant

Mechanism of Action Daclizumab is a chimeric (90% human, 10% murine) monoclonal IgG antibody produced by recombinant DNA technology. Daclizumab inhibits immune reactions by binding and blocking the alpha-chain of the interleukin-2 receptor (CD25) located on the surface of activated lymphocytes.

Pharmacodynamics/Kinetics

Distribution: V_d:

- Adults: Central compartment: 0.031 L/kg; Peripheral compartment: 0.043 L/kg
- Children: Central compartment: 0.067 L/kg; Peripheral compartment: 0.047 L/kg

Half-life elimination (estimated): Adults: Terminal: 20 days; Children: 13 days

Dosage Daclizumab is used adjunctively with other immunosuppressants (eg, cyclosporine, corticosteroids, mycophenolate mofetil, and azathioprine): I.V.:

Children: Use same weight-based dose as adults

Adults:

- Immunoprophylaxis against acute renal allograft rejection: 1 mg/kg infused over 15 minutes within 24 hours before transplantation (day 0), then every 14 days for 4 additional doses
- Treatment of graft-versus-host disease (unlabeled use, limited data): 0.5-1.5 mg/kg, repeat same dosage for transient response. Repeat doses have been administered 11-48 days following the initial dose.
- Prevention of organ rejection after heart transplant (unlabeled use): 1 mg/kg up to a maximum of 100 mg; administer within 12 hours after heart transplant and on days 8, 22, 36, and 50 post-transplant

Dosage adjustment in renal impairment: No adjustment needed.

Dosage adjustment in hepatic impairment: No data available for patients with severe impairment.

Stability Refrigerate vials at 2°C to 8°C (36°F to 46°F). Do not shake or freeze; protect undiluted solution against direct sunlight. Dose should be further diluted in 50 mL 0.9% sodium chloride solution. When mixing, gently invert bag to avoid foaming; do not shake. Do not use if solution is discolored. Diluted solution is stable for 24 hours at 4°C or for 4 hours at room temperature. Do not mix with other medications or infuse other medications through same I.V. line.

Administration For I.V. administration following dilution. Daclizumab solution should be administered within 4 hours of preparation if stored at room temperature; infuse over a 15-minute period via a peripheral or central vein.

Pregnancy Risk Factor C

Contraindications Hypersensitivity to daclizumab or any component of the formulation

Warnings/Precautions Patients on immunosuppressive therapy are at increased risk for infectious complications and secondary malignancies. Long-term effects of daclizumab on immune function are unknown. Severe hypersensitivity reactions have been rarely reported; anaphylaxis has been observed on initial exposure and following re-exposure; medications for the management of severe allergic reaction should be available for immediate use. Anti-idiotype antibodies have been measured in patients that have received daclizumab (adults 14%; children 34%); detection of antibodies may be influenced by multiple factors and may therefore be misleading.

In cardiac transplant patients, the combined use of daclizumab, cyclosporine, mycophenolate mofetil, and corticosteroids has been associated with an increased mortality. Higher mortality may be associated with the use of antilymphocyte globulin and a higher incidence of severe infections. **[U.S. Boxed**

Warning]: Should be administered under the supervision of a physician experienced in immunosuppressive therapy.

Adverse Reactions Although reported adverse events are frequent, when daclizumab is compared with placebo the incidence of adverse effects is similar between the two groups. Many of the adverse effects reported during clinical trial use of daclizumab may be related to the patient population, transplant procedure, and concurrent transplant medications. Diarrhea, fever, postoperative pain, pruritus, respiratory tract infection, urinary tract infection, and vomiting occurred more often in children than adults.

≥5%:

Cardiovascular: Chest pain, edema, hyper-/hypotension, tachycardia, thrombosis

Central nervous system: Dizziness, fatigue, fever, headache, insomnia, pain, post-traumatic pain, tremor

Dermatologic: Acne, cellulitis, wound healing impaired

Gastrointestinal: Abdominal distention, abdominal pain, constipation, diarrhea, dyspepsia, epigastric pain, nausea, pyrosis, vomiting

Genitourinary: Dysuria

Hematologic: Bleeding

Neuromuscular & skeletal: Back pain, musculoskeletal pain

Renal: Oliguria, renal tubular necrosis

Respiratory: Cough, dyspnea, pulmonary edema

Miscellaneous: Lymphocele, wound infection

≥2% to <5%:

Central nervous system: Anxiety, depression, shivering

Dermatologic: Hirsutism, pruritus, rash

Endocrine & metabolic: Dehydration, diabetes mellitus, fluid overload

Gastrointestinal: Flatulence, gastritis, hemorrhoids

Genitourinary: Urinary retention, urinary tract bleeding

Local: Application site reaction

Neuromuscular & skeletal: Arthralgia, leg cramps, myalgia, weakness

Ocular: Vision blurred

Renal: Hydronephrosis, renal damage, renal insufficiency

Respiratory: Atelectasis, congestion, hypoxia, pharyngitis, pleural effusion, rales, rhinitis

Miscellaneous: Night sweats, prickly sensation, diaphoresis

<1% (Limited to important or life-threatening): Severe hypersensitivity reactions (rare): Anaphylaxis, bronchospasm, cardiac arrest, cytokine release syndrome, hypotension, laryngeal edema, pulmonary edema, pruritus, urticaria

Overdosage/Toxicology Overdose has not been reported.

Drug Interactions

Immunosuppressants: The combined use of daclizumab, cyclosporine, mycophenolate mofetil, and corticosteroids has been associated with an increased mortality in a population of cardiac transplant recipients, particularly in patients who received antilymphocyte globulin and in patients with severe infections.

Dosage Forms Injection, solution [preservative free]: 5 mg/mL (5 mL)

References

Vincenti F, Kirkman R, Light S, et al, "Interleukin-2 Receptor Blockade With Daclizumab to Prevent Acute Rejection in Renal Transplantation. Daclizumab Triple Therapy Study Group," *N Engl J Med*, 1998, 338(3):161-5.

♦ **Dakin's Solution** *see* Sodium Hypochlorite Solution *on page 1186*
♦ **Dalacin® C (Can)** *see* Clindamycin *on page 304*
♦ **Dalacin® T (Can)** *see* Clindamycin *on page 304*
♦ **Dalacin® Vaginal (Can)** *see* Clindamycin *on page 304*
♦ **Dalmane®** *see* Flurazepam *on page 548*

Dalteparin (dal TE pa rin)

Related Information

Continuous Renal Replacement Therapy *on page 1447*
Heparin and Low Molecular Weight Heparin (LMWH) *on page 1527*

U.S. Brand Names Fragmin®

Canadian Brand Names Fragmin®

Pharmacologic Category Low Molecular Weight Heparin

Generic Available No

(Continued)

Dalteparin *(Continued)*

Use Prevention of deep vein thrombosis which may lead to pulmonary embolism, in patients requiring abdominal surgery who are at risk for thromboembolism complications (eg, patients >40 years of age, obesity, patients with malignancy, history of deep vein thrombosis or pulmonary embolism, and surgical procedures requiring general anesthesia and lasting >30 minutes); prevention of DVT in patients undergoing hip-replacement surgery; patients immobile during an acute illness; acute treatment of unstable angina or non-Q-wave myocardial infarction; prevention of ischemic complications in patients on concurrent aspirin therapy

Unlabeled/Investigational Use Active treatment of deep vein thrombosis

Mechanism of Action Low molecular weight heparin analog with a molecular weight of 4000-6000 daltons; the commercial product contains 3% to 15% heparin with a molecular weight <3000 daltons, 65% to 78% with a molecular weight of 3000-8000 daltons and 14% to 26% with a molecular weight >8000 daltons; while dalteparin has been shown to inhibit both factor Xa and factor IIa (thrombin), the antithrombotic effect of dalteparin is characterized by a higher ratio of antifactor Xa to antifactor IIa activity (ratio = 4)

Pharmacodynamics/Kinetics

Onset of action: 1-2 hours

Duration: >12 hours

Half-life elimination (route dependent): 2-5 hours

Time to peak, serum: 4 hours

Dosage Adults: SubQ:

Abdominal surgery:

Low-to-moderate DVT risk: 2500 int. units 1-2 hours prior to surgery, then once daily for 5-10 days postoperatively

High DVT risk: 5000 int. units 1-2 hours prior to surgery and then once daily for 5-10 days postoperatively

Patients undergoing total hip surgery: **Note:** Three treatment options are currently available. Dose is given for 5-10 days, although up to 14 days of treatment have been tolerated in clinical trials:

Postoperative start:

Initial: 2500 int. units 4-8 hours* after surgery

Maintenance: 5000 int. units once daily; start at least 6 hours after post-surgical dose

Preoperative (starting day of surgery):

Initial: 2500 int. units within 2 hours before surgery

Adjustment: 2500 int. units 4-8 hours* after surgery

Maintenance: 5000 int. units once daily; start at least 6 hours after post-surgical dose

Preoperative (starting evening prior to surgery):

Initial: 5000 int. units 10-14 hours before surgery

Adjustment: 5000 int. units 4-8 hours* after surgery

Maintenance: 5000 int. units once daily, allowing 24 hours between doses.

***Dose may be delayed if hemostasis is not yet achieved.**

Unstable angina or non-Q-wave myocardial infarction: 120 int. units/kg body weight (maximum dose: 10,000 int. units) every 12 hours for 5-8 days with concurrent aspirin therapy. Discontinue dalteparin once patient is clinically stable.

Immobility during acute illness: 5000 int. units once daily

Dosing adjustment in renal impairment: Half-life is increased in patients with chronic renal failure, use with caution, accumulation can be expected; specific dosage adjustments have not been recommended

Dosing adjustment in hepatic impairment: Use with caution in patients with hepatic insufficiency; specific dosage adjustments have not been recommended

Stability Store at temperatures 20°C to 25°C (68°F to 77°F).

Administration For deep SubQ injection only. May be injected in a U-shape to the area surrounding the navel, the upper outer side of the thigh, or the upper outer quadrangle of the buttock. Apply pressure to injection site; do not massage. Use thumb and forefinger to lift a fold of skin when injecting dalteparin to the navel area or thigh. Insert needle at a 45- to 90-degree angle. The entire length of needle should be inserted. Do not expel air bubble from fixed-dose syringe prior to injection. Air bubble (and extra solution, if applicable) may be expelled from graduated syringes.

Administration once daily beginning prior to surgery and continuing 5-10 days after surgery prevents deep vein thrombosis in patients at risk for thromboembolic complications. For unstable angina or non-Q-wave myocardial infarction, dalteparin is administered every 12 hours until the patient is stable (5-8 days).

Monitoring Parameters Periodic CBC including platelet count; stool occult blood tests; monitoring of PT and PTT is not necessary

Anesthesia and Critical Care Concerns/Other Considerations Many critically-ill and surgery patients require preventive measures for venous thromboembolism. LMWHs compare favorably to unfractionated heparin in the prevention and treatment of venous thromboembolism. LMWHs are associated with less thrombocytopenia, compared to heparin, and do not require routine therapeutic monitoring.

Obesity/Renal Dysfunction: There is no consensus for adjusting/correcting the weight-based dosage of LMWH for patients who are morbidly obese. Monitoring of antifactor Xa concentration 4 hours after injection may be warranted. Patients who have a reduction in calculated creatinine clearance are at risk of accumulated anticoagulant effect when they are treated with certain LMWHs. All LMWHs may not behave the same in patients with renal dysfunction. Some clinicians monitor anti-Xa levels for patients with Cl_{cr} <30 mL/minute.

Pregnancy Risk Factor B

Contraindications Hypersensitivity to dalteparin or any component of the formulation; thrombocytopenia associated with a positive *in vitro* test for antiplatelet antibodies in the presence of dalteparin; hypersensitivity to heparin or pork products; patients with active major bleeding; patients with unstable angina or non-Q-wave MI undergoing regional anesthesia; not for I.M. or I.V. use

Warnings/Precautions [U.S. Boxed Warning]: Patients with recent or anticipated neuraxial anesthesia (epidural or spinal anesthesia) are at risk of spinal or epidural hematoma and subsequent paralysis. Consider risk versus benefit prior to neuraxial anesthesia. Risk is increased by concomitant agents which may alter hemostasis, as well as traumatic or repeated epidural or spinal puncture. Patient should be observed closely for bleeding if dalteparin is administered during or immediately following diagnostic lumbar puncture, epidural anesthesia, or spinal anesthesia.

Not to be used interchangeably (unit for unit) with heparin or any other low molecular weight heparins. Use with caution in patients with known hypersensitivity to methylparaben or propylparaben. Use with caution in patients with history of heparin-induced thrombocytopenia. Monitor platelet count closely. Rare thrombocytopenia may occur. Consider discontinuation of dalteparin in any patient developing significant thrombocytopenia. Monitor patient closely for signs or symptoms of bleeding. Certain patients are at increased risk of bleeding. Risk factors include bacterial endocarditis; congenital or acquired bleeding disorders; active ulcerative or angiodysplastic GI diseases; severe uncontrolled hypertension; hemorrhagic stroke; or use shortly after brain, spinal, or ophthalmology surgery; in patient treated concomitantly with platelet inhibitors; recent GI bleeding; thrombocytopenia or platelet defects; severe liver disease; hypertensive or diabetic retinopathy; or in patients undergoing invasive procedures.

Use with caution in patients with severe renal failure (has not been studied). Safety and efficacy in pediatric patients have not been established. Rare cases of thrombocytopenia with thrombosis have occurred. Multidose vials contain benzyl alcohol and should not be used in pregnant women. Heparin can cause hyperkalemia by affecting aldosterone. Similar reactions could occur with LMWHs. Monitor for hyperkalemia.

Adverse Reactions

1% to 10%:

Hematologic: Bleeding (3% to 5%), wound hematoma (0.1% to 3%)

Local: Pain at injection site (up to 12%), injection site hematoma (0.2% to 7%)

<1% (Limited to important or life-threatening): Allergic reaction (fever, pruritus, rash, injection site reaction, bullous eruption), anaphylactoid reaction, gastrointestinal bleeding, injection site hematoma, operative site bleeding, skin necrosis, thrombocytopenia (including heparin-induced thrombocytopenia). Spinal or epidural hematomas can occur following neuraxial anesthesia or spinal puncture, resulting in paralysis. Risk is increased in patients with indwelling epidural catheters or concomitant use of other drugs affecting hemostasis, osteoporosis (3-6 month use).

(Continued)

Dalteparin *(Continued)*

Drug Interactions

Drugs which affect platelet function (eg, aspirin, NSAIDs, dipyridamole, ticlopidine, clopidogrel) may potentiate the risk of hemorrhage.

Thrombolytic agents increase the risk of hemorrhage.

Warfarin: Risk of bleeding may be increased during concurrent therapy. Dalteparin is commonly continued during the initiation of warfarin therapy to assure anticoagulation and to protect against possible transient hypercoagulability.

Ethanol/Nutrition/Herb Interactions Herb/Nutraceutical: Avoid cat's claw, dong quai, evening primrose, garlic, ginseng (all have additional antiplatelet activity).

Dosage Forms

Injection, solution [multidose vial]: Antifactor Xa 10,000 int. units per 1 mL (9.5 mL) [contains benzyl alcohol]; antifactor Xa 25,000 units per 1 mL (3.8 mL) [contains benzyl alcohol]

Injection, solution [preservative free; prefilled syringe]: Antifactor Xa 2500 int. units per 0.2 mL (0.2 mL); antifactor Xa 5000 int. units per 0.2 mL (0.2 mL); antifactor Xa 7500 int. units per 0.3 mL (0.3 mL); antifactor Xa 10,000 int. units per 1 mL (1 mL)

References

Nagge J, Crowther M, and Hirsh J, "Is Impaired Renal Function a Contraindication to the Use of Low-Molecular Weight Heparin?" *Arch Intern Med*, 2002, 162(22):2605-9.

♦ **Dantrium®** *see* Dantrolene *on page 350*

Dantrolene (DAN troe leen)

Medication Safety Issues

Sound-alike/look-alike issues:

Dantrium® may be confused with danazol, Daraprim®

U.S. Brand Names Dantrium®

Canadian Brand Names Dantrium®

Synonyms Dantrolene Sodium

Pharmacologic Category Skeletal Muscle Relaxant

Generic Available No

Use Treatment of spasticity associated with spinal cord injury, stroke, cerebral palsy, or multiple sclerosis; treatment of malignant hyperthermia

Unlabeled/Investigational Use Neuroleptic malignant syndrome (NMS)

Mechanism of Action Acts directly on skeletal muscle by interfering with release of calcium ion from the sarcoplasmic reticulum; prevents or reduces the increase in myoplasmic calcium ion concentration that activates the acute catabolic processes associated with malignant hyperthermia

Pharmacodynamics/Kinetics

Absorption: Oral: Slow and incomplete

Metabolism: Hepatic

Half-life elimination: 8.7 hours

Excretion: Feces (45% to 50%); urine (25% as unchanged drug and metabolites)

Dosage

Spasticity: Oral:

Children: Initial: 0.5 mg/kg/dose twice daily, increase frequency to 3-4 times/day at 4- to 7-day intervals, then increase dose by 0.5 mg/kg to a maximum of 3 mg/kg/dose 2-4 times/day up to 400 mg/day

Adults: 25 mg/day to start, increase frequency to 2-4 times/day, then increase dose by 25 mg every 4-7 days to a maximum of 100 mg 2-4 times/day or 400 mg/day

Malignant hyperthermia: Children and Adults:

Preoperative prophylaxis:

Oral: 4-8 mg/kg/day in 4 divided doses, begin 1-2 days prior to surgery with last dose 3-4 hours prior to surgery

I.V.: 2.5 mg/kg ~1¼ hours prior to anesthesia and infused over 1 hour with additional doses as needed and individualized

Crisis: I.V.: 2.5 mg/kg; may repeat dose up to cumulative dose of 10 mg/kg; if physiologic and metabolic abnormalities reappear, repeat regimen

Postcrisis follow-up: Oral: 4-8 mg/kg/day in 4 divided doses for 1-3 days; I.V. dantrolene may be used when oral therapy is not practical; individualize dosage beginning with 1 mg/kg or more as the clinical situation dictates

Neuroleptic malignant syndrome (unlabeled use): I.V.: 1 mg/kg; may repeat dose up to maximum cumulative dose of 10 mg/kg, then switch to oral dosage

Stability Reconstitute vial by adding 60 mL of sterile water for injection USP (**not bacteriostatic water for injection**); protect from light; use within 6 hours; avoid glass bottles for I.V. infusion

Administration I.V.: Therapeutic or emergency dose can be administered with rapid continuous I.V. push. Follow-up doses should be administered over 2-3 minutes.

Monitoring Parameters Motor performance should be monitored for therapeutic outcomes; nausea, vomiting, and liver function tests should be monitored for potential hepatotoxicity; intravenous administration requires cardiac monitor and blood pressure monitor

Pregnancy Risk Factor C

Contraindications Active hepatic disease; should not be used where spasticity is used to maintain posture or balance

Warnings/Precautions Use with caution in patients with impaired cardiac function or impaired pulmonary function. **[U.S. Boxed Warning]: Has potential for hepatotoxicity.** Overt hepatitis has been most frequently observed between the third and twelfth month of therapy. Hepatic injury appears to be greater in females and in patients >35 years of age.

Adverse Reactions

>10%:

Central nervous system: Drowsiness, dizziness, lightheadedness, fatigue
Dermatologic: Rash
Gastrointestinal: Diarrhea (mild), vomiting
Neuromuscular & skeletal: Muscle weakness

1% to 10%:

Cardiovascular: Pleural effusion with pericarditis
Central nervous system: Chills, fever, headache, insomnia, nervousness, mental depression
Gastrointestinal: Diarrhea (severe), constipation, anorexia, stomach cramps
Ocular: Blurred vision
Respiratory: Respiratory depression

<1% (Limited to important or life-threatening): Confusion, hepatic necrosis, hepatitis, seizure

Overdosage/Toxicology Symptoms of overdose include CNS depression, hypotension, nausea, and vomiting. For decontamination, lavage with activated charcoal and administer a cathartic. Do not use ipecac. Other treatment is supportive and symptomatic.

Drug Interactions Substrate of CYP3A4 (major)

CYP3A4 inducers: CYP3A4 inducers may decrease the levels/effects of dantrolene. Example inducers include aminoglutethimide, carbamazepine, nafcillin, nevirapine, phenobarbital, phenytoin, and rifamycins.

CYP3A4 inhibitors: May increase the levels/effects of dantrolene. Example inhibitors include azole antifungals, clarithromycin, diclofenac, doxycycline, erythromycin, imatinib, isoniazid, nefazodone, nicardipine, propofol, protease inhibitors, quinidine, telithromycin, and verapamil.

Increased toxicity: Estrogens (hepatotoxicity), CNS depressants (sedation), MAO inhibitors, phenothiazines, clindamycin (increased neuromuscular blockade), verapamil (hyperkalemia and cardiac depression), warfarin, clofibrate, and tolbutamide

Ethanol/Nutrition/Herb Interactions

Ethanol: Avoid ethanol (may increase CNS depression).

Herb/Nutraceutical: Avoid valerian, St John's wort, kava kava, gotu kola (may increase CNS depression).

Dosage Forms

Capsule, as sodium: 25 mg, 50 mg, 100 mg

Injection, powder for reconstitution, as sodium: 20 mg [contains mannitol 3 g]

References

Guerrero RM and Shifrar KA, "Diagnosis and Treatment of Neuroleptic Malignant Syndrome," *Clin Pharm*, 1988, 7(9):697-701.

Rosenberg MR and Green M, "Neuroleptic Malignant Syndrome. Review of Response to Therapy," *Arch Intern Med*, 1989, 149(9):1927-31.

♦ **Dantrolene Sodium** *see* Dantrolene *on page 350*

♦ **Dapcin** *see* Daptomycin *on page 352*

Daptomycin (DAP toe mye sin)

U.S. Brand Names Cubicin®

Synonyms Cidecin; Dapcin; LY146032

Pharmacologic Category Antibiotic, Cyclic Lipopeptide

Generic Available No

Use Treatment of complicated skin and skin structure infections caused by susceptible aerobic Gram-positive organisms; bacteremia, including right-sided infective endocarditis caused by MSSA or MRSA

Unlabeled/Investigational Use Treatment of severe infections caused by MRSA or VRE

Mechanism of Action Daptomycin binds to components of the cell membrane of susceptible organisms and causes rapid depolarization, inhibiting intracellular synthesis of DNA, RNA, and protein. Daptomycin is bactericidal in a concentration-dependent manner.

Pharmacodynamics/Kinetics

Distribution: 0.09 L/kg

Protein binding: 90% to 93%; 84% to 88% in patients with Cl_{cr}<30 mL/minute

Half-life elimination: 8-9 hours (up to 28 hours in renal impairment)

Excretion: Urine (78%; primarily as unchanged drug); feces (6%)

Dosage I.V.: Adults:

Skin and soft tissue: 4 mg/kg once daily for 7-14 days

Bacteremia, right-sided endocarditis caused by MSSA or MRSA: 6 mg/kg once daily for 2-6 weeks

Dosage adjustment in renal impairment: Cl_{cr} <30 mL/minute:

Skin and soft tissue infections: 4 mg/kg every 48 hours

Staphylococcal bacteremia: 6 mg/kg every 48 hours

Hemodialysis (administer after hemodialysis) and/or CAPD: Dose as in Cl_{cr} <30 mL/minute

Dosage adjustment in hepatic impairment: No adjustment required for mild-to-moderate impairment (Child-Pugh Class A or B); not evaluated in severe hepatic impairment

Stability Store under refrigeration at 2°C to 8°C (36°F to 46°F). Reconstitute vial with 10 mL NS. Should be further diluted following reconstitution in an appropriate volume of NS. Reconstituted solution (either in vial or in infusion bag) is stable for a cumulative time of 12 hours at room temperature and 48 hours if refrigerated (2°C to 8°C).

Administration Infuse over 30 minutes.

Monitoring Parameters Monitor signs and symptoms of infection. CPK should be monitored at least weekly during therapy.

Reference Range

Trough concentrations at steady-state:

4 mg/kg once daily: 5.9 ± 1.6 mcg/mL

6 mg/kg once daily: 6.7 ± 1.6 mcg/mL

Note: Trough concentrations are not predictive of efficacy/toxicity. Drug exhibits concentration-dependent bactericidal activity, so C_{max}:MIC ratios may be a more useful parameter.

Pregnancy Risk Factor B

Contraindications Hypersensitivity to daptomycin or any component of the formulation

Warnings/Precautions May be associated with an increased incidence of myopathy; discontinue in patients with signs and symptoms of myopathy in conjunction with an increase in CPK (>5 times ULN or 1000 units/L) or in asymptomatic patients with a CPK ≥10 times ULN. Myopathy may occur more frequently at dose and/or frequency in excess of recommended dosages. Use caution in patients receiving other drugs associated with myopathy (eg, HMG-CoA reductase inhibitors). Not indicated for the treatment of pneumonia (poor lung penetration). Use caution in renal impairment (dosage adjustment required). Symptoms suggestive of peripheral neuropathy have been observed with treatment; monitor for new-onset or worsening neuropathy. Superinfection by resistant strains and/or pseudomembranous colitis may be associated with use. Safety and efficacy in patients <18 years of age have not been established.

Adverse Reactions

>10%:

Cardiovascular: Anemia (2% to 13%)

Gastrointestinal: Diarrhea (5% to 12%), vomiting (3% to 12%), constipation (6% to 11%)

1% to 10%:

Cardiovascular: Peripheral edema (7%), chest pain (7%), hypertension (1% to 6%), hypotension (2% to 5%)

Central nervous system: insomnia (5% to 9%), headache (5% to7%), fever (2% to 7%), dizziness (2% to 6%), anxiety (5%)

Dermatologic: Rash (4% to 7%), pruritus (3% to 6%), erythema (5%), diaphoresis (5%)

Endocrine & metabolic: Hypokalemia (9%), hyperkalemia (5%), hyperphosphatemia (3%)

Gastrointestinal: Nausea (6% to 10%), abdominal pain (6%), dyspepsia (1% to 4%), loose stool (4%), GI hemorrhage (2%)

Genitourinary: Urinary tract infection (2% to 7%)

Hematologic: INR increased (2%)

Hepatic: Transaminases increased (2% to 3%), alkaline phosphatase increased (2%)

Local: Injection-site reaction (3% to 6%)

Neuromuscular & skeletal: Limb pain (2% to 9%), back pain (7%), CPK increased (3% to 7%), weakness (5%), arthralgia (1% to 3%)

Renal: Renal failure (2% to 6%)

Respiratory: Pharyngolaryngeal pain (8%), pleural effusion (6%), cough (3%), pneumonia (3%), dyspnea (2% to 3%)

Miscellaneous: Infection (fungal, 2% to 3%)

<1% (Limited to important or life-threatening): Anaphylaxis, atrial fibrillation, atrial flutter, cardiac arrest, dysphagia, electrolyte disturbance, eosinophilia, erythema (truncal), fatigue, flushing, hallucination, hives, hypomagnesemia, hypersensitivity, jaundice, LDH increased, leukocytosis, lymphadenopathy, mental status change, muscle cramps, muscle weakness, myalgia, osteomyelitis, paresthesia, proteinuria, prothrombin time prolonged, rhabdomyolysis, rigors, serum bicarbonate increased, stomatitis, supraventricular arrhythmia, thrombocytopenia, thrombocytosis, vertigo

Overdosage/Toxicology Treatment is symptomatic and supportive; hemodialysis removes approximately 15% in 4 hours.

Drug Interactions No clinically-significant interactions have been identified.

Dosage Forms Injection, powder for reconstitution: 500 mg

References

Cha R, Grucz RG Jr, and Rybak MJ, "Daptomycin Dose-Effect Relationship Against Resistant Gram-Positive Organisms," *Antimicrob Agents Chemother*, 2003, 47(5):1598-603.

Lai JJ and Brodeur SK, "Physical and Chemical Compatibility of Daptomycin With Nine Medications," *Ann Pharmacother*, 2004, 38(10):1612-6.

Richter SS, Kealey DE, Murray CT, et al, "The *in vitro* Activity of Daptomycin Against *Staphylococcus aureus* and *Enterococcus* species," *J Antimicrob Chemother*, 2003, 52(1):123-7.

Silverman JA, Perlmutter NG, and Shapiro HM, "Correlation of Daptomycin Bactericidal Activity and Membrane Depolarization in *Staphylococcus aureus*," *Antimicrob Agents Chemother*, 2003, 47(8):2538-44.

Darbepoetin Alfa (dar be POE e tin AL fa)

Medication Safety Issues

Sound-alike/look-alike issues:

Darbepoetin alfa may be confused with epoetin alfa

U.S. Brand Names Aranesp®

Canadian Brand Names Aranesp®

Synonyms Erythropoiesis Stimulating Protein

Pharmacologic Category Colony Stimulating Factor; Growth Factor; Recombinant Human Erythropoietin

Generic Available No

Use Treatment of anemia associated with chronic renal failure (CRF), including patients on dialysis (ESRD) and patients not on dialysis; anemia associated with chemotherapy for nonmyeloid malignancies

Mechanism of Action Induces erythropoiesis by stimulating the division and differentiation of committed erythroid progenitor cells; induces the release of reticulocytes from the bone marrow into the bloodstream, where they mature to erythrocytes. There is a dose response relationship with this effect. This results in

(Continued)

Darbepoetin Alfa *(Continued)*

an increase in reticulocyte counts followed by a rise in hematocrit and hemoglobin levels. When administered SubQ or I.V., darbepoetin's half-life is ~3 times that of epoetin alfa concentrations.

Pharmacodynamics/Kinetics

Onset of action: Increased hemoglobin levels not generally observed until 2-6 weeks after initiating treatment

Absorption: SubQ: Slow

Distribution: V_d: 0.06 L/kg

Bioavailability: CRF: SubQ: ~37% (range: 30% to 50%)

Half-life elimination: CRF: Terminal: I.V.: 21 hours, SubQ: 49 hours; cancer: SubQ: 74 hours

Note: Half-life is ~3 times as long as epoetin alfa

Time to peak: SubQ: CRF: 34 hours (range: 24-72 hours); Cancer: 90 hours (range: 71-123 hours)

Dosage Adults:

Anemia associated with CRF: I.V., SubQ: Initial: 0.45 mcg/kg once weekly; titrate to response; some patients may respond to doses given once every 2 weeks

Unlabeled dosing:

Every 2-weeks: 0.75 mcg/kg every 2 weeks

or

Every 4-weeks: 0.75 mcg/kg every 2 weeks; once titrated, multiply dose by 2 and give every 4 weeks.

Dosage adjustment:

Inadequate response: Increase dose by ~25% (not more frequently than once a month) for hemoglobin increase <1 g/dL after 4 weeks

Excessive response:

Decrease dose by ~25% when hemoglobin increases >1 g/dL in any 2-week period **or** hemoglobin increases and approaches 12 g/dL in any 2-week period

Hold dose, then decrease dose by ~25% when hemoglobin increases despite previous dose decrease (hold until hemoglobin decreases)

Anemia associated with chemotherapy: SubQ: Initial: 2.25 mcg/kg once weekly; with inadequate response after 6 weeks: 4.5 mcg/kg once weekly

or

500 mcg once every 3 weeks

Unlabeled dosing:

Every 2 weeks:

Initial: 200 mcg every 2 weeks; inadequate response: 300 mcg every 2 weeks

or

Initial: 3 mcg/kg every 2 weeks; inadequate response: 5 mcg/kg every 2 weeks

or

Every 3 weeks (front load): Initial:

4.5 mcg/kg every week until desired Hgb obtained; maintenance: 4.5 mcg/kg (or titrated dose) every 3 weeks

or

Initial: 325 mcg every week until desired Hgb obtained; maintenance: 325 mcg every 3 weeks

Dosage adjustment: Titration may be required to limit rises of Hgb to <1 g/dL over any 2-week interval and to reach a hemoglobin concentration not to exceed 12 g/dL.

Inadequate response: Increase dose up to 4.5 mcg/kg when hemoglobin increase <1 g/dL after 4-6 weeks

Excessive response:

Decrease dose by ~40% when hemoglobin increases >1 g/dL in any 2-week period **or** hemoglobin exceeds 11 g/dL in any 2-week period

Hold dose, then decrease dose by ~40% when hemoglobin increases despite previous dose decrease (hold until hemoglobin decreases) **or** when hemoglobin ≥13 g/dL (hold until hemoglobin ≤12 g/dL)

Conversion from epoetin alfa to darbepoetin alfa: See table on next page.

Dosage adjustment in renal impairment: Dosage requirements for patients with chronic renal failure who do not require dialysis may be lower than in dialysis patients. Monitor patients closely during the time period in which a dialysis regimen is initiated, dosage requirement may increase.

Conversion From Epoetin Alfa to Darbepoetin Alfa

Previous Dosage of Epoetin Alfa (units/week)	Children Darbepoetin Alfa Dosage (mcg/week)	Adults Darbepoetin Alfa Dosage (mcg/week)	Adults Darbepoetin Alfa Dosage (mcg/every 2 weeks)
<1500	Not established	6.25	12.5
1500-2499	6.25	6.25	12.5
2500-4999	10	12.5	25
5000-10,999	20	25	50
11,000-17,999	40	40	80
18,000-33,999	60	60	120
34,000-89,999	100	100	200
≥90,000	200	200	400

Note: In patients receiving epoetin alfa 2-3 times per week, darbepoetin alfa is administered once weekly. In patients receiving epoetin alfa once weekly, darbepoetin alfa is administered once every 2 weeks.

Stability Store at 2°C to 8°C (36°F to 46°F). Do not freeze or shake. Protect from light. Do not dilute or administer with other solutions.

Administration May be administered by SubQ or I.V. injection. The I.V. route is recommended in hemodialysis patients. Do not shake; vigorous shaking may denature darbepoetin alfa, rendering it biologically inactive. Do not dilute or administer in conjunction with other drug solutions. Discard any unused portion of the vial; do not pool unused portions. Discontinue immediately if signs/symptoms of anaphylaxis occur.

Monitoring Parameters Hemoglobin (weekly until maintenance dose established and after dosage changes; monitor at regular intervals once hemoglobin is stabilized); iron stores (prior to and during therapy); blood pressure

Anesthesia and Critical Care Concerns/Other Considerations Recently, a prospective, randomized, double-blind, placebo-controlled, multicenter trial was performed in critically-ill patients (Corwin, 2002) assessing the efficacy of recombinant human erythropoietin in reducing red blood cell transfusions. Patients were enrolled from December 1998 through June 2001. Over thirteen hundred ICU (medical, surgical, or medical/surgical) patients were randomized to receive placebo or 40,000 units of erythropoietin subcutaneously on ICU day 3 and then weekly for patients who remained in the hospital. Each patient's physician determined the need for red blood cell transfusion. The mean baseline hemoglobin was 9.97 g/dL in each group. Patients receiving erythropoietin were less likely to receive transfusions. The mean number of units transfused per patient in the placebo group was 3 and in the erythropoietin group was 2.4. The erythropoietin group had a 19% reduction in total units of red blood cells transfused. Mortality and adverse clinical events were not significantly different between groups. The authors concluded that weekly administration of erythropoietin in critically-ill patients reduces red blood cell transfusions and increases hemoglobin. The authors also suggest that further study is needed to determine whether use of erythropoietin results in improved clinical outcomes. In addition, data on cost effectiveness would be helpful.

A restrictive transfusion approach (Hebert, 1999) was described in a transfusion trial that was published after Corwin's trial was underway. Hebert and his group evaluated a restrictive transfusion strategy (transfuse if hemoglobin <7 g/dL to maintain between 7 and 9 g/dL) versus a liberal strategy (transfuse if hemoglobin <10 g/dL to maintain between 10 and 12 g/dL). The restrictive approach to transfusion was at least as effective as, and possibly superior to, a liberal transfusion policy in critically-ill patients. The exception to this may be patients with acute myocardial infarction and unstable angina.

Pregnancy Risk Factor C

Contraindications Hypersensitivity to darbepoetin or any component of the formulation; uncontrolled hypertension

Warnings/Precautions Erythropoietic therapies may be associated with an increased risk of cardiovascular and/or neurologic events. Darbepoetin alfa should be managed carefully; avoid hemoglobin increases >1 g/dL in any 2-week

(Continued)

Darbepoetin Alfa *(Continued)*

period, and do not exceed a target level of 12 g/dL. Prior to and during therapy, iron stores must be evaluated. Supplemental iron is recommended if serum ferritin <100 mcg/mL or serum transferrin saturation <20%. In cancer patients, the risk of thrombotic events (eg, pulmonary emboli, thrombophlebitis, thrombosis) was increased by erythropoietic therapy.

Use with caution in patients with hypertension or with a history of seizures; hypertensive encephalopathy and seizures have been reported. If hypertension is difficult to control, reduce or hold darbepoetin alpha. **Not** recommended for acute correction of severe anemia or as a substitute for transfusion. Consider discontinuing in patients who receive a renal transplant.

Prior to treatment, correct or exclude deficiencies of vitamin B_{12} and/or folate, as well as other factors which may impair erythropoiesis (aluminum toxicity, inflammatory conditions, infections). Poor response should prompt evaluation of these potential factors, as well as possible malignant processes, occult blood loss, hemolysis, and/or bone marrow fibrosis. Pure red cell aplasia (PRCA) with associated neutralizing antibodies to erythropoietin has been reported, predominantly in patients with CRF. Patients with loss of response to darbepoetin alfa should be evaluated. Discontinue treatment in patients with PRCA secondary to neutralizing antibodies to erythropoietin.

Due to the delayed onset of erythropoiesis, darbepoetin is of no value in the acute treatment of anemia. Safety and efficacy in patients with underlying hematologic diseases have not been established, including porphyria, thalassemia, hemolytic anemia, and sickle cell disease. Potentially serious allergic reactions have been reported. Do not shake solution; vigorous shaking may denature darbepoetin alfa, rendering it biologically inactive. Safety and efficacy (as initial treatment) in children have not been established; children >1 year of age with CRF have been converted from epoetin alfa to darbepoetin.

Adverse Reactions Note: Frequency of adverse events cited in patients with CRF or cancer and may be, in part, a reflection of population in which the drug is used and/or associated with dialysis procedures.

>10%:

- Cardiovascular: Hypertension (4% to 23%), hypotension (22%), edema (21%), peripheral edema (11%)
- Central nervous system: Fatigue (9% to 33%), fever (4% to 19%), headache (12% to 16%), dizziness (8% to 14%)
- Gastrointestinal: Diarrhea (16% to 22%), constipation (5% to 18%), vomiting (2% to 15%), nausea (14%), abdominal pain (12%)
- Neuromuscular & skeletal: Myalgia (8% to 21%), arthralgia (11% to 13%)
- Respiratory: Upper respiratory infection (14%), dyspnea (2% to 12%)
- Miscellaneous: Infection (27%)

1% to 10%:

- Cardiovascular: Arrhythmia (10%), angina/chest pain (6% to 8%), fluid overload (6%), CHF (6%), thrombosis (6%), MI (2%)
- Central nervous system: Seizure (≤1%), stroke (1%), TIA (1%)
- Dermatologic: Pruritus (8%), rash (7%)
- Endocrine & metabolic: Dehydration (3% to 5%)
- Local: Vascular access thrombosis (8%), injection site pain (7%), vascular access hemorrhage (6%), vascular access infection (6%)
- Neuromuscular & skeletal: Limb pain (10%), back pain (8%), weakness (5%)
- Respiratory: Cough (10%), bronchitis (6%), pneumonia (3%), pulmonary embolism (1%)
- Miscellaneous: Death (7%), flu-like symptoms (6%)

Postmarketing and/or case reports: Deep vein thrombosis, pure red cell aplasia, severe anemia (with or without other cytopenias), thromboembolism, thrombophlebitis

Overdosage/Toxicology The maximum amount of darbepoetin which may be safely administered has not been determined. However, cardiovascular and neurologic adverse events have been correlated to excessive and/or rapid rise in hemoglobin. Phlebotomy may be performed if clinically indicated.

Drug Interactions No data available

Ethanol/Nutrition/Herb Interactions Ethanol: Should be avoided due to adverse effects on erythropoiesis.

Dietary Considerations Supplemental iron intake may be required in patients with low iron stores.

Dosage Forms

Injection, solution, with human albumin 2.5 mg/mL [preservative free, single-dose vial]: 25 mcg/mL (1 mL); 40 mcg/mL (1 mL); 60 mcg/mL (1 mL); 100 mcg/mL (1 mL); 150 mcg/0.75 mL (0.75 mL); 200 mcg/mL (1 mL); 300 mcg/mL (1 mL)

Injection, solution, with human albumin 2.5 mg/mL [preservative free, prefilled syringe]: 25 mcg/0.42 mL (0.42 mL); 40 mcg/0.4 mL (0.4 mL); 60 mcg/0.3 mL (0.3 mL); 100 mcg/0.5 mL (0.5 mL); 200 mcg/0.4 mL (0.4 mL); 300 mcg/0.6 mL (0.6 mL); 500 mcg/mL (1 mL)

References

Corwin HL, Gettinger A, Pearl RG, et al, "Efficacy of Recombinant Human Erythropoietin in Critically Ill Patients, A Randomized Controlled Trial," *JAMA*, 2002, 288:2827-35.

Hebert PC, Wells G, Blajchman MA, et al, "A Multicenter, Randomized, Controlled Clinical Trial of Transfusion Requirements in Critical Care," *N Engl J Med*, 1999, 340(6):409-17.

◆ **Darvocet A500™** *see* Propoxyphene and Acetaminophen *on page 1076*
◆ **Darvocet-N® 50** *see* Propoxyphene and Acetaminophen *on page 1076*
◆ **Darvocet-N® 100** *see* Propoxyphene and Acetaminophen *on page 1076*
◆ **Darvon®** *see* Propoxyphene *on page 1074*
◆ **Darvon-N®** *see* Propoxyphene *on page 1074*
◆ **Daypro®** *see* Oxaprozin *on page 964*
◆ **DDAVP®** *see* Desmopressin *on page 363*
◆ **ddI** *see* Didanosine *on page 382*
◆ **1-Deamino-8-D-Arginine Vasopressin** *see* Desmopressin *on page 363*
◆ **Decadron®** *see* Dexamethasone *on page 366*
◆ **Decadron® Phosphate [DSC]** *see* Dexamethasone *on page 366*
◆ **Deep Sea [OTC]** *see* Sodium Chloride *on page 1183*
◆ **Dehydrobenzperidol** *see* Droperidol *on page 432*
◆ **Delta-9-tetrahydro-cannabinol** *see* Dronabinol *on page 430*
◆ **Delta-9 THC** *see* Dronabinol *on page 430*
◆ **Deltacortisone** *see* PredniSONE *on page 1050*
◆ **Deltadehydrocortisone** *see* PredniSONE *on page 1050*
◆ **Deltahydrocortisone** *see* PrednisoLONE *on page 1046*
◆ **Demadex®** *see* Torsemide *on page 1291*
◆ **Demerol®** *see* Meperidine *on page 801*
◆ **Depacon®** *see* Valproic Acid and Derivatives *on page 1329*
◆ **Depade®** *see* Naltrexone *on page 897*
◆ **Depakene®** *see* Valproic Acid and Derivatives *on page 1329*
◆ **Depakote® Delayed Release** *see* Valproic Acid and Derivatives *on page 1329*
◆ **Depakote® ER** *see* Valproic Acid and Derivatives *on page 1329*
◆ **Depakote® Sprinkle®** *see* Valproic Acid and Derivatives *on page 1329*
◆ **DepoDur™** *see* Morphine Sulfate *on page 867*
◆ **Depo-Medrol®** *see* MethylPREDNISolone *on page 830*
◆ **Deprenyl** *see* Selegiline *on page 1157*
◆ **Dermamycin® [OTC]** *see* DiphenhydrAMINE *on page 399*
◆ **Dermarest Dricort® [OTC]** *see* Hydrocortisone *on page 639*
◆ **Dermarest® Insect Bite [OTC]** *see* DiphenhydrAMINE *on page 399*
◆ **Dermarest® Plus [OTC]** *see* DiphenhydrAMINE *on page 399*
◆ **Dermtex® HC [OTC]** *see* Hydrocortisone *on page 639*

Desflurane (DES flure ane)

Medication Safety Issues

Sound-alike/look-alike issues:

Desflurane may be confused with Desferal®

Related Information

Anesthesia Considerations for Neurosurgery *on page 1401*

Inhalational Anesthetics *on page 1528*

U.S. Brand Names Suprane®

Canadian Brand Names Suprane®

Pharmacologic Category General Anesthetic, Inhalation

Generic Available No

Use Maintenance of general anesthesia

(Continued)

Desflurane *(Continued)*

Pharmacodynamics/Kinetics

Onset of action: 1-2 minutes

Duration: Emergence time: Depends on blood concentration when desflurane is discontinued

The rate of change of anesthetic concentration in the lung is more rapid with desflurane because of its low blood/gas solubility (0.42), which is similar to nitrous oxide.

Metabolism: Hepatic (0.02%)

Excretion: Exhaled gases

Dosage

Children: Maintenance: Surgical levels of anesthesia range between 5.2% to 10%

Adults: The minimum alveolar concentration (MAC), the concentration at which 50% of patients do not respond to surgical incision, ranges from 6.0% (45 years of age) to 7.3% (25 years of age). The concentration at which amnesia and loss of awareness occur (MAC - awake) is 2.4%. Surgical levels of anesthesia are achieved with concentrations between 2.5% to 8.5%.

Elderly: MAC is reduced (5.2% at 70 years of age)

Note: Because of the higher vapor pressure of desflurane, its vaporizer is heated in order to deliver a constant concentration

Administration Via desflurane-specific calibrated heated vaporizer

Monitoring Parameters Blood pressure, heart rate and rhythm, temperature, oxygen saturation, end-tidal CO_2 and end-tidal desflurane concentrations should be monitored prior to and throughout anesthesia

Anesthesia and Critical Care Concerns/Other Considerations Use of desflurane for induction of general anesthesia is not recommended due to its irritant properties and unpleasant odor which may cause breath holding and coughing.

Pregnancy Risk Factor B

Contraindications Hypersensitivity to desflurane, other halogenated agents, or any component of the formulation; severe hypotension; known or suspected history of malignant hyperthermia; patients at risk for CAD; patients in whom an increase in heart rate or blood pressure is undesirable

Warnings/Precautions Decrease in blood pressure is dose dependent, due to peripheral vasodilation, with maintenance of cardiac output. Abrupt increases in inspired concentration >1 MAC can produce a transient increase in blood pressure and heart rate due to increased plasma catecholamine levels. Hepatic blood flow is decreased. Respiration is depressed as is hypoxic pulmonary vasoconstriction, which may lead to increased pulmonary shunt. Hypoxemia-induced increase in ventilation is abolished at low desflurane concentration. It dilates the cerebral vasculature and may, in certain conditions, increase intracranial pressure. Desflurane triggers malignant hyperthermia in humans, and therefore, should not be used on patients susceptible to malignant hyperthermia. Desflurane can produce elevated carbon monoxide levels in the presence of a dry carbon dioxide absorbent within the circle breathing system of an anesthetic machine. Induction with desflurane not recommended in infants or pediatric patients because of high incidence of airway irritation (laryngospasm, coughing, breath-holding, increased secretions). May cause sensitivity hepatitis in patients who have been sensitized by previous exposure to halogenated anesthetics.

Adverse Reactions The pungency of desflurane produces laryngospasm, cough, breath-holding, increased secretions, and apnea making inhalation induction difficult. Pediatric patients have a higher incidence of these events than adults.

Frequency not defined.

Cardiovascular: Bradycardia, hyper-/hypotension, myocardial depression, nodal arrhythmia, tachycardia

Central nervous system: Emergence delirium, headache, malignant hyperthermia (rare)

Gastrointestinal: Nausea (27%), vomiting (16%)

Hepatic: Hepatitis (rare)

Ocular: Conjunctivitis

Respiratory: Airway irritation, hypoxemia, pharyngitis, respiratory depression/arrest, salivation

Miscellaneous: Shivering

Drug Interactions

Benzodiazepines: May decrease the MAC of desflurane.

Neuromuscular-blocking agents: Inhalational anesthetics may enhance the effects of NMBs.

Opioids: May decrease the MAC of desflurane.

Dosage Forms Liquid, for inhalation: 240 mL

References

Campagna JA, Miller KW, and Forman SA, "Mechanisms of Action of Inhaled Anesthetics," *N Engl J Med*, 2003, 348(21):2110-23.

Ebert TJ and Muzi M, "Sympathetic Hyperactivity During Desflurane Anesthesia in Healthy Volunteers. A Comparison With Isoflurane," *Anesthesiology*, 1993, 79(3):444-53.

Sakai EM, Connolly LA, and Klauck J, "Inhalation Anesthesiology and Volatile Liquid Anesthetics: Focus on Isoflurane, Desflurane, and Sevoflurane," *Pharmacotherapy*, 2005, 25(12):1773-88.

Yasuda N, Lockhart SH, Eger EI 2nd, et al, "Kinetics of Desflurane, Isoflurane, and Halothane in Humans," *Anesthesiology*, 1991, 74(3):489-98.

Desipramine (des IP ra meen)

Medication Safety Issues

Sound-alike/look-alike issues:

Desipramine may be confused with clomiPRAMINE, deserpidine, diphenhydrAMINE, disopyramide, imipramine, nortriptyline

Norpramin® may be confused with clomiPRAMINE, imipramine, Norpace®, nortriptyline, Tenormin®

Related Information

Antidepressant Agents *on page 1551*

Chronic Pain Management *on page 1430*

U.S. Brand Names Norpramin®

Canadian Brand Names Alti-Desipramine; Apo-Desipramine®; Norpramin®; Nu-Desipramine; PMS-Desipramine

Synonyms Desipramine Hydrochloride; Desmethylimipramine Hydrochloride

Pharmacologic Category Antidepressant, Tricyclic (Secondary Amine)

Restrictions A medication guide concerning the use of antidepressants in children and teenagers can be found on the FDA website at http://www.fda.gov/cder/Offices/ODS/labeling.htm. It should be dispensed to parents or guardians of children and teenagers receiving this medication.

Generic Available Yes

Use Treatment of depression

Unlabeled/Investigational Use Analgesic adjunct in chronic pain; peripheral neuropathies; substance-related disorders (eg, cocaine withdrawal); attention-deficit/hyperactivity disorder (ADHD); depression in children ≤12 years of age

Mechanism of Action Traditionally believed to increase the synaptic concentration of norepinephrine (and to a lesser extent, serotonin) in the central nervous system by inhibition of its reuptake by the presynaptic neuronal membrane. However, additional receptor effects have been found including desensitization of adenyl cyclase, down regulation of beta-adrenergic receptors, and down regulation of serotonin receptors.

Pharmacodynamics/Kinetics

Onset of action: 1-3 weeks; Maximum antidepressant effect: >2 weeks

Absorption: Well absorbed

Metabolism: Hepatic

Half-life elimination: Adults: 7-60 hours

Time to peak, plasma: 4-6 hours

Excretion: Urine (70%)

Dosage Oral (dose is generally administered at bedtime):

Children 6-12 years: Depression (unlabeled use): 10-30 mg/day or 1-3 mg/kg/day in divided doses; do not exceed 5 mg/kg/day

Adolescents: Depression: Initial: 25-50 mg/day; gradually increase to 100 mg/day in single or divided doses (maximum: 150 mg/day)

Adults:

Depression: Initial: 75 mg/day in divided doses; increase gradually to 150-200 mg/day in divided or single dose (maximum: 300 mg/day)

Cocaine withdrawal (unlabeled use): 50-200 mg/day in divided or single dose

Elderly: Depression: Initial dose: 10-25 mg/day; increase by 10-25 mg every 3 days for inpatients and every week for outpatients if tolerated; usual maintenance dose: 75-100 mg/day, but doses up to 150 mg/day may be necessary

Hemodialysis/peritoneal dialysis: Supplemental dose is not necessary

Monitoring Parameters Monitor blood pressure and pulse rate prior to and during initial therapy evaluate mental status; monitor weight; ECG in older adults

(Continued)

Desipramine *(Continued)*

and those patients with cardiac disease; blood levels are useful for therapeutic monitoring

Reference Range

Plasma levels do not always correlate with clinical effectiveness

Timing of serum samples: Draw trough just before next dose

Therapeutic: 50-300 ng/mL

In elderly patients the response rate is greatest with steady-state plasma concentrations >115 ng/mL

Possible toxicity: >300 ng/mL

Toxic: >1000 ng/mL

Anesthesia and Critical Care Concerns/Other Considerations Desipramine causes less sedation and anticholinergic effects than with amitriptyline or imipramine.

Pregnancy Risk Factor C

Contraindications Hypersensitivity to desipramine, drugs of similar chemical class, or any component of the formulation; use of MAO inhibitors within 14 days; use in a patient during the acute recovery phase of MI

Warnings/Precautions [U.S. Boxed Warning]: Antidepressants increase the risk of suicidal thinking and behavior in children and adolescents with major depressive disorder (MDD) and other depressive disorders; consider risk prior to prescribing. Closely monitor for clinical worsening, suicidality, or unusual changes in behavior; the child's family or caregiver should be instructed to closely observe the patient and communicate condition with healthcare provider. Such observation would generally include at least weekly face-to-face contact with patients or their family members or caregivers during the first 4 weeks of treatment, then every other week visits for the next 4 weeks, then at 12 weeks, and as clinically indicated beyond 12 weeks. Additional contact by telephone may be appropriate between face-to-face visits. Adults treated with antidepressants should be observed similarly for clinical worsening and suicidality, especially during the initial few months of a course of drug therapy, or at times of dose changes, either increases or decreases. A medication guide should be dispensed with each prescription. **Desipramine is FDA approved for the treatment of depression in adolescents.**

The possibility of a suicide attempt is inherent in major depression and may persist until remission occurs. Monitor for worsening of depression or suicidality, especially during initiation of therapy or with dose increases or decreases. Worsening depression and severe abrupt suicidality that are not part of the presenting symptoms may require discontinuation or modification of drug therapy. Use caution in high-risk patients during initiation of therapy. Prescriptions should be written for the smallest quantity consistent with good patient care. The patient's family or caregiver should be alerted to monitor patients for the emergence of suicidality and associated behaviors such as anxiety, agitation, panic attacks, insomnia, irritability, hostility, impulsivity, akathisia, hypomania, and mania; patients should be instructed to notify their healthcare provider if any of these symptoms or worsening depression occur.

May worsen psychosis in some patients or precipitate a shift to mania or hypomania in patients with bipolar disorder. Monotherapy in patients with bipolar disorder should be avoided. Patients presenting with depressive symptoms should be screened for bipolar disorder. **Desipramine is not FDA approved for the treatment of bipolar depression.**

May cause sedation, resulting in impaired performance of tasks requiring alertness (eg, operating machinery or driving). Sedative effects may be additive with other CNS depressants and/or ethanol. The degree of sedation is low-moderate relative to other antidepressants. May cause hyponatremia/SIADH. May increase the risks associated with electroconvulsive therapy. Consider discontinuing, when possible, prior to elective surgery. Therapy should not be abruptly discontinued in patients receiving high doses for prolonged periods.

May cause orthostatic hypotension (risk is moderate relative to other antidepressants) - use with caution in patients at risk of hypotension or in patients where transient hypotensive episodes would be poorly tolerated (cardiovascular disease or cerebrovascular disease). The degree of anticholinergic blockade produced by this agent is low relative to other cyclic antidepressants - however, caution should be used in patients with urinary retention, benign prostatic hyperplasia, narrow-angle glaucoma, xerostomia, visual problems, constipation, or a history of bowel obstruction.

Use with caution in patients with a history of cardiovascular disease (including previous MI, stroke, tachycardia, or conduction abnormalities). The risk conduction abnormalities with this agent is moderate relative to other antidepressants. Use caution in patients with a previous seizure disorder or condition predisposing to seizures such as brain damage, alcoholism, or concurrent therapy with other drugs which lower the seizure threshold. Use with caution in hyperthyroid patients or those receiving thyroid supplementation. Use with caution in patients with hepatic or renal dysfunction and in elderly patients.

Adverse Reactions Frequency not defined.

Cardiovascular: Arrhythmias, edema, flushing, heart block, hyper-/hypotension, MI, palpitation, stroke, tachycardia

Central nervous system: Agitation, anxiety, ataxia, confusion, delirium, disorientation, dizziness, drowsiness, drug fever, exacerbation of psychosis, extrapyramidal symptoms, fatigue, hallucinations, headache, hypomania, incoordination, insomnia, nervousness, parkinsonian syndrome, restlessness, seizure

Dermatologic: Alopecia, itching, petechiae, photosensitivity, skin rash, urticaria

Endocrine & metabolic: Breast enlargement, galactorrhea, hyper-/hypoglycemia, impotence, libido changes, SIADH

Gastrointestinal: Abdominal cramps, anorexia, black tongue, constipation, decreased lower esophageal sphincter tone may cause GE reflux, diarrhea, heartburn, nausea, paralytic ileus, stomatitis, unpleasant taste, vomiting, weight gain/loss, xerostomia

Genitourinary: Difficult urination, polyuria, sexual dysfunction, testicular edema, urinary retention

Hematologic: Agranulocytosis, eosinophilia, purpura, thrombocytopenia

Hepatic: Cholestatic jaundice, hepatitis, liver enzymes increased

Neuromuscular & skeletal: Fine muscle tremor, numbness, paresthesia of extremities, peripheral neuropathy, tingling, weakness

Ocular: Blurred vision, disturbances of accommodation, intraocular pressure increased, mydriasis

Otic: Tinnitus

Miscellaneous: Allergic reaction, diaphoresis (excessive)

Overdosage/Toxicology Symptoms of overdose include agitation, confusion, hallucinations, hypo-/hyperthermia, hypotension (severe), urinary retention, CNS depression, coma, cyanosis, dry mucous membranes, cardiac arrhythmias, and seizures. Treatment is supportive and symptom-directed. Initiate gastric decontamination (emesis is contraindicated) and ECG monitoring immediately; monitor for a minimum of 6 hours. Ventricular arrhythmias and ECG changes (eg, QRS widening) often respond with concurrent systemic alkalinization (sodium bicarbonate 0.5-2 mEq/kg I.V. or hyperventilation). Arrhythmias unresponsive to phenytoin 15-20 mg/kg (adults) may respond to lidocaine. Physostigmine (1-2 mg I.V. slowly for adults) may be indicated for reversing life-threatening cardiac arrhythmias. Dialysis and diuresis have not been proven beneficial.

Drug Interactions **Substrate** of CYP1A2 (minor), 2D6 (major); **Inhibits** CYP2A6 (moderate), 2B6 (moderate), 2D6 (moderate), 2E1 (weak), 3A4 (moderate)

Alpha- and beta-agonists: When combined with TCAs, may predispose patients to cardiac arrhythmias; may also enhance vasopressor effects; consider alternate therapy.

Altretamine: Concurrent use may cause orthostatic hypertension

Amphetamines: TCAs may enhance the effect of amphetamines; monitor for adverse CV effects

Anticholinergics: Combined use with TCAs may produce additive anticholinergic effects

Barbiturates: May decrease the levels/effects of TCAs; monitor.

Bupropion: May increase the levels of tricyclic antidepressants; based on limited information; monitor response

Carbamazepine: Tricyclic antidepressants may increase carbamazepine levels; monitor

Cholestyramine and colestipol: May bind TCAs and reduce their absorption; monitor for altered response

Clonidine: Abrupt discontinuation of clonidine may cause hypertensive crisis; amitriptyline may enhance the response

CNS depressants: Sedative effects may be additive with TCAs; monitor for increased effect; includes benzodiazepines, barbiturates, antipsychotics, ethanol, and other sedative medications

(Continued)

Desipramine *(Continued)*

CYP2A6 substrates: Desipramine may increase the levels/effects of CYP2A6 substrates. Example substrates include dexmedetomidine and ifosfamide.

CYP2B6 substrates: Desipramine may increase the levels/effects of CYP2B6 substrates. Example substrates include bupropion, cyclophosphamide, irinotecan, ketamine, promethazine, propofol, and selegiline.

CYP2D6 inhibitors: May increase the levels/effects of desipramine. Example inhibitors include chlorpromazine, delavirdine, fluoxetine, miconazole, paroxetine, pergolide, quinidine, quinine, ritonavir, and ropinirole.

CYP2D6 substrates: Desipramine may increase the levels/effects of CYP2D6 substrates. Example substrates include amphetamines, selected beta-blockers, dextromethorphan, fluoxetine, lidocaine, mirtazapine, nefazodone, paroxetine, risperidone, ritonavir, thioridazine, tricyclic antidepressants, and venlafaxine. Concurrent use with thioridazine is contraindicated.

CYP2D6 prodrug substrates: Desipramine may decrease the levels/effects of CYP2D6 prodrug substrates. Example prodrug substrates include codeine, hydrocodone, oxycodone, and tramadol.

CYP3A4 substrates: Desipramine may increase the levels/effects of CYP3A4 substrates. Example substrates include benzodiazepines, calcium channel blockers, cyclosporine, mirtazapine, nateglinide, nefazodone, sildenafil (and other PDE-5 inhibitors), tacrolimus, and venlafaxine. Selected benzodiazepines (midazolam and triazolam), cisapride, ergot alkaloids, selected HMG-CoA reductase inhibitors (lovastatin and simvastatin), and pimozide are generally contraindicated with strong CYP3A4 inhibitors.

Epinephrine (and other direct alpha-agonists): Pressor response to I.V. epinephrine, norepinephrine, and phenylephrine may be enhanced in patients receiving TCAs (**Note:** Effect is unlikely with epinephrine or levonordefrin dosages typically administered as infiltration in combination with local anesthetics)

False neurotransmitters (eg, guanadrel, methyldopa): TCAs may diminish the antihypertensive effects of false neurotransmitters.

Fenfluramine: May increase tricyclic antidepressant levels/effects

Hypoglycemic agents (including insulin): TCAs may enhance the hypoglycemic effects of tolazamide, chlorpropamide, or insulin; monitor for changes in blood glucose levels; reported with chlorpropamide, tolazamide, and insulin

Levodopa: Tricyclic antidepressants may decrease the absorption (bioavailability) of levodopa; rare hypertensive episodes have also been attributed to this combination

Linezolid: Hyperpyrexia, hypertension, tachycardia, confusion, seizures, and **deaths have been reported** with agents which inhibit MAO (serotonin syndrome); this combination should be avoided

Lithium: Concurrent use with a TCA may increase the risk for neurotoxicity

MAO inhibitors: Hyperpyrexia, hypertension, tachycardia, confusion, seizures, and **deaths have been reported** (serotonin syndrome); this combination should be avoided

Methylphenidate: Metabolism of TCAs may be decreased

Phenothiazines: Serum concentrations of some TCAs may be increased; in addition, TCAs may increase concentration of phenothiazines; monitor for altered clinical response.

Pramlintide: May increase the anticholinergic effects of TCAs.

QT_c-prolonging agents: Concurrent use of tricyclic agents with other drugs which may prolong QT_c interval may increase the risk of potentially fatal arrhythmias; includes type Ia and type III antiarrhythmics agents, selected quinolones (sparfloxacin, gatifloxacin, moxifloxacin, grepafloxacin), cisapride, and other agents

Ritonavir: Combined use of high-dose tricyclic antidepressants with ritonavir may cause serotonin syndrome in HIV-positive patients; monitor.

Serotonin modulators, SSRIs, sibutramine: Concomitant use may increase serotonergic effects; concurrent use with sibutramine is contraindicated.

Sympathomimetics, indirect-acting: Tricyclic antidepressants may result in a decreased sensitivity to indirect-acting sympathomimetics; includes dopamine and ephedrine; also see interaction with epinephrine (and direct-acting sympathomimetics)

Terbinafine: May increase the levels/effects of TCAs; monitor.

Tramadol: Tramadol's risk of seizures may be increased with TCAs

Valproic acid: May increase serum concentrations/adverse effects of some tricyclic antidepressants

Warfarin (and other oral anticoagulants): TCAs may increase the anticoagulant effect in patients stabilized on warfarin; monitor INR

Ethanol/Nutrition/Herb Interactions

Ethanol: Avoid ethanol (may increase CNS depression).

Food: Grapefruit juice may inhibit the metabolism of some TCAs and clinical toxicity may result.

Herb/Nutraceutical: Avoid valerian, St John's wort, SAMe, kava kava (may increase risk of serotonin syndrome and/or excessive sedation).

Dosage Forms Tablet, as hydrochloride: 10 mg, 25 mg, 50 mg, 75 mg, 100 mg, 150 mg

◆ **Desipramine Hydrochloride** *see* Desipramine *on page 359*
◆ **Desmethylimipramine Hydrochloride** *see* Desipramine *on page 359*

Desmopressin (des moe PRES in)

U.S. Brand Names DDAVP®; Stimate™

Canadian Brand Names Apo-Desmopressin®; DDAVP®; Minirin®; Octostim®

Synonyms 1-Deamino-8-D-Arginine Vasopressin; Desmopressin Acetate

Pharmacologic Category Antihemophilic Agent; Hemostatic Agent; Vasopressin Analog, Synthetic

Generic Available Yes

Use

Injection: Treatment of diabetes insipidus; control of bleeding in hemophilia A, and mild-to-moderate classic von Willebrand disease (type I)

Tablet, nasal solution: Treatment of diabetes insipidus; primary nocturnal enuresis

Mechanism of Action Enhances reabsorption of water in the kidneys by increasing cellular permeability of the collecting ducts; possibly causes smooth muscle constriction with resultant vasoconstriction; raises plasma levels of von Willebrand factor and factor VIII

Pharmacodynamics/Kinetics

Intranasal administration:
- Onset of increased factor VIII activity: 30 minutes (dose related)
  - Peak effect 1.5 hours
- Bioavailability: 3.2%

I.V. infusion:
- Onset of increased factor VIII activity: 30 minutes (dose related)
  - Peak effect: 1.5-2 hours
- Half-life elimination: Terminal: 3 hours (up to 9 hours in renal dysfunction)
- Excretion: Urine

Oral tablet:
- Onset of action: ADH: ~1 hour
  - Peak effect: 4-7 hours
- Bioavailability: 5% compared to intranasal; 0.16% compared to I.V.
- Half-life elimination: 1.5-2.5 hours

Dosage

Children:

Diabetes insipidus:

Intranasal (using 100 mcg/mL nasal solution): 3 months to 12 years: Initial: 5 mcg/day (0.05 mL/day) divided 1-2 times/day; range: 5-30 mcg/day (0.05-0.3 mL/day) divided 1-2 times/day; adjust morning and evening doses separately for an adequate diurnal rhythm of water turnover; doses <10 mcg should be administered using the rhinal tube system

Oral: ≥4 years: Initial: 0.05 mg twice daily; total daily dose should be increased or decreased as needed to obtain adequate antidiuresis (range: 0.1-1.2 mg divided 2-3 times/day)

Hemophilia A and von Willebrand disease (type I):

I.V.: >3 months: 0.3 mcg/kg by slow infusion; may repeat dose if needed; begin 30 minutes before procedure

Intranasal: ≥11 months: Refer to adult dosing.

Nocturnal enuresis:

Intranasal (using 100 mcg/mL nasal solution): ≥6 years: Initial: 20 mcg (0.2 mL) at bedtime; range: 10-40 mcg; it is recommended that $^1/_2$ of the dose be given in each nostril. **Note:** The nasal spray pump can only deliver doses of 10 mcg (0.1 mL) or multiples of 10 mcg (0.1 mL); if doses other than this

(Continued)

Desmopressin *(Continued)*

are needed, the rhinal tube delivery system is preferred. For 10 mcg dose, administer in one nostril.

Oral: 0.2 mg at bedtime; dose may be titrated up to 0.6 mg to achieve desired response. Patients previously on intranasal therapy can begin oral tablets 24 hours after the last intranasal dose.

Children ≥12 years and Adults:

Diabetes insipidus:

I.V., SubQ: 2-4 mcg/day (0.5-1 mL) in 2 divided doses or $^{1}/_{10}$ of the maintenance intranasal dose

Intranasal (using 100 mcg/mL nasal solution): 10-40 mcg/day (0.1-0.4 mL) divided 1-3 times/day; adjust morning and evening doses separately for an adequate diurnal rhythm of water turnover. **Note:** The nasal spray pump can only deliver doses of 10 mcg (0.1 mL) or multiples of 10 mcg (0.1 mL); if doses other than this are needed, the rhinal tube delivery system is preferred.

Oral: Initial: 0.05 mg twice daily; total daily dose should be increased or decreased as needed to obtain adequate antidiuresis (range: 0.1-1.2 mg divided 2-3 times/day)

Hemophilia A and mild to moderate von Willebrand disease (Type I):

I.V.: 0.3 mcg/kg by slow infusion, begin 30 minutes before procedure

Intranasal: Using high concentration spray (1.5 mg/mL): <50 kg: 150 mcg (1 spray); >50 kg: 300 mcg (1 spray each nostril); repeat use is determined by the patient's clinical condition and laboratory work; if using preoperatively, administer 2 hours before surgery

Dosage adjustment in renal impairment: Cl_{cr} <50 mL/minute: Use is contraindicated

Stability

DDAVP®:

Tablet, nasal spray: Store at controlled room temperature of 20°C to 25°C (68°F to 77°F). Keep nasal spray in upright position.

Rhinal tube: Store refrigerated at 2°C to 8°C (36°F to 46°F). May store at room temperature for up to 3 weeks.

Injection: Store refrigerated at 2°C to 8°C (36°F to 46°F). Dilute in 10-50 mL NS for I.V. infusion (10 mL for children ≤10 kg: 50 mL for adults and children >10 kg)

Stimate™: Store refrigerated at 2°C to 8°C (36°F to 46°F). May store at room temperature for up to 3 weeks.

Administration

I.V.: Infuse over 15-30 minutes

Intranasal:

DDAVP®: Nasal pump spray: Delivers 0.1 mL (10 mcg); for other doses which are not multiples, use rhinal tube. DDAVP® Nasal spray delivers fifty 10 mcg doses. For 10 mcg dose, administer in one nostril. Any solution remaining after 50 doses should be discarded. Pump must be primed prior to first use.

DDAVP® Rhinal tube: Insert top of dropper into tube (arrow marked end) in downward position. Squeeze dropper until solution reaches desired calibration mark. Disconnect dropper. Grasp the tube $^{3}/_{4}$inch from the end and insert tube into nostril until the fingertips reach the nostril. Place opposite end of tube into the mouth (holding breath). Tilt head back and blow with a strong, short puff into the nostril (for very young patients, an adult should blow solution into the child's nose). Reseal dropper after use.

Monitoring Parameters Blood pressure and pulse should be monitored during I.V. infusion

Diabetes insipidus: Fluid intake, urine volume, specific gravity, plasma and urine osmolality, serum electrolytes

Hemophilia A: Factor VIII coagulant activity, Factor VIII ristocetin cofactor activity, and Factor VIII antigen levels, aPTT

Von Willebrand disease: Factor VIII coagulant activity, Factor VIII ristocetin cofactor activity, and Factor VIII von Willebrand antigen levels, bleeding time

Nocturnal enuresis: Serum electrolytes if used for >7 days

Anesthesia and Critical Care Concerns/Other Considerations If desmopressin I.V. is given preoperatively, administer 30 minutes prior to surgery.

Pregnancy Risk Factor B

Contraindications Hypersensitivity to desmopressin or any component of the formulation; moderate to severe renal impairment (Cl_{cr}<50 mL/minute)

Warnings/Precautions Fluid intake should be adjusted downward in the elderly and very young patients to decrease the possibility of water intoxication and hyponatremia. Avoid overhydration especially when drug is used for its hemostatic effect. Use may rarely lead to extreme decreases in plasma osmolality, resulting in seizures and coma. Use caution with cystic fibrosis or other conditions associated with fluid and electrolyte imbalance due to potential hyponatremia. Use caution with coronary artery insufficiency or hypertensive cardiovascular disease; may increase or decrease blood pressure leading to changes in heart rate. Consider switching from nasal to intravenous solution if changes in the nasal mucosa (scarring, edema) occur leading to unreliable absorption. Use caution in patients predisposed to thrombus formation; thrombotic events (acute cerebrovascular thrombosis, acute myocardial infarction) have occurred (rare). Injection is not for use in hemophilia B, severe classic von Willebrand disease (type IIB), or in patients with factor VIII antibodies. In general, the injection is also not recommended for use in patients with ≤5% factor VIII activity level, although it may be considered in selected patients with activity levels between 2% and 5%. Some patients may demonstrate a change in response after long-term therapy (>6 months) characterized as decreased response or a shorter duration of response.

Adverse Reactions Frequency not defined (may be dose or route related).

Cardiovascular: Acute cerebrovascular thrombosis, acute MI, blood pressure increased/decreased, chest pain, edema, facial flushing, palpitation

Central nervous system: Agitation, chills, coma, dizziness, headache, insomnia, somnolence

Dermatologic: Rash

Endocrine & metabolic: Hyponatremia, water intoxication

Gastrointestinal: Abdominal cramps, dyspepsia, nausea, sore throat, vomiting

Genitourinary: Balanitis, vulval pain

Local: Injection: Burning pain, erythema, and swelling at the injection site

Ocular: Conjunctivitis, eye edema, lacrimation disorder

Respiratory: Cough, epistaxis, nasal congestion, rhinitis

Miscellaneous: Allergic reactions (rare), anaphylaxis (rare)

Overdosage/Toxicology Symptoms of overdose include drowsiness, headache, confusion, anuria, and water intoxication. In case of overdose, decrease or discontinue desmopressin.

Drug Interactions

Demeclocycline: May decrease response to endogenous antidiuretic hormone (ADH). Use caution.

Chlorpropamide: May increase response to ADH. Use caution.

Fludrocortisone: May increase response to ADH. Use caution.

Lithium: May decrease response to ADH. Use caution.

Ethanol/Nutrition/Herb Interactions Ethanol: Avoid ethanol (may decrease antidiuretic effect).

Dosage Forms

Injection, solution, as acetate (DDAVP®): 4 mcg/mL (1 mL, 10 mL)

Solution, intranasal, as acetate (DDAVP®): 100 mcg/mL (2.5 mL) [with rhinal tube]

Solution, intranasal, as acetate [spray]: 100 mcg/mL (5 mL) [delivers 10 mcg/spray]

DDAVP®: 100 mcg/mL (5 mL) [delivers 10 mcg/spray]

Stimate™: 1.5 mg/mL (2.5 mL) [delivers 150 mcg/spray]

Tablet, as acetate (DDAVP®): 0.1 mg, 0.2 mg

References

Cattaneo M, "Review of Clinical Experience of Desmopressin in Patients With Congenital and Acquired Bleeding Disorder," *Eur J Anesthesiol Suppl*, 1997, 14:10-4.

Chistolini A, Dragoni F, Ferrari A, et al, "Intranasal DDAVP®: Biological and Clinical Evaluation in Mild Factor VIII Deficiency," *Haemostasis*, 1991, 21(5):273-7.

Mannucci PM and Cattaneo M, "Desmopressin: A Nontransfusional Treatment of Hemophilia and von Willebrand Disease," *Haemostasis*, 1992, 22(5):276-80.

◆ **Desmopressin Acetate** *see* Desmopressin *on page 363*

◆ **Desyrel®** *see* Trazodone *on page 1306*

◆ **Detemir Insulin** *see* Insulin Detemir *on page 683*

◆ **Detrol®** *see* Tolterodine *on page 1285*

◆ **Detrol® LA** *see* Tolterodine *on page 1285*

Dexamethasone (deks a METH a sone)

Medication Safety Issues

Sound-alike/look-alike issues:

Dexamethasone may be confused with desoximetasone

Decadron® may be confused with Percodan®

Maxidex® may be confused with Maxzide®

Related Information

Allergic Reactions *on page 1395*

Anesthesia for Patients With Liver Disease *on page 1421*

Chronic Pain Management *on page 1430*

Corticosteroids *on page 1561*

Postoperative Nausea and Vomiting *on page 1477*

Stress Replacement of Corticosteroids *on page 1494*

U.S. Brand Names Decadron®; Decadron® Phosphate [DSC]; Dexamethasone Intensol®; DexPak® TaperPak®; Maxidex®

Canadian Brand Names Apo-Dexamethasone®; Dexasone®; Diodex®; Maxidex®; PMS-Dexamethasone

Synonyms Dexamethasone Sodium Phosphate

Pharmacologic Category Anti-inflammatory Agent; Anti-inflammatory Agent, Ophthalmic; Antiemetic; Corticosteroid, Ophthalmic; Corticosteroid, Systemic; Corticosteroid, Topical

Generic Available Yes

Use Systemically and locally for chronic swelling; allergic, hematologic, neoplastic, and autoimmune diseases; may be used in management of cerebral edema, septic shock, as a diagnostic agent, antiemetic

Unlabeled/Investigational Use General indicator consistent with depression; diagnosis of Cushing's syndrome

Mechanism of Action Decreases inflammation by suppression of neutrophil migration, decreased production of inflammatory mediators, and reversal of increased capillary permeability; suppresses normal immune response. Dexamethasone's mechanism of antiemetic activity is unknown.

Pharmacodynamics/Kinetics

Onset of action: Acetate: Prompt

Duration of metabolic effect: 72 hours; acetate is a long-acting repository preparation

Metabolism: Hepatic

Half-life elimination: Normal renal function: 1.8-3.5 hours; Biological half-life: 36-54 hours

Time to peak, serum: Oral: 1-2 hours; I.M.: ~8 hours

Excretion: Urine and feces

Dosage

Children:

Antiemetic (prior to chemotherapy): I.V. (should be given as sodium phosphate): 5-20 mg given 15-30 minutes before treatment

Anti-inflammatory immunosuppressant: Oral, I.M., I.V. (injections should be given as sodium phosphate): 0.08-0.3 mg/kg/day **or** 2.5-10 mg/m²/day in divided doses every 6-12 hours

Extubation or airway edema: Oral, I.M., I.V. (injections should be given as sodium phosphate): 0.5-2 mg/kg/day in divided doses every 6 hours beginning 24 hours prior to extubation and continuing for 4-6 doses afterwards

Cerebral edema: I.V. (should be given as sodium phosphate): Loading dose: 1-2 mg/kg/dose as a single dose; maintenance: 1-1.5 mg/kg/day (maximum: 16 mg/day) in divided doses every 4-6 hours for 5 days then taper for 5 days, then discontinue

Bacterial meningitis in infants and children >2 months: I.V. (should be given as sodium phosphate): 0.6 mg/kg/day in 4 divided doses every 6 hours for the first 4 days of antibiotic treatment; start dexamethasone at the time of the first dose of antibiotic

Physiologic replacement: Oral, I.M., I.V.: 0.03-0.15 mg/kg/day **or** 0.6-0.75 mg/m²/day in divided doses every 6-12 hours

Adults:

Antiemetic:

Prophylaxis: Oral, I.V.: 10-20 mg 15-30 minutes before treatment on each treatment day

Continuous infusion regimen: Oral or I.V.: 10 mg every 12 hours on each treatment day
Mildly emetogenic therapy: Oral, I.M., I.V.: 4 mg every 4-6 hours
Delayed nausea/vomiting: Oral: 4-10 mg 1-2 times/day for 2-4 days **or**
8 mg every 12 hours for 2 days; then
4 mg every 12 hours for 2 days **or**
20 mg 1 hour before chemotherapy; then
10 mg 12 hours after chemotherapy; then
8 mg every 12 hours for 4 doses; then
4 mg every 12 hours for 4 doses

Anti-inflammatory:
Oral, I.M., I.V. (injections should be given as sodium phosphate): 0.75-9 mg/day in divided doses every 6-12 hours
Intra-articular, intralesional, or soft tissue (as sodium phosphate): 0.4-6 mg/day
Ophthalmic:
Ointment: Apply thin coating into conjunctival sac 3-4 times/day; gradually taper dose to discontinue
Suspension: Instill 2 drops into conjunctival sac every hour during the day and every other hour during the night; gradually reduce dose to every 3-4 hours, then to 3-4 times/day
Topical: Apply 1-4 times/day. Therapy should be discontinued when control is achieved; if no improvement is seen, reassessment of diagnosis may be necessary.

Chemotherapy: Oral, I.V.: 40 mg every day for 4 days, repeated every 4 weeks (VAD regimen)

Cerebral edema: I.V. 10 mg stat, 4 mg I.M./I.V. (should be given as sodium phosphate) every 6 hours until response is maximized, then switch to oral regimen, then taper off if appropriate; dosage may be reduced after 24 days and gradually discontinued over 5-7 days

Dexamethasone suppression test (depression indicator) (unlabeled use): Oral: 1 mg at 11 PM, draw blood at 8 AM the following day for plasma cortisol determination

Cushing's syndrome, diagnostic: Oral: 1 mg at 11 PM, draw blood at 8 AM; greater accuracy for Cushing's syndrome may be achieved by the following:
Dexamethasone 0.5 mg by mouth every 6 hours for 48 hours (with 24-hour urine collection for 17-hydroxycorticosteroid excretion)
Differentiation of Cushing's syndrome due to ACTH excess from Cushing's due to other causes: Oral: Dexamethasone 2 mg every 6 hours for 48 hours (with 24-hour urine collection for 17-hydroxycorticosteroid excretion)

Multiple sclerosis (acute exacerbation): 30 mg/day for 1 week, followed by 4-12 mg/day for 1 month

Physiological replacement: Oral, I.M., I.V. (should be given as sodium phosphate): 0.03-0.15 mg/kg/day **or** 0.6-0.75 mg/m^2/day in divided doses every 6-12 hours

Treatment of shock:
Addisonian crisis/shock (ie, adrenal insufficiency/responsive to steroid therapy): I.V. (given as sodium phosphate): 4-10 mg as a single dose, which may be repeated if necessary
Unresponsive shock (ie, unresponsive to steroid therapy): I.V. (given as sodium phosphate): 1-6 mg/kg as a single I.V. dose or up to 40 mg initially followed by repeat doses every 2-6 hours while shock persists

Hemodialysis: Supplemental dose is not necessary
Peritoneal dialysis: Supplemental dose is not necessary

Stability Injection solution: Store at room temperature; protect from light and freezing.
Stability of injection of parenteral admixture at room temperature (25°C): 24 hours
Stability of injection of parenteral admixture at refrigeration temperature (4°C): 2 days; protect from light and freezing
Injection should be diluted in 50-100 mL NS or D_5W.

Administration
Oral: Administer with meals to decrease GI upset.
I.M.: Acetate injection is **not** for I.V. use.
I.V.: Administer as a 5-10 minute bolus; rapid injection is associated with a high incidence of perianal discomfort.
Topical: For external use. Do not use on open wounds. Apply sparingly to occlusive dressings. Should not be used in the presence of open or weeping lesions.

(Continued)

Dexamethasone *(Continued)*

Monitoring Parameters Hemoglobin, occult blood loss, serum potassium, and glucose

Reference Range Dexamethasone suppression test, overnight: 8 AM cortisol <6 mcg/100 mL (dexamethasone 1 mg); plasma cortisol determination should be made on the day after giving dose

Anesthesia and Critical Care Concerns/Other Considerations Dexamethasone is a long-acting corticosteroid with minimal sodium-retaining potential. Corticosteroids and muscle relaxants appear to trigger some types of ICU myopathy; avoid or administer at the lowest dose possible.

Patients will often have steroid-induced adverse effects on glucose tolerance and lipid profiles. In discontinuing steroid therapy in patients on long-term steroid supplementation, it is important that the steroid therapy be discontinued gradually. Abrupt withdrawal may result in adrenal insufficiency with hypotension and hyperkalemia. Patients on long-term steroid supplementation will require higher corticosteroid doses when subject to stress (ie, trauma, surgery, severe infection).

Oral and intravenous steroid therapy in patients with heart failure should be administered cautiously with special attention given to signs and symptoms of fluid retention.

Pregnancy Risk Factor C

Contraindications Hypersensitivity to dexamethasone or any component of the formulation; active untreated infections; ophthalmic use in viral, fungal, or tuberculosis diseases of the eye

Warnings/Precautions Use with caution in patients with hypothyroidism, cirrhosis, hypertension, CHF, ulcerative colitis, or thromboembolic disorders. Corticosteroids should be used with caution in patients with diabetes, osteoporosis, peptic ulcer, glaucoma, cataracts, or tuberculosis. Use caution following acute MI (corticosteroids have been associated with myocardial rupture). Use caution in hepatic impairment. Because of the risk of adverse effects, systemic corticosteroids should be used cautiously in the elderly in the smallest possible effective dose for the shortest duration.

May cause suppression of hypothalamic-pituitary-adrenal (HPA) axis, particularly in younger children or in patients receiving high doses for prolonged periods. Symptoms of adrenocortical insufficiency in suppressed patients may result from rapid discontinuation/withdrawal; deficits in HPA response may persist for months following discontinuation and require supplementation during metabolic stress. Patients receiving 20 mg/day of prednisone (or equivalent) may be most susceptible. Particular care is required when patients are transferred from systemic corticosteroids to inhaled products due to possible adrenal insufficiency or exacerbation of underlying disease, including an increase in allergic symptoms. Fatalities have occurred due to adrenal insufficiency in asthmatic patients during and after transfer from systemic corticosteroids to aerosol steroids; aerosol steroids do **not** provide the systemic steroid needed to treat patients having trauma, surgery, or infections. Dexamethasone does not provide adequate mineralocorticoid activity in adrenal insufficiency (may be employed as a single dose while cortisol assays are performed).

Controlled clinical studies have shown that orally-inhaled and intranasal corticosteroids may cause a reduction in growth velocity in pediatric patients. (In studies of orally-inhaled corticosteroids, the mean reduction in growth velocity was ~1 cm per year [range 0.3-1.8 cm per year] and appears to be related to dose and duration of exposure). The growth of pediatric patients receiving inhaled corticosteroids, should be monitored routinely (eg, via stadiometry). To minimize the systemic effects of orally-inhaled and intranasal corticosteroids, each patient should be titrated to the lowest effective dose.

May suppress the immune system; patients may be more susceptible to infection. Use with caution in patients with systemic infections or ocular herpes simplex. Avoid exposure to chickenpox and measles.

Adverse Reactions Frequency not defined.

Cardiovascular: Edema, hypertension, arrhythmia, cardiomyopathy, myocardial rupture (post-MI), syncope, thromboembolism, thrombophlebitis, vasculitis

Central nervous system: Insomnia, nervousness, vertigo, seizure, psychosis, pseudotumor cerebri (usually following discontinuation), headache, mood swings, delirium, hallucinations, euphoria

Dermatologic: Hirsutism, acne, skin atrophy, bruising, hyperpigmentation, pruritus (generalized), perianal pruritus (following I.V. injection), urticaria

Endocrine & metabolic: Diabetes mellitus, adrenal suppression, hyperlipidemia, Cushing's syndrome, pituitary-adrenal axis suppression, growth suppression, glucose intolerance, gynecomastia, hypokalemia, alkalosis, amenorrhea, sodium and water retention, hyperglycemia, hypercalciuria, weight gain

Gastrointestinal: Appetite increased, indigestion, peptic ulcer, nausea, vomiting, abdominal distention, ulcerative esophagitis, pancreatitis, intestinal perforation

Genitourinary: Altered (increased or decreased) spermatogenesis

Hematologic: Transient leukocytosis

Hepatic: Transaminases increased, hepatomegaly

Neuromuscular & skeletal: Arthralgia, muscle weakness, osteoporosis, fractures, myopathy (particularly in conjunction with neuromuscular disease or neuromuscular blocking agents), tendon rupture, vertebral compression fractures, neuropathy, neuritis, parasthesia

Ocular: Cataracts, glaucoma, exophthalmos, intraocular pressure increased

Miscellaneous: Infections, anaphylactoid reaction, anaphylaxis, angioedema, avascular necrosis, secondary malignancy, Kaposi's sarcoma, intractable hiccups, impaired wound healing, abnormal fat deposition, moon face

Topical: <1%: Itching, dryness, folliculitis, hypertrichosis, acneiform eruptions, hypopigmentation, perioral dermatitis, allergic contact dermatitis, skin maceration, skin atrophy, striae, miliaria, local burning, irritation. secondary infection

Overdosage/Toxicology When consumed in high doses over prolonged periods, systemic hypercorticism and adrenal suppression may occur. In these cases, discontinuation of the corticosteroid should be done judiciously.

Drug Interactions **Substrate** of CYP3A4 (minor); **Induces** CYP2A6 (weak), 2B6 (weak), 2C8 (weak), 2C9 (weak), 3A4 (weak)

Aminoglutethimide: May reduce the serum levels/effects of dexamethasone; likely via induction of microsomal isoenzymes.

Antacids: May increase the absorption of corticosteroids; separate administration by 2 hours.

Anticholinesterases: Concurrent use may lead to severe weakness in patients with myasthenia gravis.

Aprepitant: May increase the serum levels of corticosteroids; monitor.

Azole antifungals: May increase the serum levels of corticosteroids; monitor.

Bile acid sequestrants: May reduce the absorption of corticosteroids; separate administration by 2 hours.

Calcium channel blockers (nondihydropyridine): May increase the serum levels of corticosteroids; monitor.

Cyclosporine: Corticosteroids may increase the serum levels of cyclosporine. In addition, cyclosporine may increase levels of corticosteroids

Estrogens: May increase the serum levels of corticosteroids; monitor.

Fluoroquinolones: Concurrent use may increase the risk of tendon rupture, particularly in elderly patients (overall incidence rare).

Isoniazid: Serum concentrations may be decreased by corticosteroids.

Neuromuscular-blocking agents: Concurrent use with corticosteroids may increase the risk of myopathy.

Nonsteroidal anti-inflammatory drugs (NSAIDs): Concurrent use with corticosteroids may lead to an increased incidence of gastrointestinal adverse effects; use caution.

Phenytoin: Dexamethasone may decrease serum levels/effects of phenytoin; monitor.

Salicylates: Salicylates may increase the gastrointestinal adverse effects of corticosteroids.

Thalidomide: Concurrent use with corticosteroids may increase the risk of selected adverse effects (toxic epidermal necrolysis and DVT); use caution

Vaccines, toxoids: Corticosteroids may suppress the response to vaccinations. The use of live vaccines is contraindicated in immunosuppressed patients. In patients receiving high doses of systemic corticosteroids for ≥14 days, wait at least 1 month between discontinuing steroid therapy and administering immunization.

Warfarin: Corticosteroids may lead to a reduction in warfarin effect; monitor.

Ethanol/Nutrition/Herb Interactions

Ethanol: Avoid ethanol (may enhance gastric mucosal irritation).

Food: Dexamethasone interferes with calcium absorption. Limit caffeine.

Herb/Nutraceutical: Avoid cat's claw, echinacea (have immunostimulant properties).

(Continued)

Dexamethasone *(Continued)*

Dietary Considerations May be taken with meals to decrease GI upset. May need diet with increased potassium, pyridoxine, vitamin C, vitamin D, folate, calcium, and phosphorus.

Dosage Forms [DSC] = Discontinued product

Elixir, as base: 0.5 mg/5 mL (240 mL) [contains alcohol 5%; raspberry flavor]

Injection, solution, as sodium phosphate: 4 mg/mL (1 mL, 5 mL, 10 mL, 25 mL, 30 mL); 10 mg/mL (1 mL, 10 mL)

Decadron® Phosphate: 4 mg/mL (5 mL, 25 mL); 24 mg/mL (5 mL) [contains sodium bisulfite] [DSC]

Ointment, ophthalmic, as sodium phosphate: 0.05% (3.5 g)

Solution, ophthalmic, as sodium phosphate: 0.1% (5 mL)

Solution, oral: 0.5 mg/5 mL (500 mL) [cherry flavor]

Solution, oral concentrate (Dexamethasone Intensol®): 1 mg/mL (30 mL) [contains alcohol 30%]

Suspension, ophthalmic (Maxidex®): 0.1% (5 mL, 15 mL)

Tablet: 0.25 mg, 0.5 mg, 0.75 mg, 1 mg, 1.5 mg, 2 mg, 4 mg, 6 mg [some 0.5 mg tablets may contain tartrazine]

Decadron®: 0.5 mg, 0.75 mg, 4 mg

DexPak® TaperPak®: 1.5 mg [51 tablets on taper dose card]

- **Dexamethasone Intensol®** *see* Dexamethasone *on page 366*
- **Dexamethasone Sodium Phosphate** *see* Dexamethasone *on page 366*
- **Dexasone® (Can)** *see* Dexamethasone *on page 366*

Dexmedetomidine (deks MED e toe mi deen)

Medication Safety Issues

Sound-alike/look-alike issues:

Precedex™ may be confused with Peridex®

U.S. Brand Names Precedex™

Canadian Brand Names Precedex™

Synonyms Dexmedetomidine Hydrochloride

Pharmacologic Category $Alpha_2$-Adrenergic Agonist; Sedative

Generic Available No

Use Sedation of initially intubated and mechanically ventilated patients during treatment in an intensive care setting; ~~duration of infusion should not exceed 24 hours~~

Unlabeled/Investigational Use Unlabeled uses include premedication prior to anesthesia induction with thiopental; relief of pain and reduction of opioid dose following laparoscopic tubal ligation; as an adjunct anesthetic in ophthalmic surgery; treatment of shivering; premedication to attenuate the cardiostimulatory and postanesthetic delirium of ketamine

Mechanism of Action Selective $alpha_2$-adrenoceptor agonist with sedative properties; $alpha_1$ activity was observed at high doses or after rapid infusions

Pharmacodynamics/Kinetics

Onset of action: Rapid

Distribution: V_{ss}: Approximately 118 L; rapid

Protein binding: 94%

Metabolism: Hepatic via glucuronidation and CYP2A6

Half-life elimination: 6 minutes; Terminal: 2 hours

Excretion: Urine (95%); feces (4%)

Dosage Individualized and titrated to desired clinical effect

Adults: I.V.: Solution must be diluted prior to administration. Initial: Loading infusion of 1 mcg/kg over 10 minutes, followed by a maintenance infusion of 0.2-0.7 mcg/kg/hour; not indicated for infusions lasting >24 hours

Elderly (>65 years of age): Dosage reduction may need to be considered. No specific guidelines available. Dose selections should be cautious, at the low end of dosage range; titration should be slower, allowing adequate time to evaluate response.

Dosage adjustment in hepatic impairment: Dosage reduction may need to be considered. No specific guidelines available.

Stability Compatible with lactated Ringer's, 5% dextrose in water, 0.9% sodium chloride in water, 20% mannitol, thiopental, etomidate, vecuronium, pancuronium, succinylcholine, atracurium, mivacurium, glycopyrrolate, phenylephrine, atropine, midazolam, morphine, fentanyl, and a plasma substitute

May adsorb to certain types of natural rubber; use components made with synthetic or coated natural rubber gaskets whenever possible

Administration Administer using a controlled infusion device. Must be diluted in 0.9% sodium chloride solution to achieve the required concentration prior to administration. Advisable to use administration components made with synthetic or coated natural rubber gaskets. Parenteral products should be inspected visually for particulate matter and discoloration prior to administration.

Monitoring Parameters Level of sedation, heart rate, respiration, rhythm, blood pressure

Anesthesia and Critical Care Concerns/Other Considerations Unlabeled uses include premedication prior to anesthesia induction with thiopental (0.33-0.67 mcg/kg); relief of pain and reduction of opioid dose following laparoscopic tubal ligation; as an adjunct anesthetic in ophthalmic surgery; treatment of shivering; and premedication (2.5 mcg/kg) to attenuate the cardiostimulatory and postanesthetic delirium of ketamine.

Dexmedetomidine has not been reported to cause respiratory depression. Assess the patient for pain during infusion; the sedation produced by this agent is not equivalent to analgesia. Adequate pain management should be addressed.

Dexmedetomidine should not be coadministered through the same I.V. catheter with plasma or blood products (physical compatibility not established). It is compatible with lactated Ringer's, 5% dextrose in water, 0.9% sodium chloride in water, 20% mannitol, thiopental, etomidate, vecuronium, pancuronium, succinylcholine, atracurium, mivacurium, fentanyl, and a plasma substitute. Dexmedetomidine may adsorb to some types of natural rubber; administration components made with synthetic or coated natural rubber gaskets are recommended.

In a prospective, observational study of 12 ventilator-dependent patients, dexmedetomidine was assessed as a sedative. Patients received a loading dose infusion of 1 mcg/kg over 10 minutes followed by the manufacturer's recommended infusion rate (0.2-0.7 mcg/kg/hour) for up to 7 days. Some patients required higher maintenance infusion rates than recommended by the manufacturer. Mean infusion rate was 1 ± 0.7 mcg/kg/hour. The maximum rate was 2.5 mcg/kg/hour. Adverse cardiovascular events were most frequently related to the initial loading infusion. These investigators suggest using a lower loading infusion. Higher maintenance infusions may be required in some patients. Patients did not go through a withdrawal syndrome when the infusion was discontinued (Venn, 2003).

The package insert suggests that there is a potential for withdrawal with symptoms such as nervousness, agitation, headaches, and rapid rise in blood pressure.

Pregnancy Risk Factor C

Contraindications Hypersensitivity to dexmedetomidine or any component of the formulation; use outside of an intensive care setting

Warnings/Precautions Should be administered only by persons skilled in management of patients in intensive care setting. Patients should be continuously monitored. Episodes of bradycardia, hypotension, and sinus arrest have been associated with dexmedetomidine when administered rapidly I.V. (eg, bolus administration) or to patients with high vagal tone. Use caution in patients with heart block, severe ventricular dysfunction, hypovolemia, diabetes, chronic hypertension, and in the elderly. Use with caution in patients receiving vasodilators or drugs which decrease heart rate. If medical intervention is required, treatment may include stopping or decreasing the infusion; increasing the rate of I.V. fluid administration, use of pressor agents, and elevation of the lower extremities. Transient hypertension has been primarily observed during the dose in association with the initial peripheral vasoconstrictive effects of dexmedetomidine. Treatment of this is not generally necessary; however, reduction of infusion rate may be desirable.

Adverse Reactions

>10%:

Cardiovascular: Hypotension (30%)

Gastrointestinal: Nausea (11%)

1% to 10%:

Cardiovascular: Bradycardia (8%), atrial fibrillation (7%)

(Continued)

Dexmedetomidine *(Continued)*

Central nervous system: Pain (3%)
Hematologic: Anemia (3%), leukocytosis (2%)
Renal: Oliguria (2%)
Respiratory: Hypoxia (6%), pulmonary edema (2%), pleural effusion (3%)
Miscellaneous: Infection (2%), thirst (2%)

Overdosage/Toxicology In reports of overdosages where the blood concentration was 13 times the upper boundary of the therapeutic range, first-degree AV block and second degree heart block occurred. No hemodynamic compromise was noted with the AV block and the heart block resolved spontaneously within one minute. Two patients who received a 2 mcg/kg loading dose over 10 minutes experienced bradycardia and/or hypotension. One patient who received a loading dose of undiluted dexmedetomidine (19.4 mcg/kg) had cardiac arrest and was successfully resuscitated.

Drug Interactions **Substrate** of CYP2A6 (major); **Inhibits** CYP1A2 (weak), 2C9 (weak), 2D6 (strong), 3A4 (weak)

CYP2A6 inhibitors: May increase the levels/effects of dexmedetomidine. Example inhibitors include isoniazid, methoxsalen, and miconazole.

CYP2D6 substrates: Dexmedetomidine may increase the levels/effects of CYP2D6 substrates. Example substrates include amphetamines, selected beta-blockers, dextromethorphan, fluoxetine, lidocaine, mirtazapine, nefazodone, paroxetine, risperidone, ritonavir, thioridazine, tricyclic antidepressants, and venlafaxine.

CYP2D6 prodrug substrates: Dexmedetomidine may decrease the levels/effects of CYP2D6 prodrug substrates. Example prodrug substrates include codeine, hydrocodone, oxycodone, and tramadol.

Hypotension and/or bradycardia may be increased by vasodilators and heart rate-lowering agents.

Dosage Forms Injection, solution [preservative free]: 100 mcg/mL (2 mL)

References

Venn M, Newman J, and Grounds M, "A Phase II Study to Evaluate the Efficacy of Dexmedetomidine for Sedation in the Medical Intensive Care Unit," *Intensive Care Med*, 2003, 29(2):201-7.

♦ **Dexmedetomidine Hydrochloride** *see* Dexmedetomidine *on page 370*

♦ **DexPak® TaperPak®** *see* Dexamethasone *on page 366*

Dextran (DEKS tran)

Medication Safety Issues

Sound-alike/look-alike issues:

Dextran may be confused with Dexatrim®, Dexedrine®

U.S. Brand Names Gentran®; LMD®

Canadian Brand Names Gentran®

Synonyms Dextran 40; Dextran 70; Dextran, High Molecular Weight; Dextran, Low Molecular Weight

Pharmacologic Category Plasma Volume Expander

Generic Available Yes

Use Blood volume expander used in treatment of shock or impending shock when blood or blood products are not available; dextran 40 is also used as a priming fluid in cardiopulmonary bypass and for prophylaxis of venous thrombosis and pulmonary embolism in surgical procedures associated with a high risk of thromboembolic complications

Mechanism of Action Produces plasma volume expansion by virtue of its highly colloidal starch structure, similar to albumin

Pharmacodynamics/Kinetics

Onset of action: Minutes to 1 hour (depending upon the molecular weight polysaccharide administered)

Excretion: Urine (~75%) within 24 hours

Dosage I.V. (requires an infusion pump): Dose and infusion rate are dependent upon the patient's fluid status and must be individualized:

Volume expansion/shock:

Children: Total dose should not exceed 20 mL/kg during first 24 hours

Adults: 500-1000 mL at a rate of 20-40 mL/minute; maximum daily dose: 20 mL/kg for first 24 hours; 10 mL/kg/day thereafter; therapy should not be continued beyond 5 days

Pump prime (Dextran 40): Varies with the volume of the pump oxygenator; generally, the 10% solution is added in a dose of 1-2 g/kg

Prophylaxis of venous thrombosis/pulmonary embolism (Dextran 40): Begin during surgical procedure and give 50-100 g on the day of surgery; an additional 50 g (500 mL) should be administered every 2-3 days during the period of risk (up to 2 weeks postoperatively); usual maximum infusion rate for nonemergency use: 4 mL/minute

Dosing in renal and/or hepatic impairment: Use with extreme caution

Stability Store at room temperature; discard partially used containers

Administration For I.V. infusion only (use an infusion pump). Infuse initial 500 mL at a rate of 20-40 mL/minute if hypervolemic. Reduce rate for additional infusion to 4 mL/minute. **Observe patients closely for anaphylactic reaction.**

Monitoring Parameters Observe patient for signs of circulatory overload and/or monitor central venous pressure; observe patients closely during the first minute of infusion and have other means of maintaining circulation should dextran therapy result in an anaphylactoid reaction; monitor hemoglobin and hematocrit, electrolytes, serum protein

Anesthesia and Critical Care Concerns/Other Considerations Dextran should be used with extreme caution in patients with restrictive cardiovascular disease and renal or hepatic impairment. Patients should be observed closely during the first several minutes of the infusion in case anaphylactoid reaction occurs.

Dextran 40 is known as low molecular weight dextran (LMD®) and has an average molecular weight of 40,000.

Dextran 75 has an average molecular weight of 75,000.

Dextran 70 has an average molecular weight of 70,000.

Pregnancy Risk Factor C

Contraindications Hypersensitivity to dextran or any component of the formulation; marked hemostatic defects (thrombocytopenia, hypofibrinogenemia) of all types including those caused by drugs; marked cardiac decompensation; renal disease with severe oliguria or anuria

Warnings/Precautions Hypersensitivity reactions have been reported (dextran 40 rarely causes a reaction), usually early in the infusion. Monitor closely during infusion initiation for signs or symptoms of a hypersensitivity reaction. Dextran 1 is indicated for prophylaxis of serious anaphylactic reactions to dextran infusions. Administration can cause fluid or solute overload. Use caution in patients with fluid overload. Use with caution in patients with active hemorrhage. Use caution in patients receiving corticosteroids. Renal failure has been reported. Fluid status including urine output should be monitored closely. Exercise care to prevent a depression of hematocrit <30% (can cause hemodilution). Observe for signs of bleeding.

Adverse Reactions <1% (Limited to important or life-threatening): Mild hypotension, tightness of chest, wheezing

Overdosage/Toxicology Symptoms of overdose include fluid overload, pulmonary edema, increased bleeding time, and decreased platelet function. Treatment is supportive. Blood products containing clotting factors may be necessary.

Drug Interactions

Abciximab: Dextran may enhance the anticoagulant effect of abciximab. Avoid concurrent use.

Dosage Forms

Infusion [premixed in D_5W; high molecular weight]: 6% Dextran 70 (500 mL)

Infusion [premixed in D_5W; low molecular weight] (Gentran®, LMD®): 10% Dextran 40 (500 mL)

Infusion [premixed in $D_{10}W$; high molecular weight]: 32% Dextran 70 (500 mL)

Infusion [premixed in NS; high molecular weight] (Gentran®): 6% Dextran 70 (500 mL)

Infusion [premixed in NS; low molecular weight] (Gentran®, LMD®): 10% Dextran (500 mL)

♦ **Dextran 40** *see* Dextran *on page 372*
♦ **Dextran 70** *see* Dextran *on page 372*
♦ **Dextran, High Molecular Weight** *see* Dextran *on page 372*
♦ **Dextran, Low Molecular Weight** *see* Dextran *on page 372*
♦ **Dextropropoxyphene** *see* Propoxyphene *on page 1074*
♦ **DHPG Sodium** *see* Ganciclovir *on page 581*

- **Diabeta** *see* GlyBURIDE *on page 598*
- **Diaβeta®** *see* GlyBURIDE *on page 598*
- **Diamox® (Can)** *see* AcetaZOLAMIDE *on page 32*
- **Diamox® Sequels®** *see* AcetaZOLAMIDE *on page 32*
- **Diastat®** *see* Diazepam *on page 374*
- **Diastat® AcuDial™** *see* Diazepam *on page 374*
- **Diastat® Rectal Delivery System (Can)** *see* Diazepam *on page 374*
- **Diazemuls® (Can)** *see* Diazepam *on page 374*

Diazepam (dye AZ e pam)

Medication Safety Issues

Sound-alike/look-alike issues:

Diazepam may be confused with diazoxide, Ditropan®, lorazepam

Valium® may be confused with Valcyte™

Related Information

Anesthesia Considerations for Neurosurgery *on page 1401*

Anesthesia for Patients With Liver Disease *on page 1421*

Benzodiazepines *on page 1555*

Intravenous Anesthetic Agents *on page 1531*

Moderate Sedation *on page 1442*

Perioperative Management of Patients on Antiseizure Medication *on page 1458*

Sedative Agents in the Intensive Care Unit *on page 1576*

U.S. Brand Names Diastat®; Diastat® AcuDial™; Diazepam Intensol®; Valium®

Canadian Brand Names Apo-Diazepam®; Diastat®; Diastat® Rectal Delivery System; Diazemuls®; Novo-Dipam; Valium®

Pharmacologic Category Benzodiazepine

Restrictions C-IV

Generic Available Yes: Injection, tablet, solution only

Use Management of anxiety disorders, ethanol withdrawal symptoms; skeletal muscle relaxant; treatment of convulsive disorders

Orphan drug: Viscous solution for rectal administration: Management of selected, refractory epilepsy patients on stable regimens of antiepileptic drugs (AEDs) requiring intermittent use of diazepam to control episodes of increased seizure activity

Unlabeled/Investigational Use Panic disorders; preoperative sedation, light anesthesia, amnesia

Mechanism of Action Binds to stereospecific benzodiazepine receptors on the postsynaptic GABA neuron at several sites within the central nervous system, including the limbic system, reticular formation. Enhancement of the inhibitory effect of GABA on neuronal excitability results by increased neuronal membrane permeability to chloride ions. This shift in chloride ions results in hyperpolarization (a less excitable state) and stabilization.

Pharmacodynamics/Kinetics

I.V.: Status epilepticus:

Onset of action: Almost immediate

Duration: 20-30 minutes

Absorption: Oral: 85% to 100%, more reliable than I.M.

Protein binding: 98%

Metabolism: Hepatic

Half-life elimination: Parent drug: Adults: 20-50 hours; increased half-life in neonates, elderly, and those with severe hepatic disorders; Active major metabolite (desmethyldiazepam): 50-100 hours; may be prolonged in neonates

Dosage Oral absorption is more reliable than I.M.

Children:

Conscious sedation for procedures: Oral: 0.2-0.3 mg/kg (maximum: 10 mg) 45-60 minutes prior to procedure

Sedation/muscle relaxant/anxiety:

Oral: 0.12-0.8 mg/kg/day in divided doses every 6-8 hours

I.M., I.V.: 0.04-0.3 mg/kg/dose every 2-4 hours to a maximum of 0.6 mg/kg within an 8-hour period if needed

Status epilepticus:

Infants 30 days to 5 years: I.V.: 0.05-0.3 mg/kg/dose given over 2-3 minutes, every 15-30 minutes to a maximum total dose of 5 mg; repeat in 2-4 hours as needed **or** 0.2-0.5 mg/dose every 2-5 minutes to a maximum total dose of 5 mg

>5 years: I.V.: 0.05-0.3 mg/kg/dose given over 2-3 minutes every 15-30 minutes to a maximum total dose of 10 mg; repeat in 2-4 hours as needed **or** 1 mg/dose given over 2-3 minutes, every 2-5 minutes to a maximum total dose of 10 mg

Rectal: 0.5 mg/kg, then 0.25 mg/kg in 10 minutes if needed

Anticonvulsant (acute treatment): Rectal gel:

Infants <6 months: Not recommended

Children <2 years: Safety and efficacy have not been studied

Children 2-5 years: 0.5 mg/kg

Children 6-11 years: 0.3 mg/kg

Children ≥12 years: 0.2 mg/kg

Note: Dosage should be rounded upward to the next available dose, 2.5, 5, 10, 12.5, 15, 17.5, and 20 mg/dose; dose may be repeated in 4-12 hours if needed; do not use for more than 5 episodes per month or more than one episode every 5 days

Adolescents: Conscious sedation for procedures:

Oral: 10 mg

I.V.: 5 mg, may repeat with ½ dose if needed

Adults:

Anticonvulsant (acute treatment): Rectal gel: 0.2 mg/kg

Note: Dosage should be rounded upward to the next available dose, 2.5, 5, 10, 12.5, 15, 17.5, and 20 mg/dose; dose may be repeated in 4-12 hours if needed; do not use for more than 5 episodes per month or more than one episode every 5 days.

Anxiety/sedation/skeletal muscle relaxant:

Oral: 2-10 mg 2-4 times/day

I.M., I.V.: 2-10 mg, may repeat in 3-4 hours if needed

Sedation in the ICU patient: I.V.: 0.03-0.1 mg/kg every 30 minutes to 6 hours

Status epilepticus: I.V.: 5-10 mg every 10-20 minutes, up to 30 mg in an 8-hour period; may repeat in 2-4 hours if necessary

Rapid tranquilization of agitated patient (administer every 30-60 minutes): Oral: 5-10 mg; average total dose for tranquilization: 20-60 mg

Elderly:

Anticonvulsant: Rectal gel: Due to the increased half-life in elderly and debilitated patients, consider reducing dose.

Anxiety: Oral: Initial: 1-2 mg 1-2 times/day; increase gradually as needed, rarely need to use >10 mg/day (watch for hypotension and excessive sedation)

Skeletal muscle relaxant: Oral: Initial: 2-5 mg 2-4 times/day

Hemodialysis: Not dialyzable (0% to 5%); supplemental dose is not necessary

Dosing adjustment in hepatic impairment: Reduce dose by 50% in cirrhosis and avoid in severe/acute liver disease

Stability

Protect parenteral dosage form from light; potency is retained for up to 3 months when kept at room temperature; most stable at pH 4-8, hydrolysis occurs at pH <3; do not mix I.V. product with other medications

Rectal gel: Store at 25°C (77°F); excursion permitted to 15°C to 30°C (59°F to 86°F).

Administration Intensol® should be diluted before use.

In children, do not exceed 1-2 mg/minute IVP; adults 5 mg/minute

Rectal gel: Patient should be positioned on side (facing person responsible for monitoring), with top leg bent forward. Insert rectal tip (lubricated) into rectum and push in plunger gently over 3 seconds. Remove tip of rectal syringe after 3 additional seconds. Buttocks should be held together for 3 seconds after removal. Dispose of syringe appropriately.

Monitoring Parameters Respiratory, cardiovascular, and mental status; check for orthostasis

Reference Range Therapeutic: Diazepam: 0.2-1.5 mcg/mL (SI: 0.7-5.3 μmol/L); N-desmethyldiazepam (nordiazepam): 0.1-0.5 mcg/mL (SI: 0.35-1.8 μmol/L)

Anesthesia and Critical Care Concerns/Other Considerations

Oral absorption more reliable than intramuscular. Intensol® should be diluted before use. Diazepam does not have any analgesic effects. Chronic use of this agent may increase the perioperative benzodiazepine dose needed to achieve desired effect. Abrupt discontinuation after sustained use (generally >10 days)

(Continued)

Diazepam *(Continued)*

may cause withdrawal symptoms. Hypotension may result in orthostatic lightheadedness or syncope. Benzodiazepines, as a class, may depress respiration. The 2002 ACCM/SCCM guidelines for the sustained use of sedatives and analgesics in critically-ill adults recommend diazepam or midazolam for rapid sedation of acutely-agitated patients.

Status Epilepticus: A randomized, double-blind trial evaluated the efficacy of four treatments in overt status epilepticus. Treatment arms were designed based upon accepted practices of North American neurologists. The treatments were: 1) lorazepam 0.1 mg/kg, 2) diazepam 0.15 mg/kg followed by phenytoin 18 mg/kg, 3) phenytoin 18 mg/kg alone, and 4) phenobarbital 15 mg/kg. Treatment was considered successful if the seizures were terminated (clinically and by EEG) within 20 minutes of start of therapy without seizure recurrence within 60 minutes from the start of therapy. Patients who failed the first treatment received a second and a third, if necessary. Patients did not receive randomized treatments after the first one but the treating physician remained blinded. Treatment success: Lorazepam 64.9%, phenobarbital 58.2%, diazepam/phenytoin 55.8%, and phenytoin alone 43.6%. Using an "intention-to-treat" analysis, there was no statistical difference between the groups. Results of subsequent treatments in patients who failed the first therapy indicated that response rate significantly dropped regardless of treatment. Aggregate response rate to the second treatment was 7.0% and third treatment 2.3%.

Pregnancy Risk Factor D

Contraindications Hypersensitivity to diazepam or any component of the formulation (cross-sensitivity with other benzodiazepines may exist); narrow-angle glaucoma; not for use in children <6 months of age (oral, rectal gel) or <30 days of age (parenteral); pregnancy

Warnings/Precautions Diazepam has been associated with increasing the frequency of grand mal seizures. Withdrawal has also been associated with an increase in the seizure frequency. Use with caution with drugs which may decrease diazepam metabolism. Use with caution in elderly or debilitated patients, patients with hepatic disease (including alcoholics), or renal impairment. Active metabolites with extended half-lives may lead to delayed accumulation and adverse effects. Use with caution in patients with respiratory disease or impaired gag reflex.

Acute hypotension, muscle weakness, apnea, and cardiac arrest have occurred with parenteral administration. Acute effects may be more prevalent in patients receiving concurrent barbiturates, narcotics, or ethanol. Appropriate resuscitative equipment and qualified personnel should be available during administration and monitoring. Avoid use of the injection in patients with shock, coma, or acute ethanol intoxication. Intra-arterial injection or extravasation of the parenteral formulation should be avoided. Parenteral formulation contains propylene glycol, which has been associated with toxicity when administered in high dosages. Administration of rectal gel should only be performed by individuals trained to recognize characteristic seizure activity for which the product is indicated, and capable of monitoring response to determine need for additional medical intervention.

Causes CNS depression (dose-related) resulting in sedation, dizziness, confusion, or ataxia which may impair physical and mental capabilities. Patients must be cautioned about performing tasks which require mental alertness (eg, operating machinery or driving). Use with caution in patients receiving other CNS depressants or psychoactive agents. Effects with other sedative drugs or ethanol may be potentiated. The dosage of narcotics should be reduced by approximately 1/3 when diazepam is added. Benzodiazepines have been associated with falls and traumatic injury and should be used with extreme caution in patients who are at risk of these events (especially the elderly).

Use caution in patients with depression, particularly if suicidal risk may be present. Use with caution in patients with a history of drug dependence. Benzodiazepines have been associated with dependence and acute withdrawal symptoms on discontinuation or reduction in dose. Acute withdrawal, including seizures, may be precipitated in patients after administration of flumazenil to patients receiving long-term benzodiazepine therapy.

Diazepam has been associated with anterograde amnesia. Paradoxical reactions, including hyperactive or aggressive behavior, have been reported with benzodiazepines, particularly in adolescent/pediatric or psychiatric patients. Does not have analgesic, antidepressant, or antipsychotic properties.

Adverse Reactions Frequency not defined. Adverse reactions may vary by route of administration.

Cardiovascular: Hypotension, vasodilatation

Central nervous system: Agitation, amnesia, anxiety, ataxia, confusion, depression, dizziness, drowsiness, emotional lability, euphoria, fatigue, headache, incoordination, insomnia, memory impairment, paradoxical excitement or rage, seizure, slurred speech, somnolence, vertigo

Dermatologic: Rash

Endocrine & metabolic: Changes in libido

Gastrointestinal: Changes in salivation, constipation, diarrhea, nausea

Genitourinary: Incontinence, urinary retention

Hepatic: Jaundice

Local: Phlebitis, pain with injection

Neuromuscular & skeletal: Dysarthria, tremor, weakness

Ocular: Blurred vision, diplopia

Respiratory: Apnea, asthma, decrease in respiratory rate

Overdosage/Toxicology Symptoms of overdose include somnolence, confusion, coma, hypoactive reflexes, dyspnea, hypotension, slurred speech, or impaired coordination. Treatment for benzodiazepine overdose is supportive. Flumazenil has been shown to selectively block the binding of benzodiazepines to CNS receptors, resulting in a reversal of benzodiazepine-induced CNS depression, but not respiratory depression.

Drug Interactions **Substrate** of CYP1A2 (minor), 2B6 (minor), 2C9 (minor), 2C19 (major), 3A4 (major); **Inhibits** CYP2C19 (weak), 3A4 (weak)

CNS depressants: Sedative effects and/or respiratory depression may be additive with CNS depressants; includes ethanol, barbiturates, narcotic analgesics, and other sedative agents; monitor for increased effect

CYP2C19 inducers: May decrease the levels/effects of diazepam. Example inducers include aminoglutethimide, carbamazepine, phenytoin, and rifampin.

CYP2C19 inhibitors: May increase the levels/effects of diazepam. Example inhibitors include delavirdine, fluconazole, fluvoxamine, gemfibrozil, isoniazid, omeprazole, and ticlopidine.

CYP3A4 inducers: CYP3A4 inducers may decrease the levels/effects of diazepam. Example inducers include aminoglutethimide, carbamazepine, nafcillin, nevirapine, phenobarbital, phenytoin, and rifamycins.

CYP3A4 inhibitors: May increase the levels/effects of diazepam. Example inhibitors include azole antifungals, clarithromycin, diclofenac, doxycycline, erythromycin, imatinib, isoniazid, nefazodone, nicardipine, propofol, protease inhibitors, quinidine, telithromycin, and verapamil.

Levodopa: Therapeutic effects may be diminished in some patients following the addition of a benzodiazepine; limited/inconsistent data

Oral contraceptives: May decrease the clearance of some benzodiazepines (those which undergo oxidative metabolism); monitor for increased benzodiazepine effect

Theophylline: May partially antagonize some of the effects of benzodiazepines; monitor for decreased response; may require higher doses for sedation

Ethanol/Nutrition/Herb Interactions

Ethanol: Avoid ethanol (may increase CNS depression).

Food: Diazepam serum levels may be increased if taken with food. Diazepam effect/toxicity may be increased by grapefruit juice; avoid concurrent use.

Herb/Nutraceutical: St John's wort may decrease diazepam levels. Avoid valerian, St John's wort, kava kava, gotu kola (may increase CNS depression).

Test Interactions False-negative urinary glucose determinations when using Clinistix® or Diastix®

Dosage Forms

Gel, rectal:

Diastat®: Pediatric rectal tip [4.4 cm]: 5 mg/mL (2.5 mg, 5 mg) [contains ethyl alcohol 10%, sodium benzoate, benzyl alcohol 1.5%; twin pack]

Diastat® AcuDial™ delivery system:

10 mg: Pediatric/adult rectal tip [4.4 cm]: 5 mg/mL (delivers set doses of 5 mg, 7.5 mg, and 10 mg) [contains ethyl alcohol 10%, sodium benzoate, benzyl alcohol 1.5%; twin pack]

(Continued)

Diazepam *(Continued)*

20 mg: Adult rectal tip [6 cm]: 5 mg/mL (delivers set doses of 10 mg, 12.5 mg, 15 mg, 17.5 mg, and 20 mg) [contains ethyl alcohol 10%, sodium benzoate, benzyl alcohol 1.5%; twin pack]

Injection, solution: 5 mg/mL (2 mL, 10 mL) [may contain benzyl alcohol, sodium benzoate, benzoic acid]

Solution, oral: 5 mg/5 mL (5 mL, 500 mL) [wintergreen-spice flavor]

Solution, oral concentrate (Diazepam Intensol®): 5 mg/mL (30 mL)

Tablet (Valium®): 2 mg, 5 mg, 10 mg

♦ **Diazepam Intensol®** *see* Diazepam *on page 374*

Diclofenac (dye KLOE fen ak)

Medication Safety Issues

Sound-alike/look-alike issues:

Diclofenac may be confused with Diflucan®, Duphalac®

Cataflam® may be confused with Catapres®

Voltaren® may be confused with tramadol, Ultram®, Verelan®

Related Information

Chronic Pain Management *on page 1430*

U.S. Brand Names Cataflam®; Solaraze®; Voltaren®; Voltaren Ophthalmic®; Voltaren®-XR

Canadian Brand Names Apo-Diclo®; Apo-Diclo Rapide®; Apo-Diclo SR®; Cataflam®; Novo-Difenac; Novo-Difenac K; Novo-Difenac-SR; Nu-Diclo; Nu-Diclo-SR; Pennsaid®; PMS-Diclofenac; PMS-Diclofenac SR; Riva-Diclofenac; Riva-Diclofenac-K; Voltaren®; Voltaren Ophtha®; Voltaren Rapide®

Synonyms Diclofenac Potassium; Diclofenac Sodium

Pharmacologic Category Nonsteroidal Anti-inflammatory Drug (NSAID); Nonsteroidal Anti-inflammatory Drug (NSAID), Ophthalmic; Nonsteroidal Anti-inflammatory Drug (NSAID), Oral

Restrictions A medication guide should be dispensed with each prescription. A template for the required MedGuide can be found on the FDA website at http://www.fda.gov/medwatch/SAFETY/2005/safety05.htm#NSAID

Generic Available Yes: Excludes gel, ophthalmic solution

Use

Immediate release: Ankylosing spondylitis; primary dysmenorrhea; acute and chronic treatment of rheumatoid arthritis, osteoarthritis

Delayed-release tablets: Acute and chronic treatment of rheumatoid arthritis, osteoarthritis, ankylosing spondylitis

Extended-release tablets: Chronic treatment of osteoarthritis, rheumatoid arthritis

Ophthalmic solution: Postoperative inflammation following cataract extraction; temporary relief of pain and photophobia in patients undergoing corneal refractive surgery

Topical gel: Actinic keratosis (AK) in conjunction with sun avoidance

Unlabeled/Investigational Use Juvenile rheumatoid arthritis

Mechanism of Action Inhibits prostaglandin synthesis by decreasing the activity of the enzyme, cyclooxygenase, which results in decreased formation of prostaglandin precursors. Mechanism of action for the treatment of AK has not been established.

Pharmacodynamics/Kinetics

Onset of action: Cataflam® is more rapid than sodium salt (Voltaren®) because it dissolves in the stomach instead of the duodenum

Absorption: Topical gel: 10%

Protein binding: 99% to albumin

Metabolism: Hepatic to several metabolites

Half-life elimination: 2 hours

Time to peak, serum: Cataflam®: ~1 hour; Voltaren®: ~2 hours

Excretion: Urine (65%); feces (35%)

Dosage Adults:

Oral:

Analgesia/primary dysmenorrhea: Starting dose: 50 mg 3 times/day; maximum dose: 150 mg/day

Rheumatoid arthritis: 150-200 mg/day in 2-4 divided doses (100 mg/day of sustained release product)

Osteoarthritis: 100-150 mg/day in 2-3 divided doses (100-200 mg/day of sustained release product)

Ankylosing spondylitis: 100-125 mg/day in 4-5 divided doses

Ophthalmic:

Cataract surgery: Instill 1 drop into affected eye 4 times/day beginning 24 hours after cataract surgery and continuing for 2 weeks

Corneal refractive surgery: Instill 1-2 drops into affected eye within the hour prior to surgery, within 15 minutes following surgery, and then continue for 4 times/day, up to 3 days

Topical: Apply gel to lesion area twice daily for 60-90 days

Dosage adjustment in renal impairment: Not recommended in patients with advanced renal disease

Dosage adjustment in hepatic impairment: No specific dosing recommendations

Elderly: No specific dosing recommendations; elderly may demonstrate adverse effects at lower doses than younger adults, and >60% may develop asymptomatic peptic ulceration with or without hemorrhage; monitor renal function

Stability Store below 30°C (86°F); protect from moisture, store in tight container.

Administration

Oral: Do not crush tablets. Administer with food or milk to avoid gastric distress. Take with full glass of water to enhance absorption.

Ophthalmic: Wait at least 5 minutes before administering other types of eye drops.

Topical gel: Cover lesion with gel and smooth into skin gently. Do not cover lesion with occlusive dressings or apply sunscreens, cosmetics, or other medications to affected area.

Monitoring Parameters Monitor CBC, liver enzymes; monitor urine output and BUN/serum creatinine; occult blood loss, hemoglobin, hematocrit

Anesthesia and Critical Care Concerns/Other Considerations The 2002 ACCM/SCCM guidelines for analgesia (critically-ill adult) suggest that NSAIDs may be used in combination with opioids in select patients for pain management. Concern about adverse events (increased risk of renal dysfunction, altered platelet function and gastrointestinal irritation) limits its use in patients who have other underlying risks for these events.

In short-term use, NSAIDs vary considerably in their effect on blood pressure. When NSAIDs are used in patients with hypertension, appropriate monitoring of blood pressure responses should be completed and the duration of therapy, when possible, kept short. The use of NSAIDs in the treatment of patients with congestive heart failure may be associated with an increased risk for fluid accumulation and edema; may precipitate renal failure in dehydrated patients.

Pregnancy Risk Factor B (topical); C (oral)/D (3rd trimester)

Contraindications Hypersensitivity to diclofenac, aspirin, other NSAIDs, or any component of the formulation; perioperative pain in the setting of coronary artery bypass surgery (CABG); pregnancy (3rd trimester)

Warnings/Precautions [U.S. Boxed Warning]: NSAIDs are associated with an increased risk of adverse cardiovascular events, including MI, stroke, and new onset or worsening of pre-existing hypertension. Risk may be increased with duration of use or pre-existing cardiovascular risk factors or disease. Carefully evaluate individual cardiovascular risk profiles prior to prescribing. Use caution with fluid retention, CHF, or hypertension.

Use of NSAIDs can compromise existing renal function. Renal toxicity can occur in patient with impaired renal function, dehydration, heart failure, liver dysfunction, those taking diuretics and ACEI, and the elderly. Rehydrate patient before starting therapy. Monitor renal function closely. Not recommended for use in patients with advanced renal disease.

[U.S. Boxed Warning]: NSAIDs may increase risk of gastrointestinal irritation, ulceration, bleeding, and perforation. These events may occur at any time during therapy and without warning. Use caution with a history of GI disease (bleeding or ulcers), concurrent therapy with aspirin, anticoagulants and/or corticosteroids, smoking, use of alcohol, the elderly or debilitated patients.

Use the lowest effective dose for the shortest duration of time, consistent with individual patient goals, to reduce risk of cardiovascular or GI adverse events. Alternate therapies should be considered for patients at high risk.

(Continued)

Diclofenac *(Continued)*

NSAIDs may cause serious skin adverse events including exfoliative dermatitis, Stevens-Johnson syndrome (SJS), and toxic epidermal necrolysis (TEN). Anaphylactoid reactions may occur, even without prior exposure; patients with "aspirin triad" (bronchial asthma, aspirin intolerance, rhinitis) may be at increased risk. Do not use in patients who experience bronchospasm, asthma, rhinitis, or urticaria with NSAID or aspirin therapy.

Use with caution in patients with decreased hepatic function. Closely monitor patients with any abnormal LFT. Severe hepatic reactions (eg, fulminant hepatitis, liver failure) have occurred with NSAID use, rarely; discontinue if signs or symptoms of liver disease develop, or if systemic manifestations occur.

The elderly are at increased risk for adverse effects (especially peptic ulceration, CNS effects, renal toxicity) from NSAIDs even at low doses.

Withhold for at least 4-6 half-lives prior to surgical or dental procedures.

Topical gel should not be applied to the eyes, open wounds, infected areas, or to exfoliative dermatitis. Monitor patients for 1 year following application of ophthalmic drops for corneal refractive procedures. Patients using ophthalmic drops should not wear soft contact lenses. Ophthalmic drops may slow/delay healing or prolong bleeding time following surgery.

Adverse Reactions

>10%:

Local: Application site reactions (gel): Pruritus (31% to 52%), rash (35% to 46%), contact dermatitis (19% to 33%), dry skin (25% to 27%), pain (15% to 26%), exfoliation (6% to 24%), paresthesia (8% to 20%)

Ocular: Ophthalmic drops (incidence may be dependent upon indication): Lacrimation (30%), keratitis (28%), elevated IOP (15%), transient burning/stinging (15%)

1% to 10%:

Central nervous system: Headache (7%), dizziness (3%)

Dermatologic: Pruritus (1% to 3%), rash (1% to 3%)

Endocrine & metabolic: Fluid retention (1% to 3%)

Gastrointestinal: Abdominal cramps (3% to 9%), abdominal pain (3% to 9%), constipation (3% to 9%), diarrhea (3% to 9%), flatulence (3% to 9%), indigestion (3% to 9%), nausea (3% to 9%), abdominal distention (1% to 3%), peptic ulcer/GI bleed (0.6% to 2%)

Hepatic: Increased ALT/AST (2%)

Local: Application site reactions (gel): Edema (4%)

Ocular: Ophthalmic drops: Abnormal vision, acute elevated IOP, blurred vision, conjunctivitis, corneal deposits, corneal edema, corneal opacity, corneal lesions, discharge, eyelid swelling, injection, iritis, irritation, itching, lacrimation disorder, ocular allergy

Otic: Tinnitus (1% to 3%)

<1% (Limited to important or life-threatening): Oral dosage forms: Acute renal failure, agranulocytosis, allergic purpura, alopecia, anaphylactoid reactions, anaphylaxis, angioedema, aplastic anemia, aseptic meningitis, asthma, bullous eruption, cirrhosis, CHF, eosinophilia, erythema multiforme major, GI hemorrhage, hearing loss, hemolytic anemia, hepatic necrosis, hepatitis, hepatorenal syndrome, interstitial nephritis, jaundice, laryngeal edema, leukopenia, nephrotic syndrome, pancreatitis, papillary necrosis, photosensitivity, purpura, Stevens-Johnson syndrome, swelling of lips and tongue, thrombocytopenia, urticaria, visual changes, vomiting

Overdosage/Toxicology Symptoms of overdose include acute renal failure, vomiting, drowsiness, and leukocytosis. Management of NSAID intoxication is supportive and symptomatic.

Drug Interactions Substrate (minor) of CYP1A2, 2B6, 2C8, 2C9, 2C19, 2D6, 3A4; **Inhibits** CYP1A2 (moderate), 2C9 (weak), 2E1 (weak), 3A4 (strong)

ACE inhibitors: Antihypertensive effects may be decreased by concurrent therapy with NSAIDs; monitor blood pressure

Angiotensin II antagonists: Antihypertensive effects may be decreased by concurrent therapy with NSAIDs; monitor blood pressure

Anticoagulants (warfarin, heparin, LMWHs) in combination with NSAIDs can cause increased risk of bleeding.

Antiplatelet drugs (ticlopidine, clopidogrel, aspirin, abciximab, dipyridamole, eptifibatide, tirofiban) can cause an increased risk of bleeding.

Beta-blockers: NSAIDs may decrease the antihypertensive effect of beta-blockers. Monitor.

Cholestyramine (and other bile acid sequestrants): May decrease the absorption of NSAIDs. Separate by at least 2 hours.

Corticosteroids may increase the risk of GI ulceration; avoid concurrent use.

Cyclosporine: NSAIDs may increase serum creatinine, potassium, blood pressure, and cyclosporine levels; monitor cyclosporine levels and renal function carefully.

CYP1A2 substrates: Diclofenac may increase the levels/effects of CYP1A2 substrates. Example substrates include aminophylline, fluvoxamine, mexiletine, mirtazapine, ropinirole, theophylline, and trifluoperazine.

CYP3A4 substrates: Diclofenac may increase the levels/effects of CYP3A4 substrates. Example substrates include benzodiazepines, calcium channel blockers, mirtazapine, nateglinide, nefazodone, tacrolimus, and venlafaxine. Selected benzodiazepines (midazolam and triazolam), cisapride, ergot alkaloids, selected HMG-CoA reductase inhibitors (lovastatin and simvastatin), and pimozide are generally contraindicated with strong CYP3A4 inhibitors.

Gentamicin and amikacin serum concentrations are increased by indomethacin in premature infants. Results may apply to other aminoglycosides and NSAIDs.

Hydralazine's antihypertensive effect is decreased; avoid concurrent use.

Lithium levels can be increased; avoid concurrent use if possible or monitor lithium levels and adjust dose. Sulindac may have the least effect. When NSAID is stopped, lithium will need adjustment again.

Loop diuretics efficacy (diuretic and antihypertensive effect) is reduced. Indomethacin reduces this efficacy, however, it may be anticipated with any NSAID.

Methotrexate: Severe bone marrow suppression, aplastic anemia, and GI toxicity have been reported with concomitant NSAID therapy. Avoid use during moderate or high-dose methotrexate (increased and prolonged methotrexate levels). NSAID use during low-dose treatment of rheumatoid arthritis has not been fully evaluated; extreme caution is warranted.

Thiazides antihypertensive effects are decreased; avoid concurrent use.

Verapamil plasma concentration is decreased by diclofenac; avoid concurrent use.

Warfarin's INRs may be increased by piroxicam. Other NSAIDs may have the same effect depending on dose and duration. Monitor INR closely. Use the lowest dose of NSAIDs possible and for the briefest duration.

Ethanol/Nutrition/Herb Interactions

Ethanol: Avoid ethanol (may enhance gastric mucosal irritation).

Herb/Nutraceutical: Avoid alfalfa, anise, bilberry, bladderwrack, bromelain, cat's claw, celery, coleus, cordyceps, dong quai, evening primrose, feverfew, fenugreek, garlic, ginger, ginkgo biloboa, red clover, horse chestnut, grapeseed, green tea, ginseng, guggul, horse chestnut seed, horseradish, licorice, prickly ash, red clover, reishi, SAMe, sweet clover, turmeric, white willow (all have additional antiplatelet activity).

Dietary Considerations May be taken with food to decrease GI distress.

Diclofenac potassium = Cataflam®; potassium content: 5.8 mg (0.15 mEq) per 50 mg tablet

Dosage Forms [DSC] = Discontinued product

Gel, as sodium:

Solaraze®: 30 mg/g (50 g)

Solution, ophthalmic, as sodium:

Voltaren Ophthalmic®: 0.1% (2.5 mL, 5 mL)

Tablet, as potassium: 50 mg

Cataflam®: 50 mg

Tablet, delayed release, enteric coated, as sodium: 50 mg, 75 mg

Voltaren®: 25 mg [DSC], 50 mg [DSC], 75 mg

Tablet, extended release, as sodium: 100 mg

Voltaren®-XR: 100 mg

♦ **Diclofenac Potassium** *see* Diclofenac *on page 378*

♦ **Diclofenac Sodium** *see* Diclofenac *on page 378*

♦ **Di-Dak-Sol** *see* Sodium Hypochlorite Solution *on page 1186*

Didanosine (dye DAN oh seen)

Medication Safety Issues
Sound-alike/look-alike issues:
Videx® may be confused with Lidex®

U.S. Brand Names Videx®; Videx® EC

Canadian Brand Names Videx®; Videx® EC

Synonyms ddI; Dideoxyinosine

Pharmacologic Category Antiretroviral Agent, Reverse Transcriptase Inhibitor (Nucleoside)

Generic Available Yes: Delayed release capsule

Use Treatment of HIV infection; always to be used in combination with at least two other antiretroviral agents

Mechanism of Action Didanosine, a purine nucleoside (adenosine) analog and the deamination product of dideoxyadenosine (ddA), inhibits HIV replication *in vitro* in both T cells and monocytes. Didanosine is converted within the cell to the mono-, di-, and triphosphates of ddA. These ddA triphosphates act as substrate and inhibitor of HIV reverse transcriptase substrate and inhibitor of HIV reverse transcriptase thereby blocking viral DNA synthesis and suppressing HIV replication.

Pharmacodynamics/Kinetics
Absorption: Subject to degradation by acidic pH of stomach; some formulations are buffered to resist acidic pH; ≤50% reduction in peak plasma concentration is observed in presence of food. Delayed release capsules contain enteric-coated beadlets which dissolve in the small intestine.
Distribution: V_d: Children: 35.6 L/m^2; Adults: 1.08 L/kg
Protein binding: <5%
Metabolism: Has not been evaluated in humans; studies conducted in dogs show extensive metabolism with allantoin, hypoxanthine, xanthine, and uric acid being the major metabolites found in urine
Bioavailability: 42%
Half-life elimination:
Children and Adolescents: 0.8 hour
Adults: Normal renal function: 1.5 hours; active metabolite, ddATP, has an intracellular half-life >12 hours *in vitro*; Renal impairment: 2.5-5 hours
Time to peak: Buffered tablets: 0.67 hours; Delayed release capsules: 2 hours
Excretion: Urine (~55% as unchanged drug)
Clearance: Total body: Averages 800 mL/minute

Dosage Treatment of HIV infection: Oral (administer on an empty stomach):
Children:
2 weeks to 8 months: 100 mg/m^2 twice daily is recommended by the manufacturer; 50 mg/m^2 may be considered in infants 2 weeks to 4 months
>8 months: 120 mg/m^2 twice daily; dosing range: 90-150 mg/m^2 twice daily; patients with CNS disease may require higher dose
Note: At least 2 tablets per dose should be administered for adequate buffering and absorption; tablets should be chewed or dispersed (in 1 ounce of water).

Adolescents and Adults: Dosing based on patient weight:
Note: Preferred dosing frequency is twice daily for didanosine tablets/oral solution
Chewable tablets, powder for oral solution:
<60 kg: 125 mg twice daily or 250 mg once daily
≥60 kg: 200 mg twice daily or 400 mg once daily
Note: Adults should receive 2-4 tablets per dose for adequate buffering and absorption; tablets should be chewed or dispersed (in 1 ounce of water).
Delayed release capsule (Videx® EC):
<60 kg: 250 mg once daily
≥60 kg; 400 mg once daily

Dosing adjustment with tenofovir (didanosine tablets or delayed release capsules; based on tenofovir product labeling):
<60 kg: 200 mg once daily
≥60 kg: 250 mg once daily

Dosage adjustment in renal impairment: Dosing based on patient weight, creatinine clearance, and dosage form: See table on next page.
Patients requiring hemodialysis or CAPD: Dose per Cl_{cr} <10 mL/minute

Recommended Dose (mg) of Didanosine by Body Weight

Creatinine Clearance (mL/min)	≥60 kg		<60 kg	
	Tablet[1] (mg)	Delayed Release Capsule (mg)	Tablet[1] (mg)	Delayed Release Capsule (mg)
≥60	400 daily or 200 twice daily	400 daily	250 daily or 125 twice daily	250 daily
30-59	200 daily or 100 twice daily	200 daily	150 daily or 75 twice daily	125 daily
10-29	150 daily	125 daily	100 daily	125 daily
<10	100 daily	125 daily	75 daily	See footnote 2.

[1]Chewable/dispersible buffered tablet; 2 tablets must be taken with each dose; different strengths of tablets may be combined to yield the recommended dose.

[2]Not suitable for use in patients <60 kg with Cl_{cr} <10 mL/minute; use alternate formulation.

Hemodialysis: Removed by hemodialysis (40% to 60%)

Dosing adjustment in hepatic impairment: Should be considered; monitor for toxicity

Elderly patients have a higher frequency of pancreatitis (10% versus 5% in younger patients); monitor renal function and dose accordingly

Stability Tablets and delayed release capsules should be stored in tightly closed bottles at 15°C to 30°C; tablets undergo rapid degradation when exposed to an acidic environment; tablets dispersed in water are stable for 1 hour at room temperature. Reconstituted pediatric solution is stable for 30 days if refrigerated. Unbuffered powder for oral solution must be reconstituted and mixed with an equal volume of antacid at time of preparation.

Administration

Chewable/dispersible buffered tablets: The 200 mg tablet should only be used in once-daily dosing. At least 2 tablets, but no more than 4 tablets, should be taken together to allow adequate buffering. Tablets may be chewed or dispersed prior to consumption. To disperse, dissolve in 1 oz water, stir until uniform dispersion is formed, and drink immediately. May also add 1 oz of clear apple juice to initial dispersion if additional flavor is needed. The apple juice dilution is stable for 1 hour at room temperature. Do not mix with other juices.

Pediatric powder for oral solution: Prior to dispensing, the powder should be mixed with purified water USP to an initial concentration of 20 mg/mL and then further diluted with an appropriate antacid suspension to a final mixture of 10 mg/mL. Shake well prior to use.

Monitoring Parameters Serum potassium, uric acid, creatinine; hemoglobin, CBC with neutrophil and platelet count, CD4 cells; viral load; liver function tests, amylase; weight gain; perform dilated retinal exam every 6 months

Pregnancy Risk Factor B

Contraindications Hypersensitivity to didanosine or any component of the formulation

Warnings/Precautions [U.S. Boxed Warning]: Pancreatitis (sometimes fatal) has been reported; incidence is dose related. Risk factors for developing pancreatitis include a previous history of the condition, concurrent cytomegalovirus or *Mycobacterium avium-intracellulare* infection, and concomitant use of stavudine, pentamidine, or co-trimoxazole. Discontinue didanosine if clinical signs of pancreatitis occur. **[U.S. Boxed Warning]: Lactic acidosis, symptomatic hyperlactatemia, and severe hepatomegaly with steatosis (sometimes fatal) have occurred with antiretroviral nucleoside analogues, including didanosine.** Hepatotoxicity may occur even in the absence of marked transaminase elevations; suspend therapy in any patient developing clinical/laboratory findings which suggest hepatotoxicity. Pregnant women may be at increased risk of lactic acidosis and liver damage.

Peripheral neuropathy occurs in ~20% of patients receiving the drug. Retinal changes (including retinal depigmentation) and optic neuritis have been reported in adults and children using didanosine. Patients should undergo retinal examination every 6-12 months. Use with caution in patients with decreased renal or hepatic function, phenylketonuria, sodium-restricted diets, or with edema, CHF, or hyperuricemia. Twice-daily dosing is the preferred dosing frequency for didanosine tablets. Didanosine delayed release capsules are indicated for once-daily use.

(Continued)

Didanosine *(Continued)*

Adverse Reactions As reported in monotherapy studies; risk of toxicity may increase when combined with other agent.

>10%:

Gastrointestinal: Increased amylase (15% to 17%), abdominal pain (7% to 13%), diarrhea (19% to 28%)

Neuromuscular & skeletal: Peripheral neuropathy (17% to 20%)

1% to 10%:

Dermatologic: Rash, pruritus

Endocrine & metabolic: Increased uric acid

Gastrointestinal: Pancreatitis; patients >65 years of age had a higher frequency of pancreatitis than younger patients

Hepatic: Increased SGOT, increased SGPT, increased alkaline phosphatase

Postmarketing and/or case reports: Alopecia, anaphylactoid reaction, anemia, anorexia, arthralgia, diabetes mellitus, granulocytopenia, hepatitis, hyperlactatemia (symptomatic), hypersensitivity, lactic acidosis/hepatomegaly, leukopenia, liver failure, myalgia, myopathy, neuritis, optic renal impairment, pain, retinal depigmentation, rhabdomyolysis, seizure, thrombocytopenia, weakness

Overdosage/Toxicology Chronic overdose may cause pancreatitis, peripheral neuropathy, diarrhea, hyperuricemia, and hepatic impairment. There is no known antidote for didanosine overdose. Treatment is symptomatic.

Drug Interactions Drugs whose absorption depends on the level of acidity in the stomach (such as ketoconazole, itraconazole, and dapsone) should be administered at least 2 hours prior to the buffered formulations of didanosine (not affected by delayed release capsules)

Decreased effect: Buffered formulations of didanosine (tablets, pediatric oral solution) may decrease absorption of quinolones or tetracyclines, separate dosing by 2 hours; didanosine should be held during PCP treatment with pentamidine; didanosine may decrease levels of indinavir

Increased toxicity: Concomitant administration of other drugs (including hydroxyurea) which have the potential to cause peripheral neuropathy or pancreatitis may increase the risk of these toxicities

Allopurinol: May increase didanosine concentration; avoid concurrent use

Antacids: Concomitant use with buffered tablet or pediatric didanosine solution may potentiate adverse effects of aluminum- or magnesium-containing antacids

Ganciclovir: May increase didanosine concentration; monitor

Hydroxyurea: May precipitate didanosine-induced pancreatitis if added to therapy; concomitant use is not recommended

Methadone: May decrease didanosine concentration; monitor

Ribavirin: Coadministration may increase exposure to didanosine and/or its active metabolite, increasing the risk or severity of didanosine toxicities, including pancreatitis, lactic acidosis, and peripheral neuropathy. Coadministration of ribavirin with didanosine should be undertaken with caution, and patients should be monitored closely for didanosine-related toxicities; suspend therapy if signs or symptoms of toxicity are noted.

Tenofovir: Coadministration may increase exposure to didanosine and/or its active metabolite increasing the risk or severity of didanosine toxicities, including pancreatitis, hyperglycemia, lactic acidosis, and peripheral neuropathy. Some patients have experienced reduced CD4 cell counts and/or decreased virologic response. Coadministration of tenofovir with didanosine should be undertaken with caution, and patients should be monitored closely for didanosine-related toxicities; specific dosing adjustment is recommended; suspend therapy if signs or symptoms of toxicity are noted.

Ethanol/Nutrition/Herb Interactions

Ethanol: Avoid ethanol (increases risk of pancreatitis).

Food: Decreases AUC and C_{max}. Didanosine serum levels may be decreased by 55% if taken with food.

Dietary Considerations

Videx® EC: Take on an empty stomach; administer at least 1 hour before or 2 hours after eating

Chewable/dispersible tablet: Take on an empty stomach, 30 minutes before or 2 hours after eating. Chew well or mix in water; if mixed in water, may add 2 tablespoons (1 oz) apple juice for flavor. Do not use other juices. Each chewable tablet contains 36.5 mg phenylalanine and 8.6 mEq magnesium. Sodium content of buffered tablets: 264.5 mg (11.5 mEq).

Dosage Forms
Capsule, delayed release: 200 mg, 250 mg, 400 mg
Videx® EC: 125 mg, 200 mg, 250 mg, 400 mg
Powder for oral solution, pediatric (Videx®): 2 g, 4 g [makes 10 mg/mL solution after final mixing]
Tablet, buffered, chewable/dispersible (Videx®): 25 mg, 50 mg, 100 mg, 150 mg, 200 mg [all strengths contain phenylalanine 36.5 mg/tablet; orange flavor]

- ♦ **Dideoxyinosine** *see* Didanosine *on page 382*
- ♦ **Didronel®** *see* Etidronate Disodium *on page 495*
- ♦ **Diflucan®** *see* Fluconazole *on page 530*

Diflunisal (dye FLOO ni sal)

Medication Safety Issues
Sound-alike/look-alike issues:
Dolobid® may be confused with Slo-Bid®

Related Information
Acetaminophen and NSAIDS, Dosing Data *on page 1543*
Chronic Pain Management *on page 1430*

U.S. Brand Names Dolobid® [DSC]

Canadian Brand Names Apo-Diflunisal®; Novo-Diflunisal; Nu-Diflunisal

Pharmacologic Category Nonsteroidal Anti-inflammatory Drug (NSAID), Oral

Restrictions A medication guide should be dispensed with each prescription. A template for the required MedGuide can be found on the FDA website at http://www.fda.gov/medwatch/SAFETY/2005/safety05.htm#NSAID

Generic Available Yes

Use Management of inflammatory disorders usually including rheumatoid arthritis and osteoarthritis; can be used as an analgesic for treatment of mild to moderate pain

Mechanism of Action Inhibits prostaglandin synthesis by decreasing the activity of the enzyme, cyclooxygenase, which results in decreased formation of prostaglandin precursors

Pharmacodynamics/Kinetics
Onset of action: Analgesic: ~1 hour; maximal effect: 2-3 hours
Duration: 8-12 hours
Absorption: Well absorbed
Protein binding: >99%
Distribution: Enters breast milk
Metabolism: Extensively hepatic; metabolic pathways are saturable
Half-life elimination: 8-12 hours; prolonged with renal impairment
Time to peak, serum: 2-3 hours
Excretion: Urine (~3% as unchanged drug, 90% as glucuronide conjugates) within 72-96 hours

Dosage Adults: Oral:
Mild-to-moderate pain: Initial: 500-1000 mg followed by 250-500 mg every 8-12 hours; maximum daily dose: 1.5 g
Arthritis: 500-1000 mg/day in 2 divided doses; maximum daily dose: 1.5 g
Dosing adjustment in renal impairment: Use with caution; Cl_{cr} <50 mL/minute: Administer 50% of normal dose
Hemodialysis: No supplement required
CAPD: No supplement require
CAVH: Dose for GFR 10-50

Administration Tablet should be swallowed whole; do not crush or chew.

Anesthesia and Critical Care Concerns/Other Considerations The 2002 ACCM/SCCM guidelines for analgesia (critically-ill adult) suggest that NSAIDs may be used in combination with opioids in select patients for pain management. Concern about adverse events (increased risk of renal dysfunction, altered platelet function and gastrointestinal irritation) limits its use in patients who have other underlying risks for these events.

In short-term use, NSAIDs vary considerably in their effect on blood pressure. When NSAIDs are used in patients with hypertension, appropriate monitoring of blood pressure responses should be completed and the duration of therapy, when possible, kept short. The use of NSAIDs in the treatment of patients with congestive heart failure may be associated with an increased risk for fluid accumulation and edema; may precipitate renal failure in dehydrated patients.
(Continued)

Diflunisal *(Continued)*

Diflunisal is a salicylic acid derivative which is chemically different than aspirin and is not metabolized to salicylic acid. Diflunisal 500 mg is equal in analgesic efficacy to aspirin 650 mg, acetaminophen 650 mg, and acetaminophen 650 mg/ propoxyphene napsylate 100 mg, but has a longer duration of effect (8-12 hours). It is not recommended as an antipyretic. At doses ≥2 g/day, platelets are reversibly inhibited in function. Diflunisal is uricosuric at 500-750 mg/day. It causes less GI and renal toxicity than aspirin and other NSAIDs. Fecal blood loss is ½ that of aspirin at 2.6 g/day.

Pregnancy Risk Factor C (1st and 2nd trimesters)/D (3rd trimester)

Contraindications Hypersensitivity to diflunisal, aspirin, other NSAIDs, or any component of the formulation; perioperative pain in the setting of coronary artery bypass surgery (CABG); pregnancy (3rd trimester)

Warnings/Precautions [U.S. Boxed Warning]: NSAIDs are associated with an increased risk of adverse cardiovascular events, including MI, stroke, and new onset or worsening of pre-existing hypertension. Risk may be increased with duration of use or pre-existing cardiovascular risk-factors or disease. Carefully evaluate individual cardiovascular risk profiles prior to prescribing. Use caution with fluid retention, CHF, or hypertension.

[U.S. Boxed Warning]: NSAIDs may increase risk of gastrointestinal irritation, ulceration, bleeding, and perforation. These events may occur at any time during therapy and without warning. Use caution with a history of GI disease (bleeding or ulcers), concurrent therapy with aspirin, anticoagulants and/or corticosteroids, smoking, use of alcohol, the elderly or debilitated patients.

Use of NSAIDs can compromise existing renal function. Renal toxicity can occur in patient with impaired renal function, dehydration, heart failure, liver dysfunction, those taking diuretics and ACEI and the elderly. Rehydrate patient before starting therapy. Monitor renal function closely. Diflunisal is not recommended for patients with advanced renal disease.

Use the lowest effective dose for the shortest duration of time, consistent with individual patient goals, to reduce risk of cardiovascular or GI adverse events. Alternate therapies should be considered for patients at high risk.

NSAIDs may cause serious skin adverse events including exfoliative dermatitis, Stevens-Johnson syndrome (SJS), and toxic epidermal necrolysis (TEN). Anaphylactoid reactions may occur, even without prior exposure; patients with "aspirin triad" (bronchial asthma, aspirin intolerance, rhinitis) may be at increased risk. Do not use in patients who experience bronchospasm, asthma, rhinitis, or urticaria with NSAID or aspirin therapy.

A hypersensitivity syndrome has been reported; monitor for constitutional symptoms and cutaneous findings; other organ dysfunction may be involved.

Use with caution in patients with decreased hepatic function. Closely monitor patients with any abnormal LFT. Severe hepatic reactions (eg, fulminant hepatitis, liver failure) have occurred with NSAID use, rarely; discontinue if signs or symptoms of liver disease develop, or if systemic manifestations occur.

Diflunisal is a derivative of acetylsalicylic acid and therefore may be associated with Reye's syndrome. Withhold for at least 4-6 half-lives prior to surgical or dental procedures. Safety and efficacy have not been established in children <12 years of age.

Adverse Reactions

1% to 10%:

Central nervous system: Headache (3% to 9%), dizziness (1% to 3%), insomnia (1% to 3%), somnolence (1% to 3%), fatigue (1% to 3%)

Dermatologic: Rash (3% to 9%)

Gastrointestinal: Nausea (3% to 9%), dyspepsia (3% to 9%), GI pain (3% to 9%), diarrhea (3% to 9%), constipation (1% to 3%), flatulence (1% to 3%), vomiting (1% to 3%), GI ulceration

Otic: Tinnitus (1% to 3%)

<1% (Limited to important or life-threatening): Acute anaphylactic reaction, agranulocytosis, allergic reactions, angioedema, anorexia, blurred vision, bronchospasm, confusion, chest pain, cholestasis, cystitis, depression, diaphoresis, disorientation, dry mucous membranes, dyspnea, dysuria, edema, eructation, erythema multiforme, esophagitis, exfoliative dermatitis, flushing, gastritis, GI bleeding, GI perforation, hallucinations, hearing decreased, hearing loss,

hematuria, hemolytic anemia, hepatitis, hypersensitivity syndrome, hypersensitivity vasculitis, interstitial nephritis, itching, jaundice, mental depression, muscle cramps, necrotizing fasciitis, nephrotic syndrome, nervousness, palpitations, paresthesia, peptic ulcer, peripheral neuropathy, photosensitivity, proteinuria, pruritus, renal impairment, renal failure, seizure, Stevens-Johnson syndrome, stomatitis, syncope, tachycardia, thrombocytopenia, toxic epidermal necrolysis, trembling, urticaria, vasculitis, vertigo, weakness, wheezing

Overdosage/Toxicology Symptoms of overdose include drowsiness, nausea, vomiting, hyperventilation, tachycardia, tinnitus, stupor, coma, renal failure, and leukocytosis. Management of NSAID intoxication is supportive and symptomatic.

Drug Interactions

ACE inhibitors: Antihypertensive effects may be decreased by concurrent therapy with NSAIDs; monitor blood pressure.

Aminoglycosides: NSAIDs may decrease the excretion of aminoglycosides.

Angiotensin II antagonists: Antihypertensive effects may be decreased by concurrent therapy with NSAIDs; monitor blood pressure.

Anticoagulants (warfarin, heparin, LMWHs) in combination with NSAIDs can cause increased risk of bleeding.

Antiplatelet agents (ticlopidine, clopidogrel, aspirin, abciximab, dipyridamole, eptifibatide, tirofiban) can cause an increased risk of bleeding.

Beta-blockers: NSAIDs may diminish the antihypertensive effects of beta blockers.

Bisphosphonates: NSAIDs may increase the risk of gastrointestinal ulceration.

Cholestyramine (and other bile acid sequestrants): May decrease the absorption of NSAIDs. Separate by at least 2 hours.

Corticosteroids may increase the risk of GI ulceration; avoid concurrent use.

Cyclosporine: NSAIDs may increase serum creatinine, potassium, blood pressure, and cyclosporine levels; monitor cyclosporine levels and renal function carefully.

Hydralazine's antihypertensive effect is decreased; avoid concurrent use.

Lithium levels can be increased; avoid concurrent use if possible or monitor lithium levels and adjust dose.

Sulindac may have the least effect. When NSAID is stopped, lithium will need adjustment again.

Loop diuretics efficacy (diuretic and antihypertensive effect) is reduced. Indomethacin reduces this efficacy, however, it may be anticipated with any NSAID.

Methotrexate: Severe bone marrow suppression, aplastic anemia, and GI toxicity have been reported with concomitant NSAID therapy. Avoid use during moderate or high-dose methotrexate (increased and prolonged methotrexate levels). NSAID use during low-dose treatment of rheumatoid arthritis has not been fully evaluated; extreme caution is warranted.

Pemetrexed: NSAIDs may decrease the excretion of pemetrexed. Patients with Cl_{cr} 45-79 mL/minute should avoid long acting NSAIDs for 5 days before and 2 days after pemetrexed treatment.

Thiazides antihypertensive effects are decreased; avoid concurrent use.

Treprostinil: May enhance the risk of bleeding with concurrent use.

Vancomycin: NSAID©s may decrease the excretion of vancomycin.

Ethanol/Nutrition/Herb Interactions

Ethanol: Avoid ethanol (may enhance gastric mucosal irritation).

Herb/Nutraceutical: Avoid alfalfa, anise, bilberry, bladderwrack, bromelain, cat's claw, celery, coleus, cordyceps, dong quai, evening primrose, feverfew, fenugreek, garlic, ginger, ginkgo biloboa, red clover, horse chestnut, grapeseed, green tea, ginseng, guggul, horse chestnut seed, horseradish, licorice, prickly ash, red clover, reishi, SAMe, sweet clover, turmeric, white willow (all have additional antiplatelet activity).

Test Interactions Falsely elevated increase in serum salicylate levels

Dietary Considerations Should be taken with food to decrease GI distress.

Dosage Forms [DSC] = Discontinued product

Tablet: 500 mg

Dolobid®: 250 mg, 500 mg [DSC]

- **Digibind®** *see* Digoxin Immune Fab *on page 392*
- **DigiFab™** *see* Digoxin Immune Fab *on page 392*
- **Digitek®** *see* Digoxin *on page 388*

Digoxin (di JOKS in)

Medication Safety Issues

Sound-alike/look-alike issues:

Digoxin may be confused with Desoxyn®, doxepin

Lanoxin® may be confused with Lasix®, Levoxyl®, Levsinex®, Lomotil®, Lonox®, Mefoxin®, Xanax®

Related Information

Anesthesia for Patients With Liver Disease *on page 1421*
Antiarrhythmic Drugs *on page 1548*
Chronic Renal Failure *on page 1437*
Heart Failure (Systolic) *on page 1607*
Management of Postoperative Arrhythmias *on page 1451*

U.S. Brand Names Digitek®; Lanoxicaps®; Lanoxin®

Canadian Brand Names Digoxin CSD; Lanoxicaps®; Lanoxin®; Novo-Digoxin; Pediatric Digoxin CSD

Pharmacologic Category Antiarrhythmic Agent, Class IV; Cardiac Glycoside

Generic Available Yes: Excludes capsule

Use Treatment of congestive heart failure and to slow the ventricular rate in tachyarrhythmias such as atrial fibrillation, atrial flutter, and supraventricular tachycardia (paroxysmal atrial tachycardia); cardiogenic shock

Mechanism of Action

Congestive heart failure: Inhibition of the sodium/potassium ATPase pump which acts to increase the intracellular sodium-calcium exchange to increase intracellular calcium leading to increased contractility

Supraventricular arrhythmias: Direct suppression of the AV node conduction to increase effective refractory period and decrease conduction velocity - positive inotropic effect, enhanced vagal tone, and decreased ventricular rate to fast atrial arrhythmias. Atrial fibrillation may decrease sensitivity and increase tolerance to higher serum digoxin concentrations.

Pharmacodynamics/Kinetics

Onset of action: Oral: 1-2 hours; I.V.: 5-30 minutes

Peak effect: Oral: 2-8 hours; I.V.: 1-4 hours

Duration: Adults: 3-4 days both forms

Absorption: By passive nonsaturable diffusion in the upper small intestine; food may delay, but does not affect extent of absorption

Distribution:

Normal renal function: 6-7 L/kg

V_d: Extensive to peripheral tissues, with a distinct distribution phase which lasts 6-8 hours; concentrates in heart, liver, kidney, skeletal muscle, and intestines. Heart/serum concentration is 70:1. Pharmacologic effects are delayed and do not correlate well with serum concentrations during distribution phase.

Hyperthyroidism: Increased V_d

Hyperkalemia, hyponatremia: Decreased digoxin distribution to heart and muscle

Hypokalemia: Increased digoxin distribution to heart and muscles

Concomitant quinidine therapy: Decreased V_d

Chronic renal failure: 4-6 L/kg

Decreased sodium/potassium ATPase activity - decreased tissue binding

Neonates, full-term: 7.5-10 L/kg

Children: 16 L/kg

Adults: 7 L/kg, decreased with renal disease

Protein binding: 30%; in uremic patients, digoxin is displaced from plasma protein binding sites

Metabolism: Via sequential sugar hydrolysis in the stomach or by reduction of lactone ring by intestinal bacteria (in ~10% of population, gut bacteria may metabolize up to 40% of digoxin dose); metabolites may contribute to therapeutic and toxic effects of digoxin; metabolism is reduced with CHF

Bioavailability: Oral (formulation dependent): Elixir: 75% to 85%; Tablet: 70% to 80%

Half-life elimination (age, renal and cardiac function dependent):

Neonates: Premature: 61-170 hours; Full-term: 35-45 hours

Infants: 18-25 hours

Children: 35 hours

Adults: 38-48 hours

Adults, anephric: 4-6 days

Half-life elimination: Parent drug: 38 hours; Metabolites: Digoxigenin: 4 hours; Monodigitoxoside: 3-12 hours

Time to peak, serum: Oral: ~1 hour

Excretion: Urine (50% to 70% as unchanged drug)

Dosage When changing from oral (tablets or liquid) or I.M. to I.V. therapy, dosage should be reduced by 20% to 25%. Refer to the following: See table.

Dosage Recommendations for Digoxin

Age	Total Digitalizing Dose[2] (mcg/kg[1])		Daily Maintenance Dose[3] (mcg/kg[1])	
	P.O.	**I.V. or I.M.**	**P.O.**	**I.V. or I.M.**
Preterm infant[1]	20-30	15-25	5-7.5	4-6
Full-term infant[1]	25-35	20-30	6-10	5-8
1 mo - 2 y[1]	35-60	30-50	10-15	7.5-12
2-5 y[1]	30-40	25-35	7.5-10	6-9
5-10 y[1]	20-35	15-30	5-10	4-8
>10 y[1]	10-15	8-12	2.5-5	2-3
Adults	0.75-1.5 mg	0.5-1 mg	0.125-0.5 mg	0.1-0.4 mg

[1]Based on lean body weight and normal renal function for age. Decrease dose in patients with ↓ renal function; digitalizing dose often not recommended in infants and children.

[2]Give one-half of the total digitalizing dose (TDD) in the initial dose, then give one-quarter of the TDD in each of two subsequent doses at 8- to 12-hour intervals. Obtain ECG 6 hours after each dose to assess potential toxicity.

[3]Divided every 12 hours in infants and children <10 years of age. Given once daily to children >10 years of age and adults.

Dosing adjustment/interval in renal impairment:

Cl_{cr} 10-50 mL/minute: Administer 25% to 75% of dose or every 36 hours

Cl_{cr} <10 mL/minute: Administer 10% to 25% of dose or every 48 hours

Reduce loading dose by 50% in ESRD

Hemodialysis: Not dialyzable (0% to 5%)

Stability Protect elixir and injection from light; solution **compatibility**: D_5W, $D_{10}W$, NS, sterile water for injection (when diluted fourfold or greater)

Administration

I.M.: Inject no more than 2 mL per injection site. May cause intense pain.

I.V.: Inject slowly 1-5 minutes for undiluted form. May dilute up to fourfold with SWI, D_5W, or NS.

Monitoring Parameters

When to draw serum digoxin concentrations: Digoxin serum concentrations are monitored because digoxin possesses a narrow therapeutic serum range; the therapeutic endpoint is difficult to quantify and digoxin toxicity may be life-threatening. Digoxin serum levels should be drawn **at least 4 hours after an intravenous dose** and **at least 6 hours after an oral dose (optimally 12-24 hours after a dose).**

Initiation of therapy:

If a loading dose is given: Digoxin serum concentration may be drawn within 12-24 hours after the initial loading dose administration. Levels drawn this early may confirm the relationship of digoxin plasma levels and response but are of little value in determining maintenance doses.

If a loading dose is not given: Digoxin serum concentration should be obtained after 3-5 days of therapy

Maintenance therapy:

Trough concentrations should be followed just prior to the next dose or at a minimum of 4 hours after an I.V. dose and at least 6 hours after an oral dose

Digoxin serum concentrations should be obtained within 5-7 days (approximate time to steady-state) after any dosage changes. Continue to obtain digoxin serum concentrations 7-14 days after any change in maintenance dose. **Note:** In patients with end-stage renal disease, it may take 15-20 days to reach steady-state.

Additionally, patients who are receiving potassium-depleting medications such as diuretics, should be monitored for potassium, magnesium, and calcium levels

(Continued)

Digoxin *(Continued)*

Digoxin serum concentrations should be obtained whenever any of the following conditions occur:

Questionable patient compliance or to evaluate clinical deterioration following an initial good response

Changing renal function

Suspected digoxin toxicity

Initiation or discontinuation of therapy with drugs (amiodarone, quinidine, verapamil) which potentially interact with digoxin; if quinidine therapy is started; digoxin levels should be drawn within the first 24 hours after starting quinidine therapy, then 7-14 days later or empirically skip one day's digoxin dose and decrease the daily dose by 50%

Any disease changes (hypothyroidism)

Heart rate and rhythm should be monitored along with periodic ECGs to assess both desired effects and signs of toxicity

Follow closely (especially in patients receiving diuretics or amphotericin) for decreased serum potassium and magnesium or increased calcium, all of which predispose to digoxin toxicity

Assess renal function

Be aware of drug interactions

Observe patients for noncardiac signs of toxicity, confusion, and depression

Reference Range

Digoxin therapeutic serum concentrations:

Congestive heart failure: 0.5-0.8 ng/mL

Arrhythmias: 0.8-2 ng/mL

Adults: <0.5 ng/mL; probably indicates underdigitalization unless there are special circumstances

Toxic: >2.5 ng/mL

Digoxin-like immunoreactive substance (DLIS) may cross-react with digoxin immunoassay. DLIS has been found in patients with renal and liver disease, congestive heart failure, neonates, and pregnant women (3rd trimester).

Anesthesia and Critical Care Concerns/Other Considerations Elderly are at risk for toxicity due to age-related changes; volume of distribution is diminished significantly; half-life is increased as a result of decreased total body clearance. Digoxin toxicity may be potentiated in patients with hypokalemia, hypomagnesemia, and hypercalcemia. Digoxin may also rapidly approach toxic levels in patients with renal failure. For patients with renal failure, the loading dose is unchanged but maintenance doses may be adjusted and levels should be monitored very carefully. Signs of digoxin toxicity include both brady- and tachyarrhythmias. Bidirectional VT induced by digitalis toxicity indicates imminent development of ventricular fibrillation.

Digoxin has been used for many years in treatment of heart failure. Digoxin therapy is associated with a decrease in frequency in hospitalizations for exacerbations of heart failure. Digoxin use for ventricular rate control in patients with atrial fibrillation is a particularly useful strategy in those patients with coexisting systolic dysfunction. While digoxin may control ventricular response rate for atrial fibrillation at rest, the medication is less effective for rate control during exercise.

Pregnancy Risk Factor C

Contraindications Hypersensitivity to digoxin or any component of the formulation; hypersensitivity to cardiac glycosides (another may be tried); history of toxicity; ventricular tachycardia or fibrillation; idiopathic hypertrophic subaortic stenosis; constrictive pericarditis; amyloid disease; second- or third-degree heart block (except in patients with a functioning artificial pacemaker); Wolff-Parkinson-White syndrome and atrial fibrillation concurrently

Warnings/Precautions Withdrawal in CHF patients may lead to recurrence of CHF symptoms. Some arrhythmias that digoxin is used to treat may be exacerbated in digoxin toxicity. Sinus nodal disease may be worsened. Adjust doses in renal impairment and when verapamil, quinidine or amiodarone are added to a patient on digoxin. Correct hypokalemia and hypomagnesemia before initiating therapy. Calcium, especially when administered rapidly I.V., can produce serious arrhythmias. Atrial arrhythmias associated with hypermetabolic states are very difficult to treat. Rate control in atrial fibrillation may be better in a sedentary patient than an active one. Use with caution in acute MI (within 6 months). Serum concentration monitoring should be done before the next dose (patient can hold

AM dose for blood test) for an accurate assessment. Reduce or hold dose 1-2 days before elective electrical cardioversion.

Adverse Reactions Incidence of reactions are not always reported.

Cardiovascular: Heart block; first-, second- (Wenckebach), or third-degree heart block; asystole; atrial tachycardia with block; AV dissociation; accelerated junctional rhythm; ventricular tachycardia or ventricular fibrillation; PR prolongation; ST segment depression

Central nervous system: Visual disturbances (blurred or yellow vision), headache (3.2%), dizziness (4.9%), apathy, confusion, mental disturbances (4.1%), anxiety, depression, delirium, hallucinations, fever

Dermatologic: Maculopapular rash (1.6%); erythematous, scarlatiniform, papular, vesicular, or bullous rash; urticaria; pruritus; facial, angioneurotic, or laryngeal edema; shedding of fingernails or toenails; alopecia

Gastrointestinal: Nausea (3.2%), vomiting (1.6%), diarrhea (3.2%), abdominal pain

Neuromuscular & skeletal: Weakness

<1% (Limited to important or life-threatening): Abdominal pain, anorexia, eosinophilia, gynecomastia, hemorrhagic necrosis of the intestines, increased plasma estrogen and decreased serum luteinizing hormone in men and postmenopausal women and decreased plasma testosterone in men, intestinal ischemia, palpitation, sexual dysfunction, thrombocytopenia, unifocal or multiform ventricular premature contractions (especially bigeminy or trigeminy), vaginal cornification

Any arrhythmia seen in a child on digoxin should be considered as digoxin toxicity. The gastrointestinal and central nervous system symptoms are not frequently seen in children.

Overdosage/Toxicology Manifested by a wide variety of signs and symptoms difficult to distinguish from effects associated with cardiac disease. Nausea and vomiting are common early signs of toxicity and may precede or follow evidence of cardiotoxicity. Other symptoms include anorexia, diarrhea, abdominal discomfort, headache, weakness, drowsiness, visual disturbances, mental depression, confusion, restlessness, disorientation, seizures, and hallucinations. Cardiac abnormalities include ventricular tachycardia, unifocal or multifocal PVCs (bigeminal, trigeminal), paroxysmal nodal rhythms, AV dissociation, excessive slowing of the pulse, AV block of varying degree, P-R prolongation, S-T depression, and occasional atrial fibrillation. Ventricular fibrillation is a common cause of death (alterations in cardiac rate and rhythm can result in any type of known arrhythmia).

Antidote: Life-threatening digoxin toxicity is treated with Digibind®. Administer potassium except in cases of complete heart block or renal failure. Digitalis-induced arrhythmias not responsive to potassium may be treated with phenytoin or lidocaine. Cholestyramine and colestipol may decrease absorption. Other agents to consider, based on ECG and clinical assessment, include atropine, quinidine, procainamide, and propranolol. **Note:** Other antiarrhythmics appear more dangerous to use in toxicity.

Drug Interactions **Substrate** of CYP3A4 (minor)

Amiloride may reduce the inotropic response to digoxin.

Amiodarone reduces renal and nonrenal clearance of digoxin and may have additive effects on heart rate. Reduce digoxin dose by 50% with start of amiodarone.

Benzodiazepines (alprazolam, diazepam) have been associated with isolated reports of digoxin toxicity.

Beta-blocking agents (propranolol) may have additive effects on heart rate.

Calcium preparations: Rare cases of acute digoxin toxicity have been associated with parenteral calcium (bolus) administration.

Carvedilol may increase digoxin blood levels in addition to potentiating its effects on heart rate.

Cholestyramine, colestipol, kaolin-pectin may reduce digoxin absorption. Separate administration.

Cyclosporine may increase digoxin levels, possibly due to reduced renal clearance.

Erythromycin, clarithromycin, and tetracyclines may increase digoxin (not capsule form) blood levels in a subset of patients.

Indomethacin has been associated with isolated reports of increased digoxin blood levels/toxicity.

Itraconazole may increase digoxin blood levels in some patients; monitor.

(Continued)

Digoxin *(Continued)*

Levothyroxine (and other thyroid supplements) may decrease digoxin blood levels.

Metoclopramide may reduce the absorption of digoxin tablets.

Moricizine may increase the toxicity of digoxin (mechanism undefined).

Penicillamine has been associated with reductions in digoxin blood levels

Propafenone increases digoxin blood levels. Effects are highly variable; monitor closely.

Propylthiouracil (and methimazole) may increase digoxin blood levels by reducing thyroid hormone.

Quinidine increases digoxin blood levels substantially. Effect is variable (33% to 50%). Monitor digoxin blood levels/effect closely. Reduce digoxin dose by 50% with start of quinidine. Other related agents (hydroxychloroquine, quinine) should be used with caution.

Spironolactone may interfere with some digoxin assays, but may also increase blood levels directly. However, spironolactone may attenuate the inotropic effect of digoxin. Monitor effects of digoxin closely.

Succinylcholine administration to patients on digoxin has been associated with an increased risk of arrhythmias.

Verapamil diltiazem, bepridil, and nitrendipine increased serum digoxin concentrations. Other calcium channel blocking agents do not appear to share this effect. Reduce digoxin's dose with the start of verapamil.

Drugs which cause hypokalemia (thiazide and loop diuretics, amphotericin B): Hypokalemia may potentiate digoxin toxicity.

These medications have been associated with reduced digoxin blood levels which appear to be of limited clinical significance: Aminoglutethimide, aminosalicylic acid, aluminum-containing antacids, sucralfate, sulfasalazine, neomycin, ticlopidine.

These medications have been associated with increased digoxin blood levels which appear to be of limited clinical significance: Famciclovir, flecainide, ibuprofen, fluoxetine, nefazodone, cimetidine, famotidine, ranitidine, omeprazole, trimethoprim.

Ethanol/Nutrition/Herb Interactions

Food: Digoxin peak serum levels may be decreased if taken with food. Meals containing increased fiber (bran) or foods high in pectin may decrease oral absorption of digoxin.

Herb/Nutraceutical: Avoid ephedra (risk of cardiac stimulation). Avoid natural licorice (causes sodium and water retention and increases potassium loss).

Dietary Considerations Maintain adequate amounts of potassium in diet to decrease risk of hypokalemia (hypokalemia may increase risk of digoxin toxicity).

Dosage Forms [DSC] = Discontinued product

Capsule (Lanoxicaps®): 50 mcg [DSC], 100 mcg, 200 mcg [contains ethyl alcohol]

Elixir: 50 mcg/mL (2.5 mL, 5 mL, 60 mL) [contains alcohol 10%; lime flavor]

- Lanoxin® (pediatric): 50 mcg/mL (60 mL) [contains alcohol 10%; lime flavor] [DSC]

Injection: 250 mcg/mL (1 mL, 2 mL) [contains alcohol 10% and propylene glycol 40%]

- Lanoxin®: 250 mcg/mL (2 mL) [contains alcohol 10% and propylene glycol 40%]

Injection, pediatric: 100 mcg/mL (1 mL) [contains alcohol 10% and propylene glycol 40%]

Tablet: 125 mcg, 250 mcg

- Digitek®, Lanoxin®: 125 mcg, 250 mcg

♦ **Digoxin CSD (Can)** *see* Digoxin *on page 388*

Digoxin Immune Fab (di JOKS in i MYUN fab)

U.S. Brand Names Digibind®; DigiFab™

Canadian Brand Names Digibind®

Synonyms Antidigoxin Fab Fragments, Ovine

Pharmacologic Category Antidote

Generic Available No

Use Treatment of life-threatening or potentially life-threatening digoxin intoxication, including:

- acute digoxin ingestion (ie, >10 mg in adults or >4 mg in children)

- chronic ingestions leading to steady-state digoxin concentrations >6 ng/mL in adults or >4 ng/mL in children
- manifestations of digoxin toxicity due to overdose (life-threatening ventricular arrhythmias, progressive bradycardia, second- or third-degree heart block not responsive to atropine, serum potassium >5 mEq/L in adults or >6 mEq in children)

Mechanism of Action Digoxin immune antigen-binding fragments (Fab) are specific antibodies for the treatment of digitalis intoxication in carefully selected patients; binds with molecules of digoxin or digitoxin and then is excreted by the kidneys and removed from the body

Pharmacodynamics/Kinetics

Onset of action: I.V.: Improvement in 2-30 minutes for toxicity

Half-life elimination: 15-20 hours; prolonged with renal impairment

Excretion: Urine; undetectable amounts within 5-7 days

Dosage Each vial of Digibind® 38 mg or DigiFab™ 40 mg will bind ~0.5 mg of digoxin or digitoxin.

Estimation of the dose is based on the body burden of digitalis. This may be calculated if the amount ingested is known or the postdistribution serum drug level is known (round dose to the nearest whole vial). See table.

Digoxin Immune Fab

Tablets Ingested (0.25 mg)	Fab Dose (vials)
5	2
10	4
25	10
50	20
75	30
100	40
150	60
200	80

Fab dose based on serum drug level postdistribution:

Digoxin: No. of vials = level (ng/mL) x body weight (kg) divided by 100

Digitoxin: No. of vials = digitoxin (ng/mL) x body weight (kg) divided by 1000

If neither amount ingested nor drug level are known, dose empirically as follows:

For acute toxicity: 20 vials, administered in 2 divided doses to decrease the possibility of a febrile reaction, and to avoid fluid overload in small children.

For chronic toxicity: 6 vials; for infants and small children (≤20 kg), a single vial may be sufficient

Stability Should be refrigerated (2°C to 8°C). Reconstitute by adding 4 mL sterile water, resulting in 10 mg/mL for I.V. infusion. The reconstituted solution may be further diluted with NS to a convenient volume (eg, 1 mg/mL). Reconstituted solutions should be used within 4 hours if refrigerated. For very small doses, vial can be reconstituted by adding an additional 36 mL of sterile isotonic saline, to achieve a final concentration of 1 mg/mL.

Administration Continuous I.V. infusion over ≥30 minutes is preferred. May give by bolus injection if cardiac arrest is imminent. Small doses (infants/small children) may be administered using tuberculin syringe. Stopping the infusion and restarting at a slower rate may help if infusion-related reactions occur.

Monitoring Parameters Serum potassium, serum digoxin concentration prior to first dose of digoxin immune Fab; **digoxin levels will greatly increase with digoxin immune Fab use and are not an accurate determination of body stores**; standard digoxin concentration measurements may be misleading until Fab fragments are eliminated from the body.

Patients with renal failure should be monitored for a prolonged period for reintoxication with digoxin following the rerelease of bound digoxin into the blood.

Pregnancy Risk Factor C

Contraindications Hypersensitivity to sheep products or any component of the formulation

Warnings/Precautions Suicidal attempts often involve multiple drugs. Consider other drug toxicities as well. Hypersensitivity reactions can occur. Epinephrine should be immediately available. Serum potassium levels should be monitored,

(Continued)

Digoxin Immune Fab *(Continued)*

especially during the first few hours after administration. Total serum digoxin concentrations will rise precipitously following administration of this drug (has no clinical meaning - avoid monitoring serum concentrations). If digoxin was being used to treat CHF then may see exacerbation of symptoms as digoxin level is reduced. Use with caution in renal failure (experience limited) - the complex will be removed from the body more slowly. Monitor for reoccurrence of digoxin toxicity. Has reversed thrombocytopenia induced by digoxin. Failure of response to adequate treatment may call diagnosis of digitalis toxicity into question. Digoxin immune Fab is processed with papain and may cause hypersensitivity reactions in patients allergic to papaya, other papaya extracts, papain, chymopapain, or the pineapple enzyme bromelain. There may also be cross allergy with dust mite and latex allergens.

Adverse Reactions Frequency not defined.

Cardiovascular: Effects (due to withdrawal of digitalis) include exacerbation of low cardiac output states and CHF, rapid ventricular response in patients with atrial fibrillation; postural hypotension

Endocrine & metabolic: Hypokalemia

Local: Phlebitis

Miscellaneous: Allergic reactions, serum sickness

Overdosage/Toxicology Symptoms of overdose include delayed serum sickness. Treatment of serum sickness includes acetaminophen, histamine$_1$ and possibly histamine$_2$ blockers, and corticosteroids.

Drug Interactions Digoxin: Following administration of digoxin immune Fab, serum digoxin levels are markedly increased due to bound complexes (may be clinically misleading, since bound complex cannot interact with receptors).

Test Interactions Digoxin immune Fab interferes with digitalis immunoassay test leading to misleading digoxin serum concentrations until the Fab fragments are eliminated from the body. If possible, take digoxin serum levels prior to the administration of digoxin immune Fab; keeping in mind the time the last dose of digoxin was taken.

Dosage Forms Injection, powder for reconstitution:

Digibind®: 38 mg

DigiFab™: 40 mg

- **Dihydrohydroxycodeinone** *see* Oxycodone *on page 967*
- **Dihydromorphinone** *see* Hydromorphone *on page 644*
- **Dilacor® XR** *see* Diltiazem *on page 394*
- **Dilantin®** *see* Phenytoin *on page 1018*
- **Dilaudid®** *see* Hydromorphone *on page 644*
- **Dilaudid-HP®** *see* Hydromorphone *on page 644*
- **Dilaudid-HP-Plus® (Can)** *see* Hydromorphone *on page 644*
- **Dilaudid® Sterile Powder (Can)** *see* Hydromorphone *on page 644*
- **Dilaudid-XP® (Can)** *see* Hydromorphone *on page 644*
- **Diltia XT®** *see* Diltiazem *on page 394*

Diltiazem (dil TYE a zem)

Medication Safety Issues

Sound-alike/look-alike issues:

Diltiazem may be confused with Dilantin®

Cardizem® may be confused with Cardene®, Cardene SR®, Cardizem CD®, Cardizem SR®, cardiem

Cartia XT™ may be confused with Procardia XL®

Tiazac® may be confused with Tigan®, Ziac®

Related Information

Antiarrhythmic Drugs *on page 1548*

Calcium Channel Blockers *on page 1559*

Critical Care Infusion Administration Charts *on page 1514*

Hypertension *on page 1620*

Management of Postoperative Arrhythmias *on page 1451*

U.S. Brand Names Cardizem®; Cardizem® CD; Cardizem® LA; Cardizem® SR [DSC]; Cartia XT™; Dilacor® XR; Diltia XT®; Taztia XT™; Tiazac®

Canadian Brand Names Alti-Diltiazem CD; Apo-Diltiaz®; Apo-Diltiaz CD®; Apo-Diltiaz SR®; Cardizem®; Cardizem® CD; Cardizem® SR; Diltiazem HCl ER®;

Diltiazem Hydrochloride Injection; Gen-Diltiazem; Gen-Diltiazem CD; Med-Diltiazem; Novo-Diltazem; Novo-Diltazem-CD; Novo-Diltiazem HCl ER; Nu-Diltiaz; Nu-Diltiaz-CD; ratio-Diltiazem CD; Rhoxal-diltiazem CD; Rhoxal-diltiazem SR; Rhoxal-diltiazem T; Sandoz-Diltiazem CD; Sandoz-Diltiazem T; Syn-Diltiazem®; Tiazac®; Tiazac® XC

Synonyms Diltiazem Hydrochloride

Pharmacologic Category Calcium Channel Blocker

Generic Available Yes

Use

Oral: Essential hypertension; chronic stable angina or angina from coronary artery spasm

Injection: Atrial fibrillation or atrial flutter; paroxysmal supraventricular tachycardia (PSVT)

Unlabeled/Investigational Use Investigational: Therapy of Duchenne muscular dystrophy

Mechanism of Action Inhibits calcium ion from entering the "slow channels" or select voltage-sensitive areas of vascular smooth muscle and myocardium during depolarization, producing a relaxation of coronary vascular smooth muscle and coronary vasodilation; increases myocardial oxygen delivery in patients with vasospastic angina

Pharmacodynamics/Kinetics

Onset of action: Oral: Immediate release tablet: 30-60 minutes

Absorption: 70% to 80%

Distribution: V_d: 3-13 L/kg; enters breast milk

Protein binding: 70% to 80%

Metabolism: Hepatic; extensive first-pass effect; following single I.V. injection, plasma concentrations of N-monodesmethyldiltiazem and desacetyldiltiazem are typically undetectable; however, these metabolites accumulate to detectable concentrations following 24-hour constant rate infusion. N-monodesmethyldiltiazem appears to have 20% of the potency of diltiazem; desacetyldiltiazem is about 25% to 50% as potent as the parent compound.

Bioavailability: Oral: ~40%

Half-life elimination: Immediate release tablet: 3-4.5 hours, may be prolonged with renal impairment

Time to peak, serum: Immediate release tablet: 2-4 hours

Excretion: Urine and feces (primarily as metabolites)

Dosage Adults:

Oral:

Angina:

Capsule, extended release (Cardizem® CD, Cartia XT™, Dilacor® XR, Diltia XT®, Tiazac®): Initial: 120-180 mg once daily (maximum dose: 480 mg/day)

Tablet, extended release (Cardizem® LA): 180 mg once daily; may increase at 7- to 14-day intervals (maximum recommended dose: 360 mg/day)

Tablet, immediate release (Cardizem®): Usual starting dose: 30 mg 4 times/day; usual range: 180-360 mg/day

Hypertension:

Capsule, extended release (Cardizem® CD, Cartia XT™, Dilacor® XR, Diltia XT®, Tiazac®): Initial: 180-240 mg once daily; dose adjustment may be made after 14 days; usual dose range (JNC 7): 180-420 mg/day; Tiazac®: usual dose range: 120-540 mg/day

Capsule, sustained release (Cardizem® SR): Initial: 60-120 mg twice daily; dose adjustment may be made after 14 days; usual range: 240-360 mg/day

Tablet, extended release (Cardizem® LA): Initial: 180-240 mg once daily; dose adjustment may be made after 14 days; usual dose range (JNC 7): 120-540 mg/day

Note: Elderly: Patients ≥60 years may respond to a lower initial dose (ie, 120 mg once daily using extended release capsule)

I.V.: Atrial fibrillation, atrial flutter, PSVT:

Initial bolus dose: 0.25 mg/kg actual body weight over 2 minutes (average adult dose: 20 mg)

Repeat bolus dose (may be administered after 15 minutes if the response is inadequate.): 0.35 mg/kg actual body weight over 2 minutes (average adult dose: 25 mg)

Continuous infusion (requires an infusion pump; infusions >24 hours or infusion rates >15 mg/hour are not recommended.): Initial infusion rate of 10 mg/hour; rate may be increased in 5 mg/hour increments up to 15 mg/hour as needed; some patients may respond to an initial rate of 5 mg/hour.

(Continued)

Diltiazem *(Continued)*

If diltiazem injection is administered by continuous infusion for >24 hours, the possibility of decreased diltiazem clearance, prolonged elimination half-life, and increased diltiazem and/or diltiazem metabolite plasma concentrations should be considered.

Conversion from I.V. diltiazem to oral diltiazem: Start oral approximately 3 hours after bolus dose.

Oral dose (mg/day) is approximately equal to [rate (mg/hour) x 3 + 3] x 10.

3 mg/hour = 120 mg/day
5 mg/hour = 180 mg/day
7 mg/hour = 240 mg/day
11 mg/hour = 360 mg/day

Dosing comments in renal/hepatic impairment: Use with caution as extensively metabolized by the liver and excreted in the kidneys and bile.

Dialysis: Not removed by hemo- or peritoneal dialysis; supplemental dose is not necessary.

Stability

Capsule, tablet: Store at controlled room temperature.

Solution for injection: Store in refrigerator at 2°C to 8°C (36°F to 46°F). May be stored at room temperature for up to one month; do not freeze. Following dilution with $D_5$1/2NS, D_5W, or NS, solution is stable for 24 hours at room temperature or under refrigeration.

Administration

Oral: Do not crush long acting dosage forms.

Tiazac®: Capsules may be opened and sprinkled on a spoonful of applesauce. Applesauce should be swallowed without chewing, followed by drinking a glass of water.

I.V.: Bolus doses given over 2 minutes with continuous ECG and blood pressure monitoring. Continuous infusion should be via infusion pump.

Monitoring Parameters Liver function tests, blood pressure, ECG

Anesthesia and Critical Care Concerns/Other Considerations Diltiazem may be administered intravenously in the acute setting to attain ventricular rate control in patients with atrial fibrillation or flutter. Patients who respond, defined in general as at least a 20% decrease in ventricular response rate or attaining a rate <100 beats/minute, can be continued on oral therapy to maintain control. It is important to consider the potential drug interaction with digoxin, as these agents are both used in this setting. Intravenous diltiazem may be administered safely for up to 24 hours in patients with left ventricular dysfunction.

Pregnancy Risk Factor C

Contraindications Hypersensitivity to diltiazem or any component of the formulation; sick sinus syndrome; second- or third-degree AV block (except in patients with a functioning artificial pacemaker); hypotension (systolic <90 mm Hg); acute MI and pulmonary congestion

Warnings/Precautions Concomitant use with beta-blockers or digoxin can result in conduction disturbances. Avoid concurrent I.V. use of diltiazem and a beta-blocker. Use caution in left ventricular dysfunction (can exacerbate condition). Symptomatic hypotension can occur. Use with caution in hepatic or renal dysfunction.

Adverse Reactions Note: Frequencies represent ranges for various dosage forms. Patients with impaired ventricular function and/or conduction abnormalities may have higher incidence of adverse reactions.

>10%:

Cardiovascular: Edema (2% to 15%)
Central nervous system: Headache (5% to 12%)

2% to 10%:

Cardiovascular: AV block (first degree 2% to 8%), edema (lower limb, 2% to 8%), pain (6%), bradycardia (2% to 6%), hypotension (<2% to 4%), vasodilation (2% to 3%), extrasystoles (2%), flushing (1% to 2%), palpitation (1% to 2%)
Central nervous system: Dizziness (3% to 10%), nervousness (2%)
Dermatologic: Rash (1% to 4%)
Endocrine & metabolic: Gout (1% to 2%)
Gastrointestinal: Dyspepsia (1% to 6%), constipation (<2% to 4%), vomiting (2%), diarrhea (1% to 2%)
Local: Injection site reactions: Burning, itching (4%)
Neuromuscular & skeletal: Weakness (1% to 4%), myalgia (2%)

Respiratory: Rhinitis (<2% to 10%), pharyngitis (2% to 6%), dyspnea (1% to 6%), bronchitis (1% to 4%), sinus congestion (1% to 2%)

<2% (Limited to important or life-threatening): Alkaline phosphatase increased, allergic reaction, amblyopia, amnesia, arrhythmia, AV block (second or third degree), bundle branch block, CHF, depression, dysgeusia, extrapyramidal symptoms, gingival hyperplasia, hemolytic anemia, petechiae, photosensitivity, SGOT increased, SGPT increased, Stevens-Johnson syndrome, syncope, tachycardia, thrombocytopenia, tremor, toxic epidermal necrolysis

Overdosage/Toxicology Primary cardiac symptoms of calcium blocker overdose include hypotension and bradycardia. Noncardiac symptoms include confusion, stupor, nausea, vomiting, metabolic acidosis, and hyperglycemia.

Following initial gastric decontamination, if possible, repeated calcium administration may promptly reverse depressed cardiac contractility (but not sinus node depression or peripheral vasodilation). Glucagon, epinephrine, and amrinone may treat refractory hypotension. Glucagon and epinephrine also increase heart rate (outside the U.S., 4-aminopyridine may be available as an antidote). Dialysis and hemoperfusion are not effective in enhancing elimination although repeat-dose activated charcoal may serve as an adjunct with sustained-release preparations.

Drug Interactions **Substrate** of CYP2C9 (minor), 2D6 (minor), 3A4 (major); **Inhibits** CYP2C9 (weak), 2D6 (weak), 3A4 (moderate)

Alfentanil's plasma concentration is increased. Fentanyl and sufentanil may be affected similarly.

Amiodarone use may lead to bradycardia, other conduction delays, and decreased cardiac output; monitor closely if using together.

Azole antifungals may inhibit the calcium channel blocker's metabolism; avoid this combination. Try an antifungal like terbinafine (if appropriate) or monitor closely for altered effect of the calcium channel blocker.

Benzodiazepines (midazolam, triazolam) plasma concentrations are increased by diltiazem; monitor for prolonged CNS depression.

Beta-blockers may have increased pharmacodynamic interactions with diltiazem (see Warnings/Precautions).

Buspirone: Diltiazem may increase serum levels of buspirone; monitor.

Calcium may reduce the calcium channel blocker's effects, particularly hypotension.

Carbamazepine's serum concentration is increased and toxicity may result; avoid this combination.

Cimetidine reduced diltiazem's metabolism; consider an alternative H_2 antagonist.

Cyclosporine's serum concentrations are increased by diltiazem; avoid the combination. Use another calcium channel blocker or monitor cyclosporine trough levels and renal function closely.

CYP3A4 inducers: CYP3A4 inducers may decrease the levels/effects of diltiazem. Example inducers include aminoglutethimide, carbamazepine, nafcillin, nevirapine, phenobarbital, phenytoin, and rifamycins.

CYP3A4 inhibitors: May increase the levels/effects of diltiazem. Example inhibitors include azole antifungals, clarithromycin, diclofenac, doxycycline, erythromycin, imatinib, isoniazid, nefazodone, nicardipine, propofol, protease inhibitors, quinidine, telithromycin, and verapamil.

CYP3A4 substrates: Diltiazem may increase the levels/effects of CYP3A4 substrates. Example substrates include benzodiazepines, calcium channel blockers, cyclosporine, mirtazapine, nateglinide, nefazodone, sildenafil (and other PDE-5 inhibitors), tacrolimus, and venlafaxine. Selected benzodiazepines (midazolam and triazolam), cisapride, ergot alkaloids, selected HMG-CoA reductase inhibitors (lovastatin and simvastatin), and pimozide are generally contraindicated with strong CYP3A4 inhibitors.

Digoxin's serum concentration can be increased in some patients; monitor for increased effects of digoxin.

HMG-CoA reductase inhibitors (atorvastatin, lovastatin, simvastatin): Serum concentration will likely be increased; consider pravastatin/fluvastatin or a second generation dihydropyridine calcium channel blocker as an alternative.

Lithium neurotoxicity may result when diltiazem is added; monitor lithium levels.

Moricizine's serum concentration is increased; monitor clinical response closely.

Nafcillin decreases plasma concentration of diltiazem; avoid this combination.

Nitroprusside's dose required reduction in patients started on diltiazem; monitor blood pressure.

Protease inhibitor like amprenavir and ritonavir may increase diltiazem's serum concentration.

(Continued)

Diltiazem *(Continued)*

Quinidine: Diltiazem may increase serum levels of quinidine. Dosage adjustment may be required.

Rifampin increases the metabolism of calcium channel blockers; adjust the dose of the calcium channel blocker to maintain efficacy or consider an alternative to rifampin.

Sildenafil, tadalafil, vardenafil: Blood pressure-lowering effects may be additive; use caution.

Tacrolimus's serum concentrations are increased by diltiazem; avoid the combination. Use another calcium channel blocker or monitor tacrolimus trough levels and renal function closely.

Ethanol/Nutrition/Herb Interactions

Ethanol: Avoid ethanol (may increase risk of hypotension or vasodilation).

Food: Diltiazem serum levels may be elevated if taken with food. Serum concentrations were not altered by grapefruit juice in small clinical trials.

Herb/Nutraceutical: St John's wort may decrease diltiazem levels. Avoid dong quai if using for hypertension (has estrogenic activity). Avoid ephedra (may worsen arrhythmia or hypertension). Avoid yohimbe, ginseng (may worsen hypertension). Avoid garlic (may have increased antihypertensive effect).

Dosage Forms [DSC] = Discontinued product

Capsule, extended release, as hydrochloride [once-daily dosing]: 120 mg, 180 mg, 240 mg, 300 mg

Cardizem® CD: 120 mg, 180 mg, 240 mg, 300 mg, 360 mg

Cartia XT™: 120 mg, 180 mg, 240 mg, 300 mg

Dilacor® XR, Diltia XT®: 120 mg, 180 mg, 240 mg

Taztia XT™: 120 mg, 180 mg, 240 mg, 300 mg, 360 mg

Tiazac®: 120 mg, 180 mg, 240 mg, 300 mg, 360 mg, 420 mg

Capsule, sustained release, as hydrochloride [twice-daily dosing] (Cardizem® SR [DSC]): 60 mg, 90 mg, 120 mg

Injection, solution, as hydrochloride: 5 mg/mL (5 mL, 10 mL, 25 mL)

Injection, powder for reconstitution, as hydrochloride (Cardizem®): 25 mg

Tablet, as hydrochloride (Cardizem®): 30 mg, 60 mg, 90 mg, 120 mg

Tablet, extended release, as hydrochloride (Cardizem® LA): 120 mg, 180 mg, 240 mg, 300 mg, 360 mg, 420 mg

References

Karth GD, Geppert A, Neunteufl T, et al, "Amiodarone vs. Diltiazem for Rate Control in Critically Ill Patients With Atrial Tachyarrhythmias," *Crit Care Med*, 2001, 29(6):1149-53.

- **Diltiazem HCl ER® (Can)** *see* Diltiazem *on page 394*
- **Diltiazem Hydrochloride** *see* Diltiazem *on page 394*
- **Diltiazem Hydrochloride Injection (Can)** *see* Diltiazem *on page 394*
- **Dimetapp® 12-Hour Non-Drowsy Extentabs® [OTC]** *see* Pseudoephedrine *on page 1085*
- **Dimetapp® Decongestant Infant [OTC]** *see* Pseudoephedrine *on page 1085*
- **Diochloram® (Can)** *see* Chloramphenicol *on page 262*
- **Diodex® (Can)** *see* Dexamethasone *on page 366*
- **Diogent® (Can)** *see* Gentamicin *on page 589*
- **Diomycin® (Can)** *see* Erythromycin *on page 476*
- **Dionephrine® (Can)** *see* Phenylephrine *on page 1015*
- **Diopred® (Can)** *see* PrednisoLONE *on page 1046*
- **Dioptic's Atropine Solution (Can)** *see* Atropine *on page 144*
- **Diotrope® (Can)** *see* Tropicamide *on page 1320*
- **Diovan®** *see* Valsartan *on page 1334*
- **Diovol® (Can)** *see* Aluminum Hydroxide and Magnesium Hydroxide *on page 76*
- **Diovol® Ex (Can)** *see* Aluminum Hydroxide and Magnesium Hydroxide *on page 76*
- **Diphen® [OTC]** *see* DiphenhydrAMINE *on page 399*
- **Diphen® AF [OTC]** *see* DiphenhydrAMINE *on page 399*
- **Diphenhist [OTC]** *see* DiphenhydrAMINE *on page 399*

DiphenhydrAMINE (dye fen HYE dra meen)

Medication Safety Issues

Sound-alike/look-alike issues:

DiphenhydrAMINE may be confused with desipramine, dicyclomine, dimenhyDRINATE

Benadryl® may be confused with benazepril, Bentyl®, Benylin®, Caladryl®

Related Information

Allergic Reactions *on page 1395*

Contrast Media Reactions, Premedication for Prophylaxis *on page 1602*

Latex Allergy *on page 1398*

U.S. Brand Names Aler-Cap [OTC]; Aler-Dryl [OTC]; Aler-Tab [OTC]; AllerMax® [OTC]; Altaryl [OTC]; Banophen® [OTC]; Banophen® Anti-Itch [OTC]; Benadryl® Allergy [OTC]; Benadryl® Children's Allergy [OTC]; Benadryl® Children's Allergy Fastmelt® [OTC]; Benadryl® Dye-Free Allergy [OTC]; Benadryl® Injection; Benadryl® Itch Stopping [OTC]; Benadryl® Itch Stopping Extra Strength [OTC]; Compoz® Nighttime Sleep Aid [OTC]; Dermamycin® [OTC]; Dermarest® Insect Bite [OTC]; Dermarest® Plus [OTC]; Diphen® [OTC]; Diphen® AF [OTC]; Diphenhist [OTC]; Dytan™; Genahist® [OTC]; Hydramine® [OTC]; Nytol® Quick Caps [OTC]; Nytol® Quick Gels [OTC]; Q-Dryl [OTC]; Quenalin [OTC]; Siladryl® Allergy [OTC]; Siladryl® DAS [OTC]; Silphen® [OTC]; Simply Sleep® [OTC]; Sleep-ettes D [OTC]; Sleepinal® [OTC]; Sominex® [OTC]; Sominex® Maximum Strength [OTC]; Triaminic® Thin Strips™ Cough and Runny Nose [OTC]; Twilite® [OTC]; Unisom® Maximum Strength SleepGels® [OTC]

Canadian Brand Names Allerdryl®; Allernix; Benadryl®; Nytol®; Nytol® Extra Strength; PMS-Diphenhydramine; Simply Sleep®

Synonyms Diphenhydramine Citrate; Diphenhydramine Hydrochloride; Diphenhydramine Tannate

Pharmacologic Category Antihistamine

Generic Available Yes: Excludes chewable tablet, orally-disintegrating tablet, suspension, stick, strip

Use Symptomatic relief of allergic symptoms caused by histamine release which include nasal allergies and allergic dermatosis; can be used for mild nighttime sedation; prevention of motion sickness and as an antitussive; has antinauseant and topical anesthetic properties; treatment of antipsychotic-induced extrapyramidal symptoms

Mechanism of Action Competes with histamine for H_1-receptor sites on effector cells in the gastrointestinal tract, blood vessels, and respiratory tract; anticholinergic and sedative effects are also seen

Pharmacodynamics/Kinetics

Onset of action: Maximum sedative effect: 1-3 hours

Duration: 4-7 hours

Protein binding: 78%

Metabolism: Extensively hepatic; smaller degrees in pulmonary and renal systems; significant first-pass effect

Bioavailability: Oral: 40% to 60%

Half-life elimination: 2-8 hours; Elderly: 13.5 hours

Time to peak, serum: 2-4 hours

Excretion: Urine (as unchanged drug)

Dosage

Children:

Oral, I.M., I.V.:

Treatment of moderate to severe allergic reactions: 5 mg/kg/day or 150 mg/m^2/day in divided doses every 6-8 hours, not to exceed 300 mg/day

Minor allergic rhinitis or motion sickness:

2 to <6 years: 6.25 mg every 4-6 hours; maximum: 37.5 mg/day

6 to <12 years: 12.5-25 mg every 4-6 hours; maximum: 150 mg/day

≥12 years: 25-50 mg every 4-6 hours; maximum: 300 mg/day

Night-time sleep aid: 30 minutes before bedtime:

2 to <12 years: 1 mg/kg/dose; maximum: 50 mg/dose

≥12 years: 50 mg

Oral: Antitussive:

2 to <6 years: 6.25 mg every 4 hours; maximum 37.5 mg/day

6 to <12 years: 12.5 mg every 4 hours; maximum 75 mg/day

≥12 years: 25 mg every 4 hours; maximum 150 mg/day

I.M., I.V.: Treatment of dystonic reactions: 0.5-1 mg/kg/dose

(Continued)

DiphenhydrAMINE *(Continued)*

Adults:

Oral: 25-50 mg every 6-8 hours

Minor allergic rhinitis or motion sickness: 25-50 mg every 4-6 hours; maximum: 300 mg/day

Moderate to severe allergic reactions: 25-50 mg every 4 hours, not to exceed 400 mg/day

Nighttime sleep aid: 50 mg at bedtime

I.M., I.V.: 10-50 mg in a single dose every 2-4 hours, not to exceed 400 mg/day

Dystonic reaction: 50 mg in a single dose; may repeat in 20-30 minutes if necessary

Topical: For external application, not longer than 7 days

Stability Protect injection from light.

Monitoring Parameters Relief of symptoms, mental alertness

Reference Range

Antihistamine effects at levels >25 ng/mL

Drowsiness at levels 30-40 ng/mL

Mental impairment at levels >60 ng/mL

Therapeutic: Not established

Toxic: >0.1 mcg/mL

Anesthesia and Critical Care Concerns/Other Considerations Diphenhydramine's use as a sleep aid is discouraged due to its anticholinergic effects.

Pregnancy Risk Factor B

Contraindications Hypersensitivity to diphenhydramine or any component of the formulation; acute asthma; not for use in neonates

Warnings/Precautions Causes sedation, caution must be used in performing tasks which require alertness (eg, operating machinery or driving). Sedative effects of CNS depressants or ethanol are potentiated. Use with caution in patients with angle-closure glaucoma, pyloroduodenal obstruction (including stenotic peptic ulcer), urinary tract obstruction (including bladder neck obstruction and symptomatic prostatic hyperplasia), hyperthyroidism, increased intraocular pressure, and cardiovascular disease (including hypertension and tachycardia). Diphenhydramine has high sedative and anticholinergic properties, so it may not be considered the antihistamine of choice for prolonged use in the elderly. May cause paradoxical excitation in pediatric patients, and can result in hallucinations, coma, and death in overdose. Some preparations contain sodium bisulfite; syrup formulations may contain alcohol. Some preparations contain soy protein; patients with soy protein or peanut allergies should avoid.

Adverse Reactions Frequency not defined.

Cardiovascular: Hypotension, palpitation, tachycardia

Central nervous system: Sedation, sleepiness, dizziness, disturbed coordination, headache, fatigue, nervousness, paradoxical excitement, insomnia, euphoria, confusion

Dermatologic: Photosensitivity, rash, angioedema, urticaria

Gastrointestinal: Nausea, vomiting, diarrhea, abdominal pain, xerostomia, appetite increase, weight gain, dry mucous membranes, anorexia

Genitourinary: Urinary retention, urinary frequency, difficult urination

Hematologic: Hemolytic anemia, thrombocytopenia, agranulocytosis

Neuromuscular & skeletal: Tremor, paresthesia

Ocular: Blurred vision

Respiratory: Thickening of bronchial secretions

Overdosage/Toxicology Symptoms of overdose include CNS stimulation or depression; overdose may result in death in infants and children. There is no specific treatment for antihistamine overdose. Clinical toxicity is due to blockade of cholinergic receptors. For anticholinergic overdose with life-threatening symptoms, physostigmine 1-2 mg SubQ or I.V. slowly may be given to reverse these effects.

Drug Interactions **Inhibits** CYP2D6 (moderate)

Amantadine, rimantadine: Central and/or peripheral anticholinergic syndrome can occur when administered with amantadine or rimantadine

Anticholinergic agents: Central and/or peripheral anticholinergic syndrome can occur when administered with narcotic analgesics, phenothiazines and other antipsychotics (especially with high anticholinergic activity), tricyclic antidepressants, quinidine and some other antiarrhythmics, and antihistamines

Atenolol: Drugs with high anticholinergic activity may increase the bioavailability of atenolol (and possibly other beta-blockers); monitor for increased effect

Cholinergic agents: Drugs with high anticholinergic activity may antagonize the therapeutic effect of cholinergic agents; includes donepezil, rivastigmine, and tacrine

CNS depressants: Sedative effects may be additive with CNS depressants; includes ethanol, benzodiazepines, barbiturates, narcotic analgesics, and other sedative agents; monitor for increased effect

CYP2D6 substrates: Diphenhydramine may increase the levels/effects of CYP2D6 substrates. Example substrates include amphetamines, selected beta-blockers, dextromethorphan, fluoxetine, lidocaine, mirtazapine, nefazodone, paroxetine, risperidone, ritonavir, thioridazine, tricyclic antidepressants, and venlafaxine.

CYP2D6 prodrug substrates: Diphenhydramine may decrease the levels/effects of CYP2D6 prodrug substrates. Example prodrug substrates include codeine, hydrocodone, oxycodone, and tramadol.

Digoxin: Drugs with high anticholinergic activity may decrease gastric degradation and increase the amount of digoxin absorbed by delaying gastric emptying

Ethanol: Syrup should not be given to patients taking drugs that can cause disulfiram reactions (ie, metronidazole, chlorpropamide) due to high alcohol content

Levodopa: Drugs with high anticholinergic activity may increase gastric degradation and decrease the amount of levodopa absorbed by delaying gastric emptying

Neuroleptics: Drugs with high anticholinergic activity may antagonize the therapeutic effects of neuroleptics

Ethanol/Nutrition/Herb Interactions

Ethanol: Avoid ethanol (may increase CNS depression).

Herb/Nutraceutical: Avoid valerian, St John's wort, kava kava, gotu kola (may increase CNS depression).

Test Interactions May suppress the wheal and flare reactions to skin test antigens

Dietary Considerations Tablet:

Chewable, as hydrochloride: Contains phenylalanine 4.2 mg per 12.5 mg tablet

Chewable, as tannate: Contains phenylalanine 1.5 mg per 25 mg tablet

Orally-disintegrating, as citrate: Contains phenylalanine 4.5 mg per 19 mg [equivalent to diphenhydramine hydrochloride 12.5 mg] tablet; contains soy protein isolate (contraindicated in patients with soy protein allergies; use caution in peanut allergic individuals, ~10% are estimated to also have soy protein allergies)

Dosage Forms

Caplet, as hydrochloride: 25 mg, 50 mg
- Aler-Dryl, AllerMax®, Compoz® Nighttime Sleep Aid, Sleep-ettes D, Sominex® Maximum Strength, Twilite®: 50 mg
- Simply Sleep®, Nytol® Quick Caps: 25 mg

Capsule, as hydrochloride: 25 mg, 50 mg
- Aler-Cap, Banophen®, Benadryl® Allergy, Diphen®, Diphenhist, Genahist®, Q-Dryl: 25 mg
- Sleepinal®: 50 mg

Capsule, softgel, as hydrochloride: 50 mg
- Benadryl® Dye-Free Allergy: 25 mg [dye-free]
- Compoz® Nighttime Sleep Aid, Nytol® Quick Gels, Sleepinal®, Unisom® Maximum Strength SleepGels®: 50 mg

Captab, as hydrochloride (Diphenhist®): 25 mg

Cream, as hydrochloride: 2% (30 g) [contains zinc acetate 0.1%]
- Banophen® Anti-Itch: 2% (30 g) [contains zinc acetate 0.1%]
- Benadryl® Itch Stopping: 1% (30 g) [contains zinc acetate 0.1%]
- Benadryl® Itch Stopping Extra Strength: 2% (30 g) [contains zinc acetate 0.1%]
- Diphenhist®: 2% (30 g) [contains zinc acetate 0.1%]

Elixir, as hydrochloride:
- Altaryl: 12.5 mg/5 mL (120 mL, 480 mL, 3840 mL) [cherry flavor]
- Banophen®: 12.5 mg/5 mL (120 mL)
- Diphen AF: 12.5 mg/5 mL (120 mL, 240 mL, 480 mL) [alcohol free; cherry flavor]
- Q-Dryl: 12.5 mg/5 mL (480 mL) [alcohol free]

Gel, topical, as hydrochloride:
- Benadryl® Itch Stopping Extra Strength: 2% (120 mL)
- Dermarest® Plus: 2% (28 g, 42 g) [contains menthol 1%]

Injection, solution, as hydrochloride: 50 mg/mL (1 mL)

(Continued)

DiphenhydrAMINE *(Continued)*

Benadryl®: 50 mg/mL (1 mL, 10 mL)

Liquid, as hydrochloride:

AllerMax®: 12.5 mg/5 mL (120 mL)

Benadryl® Allergy: 12.5 mg/5 mL (120 mL, 240 mL) [alcohol free; contains sodium benzoate; cherry flavor]

Benadryl® Dye-Free Allergy: 12.5 mg/5 mL (120 mL) [alcohol free, dye free, sugar free; contains sodium benzoate; bubble gum flavor]

Genahist®: 12.5 mg/5 mL (120 mL) [alcohol free, sugar free; contains sodium benzoate; cherry flavor]

Hydramine®: 12.5 mg/5 mL (120 mL, 480 mL) [alcohol free]

Q-Dryl: 12.5 mg/5 mL (120 mL) [alcohol free; cherry flavor]

Quenalin: 12.5 mg/5 mL (120 mL) [fruit flavor]

Siladryl® Allergy: 12.5 mg/5 mL (120 mL, 240 mL, 480 mL) [alcohol free, sugar free; black cherry flavor]

Siladryl® DAS: 12.5 mg/5 mL (120 mL) [alcohol free, dye free, sugar free; black cherry flavor]

Liquid, topical, as hydrochloride [stick] (Benadryl® Itch Stopping Extra Strength): 2% (14 mL) [contains zinc acetate 0.1% and alcohol]

Solution, oral, as hydrochloride:

Banophen®: 12.5 mg/5mL (480 mL) [sugar free]

Diphenhist: 12.5 mg/5 mL (120 mL, 480 mL) [alcohol free; contains sodium benzoate]

Solution, topical, as hydrochloride [spray]:

Benadryl® Itch Stopping Extra Strength: 2% (60 mL) [contains zinc acetate 0.1% and alcohol]

Dermamycin®, Dermarest® Insect Bite: 2% (60 mL) [contains menthol 1%]

Strips, oral, as hydrochloride (Triaminic® Thin Strips™ Cough and Runny Nose): 12. 5 mg (16s) [grape flavor]

Suspension, as tannate (Dytan™): 25 mg/5 mL (120 mL) [strawberry flavor]

Syrup, as hydrochloride (Silphen® Cough): 12.5 mg/5 mL (120 mL, 240 mL, 480 mL) [contains alcohol; 5%; strawberry flavor]

Tablet, as hydrochloride: 25 mg, 50 mg

Aler-Tab, Benadryl® Allergy, Genahist®, Sleepinal®, Sominex®: 25 mg

Tablet, chewable, as hydrochloride (Benadryl® Children's Allergy): 12.5 mg [contains phenylalanine 4.2 mg/tablet; grape flavor]

Tablet, chewable, as tannate (Dytan™): 25 mg [contains phenylalanine; strawberry flavor]

Tablet, orally disintegrating, as citrate (Benadryl® Children's Allergy Fastmelt®): 19 mg [equivalent to diphenhydramine hydrochloride 12.5 mg; contains phenylalanine 4.5 mg/tablet and soy protein isolate; cherry flavor]

- **Diphenhydramine Citrate** *see* DiphenhydrAMINE *on page 399*
- **Diphenhydramine Hydrochloride** *see* DiphenhydrAMINE *on page 399*
- **Diphenhydramine Tannate** *see* DiphenhydrAMINE *on page 399*
- **Diphenylhydantoin** *see* Phenytoin *on page 1018*
- **Diprivan®** *see* Propofol *on page 1070*
- **Diprolene®** *see* Betamethasone *on page 169*
- **Diprolene® AF** *see* Betamethasone *on page 169*
- **Diprolene® Glycol (Can)** *see* Betamethasone *on page 169*
- **Dipropylacetic Acid** *see* Valproic Acid and Derivatives *on page 1329*
- **Diprosone® (Can)** *see* Betamethasone *on page 169*

Dipyridamole (dye peer ID a mole)

Medication Safety Issues

Sound-alike/look-alike issues:

Dipyridamole may be confused with disopyramide

Persantine® may be confused with Periactin®, Permitil®

U.S. Brand Names Persantine®

Canadian Brand Names Apo-Dipyridamole FC®; Persantine®

Pharmacologic Category Antiplatelet Agent; Vasodilator

Generic Available Yes

Use

Oral: Used with warfarin to decrease thrombosis in patients after artificial heart valve replacement

I.V.: Diagnostic agent in CAD

Unlabeled/Investigational Use Treatment of proteinuria in pediatric renal disease

Mechanism of Action Inhibits the activity of adenosine deaminase and phosphodiesterase, which causes an accumulation of adenosine, adenine nucleotides, and cyclic AMP; these mediators then inhibit platelet aggregation and may cause vasodilation; may also stimulate release of prostacyclin or PGD_2; causes coronary vasodilation

Pharmacodynamics/Kinetics

Absorption: Readily, but variable

Distribution: Adults: V_d: 2-3 L/kg

Protein binding: 91% to 99%

Metabolism: Hepatic

Half-life elimination: Terminal: 10-12 hours

Time to peak, serum: 2-2.5 hours

Excretion: Feces (as glucuronide conjugates and unchanged drug)

Dosage

Children: Oral:

Proteinuria (unlabeled use): 4-10 mg/kg/day have been used investigationally to treat proteinuria in pediatric renal disease

Mechanical prosthetic heart valves (unlabeled use): 2-5 mg/kg/day (used in combination with an oral anticoagulant in children who have systemic embolism despite adequate oral anticoagulant therapy, and used in combination with low-dose oral anticoagulation (INR 2-3) plus aspirin in children in whom full-dose oral anticoagulation is contraindicated)

Adults:

Oral: Adjunctive therapy for prophylaxis of thromboembolism with cardiac valve replacement: 75-100 mg 4 times/day

I.V.: Evaluation of coronary artery disease: 0.14 mg/kg/minute for 4 minutes; maximum dose: 60 mg

Stability I.V.: Store between 15°C to 25°C (59°F to 77°F). Do not freeze, protect from light. Prior to administration, dilute to a ≥1:2 ratio in NS, 1/2NS, or D_5W. Total volume should be ~20-50 mL.

Administration

I.V.: Infuse diluted solution over 4 minutes; following dipyridamole infusion, inject thallium-201 within 5 minutes. **Note:** Aminophylline should be available for urgent/emergent use; dosing of 50-100 mg (range: 50-250 mg) IVP over 30-60 seconds.

Tablet: Administer with water 1 hour before meals.

Monitoring Parameters Blood pressure, heart rate, ECG (stress test)

Anesthesia and Critical Care Concerns/Other Considerations For patients undergoing CABG, the Seventh American College of Chest Physicians Consensus Conference recommended against the addition of dipyridamole to aspirin therapy.

Pregnancy Risk Factor B

Contraindications Hypersensitivity to dipyridamole or any component of the formulation

Warnings/Precautions Use caution in patients with hypotension and severe cardiac disease. Use caution in patients on other antiplatelet agents or anticoagulation. Severe adverse reactions have occurred rarely with I.V. administration. Use the I.V. form with caution in patients with bronchospastic disease or unstable angina. Have aminophylline ready in case of urgency or emergency with I.V. use.

Adverse Reactions

Oral:

>10%: Dizziness (14%)

1% to 10%:

Central nervous system: Headache (2%)

Dermatologic: Rash (2%)

Gastrointestinal: Abdominal distress (6%)

Frequency not defined: Diarrhea, vomiting, flushing, pruritus, angina pectoris, liver dysfunction

Postmarketing and/or case reports: Alopecia, arthritis, cholelithiasis, dyspepsia, fatigue, hepatitis, hypersensitivity reaction, hypotension, larynx edema,

(Continued)

Dipyridamole *(Continued)*

malaise, myalgia, nausea, palpitation, paresthesia, tachycardia, thrombocytopenia

I.V.:

>10%:

Cardiovascular: Exacerbation of angina pectoris (20%)

Central nervous system: Dizziness (12%), headache (12%)

1% to 10%:

Cardiovascular: Hypotension (5%), hypertension (2%), blood pressure lability (2%), ECG abnormalities (ST-T changes, extrasystoles; 5% to 8%), pain (3%), tachycardia (3%)

Central nervous system: Flushing (3%), fatigue (1%)

Gastrointestinal: Nausea (5%)

Neuromuscular & skeletal: Paresthesia (1%)

Respiratory: Dyspnea (3%)

<1% (Limited to important or life-threatening): Abdominal pain, abnormal coordination; allergic reaction (pruritus, rash, urticaria); appetite increased; arrhythmia (ventricular tachycardia, bradycardia, AV block, SVT, atrial fibrillation, asystole); arthralgia, asthenia, back pain, breast pain, bronchospasm, cardiomyopathy, cough, depersonalization, diaphoresis, dry mouth, dysgeusia, dyspepsia, dysphagia, earache, ECG abnormalities (unspecified), edema, eructation, flatulence, hypertonia, hyperventilation, injection site reaction, intermittent claudication leg cramping, malaise, MI, myalgia, orthostatic hypotension, palpitation, perineal pain, pharyngitis, pleural pain, renal pain, rhinitis, rigor, syncope, tenesmus, thirst, tinnitus, tremor, vertigo, vision abnormalities, vomiting

Overdosage/Toxicology Symptoms of overdose include hypotension and peripheral vasodilation. Dialysis is not effective. Treatment is symptomatic and supportive.

Drug Interactions

Adenosine: Blood levels and pharmacologic effects of adenosine are increased; consider reduced doses of adenosine.

Cholinesterase inhibitors: May counteract effect of cholinesterase inhibitor and may aggravate myasthenia gravis.

Xanthine derivatives (eg, theophylline): May reduce the pharmacologic effects of dipyridamole; hold theophylline preparations for 36-48 hours before dipyridamole facilitated stress test.

Ethanol/Nutrition/Herb Interactions Herb/Nutraceutical: Avoid cat's claw, dong quai, evening primrose, feverfew, garlic, ginger, ginkgo, red clover, horse chestnut, green tea, ginseng (all have additional antiplatelet activity).

Dietary Considerations Should be taken with water 1 hour before meals.

Dosage Forms

Injection, solution: 5 mg/mL (2 mL, 10 mL)

Tablet (Persantine®): 25 mg, 50 mg, 75 mg

- **Dipyridamole and Aspirin** *see* Aspirin and Dipyridamole *on page 133*
- **Disalicylic Acid** *see* Salsalate *on page 1147*
- **Disodium Thiosulfate Pentahydrate** *see* Sodium Thiosulfate *on page 1195*
- ***d*-Isoephedrine Hydrochloride** *see* Pseudoephedrine *on page 1085*

Disopyramide (dye soe PEER a mide)

Medication Safety Issues

Sound-alike/look-alike issues:

Disopyramide may be confused with desipramine, dipyridamole

Norpace® may be confused with Norpramin®

Related Information

Antiarrhythmic Drugs *on page 1548*

U.S. Brand Names Norpace®; Norpace® CR

Canadian Brand Names Norpace®; Rythmodan®; Rythmodan®-LA

Synonyms Disopyramide Phosphate

Pharmacologic Category Antiarrhythmic Agent, Class Ia

Generic Available Yes

Use Suppression and prevention of unifocal and multifocal atrial and premature, ventricular premature complexes, coupled ventricular tachycardia; effective in the conversion of atrial fibrillation, atrial flutter, and paroxysmal atrial tachycardia to normal sinus rhythm and prevention of the recurrence of these arrhythmias after conversion by other methods

Unlabeled/Investigational Use Hypertrophic obstructive cardiomyopathy (HOCM)

Mechanism of Action Class Ia antiarrhythmic: Decreases myocardial excitability and conduction velocity; reduces disparity in refractory between normal and infarcted myocardium; possesses anticholinergic, peripheral vasoconstrictive, and negative inotropic effects

Pharmacodynamics/Kinetics

Onset of action: 0.5-3.5 hours

Duration: 1.5-8.5 hours

Absorption: 60% to 83%

Protein binding (concentration dependent): 20% to 60%

Metabolism: Hepatic to inactive metabolites

Half-life elimination: Adults: 4-10 hours; prolonged with hepatic or renal impairment

Excretion: Urine (40% to 60% as unchanged drug); feces (10% to 15%)

Dosage Oral:

Children:

<1 year: 10-30 mg/kg/24 hours in 4 divided doses

1-4 years: 10-20 mg/kg/24 hours in 4 divided doses

4-12 years: 10-15 mg/kg/24 hours in 4 divided doses

12-18 years: 6-15 mg/kg/24 hours in 4 divided doses

Adults:

<50 kg: 100 mg every 6 hours or 200 mg every 12 hours (controlled release)

>50 kg: 150 mg every 6 hours or 300 mg every 12 hours (controlled release); if no response, increase to 200 mg every 6 hours. Maximum dose required for patients with severe refractory ventricular tachycardia is 400 mg every 6 hours.

Hypertrophic obstructive cardiomyopathy (unlabeled use): Initial: Controlled release: 200 mg twice daily. If symptoms do not improve, increase by 100 mg/day at 2-week intervals to a maximum daily dose of 600 mg.

Elderly: Dose with caution, starting at the lower end of dosing range

Dosing adjustment in renal impairment: 100 mg (nonsustained release) given at the following intervals, based on creatinine clearance (mL/minute):

Cl_{cr} 30-40 mL/minute: Administer every 8 hours

Cl_{cr} 15-30 mL/minute: Administer every 12 hours

Cl_{cr} <15 mL/minute: Administer every 24 hours

or alter the dose as follows:

Cl_{cr} 30-<40 mL/minute: Reduce dose 50%

Cl_{cr} 15-30 mL/minute: Reduce dose 75%

Dialysis: Not dialyzable (0% to 5%) by hemo- or peritoneal methods; supplemental dose is not necessary.

Dosing interval in hepatic impairment: 100 mg every 6 hours or 200 mg every 12 hours (controlled release)

Stability Extemporaneously prepared suspension is stable for 4 weeks refrigerated

Administration Do not break or chew controlled release capsules. Administer around-the-clock to Administer around-the-clock rather than 4 times/day (ie, 12-6-12-6, not 9-1-5-9) to promote less variation in peak and trough serum levels

Monitoring Parameters ECG, blood pressure, urinary retention, CNS anticholinergic effects (confusion, agitation, hallucinations, etc)

Reference Range

Therapeutic concentration:

Atrial arrhythmias: 2.8-3.2 mcg/mL

Ventricular arrhythmias 3.3-7.5 mcg/mL

Toxic concentration: >7 mcg/mL

Anesthesia and Critical Care Concerns/Other Considerations In patients with pre-existing cardiovascular disease, the incidence of proarrhythmic effects and mortality may be increased with Class Ia antiarrhythmic agents. Disopyramide has significant anticholinergic effects which also limits its role in patients with cardiovascular disease.

Pregnancy Risk Factor C

Contraindications Hypersensitivity to disopyramide or any component of the formulation; cardiogenic shock; pre-existing second- or third-degree heart block

(Continued)

Disopyramide *(Continued)*

(except in patients with a functioning artificial pacemaker); congenital QT syndrome; sick sinus syndrome

Warnings/Precautions Monitor and adjust dose to prevent QT_c prolongation. Avoid concurrent use with other medications that prolong QT interval or decrease myocardial contractility. Correct hypokalemia before initiating therapy; may worsen toxicity. Watch for proarrhythmic effects. **[U.S. Boxed Warning]: In the Cardiac Arrhythmia Suppression Trial (CAST), recent (>6 days but <2 years ago) myocardial infarction patients with asymptomatic, nonlife-threatening ventricular arrhythmias did not benefit and may have been harmed by attempts to suppress the arrhythmia with flecainide or encainide. An increased mortality or nonfatal cardiac arrest rate (7.7%) was seen in the active treatment group compared with patients in the placebo group (3%). The applicability of the CAST results to other populations is unknown. Antiarrhythmic agents should be reserved for patients with life-threatening ventricular arrhythmias.** May precipitate or exacerbate CHF. Due to significant anticholinergic effects, do not use in patients with urinary retention, BPH, glaucoma, or myasthenia gravis. Reduce dosage in renal or hepatic impairment. The extended release form is not recommended for Cl_{cr} <40 mL/minute. In patients with atrial fibrillation or flutter, block the AV node before initiating. Use caution in Wolff-Parkinson-White syndrome or bundle branch block. Monitor closely for hypotension during the initiation of therapy.

Adverse Reactions The most common adverse effects are related to cholinergic blockade. The most serious adverse effects of disopyramide are hypotension and CHF.

>10%:

- Gastrointestinal: Xerostomia (32%), constipation (11%)
- Genitourinary: Urinary hesitancy (14% to 23%)

1% to 10%:

- Cardiovascular: CHF, hypotension, cardiac conduction disturbance, edema, syncope, chest pain
- Central nervous system: Fatigue, headache, malaise, dizziness, nervousness
- Dermatologic: Rash, generalized dermatoses, pruritus
- Endocrine & metabolic: Hypokalemia, elevated cholesterol, elevated triglycerides
- Gastrointestinal: Dry throat, nausea, abdominal distension, flatulence, abdominal bloating, anorexia, diarrhea, vomiting, weight gain
- Genitourinary: Urinary retention, urinary frequency, urinary urgency, impotence (1% to 3%)
- Neuromuscular & skeletal: Muscle weakness, muscular pain
- Ocular: Blurred vision, dry eyes
- Respiratory: Dyspnea

<1% (Limited to important or life-threatening): Agranulocytosis, AV block, cholestatic jaundice, depression, dysuria, creatinine increased, gynecomastia, hepatotoxicity, hypoglycemia, BUN increased, insomnia, new or worsened arrhythmia (proarrhythmic effect), paresthesia, psychotic reaction, respiratory distress, thrombocytopenia, transaminases increased. Rare cases of lupus have been reported (generally in patients previously receiving procainamide), peripheral neuropathy, psychosis, toxic cutaneous blisters

Overdosage/Toxicology Has a low toxic:therapeutic ratio and may easily produce fatal intoxication (acute toxic dose: 1 g in adults). Symptoms of overdose include sinus bradycardia, sinus node arrest or asystole, P-R, QRS, or QT interval prolongation, torsade de pointes (polymorphous ventricular tachycardia) and depressed myocardial contractility, which along with alpha-adrenergic or ganglionic blockade, may result in hypotension and pulmonary edema. Other effects are anticholinergic (dry mouth, dilated pupils, and delirium), as well as seizures, coma, and respiratory arrest.

Treatment is symptomatic and effects usually respond to conventional therapies. **Note:** Do not use other Type 1A or 1C antiarrhythmic agents to treat ventricular tachycardia. Sodium bicarbonate may treat wide QRS intervals or hypotension. Markedly impaired conduction or high degree AV block, unresponsive to bicarbonate, indicates consideration of a pacemaker.

Drug Interactions Substrate of CYP3A4 (major)

Beta-blockers may cause additive/excessive negative inotropic activity.

CYP3A4 inducers: CYP3A4 inducers may decrease the levels/effects of disopyramide. Example inducers include aminoglutethimide, carbamazepine, nafcillin, nevirapine, phenobarbital, phenytoin, and rifamycins.

CYP3A4 inhibitors: May increase the levels/effects of disopyramide. Example inhibitors include azole antifungals, clarithromycin, diclofenac, doxycycline, erythromycin, imatinib, isoniazid, nefazodone, nicardipine, propofol, protease inhibitors, quinidine, telithromycin, and verapamil.

Erythromycin and clarithromycin increase disopyramide blood levels; may cause QRS widening and/or QT interval prolongation.

Procainamide, quinidine, propafenone, or flecainide can cause increased/excessive negative inotropic effects or prolonged conduction.

Drugs which may prolong the QT interval (amiodarone, amitriptyline, bepridil, cisapride, disopyramide, erythromycin, haloperidol, imipramine, pimozide, quinidine, sotalol, and thioridazine) may be additive with disopyramide; use with caution.

Sparfloxacin, gatifloxacin, and moxifloxacin may result in additional prolongation of the QT interval; concurrent use is contraindicated.

Ethanol/Nutrition/Herb Interactions

Ethanol: Avoid ethanol (may increase CNS depression).

Herb/Nutraceutical: St John's wort may decrease disopyramide levels. Avoid ephedra (may worsen arrhythmia).

Dietary Considerations Should be taken on an empty stomach.

Dosage Forms

Capsule (Norpace®): 100 mg, 150 mg

Capsule, controlled release (Norpace® CR): 100 mg, 150 mg

- **Disopyramide Phosphate** *see* Disopyramide *on page 404*
- **Diuril®** *see* Chlorothiazide *on page 271*
- **Divalproex Sodium** *see* Valproic Acid and Derivatives *on page 1329*
- **Dixarit® (Can)** *see* Clonidine *on page 316*
- ***D*-Mannitol** *see* Mannitol *on page 790*

DOBUTamine (doe BYOO ta meen)

Medication Safety Issues

Sound-alike/look-alike issues:

DOBUTamine may be confused with DOPamine

Related Information

Critical Care Infusion Administration Charts *on page 1514*

Heart Failure (Systolic) *on page 1607*

Hemodynamic Support, Intravenous *on page 1566*

Canadian Brand Names Dobutamine Injection, USP; Dobutrex®

Synonyms Dobutamine Hydrochloride

Pharmacologic Category Adrenergic Agonist Agent

Generic Available Yes

Use Short-term management of patients with cardiac decompensation

Unlabeled/Investigational Use Positive inotropic agent for use in myocardial dysfunction of sepsis

Mechanism of Action Stimulates beta$_1$-adrenergic receptors, causing increased contractility and heart rate, with little effect on beta$_2$- or alpha-receptors

Infusion Rates of Various Dilutions of Dobutamine

Desired Delivery Rate (mcg/kg/min)	Infusion Rate (mL/kg/min)	
	500 mcg/mL[1]	1000 mcg/mL[2]
2.5	0.005	0.0025
5.0	0.01	0.005
7.5	0.015	0.0075
10.0	0.02	0.01
12.5	0.025	0.0125
15.0	0.03	0.015

[1]500 mg per liter or 250 mg per 500 mL of diluent.

[2]1000 mg per liter or 250 mg per 250 mL of diluent.

Pharmacodynamics/Kinetics

Onset of action: I.V.: 1-10 minutes

(Continued)

DOBUTamine *(Continued)*

Peak effect: 10-20 minutes

Metabolism: In tissues and hepatically to inactive metabolites

Half-life elimination: 2 minutes

Excretion: Urine (as metabolites)

Dosage Administration requires the use of an infusion pump; I.V. infusion:

Neonates: 2-15 mcg/kg/minute, titrate to desired response

Children and Adults: 2.5-20 mcg/kg/minute; maximum: 40 mcg/kg/minute, titrate to desired response. See table on previous page.

Stability Remix solution every 24 hours; store reconstituted solution under refrigeration for 48 hours or 6 hours at room temperature; pink discoloration of solution indicates slight oxidation but **no** significant loss of potency.

Stability of parenteral admixture at room temperature (25°C): 48 hours; at refrigeration (4°C): 7 days

Standard adult diluent: 250 mg/500 mL D_5W; 500 mg/500 mL D_5W

Incompatible with heparin, cefazolin, penicillin, and sodium bicarbonate; **incompatible** in alkaline solutions (sodium bicarbonate)

Compatible with dopamine, epinephrine, isoproterenol, lidocaine

Administration Use infusion device to control rate of flow; administer into large vein. Do not administer through same I.V. line as heparin, hydrocortisone sodium succinate, cefazolin, or penicillin.

To prepare for infusion:

$$\frac{6 \times \text{weight (kg)} \times \text{desired dose (mcg/kg/min)}}{\text{I.V. infusion rate (mL/h)}} = \text{mg of drug to be added to 100 mL of I.V. fluid}$$

Monitoring Parameters Blood pressure, ECG, heart rate, CVP, RAP, MAP, urine output; if pulmonary artery catheter is in place, monitor CI, PCWP, and SVR; also monitor serum potassium

Anesthesia and Critical Care Concerns/Other Considerations Septic Shock: Septic patients who have been adequately fluid resuscitated and have an adequate mean arterial pressure but low cardiac index (<2.5 L/minute/m^2) may require dobutamine. Dobutamine may help reverse tissue hypoperfusion by increasing cardiac output. Increasing cardiac output beyond the normal range has not been shown in clinical trials to improve patient outcome.

Early goal-directed therapy in the treatment of severe sepsis and septic shock provides significant survival benefits to this subset of patients. About 14% of the patients in the early goal-directed group received dobutamine. The early goal-directed patients received significantly more fluid, red-cell transfusions, and inotropic support during the initial 6 hours of their visit (Rivers, 2001). The 2004 Surviving Sepsis Campaign guidelines suggest that if central venous oxygen saturation or mixed venous oxygen saturation of 70% is not achieved (central venous pressure 8-12 mm Hg) within the first 6 hours of resuscitation, then transfuse packed red blood cells to a hematocrit of ≥30% and/or administer dobutamine (up to 20 mcg/kg/minute) to achieve this goal.

Pregnancy Risk Factor B

Contraindications Hypersensitivity to dobutamine or sulfites (some contain sodium metabisulfate), or any component of the formulation; idiopathic hypertrophic subaortic stenosis (IHSS)

Warnings/Precautions May increase heart rate. Patients with atrial fibrillation may experience an increase in ventricular response. An increase in blood pressure is more common, but occasionally a patient may become hypotensive. May exacerbate ventricular ectopy. If needed, correct hypovolemia first to optimize hemodynamics. Ineffective in the presence of mechanical obstruction such as severe aortic stenosis. Use caution post-MI (can increase myocardial oxygen demand). Use cautiously in the elderly starting at lower end of the dosage range.

Adverse Reactions Incidence of adverse events is not always reported.

Cardiovascular: Increased heart rate, increased blood pressure, increased ventricular ectopic activity, hypotension, premature ventricular beats (5%, dose related), anginal pain (1% to 3%), nonspecific chest pain (1% to 3%), palpitation (1% to 3%)

Central nervous system: Fever (1% to 3%), headache (1% to 3%), paresthesia

Endocrine & metabolic: Slight decrease in serum potassium

Gastrointestinal: Nausea (1% to 3%)

Hematologic: Thrombocytopenia (isolated cases)

Local: Phlebitis, local inflammatory changes and pain from infiltration, cutaneous necrosis (isolated cases)

Neuromuscular & skeletal: Mild leg cramps

Respiratory: Dyspnea (1% to 3%)

Overdosage/Toxicology Symptoms of overdose include fatigue, nervousness, tachycardia, hypertension, and arrhythmias. Reduce rate of administration or discontinue infusion until condition stabilizes.

Drug Interactions

Beta-blockers (nonselective ones) may increase hypertensive effect; avoid concurrent use.

Cocaine may cause malignant arrhythmias; avoid concurrent use.

Guanethidine can increase the pressor response; be aware of the patient's drug regimen.

MAO inhibitors potentiate hypertension and hypertensive crisis; avoid concurrent use.

Methyldopa can increase the pressor response; be aware of patient's drug regimen.

Reserpine increases the pressor response; be aware of patient's drug regimen.

TCAs increase the pressor response; be aware of patient's drug regimen.

Dosage Forms

Infusion, as hydrochloride [premixed in dextrose]: 1 mg/mL (250 mL, 500 mL); 2 mg/mL (250 mL); 4 mg/mL (250 mL)

Injection, solution, as hydrochloride: 12.5 mg/mL (20 mL, 40 mL, 100 mL) [contains sodium bisulfite]

References

Dellinger RP, Carlet JM, Masur H, et al, "Surviving Sepsis Campaign Guidelines for Management of Severe Sepsis and Septic Shock," *Crit Care Med*, 2004, 32(3):858-73.

Rivers E, Nguyen B, Havstad S, et al, "Early Goal-Directed Therapy in the Treatment of Severe Sepsis and Septic Shock," *N Engl J Med*, 2001, 345(19):1368-77.

"Task Force of the American College of Critical Care Medicine and Society of Critical Care Medicine. Practice Parameters for Hemodynamic Support of Sepsis in Adult Patients," *Crit Care Med*, 1999, 27(3):639-60. Available at: http://www.sccm.org/pdf/Hemodynamic%20Support.pdf.

♦ **Dobutamine Hydrochloride** *see* DOBUTamine *on page 407*

♦ **Dobutamine Injection, USP (Can)** *see* DOBUTamine *on page 407*

♦ **Dobutrex® (Can)** *see* DOBUTamine *on page 407*

Dofetilide (doe FET il ide)

U.S. Brand Names Tikosyn™

Canadian Brand Names Tikosyn™

Pharmacologic Category Antiarrhythmic Agent, Class III

Generic Available No

Use Maintenance of normal sinus rhythm in patients with chronic atrial fibrillation/atrial flutter of longer than 1-week duration who have been converted to normal sinus rhythm; conversion of atrial fibrillation and atrial flutter to normal sinus rhythm

Mechanism of Action Vaughan Williams Class III antiarrhythmic activity. Blockade of the cardiac ion channel carrying the rapid component of the delayed rectifier potassium current. Dofetilide has no effect on sodium channels, adrenergic alpha-receptors, or adrenergic beta-receptors. It increases the monophasic action potential duration due to delayed repolarization. The increase in the QT interval is a function of prolongation of both effective and functional refractory periods in the His-Purkinje system and the ventricles. Changes in cardiac conduction velocity and sinus node function have not been observed in patients with or without structural heart disease. PR and QRS width remain the same in patients with pre-existing heart block and or sick sinus syndrome.

Pharmacodynamics/Kinetics

Absorption: >90%

Distribution: V_d: 3 L/kg

Protein binding: 60% to 70%

Metabolism: Hepatic via CYP3A4, but low affinity for it; metabolites formed by N-dealkylation and N-oxidation

Bioavailability: >90%

Half-life elimination: 10 hours

Time to peak: Fasting: 2-3 hours

(Continued)

Dofetilide *(Continued)*

Excretion: Urine (80%, 80% as unchanged drug, 20% as inactive or minimally active metabolites); renal elimination consists of glomerular filtration and active tubular secretion via cationic transport system

Dosage Adults: Oral:

Note: QT or QT_c must be determined prior to first dose. If QT_c >440 msec (>500 msec in patients with ventricular conduction abnormalities), dofetilide is contraindicated (see Contraindications and Warnings/Precautions).

Initial: 500 mcg orally twice daily. Initial dosage must be adjusted in patients with estimated Cl_{cr} <60 mL/minute (see Dosage Adjustment in Renal Impairment). Dofetilide may be initiated at lower doses than recommended based on physician discretion.

Modification of dosage in response to initial dose: QT_c interval should be measured 2-3 hours after the initial dose. If the QT_c >15% of baseline, or if the QT_c is >500 msec (550 msec in patients with ventricular conduction abnormalities) dofetilide should be adjusted. If the starting dose is 500 mcg twice daily, then adjust to 250 mcg twice daily. If the starting dose was 250 mcg twice daily, then adjust to 125 mcg twice daily. If the starting dose was 125 mcg twice daily then adjust to 125 mcg every day.

Continued monitoring for doses 2-5: QT_c interval must be determined 2-3 hours after each subsequent dose of dofetilide for in-hospital doses 2-5. If the measured QT_c is >500 msec (550 msec in patients with ventricular conduction abnormalities) at any time, dofetilide should be discontinued.

Chronic therapy (following the 5th dose):

QT or QT_c and creatinine clearance should be evaluated every 3 months. If QT_c >500 msec (>550 msec in patients with ventricular conduction abnormalities), dofetilide should be discontinued.

Dosage adjustment in renal impairment:

Cl_{cr} >60 mL/minute: Administer 500 mcg twice daily.
Cl_{cr} 40-60 mL/minute: Administer 250 mcg twice daily.
Cl_{cr} 20-39 mL/minute: Administer 125 mcg twice daily.
Cl_{cr} <20 mL/minute: Contraindicated in this group.

Dosage adjustment in hepatic impairment: No dosage adjustments required in Child-Pugh Class A and B. Patients with severe hepatic impairment were not studied.

Elderly: No specific dosage adjustments are recommended based on age, however, careful assessment of renal function is particularly important in this population.

Administration Do not open capsules.

Monitoring Parameters ECG monitoring with attention to QT_c and occurrence of ventricular arrhythmias, baseline serum creatinine and changes in serum creatinine. Check serum potassium and magnesium levels if on medications where these electrolyte disturbances can occur, or if patient has a history of hypokalemia or hypomagnesemia. QT or QT_c must be monitored at specific times prior to the first dose and during the first 3 days of therapy. Thereafter, QT or QT_c and creatinine clearance must be evaluated at 3-month intervals.

Pregnancy Risk Factor C

Contraindications Hypersensitivity to dofetilide or any component of the formulation; patients with congenital or acquired long QT syndromes, do not use if a baseline QT interval or QT_c is >440 msec (500 msec in patients with ventricular conduction abnormalities); severe renal impairment (estimated Cl_{cr} <20 mL/minute); concurrent use with verapamil, cimetidine, hydrochlorothiazide (alone or in combinations), trimethoprim (alone or in combination with sulfamethoxazole), itraconazole, ketoconazole, prochlorperazine, or megestrol; baseline heart rate <50 beats/minute; other drugs that prolong QT intervals (phenothiazines, cisapride, bepridil, tricyclic antidepressants, sparfloxacin, gatifloxacin, moxifloxacin; hypokalemia or hypomagnesemia; concurrent amiodarone, clarithromycin, or erythromycin

Warnings/Precautions **[U.S. Boxed Warning]: Must be initiated (or reinitiated) in a setting with continuous monitoring and staff familiar with the recognition and treatment of life-threatening arrhythmias. Patients must be monitored with continuous ECG for a minimum of 3 days,** or for a minimum of 12 hours after electrical or pharmacological cardioversion to normal sinus rhythm, whichever is greater. Patients should be readmitted for continuous monitoring if dosage is later increased.

Reserve for patients who are highly symptomatic with atrial fibrillation/atrial flutter; torsade de pointes significantly increases with doses >500 mcg twice daily; hold class I or class III antiarrhythmics for at least three half-lives prior to starting dofetilide; use in patients on amiodarone therapy only if serum amiodarone level is <0.3 mg/L or if amiodarone was stopped for >3 months previously; correct hypokalemia or hypomagnesemia before initiating dofetilide and maintain within normal limits during treatment. Risk of hypokalemia and/or hypomagnesemia may be increased by potassium-depleting diuretics, increasing the risk of torsade de pointes. Concurrent use with other drugs known to prolong QT_c interval is not recommended.

Patients with sick sinus syndrome or with second or third-degree heart block should not receive dofetilide unless a functional pacemaker is in place. Defibrillation threshold is reduced in patients with ventricular tachycardia or ventricular fibrillation undergoing implantation of a cardioverter-defibrillator device. Safety and efficacy in children (<18 years old) have not been established. Use with caution in renal impairment; not recommended in patients receiving drugs which may compete for renal secretion via cationic transport. Use with caution in patients with severe hepatic impairment.

Adverse Reactions

Supraventricular arrhythmia patients (incidence > placebo)

>10%: Central nervous system: Headache (11%)

2% to 10%:

- Central nervous system: Dizziness (8%), insomnia (4%)
- Cardiovascular: Ventricular tachycardia (2.6% to 3.7%), chest pain (10%), torsade de pointes (3.3% in CHF patients and 0.9% in patients with a recent MI; up to 10.5% in patients receiving doses in excess of those recommended). Torsade de pointes occurs most frequently within the first 3 days of therapy.
- Dermatologic: Rash (3%)
- Gastrointestinal: Nausea (5%), diarrhea (3%), abdominal pain (3%)
- Neuromuscular & skeletal: Back pain (3%)
- Respiratory: Dyspnea (6%), respiratory tract infection (7%)
- Miscellaneous: Flu syndrome (4%)

<2% (Limited to important or life-threatening): Angioedema, AV block (0.4% to 1.5%), bundle branch block, cardiac arrest, facial paralysis, flaccid paralysis, heart block, hepatotoxicity, MI, paralysis, paresthesia, stroke, syncope, ventricular fibrillation (0% to 0.4%)

Overdosage/Toxicology The major dose-related toxicity is torsade de pointes. Treatment should be symptomatic and supportive. Watch for excessive prolongation of the QT interval in overdose situations. Continuous cardiac monitoring is necessary. A charcoal slurry is helpful when given early (15 minutes) after the overdose.

Drug Interactions **Substrate** of CYP3A4 (minor)

If dofetilide needs to be discontinued to allow dosing of other potentially interacting drug(s) (see below), a washout period of at least 2 days is needed before starting the other drug(s).

Cimetidine, a cation transport system inhibitor, inhibits dofetilide's elimination and can cause a 58% increase in dofetilide's plasma levels; concomitant use is contraindicated.

Diuretics and other drugs (aminoglycosides) which deplete potassium or magnesium may increase dofetilide toxicity (torsade de pointes). Concurrent use of hydrochlorothiazide is contraindicated.

Hydrochlorothiazide: May enhance the QT_c-prolonging effect of dofetilide. May increase serum concentration of dofetilide. Concurrent use is contraindicated.

Itraconazole: May decrease the metabolism of dofetilide. Concurrent use is contraindicated.

Ketoconazole increases dofetilide's C_{max} (53% males, 97% females) and the AUC (41% males, 69% females) when used concurrently; concomitant use is contraindicated.

QT_c-prolonging agents (including bepridil, cisapride, clarithromycin, erythromycin, tricyclic antidepressants, phenothiazines, sparfloxacin, gatifloxacin, moxifloxacin): Use is contraindicated.

Renal cationic transport inhibitors (including triamterene, metformin, amiloride, prochlorperazine, megestrol) may increase dofetilide levels; coadminister with caution.

Trimethoprim (alone or in combination with sulfamethoxazole) increases dofetilide's C_{max} (103%) and AUC (93%); concomitant use is contraindicated.

(Continued)

Dofetilide *(Continued)*

Verapamil causes an increase in dofetilide's peak plasma levels by 42%. In the supraventricular arrhythmia and a higher incidence of torsade de pointes was seen in patients on verapamil; concomitant use is contraindicated.

Ethanol/Nutrition/Herb Interactions Herb/Nutraceutical: St John's wort may decrease dofetilide levels. Avoid ephedra (may worsen arrhythmia).

Dosage Forms Capsule: 125 mcg, 250 mcg, 500 mcg

Dolasetron (dol A se tron)

Medication Safety Issues

Sound-alike/look-alike issues:

Anzemet® may be confused with Aldomet®

Dolasetron may be confused with granisetron, ondansetron, palonosetron

Related Information

Postoperative Nausea and Vomiting *on page 1477*

U.S. Brand Names Anzemet®

Canadian Brand Names Anzemet®

Synonyms Dolasetron Mesylate; MDL 73,147EF

Pharmacologic Category Antiemetic; Selective 5-HT_3 Receptor Antagonist

Generic Available No

Use Prevention of nausea and vomiting associated with emetogenic cancer chemotherapy; prevention of postoperative nausea and vomiting; treatment of postoperative nausea and vomiting (injectable form only)

Not recommended for treatment of existing chemotherapy-induced emesis (CIE).

Mechanism of Action Selective serotonin receptor (5-HT_3) antagonist, blocking serotonin both peripherally (primary site of action) and centrally at the chemoreceptor trigger zone

Pharmacodynamics/Kinetics

Absorption: Rapid and complete

Distribution: 5.8 L/kg

Protein binding: Hydrodolasetron: 69% to 77% (50% bound to $alpha_1$-acid glycoprotein)

Metabolism: Hepatic; reduction by carbonyl reductase to hydrodolasetron (active metabolite); further metabolized by CYP3A and flavin monooxygenase

Bioavailability: 75%

Half-life elimination: Dolasetron: 10 minutes; hydrodolasetron: Adults: 6-8 hours; Children: 4-6 hours

Time to peak, plasma: I.V.: 0.6 hours; Oral: 1 hour

Excretion: Urine ~67% (53% to 61% as active metabolite hydrodolasetron); feces ~33%

Dosage

Nausea and vomiting prophylaxis, chemotherapy-induced (including initial and repeat courses):

Children 2-16 years:

Oral: 1.8 mg/kg within 1 hour before chemotherapy; maximum: 100 mg/dose

I.V.: 1.8 mg/kg ~30 minutes before chemotherapy; maximum: 100 mg/dose

Adults:

Oral:100 mg single dose 1 hour prior to chemotherapy

I.V.: 1.8 mg/kg or 100 mg 30 minutes prior to chemotherapy

Prevention of postoperative nausea and vomiting:

Children 2-16 years:

Oral: 1.2 mg/kg within 2 hours before surgery; maximum: 100 mg/dose

I.V.: 0.35 mg/kg (maximum: 12.5 mg) ~15 minutes before stopping anesthesia

Adults:

Oral: 100 mg within 2 hours before surgery

I.V.: 12.5 mg ~15 minutes before stopping anesthesia

Treatment of postoperative nausea and vomiting: I.V. (only):

Children: 0.35 mg/kg (maximum: 12.5 mg) as soon as needed

Adults: 12.5 mg as soon as needed

Dosing adjustment for elderly, renal/hepatic impairment: No dosage adjustment is recommended

Stability Store intact vials and tablets at room temperature; protect from light. Stock solution (20 mg/mL) drawn into syringes is stable for 8 months at room temperature. After dilution, I.V. dolasetron is stable under normal lighting conditions at room temperature for 24 hours or under refrigeration for 48 hours with the following **compatible** intravenous fluids: 0.9% sodium chloride injection, 5% dextrose injection, 5% dextrose and 0.45% sodium chloride injection, 5% dextrose and lactated Ringer's injection, lactated Ringer's injection, and 10% mannitol injection

Administration I.V. injection may be given either undiluted IVP over 30 seconds or diluted in 50 mL of compatible fluid and infused over 15 minutes. Line should be flushed, prior to and after, dolasetron administration. Dolasetron injection may be diluted in apple or apple-grape juice and taken orally; this dilution is stable for 2 hours at room temperature.

Monitoring Parameters Liver function tests, blood pressure and pulse, and ECG in patients with cardiovascular disease

Anesthesia and Critical Care Concerns/Other Considerations Oral administration of the intravenous solution is equivalent to tablets.

Pregnancy Risk Factor B

Contraindications Hypersensitivity to dolasetron or any component of the formulation

Warnings/Precautions Administer with caution in patients who have or may develop prolongation of cardiac conduction intervals, particularly QT_c intervals. These include patients with hypokalemia or hypomagnesemia, patients taking diuretics with potential for inducing electrolyte abnormalities, patients with congenital QT syndrome, patients taking antiarrhythmic drugs or other drugs which lead to QT prolongation, and cumulative high-dose anthracycline therapy. Safety and efficacy in children <2 years of age have not been established.

Adverse Reactions Adverse events may vary according to indication

>10%:

Central nervous system: Headache (7% to 24%)

Gastrointestinal: Diarrhea (2% to 12%)

1% to 10%:

Cardiovascular: Bradycardia (5%), hypotension (5%), hypertension (2% to 3%), tachycardia (2% to 3%)

Central nervous system: Dizziness (1% to 6%), fatigue (3% to 6%), fever (3% to 5%), chills/shivering (1% to 2%), sedation (2%)

Dermatological: Pruritus (3% to 4%)

Gastrointestinal: Dyspepsia (2% to 3%), abdominal pain (3%)

Hepatic: Abnormal hepatic function (4%)

Neuromuscular & skeletal: Pain (3%)

Renal: Oliguria (1% to 3%), urinary retention (2%)

<1% (Limited to important or life-threatening): Abnormal vision, abnormal dreaming, acute renal failure, anaphylactic reaction, anemia, anorexia, ataxia, bronchospasm, confusion, constipation, diaphoresis increased, dyspnea, , edema, epistaxis, GGT increased, hematuria, hyperbilirubinemia, ischemia (peripheral), local injection site reaction, pancreatitis, photophobia, polyuria; prolonged P-R, QRS, and QT_c intervals; prothrombin time increased, purpura/hematoma, rash, sleep disorder, syncope, taste perversion, thrombocytopenia, thrombophlebitis/phlebitis, tinnitus, urticaria

Overdosage/Toxicology Prolongation of QT, AV block, severe hypotension, and dizziness have been reported. Treatment is supportive, and continuous ECG monitoring (telemetry) is recommended.

Drug Interactions Substrate (minor) of CYP2C9, 3A4; **Inhibits** CYP2D6 (weak)

Apomorphine: Due to reports of profound hypotension during concomitant therapy with ondansetron, the manufacturer of apomorphine contraindicates its use with all 5-HT_3 antagonists.

QT_c-prolonging agents (includes but may not be limited to amitriptyline, bepridil, disopyramide, erythromycin, haloperidol, imipramine, quinidine, pimozide, procainamide, sotalol, and thioridazine): Effect/toxicity of dolasetron and other QT_c-prolonging agents may be increased; use with caution.

Ethanol/Nutrition/Herb Interactions Herb/Nutraceutical: St John's wort may decrease dolasetron levels.

Dosage Forms

Injection, solution, as mesylate: 20 mg/mL (0.625 mL) [single-use ampul, Carpuject®, or vial]; 20 mg/mL (5 mL) [single-use vial]; 20 mg/mL (25 mL) [multidose vial]

(Continued)

Dolasetron *(Continued)*

Tablet, as mesylate: 50 mg, 100 mg

References

Diemunsch P, Lesser J, Feiss P, et al, "Intravenous Dolasetron Mesilate Ameliorates Postoperative Nausea and Vomiting," *Can J Anaesth*, 1997, 44(2):173-81.

Graczyk SG, McKenzie R, et al, "Intravenous Dolasetron for the Prevention of Postoperative Nausea and Vomiting After Outpatient Laparoscopic Gynecologic Surgery," *Anesth Analg*, 1997, 84(2):325-30.

Kovac AI, Scuderi PE, et al, "Treatment of Postoperative Nausea and Vomiting With Single Intravenous Doses of Dolasetron Mesylate: A Multicenter Trial," *Anesth Analg*, 1997, 85(3):546-52.

♦ **Dolasetron Mesylate** *see* Dolasetron *on page 412*
♦ **Dolobid® [DSC]** *see* Diflunisal *on page 385*
♦ **Dolophine®** *see* Methadone *on page 813*
♦ **Dom-Benzydamine (Can)** *see* Benzydamine *on page 167*
♦ **Dom-Citalopram (Can)** *see* Citalopram *on page 297*
♦ **Dom-Mefenamic Acid (Can)** *see* Mefenamic Acid *on page 795*
♦ **Dom-Methimazole (Can)** *see* Methimazole *on page 817*
♦ **Dom-Sumatriptan (Can)** *see* Sumatriptan *on page 1222*
♦ **Dom-Topiramate (Can)** *see* Topiramate *on page 1287*

DOPamine (DOE pa meen)

Medication Safety Issues
Sound-alike/look-alike issues:
DOPamine may be confused with DOBUTamine, Dopram®

Related Information
Critical Care Infusion Administration Charts *on page 1514*
Heart Failure (Systolic) *on page 1607*
Hemodynamic Support, Intravenous *on page 1566*

Synonyms Dopamine Hydrochloride; Intropin

Pharmacologic Category Adrenergic Agonist Agent

Generic Available Yes

Use Adjunct in the treatment of shock (eg, MI, open heart surgery, renal failure, cardiac decompensation) which persists after adequate fluid volume replacement

Unlabeled/Investigational Use Symptomatic bradycardia or heart block unresponsive to atropine or pacing

Mechanism of Action Stimulates both adrenergic and dopaminergic receptors, lower doses are mainly dopaminergic stimulating and produce renal and mesenteric vasodilation, higher doses also are both dopaminergic and beta$_1$-adrenergic stimulating and produce cardiac stimulation and renal vasodilation; large doses stimulate alpha-adrenergic receptors

Pharmacodynamics/Kinetics
Children: Dopamine has exhibited nonlinear kinetics in children; with medication changes, may not achieve steady-state for ~1 hour rather than 20 minutes
Onset of action: Adults: 5 minutes
Duration: Adults: <10 minutes
Metabolism: Renal, hepatic, plasma; 75% to inactive metabolites by monoamine oxidase and 25% to norepinephrine
Half-life elimination: 2 minutes
Excretion: Urine (as metabolites)
Clearance: Neonates: Varies and appears to be age related; clearance is more prolonged with combined hepatic and renal dysfunction

Dosage I.V. infusion (administration requires the use of an infusion pump):
Neonates: 1-20 mcg/kg/minute continuous infusion, titrate to desired response.
Children: 1-20 mcg/kg/minute, maximum: 50 mcg/kg/minute continuous infusion, titrate to desired response.
Adults: 1-5 mcg/kg/minute up to 20 mcg/kg/minute, titrate to desired response. Infusion may be increased by 1-4 mcg/kg/minute at 10- to 30-minute intervals until optimal response is obtained.
If dosages >20-30 mcg/kg/minute are needed, a more direct-acting pressor may be more beneficial (ie, epinephrine, norepinephrine).

The hemodynamic effects of dopamine are dose dependent:
Low-dose: 1-3 mcg/kg/minute, increased renal blood flow and urine output
Intermediate-dose: 3-10 mcg/kg/minute, increased renal blood flow, heart rate, cardiac contractility, and cardiac output

High-dose: >10 mcg/kg/minute, alpha-adrenergic effects begin to predominate, vasoconstriction, increased blood pressure

Stability Protect from light; solutions that are darker than slightly yellow should not be used; **incompatible** with alkaline solutions or iron salts; **compatible** when coadministered with dobutamine, epinephrine, isoproterenol, and lidocaine

Administration Administer into large vein to prevent the possibility of extravasation (central line administration); monitor continuously for free flow; use infusion device to control rate of flow; administration into an umbilical arterial catheter is not recommended; when discontinuing the infusion, gradually decrease the dose of dopamine (sudden discontinuation may cause hypotension).

To prepare for infusion:

$$\frac{6 \times \text{weight (kg)} \times \text{desired dose (mcg/kg/min)}}{\text{I.V. infusion rate (mL/h)}} = \text{mg of drug to be added to 100 mL of I.V. fluid}$$

Extravasation management: Due to short half-life, withdrawal of drug is often only necessary treatment. Use phentolamine as antidote. Mix 5 mg with 9 mL of NS; inject a small amount of this dilution into extravasated area. Blanching should reverse immediately. Monitor site. If blanching should recur, additional injections of phentolamine may be needed.

Monitoring Parameters Blood pressure, ECG, heart rate, CVP, RAP, MAP, urine output; if pulmonary artery catheter is in place, monitor CI, PCWP, SVR, and PVR

Anesthesia and Critical Care Concerns/Other Considerations

Low-Dose Dopamine: There is no clear evidence that low-dose dopamine confers any renal benefit. The 1999 ACCM/SCCM Practice Parameters for Hemodynamic Support of Sepsis in Adult Patients recommends against the use of low doses of dopamine to maintain renal function. Low-dose dopamine may increase renal blood flow in some patients requiring norepinephrine. Kellum and Decker (2001) reviewed 58 studies in a meta-analysis focused on determining if low-dose dopamine reduced the severity of acute renal failure, the need for dialysis, or mortality in critically-ill patients. They concluded that the use of low-dose dopamine for the treatment or prevention of acute renal failure cannot be justified. A more recent randomized, double-blind, placebo-controlled trial came to a similar conclusion (Australian and New Zealand Intensive Care Society Clinical Trials Group, 2000). This study enrolled over 300 ICU patients with clinical evidence of renal dysfunction. They were randomized to low-dose dopamine (2 mcg/kg/minute) or placebo. The investigators found no difference in serum creatinine, renal replacement therapy, intensive care length of stay, hospital stay, or mortality between the groups.

Septic Shock: In septic shock, dopamine is effective in increasing mean arterial pressure in patients who remain hypotensive after adequate volume expansion. Undesirable effects include tachycardia, increased pulmonary shunt, and decreased P_aO_2. As catecholamine stores are depleted, tachyphylaxis may occur. The 1999 ACCM/SCCM Practice Parameters for Hemodynamic Support of Sepsis in Adult Patients recommends either dopamine or norepinephrine as vasopressor therapy. Norepinephrine has a wider dosage range than dopamine.

Pregnancy Risk Factor C

Contraindications Hypersensitivity to sulfites (commercial preparation contains sodium bisulfite); pheochromocytoma; ventricular fibrillation

Warnings/Precautions Use with caution in patients with cardiovascular disease or cardiac arrhythmias or patients with occlusive vascular disease. Correct hypovolemia and electrolytes when used in hemodynamic support. May cause increases in HR and arrhythmia. Avoid infiltration - may cause severe tissue necrosis. Use with caution in post-MI patients.

Adverse Reactions Frequency not defined.

Most frequent:

- Cardiovascular: Ectopic beats, tachycardia, anginal pain, palpitation, hypotension, vasoconstriction
- Central nervous system: Headache
- Gastrointestinal: Nausea and vomiting
- Respiratory: Dyspnea

Infrequent:

- Cardiovascular: Aberrant conduction, bradycardia, widened QRS complex, ventricular arrhythmia (high dose), gangrene (high dose), hypertension
- Central nervous system: Anxiety

(Continued)

DOPamine *(Continued)*

Endocrine & metabolic: Piloerection, serum glucose increased (usually not above normal limits)

Local: Extravasation of dopamine can cause tissue necrosis and sloughing of surrounding tissues

Ocular: Intraocular pressure increased, dilated pupils

Renal: Azotemia, polyuria

Overdosage/Toxicology Symptoms of overdose include severe hypertension, cardiac arrhythmias, acute renal failure. Treat symptomatically.

Important: Antidote for peripheral ischemia: To prevent sloughing and necrosis in ischemic areas, the area should be infiltrated as soon as possible with 10-15 mL of saline solution containing 5-10 mg of Regitine (brand of phentolamine), an adrenergic blocking agent. A syringe with a fine hypodermic needle should be used, and the solution liberally infiltrated throughout the ischemic area. Sympathetic blockade with phentolamine causes immediate and conspicuous local hyperemic changes if the area is infiltrated within 12 hours. Therefore, phentolamine should be given as soon as possible after extravasation is noted.

Drug Interactions

Beta-blockers (nonselective ones) may increase hypertensive effect; avoid concurrent use.

Cocaine may cause malignant arrhythmias; avoid concurrent use.

Guanethidine's hypotensive effects may only be partially reversed; may need to use a direct-acting sympathomimetic.

MAO inhibitors potentiate hypertension and hypertensive crisis; avoid concurrent use.

Methyldopa can increase the pressor response; be aware of patient's drug regimen.

Reserpine increases the pressor response; be aware of patient's drug regimen.

TCAs increase the pressor response; be aware of patient's drug regimen.

Dosage Forms

Infusion, as hydrochloride [premixed in D_5W]: 0.8 mg/mL (250 mL, 500 mL); 1.6 mg/mL (250 mL, 500 mL); 3.2 mg/mL (250 mL)

Injection, solution, as hydrochloride: 40 mg/mL (5 mL, 10 mL); 80 mg/mL (5 mL); 160 mg/mL (5 mL) [contains sodium metabisulfite]

References

Bellomo R, Chapman M, Finfer S, et al, "Low-Dose Dopamine in Patients With Early Renal Dysfunction: A Placebo-Controlled Randomised Trial. Australian and New Zealand Intensive Care Society (ANZICS) Clinical Trials Group," *Lancet*, 2000, 356(9248):2139-43.

Dellinger RP, Carlet JM, Masur H, et al, "Surviving Sepsis Campaign Guidelines for Management of Severe Sepsis and Septic Shock," *Crit Care Med*, 2004, 32(3):858-73.

Johnson RL Jr, "Low-Dose Dopamine and Oxygen Transport by the Lung," *Circulation*, 1998, 98(2):97-9.

Kellum JA and Decker JM, "Use of Dopamine in Acute Renal Failure: A Meta-analysis," *Crit Care Med*, 2001, 29(8):1526-31.

Martin C, Papazian L, Perrin G, et al, "Norepinephrine or Dopamine for the Treatment of Hyperdynamic Septic Shock?" *Chest*, 1993, 103(6):1826-31.

"Task Force of the American College of Critical Care Medicine and Society of Critical Care Medicine. Practice Parameters for Hemodynamic Support of Sepsis in Adult Patients," *Crit Care Med*, 1999, 27(3):639-60.

van de Borne P, Oren R, and Somers VK, "Dopamine Depresses Minute Ventilation in Patients With Heart Failure," *Circulation*, 1998, 98(2):126-31.

♦ **Dopamine Hydrochloride** *see* DOPamine *on page 414*

♦ **Dopram®** *see* Doxapram *on page 418*

♦ **Doryx®** *see* Doxycycline *on page 426*

Doxacurium (doks a KYOO ri um)

Medication Safety Issues

Sound-alike/look-alike issues:

Doxacurium may be confused with doxapram, DOXOrubicin

High alert medication: The Institute for Safe Medication Practices (ISMP) includes this medication among its list of drugs which have a heightened risk of causing significant patient harm when used in error.

Related Information

Chronic Renal Failure *on page 1437*

Neuromuscular Blocking Agents *on page 1572*

U.S. Brand Names Nuromax®

Synonyms Doxacurium Chloride

Pharmacologic Category Neuromuscular Blocker Agent, Nondepolarizing

Generic Available No

Use Adjunct to general anesthesia to facilitate endotracheal intubation and to relax skeletal muscles during surgery; to facilitate mechanical ventilation in ICU patients; does not relieve pain or produce sedation; the characteristics of this agent make it especially useful in procedures requiring careful maintenance of hemodynamic stability for prolonged periods

Mechanism of Action Prevents depolarization of muscle membrane and subsequent muscle contraction by acting as a competitive antagonist to acetylcholine at the alpha subunits of the nicotinic cholinergic receptors on the motor endplates in skeletal muscle, also interferes with the mobilization of acetylcholine presynaptically; the neuromuscular blockade can be pharmacologically reversed with an anticholinesterase agent (neostigmine, edrophonium, pyridostigmine)

Pharmacodynamics/Kinetics

Onset of action: 5-11 minutes

Duration: 30 minutes (range: 12-54 minutes)

Protein binding: 30%

Excretion: Primarily urine and feces (as unchanged drug); recovery time prolonged in elderly

Dosage Administer I.V.; dose to effect; doses will vary due to interpatient variability; use ideal body weight for obese patients

Surgery:

Children >2 years: Initial: 0.03-0.05 mg/kg followed by maintenance doses of 0.005-0.01 mg/kg after 30-45 minutes

Adults: 0.05-0.08 mg/kg with thiopental/narcotic or 0.025 mg/kg after initial dose of succinylcholine for intubation; initial maintenance dose of 0.005-0.01 mg/kg after 100-160 minutes followed by repeat doses every 30-45 minutes

Pretreatment/priming: 10% of intubating dose given 3-5 minutes before initial dose

ICU: 0.05 mg/kg bolus followed by 0.025 mg/kg every 2-3 hours or 0.25-0.75 mcg/kg/minute once initial recovery from bolus dose observed

Dosing adjustment in renal impairment: Reduce initial dose and titrate carefully as duration may be prolonged

Stability Stable for 24 hours at room temperature when diluted, up to 0.1 mg/mL in dextrose 5% or normal saline; compatible with sufentanil, alfentanil, and fentanyl

Administration May be given rapid I.V. injection undiluted or via a continuous infusion using an infusion pump; use infusion solutions within 24 hours of preparation

Monitoring Parameters Blockade is monitored with a peripheral nerve stimulator, should also evaluate ECG, blood pressure, and heart rate

In the ICU setting, prolonged paralysis and generalized myopathy, following discontinuation of agent, may be minimized by appropriately monitoring degree of blockade.

Anesthesia and Critical Care Concerns/Other Considerations Doxacurium is classified as a long-acting nondepolarizing, neuromuscular blocker with virtually no cardiovascular side effects; characteristics of this agent make it especially useful in procedures requiring careful maintenance of hemodynamic stability for prolonged periods; reduce dosage in renal impairment.

Critically-Ill Adult Patients:

The 2004 Surviving Sepsis Campaign guidelines recommend avoiding use of neuromuscular blockers if at all possible in the septic patient due to the risk of prolonged neuromuscular blockade following discontinuation. If one is required, monitor carefully and observe the following recommendations.

The 2002 ACCM/SCCM/ASHP clinical practice guidelines for sustained neuromuscular blockade in the adult critically-ill patient recommend:

Optimize sedatives and analgesics prior to initiation, and monitor and adjust accordingly during course. Neuromuscular blockers do not relieve pain or produce sedation.

Protect patient's eyes from development of keratitis and corneal abrasion by administering ophthalmic ointment and taping eyelids closed or using eye patches. Reposition patient routinely to protect pressure points from breakdown. Address DVT prophylaxis.

(Continued)

Doxacurium *(Continued)*

Concurrent use of a neuromuscular blocker and corticosteroids appear to increase the risk of certain ICU myopathies; avoid or administer the corticosteroid at the lowest dose possible. Reassess need for neuromuscular blocker daily.

Using daily drug holidays (stopping neuromuscular-blocking agent until patient requires it again) may decrease the incidence of acute quadriplegic myopathy syndrome.

Tachyphylaxis can develop; switch to another neuromuscular blocker (taking into consideration the patient's organ function) if paralysis is still necessary.

Acidosis and severe hypothermia may delay the elimination of atracurium and cisatracurium.

Atracurium or cisatracurium is recommended for patients with significant hepatic or renal disease due to organ-independent Hofmann elimination.

Monitor patients clinically and via "Train of Four" (TOF) testing with a goal of adjusting the degree of blockade to 1-2 twitches or based upon the patient's clinical condition.

Pregnancy Risk Factor C

Contraindications Hypersensitivity to doxacurium or any component of the formulation

Warnings/Precautions Use with caution in the elderly, effects and duration are more variable; product contains benzyl alcohol, use with caution in newborns; use with caution in patients with renal or hepatic impairment; certain clinical conditions may result in potentiation or antagonism of neuromuscular blockade:

Potentiation: Electrolyte abnormalities, severe hyponatremia, severe hypocalcemia, severe hypokalemia, hypermagnesemia, neuromuscular diseases, acidosis, acute intermittent porphyria, renal failure, hepatic failure

Antagonism: Alkalosis, hypercalcemia, demyelinating lesions, peripheral neuropathies, diabetes mellitus

Increased sensitivity in patients with myasthenia gravis, Eaton-Lambert syndrome; resistance in burn patients (>30% of body) for period of 5-70 days postinjury; resistance in patients with muscle trauma, denervation, immobilization, infection; does not counteract bradycardia produced by anesthetics/vagal stimulation. Cross-sensitivity with other neuromuscular-blocking agents may occur; use extreme caution in patients with previous anaphylactic reactions.

Adverse Reactions <1% (Limited to important or life-threatening): Acute quadriplegic myopathy syndrome (prolonged use), diplopia, fever, hypotension, myositis ossificans (prolonged use), respiratory insufficiency and apnea, skeletal muscle weakness, urticaria, wheezing; **produces little, if any, histamine release**

Overdosage/Toxicology

Overdosage is manifested by prolonged neuromuscular blockage.

Treatment is supportive; reverse blockade with neostigmine, pyridostigmine, or edrophonium.

Drug Interactions

Decreased effect: Phenytoin, carbamazepine (decreases neuromuscular blockade)

Increased effect: Magnesium, lithium

Prolonged neuromuscular blockade: Corticosteroids, inhaled anesthetics, local anesthetics, calcium channel blockers; antiarrhythmics (eg, quinidine or procainamide); antibiotics (eg, aminoglycosides, tetracyclines, vancomycin, clindamycin); immunosuppressants (eg, cyclosporine)

Dosage Forms Injection, solution, as chloride: 1 mg/mL (5 mL) [contains benzyl alcohol]

♦ **Doxacurium Chloride** *see* Doxacurium *on page 416*

Doxapram (DOKS a pram)

Medication Safety Issues

Sound-alike/look-alike issues:

Doxapram may be confused with doxacurium, doxazosin, doxepin, Doxinate®, DOXOrubicin

Dopram® may be confused with DOPamine

U.S. Brand Names Dopram®

Synonyms Doxapram Hydrochloride

Pharmacologic Category Respiratory Stimulant; Stimulant

Generic Available Yes

Use Respiratory and CNS stimulant for respiratory depression secondary to anesthesia, drug-induced CNS depression; acute hypercapnia secondary to COPD

Mechanism of Action Stimulates respiration through action on respiratory center in medulla or indirectly on peripheral carotid chemoreceptors

Pharmacodynamics/Kinetics

Onset of action: Respiratory stimulation: I.V.: 20-40 seconds

Peak effect: 1-2 minutes

Duration: 5-12 minutes

Half-life elimination, serum: Adults: Mean: 3.4 hours

Dosage

Respiratory depression following anesthesia:

Intermittent injection: Initial: 0.5-1 mg/kg; may repeat at 5-minute intervals (only in patients who demonstrate initial response); maximum total dose: 2 mg/kg

I.V. infusion: Initial: 5 mg/minute until adequate response or adverse effects seen; decrease to 1-3 mg/minute; maximum total dose: 4 mg/kg

Drug-induced CNS depression:

Intermittent injection: Initial: Priming dose of 1-2 mg/kg, repeat after 5 minutes; may repeat at 1-2 hour intervals (until sustained consciousness); maximum: 3 g/day. May repeat in 24 hours if necessary.

I.V. infusion: Initial: Priming dose of 1-2 mg/kg, repeat after 5 minutes. If no response, wait 1-2 hours and repeat. If some stimulation is noted, initiate infusion at 1-3 mg/minute (depending on size of patient/depth of CNS depression); suspend infusion if patient begins to awaken. Infusion should not be continued for >2 hours. May reinstitute infusion as described above, including bolus, after rest interval of 30 minutes to 2 hours; maximum: 3 g/day

Acute hypercapnia secondary to COPD: I.V. infusion: Initial: Initiate infusion at 1-2 mg/minute (depending on size of patient/depth of CNS depression); may increase to maximum rate of 3 mg/minute; infusion should not be continued for >2 hours. Monitor arterial blood gases prior to initiation of infusion and at 30-minute intervals during the infusion (to identify possible development of acidosis/CO_2 retention). Additional infusions are not recommended (per manufacturer).

Stability Store at 20°C to 25°C (68°F to 77°F).

Drug-induced CNS depression or post-anesthesia: Mix doxapram 250 mg in 250 mL of D_5W, $D_{10}W$, or NS

COPD-associated hypercapnia: Mix doxapram 400 mg in 180 mL of D_5W, $D_{10}W$, or NS (final concentration: 2 mg/mL)

Administration Avoid rapid infusion.

Monitoring Parameters Monitor heart rate, blood pressure, reflexes, CNS status, ECG, arterial blood gases (COPD)

Anesthesia and Critical Care Concerns/Other Considerations Because of doxapram's transient effect, doxapram should not be used as a drug of choice to treat anesthesia-induced respiratory depression. Initial studies suggest a therapeutic range of at least 1.5 mg/L. Toxicity becomes frequent at serum levels >5 mg/L.

Pregnancy Risk Factor B

Contraindications Hypersensitivity to doxapram or any component of the formulation; cardiovascular disease, cerebral edema, cerebral vascular accident, epilepsy, head injury, hyperthyroidism, mechanical disorders of ventilation, mechanical ventilation or neuromuscular blockade, pheochromocytoma, pulmonary embolism, or severe hypertension

Warnings/Precautions Adequate airway required; consider airway protection in case of vomiting. Rapid infusion may result in hemolysis. Solution contains benzyl alcohol; not for use in neonates. If patient has received anesthesia with a volatile agent known to sensitize the myocardium to catecholamines, avoid use of doxapram until anesthetic has been eliminated. Use with caution in hepatic or renal dysfunction. Use with caution in patients with cerebral disease; lowered pCO_2 induced by hyperventilation produces cerebral vasoconstriction and decreased circulation. Use with caution in treating pulmonary disease; a pressor effect on pulmonary circulation may result in a fall in arterial pO_2. May cause severe CNS toxicity, seizures. Doxapram is neither a nonspecific CNS depressant antagonist nor an opiate antagonist. Resuscitative equipment (in addition to anticonvulsants

(Continued)

Doxapram *(Continued)*

and oxygen) should be readily available. Safety and efficacy have not been established in children <12 years of age.

Adverse Reactions Frequency not defined.

Cardiovascular: Arrhythmia, blood pressure increased, chest pain, chest tightness, flushing, heart rate changes, T waves lowered, ventricular tachycardia, ventricular fibrillation

Central nervous system: Apprehension, Babinski turns positive, disorientation, dizziness, hallucinations, headache, hyperactivity, pyrexia, seizure

Dermatologic: Burning sensation, pruritus

Gastrointestinal: Defecation urge, diarrhea, nausea, vomiting

Genitourinary: Spontaneous voiding, urinary retention

Hematologic: Hematocrit decreased, hemoglobin decreased, hemolysis, red blood cell count decreased

Local: Phlebitis

Neuromuscular & skeletal: Clonus, deep tendon reflexes increase, fasciculations, involuntary muscle movement, muscle spasm, paresthesia

Ocular: Pupillary dilatation

Renal: Albuminuria, BUN increased

Respiratory: Bronchospasm, cough, dyspnea, hiccups, hyperventilation, laryngospasm, rebound hypoventilation, tachypnea

Miscellaneous: Diaphoresis

Overdosage/Toxicology Symptoms of overdose include excessive increases in blood pressure, tachycardia, arrhythmias, muscle spasticity, dyspnea, agitation, confusion, sweating, cough, and enhanced deep tendon reflexes. Supportive care is the preferred treatment. Seizures are unlikely and can be treated with benzodiazepines. Doxapram is not dialyzable.

Drug Interactions

Inhaled anesthetics: Halothane, cyclopropane, and enflurane may sensitize the myocardium to catecholamine and epinephrine which is released at the initiation of doxapram, hence, separate discontinuation of anesthetics and start of doxapram until the volatile agent has been excreted.

MAO inhibitors: May increase increase hypertensive effect when used with doxapram.

Sympathomimetics: May increase hypertensive effect when used with doxapram.

Dosage Forms Injection, solution, as hydrochloride: 20 mg/mL (20 mL) [contains benzyl alcohol]

♦ **Doxapram Hydrochloride** *see* Doxapram *on page 418*

Doxazosin (doks AY zoe sin)

Medication Safety Issues

Sound-alike/look-alike issues:

Doxazosin may be confused with doxapram, doxepin, DOXOrubicin

Cardura® may be confused with Cardene®, Cordarone®, Cordran®, Coumadin®, K-Dur®, Ridaura®

U.S. Brand Names Cardura®; Cardura® XL

Canadian Brand Names Alti-Doxazosin; Apo-Doxazosin®; Cardura-1™; Cardura-2™; Cardura-4™; Gen-Doxazosin; Novo-Doxazosin

Synonyms Doxazosin Mesylate

Pharmacologic Category $Alpha_1$ Blocker

Generic Available Yes: Immediate release tablet

Use Treatment of hypertension alone or in conjunction with diuretics, ACE inhibitors, beta blockers, or calcium antagonists; treatment of urinary outflow obstruction and/or obstructive and irritative symptoms associated with benign prostatic hyperplasia (BPH), particularly useful in patients with troublesome symptoms who are unable or unwilling to undergo invasive procedures, but who require rapid symptomatic relief; can be used in combination with finasteride

Mechanism of Action

Hypertension: Competitively inhibits postsynaptic alpha1-adrenergic receptors which results in vasodilation of veins and arterioles and a decrease in total peripheral resistance and blood pressure; ~50% as potent on a weight by weight basis as prazosin.

BPH: Competitively inhibits postsynaptic alpha$_1$-adrenergic receptors in prostatic stromal and bladder neck tissues. This reduces the sympathetic tone-induced urethral stricture causing BPH symptoms.

Pharmacodynamics/Kinetics Not significantly affected by increased age

Duration: >24 hours

Protein binding: Extended release: 98%

Metabolism: Extensively hepatic to active metabolites; primarily via CYP3A4; secondary pathways involve CYP2D6 and 2C19

Bioavailability: Extended release relative to immediate release: 54% to 59%

Half-life elimination: 15-22 hours

Time to peak, serum: Immediate release: 2-3 hours; extended release: 8-9 hours

Excretion: Feces (63% primarily as metabolites); urine (9%)

Dosage Oral: Adults:

Immediate release: 1 mg once daily in morning or evening; may be increased to 2 mg once daily. Thereafter titrate upwards, if needed, over several weeks, balancing therapeutic benefit with doxazosin-induced postural hypotension. In the elderly, initiate at 0.5 mg once daily

Hypertension: Maximum dose: 16 mg/day

BPH: Goal: 4-8 mg/day; maximum dose: 8 mg/day

Extended release: BPH: 4 mg once daily with breakfast; titrate based on response and tolerability every 3-4 weeks to maximum recommended dose of 8 mg/day

Reintiation of therapy: If therapy is discontinued for several days, restart at 4 mg dose and titrate as before.

Conversion to extended release from immediate release: Initiate with 4 mg once daily; omit final evening dose of immediate release prior to starting morning dosing with extended release product.

Dosing adjustment in hepatic impairment: Use with caution in mild-to-moderate hepatic dysfunction. Do not use with severe impairment.

Administration Cardura ® XL: Tablets should be swallowed whole; do not crush, chew, or divide.

Monitoring Parameters Blood pressure, standing and sitting/supine; syncope may occur usually within 90 minutes of the initial dose

Pregnancy Risk Factor C

Contraindications Hypersensitivity to quinazolines (prazosin, terazosin), doxazosin, or any component of the formulation

Warnings/Precautions Can cause significant orthostatic hypotension and syncope, especially with first dose; anticipate a similar effect if therapy is interrupted for a few days, if dosage is rapidly increased, or if another antihypertensive drug (particularly vasodilators) or a PDE5 inhibitor is introduced. Patients should be cautioned about performing hazardous tasks when starting new therapy or adjusting dosage upward. Prostate cancer should be ruled out before starting for BPH. Use with caution in mild to moderate hepatic impairment; not recommended in severe dysfunction. Intraoperative floppy iris syndrome has been observed in cataract surgery patients who were on or were previously treated with alpha1 blockers. Causality has not been established and there appears to be no benefit in discontinuing alpha blocker therapy prior to surgery. Safety and efficacy in children have not been established.

The extended release formulation consists of drug within a nondeformable matrix; following drug release/absorption, the matrix/shell is expelled in the stool. The use of nondeformable products in patients with known stricture/narrowing of the GI tract has been associated with symptoms of obstruction. Use caution in patients with increased GI retention (eg, chronic constipation) as doxazosin exposure may be increased. Extended release formulation is not approved for the treatment of hypertension.

Adverse Reactions **Note:** Type and frequency of adverse reactions reflect combined data from trials with immediate release and extended release products.

>10%: Central nervous system: Dizziness (5% to 19%), headache (5% to 14%)

1% to 10%:

Cardiovascular: Orthostatic hypotension (dose related; 0.3% up to 2%), edema (3% to 4%), hypotension (2%), palpitation (1% to 2%), chest pain (1% to 2%), arrhythmia (1%), syncope (2%), flushing (1%)

Central nervous system: Fatigue (8% to 12%), somnolence (1% to 5%), nervousness (2%), pain (2%), vertigo (2% to 4%), insomnia (1%), anxiety (1%), paresthesia (1%), movement disorder (1%), ataxia (1%), hypertonia (1%), depression (1%)

Dermatologic: Rash (1%), pruritus (1%)

(Continued)

Doxazosin *(Continued)*

Endocrine & metabolic: Sexual dysfunction (2%)

Gastrointestinal: Abdominal pain (2%), diarrhea (2%), dyspepsia (1% to 2%), nausea (1% to 3%), xerostomia (1% to 2%), constipation (1%), flatulence (1%)

Genitourinary: Urinary tract infection (1%), impotence (1%), polyuria (2%), incontinence (1%)

Neuromuscular & skeletal: Back pain (2% to 3%), weakness (1% to 7%), arthritis (1%), muscle weakness (1%), myalgia (≤1%), muscle cramps (1%)

Ocular: Abnormal vision (1% to 2%), conjunctivitis (1%)

Otic: Tinnitus (1%)

Respiratory: Respiratory tract infection (5%), rhinitis (3%), dyspnea (1% to 3%), respiratory disorder (1%), epistaxis (1%)

Miscellaneous: Diaphoresis increased (1%), flu-like syndrome (1%)

<1% (Limited to important or life-threatening): Abnormal thinking, agitation, allergic reaction, amnesia, angina, anorexia, bradycardia, breast pain, bronchospasm, cataplexy, cerebrovascular accident, cholestasis, confusion, depersonalization, emotional lability, enuresis, fecal incontinence, fever, gastroenteritis, gout, hematuria, hepatitis, hypoesthesia, hypokalemia, infection, intraoperative floppy iris syndrome (cataract surgery),jaundice, leukopenia, liver function tests increased, lymphadenopathy, MI, micturition abnormality, migraine, neutropenia, nocturia, pallor, paranoia, paresis, paresthesia, parosmia, peripheral ischemia, priapism,purpura, renal calculus, rigors stroke, syncope, systemic lupus erythematosus, tachycardia, thrombocytopenia, vomiting

Overdosage/Toxicology Symptoms of overdose include severe hypotension, drowsiness, and tachycardia. Treatment is supportive and symptomatic. Lavage, activated charcoal, and fluids have shown to be effective. Dialysis not likely to benefit.

Drug Interactions

ACE inhibitors: Hypotensive effect (particularly orthostasis) may be increased.

Beta-blockers: Hypotensive effect may be increased.

Calcium channel blockers: Hypotensive effect may be increased.

Phosphodiesterase-5 (PDE5) inhibitors (eg, sildenafil, tadalafil, vardenafil): Blood pressure-lowering effects are additive. Use with caution and monitor.

Ethanol/Nutrition/Herb Interactions Herb/Nutraceutical: Avoid dong quai if using for hypertension (has estrogenic activity). Avoid ephedra, yohimbe, ginseng (may worsen hypertension). Avoid saw palmetto when used for BPH (due to limited experience with this combination). Avoid garlic (may have increased antihypertensive effect).

Dietary Considerations Cardura® XL: Take with morning meal.

Dosage Forms

Tablet, immediate release: 1 mg, 2 mg, 4 mg, 8 mg

Cardura®: 1 mg, 2 mg, 4 mg, 8 mg

Tablet, extended release:

Cardura® XL: 4 mg, 8 mg

♦ **Doxazosin Mesylate** *see* Doxazosin *on page 420*

Doxepin (DOKS e pin)

Medication Safety Issues

Sound-alike/look-alike issues:

Doxepin may be confused with digoxin, doxapram, doxazosin, Doxidan®, doxycycline

Sinequan® may be confused with saquinavir, Serentil®, Seroquel®, Singulair®

Zonalon® may be confused with Zone-A Forte®

Related Information

Antidepressant Agents *on page 1551*

Chronic Pain Management *on page 1430*

U.S. Brand Names Prudoxin™; Sinequan® [DSC]; Zonalon®

Canadian Brand Names Apo-Doxepin®; Novo-Doxepin; Sinequan®; Zonalon®

Synonyms Doxepin Hydrochloride

Pharmacologic Category Antidepressant, Tricyclic (Tertiary Amine); Topical Skin Product

Restrictions A medication guide concerning the use of antidepressants in children and teenagers can be found on the FDA website at http://www.fda.gov/cder/

Offices/ODS/labeling.htm. It should be dispensed to parents or guardians of children and teenagers receiving this medication.

Generic Available Yes: Capsule, solution

Use

Oral: Depression

Topical: Short-term (<8 days) management of moderate pruritus in adults with atopic dermatitis or lichen simplex chronicus

Unlabeled/Investigational Use Analgesic for certain chronic and neuropathic pain; anxiety

Mechanism of Action Increases the synaptic concentration of serotonin and norepinephrine in the central nervous system by inhibition of their reuptake by the presynaptic neuronal membrane

Pharmacodynamics/Kinetics

Onset of action: Peak effect: Antidepressant: Usually >2 weeks; Anxiolytic: may occur sooner

Absorption: Following topical application, plasma levels may be similar to those achieved with oral administration

Distribution: Crosses placenta; enters breast milk

Protein binding: 80% to 85%

Metabolism: Hepatic; metabolites include desmethyldoxepin (active)

Half-life elimination: Adults: 6-8 hours

Excretion: Urine

Dosage

Oral: Topical: Burning mouth syndrome (dental use): Cream: Apply 3-4 times daily

Oral (entire daily dose may be given at bedtime):

Depression or anxiety:

Children (unlabeled use): 1-3 mg/kg/day in single or divided doses

Adolescents: Initial: 25-50 mg/day in single or divided doses; gradually increase to 100 mg/day

Adults: Initial: 25-150 mg/day at bedtime or in 2-3 divided doses; may gradually increase up to 300 mg/day; single dose should not exceed 150 mg; select patients may respond to 25-50 mg/day

Elderly: Use a lower dose and adjust gradually

Chronic urticaria, angioedema, nocturnal pruritus: Adults and Elderly: 10-30 mg/day

Dosing adjustment in hepatic impairment: Use a lower dose and adjust gradually

Topical: Pruritus: Adults and Elderly: Apply a thin film 4 times/day with at least 3- to 4-hour interval between applications; not recommended for use >8 days. **Note:** Low-dose (25-50 mg) oral administration has also been used to treat pruritus, but systemic effects are increased.

Stability Protect from light

Administration

Oral: Do not mix oral concentrate with carbonated beverages (physically incompatible).

Topical: Apply thin film to affected area; use of occlusive dressings is not recommended.

Monitoring Parameters Monitor blood pressure and pulse rate prior to and during initial therapy; monitor mental status, weight; ECG in older adults; adverse effects may be increased if topical formulation is applied to >10% of body surface area

Reference Range Proposed therapeutic concentration (doxepin plus desmethyldoxepin): 110-250 ng/mL. Toxic concentration (doxepin plus desmethyldoxepin): >500 ng/mL. Utility of serum level monitoring is controversial.

Pregnancy Risk Factor B (cream); C (all other forms)

Contraindications Hypersensitivity to doxepin, drugs from similar chemical class, or any component of the formulation; narrow-angle glaucoma; urinary retention; use of MAO inhibitors within 14 days; use in a patient during acute recovery phase of MI

Warnings/Precautions **[U.S. Boxed Warning]: Antidepressants increase the risk of suicidal thinking and behavior in children and adolescents with major depressive disorder (MDD) and other depressive disorders; consider risk prior to prescribing.** Closely monitor for clinical worsening, suicidality, or unusual changes in behavior; the child's family or caregiver should be instructed to closely observe the patient and communicate condition with healthcare

(Continued)

Doxepin *(Continued)*

provider. Such observation would generally include at least weekly face-to-face contact with patients or their family members or caregivers during the first 4 weeks of treatment, then every other week visits for the next 4 weeks, then at 12 weeks, and as clinically indicated beyond 12 weeks. Additional contact by telephone may be appropriate between face-to-face visits. Adults treated with antidepressants should be observed similarly for clinical worsening and suicidality, especially during the initial few months of a course of drug therapy, or at times of dose changes, either increases or decreases. A medication guide should be dispensed with each prescription. **Doxepin is approved for treatment of depression in adolescents.**

The possibility of a suicide attempt is inherent in major depression and may persist until remission occurs. Monitor for worsening of depression or suicidality, especially during initiation of therapy or with dose increases or decreases. Worsening depression and severe abrupt suicidality that are not part of the presenting symptoms may require discontinuation or modification of drug therapy. Use caution in high-risk patients during initiation of therapy. Prescriptions should be written for the smallest quantity consistent with good patient care. The patient's family or caregiver should be alerted to monitor patients for the emergence of suicidality and associated behaviors such as anxiety, agitation, panic attacks, insomnia, irritability, hostility, impulsivity, akathisia, hypomania, and mania; patients should be instructed to notify their healthcare provider if any of these symptoms or worsening depression occur.

May worsen psychosis in some patients or precipitate a shift to mania or hypomania in patients with bipolar disorder. Monotherapy in patients with bipolar disorder should be avoided. Patients presenting with depressive symptoms should be screened for bipolar disorder. **Doxepin is not FDA approved for the treatment of bipolar depression.**

Often causes sedation, which may result in impaired performance of tasks requiring alertness (eg, operating machinery or driving). Sedative effects may be additive with other CNS depressants and/or ethanol. The degree of sedation is very high relative to other antidepressants. May increase the risks associated with electroconvulsive therapy. Consider discontinuing, when possible, prior to elective surgery. Therapy should not be abruptly discontinued in patients receiving high doses for prolonged periods.

May cause orthostatic hypotension (risk is moderate relative to other antidepressants) - use with caution in patients at risk of hypotension or in patients where transient hypotensive episodes would be poorly tolerated (cardiovascular disease or cerebrovascular disease). The degree of anticholinergic blockade produced by this agent is high relative to other cyclic antidepressants - use caution in patients with benign prostatic hyperplasia, xerostomia, visual problems, constipation, or history of bowel obstruction.

Use with caution in patients with a history of cardiovascular disease (including previous MI, stroke, tachycardia, or conduction abnormalities). The risk conduction abnormalities with this agent is moderate relative to other antidepressants. Use caution in patients with a previous seizure disorder or condition predisposing to seizures such as brain damage, alcoholism, or concurrent therapy with other drugs which lower the seizure threshold. Use with caution in hyperthyroid patients or those receiving thyroid supplementation. Use with caution in patients with hepatic or renal dysfunction and in elderly patients. Cream formulation is for external use only (not for ophthalmic, vaginal, or oral use). Do not use occlusive dressings. Use for >8 days may increase risk of contact sensitization. Doxepin is significantly absorbed following topical administration; plasma levels may be similar to those achieved with oral administration.

Adverse Reactions

Oral: Frequency not defined.

Cardiovascular: Hyper-/hypotension, tachycardia

Central nervous system: Drowsiness, dizziness, headache, disorientation, ataxia, confusion, seizure

Dermatologic: Alopecia, photosensitivity, rash, pruritus

Endocrine & metabolic: Breast enlargement, galactorrhea, SIADH, increase or decrease in blood sugar, increased or decreased libido

Gastrointestinal: Xerostomia, constipation, vomiting, indigestion, anorexia, aphthous stomatitis, nausea, unpleasant taste, weight gain, diarrhea, trouble with gums, decreased lower esophageal sphincter tone may cause GE reflux

Genitourinary: Urinary retention, testicular edema

Hematologic: Agranulocytosis, leukopenia, eosinophilia, thrombocytopenia, purpura

Neuromuscular & skeletal: Weakness, tremor, numbness, paresthesia, extrapyramidal symptoms, tardive dyskinesia

Ocular: Blurred vision

Otic: Tinnitus

Miscellaneous: Diaphoresis (excessive), allergic reactions

Topical:

>10%:

Central nervous system: Drowsiness (22%)

Dermatologic: Stinging/burning (23%)

1% to 10%:

Cardiovascular: Edema: (1%)

Central nervous system: Dizziness (2%), emotional changes (2%)

Gastrointestinal: Xerostomia (10%), taste alteration (2%)

<1% (Limited to important or life-threatening): Contact dermatitis, tongue numbness, anxiety

Overdosage/Toxicology Symptoms of overdose include confusion, hallucinations, seizures, urinary retention, hypothermia, hypotension, tachycardia, and cyanosis. Following initiation of essential overdose management, toxic symptoms should be treated symptomatically.

Drug Interactions Substrate (major) of CYP1A2, 2D6, 3A4

Altretamine: Concurrent use may cause orthostatic hypertension

Amphetamines: TCAs may enhance the effect of amphetamines; monitor for adverse CV effects

Anticholinergics: Combined use with TCAs may produce additive anticholinergic effects

Antihypertensives: TCAs may inhibit the antihypertensive response to bethanidine, clonidine, debrisoquin, guanadrel, guanethidine, guanabenz, guanfacine; monitor BP; consider alternate antihypertensive agent

Beta-agonists (nonselective): When combined with TCAs may predispose patients to cardiac arrhythmias

Bupropion: May increase the levels of tricyclic antidepressants; based on limited information; monitor response

Carbamazepine: Tricyclic antidepressants may increase carbamazepine levels; monitor

Cholestyramine and colestipol: May bind TCAs and reduce their absorption; monitor for altered response

Clonidine: Abrupt discontinuation of clonidine may cause hypertensive crisis, amitriptyline may enhance the response

CNS depressants: Sedative effects may be additive with TCAs; monitor for increased effect; includes benzodiazepines, barbiturates, antipsychotics, ethanol and other sedative medications

CYP1A2 inducers: May decrease the levels/effects of doxepin. Example inducers include aminoglutethimide, carbamazepine, phenobarbital, and rifampin.

CYP1A2 inhibitors: May increase the levels/effects of doxepin. Example inhibitors include ciprofloxacin, fluvoxamine, ketoconazole, norfloxacin, ofloxacin, and rofecoxib.

CYP2D6 inhibitors: May increase the levels/effects of doxepin. Example inhibitors include chlorpromazine, delavirdine, fluoxetine, miconazole, paroxetine, pergolide, quinidine, quinine, ritonavir, and ropinirole.

CYP3A4 inducers: CYP3A4 inducers may decrease the levels/effects of doxepin. Example inducers include aminoglutethimide, carbamazepine, nafcillin, nevirapine, phenobarbital, phenytoin, and rifamycins.

CYP3A4 inhibitors: May increase the levels/effects of doxepin. Example inhibitors include azole antifungals, clarithromycin, diclofenac, doxycycline, erythromycin, imatinib, isoniazid, nefazodone, nicardipine, propofol, protease inhibitors, quinidine, telithromycin, and verapamil.

Epinephrine (and other direct alpha-agonists): Pressor response to I.V. epinephrine, norepinephrine, and phenylephrine may be enhanced in patients receiving TCAs (**Note:** Effect is unlikely with epinephrine or levonordefrin dosages typically administered as infiltration in combination with local anesthetics)

Fenfluramine: May increase tricyclic antidepressant levels/effects

(Continued)

Doxepin *(Continued)*

Hypoglycemic agents (including insulin): TCAs may enhance the hypoglycemic effects of tolazamide, chlorpropamide, or insulin; monitor for changes in blood glucose levels; reported with chlorpropamide, tolazamide, and insulin

Levodopa: Tricyclic antidepressants may decrease the absorption (bioavailability) of levodopa; rare hypertensive episodes have also been attributed to this combination

Linezolid: Hyperpyrexia, hypertension, tachycardia, confusion, seizures, and **deaths have been reported** with agents which inhibit MAO (serotonin syndrome); this combination should be avoided

Lithium: Concurrent use with a TCA may increase the risk for neurotoxicity

MAO inhibitors: Hyperpyrexia, hypertension, tachycardia, confusion, seizures, and **deaths have been reported** (serotonin syndrome); this combination is contraindicated

Methylphenidate: Metabolism of TCAs may be decreased

Phenothiazines: Serum concentrations of some TCAs may be increased; in addition, TCAs may increase concentration of phenothiazines; monitor for altered clinical response

QT_c-prolonging agents: Concurrent use of tricyclic agents with other drugs which may prolong QT_c interval may increase the risk of potentially fatal arrhythmias; includes type Ia and type III antiarrhythmics agents, selected quinolones (sparfloxacin, gatifloxacin, moxifloxacin, grepafloxacin), cisapride, and other agents

Ritonavir: Combined use of high-dose tricyclic antidepressants with ritonavir may cause serotonin syndrome in HIV-positive patients; monitor

Sucralfate: Absorption of tricyclic antidepressants may be reduced with coadministration

Sympathomimetics, indirect-acting: Tricyclic antidepressants may result in a decreased sensitivity to indirect-acting sympathomimetics; includes dopamine and ephedrine; also see interaction with epinephrine (and direct-acting sympathomimetics)

Tramadol: Tramadol's risk of seizures may be increased with TCAs

Valproic acid: May increase serum concentrations/adverse effects of some tricyclic antidepressants

Warfarin (and other oral anticoagulants): TCAs may increase the anticoagulant effect in patients stabilized on warfarin; monitor INR

Ethanol/Nutrition/Herb Interactions

Ethanol: Avoid ethanol (may increase CNS depression).

Food: Grapefruit juice may inhibit the metabolism of some TCAs and clinical toxicity may result.

Herb/Nutraceutical: Avoid valerian, St John's wort, SAMe, kava kava (may increase risk of serotonin syndrome and/or excessive sedation).

Test Interactions Increased glucose

Dosage Forms [DSC] = Discontinued product

Capsule, as hydrochloride: 10 mg, 25 mg, 50 mg, 75 mg, 100 mg, 150 mg
  Sinequan®: 10 mg, 25 mg, 50 mg, 75 mg, 100 mg, 150 mg [DSC]

Cream, as hydrochloride:
  Prudoxin™: 5% (45 g) [contains benzyl alcohol]
  Zonalon®: 5% (30 g, 45 g) [contains benzyl alcohol]

Solution, oral concentrate, as hydrochloride (Sinequan®): 10 mg/mL (120 mL)
  Sinequan®: 10 mg/mL (120 mL) [DSC]

♦ **Doxepin Hydrochloride** *see* Doxepin *on page 422*
♦ **Doxy-100**® *see* Doxycycline *on page 426*
♦ **Doxycin (Can)** *see* Doxycycline *on page 426*

Doxycycline (doks i SYE kleen)

Medication Safety Issues

Sound-alike/look-alike issues:
  Doxycycline may be confused with dicyclomine, doxepin, doxylamine
  Doxy-100® may be confused with Doxil®
  Monodox® may be confused with Maalox®

Related Information

Prevention of Wound Infection and Sepsis in Surgical Patients *on page 1588*

U.S. Brand Names Adoxa™; Doryx®; Doxy-100®; Monodox®; Oracea™; Periostat®; Vibramycin®; Vibra-Tabs®

Canadian Brand Names Apo-Doxy®; Apo-Doxy Tabs®; Doxycin; Doxytec; Novo-Doxylin; Nu-Doxycycline; Periostat®; Vibra-Tabs®

Synonyms Doxycycline Calcium; Doxycycline Hyclate; Doxycycline Monohydrate

Pharmacologic Category Antibiotic, Tetracycline Derivative

Generic Available Yes: Excludes powder for oral solution, syrup

Use Principally in the treatment of infections caused by susceptible *Rickettsia*, *Chlamydia*, and *Mycoplasma*; alternative to mefloquine for malaria prophylaxis; treatment for syphilis, uncomplicated *Neisseria gonorrhoeae*, *Listeria*, *Actinomyces israelii*, and *Clostridium* infections in penicillin-allergic patients; used for community-acquired pneumonia and other common infections due to susceptible organisms; anthrax due to *Bacillus anthracis,* including inhalational anthrax (postexposure); treatment of infections caused by uncommon susceptible gram-negative and gram-positive organisms including *Borrelia recurrentis*, *Ureaplasma urealyticum*, *Haemophilus ducreyi*, *Yersinia pestis*, *Francisella tularensis*, *Vibrio cholerae*, *Campylobacter fetus*, *Brucella* spp, *Bartonella bacilliformis*, and *Calymmatobacterium granulomatis*; treatment of inflammatory lesions associated with rosacea

Unlabeled/Investigational Use Sclerosing agent for pleural effusion injection; vancomycin-resistant enterococci (VRE)

Mechanism of Action Inhibits protein synthesis by binding with the 30S and possibly the 50S ribosomal subunit(s) of susceptible bacteria; may also cause alterations in the cytoplasmic membrane

Periostat® capsules (proposed mechanism): Has been shown to inhibit collagenase activity *in vitro*. Also has been noted to reduce elevated collagenase activity in the gingival crevicular fluid of patients with periodontal disease. Systemic levels do not reach inhibitory concentrations against bacteria.

Pharmacodynamics/Kinetics

Absorption: Oral: Almost complete; reduced by food or milk by 20%

Distribution: Widely into body tissues and fluids including synovial, pleural, prostatic, seminal fluids, and bronchial secretions; saliva, aqueous humor, and CSF penetration is poor; readily crosses placenta; enters breast milk

Protein binding: 90%

Metabolism: Not hepatic; partially inactivated in GI tract by chelate formation

Half-life elimination: 12-15 hours (usually increases to 22-24 hours with multiple doses); End-stage renal disease: 18-25 hours

Time to peak, serum: 1.5-4 hours

Excretion: Feces (30%); urine (23%)

Dosage

Usual dosage range:

Children ≥8 years (<45 kg): Oral, I.V.: 2-5 mg/kg/day in 1-2 divided doses, not to exceed 200 mg/day

Children >8 years (>45 kg) and Adults: Oral, I.V.: 100-200 mg/day in 1-2 divided doses

Indication-specific dosing:

Children:

Anthrax: Doxycycline should be used in children if antibiotic susceptibility testing, exhaustion of drug supplies, or allergic reaction preclude use of penicillin or ciprofloxacin. For treatment, the consensus recommendation does not include a loading dose for doxycycline.

Inhalational (postexposure prophylaxis) (*MMWR*, 2001, 50:889-893): Oral, I.V. (use oral route when possible):

≤8 years: 2.2 mg/kg every 12 hours for 60 days

>8 years and ≤45 kg: 2.2 mg/kg every 12 hours for 60 days

>8 years and >45 kg: 100 mg every 12 hours for 60 days

Cutaneous (treatment): Oral: See dosing for "Inhalational (postexposure prophylaxis)"

Note: In the presence of systemic involvement, extensive edema, and/or lesions on head/neck, doxycycline should initially be administered I.V.

Inhalational/gastrointestinal/oropharyngeal (treatment): I.V.: Refer to dosing for inhalational anthrax (postexposure prophylaxis); switch to oral therapy when clinically appropriate

Note: Initial treatment should include two or more agents predicted to be effective (per CDC recommendations). Agents suggested for use in conjunction with doxycycline or ciprofloxacin include rifampin, vancomycin, imipenem, penicillin, ampicillin, chloramphenicol, clindamycin,

(Continued)

Doxycycline *(Continued)*

and clarithromycin. May switch to oral antimicrobial therapy when clinically appropriate. Continue combined therapy for 60 days

Adults:

Anthrax:

Inhalational (postexposure prophylaxis): Oral, I.V. (use oral route when possible): 100 mg every 12 hours for 60 days (*MMWR*, 2001, 50:889-93); **Note:** Preliminary recommendation, FDA review and update is anticipated.

Cutaneous (treatment): Oral: 100 mg every 12 hours for 60 days. **Note:** In the presence of systemic involvement, extensive edema, lesions on head/neck, refer to I.V. dosing for treatment of inhalational/gastrointestinal/oropharyngeal anthrax

Inhalational/gastrointestinal/oropharyngeal (treatment): I.V.: Initial: 100 mg every 12 hours; switch to oral therapy when clinically appropriate; some recommend initial loading dose of 200 mg, followed by 100 mg every 8-12 hours (*JAMA*, 1997, 278:399-411). **Note:** Initial treatment should include two or more agents predicted to be effective (per CDC recommendations). Agents suggested for use in conjunction with doxycycline or ciprofloxacin include rifampin, vancomycin, imipenem, penicillin, ampicillin, chloramphenicol, clindamycin, and clarithromycin. May switch to oral antimicrobial therapy when clinically appropriate. Continue combined therapy for 60 days

Brucellosis: Oral: 100 mg twice daily for 6 weeks with rifampin or streptomycin

Chlamydial infections, uncomplicated: Oral: 100 mg twice daily for ≥7 days

Community-acquired pneumonia, bronchitis: Oral, I.V.: 100 mg twice daily

Endometritis, salpingitis, parametritis, or peritonitis: I.V.: 100 mg twice daily with cefoxitin 2 g every 6 hours for 4 days and for ≥48 hours after patient improves; then continue with oral therapy 100 mg twice daily to complete a 10- to 14-day course of therapy

Gonococcal infection, acute (PID) in combination with another antibiotic: I.V.: 100 mg every 12 hours until improved, followed by 100 mg orally twice daily to complete 14 days

Lyme disease, Q fever, or Tularemia: Oral: 100 mg twice daily for 14-21 days

Periodontitis: Oral (Periostat®): 20 mg twice daily as an adjunct following scaling and root planing; may be administered for up to 9 months. Safety beyond 12 months of treatment and efficacy beyond 9 months of treatment have not been established.

Rickettsial disease or erlichiosis: Oral, I.V.: 100 mg twice daily for 7-14 days

Rosacea: 40 mg once daily in the morning

Sclerosing agent for pleural effusion injection (unlabeled use): Irrigation: 500 mg as a single dose in 30-50 mL of NS or SWI

Syphilis:

Early syphilis: Oral, I.V.: 200 mg/day in divided doses for 14 days

Late syphilis: Oral, I.V.: 200 mg/day in divided doses for 28 days

***Yersinia pestis* (plague):** Oral: 100 mg twice daily for 10 days

Vibrio cholerae: Oral: 300 mg as a single dose

Dosing adjustment in renal impairment: No adjustment necessary

Dialysis: Not dialyzable; 0% to 5% by hemo- and peritoneal methods or by continuous arteriovenous or venovenous hemofiltration: No supplemental dosage necessary

Stability

Capsule, tablet: Store at controlled room temperature 15°C to 30°C (59°F to 86°F); protect from light

I.V. infusion: Following reconstitution with sterile water for injection, dilute to a final concentration of 0.1-1 mg/mL using a compatible solution. Solutions for I.V. infusion may be prepared using 0.9% sodium chloride, D_5W, Ringer's injection, lactated Ringer's, D_5LR. Protect from light. Stability varies based on solution.

Administration Oral: May give with meals to decrease GI upset. Capsule and tablet: Administer with at least 8 ounces of water and have patient sit up for at least 30 minutes after taking to reduce the risk of esophageal irritation and ulceration.

Doryx® capsules and tablets are bioequivalent. Doryx® capsules may be opened and contents sprinkled on applesauce. Applesauce should be swallowed immediately; do not chew. Follow with 8 ounces of water. Applesauce should not be hot and should be soft enough to swallow without chewing.

Oracea™: Take on an empty stomach 1 hour before or 2 hours after meals.

I.V.: Infuse I.V. doxycycline over 1-4 hours; avoid extravasation

Pregnancy Risk Factor D

Contraindications Hypersensitivity to doxycycline, tetracycline or any component of the formulation; children <8 years of age, except in treatment of anthrax (including inhalational anthrax postexposure prophylaxis); severe hepatic dysfunction; pregnancy

Warnings/Precautions Do not use during pregnancy - use of tetracyclines during tooth development may cause permanent discoloration of the teeth and enamel hypoplasia; prolonged use may result in superinfection, including oral or vaginal candidiasis; photosensitivity reaction may occur with this drug; avoid prolonged exposure to sunlight or tanning equipment. Anti-anabolic effects of tetracyclines can increase BUN leading to significant renal dysfunction and hepatotoxicity in patients with pre-existing renal impairment. Autoimmune syndromes have been reported; if symptomatic conduct LFT and discontinue drug. Tetracyclines have been associated with pseudotumor cerebri. Avoid in children ≤8 years of age.

Additional specific warnings: Periostat®: Effectiveness has not been established in patients with coexistent oral candidiasis; use with caution in patients with a history or predisposition to oral candidiasis. Oracea™: Should not be used for the treatment or prophylaxis of bacterial infections, since the lower dose of drug per capsule may be subefficacious and promote resistance.

Adverse Reactions Frequency not defined.

Cardiovascular: Intracranial hypertension, pericarditis

Dermatologic: Angioneurotic edema, exfoliative dermatitis (rare), photosensitivity, rash, skin hyperpigmentation, urticaria

Endocrine & metabolic: Brown/black discoloration of thyroid gland (no dysfunction reported)

Gastrointestinal: Anorexia, diarrhea, dysphagia, enterocolitis, esophagitis (rare), esophageal ulcerations (rare), glossitis, inflammatory lesions in anogenital region, oral (mucosal) pigmentation, tooth discoloration (children)

Hematologic: Eosinophilia, hemolytic anemia, neutropenia, thrombocytopenia

Renal: Increased BUN (dose related)

Miscellaneous: Anaphylactoid purpura, anaphylaxis, bulging fontanels (infants), SLE exacerbation

Note: Adverse effects in clinical trials with Periostat® occurring at a frequency more than 1% greater than placebo included nausea, dyspepsia, joint pain, diarrhea, menstrual cramp, and pain.

Overdosage/Toxicology Symptoms of overdose include nausea, anorexia, and diarrhea. Treatment is supportive.

Drug Interactions Substrate of CYP3A4 (major); **Inhibits** CYP3A4 (moderate)

Antacids (containing aluminum, calcium, or magnesium): Decreased absorption of tetracyclines

Anticoagulants: Tetracyclines may decrease plasma thrombin activity; monitor

Barbiturates: Decreased half-life of doxycycline

Carbamazepine: Decreased half-life of doxycycline

CYP3A4 inducers: CYP3A4 inducers may decrease the levels/effects of doxycycline. Example inducers include aminoglutethimide, carbamazepine, nafcillin, nevirapine, phenobarbital, phenytoin, and rifamycins.

CYP3A4 substrates: Doxycycline may increase the levels/effects of CYP3A4 substrates. Example substrates include benzodiazepines, calcium channel blockers, mirtazapine, nateglinide, nefazodone, tacrolimus, and venlafaxine. Selected benzodiazepines (midazolam and triazolam), cisapride, ergot alkaloids, selected HMG-CoA reductase inhibitors (lovastatin and simvastatin), and pimozide are generally contraindicated with strong CYP3A4 inhibitors.

Iron-containing products: Decreased absorption of tetracyclines

Methoxyflurane: Concomitant use may cause fatal renal toxicity.

Oral contraceptives: Anecdotal reports suggesting decreased contraceptive efficacy with tetracyclines have been refuted by more rigorous scientific and clinical data.

(Continued)

Doxycycline *(Continued)*

Phenytoin: Decreased half-life of doxycycline

Ethanol/Nutrition/Herb Interactions

Ethanol: Chronic ethanol ingestion may reduce the serum concentration of doxycycline.

Food: Doxycycline serum levels may be slightly decreased if taken with food or milk. Administration with iron or calcium may decrease doxycycline absorption. May decrease absorption of calcium, iron, magnesium, zinc, and amino acids.

Herb/Nutraceutical: St John's wort may decrease doxycycline levels. Avoid dong quai, St John's wort (may also cause photosensitization).

Test Interactions False elevations of urine catecholamine levels; false-negative urine glucose using Clinistix®, Tes-Tape®

Dietary Considerations

Tetracyclines (in general): Take with food if gastric irritation occurs. While administration with food may decrease GI absorption of doxycycline by up to 20%, administration on an empty stomach is not recommended due to GI intolerance. Of currently available tetracyclines, doxycycline has the least affinity for calcium.

Oracea™: Take on an empty stomach 1 hour before or 2 hours after meals.

Doryx® 75 mg and 100 mg tablets contain sodium 4.5 mg and 6 mg, respectively.

Dosage Forms [DSC] = Discontinued product

Capsule, as hyclate: 50 mg, 100 mg
  Vibramycin®: 100 mg
Capsule, as monohydrate (Monodox®): 50 mg, 100 mg
Capsule, coated pellets, as hyclate (Doryx®): 75 mg, 100 mg [DSC]
Capsule, variable release (Oracea™): 40 mg [30 mg (immediate-release) and 10 mg (delayed-release)]
Injection, powder for reconstitution, as hyclate (Doxy-100®): 100 mg
Powder for oral suspension, as monohydrate (Vibramycin®): 25 mg/5 mL (60 mL) [raspberry flavor]
Syrup, as calcium (Vibramycin®): 50 mg/5 mL (480 mL) [contains sodium metabisulfite; raspberry-apple flavor]
Tablet, as hyclate: 100 mg
  Periostat®: 20 mg
  Vibra-Tabs®: 100 mg
Tablet, as monohydrate:
  Adoxa™: 50 mg, 75 mg, 100 mg
  Adoxa® Pak™ 1/75 [unit-dose pack]: 75 mg (31s)
  Adoxa® Pak™ 1/100 [unit-dose pack]: 100 mg (31s)
  Adoxa® Pak™ 1/150 [unit-dose pack]: 150 mg (30s)
  Adoxa® Pak™ 2/100 [unit-dose pack]: 100 mg (60s)
Tablet, delayed-release coated pellets, as hyclate (Doryx®): 75 mg [contains sodium 4.5 mg (0.196 mEq)], 100 mg [contains sodium 6 mg (0.261 mEq)]

- ♦ **Doxycycline Calcium** *see* Doxycycline *on page 426*
- ♦ **Doxycycline Hyclate** *see* Doxycycline *on page 426*
- ♦ **Doxycycline Monohydrate** *see* Doxycycline *on page 426*
- ♦ **Doxytec (Can)** *see* Doxycycline *on page 426*
- ♦ **DPA** *see* Valproic Acid and Derivatives *on page 1329*
- ♦ **DPH** *see* Phenytoin *on page 1018*
- ♦ **Dristan® Long Lasting Nasal (Can)** *see* Oxymetazoline *on page 973*
- ♦ **Drixoral® Nasal (Can)** *see* Oxymetazoline *on page 973*
- ♦ **Drixoral® ND (Can)** *see* Pseudoephedrine *on page 1085*

Dronabinol (droe NAB i nol)

Medication Safety Issues

Sound-alike/look-alike issues:
  Dronabinol may be confused with droperidol

U.S. Brand Names Marinol®

Canadian Brand Names Marinol®

Synonyms Delta-9-tetrahydro-cannabinol; Delta-9 THC; Tetrahydrocannabinol; THC

Pharmacologic Category Antiemetic; Appetite Stimulant

Restrictions C-III

Generic Available No

Use Chemotherapy-associated nausea and vomiting refractory to other antiemetic; AIDS-related anorexia

Unlabeled/Investigational Use
Cancer-related anorexia

Mechanism of Action Unknown, may inhibit endorphins in the emetic center, suppress prostaglandin synthesis, and/or inhibit medullary activity through an unspecified cortical action

Pharmacodynamics/Kinetics
Onset of action: Within 1 hour
Peak effect: 2-4 hours
Duration: 24 hours (appetite stimulation)
Absorption: Oral: 90% to 95%; 10% to 20% of dose gets into systemic circulation
Distribution: V_d: 10 L/kg; dronabinol is highly lipophilic and distributes to adipose tissue
Protein binding: 97% to 99%
Metabolism: Hepatic to at least 50 metabolites, some of which are active; 11-hydroxy-delta-9-tetrahydrocannabinol (11-OH-THC) is the major metabolite; extensive first-pass effect
Half-life elimination: Dronabinol: 25-36 hours (terminal); Dronabinol metabolites: 44-59 hours
Time to peak, serum: 0.5-4 hours
Excretion: Feces (50% as unconjugated metabolites, 5% as unchanged drug); urine (10% to 15% as acid metabolites and conjugates)

Dosage Refer to individual protocols. Oral:
Antiemetic: Children and Adults: 5 mg/m^2 1-3 hours before chemotherapy, then 5 mg/m^2/dose every 2-4 hours after chemotherapy for a total of 4-6 doses/day; increase doses in increments of 2.5 mg/m^2 to a maximum of 15 mg/m^2/dose.
Appetite stimulant: Adults: Initial: 2.5 mg twice daily (before lunch and dinner); titrate up to a maximum of 20 mg/day.

Stability Store under refrigeration (or in a cool environment) between 8°C and 15°C (46°F and 59°F); protect from freezing

Monitoring Parameters CNS effects, heart rate, blood pressure, behavioral profile

Reference Range Antinauseant effects: 5-10 ng/mL

Pregnancy Risk Factor C

Contraindications Hypersensitivity to dronabinol, cannabinoids, or any component of the formulation, or marijuana; should be avoided in patients with a history of schizophrenia

Warnings/Precautions Use with caution in patients with heart disease, hepatic disease, or seizure disorders. Reduce dosage in patients with severe hepatic impairment. May cause additive CNS effects with sedatives, hypnotics or other psychoactive agents; patients must be cautioned about performing tasks which require mental alertness (eg, operating machinery or driving).

May have potential for abuse; drug is psychoactive substance in marijuana; use caution in patients with a history of substance abuse. May cause withdrawal symptoms upon abrupt discontinuation. Use with caution in patients with mania, depression, or schizophrenia; careful psychiatric monitoring is recommended.

Adverse Reactions
>10%:
Central nervous system: Drowsiness (48%), sedation (53%), confusion (30%), dizziness (21%), detachment, anxiety, difficulty concentrating, mood change
Gastrointestinal: Appetite increased (when used as an antiemetic), xerostomia (38% to 50%)

1% to 10%:
Cardiovascular: Orthostatic hypotension, tachycardia
Central nervous system: Ataxia (4%), depression (7%), headache, vertigo, hallucinations (5%), memory lapse (4%)
Neuromuscular & skeletal: Paresthesia, weakness

<1% (Limited to important or life-threatening): Diaphoresis, diarrhea, myalgia, nightmares, syncope, tinnitus

Overdosage/Toxicology Symptoms of overdose may include tachycardia, hyper- or hypotension, behavioral disturbances, lethargy, panic reactions, seizures or motor incoordination. Benzodiazepines may be helpful for agitative behavior; Trendelenburg position and hydration may be helpful for hypotensive

(Continued)

Dronabinol *(Continued)*

effects. For other manifestations, treatment should be symptom-directed and supportive.

Drug Interactions CNS depressants: Sedative effects may be additive with CNS depressants; includes barbiturates, narcotic analgesics, and other sedative agents; monitor for increased effect

Ethanol/Nutrition/Herb Interactions

Ethanol: Avoid ethanol (may increase CNS depression).

Food: Administration with high-lipid meals may increase absorption.

Herb/Nutraceutical: St John's wort may decrease dronabinol levels.

Test Interactions Decreased FSH, LH, growth hormone, and testosterone

Dietary Considerations Capsules contain sesame oil.

Dosage Forms Capsule, gelatin: 2.5 mg, 5 mg, 10 mg [contains sesame oil]

Droperidol (droe PER i dole)

Medication Safety Issues

Sound-alike/look-alike issues:

Droperidol may be confused with dronabinol

Inapsine® may be confused with Nebcin®

Related Information

Anesthesia Considerations for Neurosurgery *on page 1401*

Moderate Sedation *on page 1442*

Postoperative Nausea and Vomiting *on page 1477*

U.S. Brand Names Inapsine®

Canadian Brand Names Droperidol Injection, USP

Synonyms Dehydrobenzperidol

Pharmacologic Category Antiemetic; Antipsychotic Agent, Typical

Generic Available Yes

Use Antiemetic in surgical and diagnostic procedures; preoperative medication in patients when other treatments are ineffective or inappropriate

Mechanism of Action Droperidol is a butyrophenone antipsychotic; antiemetic effect is a result of blockade of dopamine stimulation of the chemoreceptor trigger zone. Other effects include alpha-adrenergic blockade, peripheral vascular dilation, and reduction of the pressor effect of epinephrine resulting in hypotension and decreased peripheral vascular resistance; may also reduce pulmonary artery pressure

Pharmacodynamics/Kinetics

Onset of action: Peak effect: Parenteral: ~30 minutes

Duration: Parenteral: 2-4 hours, may extend to 12 hours

Absorption: I.M.: Rapid

Distribution: Crosses blood-brain barrier and placenta

V_d: Children: ~0.25-0.9 L/kg; Adults: ~2 L/kg

Protein binding: Extensive

Metabolism: Hepatic, to *p*-fluorophenylacetic acid, benzimidazolone, *p*-hydroxypiperidine

Half-life elimination: Adults: 2.3 hours

Excretion: Urine (75%, <1% as unchanged drug); feces (22%, 11% to 50% as unchanged drug)

Dosage Titrate carefully to desired effect

Children 2-12 years: Nausea and vomiting: I.M., I.V.: 0.05-0.06 mg/kg (maximum initial dose: 0.1 mg/kg); additional doses may be repeated to achieve effect; administer additional doses with caution

Adults: Nausea and vomiting: I.M., I.V.: Initial: 2.5 mg; additional doses of 1.25 mg may be administered to achieve desired effect; administer additional doses with caution

Stability Droperidol ampuls/vials should be stored at room temperature and protected from light. Solutions diluted in NS or D_5W are stable at room temperature for up to 7 days.

Administration Administer I.M. or I.V.; according to the manufacturer, I.V. push administration should be slow (generally regarded as 2-5 minutes); however, many clinicians administer I.V. doses rapidly (over 30-60 seconds) in an effort to reduce the incidence of EPS. The effect, if any, of rapid administration on QT prolongation is unclear. For I.V. infusion, dilute in 50-100 mL NS or D_5W; ECG monitoring for 2-3 hours after administration is recommended regardless of rate of infusion.

Monitoring Parameters To identify QT prolongation, a 12-lead ECG prior to use is recommended; continued ECG monitoring for 2-3 hours following administration is recommended. Vital signs; lipid profile, fasting blood glucose/Hgb A_{1c}, serum magnesium and potassium; BMI; mental status, abnormal involuntary movement scale (AIMS); observe for dystonias, extrapyramidal side effects, and temperature changes

Anesthesia and Critical Care Concerns/Other Considerations May cause hypotension and reflex tachycardia; this is more pronounced when the drug is given intravenously. Warnings concerning QT prolongation have altered recommendations concerning perioperative use and monitoring. Baseline 12-lead ECG screening is recommended, and continued ECG monitoring for 2-3 hours postadministration is advised. Use should be limited to patients in whom alternatives are unacceptable. Droperidol does not possess analgesic effects and has little or no amnesic properties.

Pregnancy Risk Factor C

Contraindications Hypersensitivity to droperidol or any component of the formulation; known or suspected QT prolongation, including congenital long QT syndrome (prolonged QT_c is defined as >440 msec in males or >450 msec in females)

Warnings/Precautions May alter cardiac conduction. **[U.S. Boxed Warning]: Cases of QT prolongation and torsade de pointes, including some fatal cases, have been reported.** Use extreme caution in patients with bradycardia (<50 bpm), cardiac disease, concurrent MAOI therapy, Class I and Class III antiarrhythmics or other drugs known to prolong QT interval, and electrolyte disturbances (hypokalemia or hypomagnesemia), including concomitant drugs which may alter electrolytes (diuretics).

Use with caution in patients with seizures, bone marrow suppression, or severe liver disease. May be sedating, use with caution in disorders where CNS depression is a feature. Caution in patients with hemodynamic instability, predisposition to seizures, subcortical brain damage, renal or respiratory disease. Esophageal dysmotility and aspiration have been associated with antipsychotic use - use with caution in patients at risk of pneumonia (ie, Alzheimer's disease). Caution in breast cancer or other prolactin-dependent tumors (may elevate prolactin levels). May alter temperature regulation or mask toxicity of other drugs due to antiemetic effects. May cause orthostatic hypotension - use with caution in patients at risk of this effect or those who would tolerate transient hypotensive episodes (cerebrovascular disease, cardiovascular disease, or other medications which may predispose). Significant hypotension may occur; injection contains benzyl alcohol; injection also contains sulfites which may cause allergic reaction.

May cause anticholinergic effects (confusion, agitation, constipation, xerostomia, blurred vision, urinary retention). Therefore, they should be used with caution in patients with decreased gastrointestinal motility, urinary retention, BPH, xerostomia, or visual problems. Conditions which also may be exacerbated by cholinergic blockade include narrow-angle glaucoma (screening is recommended) and worsening of myasthenia gravis. Relative to other neuroleptics, droperidol has a low potency of cholinergic blockade.

May cause extrapyramidal symptoms, including pseudoparkinsonism, acute dystonic reactions, akathisia, and tardive dyskinesia (risk of these reactions is high relative to other neuroleptics). May be associated with neuroleptic malignant syndrome (NMS) or pigmentary retinopathy. Safety in children <6 months of age has not been established.

Adverse Reactions

>10%:

- Cardiovascular: QT_c prolongation (dose dependent)
- Central nervous system: Restlessness, anxiety, extrapyramidal symptoms, dystonic reactions, pseudoparkinsonian signs and symptoms, tardive dyskinesia, seizure, altered central temperature regulation, sedation, drowsiness
- Endocrine & metabolic: Swelling of breasts
- Gastrointestinal: Weight gain, constipation

1% to 10%:

- Cardiovascular: Hypotension (especially orthostatic), tachycardia, abnormal T waves with prolonged ventricular repolarization, hypertension
- Central nervous system: Hallucinations, persistent tardive dyskinesia, akathisia
- Gastrointestinal: Nausea, vomiting

(Continued)

Droperidol *(Continued)*

Genitourinary: Dysuria

<1% (Limited to important or life-threatening): Adynamic ileus, agranulocytosis, alopecia, arrhythmia, cholestatic jaundice, decreased visual acuity (may be irreversible), heat stroke, hyperpigmentation, laryngospasm, leukopenia, neuroleptic malignant syndrome (NMS), obstructive jaundice, photosensitivity (rare), priapism, rash, respiratory depression, retinal pigmentation, tardive dystonia, torsade de pointes, urinary retention, ventricular tachycardia

Overdosage/Toxicology Symptoms of overdose include hypotension, tachycardia, hallucinations, and extrapyramidal symptoms. Following initiation of essential overdose management, toxic symptom treatment and supportive treatment should be initiated. Prolonged QT interval, seizures, and arrhythmias have been reported.

Drug Interactions

Acetylcholinesterase inhibitors (central): May increase the risk of antipsychotic-related extrapyramidal symptoms; monitor.

CNS depressants: Sedative effects may be additive with other CNS depressants; monitor for increased effect; includes benzodiazepines, barbiturates, antipsychotics, ethanol, opiates, and other sedative medications

Cyclobenzaprine: Droperidol and cyclobenzaprine may have an additive effect on prolonging the QT interval; based on limited documentation; monitor

Inhalation anesthetics: Droperidol in combination with certain forms of induction anesthesia may produce peripheral vasodilitation and hypotension

Metoclopramide: May increase extrapyramidal symptoms (EPS) or risk.

Potassium- or magnesium-depleting agents: May increase the risk of serious arrhythmias with droperidol; includes many diuretics, aminoglycosides, cyclosporine, supraphysiologic doses of corticosteroids with mineralocorticoid effects, laxatives, and amphotericin B; monitor serum potassium and magnesium levels closely.

Propofol: An increased incidence of postoperative nausea and vomiting have been reported following coadministration

QT_c-prolonging agents: May result in additive effects on cardiac conduction, potentially resulting in malignant or lethal arrhythmias; concurrent use is contraindicated. Includes cisapride, Class I and Class III antiarrhythmics (amiodarone, dofetilide, procainamide, quinidine, sotalol), pimozide, some quinolone antibiotics (moxifloxacin, sparfloxacin, gatifloxacin), tricyclic antidepressants, and some phenothiazines (mesoridazine, thioridazine).

Dosage Forms Injection, solution: 2.5 mg/mL (1 mL, 2 mL)

References

Kao LW, Kirk MA, Evers SJ, et al, "Droperidol, QT Prolongation and Sudden Death: What Is the Evidence," *Ann Emerg Med*, 2003, 41(4):546-58.

♦ **Droperidol Injection, USP (Can)** *see* Droperidol *on page 432*

Drotrecogin Alfa (dro TRE coe jin AL fa)

U.S. Brand Names Xigris®

Canadian Brand Names Xigris®

Synonyms Activated Protein C, Human, Recombinant; Drotrecogin Alfa, Activated; Protein C (Activated), Human, Recombinant

Pharmacologic Category Protein C (Activated)

Generic Available No

Use Reduction of mortality from severe sepsis (associated with organ dysfunction) in adults at high risk of death (eg, APACHE II score ≥25)

Unlabeled/Investigational Use Purpura fulminans

Mechanism of Action Inhibits factors Va and VIIIa, limiting thrombotic effects. Additional *in vitro* data suggest inhibition of plasminogen activator inhibitor-1 (PAF-1) resulting in profibrinolytic activity, inhibition of macrophage production of tumor necrosis factor, blocking of leukocyte adhesion, and limitation of thrombin-induced inflammatory responses. Relative contribution of effects on the reduction of mortality from sepsis is not completely understood.

Pharmacodynamics/Kinetics

Duration: Plasma nondetectable within 2 hours of discontinuation

Metabolism: Inactivated by endogenous plasma protease inhibitors; mean clearance: 40 L/hour; increased with severe sepsis (~50%)

Half-life elimination: 1.6 hours

Dosage I.V.:

Children and Adults: Purpura fulminans (unlabeled use): 24 mcg/kg/hour

Adults: Sepsis: 24 mcg/kg/hour for a total of 96 hours; stop infusion **immediately** if clinically-important bleeding is identified

Dosage adjustment in renal impairment: No specific adjustment recommended.

Stability Store vials under refrigeration at 2°C to 8°C (36°F to 46°F). Protect from light. Do not freeze. Reconstitute 5 mg vials with 2.5 mL and 20 mg vials with 10 mL sterile water for injection (resultant solution ~2 mg/mL). Must be further diluted (within 3 hours of reconstitution) in 0.9% sodium chloride, typically to a concentration between 100 mcg/mL and 200 mcg/mL when using infusion pump and between 100 mcg/mL and 1000 mcg/mL when infused via syringe pump. Although product information states administration must be completed within 12 hours of preparation, additional studies (data on file, Lilly Research Laboratories) show that the final solution is stable for 14 hours at 15°C to 30°C (59°F to 86°F). If not used immediately, a prepared solution may be stored in the refrigerator for up to 12 hours. The total expiration time (refrigeration and administration) should be ≤24 hours from time of preparation.

Administration Infuse separately from all other medications. Only dextrose, normal saline, dextrose/saline combinations, and lactated Ringer's solution may be infused through the same line. May administer via infusion pump. Administration of prepared solution must be completed within 12 hours of preparation. Suspend administration for 2 hours prior to invasive procedures or other procedure with significant bleeding risk; may continue treatment immediately following uncomplicated, minimally-invasive procedures, but delay for 12 hours after major invasive procedures/surgery.

Monitoring Parameters Monitor for signs and symptoms of bleeding, hemoglobin/hematocrit, PT/INR, platelet count

Anesthesia and Critical Care Concerns/Other Considerations PROWESS trial: The inclusion criteria for the PROWESS trial (Bernard, *N Engl J Med*, 2001) may help in patient selection since it is the first clinical trial evaluating a fixed dose of drotrecogin alfa in severe sepsis. The patients included had a known or suspected infection, three or more signs of systemic inflammatory syndrome (SIRS), and sepsis-induced acute organ dysfunction. Indicators of infection included: White cells in a normally sterile body fluid, perforated viscus, radiographic evidence of pneumonia in association with purulent sputum, a syndrome associated with a high risk of infection (eg, ascending cholangitis). Modified (SIRS) criteria (needed ≥3 criteria): A core temperature of ≥38°C (100.4°F) or ≤36°C (96.8°F); heart rate ≥90 bpm except in patients with a medical condition known to increase the heart rate or those receiving treatment that would prevent tachycardia; respiratory rate ≥20 breaths/minute, a $PaCO_2$ ≤32 mm Hg, or the use of mechanical ventilation; WBC count ≥12,000/mm^3, ≤4000/mm^3, or a differential count with >10% immature neutrophils. Criteria for organ dysfunction included arterial blood pressure ≤90 mm Hg or a MAP ≤70 mm Hg for at least 1 hour despite adequate fluid resuscitation, adequate intravascular volume status, or the use of vasopressors; urine output <0.5 mL/kg/hour for 1 hour despite adequate fluid resuscitation; PaO_2/FiO_2 ≤250 in the presence of other dysfunctional organ systems or ≤200 if the lung is the only dysfunctional organ; platelet count <80,000/mm^3 or acute decrease by 50%; unexplained metabolic acidosis with a high plasma lactate level.

Severe sepsis and a low risk of death: Recently a randomized, double-blind, placebo-controlled, multicenter, international trial (Abraham E, 2005) was conducted to evaluate the safety and efficacy of drotrecogin alfa in adult patients with severe sepsis and a low risk of death (APACHE II score <25 or single-organ failure). Patients were randomized to a 96 hour infusion of normal saline or drotrecogin alfa at the FDA approved dose; 2640 patients were enrolled in the study. There was no statistical difference between the groups in 28-day mortality. Hemorrhage accounted for 2 deaths (0.9%) in the placebo group and 7 deaths (2.9%) in the drotrecogin alfa group (p = 0.02) during the infusion. Drotrecogin alfa should not be used in patients with severe sepsis who are at low risk of death because of a lack of efficacy and an increased incidence of bleeding

Stability: Drotrecogin alfa has a shorter stability time than was originally suggested. This may lead to some confusion. Additional studies (data on file, Lilly Research Laboratories) show that the final solution is stable for 14 hours at controlled room temperature 15°C to 30°C (59°F to 86°F). If not used immediately, a prepared solution may be stored in the refrigerator for up to 12 hours. The

(Continued)

Drotrecogin Alfa *(Continued)*

total expiration time (refrigeration and administration) should be ≤24 hours from time of preparation. Due to brief stability consider these dilutions for infusion pumps: 5 mg/50 mL, 10 mg/100 mL, 15 mg/150 mL, 20 mg/200 mL.

Pregnancy Risk Factor C

Contraindications Hypersensitivity to drotrecogin alfa or any component of the formulation; active internal bleeding; recent hemorrhagic stroke (within 3 months); severe head trauma (within 2 months); recent intracranial or intraspinal surgery (within 2 months); intracranial neoplasm or mass lesion; evidence of cerebral herniation; presence of an epidural catheter; trauma with an increased risk of life-threatening bleeding

Warnings/Precautions Increases risk of bleeding; careful evaluation of risks and benefit is required prior to initiation (see Contraindications). Bleeding risk is increased in patients receiving concurrent therapeutic heparin, oral anticoagulants, glycoprotein IIb/IIIa antagonists, platelet aggregation inhibitors, or aspirin at a dosage of >650 mg/day (within 7 days). In addition, an increased bleeding risk is associated with prolonged INR (>3.0), gastrointestinal bleeding (within 6 weeks), decreased platelet count (<30,000/mm^3), thrombolytic therapy (within 3 days), recent ischemic stroke (within 3 months), intracranial AV malformation or aneurysm, known bleeding diathesis, severe hepatic disease (chronic), or other condition where bleeding is a significant hazard or difficult to manage due to its location. Discontinue if significant bleeding occurs (may consider continued use after stabilization). Suspend administration for 2 hours prior to invasive procedures or other procedure with significant bleeding risk; may continue treatment immediately following uncomplicated, minimally-invasive procedures, but delay for 12 hours after major invasive procedures/surgery. During treatment, aPTT cannot be used to assess coagulopathy (PT/INR not affected).

Efficacy not established in adult patients at a low risk of death (APACHE II score <25). Patients with pre-existing nonsepsis-related medical conditions with a poor prognosis (anticipated survival <28 days), patients with acute pancreatitis (no established source of infection), HIV-infected patients with a CD4 count ≤50 cells/mm^3, chronic dialysis patients, pre-existing hypercoagulable conditions, and patients who had received bone marrow, liver, lung, pancreas, or small bowel transplants were excluded from the clinical trial which established benefit. In addition, patients with a high body weight (>135 kg) were not evaluated. Safety and efficacy have not been established in pediatric patients.

Adverse Reactions As with all drugs which may affect hemostasis, bleeding is the major adverse effect associated with drotrecogin alfa. Hemorrhage may occur at virtually any site. Risk is dependent on multiple variables, including the dosage administered, concurrent use of multiple agents which alter hemostasis, and patient predisposition.

>10%:
- Dermatologic: Bruising
- Gastrointestinal: Gastrointestinal bleeding

1% to 10%: Hematologic: Bleeding (serious 2.4% during infusion vs 3.5% during 28-day study period; individual events listed as <1%)

<1% (Limited to important or life-threatening): Gastrointestinal hemorrhage, genitourinary bleeding, immune reaction (antibody production), intracranial hemorrhage (0.2%; frequencies up to 2% noted in a previous trial without placebo control), intrathoracic hemorrhage, retroperitoneal bleeding, skin/soft tissue bleeding

Overdosage/Toxicology No reported experience with overdose. Hemorrhagic complications are likely consequence of overdose. Treatment is supportive, including immediate interruption of the infusion and monitoring for hemorrhagic complications. No known antidote.

Drug Interactions No formal drug interaction studies have been conducted.

Antiplatelet agents: Aspirin (>650 mg/day), cilostazol, clopidogrel, dipyridamole, ticlopidine, or glycoprotein IIb/IIIa antagonists: Concurrent or recent use (aspirin or IIb/IIIa antagonists within 7 days) may increase risk of bleeding.

Antithrombin III: Concurrent or recent use (within 12 hours) may increase risk of bleeding.

Danaparoid: Concurrent or recent use may increase risk of bleeding.

Heparin: Concurrent use of heparin at therapeutic rates of infusion may increase the risk of bleeding. However, the use of low-dose prophylactic heparin does not appear to affect safety.

LMWHs: Concurrent or recent use (within 12 hours) may increase risk of bleeding. Primary clinical trial permitted dosages used prophylactically.

NSAIDs: Concurrent use may increase risk of bleeding. Approximately 4-6 half-lives are required for antiplatelet effects to decrease.

Thrombolytic agents: Use within 3 days of drotrecogin alfa may increase risk of bleeding.

Warfarin; Use within 7 days of drotrecogin alfa and/or elevation of INR ≥3 may increase risk of bleeding.

Ethanol/Nutrition/Herb Interactions Herb/Nutraceutical: Recent use/intake of herbs with anticoagulant or antiplatelet activity (including cat's claw, feverfew, garlic, ginkgo, ginseng, and horse chestnut seed) may increase the risk of bleeding.

Test Interactions May interfere with one-stage coagulation assays based on the aPTT (such as factor VIII, IX, and XI assays).

Dosage Forms Injection, powder for reconstitution [preservative free]: 5 mg [contains sucrose 31.8 mg], 20 mg [contains sucrose 124.9 mg]

References

Bachli EB, Vavricka SR, Walter RB, et al, "Drotecogin Alfa (Activated) for the Treatment of Meningococcal Purpura Fulminans," *Intensive Care Med*, 2003, 29(2):337.

Bernard GR, Ely EW, Wright TJ, et al, "Safety and Dose Relationship of Recombinant Human Activated Protein C for Coagulopathy in Severe Sepsis," *Crit Care Med*, 2001, 29(11):2051-9.

Bernard GR, Vincent JL, Laterre PF, et al, "Efficacy and Safety of Recombinant Human Activated Protein C for Severe Sepsis," *N Engl J Med*, 2001, 344(10):699-709.

Cone LA, B Waterbor R, Sofonio MV, "Purpura Fulminans Due to *Streptococcus pneumoniae* Sepsis Following Gastric Bypass," *Obes Surg*, 2004, 14(5):690-4.

Dellinger RP, Carlet JM, Masur H, et al, "Surviving Sepsis Campaign Guidelines for Management of Severe Sepsis and Septic Shock," *Crit Care Med*, 2004, 32(3):858-73.

Hasin T, Leibowitz D, Rot D, et al, "Early Treatment With Activated Protein C for Meningococcal Septic Shock: Case Report and Literature Review," *Intensive Care Med*, 2005, 31(7):1002-3.

Mann HJ, Demmon SL, Boelk DA, et al, "Physical and Chemical Compatibility of Drotrecogin Alfa (Activated) With 34 Drugs During Simulated Y-Site Administration," *Am J Health Syst Pharm*, 2004, 61(24):2664-71.

- **Drotrecogin Alfa, Activated** *see* Drotrecogin Alfa *on page 434*
- **Droxia®** *see* Hydroxyurea *on page 648*
- **Duocaine™** *see* Lidocaine and Bupivacaine *on page 761*
- **DuP 753** *see* Losartan *on page 778*
- **Duraclon™** *see* Clonidine *on page 316*
- **Duragesic®** *see* Fentanyl *on page 514*
- **Duralith® (Can)** *see* Lithium *on page 770*
- **Duramist® Plus [OTC]** *see* Oxymetazoline *on page 973*
- **Duramorph®** *see* Morphine Sulfate *on page 867*
- **Duration® [OTC]** *see* Oxymetazoline *on page 973*

Dutasteride (doo TAS teer ide)

U.S. Brand Names Avodart™

Canadian Brand Names Avodart™

Pharmacologic Category 5 Alpha-Reductase Inhibitor

Generic Available No

Use Treatment of symptomatic benign prostatic hyperplasia (BPH)

Unlabeled/Investigational Use Treatment of male patterned baldness

Mechanism of Action Dutasteride is a 4-azo analog of testosterone and is a competitive, selective inhibitor of both reproductive tissues (type 2) and skin and hepatic (type 1) 5α-reductase. This results in inhibition of the conversion of testosterone to dihydrotestosterone and markedly suppresses serum dihydrotestosterone levels.

Pharmacodynamics/Kinetics

Absorption: Via skin when handling capsules

Distribution: ~12% of serum concentrations partitioned into semen

Protein binding: 99% to albumin; ~97% to α_1-acid glycoprotein; >96% to semen protein

Metabolism: Hepatic via CYP3A4 isoenzyme; forms metabolites: 6-hydroxydutasteride has activity similar to parent compound, 4′-hydroxydutasteride and 1,2-dihydrodutasteride are much less potent than parent *in vitro*

Bioavailability: 60% (range: 40% to 94%)

Half-life elimination: Terminal: ~5 weeks

Time to peak: 2-3 hours

(Continued)

Dutasteride *(Continued)*

Excretion: Feces (40% as metabolites, 5% as unchanged drug); urine (<1% as unchanged drug); 55% of dose unaccounted for

Dosage Oral: Adults: Male: 0.5 mg once daily

Dosage adjustment in renal impairment: No adjustment required

Dosage adjustment in hepatic impairment: Use caution; no specific adjustments recommended

Stability Store at 25°C (77°F); excursions permitted to 15°C to 30°C (59°F to 86°F).

Administration May be administered with or without food. Capsule should be swallowed whole; should not be touched or handled by women who are pregnant or are of childbearing age.

Monitoring Parameters Objective and subjective signs of relief of benign prostatic hyperplasia, including improvement in urinary flow, reduction in symptoms of urgency, and relief of difficulty in micturition.

Pregnancy Risk Factor X

Contraindications Hypersensitivity to dutasteride, other 5α-reductase inhibitors (eg, finasteride), or any component of the formulation; not indicated for use in women or children; pregnant women or women trying to conceive should not handle the product

Warnings/Precautions Women can absorb the active ingredient through the skin and should always use caution whenever handling. Pregnant women or women trying to conceive should not handle the product. Patients with large residual urinary volume and/or severely diminished urinary flow may not benefit from this treatment. Other urological diseases including cancer should be ruled out before initiating. Men should not donate blood until ≥6 months after last dose. Use caution in hepatic impairment and with concurrent use of potent, chronic CYP3A4 inhibitors. Reduces prostate specific antigen (PSA) by 40% following 3 months of use and 50% after 6-12 months of use. If following serial PSAs, re-establish a new baseline after 3-6 months of use. If interpreting an isolated PSA value in a patient treated for 6 months, then double the PSA value for comparison.

Adverse Reactions

>10%: Endocrine & metabolic: Serum testosterone increased, thyroid-stimulating hormone increased

1% to 10%: Endocrine & metabolic: Impotence (1% to 5%), libido decreased (1% to 3%), ejaculation disorders (1%), gynecomastia (including breast tenderness, breast enlargement) (1%)

Postmarketing and/or case reports: Allergic reaction, edema (localized), pruritus, rash, urticaria

Note: Frequency of adverse events (except gynecomastia) tends to decrease with continued use (>6 months).

Overdosage/Toxicology Treatment is symptom-directed and supportive.

Drug Interactions Substrate of CYP3A4 (minor)

Calcium channel blockers, nondihydropyridine (diltiazem, verapamil): Increase in dutasteride levels with concurrent use

Ethanol/Nutrition/Herb Interactions

Ethanol: No effect or interaction noted.

Food: Maximum serum concentrations reduced by 10% to 15% when taken with food; not clinically significant.

Herb/Nutraceutical: St John's wort may decrease dutasteride levels. Avoid saw palmetto (concurrent use has not been adequately studied).

Test Interactions PSA levels decrease in treated patients. After 6 months of therapy, PSA levels stabilize to a new baseline that is ~50% of pretreatment values. If following serial PSAs in a patient, re-establish a new baseline after 3-6 months of use. If interpreting an isolated PSA value in a patient treated for 6 months, then double the PSA value for comparison.

Dietary Considerations May be taken with or without food.

Dosage Forms Capsule, softgel: 0.5 mg

- ♦ **DW286** *see* Gemifloxacin *on page 587*
- ♦ **Dynacin®** *see* Minocycline *on page 854*
- ♦ **Dyna-Hex® [OTC]** *see* Chlorhexidine Gluconate *on page 267*
- ♦ **Dytan™** *see* DiphenhydrAMINE *on page 399*
- ♦ **7E3** *see* Abciximab *on page 23*

- **EarSol® HC** *see* Hydrocortisone *on page 639*
- **Easprin®** *see* Aspirin *on page 129*
- **EC-Naprosyn®** *see* Naproxen *on page 899*
- **Econopred® Plus** *see* PrednisoLONE *on page 1046*
- **Ecotrin® [OTC]** *see* Aspirin *on page 129*
- **Ecotrin® Low Strength [OTC]** *see* Aspirin *on page 129*
- **Ecotrin® Maximum Strength [OTC]** *see* Aspirin *on page 129*
- **Ectosone (Can)** *see* Betamethasone *on page 169*
- **Edecrin®** *see* Ethacrynic Acid *on page 492*
- **Edex®** *see* Alprostadil *on page 68*

Edrophonium (ed roe FOE nee um)

Related Information

Chronic Renal Failure *on page 1437*

U.S. Brand Names Enlon®; Reversol®

Canadian Brand Names Enlon®; Tensilon®

Synonyms Edrophonium Chloride

Pharmacologic Category Antidote; Cholinergic Agonist; Diagnostic Agent

Generic Available No

Use Diagnosis of myasthenia gravis; differentiation of cholinergic crises from myasthenia crises; reversal of nondepolarizing neuromuscular blockers; adjunct treatment of respiratory depression caused by curare overdose

Mechanism of Action Inhibits destruction of acetylcholine by acetylcholinesterase. This facilitates transmission of impulses across myoneural junction and results in increased cholinergic responses such as miosis, increased tonus of intestinal and skeletal muscles, bronchial and ureteral constriction, bradycardia, and increased salivary and sweat gland secretions.

Pharmacodynamics/Kinetics

Onset of action: I.M.: 2-10 minutes; I.V.: 30-60 seconds

Duration: I.M.: 5-30 minutes: I.V.: 10 minutes

Distribution: V_d: Adults: 1.1 L/kg

Half-life elimination: Adults: 1.2-2.4 hours; Anephric patients: 2.4-4.4 hours

Excretion: Adults: Primarily urine (67%)

Dosage Usually administered I.V., however, if not possible, I.M. or SubQ may be used:

Infants:

I.M.: 0.5-1 mg

I.V.: Initial: 0.1 mg, followed by 0.4 mg if no response; total dose = 0.5 mg

Children:

Diagnosis: Initial: 0.04 mg/kg over 1 minute followed by 0.16 mg/kg if no response, to a maximum total dose of 5 mg for children <34 kg, or 10 mg for children >34 kg **or**

Alternative dosing (manufacturer's recommendation):

≤34 kg: 1 mg; if no response after 45 seconds, repeat dosage in 1 mg increments every 30-45 seconds, up to a total of 5 mg

>34 kg: 2 mg; if no response after 45 seconds, repeat dosage in 1 mg increments every 30-45 seconds, up to a total of 10 mg

I.M.:

<34 kg: 1 mg

>34 kg: 5 mg

Titration of oral anticholinesterase therapy: 0.04 mg/kg once given 1 hour after oral intake of the drug being used in treatment; if strength improves, an increase in neostigmine or pyridostigmine dose is indicated

Adults:

Diagnosis:

I.V.: 2 mg test dose administered over 15-30 seconds; 8 mg given 45 seconds later if no response is seen; test dose may be repeated after 30 minutes

I.M.: Initial: 10 mg; if no cholinergic reaction occurs, administer 2 mg 30 minutes later to rule out false-negative reaction

Titration of oral anticholinesterase therapy: 1-2 mg given 1 hour after oral dose of anticholinesterase; if strength improves, an increase in neostigmine or pyridostigmine dose is indicated

(Continued)

Edrophonium *(Continued)*

Reversal of nondepolarizing neuromuscular blocking agents (neostigmine with atropine usually preferred): I.V.: 10 mg over 30-45 seconds; may repeat every 5-10 minutes up to 40 mg

Termination of paroxysmal atrial tachycardia: I.V. rapid injection: 5-10 mg

Differentiation of cholinergic from myasthenic crisis: I.V.: 1 mg; may repeat after 1 minute. **Note:** Intubation and controlled ventilation may be required if patient has cholinergic crisis

Dosing adjustment in renal impairment: Dose may need to be reduced in patients with chronic renal failure

Administration Edrophonium is administered by direct I.V. injection; see Dosage

Monitoring Parameters Pre- and postinjection strength (cranial musculature is most useful); heart rate, respiratory rate, blood pressure

Anesthesia and Critical Care Concerns/Other Considerations Atropine should be administered along with edrophonium when reversing the effects of nondepolarizing agents to antagonize the cholinergic effects at the muscarinic receptors, especially bradycardia; important to recognize the difference in dose for diagnosis of myasthenia gravis versus reversal of muscle relaxant, a much larger dose is needed for desired effect of reversal of muscle paralysis

Pregnancy Risk Factor C

Contraindications Hypersensitivity to edrophonium, sulfites, or any component of the formulation; GI or GU obstruction

Warnings/Precautions Use with caution in patients with bronchial asthma and those receiving a cardiac glycoside; atropine sulfate should always be readily available as an antagonist. Overdosage can cause cholinergic crisis which may be fatal. I.V. atropine should be readily available for treatment of cholinergic reactions.

Adverse Reactions Frequency not defined.

Cardiovascular: Arrhythmias (especially bradycardia), hypotension, decreased carbon monoxide, tachycardia, AV block, nodal rhythm, nonspecific ECG changes, cardiac arrest, syncope, flushing

Central nervous system: Convulsions, dysarthria, dysphonia, dizziness, loss of consciousness, drowsiness, headache

Dermatologic: Skin rash, thrombophlebitis (I.V.), urticaria

Gastrointestinal: Hyperperistalsis, nausea, vomiting, salivation, diarrhea, stomach cramps, dysphagia, flatulence

Genitourinary: Urinary urgency

Neuromuscular & skeletal: Weakness, fasciculations, muscle cramps, spasms, arthralgia

Ocular: Small pupils, lacrimation

Respiratory: Increased bronchial secretions, laryngospasm, bronchiolar constriction, respiratory muscle paralysis, dyspnea, respiratory depression, respiratory arrest, bronchospasm

Miscellaneous: Diaphoresis (increased), anaphylaxis, allergic reactions

Overdosage/Toxicology Symptoms of overdose include muscle weakness, nausea, vomiting, miosis, bronchospasm, and respiratory paralysis. Maintain an adequate airway. For muscarinic symptoms, the antidote is atropine 0.4-0.5 mg I.V. repeated every 3-10 minutes (initial doses as high as 1.2 mg have been administered). Skeletal muscle effects of edrophonium are not alleviated by atropine.

Drug Interactions

Decreased effect: Atropine, nondepolarizing muscle relaxants, procainamide, quinidine

Increased effect: Succinylcholine, digoxin, I.V. acetazolamide, neostigmine, physostigmine

Test Interactions Increased aminotransferase [ALT (SGPT)/AST (SGOT)] (S), amylase (S)

Dosage Forms Injection, solution, as chloride:

Enlon®: 10 mg/mL (15 mL) [contains sodium sulfite]

Reversol®: 10 mg/mL (10 mL) [contains sodium sulfite]

- **Edrophonium Chloride** *see* Edrophonium *on page 439*
- **E.E.S.®** *see* Erythromycin *on page 476*

Efavirenz (e FAV e renz)

U.S. Brand Names Sustiva®

Canadian Brand Names Sustiva®

Pharmacologic Category Antiretroviral Agent, Reverse Transcriptase Inhibitor (Non-nucleoside)

Generic Available No

Use Treatment of HIV-1 infections in combination with at least two other antiretroviral agents

Mechanism of Action As a non-nucleoside reverse transcriptase inhibitor, efavirenz has activity against HIV-1 by binding to reverse transcriptase. It consequently blocks the RNA-dependent and DNA-dependent DNA polymerase activities including HIV-1 replication. It does not require intracellular phosphorylation for antiviral activity.

Pharmacodynamics/Kinetics

Absorption: Increased by fatty meals

Distribution: CSF concentrations exceed free fraction in serum

Protein binding: >99%, primarily to albumin

Metabolism: Hepatic via CYP3A4 and 2B6; may induce its own metabolism

Half-life elimination: Single dose: 52-76 hours; Multiple doses: 40-55 hours

Time to peak: 3-8 hours

Excretion: Feces (16% to 41% primarily as unchanged drug); urine (14% to 34% as metabolites)

Dosage Oral: Dosing at bedtime is recommended to limit central nervous system effects; should not be used as single-agent therapy

Children ≥3 years: Dosage is based on body weight

- 10 kg to <15 kg: 200 mg once daily
- 15 kg to <20 kg: 250 mg once daily
- 20 kg to <25 kg: 300 mg once daily
- 25 kg to <32.5 kg: 350 mg once daily
- 32.5 kg to <40 kg: 400 mg once daily
- ≥40 kg: 600 mg once daily

Adults: 600 mg once daily

Dosing adjustment in renal impairment: None recommended

Dosing comments in hepatic impairment: Limited clinical experience, use with caution

Stability Store below 25°C (77°F).

Administration Administer on an empty stomach. Capsules may be opened and added to liquids or small amounts of food.

Monitoring Parameters Serum transaminases (discontinuation of treatment should be considered for persistent elevations greater than five times the upper limit of normal), cholesterol, triglycerides, signs and symptoms of infection

Pregnancy Risk Factor D

Contraindications Clinically-significant hypersensitivity to efavirenz or any component of the formulation; concurrent use of cisapride, midazolam, triazolam, voriconazole, or ergot alkaloids (includes dihydroergotamine, ergotamine, ergonovine, methylergonovine); pregnancy

Warnings/Precautions Do not use as single-agent therapy; avoid pregnancy; women of childbearing potential should undergo pregnancy testing prior to initiation of therapy; use caution with other agents metabolized by cytochrome P450 isoenzyme 3A4 (see Contraindications); use caution with history of mental illness/drug abuse (predisposition to psychological reactions); may cause CNS and psychiatric symptoms, which include impaired concentration, dizziness or drowsiness (avoid potentially hazardous tasks such as driving or operating machinery if these effects are noted); serious psychiatric side effects have been associated with efavirenz, including severe depression, suicide, paranoia, and mania; discontinue if severe rash (involving blistering, desquamation, mucosal involvement or fever) develops. Children are more susceptible to development of rash; prophylactic antihistamines may be used. Caution in patients with known or suspected hepatitis B or C infection (monitoring of liver function is recommended); hepatic impairment. Persistent elevations of serum transaminases >5 times the upper limit of normal should prompt evaluation - benefit of continued therapy should be weighed against possible risk of hepatotoxicity. Concomitant use with St John's wort is not recommended.

(Continued)

Efavirenz *(Continued)*

Adverse Reactions

>10%:

Central nervous system: Dizziness* (2% to 28%), depression (1% to 16%), insomnia (6% to 16%), anxiety (1% to 11%), pain* (1% to 13%)

Dermatologic: Rash* (NCI grade 1: 9% to 11%, NCI grade 2: 15% to 32%, NCI grade 3 or 4: <1%); 26% experienced new rash vs 17% in control groups; up to 46% of pediatric patients experience rash (median onset: 8 days)

Endocrine & metabolic: HDL increased (25% to 35%), total cholesterol increased (20% to 40%)

Gastrointestinal: Diarrhea* (3% to 14%), nausea* (2% to 12%)

1% to 10%:

Central nervous system: Impaired concentration (2% to 8%), headache* (2% to 7%), somnolence (2% to 7%), fatigue (2% to 7%), abnormal dreams (1% to 6%), nervousness (2% to 6%), severe depression (2%), hallucinations (1%)

Dermatologic: Pruritus (1% to 9%)

Gastrointestinal: Vomiting* (6% to 7%), dyspepsia (3%), abdominal pain (1% to 3%), anorexia (1% to 2%)

Miscellaneous: Diaphoresis increased (1% to 2%)

*Adverse effect reported in ≥10% of patients 3-16 years of age

<1% (Limited to important or life-threatening): Aggressive reaction, agitation, allergic reaction, body fat accumulation/redistribution, convulsions, liver failure, manic reaction, neuropathy, paranoid reaction, Stevens-Johnson syndrome, suicide, visual abnormality

Overdosage/Toxicology Increased central nervous system symptoms and involuntary muscle contractions have been reported in accidental overdose. Treatment is supportive. Activated charcoal may enhance elimination; dialysis is unlikely to remove the drug.

Drug Interactions Substrate (major) of CYP2B6, 3A4; **Inhibits** CYP2C9 (moderate), 2C19 (moderate), 3A4 (moderate); **Induces** CYP2B6 (weak), 3A4 (strong)

Amprenavir: AUC of amprenavir may be decreased by 36%.

Atazanavir: Serum concentration of atazanavir may be reduced by efavirenz; dosage adjustment of atazanavir is recommended.

Benzodiazepines: Toxicity of some benzodiazepines may be increased by efavirenz; concurrent use of midazolam and triazolam is contraindicated.

Cisapride: Toxicity is significantly increased by efavirenz; concurrent use is contraindicated.

Clarithromycin: Serum concentrations of clarithromycin are decreased by efavirenz, clinical significance unknown; rash reported with concomitant use (46%); azithromycin or other alternative agent should be considered.

CYP2B6 inducers: May decrease the levels/effects of efavirenz. Example inducers include carbamazepine, nevirapine, phenobarbital, phenytoin, and rifampin.

CYP2C9 Substrates: Efavirenz may increase the levels/effects of CYP2C9 substrates. Example substrates include bosentan, dapsone, fluoxetine, glimepiride, glipizide, losartan, montelukast, nateglinide, paclitaxel, phenytoin, warfarin, and zafirlukast.

CYP2C19 substrates: Efavirenz may increase the levels/effects of CYP2C19 substrates. Example substrates include citalopram, diazepam, methsuximide, phenytoin, propranolol, and sertraline.

CYP3A4 inducers: CYP3A4 inducers may decrease the levels/effects of efavirenz. Example inducers include aminoglutethimide, carbamazepine, nafcillin, nevirapine, phenobarbital, phenytoin, and rifamycins.

CYP3A4 substrates: Efavirenz may alter the levels/effects of CYP3A4 substrates. Example substrates include benzodiazepines, calcium channel blockers, ergot derivatives, mirtazapine, nateglinide, nefazodone, tacrolimus, and venlafaxine.

Ergot alkaloids (dihydroergotamine, ergotamine, ergonovine, methylergonovine): Toxicity is significantly increased by efavirenz; concurrent use is contraindicated.

Estrogens (ethinyl estradiol): Serum concentrations of ethinyl estradiol. are increased by efavirenz; clinical significance not known, barrier contraception is recommended.

Indinavir: AUC of indinavir is decreased by 31%; dose of indinavir should be increased.

Lopinavir/ritonavir: Serum concentration of lopinavir are decreased; increase dosage of lopinavir/ritonavir to 533 mg/133 mg twice daily.
Methadone: Serum concentrations of methadone are decreased by efavirenz; stable patients should be monitored for withdrawal.
Nelfinavir: AUC of nelfinavir is increased by 20%.
Rifabutin: Serum concentrations of rifabutin are decreased by efavirenz; rifabutin dose should be increased.
Rifampin: Serum concentrations of efavirenz are decreased by rifampin.
Ritonavir: AUC of both agents are increased by ~20%; associated with increased adverse effects and laboratory abnormalities; monitoring of liver enzymes is recommended.
Saquinavir: AUC of saquinavir is decreased by ~60%; do not use saquinavir as sole protease inhibitor.
Sertraline: Serum concentrations may be decreased by efavirenz.
St John's wort: Specific drug interaction studies have not been conducted; serum concentrations of efavirenz are expected to significantly decrease.
Voriconazole: Serum levels may be reduced by efavirenz; concurrent use is contraindicated.
Warfarin: Serum concentrations of warfarin may be increased or decreased; monitor.

Ethanol/Nutrition/Herb Interactions
Ethanol: Avoid ethanol (hepatic and CNS adverse effects).
Food: Avoid high-fat meals (increase the absorption of efavirenz).
Herb/Nutraceutical: St John's wort may decrease efavirenz serum levels. Avoid concurrent use.

Test Interactions False positive test for cannabinoids have been reported when the CEDIA DAU Multilevel THC assay is used. False positive results with other assays for cannabinoids have not been observed.

Dietary Considerations Should be taken on an empty stomach.

Dosage Forms
Capsule: 50 mg, 100 mg, 200 mg
Tablet: 600 mg

- **Effexor®** *see* Venlafaxine *on page 1347*
- **Effexor® XR** *see* Venlafaxine *on page 1347*
- **EHDP** *see* Etidronate Disodium *on page 495*
- **Elavil** *see* Amitriptyline *on page 89*
- **Eldepryl®** *see* Selegiline *on page 1157*

Eletriptan (el e TRIP tan)

U.S. Brand Names Relpax®
Canadian Brand Names Relpax®
Synonyms Eletriptan Hydrobromide
Pharmacologic Category Serotonin $5\text{-}HT_{1B,\ 1D}$ Receptor Agonist
Generic Available No
Use Acute treatment of migraine, with or without aura
Mechanism of Action Selective agonist for serotonin ($5\text{-}HT_{1B}$, $5\text{-}HT_{1D}$, $5\text{-}HT_{1F}$ receptors) in cranial arteries; causes vasoconstriction and reduce sterile inflammation associated with antidromic neuronal transmission correlating with relief of migraine

Pharmacodynamics/Kinetics
Absorption: Well absorbed
Distribution: V_d: 138 L
Protein binding: ~85%
Metabolism: Hepatic via CYP3A4; forms one metabolite (active)
Bioavailability: ~50%, increased with high-fat meal
Half-life elimination: 4 hours (Elderly: 4.4-5.7 hours); Metabolite: ~13 hours
Time to peak, plasma: 1.5-2 hours

Dosage Oral: Adults: Acute migraine: 20-40 mg; if the headache improves but returns, dose may be repeated after 2 hours have elapsed since first dose; maximum 80 mg/day.
Note: If the first dose is ineffective, diagnosis needs to be re-evaluated. Safety of treating >3 headaches/month has not been established.
Dosage adjustment in renal impairment: No dosing adjustment needed; monitor for increased blood pressure
(Continued)

Eletriptan *(Continued)*

Dosage adjustment in hepatic impairment:
Mild to moderate impairment: No adjustment necessary
Severe impairment: Use is contraindicated

Stability Store at 25°C (77°F); excursions permitted to 15°C to 30°C (59°F to 86°F)

Pregnancy Risk Factor C

Contraindications Hypersensitivity to eletriptan or any component of the formulation; ischemic heart disease or signs or symptoms of ischemic heart disease (including Prinzmetal's angina, angina pectoris, MI, silent myocardial ischemia); cerebrovascular syndromes (including strokes, transient ischemic attacks); peripheral vascular syndromes (including ischemic bowel disease); uncontrolled hypertension; use within 24 hours of ergotamine derivatives; use within 24 hours of another 5-HT_1 agonist; use within 72 hours of potent CYP3A4 inhibitors; management of hemiplegic or basilar migraine; prophylactic treatment of migraine; severe hepatic impairment

Warnings/Precautions Eletriptan is indicated only in patients ≥18 years of age with a clear diagnosis of migraine headache. If a patient does not respond to the first dose, the diagnosis of migraine should be reconsidered. Do not give to patients with risk factors for CAD until a cardiovascular evaluation has been performed; if evaluation is satisfactory, the healthcare provider should administer the first dose and cardiovascular status should be periodically evaluated. Cardiac events (coronary artery vasospasm, transient ischemia, MI, ventricular tachycardia/fibrillation, cardiac arrest, and death), cerebral/subarachnoid hemorrhage, stroke, peripheral vascular ischemia, and colonic ischemia have been reported with 5-HT_1 agonist administration. Significant elevation in blood pressure, including hypertensive crisis, has also been reported on rare occasions in patients with and without a history of hypertension. Use with caution with renal or mild to moderate hepatic impairment. Safety and efficacy in pediatric patients have not been established.

Adverse Reactions

1% to 10%:
Cardiovascular: Chest pain/tightness (1% to 4%; placebo 1%), palpitation
Central nervous system: Dizziness (3% to 7%; placebo 3%), somnolence (3% to 7%; placebo 4%), headache (3% to 4%; placebo 3%), chills, pain, vertigo
Gastrointestinal: Nausea (4% to 8%; placebo 5%), xerostomia (2% to 4%, placebo 2%), dysphagia (1% to 2%), abdominal pain/discomfort (1% to 2%; placebo 1%), dyspepsia (1% to 2%; placebo 1%)
Neuromuscular & skeletal: Weakness (4% to 10%), paresthesia (3% to 4%), back pain, hypertonia, hypoesthesia
Respiratory: Pharyngitis
Miscellaneous: Diaphoresis

<1% (Limited to important or life-threatening): Agitation, allergic reaction, angina, arrhythmia, ataxia, confusion, constipation, CPK increased, depersonalization, depression, diarrhea, dreams (abnormal), dyspnea, edema, emotional lability, esophagitis, euphoria, hyperesthesia, hyperkinesia, hypertension, impotence, incoordination, insomnia, lacrimation disorder, liver function tests abnormal, myalgia, myasthenia, nervousness, peripheral vascular disorder, photophobia, polyuria, pruritus, rash, salivation increased, shock, speech disorder, stupor, tachycardia, taste perversion, thrombophlebitis, tinnitus, tongue edema, tremor, urinary frequency, vasospasm, vision abnormal

Overdosage/Toxicology Hypertension or more serious cardiovascular symptoms may occur. Clinical and electrocardiographic monitoring needed for at least 20 hours even if patient is asymptomatic. Treatment is symptom-directed and supportive.

Drug Interactions Substrate of CYP3A4 (major)

CYP3A4 inhibitors: May increase the levels/effects of eletriptan. Example inhibitors include azole antifungals, clarithromycin, diclofenac, doxycycline, erythromycin, imatinib, isoniazid, nefazodone, nicardipine, propofol, protease inhibitors, quinidine, telithromycin, and verapamil.

Ergot-containing drugs: Prolong vasospastic reactions; do not use eletriptan or ergot-containing drugs within 24 hours of each other.

Ethanol/Nutrition/Herb Interactions Food: High-fat meal increases bioavailability.

Dosage Forms Tablet, as hydrobromide: 20 mg, 40 mg [as base]

Emtricitabine (em trye SYE ta been)

U.S. Brand Names Emtriva®

Canadian Brand Names Emtriva®

Synonyms BW524W91; Coviracil; FTC

Pharmacologic Category Antiretroviral Agent, Reverse Transcriptase Inhibitor (Nucleoside)

Generic Available No

Use Treatment of HIV infection in combination with at least two other antiretroviral agents

Unlabeled/Investigational Use Hepatitis B (with HIV coinfection)

Mechanism of Action Nucleoside reverse transcriptase inhibitor; emtricitabine is a cytosine analogue which is phosphorylated intracellularly to emtricitabine 5'-triphosphate which interferes with HIV viral RNA dependent DNA polymerase resulting in inhibition of viral replication.

Pharmacodynamics/Kinetics

Absorption: Rapid, extensive

Protein binding: <4%

Metabolism: Limited, via oxidation and conjugation (not via CYP isoenzymes)

Bioavailability: Capsule: 93%; solution: 75%

Half-life elimination: Normal renal function: Adults: 10 hours; children: 5-18 hours

Time to peak, plasma: 1-2 hours

Excretion: Urine (86% primarily as unchanged drug, 13% as metabolites); feces (14%)

Dosage Oral:

Children: 3 months to 17 years:

Capsule: Children >33 kg: 200 mg once daily

Solution: 6 mg/kg once daily; maximum: 240 mg/day

Adults:

Capsule: 200 mg once daily

Solution: 240 mg once daily

Dosage adjustment in renal impairment: Adults (consider similar adjustments in children):

Cl_{cr} 30-49 mL/minute: Capsule: 200 mg every 48 hours; solution: 120 mg every 24 hours

Cl_{cr} 15-29 mL/minute: Capsule: 200 mg every 72 hours; solution: 80 mg every 24 hours

Cl_{cr} <15 mL/minute (including hemodialysis patients): Capsule: 200 mg every 96 hours; solution: 60 mg every 24 hours; administer after dialysis on dialysis days

Dosage adjustment in hepatic impairment: No adjustment required.

Stability Store capsules at 15°C to 30°C (59°F to 86°F). Solution should be stored under refrigeration at 2°C to 8°C (36°F to 46°F); once dispensed, may be stored at 15°C to 30°C (59°F to 86°F) if used within 3 months.

Administration May be administered with or without food.

Monitoring Parameters Viral load, CD4, liver function tests; hepatitis B testing is recommended prior to initiation of therapy

Pregnancy Risk Factor B

Contraindications Hypersensitivity to emtricitabine or any component of the formulation

Warnings/Precautions **[U.S. Boxed Warning]: Lactic acidosis, severe hepatomegaly, and hepatic failure have occurred rarely with emtricitabine (similar to other nucleoside analogues).** Some cases have been fatal; stop treatment if lactic acidosis or hepatotoxicity occur. Prior liver disease, obesity,
(Continued)

Emtricitabine *(Continued)*

extended duration of therapy, and female gender may represent risk factors for severe hepatic reactions. Testing for hepatitis B is recommended prior to the initiation of therapy; **[U.S. Boxed Warnings]: Hepatitis B may be exacerbated following discontinuation of emtricitabine; not indicated for treatment of chronic hepatitis B; safety and efficacy in HIV/HBV co-infected patients not established.** Immune reconstitution syndrome may develop resulting in the occurrence of an inflammatory response to an indolent or residual opportunistic infection; further evaluation and treatment may be required. Use caution in patients with renal impairment (dosage adjustment required). Safety and efficacy in children ≤3 years of age have not been established.

Adverse Reactions Clinical trials were conducted in patients receiving other antiretroviral agents, and it is not possible to correlate frequency of adverse events with emtricitabine alone. The range of frequencies of adverse events is generally comparable to comparator groups, with the exception of hyperpigmentation, which occurred more frequently in patients receiving emtricitabine. Unless otherwise noted, percentages are as reported in adults.

>10%:

Central nervous system: Dizziness (4% to 25%), headache (13% to 22%), fever (children 18%), insomnia (7% to 16%), abnormal dreams (2% to 11%)

Dermatologic: Hyperpigmentation (adults 2% to 4%; children 32%; primarily of palms and/or soles but may include tongue, arms, lip and nails; generally mild and nonprogressive without associated local reactions such as pruritus or rash); rash (17% to 30%; includes pruritus, maculopapular rash, vesiculobullous rash, pustular rash, and allergic reaction)

Gastrointestinal: Diarrhea (adults 23%; children 20%), vomiting (adults 9%; children 23%), nausea (13% to 18%), abdominal pain (8% to 14%), gastroenteritis (children 11%)

Neuromuscular & skeletal: Weakness (12% to 16%), CPK increased (11% to 12%)

Otic: Otitis media (children 23%)

Respiratory: Cough (adults 14%; children 28%), rhinitis (adults 12% to 18%; children 20%), pneumonia (children 15%)

Miscellaneous: Infection (children 44%)

1% to 10%:

Central nervous system: Depression (6% to 9%), neuropathy/neuritis (4%)

Endocrine & metabolic: Serum triglycerides increased (9% to 10%), disordered glucose homeostasis (2% to 3%), serum amylase increased (adults 2% to 5%; children 9%), serum lipase increased (≤1%)

Gastrointestinal: Dyspepsia (4% to 8%)

Hematologic: Anemia (children: 7%)

Hepatic: Transaminases increased (2% to 6%), bilirubin increased (1%)

Neuromuscular & skeletal: Myalgia (4% to 6%), paresthesia (5% to 6%), arthralgia (3% to 5%)

Overdosage/Toxicology Treatment is supportive and symptom-directed. Approximately 30% of a dose is removed by hemodialysis.

Drug Interactions Note: Limited drug interaction data available. No evidence of a clinically-significant interaction when administered with tenofovir, indinavir, famciclovir, zidovudine, or stavudine.

Ribavirin: Concomitant use of ribavirin and nucleoside analogues may increase the risk of developing lactic acidosis.

Ethanol/Nutrition/Herb Interactions Food: Food decreases peak plasma concentrations, but does not alter the extent of absorption or overall systemic exposure.

Dietary Considerations May be taken with or without food.

Dosage Forms

Capsule: 200 mg

Solution: 10 mg/mL (170 mL) [cotton candy flavor]

♦ **Emtriva®** *see* Emtricitabine *on page 445*

Enalapril (e NAL a pril)

Medication Safety Issues

Sound-alike/look-alike issues:

Enalapril may be confused with Anafranil®, Elavil®, Eldepryl®, nafarelin, ramipril

Related Information

Angiotensin Agents *on page 1544*
Heart Failure (Systolic) *on page 1607*
Hypertension *on page 1620*
Postoperative Hypertension *on page 1471*
Preoperative Evaluation of the Cardiac Patient for Noncardiac Surgery *on page 1485*

U.S. Brand Names Vasotec®

Canadian Brand Names Vasotec®

Synonyms Enalaprilat; Enalapril Maleate

Pharmacologic Category Angiotensin-Converting Enzyme (ACE) Inhibitor

Generic Available Yes

Use Management of mild to severe hypertension; treatment of congestive heart failure, left ventricular dysfunction after myocardial infarction

Unlabeled/Investigational Use

Unlabeled: Hypertensive crisis, diabetic nephropathy, rheumatoid arthritis, diagnosis of anatomic renal artery stenosis, hypertension secondary to scleroderma renal crisis, diagnosis of aldosteronism, idiopathic edema, Bartter's syndrome, postmyocardial infarction for prevention of ventricular failure

Investigational: Severe congestive heart failure in infants, neonatal hypertension, acute pulmonary edema

Mechanism of Action Competitive inhibitor of angiotensin-converting enzyme (ACE); prevents conversion of angiotensin I to angiotensin II, a potent vasoconstrictor; results in lower levels of angiotensin II which causes an increase in plasma renin activity and a reduction in aldosterone secretion

Pharmacodynamics/Kinetics

Onset of action: Oral: ~1 hour
Duration: Oral: 12-24 hours
Absorption: Oral: 55% to 75%
Protein binding: 50% to 60%
Metabolism: Prodrug, undergoes hepatic biotransformation to enalaprilat
Half-life elimination:
  Enalapril: Adults: Healthy: 2 hours; Congestive heart failure: 3.4-5.8 hours
  Enalaprilat: Infants 6 weeks to 8 months old: 6-10 hours; Adults: 35-38 hours
Time to peak, serum: Oral: Enalapril: 0.5-1.5 hours; Enalaprilat (active): 3-4.5 hours
Excretion: Urine (60% to 80%); some feces

Dosage Use lower listed initial dose in patients with hyponatremia, hypovolemia, severe congestive heart failure, decreased renal function, or in those receiving diuretics.

Oral: **Enalapril**: Children 1 month to 16 years: Hypertension: Initial: 0.08 mg/kg (up to 5 mg) once daily; adjust dosage based on patient response; doses >0.58 mg/kg (40 mg) have not been evaluated in pediatric patients

Investigational: Congestive heart failure: Initial oral doses of **enalapril**: 0.1 mg/kg/day increasing as needed over 2 weeks to 0.5 mg/kg/day have been used in infants

Investigational: Neonatal hypertension: I.V. doses of **enalaprilat**: 5-10 mcg/kg/dose administered every 8-24 hours have been used; monitor patients carefully; select patients may require higher doses

Adults:

Oral: **Enalapril:**

Hypertension: 2.5-5 mg/day then increase as required, usually at 1- to 2-week intervals; usual dose range (JNC 7): 2.5-40 mg/day in 1-2 divided doses. **Note:** Initiate with 2.5 mg if patient is taking a diuretic which cannot be discontinued. May add a diuretic if blood pressure cannot be controlled with enalapril alone.

Heart failure: Initial: 2.5 mg once or twice daily (usual range: 5-40 mg/day in 2 divided doses). Titrate slowly at 1- to 2-week intervals. Target dose: 10-20 mg twice daily (ACC/AHA 2005 Heart Failure Guidelines)

Asymptomatic left ventricular dysfunction: 2.5 mg twice daily, titrated as tolerated to 20 mg/day

I.V.: **Enalaprilat:**

Hypertension: 1.25 mg/dose, given over 5 minutes every 6 hours; doses as high as 5 mg/dose every 6 hours have been tolerated for up to 36 hours. **Note:** If patients are concomitantly receiving diuretic therapy, begin with 0.625 mg I.V. over 5 minutes; if the effect is not adequate after 1 hour,

(Continued)

Enalapril *(Continued)*

repeat the dose and administer 1.25 mg at 6-hour intervals thereafter; if adequate, administer 0.625 mg I.V. every 6 hours.

Heart failure: Avoid I.V. administration in patients with unstable heart failure or those suffering acute myocardial infarction.

Conversion from I.V. to oral therapy if not concurrently on diuretics: 5 mg once daily; subsequent titration as needed; if concurrently receiving diuretics and responding to 0.625 mg I.V. every 6 hours, initiate with 2.5 mg/day.

Dosing adjustment in renal impairment:

Oral: Enalapril:

Cl_{cr} 30-80 mL/minute: Administer 5 mg/day titrated upwards to maximum of 40 mg.

Cl_{cr} <30 mL/minute: Administer 2.5 mg day; titrated upward until blood pressure is controlled.

For heart failure patients with sodium <130 mEq/L or serum creatinine >1.6 mg/dL, initiate dosage with 2.5 mg/day, increasing to twice daily as needed. Increase further in increments of 2.5 mg/dose at >4-day intervals to a maximum daily dose of 40 mg.

I.V.: Enalaprilat:

Cl_{cr} >30 mL/minute: Initiate with 1.25 mg every 6 hours and increase dose based on response.

Cl_{cr} <30 mL/minute: Initiate with 0.625 mg every 6 hours and increase dose based on response.

Hemodialysis: Moderately dialyzable (20% to 50%); administer dose postdialysis (eg, 0.625 mg I.V. every 6 hours) or administer 20% to 25% supplemental dose following dialysis; Clearance: 62 mL/minute.

Peritoneal dialysis: Supplemental dose is not necessary, although some removal of drug occurs.

Dosing adjustment in hepatic impairment: Hydrolysis of enalapril to enalaprilat may be delayed and/or impaired in patients with severe hepatic impairment, but the pharmacodynamic effects of the drug do not appear to be significantly altered; no dosage adjustment.

Stability Enalaprilat: Clear, colorless solution which should be stored at <30°C; I.V. is 24 hours at room temperature in D_5W or NS

Administration Administer direct IVP over at least 5 minutes or dilute up to 50 mL and infuse; discontinue diuretic, if possible, for 2-3 days before beginning enalapril therapy

Monitoring Parameters Blood pressure, renal function, WBC, serum potassium; blood pressure monitor required during intravenous administration

Anesthesia and Critical Care Concerns/Other Considerations Severe hypotension may occur in patients who are sodium and/or volume depleted, initiate lower doses and monitor closely when starting therapy in these patients

ACE inhibitors decrease morbidity and mortality in patients with asymptomatic and symptomatic left ventricular dysfunction. In this situation, they decrease hospitalizations for, and retard progression to, congestive heart failure. ACE inhibitors are also indicated in patients postmyocardial infarction in whom left ventricular ejection fraction is <40%. When used in patients with heart failure, the target dose of 10 mg twice daily should be achieved, if possible. Lower daily doses of ACE inhibitors have not demonstrated the same cardioprotective effects.

ACE inhibitor therapy may elicit rapid increases in potassium and creatinine, especially when used in patients with bilateral renal artery stenosis. When ACE inhibition is introduced in patients with pre-existing diuretic therapy who are hypovolemic, the ACE inhibitor may induce acute hypotension.

Pregnancy Risk Factor C (1st trimester)/D (2nd and 3rd trimesters)

Contraindications Hypersensitivity to enalapril or enalaprilat; angioedema related to previous treatment with an ACE inhibitor; patients with idiopathic or hereditary angioedema; bilateral renal artery stenosis; pregnancy (2nd and 3rd trimesters)

Warnings/Precautions Anaphylactic reactions can occur. Angioedema can occur at any time during treatment (especially following first dose). It may involve head and neck (potentially affecting the airway) or the intestine (presenting with abdominal pain). Prolonged monitoring may be required especially if tongue, glottis, or larynx are involved as they are associated with airway obstruction. Those with a history of airway surgery in this situation have a higher risk. Careful blood pressure monitoring with first dose (hypotension can occur especially in volume-depleted patients). **[U.S. Boxed Warning]: Based on human data, ACEIs can cause injury and death to the developing fetus when used in the second and third trimesters. ACEIs should be discontinued as soon as possible once pregnancy is detected.** Dosage adjustment needed in renal impairment. Use with caution in hypovolemia; collagen vascular diseases; valvular stenosis (particularly aortic stenosis); hyperkalemia; or before, during, or immediately after anesthesia. Avoid rapid dosage escalation which may lead to renal insufficiency.

Rare toxicities associated with ACE inhibitors include cholestatic jaundice (which may progress to hepatic necrosis) and neutropenia/agranulocytosis with myeloid hyperplasia. Hypersensitivity reactions may be seen during hemodialysis with high-flux dialysis membranes (eg, AN69). Hyperkalemia may rarely occur. If patient has renal impairment then a baseline WBC with differential and serum creatinine should be evaluated and monitored closely during the first 3 months of therapy. Use with caution in unilateral renal artery stenosis and pre-existing renal insufficiency.

Adverse Reactions Note: Frequency ranges include data from hypertension and heart failure trials. Higher rates of adverse reactions have generally been noted in patients with CHF. However, the frequency of adverse effects associated with placebo is also increased in this population.

1% to 10%:

- Cardiovascular: Hypotension (0.9% to 6.7%), chest pain (2%), syncope (0.5% to 2%), orthostasis (2%), orthostatic hypotension (2%)
- Central nervous system: Headache (2% to 5%), dizziness (4% to 8%), fatigue (2% to 3%)
- Dermatologic: Rash (1.5%)
- Gastrointestinal: Abnormal taste, abdominal pain, vomiting, nausea, diarrhea, anorexia, constipation
- Neuromuscular & skeletal: Weakness
- Renal: Increased serum creatinine (0.2% to 20%), worsening of renal function (in patients with bilateral renal artery stenosis or hypovolemia)
- Respiratory (1% to 2%): Bronchitis, cough, dyspnea

<1% (Limited to important or life-threatening): Agranulocytosis, alopecia, angina pectoris, angioedema, ataxia, bronchospasm, cardiac arrest, cerebral vascular accident, depression, erythema multiforme, exfoliative dermatitis, giant cell arteritis, gynecomastia, hallucinations, hemolysis with G6PD, Henoch-Schönlein purpura, hepatitis, ileus, impotence, jaundice, lichen-form reaction, MI, neutropenia, ototoxicity, pancreatitis, paresthesia, pemphigus, pemphigus foliaceus, photosensitivity, psychosis, pulmonary edema, sicca syndrome, Stevens-Johnson syndrome, systemic lupus erythematosus, toxic epidermal necrolysis, toxic pustuloderma, vertigo. Worsening of renal function may occur in patients with bilateral renal artery stenosis or in hypovolemic patients. A syndrome which may include fever, myalgia, arthralgia, interstitial nephritis, vasculitis, rash, eosinophilia and positive ANA, and elevated ESR has been reported for enalapril and other ACE inhibitors.

Overdosage/Toxicology Mild hypotension has been the primary toxic effect seen with acute overdose. Bradycardia may also occur. Hyperkalemia occurs even with therapeutic doses, especially in patients with renal insufficiency and those taking NSAIDs. Following initiation of essential overdose management, toxic symptom treatment and supportive treatment should be initiated.

Drug Interactions Substrate of CYP3A4 (major)

- $Alpha_1$ blockers: Hypotensive effect increased.
- Aspirin: The effects of ACE inhibitors may be blunted by aspirin administration, particularly at higher dosages and/or increase adverse renal effects.
- CYP3A4 inducers: CYP3A4 inducers may decrease the levels/effects of enalapril. Example inducers include aminoglutethimide, carbamazepine, nafcillin, nevirapine, phenobarbital, phenytoin, and rifamycins.
- Diuretics: Hypovolemia due to diuretics may precipitate acute hypotensive events or acute renal failure.
- Insulin: Risk of hypoglycemia may be increased.
- Lithium: Risk of lithium toxicity may be increased; monitor lithium levels, especially in the first 4 weeks of therapy.
- Mercaptopurine: Risk of neutropenia may be increased.

(Continued)

Enalapril *(Continued)*

NSAIDs: May attenuate hypertensive efficacy; effect has been seen with captopril and may occur with other ACE inhibitors; monitor blood pressure. May increase risk of renal adverse effects.

Potassium-sparing diuretics (amiloride, spironolactone, triamterene): Increased risk of hyperkalemia.

Potassium supplements may increase the risk of hyperkalemia.

Trimethoprim (high dose) may increase the risk of hyperkalemia.

Ethanol/Nutrition/Herb Interactions Herb/Nutraceutical: St John's wort may decrease enalapril levels. Avoid dong quai if using for hypertension (has estrogenic activity). Avoid ephedra, yohimbe, ginseng (may worsen hypertension). Avoid natural licorice (causes sodium and water retention and increases potassium loss). Avoid garlic (may have increased antihypertensive effect).

Test Interactions Positive Coombs' [direct]; may cause false-positive results in urine acetone determinations using sodium nitroprusside reagent

Dietary Considerations Limit salt substitutes or potassium-rich diet.

Dosage Forms

Injection, solution, as enalaprilat: 1.25 mg/mL (1 mL, 2 mL) [contains benzyl alcohol]

Tablet, as maleate (Vasotec®): 2.5 mg, 5 mg, 10 mg, 20 mg

References

Erstad BL and Barletta JF, "Treatment of Hypertension in the Perioperative Patient," *Ann Pharmacother*, 2000, 34(1):66-79.

- **Enalaprilat** *see* Enalapril *on page 446*
- **Enalapril Maleate** *see* Enalapril *on page 446*
- **Encort™** *see* Hydrocortisone *on page 639*
- **Endantadine® (Can)** *see* Amantadine *on page 77*
- **Endocet®** *see* Oxycodone and Acetaminophen *on page 969*
- **Endodan® [DSC]** *see* Oxycodone and Aspirin *on page 971*
- **Endo®-Levodopa/Carbidopa (Can)** *see* Levodopa and Carbidopa *on page 743*
- **Enerjets [OTC]** *see* Caffeine *on page 211*

Enflurane (EN floo rane)

Medication Safety Issues

Sound-alike/look-alike issues:

Enflurane may be confused with isoflurane

Related Information

Anesthesia Considerations for Neurosurgery *on page 1401*

Chronic Renal Failure *on page 1437*

Inhalational Anesthetics *on page 1528*

U.S. Brand Names Compound 347™; Ethrane®

Pharmacologic Category General Anesthetic, Inhalation

Generic Available No

Use Maintenance of general anesthesia

Pharmacodynamics/Kinetics

Onset of action: 7-10 minutes

Duration: Emergence time: Depends on blood concentration when enflurane is discontinued

Metabolism: Hepatic (2% to 10%)

Excretion: Exhaled gases

Dosage Minimum alveolar concentration (MAC), the concentration at which 50% of patients do not respond to surgical incision, is 1.6% for enflurane. The concentration at which amnesia and loss of awareness occur (MAC - awake) is 0.4%. Surgical levels of anesthesia are achieved with concentrations between 0.5% to 3%. MAC is reduced in the elderly.

Administration Via enflurane-specific calibrated vaporizers

Monitoring Parameters Blood pressure, heart rate and rhythm, temperature, oxygen saturation, end-tidal CO_2 and end-tidal enflurane concentrations should be monitored prior to and throughout anesthesia

Anesthesia and Critical Care Concerns/Other Considerations Use of enflurane for induction of general anesthesia is not recommended due to its airway irritant properties and unpleasant odor which may cause breath holding and coughing.

Contraindications Hypersensitivity to enflurane or any component of the formulation; known or suspected history of malignant hyperthermia

Warnings/Precautions Decrease in blood pressure is dose dependent, primarily due to peripheral vasodilation. Enflurane does not depress cardiac conduction nor does it sensitize the myocardium to catecholamine-induced arrhythmias like halothane. Respiration is depressed with a $PaCO_2$ of 55 mm Hg at 1 MAC. Hypoxic pulmonary vasoconstriction is blunted. EEG seizure complexes have been seen with higher doses especially associated with hypocarbia; therefore, it is not recommended for use in patients with seizure history. Hypoxia induced increase in ventilation is abolished at low enflurane concentration. Enflurane dilates the cerebral vasculature and may, in certain conditions, increase intracranial pressure. Renal, splenic, and hepatic blood flow are reduced. Enflurane is a trigger of malignant hyperthermia.

Adverse Reactions Frequency not defined.

Cardiovascular: Hypotension, myocardial depression, tachycardia

Central nervous system: Seizure activity during or after emergence from enflurane anesthesia; motor activity and/or seizure, especially with hypocapnia

Gastrointestinal: Nausea, vomiting

Hepatic: Hepatic injury, hepatic failure (rare)

Renal: Renal dysfunction, nephrotoxicity

Respiratory: Respiratory depression/arrest, hypoxemia, breath holding, cough

Miscellaneous: Shivering

Drug Interactions Substrate of CYP2E1 (major)

Aminoglycosides: Concomitant use may increase risk of nephrotoxicity.

Antihypertensives: Excessive hypotension may occur with combined use.

Benzodiazepines, opioids: Concurrent use of opioids and/or benzodiazepines decreases the MAC of enflurane.

CYP2E1 inhibitors: May increase the levels/effects of enflurane. Example inhibitors include disulfiram, isoniazid, and miconazole.

Neuromuscular-blocking agents (nondepolarizing): Enflurane may potentiate the action of nondepolarizing, neuromuscular-blocking agents.

Dosage Forms Liquid, for inhalation: >99.9% (250 mL)

References

Campagna JA, Miller KW, and Forman SA, "Mechanisms of Action of Inhaled Anesthetics," *N Engl J Med*, 2003, 348(21):2110-23.

Cousins MJ, Greenstein LR, Hitt BA, et al, "Metabolism and Renal Effects of Enflurane in Man," *Anesthesiology*, 1976, 44(1):44-53.

Gion H and Saidman LJ, "The Minimum Alveolar Concentration of Enflurane in Man," *Anesthesiology*, 1971, 35(4):361-4.

♦ **Engerix-B®** *see* Hepatitis B Vaccine *on page 620*

♦ **Engerix-B® and Havrix®** *see* Hepatitis A Inactivated and Hepatitis B (Recombinant) Vaccine *on page 615*

♦ **Enlon®** *see* Edrophonium *on page 439*

Enoxaparin (ee noks a PA rin)

Medication Safety Issues

Sound-alike/look-alike issues:

Lovenox® may be confused with Lotronex®, Protonix®

High alert medication: The Institute for Safe Medication Practices (ISMP) includes this medication among its list of drugs which have a heightened risk of causing significant patient harm when used in error.

Related Information

Heparin and Low Molecular Weight Heparin (LMWH) *on page 1527*

U.S. Brand Names Lovenox®

Canadian Brand Names Enoxaparin Injection; Lovenox®; Lovenox® HP

Synonyms Enoxaparin Sodium

Pharmacologic Category Low Molecular Weight Heparin

Generic Available No

Use

DVT Treatment (acute): Inpatient treatment (patients with and without pulmonary embolism) and outpatient treatment (patients without pulmonary embolism)

(Continued)

Enoxaparin *(Continued)*

DVT prophylaxis: Following hip or knee replacement surgery, abdominal surgery, or in medical patients with severely-restricted mobility during acute illness in patients at risk of thromboembolic complications

Note: High-risk patients include those with one or more of the following risk factors: >40 years of age, obesity, general anesthesia lasting >30 minutes, malignancy, history of deep vein thrombosis or pulmonary embolism

Unstable angina and non-Q-wave myocardial infarction (to prevent ischemic complications)

Unlabeled/Investigational Use Prophylaxis and treatment of thromboembolism in children

Mechanism of Action Standard heparin consists of components with molecular weights ranging from 4000-30,000 daltons with a mean of 16,000 daltons. Heparin acts as an anticoagulant by enhancing the inhibition rate of clotting proteases by antithrombin III impairing normal hemostasis and inhibition of factor Xa. Low molecular weight heparins have a small effect on the activated partial thromboplastin time and strongly inhibit factor Xa. Enoxaparin is derived from porcine heparin that undergoes benzylation followed by alkaline depolymerization. The average molecular weight of enoxaparin is 4500 daltons which is distributed as (≤20%) 2000 daltons (≥68%) 2000-8000 daltons, and (≤15%) >8000 daltons. Enoxaparin has a higher ratio of antifactor Xa to antifactor IIa activity than unfractionated heparin.

Pharmacodynamics/Kinetics

Onset of action: Peak effect: SubQ: Antifactor Xa and antithrombin (antifactor IIa): 3-5 hours

Duration: 40 mg dose: Antifactor Xa activity: ~12 hours

Metabolism: Hepatic, to lower molecular weight fragments (little activity)

Protein binding: Does not bind to heparin binding proteins

Half-life elimination, plasma: 2-4 times longer than standard heparin, independent of dose; based on anti-Xa activity: 4.5-7 hours

Excretion: Urine (40% of dose; 10% as active fragments)

Dosage SubQ:

Infants and Children (unlabeled use):

Infants <2 months: Initial:

Prophylaxis: 0.75 mg/kg every 12 hours

Treatment: 1.5 mg/kg every 12 hours

Infants >2 months and Children ≤18 years: Initial:

Prophylaxis: 0.5 mg/kg every 12 hours

Treatment: 1 mg/kg every 12 hours

Maintenance: See **Dosage Titration** table:

Enoxaparin Pediatric Dosage Titration

Antifactor Xa	Dose Titration	Time to Repeat Antifactor Xa Level
<0.35 units/mL	Increase dose by 25%	4 h after next dose
0.35-0.49 units/mL	Increase dose by 10%	4 h after next dose
0.5-1 unit/mL	Keep same dosage	Next day, then 1 wk later, then monthly (4 h after dose)
1.1-1.5 units/mL	Decrease dose by 20%	Before next dose
1.6-2 units/mL	Hold dose for 3 h and decrease dose by 30%	Before next dose, then 4 h after next dose
>2 units/mL	Hold all doses until antifactor Xa is 0.5 units/mL, then decrease dose by 40%	Before next dose and every 12 h until antifactor Xa <0.5 units/mL

Modified from Monagle P, Michelson AD, Bovill E, et al, "Antithrombotic Therapy in Children," *Chest*, 2001, 119:344S-70S.

Adults:

DVT prophylaxis:

Hip replacement surgery:

Twice-daily dosing: 30 mg twice daily, with initial dose within 12-24 hours after surgery, and every 12 hours until risk of DVT has diminished or the patient is adequately anticoagulated on warfarin.

Once-daily dosing: 40 mg once daily, with initial dose within 9-15 hours before surgery, and daily until risk of DVT has diminished or the patient is adequately anticoagulated on warfarin.

Knee replacement surgery: 30 mg twice daily, with initial dose within 12-24 hours after surgery, and every 12 hours until risk of DVT has diminished (usually 7-10 days).

Abdominal surgery: 40 mg once daily, with initial dose given 2 hours prior to surgery; continue until risk of DVT has diminished (usual 7-10 days).

Medical patients with severely-restricted mobility during acute illness: 40 mg once daily; continue until risk of DVT has diminished

DVT treatment (acute): **Note:** Start warfarin within 72 hours and continue enoxaparin until INR is between 2.0 and 3.0 (usually 7 days).

Inpatient treatment (with or without pulmonary embolism): 1 mg/kg/dose every 12 hours or 1.5 mg/kg once daily.

Outpatient treatment (without pulmonary embolism): 1 mg/kg/dose every 12 hours.

Unstable angina or non-Q-wave MI: 1 mg/kg twice daily in conjunction with oral aspirin therapy (100-325 mg once daily); continue until clinical stabilization (a minimum of at least 2 days)

Elderly: Increased incidence of bleeding with doses of 1.5 mg/kg/day or 1 mg/kg every 12 hours; injection-associated bleeding and serious adverse reactions are also increased in the elderly. Careful attention should be paid to elderly patients <45 kg.

Dosing adjustment in renal impairment: SubQ:

Cl_{cr} ≥30 mL/minute: No specific adjustment recommended (per manufacturer); monitor closely for bleeding

Cl_{cr} <30 mL/minute:

DVT prophylaxis in abdominal surgery, hip replacement, knee replacement, or in medical patients during acute illness: 30 mg once daily

DVT treatment (inpatient or outpatient treatment in conjunction with warfarin): 1 mg/kg once daily

Unstable angina, non-Q-wave MI (with ASA): 1 mg/kg once daily

Dialysis: Enoxaparin has not been FDA approved for use in dialysis patients. It's elimination is primarily via the renal route. Serious bleeding complications have been reported with use in patients who are dialysis dependent or have severe renal failure. LMWH administration at fixed doses without monitoring has greater unpredictable anticoagulant effects in patients with chronic kidney disease. If used, dosages should be reduced and anti-Xa activity frequently monitored, as accumulation may occur with repeated doses. Many clinicians would not use enoxaparin in this population especially without timely anti-Xa activity assay results.

Hemodialysis: Supplemental dose is not necessary.

Peritoneal dialysis: Significant drug removal is unlikely based on physiochemical characteristics.

Stability Store at 15°C to 25°C (59°F to 77°F); do not freeze; do not mix with other injections or infusions

Administration Should be administered by deep SubQ injection to the left or right anterolateral and left or right posterolateral abdominal wall. To avoid loss of drug from the 30 mg and 40 mg syringes, do not expel the air bubble from the syringe prior to injection. In order to minimize bruising, do not rub injection site. An automatic injector (Lovenox EasyInjector™) is available with the 30 mg and 40 mg syringes to aid the patient with self-injections. **Note:** Enoxaparin is available in 100 mg/mL and 150 mg/mL concentrations.

Monitoring Parameters Platelets, occult blood, and anti-Xa activity, if available; the monitoring of PT and/or aPTT is not necessary

Anesthesia and Critical Care Concerns/Other Considerations Many critically-ill and surgical patients require preventative measures for venous thromboembolism. Low molecular weight heparins (LMWHs) compare favorably to unfractionated heparin in the prevention and treatment of venous thromboembolism. LMWHs are associated with less thrombocytopenia, compared to heparin, and do not require routine therapeutic monitoring.

Obesity/Renal Dysfunction: There is no consensus for adjusting/correcting the weight-based dosage of LMWH for patients who are morbidly obese. Monitoring of antifactor Xa concentration 4 hours after injection may be warranted. Patients who have a reduction in calculated creatinine clearance are at risk of accumulated anticoagulant effect when they are treated with certain LMWHs. All LMWHs

(Continued)

Enoxaparin *(Continued)*

may not behave the same in patients with renal dysfunction. Some clinicians monitor anti-Xa levels in patients with Cl_{cr} <30 mL/minute.

Pregnancy Risk Factor B

Contraindications Hypersensitivity to enoxaparin, heparin, or any component of the formulation; thrombocytopenia associated with a positive *in vitro* test for antiplatelet antibodies in the presence of enoxaparin; hypersensitivity to pork products; active major bleeding; not for I.M. or I.V. use

Warnings/Precautions

[U.S. Boxed Warning]: Patients with recent or anticipated neuraxial anesthesia (epidural or spinal anesthesia) are at risk of spinal or epidural hematoma and subsequent paralysis. Consider risk versus benefit prior to neuraxial anesthesia; risk is increased by concomitant agents which may alter hemostasis, as well as traumatic or repeated epidural or spinal puncture. Patient should be observed closely for bleeding if enoxaparin is administered during or immediately following diagnostic lumbar puncture, epidural anesthesia, or spinal anesthesia.

Do not administer intramuscularly. Not recommended for thromboprophylaxis in patients with prosthetic heart valves (especially pregnant women). Not to be used interchangeably (unit for unit) with heparin or any other low molecular weight heparins. Use caution in patients with history of heparin-induced thrombocytopenia. Monitor patient closely for signs or symptoms of bleeding. Certain patients are at increased risk of bleeding. Risk factors include bacterial endocarditis; congenital or acquired bleeding disorders; active ulcerative or angiodysplastic GI diseases; severe uncontrolled hypertension; hemorrhagic stroke; use shortly after brain, spinal, or ophthalmology surgery; patients treated concomitantly with platelet inhibitors; recent GI bleeding; thrombocytopenia or platelet defects; severe liver disease; hypertensive or diabetic retinopathy; or in patients undergoing invasive procedures. Monitor platelet count closely. Rare cases of thrombocytopenia have occurred. Manufacturer recommends discontinuation of therapy if platelets are <100,000/mm^3. Risk of bleeding may be increased in women <45 kg and in men <57 kg. Use caution in patients with renal failure; dosage adjustment needed if Cl_{cr} <30 mL/minute. Safety and efficacy in pediatric patients have not been established. Use with caution in the elderly (delayed elimination may occur). Heparin can cause hyperkalemia by affecting aldosterone. Similar reactions could occur with LMWHs. Monitor for hyperkalemia. Multiple-dose vials contain benzyl alcohol (use caution in pregnant women).

Adverse Reactions As with all anticoagulants, bleeding is the major adverse effect of enoxaparin. Hemorrhage may occur at virtually any site. Risk is dependent on multiple variables. At the recommended doses, single injections of enoxaparin do not significantly influence platelet aggregation or affect global clotting time (ie, PT or aPTT).

1% to 10%:

- Central nervous system: Fever (5% to 8%), confusion, pain
- Dermatologic: Erythema, bruising
- Gastrointestinal: Nausea (3%), diarrhea
- Hematologic: Hemorrhage (5% to 13%), thrombocytopenia (2%), hypochromic anemia (2%)
- Hepatic: Increased ALT/AST
- Local: Injection site hematoma (9%), local reactions (irritation, pain, ecchymosis, erythema)

<1% (Limited to important or life-threatening): Allergic reaction, anaphylactoid reaction, eczematous plaques, hyperlipidemia, hypersensitivity cutaneous vasculitis, hypertriglyceridemia, itchy erythematous patches. pruritus, purpura, skin necrosis, thrombocytosis, urticaria, vesicobullous rash. Retroperitoneal or intracranial bleed (some fatal). Spinal or epidural hematomas can occur following neuraxial anesthesia or spinal puncture, resulting in paralysis. Risk is increased in patients with indwelling epidural catheters or concomitant use of other drugs affecting hemostasis. Cases of heparin-induced thrombocytopenia with thrombosis (some complicated by organ infarction, limb ischemia, or death) have been reported. Prosthetic valve thrombosis, including fatal cases, has been reported in pregnant women receiving enoxaparin as thromboprophylaxis.

Overdosage/Toxicology Symptoms of overdose include hemorrhage. Protamine sulfate has been used to reverse effects (protamine 1 mg neutralizes enoxaparin 1 mg). Monitor aPTT 2-4 hours after first infusion; consider readministration of protamine (50% of original dose). Note: anti-Xa activity is never completely neutralized (maximum of 60% to 75%). Avoid overdose of protamine.

Drug Interactions

Drugs which affect platelet function (eg, aspirin, NSAIDs, dipyridamole, ticlopidine, clopidogrel) may potentiate the risk of hemorrhage.

Thrombolytic agents increase the risk of hemorrhage.

Warfarin: Risk of bleeding may be increased during concurrent therapy. Enoxaparin is commonly continued during the initiation of warfarin therapy to assure anticoagulation and to protect against possible transient hypercoagulability.

Ethanol/Nutrition/Herb Interactions Herb/Nutraceutical: Avoid cat's claw, dong quai, evening primrose, feverfew, garlic, ginger, ginkgo, red clover, horse chestnut, green tea, ginseng (all have additional antiplatelet activity).

Dosage Forms

Injection, solution, as sodium [graduated prefilled syringe; preservative free]: 60 mg/0.6 mL (0.6 mL); 80 mg/0.8 mL (0.8 mL); 100 mg/mL (1 mL); 120 mg/0.8 mL (0.8 mL); 150 mg/mL (1 mL)

Injection, solution, as sodium [multidose vial]: 100 mg/mL (3 mL) [contains benzyl alcohol]

Injection, solution, as sodium [prefilled syringe; preservative free]: 30 mg/0.3 mL (0.3 mL); 40 mg/0.4 mL (0.4 mL)

References

Nagge J, Crowther M, and Hirsh J, "Is Impaired Renal Function a Contraindication to the Use of Low-Molecular Weight Heparin?" *Arch Intern Med*, 2002, 162(22):2605-9.

- **Enoxaparin Injection (Can)** *see* Enoxaparin *on page 451*
- **Enoxaparin Sodium** *see* Enoxaparin *on page 451*
- **Entrophen® (Can)** *see* Aspirin *on page 129*
- **Entsol® [OTC]** *see* Sodium Chloride *on page 1183*
- **Enulose®** *see* Lactulose *on page 724*

Ephedrine (e FED rin)

Medication Safety Issues

Sound-alike/look-alike issues:

Ephedrine may be confused with Epifrin®, epinephrine

Related Information

Contrast Media Reactions, Premedication for Prophylaxis *on page 1602*

U.S. Brand Names Pretz-D® [OTC]

Synonyms Ephedrine Sulfate

Pharmacologic Category Alpha/Beta Agonist

Generic Available Yes

Use Treatment of bronchial asthma, nasal congestion, acute bronchospasm, idiopathic orthostatic hypotension, hypotension induced by spinal anesthesia

Mechanism of Action Releases tissue stores of epinephrine and thereby produces an alpha- and beta-adrenergic stimulation; longer-acting and less potent than epinephrine

Pharmacodynamics/Kinetics

Onset of action: Oral: Bronchodilation: 0.25-1 hour

Duration: Oral: 3-6 hours

Distribution: Crosses placenta; enters breast milk

Metabolism: Minimally hepatic

Half-life elimination: 2.5-3.6 hours

Excretion: Urine (60% to 77% as unchanged drug) within 24 hours

Dosage

Children:

Oral, SubQ: 3 mg/kg/day or 25-100 mg/m^2/day in 4-6 divided doses every 4-6 hours

I.M., slow I.V. push: 0.2-0.3 mg/kg/dose every 4-6 hours

Adults:

Oral: 25-50 mg every 3-4 hours as needed

I.M., SubQ: 25-50 mg, parenteral adult dose should not exceed 150 mg in 24 hours

I.M.: Hypotension induced by anesthesia: 25 mg

I.V.: 5-25 mg/dose slow I.V. push repeated after 5-10 minutes as needed, then every 3-4 hours not to exceed 150 mg/24 hours

(Continued)

Ephedrine *(Continued)*

Nasal spray:

Children 6-12 years: 1-2 sprays into each nostril, not more frequently than every 4 hours

Children ≥12 years and Adults: 2-3 sprays into each nostril, not more frequently than every 4 hours

Stability Protect all dosage forms from light

Monitoring Parameters Injection solution: Monitor blood pressure, pulse

Anesthesia and Critical Care Concerns/Other Considerations For I.V. administration, give the undiluted injection slowly. Additional I.V. doses may be given every 5-10 minutes if needed. Do not exceed adult parenteral dose of 150 mg/24 hours. Do not exceed pediatric dose of 3 mg/kg/24 hours. Use the smallest effective dose. Anesthesiologists may administer to treat nausea and vomiting that has failed traditional antiemetic therapy and might be caused by hypotension.

Pregnancy Risk Factor C

Contraindications Hypersensitivity to ephedrine or any component of the formulation; cardiac arrhythmias; angle-closure glaucoma; concurrent use of other sympathomimetic agents

Warnings/Precautions Blood volume depletion should be corrected before ephedrine therapy is instituted; use caution in patients with unstable vasomotor symptoms, diabetes, hyperthyroidism, prostatic hyperplasia, or a history of seizures; also use caution in the elderly and those patients with cardiovascular disorders such as coronary artery disease, arrhythmias, and hypertension. Ephedrine may cause hypertension resulting in intracranial hemorrhage. Long-term use may cause anxiety and symptoms of paranoid schizophrenia. Avoid as a bronchodilator; generally not used as a bronchodilator since new $beta_2$ agents are less toxic. Use with caution in the elderly, since it crosses the blood-brain barrier and may cause confusion.

Adverse Reactions Frequency not defined.

Cardiovascular: Hypertension, tachycardia, palpitation, elevation or depression of blood pressure, unusual pallor, chest pain, arrhythmia

Central nervous system: CNS stimulating effects, nervousness, anxiety, apprehension, fear, tension, agitation, excitation, restlessness, irritability, insomnia, hyperactivity, dizziness, headache

Gastrointestinal: Xerostomia, nausea, anorexia, GI upset, vomiting

Genitourinary: Painful urination

Neuromuscular & skeletal: Trembling, tremor (more common in the elderly), weakness

Respiratory: Dyspnea

Miscellaneous: Diaphoresis (increased)

Overdosage/Toxicology Symptoms of overdose include dysrhythmias, CNS excitation, respiratory depression, vomiting, and convulsions. There is no specific antidote for ephedrine intoxication and treatment is primarily supportive.

Drug Interactions

Alpha- and beta-adrenergic-blocking agents decrease ephedrine vasopressor effects.

Cardiac glycosides or general anesthetics may increase cardiac stimulation.

MAO inhibitors or atropine may increase blood pressure

Sympathomimetic agents: Additive cardiostimulation with other sympathomimetic agents.

Theophylline may lead to cardiostimulation.

Ethanol/Nutrition/Herb Interactions Herb/Nutraceutical: Avoid ephedra, yohimbe (may cause CNS stimulation).

Test Interactions Can cause a false-positive amphetamine EMIT assay

Dosage Forms

Capsule, as sulfate: 25 mg

Injection, solution, as sulfate: 50 mg/mL (1 mL, 10 mL)

Solution, intranasal spray, as sulfate (Pretz-D®): 0.25% (50 mL)

References

Pickup ME, May CS, Sendagire R, et al, "The Pharmacokinetics of Ephedrine After Oral Dosage in Asthmatics Receiving Acute and Chronic Treatment," *Br J Clin Pharmacol*, 1976, 3(1):123-34.

Stein GC, "Requirements for Pharmacists Dispensing Ephedrine Products," *Am J Health Syst Pharm*, 1995, 52(15):1630.

♦ **Ephedrine Sulfate** *see* Ephedrine *on page 455*

Epinephrine (ep i NEF rin)

Medication Safety Issues

Sound-alike/look-alike issues:

Epinephrine may be confused with ephedrine

Epifrin® may be confused with ephedrine, EpiPen®

EpiPen® may be confused with Epifrin®

Medication errors have occurred due to confusion with epinephrine products expressed as ratio strengths (eg, 1:1000 vs 1:10,000).

Epinephrine 1:1000 = 1 mg/mL and is most commonly used SubQ.

Epinephrine 1:10,000 = 0.1 mg/mL and is used I.V.

Related Information

Allergic Reactions *on page 1395*

Critical Care Infusion Administration Charts *on page 1514*

Hemodynamic Support, Intravenous *on page 1566*

U.S. Brand Names Adrenalin®; EpiPen®; EpiPen® Jr; Primatene® Mist [OTC]; Raphon [OTC]; S2® [OTC]; Twinject™

Canadian Brand Names Adrenalin®; EpiPen®; EpiPen® Jr

Synonyms Adrenaline; Epinephrine Bitartrate; Epinephrine Hydrochloride; Racepinephrine

Pharmacologic Category Alpha/Beta Agonist; Antidote

Generic Available Yes: Solution for injection

Use Treatment of bronchospasms, bronchial asthma, nasal congestion, viral croup, anaphylactic reactions, cardiac arrest; added to local anesthetics to decrease systemic absorption of local anesthetics and increase duration of action; decrease superficial hemorrhage

Unlabeled/Investigational Use ACLS guidelines: Ventricular fibrillation (VF) or pulseless ventricular tachycardia (VT) unresponsive to initial defibrillatory shocks; pulseless electrical activity, asystole, hypotension unresponsive to volume resuscitation; symptomatic bradycardia or hypotension unresponsive to atropine or pacing; inotropic support

Mechanism of Action Stimulates alpha-, beta$_1$-, and beta$_2$-adrenergic receptors resulting in relaxation of smooth muscle of the bronchial tree, cardiac stimulation, and dilation of skeletal muscle vasculature; small doses can cause vasodilation via beta$_2$-vascular receptors; large doses may produce constriction of skeletal and vascular smooth muscle

Pharmacodynamics/Kinetics

Onset of action: Bronchodilation: SubQ: ~5-10 minutes; Inhalation: ~1 minute

Distribution: Crosses placenta

Metabolism: Taken up into the adrenergic neuron and metabolized by monoamine oxidase and catechol-o-methyltransferase; circulating drug hepatically metabolized

Excretion: Urine (as inactive metabolites, metanephrine, and sulfate and hydroxy derivatives of mandelic acid, small amounts as unchanged drug)

Dosage

Neonates: Cardiac arrest: I.V.: 0.01-0.03 mg/kg (0.1-0.3 mL/kg of **1:10,000** solution) every 3-5 minutes as needed. Although I.V. route is preferred, may consider administration of doses up to 0.1 mg/kg through the endotracheal tube until I.V. access established; dilute intratracheal doses to 1-2 mL with normal saline.

Infants and Children:

Asystole/pulseless arrest, bradycardia, VT/VF (after failed defibrillations):

I.V., I.O.: 0.01 mg/kg (0.1 mL/kg of **1:10,000** solution) every 3-5 minutes as needed (maximum: 1 mg)

Intratracheal: 0.1 mg/kg (0.1 mL/kg of **1:1000** solution) every 3-5 minutes (maximum: 10 mg)

Continuous I.V. infusion: 0.1-1 mcg/kg/; doses <0.3 mcg/kg/minute generally produce β-adrenergic effects and higher doses generally produce α-adrenergic vasoconstriction; titrate dosage to desired effect

Bronchodilator: SubQ: 0.01 mg/kg (0.01 mL/kg of **1:1000**) (single doses not to exceed 0.5 mg) every 20 minutes for 3 doses

Nebulization: 1-3 inhalations up to every 3 hours using solution prepared with 10 drops of 1:100

(Continued)

Epinephrine *(Continued)*

Children <4 years: S2® (racepinephrine, OTC labeling): Croup: 0.05 mL/kg (max 0.5 mL/dose); dilute in NS 3 mL. Administer over ~15 minutes; do not administer more frequently than every 2 hours.

Inhalation: Children ≥4 years: Primatene® Mist: Refer to Adults dosing.

Decongestant: Children ≥6 years: Refer to Adults dosing

Hypersensitivity reaction:

SubQ, I.V.: 0.01 mg/kg every 20 minutes; larger doses or continuous infusion may be needed for some anaphylactic reactions

SubQ, I.M.:

15-30 kg: Twinject™: 0.15 mg (for self-administration following severe allergic reactions to insect stings, food, etc)

>30 kg: Refer to Adults dosing

I.M.:

<30 kg: Epipen® Jr: 0.15 mg (for self-administration following severe allergic reactions to insect stings, food, etc)

>30 kg: Refer to Adults dosing

Adults:

Asystole/pulseless arrest, bradycardia, VT/VF:

I.V., I.O.: 1 mg every 3-5 minutes; if this approach fails, higher doses of epinephrine (up to 0.2 mg/kg) may be indicated for treatment of specific problems (eg, beta-blocker or calcium channel blocker overdose)

Intratracheal: Administer 2-2.5 mg for VF or pulseless VT if I.V./I.O. access is delayed or cannot be established; dilute in 5-10 mL NS or distilled water. **Note:** Absorption is greater with distilled water, but causes more adverse effects on PaO_2.

Bradycardia (symptomatic) or hypotension (not responsive to atropine or pacing): I.V. infusion: 2-10 mcg/minute; titrate to desired effect

Bronchodilator:

SubQ: 0.3-0.5 mg **(1:1000)** every 20 minutes for 3 doses

Nebulization: 1-3 inhalations up to every 3 hours using solution prepared with 10 drops of the **1:100** product

S2® (racepinephrine, OTC labeling): 0.5 mL (~10 drops). Dose may be repeated not more frequently than very 3-4 hours if needed. Solution should be diluted if using jet nebulizer.

Inhalation: Primatene® Mist (OTC labeling): One inhalation, wait at least 1 minute; if relieved, may use once more. Do not use again for at least 3 hours.

Decongestant: Intranasal: Apply 1:1000 locally as drops or spray or with sterile swab

Hypersensitivity reaction:

I.M., SubQ: 0.3-0.5 mg (1:1000) every 15-20 minutes if condition requires (I.M route is preferred)

>30 kg: Twinject™: 0.3 mg (for self-administration following severe allergic reactions to insect stings, food, etc)

I.M.: >30 kg: Epipen®: 0.3 mg (for self-administration following severe allergic reactions to insect stings, food, etc)

I.V.: 0.1 mg (1:10,000) over 5 minutes. May infuse at 1-4 mcg/minute to prevent the need to repeat injections frequently.

Stability

Epinephrine is sensitive to light and air; protection from light is recommended. Oxidation turns drug pink, then a brown color. **Solutions should not be used if they are discolored or contain a precipitate.**

Adrenalin®: Store between 15°C to 25°C (59°F to 77°F); protect from light and freezing. The 1:1000 solution should be discarded 30 days after initial use.

Raphon: Store between 2°C to 25°C (36°F to 77°F). Refrigerate after opening.

Twinject™: Store between 20°C to 25°C (68°F to 77°F); protect from light and freezing. Do not refrigerate.

Stability of injection of parenteral admixture at room temperature (25°C) or refrigeration (4°C): 24 hours

Standard I.V. diluent: 1 mg/250 mL NS

Preparation of adult I.V. infusion: Dilute 1 mg in 250 mL of D_5W or NS (4 mcg/mL). Administer at an initial rate of 1 mcg/minute and increase to desired effects. At 20 mcg/minute pure alpha effects occur.

S2®: Dilution not required when administered via hand-nebulizer; dilute with NS 3-5 mL if using jet nebulizer

Administration Central line administration only. I.V. infusions require an infusion pump. Epinephrine solutions for injection can be administered SubQ, I.M., I.V., I.O.; I.M. administration into the buttocks should be avoided.

Inhalation: S2®: Administer over ~15 minutes; must be diluted if using jet nebulizer

Intratracheal: Dilute in NS or distilled water. Absorption is greater with distilled water, but causes more adverse effects on PaO_2. Pass catheter beyond tip of tracheal tube, stop compressions, spray drug quickly down tube. Follow immediately with several quick insufflations and continue chest compressions.

Extravasation management: Use phentolamine as antidote. Mix 5 mg with 9 mL of NS. Inject a small amount of this dilution into extravasated area. Blanching should reverse immediately. Monitor site. If blanching should recur, additional injections of phentolamine may be needed.

Monitoring Parameters Pulmonary function, heart rate, blood pressure, site of infusion for blanching, extravasation; cardiac monitor and blood pressure monitor required. If using to treat hypotension, assess intravascular volume and support as needed.

Reference Range Therapeutic: 31-95 pg/mL (SI: 170-520 pmol/L)

Anesthesia and Critical Care Concerns/Other Considerations

Septic Shock: Epinephrine's use may be limited by its effects on renal and gastric blood flow and its propensity to increase lactic acid concentrations.

Cardiac Arrest: Epinephrine can be given by endotracheal route during cardiac resuscitation. High-intravenous dose epinephrine (0.1 mg/kg) has not shown to improve survival or neurological outcomes. May have more postresuscitation complications than survivors who receive standard dose epinephrine. Eight randomized clinical studies (>9000 patients) have found no improvement in survival to hospital discharge or neurological outcomes compared with standard epinephrine.

A prospective, multicenter, double-blind randomized, controlled trial evaluated the efficacy of vasopressin or epinephrine when administered to adult patients who suffered an out-of-hospital cardiac arrest (Wenzel V, 2004). For inclusions, patients presented with ventricular fibrillation, pulseless electrical activity, or asystole. They were excluded if they were successfully defibrillated without the administration of a vasopressor, had a terminal illness or had a DNR order, a lack of intravenous access, hemorrhagic shock, pregnancy, cardiac arrest due to trauma, or were <18 years of age. Eligible patients were randomized to intravenous vasopressin (40 units) or epinephrine (1 mg). Each patient received an injection of the study drug, if spontaneous circulation was not restored in 3 minutes they received a second dose (same amount) of the same study drug. If there was no response, the managing physician had the option of giving epinephrine. Patients with ventricular fibrillation were randomized after the first three attempts at defibrillation failed; all others were randomized immediately. The primary endpoint was survival to hospital admission; the secondary endpoint was survival to hospital discharge. Five hundred and eighty-nine patients were randomized to vasopressin and five hundred and ninety-seven patients were randomized to epinephrine. There was no significant difference in the rate of hospital admission between the vasopressin group and the epinephrine group if they had ventricular fibrillation (46.2% vs 43% respectively, p: 0.48) or pulseless electrical activity (33.7% vs 30.5% respectively, p: 0.65). Patients with asystole responded significantly better to vasopressin; having higher rates of hospital admission (29% vs 20.3% in the epinephrine group, p: 0.02) and hospital discharge (4.7% vs 1.5% in the epinephrine group, p: 0.04). Patients who failed vasopressin therapy and received additional epinephrine had significant improvement in survival to hospital admission (25.7% vs 16.4% in the epinephrine group, p: 0.002) and discharge (6.2% vs 1.7%, p: 0.002). Similar patients who were randomized to epinephrine and failed to respond did not improve with additional epinephrine. Cerebral performance among all patients who survived to discharge was similar in both groups. In this trial, vasopressin was superior to epinephrine in patients with asystole. Vasopressin followed by epinephrine may be more effective than epinephrine alone in refractory out-of-hospital cardiac arrest.

A small in-hospital cardiac arrest study evaluated the efficacy of vasopressin or epinephrine in 200 patients. These investigators did not find any differences between the two treatment groups with regard to survival, discharge, or cerebral performance (Stiell I, 2001).

Pregnancy Risk Factor C

(Continued)

Epinephrine *(Continued)*

Contraindications Hypersensitivity to epinephrine or any component of the formulation; cardiac arrhythmias; angle-closure glaucoma

Warnings/Precautions Use with caution in elderly patients, patients with diabetes mellitus, cardiovascular diseases (angina, tachycardia, myocardial infarction), thyroid disease, or cerebral arteriosclerosis, Parkinson's; some products contain sulfites as preservatives. Rapid I.V. infusion may cause death from cerebrovascular hemorrhage or cardiac arrhythmias. Oral inhalation of epinephrine is **not** the preferred route of administration. Avoid topical application where reduced perfusion could lead to ischemic tissue damage (eg, penis, ears, digits).

Adverse Reactions Frequency not defined.

Cardiovascular: Angina, cardiac arrhythmia, chest pain, flushing, hypertension, increased myocardial oxygen consumption, pallor, palpitation, sudden death, tachycardia (parenteral), vasoconstriction, ventricular ectopy

Central nervous system: Anxiety, dizziness, headache, insomnia, lightheadedness, nervousness, restlessness

Gastrointestinal: Dry throat, nausea, vomiting, xerostomia

Genitourinary: Acute urinary retention in patients with bladder outflow obstruction

Neuromuscular & skeletal: Trembling, weakness

Ocular: Allergic lid reaction, burning, eye pain, ocular irritation, precipitation of or exacerbation of narrow-angle glaucoma, transient stinging

Renal: Decreased renal and splanchnic blood flow

Respiratory: Dyspnea, wheezing

Miscellaneous: Diaphoresis (increased)

Overdosage/Toxicology Symptoms of overdose include arrhythmias, unusually large pupils, pulmonary edema, renal failure, metabolic acidosis; and hypertension, which may result in subarachnoid hemorrhage and hemiplegia. There is no specific antidote for epinephrine intoxication and treatment is primarily supportive.

Drug Interactions Increased toxicity: Increased cardiac irritability if administered concurrently with halogenated inhalational anesthetics, beta-blocking agents, alpha-blocking agents

Ethanol/Nutrition/Herb Interactions Herb/Nutraceutical: Avoid ephedra, yohimbe (may cause CNS stimulation).

Test Interactions Increased bilirubin (S), catecholamines (U), glucose, uric acid (S)

Dosage Forms

Aerosol for oral inhalation:

Primatene® Mist: 0.22 mg/inhalation (15 mL, 22.5 mL) [contains CFCs]

Injection, solution [prefilled auto injector]:

EpiPen®: 0.3 mg/0.3 mL [1:1000] (2 mL) [contains sodium metabisulfite; available as single unit or in double-unit pack with training unit]

EpiPen® Jr: 0.15 mg/0.3 mL [1:2000] (2 mL) [contains sodium metabisulfite; available as single unit or in double-unit pack with training unit]

Twinject™: 0.15 mg/0.15 mL [1:1000] (1.1 mL) [contains sodium bisulfite; two 0.15 mg doses per injector]; 0.3 mg/0.3 mL [1:1000] (1.1 mL) [contains sodium bisulfite; two 0.3 mg doses per injector]

Injection, solution, as hydrochloride: 0.1 mg/mL [1:10,000] (10 mL); 1 mg/mL [1:1000] (1 mL) [products may contain sodium metabisulfite]

Adrenalin®: 1 mg/mL [1:1000] (1 mL, 30 mL) [contains sodium bisulfite]

Solution for oral inhalation, as hydrochloride:

Adrenalin®: 1% [10 mg/mL, 1:100] (7.5 mL) [contains sodium bisulfite]

Solution for oral inhalation [racepinephrine]:

S2®: 2.25% (0.5 mL, 15 mL) [as d-epinephrine 1.125% and l-epinephrine 1.125%; contains metabisulfites]

Solution, topical [racepinephrine]:

Raphon: 2.25% (15 mL) [as d-epinephrine 1.125% and l-epinephrine 1.125%; contains metabisulfites]

References

American Heart Association and the International Liaison Committee on Resuscitation (ILCOR), "Guidelines 2000 Conference for Cardiopulmonary Resuscitation and Emergency Cardiovascular Care: International Consensus on Science," *Circulation*, 2000, 102(8):I1-252.

Mokhlesi B, Leikin JB, Murray P, et al, "Adult Toxicology in Critical Care. Part 11: Specific Poisonings," *Chest*, 2003, 123(3):897-922.

Murphy FT, Manown TJ, Knutson SW, et al, "Epinephrine-Induced Lactic Acidosis in the Setting of Status Asthmaticus," *South Med J*, 1995, 88(5):577-9.

Stiell IG, Hebert PC, Wells GA, et al, "Vasopressin Versus Epinephrine for in Hospital Cardiac Arrest: A Randomised Controlled Trial," *Lancet*, 2001, 358(9276):105-9.

Wenzel V, Krismer AC, Arntz HR, et al, "A Comparison of Vasopressin and Epinephrine for Out-of-Hospital Cardiopulmonary Resuscitation," *N Engl J Med*, 2004, 350(2):105-13.

- **Epinephrine Bitartrate** *see* Epinephrine *on page 457*
- **Epinephrine Hydrochloride** *see* Epinephrine *on page 457*
- **EpiPen®** *see* Epinephrine *on page 457*
- **EpiPen® Jr** *see* Epinephrine *on page 457*
- **Epitol®** *see* Carbamazepine *on page 225*
- **Epival® I.V. (Can)** *see* Valproic Acid and Derivatives *on page 1329*
- **Epivir®** *see* Lamivudine *on page 725*
- **Epivir-HBV®** *see* Lamivudine *on page 725*

Eplerenone (e PLER en one)

Medication Safety Issues
Sound-alike/look-alike issues:
Inspra™ may be confused with Spiriva®

U.S. Brand Names Inspra™

Pharmacologic Category Diuretic, Potassium-Sparing; Selective Aldosterone Blocker

Generic Available No

Use Treatment of hypertension (may be used alone or in combination with other antihypertensive agents); treatment of CHF following acute MI

Mechanism of Action Aldosterone increases blood pressure primarily by inducing sodium reabsorption. Eplerenone reduces blood pressure by blocking aldosterone binding at mineralocorticoid receptors found in the kidney, heart, blood vessels and brain.

Pharmacodynamics/Kinetics
Distribution: V_d: 43-90 L
Protein binding: ~50%; primarily to $alpha_1$-acid glycoproteins
Metabolism: Primarily hepatic via CYP3A4; metabolites inactive
Half-life elimination: 4-6 hours
Time to peak, plasma: 1.5 hours; may take up to 4 weeks for full therapeutic effect
Excretion: Urine (67%; <5% as unchanged drug), feces (32%)

Dosage Oral: Adults:
Hypertension: Initial: 50 mg once daily; may increase to 50 mg twice daily if response is not adequate; may take up to 4 weeks for full therapeutic response. Doses >100 mg/day are associated with increased risk of hyperkalemia and no greater therapeutic effect.
Concurrent use with moderate CYP3A4 inhibitors: Initial: 25 mg once daily
Congestive heart failure (post-MI): Initial: 25 mg once daily; dosage goal: titrate to 50 mg once daily within 4 weeks, as tolerated
Dosage adjustment per serum potassium concentrations for CHF:
<5.0 mEq/L:
Increase dose from 25 mg every other day to 25 mg daily **or**
Increase dose from 25 mg daily to 50 mg daily
5.0-5.4 mEq/L: No adjustment needed
5.5-5.9 mEq/L:
Decrease dose from 50 mg daily to 25 mg daily **or**
Decrease dose from 25 mg daily to 25 mg every other day **or**
Decrease does from 25 mg every other day to withhold medication
≥6.0 mEq/L: Withhold medication until potassium <5.5 mEq/L, then restart at 25 mg every other day

Dosage adjustment in renal impairment:
Patients with hypertension with Cl_{cr} <50 mL/minute or serum creatinine >2.0 mg/dL in males or >1.8 mg/dL in females: Use is contraindicated; risk of hyperkalemia increases with declining renal function
Patients with CHF post-MI: Use with caution

Dosage adjustment in hepatic impairment: No dosage adjustment needed for mild-to-moderate impairment; safety and efficacy not established for severe impairment

Stability Store at controlled room temperature of 25°C (77°F).

Administration May be administered with or without food.

Monitoring Parameters Blood pressure; serum potassium (levels monitored every 2 weeks for the first 1-2 months, then monthly in clinical trials); renal function

(Continued)

Eplerenone *(Continued)*

Pregnancy Risk Factor B

Contraindications Hypersensitivity to eplerenone or any component of the formulation; serum potassium >5.5 mEq/L; Cl_{cr} ≤30 mL/minute; concomitant use of strong CYP3A4 inhibitors (see Drug Interactions for details)

The following additional contraindications apply to patients with hypertension: Type 2 diabetes mellitus (noninsulin dependent, NIDDM) with microalbuminuria; serum creatinine >2.0 mg/dL in males or >1.8 mg/dL in females; Cl_{cr} <50 mL/minute; concomitant use with potassium supplements or potassium-sparing diuretics

Warnings/Precautions Dosage adjustment needed for patients on moderate CYP3A4 inhibitors (see Drug Interactions for details). Monitor closely for hyperkalemia; increases in serum potassium were dose related during clinical trials and rates of hyperkalemia also increased with declining renal function. Safety and efficacy have not been established in pediatric patients or in patients with severe hepatic impairment. Use with caution in CHF patients post-MI with diabetes.

Adverse Reactions

>10%: Endocrine & metabolic: Hypertriglyceridemia (1% to 15%, dose related)

1% to 10%:

- Central nervous system: Dizziness (3%), fatigue (2%)
- Endocrine & metabolic: Breast pain (males <1% to 1%), creatinine increased (6% in CHF), gynecomastia (males <1% to 1%), hyponatremia (2%, dose related), hypercholesterolemia (<1% to 1%); hyperkalemia (mild-to-moderate hypertension <1%; left ventricular dysfunction ~6% had serum potassium ≥6 mEq/L)
- Gastrointestinal: Diarrhea (2%), abdominal pain (1%)
- Genitourinary: Abnormal vaginal bleeding (<1% to 2%)
- Renal: Albuminuria (1%)
- Respiratory: Cough (2%)
- Miscellaneous: Flu-like syndrome (2%)

<1% (Limited to important or life-threatening): BUN increased, liver function tests increased, serum creatinine increased, uric acid increased

Overdosage/Toxicology Cases of human overdose have not been reported; hypotension or hyperkalemia would be expected. Treatment should be symptom-directed and supportive. Eplerenone is not removed by hemodialysis; binds extensively to charcoal.

Drug Interactions **Substrate** of CYP3A4 (major)

ACE inhibitors: Concomitant use increases serum potassium, use of ACE inhibitors and another mineralocorticoid receptor blocker has led to clinically relevant hyperkalemia. Use with caution; monitoring of potassium levels recommended.

Angiotensin II receptor antagonists: Concomitant use increases serum potassium, use of angiotensin II receptor antagonists and another mineralocorticoid receptor blocker has led to clinically relevant hyperkalemia. Use with caution; monitoring of potassium levels recommended.

CYP3A4 inducers: CYP3A4 inducers may decrease the levels/effects of eplerenone. Example inducers include aminoglutethimide, carbamazepine, nafcillin, nevirapine, phenobarbital, phenytoin, and rifamycins.

CYP3A4 inhibitors: May increase the levels/effects of eplerenone. Example inhibitors include azole antifungals, ciprofloxacin, clarithromycin, diclofenac, doxycycline, erythromycin, imatinib, isoniazid, nefazodone, nicardipine, propofol, protease inhibitors, quinidine, and verapamil.

Lithium: Interaction studies have not been conducted, however, monitoring of lithium levels is recommended.

NSAIDs: Interaction studies have not been conducted, however, NSAIDs may decrease the antihypertensive effects and cause hyperkalemia in patients with impaired renal function. Blood pressure should be monitored closely.

Potassium-sparing diuretics (amiloride, spironolactone, triamterene): Increase risk of hyperkalemia; concurrent use is contraindicated.

Potassium supplements: Increase risk of hyperkalemia; concurrent use is contraindicated.

Ethanol/Nutrition/Herb Interactions

Food: Grapefruit juice increases eplerenone AUC ~25%.

Herb/Nutraceutical: St John's wort decreases eplerenone AUC ~30%.

Dietary Considerations May be taken with or without food. Do not use salt substitutes containing potassium.

Dosage Forms Tablet: 25 mg, 50 mg

♦ **EPO** *see* Epoetin Alfa *on page 463*

Epoetin Alfa (e POE e tin AL fa)

Medication Safety Issues

Sound-alike/look-alike issues:

Epoetin alfa may be confused with darbepoetin alfa

U.S. Brand Names Epogen®; Procrit®

Canadian Brand Names Eprex®

Synonyms EPO; Erythropoietin; NSC-724223; *r*HuEPO-α

Pharmacologic Category Colony Stimulating Factor

Generic Available No

Use Treatment of anemia related to HIV therapy, chronic renal failure, antineoplastic therapy (for nonmyeloid malignancies); reduction of allogeneic blood transfusion for elective, noncardiac, nonvascular surgery

Unlabeled/Investigational Use Anemia associated with rheumatic disease; hypogenerative anemia of Rh hemolytic disease; sickle cell anemia; acute renal failure; Gaucher's disease; Castleman's disease; paroxysmal nocturnal hemoglobinuria; anemia of critical illness (limited documentation); anemia of prematurity

Mechanism of Action Induces erythropoiesis by stimulating the division and differentiation of committed erythroid progenitor cells; induces the release of reticulocytes from the bone marrow into the bloodstream, where they mature to erythrocytes. There is a dose response relationship with this effect. This results in an increase in reticulocyte counts followed by a rise in hematocrit and hemoglobin levels.

Pharmacodynamics/Kinetics

Onset of action: Several days

Peak effect: 2-3 weeks

Distribution: V_d: 9 L; rapid in the plasma compartment; concentrated in liver, kidneys, and bone marrow

Metabolism: Some degradation does occur

Bioavailability: SubQ: ~21% to 31%; intraperitoneal epoetin: 3% (a few patients)

Half-life elimination: Cancer: SubQ: 16-67 hours; Chronic renal failure: 4-13 hours

Time to peak, serum: Chronic renal failure: 5-13 hours

Excretion: Feces (majority); urine (small amounts, 10% unchanged in normal volunteers)

Dosage

Chronic renal failure patients: I.V., SubQ:

Children: Initial dose: 50 units/kg 3 times/week

Adults: Initial dose: 50-100 units/kg 3 times/week

Dose adjustment: Children and Adults: Reduce dose by 25% when hemoglobin approaches 12 g/dL **or** hemoglobin increases 1 g/dL in any 2-week period. Increase dose by 25% if hemoglobin does not increase by 2 g/dL after 8 weeks of therapy (with adequate iron stores, may increase dose by 25% if hemoglobin increase <1 g/dL over 4 weeks) and hemoglobin is below suggested target range. Suggested target hemoglobin range: 10-12 g/dL. Do not increase dose more frequently than at 4-week intervals.

Maintenance dose: Individualize to target range; limit additional dosage increases to every 4 weeks (or longer)

Dialysis patients: Median dose:

Children: 167 units/kg/week (hemodialysis) **or** 76 units/kg/week (peritoneal dialysis)

Adults: 75 units/kg 3 times/week

Nondialysis patients:

Children: Dosing range: 50-250 units/kg 1-3 times/week

Adults: Median dose: 75-150 units/kg/week

Zidovudine-treated, HIV-infected patients (patients with erythropoietin levels >500 mU/mL are **unlikely** to respond): I.V., SubQ:

Children: Initial dose: Reported dosing range: 50-400 units/kg 2-3 times/week

Adults: 100 units/kg 3 times/week for 8 weeks. **Dose adjustment:** Increase dose by 50-100 units/kg 3 times/week if response is not satisfactory in terms of reducing transfusion requirements or increasing hemoglobin after 8 weeks of therapy. Evaluate response every 4-8 weeks thereafter and adjust the dose accordingly by 50-100 units/kg increments 3 times/week. If patient has not responded satisfactorily to a 300 unit/kg dose 3 times/week, a response to higher doses is unlikely. Stop dose if hemoglobin exceeds 13 g/dL and

(Continued)

Epoetin Alfa *(Continued)*

resume treatment at a 25% dose reduction when hemoglobin drops to 12 g/dL.

Cancer patient on chemotherapy: Treatment of patients with erythropoietin levels >200 mU/mL is **not recommended**

Children: I.V.: 600 units/kg once weekly (maximum: 40,000 units)

Adults: SubQ: Initial dose: 150 units/kg 3 times/week or 40,000 units once weekly; commonly used doses range from 10,000 units 3 times/week to 40,000-60,000 units once weekly.

Dose adjustment: Children and Adults: If response is not satisfactory after a sufficient period of evaluation (8 weeks of 3 times/week and 4 weeks of once-weekly therapy), the dose may be increased every 4 weeks (or longer) up to 300 units/kg 3 times/week, **or** when dosed weekly, increased all at once to 60,000 units weekly (adults) or 900 units/kg/week; maximum 60,000 units (pediatrics). If patient does not respond, a response to higher doses is unlikely. Stop dose if hemoglobin exceeds 13 g/dL and resume treatment at a 25% dose reduction when hemoglobin drops to 12 g/dL; reduce dose by 25% if hemoglobin increases by 1 g/dL in any 2-week period, or if hemoglobin approaches 12 g/dL.

Alternative dose (unlabeled dosing): Adults: SubQ: Initial dose: 60,000 units once weekly for 8 weeks. **Dose adjustment:** If patient does not respond, a response to higher doses is unlikely. If response is adequate (hemoglobin increases >2 g/dL after 8 weeks), begin maintenance dose of 120,000 units, to be given once every 3 weeks. During any point of initial or maintenance therapy, if the hemoglobin increases 1.3 g/dL in a 2-week period, decrease dose to 40,000 units once weekly. Stop dose if hemoglobin exceeds 15 g/dL and resume treatment at 20,000 units once-weekly when hemoglobin drops to 13 g/dL.

Surgery patients: Prior to initiating treatment, obtain a hemoglobin to establish that is >10 mg/dL or ≤13 mg/dL: Adults: SubQ: Initial dose: 300 units/kg/day for 10 days before surgery, on the day of surgery, and for 4 days after surgery

Alternative dose: 600 units/kg in once weekly doses (21, 14, and 7 days before surgery) plus a fourth dose on the day of surgery

Anemia of critical illness (unlabeled use): Adults: SubQ: 40,000 units once weekly

Anemia of prematurity (unlabeled use): Infants: I.V., SubQ: Dosing range: 500-1250 units/kg/week; commonly used dose: 250 units/kg 3 times/week; supplement with oral iron therapy 3-8 mg/kg/day

Dosage adjustment in renal impairment:

Hemodialysis: Supplemental dose is not necessary.

Peritoneal dialysis: Supplemental dose is not necessary.

Stability

Vials should be stored at 2°C to 8°C (36°F to 46°F); **do not freeze or shake.**

Single-dose 1 mL vial contains no preservative: Use one dose per vial; do not re-enter vial; discard unused portions.

Single-dose vials (except 40,000 units/mL vial) are stable for 2 weeks at room temperature; single-dose 40,000 units/mL vial is stable for 1 week at room temperature.

Multidose 1 mL or 2 mL vial contains preservative; store at 2°C to 8°C after initial entry and between doses; discard 21 days after initial entry.

Multidose vials (with preservative) are stable for 1 week at room temperature.

Prefilled syringes containing the 20,000 units/mL formulation with preservative are stable for 6 weeks refrigerated (2°C to 8°C).

Dilutions of 1:10 and 1:20 (1 part epoetin:19 parts sodium chloride) are stable for 18 hours at room temperature.

Prior to SubQ administration, preservative free solutions may be mixed with bacteriostatic NS containing benzyl alcohol 0.9% in a 1:1 ratio. Dilutions of 1:10 in $D_{10}W$ with human albumin 0.05% or 0.1% are stable for 24 hours.

Administration SubQ, I.M. (I.V. not recommended unless on hemodialysis; I.V. administration may require up to 40% more drug as SubQ/I.M. administration to achieve the same therapeutic result)

Patients with CRF on dialysis: I.V. route preferred; may be administered I.V. bolus into the venous line after dialysis.

Patients with CRF not on dialysis: May be administered I.V. or SubQ

Monitoring Parameters Blood pressure; hematocrit/hemoglobin, CBC with differential and platelets, transferring saturation and ferritin

Suggested tests to be monitored and their frequency: See table.

Test	Initial Phase Frequency	Maintenance Phase Frequency
Hematocrit/hemoglobin	2 x/week	2-4 x/month
Blood pressure	3 x/week	3 x/week
Serum ferritin	Monthly	Quarterly
Transferrin saturation	Monthly	Quarterly
Serum chemistries including CBC with differential, creatinine, blood urea nitrogen, potassium, phosphorous	Regularly per routine	Regularly per routine

Hematocrit should be determined twice weekly until stabilization within the target range (30% to 36%), and twice weekly for at least 2-6 weeks after a dose increase.

Reference Range Guidelines should be based on the following figure or published literature

Guidelines for estimating appropriateness of endogenous EPO levels for varying levels of anemia via the EIA assay method: See figure. The reference range for erythropoietin in serum, for subjects with normal hemoglobin and hematocrit, is 4.1-22.2 mU/mL by the EIA method. Erythropoietin levels are typically inversely related to hemoglobin (and hematocrit) levels in anemias not attributed to impaired erythropoietin production.

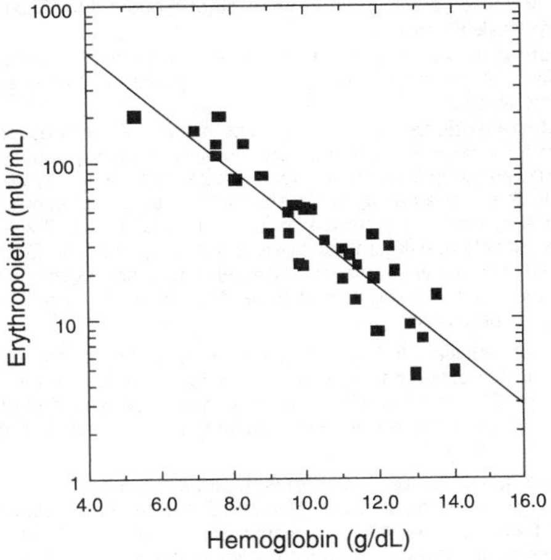

Zidovudine-treated HIV patients: Available evidence indicates patients with endogenous serum erythropoietin levels >500 mU/mL are unlikely to respond

Cancer chemotherapy patients: Treatment of patients with endogenous serum erythropoietin levels >200 mU/mL is not recommended

Serum EPO levels can be ordered routinely from clinical chemistry (red top serum separator tube).

Anesthesia and Critical Care Concerns/Other Considerations Recently a prospective, randomized, double-blind, placebo-controlled, multicenter trial was performed with critically-ill patients (Corwin, 2002), assessing the efficacy of recombinant human erythropoietin in reducing red blood cell transfusions. Patients were enrolled from December 1998 through June 2001. Over 1300 ICU (medical, surgical, or medical/surgical) patients were randomized to receive placebo or 40,000 units of erythropoietin subcutaneously on ICU day 3 and then weekly for patients who remained in the hospital. Inclusion criteria included ICU stay for 3 days, age >18 years, and hematocrit <38%. Exclusion criteria included acute ischemic heart disease. Each patient's physician determined the need for red blood cell transfusion. Results: The mean baseline hemoglobin was 9.97 g/dL (Continued)

Epoetin Alfa *(Continued)*

in each group. Patients receiving erythropoietin were less likely to receive transfusions. The median number of units transfused per patient in the placebo group was 2 and in the erythropoietin group was 1 (P <0.001). The erythropoietin group had a 19% reduction in total units of red blood cells transfused per days alive (P=0.04; confidence interval [CI] 0.79-0.83). Mortality and adverse clinical events were not significantly different between groups. The authors concluded that weekly administration of erythropoietin in critically-ill patients reduces red blood cell transfusions and increases hemoglobin. The authors also suggest that further study is needed to determine whether use of erythropoietin results in improved clinical outcomes. In addition, data on cost effectiveness would be helpful.

A restrictive transfusion approach (Hebert, 1999) was described in a transfusion trial that was published after Corwin's trial was underway. Hebert and his group evaluated a restrictive transfusion strategy (transfuse if hemoglobin <7 g/dL to maintain between 7 and 9 g/dL) versus a liberal strategy (transfuse if hemoglobin <10 g/dL to maintain between 10 and 12 g/dL). Inclusion criteria included anticipated ICU stay >24 hours, hemoglobin ≤9 g/dL with 72 hours of ICU admission, and euvolemia after initial treatment. Exclusion criteria included chronic anemia, active bleeding, or admission after a routine cardiac surgical procedure. The restrictive approach to transfusion was at least as effective as and possibly superior to a liberal transfusion policy in critically-ill patients. The exception to this may be patients with acute myocardial infarction and unstable angina.

The 2004 Surviving Sepsis Campaign guidelines do not recommend erythropoietin as a treatment for anemia associated with severe sepsis but suggest that it may be used when septic patients have other therapeutic indications.

Pregnancy Risk Factor C

Contraindications Hypersensitivity to erythropoietin, albumin (human) or mammalian cell-derived products, or any component of the formulation; uncontrolled hypertension

Warnings/Precautions Use caution with history of seizures or hypertension; blood pressure should be controlled prior to start of therapy and monitored closely throughout treatment. Excessive rate of rise of hematocrit may be possibly associated with the exacerbation of hypertension or seizures; decrease the epoetin dose if the hemoglobin increase exceeds 1 g/dL in any 2-week period. Use caution in patients at risk for thrombosis or with history of cardiovascular disease. Increased mortality has been observed when aggressive dosing is used in CHF or anginal patients undergoing hemodialysis. Multidose vials contain benzyl alcohol; do not use in premature infants.

Pure red cell aplasia (PRCA) with neutralizing antibodies to erythropoietin has been reported in patients treated with recombinant products; may occur more in patients with CRF. Patients should be evaluated for any loss of effect to therapy and treatment discontinued with evidence of PRCA. Response to therapy may be limited by multiple factors.

Prior to and during therapy, iron stores must be evaluated; iron supplementation should be given during therapy. Use caution with porphyria, exacerbation of porphyria has been reported in patients with chronic renal failure. Not recommended for acute correction of severe anemia or as a substitute for transfusion. Safety and efficacy in children <1 month of age have not been established.

Adverse Reactions Note: Adverse drug reaction incidences vary based on condition being treated and dose administered.

>10%:

- Cardiovascular: Hypertension (5% to 24%), edema (6% to 17%)
- Central nervous system: Fever (29% to 51%), dizziness (<7% to 21%), insomnia (13% to 21%), headache (10% to 19%)
- Dermatologic: Pruritus (14% to 22%), skin pain (4% to 18%), rash (≤16%)
- Gastrointestinal: Nausea (11% to 58%), constipation (42% to 53%), vomiting (8% to 29%), diarrhea (9% to 21%), dyspepsia (7% to 11%)
- Genitourinary: Urinary tract infection (3% to 12%)
- Local: Injection-site reaction (<10% to 29%)
- Neuromuscular & skeletal: Arthralgia (11%), paresthesia (11%)
- Respiratory: Cough (18%), congestion (15%), dyspnea (13% to 14%), upper respiratory infection (11%)

1% to 10%:

- Cardiovascular: Deep vein thrombosis (3% to 10%)
- Central nervous system: Seizure (1% to 3%)

Local: Clotted vascular access (7%)

<1% (Limited to important or life-threatening): Allergic reaction, anemia (severe; with or without other cytopenias), CVA, flu-like syndrome, hyperkalemia, hypersensitivity reactions, hypertensive encephalopathy, microvascular thrombosis, MI, myalgia, neutralizing antibodies, pulmonary embolism, pure red cell aplasia, thrombophlebitis, tachycardia, thrombosis, TIA, urticaria

Overdosage/Toxicology Symptoms of overdose include erythrocytosis and polycythemia. Doses of up to 1500 units/kg 3 times a week for 3-4 weeks have been administered to adults. Phlebotomy may be indicated for polycythemia; treatment is otherwise symptom-directed and supportive.

Dosage Forms

Injection, solution [preservative free]: 2000 units/mL (1 mL); 3000 units/mL (1 mL); 4000 units/mL (1 mL); 10,000 units/mL (1 mL); 40,000 units/mL (1 mL) [contains human albumin]

Injection, solution [with preservative]: 10,000 units/mL (2 mL); 20,000 units/mL (1 mL) [contains human albumin and benzyl alcohol]

References

Corwin HL, Gettinger A, Pearl RG, et al, "Efficacy of Recombinant Human Erythropoietin in Critically Ill Patients, A Randomized Controlled Trial," *JAMA*, 2002, 288:2827-35.

Dellinger RP, Carlet JM, Masur H, et al, "Surviving Sepsis Campaign Guidelines for Management of Severe Sepsis and Septic Shock," *Crit Care Med*, 2004, 32(3):858-73.

Hebert PC, Wells G, Blajchman MA, et al, "A Multicenter, Randomized, Controlled Clinical Trial of Transfusion Requirements in Critical Care," *N Engl J Med*, 1999, 340(6):409-17.

♦ **Epogen®** *see* Epoetin Alfa *on page 463*

Epoprostenol (e poe PROST en ole)

Related Information

Continuous Renal Replacement Therapy *on page 1447*

U.S. Brand Names Flolan®

Canadian Brand Names Flolan®

Synonyms Epoprostenol Sodium; PGI_2; PGX; Prostacyclin

Pharmacologic Category Prostaglandin

Restrictions Orders for epoprostenol are distributed by two sources in the United States. Information on orders or reimbursement assistance may be obtained from either Accredo Health, Inc (1-800-935-6526) or TheraCom, Inc (1-877-356-5264).

Generic Available No

Use Treatment of idiopathic pulmonary arterial hypertension [IPAH]; pulmonary hypertension associated with the scleroderma spectrum of disease [SSD] in NYHA Class III and Class IV patients who do not respond adequately to conventional therapy

Mechanism of Action Epoprostenol is also known as prostacyclin and PGI_2. It is a strong vasodilator of all vascular beds. In addition, it is a potent endogenous inhibitor of platelet aggregation. The reduction in platelet aggregation results from epoprostenol's activation of intracellular adenylate cyclase and the resultant increase in cyclic adenosine monophosphate concentrations within the platelets. Additionally, it is capable of decreasing thrombogenesis and platelet clumping in the lungs by inhibiting platelet aggregation.

Pharmacodynamics/Kinetics

Metabolism: Rapidly hydrolyzed; subject to some enzymatic degradation; forms one active metabolite and 13 inactive metabolites

Half-life elimination: 6 minutes

Excretion: Urine (84%); feces (4%)

Dosage Children (unlabeled use) and Adults: I.V.: Initial: 1-2 ng/kg/minute, increase dose in increments of 1-2 ng/kg/minute every 15 minutes or longer until dose-limiting side effects are noted or tolerance limit to epoprostenol is observed

Dose adjustment:

Increase dose in 1-2 ng/kg/minute increments at intervals of at least 15 minutes if symptoms persist or recur following improvement. In clinical trials, dosing increases occurred at intervals of 24-48 hours.

Decrease dose in 2 ng/kg/minute decrements at intervals of at least 15 minutes in case of dose-limiting pharmacologic events. Avoid abrupt withdrawal or sudden large dose reductions.

Lung transplant: In patients receiving lung transplants, epoprostenol was tapered after the initiation of cardiopulmonary bypass.

(Continued)

Epoprostenol *(Continued)*

Stability Prior to use, store vials at 15°C to 25°C (59°F to 77°F); protect from light, do not freeze. Reconstitute only with provided sterile diluent. Following reconstitution, solution must be stored under refrigeration at 2°C to 8°C (36°F to 46°F) if not used immediately; protect from light, do not freeze; discard if refrigerated for >48 hours. See table. During use, a single reservoir of solution may be used at room temperature for a total duration of 8 hours, or used with a cold pouch for administration up to 24 hours. Cold packs should be changed every 12 hours.

Preparation of Epoprostenol Infusion

To make 100 mL of solution with concentration:	Directions
3000 ng/mL	Dissolve one 0.5 mg vial with 5 mL supplied diluent, withdraw 3 mL, and add to sufficient diluent to make a total of 100 mL.
5000 ng/mL	Dissolve one 0.5 mg vial with 5 mL supplied diluent, withdraw entire vial contents, and add a sufficient volume of diluent to make a total of 100 mL.
10,000 ng/mL	Dissolve two 0.5 mg vials each with 5 mL supplied diluent, withdraw entire vial contents, and add a sufficient volume of diluent to make a total of 100 mL.
15,000 ng/mL	Dissolve one 1.5 mg vial with 5 mL supplied diluent, withdraw entire vial contents, and add a sufficient volume of diluent to make a total of 100 mL.

Administration

The ambulatory infusion pump should be small and lightweight, be able to adjust infusion rates in 2 ng/kg/minute increments, have occlusion, end of infusion, and low battery alarms, have ± 6% accuracy of the programmed rate, and have positive continuous or pulsatile pressure with intervals ≤3 minutes between pulses. The reservoir should be made of polyvinyl chloride, polypropylene, or glass. The infusion pump used in the most recent clinical trial was CADD-1 HFX 5100 (Pharmacia Deltec).

Monitoring Parameters Monitor for improvements in pulmonary function, decreased exertional dyspnea, fatigue, syncope and chest pain, pulmonary vascular resistance, pulmonary arterial pressure and quality of life. In addition, the pump device and catheters should be monitored frequently to avoid "system" related failure. Monitor arterial pressure; assess all vital functions. Hypoxia, flushing, and tachycardia may indicate overdose.

Pregnancy Risk Factor B

Contraindications Hypersensitivity to epoprostenol or to structurally-related compounds; chronic use in patients with CHF due to severe left ventricular systolic dysfunction; patients who develop pulmonary edema during dose initiation

Warnings/Precautions Abrupt interruptions or large sudden reductions in dosage may result in rebound pulmonary hypertension; some patients with primary pulmonary hypertension have developed pulmonary edema during dose ranging, which may be associated with pulmonary veno-occlusive disease; during chronic use, unless contraindicated, anticoagulants should be coadministered to reduce the risk of thromboembolism

Adverse Reactions

Note: Adverse events reported during dose initiation and escalation include flushing (58%), headache (49%), nausea/vomiting (32%), hypotension (16%), anxiety/nervousness/agitation (11%), chest pain (11%); abdominal pain, back pain, bradycardia, diaphoresis, dizziness, dyspepsia, dyspnea, hypoesthesia/paresthesia, musculoskeletal pain, and tachycardia are also reported. The following adverse events have been reported during chronic administration for IPAH. Although some may be related to the underlying disease state, anxiety, diarrhea, flu-like symptoms, flushing, headache, jaw pain, nausea, nervousness, and vomiting are clearly contributed to epoprostenol.

>10%:

Cardiovascular: Chest pain (67%), palpitation (63%), flushing (42%), tachycardia (35%), arrhythmia (27%), hemorrhage (19%), bradycardia (15%)

Central nervous system: Dizziness (83%), headache (83%), chills/fever/sepsis/flu-like symptoms (25%), anxiety/nervousness/tremor (21%)
Gastrointestinal: Nausea/vomiting (67%), diarrhea (37%)
Genitourinary: Weight loss (27%)
Local: Injection-site reactions: Infection (21%), pain (13%)
Neuromuscular & skeletal: Weakness (87%), jaw pain (54%), myalgia (44%), musculoskeletal pain (35%; predominantly involving legs and feet), hypoesthesia/hyperparesthesia/paresthesia (12%)
Respiratory: Dyspnea (90%)

1% to 10%:
Cardiovascular: Supraventricular tachycardia (8%), cerebrovascular accident (4%)
Central nervous system: Convulsion (4%)
Dermatologic: Rash (10%; conventional therapy 13%), pruritus (4%)
Endocrine & metabolic: Hypokalemia (6%)
Gastrointestinal: Constipation (6%), weight gain (6%)
Neuromuscular & skeletal: Arthralgia (6%)
Ocular: Amblyopia (8%), vision abnormality (4%)
Respiratory: Epistaxis (4%), pleural effusion (4%)

<1% (Limited to important or life-threatening): Anemia, ascites, hypersplenism, hyperthyroidism, pancytopenia, splenomegaly, thrombocytopenia

Overdosage/Toxicology Symptoms of overdose include headache, hypotension, tachycardia, nausea, vomiting, diarrhea, and flushing. If any of these symptoms occur, reduce the infusion rate until symptoms subside. If symptoms do not subside, consider drug discontinuation. Fatal cases of hypoxemia, hypotension, and respiratory arrest have been reported. Long-term overdose may lead to high output cardiac failure.

Drug Interactions

Antihypertensive agents: The hypotensive effects of epoprostenol may be exacerbated by other vasodilators, diuretics, or by using acetate in dialysis fluids.
Antiplatelet agents (aspirin, IIb/IIIa antagonists, clopidogrel, ticlopidine): Risk of bleeding may be increased
Digoxin: Serum levels may be increased; clearance decreased by 15%; monitor
Furosemide: Serum levels may be increased; clinical significance low; clearance decreased by 13%
Heparin (including low molecular weight heparins): Risk of bleeding may be increased
Warfarin: Risk of bleeding may be increased

Dosage Forms Injection, powder for reconstitution, as sodium: 0.5 mg, 1.5 mg [provided with 50 mL sterile diluent]

♦ **Epoprostenol Sodium** *see* Epoprostenol *on page 467*

♦ **Eprex® (Can)** *see* Epoetin Alfa *on page 463*

Eprosartan (ep roe SAR tan)

Related Information

Angiotensin Agents *on page 1544*

U.S. Brand Names Teveten®

Canadian Brand Names Teveten®

Pharmacologic Category Angiotensin II Receptor Blocker

Generic Available No

Use Treatment of hypertension; may be used alone or in combination with other antihypertensives

Mechanism of Action Angiotensin II is formed from angiotensin I in a reaction catalyzed by angiotensin-converting enzyme (ACE, kininase II). Angiotensin II is the principal pressor agent of the renin-angiotensin system, with effects that include vasoconstriction, stimulation of synthesis and release of aldosterone, cardiac stimulation, and renal reabsorption of sodium. Eprosartan blocks the vasoconstrictor and aldosterone-secreting effects of angiotensin II by selectively blocking the binding of angiotensin II to the AT1 receptor in many tissues, such as vascular smooth muscle and the adrenal gland. Its action is therefore independent of the pathways for angiotensin II synthesis. Blockade of the renin-angiotensin system with ACE inhibitors, which inhibit the biosynthesis of angiotensin II from angiotensin I, is widely used in the treatment of hypertension. ACE inhibitors also inhibit the degradation of bradykinin, a reaction also catalyzed by ACE. Because eprosartan does not inhibit ACE (kininase II), it does not affect
(Continued)

Eprosartan *(Continued)*

the response to bradykinin. Whether this difference has clinical relevance is not yet known. Eprosartan does not bind to or block other hormone receptors or ion channels known to be important in cardiovascular regulation.

Pharmacodynamics/Kinetics

Protein binding: 98%

Metabolism: Minimally hepatic

Bioavailability: 300 mg dose: 13%

Half-life elimination: Terminal: 5-9 hours

Time to peak, serum: Fasting: 1-2 hours

Excretion: Feces (90%); urine (7%, mostly as unchanged drug)

Clearance: 7.9 L/hour

Dosage Adults: Oral: Dosage must be individualized; can administer once or twice daily with total daily doses of 400-800 mg. Usual starting dose is 600 mg once daily as monotherapy in patients who are euvolemic. Limited clinical experience with doses >800 mg.

Dosage adjustment in renal impairment: No starting dosage adjustment is necessary; however, carefully monitor the patient

Dosage adjustment in hepatic impairment: No starting dosage adjustment is necessary; however, carefully monitor the patient

Elderly: No starting dosage adjustment is necessary; however, carefully monitor the patient

Anesthesia and Critical Care Concerns/Other Considerations The angiotensin II receptor antagonists appear to have similar indications as the ACE inhibitors. In heart failure, the angiotensin II antagonists are especially useful in providing an alternative therapy in those patients who have intractable cough in response to ACE inhibitor therapy. Candesartan has been studied as an alternative therapy in chronic heart failure patients who cannot tolerate an ACE-I (CHARM-Alternative) and as an added therapy in heart failure patients who are maintained on an ACE-I (CHARM-Added). In both studies the combined endpoint of cardiovascular death or heart failure hospitalizations was significantly improved over the placebo treated group. Similar to ACE inhibitors, pre-existing volume depletion caused by diuretic therapy may potentiate hypotension in response to angiotensin II antagonists. Concomitant NSAID therapy may attenuate blood pressure control; use of NSAIDs should be avoided or limited, with monitoring of blood pressure control. In the setting of heart failure, NSAID use may be associated with an increased risk for fluid accumulation and edema.

Pregnancy Risk Factor C (1st trimester); D (2nd and 3rd trimesters)

Contraindications Hypersensitivity to eprosartan or any component of the formulation; sensitivity to other A-II receptor antagonists; bilateral renal artery stenosis; pregnancy (2nd and 3rd trimesters)

Warnings/Precautions [U.S. Boxed Warning]: Based on human data, drugs that act on the angiotensin system can cause injury and death to the developing fetus when used in the second and third trimesters. Angiotensin receptor blockers should be discontinued as soon as possible once pregnancy is detected. Avoid use or use a smaller dose in patients who are volume depleted; correct depletion first. Deterioration in renal function can occur with initiation. Use with caution in unilateral renal artery stenosis and pre-existing renal insufficiency; significant aortic/mitral stenosis. Safety and efficacy not established in pediatric patients.

Adverse Reactions

1% to 10%:

Central nervous system: Fatigue (2%), depression (1%)

Endocrine & metabolic: Hypertriglyceridemia (1%)

Gastrointestinal: Abdominal pain (2%)

Genitourinary: Urinary tract infection (1%)

Respiratory: Upper respiratory tract infection (8%), rhinitis (4%), pharyngitis (4%), cough (4%)

Miscellaneous: Viral infection (2%), injury (2%)

<1% (Limited to important or life-threatening): Abnormal ECG, angina, arthritis, asthma, ataxia, bradycardia, BUN increased, creatinine increased, eczema, edema, esophagitis, ethanol intolerance, gingivitis, gout, hypotension, influenza-like symptoms, leg cramps, leukopenia, maculopapular rash, migraine, neuritis, neutropenia, orthostasis, palpitation, paresthesia, peripheral ischemia,

purpura, renal calculus, somnolence, tachycardia, tendonitis, thrombocytopenia, tinnitus, tremor, urinary incontinence, vertigo; rhabdomyolysis has been reported (rarely) with angiotensin-receptor antagonists.

Overdosage/Toxicology The most likely manifestations of overdose would be hypotension and tachycardia. Initiate supportive care for symptomatic hypotension.

Drug Interactions Inhibits CYP2C9 (weak)

Lithium: Risk of toxicity may be increased by eprosartan; monitor lithium levels.

NSAIDs: May decrease angiotensin II antagonist efficacy; effect has been seen with losartan, but may occur with other medications in this class; monitor blood pressure

Potassium-sparing diuretics (amiloride, potassium, spironolactone, triamterene): Increased risk of hyperkalemia.

Potassium supplements may increase the risk of hyperkalemia.

Trimethoprim (high dose) may increase the risk of hyperkalemia.

Ethanol/Nutrition/Herb Interactions Herb/Nutraceutical: Avoid dong quai if using for hypertension (has estrogenic activity). Avoid ephedra, yohimbe, ginseng (may worsen hypertension). Avoid garlic (may have increased antihypertensive effect).

Dosage Forms Tablet: 400 mg, 600 mg

♦ **Epsilon Aminocaproic Acid** *see* Aminocaproic Acid *on page 81*

♦ **Epsom Salts** *see* Magnesium Sulfate *on page 787*

♦ **Eptacog Alfa (Activated)** *see* Factor VIIa (Recombinant) *on page 501*

Eptifibatide (ep TIF i ba tide)

U.S. Brand Names Integrilin®

Canadian Brand Names Integrilin®

Synonyms Intrifiban

Pharmacologic Category Antiplatelet Agent, Glycoprotein IIb/IIIa Inhibitor

Generic Available No

Use Treatment of patients with acute coronary syndrome (unstable angina/non-Q wave myocardial infarction [UA/NQMI]), including patients who are to be managed medically and those undergoing percutaneous coronary intervention (PCI including angioplasty, intracoronary stenting)

Mechanism of Action Eptifibatide is a cyclic heptapeptide which blocks the platelet glycoprotein IIb/IIIa receptor, the binding site for fibrinogen, von Willebrand factor, and other ligands. Inhibition of binding at this final common receptor reversibly blocks platelet aggregation and prevents thrombosis.

Pharmacodynamics/Kinetics

Onset of action: Within 1 hour

Duration: Platelet function restored ~4 hours following discontinuation

Protein binding: ~25%

Half-life elimination: 2.5 hours

Excretion: Primarily urine (as eptifibatide and metabolites); significant renal impairment may alter disposition of this compound

Clearance: Total body: 55-58 mL/kg/hour; Renal: ~50% of total in healthy subjects

Dosage I.V.: Adults:

Acute coronary syndrome: Bolus of 180 mcg/kg (maximum: 22.6 mg) over 1-2 minutes, begun as soon as possible following diagnosis, followed by a continuous infusion of 2 mcg/kg/minute (maximum: 15 mg/hour) until hospital discharge or initiation of CABG surgery, up to 72 hours. Concurrent aspirin and heparin therapy (target aPTT 50-70 seconds) are recommended.

Percutaneous coronary intervention (PCI) with or without stenting: Bolus of 180 mcg/kg (maximum: 22.6 mg) administered immediately before the initiation of PCI, followed by a continuous infusion of 2 mcg/kg/minute (maximum: 15 mg/hour). A second 180 mcg/kg bolus (maximum: 22.6 mg) should be administered 10 minutes after the first bolus. Infusion should be continued until hospital discharge or for up to 18-24 hours, whichever comes first. Concurrent aspirin (160-325 mg 1-24 hours before PCI and daily thereafter) and heparin therapy (ACT 200-300 seconds during PCI) are recommended. Heparin infusion after PCI is discouraged. In patients who undergo coronary artery bypass graft surgery, discontinue infusion prior to surgery.

(Continued)

Eptifibatide *(Continued)*

Elderly: No dosing adjustment for the elderly appears to be necessary; adjust carefully to renal function.

Dosing adjustment in renal impairment: Dialysis is a contraindication to use.

Acute coronary syndrome: Cl_{cr} <50 mL/minute: Use 180 mcg/kg bolus (maximum: 22.6 mg) and 1 mcg/kg/minute infusion (maximum: 7.5 mg/hour)

Percutaneous coronary intervention (PCI) with or without stenting: Cl_{cr} <50 mL/minute: Use 180 mcg/kg bolus (maximum: 22.6 mg) administered immediately before the initiation of PCI and followed by a continuous infusion of 1 mcg/kg/minute (maximum: 7.5 mg/hour). A second 180 mcg/kg (maximum: 22.6 mg) bolus should be administered 10 minutes after the first bolus.

Stability Vials should be stored refrigerated at 2°C to 8°C (36°F to 46°F). Vials can be kept at room temperature for 2 months. Protect from light until administration. Do not use beyond the expiration date. Discard any unused portion left in the vial.

May be administered in same I.V. line as alteplase, atropine, dobutamine, heparin, lidocaine, meperidine, metoprolol, midazolam, morphine, nitroglycerin, verapamil, normal saline (infusion may contain up to 60 mEq/L KCl), or normal saline/D_5W (infusion may contain up to 60 mEq/L KCl).

Administration Do not shake vial. Visually inspect for discoloration or particulate matter prior to administration. The bolus dose should be withdrawn from the 10 mL vial into a syringe and administered by I.V. push over 1-2 minutes. Begin continuous infusion immediately following bolus administration, administered directly from the 100 mL vial. The 100 mL vial should be spiked with a vented infusion set.

Monitoring Parameters Coagulation parameters, signs/symptoms of excessive bleeding. Laboratory tests at baseline and monitoring during therapy: hematocrit and hemoglobin, platelet count, serum creatinine, PT/aPTT (maintain aPTT between 50-70 seconds unless PCI is to be performed), and ACT with PCI (maintain ACT between 200-300 seconds during PCI).

Assess sheath insertion site and distal pulses of affected leg every 15 minutes for the first hour and then every 1 hour for the next 6 hours. Arterial access site care is important to prevent bleeding. Care should be taken when attempting vascular access that only the anterior wall of the femoral artery is punctured, avoiding a Seldinger (through and through) technique for obtaining sheath access. Femoral vein sheath placement should be avoided unless needed. While the vascular sheath is in place, patients should be maintained on complete bed rest with the head of the bed at a 30° angle and the affected limb restrained in a straight position.

Observe patient for mental status changes, hemorrhage, assess nose and mouth mucous membranes, puncture sites for oozing, ecchymosis and hematoma formation, and examine urine, stool and emesis for presence of occult or frank blood; gentle care should be provided when removing dressings.

Anesthesia and Critical Care Concerns/Other Considerations Eptifibatide has a short duration of action and hemostasis is restored within about 4 hours after discontinuation in patients with normal renal function. Acute profound thrombocytopenia has been associated with eptifibatide use.

Pregnancy Risk Factor B

Contraindications Hypersensitivity to eptifibatide or any component of the product; active abnormal bleeding or a history of bleeding diathesis within the previous 30 days; history of CVA within 30 days or a history of hemorrhagic stroke; severe hypertension (systolic blood pressure >200 mm Hg or diastolic blood pressure >110 mm Hg) not adequately controlled on antihypertensive therapy; major surgery within the preceding 6 weeks; current or planned administration of another parenteral GP IIb/IIIa inhibitor; thrombocytopenia; dependency on renal dialysis

Warnings/Precautions Bleeding is the most common complication. Most major bleeding occurs at the arterial access site where the cardiac catheterization was done. When bleeding can not be controlled with pressure, discontinue infusion and heparin. Use caution in patients with hemorrhagic retinopathy or with other drugs that affect hemostasis. Concurrent use with thrombolytics has not been established as safe. Minimize other procedures including arterial and venous punctures, I.M. injections, nasogastric tubes, etc. Sheath should not be removed unless the aPTT <45 sec or the ACT <150 sec. Use caution in renal dysfunction (estimated Cl_{cr} <50 mL/minute); dosage adjustment required. Safety and efficacy in pediatric patients have not been determined.

Adverse Reactions Bleeding is the major drug-related adverse effect. Access site is often primary source of bleeding complications. Incidence of bleeding is also related to heparin intensity. Patients weighing <70 kg may have an increased risk of major bleeding.

>10%: Hematologic: Bleeding (major: 1% to 11%; minor: 3% to 14%; transfusion required: 2% to 13%)

1% to 10%:
- Cardiovascular: Hypotension (up to 7%)
- Hematologic: Thrombocytopenia (1% to 3%)
- Local: Injection site reaction

<1% (Limited to important or life-threatening): Acute profound thrombocytopenia, anaphylaxis, fatal bleeding events, GI hemorrhage, intracranial hemorrhage (0.5% to 0.7%), pulmonary hemorrhage, stroke

Overdosage/Toxicology Two cases of human overdose have been reported; neither case was eventful or associated with major bleeding. Symptoms of overdose in animal studies include loss of righting reflex, dyspnea, ptosis, decreased muscle tone, and petechial hemorrhage. Treatment is supportive. Dialysis may be beneficial.

Drug Interactions

Cephalosporins which contain the MTT side chain may theoretically increase the risk of hemorrhage

Drotrecogin alfa: Antiplatelet agents (eg, eptifibatide) may enhance the adverse/toxic effect of drotrecogin alfa; bleeding may occur.

Drugs which affect platelet function (eg, aspirin, NSAIDs, dipyridamole, ticlopidine, clopidogrel) may potentiate the risk of hemorrhage; use with caution

Heparin and aspirin: Use with aspirin and heparin may increase bleeding over aspirin and heparin alone. However, aspirin and heparin were used concurrently in the majority of patients in the major clinical studies of eptifibatide

Thrombolytic agents theoretically may increase the risk of hemorrhage; use with caution

Warfarin and oral anticoagulants: Risk of bleeding may be increased during concurrent therapy

Other IIb/IIIa antagonists: Avoid concomitant use of other glycoprotein IIb/IIIa antagonists (see Contraindications)

Ethanol/Nutrition/Herb Interactions Herb/Nutraceutical: Avoid alfalfa, anise, bilberry, bladderwrack, bromelain, cat's claw, celery, coleus, cordyceps, dong quai, evening primrose oil, fenugreek, feverfew, garlic, ginger, ginkgo biloba, ginseng (American), ginseng (Panax), ginseng (Siberian), grape seed, green tea, guggul, horse chestnut seed, horseradish, licorice, prickly ash, red clover, reishi, same (s-adenosylmethionine), sweet clover, turmeric, and white willow (all have additional antiplatelet activity).

Dosage Forms Injection, solution: 0.75 mg/mL (100 mL); 2 mg/mL (10 mL, 100 mL)

♦ **Equetro™** *see* Carbamazepine *on page 225*

Ertapenem (er ta PEN em)

Medication Safety Issues

Sound-alike/look-alike issues:

Invanz® may be confused with Avinza™

U.S. Brand Names Invanz®

Canadian Brand Names Invanz®

Synonyms Ertapenem Sodium; L-749,345; MK0826

Pharmacologic Category Antibiotic, Carbapenem

Generic Available No

Use Treatment of the following moderate-severe infections: Complicated intra-abdominal infections, complicated skin and skin structure infections (including diabetic foot infections without osteomyelitis), complicated UTI (including pyelonephritis), acute pelvic infections, and community-acquired pneumonia. Antibacterial coverage includes aerobic gram-positive organisms, aerobic gram-negative organisms, anaerobic organisms.

Note: Methicillin-resistant *Staphylococcus*, *Enterococcus* spp, penicillin-resistant strains of *Streptococcus pneumoniae*, beta-lactamase-positive strains of

(Continued)

Ertapenem *(Continued)*

Haemophilus influenzae are **resistant** to ertapenem, as are most *Pseudomonas aeruginosa*.

Mechanism of Action Inhibits bacterial cell wall synthesis by binding to one or more of the penicillin binding proteins; which in turn inhibits the final transpeptidation step of peptidoglycan synthesis in bacterial cell walls, thus inhibiting cell wall biosynthesis. Bacteria eventually lyse due to ongoing activity of cell wall autolytic enzymes (autolysins and murein hydrolases) while cell wall assembly is arrested.

Pharmacodynamics/Kinetics

Absorption: I.M.: Almost complete

Distribution: V_{dss}:

Children 3 months to 12 years: 0.2 L/kg

Children 13-17 years: 0.16 L/kg

Adults: 0.12 L/kg

Protein binding (concentration dependent): 85% at 300 mcg/mL, 95% at <100 mcg/mL

Metabolism: Hydrolysis to inactive metabolite

Bioavailability: I.M.: 90%

Half-life elimination:

Children 3 months to 12 years: 2.5 hours

Children ≥13 years and Adults: 4 hours

Time to peak: I.M.: 2.3 hours

Excretion: Urine (80% as unchanged drug and metabolite); feces (10%)

Dosage

Usual dosage ranges:

Children 3 months to 12 years: I.M., I.V.: 15 mg/kg twice daily (maximum: 1 g)

Children ≥13 years and Adults: I.M., I.V.: 1 g/day

Indication-specific dosing:

Children 3 months to 12 years: I.M., I.V.:

Community-acquired pneumonia, urinary tract infections/pyelonephritis: 15 mg/kg twice daily (maximum: 1 g/day); duration of total antibiotic treatment: 10-14 days (**Note:** Duration includes possible switch to appropriate oral therapy after at least 3 days of parenteral treatment, once clinical improvement demonstrated.)

Intra-abdominal infection: 15 mg/kg twice daily (maximum: 1 g/day) for 5-14 days

Pelvic infections (acute): 15 mg/kg twice daily (maximum: 1 g/day) for 3-10 days

Skin and skin structure infections: 15 mg/kg twice daily (maximum: 1 g/day) for 7-14 days

Children ≥13 years and Adults: I.M., I.V.:

Community-acquired pneumonia, urinary tract infections/pyelonephritis: 1 g/day; duration of total antibiotic treatment: 10-14 days (**Note:** Duration includes possible switch to appropriate oral therapy after at least 3 days of parenteral treatment, once clinical improvement demonstrated.)

Intra-abdominal infection: 1 g/day for 5-14 days

Pelvic infections (acute): 1 g/day for 3-10 days

Skin and skin structure infections (including diabetic foot infections): 1 g/day for 7-14 days

Elderly: Refer to adult dosing.

Dosage adjustment in renal impairment:

Children: No data available for pediatric patients with renal insufficiency.

Adults: Cl_{cr} <30 mL/minute and ESRD: 500 mg/day

Hemodialysis: Adults: When the daily dose is given within 6 hours prior to hemodialysis, a supplementary dose of 150 mg is required following hemodialysis.

Dosage adjustment in hepatic impairment: Adjustments cannot be recommended (lack of experience and research in this patient population).

Stability Before reconstitution store at ≤25°C (77°F).

I.M.: Reconstitute 1 g vial with 3.2 mL of 1% lidocaine HCl injection (without epinephrine). Shake well. Use within 1 hour after preparation.

I.V.: Reconstitute 1 g vial with 10 mL of water for injection, 0.9% sodium chloride injection, or bacteriostatic water for injection. Shake well. For adults, transfer dose to 50 mL of 0.9% sodium chloride injection; for children, dilute dose with NS to a final concentration of ≤20 mg/mL. Reconstituted I.V. solution may be stored at room temperature and used within 6 hours **or** refrigerated, stored for up to 24 hours and used within 4 hours after removal from refrigerator. Do not freeze.

Administration

I.M.: Avoid injection into a blood vessel. Make sure patient does not have an allergy to lidocaine or another anesthetic of the amide type. Administer by deep I.M. injection into a large muscle mass (eg, gluteal muscle or lateral part of the thigh). Do not administer I.M. preparation or drug reconstituted for I.M. administration intravenously.

I.V.: Infuse over 30 minutes

Monitoring Parameters Periodic renal, hepatic, and hematopoietic assessment during prolonged therapy; neurological assessment

Pregnancy Risk Factor B

Contraindications Hypersensitivity to ertapenem, other carbapenems, or any component of the formulation; anaphylactic reactions to beta-lactam antibiotics. If using intramuscularly, known hypersensitivity to local anesthetics of the amide type (lidocaine is the diluent).

Warnings/Precautions Use caution with renal impairment. Dosage adjustment required in patients with moderate-to-severe renal dysfunction; elderly patients often require lower doses (based upon renal function). Prolonged use may result in superinfection. Has been associated with CNS adverse effects, including confusional states and seizures; use caution with CNS disorders (eg, brain lesions, history of seizures). Serious hypersensitivity reactions, including anaphylaxis, have been reported (some without a history of previous allergic reactions to beta-lactams). Doses for I.M. administration are mixed with lidocaine; consult Lidocaine *on page 755* information for associated Warnings/Precautions. Safety and efficacy in patients <3 months of age have not been established.

Adverse Reactions Note: Percentages reported in adults.

1% to 10%:

Cardiovascular: Swelling/edema (3%), chest pain (1%), hypertension (0.7% to ≤2%), hypotension (1% to 2%), tachycardia (1% to 2%)

Central nervous system: Headache (6% to 7%), altered mental status (ie, agitation, confusion, disorientation, decreased mental acuity, changed mental status, somnolence, stupor) (3% to 5%), fever (2% to 5%), insomnia (3%), dizziness (2%), fatigue (1%), anxiety (0.8% to ≤1%)

Dermatologic: Rash (2% to 3%), pruritus (1% to 2%), erythema (1% to 2%)

Gastrointestinal: Diarrhea (9% to 10%), nausea (6% to 9%), abdominal pain (4%), vomiting (4%), constipation (3% to 4%), acid regurgitation (1% to 2%), dyspepsia (1%), oral candidiasis (0.1% to ≤1%)

Genitourinary: Vaginitis (1% to 3%)

Hematologic: Platelet count increased (4% to 7%), eosinophils increased (1% to 2%)

Hepatic: Hepatic enzyme elevations (7% to 9%), alkaline phosphatase increase (4% to 7%)

Local: Infused vein complications (5% to 7%), phlebitis/thrombophlebitis (2%), extravasation (0.7% to ≤2%)

Neuromuscular & skeletal: Leg pain (0.4% to 1%)

Respiratory: Dyspnea (1% to 3%), cough (1% to 2%), pharyngitis (0.7% to ≤1%), rales/rhonchi (0.5% to ≤1%), respiratory distress (0.2% to ≤1%)

<1% (Limited to important or life-threatening): Anaphylaxis, arrhythmia, asthma, asystole, atrial fibrillation, bradycardia, cardiac arrest, cholelithiasis, epistaxis, gastrointestinal hemorrhage, gout, hallucinations, heart failure, heart murmur, hypoxemia, ileus, pancreatitis, pseudomembranous colitis, pyloric stenosis, seizure (0.5%), subdural hemorrhage, syncope, urticaria, ventricular tachycardia, vertigo

Overdosage/Toxicology Treatment is symptom-directed and supportive. Ertapenem is removed by hemodialysis (plasma clearance increased by 30% following 4-hour session).

Drug Interactions

Probenecid: Serum concentrations of ertapenem may be increased; use caution.

Valproic acid: Ertapenem may decrease valproic acid serum concentrations to subtherapeutic levels; monitor.

Dietary Considerations Sodium content: 137 mg (~6 mEq) per gram of ertapenem

Dosage Forms Injection, powder for reconstitution: 1 g [contains sodium 137 mg/g (~6 mEq/g)]

♦ **Ertapenem Sodium** *see* Ertapenem *on page 473*

- **Erybid™ (Can)** *see* Erythromycin *on page 476*
- **Eryc®** *see* Erythromycin *on page 476*
- **Eryderm®** *see* Erythromycin *on page 476*
- **Erygel®** *see* Erythromycin *on page 476*
- **EryPed®** *see* Erythromycin *on page 476*
- **Ery-Tab®** *see* Erythromycin *on page 476*
- **Erythrocin®** *see* Erythromycin *on page 476*

Erythromycin (er ith roe MYE sin)

Medication Safety Issues

Sound-alike/look-alike issues:

Erythromycin may be confused with azithromycin, clarithromycin, Ethmozine®
Akne-Mycin® may be confused with AK-Mycin®
E.E.S.® may be confused with DES®
Eryc® may be confused with Emcyt®, Ery-Tab®
Ery-Tab® may be confused with Eryc®
Erythrocin® may be confused with Ethmozine®

Related Information

Anesthesia for Patients With Liver Disease *on page 1421*
Prevention of Wound Infection and Sepsis in Surgical Patients *on page 1588*

U.S. Brand Names Akne-Mycin®; A/T/S®; E.E.S.®; Eryc®; Eryderm®; Erygel®; EryPed®; Ery-Tab®; Erythrocin®; PCE®; Romycin®; Staticin® [DSC]; Theramycin Z®; T-Stat® [DSC]

Canadian Brand Names Apo-Erythro Base®; Apo-Erythro E-C®; Apo-Erythro-ES®; Apo-Erythro-S®; Diomycin®; EES®; Erybid™; Eryc®; Novo-Rythro Estolate; Novo-Rythro Ethylsuccinate; Nu-Erythromycin-S; PCE®; PMS-Erythromycin; Sans Acne®

Synonyms Erythromycin Base; Erythromycin Estolate; Erythromycin Ethylsuccinate; Erythromycin Gluceptate; Erythromycin Lactobionate; Erythromycin Stearate

Pharmacologic Category Antibiotic, Macrolide; Antibiotic, Ophthalmic; Antibiotic, Topical; Topical Skin Product; Topical Skin Product, Acne

Generic Available Yes

Use

Systemic: Treatment of susceptible bacterial infections including *S. pyogenes*, some *S. pneumoniae*, some *S. aureus*, *M. pneumoniae*, *Legionella pneumophila*, diphtheria, pertussis, chancroid, *Chlamydia*, erythrasma, *N. gonorrhoeae*, *E. histolytica*, syphilis and nongonococcal urethritis, and *Campylobacter* gastroenteritis; used in conjunction with neomycin for decontaminating the bowel

Ophthalmic: Treatment of superficial eye infections involving the conjunctiva or cornea; neonatal ophthalmia

Topical: Treatment of acne vulgaris

Unlabeled/Investigational Use Systemic: Treatment of gastroparesis

Mechanism of Action Inhibits RNA-dependent protein synthesis at the chain elongation step; binds to the 50S ribosomal subunit resulting in blockage of transpeptidation

Pharmacodynamics/Kinetics

Absorption: Oral: Variable but better with salt forms than with base form; 18% to 45%; ethylsuccinate may be better absorbed with food

Distribution: Crosses placenta; enters breast milk

Relative diffusion from blood into CSF: Minimal even with inflammation

CSF:blood level ratio: Normal meninges: 1% to 12%; Inflamed meninges: 7% to 25%

Protein binding: 75% to 90%

Metabolism: Hepatic via demethylation

Half-life elimination: Peak: 1.5-2 hours; End-stage renal disease: 5-6 hours

Time to peak, serum: Base: 4 hours; Ethylsuccinate: 0.5-2.5 hours; delayed with food due to differences in absorption

Excretion: Primarily feces; urine (2% to 15% as unchanged drug)

Dosage

Usual dosage range:

Neonates: Ophthalmic: Prophylaxis of neonatal gonococcal or chlamydial conjunctivitis: 0.5-1 cm ribbon of ointment should be instilled into each conjunctival sac

Infants and Children:

Oral: (**Note:** Due to differences in absorption, 400 mg erythromycin ethylsuccinate produces the same serum levels as 250 mg erythromycin base, sterate or estolate)

Base: 30-50 mg/kg/day in 2-4 divided doses; do not exceed 2 g/day

Estolate: 30-50 mg/kg/day in 2-4 divided doses; do not exceed 2 g/day

Ethylsuccinate: 30-50 mg/kg/day in 2-4 divided doses; do not exceed 3.2 g/day

Stearate: 30-50 mg/kg/day in 2-4 divided doses; do not exceed 2 g/day

I.V.: Lactobionate: 15-50 mg/kg/day divided every 6 hours, not to exceed 4 g/day

Children and Adults:

Ophthalmic: Instill ½" (1.25 cm) 2-6 times/day depending on the severity of the infection

Topical: Apply over the affected area twice daily after the skin has been thoroughly washed and patted dry

Adults:

Oral:

Base: 250-500 mg every 6-12 hours

Ethylsuccinate: 400-800 mg every 6-12 hours

I.V.: Lactobionate: 15-20 mg/kg/day divided every 6 hours or 500 mg to 1 g every 6 hours, or given as a continuous infusion over 24 hours (maximum: 4 g/24 hours)

Indication-specific dosing:

Children: Oral:

Acne vulgaris (unlabeled use): 250-1500 mg/day in 2 divided doses; therapy may be continued for 4-6 weeks at lowest possible dose

Pharyngitis: 40 mg/kg/day in 2 doses; maximum: 1600 mg/day; short-course therapy for 5 days may be considered

Pertussis (CDC guidelines): 40-50 mg/kg/day in 4 divided doses for 14 days; maximum 2 g/day (not preferred agent for infants <1 month)

Preop bowel preparation: 20 mg/kg erythromycin base at 1, 2, and 11 PM on the day before surgery combined with mechanical cleansing of the large intestine and oral neomycin

Adults:

Cervicitis: Oral: 500 mg 4 times/day for 7 days

Chancroid (unlabeled use; not a preferred agent): Oral: 500 mg 4 times/day for 7 days

Community-acquired pneumonia, bronchitis: Oral, I.V.: 500-1000 mg 4 times/day for 10-14 days. If *Legionella* is suspected/confirmed, 750-1000 mg 4 times/day for 21 days or more may be recommended. **Note:** Other macrolides and/or fluoroquinolones may be preferred and better tolerated.

Lymphogranuloma venereum: Oral: 500 mg 4 times/day for 21 days

Nongonococcal urethritis (recurrent): Oral: CDC Guidelines for the Treatment of Sexually Transmitted Diseases recommendation: Metronidazole (2 g as a single dose) plus 7 days of erythromycin base (500 mg 4 times/day) or erythromycin ethylsuccinate (800 mg 4 times/day)

Pertussis (CDC guidelines): 500 mg every 6 hours for 14 days

Preop bowel preparation (unlabeled use): Oral: 1 g erythromycin base at 1, 2, and 11 PM on the day before surgery combined with mechanical cleansing of the large intestine and oral neomycin

Gastrointestinal prokinetic (unlabeled use): Oral: Erythromycin has been used as a prokinetic agent to improve gastric emptying time and intestinal motility. In adults, 200 mg was infused I.V. initially followed by 250 mg orally 3 times/day 30 minutes before meals. Lower dosages have been used in some trials.

Dosage adjustment in renal impairment: Dialysis: Slightly dialyzable (5% to 20%); no supplemental dosage necessary in hemo- or peritoneal dialysis or in continuous arteriovenous or venovenous hemofiltration

Stability

Injection:

Erythromycin lactobionate should be reconstituted with sterile water for injection without preservatives to avoid gel formation; the reconstituted solution is stable for 2 weeks when refrigerated or for 24 hours at room temperature

Erythromycin I.V. infusion solution is stable at pH 6-8. Stability of lactobionate is pH dependent; I.V. form has the longest stability in 0.9% sodium chloride (NS) and should be prepared in this base solution whenever possible. Do not

(Continued)

Erythromycin *(Continued)*

use D_5W as a diluent unless sodium bicarbonate is added to solution. If I.V. must be prepared in D_5W, 0.5 mL of the 8.4% sodium bicarbonate solution should be added per each 100 mL of D_5W.

Stability of parenteral admixture at room temperature (25°C) and at refrigeration temperature (4°C): 24 hours

Standard diluent: 500 mg/250 mL D_5W/NS; 750 mg/250 mL D_5W/NS; 1 g/250 mL D_5W/NS

Oral suspension:

Granules: After mixing, store under refrigeration and use within 10 days.

Powder: Refrigerate to preserve taste. Erythromycin ethylsuccinate may be stored at room temperature if used within 14 days. EryPed® drops should be used within 35 days following reconstitution; may store at room temperature or under refrigeration.

Topical and ophthalmic formulations: Store at room temperature.

Administration

Oral: Do not crush enteric coated drug product. GI upset, including diarrhea, is common. May be administered with food to decrease GI upset. Do not give with milk or acidic beverages.

I.V.: Infuse 1 g over 20-60 minutes. I.V. infusion may be very irritating to the vein. If phlebitis/pain occurs with used dilution, consider diluting further (eg, 1:5) if fluid status of the patient will tolerate, or consider administering in larger available vein. The addition of lidocaine or bicarbonate does not decrease the irritation of erythromycin infusions.

Ophthalmic: Avoid contact of tip of ophthalmic ointment tube with affected eye

Anesthesia and Critical Care Concerns/Other Considerations Erythromycin, when used with drugs that affect the QT interval (eg, cisapride, ergot derivatives, pimozide) or when administered to patients with a prolonged QT interval, may further increase the QT interval and the risk of torsade de pointes (proarrhythmias).

Pregnancy Risk Factor B

Contraindications Hypersensitivity to erythromycin or any component of the formulation

Systemic: Pre-existing liver disease (erythromycin estolate); concomitant use with ergot derivatives, pimozide, or cisapride

Warnings/Precautions Systemic: Use caution with hepatic impairment with or without jaundice has occurred, it may be accompanied by malaise, nausea, vomiting, abdominal colic, and fever; discontinue use if these occur; avoid using erythromycin lactobionate in neonates since formulations may contain benzyl alcohol which is associated with toxicity in neonates; observe for superinfections. Use in infants has been associated with infantile hypertrophic pyloric stenosis (IHPS). Macrolides have been associated with rare QT prolongation and ventricular arrhythmias, including torsade de pointes. Elderly may be at increased risk of adverse events, including hearing loss and/or torsade de pointes when dosage ≥4 g/day, particularly if concurrent renal/hepatic impairment.

Adverse Reactions

Systemic:

Cardiovascular: Ventricular arrhythmia, QT_c prolongation, torsade de pointes (rare), ventricular tachycardia (rare)

Central nervous system: Headache (8%), pain (2%), fever, seizure

Dermatitis: Rash (3%), pruritus (1%)

Gastrointestinal: Abdominal pain (8%), cramping, nausea (8%), oral candidiasis, vomiting (3%), diarrhea (7%), dyspepsia (2%), flatulence (2%), anorexia, pseudomembranous colitis, hypertrophic pyloric stenosis (including cases in infants or IHPS), pancreatitis

Hematologic: Eosinophilia (1%)

Hepatic: Cholestatic jaundice (most common with estolate), increased liver function tests (2%)

Local: Phlebitis at the injection site, thrombophlebitis

Neuromuscular & skeletal: Weakness (2%)

Respiratory: Dyspnea (1%), cough (3%)

Miscellaneous: Hypersensitivity reactions, allergic reactions

Topical: 1% to 10%: Dermatologic: Erythema, desquamation, dryness, pruritus

Overdosage/Toxicology Symptoms of overdose include nausea, vomiting, diarrhea, prostration, reversible pancreatitis, hearing loss with or without tinnitus or vertigo. Care is general and supportive only.

Drug Interactions Substrate of CYP2B6 (minor), 3A4 (major); **Inhibits** CYP1A2 (weak), 3A4 (moderate)

Alfentanil (and possibly other narcotic analgesics): Serum levels may be increased by erythromycin; monitor for increased effect.

Antipsychotic agents (particularly mesoridazine and thioridazine): Risk of QT_c prolongation and malignant arrhythmias may be increased.

Benzodiazepines (those metabolized by CYP3A4, including alprazolam and triazolam): Serum levels may be increased by erythromycin; somnolence and confusion have been reported.

Bromocriptine: Serum levels may be increased by erythromycin; monitor for increased effect.

Buspirone: Serum levels may be increased by erythromycin; monitor.

Calcium channel blockers (felodipine, verapamil, and potentially others metabolized by CYP3A4): Serum levels may be increased by erythromycin; monitor.

Carbamazepine: Serum levels may be increased by erythromycin; monitor.

Cilostazol: Serum levels may be increased by erythromycin.

Cisapride: Serum levels may be increased by erythromycin; serious arrhythmias have occurred; concurrent use contraindicated.

Clindamycin (and lincomycin): Use with erythromycin may result in pharmacologic antagonism; manufacturer recommends avoiding this combination.

Clozapine: Serum levels may be increased by erythromycin; monitor.

Colchicine: serum levels/toxicity may be increased by erythromycin; monitor. Avoid use, if possible.

Cyclosporine: Serum levels may be increased by erythromycin; monitor serum levels.

CYP3A4 inducers: CYP3A4 inducers may decrease the levels/effects of erythromycin. Example inducers include aminoglutethimide, carbamazepine, nafcillin, nevirapine, phenobarbital, phenytoin, and rifamycins.

CYP3A4 inhibitors: May increase the levels/effects of erythromycin. Example inhibitors include azole antifungals, clarithromycin, diclofenac, doxycycline, imatinib, isoniazid, nefazodone, nicardipine, propofol, protease inhibitors, quinidine, telithromycin, and verapamil.

CYP3A4 substrates: Erythromycin may increase the levels/effects of CYP3A4 substrates. Example substrates include benzodiazepines, calcium channel blockers, cyclosporine, mirtazapine, nateglinide, nefazodone, sildenafil (and other PDE-5 inhibitors), tacrolimus, and venlafaxine. Selected benzodiazepines (midazolam and triazolam), cisapride, ergot alkaloids, selected HMG-CoA reductase inhibitors (lovastatin and simvastatin), and pimozide are generally contraindicated with strong CYP3A4 inhibitors.

Delavirdine: Serum levels of erythromycin may be increased; also, serum levels of delavirdine may increased by erythromycin (low risk); monitor.

Digoxin: Serum levels may be increased by erythromycin; monitor digoxin levels.

Disopyramide: Serum levels may be increased by erythromycin; in addition, QT_c prolongation and risk of malignant arrhythmia may be increased; avoid combination.

Ergot alkaloids: Concurrent use may lead to acute ergot toxicity (severe peripheral vasospasm and dysesthesia).

HMG-CoA reductase inhibitors (atorvastatin, lovastatin, and simvastatin); Erythromycin may increase serum levels of "statins" metabolized by CYP3A4, increasing the risk of myopathy/rhabdomyolysis (does not include fluvastatin and pravastatin). Switch to pravastatin/fluvastatin or suspend treatment during course of erythromycin therapy.

Loratadine: Serum levels may be increased by erythromycin; monitor.

Methylprednisolone: Serum levels may be increased by erythromycin; monitor.

Neuromuscular-blocking agents: May be potentiated by erythromycin (case reports).

Phenytoin: Serum levels may be increased by erythromycin; other evidence suggested phenytoin levels may be decreased in some patients; monitor.

Pimozide: Serum levels may be increased, leading to malignant arrhythmias; concomitant use is contraindicated.

Protease inhibitors (amprenavir, nelfinavir, and ritonavir): May increase serum levels of erythromycin.

QT_c-prolonging agents: Concomitant use may increase the risk of malignant arrhythmias.

Quinidine: Serum levels may be increased by erythromycin; in addition, the risk of QT_c prolongation and malignant arrhythmias may be increased during concurrent use.

(Continued)

Erythromycin *(Continued)*

Quinolone antibiotics (sparfloxacin, gatifloxacin, and moxifloxacin): Concurrent use may increase the risk of malignant arrhythmias.
Rifabutin: Serum levels may be increased by erythromycin; monitor.
Sildenafil, tadalafil, vardenafil: Serum concentration may be substantially increased by erythromycin. Do not exceed single sildenafil doses of 25 mg in 48 hours, a single tadalafil dose of 10 mg in 72 hours, or a single vardenafil dose of 2.5 mg in 24 hours.
Tacrolimus: Serum levels may be increased by erythromycin; monitor serum concentration.
Theophylline: Serum levels may be increased by erythromycin; monitor.
Valproic acid (and derivatives): Serum levels may be increased by erythromycin; monitor.
Vinblastine (and vincristine): Serum levels may be increased by erythromycin.
Warfarin: Effects may be potentiated; monitor INR closely and adjust warfarin dose as needed or choose another antibiotic.
Zafirlukast: Serum levels may be decreased by erythromycin; monitor.
Zopiclone: Serum levels may be increased by erythromycin; monitor.

Ethanol/Nutrition/Herb Interactions
Ethanol: Avoid ethanol (may decrease absorption of erythromycin or enhance ethanol effects).
Food: Increased drug absorption with meals; erythromycin serum levels may be altered if taken with food.
Herb/Nutraceutical: St John's wort may decrease erythromycin levels.

Test Interactions False-positive urinary catecholamines

Dietary Considerations Systemic: Drug may cause GI upset; may take with food.

Dosage Forms [DSC] = Discontinued product; [CAN] = Canadian brand name
Capsule, delayed release, enteric-coated pellets, as base (Eryc®): 250 mg
Gel, topical: 2% (30 g, 60 g)
  A/T/S®: 2% (30 g) [contains alcohol 92%]
  Erygel®: 2% (30 g, 60 g) [contains alcohol 92%]
Granules for oral suspension, as ethylsuccinate (E.E.S.®): 200 mg/5 mL (100 mL, 200 mL) [cherry flavor]
Injection, powder for reconstitution, as lactobionate (Erythrocin®): 500 mg, 1 g
Ointment, ophthalmic: 0.5% [5 mg/g] (1 g, 3.5 g)
  Romycin®: 0.5% [5 mg/g] (3.5 g)
Ointment, topical (Akne-Mycin®): 2% (25 g)
Powder for oral suspension, as ethylsuccinate (EryPed®): 200 mg/5 mL (100 mL, 200 mL) [fruit flavor]; 400 mg/5 mL (100 mL, 200 mL) [banana flavor]
Powder for oral suspension, as ethylsuccinate [drops] (EryPed®): 100 mg/2.5 mL (50 mL) [fruit flavor]
Solution, topical: 2% (60 mL)
  A/T/S®: 2% (60 mL) [contains alcohol 66%]
  Eryderm®, T-Stat® [DSC], Theramycin Z®: 2% (60 mL) [contain alcohol]
  Sans Acne® [CAN]: 2% (60 mL) [contains ethyl alcohol 44%; not available in U.S.]
  Staticin®: 1.5% (60 mL) [DSC]
Suspension, oral, as estolate: 125 mg/5 mL (480 mL); 250 mg/5 mL (480 mL)
Suspension, oral, as ethylsuccinate: 200 mg/5 mL (480 mL); 400 mg/5 mL (480 mL)
  E.E.S.®: 200 mg/5 mL (100 mL, 480 mL) [fruit flavor]; 400 mg/5 mL (100 mL, 480 mL) [orange flavor]
Swab (T-Stat® [DSC]): 2% (60s)
Tablet, chewable, as ethylsuccinate (EryPed®): 200 mg [fruit flavor] [DSC]
Tablet, delayed release, enteric coated, as base (Ery-Tab®): 250 mg, 333 mg, 500 mg
Tablet, as base: 250 mg, 500 mg
Tablet, as ethylsuccinate (E.E.S.®): 400 mg
Tablet, as stearate: 250 mg
  Erythrocin®: 250 mg, 500 mg
Tablet [polymer-coated particles], as base (PCE®): 333 mg, 500 mg

References
"Antimicrobial Prophylaxis for Surgery," *Treat Guidel Med Lett*, 2004, 2(20):27-32.

♦ **Erythromycin Base** *see* Erythromycin *on page 476*
♦ **Erythromycin Estolate** *see* Erythromycin *on page 476*

- **Erythromycin Ethylsuccinate** *see* Erythromycin *on page 476*
- **Erythromycin Gluceptate** *see* Erythromycin *on page 476*
- **Erythromycin Lactobionate** *see* Erythromycin *on page 476*
- **Erythromycin Stearate** *see* Erythromycin *on page 476*
- **Erythropoiesis Stimulating Protein** *see* Darbepoetin Alfa *on page 353*
- **Erythropoietin** *see* Epoetin Alfa *on page 463*
- **Eserine® (Can)** *see* Physostigmine *on page 1026*
- **Eserine Salicylate** *see* Physostigmine *on page 1026*
- **Eskalith® [DSC]** *see* Lithium *on page 770*
- **Eskalith CR®** *see* Lithium *on page 770*

Esmolol (ES moe lol)

Medication Safety Issues

Sound-alike/look-alike issues:

Esmolol may be confused with Osmitrol®

Brevibloc® may be confused with bretylium, Brevital®, Bumex®, Buprenex®

Related Information

Anesthesia for Patients With Liver Disease *on page 1421*

Antiarrhythmic Drugs *on page 1548*

Beta-Blockers *on page 1557*

Hypertension *on page 1620*

Management of Postoperative Arrhythmias *on page 1451*

Postoperative Hypertension *on page 1471*

Preoperative Evaluation of the Cardiac Patient for Noncardiac Surgery *on page 1485*

U.S. Brand Names Brevibloc®

Canadian Brand Names Brevibloc®

Synonyms Esmolol Hydrochloride

Pharmacologic Category Antiarrhythmic Agent, Class II; Beta Blocker, $Beta_1$ Selective

Generic Available Yes: Excludes infusion

Use Treatment of supraventricular tachycardia (SVT) and atrial fibrillation/flutter (control ventricular rate); treatment of tachycardia and/or hypertension (especially intraoperative or postoperative); treatment of noncompensatory sinus tachycardia

Unlabeled/Investigational Use In children, for SVT and postoperative hypertension

Mechanism of Action Class II antiarrhythmic: Competitively blocks response to $beta_1$-adrenergic stimulation with little or no effect of $beta_2$-receptors except at high doses, no intrinsic sympathomimetic activity, no membrane stabilizing activity

Pharmacodynamics/Kinetics

Onset of action: Beta-blockade: I.V.: 2-10 minutes (quickest when loading doses are administered)

Duration of hemodynamic effects: 10-30 minutes; prolonged following higher cumulative doses, extended duration of use

Protein binding: 55%

Metabolism: In blood by red blood cell esterases

Half-life elimination: Adults: 9 minutes; elimination of metabolite decreases with end stage renal disease

Excretion: Urine (~69% as metabolites, 2% unchanged drug)

Dosage I.V. infusion requires an infusion pump (must be adjusted to individual response and tolerance):

Children:

SVT (unlabeled use): A limited amount of information regarding esmolol use in pediatric patients is currently available. Some centers have utilized doses of 100-500 mcg/kg given over 1 minute for control of supraventricular tachycardias.

Postoperative hypertension (unlabeled use): Loading doses of 500 mcg/kg/minute over 1 minute with maximal doses of 50-250 mcg/kg/minute (mean = 173) have been used in addition to nitroprusside to treat postoperative hypertension after coarctation of aorta repair.

Adults:

Intraoperative tachycardia and/or hypertension (immediate control): Initial bolus: 80 mg (~1 mg/kg) over 30 seconds, followed by a 150 mcg/kg/minute

(Continued)

Esmolol *(Continued)*

infusion, if necessary. Adjust infusion rate as needed to maintain desired heart rate and/or blood pressure, up to 300 mcg/kg/minute.

For control of postoperative hypertension, as many as one-third of patients may require higher doses (250-300 mcg/kg/minute) to control blood pressure; the safety of doses >300 mcg/kg/minute has not been studied.

Supraventricular tachycardia or gradual control of postoperative tachycardia/hypertension: Loading dose: 500 mcg/kg over 1 minute; follow with a 50 mcg/kg/minute infusion for 4 minutes; response to this initial infusion rate may be a rough indication of the responsiveness of the ventricular rate.

Infusion may be continued at 50 mcg/kg/minute or, if the response is inadequate, titrated upward in 50 mcg/kg/minute increments (increased no more frequently than every 4 minutes) to a maximum of 200 mcg/kg/minute.

To achieve more rapid response, following the initial loading dose and 50 mcg/kg/minute infusion, rebolus with a second 500 mcg/kg loading dose over 1 minute, and increase the maintenance infusion to 100 mcg/kg/minute for 4 minutes. If necessary, a third (and final) 500 mcg/kg loading dose may be administered, prior to increasing to an infusion rate of 150 mcg/minute. After 4 minutes of the 150 mcg/kg/minute infusion, the infusion rate may be increased to a maximum rate of 200 mcg/kg/minute (without a bolus dose).

Usual dosage range (SVT): 50-200 mcg/kg/minute with average dose of 100 mcg/kg/minute.

Guidelines for transfer to oral therapy (beta blocker, calcium channel blocker):

Infusion should be reduced by 50% 30 minutes following the first dose of the alternative agent

Manufacturer suggests following the second dose of the alternative drug, patient's response should be monitored and if control is adequate for the first hours, esmolol may be discontinued.

Dialysis: Not removed by hemo- or peritoneal dialysis; supplemental dose is not necessary.

Stability Clear, colorless to light yellow solution which should be stored at 15°C to 30°C (59°F to 85°F); protect from freezing and excessive heat.

Stability of parenteral admixture at room temperature (25°C) is 24 hours.

Administration Infusions must be administered with an infusion pump. The concentrate (250 mg/mL ampul) is **not** for direct I.V. injection, but rather must first be diluted to a final concentration of 10 mg/mL (ie, 2.5 g in 250 mL or 5 g in 500 mL). Concentrations >10 mg/mL or infusion into small veins or through a butterfly catheter should be avoided (can cause thrombophlebitis). Decrease or discontinue infusion if hypotension or congestive heart failure occur. Medication port of premixed bags should be used to withdraw only the initial bolus, if necessary (not to be used for withdrawal of additional bolus doses).

Monitoring Parameters Blood pressure, heart rate, MAP, ECG, respiratory rate, I.V. site; cardiac monitor and blood pressure monitor required

Anesthesia and Critical Care Concerns/Other Considerations Esmolol 250 mg/mL contains propylene glycol 258 mg/mL (25% v/v).

This agent is also used to blunt sympathetic response during intubation, in "at-risk" patients such as those with coronary artery disease (CAD), angina, uncontrolled hypertension, and hyperthyroidism. Esmolol may lose $beta_1$-specificity after higher doses. It should be used with caution in patients with pulmonary disease and diabetes.

Esmolol provides an important mechanism for close titration of rate control in patients with atrial fibrillation; may also be beneficial in allowing close blood pressure control. Esmolol should only be administered in intensive care or closely monitored situations. Potential adverse effects include hypotension and bradyarrhythmias (usually short-lived due to short half-life of 9 minutes).

Pregnancy Risk Factor C (manufacturer); D (2nd and 3rd trimesters - expert analysis)

Contraindications Hypersensitivity to esmolol or any component of the formulation; sinus bradycardia; heart block greater than first degree (except in patients with a functioning artificial pacemaker); cardiogenic shock; bronchial asthma (relative); uncompensated cardiac failure; hypotension; pregnancy (2nd and 3rd trimesters)

Warnings/Precautions Hypotension is common; patients need close blood pressure monitoring. Administer cautiously in compensated heart failure and monitor for a worsening of the condition. Use caution in patients with PVD (can aggravate arterial insufficiency). Use caution with concurrent use of beta-blockers and either verapamil or diltiazem; bradycardia or heart block can occur. Avoid concurrent I.V. use of both agents. Use beta-blockers cautiously in patients with bronchospastic disease; monitor pulmonary status closely. Use cautiously in diabetics because it can mask prominent hypoglycemic symptoms. Can mask signs of thyrotoxicosis. Can cause fetal bradycardia when administered in the 3rd trimester of pregnancy or at delivery. Use caution in patients with renal dysfunction (active metabolite retained). Do not use in the treatment of hypertension associated with vasoconstriction related to hypothermia. Concentrations >10 mg/mL or infusion into small veins or through a butterfly catheter should be avoided (can cause thrombophlebitis). Extravasation can lead to skin necrosis and sloughing.

Adverse Reactions

>10%:

Cardiovascular: Asymptomatic hypotension (dose-related: 25% to 38%), symptomatic hypotension (dose-related: 12%)

Miscellaneous: Diaphoresis (10%)

1% to 10%:

Cardiovascular: Peripheral ischemia (1%)

Central nervous system: Dizziness (3%), somnolence (3%), confusion (2%), headache (2%), agitation (2%), fatigue (1%)

Gastrointestinal: Nausea (7%), vomiting (1%)

Local: Pain on injection (8%), infusion site reaction

<1% (Limited to important or life-threatening): Alopecia, bronchospasm, chest pain, CHF, depression, dyspnea, edema, exfoliative dermatitis, heart block, infusion site reactions, paresthesia, pruritus, pulmonary edema, rigors, seizure, severe bradycardia/asystole (rare), skin necrosis (from extravasation), syncope, thrombophlebitis, urinary retention

Overdosage/Toxicology Symptoms of overdose include hypotension, bradycardia, bronchospasm, congestive heart failure, and heart block. Initially, a decrease/discontinuation of the esmolol infusion and administration of fluids may be the best treatment for hypotension. Sympathomimetics (eg, epinephrine or dopamine), glucagon, or an anticholinergic or a pacemaker can be used to treat the toxic bradycardia, asystole, and/or hypotension.

Drug Interactions

Acetylcholinesterase Inhibitors: May enhance the bradycardic effect of beta-blockers.

Alpha/beta agonists (direct acting): Beta blockers may enhance the vasopressor effect of alpha/beta agonists (direct-acting). Epinephrine used as a local anesthetic for dental procedures will not likely cause clinically-relevant problems.

$Alpha_1$-blockers: Beta blockers may enhance the orthostatic effect of $alpha_1$ blockers. The risk associated with ophthalmic products is probably less than systemic products.

$Alpha_2$ agonists: Beta blockers may enhance the rebound hypertensive effect of $alpha_2$ agonists. This effect can occur when the $alpha_2$ agonist is abruptly withdrawn.

Amiodarone: May enhance the bradycardic effect of beta-blockers. Possibly to the point of cardiac arrest. Consider therapy modification.

$Beta_2$ agonists: May diminish the bradycardic effect of beta-blockers ($beta_1$ selective); of concern with high doses of some beta-blockers.

Calcium channel blockers (nondihydropyridine): May enhance the hypotensive effect of beta-blockers. Bradycardia and signs of heart failure have also been reported.

Cardiac glycosides: Beta-blockers may enhance the bradycardic effect of cardiac glycosides.

Disopyramide; May enhance the bradycardic effect of beta-blockers. Use caution if coadministering disopyramide and a beta-blocker (especially if both are I.V.).

Insulin preparations: Beta-blockers may enhance the hypoglycemic effect of insulin preparations.

NSAIDs: May diminish the antihypertensive effect of beta-blockers.

Sulfonylureas: Beta-blockers may enhance the hypoglycemic effect of sulfonylureas. Cardioselective beta-blockers (eg, esmolol) may be safer than nonselective beta-blockers. All beta-blockers appear to mask tachycardia as an initial symptom of hypoglycemia.

(Continued)

Esmolol *(Continued)*

Test Interactions Increases cholesterol (S), glucose

Dosage Forms

Infusion [premixed in sodium chloride; preservative free] (Brevibloc®): 2000 mg (100 mL) [20 mg/mL; double strength]; 2500 mg (250 mL) [10 mg/mL]

Injection, solution, as hydrochloride: 10 mg/mL (10 mL) [premixed in sodium chloride]

Brevibloc®: 10 mg/mL (10 mL) [alcohol free; premixed in sodium chloride]; 20 mg/mL (5 mL, 100 mL) [alcohol free; double strength; premixed in sodium chloride]; 250 mg/mL (10 mL) [contains alcohol 25%, propylene glycol 25%; concentrate]

References

Antman EM, Anbe SC, Alpert JS, et al, "ACC/AHA Guidelines for the Management of Patients With ST-Elevation Myocardial Infarction - Executive Summary: A Report of the American College of Cardiology/American Heart Association Task Force on Practice Guidelines (Writing Committee to Revise the 1999 Guidelines for the Management of Patients With Acute Myocardial Infarction)," *Circulation*, 2004, 110:588-636. Available at: http://www.circulationaha.org/cgi/content/full/110/5/588. Last accessed August 26, 2004.

Braunwald E, Antman EM, Beasley JW, et al, "ACC/AHA 2002 Guideline Update for the Management of Patients With Unstable Angina and Non-ST-Segment Elevation Myocardial Infarction - Summary Article: A Report of the American College of Cardiology/American Heart Association Task Force on Practice Guidelines (Committee on the Management of Patients With Unstable Angina)," *J Am Coll Cardiol*, 2002, 40(7):1366-74. Available at: http://www.acc.org/clinical/guidelines/unstable/incorporated/index.htm. Accessed May 20, 2003.

Chobanian AV, Bakris GL, Black HR, et al, "The Seventh Report of the Joint National Committee on Prevention, Detection, Evaluation, and Treatment of High Blood Pressure," *JAMA*, 2003, 289(19):2560-72.

Erstad BL and Barletta JF, "Treatment of Hypertension in the Perioperative Patient," *Ann Pharmacother*, 2000, 34(1):66-79.

Mokhlesi B, Leikin JB, Murray P, et al, "Adult Toxicology in Critical Care. Part 11: Specific Poisonings," *Chest*, 2003, 123(3):897-922.

♦ **Esmolol Hydrochloride** *see* Esmolol *on page 481*

Esomeprazole (es oh ME pray zol)

U.S. Brand Names Nexium®

Canadian Brand Names Nexium®

Synonyms Esomeprazole Magnesium

Pharmacologic Category Proton Pump Inhibitor; Substituted Benzimidazole

Generic Available No

Use

Oral: Short-term (4-8 weeks) treatment of erosive esophagitis; maintaining symptom resolution and healing of erosive esophagitis; treatment of symptomatic gastroesophageal reflux disease (GERD); as part of a multidrug regimen for *Helicobacter pylori* eradication in patients with duodenal ulcer disease (active or history of within the past 5 years); prevention of gastric ulcers in patients at risk (age ≥60 years and/or history of gastric ulcer) associated with continuous NSAID therapy

I.V.: Short-term (≤10 weeks) treatment of gastroesophageal reflux disease (GERD) when oral therapy is not possible or appropriate

Mechanism of Action Proton pump inhibitor suppresses gastric acid secretion by inhibition of the H^+/K^+-ATPase in the gastric parietal cell

Pharmacodynamics/Kinetics

Distribution: V_{dss}: 16 L

Protein binding: 97%

Metabolism: Hepatic via CYP2C19 and 3A4 enzymes to hydroxy, desmethyl, and sulfone metabolites (all inactive)

Bioavailability: 90% with repeat dosing

Half-life elimination: 1-1.5 hours

Time to peak: 1.5 hours

Excretion: Urine (80%); feces (20%)

Dosage Note: Delayed-release capsules should be swallowed whole and taken at least 1 hour before eating

Adolescents 12-17 years: Oral: GERD: 20-40 mg once daily for up to 8 weeks

Adults:

Oral:

Erosive esophagitis (healing): Initial: 20-40 mg once daily for 4-8 weeks; if incomplete healing, may continue for an additional 4-8 weeks; maintenance: 20 mg once daily

Symptomatic GERD: 20 mg once daily for 4 weeks; may continue an additional 4 weeks if symptoms persist

Helicobacter pylori eradication: 40 mg once daily for 10 days; requires combination therapy

Prevention of NSAID-induced gastric ulcers: 20-40 mg once daily for up to 6 months

I.V.: GERD: 20 mg or 40 mg once daily for ≤10 days; change to oral therapy as soon as appropriate

Elderly: No dosage adjustment needed

Dosage adjustment in renal impairment: No dosage adjustment needed

Dosage adjustment in hepatic impairment:

Mild-to-moderate hepatic impairment (Child-Pugh Class A or B): No dosage adjustment needed

Severe hepatic impairment (Child-Pugh Class C): Dose should not exceed 20 mg/day

Stability Capsule: Store at 15°C to 30°C (59°F to 86°F); keep container tightly closed

Powder for injection: Store at 15°C to 30°C (59°F to 86°F); protect from light.

For I.V. injection: Reconstitute powder with 5 mL NS.

For I.V. infusion: Initially reconstitute powder with 5 mL of NS, LR, or D_5W, then further dilute to a final volume of 50 mL.

Following reconstitution, solution for injection prepared in NS, and solution for infusion prepared in NS or LR should be used within 12 hours. Following reconstitution, solution for infusion prepared in D_5W should be used within 6 hours. Refrigeration is not required following reconstitution.

Administration

Oral: Capsule should be swallowed whole and taken at least 1 hour before eating (best if taken before breakfast). For patients with difficulty swallowing, open capsule and mix contents with 1 tablespoon of applesauce. Swallow immediately; mixture should not be chewed or warmed. The mixture should not be stored for future use.

I.V.: May be administered by injection (≥3 minutes) or infusion (10-30 minutes). Flush line prior to and after administration with NS, LR, or D_5W.

Nasogastric tube: Open capsule and place intact granules into a 60 mL syringe; mix with 50 mL of water. Replace plunger and shake vigorously for 15 seconds. Ensure that no granules remain in syringe tip. Do not administer if pellets dissolve or disintegrate. After administration, flush nasogastric tube with additional water. Use suspension immediately after preparation.

Monitoring Parameters Susceptibility testing recommended in patients who fail *H. pylori* eradication regimen (esomeprazole, clarithromycin, and amoxicillin)

Anesthesia and Critical Care Concerns/Other Considerations The contents of the capsule remain intact when exposed to tap water, orange juice, apple juice, and yogurt.

For administration into a nasogastric tube: Open capsule and place intact granules into a 60 mL syringe; mix with 50 mL of water. Replace plunger and shake vigorously for 15 seconds. Do not administer if pellets dissolve or disintegrate. After administration, flush nasogastric tube with additional water. Use suspension immediately after preparation.

Pregnancy Risk Factor B

Contraindications Hypersensitivity to esomeprazole, substituted benzimidazoles (ie, lansoprazole, omeprazole, pantoprazole, rabeprazole), or any component of the formulation

Warnings/Precautions Relief of symptoms does not preclude the presence of a gastric malignancy. Atrophic gastritis (by biopsy) has been noted with long-term omeprazole therapy; this may also occur with esomeprazole. No reports of enterochromaffin-like (ECL) cell carcinoids, dysplasia, or neoplasia has occurred. No reports of enterochromaffin-like (ECL) cell carcinoids, dysplasia, or neoplasia has occurred. Safety and efficacy in children <12 years of age have not been established.

Adverse Reactions Unless otherwise specified, percentages represent adverse reactions identified in clinical trials evaluating the intravenous formulation.

>10%: Central nervous system: Headache (I.V. 11%; oral 4% to 8%)

1% to 10%:

Central nervous system: Dizziness (3%)

Dermatologic: Pruritus (≤1%)

(Continued)

Esomeprazole *(Continued)*

Gastrointestinal: Flatulence (10%), nausea (2% to 6%), abdominal pain (6%; oral 3% to 4%), diarrhea (4%), xerostomia (2% to 4%), dyspepsia (<1% to 6%), constipation (3%)

Local: Injection site reaction (2%)

Respiratory: Sinusitis (≤2%), respiratory infection (1%)

<1% (Limited to important or life-threatening): Agranulocytosis, albuminuria, alkaline phosphatase increased, allergic reactions, alopecia, anaphylactic shock, anaphylaxis, anemia, angioedema, arthritis exacerbation, arthropathy, asthenia, asthma exacerbation, Barrett's esophagus, benign polyps/nodules, bilirubinemia, blurred vision, cervical lymphadenopathy, chest pain, confusion, creatinine increased, cystitis, depression/depression exacerbation, dermatitis, duodenitis, dysmenorrhea, dysphagia, dyspnea, epigastric pain, epistaxis, erythema multiforme, esophageal stricture, esophageal ulceration, esophageal varices, esophagitis, facial edema, fever, fibromyalgia syndrome, flu-like syndrome, flushing, fungal infection, gastric ulcer, gastritis, gastroenteritis, genital moniliasis, GI dysplasia, GI hemorrhage, glycosuria, goiter, hematuria, hepatic enzymes increased, hepatitis, hernia, hot flushes, hypertension, hypertonia, hyperuricemia, hypochromic anemia, hypoesthesia, hyponatremia, jaundice, larynx edema, leukocytosis, leukopenia, maculopapular rash, migraine, myalgia, pain, pancreatitis, pancytopenia, paresthesia, parosmia, peripheral edema, polymyalgia rheumatica, polyuria, pruritus ani, rash, rigors, serum gastrin increased, Stevens-Johnson syndrome, substernal chest pain, tachycardia, thrombocytopenia, thyroid stimulating hormone increased, tinnitus, tongue edema, total bilirubin increased, toxic epidermal necrolysis, tremor, ulcerative stomatitis, urticaria, vaginitis, vertigo, vision change, vitamin B_{12} deficiency, vomiting

Overdosage/Toxicology Doses up to 2400 mg have been reported. Symptoms of overdose may include confusion, drowsiness, blurred vision, tachycardia, nausea, sweating, headache or dry mouth. Treatment is symptom-directed and supportive; not dialyzable.

Drug Interactions **Substrate** of CYP2C19 (major), 3A4 (minor); **Inhibits** CYP2C19 (moderate)

Benzodiazepines metabolized by oxidation (eg, diazepam, midazolam, triazolam): Esomeprazole and omeprazole may increase levels of benzodiazepines metabolized by oxidation.

Carbamazepine: Esomeprazole and omeprazole may increase carbamazepine levels. Carbamazepine may decrease the effects of esomeprazole.

CYP2C19 inducers: May decrease the levels/effects of esomeprazole. Example inducers include aminoglutethimide, carbamazepine, phenytoin, and rifampin.

CYP2C19 substrates: Esomeprazole may increase the levels/effects of CYP2C19 substrates. Example substrates include citalopram, diazepam, methsuximide, phenytoin, propranolol, and sertraline.

HMG-CoA reductase inhibitors: Esomeprazole may increase the levels/effects; monitor.

Iron salts: Esomeprazole may decrease the absorption of orally-administered iron salts.

Itraconazole and ketoconazole: Proton pump inhibitors may decrease the absorption of itraconazole and ketoconazole.

Protease inhibitors: Proton pump inhibitors may decrease absorption of some protease inhibitors (atazanavir and indinavir).

Ethanol/Nutrition/Herb Interactions Food: Absorption is decreased by 43% to 53% when taken with food.

Dietary Considerations Take at least 1 hour before meals; best if taken before breakfast. The contents of the capsule may be mixed in applesauce or water; pellets also remain intact when exposed to orange juice, apple juice, and yogurt.

Dosage Forms

Capsule, delayed release:

Nexium®: 20 mg, 40 mg

Injection, powder for reconstitution:

Nexium®: 20 mg, 40 mg [contains edetate sodium]

◆ **Esomeprazole Magnesium** *see* Esomeprazole *on page 484*

Estazolam (es TA zoe lam)

Medication Safety Issues

Sound-alike/look-alike issues:

ProSom® may be confused with PhosLo®, Proscar®, Pro-Sof® Plus, Prozac®, Psorcon®

Related Information

Benzodiazepines *on page 1555*

U.S. Brand Names ProSom®

Pharmacologic Category Benzodiazepine

Restrictions C-IV

Generic Available Yes

Use Short-term management of insomnia

Mechanism of Action Binds to stereospecific benzodiazepine receptors on the postsynaptic GABA neuron at several sites within the central nervous system, including the limbic system, reticular formation. Enhancement of the inhibitory effect of GABA on neuronal excitability results by increased neuronal membrane permeability to chloride ions. This shift in chloride ions results in hyperpolarization (a less excitable state) and stabilization.

Pharmacodynamics/Kinetics

Onset of action: ~1 hour

Duration: Variable

Metabolism: Extensively hepatic

Half-life elimination: 10-24 hours (no significant changes in elderly)

Time to peak, serum: 0.5-1.6 hours

Excretion: Urine (<5% as unchanged drug)

Dosage Adults: Oral: 1 mg at bedtime, some patients may require 2 mg; start at doses of 0.5 mg in debilitated or small elderly patients

Dosing adjustment in hepatic impairment: May be necessary

Monitoring Parameters Respiratory and cardiovascular status

Anesthesia and Critical Care Concerns/Other Considerations Abrupt discontinuation after sustained use (generally >10 days) may cause withdrawal symptoms.

Pregnancy Risk Factor X

Contraindications Hypersensitivity to estazolam or any component of the formulation (cross-sensitivity with other benzodiazepines may exist); pregnancy

Note: Manufacturer states concurrent therapy with itraconazole or ketoconazole is contraindicated.

Warnings/Precautions As a hypnotic, should be used only after evaluation of potential causes of sleep disturbance. Failure of sleep disturbance to resolve after 7-10 days may indicate psychiatric or medical illness. Use is not recommended in patients with depressive disorders or psychoses. Avoid use in patients with sleep apnea. Use with caution in patients receiving concurrent CYP3A4 inhibitors, particularly when these agents are added to therapy. Use with caution in elderly or debilitated patients, patients with hepatic disease (including alcoholics), renal impairment, respiratory disease, impaired gag reflex, or obese patients.

Causes CNS depression (dose-related) which may impair physical and mental capabilities. Use with caution in patients receiving other CNS depressants or psychoactive agents. Benzodiazepines have been associated with falls and traumatic injury and should be used with extreme caution in patients who are at risk of these events (especially the elderly). May cause physical or psychological dependence - use with caution in patients with a history of drug dependence.

Benzodiazepines have been associated with anterograde amnesia. Paradoxical reactions, including hyperactive or aggressive behavior, have been reported with benzodiazepines, particularly in adolescent/pediatric or psychiatric patients. Does not have analgesic, antidepressant, or antipsychotic properties.

Adverse Reactions

>10%:

Central nervous system: Somnolence

Neuromuscular & skeletal: Weakness

1% to 10%:

Cardiovascular: Flushing, palpitation

(Continued)

Estazolam *(Continued)*

Central nervous system: Anxiety, confusion, dizziness, hypokinesia, abnormal coordination, hangover effect, agitation, amnesia, apathy, emotional lability, euphoria, hostility, seizure, sleep disorder, stupor, twitch
Dermatologic: Dermatitis, pruritus, rash, urticaria
Gastrointestinal: Xerostomia, constipation, decreased appetite, flatulence, gastritis, increased appetite, perverse taste
Genitourinary: Frequent urination, menstrual cramps, urinary hesitancy, urinary frequency, vaginal discharge/itching
Neuromuscular & skeletal: Paresthesia
Ocular: Photophobia, eye pain, eye swelling
Respiratory: Cough, dyspnea, asthma, rhinitis, sinusitis
Miscellaneous: Diaphoresis

<1% (Limited to important or life-threatening): Allergic reactions, chills, drug dependence, fever, muscle spasm, myalgia, neck pain

Overdosage/Toxicology Symptoms of overdose include respiratory depression, hypoactive reflexes, unsteady gait, and hypotension. Treatment for benzodiazepine overdose is supportive. Flumazenil has been shown to selectively block the binding of benzodiazepines to CNS receptors, resulting in a reversal of benzodiazepine-induced sedation; however, its use may not reverse respiratory depression.

Drug Interactions **Substrate** of CYP3A4 (minor)

CNS depressants: Sedative effects and/or respiratory depression may be additive with CNS depressants; includes ethanol, barbiturates, narcotic analgesics, and other sedative agents; monitor for increased effect
Itraconazole, ketoconazole: Concurrent use is contraindicated (per manufacturer); however, estazolam is a minor CYP3A4 substrate and an effect has not been documented in clinical studies.
Levodopa: Therapeutic effects may be diminished in some patients following the addition of a benzodiazepine; limited/inconsistent data
Oral contraceptives: May decrease the clearance of some benzodiazepines (those which undergo oxidative metabolism); monitor for increased benzodiazepine effect
Theophylline: May partially antagonize some of the effects of benzodiazepines; monitor for decreased response; may require higher doses for sedation

Ethanol/Nutrition/Herb Interactions

Ethanol: Avoid ethanol (may increase CNS depression).
Food: Serum levels and/or toxicity may be increased by grapefruit juice.

Dosage Forms Tablet: 1 mg, 2 mg

♦ **Estrogenic Substances, Conjugated** *see* Estrogens (Conjugated/Equine) *on page 488*

Estrogens (Conjugated/Equine)

(ES troe jenz KON joo gate ed, EE kwine)

Medication Safety Issues

Sound-alike/look-alike issues:
Premarin® may be confused with Primaxin®, Provera®, Remeron®

U.S. Brand Names Premarin®

Canadian Brand Names Cenestin; C.E.S.®; Premarin®

Synonyms CEE; C.E.S.; Estrogenic Substances, Conjugated

Pharmacologic Category Estrogen Derivative

Generic Available No

Use Treatment of moderate to severe vasomotor symptoms associated with menopause; treatment of vulvar and vaginal atrophy; hypoestrogenism (due to hypogonadism, castration, or primary ovarian failure); prostatic cancer (palliation); breast cancer (palliation); osteoporosis (prophylaxis, postmenopausal women at significant risk only); abnormal uterine bleeding

Unlabeled/Investigational Use Uremic bleeding

Mechanism of Action Conjugated estrogens contain a mixture of estrone sulfate, equilin sulfate, 17 alpha-dihydroequilin, 17 alpha-estradiol and 17 beta-dihydroequilin. Estrogens are responsible for the development and maintenance of the female reproductive system and secondary sexual characteristics. Estradiol is the principle intracellular human estrogen and is more potent than estrone and estriol at the receptor level; it is the primary estrogen secreted prior to menopause. Following menopause, estrone and estrone sulfate are more highly produced. Estrogens modulate the pituitary secretion of gonadotropins, luteinizing hormone, and follicle-stimulating hormone through a negative feedback system; estrogen replacement reduces elevated levels of these hormones in postmenopausal women.

Pharmacodynamics/Kinetics

Absorption: Well absorbed

Metabolism: Hepatic via CYP3A4; estradiol is converted to estrone and estriol; also undergoes enterohepatic recirculation; estrone sulfite is the main metabolite in postmenopausal women

Excretion: Urine (primarily estriol, also as estradiol, estrone, and conjugates

Dosage Adults:

Male: Androgen-dependent prostate cancer palliation: Oral: 1.25-2.5 mg 3 times/day

Female:

Prevention of postmenopausal osteoporosis: Oral: Initial: 0.3 mg/day cyclically* or daily, depending on medical assessment of patient. Dose may be adjusted based on bone mineral density and clinical response. The lowest effective dose should be used.

Moderate to severe vasomotor symptoms associated with menopause: Oral: Initial: 0.3 mg/day, cyclically* or daily, depending on medical assessment of patient. The lowest dose that will control symptoms should be used. Medication should be discontinued as soon as possible.

Vulvar and vaginal atrophy:

Oral: Initial: 0.3 mg/day; the lowest dose that will control symptoms should be used. May be given cyclically* or daily, depending on medical assessment of patient. Medication should be discontinued as soon as possible.

Vaginal cream: Intravaginal: ½ to 2 g/day given cyclically*

Abnormal uterine bleeding:

Acute/heavy bleeding:

Oral (unlabeled route): 1.25 mg, may repeat every 4 hours for 24 hours, followed by 1.25 mg once daily for 7-10 days

I.M., I.V.: 25 mg, may repeat in 6-12 hours if needed

Note: Treatment should be followed by a low-dose oral contraceptive; medroxyprogesterone acetate along with or following estrogen therapy can also be given

Nonacute/lesser bleeding: Oral (unlabeled route): 1.25 mg once daily for 7-10 days

Female hypogonadism: Oral: 0.3-0.625 mg/day given cyclically*; dose may be titrated in 6- to 12-month intervals; progestin treatment should be added to maintain bone mineral density once skeletal maturity is achieved.

Female castration, primary ovarian failure: Oral: 1.25 mg/day given cyclically*; adjust according to severity of symptoms and patient response. For maintenance, adjust to the lowest effective dose.

***Cyclic administration:** Either 3 weeks on, 1 week off **or** 25 days on, 5 days off

Male and Female:

Breast cancer palliation, metastatic disease in selected patients: Oral: 10 mg 3 times/day for at least 3 months

Uremic bleeding (unlabeled use): I.V.: 0.6 mg/kg/day for 5 days

Elderly: Refer to Adults dosing; a higher incidence of stroke and invasive breast cancer was observed in women >75 years in a WHI substudy.

Stability

Injection: Refrigerate at 2°C to 8°C (36°F to 46°F) prior to reconstitution. Reconstitute using provided diluent; do not shake violently. Following reconstitution, solution may be stored under refrigeration for up to 60 days. Do not use if darkening or precipitation occurs.

Tablets, vaginal cream: Store at room temperature (25°C)

Administration

Injection: May also be administered intramuscularly; when administered I.V., drug should be administered slowly to avoid the occurrence of a flushing reaction

Oral tablet, vaginal cream: Administer at bedtime to minimize adverse effects.

Monitoring Parameters Yearly physical examination that includes blood pressure and Papanicolaou smear, breast exam, mammogram. Monitor for signs of endometrial cancer in female patients with uterus. Adequate diagnostic measures, including endometrial sampling, if indicated, should be performed to

(Continued)

Estrogens (Conjugated/Equine) *(Continued)*

rule out malignancy in all cases of undiagnosed abnormal vaginal bleeding. Monitor for loss of vision, sudden onset of proptosis, diplopia, migraine; signs and symptoms of thromboembolic disorders; glycemic control in diabetics; lipid profiles in patients being treated for hyperlipidemias; thyroid function in patients on thyroid hormone replacement therapy.

Menopausal symptoms: Assess need for therapy at 3- to 6-month intervals

Prevention of osteoporosis: Bone density measurement

Reference Range

Children: <10 mcg/24 hours (SI: <35 μmol/day) (values at Mayo Medical Laboratories)

Adults:

Male: 15-40 mcg/24 hours (SI: 52-139 μmol/day)

Female:

Menstruating: 15-80 mcg/24 hours (SI: 52-277 μmol/day)

Postmenopausal: <20 mcg/24 hours (SI: <69 μmol/day)

Pregnancy Risk Factor X

Contraindications Hypersensitivity to estrogens or any component of the formulation; undiagnosed abnormal vaginal bleeding; history of or current thrombophlebitis or venous thromboembolic disorders (including DVT, PE); active or recent (within 1 year) arterial thromboembolic disease (eg, stroke, MI); carcinoma of the breast (except in appropriately selected patients being treated for metastatic disease); estrogen-dependent tumor; hepatic dysfunction or disease; pregnancy

Warnings/Precautions

Cardiovascular-related considerations: **[U.S. Boxed Warning]: Estrogens with or without progestin should not be used to prevent coronary heart disease.** Use caution with cardiovascular disease or dysfunction. May increase the risks of hypertension, myocardial infarction (MI), stroke, pulmonary emboli (PE), and deep vein thrombosis; incidence of these effects was shown to be significantly increased in postmenopausal women using conjugated equine estrogens (CEE) in combination with medroxyprogesterone acetate (MPA). Nonfatal MI, PE, and thrombophlebitis have also been reported in males taking high doses of CEE (eg, for prostate cancer). Estrogen compounds are generally associated with lipid effects such as increased HDL-cholesterol and decreased LDL-cholesterol. Triglycerides may also be increased; use with caution in patients with familial defects of lipoprotein metabolism. Whenever possible, estrogens should be discontinued at least 4 weeks prior to and for 2 weeks following elective surgery associated with an increased risk of thromboembolism or during periods of prolonged immobilization.

Neurological considerations: **[U.S. Boxed Warning]: The risk of dementia may be increased in postmenopausal women;** increased incidence was observed in women ≥65 years of age taking CEE alone or in combination with MPA.

Cancer-related considerations: **[U.S. Boxed Warning]: Unopposed estrogens may increase the risk of endometrial carcinoma in postmenopausal women.** Estrogens may exacerbate endometriosis. Malignant transformation of residual endometrial implants has been reported post-hysterectomy with estrogen only therapy. Consider adding a progestin in women with residual endometriosis post-hysterectomy. Estrogens may increase the risk of breast cancer. An increased risk of invasive breast cancer was observed in postmenopausal women using CEE in combination with MPA; a smaller increase in risk was seen with estrogen therapy alone in observational studies. An increase in abnormal mammograms has also been reported with estrogen and progestin therapy. Estrogen use may lead to severe hypercalcemia in patients with breast cancer and bone metastases; discontinue estrogen if hypercalcemia occurs.

Estrogens may cause retinal vascular thrombosis; discontinue permanently if papilledema or retinal vascular lesions are observed on examination. Use with caution in patients with diseases which may be exacerbated by fluid retention, including asthma, epilepsy, migraine, diabetes or renal dysfunction. Use with caution in patients with a history of severe hypocalcemia, SLE, hepatic hemangiomas, porphyria, endometriosis, and gallbladder disease. Use caution with history of cholestatic jaundice associated with past estrogen use or pregnancy. Safety and efficacy in pediatric patients have not been established. Prior to puberty, estrogens may cause premature closure of the epiphyses, premature breast development in girls or gynecomastia in boys. Vaginal bleeding and vaginal cornification may also be induced in girls.

Before prescribing estrogen therapy to postmenopausal women, the risks and benefits must be weighed for each patient. Women should be informed of these risks and benefits, as well as possible effects of progestin when added to estrogen therapy. Estrogens with or without progestin should be used for shortest duration possible consistent with treatment goals. Conduct periodic risk:benefit assessments.

When used solely for prevention of osteoporosis in women at significant risk, nonestrogen treatment options should be considered. When used solely for the treatment of vulvar and vaginal atrophy, topical vaginal products should be considered. Use caution applying topical products to severely atrophic vaginal mucosa.

Adverse Reactions

Note: Percentages reported in postmenopausal women.

>10%:

- Central nervous system: Headache (26% to 32%; placebo 28%)
- Endocrine & metabolic: Breast pain (7% to 12%; placebo 9%)
- Gastrointestinal: Abdominal pain (15% to 17%)
- Genitourinary: Vaginal hemorrhage (2% to 14%)
- Neuromuscular & skeletal: Back pain (13% to 14%)

1% to 10%:

- Central nervous system: Nervousness (2% to 5%)
- Endocrine & metabolic: Leukorrhea (4% to 7%)
- Gastrointestinal: Flatulence (6% to 7%)
- Genitourinary: Vaginitis (5% to 7%), vaginal moniliasis (5% to 6%)
- Neuromuscular & skeletal: Weakness (7% to 8%), leg cramps (3% to 7%)

In addition, the following have been reported with estrogen and/or progestin therapy:

Cardiovascular: Edema, hypertension, MI, stroke, venous thromboembolism

Central nervous system: Dizziness, epilepsy exacerbation, headache, irritability, mental depression, migraine, mood disturbances, nervousness

Dermatologic: Angioedema, chloasma, erythema multiforme, erythema nodosum, hemorrhagic eruption, hirsutism, loss of scalp hair, melasma, pruritus, rash, urticaria

Endocrine & metabolic: Breast cancer, breast enlargement, breast tenderness, libido (changes in), increased thyroid-binding globulin, increased total thyroid hormone (T_4), increased serum triglycerides/phospholipids, increased HDL-cholesterol, decreased LDL-cholesterol, impaired glucose tolerance, hypercalcemia, hypocalcemia

Gastrointestinal: Abdominal cramps, bloating, cholecystitis, cholelithiasis, gallbladder disease, nausea, pancreatitis, vomiting, weight gain/loss

Genitourinary: Alterations in frequency and flow of menses, changes in cervical secretions, endometrial cancer, endometrial hyperplasia, increased size of uterine leiomyomata, vaginal candidiasis

Hematologic: Aggravation of porphyria, decreased antithrombin III and antifactor Xa, increased levels of fibrinogen, increased platelet aggregability and platelet count; increased prothrombin and factors VII, VIII, IX, X

Hepatic: Cholestatic jaundice, hepatic hemangiomas enlarged

Neuromuscular & skeletal: Arthralgias, chorea, leg cramps

Local: Thrombophlebitis

Ocular: Intolerance to contact lenses, retinal vascular thrombosis, steeping of corneal curvature

Respiratory: Asthma exacerbation, pulmonary thromboembolism

Miscellaneous: Anaphylactoid/anaphylactic reactions, carbohydrate intolerance

Overdosage/Toxicology Toxicity is unlikely following single exposures of excessive doses, any treatment following emesis and charcoal administration should be supportive and symptomatic. Effects noted after large doses include headache, nausea, and vomiting. Bleeding may occur in females.

Drug Interactions

Based on estradiol and estrone: **Substrate** of CYP1A2 (major), 2A6 (minor), 2B6 (minor), 2C9 (minor), 2C19 (minor), 2D6 (minor), 2E1 (minor), 3A4 (major); **Inhibits** CYP1A2 (weak), 2C8 (weak); **Induces** CYP3A4 (weak)

Anticoagulants: Increase potential for thromboembolic events

Cyclosporine: Estrogen derivatives may enhance the hepatotoxic effect of cyclosporine. Estrogen derivatives may increase the serum concentration of cyclosporine.

(Continued)

Estrogens (Conjugated/Equine) *(Continued)*

CYP1A2 inducers: May decrease the levels/effects of estrogens. Example inducers include aminoglutethimide, carbamazepine, phenobarbital, and rifampin.

CYP3A4 inducers: CYP3A4 inducers may decrease the levels/effects of estrogens. Example inducers include aminoglutethimide, carbamazepine, nafcillin, nevirapine, phenobarbital, phenytoin, and rifamycins.

Thyroid products: Estrogen derivatives may diminish the therapeutic effect of thyroid products; monitor.

Ethanol/Nutrition/Herb Interactions

Ethanol: Avoid ethanol (routine use increases estrogen level and risk of breast cancer). Ethanol may also increase the risk of osteoporosis.

Food: Folic acid absorption may be decreased.

Herb/Nutraceutical: St John's wort may decrease levels. Herbs with estrogenic properties may enhance the adverse/toxic effect of estrogen derivatives; examples include alfalfa, black cohosh, bloodroot, hops, kudzu, licorice, red clover, saw palmetto, soybean, thyme, wild yam, yucca.

Test Interactions Pathologist should be advised of estrogen/progesterone therapy when specimens are submitted. Reduced response to metyrapone test.

Dietary Considerations Ensure adequate calcium and vitamin D intake when used for the prevention of osteoporosis. Powder for reconstitution for injection (25 mg) contains lactose 200 mg.

Dosage Forms

Cream, vaginal: 0.625 mg/g (42.5 g)

Injection, powder for reconstitution: 25 mg [contains lactose 200 mg; diluent contains benzyl alcohol]

Tablet: 0.3 mg, 0.45 mg, 0.625 mg, 0.9 mg, 1.25 mg

♦ **Ethacrynate Sodium** *see* Ethacrynic Acid *on page 492*

Ethacrynic Acid (eth a KRIN ik AS id)

Medication Safety Issues

Sound-alike/look-alike issues:

Edecrin® may be confused with Eulexin®, Ecotrin®

Related Information

Diuretics, Loop *on page 1565*

Heart Failure (Systolic) *on page 1607*

U.S. Brand Names Edecrin®

Canadian Brand Names Edecrin®

Synonyms Ethacrynate Sodium

Pharmacologic Category Diuretic, Loop

Generic Available No

Use Management of edema associated with congestive heart failure; hepatic cirrhosis or renal disease; short-term management of ascites due to malignancy, idiopathic edema, and lymphedema

Mechanism of Action Inhibits reabsorption of sodium and chloride in the ascending loop of Henle and distal renal tubule, interfering with the chloride-binding cotransport system, thus causing increased excretion of water, sodium, chloride, magnesium, and calcium

Pharmacodynamics/Kinetics

Onset of action: Diuresis: Oral: ~30 minutes; I.V.: 5 minutes

Peak effect: Oral: 2 hours; I.V.: 30 minutes

Duration: Oral: 12 hours; I.V.: 2 hours

Absorption: Oral: Rapid

Protein binding: >90%

Metabolism: Hepatic (35% to 40%) to active cysteine conjugate

Half-life elimination: Normal renal function: 2-4 hours

Excretion: Feces and urine (30% to 60% as unchanged drug)

Dosage I.V. formulation should be diluted in D_5W or NS (1 mg/mL) and infused over several minutes.

Children: Oral: 1 mg/kg/dose once daily; increase at intervals of 2-3 days as needed, to a maximum of 3 mg/kg/day.

Adults:

Oral: 50-200 mg/day in 1-2 divided doses; may increase in increments of 25-50 mg at intervals of several days; doses up to 200 mg twice daily may be required with severe, refractory edema.

I.V.: 0.5-1 mg/kg/dose (maximum: 100 mg/dose); repeat doses not routinely recommended; however, if indicated, repeat doses every 8-12 hours.

Dosing adjustment/comments in renal impairment: Cl_{cr} <10 mL/minute: Avoid use.

Dialysis: Not removed by hemo- or peritoneal dialysis; supplemental dose is not necessary.

Administration Injection should **not** be given SubQ or I.M. due to local pain and irritation; single I.V. doses should not exceed 100 mg; if a second dose is needed, use a new injection site to avoid possible thrombophlebitis

Monitoring Parameters Blood pressure, renal function, serum electrolytes, and fluid status closely, including weight and I & O daily; hearing

Anesthesia and Critical Care Concerns/Other Considerations Ethacrynic acid has limited use over other loop diuretics because of increased risk of ototoxicity. If given the morning of surgery, it may render the patient volume depleted and blood pressure may be labile during general anesthesia.

Pregnancy Risk Factor B

Contraindications Hypersensitivity to ethacrynic acid or any component of the formulation; anuria; history of severe watery diarrhea caused by this product; infants

Warnings/Precautions Adjust dose to avoid dehydration. In cirrhosis, avoid electrolyte and acid/base imbalances that might lead to hepatic encephalopathy. Ototoxicity is associated with rapid I.V. administration, renal impairment, excessive doses, and concurrent use of other ototoxins. Has been associated with a higher incidence of ototoxicity than other loop diuretics. Hypersensitivity reactions can rarely occur, however, ethacrynic acid has no cross-reactivity to sulfonamides or sulfonylureas. Monitor fluid status and renal function in an attempt to prevent oliguria, azotemia, and reversible increases in BUN and creatinine. Close medical supervision of aggressive diuresis required. Watch for and correct electrolyte disturbances. Coadministration of antihypertensives may increase the risk of hypotension. Increased risk of gastric hemorrhage associated with corticosteroid therapy.

Adverse Reactions Frequency not defined.

Central nervous system: Headache, fatigue, apprehension, confusion, fever, chills, encephalopathy (patients with pre-existing liver disease); vertigo

Dermatologic: Skin rash, Henoch-Schönlein purpura (in patient with rheumatic heart disease)

Endocrine & metabolic: Hyponatremia, hyperglycemia, variations in phosphorus, CO_2 content, bicarbonate, and calcium; reversible hyperuricemia, gout, hyperglycemia, hypoglycemia (occurred in two uremic patients who received doses above those recommended)

Gastrointestinal: Anorexia, malaise, abdominal discomfort or pain, dysphagia, nausea, vomiting, and diarrhea, gastrointestinal bleeding, acute pancreatitis (rare)

Genitourinary: Hematuria

Hepatic: Jaundice, abnormal liver function tests

Hematology: Agranulocytosis, severe neutropenia, thrombocytopenia

Local: Thrombophlebitis (with intravenous use), local irritation and pain

Ocular: Blurred vision

Otic: Tinnitus, temporary or permanent deafness

Renal: Increased serum creatinine

Overdosage/Toxicology Symptoms of overdose include electrolyte depletion, volume depletion, dehydration, and circulatory collapse. Treatment is supportive.

Drug Interactions

ACE inhibitors: Hypotensive effects and/or renal effects are potentiated by hypovolemia.

Antidiabetic agents: Glucose tolerance may be decreased.

Antihypertensive agents: Hypotensive effects may be enhanced.

Cephaloridine or cephalexin: Nephrotoxicity may occur.

Cholestyramine or colestipol may reduce bioavailability of ethacrynic acid.

Clofibrate: Protein binding may be altered in hypoalbuminemic patients receiving ethacrynic acid, potentially increasing toxicity.

Digoxin: Ethacrynic acid-induced hypokalemia may predispose to digoxin toxicity; monitor potassium.

(Continued)

Ethacrynic Acid *(Continued)*

Indomethacin (and other NSAIDs) may reduce natriuretic and hypotensive effects of diuretics.

Lithium: Renal clearance may be reduced. Isolated reports of lithium toxicity have occurred; monitor lithium levels.

NSAIDs: Risk of renal impairment may increase when used in conjunction with diuretics.

Ototoxic drugs (aminoglycosides, cis-platinum): Concomitant use of ethacrynic acid may increase risk of ototoxicity, especially in patients with renal dysfunction.

Peripheral adrenergic-blocking drugs or ganglionic blockers: Effects may be increased.

Salicylates (high-dose) with diuretics may predispose patients to salicylate toxicity due to reduced renal excretion or alter renal function.

Thiazides: Synergistic diuretic effects occur.

Dietary Considerations This product may cause a potassium loss. Your healthcare provider may prescribe a potassium supplement, another medication to help prevent the potassium loss, or recommend that you eat foods high in potassium, especially citrus fruits. Do not change your diet on your own while taking this medication, especially if you are taking potassium supplements or medications to reduce potassium loss. Too much potassium can be as harmful as too little.

Dosage Forms

Injection, powder for reconstitution, as ethacrynate sodium: 50 mg

Tablet: 25 mg

♦ **Ethamolin®** *see* Ethanolamine Oleate *on page 494*

♦ **Ethanol** *see* Alcohol (Ethyl) *on page 53*

Ethanolamine Oleate (ETH a nol a meen OH lee ate)

Medication Safety Issues

Sound-alike/look-alike issues:

Ethamolin® may be confused with ethanol

U.S. Brand Names Ethamolin®

Synonyms Monoethanolamine

Pharmacologic Category Sclerosing Agent

Generic Available No

Use Orphan drug: Sclerosing agent used for bleeding esophageal varices

Mechanism of Action Derived from oleic acid and similar in physical properties to sodium morrhuate; however, the exact mechanism of the hemostatic effect used in endoscopic injection sclerotherapy is not known. Intravenously injected ethanolamine oleate produces a sterile inflammatory response resulting in fibrosis and occlusion of the vein; a dose-related extravascular inflammatory reaction occurs when the drug diffuses through the venous wall. Autopsy results indicate that variceal obliteration occurs secondary to mural necrosis and fibrosis. Thrombosis appears to be a transient reaction.

Dosage Adults: 1.5-5 mL per varix, up to 20 mL total or 0.4 mL/kg for a 50 kg patient; doses should be decreased in patients with severe hepatic dysfunction and should receive less than recommended maximum dose

Administration Use care to use acceptable technique to avoid necrosis

Pregnancy Risk Factor C

Contraindications Hypersensitivity to agent or oleic acid

Warnings/Precautions Fatal anaphylactic shock has been reported following administration; use with caution and decrease doses in patients with significant liver dysfunction (Child class C), with concomitant cardiorespiratory disease, or in the elderly or critically-ill

Adverse Reactions

1% to 10%:

Central nervous system: Pyrexia (1.8%)

Gastrointestinal: Esophageal ulcer (2%), esophageal stricture (1.3%)

Respiratory: Pleural effusion (2%), pneumonia (1.2%)

Miscellaneous: Retrosternal pain (1.6%)

<1% (Limited to important or life-threatening): Acute renal failure, anaphylaxis, esophagitis, injection necrosis, perforation

Overdosage/Toxicology Anaphylaxis after administration of larger than normal volumes, severe intramural necrosis. Treatment is supportive with epinephrine, corticosteroids, fluids, and pressors.

Drug Interactions No data reported

Dosage Forms Injection, solution: 5% [50 mg/mL] (2 mL) [contains benzyl alcohol]

- **Ethmozine®** *see* Moricizine *on page 866*
- **Ethoxynaphthamido Penicillin Sodium** *see* Nafcillin *on page 890*
- **Ethrane®** *see* Enflurane *on page 450*
- **Ethyl Alcohol** *see* Alcohol (Ethyl) *on page 53*

Etidronate Disodium (e ti DROE nate dye SOW dee um)

Medication Safety Issues

Sound-alike/look-alike issues:

Etidronate may be confused with etidocaine, etomidate, etretinate

U.S. Brand Names Didronel®

Canadian Brand Names Apo-Etidronate®; Didronel®; Gen-Etidronate

Synonyms EHDP; Sodium Etidronate

Pharmacologic Category Bisphosphonate Derivative

Generic Available No

Use Symptomatic treatment of Paget's disease; prevention and treatment of heterotopic ossification due to spinal cord injury or after total hip replacement

Unlabeled/Investigational Use Postmenopausal osteoporosis

Mechanism of Action Decreases bone resorption by inhibiting osteocystic osteolysis; decreases mineral release and matrix or collagen breakdown in bone

Pharmacodynamics/Kinetics

Onset of action: 1-3 months

Duration: Can persist for 12 months without continuous therapy

Absorption: ~3%

Metabolism: None

Half-life elimination: 1-6 hours

Excretion: Primarily urine (as unchanged drug); feces (as unabsorbed drug)

Dosage Oral: Adults:

Paget's disease:

Initial: 5-10 mg/kg/day (not to exceed 6 months) or 11-20 mg/kg/day (not to exceed 3 months). Doses >20 mg/kg/day are **not** recommended.

Retreatment: Initiate only after etidronate-free period ≥90 days. Monitor patients every 3-6 months. Retreatment regimens are the same as for initial treatment.

Heterotopic ossification:

Caused by spinal cord injury: 20 mg/kg/day for 2 weeks, then 10 mg/kg/day for 10 weeks; total treatment period: 12 weeks

Complicating total hip replacement: 20 mg/kg/day for 1 month preoperatively then 20 mg/kg/day for 3 months postoperatively; total treatment period is 4 months

Postmenopausal osteoporosis (unlabeled use): Oral: 400 mg/day for 2 weeks, followed by 13-week period with no etidronate, then repeat cycle. Maintain adequate calcium and vitamin D intake during the entire 15-week treatment cycle

Dosing adjustment in renal impairment: Use with caution; specific guidelines are not available, however consider dose reduction.

Stability Store at controlled room temperature of 15°C to 30°C (59°F to 86°F).

Administration Administer tablet should be administered on an empty stomach 2 hours before food.

Monitoring Parameters Serum calcium and phosphorous; serum creatinine and BUN

Reference Range Calcium (total): Adults: 9.0-11.0 mg/dL

Pregnancy Risk Factor C

Contraindications Hypersensitivity to bisphosphonates or any component of the formulation; overt osteomalacia

Warnings/Precautions Ensure adequate calcium and vitamin D intake. Etidronate may retard mineralization of bone; treatment may need delayed or interrupted until callus is present. Use caution in patients with renal impairment. Use caution with enterocolitis; diarrhea has been reported at high doses and therapy may need to be withheld.

(Continued)

Etidronate Disodium *(Continued)*

Bisphosphonate therapy has been associated with osteonecrosis, primarily of the jaw; this has been observed mostly in cancer patients, but also in patients with postmenopausal osteoporosis and other diagnoses. Risk factors include a diagnosis of cancer, with concomitant chemotherapy, radiotherapy or corticosteroids; anemia, coagulopathy, infection or pre-existing dental disease. Symptoms included nonhealing extraction socket or an exposed jawbone. There are no data addressing whether discontinuation of therapy reduces the risk of developing osteonecrosis. However, as a precautionary measure, dental exams and preventative dentistry should be performed prior to placing patients with risk factors on chronic bisphosphonate therapy. Invasive dental procedures should be avoided during treatment.

Severe and potentially incapacitating musculoskeletal pain has been observed with bisphosphonates, with onset ranging from one day to several months after beginning therapy. Symptoms usually abate upon discontinuation, but may recur upon reinitiation of bisphosphonate treatment.

Safety and efficacy in pediatric patients have not been established.

Adverse Reactions Frequency not defined.

Gastrointestinal: Diarrhea, nausea

Neuromuscular & skeletal: Bone pain

Postmarketing and/or case reports: Agranulocytosis, alopecia, amnesia, angioedema, arthralgia, arthritis, asthma exacerbation, bone fracture, confusion, depression, esophagitis, follicular eruption, gastritis, glossitis, hallucination, headache, hypersensitivity reactions, leg cramps, leukopenia, macular rash, maculopapular rash, musculoskeletal pain, osteomalacia, pancytopenia, paresthesia, peptic ulcer disease exacerbation, pruritus, Stevens-Johnson syndrome, urticaria

Overdosage/Toxicology Hypocalcemia, vomiting, paresthesia, diarrhea, and hematologic abnormalities may be expected following acute overdose. Nephrotic syndrome and fracture may be observed with chronic overdose. Intravenous calcium may be used to treat hypocalcemia.

Drug Interactions

Aminoglycosides: May lower serum calcium levels with prolonged administration. Concomitant use may have an additive hypocalcemic effect.

Antacids: May decrease the absorption of bisphosphonate derivatives; should be administered at a different time of the day. Antacids containing aluminum, calcium, or magnesium are of specific concern.

Calcium salts: May decrease the absorption of bisphosphonate derivatives. Separate oral dosing in order to minimize risk of interaction.

Iron salts: May decrease the absorption of bisphosphonate derivatives. Only oral iron salts and oral bisphosphonates are of concern.

Magnesium salts: May decrease the absorption of bisphosphonate derivatives. Only oral magnesium salts and oral bisphosphonates are of concern.

Nonsteroidal anti-inflammatory drugs (NSAIDs): May enhance the gastrointestinal adverse/toxic effects (increased incidence of GI ulcers) of bisphosphonate derivatives.

Phosphate supplements: Bisphosphonate derivatives may enhance the hypocalcemic effect of phosphate supplements.

Ethanol/Nutrition/Herb Interactions Food: Food decreases the absorption and bioavailability of the drug.

Test Interactions Bisphosphonates may interfere with diagnostic imaging agents such as technetium-99m-diphosphonate in bone scans.

Dietary Considerations Administer tablet with water or fruit juice on an empty stomach; avoid administering foods/supplements with calcium, iron, or magnesium within 2 hours of drug; maintain adequate intake of calcium and vitamin D.

Dosage Forms Tablet: 200 mg, 400 mg

Etodolac (ee toe DOE lak)

Medication Safety Issues

Sound-alike/look-alike issues:

Lodine® may be confused with codeine, iodine, Iopidine®, Lopid®

Related Information

Acetaminophen and NSAIDS, Dosing Data *on page 1543*
Chronic Pain Management *on page 1430*

U.S. Brand Names Lodine® [DSC]; Lodine® XL [DSC]

Canadian Brand Names Apo-Etodolac®; Lodine®; Utradol™

Synonyms Etodolic Acid

Pharmacologic Category Nonsteroidal Anti-inflammatory Drug (NSAID), Oral

Restrictions A medication guide should be dispensed with each prescription. A template for the required MedGuide can be found on the FDA website at http://www.fda.gov/medwatch/SAFETY/2005/safety05.htm#NSAID

Generic Available Yes

Use Acute and long-term use in the management of signs and symptoms of osteoarthritis; rheumatoid arthritis and juvenile rheumatoid arthritis; management of acute pain

Mechanism of Action Inhibits prostaglandin synthesis by decreasing the activity of the enzyme, cyclooxygenase, which results in decreased formation of prostaglandin precursors

Pharmacodynamics/Kinetics

Onset of action: Analgesic: 2-4 hours; Maximum anti-inflammatory effect: A few days

Absorption: ≥80%

Distribution: V_d:

Immediate release: Adults:0.4 L/kg

Extended release: Adults: 0.57 L/kg; Children (6-16 years): 0 .08 L/kg

Protein binding: ≥99%, primarily albumin

Metabolism: Hepatic

Half-life elimination: Terminal: Adults: 5-8 hours

Extended release: Children (6-16 years): 12 hours

Time to peak, serum:

Immediate release: Adults: 1-2 hours

Extended release: Extended release: 5-7 hours, increased 1.4-3.8 hours with food

Excretion: Urine 73% (1% unchanged); feces 16%

Dosage Note: For chronic conditions, response is usually observed within 2 weeks.

Children 6-16 years: Oral: Juvenile rheumatoid arthritis (Lodine® XL):

20-30 kg: 400 mg once daily

31-45 kg: 600 mg once daily

46-60 kg: 800 mg once daily

>60 kg: 1000 mg once daily

Adults: Oral:

Acute pain: 200-400 mg every 6-8 hours, as needed, not to exceed total daily doses of 1000 mg

Rheumatoid arthritis, osteoarthritis: 400 mg 2 times/day **or** 300 mg 2-3 times/day **or** 500 mg 2 times/day (doses >1000 mg/day have not been evaluated)

Lodine® XL: 400-1000 mg once daily

Elderly: Refer to adult dosing; in patients ≥65 years, no dosage adjustment required based on pharmacokinetics. The elderly are more sensitive to antiprostaglandin effects and may need dosage adjustments.

Dosage adjustment in renal impairment:

Mild to moderate: No adjustment required

Severe: Use not recommended; use with caution

Hemodialysis: Not removed

Dosage adjustment in hepatic impairment: No adjustment required.

Stability Store at 20°C to 25°C (68°F to 77°F); protect from moisture

Monitoring Parameters Monitor CBC and chemistry profile, liver enzymes; in patients with an increased risk for renal failure (CHF or decreased renal function, taking ACE inhibitors or diuretics, elderly), monitor urine output and BUN/serum creatinine

Anesthesia and Critical Care Concerns/Other Considerations The 2002 ACCM/SCCM guidelines for analgesia (critically-ill adult) suggest that NSAIDs may be used in combination with opioids in select patients for pain management. Concern about adverse events (increased risk of renal dysfunction, altered platelet function and gastrointestinal irritation) limits its use in patients who have other underlying risks for these events.

In short-term use, NSAIDs vary considerably in their effect on blood pressure. When NSAIDs are used in patients with hypertension, appropriate monitoring of blood pressure responses should be completed and the duration of therapy, when

(Continued)

Etodolac *(Continued)*

possible, kept short. The use of NSAIDs in the treatment of patients with congestive heart failure may be associated with an increased risk for fluid accumulation and edema. May precipitate renal failure in dehydrated patients.

Pregnancy Risk Factor C/D (3rd trimester)

Contraindications Hypersensitivity to etodolac, aspirin, other NSAIDs, or any component of the formulation; perioperative pain in the setting of coronary artery bypass surgery (CABG); pregnancy

Warnings/Precautions **[U.S. Boxed Warning]: NSAIDs are associated with an increased risk of adverse cardiovascular events, including MI, stroke, and new onset or worsening of pre-existing hypertension.** Risk may be increased with duration of use or pre-existing cardiovascular risk-factors or disease. Carefully evaluate individual cardiovascular risk profiles prior to prescribing. Use caution with fluid retention, CHF, or hypertension.

[U.S. Boxed Warning]: NSAIDs may increase risk of gastrointestinal irritation, ulceration, bleeding, and perforation. These events may occur at any time during therapy and without warning. Use caution with a history of GI disease (bleeding or ulcers), concurrent therapy with aspirin, anticoagulants and/or corticosteroids, smoking, use of alcohol, the elderly or debilitated patients.

Use of NSAIDs can compromise existing renal function. Renal toxicity can occur in patient with impaired renal function, dehydration, heart failure, liver dysfunction, those taking diuretics and ACE inhibitors and the elderly. Rehydrate patient before starting therapy. Monitor renal function closely. Etodolac is not recommended for patients with advanced renal disease.

Use the lowest effective dose for the shortest duration of time, consistent with individual patient goals, to reduce risk of cardiovascular or GI adverse events. Alternate therapies should be considered for patients at high risk.

NSAIDs may cause serious skin adverse events including exfoliative dermatitis, Stevens-Johnson syndrome (SJS), and toxic epidermal necrolysis (TEN). Anaphylactoid reactions may occur, even without prior exposure; patients with "aspirin triad" (bronchial asthma, aspirin intolerance, rhinitis) may be at increased risk. Do not use in patients who experience bronchospasm, asthma, rhinitis, or urticaria with NSAID or aspirin therapy.

Use with caution in patients with decreased hepatic function. Closely monitor patients with any abnormal LFT. Severe hepatic reactions (eg, fulminant hepatitis, liver failure) have occurred with NSAID use, rarely; discontinue if signs or symptoms of liver disease develop, or if systemic manifestations occur. The elderly are at increased risk for adverse effects (especially peptic ulceration, CNS effects, renal toxicity) from NSAIDs even at low doses.

Withhold for at least 4-6 half-lives prior to surgical or dental procedures.

Use of extended release product consisting of a nondeformable matrix should be avoided in patients with stricture/narrowing of the GI tract; symptoms of obstruction have been associated with nondeformable products.

Adverse Reactions

1% to 10%:

Central nervous system: Dizziness (3% to 9 %), chills/fever (1% to 3%), depression (1% to 3%), nervousness (1% to 3%)

Dermatologic: Rash (1% to 3%), pruritus (1% to 3%)

Gastrointestinal: Abdominal cramps (3% to 9%), nausea (3% to 9%), vomiting (1% to 3%), dyspepsia (10%), diarrhea (3% to 9%), constipation (1% to 3%), flatulence (3% to 9%), melena (1% to 3%), gastritis (1% to 3%)

Genitourinary: Dysuria (1% to 3%)

Neuromuscular & skeletal: Weakness (3% to 9%)

Ocular: Blurred vision (1% to 3%)

Otic: Tinnitus (1% to 3%)

Renal: Polyuria (1% to 3%)

<1% (Limited to important or life-threatening): Agranulocytosis, allergic reaction, allergic/necrotizing vasculitis, alopecia, anaphylactic/anaphylactoid reactions, anemia, angioedema, anorexia, arrhythmia, aseptic meningitis, asthma, bleeding time increased, CHF, confusion, conjunctivitis, CVA, cystitis, duodenitis, dyspnea, ecchymosis, edema, erythema multiforme, esophagitis (+/- stricture or cardiospasm), exfoliative dermatitis, GI ulceration, hallucinations,

headache, hearing decreased, hematemesis, hematuria, hepatic failure, hepatitis, hyperglycemia (in controlled diabetics), hyperpigmentation, hypertension, infection, insomnia, interstitial nephritis, irregular uterine bleeding, jaundice, LFTs increased, leukopenia, MI, palpitations, pancreatitis, pancytopenia, paresthesia, peptic ulcer (+/- bleeding/perforation), peripheral neuropathy, photophobia, photosensitivity, pulmonary infiltration (eosinophilia), rectal bleeding, renal calculus, renal failure, renal insufficiency, shock, Stevens-Johnson syndrome, syncope, thrombocytopenia, toxic epidermal necrolysis, ulcerative stomatitis, urticaria, vesiculobullous rash, renal papillary necrosis, visual disturbances

Overdosage/Toxicology Symptoms of overdose include acute renal failure, vomiting, drowsiness, leukocytosis. Management of NSAID intoxication is supportive and symptomatic. Emesis and/or activated charcoal and/or osmotic cathartic may be considered when overdoses are large (5-10 times usual dose) or recent (within 4 hours). Diuresis, urine alkalinization, hemodialysis, and hemoperfusion are not likely to be useful.

Drug Interactions

ACE inhibitors: Antihypertensive effects may be decreased by concurrent therapy with NSAIDs; monitor blood pressure.

Aminoglycosides: NSAIDs may decrease the excretion of aminoglycosides.

Angiotensin II antagonists: Antihypertensive effects may be decreased by concurrent therapy with NSAIDs; monitor blood pressure.

Anticoagulants (warfarin, heparin, LMWHs) in combination with NSAIDs can cause increased risk of bleeding.

Antiplatelet agents (ticlopidine, clopidogrel, aspirin, abciximab, dipyridamole, eptifibatide, tirofiban) can cause an increased risk of bleeding.

Beta-blockers: NSAIDs may diminish the antihypertensive effects of beta-blockers.

Bisphosphonates: NSAIDs may increase the risk of gastrointestinal ulceration.

Cholestyramine and colestipol reduce the bioavailability of some NSAIDs; separate administration times.

Corticosteroids may increase the risk of GI ulceration; avoid concurrent use.

Cyclosporine: NSAIDs may increase serum creatinine, potassium, blood pressure, and cyclosporine levels; monitor cyclosporine levels and renal function carefully.

Hydralazine's antihypertensive effect is decreased; avoid concurrent use.

Lithium levels can be increased; avoid concurrent use if possible or monitor lithium levels and adjust dose. Sulindac may have the least effect. When NSAID is stopped, lithium will need adjustment again.

Loop diuretics efficacy (diuretic and antihypertensive effect) is reduced. Indomethacin reduces this efficacy, however, it may be anticipated with any NSAID.

Methotrexate: Severe bone marrow suppression, aplastic anemia, and GI toxicity have been reported with concomitant NSAID therapy. Avoid use during moderate or high-dose methotrexate (increased and prolonged methotrexate levels). NSAID use during low-dose treatment of rheumatoid arthritis has not been fully evaluated; extreme caution is warranted.

Pemetrexed: NSAIDs may decrease the excretion of pemetrexed. Patients with Cl_{cr} 45-79 mL/minute should avoid short acting NSAIDs for 2 days before and 2 days after pemetrexed treatment.

Thiazides antihypertensive effects are decreased; avoid concurrent use.

Treprostinil: May enhance the risk of bleeding with concurrent use.

Vancomycin: NSAIDs may decrease the excretion of vancomycin. Avoid concurrent use.

Verapamil plasma concentration is decreased by some NSAIDs; avoid concurrent use.

Ethanol/Nutrition/Herb Interactions

Ethanol: Avoid ethanol (may enhance gastric mucosal irritation).

Food: Etodolac peak serum levels may be decreased if taken with food.

Herb/Nutraceutical: Avoid alfalfa, anise, bilberry, bladderwrack, bromelain, cat's claw, celery, coleus, cordyceps, dong quai, evening primrose, feverfew, fenugreek, garlic, ginger, ginkgo biloba, red clover, horse chestnut, grapeseed, green tea, ginseng, guggul, horse chestnut seed, horseradish, licorice, prickly ash, red clover, reishi, SAMe, sweet clover, turmeric, white willow (all have additional antiplatelet activity)

Test Interactions False-positive for urinary bilirubin and ketone

Dietary Considerations May be taken with food to decrease GI distress.

Dosage Forms [DSC] = Discontinued product

(Continued)

Etodolac *(Continued)*

Capsule: 200 mg, 300 mg
  Lodine®: 200 mg, 300 mg [DSC]
Tablet: 400 mg, 500 mg
Tablet, extended release (Lodine® XL): 400 mg, 500 mg [DSC]

- **Etodolic Acid** *see* Etodolac *on page 496*
- **EtOH** *see* Alcohol (Ethyl) *on page 53*

Etomidate (e TOM i date)

Medication Safety Issues
Sound-alike/look-alike issues:
Etomidate may be confused with etidronate

Related Information
Anesthesia Considerations for Neurosurgery *on page 1401*
Intravenous Anesthetic Agents *on page 1531*

U.S. Brand Names Amidate®

Canadian Brand Names Amidate®

Pharmacologic Category General Anesthetic

Generic Available Yes

Use Induction and maintenance of general anesthesia

Unlabeled/Investigational Use Sedation for diagnosis of seizure foci

Mechanism of Action Ultrashort-acting nonbarbiturate hypnotic (benzylimidazole) used for the induction of anesthesia; chemically, it is a carboxylated imidazole which produces a rapid induction of anesthesia with minimal cardiovascular effects; produces EEG burst suppression at high doses

Pharmacodynamics/Kinetics
Onset of action: 30-60 seconds
  Peak effect: 1 minute
Duration: 3-5 minutes; terminated by redistribution
Distribution: V_d: 2-4.5 L/kg
Protein binding: 76%;
Metabolism: Hepatic and plasma esterases
Half-life elimination: Terminal: 2.6 hours

Dosage Children >10 years and Adults: I.V.: Initial: 0.2-0.6 mg/kg over 30-60 seconds for induction of anesthesia; maintenance: 5-20 mcg/kg/minute

Stability Store at room temperature.

Administration Administer I.V. push over 30-60 seconds. Solution is highly irritating; avoid administration into small vessels; in some cases, preadministration of lidocaine may be considered.

Monitoring Parameters Cardiac monitoring and blood pressure required

Anesthesia and Critical Care Concerns/Other Considerations Etomidate 2 mg/mL contains propylene glycol 362.6 mg/mL (35% v/v).

Etomidate decreases cerebral metabolism and cerebral blood flow while maintaining perfusion pressure; can enhance somatosensory evoked potential recordings. Premedication with opioids or benzodiazepines can decrease myoclonus. Etomidate is a relatively safe anesthetic for use in patients with stable cardiovascular disease.

Pregnancy Risk Factor C

Contraindications Hypersensitivity to etomidate or any component of the formulation

Warnings/Precautions Etomidate inhibits 11-B-hydroxylase, an enzyme important in adrenal steroid production. A single induction dose blocks the normal stress-induced increase in adrenal cortisol production for 4-8 hours, up to 24 hours in elderly and debilitated patients. Continuous infusion of etomidate for sedation in the ICU may increase mortality because patients may not be able to respond to stress. No problem has been identified with a single dose for induction of anesthesia. Consider exogenous corticosteroid replacement in patients undergoing severe stress.

Adverse Reactions
>10%:
  Gastrointestinal: Nausea, vomiting on emergence from anesthesia
  Local: Pain at injection site (30% to 80%)

Neuromuscular & skeletal: Myoclonus (33%), transient skeletal movements, uncontrolled eye movements

1% to 10%: Hiccups

<1% (Limited to important or life-threatening): Apnea, arrhythmia, bradycardia, decreased cortisol synthesis, hypertension, hyperventilation, hypotension, hypoventilation, laryngospasm, tachycardia

Overdosage/Toxicology Symptoms of overdose include respiratory arrest and coma. Treatment is supportive.

Drug Interactions

Fentanyl: Decreases etomidate elimination

Verapamil: May increase the anesthetic and respiratory depressant effects of etomidate

Dosage Forms Injection, solution: 2 mg/mL (10 mL, 20 mL) [contains propylene glycol 35% v/v]

- **Euglucon® (Can)** *see* GlyBURIDE *on page 598*
- **Evoclin™** *see* Clindamycin *on page 304*
- **Exubera®** *see* Insulin Inhalation *on page 686*
- **EZ-Char™ [OTC]** *see* Charcoal *on page 259*
- **Factive®** *see* Gemifloxacin *on page 587*

Factor VIIa (Recombinant) (FAK ter SEV en ree KOM be nant)

Medication Safety Issues

Sound-alike/look-alike issues:

NovoSeven® may be confused with Novacet®

U.S. Brand Names NovoSeven®

Canadian Brand Names Niastase®

Synonyms Coagulation Factor VIIa; Eptacog Alfa (Activated); rFVIIa

Pharmacologic Category Antihemophilic Agent; Blood Product Derivative

Generic Available No

Use Treatment of bleeding episodes and prevention of bleeding in surgical interventions in patients with hemophilia A or B with inhibitors to factor VIII or factor IX and in patients with congenital factor VII deficiency

Mechanism of Action Recombinant factor VIIa, a vitamin K-dependent glycoprotein, promotes hemostasis by activating the extrinsic pathway of the coagulation cascade. It replaces deficient activated coagulation factor VII, which complexes with tissue factor and may activate coagulation factor X to Xa and factor IX to IXa. When complexed with other factors, coagulation factor Xa converts prothrombin to thrombin, a key step in the formation of a fibrin-platelet hemostatic plug.

Pharmacodynamics/Kinetics

Distribution: V_d: 103 mL/kg (78-139)

Half-life elimination: 2.3 hours (1.7-2.7)

Excretion: Clearance: 33 mL/kg/hour (27-49)

Dosage Children and Adults: I.V. administration only: Hemophilia A or B with inhibitors:

Bleeding episodes: 90 mcg/kg every 2 hours until hemostasis is achieved or until the treatment is judged ineffective. The dose and interval may be adjusted based upon the severity of bleeding and the degree of hemostasis achieved. For patients experiencing severe bleeds, dosing should be continued at 3- to 6-hour intervals after hemostasis has been achieved and the duration of dosing should be minimized.

Surgical interventions: 90 mcg/kg immediately before surgery, repeat at 2-hour intervals for the duration of surgery. Continue every 2 hours for 48 hours, then every 2-6 hours until healed for minor surgery; continue every 2 hours for 5 days, then every 4 hours until healed for major surgery.

Congenital factor VII deficiency: Bleeding episodes and surgical interventions: 15-30 mcg/kg every 4-6 hours until hemostasis. Doses as low as 10 mcg/kg have been effective.

Stability Store under refrigeration at 2°C to 8°C (36°F to 46°F); protect from light. Prior to reconstitution, bring vials to room temperature. Reconstitute each vial to a final concentration of 0.6 mg/mL as follows:

1.2 mg vial: 2.2 mL sterile water

2.4 mg vial: 4.3 mL sterile water

4.8 mg vial: 8.5 mL sterile water

(Continued)

Factor VIIa (Recombinant) *(Continued)*

Add diluent along wall of vial, do not inject directly into powder. Gently swirl until dissolved.

Reconstituted solutions may be stored at room temperature or under refrigeration, but must be infused within 3 hours of reconstitution. Do not freeze reconstituted solutions. Do not store reconstituted solutions in syringes.

Administration I.V. administration only; bolus over 2-5 minutes; administer within 3 hours after reconstitution

Monitoring Parameters Monitor for evidence of hemostasis; although the prothrombin time, aPTT, and factor VII clotting activity have no correlation with achieving hemostasis, these parameters may be useful as adjunct tests to evaluate efficacy and guide dose or interval adjustments

Anesthesia and Critical Care Concerns/Other Considerations A number of patient-specific factors may influence the potential efficacy of factor VIIa including hypothermia, thrombocytopenia, acidic arterial pH, and the amount of blood products transfused prior to administration. Factor VIIa exerts its mechanism of action at the site of vascular injury where tissue factor is expressed and activated platelets are found. Factor VIIa binds directly to the surface of activated platelets and activates factor X to Xa and generates thrombin as a result. Adequate platelets may be required for factor VIIa to properly induce coagulation.

Pregnancy Risk Factor C

Contraindications Hypersensitivity to factor VII or any component of the formulation; hypersensitivity to mouse, hamster, or bovine proteins

Warnings/Precautions Patients should be monitored for signs and symptoms of activation of the coagulation system or thrombosis. Thrombotic events may be increased in patients with disseminated intravascular coagulation (DIC), advanced atherosclerotic disease, sepsis, crush injury, or concomitant treatment with prothrombin complex concentrates. Decreased dosage or discontinuation is warranted in confirmed DIC. Efficacy with prolonged infusions and data evaluating this agent's long-term adverse effects are limited.

Adverse Reactions

1% to 10%:

Cardiovascular: Hypertension

Central nervous system: Fever

Hematologic: Hemorrhage, decreased plasma fibrinogen

Neuromuscular & skeletal: Hemarthrosis

<1% (Limited to important or life-threatening): Abnormal renal function, allergic reaction, anaphylactic reaction, arterial thrombosis, arthrosis, bradycardia, cerebral infarction and/or ischemia, coagulation disorder, consumptive coagulopathy, decreased therapeutic response, deep vein thrombosis, disseminated intravascular coagulation (DIC), edema, fibrinolysis increased, gastrointestinal bleeding, headache, hypersensitivity, hypotension, injection-site reactions, intracranial hemorrhage, localized phlebitis, MI, myocardial ischemia, pain, pneumonia, prothrombin decreased, pruritus, pulmonary embolism, purpura, rash, splenic hematoma, thrombophlebitis, thrombosis, vomiting

Overdosage/Toxicology Experience with overdose in humans is limited; an increased risk of thrombotic events may occur in overdosage. Treatment is symptomatic and supportive.

Dietary Considerations Contains sodium 0.44 mEq/mg rFVIIa

Dosage Forms Injection, powder for reconstitution [preservative free]: 1.2 mg, 2.4 mg, 4.8 mg [latex free; contains sodium 0.44 mEq/mg rFVIIa, polysorbate 80]

References

Mayer SA, Brun NC, Begtrup K, et al, "Recombinant Activated Factor VII for Acute Intracerebral Hemorrhage," *N Engl J Med*, 2005, 352(8):777-85.

Mohr AM, Holcomb JB, Dutton RP, et al, "Recombinant Activated Factor VIIa and Hemostasis in Critical Care: A Focus on Trauma," *Crit Care*, 2005, 9 (Suppl 5):37-42.

♦ **Factor VIII (Recombinant)** *see* Antihemophilic Factor (Recombinant) *on page 113*

Factor IX (FAK ter nyne)

U.S. Brand Names AlphaNine® SD; BeneFix®; Mononine®

Canadian Brand Names BeneFix®; Immunine® VH; Mononine®

Pharmacologic Category Antihemophilic Agent; Blood Product Derivative

Generic Available No

Use Control bleeding in patients with factor IX deficiency (hemophilia B or Christmas disease)

Mechanism of Action Replaces deficient clotting factor IX; concentrate of factor IX; hemophilia B, or Christmas disease, is an X-linked inherited disorder of blood coagulation characterized by insufficient or abnormal synthesis of the clotting protein factor IX. Factor IX is a vitamin K-dependent coagulation factor which is synthesized in the liver. Factor IX is activated by factor XIa in the intrinsic coagulation pathway. Activated factor IX (IXa), in combination with factor VII:C activates factor X to Xa, resulting ultimately in the conversion of prothrombin to thrombin and the formation of a fibrin clot. The infusion of exogenous factor IX to replace the deficiency present in hemophilia B temporarily restores hemostasis.

Pharmacodynamics/Kinetics Half-life elimination: IX component: 23-31 hours

Dosage Dosage is expressed in units of factor IX activity and must be individualized. I.V. only:

Formula for units required to raise blood level %:

AlphaNine® SD, Mononine®: Children and Adults:

Number of Factor IX Units Required = body weight (in kg) x desired Factor IX level increase (% normal) x 1 unit/kg

For example, for a 100% level a patient who has an actual level of 20%: Number of Factor IX Units needed = 70 kg x 80% x 1 Unit/kg = 5600 Units

BeneFix®:

Children <15 years:

Number of Factor IX Units Required = body weight (in kg) x desired Factor IX level increase (% normal) x 1.4 units/kg

Adults:

Number of Factor IX Units Required = body weight (in kg) x desired Factor IX level increase (% normal) x 1.2 units/kg

Guidelines: As a general rule, the level of factor IX required for treatment of different conditions is listed below:

Minor spontaneous hemorrhage, prophylaxis:

Desired levels of factor IX for hemostasis: 15% to 25%

Initial loading dose to achieve desired level: 20-30 units/kg

Frequency of dosing: Every 12-24 hours if necessary

Duration of treatment: 1-2 days

Moderate hemorrhage:

Desired levels of factor IX for hemostasis: 25% to 50%

Initial loading dose to achieve desired level: 25-50 units/kg

Frequency of dosing: Every 12-24 hours

Duration of treatment: 2-7 days

Major hemorrhage:

Desired levels of factor IX for hemostasis: >50%

Initial loading dose to achieve desired level: 30-50 units/kg

Frequency of dosing: Every 12-24 hours, depending on half-life and measured factor IX levels (after 3-5 days, maintain at least 20% activity)

Duration of treatment: 7-10 days, depending upon nature of insult

Surgery:

Desired levels of factor IX for hemostasis: 50% to 100%

Initial loading dose to achieve desired level: 50-100 units/kg

Frequency of dosing: Every 12-24 hours, depending on half-life and measured factor IX levels

Duration of treatment: 7-10 days, depending upon nature of insult

Stability When stored at refrigerator temperature, 2°C to 8°C (36°F to 46°F), coagulation factor IX is stable for the period indicated by the expiration date on its label. Avoid freezing which may damage container for the diluent.

AlphaNine® SD: May also be stored at ≤30°C (≤86°F) for up to 3 months.

BeneFix®: May also be stored at ≤25°C (≤77°F) for up to 6 months.

Mononine®: May also be stored at ≤30°C (≤86°F) for up to 1 month. When reconstituted to ~100 int. units/mL, infusion rate should be up to 225 units/minute (2 mL/minute).

Stability of parenteral admixture at room temperature (25°C): 3 hours

Administration Solution should be infused at room temperature

I.V. administration only: Should be infused **slowly**: The rate of administration should be determined by the response and comfort of the patient.

Mononine®: Intravenous dosage administration rates of up to 225 units/minute (~2 mL/minute) have been regularly tolerated without incident. **Infuse at a rate not exceeding 2 mL/minute**.

(Continued)

Factor IX *(Continued)*

Monitoring Parameters Levels of factors IX, PTT

Reference Range Average normal factor IX levels are 50% to 150%; patients with severe hemophilia will have levels <1%, often undetectable. Moderate forms of the disease have levels of 1% to 10% while some mild cases may have 11% to 49% of normal factor IX.

Maintain factor IX plasma level at least 20% until hemostasis achieved after acute joint or muscle bleeding

In preparation for and following surgery:

- Level to prevent spontaneous hemorrhage: 5%
- Minimum level for hemostasis following trauma and surgery: 30% to 50%
- Severe hemorrhage: >60%
- Major surgery: ≥50% prior to procedure, 30% to 50% for several days after surgery, and >20% for 10-14 days thereafter

Pregnancy Risk Factor C

Contraindications Hypersensitivity to mouse protein (Mononine®), hamster protein (BeneFix®), or any component of the formulation

Warnings/Precautions Use with caution in patients with liver dysfunction; some products prepared from pooled human plasma - the risk of viral transmission is not totally eradicated; monitor patients who receive repeated doses twice daily with PTT and level of factor being replaced (eg, IX). Observe closely for signs or symptoms of intravascular coagulation or thrombosis. Caution should be exercised when administering to patients with liver disease, postoperatively, neonates, or patients at risk of thromboembolic phenomena or disseminated intravascular coagulation because of the potential risk of thromboembolic complications.

AlphaNine® SD, Mononine® contain **nondetectable levels of factors II, VII, and X** (<0.0025 units per factor IX unit using standard coagulation assays) and are, therefore, **NOT INDICATED** for replacement therapy of any of these clotting factors.

BeneFix®, Mononine® are **NOT INDICATED** in the treatment or reversal of coumarin-induced anticoagulation or in a hemorrhagic state caused by hepatitis-induced lack of production of liver dependent coagulation factors.

Adverse Reactions Frequency not defined.

- Cardiovascular: Angioedema, cyanosis, flushing, hypotension, tightness in chest, tightness in neck, thrombosis (following high dosages because of presence of activated clotting factors)
- Central nervous system: Fever, headache, chills, somnolence, dizziness, drowsiness, lightheadedness
- Dermatologic: Urticaria, rash
- Gastrointestinal: Nausea, vomiting, abnormal taste
- Hematologic: Disseminated intravascular coagulation (DIC)
- Local: Injection site discomfort
- Neuromuscular & skeletal: Tingling
- Respiratory: Dyspnea, laryngeal edema, allergic rhinitis
- Miscellaneous: Transient fever (following rapid administration), anaphylaxis, burning sensation in jaw/skull

Overdosage/Toxicology Symptoms of overdose include disseminated intravascular coagulation (DIC).

Drug Interactions Increased toxicity: Do not coadminister with aminocaproic acid; may increase the risk for thrombosis.

Dosage Forms Injection, powder for reconstitution (**Note:** Exact potency labeled on each vial):

- AlphaNine® SD [human derived; solvent detergent treated; virus filtered; contains nondetectable levels of factors II, VII, X; supplied with diluent]
- BeneFix® [recombinant formulation; supplied with diluent]
- Mononine® [human derived; monoclonal antibody purified; contains nondetectable levels of factors II, VII, X; supplied with diluent]

Factor IX Complex (Human) (FAK ter nyne KOM pleks HYU man)

U.S. Brand Names Bebulin® VH; Profilnine® SD; Proplex® T

Synonyms Prothrombin Complex Concentrate

Pharmacologic Category Antihemophilic Agent; Blood Product Derivative

Generic Available No

Use

Control bleeding in patients with factor IX deficiency (hemophilia B or Christmas disease) **Note:** Factor IX concentrate containing **only** factor IX is also available and preferable for this indication.

Prevention/control of bleeding in hemophilia A patients with inhibitors to factor VIII

Prevention/control of bleeding in patients with factor VII deficiency

Emergency correction of the coagulopathy of warfarin excess in critical situations.

Mechanism of Action Replaces deficient clotting factor including factor X; hemophilia B, or Christmas disease, is an X-linked recessively inherited disorder of blood coagulation characterized by insufficient or abnormal synthesis of the clotting protein factor IX. Factor IX is a vitamin K-dependent coagulation factor which is synthesized in the liver. Factor IX is activated by factor XIa in the intrinsic coagulation pathway. Activated factor IX (IXa), in combination with factor VII:C activates factor X to Xa, resulting ultimately in the conversion of prothrombin to thrombin and the formation of a fibrin clot. The infusion of exogenous factor IX to replace the deficiency present in hemophilia B temporarily restores hemostasis.

Pharmacodynamics/Kinetics

Half-life elimination:

VII component: Initial: 4-6 hours; Terminal: 22.5 hours

IX component: 24 hours

Dosage Children and Adults: Dosage is expressed in units of factor IX activity and must be individualized. I.V. only:

Formula for units required to raise blood level %:

Total blood volume (mL blood/kg) = 70 mL/kg (adults), 80 mL/kg (children)

Plasma volume = total blood volume (mL) x [1 - Hct (in decimals)]

For example, for a 70 kg adult with a Hct = 40%: Plasma volume = [70 kg x 70 mL/kg] x [1 - 0.4] = 2940 mL

To calculate number of units needed to increase level to desired range (highly individualized and dependent on patient's condition): Number of units = desired level increase [desired level - actual level] x plasma volume (in mL)

For example, for a 100% level in the above patient who has an actual level of 20%: Number of units needed = [1 (for a 100% level) - 0.2] x 2940 mL = 2352 units

As a general rule, the level of factor IX required for treatment of different conditions is listed below:

Minor Spontaneous Hemorrhage, Prophylaxis:

Desired levels of factor IX for hemostasis: 15% to 25%

Initial loading dose to achieve desired level: <20-30 units/kg

Frequency of dosing: Once; repeated in 24 hours if necessary

Duration of treatment: Once; repeated if necessary

Major Trauma or Surgery:

Desired levels of factor IX for hemostasis: 25% to 50%

Initial loading dose to achieve desired level: <75 units/kg

Frequency of dosing: Every 18-30 hours, depending on half-life and measured factor IX levels

Duration of treatment: Up to 10 days, depending upon nature of insult

Factor VIII inhibitor patients: 75 units/kg/dose; may be given every 6-12 hours

Anticoagulant overdosage: I.V.: 15 units/kg

Stability When stored at refrigerator temperature, 2°C to 8°C (36°F to 46°F), coagulation factor IX is stable for the period indicated by the expiration date on its label. Avoid freezing which may damage container for the diluent. Once diluted should be used promptly; stable for up to 3 hours.

For reconstitution, refer to instructions for individual products. Diluent and factor IX complex should come to room temperature before combining. Diluent vial should be inverted over concentrate vial. After diluent is pulled, disconnect. The provided filter needle should be used to withdraw concentrate. Remove needle and attach to infusion set or replace needle for infusion.

Administration I.V. administration only; should be infused **slowly**. Rate should not exceed 2 mL/minute for Bebulin® VH, 3 mL/minute for Proplex® T, or 10 mL/minute for Profilnine® SD.

Monitoring Parameters Levels of factors being replaced (eg, VII or IX), PT, PTT

Reference Range Average normal factor VII and factor IX levels are 50% to 150%; patients with severe hemophilia will have levels <1%, often undetectable. Moderate forms of the disease have levels of 1% to 10% while some mild cases may have 11% to 49% of normal factor IX.

(Continued)

Factor IX Complex (Human) *(Continued)*

Maintain factor IX plasma level at least 20% until hemostasis achieved after acute joint or muscle bleeding

In preparation for and following surgery:

Level to prevent spontaneous hemorrhage: 5%

Minimum level for hemostasis following trauma and surgery: 30% to 50%

Severe hemorrhage: >60%

Major surgery: >60% prior to procedure, 30% to 50% for several days after surgery, and >20% for 7-10 days thereafter

Pregnancy Risk Factor C

Contraindications Liver disease with signs of intravascular coagulation or fibrinolysis, not for use in factor VII deficiencies, patients undergoing elective surgery

Warnings/Precautions Use with caution in patients with liver dysfunction. Prepared from pooled human plasma - the risk of viral transmission is not totally eradicated. Thromboembolic complications rarely occur; more likely to occur during postoperative period or in patients with risk factors. Treatment should stop if respiratory distress or any changes in blood pressure or pulse rate occur.

Adverse Reactions

1% to 10%:

Central nervous system: Fever, headache, chills

Neuromuscular & skeletal: Tingling

Miscellaneous: Following rapid administration: Transient fever

<1% (Limited to important or life-threatening): Disseminated intravascular coagulation (DIC), flushing, nausea, somnolence, thrombosis following high dosages because of presence of activated clotting factors, tightness in chest, tightness in neck, urticaria, vomiting

Overdosage/Toxicology Symptoms of overdose include disseminated intravascular coagulation (DIC).

Drug Interactions Increased toxicity: Do not coadminister with aminocaproic acid may increase risk for thrombosis

Dosage Forms Injection, powder for reconstitution (**Note:** Exact potency labeled on each vial):

Bebulin® VH [single-dose vial; vapor heated; supplied with sterile water for injection]

Profilnine® SD [single-dose vial; solvent detergent treated]

Proplex® T [single-dose vial; heat treated; supplied with sterile water for injection]

Famotidine (fa MOE ti deen)

U.S. Brand Names Fluxid™; Pepcid®; Pepcid® AC [OTC]

Canadian Brand Names Apo-Famotidine®; Famotidine Omega; Gen-Famotidine; Novo-Famotidine; Nu-Famotidine; Pepcid®; Pepcid® AC; Pepcid® I.V.; ratio-Famotidine; Riva-Famotidine; Ulcidine

Pharmacologic Category Histamine H_2 Antagonist

Generic Available Yes: Injection, tablet

Use Therapy and treatment of duodenal ulcer, gastric ulcer, control gastric pH in critically-ill patients, symptomatic relief in gastritis, gastroesophageal reflux, active benign ulcer, and pathological hypersecretory conditions

OTC labeling: Relief of heartburn, acid indigestion, and sour stomach

Unlabeled/Investigational Use Part of a multidrug regimen for *H. pylori* eradication to reduce the risk of duodenal ulcer recurrence

Mechanism of Action Competitive inhibition of histamine at H_2 receptors of the gastric parietal cells, which inhibits gastric acid secretion

Pharmacodynamics/Kinetics

Onset of action: GI: Oral: Within 1-3 hour

Duration: 10-12 hours

Protein binding: 15% to 20%

Bioavailability: Oral: 40% to 50%

Half-life elimination:

Injection, oral suspension, tablet: 2.5-3.5 hours; prolonged with renal impairment; Oliguria: 20 hours

Orally-disintegrating tablet: 2.5-5 hours

Time to peak, serum: Oral: ~1-3 hours

Excretion: Urine (as unchanged drug)

Dosage

Children: Treatment duration and dose should be individualized

Peptic ulcer: 1-16 years:

Oral: 0.5 mg/kg/day at bedtime or divided twice daily (maximum dose: 40 mg/day); doses of up to 1 mg/kg/day have been used in clinical studies

I.V.: 0.25 mg/kg every 12 hours (maximum dose: 40 mg/day); doses of up to 0.5 mg/kg have been used in clinical studies

GERD: Oral:

<3 months: 0.5 mg/kg once daily

3-12 months: 0.5 mg/kg twice daily

1-16 years: 1 mg/kg/day divided twice daily (maximum dose: 40 mg twice daily); doses of up to 2 mg/kg/day have been used in clinical studies

Children ≥12 years and Adults: Heartburn, indigestion, sour stomach: OTC labeling: Oral: 10-20 mg every 12 hours; dose may be taken 15-60 minutes before eating foods known to cause heartburn

Adults:

Duodenal ulcer: Oral: Acute therapy: 40 mg/day at bedtime for 4-8 weeks; maintenance therapy: 20 mg/day at bedtime

Helicobacter pylori eradication (unlabeled use): 40 mg once daily; requires combination therapy with antibiotics

Gastric ulcer: Oral: Acute therapy: 40 mg/day at bedtime

Hypersecretory conditions: Oral: Initial: 20 mg every 6 hours, may increase in increments up to 160 mg every 6 hours

GERD: Oral: 20 mg twice daily for 6 weeks

Esophagitis and accompanying symptoms due to GERD: Oral: 20 mg or 40 mg twice daily for up to 12 weeks

Patients unable to take oral medication: I.V.: 20 mg every 12 hours

Dosing adjustment in renal impairment: Cl_{cr} <50 mL/minute: Manufacturer recommendation: Administer 50% of dose **or** increase the dosing interval to every 36-48 hours (to limit potential CNS adverse effects).

Stability

Oral:

Powder for oral suspension: Prior to mixing, dry powder should be stored at room temperature of 25°C (77°F). Reconstituted oral suspension is stable for 30-days at room temperature. Do not freeze

Tablet: Store at 20°C (77°F); excursions permitted between 15°C to 30°C (59°F to 86°F); protect from moisture

Orally-disintegrating tablet: Store at 20°C to 25°C (68°F to 77°F); excursions permitted between 15°C to 30°C (59°F to 86°F); protect from moisture

I.V.:

Solution for injection: Prior to use, store at 2°C to 8°C (36°F to 46°F). If solution freezes, allow to solubilize at room temperature.

I.V. push: Dilute famotidine with NS (or another compatible solution) to a total of 5-10 mL (some centers also administer undiluted). Following reconstitution, solutions for I.V. push should be used immediately, or may be stored in refrigerator and used within 48 hours.

Infusion: Dilute with D_5W 100 mL or another compatible solution. Following reconstitution, solutions for infusion are stable for 7 days at room temperature.

Solution for injection, premixed bags: Store at room temperature of 25°C (77°F). Avoid excessive heat.

Administration

Oral:

Suspension: Shake vigorously before use. May be taken with or without food.

Tablet: May be taken with or without food.

Orally-disintegrating tablet: Place tablet on tongue with dry hands; tablet dissolves rapidly in saliva. May be taken with or without liquid or food; do not break tablet

I.V.:

I.V. push: Inject over at least 2 minutes

Solution for infusion: Administer over 15-30 minutes

Pregnancy Risk Factor B

Contraindications Hypersensitivity to famotidine, other H_2 antagonists, or any component of the formulation

(Continued)

Famotidine *(Continued)*

Warnings/Precautions Modify dose in patients with renal impairment; chewable tablets contain phenylalanine; multidose vials contain benzyl alcohol

OTC labeling: When used for self-medication, patients should be instructed not to use if they have difficulty swallowing, have vomiting with blood, or bloody or black stools. Not for use with other acid reducers.

Adverse Reactions

Note: Agitation and vomiting have been reported in up to 14% of pediatric patients <1 year of age.

1% to 10%:

Central nervous system: Dizziness (1%), headache (5%)

Gastrointestinal: Constipation (1%), diarrhea (2%)

<1% (Limited to important or life-threatening): Abdominal discomfort, acne, agranulocytosis, allergic reaction, alopecia, anaphylaxis, angioedema, anorexia, arrhythmia, AST/ALT increased, bradycardia, bronchospasm, BUN/creatinine increased, drowsiness, fatigue, fever, hypertension, insomnia, jaundice, neutropenia, palpitation, paresthesia, proteinuria, pruritus, psychic disturbances, rash, seizure, tachycardia, thrombocytopenia, toxic epidermal necrolysis, urticaria, vomiting, weakness

Overdosage/Toxicology Symptoms of overdose include hypotension, tachycardia, vomiting, and drowsiness. Treatment is symptomatic and supportive.

Drug Interactions

Cefpodoxime: Histamine H_2 antagonists may decrease the absorption of cefpodoxime; separate oral doses by at least 2 hours. Risk: Moderate

Cefuroxime: Histamine H_2 antagonists may decrease the absorption of cefuroxime; separate oral doses by at least 2 hours. Risk: Moderate

Cyclosporine: Histamine H_2 antagonists may increase the serum concentration of cyclosporine; monitor

Delavirdine: Delavirdine's absorption is decreased; avoid concurrent use with H_2 antagonists

Itraconazole: Histamine H_2 antagonists may decrease the absorption of itraconazole; monitor

Ketoconazole: Histamine H_2 antagonists may decrease the absorption of ketoconazole; monitor

Ethanol/Nutrition/Herb Interactions

Ethanol: Avoid ethanol (may cause gastric mucosal irritation).

Food: Famotidine bioavailability may be increased if taken with food.

Dietary Considerations Phenylalanine content: Pepcid® AC chewable: Each 10 mg tablet contains phenylalanine 1.4 mg

Dosage Forms [DSC] = Discontinued product

Gelcap (Pepcid® AC): 10 mg

Infusion [premixed in NS] (Pepcid®): 20 mg (50 mL)

Injection, solution: 10 mg/mL (4 mL, 20 mL, 50 mL) [contains benzyl alcohol]

Pepcid®: 10 mg/mL (4 mL [DSC], 20 mL)

Injection, solution [preservative free] (Pepcid®): 10 mg/mL (2 mL)

Powder for oral suspension (Pepcid®): 40 mg/5 mL (50 mL) [contains sodium benzoate; cherry-banana-mint flavor]

Tablet: 10 mg [OTC], 20 mg, 40 mg

Pepcid®: 20 mg, 40 mg

Pepcid® AC: 10 mg, 20 mg

Tablet, chewable (Pepcid® AC): 10 mg [contains phenylalanine 1.4 mg/tablet; mint flavor]

Tablet, orally disintegrating (Fluxid™): 20 mg, 40 mg [cherry flavor]

♦ **Famotidine Omega (Can)** *see* Famotidine *on page 506*

♦ **Faslodex®** *see* Fulvestrant *on page 571*

Fat Emulsion (fat e MUL shun)

U.S. Brand Names Intralipid®; Liposyn® III

Canadian Brand Names Intralipid®; Liposyn® II

Synonyms Intravenous Fat Emulsion

Pharmacologic Category Caloric Agent

Generic Available No

Use Source of calories and essential fatty acids for patients requiring parenteral nutrition of extended duration

Mechanism of Action Essential for normal structure and function of cell membranes

Pharmacodynamics/Kinetics

Metabolism: Undergoes lipolysis to free fatty acids which are utilized by reticuloendothelial cells

Half-life elimination: 0.5-1 hour

Dosage Fat emulsion should not exceed 60% of the total daily calories

Premature Infants: Initial dose: 0.25-0.5 g/kg/day, increase by 0.25-0.5 g/kg/day to a maximum of 3 g/kg/day depending on needs/nutritional goals; limit to 1 g/kg/day if on phototherapy; maximum rate of infusion: 0.15 g/kg/hour (0.75 mL/kg/hour of 20% solution)

Infants and Children: Initial dose: 0.5-1 g/kg/day, increase by 0.5 g/kg/day to a maximum of 3 g/kg/day depending on needs/nutritional goals; maximum rate of infusion: 0.25 g/kg/hour (1.25 mL/kg/hour of 20% solution)

Adolescents and Adults: Initial dose: 1 g/kg/day, increase by 0.5-1 g/kg/day to a maximum of 2.5 g/kg/day of 10% and 3 g/kg/day of 20% depending on needs/nutritional goals; maximum rate of infusion: 0.25 g/kg/hour (1.25 mL/kg/hour of 20% solution); do not exceed 50 mL/hour (20%) or 100 mL/hour (10%)

Prevention of essential fatty acid deficiency (8% to 10% of total caloric intake): 0.5-1 g/kg/24 hours

Children: 5-10 mL/kg/day at 0.1 mL/minute then up to 100 mL/hour

Adults: 500 mL (10%) twice weekly at rate of 1 mL/minute for 30 minutes, then increase to 42 mL/hour (500 mL over 12 hours)

Note: At the onset of therapy, the patient should be observed for any immediate allergic reactions such as dyspnea, cyanosis, and fever; slower initial rates of infusion may be used for the first 10-15 minutes of the infusion (eg, 0.1 mL/minute of 10% or 0.05 mL/minute of 20% solution)

Stability May be stored at room temperature; do not store partly used bottles for later use; do not use if emulsion appears to be oiling out

Administration May be simultaneously infused with amino acid dextrose mixtures by means of Y-connector located near infusion site. The 10% isotonic solution which has 1.1 cal/mL (10%) and may be administered peripherally; the 20% (2 cal/mL) is not recommended for use in low birth weight infants.

Monitoring Parameters Serum triglycerides; before initiation of therapy and at least weekly during therapy. Frequent (some advise daily) platelet counts should be performed in neonatal patients receiving parenteral lipids.

Pregnancy Risk Factor C

Contraindications Hypersensitivity to fat emulsion or any component of the formulation; severe egg or legume (soybean) allergies; pathologic hyperlipidemia, lipoid nephrosis pancreatitis with hyperlipemia

Warnings/Precautions Use caution in patients with severe liver damage, pulmonary disease, anemia, or blood coagulation disorder; use with caution in jaundiced, premature, and low birth weight children. Some formulations may contain aluminum which may accumulate following prolonged administration in renally-impaired patients. Due to immature renal function, premature neonates are at higher risk of accumulation/toxicity from aluminum. To avoid hyperlipidemia and/or fat deposition, do not exceed recommended daily doses. Monitor by appropriate laboratory evaluation (e.g., triglycerides).

[U.S. Boxed Warning]: Deaths have been reported in preterm infants in association with fat emulsion infusion; fat accumulation in the lungs has been noted on autopsy. Infusion rate should not exceed 1g fat/kg in four hours; strict monitoring of metabolic tolerance and elimination of infused fat from the circulation must occur. Allow lipemia to resolve between daily infusions.

Adverse Reactions Frequency not defined.

Cardiovascular: Cyanosis, flushing, chest pain

Central nervous system: Headache, dizziness

Endocrine & metabolic: Hyperlipemia, hypertriglyceridemia

Gastrointestinal: Nausea, vomiting, diarrhea

Hematologic: Hypercoagulability, thrombocytopenia in neonates (rare)

Hepatic: Hepatomegaly, pancreatitis

Local: Thrombophlebitis

Respiratory: Dyspnea

Miscellaneous: Sepsis, diaphoresis, brown pigment deposition in the reticuloendothelial system (significance unknown)

(Continued)

Fat Emulsion *(Continued)*

Overdosage/Toxicology Rapid administration results in fluid or fat overload causing dilution of serum electrolytes, overhydration, pulmonary edema, impaired pulmonary diffusion capacity, and metabolic acidosis. Treatment is supportive.

Dosage Forms Injection, emulsion [soybean oil]:

Intralipid®: 10% [100 mg/mL] (100 mL, 250 mL, 500 mL); 20% [200 mg/mL] (50 mL, 100 mL, 250 mL, 500 mL, 1000 mL); 30% [300 mg/mL] (500 mL)

Liposyn® III: 10% [100 mg/mL] (200 mL, 500 mL); 20% [200 mg/mL] (200 mL, 500 mL); 30% [300 mg/mL] (500 mL)

♦ **Feldene®** *see* Piroxicam *on page 1032*

Fenoldopam (fe NOL doe pam)

Related Information

Chronic Renal Failure *on page 1437*
Hypertension *on page 1620*
Postoperative Hypertension *on page 1471*

U.S. Brand Names Corlopam®

Canadian Brand Names Corlopam®

Synonyms Fenoldopam Mesylate

Pharmacologic Category Dopamine Agonist

Generic Available Yes

Use Treatment of severe hypertension (up to 48 hours in adults), including in patients with renal compromise; short-term (up to 4 hours) blood pressure reduction in pediatric patients

Mechanism of Action A selective postsynaptic dopamine agonist (D_1-receptors) which exerts hypotensive effects by decreasing peripheral vasculature resistance with increased renal blood flow, diuresis, and natriuresis; 6 times as potent as dopamine in producing renal vasodilitation; has minimal adrenergic effects

Pharmacodynamics/Kinetics

Onset of action: I.V.: 10 minutes
Duration: I.V.: 1 hour
Distribution: V_d: 0.6 L/kg
Half-life elimination: I.V.: Children: 3-5 minutes; Adults: ~5 minutes
Metabolism: Hepatic via methylation, glucuronidation, and sulfation; the 8-sulfate metabolite may have some activity; extensive first-pass effect
Excretion: Urine (90%); feces (10%)

Dosage I.V.: Hypertension, severe:

Children: Initial: 0.2 mcg/kg/minute; may be increased to dosages of 0.3-0.5 mcg/kg/minute every 20-30 minutes (maximum dose: 0.8 mcg/kg/minute); limited to short-term (4 hours) use

Adults: Initial: 0.1-0.3 mcg/kg/minute (lower initial doses may be associated with less reflex tachycardia); may be increased in increments of 0.05-0.1 mcg/kg/minute every 15 minutes until target blood pressure is reached; the maximal infusion rate reported in clinical studies was 1.6 mcg/kg/minute

Dosing adjustment in renal impairment: None required

Dosing adjustment in hepatic impairment: None published

Stability Store at 2°C to 30°C (35°F to 86°F). Must be diluted prior to infusion; compatible with NS or D_5W. Final dilution for children is 60 mcg/mL and for adults is 40 mcg/mL. Following dilution, store at room temperature and use solution within 24 hours.

Administration For I.V. infusion using an infusion pump.

Monitoring Parameters Blood pressure, heart rate, ECG, renal/hepatic function tests

Reference Range Mean plasma fenoldopam levels after a 2 hour infusion (at 0.5 mcg/kg/minute) and a 100 mg dose is approximately 13 ng/mL and 50 ng/mL

Anesthesia and Critical Care Concerns/Other Considerations Suitable for use in patients whose condition is unstable or rapidly changing because the effects of the drug are predictable and easily reversible; it has been found to safely control blood pressure in patients with a variety of pre-existing conditions including kidney disease, liver disease, and heart failure. (Clinical benefit other than blood pressure reduction has not been established.) Dosage adjustment is not required in any of these situations. The drug is quickly metabolized into inactive substances before it is excreted. Unlike the situation with some other intravenous antihypertensives, the patient does not need an arterial line for blood pressure monitoring; a blood pressure cuff is sufficient. Since the drug induces natriuresis, diuresis, and increased creatinine clearance, it may have an advantage over nitroprusside, especially in patients with severe renal insufficiency and in volume-overloaded patients.

Contrast Nephropathy: Fenoldopam is ineffective in the prevention of contrast-induced nephropathy.

Pregnancy Risk Factor B

Contraindications Hypersensitivity of fenoldopam or any component of the formulation

Warnings/Precautions Use caution in patients with glaucoma or intraocular hypertension. A dose-related tachycardia can occur, especially at infusion rates >0.1 mcg/kg/minute. Use caution in angina patients (can increase myocardial oxygen demand with tachycardia). Close monitoring of blood pressure is necessary (hypotension can occur). Monitor for hypokalemia at intervals of 6 hours during infusion. For continuous infusion only (no bolus doses). The effects of hemodialysis on the pharmacokinetics of fenoldopam have not been evaluated. Use caution with increased intracranial pressure. Contains sulfites; may cause allergic reaction in susceptible individuals.

Adverse Reactions Frequency not always defined.

Cardiovascular: Angina, asymptomatic T wave flattening on ECG, chest pain, edema, facial flushing (>5%), fibrillation (atrial), flutter (atrial), hypotension (>5%), tachycardia

Central nervous system: Dizziness, headache (>5%)

Endocrine & metabolic: Hypokalemia

Gastrointestinal: Abdominal pain/fullness, diarrhea, nausea (>5%), vomiting, xerostomia

Local: Injection site reactions

Ocular: Intraocular pressure (increased), blurred vision

Hepatic: Increases in portal pressure in cirrhotic patients

Drug Interactions

Concurrent acetaminophen may increase fenoldopam levels (30% to 70%).

Beta-blockers increase the risk of hypotension. Avoid concurrent use; if used concurrently, close monitoring is recommended.

Dosage Forms Injection, solution: 10 mg/mL (1 mL, 2 mL) [contains sodium metabisulfite and propylene glycol]

References

Allaqaband S, Tumuluri R, Malik AM, et al, "Prospective Randomized Study of N-acetylcysteine, Fenoldopam, and Saline for Prevention of Radiocontrast-Induced Nephropathy," *Catheter Cardiovascular Interv*, 2002, 57(3):279-83.

Erstad BL and Barletta JF, "Treatment of Hypertension in the Perioperative Patient," *Ann Pharmacother*, 2000, 34(1):66-79.

Stone GW, McCullough PA, Tumlin JA, et al, "Fenoldopam Mesylate for the Prevention of Contrast-Induced Nephropathy: A Randomized Controlled Trial," *JAMA*, 2003, 290(17):2284-91.

♦ **Fenoldopam Mesylate** *see* Fenoldopam *on page 510*

Fenoprofen (fen oh PROE fen)

Medication Safety Issues

Sound-alike/look-alike issues:

Fenoprofen may be confused with flurbiprofen

Nalfon® may be confused with Naldecon®

Related Information

Acetaminophen and NSAIDS, Dosing Data *on page 1543*

Chronic Pain Management *on page 1430*

U.S. Brand Names Nalfon®

Canadian Brand Names Nalfon®

Synonyms Fenoprofen Calcium

Pharmacologic Category Nonsteroidal Anti-inflammatory Drug (NSAID), Oral

Restrictions A medication guide should be dispensed with each prescription. A template for the required MedGuide can be found on the FDA website at http://www.fda.gov/medwatch/SAFETY/2005/safety05.htm#NSAID

Generic Available Yes: Tablet

Use Symptomatic treatment of acute and chronic rheumatoid arthritis and osteoarthritis; relief of mild to moderate pain

(Continued)

Fenoprofen *(Continued)*

Mechanism of Action Inhibits prostaglandin synthesis by decreasing the activity of the enzyme, cyclooxygenase, which results in decreased formation of prostaglandin precursors

Pharmacodynamics/Kinetics

Onset of action: A few days

Absorption: Rapid, 80%

Distribution: Does not cross the placenta

Protein binding: 99%

Metabolism: Extensively hepatic

Half-life elimination: 2.5-3 hours

Time to peak, serum: ~2 hours

Excretion: Urine (2% to 5% as unchanged drug); feces (small amounts)

Dosage Adults: Oral:

Rheumatoid arthritis: 300-600 mg 3-4 times/day up to 3.2 g/day

Mild to moderate pain: 200 mg every 4-6 hours as needed

Dosage adjustment in renal impairment: Not recommended in patients with advanced renal disease

Administration Do not crush tablets. Swallow whole with a full glass of water. Take with food to minimize stomach upset.

Monitoring Parameters Monitor CBC, liver enzymes; monitor urine output and BUN/serum creatinine in patients receiving diuretics

Reference Range Therapeutic: 20-65 mcg/mL (SI: 82-268 μmol/L)

Anesthesia and Critical Care Concerns/Other Considerations The 2002 ACCM/SCCM guidelines for analgesia (critically-ill adult) suggest that NSAIDs may be used in combination with opioids in select patients for pain management. Concern about adverse events (increased risk of renal dysfunction, altered platelet function and gastrointestinal irritation) limits its use in patients who have other underlying risks for these events.

In short-term use, NSAIDs vary considerably in their effect on blood pressure. When NSAIDs are used in patients with hypertension, appropriate monitoring of blood pressure responses should be completed and the duration of therapy, when possible, kept short. The use of NSAIDs in the treatment of patients with congestive heart failure may be associated with an increased risk for fluid accumulation and edema. May precipitate renal failure in dehydrated patients.

Pregnancy Risk Factor C/D (3rd trimester)

Contraindications Hypersensitivity to fenoprofen, aspirin, or other NSAIDs, or any component of the formulation; perioperative pain in the setting of coronary artery bypass surgery (CABG); significant renal dysfunction; pregnancy (3rd trimester)

Warnings/Precautions [U.S. Boxed Warning]: NSAIDs are associated with an increased risk of adverse cardiovascular events, including MI, stroke, and new onset or worsening of pre-existing hypertension. Risk may be increased with duration of use or pre-existing cardiovascular risk-factors or disease. Carefully evaluate individual cardiovascular risk profiles prior to prescribing. Use caution with fluid retention, CHF, or hypertension.

Use of NSAIDs can compromise existing renal function. Renal toxicity can occur in patient with impaired renal function, dehydration, heart failure, liver dysfunction, those taking diuretics and ACEI, and the elderly. Rehydrate patient before starting therapy. Monitor renal function closely. Not recommended for use in patients with advanced renal disease.

[U.S. Boxed Warning]: NSAIDs may increase risk of gastrointestinal irritation, ulceration, bleeding, and perforation. These events may occur at any time during therapy and without warning. Use caution with a history of GI disease (bleeding or ulcers), concurrent therapy with aspirin, anticoagulants and/or corticosteroids, smoking, use of alcohol, the elderly or debilitated patients.

Use the lowest effective dose for the shortest duration of time, consistent with individual patient goals, to reduce risk of cardiovascular or GI adverse events. Alternate therapies should be considered for patients at high risk.

NSAIDs may cause serious skin adverse events including exfoliative dermatitis, Stevens-Johnson syndrome (SJS), and toxic epidermal necrolysis (TEN). Anaphylactoid reactions may occur, even without prior exposure; patients with "aspirin triad" (bronchial asthma, aspirin intolerance, rhinitis) may be at increased risk. Do not use in patients who experience bronchospasm, asthma, rhinitis, or urticaria with NSAID or aspirin therapy.

Use with caution in patients with decreased hepatic function. Closely monitor patients with any abnormal LFT. Severe hepatic reactions (eg, fulminant hepatitis, liver failure) have occurred with NSAID use, rarely; discontinue if signs or symptoms of liver disease develop, or if systemic manifestations occur.

The elderly are at increased risk for adverse effects (especially peptic ulceration, CNS effects, renal toxicity) from NSAIDs even at low doses.

Withhold for at least 4-6 half-lives prior to surgical or dental procedures. Safety and efficacy have not been established in children <18 years of age.

Adverse Reactions

>10%:

Central nervous system: Dizziness (7% to 15%), somnolence (9% to 15%)

Gastrointestinal: Abdominal cramps (2% to 4%), heartburn, indigestion, nausea (8% to 14%), dyspepsia (10% to 14%), flatulence (14%), anorexia (14%), constipation (7% to 14%), occult blood in stool (14%), vomiting (3% to 14%), diarrhea (2% to 14%)

1% to 10%:

Central nervous system: Headache (9%)

Dermatologic: Itching

Endocrine & metabolic: Fluid retention

<1% (Limited to important or life-threatening): Agranulocytosis, anemia, angioedema, arrhythmia, bone marrow depression, CHF, dyspnea, erythema multiforme, GI ulceration, hemolytic anemia, hepatitis, hypertension, leukopenia, polyuria, renal failure (acute), Stevens-Johnson syndrome, thrombocytopenia, tachycardia, toxic epidermal necrolysis

Overdosage/Toxicology Symptoms of overdose include acute renal failure, vomiting, drowsiness, and leukocytosis. Management of NSAID intoxication is supportive and symptomatic.

Drug Interactions

ACE inhibitors: Antihypertensive effects may be decreased by concurrent therapy with NSAIDs; monitor blood pressure.

Angiotensin II antagonists: Antihypertensive effects may be decreased by concurrent therapy with NSAIDs; monitor blood pressure.

Anticoagulants (warfarin, heparin, LMWHs) in combination with NSAIDs can cause increased risk of bleeding.

Antiplatelet drugs (ticlopidine, clopidogrel, aspirin, abciximab, dipyridamole, eptifibatide, tirofiban) can cause an increased risk of bleeding.

Beta-blockers: NSAIDs may decrease the antihypertensive effect of beta-blockers. Monitor.

Cholestyramine (and other bile acid sequestrants): May decrease the absorption of NSAIDs. Separate by at least 2 hours.

Corticosteroids may increase the risk of GI ulceration; avoid concurrent use.

Cyclosporine: NSAIDs may increase serum creatinine, potassium, blood pressure, and cyclosporine levels; monitor cyclosporine levels and renal function carefully.

Gentamicin and amikacin serum concentrations are increased by indomethacin in premature infants. Results may apply to other aminoglycosides and NSAIDs.

Hydralazine's antihypertensive effect is decreased; avoid concurrent use.

Lithium levels can be increased; avoid concurrent use if possible or monitor lithium levels and adjust dose. Sulindac may have the least effect. When NSAID is stopped, lithium will need adjustment again.

Loop diuretics efficacy (diuretic and antihypertensive effect) is reduced. Indomethacin reduces this efficacy, however, it may be anticipated with any NSAID.

Methotrexate: Severe bone marrow suppression, aplastic anemia, and GI toxicity have been reported with concomitant NSAID therapy. Avoid use during moderate or high-dose methotrexate (increased and prolonged methotrexate levels). NSAID use during low-dose treatment of rheumatoid arthritis has not been fully evaluated; extreme caution is warranted.

Thiazide efficacy (diuretic and antihypertensive effect) may be reduced. Indomethacin may reduce this efficacy and it may be anticipated with any NSAID.

Verapamil plasma concentration is decreased by diclofenac; avoid concurrent use.

Warfarin's INRs may be increased by piroxicam. Other NSAIDs may have the same effect depending on dose and duration. Monitor INR closely. Use the lowest dose of NSAIDs possible and for the briefest duration.

(Continued)

Fenoprofen *(Continued)*

Ethanol/Nutrition/Herb Interactions

Ethanol: Avoid ethanol (may enhance gastric mucosal irritation).

Food: Fenoprofen peak serum levels may be decreased if taken with food.

Herb/Nutraceutical: Avoid alfalfa, anise, bilberry, bladderwrack, bromelain, cat's claw, celery, coleus, cordyceps, dong quai, evening primrose, feverfew, fenugreek, garlic, ginger, ginkgo biloboa, red clover, horse chestnut, grapeseed, green tea, ginseng, guggul, horse chestnut seed, horseradish, licorice, prickly ash, red clover, reishi, SAMe, sweet clover, turmeric, white willow (all have additional antiplatelet activity).

Test Interactions Increased chloride (S), increased sodium (S)

Dietary Considerations May be taken with food to decrease GI distress.

Dosage Forms

Capsule, as calcium (Nalfon®): 200 mg, 300 mg

Tablet, as calcium: 600 mg

♦ **Fenoprofen Calcium** *see* Fenoprofen *on page 511*

Fentanyl (FEN ta nil)

Medication Safety Issues

Sound-alike/look-alike issues:

Fentanyl may be confused with alfentanil, sufentanil

New patch dosage form of Duragesic®-12 actually delivers 12.5 mcg/hour of fentanyl. Use caution, as orders may be written as "Duragesic 12.5" which can be erroneously interpreted as a 125 mcg dose.

Iontophoretic transdermal system (Ionsys™) may contain conducting metal (eg, aluminum); remove patch prior to MRI. Transdermal patch (eg, Duragesic®) does not contain any metal-based compounds; however, the printed ink used to indicate strength on the outer surface of the patch does contain titanium dioxide, but the amount is minimal.

Related Information

Acute Postoperative Pain *on page 1388*
Anesthesia Considerations for Neurosurgery *on page 1401*
Anesthesia for Patients With Liver Disease *on page 1421*
Chronic Pain Management *on page 1430*
Chronic Renal Failure *on page 1437*
Moderate Sedation *on page 1442*
Narcotic / Opioid Analgesics *on page 1568*
Opioids *on page 1535*
Substance Abuse and Anesthesia *on page 1496*

U.S. Brand Names Actiq®; Duragesic®; Ionsys™; Sublimaze®

Canadian Brand Names Actiq®; Duragesic®; Fentanyl Citrate Injection, USP

Synonyms Fentanyl Citrate; Fentanyl Hydrocholoride

Pharmacologic Category Analgesic, Narcotic; General Anesthetic

Restrictions C-II

Generic Available Yes: Excludes lozenge and iontophoretic transdermal system

Use

Injection: Sedation, relief of pain, preoperative medication, adjunct to general or regional anesthesia

Iontophoretic transdermal system (Ionsys™): Short-term in-hospital management of acute post-operative pain

Transdermal patch (eg, Duragesic®): Management of moderate-to-severe chronic pain

Transmucosal (Actiq®): Management of breakthrough cancer pain

Mechanism of Action Binds with stereospecific receptors at many sites within the CNS, increases pain threshold, alters pain reception, inhibits ascending pain pathways

Pharmacodynamics/Kinetics

Onset of action: Analgesic: I.M.: 7-15 minutes; I.V.: Almost immediate; Transmucosal: 5-15 minutes

Peak effect: Transmucosal: Analgesic: 20-30 minutes

Duration: I.M.: 1-2 hours; I.V.: 0.5-1 hour; Transmucosal: Related to blood level; respiratory depressant effect may last longer than analgesic effect

Absorption:

Transmucosal: Rapid, ~25% from the buccal mucosa; 75% swallowed with saliva and slowly absorbed from GI tract

Iontophoretic transdermal system (Ionsys™): Fentanyl levels continue to rise for 5 minutes after the completion of each 10-minute dose

Distribution: Highly lipophilic, redistributes into muscle and fat

Metabolism: Hepatic, primarily via CYP3A4

Bioavailability: Transmucosal: ~50% (range: 36% to 71%)

Half-life elimination: 2-4 hours

Iontophoretic transdermal system (Ionsys™): 11 hours

Transdermal patch: 17 hours (half-life is influenced by absorption rate)

Transmucosal: 6.6 hours (range: 5-15 hours)

Time to peak: Transdermal patch: 24-72 hours

Excretion: Urine (primarily as metabolites, 10% as unchanged drug)

Dosage Note: These are guidelines and do not represent the maximum doses that may be required in all patients. Doses should be titrated to pain relief/prevention. Monitor vital signs routinely. Single I.M. doses have a duration of 1-2 hours, single I.V. doses last 0.5-1 hour.

Sedation for minor procedures/analgesia:

Children 1-12 years:

Sedation for minor procedures/analgesia: I.M., I.V.: 1-2 mcg/kg/dose; may repeat at 30- to 60-minute intervals. **Note:** Children 18-36 months of age may require 2-3 mcg/kg/dose

Continuous sedation/analgesia: Initial I.V. bolus: 1-2 mcg/kg; then 1-3 mcg/kg/hour to a maximum dose of 5 mcg/kg/hour

Children >12 years and Adults: I.V.: 25-50 mcg; may repeat every 3-5 minutes to desired effect or adverse event; maximum dose of 500 mcg/4 hours; higher doses are used for major procedures

Surgery: Adults:

Premedication: I.M., slow I.V.: 25-100 mcg/dose 30-60 minutes prior to surgery

Adjunct to regional anesthesia: Slow I.V.: 25-100 mcg/dose over 1-2 minutes. **Note:** An I.V. should be in place with regional anesthesia so the I.M. route is rarely used but still maintained as an option in the package labeling.

Adjunct to general anesthesia: Slow I.V.:

Low dose: 0.5-2 mcg/kg/dose depending on the indication. For example, 0.5 mcg/kg will provide analgesia or reduce the amount of propofol needed for laryngeal mask airway insertion with minimal respiratory depression. However, to blunt the hemodynamic response to intubation 2 mcg/kg is often necessary.

Moderate dose: Initial: 2-15 mcg/kg/dose; Maintenance (bolus or infusion): 1-2 mcg/kg/hour. Discontinuing fentanyl infusion 30-60 minutes prior to the end of surgery will usually allow adequate ventilation upon emergence from anesthesia. For "fast-tracking" and early extubation following major surgery, total fentanyl doses are limited to 10-15 mcg/kg.

High dose: **Note:** High-dose (20-50 mcg/kg/dose) fentanyl is rarely used, but is still maintained in the package labeling.

Acute pain management: Adults:

Severe: I.M, I.V.: 50-100 mcg/dose every 1-2 hours as needed; patients with prior opiate exposure may tolerate higher initial doses

Patient-controlled analgesia (PCA): I.V.: Usual concentration: 10 mcg/mL

Demand dose: Usual: 10 mcg; range: 10-50 mcg

Lockout interval: 5-8 minutes

Mechanically-ventilated patients (based on 70 kg patient): Slow I.V.: 0.35-1.5 mcg/kg every 30-60 minutes as needed; infusion: 0.7-10 mcg/kg/hour

Iontophoretic transdermal system: 40 mcg per activation on-demand (maximum: 6 doses/hour). **Note:** Patient's pain should be controlled prior to initiating system. Instruct patient how to operate system. Only the patient should initiate system. Each system operates for 24 hours or until 80 doses have been administered, whichever comes first.

Breakthrough cancer pain:

Adults: Transmucosal: Actiq® dosing should be individually titrated to provide adequate analgesia with minimal side effects. For patients who are tolerant to and currently receiving opioid therapy for persistent cancer pain. Initial starting dose: 200 mcg; the second dose may be started 15 minutes after completion of the first dose. Consumption should be limited to 4 units/day or

(Continued)

Fentanyl *(Continued)*

less. Patients needing more than 4 units/day should have the dose of their long-term opioid re-evaluated.

Elderly >65 years: Transmucosal: Actiq®: Dose should be reduced to 2.5-5 mcg/kg

Chronic pain management: Children ≥2 years and Adults (opioid-tolerant patients): Transdermal patch (eg, Duragesic®):

Initial: To convert patients from oral or parenteral opioids to transdermal patch, a 24-hour analgesic requirement should be calculated (based on prior opiate use). Using the tables, the appropriate initial dose can be determined. The initial fentanyl dosage may be approximated from the 24-hour morphine dosage and titrated to minimize adverse effects and provide analgesia. With the initial application, the absorption of transdermal fentanyl requires several hours to reach plateau; therefore transdermal fentanyl is inappropriate for management of acute pain. Change patch every 72 hours.

Conversion from continuous infusion of fentanyl: In patients who have adequate pain relief with a fentanyl infusion, fentanyl may be converted to transdermal dosing at a rate equivalent to the intravenous rate. A two-step taper of the infusion to be completed over 12 hours has been recommended after the patch is applied. The infusion is decreased to 50% of the original rate six hours after the application of the first patch, and subsequently discontinued twelve hours after application.

Titration: Short-acting agents may be required until analgesic efficacy is established and/or as supplements for "breakthrough" pain. The amount of supplemental doses should be closely monitored. Appropriate dosage increases may be based on daily supplemental dosage using the ratio of 45 mg/24 hours of oral morphine to a 12.5 mcg/hour increase in fentanyl dosage.

Frequency of adjustment: The dosage should not be titrated more frequently than every 3 days after the initial dose or every 6 days thereafter. Patients should wear a consistent fentanyl dosage through two applications (6 days) before dosage increase based on supplemental opiate dosages can be estimated.

Frequency of application: The majority of patients may be controlled on every 72-hour administration; however, a small number of patients require every 48-hour administration.

Dose conversion guidelines for transdermal fentanyl [1] (see tables).

Recommended Initial Duragesic® Dose Based Upon Daily Oral Morphine Dose[1]

Oral 24-Hour Morphine (mg/d)	Duragesic® Dose (mcg/h)
60-134[2]	25
135-224	50
225-314	75
315-404	100
405-494	125
495-584	150
585-674	175
675-764	200
765-854	225
855-944	250
945-1034	275
1035-1124	300

[1]The table should NOT be used to convert from transdermal fentanyl (eg, Duragesic®) to other opioid analgesics. Rather, following removal of the patch, titrate the dose of the new opioid until adequate analgesia is achieved.

[2]Pediatric patients initiating therapy on a 25 mcg/hour Duragesic® system should be opioid-tolerant and receiving at least 60 mg oral morphine equivalents per day.

Dosing Conversion Guidelines[1,2]

Current Analgesic	Daily Dosage (mg/day)			
Morphine (I.M./I.V.)	10-22	23-37	38-52	53-67
Oxycodone (oral)	30-67	67.5-112	112.5-157	157.5-202
Oxycodone (I.M./I.V.)	15-33	33.1-56	56.1-78	78.1-101
Codeine (oral)	150-447	448-747	748-1047	1048-1347
Hydromorphone (oral)	8-17	17.1-28	28.1-39	39.1-51
Hydromorphone (I.V.)	1.5-3.4	3.5-5.6	5.7-7.9	8-10
Meperidine (I.M.)	75-165	166-278	279-390	391-503
Methadone (oral)	20-44	45-74	75-104	105-134
Methadone (I.M.)	10-22	23-37	38-52	53-67
Fentanyl transdermal recommended dose (mcg/h)	**25 mcg/h**	**50 mcg/h**	**75 mcg/h**	**100 mcg/h**

[1]The table should NOT be used to convert from transdermal fentanyl (eg, Duragesic®) to other opioid analgesics. Rather, following removal of the patch, titrate the dose of the new opioid until adequate analgesia is achieved.

[2] Duragesic® product insert, Janssen Pharmaceutica, Feb 2005.

Opioid Analgesics Initial Oral Dosing Commonly Used for Severe Pain

Drug	Equianalgesic Dose (mg)		Initial Oral Dose	
	Oral[1]	Parenteral[2]	Children (mg/kg)	Adults (mg)
Buprenorphine	—	0.4	—	—
Butorphanol	—	2	—	—
Hydromorphone	7.5	1.5	0.06	4-8
Levorphanol	4 (acute) 1 (chronic)	2 (acute) 1 (chronic)	0.04	2-4
Meperidine	300	75	Not Recommended	
Methadone	10	5	0.2	0.2
Morphine	30	10	0.3	15-30
Nalbuphine	—	10	—	—
Pentazocine	50	30	—	—
Oxycodone	20	—	0.3	10-20
Oxymorphone	1	—	—	—

From "Principles of Analgesic Use in the Treatment of Acute Pain and Cancer Pain," *Am Pain Soc*, Fifth Ed.

[1]Elderly: Starting dose should be lower for this population group

[2]Standard parenteral doses for acute pain in adults; can be used to doses for I.V. infusions and repeated small I.V. boluses. Single I.V. boluses, use half the I.M. dose. Children >6 months: I.V. dose = parenteral equianalgesic dose x weight (kg)/100

Dosing adjustment in hepatic impairment: Actiq®: Although fentanyl kinetics may be altered in hepatic disease, Actiq® can be used successfully in the management of breakthrough cancer pain. Doses should be titrated to reach clinical effect with careful monitoring of patients with severe hepatic disease.

(Continued)

Fentanyl *(Continued)*

Stability

Injection formulation: Store at controlled room temperature of 15°C to 25°C (59°F to 86°F); protect from light

Ionophoretic transdermal system: Store at 15°C to 30°C (59°F to 86°F)

Transdermal patch: Do not store above 25°C (77°F)

Transmucosal: Store at controlled room temperature of 15°C to 30°C (59°F to 86°F)

Administration

I.V.: Muscular rigidity may occur with rapid I.V. administration.

Transdermal patch (eg, Duragesic®): Apply to nonirritated and nonirradiated skin, such as chest, back, flank, or upper arm. Do not shave skin; hair at application site should be clipped. Prior to application, clean site with clear water and allow to dry completely. Do not use damaged or cut patches; a rapid release of fentanyl and increased systemic absorption may occur. Firmly press in place and hold for 30 seconds. Change patch every 72 hours. Do **not** use soap, alcohol, or other solvents to remove transdermal gel if it accidentally touches skin; use copious amounts of water. Avoid exposing application site to external heat sources (eg, heating pad, electric blanket, heat lamp, hot tub).

Iontophoretic transdermal system: System should be tested and applied by healthcare professional. The sticker on the back of the pouch is intended for use by the registered nurse. The sticker should be removed and applied to the Ionsys™ system with a date and time of application so that subsequent health-care providers will know when the system expires (24 hours after application). Apply to intact, nonirritated, nonirradiated skin on chest or upper outer arm. Do not apply scarred, burned, or tattooed areas. Any excessive hair at application site should be clipped; do not shave. Remove clear, plastic release liner before placement on skin. Avoid pulling on red tab. To administer a dose, the patient must press the button twice firmly within 3 seconds. An audible tone (beep) indicates the start of the delivery of the dose; red light remains on throughout the 10-minute dosing period. Each system operates for 24 hours or until 80 doses have been used (whichever comes first). Rotate skin site if another system is required after the first one is finished. If the hydrogel (where fentanyl is housed) becomes separated from the delivery system during removal, use gloves or tweezers to remove the hydrogel from skin. Do not use soap, alcohol, or other solvents to remove the hydrogel as they can increase absorption of fentanyl. Apply to intact, nonirritated, nonirradiated skin on chest or upper outer arm. Once a system has been removed, the same system can not be reapplied.

Transmucosal: Foil overwrap should be removed just prior to administration. Place the unit in mouth and allow it to dissolve. Do **not** chew. Actiq® units may be moved from one side of the mouth to the other. The unit should be consumed over a period of 15 minutes. Unit should be removed after it is consumed or if patient has achieved an adequate response and/or shows signs of respiratory depression. For patients who have received transmucosal product within 6-12 hours, it is recommended that if other narcotics are required, they should be used at starting doses $1/4$ to $1/3$ those usually recommended.

Monitoring Parameters Respiratory and cardiovascular status, blood pressure, heart rate; signs of misuse, abuse, or addiction

Transdermal patch: Monitor for 24 hours after application of first dose

Anesthesia and Critical Care Concerns/Other Considerations When developing a therapeutic plan for pain control, scheduled, intermittent opioid dosing or continuous infusion is preferred over the "as needed" regimen. The 2002 ACCM/SCCM guidelines for analgesia (critically-ill adult) recommend fentanyl in patients who need immediate pain relief because of its rapid onset of action. Repeated doses or a continuous infusion of fentanyl may cause accumulation. Fentanyl or hydromorphone is preferred in patients who are hypotensive or have renal dysfunction. Morphine or hydromorphone is recommended for intermittent, scheduled therapy. Both have a longer duration of action requiring less frequent administration. Fentanyl is great to prevent pain during a procedure and can be dosed intermittently for such an application. Prolonged analgesia requires an infusion.

Fentanyl is 50-100 times as potent as morphine; morphine 10 mg I.M. is equivalent to fentanyl 0.1-0.2 mg I.M.; fentanyl has less hypotensive effects than morphine due to lack of histamine release. However, fentanyl may cause rigidity with high doses. If the patient has required high-dose analgesia or has used for a prolonged period (~7 days), taper dose to prevent withdrawal; monitor for signs and symptoms of withdrawal.

Pregnancy Risk Factor C/D (prolonged use or high doses at term)

Contraindications Hypersensitivity to fentanyl or any component of the formulation; increased intracranial pressure; severe respiratory disease or depression including acute asthma (unless patient is mechanically ventilated); paralytic ileus; severe liver or renal insufficiency; pregnancy (prolonged use or high doses near term)

Iontophoretic transdermal system (Ionsys™): Hypersensitivity to fentanyl, cetylpyridinium chloride (eg, Cepacol®) or any component of Ionsys™ system

Transmucosal lozenges (Actiq®) or transdermal patches (eg, Duragesic®) must not be used in patients who are not opioid tolerant. Patients are considered opioid-tolerant if they are taking at least 60 mg morphine/day, 30 mg oral oxycodone/day, 8 mg oral hydromorphone/day, 25 mcg transdermal fentanyl/hour, or an equivalent dose of another opioid for ≥1 week. Transdermal patches are not for use in acute pain, mild pain, intermittent pain, or postoperative pain management.

Warnings/Precautions An opioid-containing analgesic regimen should be tailored to each patient's needs and based upon the type of pain being treated (acute versus chronic), the route of administration, degree of tolerance for opioids (naive versus chronic user), age, weight, and medical condition. The optimal analgesic dose varies widely among patients. Doses should be titrated to pain relief/prevention. When using with other CNS depressants, reduce dose of one or both agents. Fentanyl shares the toxic potentials of opiate agonists, and precautions of opiate agonist therapy should be observed; use with caution in patients with bradycardia; rapid I.V. infusion may result in skeletal muscle and chest wall rigidity leading to respiratory distress and/or apnea, bronchoconstriction, laryngospasm; inject slowly over 3-5 minutes. Tolerance or drug dependence may result from extended use. Use caution in patients with a history of drug dependence or abuse. The elderly may be particularly susceptible to the CNS depressant and constipating effects of narcotics. Use extreme caution in patients with COPD or other chronic respiratory conditions

Actiq®: **[U.S. Boxed Warning]: Should be used only for the care of cancer patients and is intended for use by specialists who are knowledgeable in treating cancer pain.** For patients who have received transmucosal product within 6-12 hours, it is recommended that if other narcotics are required, they should be used at starting doses 1/4 to 1/3 those usually recommended. **[U.S. Boxed Warning]:Actiq® preparations contain an amount of medication that can be fatal to children.** Keep all units out of the reach of children and discard any open units properly.. Patients and caregivers should be counseled on the dangers to children including the risk of exposure to partially-consumed units

Transdermal patches (eg, Duragesic®): **[U.S. Boxed Warning]: Serious or life-threatening hypoventilation may occur, even in opioid-tolerant patients.** Serum fentanyl concentrations may increase approximately one-third for patients with a body temperature of 40°C secondary to a temperature-dependent increase in fentanyl release from the patch and increased skin permeability. Avoid exposure of application site to direct external heat sources. Patients who experience adverse reactions should be monitored for at least 24 hours after removal of the patch. Transdermal patch does not contain any metal-based compounds; the printed ink used to indicate strength on the outer surface of the patch does contain titanium dioxide but the amount is minimal; adverse events have not been reported while wearing during an MRI. **[U.S. Boxed Warning]: Safety and efficacy of transdermal patch have been limited to children ≥2 years of age who are opioid tolerant.**

Iontophoretic transdermal system (Ionsys™): **[U.S. Boxed Warning]: Should only be used for the treatment of hospitalized patients. To avoid overdose, the patient should be the only one to activate the system. Unintended exposure to fentanyl hydrogel could lead to absorption of fatal dose; hydrogel should not come in contact with fingers or mouth.** Should be used only in patients who are able to understand and follow instructions to operate the system. The error detection circuit uses a series of audible signals to alert the patient when a dose is not being delivered; use caution in patients who have high frequency hearing impairment. Ionsys™ contains metal parts; remove prior to MRI procedure, cardioversion, or defibrillation. May interfere with radiographic image or CAT scan as system contains radiopaque components. Patients on chronic

(Continued)

Fentanyl *(Continued)*

opioids or with a history of opioid abuse may require higher analgesic doses than Ionsys™ is able to provide. Prior to patient's hospital discharge, the system must be removed and disposed of in accordance with State and Federal regulations for a C-II substance. **[U.S. Boxed Warning]: Even if all 80 doses are used, a significant amount of fentanyl remains in the iontophoretic transdermal system and requires proper removal and disposal to avoid misuse, abuse, or diversion.** Safety and efficacy of iontophoretic transdermal system have not been established in children <18 years of age.

Adverse Reactions

>10%:

Cardiovascular: Hypotension, bradycardia

Central nervous system: CNS depression, confusion, drowsiness, sedation

Gastrointestinal: Nausea, vomiting, constipation, xerostomia

Local: Application-site reaction (iontophoretic system 14%)

Neuromuscular & skeletal: Chest wall rigidity (high dose I.V.), weakness

Ocular: Miosis

Respiratory: Respiratory depression

Miscellaneous: Diaphoresis

1% to 10%:

Cardiovascular: Cardiac arrhythmia, edema, orthostatic hypotension, hypertension, syncope, tachycardia

Central nervous system: Abnormal dreams, abnormal thinking, agitation, amnesia, anxiety, dizziness, euphoria, fatigue, fever, hallucinations, headache, insomnia, nervousness, paranoid reaction

Dermatologic: Erythema, papules, pruritus (iontophoretic system 6%), rash

Gastrointestinal: Abdominal pain, anorexia, biliary tract spasm, diarrhea, dyspepsia, flatulence, ileus

Genitourinary: Urinary retention (iontophoretic transdermal system 3%)

Hematologic: Anemia

Neuromuscular & skeletal: Abnormal coordination, abnormal gait, back pain, paresthesia, rigors, tremor

Respiratory: Apnea, bronchitis, dyspnea, hemoptysis, hypoxia, pharyngitis, rhinitis, sinusitis, upper respiratory infection

Miscellaneous: Hiccups, flu-like syndrome, speech disorder

<1% (Limited to important or life-threatening): Amblyopia, anorgasmia, aphasia, bradycardia, bronchospasm, circulatory depression, CNS excitation or delirium, convulsions, dental caries (Actiq®), depersonalization, dysesthesia, ejaculatory difficulty, exfoliative dermatitis, gum line erosion (Actiq®), hyper-/hypotonia, laryngospasm, paradoxical dizziness, physical and psychological dependence with prolonged use, stertorous breathing, stupor, tachycardia, tooth loss (Actiq®), urinary tract spasm, urticaria, vertigo

Overdosage/Toxicology Symptoms of overdose include CNS depression, respiratory depression, and miosis; muscle and chest wall rigidity (may require nondepolarizing skeletal muscle relaxant). Treatment is supportive. If overdose from transdermal patch (eg, Duragesic®), remove system from patient's skin. Naloxone, 2 mg I.V. with repeat administration as necessary up to a total of 10 mg, can also be used to reverse toxic effects of the opiate. Patients who experience adverse reactions during use of transdermal patch (eg, Duragesic®) should be monitored for at least 24 hours after removal of the patch.

Drug Interactions Substrate of CYP3A4 (major); **Inhibits** CYP3A4 (weak)

Antipsychotic agents (phenothiazines): May enhance the hypotensive effect of analgesics (narcotic).

CNS depressants: Increased sedation with CNS depressants.;

CYP3A4 inhibitors: May increase the levels/effects of fentanyl. Potentially fatal respiratory depression may occur when a potent inhibitor is used in a patient receiving chronic fentanyl (eg, transdermal patch). Example inhibitors include azole antifungals, clarithromycin, diclofenac, doxycycline, erythromycin, imatinib, isoniazid, nefazodone, nicardipine, propofol, protease inhibitors, quinidine, telithromycin, and verapamil.

MAO inhibitors: Not recommended to use Actiq® within 14 days. Severe and unpredictable potentiation by MAO inhibitors has been reported with opioid analgesics.

Pegvisomant: Analgesics (narcotic) may diminish the therapeutic effect of pegvisomant.

Protease inhibitors: May decrease the metabolism, via CYP isoenzymes, of fentanyl.

Selective serotonin reuptake inhibitors (SSRIs): Analgesics (narcotic) may enhance the serotonergic effect of SSRIs. This may cause serotonin syndrome.

Sibutramine: Fentanyl may enhance the serotonergic effect of sibutramine.

Ethanol/Nutrition/Herb Interactions

Ethanol: Avoid ethanol (may increase CNS depression).

Food: Glucose may cause hyperglycemia.

Herb/Nutraceutical: St John's wort may decrease fentanyl levels. Avoid valerian, St John's wort, kava kava, gotu kola (may increase CNS depression).

Dietary Considerations Actiq® contains 2 g sugar per unit.

Dosage Forms

Infusion [premixed in NS]: 0.05 mg (10 mL); 1 mg (100 mL); 1.25 mg (250 mL); 2 mg (100 mL); 2.5 mg (250 mL)

Injection, solution, as citrate [preservative free]: 0.05 mg/mL (2 mL, 5 mL, 10 mL, 20 mL, 30 mL, 50 mL)

Sublimaze®: 0.05 mg/mL (2 mL, 5 mL, 10 mL, 20 mL)

Lozenge, oral transmucosal, as citrate:

Actiq®: 200 mcg, 400 mcg, 600 mcg, 800 mcg, 1200 mcg, 1600 mcg [mounted on a plastic radiopaque handle; raspberry flavor]

Transdermal patch: 25 mcg/hour [6.25 cm^2] (5s); 50 mcg/hour [12.5 cm^2] (5s); 75 mcg/hour [18.75 cm^2]; 100 mcg/hour [25 cm^2] (5s)

Duragesic®: 12 [delivers 12.5 mcg/hour; 5 cm^2; contains alcohol 0.1 mL/10 cm^2] (5s); 25 [delivers 25 mcg/hour; 10 cm^2; contains alcohol 0.1 mL/10 cm^2] (5s); 50 [delivers 50 mcg/hour; 20 cm^2; contains alcohol 0.1 mL/10 cm^2] (5s); 75 [delivers 75 mcg/hour; 30 cm^2; contains alcohol 0.1 mL/10 cm^2]; 100 [delivers 100 mcg/hour; 40 cm^2; contains alcohol 0.1 mL/10 cm^2] (5s)

Transdermal iontophoretic system:

Ionsys™: Fentanyl hydrochloride 40 mcg/dose [80 doses/patch; contains 3-volt lithium battery]

References

Bedforth NM and Lockey DJ, "Raynaud's Syndrome Following Intravenous Induction of Anaesthesia," *Anaesthesia*, 1995, 50(3):248-9.

Bennett MR and Adams AP, "Postoperative Respiratory Complications of Opiates," *Clin Anaesthesiol*, 1983, 1:41-56.

Carr DB, Jacox AK, Chapman RC, et al, "Acute Pain Management," Guideline Technical Report, No. 1. Rockville, MD: U.S. Department of Health and Human Services, Public Health Service, Agency for Health Care Policy and Research. AHCPR Publication No. 95-0034. February 1995.

Furuya H and Okumura F, "Hemolysis After Administration of High Dose Fentanyl," *Anesth Analg*, 1986, 65(2):207-8.

Jacobi J, Fraser GL, Coursin DB, et al, "Clinical Practice Guidelines for the Sustained Use of Sedatives and Analgesics in the Critically Ill Adult," *Crit Care Med*, 2002, 30(1):119-41. Available at: http://www.sccm.org/pdf/sedatives.pdf.

Katz R, Kelly HW, and Hsi A, "Prospective Study on the Occurrence of Withdrawal in Critically Ill Children Who Receive Fentanyl by Continuous Infusion," *Crit Care Med*, 1994, 22(5):763-7.

Mokhlesi B, Leikin JB, Murray P, et al, "Adult Toxicology in Critical Care. Part 11: Specific Poisonings," *Chest*, 2003, 123(3):897-922.

◆ **Fentanyl Citrate** *see* Fentanyl *on page 514*

◆ **Fentanyl Citrate Injection, USP (Can)** *see* Fentanyl *on page 514*

◆ **Fentanyl Hydrocholoride** *see* Fentanyl *on page 514*

◆ **Ferric (III) Hexacyanoferrate (II)** *see* Ferric Hexacyanoferrate *on page 521*

Ferric Hexacyanoferrate (FER ik hex a SYE an oh fer ate)

U.S. Brand Names Radiogardase™

Synonyms Ferric (III) Hexacyanoferrate (II); Insoluble Prussian Blue; Prussian Blue

Pharmacologic Category Antidote

Generic Available No

Use Treatment of known or suspected internal contamination with radioactive cesium and/or radioactive or nonradioactive thallium

Mechanism of Action Binds to cesium and thallium isotopes in the gastrointestinal tract following their ingestion or excretion in the bile; reduces their gastrointestinal reabsorption (enterohepatic circulation)

Pharmacodynamics/Kinetics

Absorption: Ferric hexacyanoferrate: Oral: None

(Continued)

Ferric Hexacyanoferrate *(Continued)*

Half-life elimination:

Cesium-137: Effective: Adults: 80 days, decreased by 69% with ferric hexacyanoferrate; adolescents: 62 days, decreased by 46% with ferric hexacyanoferrate; children: 42 days, decreased by 43% with ferric hexacyanoferrate

Nonradioactive thallium: Biological: 8-10 days; with ferric hexacyanoferrate: 3 days

Excretion:

Cesium-137: Without ferric hexacyanoferrate: Urine (~80%); feces (~20%)

Thallium: Without ferric hexacyanoferrate: Fecal to urine excretion ration: 2:1

Ferric hexacyanoferrate: Feces (99%, unchanged)

Dosage Oral: Internal contamination with radioactive cesium and/or radioactive or nonradioactive thallium:

Children 2-12 years: 1 g 3 times/day; treatment should begin as soon as possible following exposure, but is also effective if therapy is delayed

Children >12 years and Adults: 3 g 3 times/day; treatment should begin as soon as possible following exposure, but is also effective if therapy is delayed

Note: Cesium exposure: Once internal radioactivity is substantially decreased, dosage may be reduced to 1-2 g 3 times/day to improve gastrointestinal tolerance

Elderly: Refer to Adults dosing

Dosage adjustment in renal impairment: Studies have not been conducted; however, ferric hexacyanoferrate is not renally eliminated.

Dosage adjustment in hepatic impairment: Studies have not been conducted; however, effectiveness may be decreased due to decreased bile excretion of cesium and thallium.

Stability Store in the dark at controlled room temperature of 15°C to 30°C (59°F to 86°F).

Administration Capsules may be opened and mixed with bland food or liquid (instruct patients that mouth and teeth may become blue). Administer with food to stimulate excretion of cesium or thallium. Increase dietary fiber or take with fiber laxative to decrease constipation.

Monitoring Parameters

Bowel movements; CBC and electrolytes weekly

Baseline cesium and/or thallium exposure (whole body counting and/or bioassay, feces or urine sample); urine and fecal cesium and/or thallium weekly during therapy; residual whole body radioactivity after 30 days of treatment

Pregnancy Risk Factor C

Contraindications None known

Warnings/Precautions Ferric hexacyanoferrate increases the rate of elimination of thallium and cesium; it does not treat complications of radiation exposure. Supportive treatment for radiation toxicity should be given concomitantly. Use caution with decreased gastric motility; constipation should be avoided to prevent increased radiation absorption from the gastrointestinal tract. Use caution with pre-existing cardiac arrhythmias or electrolyte imbalances. Patients should be instructed to minimize radiation exposure to others. Additional decontamination and/or treatment may be needed if exposure to other radioactive isotopes is known or suspected.

Adverse Reactions

>10%: Gastrointestinal: Constipation (24%)

1% to 10%: Endocrine & metabolic: Hypokalemia (7%)

Frequency not defined: Gastrointestinal: Gastric distress, fecal discoloration (blue)

Overdosage/Toxicology Effects of overdose are not known. Severe constipation, GI obstruction,or severe electrolyte depletion may be expected.

Drug Interactions Specific drug interaction studies have not been conducted. May bind with medications.

Ethanol/Nutrition/Herb Interactions Food: May increase effectiveness by stimulating bile secretion and thereby increasing the amount of cesium or thallium available to bind with ferric hexacyanoferrate. May bind with essential nutrients.

Dietary Considerations Take with food to stimulate excretion of cesium or thallium. A high-fiber diet or fiber laxative is recommended to avoid constipation.

Dosage Forms Capsule: 0.5 g

♦ **FeverALL® [OTC]** *see* Acetaminophen *on page 26*

Fibrin Sealant Kit (FI brin SEEL ent kit)

U.S. Brand Names Crosseal™; Tisseel® VH
Canadian Brand Names Tisseel® VH
Synonyms FS
Pharmacologic Category Hemostatic Agent
Generic Available No
Use

Crosseal™: Adjunct to hemostasis in liver surgery

Tisseel® VH: Adjunct to hemostasis in cardiopulmonary bypass surgery and splenic injury (due to blunt or penetrating trauma to the abdomen) when the control of bleeding by conventional surgical techniques is ineffective or impractical; adjunctive sealant for closure of colostomies; hemostatic agent in heparinized patients undergoing cardiopulmonary bypass

Mechanism of Action Formation of a biodegradable adhesive is done by duplicating the last step of the coagulation cascade, the formation of fibrin from fibrinogen. Fibrinogen is the main component of the sealant solution. The solution also contains thrombin, which transforms fibrinogen from the sealer protein solution into fibrin, and fibrinolysis inhibitor (aprotinin), which prevents the premature degradation of fibrin. When mixed as directed, a viscous solution forms that sets into an elastic coagulum.

Pharmacodynamics/Kinetics Onset of action:

Crosseal™: Time to hemostasis: 5.3 minutes

Tisseel® VH: Time to hemostasis: 5 minutes (65% of patients); Final prepared sealant: 70% strength: ~10 minutes; Full strength: ~2 hours

Dosage Adjunct to hemostasis: Apply topically; actual dose is based on size of surface to be covered:

Crosseal™: Children and Adults: To cover a layer of 1 mm thickness:

Maximum area to be sealed: 20 cm^2
Required size of Crosseal™ kit: 1 mL
Maximum area to be sealed: 40 cm^2
Required size of Crosseal™ kit: 2 mL
Maximum area to be sealed: 100 cm^2
Required size of Crosseal™ kit: 5 mL
Note: If hemostatic effect is not complete, apply a second layer.

Tisseel® VH: Adults:

Maximum area to be sealed: 4 cm^2
Required size of Tisseel® VH kit: 0.5 mL
Maximum area to be sealed: 8 cm^2
Required size of Tisseel® VH kit: 1 mL
Maximum area to be sealed: 16 cm^2
Required size of Tisseel® VH kit: 2 mL
Maximum area to be sealed: 40 cm^2
Required size of Tisseel® VH kit: 5 mL

Apply in thin layers to avoid excess formation of granulation tissue and slow absorption of the sealant. Following application, hold the sealed parts in the desired position for 3-5 minutes. To prevent sealant from adhering to gloves or surgical instruments, wet them with saline prior to contact.

Stability

Crosseal™: Store frozen at or below -18°C; unopened vials may be stored at 2°C to 8°C (35°F to 46°F) for up to 30 days or up to 24 hours at room temperature. Store application device at room temperature. Vials should be thawed prior to use.

Tisseel® VH: Store at 2°C to 8°C (35°F to 46°F). Do not freeze. Solution may be prepared by reconstituting the freeze-dried sealer protein concentrate using the Fibrinotherm® (preferred method), a water bath, or an incubator. The thrombin solution is prepared separately. The two solutions are then transferred to the sterile field and applied to the affected area using the Duploject® syringe system. Application must be done within 4 hours of preparing the solution. Total reconstitution time may take up to 40 minutes.

To reconstitute the sealer protein: Fibrinotherm® method: The Fibrinotherm® is a combined heating and stirring device that can be obtained from the manufacturer. After removing the caps from the sealer concentrate and the fibrinolysis inhibitor solution, disinfect with a germicidal solution that does **not** contain iodine. Turn on the stirring switch of the Fibrinotherm® and insert

(Continued)

Fibrin Sealant Kit *(Continued)*

each vial into the appropriate openings. Turn on the heating switch. The vials will automatically preheat at 37°C for 10 minutes. Transfer the fibrinolysis inhibitor solution into the vial of sealer protein concentrate. Use the adapter to insert the vial into the largest opening of the Fibrinotherm®. Stir contents for 8-10 minutes. If total dissolution has not occurred within 20 minutes, discard and prepare a fresh kit. If not used promptly, keep the solution at 37°C. Stir again shortly before drawing up solution.

Preparation of thrombin solution: After removing the caps from the calcium chloride and thrombin vials, disinfect with a germicidal solution that does **not** contain iodine. Add the calcium chloride to the thrombin vial. Swirl briefly. Keep the prepared solution at 37°C until use.

Note: Prior to application, the sealer protein solution and the thrombin solution should be transferred to a sterile field. To do this, the scrub nurse should withdraw the solution into the provided syringes, while the circulating nurse holds the vials. Withdraw solutions slowly to reduce the possible formation of large air bubbles.

Preparation of the final solution: The two resulting solutions are then placed into the Duploject® system, comprised of two identical disposable syringes, provided in the kit. The syringes have a common plunger, which allows equal volumes of both solutions to be fed through a joining piece, mixed, and ejected through a common application needle. Both syringes should contain equal volumes of solution. Do not expel any air bubbles (may clog). If the application process is interrupted, immediately prior to resuming application, replace the needle with one of the 3 spare needles provided in the kit. Discard any remaining solution.

Administration

Crosseal™: Solution should be sprayed or dripped on the tissue to produce an even, thin layer. Application with provided device allows for the simultaneous application of both solutions.

Tisseel® VH: Apply in thin layers to avoid excess formation of granulation tissue and slow absorption of the sealant. Following application, hold the sealed parts in the desired position for 3-5 minutes. To prevent sealant from adhering to gloves or surgical instruments, wet them with saline prior to contact.

Pregnancy Risk Factor C

Contraindications Hypersensitivity to any component of the formulations in the kit; massive and brisk arterial bleeding

Crosseal™: Hypersensitivity to human blood products; not for use in surgical situations where contact with CSF or dura mater may occur

Tisseel® VH: Hypersensitivity to human blood products or bovine protein; aprotinin

Warnings/Precautions For topical use only; do not inject into a vessel or tissue. Components of the kit made from human plasma may potentially transmit disease. Any infection suspected of being transmitted by this product should be reported to the manufacturer.

Tisseel® VH: Do not apply to wound surface containing alcohol, iodine, or heavy-metal ions. Do not use with oxycellulose-containing preparations. Safety and efficacy in pediatric patients have not been established.

Adverse Reactions May be related to aprotinin contained in some products.

<1%: Hypersensitivity including anaphylactoid or anaphylactic reactions (0.5/100,000 exposures), hypotension

Drug Interactions

Alcohol, heavy-metal ions, iodine: May denature the sealer protein and thrombin solution in the Tisseel® VH kit; wound surface should be cleaned to remove these products prior to application of fibrin sealant

Oxycellulose preparations: Reduce efficacy of Tisseel®; do not use as a carrier

Dosage Forms Topical: Kit [each kit contains]:

Crosseal™: Fibrinogen 40-60 mg/mL [human; also contains tranexamic acid]; thrombin 800-1200 int. units/mL [human; also contains human albumin and mannitol]; spray application device (1 mL, 2 mL, 5 mL)

Tisseel® VH: Fibrinogen 75-115 mg/mL [sealer protein concentrate, human]; aprotinin 3000 KIU/mL [fibrinolysis inhibitor solution, bovine]; thrombin 500 int. units/mL [human]; calcium chloride solution 40 micromoles/mL (0.5 mL, 1 mL, 2 mL, 5 mL)

Filgrastim (fil GRA stim)

Medication Safety Issues

Sound-alike/look-alike issues:

Neupogen® may be confused with Epogen®, Neumega®, Nutramigen®

U.S. Brand Names Neupogen®

Canadian Brand Names Neupogen®

Synonyms G-CSF; Granulocyte Colony Stimulating Factor

Pharmacologic Category Colony Stimulating Factor

Generic Available No

Use Stimulation of granulocyte production in chemotherapy-induced neutropenia (nonmyeloid malignancies, acute myeloid leukemia, and bone marrow transplantation); severe chronic neutropenia (SCN); patients undergoing peripheral blood progenitor cell (PBPC) collection

Mechanism of Action Stimulates the production, maturation, and activation of neutrophils; filgrastim activates neutrophils to increase both their migration and cytotoxicity. See table.

Comparative Effects — Filgrastim vs Sargramostim

Proliferation/Differentiation	Filgrastim	Sargramostim
Neutrophils	Yes	Yes
Eosinophils	No	Yes
Macrophages	No	Yes
Neutrophil migration	Enhanced	Inhibited

Pharmacodynamics/Kinetics

Onset of action: ~24 hours; plateaus in 3-5 days

Duration: ANC decreases by 50% within 2 days after discontinuing filgrastim; white counts return to the normal range in 4-7 days; peak plasma levels can be maintained for up to 12 hours

Absorption: SubQ: 100%

Distribution: V_d: 150 mL/kg; no evidence of drug accumulation over a 11- to 20-day period

Metabolism: Systemically degraded

Half-life elimination: 1.8-3.5 hours

Time to peak, serum: SubQ: 2-6 hours

Dosage Refer to individual protocols.

Dosing, even in morbidly obese patients, should be based on actual body weight. Rounding doses to the nearest vial size often enhances patient convenience and reduces costs without compromising clinical response.

SubQ, I.V.:

Myelosuppressive therapy: 5 mcg/kg/day; doses may be increased by 5 mcg/kg according to the duration and severity of the neutropenia; continue for up to 14 days or until the ANC reaches 10,000/mm^3

Bone marrow transplantation: 10 mcg/kg/day; doses may be increased by 5 mcg/kg according to the duration and severity of neutropenia; recommended steps based on neutrophil response:

When ANC >1000/mm^3 for 3 consecutive days: Reduce filgrastim dose to 5 mcg/kg/day

If ANC remains >1000/mm^3 for 3 more consecutive days: Discontinue filgrastim

If ANC decreases to <1000/mm^3: Resume at 5 mcg/kg/day

If ANC decreases <1000/mm^3 during the 5 mcg/kg/day dose, increase filgrastim to 10 mcg/kg/day and follow the above steps

SubQ:

Peripheral blood progenitor cell (PBPC) collection: 10 mcg/kg/day **or** 5-8 mcg/kg twice daily in donors. Begin at least 4 days before the first leukopheresis and continue until the last leukopheresis; the optimal timing and duration of growth factor stimulation has not been determined.

Severe chronic neutropenia:

Congenital: 6 mcg/kg twice daily

Idiopathic/cyclic: 5 mcg/kg/day

Stability Intact vials and prefilled syringes should be stored under refrigeration at 2°C to 8°C (36°F to 46°F) and protected from direct sunlight. Filgrastim should be

(Continued)

Filgrastim *(Continued)*

protected from freezing and temperatures >30°C to avoid aggregation. If inadvertently frozen, thaw in a refrigerator and use within 24 hours; do not use if frozen >24 hours or frozen more than once. The solution should not be shaken since bubbles and/or foam may form. If foaming occurs, the solution should be left undisturbed for a few minutes until bubbles dissipate.

Filgrastim vials and prefilled syringes are stable for 7 days at 9°C to 30°C (47°F to 86°F), however, the manufacturer recommends discarding after 24 hours because of microbiological concerns. The product is packaged without a preservative.

Undiluted filgrastim is stable for 24 hours at 15°C to 30°C and for 2 weeks at 2°C to 8°C (36°F to 46°F) in tuberculin syringes. However, the manufacturer recommends to use immediately because of concern for bacterial contamination.

Do not dilute with saline at any time; product may precipitate. Filgrastim may be diluted in dextrose 5% in water to a concentration 5-15 mcg/mL for I.V. infusion administration (minimum concentration: 5 mcg/mL). This diluted solution is stable for 7 days at 2°C to 8°C (36°F to 46°F). Dilution to <5 mcg/mL is not recommended. Concentrations 5-15 mcg/mL require addition of albumin (final concentration of 2 mg/mL) to the bag to prevent absorption to plastics. Compatible with glass bottles, PVC and polyolefin I.V. bags, and polypropylene syringes when diluted in 5% dextrose or 5% dextrose with albumin.

Administration May be administered undiluted by SubQ injection. May also be administered by I.V. bolus over 15-30 minutes in D_5W, or by continuous SubQ or I.V. infusion. Do not administer earlier than 24 hours after or in the 24 hours prior to cytotoxic chemotherapy.

Monitoring Parameters CBC with differential prior to treatment and twice weekly during filgrastim treatment for chemotherapy-induced neutropenia (3 times a week following marrow transplantation). For severe chronic neutropenia, monitor CBC twice weekly during the first month of therapy and for 2 weeks following dose adjustments; monthly thereafter. Leukocytosis (white blood cell counts ≥100,000/mm^3) has been observed in ~2% of patients receiving filgrastim at doses >5 mcg/kg/day.

Reference Range No clinical benefit seen with ANC >10,000/mm^3

Anesthesia and Critical Care Concerns/Other Considerations

Reimbursement Hotline: 1-800-272-9376

Professional Services [AMGEN]: 1-800-77-AMGEN

Pregnancy Risk Factor C

Contraindications Hypersensitivity to filgrastim, *E. coli*-derived proteins, or any component of the formulation

Warnings/Precautions Do not use filgrastim in the period 24 hours before to 24 hours after administration of cytotoxic chemotherapy because of the potential sensitivity of rapidly dividing myeloid cells to cytotoxic chemotherapy. Precaution should be exercised in the usage of filgrastim in any malignancy with myeloid characteristics. Filgrastim can potentially act as a growth factor for any tumor type, particularly myeloid malignancies. Tumors of nonhematopoietic origin may have surface receptors for filgrastim. Safety and efficacy have not been established with patients receiving radiation therapy, or with chemotherapy associated with delayed myelosuppression (eg, nitrosoureas, mitomycin C).

Allergic-type reactions have occurred with first or later doses. Reactions tended to occur more frequently with intravenous administration and within 30 minutes of infusion. Rare cases of splenic rupture or adult respiratory distress syndrome have been reported in association with filgrastim; patients must be instructed to report left upper quadrant pain or shoulder tip pain or respiratory distress. Use caution in patients with sickle cell diseases; sickle cell crises have been reported following filgrastim therapy.

Adverse Reactions

>10%:

Central nervous system: Fever (12%)

Dermatologic: Petechiae (17%), rash (12%)

Gastrointestinal: Splenomegaly (≤33% of patients with cyclic neutropenia/congenital agranulocytosis receiving filgrastim for ≥14 days; rare in other patients)

Hepatic: Alkaline phosphatase increased (21%)

Neuromuscular & skeletal: Bone pain (22% to 33%), commonly in the lower back, posterior iliac crest, and sternum

Respiratory: Epistaxis (9% to 15%)

1% to 10%:

Cardiovascular: Hyper-/hypotension (4%), S-T segment depression (3%), myocardial infarction/arrhythmias (3%)

Central nervous system: Headache (7%)

Gastrointestinal: Nausea (10%), vomiting (7%), peritonitis (2%)

Hematologic: Leukocytosis (2%)

<1% (Limited to important or life-threatening): Adult respiratory distress syndrome, allergic reactions, alopecia, arthralgia, cutaneous vasculitis, dyspnea, edema (facial), erythema nodosum, hematuria, hepatomegaly, hypersensitivity reaction, injection-site reaction, pericarditis, proteinuria, psoriasis exacerbation, splenic rupture, tachycardia, transient supraventricular arrhythmia, thrombophlebitis, urticaria, wheezing

Overdosage/Toxicology No clinical adverse effects have been seen with high doses producing ANC >10,000/mm^3. Filgrastim discontinuation should result in a 50% decrease in circulating neutrophils within 1-2 days and a return to pretreatment levels in 1-7 days.

Dietary Considerations Injection solution contains sodium 0.035 mg/mL and sorbitol.

Dosage Forms

Injection, solution [preservative free]: 300 mcg/mL (1 mL, 1.6 mL) [vial; contains sodium 0.035 mg/mL and sorbitol]

Injection, solution [preservative free]: 600 mcg/mL (0.5 mL, 0.8 mL) [prefilled Singleject® syringe; contains sodium 0.035 mg/mL and sorbitol]

- **Fioricet® with Codeine** *see* Butalbital, Acetaminophen, Caffeine, and Codeine *on page 207*
- **FK506** *see* Tacrolimus *on page 1225*
- **Flagyl®** *see* Metronidazole *on page 842*
- **Flagyl ER®** *see* Metronidazole *on page 842*
- **Flagyl® I.V. RTU™** *see* Metronidazole *on page 842*
- **Flamazine® (Can)** *see* Silver Sulfadiazine *on page 1173*

Flecainide (fle KAY nide)

Medication Safety Issues

Sound-alike/look-alike issues:

Flecainide may be confused with fluconazole

Tambocor™ may be confused with tamoxifen

Related Information

Antiarrhythmic Drugs *on page 1548*

U.S. Brand Names Tambocor™

Canadian Brand Names Apo-Flecainide®; Tambocor™

Synonyms Flecainide Acetate

Pharmacologic Category Antiarrhythmic Agent, Class Ic

Generic Available Yes

Use Prevention and suppression of documented life-threatening ventricular arrhythmias (eg, sustained ventricular tachycardia); controlling symptomatic, disabling supraventricular tachycardias in patients without structural heart disease in whom other agents fail

Mechanism of Action Class Ic antiarrhythmic; slows conduction in cardiac tissue by altering transport of ions across cell membranes; causes slight prolongation of refractory periods; decreases the rate of rise of the action potential without affecting its duration; increases electrical stimulation threshold of ventricle, His-Purkinje system; possesses local anesthetic and moderate negative inotropic effects

Pharmacodynamics/Kinetics

Absorption: Oral: Rapid

Distribution: Adults: V_d: 5-13.4 L/kg

Protein binding: Alpha$_1$ glycoprotein: 40% to 50%

Metabolism: Hepatic

Bioavailability: 85% to 90%

(Continued)

Flecainide *(Continued)*

Half-life elimination: Infants: 11-12 hours; Children: 8 hours; Adults: 7-22 hours, increased with congestive heart failure or renal dysfunction; End-stage renal disease: 19-26 hours

Time to peak, serum: ~1.5-3 hours

Excretion: Urine (80% to 90%, 10% to 50% as unchanged drug and metabolites)

Dosage Oral:

Children:

Initial: 3 mg/kg/day or 50-100 mg/m²/day in 3 divided doses

Usual: 3-6 mg/kg/day or 100-150 mg/m²/day in 3 divided doses; up to 11 mg/kg/day or 200 mg/m²/day for uncontrolled patients with subtherapeutic levels

Adults:

Life-threatening ventricular arrhythmias:

Initial: 100 mg every 12 hours

Increase by 50-100 mg/day (given in 2 doses/day) every 4 days; maximum: 400 mg/day.

Use of higher initial doses and more rapid dosage adjustments have resulted in an increased incidence of proarrhythmic events and congestive heart failure, particularly during the first few days. Do not use a loading dose. Use very cautiously in patients with history of congestive heart failure or myocardial infarction.

Prevention of paroxysmal supraventricular arrhythmias in patients with disabling symptoms but no structural heart disease:

Initial: 50 mg every 12 hours

Increase by 50 mg twice daily at 4-day intervals; maximum: 300 mg/day.

Dosing adjustment in severe renal impairment: Cl_{cr} <35 mL/minute: Decrease initial dose to 50 mg every 12 hours; increase doses at intervals >4 days monitoring ECG levels closely.

Dialysis: Not dialyzable (0% to 5%) via hemo- or peritoneal dialysis; no supplemental dose necessary.

Dosing adjustment/comments in hepatic impairment: Monitoring of plasma levels is recommended because of significantly increased half-life.

When transferring from another antiarrhythmic agent, allow for 2-4 half-lives of the agent to pass before initiating flecainide therapy.

Administration Administer around-the-clock to promote less variation in peak and trough serum levels

Monitoring Parameters ECG, blood pressure, pulse, periodic serum concentrations, especially in patients with renal or hepatic impairment

Reference Range Therapeutic: 0.2-1 mcg/mL; pediatric patients may respond at the lower end of the recommended therapeutic range

Anesthesia and Critical Care Concerns/Other Considerations Based on adverse outcomes noted with flecainide in the CAST trial, the FDA recommends that use of flecainide be limited to patients with life-threatening ventricular arrhythmias.

Pregnancy Risk Factor C

Contraindications Hypersensitivity to flecainide or any component of the formulation; pre-existing second- or third-degree AV block or with right bundle branch block when associated with a left hemiblock (bifascicular block) (except in patients with a functioning artificial pacemaker); cardiogenic shock; coronary artery disease (based on CAST study results); concurrent use of ritonavir or amprenavir

Warnings/Precautions **[U.S. Boxed Warning]: In the Cardiac Arrhythmia Suppression Trial (CAST), recent (>6 days but <2 years ago) myocardial infarction patients with asymptomatic, nonlife-threatening ventricular arrhythmias did not benefit and may have been harmed by attempts to suppress the arrhythmia with flecainide or encainide. An increased mortality or nonfatal cardiac arrest rate (7.7%) was seen in the active treatment group compared with patients in the placebo group (3%). The applicability of the CAST results to other populations is unknown. The risks of class 1C agents and the lack of improved survival make use in patients without life-threatening arrhythmias generally unacceptable. Not recommended for patients with chronic atrial fibrillation; may have proarrhythmic effects. When treating atrial flutter, 1:1 atrioventricular conduction may occur; pre-emptive negative chronotropic therapy (eg, digoxin, beta-blockers) may lower the risk.** Pre-existing hypokalemia or hyperkalemia should be corrected before initiation (can alter drug's effect). A worsening or new arrhythmia may occur (proarrhythmic effect). Use caution in heart failure (may precipitate or exacerbate CHF). Dose-related increases in PR, QRS, and QT intervals occur. Use with caution in sick sinus syndrome or with permanent pacemakers or temporary pacing wires (can increase endocardial pacing thresholds). Cautious use in significant hepatic impairment.

Adverse Reactions

>10%:

Central nervous system: Dizziness (19% to 30%)

Ocular: Visual disturbances (16%)

Respiratory: Dyspnea (~10%)

1% to 10%:

Cardiovascular: Palpitations (6%), chest pain (5%), edema (3.5%), tachycardia (1% to 3%), proarrhythmic (4% to 12%), sinus node dysfunction (1.2%), syncope

Central nervous system: Headache (4% to 10%), fatigue (8%), nervousness (5%) additional symptoms occurring at a frequency between 1% and 3%: fever, malaise, hypoesthesia, paresis, ataxia, vertigo, somnolence, tinnitus, anxiety, insomnia, depression

Dermatologic: Rash (1% to 3%)

Gastrointestinal: Nausea (9%), constipation (1%), abdominal pain (3%), anorexia (1% to 3%), diarrhea (0.7% to 3%)

Neuromuscular & skeletal: Tremor (5%), weakness (5%), paresthesia (1%)

Ocular: Diplopia (1% to 3%), blurred vision

<1% (Limited to important or life-threatening): Alopecia, alters pacing threshold, amnesia, angina, AV block, bradycardia, bronchospasm, CHF, corneal deposits, depersonalization, euphoria, exfoliative dermatitis, granulocytopenia, heart block, increased P-R, leukopenia, metallic taste, neuropathy, paradoxical increase in ventricular rate in atrial fibrillation/flutter, paresthesia, photophobia, pneumonitis, pruritus, QRS duration, swollen lips/tongue/mouth, tardive dyskinesia, thrombocytopenia, urinary retention, urticaria, ventricular arrhythmia

Overdosage/Toxicology Flecainide has a narrow therapeutic index and severe toxicity may occur slightly above the therapeutic range, especially if combined with other antiarrhythmic drugs. (Acute single ingestion of twice the daily therapeutic dose is life-threatening). Symptoms of overdose include increase in P-R, QRS, or QT intervals and amplitude of the T wave, AV block, bradycardia, hypotension, ventricular arrhythmias (monomorphic or polymorphic ventricular tachycardia), and asystole. Other symptoms include dizziness, blurred vision, headache, and GI upset. Treatment is supportive.

Drug Interactions **Substrate** of CYP1A2 (minor), 2D6 (major); **Inhibits** CYP2D6 (weak)

Amiodarone increases in flecainide plasma levels; consider reducing flecainide dose by 25% to 33% with concurrent use.

Amprenavir and ritonavir may increase cardiotoxicity of flecainide (decrease metabolism).

Cimetidine may decrease flecainide's metabolism; monitor cardiac status or use an alternative H_2 antagonist.

CYP2D6 inhibitors: May increase the levels/effects of flecainide. Example inhibitors include chlorpromazine, delavirdine, fluoxetine, miconazole, paroxetine, pergolide, quinidine, quinine, ritonavir, and ropinirole.

Digoxin's serum concentration may increase slightly.

Propranolol (and possibly other beta-blockers) increases flecainide blood levels, and propranolol blood levels are increased with concurrent use; monitor for excessive negative inotropic effects.

Quinidine may decrease flecainide's metabolism; monitor cardiac status.

Urinary alkalinizers (antacids, sodium bicarbonate, acetazolamide) may increase flecainide blood levels.

Ethanol/Nutrition/Herb Interactions Food: Clearance may be decreased in patients following strict vegetarian diets due to urinary pH ≥8. Dairy products (milk, infant formula, yogurt) may interfere with the absorption of flecainide in infants; there is one case report of a neonate (GA 34 weeks PNA >6 days) who required extremely large doses of oral flecainide when administered every 8 hours with feedings ("milk feeds"); changing the feedings from "milk feeds" to 5% glucose feeds alone resulted in a doubling of the flecainide serum concentration and toxicity.

Dosage Forms Tablet, as acetate: 50 mg, 100 mg, 150 mg

♦ **Flecainide Acetate** *see* Flecainide *on page 527*

- **Fleet® Accu-Prep® [OTC]** *see* Sodium Phosphates *on page 1189*
- **Fleet® Enema [OTC]** *see* Sodium Phosphates *on page 1189*
- **Fleet® Phospho-Soda® [OTC]** *see* Sodium Phosphates *on page 1189*
- **Fleet® Phospho-Soda® Oral Laxative (Can)** *see* Sodium Phosphates *on page 1189*
- **Flexbumin** *see* Albumin *on page 48*
- **Flolan®** *see* Epoprostenol *on page 467*
- **Flomax®** *see* Tamsulosin *on page 1233*
- **Flomax® CR (Can)** *see* Tamsulosin *on page 1233*
- **Florazole® ER (Can)** *see* Metronidazole *on page 842*
- **Florinef®** *see* Fludrocortisone *on page 533*
- **Floxin®** *see* Ofloxacin *on page 950*
- **Floxin Otic Singles** *see* Ofloxacin *on page 950*
- **Flubenisolone** *see* Betamethasone *on page 169*

Fluconazole (floo KOE na zole)

Medication Safety Issues

Sound-alike/look-alike issues:

Fluconazole may be confused with flecainide

Diflucan® may be confused with diclofenac, Diprivan®, disulfiram

Related Information

Antifungal Agents *on page 1554*

U.S. Brand Names Diflucan®

Canadian Brand Names Apo-Fluconazole®; Diflucan®; Fluconazole Injection; Fluconazole Omega; Gen-Fluconazole; GMD-Fluconazole; Novo-Fluconazole; Riva-Fluconazole

Pharmacologic Category Antifungal Agent, Oral; Antifungal Agent, Parenteral

Generic Available Yes

Use Treatment of candidiasis (vaginal, oropharyngeal, esophageal, urinary tract infections, peritonitis, pneumonia, and systemic infections); cryptococcal meningitis; antifungal prophylaxis in allogeneic bone marrow transplant recipients

Mechanism of Action Interferes with cytochrome P450 activity, decreasing ergosterol synthesis (principal sterol in fungal cell membrane) and inhibiting cell membrane formation

Pharmacodynamics/Kinetics

Distribution: Widely throughout body with good penetration into CSF, eye, peritoneal fluid, sputum, skin, and urine

Relative diffusion blood into CSF: Adequate with or without inflammation (exceeds usual MICs)

CSF:blood level ratio: Normal meninges: 70% to 80%; Inflamed meninges: >70% to 80%

Protein binding, plasma: 11% to 12%

Bioavailability: Oral: >90%

Half-life elimination: Normal renal function: ~30 hours

Time to peak, serum: Oral: 1-2 hours

Excretion: Urine (80% as unchanged drug)

Dosage The daily dose of fluconazole is the same for oral and I.V. administration

Usual dosage ranges:

Neonates: First 2 weeks of life, especially premature neonates: Same dose as older children every 72 hours

Children: Loading dose: 6-12 mg/kg; maintenance: 3-12 mg/kg/day; duration and dosage depends on severity of infection

Adults: 200-400 mg/day; duration and dosage depends on severity of infection

Indication-specific dosing:

Children:

Candidiasis:

Oropharyngeal: Loading dose: 6 mg/kg; maintenance: 3 mg/kg/day for 2 weeks

Esophageal: Loading dose: 6 mg/kg; maintenance: 3-12 mg/kg/day for 21 days and at least 2 weeks following resolution of symptoms

Systemic infection: 6 mg/kg every 12 hours for 28 days

Meningitis, cryptococcal: Loading dose: 12 mg/kg; maintenance: 6-12 mg/kg/day for 10-12 weeks following negative CSF culture; relapse suppression: 6 mg/kg/day

Adults:

Candidiasis:

Candidemia, primary therapy, non-neutropenic: 400-800 mg/day for 14 days after last positive blood culture and resolution of signs/symptoms

Alternate therapy: 800 mg/day with amphotericin B for 4-7 days followed by 800 mg/day for 14 days after last positive blood culture and resolution of signs/symptoms

Candidemia, secondary, neutropenic: 6-12 mg/kg/day for 14 days after last positive blood culture and resolution of signs/symptoms

Chronic, disseminated: 6 mg/kg/day for 3-6 months

Oropharyngeal (long-term suppression): 200 mg/day; chronic therapy is recommended in immunocompromised patients with history of oropharyngeal candidiasis (OPC)

Osteomyelitis: 6 mg/kg/day for 6-12 months

Esophageal: 200 mg on day 1, then 100-200 mg/day for 2-3 weeks after clinical improvement

Prophylaxis in bone marrow transplant: 400 mg/day; begin 3 days before onset of neutropenia and continue for 7 days after neutrophils >1000 cells/mm^3

Urinary: 200 mg/day for 1-2 weeks

Vaginal: 150 mg as a single dose

Coccidiomycosis: 400 mg/day; doses of 800-1000 mg/day have been used for meningeal disease; usual duration of therapy ranges from 3-6 months for primary uncomplicated infections and up to 1 year for pulmonary (chronic and diffuse) infection

Endocarditis, prosthetic valve, early: 6-12 mg/kg/day for 6 weeks after valve replacement

Endophthalmitis: 6-12 mg/kg/day or 400-800 mg/day for 6-12 weeks after surgical intervention. **Note:** *C. krusei* and *C. galbrata* infection acquired exogenously should be treated with voriconazole.

Meningitis, cryptococcal: 400-800 mg/day for 10-12 weeks or with flucytosine 100-150 mg/day for 6 weeks; maintenance: 200-400 mg/day

Pneumonia, cryptococcal (mild-to-moderate): 200-400 mg/day for 6-12 months (life-long in HIV-positive patients)

Dosing adjustment/interval in renal impairment:

No adjustment for vaginal candidiasis single-dose therapy

For multiple dosing, administer usual load then adjust daily doses

Cl_{cr} ≤50 mL/minute (no dialysis): Administer 50% of recommended dose or administer every 48 hours.

Hemodialysis: 50% is removed by hemodialysis; administer 100% of daily dose (according to indication) after each dialysis treatment.

Continuous arteriovenous or venovenous hemofiltration: Dose as for Cl_{cr} 10-50 mL/minute.

Stability

Powder for oral suspension: Store dry powder at ≤30°C (86°F). Following reconstitution, store at 5°C to 30°C (41°F to 86°F). Discard unused portion after 2 weeks. Do not freeze.

Injection: Store injection in glass at 5°C to 30°C (41°F to 86°F). Store injection in Viaflex® at 5°C to 25°C (41°F to 77°F). Protect from freezing. Do not unwrap unit until ready for use.

Administration I.V.: Infuse over approximately 1-2 hours; do not exceed 200 mg/hour

Oral: May be administred with or without food

Monitoring Parameters Periodic liver function tests (AST, ALT, alkaline phosphatase) and renal function tests, potassium

Anesthesia and Critical Care Concerns/Other Considerations Do not use if cloudy or precipitated. If administered by I.V. infusion, give over 1-2 hours.

Pregnancy Risk Factor C

Contraindications Hypersensitivity to fluconazole, other azoles, or any component of the formulation; concomitant administration with cisapride

Warnings/Precautions Should be used with caution in patients with renal and hepatic dysfunction or previous hepatotoxicity from other azole derivatives. Patients who develop abnormal liver function tests during fluconazole therapy

(Continued)

Fluconazole *(Continued)*

should be monitored closely and discontinued if symptoms consistent with liver disease develop. Use caution in patients at risk of proarrhythmias.

Adverse Reactions Frequency not always defined.

Cardiovascular: Angioedema, pallor, QT prolongation, torsade de pointes

Central nervous system: Headache (2% to 13%), seizure, dizziness

Dermatologic: Rash (2%), alopecia, toxic epidermal necrolysis, Stevens-Johnson syndrome

Endocrine & metabolic: Hypercholesterolemia, hypertriglyceridemia, hypokalemia

Gastrointestinal: Nausea (4% to 7%), vomiting (2%), abdominal pain (2% to 6%), diarrhea (2% to 3%), taste perversion, dyspepsia

Hematologic: Agranulocytosis, leukopenia, neutropenia, thrombocytopenia

Hepatic: Hepatic failure (rare), hepatitis, cholestasis, jaundice, increased ALT/AST, increased alkaline phosphatase

Respiratory: Dyspnea

Miscellaneous: Anaphylactic reactions (rare)

Overdosage/Toxicology Symptoms of overdose include decreased lacrimation, salivation, respiration and motility, urinary incontinence, and cyanosis. Treatment includes supportive measures. A 3-hour hemodialysis will remove 50%.

Drug Interactions Inhibits CYP1A2 (weak), 2C9 (strong), 2C19 (strong), 3A4 (moderate)

Benzodiazepines (metabolized by oxidation, eg, alprazolam, triazolam, midazolam, diazepam) serum concentrations are increased by fluconazole which may cause increased CNS sedation. Consider a benzodiazepine not metabolized by CYP3A4 or another antifungal.

Caffeine's metabolism is decreased; monitor for tachycardia, nervousness, and anxiety.

Calcium channel blockers may have increased serum concentrations; consider another agent instead of a calcium channel blocker, another antifungal, or reduce the dose of the calcium channel blocker. Monitor blood pressure.

Cisapride's serum concentration is increased which may lead to malignant arrhythmias; concurrent use is contraindicated.

Cyclosporine's serum concentration is increased; monitor cyclosporine's serum concentration and renal function.

CYP2C9 Substrates: Fluconazole may increase the levels/effects of CYP2C9 substrates. Example substrates include bosentan, dapsone, fluoxetine, glimepiride, glipizide, losartan, montelukast, nateglinide, paclitaxel, phenytoin, warfarin, and zafirlukast.

CYP2C19 substrates: Fluconazole may increase the levels/effects of CYP2C19 substrates. Example substrates include citalopram, diazepam, methsuximide, phenytoin, propranolol, and sertraline.

CYP3A4 substrates: Fluconazole may increase the levels/effects of CYP3A4 substrates. Example substrates include benzodiazepines, calcium channel blockers, cyclosporine, mirtazapine, nateglinide, nefazodone, sildenafil (and other PDE-5 inhibitors), tacrolimus, and venlafaxine. Selected benzodiazepines (midazolam and triazolam), cisapride, ergot alkaloids, selected HMG-CoA reductase inhibitors (lovastatin and simvastatin), and pimozide are generally contraindicated with strong CYP3A4 inhibitors.

HMG-CoA reductase inhibitors (except pravastatin and fluvastatin) have increased serum concentrations; switch to pravastatin/fluvastatin or monitor for development of myopathy.

Losartan's active metabolite is reduced in concentration; consider another antihypertensive agent unaffected by the azole antifungals, another antifungal, or monitor blood pressure closely.

Phenytoin's serum concentration is increased; monitor phenytoin levels and adjust dose as needed.

Rifampin decreases fluconazole's serum concentration; monitor infection status.

Tacrolimus's serum concentration is increased; monitor tacrolimus's serum concentration and renal function.

Warfarin's effects are increased; monitor INR and adjust warfarin's dose as needed.

Dietary Considerations Take with or without regard to food.

Dosage Forms

Infusion [premixed in sodium chloride]: 2 mg/mL (100 mL, 200 mL)

Diflucan® [premixed in sodium chloride or dextrose] 2 mg/mL (100 mL, 200 mL)

Powder for oral suspension (Diflucan®): 10 mg/mL (35 mL); 40 mg/mL (35 mL) [contains sodium benzoate; orange flavor]

Tablet (Diflucan®): 50 mg, 100 mg, 150 mg, 200 mg

References

Pappas PG, Rex JH, Sobel JD, et al, "Guidelines for Treatment of Candidiasis," *Clin Infect Dis*, 2004, 38(2):161-89.

Peltz RK, Hendrix CW, Swoboda SM, et al, "Double-Blind Placebo-Controlled Trial of Fluconazole to Prevent Candidal Infections in Critically Ill Surgical Patients," *Ann Surg*, 2001, 233(4):542-8.

Rex JH, Walsh TJ, Sobel JD, et al, "Practice Guidelines for the Treatment of Candidiasis," *Clin Infect Dis*, 2000, 30(4):662-78.

Valtonen M, Tiula E, and Neuvonen PJ, "Effect of Continuous Veno-Venous Haemofiltration and Haemodiafiltration on the Elimination of Fluconazole in Patients With Acute Renal Failure," *J Antimicrob Chemother*, 1997, 40(5):695-700.

♦ **Fluconazole Injection (Can)** *see* Fluconazole *on page 530*

♦ **Fluconazole Omega (Can)** *see* Fluconazole *on page 530*

Fludrocortisone (floo droe KOR ti sone)

Medication Safety Issues

Sound-alike/look-alike issues:

Florinef® may be confused with Fiorinal®

Related Information

Corticosteroids *on page 1561*

U.S. Brand Names Florinef®

Canadian Brand Names Florinef®

Synonyms 9α-Fluorohydrocortisone Acetate; Fludrocortisone Acetate; Fluohydrisone Acetate; Fluohydrocortisone Acetate

Pharmacologic Category Corticosteroid, Systemic

Generic Available Yes

Use Partial replacement therapy for primary and secondary adrenocortical insufficiency in Addison's disease; treatment of salt-losing adrenogenital syndrome

Mechanism of Action Promotes increased reabsorption of sodium and loss of potassium from renal distal tubules

Pharmacodynamics/Kinetics

Absorption: Rapid and complete

Protein binding: 42%

Metabolism: Hepatic

Half-life elimination, plasma: 30-35 minutes; Biological: 18-36 hours

Time to peak, serum: ~1.7 hours

Dosage Oral:

Infants and Children: 0.05-0.1 mg/day

Adults: 0.1-0.2 mg/day with ranges of 0.1 mg 3 times/week to 0.2 mg/day

Addison's disease: Initial: 0.1 mg/day; if transient hypertension develops, reduce the dose to 0.05 mg/day. Preferred administration with cortisone (10-37.5 mg/day) or hydrocortisone (10-30 mg/day).

Salt-losing adrenogenital syndrome: 0.1-0.2 mg/day

Administration Administration in conjunction with a glucocorticoid is preferable

Monitoring Parameters Monitor blood pressure and signs of edema when patient is on chronic therapy; very potent mineralocorticoid with high glucocorticoid activity; monitor serum electrolytes, serum renin activity, and blood pressure; monitor for evidence of infection; stop treatment if a significant increase in weight or blood pressure, edema, or cardiac enlargement occurs

Anesthesia and Critical Care Concerns/Other Considerations In patients with salt-losing forms of congenital adrenogenital syndrome, use along with cortisone or hydrocortisone. Fludrocortisone 0.1 mg has sodium retention activity equal to DOCA® 1 mg.

Adrenal Insufficiency: Patients on long-term steroid supplementation will require higher corticosteroid doses when subject to stress (ie, trauma, surgery, severe infection). This agent has significant mineralocorticoid activity with consequent hemodynamic effects. Fludrocortisone has been used to treat severe orthostatic hypotension. Abrupt withdrawal may result in adrenal insufficiency with hypotension and hyperkalemia. A recent randomized, double-blind, placebo controlled trial assessed whether low dose corticosteroid administration could improve 28-day survival in patients with septic shock and acquired adrenal insufficiency. A lack of adrenal reserves is defined by an increase in serum cortisol of ≤9 mcg/dL in response to corticotropin administration. Cortisol levels were drawn immediately before corticotropin administration and 30 to 60 minutes afterwards.

(Continued)

Fludrocortisone *(Continued)*

Three hundred adult septic shock patients requiring mechanical ventilation and vasopressor support were randomized to either hydrocortisone (50 mg IVP every 6 hours) and fludrocortisone (50 mcg tablet daily via nasogastric tube) or matching placebos for 7 days. Patients included had severe sepsis requiring vasopressor support and mechanical ventilation. In patients who did not appropriately respond to corticotropin (nonresponders), there were significantly fewer deaths in the active treatment group. Vasopressor therapy was withdrawn more frequently in this subset of the active treatment group. Adverse events were similar in both groups. Patients who lack adrenal reserve and thus have acquired adrenal insufficiency during the stress of septic shock may benefit from physiologic steroid replacement. Further study is required to better characterize the patient populations who may benefit.

Pregnancy Risk Factor C

Contraindications Hypersensitivity to fludrocortisone or any component of the formulation; systemic fungal infections

Warnings/Precautions Taper dose gradually when therapy is discontinued; use with caution with Addison's disease, sodium retention and potassium loss

Adverse Reactions Frequency not defined.

Cardiovascular: Hypertension, edema, CHF

Central nervous system: Convulsions, headache, dizziness

Dermatologic: Acne, rash, bruising

Endocrine & metabolic: Hypokalemic alkalosis, suppression of growth, hyperglycemia, HPA suppression

Gastrointestinal: Peptic ulcer

Neuromuscular & skeletal: Muscle weakness

Ocular: Cataracts

Miscellaneous: Diaphoresis, anaphylaxis (generalized)

Overdosage/Toxicology Symptoms of overdose include hypertension, edema, hypokalemia, excessive weight gain. When consumed in excessive quantities, systemic hypercorticism and adrenal suppression may occur. In those cases, discontinuation of the corticosteroid should be done judiciously.

Drug Interactions Decreased effect:

Anticholinesterases effects are antagonized

Decreased corticosteroid effects by rifampin, barbiturates, and hydantoins

Decreased salicylate levels

Dietary Considerations Systemic use of mineralocorticoids/corticosteroids may require a diet with increased potassium, vitamins A, B_6, C, D, folate, calcium, zinc, and phosphorus, and decreased sodium. With fludrocortisone, a decrease in dietary sodium is often not required as the increased retention of sodium is usually the desired therapeutic effect.

Dosage Forms Tablet, as acetate: 0.1 mg

References

Abraham E and Evans T, "Corticosteroids and Septic Shock (editorial)," *JAMA*, 2002, 288(7):886-7.

Annane D, Sebille V, Charpentier C, et al, "Effect of Treatment With Low Doses of Hydrocortisone and Fludrocortisone on Mortality in Patients With Septic Shock," *JAMA*, 2002, 288(7):862-71.

Coursin DB and Wood KE, "Corticosteroid Supplementation for Adrenal Insufficiency," *JAMA*, 2002, 287(2):236-40.

Cooper MS and Stewart PM, "Corticosteroid Insufficiency in Acutely Ill Patients," *N Engl J Med*, 2003, 348(8):727-34.

Dellinger RP, Carlet JM, Masur H, et al, "Surviving Sepsis Campaign Guidelines for Management of Severe Sepsis and Septic Shock," *Crit Care Med*, 2004, 32(3):858-73.

Hotchkiss RS and Karl IE, "The Pathophysiology and Treatment of Sepsis," *N Engl J Med*, 2003, 348(2):138-50.

♦ **Fludrocortisone Acetate** *see* Fludrocortisone *on page 533*

Flumazenil (FLOO may ze nil)

Related Information

Anesthesia for Patients With Liver Disease *on page 1421*

U.S. Brand Names Romazicon®

Canadian Brand Names Anexate®; Flumazenil Injection; Flumazenil Injection, USP; Romazicon®

Pharmacologic Category Antidote

Generic Available Yes

Use Benzodiazepine antagonist; reverses sedative effects of benzodiazepines used in conscious sedation and general anesthesia; treatment of benzodiazepine overdose

Mechanism of Action Competitively inhibits the activity at the benzodiazepine recognition site on the GABA/benzodiazepine receptor complex. Flumazenil does not antagonize the CNS effect of drugs affecting GABA-ergic neurons by means other than the benzodiazepine receptor (ethanol, barbiturates, general anesthetics) and does not reverse the effects of opioids

Pharmacodynamics/Kinetics

Onset of action: 1-3 minutes; 80% response within 3 minutes

Peak effect: 6-10 minutes

Duration: Resedation: ~1 hour; duration related to dose given and benzodiazepine plasma concentrations; reversal effects of flumazenil may wear off before effects of benzodiazepine

Distribution: Initial V_d: 0.5 L/kg; V_{dss} 0.77-1.6 L/kg

Protein binding: 40% to 50%

Metabolism: Hepatic; dependent upon hepatic blood flow

Half-life elimination: Adults: Alpha: 7-15 minutes; Terminal: 41-79 minutes

Excretion: Feces; urine (0.2% as unchanged drug)

Dosage

Children and Adults: I.V.: See table.

Flumazenil

Pediatric Dosage (further studies needed) Pediatric dosage for **reversal of conscious sedation and general anesthesia:**	
Initial dose	0.01 mg/kg over 15 seconds (maximum: 0.2 mg)
Repeat doses (maximum: 4 doses)	0.005-0.01 mg/kg (maximum: 0.2 mg) repeated at 1-minute intervals
Maximum total cumulative dose	1 mg or 0.05 mg/kg (whichever is lower)
Adult Dosage Adult dosage for **reversal of conscious sedation and general anesthesia:**	
Initial dose	0.2 mg intravenously over 15 seconds
Repeat doses	If desired level of consciousness is not obtained, 0.2 mg may be repeated at 1-minute intervals.
Maximum total cumulative dose	1 mg (usual dose: 0.6-1 mg) **In the event of resedation:** Repeat doses may be given at 20-minute intervals with maximum of 1 mg/dose and 3 mg/hour.
Adult dosage for **suspected benzodiazepine overdose:**	
Initial dose	0.2 mg intravenously over 30 seconds; if the desired level of consciousness is not obtained, 0.3 mg can be given over 30 seconds
Repeat doses	0.5 mg over 30 seconds repeated at 1-minute intervals
Maximum total cumulative dose	3 mg (usual dose 1-3 mg) Patients with a partial response at 3 mg may require additional titration up to a total dose of 5 mg. If a patient has not responded 5 minutes after cumulative dose of 5 mg, the major cause of sedation is not likely due to benzodiazepines. **In the event of resedation:** May repeat doses at 20-minute intervals with maximum of 1 mg/dose and 3 mg/hour.

Resedation: Repeated doses may be given at 20-minute intervals as needed; repeat treatment doses of 1 mg (at a rate of 0.5 mg/minute) should be given at any time and no more than 3 mg should be given in any hour. After intoxication with high doses of benzodiazepines, the duration of a single dose of flumazenil is not expected to exceed 1 hour; if desired, the period of wakefulness may be prolonged with repeated low intravenous doses of flumazenil, or by an infusion of 0.1-0.4 mg/hour. Most patients with benzodiazepine overdose will respond to a cumulative dose of 1-3 mg and doses >3 mg do not reliably produce additional effects. Rarely, patients with a partial response at 3 mg may require additional titration up to a total dose of 5 mg. **If a patient has not responded 5 minutes after receiving a cumulative dose of 5 mg, the major cause of sedation is not likely to be due to benzodiazepines.**

Elderly: No differences in safety or efficacy have been reported. However, increased sensitivity may occur in some elderly patients.

(Continued)

Flumazenil *(Continued)*

Dosing in renal impairment: Not significantly affected by renal failure (Cl_{cr} <10 mL/minute) or hemodialysis beginning 1 hour after drug administration

Dosing in hepatic impairment: Initial dose of flumazenil used for initial reversal of benzodiazepine effects is not changed; however, subsequent doses in liver disease patients should be reduced in size or frequency

Stability Store at 15°C to 30°C (59°F to 86°F). For I.V. use only; **compatible** with D_5W, lactated Ringer's, or normal saline; once drawn up in the syringe or mixed with solution use within 24 hours; discard any unused solution after 24 hours

Administration I.V.: Administer in freely-running I.V. into large vein. Inject over 15 seconds for conscious sedation and general anesthesia and over 30 seconds for overdose.

Monitoring Parameters Monitor patients for return of sedation or respiratory depression

Anesthesia and Critical Care Concerns/Other Considerations Flumazenil does **not** antagonize the CNS effects of other GABA agonists (such as ethanol, barbiturates, or general anesthetics), nor does it reverse narcotics.

Pregnancy Risk Factor C

Contraindications Hypersensitivity to flumazenil, benzodiazepines, or any component of the formulation; patients given benzodiazepines for control of potentially life-threatening conditions (eg, control of intracranial pressure or status epilepticus); patients who are showing signs of serious cyclic-antidepressant overdosage

Warnings/Precautions **[U.S. Boxed Warning]: Benzodiazepine reversal may result in seizures in some patients.** Patients who may develop seizures include patients on benzodiazepines for long-term sedation, tricyclic antidepressant overdose patients, concurrent major sedative-hypnotic drug withdrawal, recent therapy with repeated doses of parenteral benzodiazepines, myoclonic jerking or seizure activity prior to flumazenil administration. Flumazenil does not reverse respiratory depression/hypoventilation or cardiac depression. Resedation occurs more frequently in patients where a large single dose or cumulative dose of a benzodiazepine is administered along with a neuromuscular blocking agent and multiple anesthetic agents. Flumazenil should be used with caution in the intensive care unit because of increased risk of unrecognized benzodiazepine dependence in such settings. Should not be used to diagnose benzodiazepine-induced sedation. Reverse neuromuscular blockade before considering use. Flumazenil does not antagonize the CNS effects of other GABA agonists (such as ethanol, barbiturates, or general anesthetics); nor does it reverse narcotics. Use with caution in patients with a history of panic disorder; may provoke panic attacks. Use caution in drug and ethanol-dependent patients; these patients may also be dependent on benzodiazepines. Not recommended for treatment of benzodiazepine dependence. Use with caution in head injury patients. Use caution in patients with mixed drug overdoses; toxic effects of other drugs taken may emerge once benzodiazepine effects are reversed. Flumazenil does not consistently reverse amnesia; patient may not recall verbal instructions after procedure. Use caution in severe hepatic dysfunction and in patients relying on a benzodiazepine for seizure control. Safety and efficacy have not been established in children >1 year of age.

Adverse Reactions

>10%: Gastrointestinal: Vomiting, nausea

1% to 10%:

- Cardiovascular: Palpitations
- Central nervous system: Headache, anxiety, nervousness, insomnia, abnormal crying, euphoria, depression, agitation, dizziness, emotional lability, ataxia, depersonalization, increased tears, dysphoria, paranoia, fatigue, vertigo
- Endocrine & metabolic: Hot flashes
- Gastrointestinal: Xerostomia
- Local: Pain at injection site
- Neuromuscular & skeletal: Tremor, weakness, paresthesia
- Ocular: Abnormal vision, blurred vision
- Respiratory: Dyspnea, hyperventilation
- Miscellaneous: Diaphoresis

<1% (Limited to important or life-threatening): Bradycardia, chest pain, confusion, fear, generalized convulsions, hypertension, junctional tachycardia, panic attacks, tachycardia, ventricular tachycardia, withdrawal syndrome

Overdosage/Toxicology Excessively high doses may cause anxiety, agitation, increased muscle tone, hyperesthesia and seizures.

Drug Interactions

Nonbenzodiazepine hypnotics (zaleplon, zolpidem, zopiclone): Flumazenil reverses the effects of these hypnotics.

Dosage Forms Injection, solution: 0.1 mg/mL (5 mL, 10 mL) [contains edetate sodium]

References

Mokhlesi B, Leikin JB, Murray P, et al, "Adult Toxicology in Critical Care. Part 11: Specific Poisonings," *Chest*, 2003, 123(3):897-922.

Trujillo MH, Guerrero J, Fragachan C, et al, "Pharmacologic Antidotes in Critical Care Medicine: A Practical Guide for Administration," *Crit Care Med*, 1998, 26(2):377-91.

♦ **Flumazenil Injection (Can)** *see* Flumazenil *on page 534*
♦ **Flumazenil Injection, USP (Can)** *see* Flumazenil *on page 534*

Flunisolide (floo NISS oh lide)

Medication Safety Issues

Sound-alike/look-alike issues:

Flunisolide may be confused with Flumadine®, fluocinonide
Nasarel® may be confused with Nizoral®

Related Information

Asthma *on page 1594*
Corticosteroids *on page 1561*

U.S. Brand Names AeroBid®; AeroBid®-M; Aerospan™; Nasarel®

Canadian Brand Names Alti-Flunisolide; Apo-Flunisolide®; Nasalide®; PMS-Flunisolide; Rhinalar®

Pharmacologic Category Corticosteroid, Inhalant (Oral); Corticosteroid, Nasal

Generic Available Yes: Nasal spray

Use Steroid-dependent asthma; nasal solution is used for seasonal or perennial rhinitis

Mechanism of Action Decreases inflammation by suppression of migration of polymorphonuclear leukocytes and reversal of increased capillary permeability; does not depress hypothalamus

Pharmacodynamics/Kinetics

Absorption: Nasal inhalation: ~50%
Metabolism: Rapidly hepatic to active metabolites
Bioavailability: 40% to 50%
Half-life elimination: 1.8 hours
Excretion: Urine and feces (equal amounts)

Dosage Note: AeroBid® and Aerospan™ are not interchangeable; dosing changes when switching from one to another.

Oral Inhalation: Asthma:

AeroBid®:

Children 6-15 years: 2 inhalations twice daily (morning and evening); up to 4 inhalations/day

Children ≥16 years and Adults: 2 inhalations twice daily (morning and evening); up to 8 inhalations/day maximum

Aerospan™:

Children 6-11 years: 1 inhalation twice daily; up to 4 inhalations/day

Children ≥12 years and Adults: 2 inhalations twice daily; up to 8 inhalations/day

Intranasal: Rhinitis:

Children 6-14 years: 1 spray each nostril 3 times daily **or** 2 sprays in each nostril twice daily; not to exceed 4 sprays/day in each nostril (200 mcg/day)

Children ≥15 years and Adults: 2 sprays each nostril twice daily (morning and evening); may increase to 2 sprays 3 times daily; maximum dose: 8 sprays/day in each nostril (400 mcg/day)

Stability

Aerospan™: Store at 15°C to 30°C (59°F to 86°F). Do not store near heat or flame. Protect from freezing and sunlight.

AeroBid®: Store below 49°C (below 120°F).

Administration Inhalation: Shake well before using. Rinse mouth following use of oral inhalers.

(Continued)

Flunisolide *(Continued)*

Aerospan™: Has a self-contained spacer; do not use with another spacer. Prime inhaler prior to first use. Begin inhalation immediately prior to actuation; a delay may reduce dose by ≥75%.

Pregnancy Risk Factor C

Contraindications Hypersensitivity to flunisolide or any component of the formulation; acute status asthmaticus; viral, tuberculosis, fungal, or bacterial respiratory infections; infections of the nasal mucosa

Warnings/Precautions Use with caution in patients with hypothyroidism, cirrhosis, hypertension, CHF, ulcerative colitis, thromboembolic disorders

May cause suppression of hypothalamic-pituitary-adrenal (HPA) axis, particularly in younger children or in patients receiving high doses for prolonged periods. Particular care is required when patients are transferred from systemic corticosteroids to inhaled products due to possible adrenal insufficiency or withdrawal from steroids, including an increase in allergic symptoms. Patients receiving 20 mg per day of prednisone (or equivalent) may be most susceptible. Fatalities have occurred due to adrenal insufficiency in asthmatic patients during and after transfer from systemic corticosteroids to aerosol steroids; aerosol steroids do **not** provide the systemic steroid needed to treat patients having trauma, surgery, or infections. Withdrawal and discontinuation of the corticosteroid should be done slowly and carefully

Controlled clinical studies have shown that orally-inhaled and intranasal corticosteroids may cause a reduction in growth velocity in pediatric patients. (In studies of orally-inhaled corticosteroids, the mean reduction in growth velocity was approximately 1 centimeter per year [range 0.3-1.8 cm per year] and appears to be related to dose and duration of exposure.) The growth of pediatric patients receiving inhaled corticosteroids, should be monitored routinely (eg, via stadiometry). To minimize the systemic effects of orally-inhaled and intranasal corticosteroids, each patient should be titrated to the lowest effective dose.

May suppress the immune system, patients may be more susceptible to infection. Use with caution in patients with systemic infections or ocular herpes simplex. Avoid exposure to chickenpox and measles.

Adverse Reactions

>10%:
- Central nervous system: Headache (intranasal <5%; oral 9% to 25%)
- Gastrointestinal: Aftertaste (10% to 17%)
- Respiratory: Nasal burning (intranasal 45%), pharyngitis (14% to 20%), rhinitis (<15%), nasal irritation (>1% to 13%)

1% to 10%:
- Cardiovascular: Chest pain (1% to 3%), edema (1% to 3%), chest tightness, hypertension, palpitations, tachycardia
- Central nervous system: Fever (1% to 9%), dizziness (1% to 3%), insomnia (1% to 3%), migraine (1% to 3%), chills, malaise, irritability, shakiness, anxiety, depression, faintness, fatigue, moodiness, vertigo
- Dermatologic: Erythema multiform (1% to 3%), acne, eczema, pruritus, urticaria
- Endocrine & metabolic: Dysmenorrhea (1% to 3%)
- Gastrointestinal: Dyspepsia (2% to 4%), abdominal pain (1% to 3%), diarrhea (1% to 10%), gastroenteritis (1% to 3%), nausea (Aerospan™: 1% to 3%), oral candidiasis (1% to 3%), taste perversion (1% to 3%), abdominal fullness, constipation, gas, heartburn, sore throat, dry throat, mouth discomfort, throat irritation
- Genitourinary: Vaginitis (1% to 3%), urinary tract infection (1% to 4%)
- Neuromuscular & skeletal: Myalgia (1% to 3%), neck pain (1% to 3%), numbness, weakness
- Ocular: Conjunctivitis (1% to 3%), blurred vision
- Renal: Laryngitis (1% to 3%)
- Respiratory: Sinusitis (<9%), epistaxia (<3%), bronchospasm, cough increased, dyspnea, hoarseness, nasal ulcer, sneezing, wheezing
- Miscellaneous: Allergy (4% to 5%), infection (3% to 9%), loss of smell, voice alteration (1% to 3%), flu-like syndrome, diaphoresis

<1% (Limited to important or life-threatening): Adrenal suppression

Overdosage/Toxicology When consumed in high doses over prolonged periods, systemic hypercorticism and adrenal suppression may occur. In those cases, discontinuation of the corticosteroid should be done judiciously.

Drug Interactions Expected interactions similar to other corticosteroids

Salmeterol: The addition of salmeterol has been demonstrated to improve response to inhaled corticosteroids (as compared to increasing steroid dosage).

Dosage Forms

Aerosol for oral inhalation:

AeroBid®: 250 mcg/actuation (7 g) [100 metered inhalations; contains CFCs]

AeroBid®-M: 250 mcg/actuation (7 g) [100 metered inhalations; contains CFCs; menthol flavor]

Aerospan™: 80 mcg/actuation (5.1 g) [60 metered inhalations; CFC free]; 80 mcg/actuation (8.9 g) [120 metered inhalations; CFC free]

Solution, intranasal [spray]: 29 mcg/actuation (25 mL) [200 sprays]

Nasarel®: 29 mcg/actuation (25 mL) [200 sprays; contains benzalkonium chloride]

- **Fluohydrisone Acetate** *see* Fludrocortisone *on page 533*
- **Fluohydrocortisone Acetate** *see* Fludrocortisone *on page 533*
- **9α-Fluorohydrocortisone Acetate** *see* Fludrocortisone *on page 533*

Fluoxetine (floo OKS e teen)

Medication Safety Issues

Sound-alike/look-alike issues:

Fluoxetine may be confused with duloxetine, fluvastatin

Prozac® may be confused with Prilosec®, Proscar®, ProSom®, ProStep®

Sarafem® may be confused with Serophene®

Related Information

Antidepressant Agents *on page 1551*

Chronic Pain Management *on page 1430*

U.S. Brand Names Prozac®; Prozac® Weekly™; Sarafem®

Canadian Brand Names Alti-Fluoxetine; Apo-Fluoxetine®; BCI-Fluoxetine; CO Fluoxetine; FXT; Gen-Fluoxetine; Novo-Fluoxetine; Nu-Fluoxetine; PMS-Fluoxetine; Prozac®; Rhoxal-fluoxetine; Sandoz-Fluoxetine

Synonyms Fluoxetine Hydrochloride

Pharmacologic Category Antidepressant, Selective Serotonin Reuptake Inhibitor

Restrictions A medication guide concerning the use of antidepressants in children and teenagers can be found on the FDA website at http://www.fda.gov/cder/Offices/ODS/labeling.htm. It should be dispensed to parents or guardians of children and teenagers receiving this medication.

Generic Available Yes: Excludes delayed release capsule

Use Treatment of major depressive disorder (MDD); treatment of binge-eating and vomiting in patients with moderate-to-severe bulimia nervosa; obsessive-compulsive disorder (OCD); premenstrual dysphoric disorder (PMDD); panic disorder with or without agoraphobia

Unlabeled/Investigational Use Selective mutism

Mechanism of Action Inhibits CNS neuron serotonin reuptake; minimal or no effect on reuptake of norepinephrine or dopamine; does not significantly bind to alpha-adrenergic, histamine, or cholinergic receptors

Pharmacodynamics/Kinetics

Absorption: Well absorbed; delayed 1-2 hours with weekly formulation

Protein binding: 95%

Metabolism: Hepatic to norfluoxetine (activity equal to fluoxetine)

Half-life elimination: Adults:

Parent drug: 1-3 days (acute), 4-6 days (chronic), 7.6 days (cirrhosis)

Metabolite (norfluoxetine): 9.3 days (range: 4-16 days), 12 days (cirrhosis)

Time to peak: 6-8 hours

Excretion: Urine (10% as norfluoxetine, 2.5% to 5% as fluoxetine)

Note: Weekly formulation results in greater fluctuations between peak and trough concentrations of fluoxetine and norfluoxetine compared to once-daily dosing (24% daily/164% weekly; 17% daily/43% weekly, respectively). Trough concentrations are 76% lower for fluoxetine and 47% lower for norfluoxetine than the concentrations maintained by 20 mg once-daily dosing. Steady-state fluoxetine concentrations are ~50% lower following the once-weekly regimen compared to 20 mg once daily. Average steady-state concentrations of once-daily dosing were highest in children ages 6 to <13 (fluoxetine 171 ng/mL; norfluoxetine 195 ng/mL), followed by adolescents ages 13 to <18 (fluoxetine 86 ng/mL; norfluoxetine 113

(Continued)

Fluoxetine *(Continued)*

ng/mL); concentrations were considered to be within the ranges reported in adults (fluoxetine 91-302 ng/mL; norfluoxetine 72-258 ng/mL).

Dosage Oral: **Note:** Upon discontinuation of fluoxetine therapy, gradually taper dose. If intolerable symptoms occur following a dose reduction, consider resuming the previously prescribed dose and/or decrease dose at a more gradual rate.

Children:

Depression: 8-18 years: 10-20 mg/day; lower-weight children can be started at 10 mg/day, may increase to 20 mg/day after 1 week if needed

OCD: 7-18 years: Initial: 10 mg/day; in adolescents and higher-weight children, dose may be increased to 20 mg/day after 2 weeks. Range: 10-60 mg/day

Selective mutism (unlabeled use):

<5 years: No dosing information available

5-18 years: Initial: 5-10 mg/day; titrate upwards as needed (usual maximum dose: 60 mg/day)

Adults: 20 mg/day in the morning; may increase after several weeks by 20 mg/day increments; maximum: 80 mg/day; doses >20 mg may be given once daily or divided twice daily. **Note:** Lower doses of 5-10 mg/day have been used for initial treatment.

Usual dosage range:

Bulimia nervosa: 60-80 mg/day

Depression: 20-40 mg/day; patients maintained on Prozac® 20 mg/day may be changed to Prozac® Weekly™ 90 mg/week, starting dose 7 days after the last 20 mg/day dose

OCD: 40-80 mg/day

Panic disorder: Initial: 10 mg/day; after 1 week, increase to 20 mg/day; may increase after several weeks; doses >60 mg/day have not been evaluated

PMDD (Sarafem™): 20 mg/day continuously, **or** 20 mg/day starting 14 days prior to menstruation and through first full day of menses (repeat with each cycle)

Elderly: Depression: Some patients may require an initial dose of 10 mg/day with dosage increases of 10 and 20 mg every several weeks as tolerated; should not be taken at night unless patient experiences sedation

Dosing adjustment in renal impairment:

Single dose studies: Pharmacokinetics of fluoxetine and norfluoxetine were similar among subjects with all levels of impaired renal function, including anephric patients on chronic hemodialysis

Chronic administration: Additional accumulation of fluoxetine or norfluoxetine may occur in patients with severely impaired renal function

Hemodialysis: Not removed by hemodialysis; use of lower dose or less frequent dosing is not usually necessary.

Dosing adjustment in hepatic impairment: Elimination half-life of fluoxetine is prolonged in patients with hepatic impairment; a lower or less frequent dose of fluoxetine should be used in these patients

Cirrhosis patients: Administer a lower dose or less frequent dosing interval

Compensated cirrhosis without ascites: Administer 50% of normal dose

Stability All dosage forms should be stored at controlled room temperature of 15°C to 30°C (50°F to 86°F); oral liquid should be dispensed in a light-resistant container

Monitoring Parameters Mental status for depression, suicidal ideation, anxiety, social functioning, mania, panic attacks; akathisia, sleep

Reference Range Therapeutic levels have not been well established

Therapeutic: Fluoxetine: 100-800 ng/mL (SI: 289-2314 nmol/L); Norfluoxetine: 100-600 ng/mL (SI: 289-1735 nmol/L)

Toxic: Fluoxetine plus norfluoxetine: >2000 ng/mL

Anesthesia and Critical Care Concerns/Other Considerations SSRIs are relatively safe compared to other antidepressants in patients with cardiovascular disease.

Buspirone and cyproheptadine, may be useful in treatment of sexual dysfunction during treatment with a selective serotonin reuptake inhibitor.

Weekly capsules are a delayed release formulation containing enteric-coated pellets of fluoxetine hydrochloride, equivalent to 90 mg fluoxetine. Therapeutic equivalence of weekly formulation with daily formulation for delaying time to relapse has not been established.

Pregnancy Risk Factor C

Contraindications Hypersensitivity to fluoxetine or any component of the formulation; patients currently receiving MAO inhibitors, pimozide, or thioridazine

Note: MAO inhibitor therapy must be stopped for 14 days before fluoxetine is initiated. Treatment with MAO inhibitors, thioridazine, or mesoridazine should not be initiated until 5 weeks after the discontinuation of fluoxetine.

Warnings/Precautions

Major psychiatric warnings:

- **[U.S. Boxed Warning]: Antidepressants increase the risk of suicidal thinking and behavior in children and adolescents with major depressive disorder (MDD) and other depressive disorders;** consider risk prior to prescribing. Closely monitor for clinical worsening, suicidality, or unusual changes in behavior; the child's family or caregiver should be instructed to closely observe the patient and communicate condition with healthcare provider. A medication guide concerning the use of antidepressants in children and teenagers should be dispensed with each prescription. **Fluoxetine is FDA approved for the treatment of OCD in children ≥7 years of age and MDD in children ≥8 years of age.**
- The possibility of a suicide attempt is inherent in major depression and may persist until remission occurs. Patients treated with antidepressants should be observed for clinical worsening and suicidality, especially during the initial few months of a course of drug therapy, or at times of dose changes, either increases or decreases. Worsening depression and severe abrupt suicidality that are not part of the presenting symptoms may require discontinuation or modification of drug therapy. Use caution in high-risk patients during initiation of therapy.
- Prescriptions should be written for the smallest quantity consistent with good patient care. The patient's family or caregiver should be alerted to monitor patients for the emergence of suicidality and associated behaviors such as anxiety, agitation, panic attacks, insomnia, irritability, hostility, impulsivity, akathisia, hypomania, and mania; patients should be instructed to notify their healthcare provider if any of these symptoms or worsening depression or psychosis occur.
- May worsen psychosis in some patients or precipitate a shift to mania or hypomania in patients with bipolar disorder. Monotherapy in patients with bipolar disorder should be avoided. Patients presenting with depressive symptoms should be screened for bipolar disorder. **Fluoxetine is not FDA approved for the treatment of bipolar depression.** Safety and efficacy in children <8 years of age (major depressive disorder) and <7 years of age (OCD) have not been established.

Key adverse effects:

- Allergic events and rash: Fluoxetine use has been associated with occurrences of significant rash and allergic events, including vasculitis, lupus-like syndrome, laryngospasm, anaphylactoid reactions, and pulmonary inflammatory disease. Discontinue if underlying cause of rash cannot be identified.
- Anticholinergic effects: Relatively devoid of these side effects
- CNS depression: Has a low potential to impair cognitive or motor performance; caution operating hazardous machinery or driving.
- CNS effects: May cause insomnia, anxiety, nervousness or anorexia.
- SIADH and hyponatremia: Has been associated with the development of SIADH; hyponatremia has been reported rarely, predominately in the elderly.

Concurrent disease:

- Diabetes: May alter glycemic control in patients with diabetes.
- Hepatic impairment: Use caution; clearance is decreased and plasma concentrations are increased; a lower dosage may be needed.
- Platelet aggregation: May impair platelet aggregation, resulting in bleeding.
- Renal impairment: Use caution; clearance is decreased and plasma concentrations are increased; a lower dosage may be needed.
- Seizure disorders: Use caution with a previous seizure disorder or condition predisposing to seizures such as brain damage or alcoholism.
- Sexual dysfunction: May cause or exacerbate sexual dysfunction.
- Weight loss: May cause weight loss. Use caution in patients where weight loss is undesirable.

Concurrent drug therapy:

- Agents which lower seizure threshold: Use caution with concurrent therapy.
- Anticoagulants/Antiplatelets: Use caution with concomitant use of NSAIDs, ASA, or other drugs that affect coagulation; the risk of bleeding is potentiated.

(Continued)

Fluoxetine *(Continued)*

- Cardiovascular: Use caution with history of MI or unstable heasrt disease; use in these patients is limited
- CNS depressants: Use caution with concomitant therapy.
- MAO inhibitors: Potential for severe reaction when used with MAO inhibitors; autonomic instability, coma, death, delirium, diaphoresis, hyperthermia, mental status changes/agitation, muscular rigidity, myoclonus, neuroleptic malignant syndrome features, and seizures may occur.
- Thioridazine: Fluoxetine may elevate plasma levels of thioridazine; increasing risk of QTc interval prolongation; this may lead to serious ventricular arrhythmias such as torsade de pointes-type arrhythmias and sudden death. **Concurrent use is contraindicated.**

Special populations:

- Elderly: Use caution in elderly patients.

Special notes:

- Electroconvulsive therapy: May increase the risks associated with electroconvulsive therapy; consider discontinuing, when possible, prior to ECT treatment.
- Long half-life: Due to the long half-life of fluoxetine and its metabolites, the effects and interactions noted may persist for prolonged periods following discontinuation.
- Withdrawal syndrome: May cause dysphoric mood, irritability, agitation, dizziness, sensory disturbances, anxiety, confusion, headache, lethargy, emotional lability, insomnia, hypomania, tinnitus, and seizures. Upon discontinuation of fluoxetine therapy, gradually taper dose. If intolerable symptoms occur following a decrease in dosage or upon discontinuation of therapy, then resuming the previous dose with a more gradual taper should be considered.

Adverse Reactions Percentages listed for adverse effects as reported in placebo-controlled trials and were generally similar in adults and children; actual frequency may be dependent upon diagnosis and in some cases the range presented may be lower than or equal to placebo for a particular disorder.

>10%:

Central nervous system: Insomnia (10% to 33%), headache (21%), anxiety (6% to 15%), nervousness (8% to 14%), somnolence (5% to 17%)

Endocrine & metabolic: Libido decreased (1% to 11%)

Gastrointestinal: Nausea (12% to 29%), diarrhea (8% to 18%), anorexia (4% to 11%), xerostomia (4% to 12%)

Neuromuscular & skeletal: Weakness (7% to 21%), tremor (3% to 13%)

Respiratory: Pharyngitis (3% to 11%), yawn (<1% to 11%)

1% to 10%:

Cardiovascular: Vasodilation (1% to 5%), fever (2%), chest pain, hemorrhage, hypertension, palpitation

Central nervous system: Dizziness (9%), dream abnormality (1% to 5%), thinking abnormality (2%), agitation, amnesia, chills, confusion, emotional lability, sleep disorder

Dermatologic: Rash (2% to 6%), pruritus (4%)

Endocrine & metabolic: Ejaculation abnormal (<1% to 7%), impotence (<1% to 7%)

Gastrointestinal: Dyspepsia (6% to 10%), constipation (5%), flatulence (3%), vomiting (3%), weight loss (2%), appetite increased, taste perversion, weight gain

Genitourinary: Urinary frequency

Ocular: Vision abnormal (2%)

Otic: Ear pain, tinnitus

Respiratory: Sinusitis (1% to 6%)

Miscellaneous: Flu-like syndrome (3% to 10%), diaphoresis (2% to 8%)

<1% (Limited to important or life-threatening): Allergies, alopecia, anaphylactoid reactions, angina, arrhythmia, asthma, cataract, CHF, cholelithiasis, cholestatic jaundice, colitis, dyskinesia, dysphagia, eosinophilic pneumonia, erythema nodosum, esophagitis, euphoria, exfoliative dermatitis, extrapyramidal symptoms (rare), gout, hallucinations, hepatic failure/necrosis, hemorrhage, hyperprolactinemia, hyponatremia (possibly in association with SIADH), immune-related hemolytic anemia, laryngospasm, lupus-like syndrome, MI, neuroleptic malignant syndrome (NMS), optic neuritis, pancreatitis, pancytopenia, photosensitivity reaction, postural hypotension, priapism, pulmonary embolism, pulmonary fibrosis, pulmonary hypertension, QT prolongation, renal

failure, serotonin syndrome, Stevens-Johnson syndrome, syncope, thrombocytopenia, thrombocytopenic purpura, vasculitis, ventricular tachycardia (including torsade de pointes)

Overdosage/Toxicology Among 633 adult patients who overdosed on fluoxetine alone, 34 resulted in a fatal outcome. Symptoms of overdose include ataxia, sedation, coma, and ECG abnormalities (QT prolongation, torsade de pointes). Respiratory depression may occur, especially with coingestion of ethanol or other drugs. Seizures rarely occur. Treatment is symptom-directed and supportive. Forced diuresis and dialysis are not likely to benefit.

Drug Interactions Substrate of CYP1A2 (minor), 2B6 (minor), 2C9 (major), 2C19 (minor), 2D6 (major), 2E1 (minor), 3A4 (minor); **Inhibits** CYP1A2 (moderate), 2B6 (weak), 2C9 (weak), 2C19 (moderate), 2D6 (strong), 3A4 (weak)

Amphetamines: SSRIs may increase the sensitivity to amphetamines, and amphetamines may increase the risk of serotonin syndrome.

Benzodiazepines: Fluoxetine may inhibit the metabolism of alprazolam and diazepam resulting in elevated serum levels; monitor for increased sedation and psychomotor impairment.

Beta-blockers: Fluoxetine may inhibit the metabolism of metoprolol and propranolol resulting in cardiac toxicity; monitor for bradycardia, hypotension, and heart failure if combination is used; not established for all beta-blockers (unlikely with atenolol or nadolol due to renal elimination).

Buspirone: Fluoxetine inhibits the reuptake of serotonin; combined use with a serotonin agonist (buspirone) may cause serotonin syndrome.

Carbamazepine: Fluoxetine may inhibit the metabolism of carbamazepine resulting in increased carbamazepine levels and toxicity; monitor for altered carbamazepine response.

Carvedilol: Serum concentrations may be increased; monitor carefully for increased carvedilol effect (hypotension and bradycardia).

Clozapine: Fluoxetine may increase serum levels of clozapine; levels may increase by 76%; monitor for increased effect/toxicity.

Cyclosporine: Fluoxetine may increase serum levels of cyclosporine (and possibly tacrolimus); monitor.

CYP1A2 substrates: Fluoxetine may increase the levels/effects of CYP1A2 substrates. Example substrates include aminophylline, fluvoxamine, mexiletine, mirtazapine, ropinirole, theophylline, and trifluoperazine.

CYP2C9 inducers: May decrease the levels/effects of fluoxetine. Example inducers include carbamazepine, phenobarbital, phenytoin, rifampin, rifapentine, and secobarbital.

CYP2C9 Inhibitors may increase the levels/effects of fluoxetine. Example inhibitors include delavirdine, fluconazole, gemfibrozil, ketoconazole, nicardipine, NSAIDs, sulfonamides and tolbutamide.

CYP2C19 substrates: Fluoxetine may increase the levels/effects of CYP2C19 substrates. Example substrates include citalopram, diazepam, methsuximide, phenytoin, propranolol, and sertraline.

CYP2D6 inhibitors: May increase the levels/effects of fluoxetine. Example inhibitors include chlorpromazine, delavirdine, miconazole, paroxetine, pergolide, quinidine, quinine, ritonavir, and ropinirole.

CYP2D6 substrates: Fluoxetine may increase the levels/effects of CYP2D6 substrates. Example substrates include amphetamines, selected beta-blockers, dextromethorphan, lidocaine, mirtazapine, nefazodone, paroxetine, risperidone, ritonavir, thioridazine, tricyclic antidepressants, and venlafaxine.

CYP2D6 prodrug substrates: Fluoxetine may decrease the levels/effects of CYP2D6 prodrug substrates. Example prodrug substrates include codeine, hydrocodone, oxycodone, and tramadol.

Cyproheptadine: May inhibit the effects of serotonin reuptake inhibitors (fluoxetine); monitor for altered antidepressant response; cyproheptadine acts as a serotonin agonist.

Dextromethorphan: Fluoxetine inhibits the metabolism of dextromethorphan; visual hallucinations occurred in a patient receiving this combination; monitor for serotonin syndrome.

Digoxin: Fluoxetine may increase serum levels of digoxin; monitor.

Haloperidol: Fluoxetine may inhibit the metabolism of haloperidol and cause extrapyramidal symptoms (EPS); monitor patients for EPS if combination is utilized.

HMG-CoA reductase inhibitors: Fluoxetine may inhibit the metabolism of lovastatin and simvastatin resulting in myositis and rhabdomyolysis; these combinations are best avoided.

(Continued)

Fluoxetine *(Continued)*

Lithium: Reports of both increased and decreased lithium levels when used concomitantly with fluoxetine. Patients receiving fluoxetine and lithium have developed neurotoxicity. If combination is used; monitor lithium levels and for neurotoxicity.

Loop diuretics: Fluoxetine may cause hyponatremia; additive hyponatremic effects may be seen with combined use of a loop diuretic (bumetanide, furosemide, torsemide); monitor for hyponatremia.

MAO inhibitors: Combined use of fluoxetine with nonselective MAOIs (ie, isocarboxazid, phenelzine) is contraindicated; fatal reactions have been reported; wait 5 weeks after stopping fluoxetine before starting an MAO inhibitor and 2 weeks after stopping an MAO inhibitor before starting fluoxetine.

Meperidine: Combined use with fluoxetine theoretically may increase the risk of serotonin syndrome.

Nefazodone: May increase the risk of serotonin syndrome with SSRIs; monitor.

NSAIDs: Concomitant use of fluoxetine and NSAIDs, aspirin, or other drugs affecting coagulation has been associated with an increased risk of bleeding; monitor.

Phenytoin: Fluoxetine inhibits the metabolism of phenytoin and may result in phenytoin toxicity; monitor for phenytoin toxicity (ataxia, confusion, dizziness, nystagmus, involuntary muscle movement).

Pimozide: Due to potential QT_c interval prolongation, concomitant use is contraindicated.

Propafenone: Serum concentrations and/or toxicity may be increased by fluoxetine; avoid concurrent administration.

Ritonavir: Combined use of fluoxetine with ritonavir may cause serotonin syndrome in HIV-positive patients; monitor.

Selegiline: Fluoxetine has been reported to cause mania or hypertension when combined with selegiline; this combination is best avoided. Concurrent use with SSRIs has also been reported to cause serotonin syndrome. As a MAO type B inhibitor, the risk of serotonin syndrome may be less than with nonselective MAO inhibitors.

Sibutramine: May increase the risk of serotonin syndrome with SSRIs; avoid coadministration.

SSRIs: Fluoxetine inhibits the reuptake of serotonin; combined use with other drugs which inhibit the reuptake may cause serotonin syndrome.

Sumatriptan (and other serotonin agonists): Concurrent use may result in toxicity; weakness, hyper-reflexia, and incoordination have been observed with sumatriptan and SSRIs. In addition, concurrent use may theoretically increase the risk of serotonin syndrome; includes sumatriptan, naratriptan, rizatriptan, and zolmitriptan.

Sympathomimetics: May increase the risk of serotonin syndrome with SSRIs.

Thioridazine: Fluoxetine may inhibit the metabolism of thioridazine, resulting in increased plasma levels and increasing the risk of QT_c interval prolongation. This may lead to serious ventricular arrhythmias, such as torsade de pointes-type arrhythmias and sudden death. Do not use together. Wait at least 5 weeks after discontinuing fluoxetine prior to starting thioridazine.

Tramadol: Fluoxetine combined with tramadol (serotonergic effects) may cause serotonin syndrome; monitor.

Trazodone: Fluoxetine may inhibit the metabolism of trazodone resulting in increased toxicity; monitor.

Tricyclic antidepressants: Fluoxetine inhibits the metabolism of tricyclic antidepressants (amitriptyline, desipramine, imipramine, nortriptyline) resulting is elevated serum levels; if combination is warranted, a low dose of TCA (10-25 mg/day) should be utilized.

Tryptophan: Fluoxetine inhibits the reuptake of serotonin; combination with tryptophan, a serotonin precursor, may cause agitation and restlessness; this combination is best avoided.

Valproic acid: Fluoxetine may increase serum levels of valproic acid; monitor.

Venlafaxine: Fluoxetine may increase the risk of serotonin syndrome.

Warfarin: Fluoxetine may alter the hypoprothrombinemic response to warfarin; monitor.

Ethanol/Nutrition/Herb Interactions

Ethanol: Avoid ethanol (may increase CNS depression). Depressed patients should avoid/limit intake.

Herb/Nutraceutical: Avoid valerian, St John's wort, kava kava, gotu kola (may increase CNS depression).

Dietary Considerations May be taken with or without food.

Dosage Forms [DSC] = Discontinued product

Capsule, as hydrochloride: 10 mg, 20 mg, 40 mg
- Prozac®: 10 mg, 20 mg, 40 mg
- Sarafem®: 10 mg, 20 mg

Capsule, delayed release, as hydrochloride (Prozac® Weekly™): 90 mg

Solution, oral, as hydrochloride (Prozac®): 20 mg/5 mL (120 mL) [contains alcohol 0.23% and benzoic acid; mint flavor]

Tablet, as hydrochloride: 10 mg, 20 mg
- Prozac® [scored]: 10 mg [DSC]

♦ **Fluoxetine Hydrochloride** *see* Fluoxetine *on page 539*

Fluphenazine (floo FEN a zeen)

Medication Safety Issues

Sound-alike/look-alike issues:
- Prolixin® may be confused with Proloprim®

U.S. Brand Names Prolixin® [DSC]; Prolixin Decanoate®

Canadian Brand Names Apo-Fluphenazine®; Apo-Fluphenazine Decanoate®; Modecate®; Modecate® Concentrate; PMS-Fluphenazine Decanoate

Synonyms Fluphenazine Decanoate

Pharmacologic Category Antipsychotic Agent, Typical, Phenothiazine

Generic Available Yes: Injection, tablet

Use Management of manifestations of psychotic disorders and schizophrenia; depot formulation may offer improved outcome in individuals with psychosis who are nonadherent with oral antipsychotics

Unlabeled/Investigational Use Pervasive developmental disorder

Mechanism of Action Fluphenazine is a piperazine phenothiazine antipsychotic which blocks postsynaptic mesolimbic dopaminergic D_1 and D_2 receptors in the brain; depresses the release of hypothalamic and hypophyseal hormones; believed to depress the reticular activating system thus affecting basal metabolism, body temperature, wakefulness, vasomotor tone, and emesis

Pharmacodynamics/Kinetics

Onset of action: I.M., SubQ (derivative dependent): Hydrochloride salt: ~1 hour
- Peak effect: Neuroleptic: Decanoate: 48-96 hours

Duration: Hydrochloride salt: 6-8 hours; Decanoate: 24-72 hours

Absorption: Oral: Erratic and variable

Distribution: Crosses placenta; enters breast milk

Protein binding: 91% and 99%

Metabolism: Hepatic

Half-life elimination (derivative dependent): Hydrochloride: 33 hours; Decanoate: 163-232 hours

Excretion: Urine (as metabolites)

Dosage

Children: Oral: Childhood-onset pervasive developmental disorder (unlabeled use): 0.04 mg/kg/day

Adults: Psychoses:
- Oral: 0.5-10 mg/day in divided doses at 6- to 8-hour intervals; some patients may require up to 40 mg/day
- I.M.: 2.5-10 mg/day in divided doses at 6- to 8-hour intervals (parenteral dose is $\frac{1}{3}$ to $\frac{1}{2}$ the oral dose for the hydrochloride salts)
- I.M. (decanoate): 12.5 mg every 2 weeks
  - Conversion from hydrochloride to decanoate I.M. 0.5 mL (12.5 mg) decanoate every 3 weeks is approximately equivalent to 10 mg hydrochloride/day

Hemodialysis: Not dialyzable (0% to 5%)

Stability Avoid freezing; protect all dosage forms from light; clear or slightly yellow solutions may be used; should be dispensed in amber or opaque vials/bottles. Solutions may be diluted or mixed with fruit juices or other liquids but must be administered immediately after mixing; do not prepare bulk dilutions or store bulk dilutions.

Administration Avoid contact of oral solution or injection with skin (contact dermatitis). Oral liquid should be diluted in the following **only**: Water, saline,

(Continued)

Fluphenazine *(Continued)*

homogenized milk, carbonated orange beverages, pineapple, apricot, prune, orange, tomato, and grapefruit juices. Do **not** dilute in beverages containing caffeine, tannics, or pectinate. Watch for hypotension when administering I.M.

Monitoring Parameters Vital signs; lipid profile, fasting blood glucose/Hgb A_{1c}; BMI; mental status, abnormal involuntary movement scale (AIMS), extrapyramidal symptoms (EPS)

Reference Range Therapeutic: 0.3-3 ng/mL (SI: 0.6-6.0 nmol/L); correlation of serum concentrations and efficacy is controversial; most often dosed to best response

Anesthesia and Critical Care Concerns/Other Considerations Less sedative and hypotensive effects than chlorpromazine

Pregnancy Risk Factor C

Contraindications Hypersensitivity to fluphenazine or any component of the formulation (cross-reactivity between phenothiazines may occur); severe CNS depression; coma; subcortical brain damage; blood dyscrasias; hepatic disease

Warnings/Precautions May be sedating, use with caution in disorders where CNS depression is a feature. Use with caution in Parkinson's disease. Caution in patients with hemodynamic instability; bone marrow suppression; predisposition to seizures; severe cardiac, renal, or respiratory disease. Esophageal dysmotility and aspiration have been associated with antipsychotic use - use with caution in patients at risk of pneumonia (ie, Alzheimer's disease). Caution in breast cancer or other prolactin-dependent tumors (may elevate prolactin levels). May alter temperature regulation or mask toxicity of other drugs due to antiemetic effects. May alter cardiac conduction; life-threatening arrhythmias have occurred with therapeutic doses of phenothiazines. Hypotension may occur, particularly with I.M. administration. May cause orthostatic hypotension - use with caution in patients at risk of this effect or those who would tolerate transient hypotensive episodes (cerebrovascular disease, cardiovascular disease, or other medications which may predispose). Adverse effects of depot injections may be prolonged.

Phenothiazines may cause anticholinergic effects (confusion, agitation, constipation, xerostomia, blurred vision, urinary retention). Therefore, they should be used with caution in patients with decreased gastrointestinal motility, urinary retention, BPH, xerostomia, or visual problems. Conditions which also may be exacerbated by cholinergic blockade include narrow-angle glaucoma (screening is recommended) and worsening of myasthenia gravis. Relative to other antipsychotics, fluphenazine has a low potency of cholinergic blockade.

May cause extrapyramidal symptoms, including pseudoparkinsonism, acute dystonic reactions, akathisia and tardive dyskinesia (risk of these reactions is high relative to other antipsychotics). May be associated with neuroleptic malignant syndrome (NMS) or pigmentary retinopathy.

Adverse Reactions Frequency not defined.

Cardiovascular: Tachycardia, fluctuations in blood pressure, hyper-/hypotension, arrhythmia, edema

Central nervous system: Parkinsonian symptoms, akathisia, dystonias, tardive dyskinesia, dizziness, hyper-reflexia, headache, cerebral edema, drowsiness, lethargy, restlessness, excitement, bizarre dreams, EEG changes, depression, seizure, NMS, altered central temperature regulation

Dermatologic: Dermatitis, eczema, erythema, itching, photosensitivity, rash, seborrhea, skin pigmentation, urticaria

Endocrine & metabolic: Changes in menstrual cycle, breast pain, amenorrhea, galactorrhea, gynecomastia, libido (changes in), elevated prolactin, SIADH

Gastrointestinal: Weight gain, loss of appetite, salivation, xerostomia, constipation, paralytic ileus, laryngeal edema

Genitourinary: Ejaculatory disturbances, impotence, polyuria, bladder paralysis, enuresis

Hematologic: Agranulocytosis, leukopenia, thrombocytopenia, nonthrombocytopenic purpura, eosinophilia, pancytopenia

Hepatic: Cholestatic jaundice, hepatotoxicity

Neuromuscular & skeletal: Trembling of fingers, SLE, facial hemispasm

Ocular: Pigmentary retinopathy, cornea and lens changes, blurred vision, glaucoma

Respiratory: Nasal congestion, asthma

Overdosage/Toxicology Symptoms of overdose include deep sleep, hypo- or hypertension, dystonia, seizures, extrapyramidal symptoms, and respiratory failure. Following initiation of essential overdose management, toxic symptom treatment and supportive treatment should be initiated.

Drug Interactions Substrate of CYP2D6 (major); **Inhibits** CYP1A2 (weak), 2C9 (weak), 2D6 (weak), 2E1 (weak)

Acetylcholinesterase inhibitors (central): May increase the risk of antipsychotic-related extrapyramidal symptoms; monitor.

Aluminum salts: May decrease the absorption of phenothiazines; monitor

Amphetamines: Efficacy may be diminished by antipsychotics; in addition, amphetamines may increase psychotic symptoms. Avoid concurrent use

Anticholinergics: May inhibit the therapeutic response to phenothiazines and excess anticholinergic effects may occur; includes benztropine, trihexyphenidyl, biperiden, and drugs with significant anticholinergic activity (TCAs, antihistamines, disopyramide)

Antihypertensives: Concurrent use of phenothiazines with an antihypertensive may produce additive hypotensive effects (particularly orthostasis)

Bromocriptine: Phenothiazines inhibit the ability of bromocriptine to lower serum prolactin concentrations

CNS depressants: Sedative effects may be additive with phenothiazines; monitor for increased effect; includes barbiturates, benzodiazepines, narcotic analgesics, ethanol, and other sedative agents

CYP2D6 inhibitors: May increase the levels/effects of fluphenazine. Example inhibitors include chlorpromazine, delavirdine, fluoxetine, miconazole, paroxetine, pergolide, quinidine, quinine, ritonavir, and ropinirole.

Epinephrine: Chlorpromazine (and possibly other low potency antipsychotics) may diminish the pressor effects of epinephrine

Guanethidine and guanadrel: Antihypertensive effects may be inhibited by phenothiazines

Levodopa: Phenothiazines may inhibit the antiparkinsonian effect of levodopa; avoid this combination

Lithium: Phenothiazines may produce neurotoxicity with lithium; this is a rare effect

Metoclopramide: May increase extrapyramidal symptoms (EPS) or risk.

Phenytoin: May reduce serum levels of phenothiazines; phenothiazines may increase phenytoin serum levels

Propranolol: Serum concentrations of phenothiazines may be increased; propranolol also increases phenothiazine concentrations

Polypeptide antibiotics: Rare cases of respiratory paralysis have been reported with concurrent use of phenothiazines

QT_c-prolonging agents: Effects on QT_c interval may be additive with phenothiazines, increasing the risk of malignant arrhythmias; includes type Ia antiarrhythmics, TCAs, and some quinolone antibiotics (sparfloxacin, moxifloxacin and gatifloxacin)

Sulfadoxine-pyrimethamine: May increase phenothiazine concentrations

Tricyclic antidepressants: Concurrent use may produce increased toxicity or altered therapeutic response

Trazodone: Phenothiazines and trazodone may produce additive hypotensive effects

Valproic acid: Serum levels may be increased by phenothiazines

Ethanol/Nutrition/Herb Interactions

Ethanol: Avoid ethanol (may increase CNS depression).

Herb/Nutraceutical: Avoid dong quai, St John's wort (may also cause photosensitization). Avoid kava kava, gotu kola, valerian, St John's wort (may increase CNS depression).

Dosage Forms [DSC] = Discontinued product

Elixir, as hydrochloride (Prolixin®): 2.5 mg/5 mL (60 mL) [contains alcohol 14% and sodium benzoate] [DSC]

Injection, oil, as decanoate: 25 mg/mL (5 mL) [may contain benzyl alcohol, sesame oil]

Prolixin Decanoate®: 25 mg/mL (5 mL) [contains benzyl alcohol, sesame oil]

Injection, solution, as hydrochloride (Prolixin® [DSC]): 2.5 mg/mL (10 mL)

Solution, oral concentrate, as hydrochloride (Prolixin®): 5 mg/mL (120 mL) [contains alcohol 14%] [DSC]

Tablet, as hydrochloride: 1 mg, 2.5 mg, 5 mg, 10 mg

Prolixin®: 1 mg, 2.5 mg, 5 mg [contains tartrazine], 10 mg [DSC]

♦ **Fluphenazine Decanoate** *see* Fluphenazine *on page 545*

Flurazepam (flure AZ e pam)

Medication Safety Issues
Sound-alike/look-alike issues:
Flurazepam may be confused with temazepam
Dalmane® may be confused with Demulen®, Dialume®

Related Information
Anesthesia Considerations for Neurosurgery *on page 1401*
Benzodiazepines *on page 1555*

U.S. Brand Names Dalmane®

Canadian Brand Names Apo-Flurazepam®; Dalmane®; Som Pam

Synonyms Flurazepam Hydrochloride

Pharmacologic Category Hypnotic, Benzodiazepine

Restrictions C-IV

Generic Available Yes

Use Short-term treatment of insomnia

Mechanism of Action Binds to stereospecific benzodiazepine receptors on the postsynaptic GABA neuron at several sites within the central nervous system, including the limbic system, reticular formation. Enhancement of the inhibitory effect of GABA on neuronal excitability results by increased neuronal membrane permeability to chloride ions. This shift in chloride ions results in hyperpolarization (a less excitable state) and stabilization.

Pharmacodynamics/Kinetics
Onset of action: Hypnotic: 15-20 minutes
Peak effect: 3-6 hours
Duration: 7-8 hours
Metabolism: Hepatic to N-desalkylflurazepam (active)
Half-life elimination: Desalkylflurazepam:
Adults: Single dose: 74-90 hours; Multiple doses: 111-113 hours
Elderly (61-85 years): Single dose: 120-160 hours; Multiple doses: 126-158 hours

Dosage Oral:
Children: Insomnia:
≤15 years: Dose not established
>15 years: 15 mg at bedtime
Adults: Insomnia: 15-30 mg at bedtime
Elderly: Insomnia: Oral: 15 mg at bedtime; avoid use if possible

Stability Store in light-resistant containers

Administration Give 30 minutes to 1 hour before bedtime on an empty stomach with full glass of water. May be taken with food if GI distress occurs.

Monitoring Parameters Respiratory and cardiovascular status

Reference Range Therapeutic: 0-4 ng/mL (SI: 0-9 nmol/L); Metabolite N-desalkylflurazepam: 20-110 ng/mL (SI: 43-240 nmol/L); Toxic: >0.12 mcg/mL

Anesthesia and Critical Care Concerns/Other Considerations Chronic use of this agent may increase the perioperative benzodiazepine dose needed to achieve desired effect. Abrupt discontinuation after sustained use (generally >10 days) may cause withdrawal symptoms.

Pregnancy Risk Factor X

Contraindications Hypersensitivity to flurazepam or any component of the formulation (cross-sensitivity with other benzodiazepines may exist); narrow-angle glaucoma; pregnancy

Warnings/Precautions Use with caution in elderly or debilitated patients, patients with hepatic disease (including alcoholics), or renal impairment. Active metabolites with extended half-lives may lead to delayed accumulation and adverse effects. Use with caution in patients with respiratory disease, or impaired gag reflex. Avoid use in patients with sleep apnea.

Causes CNS depression (dose-related) resulting in sedation, dizziness, confusion, or ataxia which may impair physical and mental capabilities. Patients must be cautioned about performing tasks which require mental alertness (eg, operating machinery or driving). Use with caution in patients receiving other CNS depressants or psychoactive agents. Effects with other sedative drugs or ethanol may be potentiated. Benzodiazepines have been associated with falls and traumatic injury and should be used with extreme caution in patients who are at risk of these events (especially the elderly).

Use caution in patients with depression, particularly if suicidal risk may be present. Use with caution in patients with a history of drug dependence. Benzodiazepines have been associated with dependence and acute withdrawal symptoms on discontinuation or reduction in dose (may occur after as little as 10 days of use). Acute withdrawal, including seizures, may be precipitated in patients after administration of flumazenil to patients receiving long-term benzodiazepine therapy.

As a hypnotic, should be used only after evaluation of potential causes of sleep disturbance. Failure of sleep disturbance to resolve after 7-10 days may indicate psychiatric or medical illness. A worsening of insomnia or the emergence of new abnormalities of thought or behavior may represent unrecognized psychiatric or medical illness and requires immediate and careful evaluation.

Benzodiazepines have been associated with anterograde amnesia. Paradoxical reactions, including hyperactive or aggressive behavior have been reported with benzodiazepines, particularly in adolescent/pediatric or psychiatric patients. Does not have analgesic, antidepressant, or antipsychotic properties.

Adverse Reactions Frequency not defined.

Cardiovascular: Palpitations, chest pain

Central nervous system: Drowsiness, ataxia, lightheadedness, memory impairment, depression, headache, hangover effect, confusion, nervousness, dizziness, falling, apprehension, irritability, euphoria, slurred speech, restlessness, hallucinations, paradoxical reactions, talkativeness

Dermatologic: Rash, pruritus

Gastrointestinal: Xerostomia, constipation, increased/excessive salivation, heartburn, upset stomach, nausea, vomiting, diarrhea, increased or decreased appetite, bitter taste, weight gain/loss

Hematologic: Euphoria, granulocytopenia

Hepatic: Elevated SGOT/SGPT, total bilirubin, alkaline phosphatase; cholestatic jaundice

Neuromuscular & skeletal: Dysarthria, body/joint pain, reflex slowing, weakness

Ocular: Blurred vision, burning eyes, difficulty focusing

Otic: Tinnitus

Respiratory: Apnea, dyspnea

Miscellaneous: Diaphoresis, drug dependence

Overdosage/Toxicology Symptoms of overdose include respiratory depression, hypoactive reflexes, unsteady gait, and hypotension. Treatment for benzodiazepine overdose is supportive. Flumazenil has been shown to selectively block the binding of benzodiazepines to CNS receptors, resulting in a reversal of benzodiazepine-induced CNS depression. Respiratory depression may not be reversed.

Drug Interactions **Substrate** of CYP3A4 (major); **Inhibits** CYP2E1 (weak)

CNS depressants: Sedative effects and/or respiratory depression may be additive with CNS depressants; includes ethanol, barbiturates, narcotic analgesics, and other sedative agents; monitor for increased effect

CYP3A4 inducers: CYP3A4 inducers may decrease the levels/effects of flurazepam. Example inducers include aminoglutethimide, carbamazepine, nafcillin, nevirapine, phenobarbital, phenytoin, and rifamycins.

CYP3A4 inhibitors: May increase the levels/effects of flurazepam. Example inhibitors include azole antifungals, clarithromycin, diclofenac, doxycycline, erythromycin, imatinib, isoniazid, nefazodone, nicardipine, propofol, protease inhibitors, quinidine, telithromycin, and verapamil.

Levodopa: Therapeutic effects may be diminished in some patients following the addition of a benzodiazepine; limited/inconsistent data

Oral contraceptives: May decrease the clearance of some benzodiazepines (those which undergo oxidative metabolism); monitor for increased benzodiazepine effect

Theophylline: May partially antagonize some of the effects of benzodiazepines; monitor for decreased response; may require higher doses for sedation

Ethanol/Nutrition/Herb Interactions

Ethanol: Avoid ethanol (may increase CNS depression).

Food: Serum levels and response to flurazepam may be increased by grapefruit juice, but unlikely because of flurazepam's high oral bioavailability.

Herb/Nutraceutical: Avoid valerian, St John's wort, kava kava, gotu kola (may increase CNS depression).

Dosage Forms Capsule, as hydrochloride: 15 mg, 30 mg

♦ **Flurazepam Hydrochloride** *see* Flurazepam *on page 548*

Flurbiprofen (flure BI proe fen)

Medication Safety Issues

Sound-alike/look-alike issues:

Flurbiprofen may be confused with fenoprofen

Ansaid® may be confused with Asacol®, Axid®

Ocufen® may be confused with Ocuflox®, Ocupress®

Related Information

Chronic Pain Management *on page 1430*

U.S. Brand Names Ansaid® [DSC]; Ocufen®

Canadian Brand Names Alti-Flurbiprofen; Ansaid®; Apo-Flurbiprofen®; Froben®; Froben-SR®; Novo-Flurprofen; Nu-Flurprofen; Ocufen®

Synonyms Flurbiprofen Sodium

Pharmacologic Category Nonsteroidal Anti-inflammatory Drug (NSAID), Ophthalmic; Nonsteroidal Anti-inflammatory Drug (NSAID), Oral

Restrictions A medication guide should be dispensed with each prescription. A template for the required MedGuide can be found on the FDA website at: http://www.fda.gov/medwatch/SAFETY/2005/safety05.htm#NSAID

Generic Available Yes

Use

Oral: Treatment of rheumatoid arthritis and osteoarthritis

Ophthalmic: Inhibition of intraoperative miosis

Mechanism of Action Inhibits prostaglandin synthesis by decreasing the activity of the enzyme, cyclooxygenase, which results in decreased formation of prostaglandin precursors

Pharmacodynamics/Kinetics

Onset of action: ~1-2 hours

Distribution: V_d: 0.12 L/kg

Protein binding: 99%, primarily albumin

Metabolism: Hepatic via CYP2C9; forms metabolites such as 4-hydroxy-flurbiprofen (inactive)

Half-life elimination: 5.7 hours

Time to peak: 1.5 hours

Excretion: Urine (primarily as metabolites)

Dosage

Oral:

Rheumatoid arthritis and osteoarthritis: 200-300 mg/day in 2-, 3-, or 4 divided doses; do not administer more than 100 mg for any single dose; maximum: 300 mg/day

Dental: Management of postoperative pain: 100 mg every 12 hours

Ophthalmic: Instill 1 drop every 30 minutes, beginning 2 hours prior to surgery (total of 4 drops in each affected eye)

Dosage adjustment in renal impairment: Not recommended in patients with advanced renal disease

Administration Tablet: Take with a full glass of water.

Anesthesia and Critical Care Concerns/Other Considerations The 2002 ACCM/SCCM guidelines for analgesia (critically-ill adult) suggest that NSAIDs may be used in combination with opioids in select patients for pain management. Concern about adverse events (increased risk of renal dysfunction, altered platelet function and gastrointestinal irritation) limits its use in patients who have other underlying risks for these events.

In short-term use, NSAIDs vary considerably in their effect on blood pressure. When NSAIDs are used in patients with hypertension, appropriate monitoring of blood pressure responses should be completed and the duration of therapy, when possible, kept short. The use of NSAIDs in the treatment of patients with congestive heart failure may be associated with an increased risk for fluid accumulation and edema; may precipitate renal failure in dehydrated patients.

Pregnancy Risk Factor C/D (3rd trimester)

Contraindications Hypersensitivity to flurbiprofen, aspirin, other NSAIDs, or any component of the formulation; perioperative pain in the setting of coronary artery bypass surgery (CABG); dendritic keratitis; pregnancy (3rd trimester)

Warnings/Precautions [U.S. Boxed Warning]: NSAIDs are associated with an increased risk of adverse cardiovascular events, including MI, stroke, and new onset or worsening of pre-existing hypertension. Risk may be increased with duration of use or pre-existing cardiovascular risk-factors or disease. Carefully evaluate individual cardiovascular risk profiles prior to prescribing. Use caution with fluid retention, CHF, or hypertension.

Use of NSAIDs can compromise existing renal function. Renal toxicity can occur in patient with impaired renal function, dehydration, heart failure, liver dysfunction, those taking diuretics and ACEI, and the elderly. Rehydrate patient before starting therapy. Monitor renal function closely. Not recommended for use in patients with advanced renal disease.

[U.S. Boxed Warning]: NSAIDs may increase risk of gastrointestinal irritation, ulceration, bleeding, and perforation. These events may occur at any time during therapy and without warning. Use caution with a history of GI disease (bleeding or ulcers), concurrent therapy with aspirin, anticoagulants and/or corticosteroids, smoking, use of alcohol, the elderly or debilitated patients.

Use the lowest effective dose for the shortest duration of time, consistent with individual patient goals, to reduce risk of cardiovascular or GI adverse events. Alternate therapies should be considered for patients at high risk.

NSAIDs may cause serious skin adverse events including exfoliative dermatitis, Stevens-Johnson syndrome (SJS), and toxic epidermal necrolysis (TEN). Anaphylactoid reactions may occur, even without prior exposure; patients with "aspirin triad" (bronchial asthma, aspirin intolerance, rhinitis) may be at increased risk. Do not use in patients who experience bronchospasm, asthma, rhinitis, or urticaria with NSAID or aspirin therapy.

Use with caution in patients with decreased hepatic function. Closely monitor patients with any abnormal LFT. Severe hepatic reactions (eg, fulminant hepatitis, liver failure) have occurred with NSAID use, rarely; discontinue if signs or symptoms of liver disease develop, or if systemic manifestations occur.

The elderly are at increased risk for adverse effects (especially peptic ulceration, CNS effects, renal toxicity) from NSAIDs even at low doses.

Withhold for at least 4-6 half-lives prior to surgical or dental procedures. Safety and efficacy have not been established in children <18 years of age.

Adverse Reactions

Ophthalmic: Frequency not defined: Ocular: Slowing of corneal wound healing, mild ocular stinging, itching and burning, ocular irritation, fibrosis, miosis, mydriasis, bleeding tendency increased

Oral:

>1%:

Cardiovascular: Edema

Central nervous system: Amnesia, anxiety, depression, dizziness, headache, insomnia, malaise, nervousness, somnolence

Dermatologic: Rash

Gastrointestinal: Abdominal pain, constipation, diarrhea, dyspepsia, flatulence, GI bleeding, nausea, vomiting, weight changes

Hepatic: Liver enzymes elevated

Neuromuscular & skeletal: Reflexes increased, tremor, vertigo, weakness

Ocular: Vision changes

Otic: Tinnitus

Respiratory: Rhinitis

<1% (Limited to important or life-threatening): Anaphylactic reaction, anemia, angioedema, asthma, bruising, cerebrovascular ischemia, CHF, confusion, eczema, eosinophilia, epistaxis, exfoliative dermatitis, fever, gastric/peptic ulcer, hematocrit decreased, hematuria, hemoglobin decreased, hepatitis, hypertension, hyperuricemia, interstitial nephritis, jaundice, leukopenia, paresthesia, parosmia, photosensitivity, pruritus, purpura, renal failure, stomatitis, thrombocytopenia, toxic epidermal necrolysis, urticaria, vasodilation

Overdosage/Toxicology Symptoms of overdose include apnea, metabolic acidosis, coma, nystagmus, leukocytosis, and renal failure. Management of NSAID intoxication is supportive and symptomatic. Since many NSAIDs undergo enterohepatic cycling, multiple doses of charcoal may be needed to reduce the potential for delayed toxicities.

Drug Interactions Substrate of CYP2C9 (minor); **Inhibits** CYP2C9 (strong)

ACE inhibitors: Antihypertensive effects may be decreased by concurrent therapy with NSAIDs; monitor blood pressure.

Angiotensin II antagonists: Antihypertensive effects may be decreased by concurrent therapy with NSAIDs; monitor blood pressure.

(Continued)

Flurbiprofen *(Continued)*

Anticoagulants (warfarin, heparin, LMWHs) in combination with NSAIDs can cause increased risk of bleeding.

Antiplatelet drugs (ticlopidine, clopidogrel, aspirin, abciximab, dipyridamole, eptifibatide, tirofiban) can cause an increased risk of bleeding.

Beta-blockers: NSAIDs may decrease the antihypertensive effect of beta-blockers. Monitor.

Cholestyramine (and other bile acid sequestrants): May decrease the absorption of NSAIDs. Separate by at least 2 hours.

Corticosteroids may increase the risk of GI ulceration; avoid concurrent use.

Cyclosporine: NSAIDs may increase serum creatinine, potassium, blood pressure, and cyclosporine levels; monitor cyclosporine levels and renal function carefully.

CYP2C9 Substrates: Flurbiprofen may increase the levels/effects of CYP2C9 substrates. Example substrates include bosentan, dapsone, fluoxetine, glimepiride, glipizide, losartan, montelukast, nateglinide, paclitaxel, phenytoin, warfarin, and zafirlukast.

Gentamicin and amikacin serum concentrations are increased by indomethacin in premature infants. Results may apply to other aminoglycosides and NSAIDs.

Hydralazine's antihypertensive effect is decreased; avoid concurrent use.

Lithium levels can be increased; avoid concurrent use if possible or monitor lithium levels and adjust dose. Sulindac may have the least effect. When NSAID is stopped, lithium will need adjustment again.

Loop diuretics efficacy (diuretic and antihypertensive effect) is reduced. Indomethacin reduces this efficacy, however, it may be anticipated with any NSAID.

Methotrexate: Severe bone marrow suppression, aplastic anemia, and GI toxicity have been reported with concomitant NSAID therapy. Avoid use during moderate or high-dose methotrexate (increased and prolonged methotrexate levels). NSAID use during low-dose treatment of rheumatoid arthritis has not been fully evaluated; extreme caution is warranted.

Thiazides antihypertensive effects are decreased; avoid concurrent use.

Warfarin's INRs may be increased by piroxicam. Other NSAIDs may have the same effect depending on dose and duration. Monitor INR closely. Use the lowest dose of NSAIDs possible and for the briefest duration.

Verapamil plasma concentration is decreased by some NSAIDs; avoid concurrent use.

Ethanol/Nutrition/Herb Interactions

Ethanol: Avoid ethanol (may enhance gastric mucosal irritation).

Food: Food may decrease the rate but not the extent of absorption.

Herb/Nutraceutical: Avoid alfalfa, anise, bilberry, bladderwrack, bromelain, cat's claw, celery, coleus, cordyceps, dong quai, evening primrose, feverfew, fenugreek, garlic, ginger, ginkgo biloboa, red clover, horse chestnut, grapeseed, green tea, ginseng, guggul, horse chestnut seed, horseradish, licorice, prickly ash, red clover, reishi, SAMe, sweet clover, turmeric, white willow (all have additional antiplatelet activity).

Dietary Considerations Tablet may be taken with food, milk, or antacid to decrease GI effects.

Dosage Forms [DSC] = Discontinued product

Solution, ophthalmic, as sodium (Ocufen®): 0.03% (2.5 mL) [contains thimerosal]

Tablet: 50 mg, 100 mg

Ansaid®: 50 mg, 100 mg [DSC]

♦ **Flurbiprofen Sodium** *see* Flurbiprofen *on page 550*

Fluvastatin (FLOO va sta tin)

Medication Safety Issues

Sound-alike/look-alike issues:

Fluvastatin may be confused with fluoxetine

Related Information

Hyperlipidemia Management *on page 1614*

U.S. Brand Names Lescol®; Lescol® XL

Canadian Brand Names Lescol®; Lescol® XL

Pharmacologic Category Antilipemic Agent, HMG-CoA Reductase Inhibitor

Generic Available No

Use To be used as a component of multiple risk factor intervention in patients at risk for atherosclerosis vascular disease due to hypercholesterolemia

Adjunct to dietary therapy to reduce elevated total cholesterol (total-C), LDL-C, triglyceride, and apolipoprotein B (apo-B) levels and to increase HDL-C in primary hypercholesterolemia and mixed dyslipidemia (Fredrickson types IIa and IIb); to slow the progression of coronary atherosclerosis in patients with coronary heart disease; reduce risk of coronary revascularization procedures in patients with coronary heart disease

Mechanism of Action Acts by competitively inhibiting 3-hydroxyl-3-methylglutaryl-coenzyme A (HMG-CoA) reductase, the enzyme that catalyzes the reduction of HMG-CoA to mevalonate; this is an early rate-limiting step in cholesterol biosynthesis. HDL is increased while total, LDL and VLDL cholesterols, apolipoprotein B, and plasma triglycerides are decreased.

Pharmacodynamics/Kinetics

Onset: Peak effect: Maximal LDL-C reductions achieved within 4 weeks
Distribution: V_d: 0.35 L/kg
Protein binding: >98%
Metabolism: To inactive and active metabolites (oxidative metabolism via CYP2C9 [75%], 2C8 [~5%], and 3A4 [~20%] isoenzymes); active forms do not circulate systemically; extensive (saturable) first-pass hepatic extraction
Bioavailability: Absolute: Capsule: 24%; Extended release tablet: 29%
Half-life elimination: Capsule: <3 hours; Extended release tablet: 9 hours
Time to peak: Capsule: 1 hour; Extended release tablet: 3 hours
Excretion: Feces (90%): urine (5%)

Dosage

Adolescents 10-16 years: Oral: Heterozygous familial hypercholesterolemia: Initial: 20 mg once daily; may increase every 6 weeks based on tolerability and response to a maximum recommended dose of 80 mg/day, given in 2 divided doses (immediate release capsule) or as a single daily dose (extended release tablet)

Note: Indicated only for adjunctive therapy when diet alone cannot reduce LDL-C below 190 mg/dL, or 160 mg/dL (with cardiovascular risk factors). Female patients must be 1 year postmenarche.

Adults: Oral:

Patients requiring ≥25% decrease in LDL-C: 40 mg capsule once daily in the evening, 80 mg extended release tablet once daily (anytime), or 40 mg capsule twice daily

Patients requiring <25% decrease in LDL-C: Initial: 20 mg capsule once daily in the evening; may increase based on tolerability and response to a maximum recommended dose of 80 mg/day, given in 2 divided doses (immediate release capsule) or as a single daily dose (extended release tablet)

Dosage adjustment in renal impairment: Less than 6% excreted renally; no dosage adjustment needed with mild-to-moderate renal impairment; use with caution in severe impairment

Dosage adjustment in hepatic impairment: Levels may accumulate in patients with liver disease (increased AUC and C_{max}); use caution with severe hepatic impairment or heavy ethanol ingestion; contraindicated in active liver disease or unexplained transaminase elevations; decrease dose and monitor effects carefully in patients with hepatic insufficiency

Elderly: No dosage adjustment necessary based on age

Stability Store at 15°C to 30°C (59°F to 86°F); protect from light

Administration Patient should be placed on a standard cholesterol-lowering diet before and during treatment; fluvastatin may be taken without regard to meals; adjust dosage as needed in response to periodic lipid determinations during the first 4 weeks after a dosage change; lipid-lowering effects are additive when fluvastatin is combined with a bile-acid binding resin or niacin, however, it must be administered at least 2 hours following these drugs. Do not break, chew, or crush extended release tablets; do not open capsules.

Monitoring Parameters Obtain baseline LFTs and total cholesterol profile; repeat tests at 12 weeks after initiation of therapy or elevation in dose, and periodically thereafter. Monitor LDL-C at intervals no less than 4 weeks.

Anesthesia and Critical Care Concerns/Other Considerations Statin therapy should be held temporarily in patients with conditions (ie, sepsis; hypotension; major surgery; trauma; severe metabolic, endocrine or electrolyte disorders; uncontrolled seizures) that predispose them to acute renal failure secondary to rhabdomyolysis.

(Continued)

Fluvastatin *(Continued)*

Myopathy: Currently marketed HMG-CoA reductase inhibitors appear to have a similar potential for causing myopathy. Incidence of severe myopathy is about 0.08% to 0.09%. The factors that increase risk include advanced age (especially >80 years of age), women more frequently than men, small body frame, frailty, multisystem disease (eg, chronic renal insufficiency especially due to diabetes), multiple medications, perioperative periods (higher risk when continued during hospitalization for major surgery), drug interactions (use with caution or avoid). The combination of a HMG-CoA reductase inhibitor plus nicotinic acid seems to carry a lower risk of myopathy than does a HMG-CoA reductase inhibitor plus a fibrate. Other medications, when used concurrently, may enhance the risk of myopathy associated with statins; these include drugs that inhibit CYP3A4 isoenzymes (lovastatin, simvastatin, atorvastatin) or CYP2C9 isoenzymes (fluvastatin). HMG-CoA reductase inhibitors may exacerbate exercise-induced skeletal muscle injury. Many experts favor getting a baseline creatine kinase (CK) measurement before initiating therapy (asymptomatic CK elevations are common). Obtain a CK measurement if patient complains of muscle soreness, tenderness, or pain.

Pregnancy Risk Factor X

Contraindications Hypersensitivity to fluvastatin or any component of the formulation; active liver disease; unexplained persistent elevations of serum transaminases; pregnancy; breast-feeding

Warnings/Precautions Secondary causes of hyperlipidemia should be ruled out prior to therapy. Liver function must be monitored by periodic laboratory assessment. Rhabdomyolysis with acute renal failure has occurred with fluvastatin and other HMG-CoA reductase inhibitors. Risk may be increased with concurrent use of other drugs which may cause rhabdomyolysis (including gemfibrozil, fibric acid derivatives, or niacin at doses ≥1 g/day). Temporarily discontinue in any patient experiencing markedly elevated CPK levels, myopathy, or an acute/serious condition predisposing to renal failure secondary to rhabdomyolysis. Use caution in patients with previous liver disease or heavy ethanol use. Use caution in patients with concurrent medications or conditions which reduce steroidogenesis. Efficacy and safety in children <10 years of age have not been established.

Adverse Reactions As reported with fluvastatin capsules; in general, adverse reactions reported with fluvastatin extended release tablet were similar, but the incidence was less.

1% to 10%:

- Central nervous system: Headache (9%), fatigue (3%), insomnia (3%)
- Gastrointestinal: Dyspepsia (8%), diarrhea (5%), abdominal pain (5%), nausea (3%)
- Genitourinary: Urinary tract infection (2%)
- Neuromuscular & skeletal: Myalgia (5%)
- Respiratory: Sinusitis (3%), bronchitis (2%)

<1% (Limited to important or life-threatening) including additional class-related events (not necessarily reported with fluvastatin therapy): Alopecia, anaphylaxis, angioedema, arthralgia, arthritis, cataracts, cholestatic jaundice, cirrhosis, CPK increased (>10x normal), depression, dermatomyositis, dyspnea, eosinophilia, erectile dysfunction, erythema multiforme, ESR increased, facial paresis, fatty liver, fever, fulminant hepatic necrosis, gynecomastia, hemolytic anemia, hepatitis, hepatoma, hypersensitivity reaction, impotence, leukopenia, memory loss, muscle cramps, myopathy, nodules, ophthalmoplegia, pancreatitis, paresthesia, peripheral nerve palsy, peripheral neuropathy, photosensitivity, polymyalgia rheumatica, positive ANA, pruritus, psychic disturbance, purpura, rash, renal failure (secondary to rhabdomyolysis), rhabdomyolysis, skin discoloration, Stevens-Johnson syndrome, systemic lupus erythematosus-like syndrome, taste alteration, thrombocytopenia, thyroid dysfunction, toxic epidermal necrolysis, transaminases increased, tremor, urticaria, vasculitis, vertigo

Overdosage/Toxicology GI complaints and elevated SGOT and SGPT have been reported following large doses of the extended release tablets. In case of overdose, treatment should be symptom-directed and supportive; dialyzability is not known, but given high protein binding not likely to benefit.

Drug Interactions Substrate of CYP2C9 (major), 2C8 (minor), 2D6 (minor), 3A4 (minor); **Inhibits** CYP1A2 (weak), 2C8 (weak), 2C9 (moderate), 2D6 (weak), 3A4 (weak)

Cholestyramine: Cholestyramine may decrease the absorption of fluvastatin. Separate administration times by at least 4 hours. Cholestyramine may increase the therapeutic effects of fluvastatin.

CYP2C9 inhibitors: May increase the levels/effects of fluvastatin. Example inhibitors include delavirdine, fluconazole, gemfibrozil, ketoconazole, nicardipine, NSAIDs, sulfonamides, and tolbutamide.

CYP2C9 substrates: Fluvastatin may increase levels/effects of CYP2C9 substrates. Example substrates include bosentan, dapsone, fluoxetine, glimepiride, glipizide, losartan, montelukast, nateglinide, paclitaxel, phenytoin, warfarin, and zafirlukast.

Fibric acid derivatives: May increase the risk of myopathy and rhabdomyolysis.

Fluconazole: May increase the levels/effects of fluvastatin; monitor.

Glyburide: C_{max} and AUC of both fluvastatin and glyburide may increase; half-life of glyburide may also increase; monitor

Omeprazole: Omeprazole may increase serum concentrations of fluvastatin

Phenytoin: C_{max} and AUC of both phenytoin and fluvastatin may be increased when given together; monitor phenytoin when fluvastatin is initiated, modified, or discontinued

Rifamycin derivatives: May decrease serum concentrations of fluvastatin

Warfarin: Fluvastatin may increase hypoprothrombinemic effects of warfarin; monitor INR closely when fluvastatin is initiated, modified, or discontinued

Ethanol/Nutrition/Herb Interactions

Ethanol: Avoid excessive ethanol consumption (due to potential hepatic effects).

Food: Reduces rate but not the extent of absorption. Red yeast rice contains an estimated 2.4 mg lovastatin per 600 mg rice.

Dietary Considerations Generally, patients should be placed on a standard cholesterol-lowering diet and other lifestyle modifications for 3-6 months prior to the initiation of drug therapy. The diet should be continued during drug therapy. However, for patients with advanced risk factors (eg, known coronary heart disease), drug therapy may be initiated concurrently with diet modification. May be taken without regard to meals. Red yeast rice contains an estimated 2.4 mg lovastatin per 600 mg rice.

Dosage Forms

Capsule (Lescol®): 20 mg, 40 mg

Tablet, extended release (Lescol® XL): 80 mg

- **Fluxid™** *see* Famotidine *on page 506*
- **Folinic Acid** *see* Leucovorin *on page 738*

Fomepizole (foe ME pi zole)

U.S. Brand Names Antizol®

Synonyms 4-Methylpyrazole; 4-MP

Pharmacologic Category Antidote

Generic Available No

Use Orphan drug: Treatment of methanol or ethylene glycol poisoning alone or in combination with hemodialysis

Unlabeled/Investigational Use Known or suspected propylene glycol toxicity

Mechanism of Action Fomepizole competitively inhibits alcohol dehydrogenase, an enzyme which catalyzes the metabolism of ethanol, ethylene glycol, and methanol to their toxic metabolites. Ethylene glycol is metabolized to glycoaldehyde, then oxidized to glycolate, glyoxylate, and oxalate. Glycolate and oxalate are responsible for metabolic acidosis and renal damage. Methanol is metabolized to formaldehyde, then oxidized to formic acid. Formic acid is responsible for metabolic acidosis and visual disturbances.

Pharmacodynamics/Kinetics

Onset of effect: Peak effect: Maximum: 1.5-2 hours

Absorption: Oral: Readily absorbed

Distribution: V_d: 0.6-1.02 L/kg; rapidly into total body water

Protein binding: Negligible

Metabolism: Hepatic to 4-carboxypyrazole (80% to 85% of dose), 4-hydroxymethylpyrazole, and their N-glucuronide conjugates; following multiple doses, induces its own metabolism via CYP oxidases after 30-40 hours

Half-life elimination: Has not been calculated; varies with dose

Excretion: Urine (1% to 3.5% as unchanged drug and metabolites)

Dosage Adults: Ethylene glycol and methanol toxicity: I.V.: A loading dose of 15 mg/kg should be administered, followed by doses of 10 mg/kg every 12 hours for 4 doses, then 15 mg/kg every 12 hours thereafter until ethylene glycol levels have been reduced <20 mg/dL and patient is asymptomatic with normal pH

(Continued)

Fomepizole *(Continued)*

Dosage adjustment in renal impairment: Fomepizole and its metabolites are excreted in the urine; dialysis should be considered in addition to fomepizole in the case of renal failure, significant or worsening metabolic acidosis, or a measured ethylene glycol level of ≥50 mg/dL. Patients should be dialyzed to correct metabolic abnormalities and to lower the ethylene glycol level <50 mg/dL; fomepizole is dialyzable and the frequency of dosing should be increased to every 4 hours during hemodialysis

Fomepizole is dialyzable and the frequency of dosing should be increased to every 4 hours during hemodialysis

Dose at the beginning of hemodialysis:

If <6 hours since last fomepizole dose: Do not administer dose

If ≥6 hours since last fomepizole dose: Administer next scheduled dose

Dosing during hemodialysis: Dose every 4 hours

Dosing at the time hemodialysis is complete, based on time between last dose and the end of hemodialysis:

<1 hour: Do not administer dose at the end of hemodialysis

1-3 hours: Administer 1/2 of next scheduled dose

>3 hours: Administer next scheduled dose

Maintenance dose when off hemodialysis: Give next scheduled dose 12 hours from last dose administered.

Dosage adjustment in hepatic impairment: Fomepizole is metabolized in the liver; specific dosage adjustments have not been determined in patients with hepatic impairment

Stability Fomepizole diluted in 0.9% sodium chloride injection or dextrose 5% injection is stable for at least 24 hours when stored refrigerated or at room temperature; although, it is chemically and physically stable when diluted as recommended, sterile precautions should be observed because diluents generally do not contain preservatives.

After dilution, do not use beyond 24 hours. Fomepizole solidifies at temperatures <25°C (77°F). If the fomepizole solution has become solid in the vial, the solution should carefully be warmed by running the vial under warm water or by holding in the hand. Solidification does not affect the efficacy, safety, or stability of the drug.

Administration The appropriate dose of fomepizole should be drawn from the vial with a syringe and injected into at least 100 mL of sterile 0.9% sodium chloride injection or dextrose 5% injection. All doses should be administered as a slow intravenous infusion (IVPB) over 30 minutes.

Monitoring Parameters Fomepizole plasma levels should be monitored; response to fomepizole; monitor plasma/urinary ethylene glycol or methanol levels, urinary oxalate (ethylene glycol), plasma/urinary osmolality, renal/hepatic function, serum electrolytes, arterial blood gases; anion and osmolar gaps, resolution of clinical signs and symptoms of ethylene glycol or methanol intoxication

Reference Range

Fomepizole: Concentrations 100-300 µmol/L (8.2-24.6 mg/L) should result in enzyme inhibition of alcohol dehydrogenase

Ethylene glycol: Lethal dose is ~1.4 mL/kg

Methanol: Lethal dose is ~1-2 mL/kg

Anesthesia and Critical Care Concerns/Other Considerations Alternate therapies, including ethanol and hemodialysis, are difficult to use in children. Fomepizole's affinity for alcohol dehydrogenase is 8000 times greater than ethanol.

Pregnancy Risk Factor C

Contraindications Documented serious hypersensitivity reaction to fomepizole or other pyrazoles; hypersensitivity to any component of the formulation

Warnings/Precautions Should not be given undiluted or by bolus injection; fomepizole is metabolized in the liver and excreted in the urine, use caution with hepatic or renal impairment; hemodialysis should be used in patients with renal failure, significant or worsening metabolic acidosis, or ethylene glycol/methanol levels ≥50 mg/dL; monitor and manage adverse events of intoxication (respiratory distress syndrome, visual disturbances, hypocalcemia); safety and efficacy in pediatric patients have not been established

Adverse Reactions

>10%:

Central nervous system: Headache (14%)

Gastrointestinal: Nausea (11%)

1% to 10% (≤3% unless otherwise noted):

Cardiovascular: Bradycardia, facial flush, hypotension, phlebosclerosis, shock, tachycardia

Central nervous system: Dizziness (6%), increased drowsiness (6%), agitation, anxiety, lightheadedness, seizure, vertigo

Dermatologic: Rash

Endocrine & metabolic: Increased liver function tests

Gastrointestinal: Bad/metallic taste (6%), abdominal pain, decreased appetite, diarrhea, heartburn, vomiting

Hematologic: Anemia, disseminated intravascular coagulation, eosinophilia, lymphangitis

Local: Application site reaction, inflammation at the injection site, pain during injection, phlebitis

Neuromuscular & skeletal: Backache

Ocular: Nystagmus, transient blurred vision, visual disturbances

Renal: Anuria

Respiratory: Abnormal smell, hiccups, pharyngitis

Miscellaneous: Multiorgan failure, speech disturbances

<1% (Limited to important or life-threatening): Mild allergic reactions (mild rash, eosinophilia)

Overdosage/Toxicology

Nausea, dizziness, and vertigo were noted in healthy volunteers receiving 3-6 times the recommended dose. This dose-dependent CNS effect was short-lived in most subjects and lasted up to 30 hours in one subject.

Because fomepizole is dialyzable, dialysis may be useful in treating cases of overdosage

Ethanol/Nutrition/Herb Interactions Ethanol: Ethanol decreases the rate of fomepizole elimination by ~50%; conversely, fomepizole decreases the rate of elimination of ethanol by ~40%.

Dosage Forms Injection, solution [preservative free]: 1 g/mL (1.5 mL)

References

"American Academy of Clinical Toxicology Practice Guidelines on the Treatment of Methanol Poisoning," *J Toxicol Clin Toxicol*, 2002, 40(4):415-46.

Brent J, McMartin K, Phillips S, et al, "Fomepizole for the Treatment of Methanol Poisoning," *N Engl J Med*, 2001, 344(6):424-9.

Mokhlesi B, Leikin JB, Murray P, et al, "Adult Toxicology in Critical Care. Part 11: Specific Poisonings," *Chest*, 2003, 123(3):897-922.

Fondaparinux (fon da PARE i nuks)

U.S. Brand Names Arixtra®

Canadian Brand Names Arixtra®

Synonyms Fondaparinux Sodium

Pharmacologic Category Factor Xa Inhibitor

Generic Available No

Use Prophylaxis of deep vein thrombosis (DVT) in patients undergoing surgery for hip replacement, knee replacement, hip fracture (including extended prophylaxis following hip fracture surgery), or abdominal surgery (in patients at risk for thromboembolic complications); treatment of acute pulmonary embolism (PE); treatment of acute DVT without PE

Mechanism of Action Fondaparinux is a synthetic pentasaccharide that causes an antithrombin III-mediated selective inhibition of factor Xa. Neutralization of factor Xa interrupts the blood coagulation cascade and inhibits thrombin formation and thrombus development.

Pharmacodynamics/Kinetics

Absorption: Rapid and complete

Distribution: V_d: 7-11 L; mainly in blood

Protein binding: ≥94% to antithrombin III

Bioavailability: 100%

Half-life elimination: 17-21 hours; prolonged with worsening renal impairment

Time to peak: 2-3 hours

Excretion: Urine (as unchanged drug); decreased clearance in patients <50 kg

Dosage SubQ:

DVT prophylaxis: Adults ≥50 kg: 2.5 mg once daily. **Note:** Initiate dose after hemostasis has been established, 6-8 hours postoperatively.

Usual duration: 5-9 days (up to 10 days following abdominal surgery or up to 11 days following hip replacement or knee replacement)

(Continued)

Fondaparinux *(Continued)*

Extended prophylaxis is recommended following hip fracture surgery (has been tolerated for up to 32 days).

Acute DVT/PE treatment: SubQ: Adults: **Note:** Concomitant treatment with warfarin sodium should be initiated as soon as possible, usually within 72 hours:

<50 kg: 5 mg once daily

50-100 kg: 7.5 mg once daily

>100 kg: 10 mg once daily

Usual duration: 5-9 days (has been administered up to 26 days)

Dosage adjustment in renal impairment:

Cl_{cr} 30-50 mL/minute: Use caution

Cl_{cr} <30 mL/minute: Contraindicated

Stability Store at 15°C to 30°C (59°F to 86°F).

Administration Do not administer I.M.; for SubQ administration only. Do not mix with other injections or infusions. Do not expel air bubble from syringe before injection. Administer according to recommended regimen; early initiation (before 6 hours after surgery) has been associated with increased bleeding.

Monitoring Parameters Periodic monitoring of CBC, serum creatinine, occult blood testing of stools recommended. Antifactor Xa activity of fondaparinux can be measured by the assay if fondaparinux is used as the calibrator. PT and aPTT are insensitive measures of fondaparinux activity.

Pregnancy Risk Factor B

Contraindications Hypersensitivity to fondaparinux or any component of the formulation; severe renal impairment (Cl_{cr} <30 mL/minute); body weight <50 kg (prophylaxis); active major bleeding; bacterial endocarditis; thrombocytopenia associated with a positive *in vitro* test for antiplatelet antibody in the presence of fondaparinux

Warnings/Precautions [U.S. Boxed Warning]: Patients with recent or anticipated neuraxial anesthesia (epidural or spinal anesthesia) are at risk of spinal or epidural hematoma and subsequent paralysis. Consider risk versus benefit prior to neuraxial anesthesia; risk is increased by concomitant agents which may alter hemostasis, as well as traumatic or repeated epidural or spinal puncture. Patient should be observed closely for bleeding if administered during or immediately following diagnostic lumbar puncture, epidural anesthesia, or spinal anesthesia.

Not to be used interchangeably (unit-for-unit) with heparin, low molecular weight heparins (LMWHs), or heparinoids. Use caution in patients with moderate renal dysfunction (Cl_{cr} 30-50 mL/minute). Patients with serum creatinine >2 mg/dL were excluded from clinical trials. Periodically monitor renal function; discontinue if severe dysfunction or labile function develops.

Use caution in conditions with increased risk of hemorrhage such as congenital or acquired bleeding disorders; active ulcerative or angiodysplastic gastrointestinal disease; hemorrhagic stroke; shortly after brain, spinal, or ophthalmologic surgery; or in patients taking platelet inhibitors. Risk of major bleeding may be increased if initial dose is administered earlier then recommended (initiation recommended at 6-8 hours following surgery). Discontinue agents that may enhance the risk of hemorrhage if possible. If thrombocytopenia occurs, discontinue fondaparinux. Use caution in the elderly, patients with a history of heparin-induced thrombocytopenia, patients with a bleeding diathesis, uncontrolled hypertension, recent gastrointestinal ulceration, diabetic retinopathy, and hemorrhage. Use caution in patients <50 kg who are being treated for DVT/PE; fondaparinux clearance may be decreased. Safety and efficacy in pediatric patients have not been established.

Adverse Reactions As with all anticoagulants, bleeding is the major adverse effect. Hemorrhage may occur at any site. Risk appears increased by a number of factors including renal dysfunction, age (>75 years), and weight (<50 kg).

>10%:

Central nervous system: Fever (4% to 14%)

Gastrointestinal: Nausea (11%)

Hematologic: Anemia (20%)

1% to 10%:

Cardiovascular: Edema (9%), hypotension (4%), confusion (3%)

Central nervous system: Insomnia (5%), dizziness (4%), headache (2% to 5%), pain (2%)

Dermatologic: Rash (8%), purpura (4%), bullous eruption (3%)
Endocrine & metabolic: Hypokalemia (1% to 4%)
Gastrointestinal: Constipation (5% to 9%), vomiting (6%), diarrhea (3%), dyspepsia (2%)
Genitourinary: Urinary tract infection (4%), urinary retention (3%)
Hematologic: Moderate thrombocytopenia (50,000-100,000/mm^3: 3%), major bleeding (1% to 3%), minor bleeding (2% to 4%), hematoma (3%); risk of major bleeding increased as high as 5% in patients receiving initial dose <6 hours following surgery
Hepatic: SGOT increased (2%), SGPT increased (3%)
Local: Injection site reaction (bleeding, rash, pruritus)
Miscellaneous: Wound drainage increased (5%)

<1% (Limited to important or life-threatening): Hepatic enzymes increased, severe thrombocytopenia (<50,000/mm^3)

Overdosage/Toxicology Treatment is symptom-directed and supportive. Hemodialysis may increase clearance by 20%.

Drug Interactions

Anticoagulants: May enhance the effects of other anticoagulants.
Antiplatelet agents (including abciximab, anagrelide, cilostazol, clopidogrel, dipyridamole, eptifibatide, ticlopidine, tirofiban): May enhance the anticoagulant effect of fondaparinux.
Drotrecogin alfa: May enhance the bleeding potential with drotrecogin alfa.
NSAIDs: May enhance the anticoagulant effect of fondaparinux.
Salicylates: May enhance the anticoagulant effect of fondaparinux.
Thrombolytic agents: Increase the risk of hemorrhage.

Ethanol/Nutrition/Herb Interactions Herb/Nutraceutical: Avoid alfalfa, anise, bilberry, bladderwrack, bromelain, cat's claw, celery, coleus, cordyceps, dong quai, evening primrose oil, fenugreek, feverfew, garlic, ginger, ginkgo biloba, ginseng (American/Panax/Siberian), grape seed, green tea, guggul, horse chestnut seed, horseradish, licorice, prickly ash, red clover, reishi, sweet clover, turmeric, white willow (all possess anticoagulant or antiplatelet activity and as such, may enhance the anticoagulant effects of fondaparinux).

Test Interactions International standards of heparin or LMWH are not the appropriate calibrators for antifactor Xa activity of fondaparinux.

Dosage Forms Injection, solution, as sodium [preservative free]: 2.5 mg/0.5 mL (0.5 mL); 5 mg/0.4 mL (0.4 mL); 7.5 mg/0.6 mL (0.6 mL); 10 mg/0.8 mL (0.8 mL) [prefilled syringe]

References

Bauer KA, "Fondaparinux Sodium: A Selective Inhibitor of Factor Xa," *Am J Health-Syst Pharm*, 2001, 58(Suppl 2):14-7.

Bauer KA, Eriksson BI, Lassen MR, et al, "Fondaparinux Compared With Enoxaparin for the Prevention of Venous Thromboembolism After Elective Major Knee Surgery," *N Engl J Med*, 2001, 345(18):1305-10.

Eriksson BI, Bauer KA, Lassen MR, et al, "Fondaparinux Compared With Enoxaparin for the Prevention of Venous Thromboembolism After Hip-Fracture Surgery," *N Engl J Med*, 2001, 345(18):1298-304.

♦ **Fondaparinux Sodium** *see* Fondaparinux *on page 557*
♦ **Foradil® (Can)** *see* Formoterol *on page 559*
♦ **Foradil® Aerolizer™** *see* Formoterol *on page 559*
♦ **Forane®** *see* Isoflurane *on page 702*

Formoterol (for MOH te rol)

Medication Safety Issues

Sound-alike/look-alike issues:
Foradil® may be confused with Toradol®
Foradil® capsules for inhalation are for administration via Aerolizer™ inhaler and are not for oral use.

U.S. Brand Names Foradil® Aerolizer™

Canadian Brand Names Foradil®; Oxeze® Turbuhaler®

Synonyms Formoterol Fumarate

Pharmacologic Category Beta$_2$-Adrenergic Agonist

Generic Available No

Use Maintenance treatment of asthma and prevention of bronchospasm in patients ≥5 years of age with reversible obstructive airway disease, including patients with symptoms of nocturnal asthma, who require regular treatment with inhaled, short-acting beta$_2$ agonists; maintenance treatment of bronchoconstriction in (Continued)

Formoterol *(Continued)*

patients with COPD; prevention of exercise-induced bronchospasm in patients ≥5 years of age

Note: Oxeze® is also approved in Canada for acute relief of symptoms ("on demand" treatment) in patients ≥6 years of age.

Mechanism of Action Relaxes bronchial smooth muscle by selective action on $beta_2$ receptors with little effect on heart rate. Formoterol has a long-acting effect.

Pharmacodynamics/Kinetics

Onset: Within 3 minutes

Peak effect: 80% of peak effect within 15 minutes

Duration: Improvement in FEV_1 observed for 12 hours in most patients

Absorption: Rapidly into plasma

Protein binding: 61% to 64% *in vitro* at higher concentrations than achieved with usual dosing

Metabolism: Hepatic via direct glucuronidation and O-demethylation; CYP2D6, CYP2C8/9, CYP2C19, CYP2A6 involved in O-demethylation

Half-life elimination: ~10-14 hours

Time to peak: Maximum improvement in FEV_1 in 1-3 hours

Excretion:

Children 5-12 years: Urine (7% to 9% as direct glucuronide metabolites, 6% as unchanged drug)

Adults: Urine (15% to 18% as direct glucuronide metabolites, 10% as unchanged drug)

Dosage

Asthma maintenance treatment: Children ≥5 years and Adults: Inhalation: 12 mcg capsule every 12 hours

Oxeze® (CAN): **Note:** Not labeled for use in the U.S.: Children ≥6 years and Adults: Inhalation: 6 mcg or 12 mcg every 12 hours. Maximum dose: Children: 24 mcg/day; Adults: 48 mcg/day

Prevention of exercise-induced bronchospasm: Children ≥5 years and Adults: Inhalation: 12 mcg capsule at least 15 minutes before exercise on an "as needed" basis; additional doses should not be used for another 12 hours. **Note:** If already using for asthma maintenance then should not use additional doses for exercise-induced bronchospasm.

Oxeze® (CAN): **Note:** Not labeled for use in the U.S.: Children ≥6 years and Adults: Inhalation: 6 mcg or 12 mcg at least 15 minutes before exercise.

COPD maintenance treatment: Adults: Inhalation: 12 mcg capsule every 12 hours

Additional indication for Oxeze® (approved in Canada): Acute ("on demand") relief of bronchoconstriction: Children ≥12 years and Adults: 6 mcg or 12 mcg as a single dose (maximum dose: 72 mcg in any 24-hour period). The prolonged use of high dosages (48 mcg/day for ≥3 consecutive days) may be a sign of suboptimal control, and should prompt the re-evaluation of therapy.

Stability Prior to dispensing, store in refrigerator at 2°C to 8°C (36°F to 46°F); after dispensing, store at room temperature at 20°C to 25°C (68°F to 77°F). Protect from heat and moisture. Capsules should always be stored in the blister and only removed immediately before use. Always check expiration date. Use within 4 months of purchase date or product expiration date, whichever comes first.

Administration Remove capsule from foil blister **immediately** before use. Place capsule in the capsule-chamber in the base of the Aerolizer™ Inhaler. Must only use the Aerolizer™ Inhaler. Press both buttons **once only** and then release. Keep inhaler in a level, horizontal position. Exhale fully. Do not exhale into inhaler. Tilt head slightly back and inhale (rapidly, steadily, and deeply). Hold breath as long as possible. If any powder remains in capsule, exhale and inhale again. Repeat until capsule is empty. Throw away empty capsule; do not leave in inhaler. Do not use a spacer with the Aerolizer™ Inhaler. Always keep capsules and inhaler dry.

Monitoring Parameters FEV_1, peak flow, and/or other pulmonary function tests; blood pressure, heart rate; CNS stimulation; serum glucose, serum potassium

Pregnancy Risk Factor C

Contraindications Hypersensitivity to adrenergic amines, formoterol, or any component of the formulation

Note: The approved U.S. labeling lists the need for acute bronchodilation as a contraindication; however, a formulation (Oxeze®) is approved for acute treatment in other countries (ie, Canada).

Warnings/Precautions Optimize anti-inflammatory treatment before initiating maintenance treatment with formoterol. Do not use as a component of chronic therapy without an anti-inflammatory agent. Patient must be instructed to seek medical attention in cases where acute symptoms are not relieved by rapid-onset beta-agonist or when a previous level of response is diminished. Treatment must not be delayed. Rarely, paradoxical bronchospasm may occur with use of inhaled bronchodilating agents; this should be distinguished from inadequate response.

Acute episodes should be treated with rapid-onset $beta_2$ agonist. The approved U.S. labeling states that formoterol is not meant to relieve acute asthmatic symptoms. Although, a formulation of formoterol (Oxeze®) is approved for acute treatment outside the U.S. (ie, Canada).

Do not exceed recommended dose; serious adverse events (including fatalities) have been associated with excessive use of inhaled sympathomimetics. $Beta_2$ agonists may increase risk of arrhythmias, decrease serum potassium, prolong QT_c interval, or increase serum glucose. These effects may be exacerbated in hypoxemia. Use caution in patients with cardiovascular disease (arrhythmia or hypertension or CHF), convulsive disorders, diabetes, glaucoma, hyperthyroidism, or hypokalemia. Beta agonists may cause elevation in blood pressure, heart rate, and result in CNS stimulation/excitation. Safety and efficacy have not been established in children <5 years of age.

Adverse Reactions Children are more likely to have infection, inflammation, abdominal pain, nausea, and dyspepsia.

>10%:

- Endocrine & metabolic: Serum glucose increased, serum potassium decreased
- Miscellaneous: Viral infection (17%)

1% to 10%:

- Cardiovascular: Chest pain (2%)
- Central nervous system: Tremor (2%), dizziness (2%), insomnia (2%), dysphonia (1%)
- Dermatologic: Rash (1%)
- Respiratory: Bronchitis (5%), infection (3%), dyspnea (2%), tonsillitis (1%)

<1% (Limited to important or life-threatening): Anaphylactic reactions (severe hypotension, angioedema), asthma exacerbation

Overdosage/Toxicology Symptoms of overdose include tachycardia, tremor, hypertension, angina, and seizures. Hypokalemia also may occur. Cardiac arrest and death may be associated with abuse of beta-agonist bronchodilators. Treatment includes immediate discontinuation and symptomatic and supportive therapies. Cautious use of beta-adrenergic blocking agents may be considered in severe cases.

Drug Interactions **Substrate** (minor) of CYP2A6, 2C9, 2C19, 2D6

Adrenergic agonist: Additive adrenergic stimulation may occur with concurrent use

Antidepressants, tricyclic: Concurrent use may potentiate cardiovascular side effects

Beta blockers: May block therapeutic effects of formoterol; may produce bronchospasm. If use is necessary, cautiously consider a cardioselective beta-blocker. Monitor closely.

Corticosteroids: May potentiate hypokalemia

Diuretics (thiazide or loops): May potentiate hypokalemia

MAO inhibitors: Concurrent use may potentiate cardiovascular side effects.

QT_c-prolonging agents: Concurrent use may potentiate cardiovascular side effects; includes dofetilide, type Ia antiarrhythmics (quinidine, procainamide), pimozide, some quinolone antibiotics (moxifloxacin, sparfloxacin, gatifloxacin), sotalol, mesoridazine, and thioridazine

Theophylline derivatives: May potentiate hypokalemia

Dosage Forms [CAN] = Canadian brand name

Powder for oral inhalation, as fumarate:

- Foradil® Aerolizer™ [capsule]: 12 mcg (12s, 60s) [contains lactose 25 mg]
- Oxeze® Turbuhaler® [CAN]: 6 mcg/inhalation [delivers 60 metered doses; contains lactose 600 mcg/dose]; 12 mcg/inhalation [delivers 60 metered doses; contains lactose 600 mcg/dose] [not available in the U.S.]

- ♦ **Formoterol Fumarate** *see* Formoterol *on page 559*
- ♦ **Formulation R™ [OTC]** *see* Phenylephrine *on page 1015*
- ♦ **5-Formyl Tetrahydrofolate** *see* Leucovorin *on page 738*
- ♦ **Fortamet™** *see* Metformin *on page 810*
- ♦ **Fortaz®** *see* Ceftazidime *on page 246*
- ♦ **Fortovase® [DSC]** *see* Saquinavir *on page 1149*

Fosinopril (foe SIN oh pril)

Medication Safety Issues

Sound-alike/look-alike issues:

Fosinopril may be confused with lisinopril

Monopril® may be confused with Accupril®, minoxidil, moexipril, Monoket®, Monurol™, ramipril

Related Information

Angiotensin Agents *on page 1544*

Heart Failure (Systolic) *on page 1607*

Preoperative Evaluation of the Cardiac Patient for Noncardiac Surgery *on page 1485*

U.S. Brand Names Monopril®

Canadian Brand Names Apo-Fosinopril®; Monopril®; Novo-Fosinopril; ratio-Fosinopril; Riva-Fosinopril

Synonyms Fosinopril Sodium

Pharmacologic Category Angiotensin-Converting Enzyme (ACE) Inhibitor

Generic Available Yes

Use Treatment of hypertension, either alone or in combination with other antihypertensive agents; treatment of congestive heart failure, left ventricular dysfunction after myocardial infarction

Mechanism of Action Competitive inhibitor of angiotensin-converting enzyme (ACE); prevents conversion of angiotensin I to angiotensin II, a potent vasoconstrictor; results in lower levels of angiotensin II which causes an increase in plasma renin activity and a reduction in aldosterone secretion; a CNS mechanism may also be involved in hypotensive effect as angiotensin II increases adrenergic outflow from CNS; vasoactive kallikreins may be decreased in conversion to active hormones by ACE inhibitors, thus reducing blood pressure

Pharmacodynamics/Kinetics

Onset of action: 1 hour

Duration: 24 hours

Absorption: 36%

Protein binding: 95%

Metabolism: Prodrug, hydrolyzed to its active metabolite fosinoprilat by intestinal wall and hepatic esterases

Bioavailability: 36%

Half-life elimination, serum (fosinoprilat): 12 hours

Time to peak, serum: ~3 hours

Excretion: Urine and feces (as fosinoprilat and other metabolites in roughly equal proportions, 45% to 50%)

Dosage Oral:

Children >50 kg: Hypertension: Initial: 5-10 mg once daily

Adults:

Hypertension: Initial: 10 mg/day; most patients are maintained on 20-40 mg/day. May need to divide the dose into two if trough effect is inadequate; discontinue the diuretic, if possible 2-3 days before initiation of therapy; resume diuretic therapy carefully, if needed.

Heart failure: Initial: 10 mg/day (5 mg if renal dysfunction present) and increase, as needed, to a maximum of 40 mg once daily over several weeks; usual dose: 20-40 mg/day. If hypotension, orthostasis, or azotemia occur during titration, consider decreasing concomitant diuretic dose, if any.

Dosing adjustment/comments in renal impairment: None needed since hepatobiliary elimination compensates adequately diminished renal elimination.

Hemodialysis: Moderately dialyzable (20% to 50%)

Stability Store at 25°C (77°F); excursions permitted to 15°C to 30°C (59°F to 86°F). Protect from moisture by keeping bottle tightly closed.

Monitoring Parameters Blood pressure (supervise for at least 2 hours after the initial dose or any increase for significant orthostasis); serum potassium, creatinine, BUN, WBC

Anesthesia and Critical Care Concerns/Other Considerations ACE inhibitor therapy may elicit rapid increases in potassium and creatinine, especially when used in patients with bilateral renal artery stenosis. When ACE inhibition is introduced in patients with pre-existing diuretic therapy who are hypovolemic, the ACE inhibitor may induce acute hypotension. Concomitant NSAID therapy may attenuate blood pressure control; use of NSAIDs should be avoided or limited, with monitoring of blood pressure control. Because of the potent teratogenic effects of ACE inhibitors, these drugs should be avoided, if possible, when treating women of childbearing potential not on effective birth control measures.

ACE inhibitors decrease morbidity and mortality in patients with asymptomatic and symptomatic left ventricular dysfunction. ACE inhibitors are also indicated in patients postmyocardial infarction in whom left ventricular ejection fraction is <40%. ACE inhibitors have renal protective effects in patients with proteinuria and possibly cardioprotective effects in high-risk patients.

Pregnancy Risk Factor C (1st trimester)/D (2nd and 3rd trimesters)

Contraindications Hypersensitivity to fosinopril or any component of the formulation; angioedema related to previous treatment with an ACE inhibitor; idiopathic or hereditary angioedema; bilateral renal artery stenosis; pregnancy (2nd and 3rd trimesters)

Warnings/Precautions Anaphylactic reactions can occur. Angioedema can occur at any time during treatment (especially following first dose). It may involve head and neck (potentially affecting the airway) or the intestine (presenting with abdominal pain). Prolonged monitoring may be required especially if tongue, glottis, or larynx are involved as they are associated with airway obstruction. Those with a history of airway surgery in this situation have a higher risk. Careful blood pressure monitoring (hypotension can occur especially in volume-depleted patients). **[U.S. Boxed Warning]: Based on human data, ACEIs can cause injury and death to the developing fetus when used in the second and third trimesters. ACEIs should be discontinued as soon as possible once pregnancy is detected.** Dosage adjustment needed in severe renal impairment (Cl_{cr} <10 mL/minute). Use with caution in hypovolemia; collagen vascular diseases; valvular stenosis (particularly aortic stenosis); hyperkalemia; or before, during, or immediately after anesthesia. Avoid rapid dosage escalation which may lead to renal insufficiency. Rare toxicities associated with ACE inhibitors include cholestatic jaundice (which may progress to hepatic necrosis) and neutropenia/agranulocytosis with myeloid hyperplasia. Hypersensitivity reactions may be seen during hemodialysis with high-flux dialysis membranes (eg, AN69). Hyperkalemia may rarely occur. If patient has renal impairment, then a baseline WBC with differential and serum creatinine should be evaluated and monitored closely during initial therapy. Use with caution in unilateral renal artery stenosis and pre-existing renal insufficiency.

Adverse Reactions Note: Frequency ranges include data from hypertension and heart failure trials. Higher rates of adverse reactions have generally been noted in patients with CHF. However, the frequency of adverse effects associated with placebo is also increased in this population.

>10%: Central nervous system: Dizziness (1.6% to 11.9%)

1% to 10%:

- Cardiovascular: Orthostatic hypotension (1.4% to 1.9%), palpitation (1.4%)
- Central nervous system: Dizziness (1% to 2%; up to 12% in CHF patients), headache (3.2%), fatigue (1% to 2%)
- Endocrine & metabolic: Hyperkalemia (2.6%)
- Gastrointestinal: Diarrhea (2.2%), nausea/vomiting (1.2% to 2.2%)
- Hepatic: Transaminases increased
- Neuromuscular & skeletal: Musculoskeletal pain (<1% to 3.3%), noncardiac chest pain (<1% to 2.2%), weakness (1.4%)
- Renal: Increased serum creatinine, worsening of renal function (in patients with bilateral renal artery stenosis or hypovolemia)
- Respiratory: Cough (2.2% to 9.7%)
- Miscellaneous: Upper respiratory infection (2.2%)

>1% but ≤ frequency in patients receiving placebo: Sexual dysfunction, fever, flu-like syndrome, dyspnea, rash, headache, insomnia

<1% (Limited to important or life-threatening): Anaphylactoid reaction, angina, angioedema, arthralgia, bronchospasm, cerebral infarction, cerebrovascular accident, gout, hepatitis, hepatomegaly, myalgia, MI, pancreatitis, paresthesia, photosensitivity, pleuritic chest pain, pruritus, rash, renal insufficiency, shock, sudden death, syncope, TIA, tinnitus, urticaria, vertigo. In a small number of patients, a symptom complex of cough, bronchospasm, and eosinophilia has been observed with fosinopril.

Other events reported with ACE inhibitors: Acute renal failure, agranulocytosis, anemia, aplastic anemia, bullous pemphigus, cardiac arrest, eosinophilic pneumonitis, exfoliative dermatitis, gynecomastia, hemolytic anemia, hepatic failure, jaundice, neutropenia, pancytopenia, Stevens-Johnson syndrome, symptomatic hyponatremia, thrombocytopenia. In addition, a syndrome which may

(Continued)

Fosinopril *(Continued)*

include fever, myalgia, arthralgia, interstitial nephritis, vasculitis, rash, eosinophilia and positive ANA, and elevated ESR has been reported for other ACE inhibitors.

Overdosage/Toxicology Mild hypotension has been the primary toxic effect seen with acute overdose. Bradycardia may also occur; hyperkalemia occurs even with therapeutic doses, especially in patients with renal insufficiency and those taking NSAIDs. Treatment is symptom-directed and supportive.

Drug Interactions

Alpha$_1$ blockers: Hypotensive effect increased.

Antacids (aluminum hydroxide, magnesium hydroxide and simethicone): Absorption of fosinopril impaired; separate dose by 2 hours.

Aspirin: The effects of ACE inhibitors may be blunted by aspirin administration, particularly at higher dosages and/or increase adverse renal effects.

Diuretics: Hypovolemia due to diuretics may precipitate acute hypotensive events or acute renal failure.

Insulin: Risk of hypoglycemia may be increased.

Lithium: Risk of lithium toxicity may be increased; monitor lithium levels, especially the first 4 weeks of therapy.

Mercaptopurine: Risk of neutropenia may be increased.

NSAIDs: May attenuate hypertensive efficacy; effect has been seen with captopril and may occur with other ACE inhibitors; monitor blood pressure. May increase risk of adverse renal effects.

Potassium-sparing diuretics (amiloride, spironolactone, triamterene): Increased risk of hyperkalemia.

Potassium supplements may increase the risk of hyperkalemia.

Trimethoprim (high dose) may increase the risk of hyperkalemia.

Ethanol/Nutrition/Herb Interactions Herb/Nutraceutical: Avoid dong quai if using for hypertension (has estrogenic activity). Avoid ephedra, garlic, yohimbe, ginseng (may worsen hypertension).

Test Interactions Positive Coombs' [direct]; may cause false-positive results in urine acetone determinations using sodium nitroprusside reagent

Dietary Considerations Should not take a potassium salt supplement without the advice of healthcare provider.

Dosage Forms Tablet, as sodium: 10 mg, 20 mg, 40 mg

♦ **Fosinopril Sodium** *see* Fosinopril *on page 562*

Fosphenytoin (FOS fen i toyn)

Medication Safety Issues

Sound-alike/look-alike issues:

Cerebyx® may be confused with Celebrex®, Celexa™, Cerezyme®

Related Information

Perioperative Management of Patients on Antiseizure Medication *on page 1458*

U.S. Brand Names Cerebyx®

Canadian Brand Names Cerebyx®

Synonyms Fosphenytoin Sodium

Pharmacologic Category Anticonvulsant, Hydantoin

Generic Available No

Use Used for the control of generalized convulsive status epilepticus and prevention and treatment of seizures occurring during neurosurgery; indicated for short-term parenteral administration when other means of phenytoin administration are unavailable, inappropriate or deemed less advantageous (the safety and effectiveness of fosphenytoin in this use has not been systematically evaluated for more than 5 days)

Mechanism of Action Diphosphate ester salt of phenytoin which acts as a water soluble prodrug of phenytoin; after administration, plasma esterases convert fosphenytoin to phosphate, formaldehyde and phenytoin as the active moiety; phenytoin works by stabilizing neuronal membranes and decreasing seizure activity by increasing efflux or decreasing influx of sodium ions across cell membranes in the motor cortex during generation of nerve impulses

Pharmacodynamics/Kinetics Also refer to Phenytoin monograph for additional information.

Protein binding: Fosphenytoin: 95% to 99% to albumin; can displace phenytoin and increase free fraction (up to 30% unbound) during the period required for conversion of fosphenytoin to phenytoin

Metabolism: Fosphenytoin is rapidly converted via hydrolysis to phenytoin; phenytoin is metabolized in the liver and forms metabolites

Bioavailability: I.M.: Fosphenytoin: 100%

Half-life elimination:

Fosphenytoin: 15 minutes

Phenytoin: Variable (mean: 12-29 hours); kinetics of phenytoin are saturable

Time to peak: Conversion to phenytoin: Following I.V. administration (maximum rate of administration): 15 minutes; following I.M. administration, peak phenytoin levels are reached in 3 hours

Excretion: Phenytoin: Urine (as inactive metabolites)

Dosage The dose, concentration in solutions, and infusion rates for fosphenytoin are expressed as phenytoin sodium equivalents (PE); fosphenytoin should always be prescribed and dispensed in phenytoin sodium equivalents (PE)

Infants and Children (unlabeled use): I.V.:

Loading dose: 10-20 mg PE/kg for the treatment of generalized convulsive status epilepticus

Maintenance dosing: Phenytoin dosing guidelines in pediatric patients are used when dosing fosphenytoin using doses in PE equal to the phenytoin doses (ie, phenytoin 1 mg = fosphenytoin 1 PE); maintenance doses may be started 8-12 hours after a loading dose

Adults:

Status epilepticus: I.V.: Loading dose: 15-20 mg PE/kg I.V. administered at 100-150 mg PE/minute

Nonemergent loading and maintenance dosing: I.V. or I.M.:

Loading dose: 10-20 mg PE/kg I.V. or I.M. (maximum I.V. rate: 150 mg PE/minute)

Initial daily maintenance dose: 4-6 mg PE/kg/day I.V. or I.M.

I.M. or I.V. substitution for oral phenytoin therapy: May be substituted for oral phenytoin sodium at the same total daily dose; however, Dilantin® capsules are ~90% bioavailable by the oral route; phenytoin, supplied as fosphenytoin, is 100% bioavailable by both the I.M. and I.V. routes; for this reason, plasma phenytoin concentrations may increase when I.M. or I.V. fosphenytoin is substituted for oral phenytoin sodium therapy; in clinical trials I.M. fosphenytoin was administered as a single daily dose utilizing either 1 or 2 injection sites; some patients may require more frequent dosing

Dosing adjustments in renal/hepatic impairment: Phenytoin clearance may be substantially reduced in cirrhosis and plasma level monitoring with dose adjustment advisable; free phenytoin levels should be monitored closely in patients with renal or hepatic disease or in those with hypoalbuminemia; furthermore, fosphenytoin clearance to phenytoin may be increased without a similar increase in phenytoin in these patients leading to increase frequency and severity of adverse events

Stability Refrigerate at 2°C to 8°C (36°F to 46°F). Do not store at room temperature for more than 48 hours. Do not use vials that develop particulate matter. Must be diluted to concentrations 1.5-25 mg PE/mL, in normal saline or D_5W, for I.V. infusion.

Administration

I.M.: May be administered as a single daily dose using either 1 or 2 injection sites.

I.V.: Rates of infusion:

Children: 1-3 mg PE/kg/minute

Adults: Should not exceed 150 mg PE/minute

Monitoring Parameters Continuous blood pressure, ECG, and respiratory function monitoring with loading dose and for 10-20 minutes following infusion; vital signs, CBC, liver function tests, plasma level monitoring (plasma levels should not be measured until conversion to phenytoin is complete, ~2 hours after an I.V. infusion or ~4 hours after an I.M. injection)

Reference Range

Therapeutic: 10-20 mcg/mL (SI: 40-79 μmol/L); toxicity is measured clinically, and some patients require levels outside the suggested therapeutic range

Toxic: 30-50 mcg/mL (SI: 120-200 μmol/L)

Lethal: >100 mcg/mL (SI: >400 μmol/L)

(Continued)

Fosphenytoin *(Continued)*

Manifestations of toxicity:
- Nystagmus: 20 mcg/mL (SI: 79 μmol/L)
- Ataxia: 30 mcg/mL (SI: 118.9 μmol/L)
- Decreased mental status: 40 mcg/mL (SI: 159 μmol/L)
- Coma: 50 mcg/mL (SI: 200 μmol/L)

Peak serum phenytoin level after a 375 mg I.M. fosphenytoin dose in healthy males: 5.7 mcg/mL

Peak serum fosphenytoin levels and phenytoin levels after a 1.2 g infusion (I.V.) in healthy subjects over 30 minutes were 129 mcg/mL and 17.2 mcg/mL respectively

Anesthesia and Critical Care Concerns/Other Considerations Fosphenytoin 1.5 mg is approximately equivalent to phenytoin 1 mg.

Fosphenytoin is compatible with all diluents; does not require propylene glycol or ethanol for solubility. Since there is no precipitation problem with fosphenytoin, no I.V. filter is required. Formaldehyde production is not expected to be clinically consequential (about 200 mg) if used for 1 week. As with phenytoin, fosphenytoin, when given I.V., can cause marked and dramatic hypotension and reflex tachycardia. Fosphenytoin administration is safer, in that the risk of hypotension may be somewhat less, and there are no adverse effects of extravasation. Avoid rapid I.V. infusion of fosphenytoin (infusion rates >150 mg of phenytoin equivalent per minute). Pruritus can be severe, requiring discontinuation of infusion.

Pregnancy Risk Factor D

Contraindications Hypersensitivity to phenytoin, other hydantoins, or any component of the formulation; patients with sinus bradycardia, sinoatrial block, second- and third-degree AV block, or Adams-Stokes syndrome; occurrence of rash during treatment (should not be resumed if rash is exfoliative, purpuric, or bullous); treatment of absence seizures

Warnings/Precautions Doses of fosphenytoin are expressed as their phenytoin sodium equivalent (PE). Antiepileptic drugs should not be abruptly discontinued. Hypotension may occur, especially after I.V. administration at high doses and high rates of administration. Administration of phenytoin has been associated with atrial and ventricular conduction depression and ventricular fibrillation. Careful cardiac monitoring is needed when administering I.V. loading doses of fosphenytoin. Acute hepatotoxicity associated with a hypersensitivity syndrome characterized by fever, skin eruptions, and lymphadenopathy has been reported to occur within the first 2 months of treatment. Discontinue if skin rash or lymphadenopathy occurs. Use with caution in patients with hypotension, severe myocardial insufficiency, diabetes mellitus, porphyria, hypoalbuminemia, hypothyroidism, fever, or hepatic or renal dysfunction.

Adverse Reactions The more important adverse clinical events caused by the I.V. use of fosphenytoin or phenytoin are cardiovascular collapse and/or central nervous system depression. Hypotension can occur when either drug is administered rapidly by the I.V. route. Do not exceed a rate of 150 mg phenytoin equivalent/minute when administering fosphenytoin.

The adverse clinical events most commonly observed with the use of fosphenytoin in clinical trials were nystagmus, dizziness, pruritus, paresthesia, headache, somnolence, and ataxia. Paresthesia and pruritus were seen more often following fosphenytoin (versus phenytoin) administration and occurred more often with I.V. fosphenytoin than with I.M. administration. These events were dose- and rate-related (doses ≥15 mg/kg at a rate of 150 mg/minute). These sensations, generally described as itching, burning, or tingling are usually not at the infusion site. The location of the discomfort varied with the groin mentioned most frequently. The paresthesia and pruritus were transient events that occurred within several minutes of the start of infusion and generally resolved within 10 minutes after completion of infusion.

Transient pruritus, tinnitus, nystagmus, somnolence, and ataxia occurred 2-3 times more often at doses ≥15 mg/kg and rates ≥150 mg/minute.

I.V. administration (maximum dose/rate):

>10%:
- Central nervous system: Nystagmus, dizziness, somnolence, ataxia
- Dermatologic: Pruritus

1% to 10%:
- Cardiovascular: Hypotension, vasodilation, tachycardia

Central nervous system: Stupor, incoordination, paresthesia, extrapyramidal syndrome, tremor, agitation, hypoesthesia, dysarthria, vertigo, brain edema, headache
Gastrointestinal: Nausea, tongue disorder, dry mouth, vomiting
Neuromuscular & skeletal: Pelvic pain, muscle weakness, back pain
Ocular: Diplopia, amblyopia
Otic: Tinnitus, deafness
Miscellaneous: Taste perversion

I.M. administration (substitute for oral phenytoin):

1% to 10%:
Central nervous system: Nystagmus, tremor, ataxia, headache, incoordination, somnolence, dizziness, paresthesia, reflexes decreased
Dermatologic: Pruritus
Gastrointestinal: Nausea, vomiting
Hematologic/lymphatic: Ecchymosis
Neuromuscular & skeletal: Muscle weakness

<1% (Limited to important or life-threatening): Acidosis, acute hepatic failure, acute hepatotoxicity, alkalosis, anemia, atrial flutter, bundle branch block, cardiac arrest, cardiomegaly, cerebral hemorrhage, cerebral infarct, CHF, cyanosis, dehydration, hyperglycemia, hyperkalemia, hypertension, hypochromic anemia, hypokalemia, hypophosphatemia, ketosis, leukocytosis, leukopenia, lymphadenopathy, palpitation, postural hypotension, pulmonary embolus, QT interval prolongation, sinus bradycardia, syncope, thrombocytopenia, thrombophlebitis, ventricular extrasystoles

Overdosage/Toxicology Symptoms of fosphenytoin overdose include bradycardia, asystole, cardiac arrest, hypotension, vomiting, metabolic acidosis, and lethargy. Treatment is supportive for hypotension.

Drug Interactions As phenytoin: **Substrate** of CYP2C9 (major), 2C19 (major), 3A4 (minor); **Induces** CYP2B6 (strong), 2C8 (strong), 2C9 (strong), 2C19 (strong), 3A4 (strong)

Acetaminophen: Phenytoin may enhance the hepatotoxic potential of acetaminophen overdoses

Acetazolamide: Concurrent use with phenytoin may result in an increased risk of osteomalacia

Acyclovir: May decrease phenytoin serum levels; limited documentation; monitor

Allopurinol: May increase phenytoin serum concentrations; monitor

Antiarrhythmics: Phenytoin may increase the metabolism of antiarrhythmics, decreasing their clinical effect; includes disopyramide, propafenone, and quinidine; amiodarone also may increase phenytoin concentrations (see CYP inhibitors)

Anticonvulsants: Phenytoin may increase the metabolism of anticonvulsants; includes barbiturates, carbamazepine, ethosuximide, felbamate, lamotrigine, tiagabine, topiramate, and zonisamide; does not appear to affect gabapentin or levetiracetam; felbamate and gabapentin may increase phenytoin levels; monitor

Antineoplastics: Several chemotherapeutic agents have been associated with a decrease in serum phenytoin levels; includes cisplatin, bleomycin, carmustine, methotrexate, and vinblastine; monitor phenytoin serum levels. Limited evidence also suggest that enzyme-inducing anticonvulsant therapy may reduce the effectiveness of some chemotherapy regimens (specifically in ALL). Teniposide and methotrexate may be cleared more rapidly in these patients.

Antipsychotics: Phenytoin may enhance the metabolism (decrease the efficacy) of antipsychotics; monitor for altered response; dose adjustment may be needed; also see note on clozapine

Benzodiazepines: Phenytoin may decrease the serum concentrations of some benzodiazepines; monitor for decreased benzodiazepine effect

Beta-blockers: Metabolism of beta-blockers may be increased and clinical effect decreased; atenolol and nadolol are unlikely to interact given their renal elimination

Calcium channel blockers: Phenytoin may enhance the metabolism of calcium channel blockers, decreasing their clinical effect; calcium channel blockers (diltiazem, nifedipine) have been reported to increase phenytoin levels (case report); monitor

Capecitabine: May increase the serum concentrations of phenytoin; monitor

Chloramphenicol: Phenytoin may increase the metabolism of chloramphenicol and chloramphenicol may inhibit phenytoin metabolism; monitor for altered response

(Continued)

Fosphenytoin *(Continued)*

Cimetidine: May increase the serum concentrations of phenytoin; monitor.

Ciprofloxacin: Case reports indicate ciprofloxacin may increase or decrease serum phenytoin concentrations; monitor

Clozapine: May decrease phenytoin serum concentrations; monitor

CNS depressants: Sedative effects may be additive with other CNS depressants; monitor for increased effect; includes ethanol, barbiturates, sedatives, antidepressants, narcotic analgesics, and benzodiazepines

Corticosteroids: Phenytoin may increase the metabolism of corticosteroids, decreasing their clinical effect; also see dexamethasone

Cyclosporine and tacrolimus: Levels may be decreased by phenytoin; monitor

CYP2B6 substrates: Phenytoin may decrease the levels/effects of CYP2B6 substrates. Example substrates include bupropion, efavirenz, promethazine, selegiline, and sertraline.

CYP2C9 inducers: May decrease the levels/effects of phenytoin. Example inducers include carbamazepine, phenobarbital, rifampin, rifapentine, and secobarbital.

CYP2C9 Inhibitors may increase the levels/effects of phenytoin. Example inhibitors include delavirdine, fluconazole, gemfibrozil, ketoconazole, nicardipine, NSAIDs, sulfonamides and tolbutamide.

CYP2C8 Substrates: Phenytoin may decrease the levels/effects of CYP2C8 substrates. Example substrates include amiodarone, paclitaxel, pioglitazone, repaglinide, and rosiglitazone.

CYP2C9 Substrates: Phenytoin may decrease the levels/effects of CYP2C9 substrates. Example substrates include bosentan, celecoxib, dapsone, fluoxetine, glimepiride, glipizide, losartan, montelukast, nateglinide, paclitaxel, sulfonamides, trimethoprim, warfarin, and zafirlukast.

CYP2C19 inducers: May decrease the levels/effects of phenytoin. Example inducers include aminoglutethimide, carbamazepine, phenytoin, and rifampin.

CYP2C19 inhibitors: May increase the levels/effects of phenytoin. Example inhibitors include delavirdine, fluconazole, fluvoxamine, gemfibrozil, isoniazid, omeprazole, and ticlopidine.

CYP2C19 substrates: Phenytoin may decrease the levels/effects of CYP2C19 substrates. Example substrates include citalopram, diazepam, methsuximide, phenytoin, propranolol, proton pump inhibitors, sertraline, and voriconazole

CYP3A4 substrates: Phenytoin may decrease the levels/effects of CYP3A4 substrates. Example substrates include benzodiazepines, calcium channel blockers, clarithromycin, cyclosporine, erythromycin, estrogens, mirtazapine, nateglinide, nefazodone, nevirapine, protease inhibitors, tacrolimus, and venlafaxine

Dexamethasone: May decrease serum phenytoin due to increased metabolism; monitor

Digoxin: Effects and/or levels of digitalis glycosides may be decreased by phenytoin

Disulfiram: May increase serum phenytoin concentrations; monitor

Dopamine: Phenytoin (I.V.) may increase the effect of dopamine (enhanced hypotension)

Doxycycline: Phenytoin may enhance the metabolism of doxycycline, decreasing its clinical effect; higher dosages may be required

Estrogens: Phenytoin may increase the metabolism of estrogens, decreasing their clinical effect; monitor

Folic acid: Replacement of folic acid has been reported to increase the metabolism of phenytoin, decreasing its serum concentrations and/or increasing seizures

HMG-CoA reductase inhibitors: Phenytoin may increase the metabolism of these agents, reducing their clinical effect; monitor

Itraconazole: Phenytoin may decrease the effect of itraconazole

Levodopa: Phenytoin may inhibit the anti-Parkinson effect of levodopa

Lithium: Concurrent use of phenytoin and lithium has resulted in lithium intoxication

Methadone: Phenytoin may enhance the metabolism of methadone resulting in methadone withdrawal

Methylphenidate: May increase serum phenytoin concentrations; monitor

Metronidazole: May increase the serum concentrations of phenytoin; monitor.

Neuromuscular-blocking agents: Duration of effect may be decreased by phenytoin

Omeprazole: May increase serum phenytoin concentrations; monitor
Oral contraceptives: Phenytoin may enhance the metabolism of oral contraceptives, decreasing their clinical effect; an alternative method of contraception should be considered
Primidone: Phenytoin enhances the conversion of primidone to phenobarbital resulting in elevated phenobarbital serum concentrations
Quetiapine: Serum concentrations may be substantially reduced by phenytoin, potentially resulting in a loss of efficacy; limited documentation; monitor
SSRIs: May increase phenytoin serum concentrations; fluoxetine and fluvoxamine are known to inhibit metabolism via CYP enzymes; sertraline and paroxetine have also been shown to increase concentrations in some patients; monitor
Theophylline: Phenytoin may increase metabolism of theophylline derivatives and decrease their clinical effect; theophylline may also increase phenytoin concentrations
Thyroid hormones (including levothyroxine): Phenytoin may alter the metabolism of thyroid hormones, reducing its effect; there is limited documentation of this interaction, but monitoring should be considered
Ticlopidine: May increase serum phenytoin concentrations and/or toxicity; monitor
Tricyclic antidepressants: Phenytoin may increase metabolism of tricyclic antidepressants and decrease their clinical effect; sedative effects may be additive; tricyclics may also increase phenytoin concentrations
Topiramate: Phenytoin may decrease serum levels of topiramate; topiramate may increase the effect of phenytoin
Trazodone: Serum levels of phenytoin may be increased; limited documentation; monitor
Trimethoprim: May increase serum phenytoin concentrations; monitor
Valproic acid (and sulfisoxazole): May displace phenytoin from binding sites; valproic acid may increase, decrease, or have no effect on phenytoin serum concentrations
Vigabatrin: May reduce phenytoin serum concentrations; monitor
Warfarin: Phenytoin transiently increased the hypothrombinemia response to warfarin initially; this is followed by an inhibition of the hypoprothrombinemic response

Ethanol/Nutrition/Herb Interactions

Ethanol:

Acute use: Avoid or limit ethanol (inhibits metabolism of phenytoin); watch for sedation.

Chronic use: Avoid or limit ethanol (stimulates metabolism of phenytoin).

Test Interactions Increased glucose, alkaline phosphatase (S); decreased thyroxine (S), calcium (S); serum sodium increased in overdose setting

Dietary Considerations Provides phosphate 0.0037 mmol/mg PE fosphenytoin

Dosage Forms Injection, solution, as sodium: 75 mg/mL [equivalent to phenytoin sodium 50 mg/mL] (2 mL, 10 mL)

References

Chapman MG, Smith M, and Hirsch NP, "Status Epilepticus," *Anaesthesia*, 2001, 56(7):648-59.
Manno EM, "New Management Strategies in the Treatment of Status Epilepticus," *Mayo Clin Proc*, 2003, 78(4):508-18.

- **Fosphenytoin Sodium** *see* Fosphenytoin *on page 564*
- **Fragmin®** *see* Dalteparin *on page 347*
- **Fraxiparine™ (Can)** *see* Nadroparin *on page 888*
- **Fraxiparine™ Forte (Can)** *see* Nadroparin *on page 888*
- **Froben® (Can)** *see* Flurbiprofen *on page 550*
- **Froben-SR® (Can)** *see* Flurbiprofen *on page 550*
- **Frova®** *see* Frovatriptan *on page 569*

Frovatriptan (froe va TRIP tan)

U.S. Brand Names Frova®

Synonyms Frovatriptan Succinate

Pharmacologic Category Antimigraine Agent; Serotonin 5-$HT_{1B, 1D}$ Receptor Agonist

Generic Available No

Use Acute treatment of migraine with or without aura in adults

(Continued)

Frovatriptan *(Continued)*

Mechanism of Action Selective agonist for serotonin ($5\text{-}HT_{1B}$ and $5\text{-}HT_{1D}$ receptor) in cranial arteries to cause vasoconstriction and reduces sterile inflammation associated with antidromic neuronal transmission correlating with relief of migraine.

Pharmacodynamics/Kinetics

Distribution: Male: 4.2 L/kg; Female: 3.0 L/kg

Protein binding: 15%

Metabolism: Primarily hepatic via CYP1A2

Bioavailability: 20% to 30%

Half-life elimination: 26 hours

Time to peak: 2-4 hours

Excretion: Feces (62%); urine (32%)

Dosage Oral: Adults: Migraine: 2.5 mg; if headache recurs, a second dose may be given if first dose provided some relief and at least 2 hours have elapsed since the first dose (maximum daily dose: 7.5 mg)

Dosage adjustment in renal impairment: No adjustment necessary

Dosage adjustment in hepatic impairment: No adjustment necessary in mild to moderate hepatic impairment; use with caution in severe impairment

Stability Store at room temperature of 25°C (77°F); protect from moisture and light.

Administration Administer with fluids.

Pregnancy Risk Factor C

Contraindications Hypersensitivity to frovatriptan or any component of the formulation; patients with ischemic heart disease or signs or symptoms of ischemic heart disease (including Prinzmetal's angina, angina pectoris, myocardial infarction, silent myocardial ischemia); cerebrovascular syndromes (including strokes, transient ischemic attacks); peripheral vascular syndromes (including ischemic bowel disease); uncontrolled hypertension; use within 24 hours of ergotamine derivatives; use within 24 hours of another $5\text{-}HT_1$ agonist; management of hemiplegic or basilar migraine; prophylactic treatment of migraine; severe hepatic impairment

Warnings/Precautions Not intended for migraine prophylaxis, or treatment of cluster headaches, hemiplegic or basilar migraines. Cardiac, cerebral/subarachnoid hemorrhage, and stroke have been reported with $5\text{-}HT_1$ agonist administration. May cause vasospastic reactions resulting in colonic, peripheral, or coronary ischemia. Do not give to patients with risk factors for CAD until a cardiovascular evaluation has been performed; if evaluation is satisfactory, the healthcare provider should administer the first dose and cardiovascular status should be periodically evaluated. Significant elevation in blood pressure, including hypertensive crisis, has also been reported on rare occasions in patients using other $5\text{-}HT_{1D}$ agonists with and without a history of hypertension. Use with caution in patients with history of seizure disorder. Safety and efficacy in pediatric patients have not been established.

Adverse Reactions

1% to 10%:

Cardiovascular: Chest pain (2%), flushing (4%), palpitation (1%)

Central nervous system: Dizziness (8%), fatigue (5%), headache (4%), hot or cold sensation (3%), anxiety (1%), dysesthesia (1%), hypoesthesia (1%), insomnia (1%), pain (1%)

Gastrointestinal: Hyposalivation (3%), dyspepsia (2%), abdominal pain (1%), diarrhea (1%), vomiting (1%)

Neuromuscular & skeletal: Paresthesia (4%), skeletal pain (3%)

Ocular: Visual abnormalities (1%)

Otic: Tinnitus (1%)

Respiratory: Rhinitis (1%), sinusitis (1%)

Miscellaneous: Diaphoresis (1%)

<1% (Limited to important or life-threatening): Abnormal dreaming, abnormal gait, abnormal lacrimation, abnormal reflexes, abnormal urine, agitation, amnesia, arthralgia, arthrosis, ataxia, back pain, bradycardia, bullous eruption, cheilitis, confusion, conjunctivitis, constipation, dehydration, depersonalization, depression, dysphagia, dyspnea, earache, ECG changes, emotional lability, epistaxis, eructation, esophagospasm, euphoria, eye pain, fever, gastroesophageal reflux, hiccup, hot flushes, hyperacusis, hyperesthesia, hypertonia, hyperventilation, hypocalcemia, hypoglycemia, hypotonia, impaired concentration, involuntary muscle contractions, laryngitis, leg cramps, malaise, micturition, muscle

weakness, myalgia, nervousness, nocturia, peptic ulcer, personality disorder, pharyngitis, polyuria, pruritus, purpura, renal pain, rigors, saliva increased, salivary gland pain, speech disorder, stomatitis, syncope, tachycardia, taste perversion, thirst, tongue paralysis, toothache, tremor, unspecified pain, urinary frequency, vertigo, weakness

Overdosage/Toxicology Single oral doses of up to 100 mg have been reported without adverse effects. Treatment of overdose should be supportive and symptomatic. Monitor for at least 48 hours or until signs and symptoms subside. It is not known if hemodialysis or peritoneal dialysis is effective.

Drug Interactions **Substrate** of CYP1A2 (minor)

Ergot derivatives: Ergot derivatives may cause prolonged vasospastic reactions, creating additive toxicity with frovatriptan. Do not use within 24 hours of each other.

Estrogens (oral contraceptives): Estradiol may increase serum concentrations of frovatriptan

Propranolol: Propranolol may increase serum concentrations of frovatriptan

Selective serotonin reuptake inhibitors (SSRIs): Frovatriptan may increase SSRI toxicity (eg, weakness, hyper-reflexia, incoordination)

Serotonin agonists: May exhibit additive toxicity with other serotonin agonists (eg, antidepressants, dextromethorphan, tramadol), leading to serotonin syndrome.

Ethanol/Nutrition/Herb Interactions Food: Food does not affect frovatriptan bioavailability.

Dosage Forms Tablet, as base: 2.5 mg

- **Frovatriptan Succinate** *see* Frovatriptan *on page 569*
- **Frusemide** *see* Furosemide *on page 572*
- **FS** *see* Fibrin Sealant Kit *on page 523*
- **FTC** *see* Emtricitabine *on page 445*
- **Fucidin® (Can)** *see* Fusidic Acid *on page 575*
- **Fucithalmic® (Can)** *see* Fusidic Acid *on page 575*

Fulvestrant (fool VES trant)

U.S. Brand Names Faslodex®

Synonyms ICI-182,780; Zeneca 182,780; ZM-182,780

Pharmacologic Category Antineoplastic Agent, Estrogen Receptor Antagonist

Generic Available No

Use Treatment of hormone receptor positive metastatic breast cancer in postmenopausal women with disease progression following antiestrogen therapy.

Unlabeled/Investigational Use Endometriosis; uterine bleeding

Mechanism of Action Steroidal compound which competitively binds to estrogen receptors on tumors and other tissue targets, producing a nuclear complex that decreases DNA synthesis and inhibits estrogen effects. Fulvestrant has no estrogen-receptor agonist activity. Causes down-regulation of estrogen receptors and inhibits tumor growth.

Pharmacodynamics/Kinetics

Duration: I.M.: Plasma levels maintained for at least 1 month

Distribution: V_d: 3-5 L/kg

Protein binding: 99%

Metabolism: Hepatic via multiple pathways (CYP3A4 substrate, relative contribution to metabolism unknown)

Bioavailability: Oral: Poor

Half-life elimination: ~40 days

Time to peak, plasma: I.M.: 7-9 days

Excretion: Feces (>90%); urine (<1%)

Dosage I.M.: Adults (postmenopausal women): 250 mg at 1-month intervals

Dosage adjustment in renal impairment: No adjustment required.

Dosage adjustment in hepatic impairment: Use in moderate to severe hepatic impairment has not been evaluated; use caution.

Stability Store under refrigeration at 2°C to 8°C (36°F to 46°F).

Administration I.M. injection into a relatively large muscle (ie, buttock); do not administer I.V., SubQ, or intra-arterially. May be administered as a single 5 mL injection or two concurrent 2.5 mL injections.

Pregnancy Risk Factor D

(Continued)

Fulvestrant *(Continued)*

Contraindications Hypersensitivity to fulvestrant or any component of the formulation; contraindications to I.M. injections (bleeding diatheses, thrombocytopenia, or therapeutic anticoagulation); pregnancy

Warnings/Precautions Use caution in hepatic impairment.

Adverse Reactions

>10%:

Cardiovascular: Vasodilation (18%)

Central nervous system: Pain (19%), headache (15%)

Endocrine & metabolic: Hot flushes (19% to 24%)

Gastrointestinal: Nausea (26%), vomiting (13%), constipation (13%), diarrhea (12%), abdominal pain (12%)

Local: Injection site reaction (11%)

Neuromuscular & skeletal: Weakness (23%), bone pain (16%), back pain (14%)

Respiratory: Pharyngitis (16%), dyspnea (15%)

1% to 10%:

Cardiovascular: Edema (9%), chest pain (7%)

Central nervous system: Dizziness (7%), insomnia (7%), paresthesia (6%), fever (6%), depression (6%), anxiety (5%)

Dermatologic: Rash (7%)

Gastrointestinal: Anorexia (9%), weight gain (1% to 2%)

Genitourinary: Pelvic pain (10%), urinary tract infection (6%), vaginitis (2% to 3%)

Hematologic: Anemia (5%)

Neuromuscular and skeletal: Arthritis (3%)

Respiratory: Cough (10%)

Miscellaneous: Diaphoresis increased (5%)

<1% (limited to important or life-threatening): Angioedema, hypersensitivity reactions, leukopenia, myalgia, thrombosis, urticaria, vaginal bleeding, vertigo

Overdosage/Toxicology No specific experience in overdose. Treatment is supportive.

Drug Interactions Substrate of CYP3A4 (minor)

Dosage Forms Injection, solution: 50 mg/mL (2.5 mL, 5 mL) [prefilled syringe; contains alcohol, benzyl alcohol, benzyl stearate, castor oil]

- **Fungizone® (Can)** *see* Amphotericin B (Conventional) *on page 96*
- **Furadantin®** *see* Nitrofurantoin *on page 927*
- **Furazosin** *see* Prazosin *on page 1044*

Furosemide (fyoor OH se mide)

Medication Safety Issues

Sound-alike/look-alike issues:

Furosemide may be confused with torsemide

Lasix® may be confused with Esidrix®, Lanoxin®, Lidex®, Lomotil®, Luvox®, Luxiq®

Related Information

Anesthesia for Patients With Liver Disease *on page 1421*

Diuretics, Loop *on page 1565*

Heart Failure (Systolic) *on page 1607*

Hemodynamic Support, Intravenous *on page 1566*

U.S. Brand Names Lasix®

Canadian Brand Names Apo-Furosemide®; Furosemide Injection, USP; Furosemide Special; Lasix®; Lasix® Special; Novo-Semide

Synonyms Frusemide

Pharmacologic Category Diuretic, Loop

Generic Available Yes

Use Management of edema associated with congestive heart failure and hepatic or renal disease; alone or in combination with antihypertensives in treatment of hypertension

Mechanism of Action Inhibits reabsorption of sodium and chloride in the ascending loop of Henle and distal renal tubule, interfering with the chloride-binding cotransport system, thus causing increased excretion of water, sodium, chloride, magnesium, and calcium

Pharmacodynamics/Kinetics

Onset of action: Diuresis: Oral: 30-60 minutes; I.M.: 30 minutes; I.V.: ~5 minutes

Peak effect: Oral: 1-2 hours

Duration: Oral: 6-8 hours; I.V.: 2 hours

Absorption: Oral: 60% to 67%

Protein binding: >98%

Metabolism: Minimally hepatic

Half-life elimination: Normal renal function: 0.5-1.1 hours; End-stage renal disease: 9 hours

Excretion: Urine (Oral: 50%, I.V.: 80%) within 24 hours; feces (as unchanged drug); nonrenal clearance prolonged in renal impairment

Dosage

Infants and Children:

Oral: 1-2 mg/kg/dose increased in increments of 1 mg/kg/dose with each succeeding dose until a satisfactory effect is achieved to a maximum of 6 mg/kg/dose no more frequently than 6 hours.

I.M., I.V.: 1 mg/kg/dose, increasing by each succeeding dose at 1 mg/kg/dose at intervals of 6-12 hours until a satisfactory response up to 6 mg/kg/dose.

Adults:

Oral: 20-80 mg/dose initially increased in increments of 20-40 mg/dose at intervals of 6-8 hours; usual maintenance dose interval is twice daily or every day; may be titrated up to 600 mg/day with severe edematous states.

Hypertension (JNC 7): 20-80 mg/day in 2 divided doses

I.M., I.V.: 20-40 mg/dose, may be repeated in 1-2 hours as needed and increased by 20 mg/dose until the desired effect has been obtained. Usual dosing interval: 6-12 hours; for acute pulmonary edema, the usual dose is 40 mg I.V. over 1-2 minutes. If not adequate, may increase dose to 80 mg. **Note:** ACC/AHA 2005 guidelines for chronic congestive heart failure recommend a maximum single dose of 160-200 mg.

Continuous I.V. infusion: Initial I.V. bolus dose of 20-40 mg followed by continuous I.V. infusion doses of 10-40 mg/hour. Double as necessary to a maximum of 80-160 mg/hour if urine output is <1 mL/kg/hour. Continuous infusions have been found to be effective and result in a lower daily requirement of furosemide than with intermittent dosing. Other studies have used a rate of ≤4 mg/minute as a continuous I.V. infusion. **Note:** ACC/AHA 2005 guidelines for chronic congestive heart failure recommend 40 mg I.V. load then 10-40 mg/hour infusion.

Refractory heart failure: Oral, I.V.: Doses up to 8 g/day have been used.

Elderly: Oral, I.M., I.V.: Initial: 20 mg/day; increase slowly to desired response.

Dosing adjustment/comments in renal impairment: Acute renal failure: High doses (up to 1-3 g/day - oral/I.V.) have been used to initiate desired response; avoid use in oliguric states.

Dialysis: Not removed by hemo- or peritoneal dialysis; supplemental dose is not necessary.

Dosing adjustment/comments in hepatic disease: Diminished natriuretic effect with increased sensitivity to hypokalemia and volume depletion in cirrhosis; monitor effects, particularly with high doses.

Stability

Furosemide injection should be stored at controlled room temperature and protected from light

Exposure to light may cause discoloration; do not use furosemide solutions if they have a yellow color

Refrigeration may result in precipitation or crystallization, however, resolubilization at room temperature or warming may be performed without affecting the drug's stability

Furosemide solutions are unstable in acidic media but very stable in basic media

I.V. infusion solution mixed in NS or D_5W solution is stable for 24 hours at room temperature. May also be diluted for infusion 1-2 mg/mL (maximum: 10 mg/mL) over 10-15 minutes (following infusion rate parameters).

Administration

I.V.: I.V. injections should be given slowly. In adults, undiluted direct I.V. injections may be administered at a rate of 40 mg over 1-2 minutes; maximum rate of administration for IVPB or continuous infusion: 4 mg/minute. In children, a maximum rate of 0.5 mg/kg/minute has been recommended.

Oral: May be taken with or without food.

Monitoring Parameters Monitor weight and I & O daily; blood pressure, orthostasis, serum electrolytes, renal function; in high doses, monitor hearing

Anesthesia and Critical Care Concerns/Other Considerations It is important that patients be closely followed for hypokalemia, hypomagnesemia, and

(Continued)

Furosemide *(Continued)*

volume depletion because of significant diuresis. If given the morning of surgery, it may render the patient volume depleted and blood pressure may be labile during general anesthesia.

Pregnancy Risk Factor C

Contraindications Hypersensitivity to furosemide, any component, or sulfonylureas; anuria; patients with hepatic coma or in states of severe electrolyte depletion until the condition improves or is corrected

Warnings/Precautions Adjust dose to avoid dehydration. In cirrhosis, avoid electrolyte and acid/base imbalances that might lead to hepatic encephalopathy. Ototoxicity is associated with rapid I.V. administration, renal impairment, excessive doses, and concurrent use of other ototoxins. Hypersensitivity reactions can rarely occur. Monitor fluid status and renal function in an attempt to prevent oliguria, azotemia, and reversible increases in BUN and creatinine. Close medical supervision of aggressive diuresis required. Monitor closely for electrolyte imbalances particularly hypokalemia. Watch for and correct electrolyte disturbances. Coadministration of antihypertensives may increase the risk of hypotension. Avoid use of medications in which the toxicity is enhanced by hypokalemia (including quinolones with QT prolongation).

Chemical similarities are present among sulfonamides, sulfonylureas, carbonic anhydrase inhibitors, thiazides, and loop diuretics (except ethacrynic acid). Use in patients with sulfonylurea allergy is specifically contraindicated in product labeling, however, a risk of cross-reaction exists in patients with allergy to any of these compounds; avoid use when previous reaction has been severe.

Adverse Reactions Frequency not defined.

Cardiovascular: Orthostatic hypotension, necrotizing angiitis, thrombophlebitis, chronic aortitis, acute hypotension, sudden death from cardiac arrest (with I.V. or I.M. administration)

Central nervous system: Paresthesias, vertigo, dizziness, lightheadedness, headache, blurred vision, xanthopsia, fever, restlessness

Dermatologic: Exfoliative dermatitis, erythema multiforme, purpura, photosensitivity, urticaria, rash, pruritus, cutaneous vasculitis

Endocrine & metabolic: Hyperglycemia, hyperuricemia, hypokalemia, hypochloremia, metabolic alkalosis, hypocalcemia, hypomagnesemia, gout, hyponatremia

Gastrointestinal: Nausea, vomiting, anorexia, oral and gastric irritation, cramping, diarrhea, constipation, pancreatitis, intrahepatic cholestatic jaundice, ischemia hepatitis

Genitourinary: Urinary bladder spasm, urinary frequency

Hematological: Aplastic anemia (rare), thrombocytopenia, agranulocytosis (rare), hemolytic anemia, leukopenia, anemia, purpura

Neuromuscular & skeletal: Muscle spasm, weakness

Otic: Hearing impairment (reversible or permanent with rapid I.V. or I.M. administration), tinnitus, reversible deafness (with rapid I.V. or I.M. administration)

Renal: Vasculitis, allergic interstitial nephritis, glycosuria, fall in glomerular filtration rate and renal blood flow (due to overdiuresis), transient rise in BUN

Miscellaneous: Anaphylaxis (rare), exacerbate or activate systemic lupus erythematosus

Overdosage/Toxicology Symptoms of overdose include electrolyte depletion, volume depletion, hypotension, dehydration, and circulatory collapse. Treatment is supportive.

Drug Interactions

ACE inhibitors: Hypotensive effects and/or renal effects are potentiated by hypovolemia.

Antidiabetic agents: Glucose tolerance may be decreased.

Antihypertensive agents: Hypotensive effects may be enhanced.

Cephaloridine or cephalexin: Nephrotoxicity may occur.

Cholestyramine or colestipol may reduce bioavailability of furosemide.

Digoxin: Furosemide-induced hypokalemia may predispose to digoxin toxicity. Monitor potassium.

Fibric acid derivatives: Blood levels of furosemide and fibric acid derivatives (ie, clofibrate and fenofibrate) may be increased during concurrent dosing (particularly in hypoalbuminemia). Limited documentation; monitor for increased effect/toxicity.

Indomethacin (and other NSAIDs) may reduce natriuretic and hypotensive effects of furosemide.

Lithium: Renal clearance may be reduced. Isolated reports of lithium toxicity have occurred; monitor lithium levels.

Metformin may decrease furosemide concentrations.

Metformin blood levels may be increased by furosemide.

NSAIDs: Risk of renal impairment may increase when used in conjunction with furosemide.

Ototoxic drugs (aminoglycosides, cis-platinum): Concomitant use of furosemide may increase risk of ototoxicity, especially in patients with renal dysfunction.

Peripheral adrenergic-blocking drugs or ganglionic blockers: Effects may be increased.

Phenobarbital or phenytoin may reduce diuretic response to furosemide.

Salicylates (high-dose) with furosemide may predispose patients to salicylate toxicity due to reduced renal excretion or alter renal function.

Succinylcholine: Action may be potentiated by furosemide.

Sucralfate may limit absorption of furosemide, effects may be significantly decreased; separate oral administration by 2 hours.

Thiazides: Synergistic diuretic effects occur.

Tubocurarine: The skeletal muscle-relaxing effect may be attenuated by furosemide.

Ethanol/Nutrition/Herb Interactions

Food: Furosemide serum levels may be decreased if taken with food.

Herb/Nutraceutical: Avoid dong quai if using for hypertension (has estrogenic activity). Avoid ephedra, yohimbe, ginseng (may worsen hypertension). Limit intake of natural licorice. Avoid garlic (may have increased antihypertensive effect).

Dietary Considerations May cause a potassium loss; potassium supplement or dietary changes may be required. Administer on an empty stomach. May be administered with food or milk if GI distress occurs. Do not mix with acidic solutions.

Dosage Forms

Injection, solution: 10 mg/mL (2 mL, 4 mL, 8 mL, 10 mL)

Solution, oral: 10 mg/mL (60 mL, 120 mL) [orange flavor]; 40 mg/5 mL (5 mL, 500 mL) [pineapple-peach flavor]

Tablet (Lasix®): 20 mg, 40 mg, 80 mg

♦ **Furosemide Injection, USP (Can)** *see* Furosemide *on page 572*

♦ **Furosemide Special (Can)** *see* Furosemide *on page 572*

Fusidic Acid (fyoo SI dik AS id)

Canadian Brand Names Fucidin®; Fucithalmic®

Synonyms Sodium Fusidate

Pharmacologic Category Antibiotic, Miscellaneous

Restrictions Not available in U.S.

Generic Available No

Use

Systemic: Treatment of skin and soft tissue infections, or osteomyelitis, caused by susceptible organisms, including *Staphylococcus aureus* (penicillinase-producing or nonpenicillinase strains); may be used in the treatment of pneumonia, septicemia, endocarditis, burns, and cystic fibrosis caused by susceptible organisms when other antibiotics have failed

Topical: Treatment of primary and secondary skin infections caused by susceptible organisms

Ophthalmic: Treatment of superficial infections of the eye and conjunctiva caused by susceptible organisms

Mechanism of Action Inhibits protein synthesis by blocking aminoacyl-sRNA transfer to protein in susceptible bacteria.

Pharmacodynamics/Kinetics

Protein binding: 97%

Metabolism: Hepatic, to multiple metabolites

Half-life elimination: 5-6 hours

Time to peak, serum: Oral: 2-4 hours

Excretion: Feces (~100%, via bile)

Dosage

I.V.:

Children ≤12 years: 20 mg/kg/day in 3 divided doses

Children >12 years and Adults: 500 mg sodium fusidate 3 times/day

(Continued)

Fusidic Acid *(Continued)*

Ophthalmic: Children ≥2 years and Adults: Instill 1 drop in each eye every 12 hours for 7 days

Topical: Children and Adults: Apply to affected area 3-4 times/day until favorable results are achieved. If a gauze dressing is used, frequency of application may be reduced to 1-2 times/day.

Oral: Adults: 500 mg sodium fusidate 3 times/day. (**Note:** Oral dosage may be increased to 1000 mg 3 times/day in fulminating infections.)

Dosage adjustment in renal impairment: No dosage adjustment required

Dosage adjustment in hepatic impairment: Oral, I.V.: Use with extreme caution in patients with hepatic impairment; monitor liver function periodically during therapy

Stability

Cream: Store below 25°C.

Injection, powder for reconstitution: Store below 25°C. Reconstitute 500 mg vial of powder for injection by adding 10 mL of supplied diluent containing phosphate/citrate buffer. Reconstituted solution may be further diluted with NS or D_5W; should be used within 24 hours. Add to NS or D_5W to produce a final concentration of 1-2 mg/mL. For patients weighing <50 kg, reconstituted drug should be diluted at least 10-fold in a compatible solution. Discard solution if opalescence is observed. Compatible in NS, D_5W, or LR. Do not administer with whole blood or amino acid solutions. Incompatible with calcium solutions, carbenicillin, gentamicin, or kanamycin.

Ointment: Store below 30°C.

Ophthalmic suspension: Store at 2°C to 25°C. Discard multidose vials 1 month after opening.

Administration I.V.: Should not be administered I.M. or SubQ. Intravenous administration should be via a large bore vein with good blood flow. Administer over 2 hours or more. Do not administer with whole blood or amino acid solutions.

Monitoring Parameters Monitor liver function tests, including bilirubin periodically during systemic therapy

Contraindications Hypersensitivity to fusidic acid or any component of the formulation

Warnings/Precautions Use with extreme caution in hepatic impairment; monitor liver function regularly during treatment. Intravenous formulation contains phosphate/citrate buffer; excessive amounts may lead to hypocalcemia. Use with extreme caution in patients with pre-existing hypocalcemia. Should not be administered I.M. or SubQ; local tissue injury may occur.

Adverse Reactions

Cardiovascular: Edema (leg), thrombophlebitis, venospasm

Central nervous system: Dizziness, headache, psychic disturbance

Dermatologic: Pruritus, rash

Gastrointestinal: Anorexia, dyspepsia, diarrhea, epigastric distress, nausea, vomiting

Hepatic: Jaundice

Local: Injection site reaction (redness, irritation)

Ocular: Blurred vision

Ophthalmic suspension: Ocular: Transient stinging, tearing, eyelid edema, temporary blurred vision

Overdosage/Toxicology Limited experience in overdose. Symptoms may include gastrointestinal distress, diarrhea, jaundice, and hepatic injury. Large amounts of intravenous solution may lead to hypophosphatemia (due to phosphate/citrate buffer). Not significantly removed by dialysis.

Drug Interactions

Rifampin: Concurrent administration may increase the risk of jaundice.

Note: Drugs with extensive biliary excretion may increase the risk of jaundice, due to competition for secretion pathway.

Dietary Considerations May take tablets with food to minimize gastrointestinal upset.

Dosage Forms [CAN] = Canadian brand name

Cream, as fusidic acid:

Fucidin®: 2% (15 g, 30 g)

Injection, powder for reconstitution, as sodium fusidate:

Fucidin®: 500 mg [packaged with 10 mL diluent/buffer solution]

Ointment, topical, as sodium fusidate:
Fucidin®: 2% (15 g, 30 g) [contains lanolin]
Suspension, ophthalmic, as fusidic acid:
Fucithalmic®: 10 mg/g [1%] (0.2 g) [unit-dose, without preservative]; (3 g, 5 g) [multidose, contains benzalkonium chloride]
Tablet, as sodium fusidate:
Fucidin®: 250 mg

♦ **FXT (Can)** *see* Fluoxetine *on page 539*

Gabapentin (GA ba pen tin)

Medication Safety Issues
Sound-alike/look-alike issues:
Neurontin® may be confused with Neoral®, Noroxin®

Related Information
Chronic Pain Management *on page 1430*
Perioperative Management of Patients on Antiseizure Medication *on page 1458*

U.S. Brand Names Neurontin®

Canadian Brand Names Apo-Gabapentin®; BCI-Gabapentin; Gen-Gabapentin; Neurontin®; Novo-Gabapentin; Nu-Gabapentin; PMS-Gabapentin

Pharmacologic Category Anticonvulsant, Miscellaneous

Generic Available Yes: Capsule, tablet

Use Adjunct for treatment of partial seizures with and without secondary generalized seizures in patients >12 years of age with epilepsy; adjunct for treatment of partial seizures in pediatric patients 3-12 years of age; management of postherpetic neuralgia (PHN) in adults

Unlabeled/Investigational Use Social phobia; chronic pain

Mechanism of Action Gabapentin is structurally related to GABA. However, it does not bind to $GABA_A$ or $GABA_B$ receptors, and it does not appear to influence synthesis or uptake of GABA. High affinity gabapentin binding sites have been located throughout the brain; these sites correspond to the presence of voltage-gated calcium channels specifically possessing the alpha-2-delta-1 subunit. This channel appears to be located presynaptically, and may modulate the release of excitatory neurotransmitters which participate in epileptogenesis and nociception.

Pharmacodynamics/Kinetics
Absorption: 50% to 60% from proximal small bowel by L-amino transport system
Distribution: V_d: 0.6-0.8 L/kg
Protein binding: <3%
Bioavailability: Inversely proportional to dose due to saturable absorption:
900 mg/day: 60%
1200 mg/day: 47%
2400 mg/day: 34%
3600 mg/day: 33%
4800 mg/day: 27%
Half-life elimination: 5-7 hours; anuria 132 hours; during dialysis 3.8 hours
Excretion: Proportional to renal function; urine (as unchanged drug)

Dosage Oral:
Children: Anticonvulsant:
3-12 years: Initial: 10-15 mg/kg/day in 3 divided doses; titrate to effective dose over ~3 days; dosages of up to 50 mg/kg/day have been tolerated in clinical studies
3-4 years: Effective dose: 40 mg/kg/day in 3 divided doses
≥5-12 years: Effective dose: 25-35 mg/kg/day in 3 divided doses
See "Note" in Adults dosing.
Children >12 years and Adults:
Anticonvulsant: Initial: 300 mg 3 times/day; if necessary the dose may be increased up to 1800 mg/day. Doses of up to 2400 mg/day have been tolerated in long-term clinical studies; up to 3600 mg/day has been tolerated in short-term studies.
Note: If gabapentin is discontinued or if another anticonvulsant is added to therapy, it should be done slowly over a minimum of 1 week
Pain (unlabeled use): 300-1800 mg/day given in 3 divided doses has been the most common dosage range

(Continued)

Gabapentin *(Continued)*

Adults: Postherpetic neuralgia or neuropathic pain: Day 1: 300 mg, Day 2: 300 mg twice daily, Day 3: 300 mg 3 times/day; dose may be titrated as needed for pain relief (range: 1800-3600 mg/day, daily doses >1800 mg do not generally show greater benefit)

Elderly: Studies in elderly patients have shown a decrease in clearance as age increases. This is most likely due to age-related decreases in renal function; dose reductions may be needed.

Dosing adjustment in renal impairment: Children ≥12 years and Adults: See table.

Hemodialysis: Dialyzable

Gabapentin Dosing Adjustments in Renal Impairment

Creatinine Clearance (mL/min)	Daily Dose Range
≥60	300-1200 mg tid
>30-59	200-700 mg bid
>15-29	200-700 mg daily
15[1]	100-300 mg daily
Hemodialysis[2]	125-350 mg

[1]Cl_{cr}<15 mL/minute: Reduce daily dose in proportion to creatinine clearance.

[2]Single supplemental dose administered after each 4 hours of hemodialysis

Stability Store at 25°C (77°F); excursions permitted to 15°C to 30°C (59°F to 86°F).

Administration Administer first dose on first day at bedtime to avoid somnolence and dizziness. Dosage must be adjusted for renal function; when given 3 times daily, the maximum time between doses should not exceed 12 hours.

Monitoring Parameters Monitor serum levels of concomitant anticonvulsant therapy

Anesthesia and Critical Care Concerns/Other Considerations CSF level is 20% of blood concentration. Gabapentin is not recommended for children <3 years of age.

Pregnancy Risk Factor C

Contraindications Hypersensitivity to gabapentin or any component of the formulation

Warnings/Precautions Avoid abrupt withdrawal, may precipitate seizures; use cautiously in patients with severe renal dysfunction; male rat studies demonstrated an association with pancreatic adenocarcinoma (clinical implication unknown). May cause CNS depression, which may impair physical or mental abilities. Patients must be cautioned about performing tasks which require mental alertness (eg, operating machinery or driving). Effects with other sedative drugs or ethanol may be potentiated. Pediatric patients (3-12 years of age) have shown increased incidence of CNS-related adverse effects, including emotional lability, hostility, thought disorder, and hyperkinesia. Safety and efficacy in children <3 years of age have not been established.

Adverse Reactions As reported in patients >12 years of age, unless otherwise noted in children (3-12 years)

>10%:

Central nervous system: Somnolence (20%; children 8%), dizziness (17% to 28%; children 3%), ataxia (13%), fatigue (11%)

Miscellaneous: Viral infection (children 11%)

1% to 10%:

Cardiovascular: Peripheral edema (2% to 8%), vasodilatation (1%)

Central nervous system: Fever (children 10%), hostility (children 8%), emotional lability (children 4%), fatigue (children 3%), headache (3%), ataxia (3%), abnormal thinking (2% to 3%; children 2%), amnesia (2%), depression (2%), dysarthria (2%), nervousness (2%), abnormal coordination (1% to 2%), twitching (1%), hyperesthesia (1%)

Dermatologic: Pruritus (1%), rash (1%)

Endocrine & metabolic: Hyperglycemia (1%)

Gastrointestinal: Diarrhea (6%), nausea/vomiting (3% to 4%; children 8%), abdominal pain (3%), weight gain (adults and children 2% to 3%), dyspepsia (2%), flatulence (2%), dry throat (2%), xerostomia (2% to 5%), constipation (2% to 4%), dental abnormalities (2%), appetite stimulation (1%)

Genitourinary: Impotence (2%)

Hematologic: Leukopenia (1%), decreased WBC (1%)

Neuromuscular & skeletal: Tremor (7%), weakness (6%), hyperkinesia (children 3%), abnormal gait (2%), back pain (2%), myalgia (2%), fracture (1%)

Ocular: Nystagmus (8%), diplopia (1% to 6%), blurred vision (3% to 4%), conjunctivitis (1%)

Otic: Otitis media (1%)

Respiratory: Rhinitis (4%), bronchitis (children 3%), respiratory infection (children 3%), pharyngitis (1% to 3%), cough (2%)

Miscellaneous: Infection (5%)

Postmarketing and additional clinical reports (limited to important or life-threatening): Acute renal failure, anemia, angina, angioedema, aphasia, arrhythmias (various), aspiration pneumonia, blindness, bradycardia, bronchospasm, cerebrovascular accident, CNS tumors, coagulation defect, colitis, Cushingoid appearance, dyspnea, encephalopathy, facial paralysis, fecal incontinence, glaucoma, glycosuria, heart block, hearing loss, hematemesis, hematuria, hemiplegia, hemorrhage, hepatitis, hepatomegaly, hyper-/hypotension, hyperlipidemia, hyper-/hypothyroidism, hyper-/hypoventilation, gastroenteritis, heart failure, leukocytosis, liver function tests increased, local myoclonus, lymphadenopathy, lymphocytosis, meningismus, MI, migraine, nephrosis, nerve palsy, non-Hodgkin's lymphoma, ovarian failure, pulmonary thrombosis, pericardial rub, pulmonary embolus, pericardial effusion, pericarditis, pancreatitis, peptic ulcer, purpura, paresthesia, palpitation, peripheral vascular disorder, pneumonia, psychosis, renal stone, retinopathy, skin necrosis, status epilepticus, subdural hematoma, syncope, tachycardia, thrombocytopenia, thrombophlebitis

Overdosage/Toxicology Acute oral overdoses of up to 49 g have been reported; double vision, slurred speech, drowsiness, lethargy, and diarrhea were observed. Patients recovered with supportive care. Decontaminate using lavage/activated charcoal with cathartic. Multiple dosing of activated charcoal may be useful; hemodialysis may be useful.

Drug Interactions CNS depressants: Sedative effects may be additive with CNS depressants; includes ethanol, barbiturates, narcotic analgesics, and other sedative agents. Monitor for increased effect.

Ethanol/Nutrition/Herb Interactions

Ethanol: Avoid ethanol (may increase CNS depression).

Food: Does not change rate or extent of absorption.

Herb/Nutraceutical: Avoid evening primrose (seizure threshold decreased). Avoid valerian, St John's wort, kava kava, gotu kola (may increase CNS depression).

Test Interactions False positives have been reported with the Ames N-Multistix SG® dipstick test for urine protein

Dietary Considerations May be taken without regard to meals.

Dosage Forms

Capsule (Neurontin®): 100 mg, 300 mg, 400 mg

Solution, oral (Neurontin®): 250 mg/5 mL (480 mL) [cool strawberry anise flavor]

Tablet: 100 mg, 300 mg, 400 mg

Neurontin®: 600 mg, 800 mg

References

Dierking G, Duedahl TH, Rasmussen ML, et al, "Effects of Gabapentin on Postoperative Morphine Consumption and Pain After Abdominal Hysterectomy: A Randomized, Double-Blind Trial," *Acta Anaesthesiol Scand*, 2004, 48(3):322-7.

Dirks J, Fredensborg BB, Christensen D, et al, "A Randomized Study of the Effects of Single-Dose Gabapentin Versus Placebo on Postoperative Pain and Morphine Consumption After Mastectomy," *Anesthesiology*, 2002, 97(3):560-4.

Pandey CK, Priye S, Singh S, et al, "Preemptive Use of Gabapentin Significantly Decreases Postoperative Pain and Rescue Analgesic Requirements in Laparoscopic Cholecystectomy," *Can J Anaesth*, 2004, 51(4):358-63.

Rorarius MG, Mennander S, Suominen P, et al, "Gabapentin for the Prevention of Postoperative Pain After Vaginal Hysterectomy," *Pain*, 2004, 110(1-2):175-81.

Turan A, Memis D, Karamanlioglu B, et al, "The Analgesic Effects of Gabapentin in Monitored Anesthesia Care for Ear-Nose-Throat Surgery," *Anesth Analg*, 2004, 99(2):375-8, table of contents.

◆ **Gabitril®** *see* Tiagabine *on page 1262*

Gallium Nitrate (GAL ee um NYE trate)

U.S. Brand Names Ganite™

Synonyms NSC-15200

Pharmacologic Category Calcium-Lowering Agent

Generic Available No

Use Treatment of hypercalcemia

Mechanism of Action Inhibits bone resorption by inhibiting osteoclast function

Pharmacodynamics/Kinetics

Onset of calcium lowering: Seen within 24-48 hours of beginning therapy, with normocalcemia achieved within 4-7 days of beginning therapy

Bioavailability: Oral: 5%

Distribution: Tissue concentrations were determined postmortem in one patient and concentrations were higher in liver and kidney than in lung, skin, muscle, heart, and cervix tumor; in dogs, tissue gallium concentrations were higher in renal cortex, bone, bone marrow, small intestine, and liver than in skeletal muscle and brain

Half-life elimination: Alpha: 1.25 hours; Beta: ~24 hours

Elimination half-life varies with method of administration (72-115 hours with prolonged intravenous infusion versus 24 hours with bolus administration); long elimination half-life may be related to slow release from tissue such as bone

Excretion: Primarily renal with no prior metabolism in the liver or kidney

Dosage I.V.: Adults: 200 mg/m^2/day for 5 days; duration may be shortened during a course if normocalcemia is achieved. If hypercalcemia is mild and with very few symptoms, 100 mg/m^2/day may be used.

Dosage adjustment in renal impairment:

Serum creatinine >2.5 mg/dL: Contraindicated

Serum creatinine 2 to <2.5 mg/dL: No guidelines exist; frequent monitoring is recommended

Stability

Store unopened vials (25 mg/mL) at room temperature of 15°C to 30°C (59°F to 86°F); not light sensitive. Dilute in 250-1000 mL NS or D_5W for infusion. Solutions in 0.9% NaCl or D_5W are stable for 48 hours at room temperature or for 7 days under refrigeration at 2°C to 8°C (36°F to 46°F).

Administration I.V. infusion over 30 minutes to 24 hours

Monitoring Parameters Renal function, serum calcium (daily), serum phosphorus (twice weekly)

Pregnancy Risk Factor C

Contraindications Hypersensitivity to gallium nitrate or any component of the formulation; severe renal dysfunction (creatinine >2.5 mg/dL)

Warnings/Precautions Hazardous agent - use appropriate precautions for handling and disposal. **[U.S. Boxed Warning]: Use caution with renal impairment or when administering other nephrotoxic drugs (eg, aminoglycosides, amphotericin B);** consider discontinuing gallium nitrate during treatment with nephrotoxic drugs. Maintain adequate hydration. Safety and efficacy in pediatric patients have not been established.

Adverse Reactions Not all frequencies defined.

Cardiovascular: Hypotension, tachycardia, edema of lower extremities

Central nervous system: Lethargy, confusion, dreams, hallucinations, hypothermia, fever

Dermatologic: Rash

Endocrine & metabolic: Hypophosphatemia (>50%, usually asymptomatic); hypocalcemia; mild respiratory alkalosis with hyperchloremia

Hematologic: Anemia, leukopenia

Gastrointestinal: Nausea (14%, generally mild), vomiting, diarrhea, constipation

Neuromuscular & skeletal: Paresthesia

Renal: Nephrotoxicity (>10%, generally reversible and reported to be minimized with adequate hydration and urine output)

Respiratory: Dyspnea, rales, rhonchi, pleural effusion, pulmonary infiltrates

Note: Toxicities reported with doses higher than those used to treat hypercalcemia (ie, in trials evaluating anticancer effect): Optic neuritis, tinnitus, hearing acuity decreased, metallic taste, hypomagnesemia, encephalopathy

Overdosage/Toxicology Symptoms of overdose include nausea, vomiting, and increased risk of nephrotoxicity.

Drug Interactions

Cyclophosphamide: Concurrent use of low dose gallium nitrate has been associated with dyspnea, stomatitis, asthenia, and rarely interstitial pneumonitis.

Nephrotoxic drugs (eg, aminoglycosides, amphotericin B): Concurrent use with gallium nitrate may increase nephrotoxic effects.

Dosage Forms Injection, solution [preservative free]: 25 mg/mL (20 mL)

- **Gamimune® N (Can)** *see* Immune Globulin (Intravenous) *on page 666*
- **Gammagard® Liquid** *see* Immune Globulin (Intravenous) *on page 666*
- **Gammagard® S/D** *see* Immune Globulin (Intravenous) *on page 666*
- **Gamma Hydroxybutyric Acid** *see* Sodium Oxybate *on page 1187*
- **Gammar®-P I.V.** *see* Immune Globulin (Intravenous) *on page 666*
- **Gamunex®** *see* Immune Globulin (Intravenous) *on page 666*

Ganciclovir (gan SYE kloe veer)

Medication Safety Issues

Sound-alike/look-alike issues:

Cytovene® may be confused with Cytosar®, Cytosar-U®

U.S. Brand Names Cytovene®; Vitrasert®

Canadian Brand Names Cytovene®; Vitrasert®

Synonyms DHPG Sodium; GCV Sodium; Nordeoxyguanosine

Pharmacologic Category Antiviral Agent

Generic Available Yes: Capsule

Use

Parenteral: Treatment of CMV retinitis in immunocompromised individuals, including patients with acquired immunodeficiency syndrome; prophylaxis of CMV infection in transplant patients

Oral: Alternative to the I.V. formulation for maintenance treatment of CMV retinitis in immunocompromised patients, including patients with AIDS, in whom retinitis is stable following appropriate induction therapy and for whom the risk of more rapid progression is balanced by the benefit associated with avoiding daily I.V. infusions.

Implant: Treatment of CMV retinitis

Unlabeled/Investigational Use May be given in combination with foscarnet in patients who relapse after monotherapy with either drug

Mechanism of Action Ganciclovir is phosphorylated to a substrate which competitively inhibits the binding of deoxyguanosine triphosphate to DNA polymerase resulting in inhibition of viral DNA synthesis

Pharmacodynamics/Kinetics

Distribution: V_d: 15.26 L/1.73 m^2; widely to all tissues including CSF and ocular tissue

Protein binding: 1% to 2%

Bioavailability: Oral: Fasting: 5%; Following food: 6% to 9%; Following fatty meal: 28% to 31%

Half-life elimination: 1.7-5.8 hours; prolonged with renal impairment; End-stage renal disease: 5-28 hours

Excretion: Urine (80% to 99% as unchanged drug)

Dosage

CMV retinitis: Slow I.V. infusion (dosing is based on total body weight):

Children >3 months and Adults:

Induction therapy: 5 mg/kg/dose every 12 hours for 14-21 days followed by maintenance therapy

Maintenance therapy: 5 mg/kg/day as a single daily dose for 7 days/week or 6 mg/kg/day for 5 days/week

CMV retinitis: Oral: 1000 mg 3 times/day with food **or** 500 mg 6 times/day with food

Prevention of CMV disease in patients with advanced HIV infection and normal renal function: Oral: 1000 mg 3 times/day with food

Prevention of CMV disease in transplant patients: Same initial and maintenance dose as CMV retinitis except duration of initial course is 7-14 days, duration of maintenance therapy is dependent on clinical condition and degree of immunosuppression

Intravitreal implant: One implant for 5- to 8-month period; following depletion of ganciclovir, as evidenced by progression of retinitis, implant may be removed and replaced

(Continued)

Ganciclovir *(Continued)*

Elderly: Refer to adult dosing; in general, dose selection should be cautious, reflecting greater frequency of organ impairment

Dosing adjustment in renal impairment:

I.V. (Induction):

Cl_{cr} 50-69 mL/minute: Administer 2.5 mg/kg/dose every 12 hours

Cl_{cr} 25-49 mL/minute: Administer 2.5 mg/kg/dose every 24 hours

Cl_{cr} 10-24 mL/minute: Administer 1.25 mg/kg/dose every 24 hours

Cl_{cr} <10 mL/minute: Administer 1.25 mg/kg/dose 3 times/week following hemodialysis

I.V. (Maintenance):

Cl_{cr} 50-69 mL/minute: Administer 2.5 mg/kg/dose every 24 hours

Cl_{cr} 25-49 mL/minute: Administer 1.25 mg/kg/dose every 24 hours

Cl_{cr} 10-24 mL/minute: Administer 0.625 mg/kg/dose every 24 hours

Cl_{cr} <10 mL/minute: Administer 0.625 mg/kg/dose 3 times/week following hemodialysis

Oral:

Cl_{cr} 50-69 mL/minute: Administer 1500 mg/day or 500 mg 3 times/day

Cl_{cr} 25-49 mL/minute: Administer 1000 mg/day or 500 mg twice daily

Cl_{cr} 10-24 mL/minute: Administer 500 mg/day

Cl_{cr} <10 mL/minute: Administer 500 mg 3 times/week following hemodialysis

Hemodialysis effects: Dialyzable (50%) following hemodialysis; administer dose postdialysis. During peritoneal dialysis, dose as for Cl_{cr} <10 mL/minute. During continuous arteriovenous or venovenous hemofiltration, administer 2.5 mg/kg/dose every 24 hours.

Stability Intact vials should be stored at room temperature and protected from temperatures >40°C Reconstitute powder with unpreserved sterile water **not** bacteriostatic water because parabens may cause precipitation; dilute in 250-1000 mL D_5W or NS to a concentration ≤10 mg/mL for infusion.

Reconstituted solution is stable for 12 hours at room temperature, however, conflicting data indicates that reconstituted solution is stable for 60 days under refrigeration (4°C). Stability of parenteral admixture at room temperature (25°C) and at refrigeration temperature (4°C) is 5 days.

Administration Oral: Should be administered with food.

I.V.: Should not be administered by I.M., SubQ, or rapid IVP; administer by slow I.V. infusion over at least 1 hour

Monitoring Parameters CBC with differential and platelet count, serum creatinine, ophthalmologic exams

Pregnancy Risk Factor C

Contraindications Hypersensitivity to ganciclovir, acyclovir, or any component of the formulation; absolute neutrophil count <500/mm^3; platelet count <25,000/mm^3

Warnings/Precautions Hazardous agent - use appropriate precautions for handling and disposal. Dosage adjustment or interruption of ganciclovir therapy may be necessary in patients with neutropenia and/or thrombocytopenia and patients with impaired renal function. Use with extreme caution in children since long-term safety has not been determined and due to ganciclovir's potential for long-term carcinogenic and adverse reproductive effects; ganciclovir may adversely affect spermatogenesis and fertility; due to its mutagenic potential, contraceptive precautions for female and male patients need to be followed during and for at least 90 days after therapy with the drug; take care to administer only into veins with good blood flow.

Adverse Reactions

>10%:

Central nervous system: Fever (38% to 48%)

Dermatologic: Rash (15% oral, 10% I.V.)

Gastrointestinal: Abdominal pain (17% to 19%), diarrhea (40%), nausea (25%), anorexia (15%), vomiting (13%)

Hematologic: Anemia (20% to 25%), leukopenia (30% to 40%)

1% to 10%:

Central nervous system: Confusion, neuropathy (8% to 9%), headache (4%)

Dermatologic: Pruritus (5%)

Hematologic: Thrombocytopenia (6%), neutropenia with ANC <500/mm^3 (5% oral, 14% I.V.)

Neuromuscular & skeletal: Paresthesia (6% to 10%), weakness (6%)

Ocular: Retinal detachment (8% oral, 11% I.V.; relationship to ganciclovir not established)

Miscellaneous: Sepsis (4% oral, 15% I.V.)

<1% (Limited to important or life-threatening): Alopecia, arrhythmia, ataxia, bronchospasm, coma, dyspnea, encephalopathy, eosinophilia, exfoliative dermatitis, extrapyramidal symptoms, hemorrhage, nervousness, pancytopenia, psychosis, renal failure, seizure, SIADH, Stevens-Johnson syndrome, torsade de pointes, urticaria, visual loss

Overdosage/Toxicology Symptoms of overdose include neutropenia, vomiting, hypersalivation, bloody diarrhea, cytopenia, and testicular atrophy. Treatment is supportive. Hemodialysis removes 50% of the drug. Hydration may be of some benefit.

Drug Interactions

Decreased effect: Didanosine: A decrease in steady-state ganciclovir AUC may occur

Increased toxicity:

Immunosuppressive agents may increase cytotoxicity of ganciclovir

Imipenem/cilastatin may increase seizure potential

Zidovudine: Oral ganciclovir increased the AUC of zidovudine, although zidovudine decreases steady state levels of ganciclovir. Since both drugs have the potential to cause neutropenia and anemia, some patients may not tolerate concomitant therapy with these drugs at full dosage.

Probenecid: The renal clearance of ganciclovir is decreased in the presence of probenecid

Didanosine levels are increased with concurrent ganciclovir

Other nephrotoxic drugs (eg, amphotericin and cyclosporine) may have additive nephrotoxicity with ganciclovir

Dietary Considerations Sodium content of 500 mg vial: 46 mg

Dosage Forms [DSC] = Discontinued product

Capsule: 250 mg, 500 mg

Cytovene®: 250 mg, 500 mg [DSC]

Implant, intravitreal (Vitrasert®): 4.5 mg [released gradually over 5-8 months]

Injection, powder for reconstitution, as sodium (Cytovene®): 500 mg

- **Ganite™** *see* Gallium Nitrate *on page 580*
- **Garamycin® (Can)** *see* Gentamicin *on page 589*

Gatifloxacin (gat i FLOKS a sin)

U.S. Brand Names Tequin® [DSC]; Zymar™

Canadian Brand Names Tequin®; Zymar™

Pharmacologic Category Antibiotic, Ophthalmic; Antibiotic, Quinolone

Generic Available No

Use

Oral, I.V.: Treatment of the following infections when caused by susceptible bacteria: Acute bacterial exacerbation of chronic bronchitis; acute sinusitis; community-acquired pneumonia including pneumonia caused by multidrug-resistant *S. pneumoniae* (MDRSP); uncomplicated skin and skin structure infection; uncomplicated urinary tract infections (cystitis); complicated urinary tract infections; pyelonephritis; uncomplicated urethral and cervical gonorrhea; acute, uncomplicated rectal infections in women

Ophthalmic: Bacterial conjunctivitis

Mechanism of Action Gatifloxacin is a DNA gyrase inhibitor, and also inhibits topoisomerase IV. DNA gyrase (topoisomerase II) is an essential bacterial enzyme that maintains the superhelical structure of DNA. DNA gyrase is required for DNA replication and transcription, DNA repair, recombination, and transposition; inhibition is bactericidal.

Pharmacodynamics/Kinetics

Absorption: Oral: Well absorbed; Ophthalmic: Not measurable

Distribution: V_d: 1.5-2.0 L/kg; concentrates in alveolar macrophages and lung parenchyma

Protein binding: 20%

Metabolism: Only 1%; no interaction with CYP

Bioavailability: 96%

Half-life elimination: 7.1-13.9 hours; ESRD/CAPD: 30-40 hours

Time to peak: Oral: 1 hour

Excretion: Urine (70% as unchanged drug, <1% as metabolites); feces (5%)

(Continued)

Gatifloxacin *(Continued)*

Dosage

Usual dosage range:

Adults: Oral, I.V.: 400 mg once daily

Indication-specific dosing:

Children ≥1 year and Adults:

Bacterial conjunctivitis: Ophthalmic:

Days 1 and 2: Instill 1 drop into affected eye(s) every 2 hours while awake (maximum: 8 times/day)

Days 3-7: Instill 1 drop into affected eye(s) up to 4 times/day while awake

Adults: Oral, I.V.:

Acute bacterial exacerbation of chronic bronchitis: 400 mg every 24 hours for 5 days

Acute sinusitis: 400 mg every 24 hours for 10 days

Community-acquired pneumonia (including atypical organisms): 400 mg every 24 hours for 7-14 days

Pyelonephritis (acute): 400 mg every 24 hours for 7-10 days

Skin/skin structure infections (uncomplicated): 400 mg every 24 hours for 7-10 days

Traveler's diarrhea (unlabeled use): 400 mg once daily for 3 days

Urinary tract infections:

Complicated: 400 mg every 24 hours for 7-10 days

Uncomplicated, cystitis: 400 mg single dose or 200 mg every 24 hours for 3 days

Urethral gonorrhea in men (uncomplicated), cervical or rectal gonorrhea in women and pharyngitis (gonococcal): 400 mg single dose

Elderly: No dosage adjustment is required based on age, however, assessment of renal function is particularly important in this population.

Dosage adjustment in renal impairment: Creatinine clearance <40 mL/minute (or patients on hemodialysis/CAPD) should receive an initial dose of 400 mg, followed by a subsequent dose of 200 mg every 24 hours. Patients receiving single-dose or 3-day therapy for appropriate indications do not require dosage adjustment. Administer after hemodialysis.

Dosage adjustment in hepatic impairment: No dosage adjustment is required in mild-moderate hepatic disease. No data are available in severe hepatic impairment (Child-Pugh Class C).

Stability

Ophthalmic solution: Store between 15°C to 25°C (59°F to 77°F). Do not freeze.

Solution for injection: Store at 25°C (77°F). Do not freeze. Single-use vials must be diluted to a concentration of 2 mg/mL prior to administration; may be diluted with D_5W, NS, D_5NS, D_5LR, 5% sodium bicarbonate, or Plasma-Lyte® 56/D_5W, or $D_5$1/2NS with 20 mEq KCl. Do not dilute with SWFI (a hypotonic solution results). Following dilution, stable for 14 days when stored between 20°C to 25°C or 2° to 8°C. Diluted solutions (except those prepared in 5% sodium bicarbonate) may also be frozen for up to 6 months when stored at -25°C to -10°C (-13°F to 14°F). Solutions may then be thawed at room temperature and should be used within 14 days (store between 20°C to 25°C or 2°C to 8°C); do not refreeze.

Tablet: Store at 25°C (77°F).

Administration

Oral: May be administered with or without food, milk, or calcium supplements. Gatifloxacin should be taken 4 hours before supplements (including multivitamins) containing iron, zinc, or magnesium.

I.V.: For I.V. infusion only. Concentrated injection (10 mg/mL) must be diluted to 2 mg/mL prior to administration. No further dilution is required for premixed 100 mL and 200 mL solutions. Infuse over 60 minutes. Avoid rapid or bolus infusions.

Monitoring Parameters WBC, signs of infection; signs or symptoms of hypo-/hyperglycemia

Anesthesia and Critical Care Concerns/Other Considerations Gatifloxacin causes a dose-dependent QT prolongation. Coadministration of gatifloxacin with other drugs that also prolong the QT interval or induce bradycardia (eg, beta-blockers, amiodarone) should be done cautiously. Careful consideration should be given in the use of gatifloxacin in patients with cardiovascular disease, particularly in those with conduction abnormalities.

Pregnancy Risk Factor C

Contraindications Hypersensitivity to gatifloxacin, other quinolone antibiotics, or any component of the formulation; diabetes mellitus

Warnings/Precautions Use with caution in patients with significant bradycardia or acute myocardial ischemia. May prolong QT interval (concentration related). Use caution in patients with known prolongation of QT interval, uncorrected hypokalemia, or concurrent administration of other medications known to prolong the QT interval (including Class Ia and Class III antiarrhythmics, cisapride, erythromycin, antipsychotics, and tricyclic antidepressants). May cause increased CNS stimulation, increased intracranial pressure, convulsions, or psychosis. Use with caution in individuals at risk of seizures (CNS disorders or concurrent therapy with medications which may lower seizure threshold). Potential for seizures, although very rare, may be increased with concomitant NSAID therapy. Discontinue in patients who experience significant CNS adverse effects (dizziness, hallucinations, suicidal ideation or actions). Use caution in renal dysfunction (dosage adjustment required) and in severe hepatic insufficiency (no data available). Serious disruptions in glucose regulation (including hyperglycemia and severe hypoglycemia) may occur, usually (but not always) in patients with diabetes. Other risk factors for glucose dysregulation include advanced age, renal insufficiency, and use of concurrent medications which alter glucose utilization. Hypoglycemia may be more prevalent in the initial 3 days of therapy while a greater risk of hyperglycemia may be present after the initial 3 days (particularly days 4-10). Monitor closely and discontinue if hyper- or hypoglycemia occur. Tendon inflammation and/or rupture has been reported with this and other quinolone antibiotics. Risk may be increased with concurrent corticosteroids, particularly in the elderly. Discontinue at first signs or symptoms of tendon or pain.

Severe hypersensitivity reactions, including anaphylaxis, have occurred with quinolone therapy. If an allergic reaction occurs (itching, urticaria, dyspnea, facial edema, loss of consciousness, tingling, cardiovascular collapse) discontinue drug immediately. Prolonged use may result in superinfection; pseudomembranous colitis may occur and should be considered in all patients who present with diarrhea. Quinolones may exacerbate myasthenia gravis, use with caution (rare, potentially life-threatening weakness of respiratory muscles may occur). May cause peripheral neuropathy (rare); discontinue if symptoms of sensory or sensorimotor neuropathy occur. Do not inject ophthalmic solution subconjunctivally or introduce directly into the anterior chamber of the eye.

Safety and efficacy for ophthalmic use have not been established in children <1 year of age. Safety and efficacy for systemic use have not been established in patients <18 years of age.

Adverse Reactions

Systemic therapy:

3% to 10%:

Central nervous system: Headache (3%), dizziness (3%)
Gastrointestinal: Nausea (8%), diarrhea (4%)
Genitourinary: Vaginitis (6%)
Local: Injection site reactions (5%)

0.1% to ≤3%: Abdominal pain, abnormal dreams, abnormal vision, agitation, alkaline phosphatase increased, allergic reaction, anorexia, anxiety, arthralgia, back pain, chest pain, chills, confusion, constipation, diaphoresis, dry skin, dyspepsia, dyspnea, dysuria, electrolyte abnormalities, facial edema, fever, flatulence, gastritis, glossitis, hematuria, hyperglycemia, hypertension, insomnia, leg cramps, mouth ulceration, nervousness, neutropenia, oral candidiasis, palpitation, paresthesia, peripheral edema, pharyngitis, pruritus, rash, serum amylase increased, serum bilirubin increased, serum transaminases increased, somnolence, stomatitis, taste perversion, thirst, tinnitus, tremor, weakness, vasodilation, vertigo, vomiting

<0.1% (Limited to important or life-threatening): Abnormal thinking, acute renal failure, anaphylactic reaction, angioneurotic edema, arthritis, asthenia, ataxia, bone pain, bradycardia, breast pain, bronchospasm, cheilitis, colitis, cyanosis, depersonalization, depression, diabetes mellitus, dysphagia, ear pain, ecchymosis, edema, epistaxis, ethanol intolerance, euphoria, eye pain, gastrointestinal hemorrhage, gingivitis, halitosis, hallucination, hematemesis, hematuria, hepatitis, hostility, hyperesthesia, hyperglycemia (severe; including nonketotic hyperglycemia), hypertonia, hyperventilation, hypoglycemia (severe; including hypoglycemic coma), increased INR, increased prothrombin time, lymphadenopathy, maculopapular rash, metrorrhagia, migraine, myalgia, myasthenia, neck pain, nonketotic hyperglycemia, pancreatitis, panic attacks, paranoia,

(Continued)

Gatifloxacin *(Continued)*

parosmia, peripheral neuropathy, photophobia, pseudomembranous colitis, psychosis, ptosis, rectal hemorrhage, seizure, severe hyper-/hypoglycemia, Stevens-Johnson syndrome, stress, syncope, tachycardia, taste disturbance, tendon rupture, rupture, thrombocytopenia, torsade de pointes, tongue edema, vesiculobullous rash

Ophthalmic therapy:

5% to 10%: Ocular: Conjunctival irritation, keratitis, lacrimation increased, papillary conjunctivitis

1% to 4%:

Central nervous system: Headache

Gastrointestinal: Taste disturbance

Ocular: Chemosis, conjunctival hemorrhage, discharge, dry eye, edema, irritation, pain, visual acuity decreased

Overdosage/Toxicology Potential symptoms of overdose may include CNS excitation, seizures, QT prolongation, and arrhythmias (including torsade de pointes). Patients should be monitored by continuous ECG in the event of an overdose. Management is supportive and symptomatic. Not removed by dialysis.

Drug Interactions

Atypical antipsychotics and protease inhibitors: May cause hyperglycemia; use with caution and monitor.

Corticosteroids: Concurrent use may increase the risk of tendon rupture, particularly in elderly patients (overall incidence rare).

Hypoglycemic agents: Gatifloxacin may alter glucose control in patients receiving hypoglycemic agents with or without insulin. Cases of severe disturbances (including symptomatic hypoglycemia) have been reported, typically within 1-3 days of gatifloxacin initiation.

Metal cations (aluminum, calcium, iron, magnesium, and zinc) bind quinolones in the gastrointestinal tract and inhibit absorption. Concurrent administration of most antacids (not calcium carbonate), oral electrolyte supplements, quinapril, sucralfate, some didanosine formulations (chewable/buffered tablets and pediatric powder for oral suspension), and other highly-buffered oral drugs, should be avoided. Gatifloxacin should be administered 4 hours before these agents.

Probenecid: May decrease renal secretion of quinolones.

QT_c-prolonging agents: Effects may be additive with gatifloxacin. Use caution with Class Ia and Class III antiarrhythmics, erythromycin, cisapride, antipsychotics, and cyclic antidepressants.

Warfarin: The hypoprothrombinemic effect of warfarin may be enhanced by some quinolone antibiotics; monitor INR.

Ethanol/Nutrition/Herb Interactions

Ethanol: Caution with ethanol (may cause hypoglycemia).

Herb/Nutraceutical: Avoid dong quai, St John's wort (may also cause photosensitization); caution with chromium, garlic, gymnema (may cause hypoglycemia).

Test Interactions Some quinolones may produce a false-positive urine screening result for opiates using commercially-available immunoassay kits. This has been demonstrated most consistently for levofloxacin and ofloxacin, but other quinolones have shown cross-reactivity in certain assay kits. Confirmation of positive opiate screens by more specific methods should be considered.

Dietary Considerations May take tablets with or without food, milk, or calcium supplements. Gatifloxacin should be taken 4 hours before supplements (including multivitamins) containing iron, zinc, or magnesium.

Dosage Forms [DSC] = Discontinued product

Injection, infusion [premixed in D_5W]:

Tequin®: 200 mg (100 mL), 400 mg (200 mL) [DSC]

Injection, solution [preservative free]:

Tequin®: 10 mg/mL (40 mL) [DSC]

Solution, ophthalmic:

Zymar™: 0.3% (2.5 mL, 5 mL) [contains benzalkonium chloride]

Tablet:

Tequin®: 200 mg, 400 mg [DSC]

Tequin® Teq-paq™ [unit-dose pack]: 400 mg (5s) [DSC]

- **G-CSF** *see* Filgrastim *on page 525*
- **GCV Sodium** *see* Ganciclovir *on page 581*
- **Gelusil® Extra Strength (Can)** *see* Aluminum Hydroxide and Magnesium Hydroxide *on page 76*

Gemifloxacin (je mi FLOKS a sin)

U.S. Brand Names Factive®

Synonyms DW286; Gemifloxacin Mesylate; LA 20304a; SB-265805

Pharmacologic Category Antibiotic, Quinolone

Generic Available No

Use Treatment of acute exacerbation of chronic bronchitis; treatment of community-acquired pneumonia, including pneumonia caused by multidrug-resistant strains of *S. pneumoniae* (MDRSP)

Unlabeled/Investigational Use Acute sinusitis, uncomplicated urinary tract infection

Mechanism of Action Gemifloxacin is a DNA gyrase inhibitor and also inhibits topoisomerase IV. DNA gyrase (topoisomerase IV) is an essential bacterial enzyme that maintains the superhelical structure of DNA. DNA gyrase is required for DNA replication and transcription, DNA repair, recombination, and transposition; bactericidal

Pharmacodynamics/Kinetics

Absorption: Well absorbed from the GI tract

Bioavailability: 71%

Metabolism: Hepatic (minor); forms metabolites (CYP isoenzymes are not involved)

Time to peak, plasma: 1-2 hours

Protein binding: 60% to 70%

Half-life elimination: 7 hours (range 4-12 hours)

Excretion: Urine (30% to 40%); feces (60%)

Dosage

Usual dosage range:

Adults: Oral: 320 mg once daily

Indication-specific dosing:

Adults: Oral:

Acute exacerbations of chronic bronchitis: 320 mg once daily for 5 days

Community-acquired pneumonia (mild to moderate): 320 mg once daily for 7 days

Sinusitis (unlabeled use): 320 mg once daily for 10 days

Dosage adjustment in renal impairment: Cl_{cr} ≤40 mL/minute (or patients on hemodialysis/CAPD): 160 mg once daily (administer dose following hemodialysis)

Dosage adjustment in hepatic impairment: No adjustment required.

Stability Store at 25°C (77°F); excursions permitted to 15°C to 30°C (59°F to 86°F); protect from light

Administration May be administered with or without food, milk, or calcium supplements. Gemifloxacin should be taken 3 hours before or 2 hours after supplements (including multivitamins) containing iron, zinc, or magnesium.

Monitoring Parameters WBC, signs/symptoms of infection

Pregnancy Risk Factor C

Contraindications Hypersensitivity to gemifloxacin, other fluoroquinolones, or any component of the formulation

Warnings/Precautions Fluoroquinolones may prolong QT_c interval; avoid use of gemifloxacin in patients with uncorrected hypokalemia, hypomagnesemia, or concurrent administration of other medications known to prolong the QT interval (including Class Ia and Class III antiarrhythmics, cisapride, erythromycin, antipsychotics, and tricyclic antidepressants). Use with caution in patients with significant bradycardia or acute myocardial ischemia. Use with caution in individuals at risk of seizures (CNS disorders or concurrent therapy with medications which may lower seizure threshold). Potential for seizures, although very rare, may be increased with concomitant NSAID therapy. Discontinue in patients who experience significant CNS adverse effects (dizziness, hallucinations, suicidal ideation or actions). Use caution in renal dysfunction (dosage adjustment required).

Severe hypersensitivity reactions, including anaphylaxis, have occurred with quinolone therapy. If an allergic reaction occurs (itching, urticaria, dyspnea or facial edema, loss of consciousness, tingling, cardiovascular collapse), discontinue drug immediately. Prolonged use may result in superinfection; pseudomembranous colitis may occur and should be considered in all patients who present with diarrhea. Tendon inflammation and/or rupture has been reported with other

(Continued)

Gemifloxacin *(Continued)*

quinolone antibiotics; risk may increase with concurrent corticosteroids, particularly in the elderly. Discontinue at first sign of tendon inflammation or pain. Peripheral neuropathy has been linked to the use of quinolones; these cases were rare. Experience with quinolones in immature animals has resulted in permanent arthropathy. Safety and effectiveness in pediatric patients (<18 years of age) have not been established.

Adverse Reactions

1% to 10%:

Central nervous system: Headache (1%), dizziness (1%)
Dermatologic: Rash (3%)
Gastrointestinal: Diarrhea (4%), nausea (3%), abdominal pain (1%), vomiting (1%)
Hepatic: Transaminases increased (1% to 2%)

<1% (Limited to important or life-threatening): Abnormal vision, anemia, anorexia, arthralgia, asthenia, back pain, bilirubin increased, constipation, CPK increased, cramps (leg), dermatitis, dry mouth, dyspepsia, dyspnea, eczema, eosinophilia, fatigue, flatulence, fungal infection, gastritis, genital moniliasis, GGT increased, granulocytopenia, hyperglycemia, insomnia, leukopenia, moniliasis, myalgia, nervousness, pharyngitis, photosensitivity, pruritus, somnolence, taste perversion, thrombocythemia, thrombocytopenia, tremor, urticaria, vaginitis, vertigo

Important adverse effects reported with other agents in this drug class include (not reported for gemifloxacin): Allergic reactions, CNS stimulation, hepatitis, jaundice, peripheral neuropathy, pneumonitis (eosinophilic), seizure; sensorimotor-axonal neuropathy (paresthesia, hypoesthesias, dysesthesias, weakness); severe dermatologic reactions (toxic epidermal necrolysis, Stevens-Johnson syndrome); tendon rupture, torsade de pointes, vasculitis

Overdosage/Toxicology Treatment should be symptom-directed and supportive; 20% to 30% removed by hemodialysis.

Drug Interactions

Corticosteroids: Concurrent use may increase the risk of tendon rupture, particularly in elderly patients (overall incidence rare).

Glyburide: Quinolones may increase the effect of glyburide; monitor.

Metal cations (aluminum, calcium, iron, magnesium, and zinc) bind quinolones in the gastrointestinal tract and inhibit absorption. Concurrent administration of most antacids (not calcium carbonate), oral electrolyte supplements, quinapril, sucralfate, some didanosine formulations (chewable/buffered tablets and pediatric powder for oral suspension), and other highly-buffered oral drugs, should be avoided. Gemifloxacin should be administered 2 hours before or 3 hours after these agents.

Probenecid: May decrease renal secretion of quinolones.

QT_c-prolonging agents: Effects may be additive with gemifloxacin. Avoid concurrent use with Class Ia and Class III antiarrhythmics, erythromycin, cisapride, antipsychotics, and cyclic antidepressants.

Warfarin: The hypoprothrombinemic effect of warfarin may be enhanced by some quinolone antibiotics; monitor INR.

Ethanol/Nutrition/Herb Interactions Herb/Nutraceutical: Avoid dong quai, St John's wort (may also cause photosensitization).

Dietary Considerations May take tablets with or without food, milk, or calcium supplements. Gemifloxacin should be taken 3 hours before or 2 hours after supplements (including multivitamins) containing iron, zinc, or magnesium.

Dosage Forms Tablet, as mesylate: 320 mg

- **Gemifloxacin Mesylate** *see* Gemifloxacin *on page 587*
- **Gen-Acyclovir (Can)** *see* Acyclovir *on page 39*
- **Genahist® [OTC]** *see* DiphenhydrAMINE *on page 399*
- **Gen-Alprazolam (Can)** *see* Alprazolam *on page 65*
- **Gen-Amiodarone (Can)** *see* Amiodarone *on page 83*
- **Genapap™ [OTC]** *see* Acetaminophen *on page 26*
- **Genapap™ Children [OTC]** *see* Acetaminophen *on page 26*
- **Genapap™ Extra Strength [OTC]** *see* Acetaminophen *on page 26*
- **Genapap™ Infant [OTC]** *see* Acetaminophen *on page 26*
- **Genaphed® [OTC]** *see* Pseudoephedrine *on page 1085*
- **Genasal [OTC]** *see* Oxymetazoline *on page 973*

- ♦ **Gen-Atenolol (Can)** *see* Atenolol *on page 136*
- ♦ **Gen-Azathioprine (Can)** *see* Azathioprine *on page 148*
- ♦ **Gen-Baclofen (Can)** *see* Baclofen *on page 156*
- ♦ **Gen-Beclo (Can)** *see* Beclomethasone *on page 161*
- ♦ **Gen-Buspirone (Can)** *see* BusPIRone *on page 205*
- ♦ **Gen-Captopril (Can)** *see* Captopril *on page 221*
- ♦ **Gen-Carbamazepine CR (Can)** *see* Carbamazepine *on page 225*
- ♦ **Gen-Cimetidine (Can)** *see* Cimetidine *on page 281*
- ♦ **Gen-Ciprofloxacin (Can)** *see* Ciprofloxacin *on page 285*
- ♦ **Gen-Citalopram (Can)** *see* Citalopram *on page 297*
- ♦ **Gen-Clomipramine (Can)** *see* ClomiPRAMINE *on page 309*
- ♦ **Gen-Clonazepam (Can)** *see* Clonazepam *on page 313*
- ♦ **Gen-Diltiazem (Can)** *see* Diltiazem *on page 394*
- ♦ **Gen-Diltiazem CD (Can)** *see* Diltiazem *on page 394*
- ♦ **Gen-Divalproex (Can)** *see* Valproic Acid and Derivatives *on page 1329*
- ♦ **Gen-Doxazosin (Can)** *see* Doxazosin *on page 420*
- ♦ **Genebs [OTC]** *see* Acetaminophen *on page 26*
- ♦ **Genebs Extra Strength [OTC]** *see* Acetaminophen *on page 26*
- ♦ **Generlac** *see* Lactulose *on page 724*
- ♦ **Gen-Etidronate (Can)** *see* Etidronate Disodium *on page 495*
- ♦ **Gen-Famotidine (Can)** *see* Famotidine *on page 506*
- ♦ **Gen-Fluconazole (Can)** *see* Fluconazole *on page 530*
- ♦ **Gen-Fluoxetine (Can)** *see* Fluoxetine *on page 539*
- ♦ **Gen-Gabapentin (Can)** *see* Gabapentin *on page 577*
- ♦ **Gen-Glybe (Can)** *see* GlyBURIDE *on page 598*
- ♦ **Gengraf®** *see* CycloSPORINE *on page 337*
- ♦ **Gen-Hydroxyurea (Can)** *see* Hydroxyurea *on page 648*
- ♦ **Gen-Ipratropium (Can)** *see* Ipratropium *on page 698*
- ♦ **Gen-Lamotrigine (Can)** *see* Lamotrigine *on page 727*
- ♦ **Gen-Levothyroxine (Can)** *see* Levothyroxine *on page 751*
- ♦ **Gen-Lovastatin (Can)** *see* Lovastatin *on page 782*
- ♦ **Gen-Meloxicam (Can)** *see* Meloxicam *on page 798*
- ♦ **Gen-Metformin (Can)** *see* Metformin *on page 810*
- ♦ **Gen-Minocycline (Can)** *see* Minocycline *on page 854*
- ♦ **Gen-Nabumetone (Can)** *see* Nabumetone *on page 883*
- ♦ **Gen-Naproxen EC (Can)** *see* Naproxen *on page 899*
- ♦ **Gen-Nitro (Can)** *see* Nitroglycerin *on page 928*
- ♦ **Gen-Nizatidine (Can)** *see* Nizatidine *on page 935*
- ♦ **Gen-Nortriptyline (Can)** *see* Nortriptyline *on page 938*
- ♦ **Genoptic® [DSC]** *see* Gentamicin *on page 589*
- ♦ **Genotropin®** *see* Human Growth Hormone *on page 625*
- ♦ **Genotropin Miniquick®** *see* Human Growth Hormone *on page 625*
- ♦ **Gen-Paroxetine (Can)** *see* Paroxetine *on page 988*
- ♦ **Gen-Piroxicam (Can)** *see* Piroxicam *on page 1032*
- ♦ **Genpril® [OTC]** *see* Ibuprofen *on page 651*
- ♦ **Gen-Ranidine (Can)** *see* Ranitidine *on page 1105*
- ♦ **Gen-Salbutamol (Can)** *see* Albuterol *on page 50*
- ♦ **Gen-Selegiline (Can)** *see* Selegiline *on page 1157*
- ♦ **Gen-Sertraline (Can)** *see* Sertraline *on page 1161*
- ♦ **Gen-Simvastatin (Can)** *see* Simvastatin *on page 1174*
- ♦ **Gen-Sotalol (Can)** *see* Sotalol *on page 1198*
- ♦ **Gen-Sumatriptan (Can)** *see* Sumatriptan *on page 1222*
- ♦ **Gentak®** *see* Gentamicin *on page 589*

Gentamicin (jen ta MYE sin)

Medication Safety Issues

Sound-alike/look-alike issues:

Gentamicin may be confused with kanamycin

Garamycin® may be confused with kanamycin, Terramycin®

(Continued)

Gentamicin *(Continued)*

Related Information

Anesthesia for Patients With Liver Disease *on page 1421*
Prevention of Bacterial Endocarditis *on page 1583*
Prevention of Wound Infection and Sepsis in Surgical Patients *on page 1588*

U.S. Brand Names Genoptic® [DSC]; Gentak®

Canadian Brand Names Alcomicin®; Diogent®; Garamycin®; Gentamicin Injection, USP; SAB-Gentamicin

Synonyms Gentamicin Sulfate

Pharmacologic Category Antibiotic, Aminoglycoside; Antibiotic, Ophthalmic; Antibiotic, Topical

Generic Available Yes

Use Treatment of susceptible bacterial infections, normally gram-negative organisms including *Pseudomonas*, *Proteus*, *Serratia*, and gram-positive *Staphylococcus*; treatment of bone infections, respiratory tract infections, skin and soft tissue infections, as well as abdominal and urinary tract infections, endocarditis, and septicemia; used topically to treat superficial infections of the skin or ophthalmic infections caused by susceptible bacteria; prevention of bacterial endocarditis prior to dental or surgical procedures

Mechanism of Action Interferes with bacterial protein synthesis by binding to 30S and 50S ribosomal subunits resulting in a defective bacterial cell membrane

Pharmacodynamics/Kinetics

Absorption: Oral: None

Distribution: Crosses placenta

V_d: Increased by edema, ascites, fluid overload; decreased with dehydration (see table)

Aminoglycoside Penetration Into Various Tissues

Site	Extent of Distribution
Eye	Poor
CNS	Poor (<25%)
Pleural	Excellent
Bronchial secretions	Poor
Sputum	Fair (10%-50%)
Pulmonary tissue	Excellent
Ascitic fluid	Variable (43%-132%)
Peritoneal fluid	Poor
Bile	Variable (25%-90%)
Bile with obstruction	Poor
Synovial fluid	Excellent
Bone	Poor
Prostate	Poor
Urine	Excellent
Renal tissue	Excellent

Neonates: 0.4-0.6 L/kg
Children: 0.3-0.35 L/kg
Adults: 0.2-0.3 L/kg

Relative diffusion from blood into CSF: Minimal even with inflammation

CSF:blood level ratio: Normal meninges: Nil; Inflamed meninges: 10% to 30%

Protein binding: <30%

Half-life elimination

Infants: <1 week old: 3-11.5 hours; 1 week to 6 months old: 3-3.5 hours

Adults: 1.5-3 hours; End-stage renal disease: 36-70 hours

Time to peak, serum: I.M.: 30-90 minutes; I.V.: 30 minutes after 30-minute infusion

Excretion: Urine (as unchanged drug)

Clearance: Directly related to renal function

Dosage Note: Dosage Individualization is **critical** because of the low therapeutic index.

Use of ideal body weight (IBW) for determining the mg/kg/dose appears to be more accurate than dosing on the basis of total body weight (TBW). In morbid obesity, dosage requirement may best be estimated using a dosing weight of IBW + 0.4 (TBW - IBW).

Initial and periodic plasma drug levels (eg, peak and trough with conventional dosing) should be determined, particularly in critically-ill patients with serious infections or in disease states known to significantly alter aminoglycoside pharmacokinetics (eg, cystic fibrosis, burns, or major surgery).

Usual dosage ranges:

Infants and Children <5 years: I.M., I.V.: 2.5 mg/kg/dose every 8 hours*

Children ≥5 years: I.M., I.V.: 2-2.5 mg/kg/dose every 8 hours*

***Note:** Higher individual doses and/or more frequent intervals (eg, every 6 hours) may be required in selected clinical situations (cystic fibrosis) or serum levels document the need

Children and Adults:

Intrathecal: 4-8 mg/day

Ophthalmic:

Ointment: Instill 1/2" (1.25 cm) 2-3 times/day to every 3-4 hours

Solution: Instill 1-2 drops every 2-4 hours, up to 2 drops every hour for severe infections

Topical: Apply 3-4 times/day to affected area

Adults: I.M., I.V.:

Conventional: 1-2.5 mg/kg/dose every 8-12 hours; to ensure adequate peak concentrations early in therapy, higher initial dosage may be considered in selected patients when extracellular water is increased (edema, septic shock, postsurgical, or trauma)

Once daily: 4-7 mg/kg/dose once daily; some clinicians recommend this approach for all patients with normal renal function; this dose is at least as efficacious with similar, if not less, toxicity than conventional dosing

Indication-specific dosing:

Neonates: I.V.:

Meningitis:

0-7 days of age: <2000 g: 2.5 mg/kg every 18-24 hours; >2000 g: 2.5 mg/kg every 12 hours

8-28 days of age: <2000 g: 2.5 mg/kg every 8-12 hours; >2000 g: 2.5 mg/kg every 8 hours

Adults: I.M., I.V.:

Brucellosis: 240 mg (I.M.) daily or 5 mg/kg (I.V.) daily for 7 days; either regimen recommended in combination with doxycycline

Cholangitis: 4-6 mg/kg once daily with ampicillin

Diverticulitis (complicated): 1.5-2 mg/kg every 8 hours (with ampicillin and metronidazole)

Endocarditis prophylaxis: Dental, oral, upper respiratory procedures, GI/GU procedures: 1.5 mg/kg with ampicillin (50 mg/kg) 30 minutes prior to procedure

Endocarditis or synergy (for Gram-positive infections): 1 mg/kg every 8 hours (with ampicillin)

Meningitis:

(Enterococcus sp or *Pseudomonas aeruginosa)*: Loading dose 2 mg/kg, then 1.7 mg/kg/dose every 8 hours (administered with another bacteriocidal drug)

Listeria: 5-7 mg/kg/day (with penicillin) for 1 week

Pelvic inflammatory disease: Loading dose: 2 mg/kg, then 1.5 mg/kg every 8 hours

Alternate therapy: 4.5 mg/kg once daily

Plague (*Yersinia pestis*): Treatment: 5 mg/kg/day, followed by postexposure prophylaxis with doxycycline

Pneumonia, hospital- or ventilator-associated: 7 mg/kg/day (with antipseudomonal beta-lactam or carbapenem)

Tularemia: 5 mg/kg/day divided every 8 hours for 1-2 weeks

Urinary tract infection: 1.5 mg/kg/dose every 8 hours

Dosing interval in renal impairment:

Conventional dosing:

Cl_{cr} ≥60 mL/minute: Administer every 8 hours

Cl_{cr} 40-60 mL/minute: Administer every 12 hours

Cl_{cr} 20-40 mL/minute: Administer every 24 hours

Cl_{cr} <20 mL/minute: Loading dose, then monitor levels

(Continued)

Gentamicin *(Continued)*

High-dose therapy: Interval may be extended (eg, every 48 hours) in patients with moderate renal impairment (Cl_{cr} 30-59 mL/minute) and/or adjusted based on serum level determinations.

Hemodialysis: Dialyzable; removal by hemodialysis: 30% removal of aminoglycosides occurs during 4 hours of HD; administer dose after dialysis and follow levels

Removal by continuous ambulatory peritoneal dialysis (CAPD):

Administration via CAPD fluid:

Gram-negative infection: 4-8 mg/L (4-8 mcg/mL) of CAPD fluid

Gram-positive infection (eg, synergy): 3-4 mg/L (3-4 mcg/mL) of CAPD fluid

Administration via I.V., I.M. route during CAPD: Dose as for Cl_{cr} <10 mL/minute and follow levels

Removal via continuous arteriovenous or venovenous hemofiltration: Dose as for Cl_{cr} 10-40 mL/minute and follow levels

Dosing adjustment/comments in hepatic disease: Monitor plasma concentrations

Stability

Gentamicin is a colorless to slightly yellow solution which should be stored between 2°C to 30°C, but refrigeration is not recommended

I.V. infusion solutions mixed in NS or D_5W solution are stable for 24 hours at room temperature and refrigeration

Premixed bag: Manufacturer expiration date

Out of overwrap stability: 30 days

Administration

I.M.: Administer by deep I.M. route if possible. Slower absorption and lower peak concentrations, probably due to poor circulation in the atrophic muscle, may occur following I.M. injection; in paralyzed patients, suggest I.V. route.

Ophthalmic: Administer any other ophthalmics 10 minutes before or after gentamicin preparations.

Some penicillins (eg, carbenicillin, ticarcillin and piperacillin) have been shown to inactivate aminoglycosides *in vitro*. This has been observed to a greater extent with tobramycin and gentamicin, while amikacin has shown greater stability against inactivation. Concurrent use of these agents may pose a risk of reduced antibacterial efficacy *in vivo*, particularly in the setting of profound renal impairment. However, definitive clinical evidence is lacking. If combination penicillin/aminoglycoside therapy is desired in a patient with renal dysfunction, separation of doses (if feasible), and routine monitoring of aminoglycoside levels, CBC, and clinical response should be considered.

Monitoring Parameters Urinalysis, urine output, BUN, serum creatinine; hearing should be tested before, during, and after treatment; particularly in those at risk for ototoxicity or who will be receiving prolonged therapy (>2 weeks)

Some penicillin derivatives may accelerate the degradation of aminoglycosides*in vitro*. This may be clinically-significant for certain penicillin (ticarcillin, piperacillin, carbenicillin) and aminoglycoside (gentamicin, tobramycin) combination therapy in patients with significant renal impairment. Close monitoring of aminoglycoside levels is warranted.

Reference Range

Timing of serum samples: Draw peak 30 minutes after 30-minute infusion has been completed or 1 hour after I.M. injection; draw trough immediately before next dose

Sample size: 0.5-2 mL blood (red top tube) or 0.1-1 mL serum (separated)

Therapeutic levels:

Peak:

Serious infections: 6-8 mcg/mL (12-17 μmol/L)

Life-threatening infections: 8-10 mcg/mL (17-21 μmol/L)

Urinary tract infections: 4-6 mcg/mL

Synergy against gram-positive organisms: 3-5 mcg/mL

Trough:

Serious infections: 0.5-1 mcg/mL

Life-threatening infections: 1-2 mcg/mL

The American Thoracic Society (ATS) recommends trough levels of <1 mcg/mL for patients with hospital-acquired pneumonia.

Obtain drug levels after the third dose unless renal dysfunction/toxicity suspected

Anesthesia and Critical Care Concerns/Other Considerations Gentamicin is the only aminoglycoside that is commercially available in a preservative-free solution for injection.

Pregnancy Risk Factor C

Contraindications Hypersensitivity to gentamicin or other aminoglycosides

Warnings/Precautions [U.S. Boxed Warning]: Aminoglycosides may cause neurotoxicity and/or nephrotoxicity; usual risk factors include prexisiting renal impairment, concomitant neuro-/nephrotoxic medications, advanced age and dehydration. Ototoxicity may be directly proportional to the amount of drug given and the duration of treatment; tinnitus or vertigo are indications of vestibular injury and impending hearing loss; renal damage is usually reversible

Not intended for long-term therapy due to toxic hazards associated with extended administration; use caution in pre-existing renal insufficiency, vestibular or cochlear impairment, myasthenia gravis, hypocalcemia, conditions which depress neuromuscular transmission. Dosage modification required in patients with impaired renal function

Adverse Reactions

>10%:

Central nervous system: Neurotoxicity (vertigo, ataxia)

Neuromuscular & skeletal: Gait instability

Otic: Ototoxicity (auditory), ototoxicity (vestibular)

Renal: Nephrotoxicity, decreased creatinine clearance

1% to 10%:

Cardiovascular: Edema

Dermatologic: Skin itching, reddening of skin, rash

<1% (Limited to important or life-threatening): Agranulocytosis, allergic reaction, dyspnea, granulocytopenia, photosensitivity, pseudomotor cerebri, thrombocytopenia

Overdosage/Toxicology Symptoms of overdose include ototoxicity, nephrotoxicity, and neuromuscular toxicity. Serum level monitoring is recommended. The treatment of choice, following a single acute overdose, appears to be maintenance of urine output of at least 3 mL/kg/hour during the acute treatment phase. Dialysis is of questionable value in enhancing aminoglycoside elimination.

Drug Interactions

Increased toxicity:

Aminoglycosides may potentiate the effects of neuromuscular-blocking agents.

Penicillins, cephalosporins, amphotericin B, loop diuretics may increase nephrotoxic potential

Decreased effect: Gentamicin's efficacy reduced when given concurrently with carbenicillin, ticarcillin, or piperacillin to patients with severe renal impairment (inactivation). Separate administration.

Test Interactions

Some penicillin derivatives may accelerate the degradation of aminoglycosides *in vitro*, leading to a potential underestimation of aminoglycoside serum concentration.

Dietary Considerations Calcium, magnesium, potassium: Renal wasting may cause hypocalcemia, hypomagnesemia, and/or hypokalemia.

Dosage Forms [DSC] = Discontinued product

Cream, topical, as sulfate: 0.1% (15 g, 30 g)

Infusion, as sulfate [premixed in NS]: 40 mg (50 mL); 60 mg (50 mL, 100 mL); 70 mg (50 mL); 80 mg (50 mL, 100 mL); 90 mg (100 mL); 100 mg (50 mL, 100 mL); 120 mg (100 mL)

Injection, solution, as sulfate [ADD-Vantage® vial]: 10 mg/mL (6 mL, 8 mL, 10 mL)

Injection, solution, as sulfate: 40 mg/mL (2 mL, 20 mL) [may contain sodium metabisulfite]

Injection, solution, pediatric, as sulfate: 10 mg/mL (2 mL) [may contain sodium metabisulfite]

Injection, solution, pediatric, as sulfate [preservative free]: 10 mg/mL (2 mL)

Ointment, ophthalmic, as sulfate (Gentak®): 0.3% [3 mg/g] (3.5 g)

Ointment, topical, as sulfate: 0.1% (15 g, 30 g)

Solution, ophthalmic, as sulfate: 0.3% (5 mL, 15 mL) [contains benzalkonium chloride]

Genoptic®: 0.3% (1 mL) [contains benzalkonium chloride] [DSC]

Gentak®: 0.3% (5 mL; 15 mL [DSC]) [contains benzalkonium chloride]

(Continued)

Gentamicin *(Continued)*

References

American Thoracic Society and Infectious Diseases Society of America, "Guidelines for the Management of Adults With Hospital-Acquired, Ventilator-Associated, and Healthcare-Associated Pneumonia," *Am J Respir Crit Care Med*, 2005, 171(4):388-416.

Gilbert DN, Moellering RC, Eliopoulos GM, et al, eds, *The Sanford Guide To Antimicrobial Therapy*, 2006, 36th ed, Hyde Park, VT: Antimicrobial Therapy, Inc, 2006, 6-7.

Tunkel AR, Hartman BJ, Kaplan SL, et al, "Practice Guidelines for the Management of Bacterial Meningitis," *Clin Infect Dis*, 2004, 39(9):1267-84.

◆ **Gentamicin Injection, USP (Can)** *see* Gentamicin *on page 589*
◆ **Gentamicin Sulfate** *see* Gentamicin *on page 589*
◆ **Gen-Temazepam (Can)** *see* Temazepam *on page 1239*
◆ **Gen-Ticlopidine (Can)** *see* Ticlopidine *on page 1266*
◆ **Gen-Timolol (Can)** *see* Timolol *on page 1268*
◆ **Gen-Topiramate (Can)** *see* Topiramate *on page 1287*
◆ **Gentran®** *see* Dextran *on page 372*
◆ **Gen-Trazodone (Can)** *see* Trazodone *on page 1306*
◆ **Gen-Triazolam (Can)** *see* Triazolam *on page 1316*
◆ **Gen-Verapamil (Can)** *see* Verapamil *on page 1352*
◆ **Gen-Verapamil SR (Can)** *see* Verapamil *on page 1352*
◆ **Gen-Warfarin (Can)** *see* Warfarin *on page 1362*
◆ **Geodon®** *see* Ziprasidone *on page 1374*
◆ **GF196960** *see* Tadalafil *on page 1230*
◆ **GHB** *see* Sodium Oxybate *on page 1187*
◆ **GI87084B** *see* Remifentanil *on page 1109*
◆ **Glargine Insulin** *see* Insulin Glargine *on page 684*
◆ **Glibenclamide** *see* GlyBURIDE *on page 598*

GlipiZIDE (GLIP i zide)

Medication Safety Issues

Sound-alike/look-alike issues:

GlipiZIDE may be confused with glimepiride, glyBURIDE
Glucotrol® may be confused with Glucophage®, Glucotrol® XL, glyBURIDE
Glucotrol® XL may be confused with Glucotrol®

Related Information

Thiazolidinediones *on page 1577*
Perioperative Management of the Diabetic Patient *on page 1464*

U.S. Brand Names Glucotrol®; Glucotrol® XL

Synonyms Glydiazinamide

Pharmacologic Category Antidiabetic Agent, Sulfonylurea

Generic Available Yes

Use Management of type 2 diabetes mellitus (noninsulin dependent, NIDDM)

Mechanism of Action Stimulates insulin release from the pancreatic beta cells; reduces glucose output from the liver; insulin sensitivity is increased at peripheral target sites

Pharmacodynamics/Kinetics

Onset of action: Peak effect: Blood glucose reductions: 1.5-2 hours
Duration: 12-24 hours
Absorption: Delayed with food
Protein binding: 92% to 99%
Metabolism: Hepatic with metabolites
Half-life elimination: 2-4 hours
Excretion: Urine (60% to 80%, 91% to 97% as metabolites); feces (11%)

Dosage Oral (allow several days between dose titrations): Adults: Initial: 5 mg/day; adjust dosage at 2.5-5 mg daily increments as determined by blood glucose response at intervals of several days.

Immediate release tablet: Maximum recommended once-daily dose: 15 mg; maximum recommended total daily dose: 40 mg

Extended release tablet (Glucotrol® XL): Maximum recommended dose: 20 mg

When transferring from insulin to glipizide:

Current insulin requirement ≤20 units: Discontinue insulin and initiate glipizide at usual dose

Current insulin requirement >20 units: Decrease insulin by 50% and initiate glipizide at usual dose; gradually decrease insulin dose based on patient response. Several days should elapse between dosage changes.

Elderly: Initial: 2.5 mg/day; increase by 2.5-5 mg/day at 1- to 2-week intervals

Dosing adjustment/comments in renal impairment: Cl_{cr} <10 mL/minute: Some investigators recommend not using

Dosing adjustment in hepatic impairment: Initial dosage should be 2.5 mg/day

Administration Administer immediate release tablets 30 minutes before a meal to achieve greatest reduction in postprandial hyperglycemia. Extended release tablets should be given with breakfast. Patients who are NPO may need to have their dose held to avoid hypoglycemia.

Monitoring Parameters Urine for glucose and ketones; monitor for signs and symptoms of hypoglycemia (fatigue, excessive hunger, profuse sweating, numbness of extremities), fasting blood glucose, hemoglobin A_{1c}, fructosamine

Reference Range Target range: Adults:

Fasting blood glucose: <120 mg/dL

Glycosylated hemoglobin: <7%

Anesthesia and Critical Care Concerns/Other Considerations The possibility of higher doses of sulfonylureas eliciting an increase in cardiovascular events, because of their effects on blocking potassium sensitive ATP channels, has been raised. Longer-term prospective trials of sulfonylurea therapy, such as the UKPDS, do not reveal any increased cardiovascular mortality.

Pregnancy Risk Factor C

Contraindications Hypersensitivity to glipizide or any component of the formulation, other sulfonamides; type 1 diabetes mellitus (insulin dependent, IDDM)

Warnings/Precautions Use with caution in patients with severe hepatic disease.

Chemical similarities are present among sulfonamides, sulfonylureas, carbonic anhydrase inhibitors, thiazides, and loop diuretics (except ethacrynic acid). Use in patients with sulfonamide allergy is specifically contraindicated in product labeling, however, a risk of cross-reaction exists in patients with allergy to any of these compounds; avoid use when previous reaction has been severe.

The extended release formulation consists of drug within a nondeformable matrix; following drug release/absorption, the matrix/shell is expelled in the stool. The use of nondeformable products in patients with known stricture/narrowing of the GI tract has been associated with symptoms of obstruction. Avoid use of extended release tablets (Glucotrol® XL) in patients with severe gastrointestinal narrowing or esophageal dysmotility.

Product labeling states oral hypoglycemic drugs may be associated with an increased cardiovascular mortality as compared to treatment with diet alone or diet plus insulin. Data to support this association are limited, and several studies, including a large prospective trial (UKPDS) have not supported an association.

Adverse Reactions Frequency not defined.

Cardiovascular: Edema, syncope

Central nervous system: Anxiety, depression, dizziness, headache, insomnia, nervousness

Dermatologic: Rash, urticaria, photosensitivity, pruritus

Endocrine & metabolic: Hypoglycemia, hyponatremia, SIADH (rare)

Gastrointestinal: Anorexia, nausea, vomiting, diarrhea, epigastric fullness, constipation, heartburn, flatulence

Hematologic: Blood dyscrasias, aplastic anemia, hemolytic anemia, bone marrow suppression, thrombocytopenia, agranulocytosis

Hepatic: Cholestatic jaundice, hepatic porphyria

Neuromuscular & skeletal: Arthralgia, leg cramps, myalgia, tremor

Ocular: Blurred vision

Renal: Diuretic effect (minor)

Miscellaneous: Diaphoresis, disulfiram-like reaction

Postmarketing and/or case reports: Abdominal pain

Overdosage/Toxicology Symptoms of overdose include low blood sugar, tingling of lips and tongue, nausea, yawning, confusion, agitation, tachycardia, sweating, convulsions, stupor, and coma. Intoxication with sulfonylureas can cause hypoglycemia and are best managed with glucose administration (oral for milder hypoglycemia or by injection in more severe forms).

Drug Interactions **Substrate** of 2C8/9 (major)

Anabolic steroids may increase hypoglycemic effect; monitor blood glucose.

ACE inhibitors may increase hypoglycemic effect; monitor blood glucose.

(Continued)

GlipiZIDE *(Continued)*

Beta-blockers decrease hypoglycemic effect, mask most hypoglycemic symptoms, decrease glycogenolysis; avoid use in diabetics with frequent hypoglycemic episodes.

Cholestyramine decreases glipizide's absorption; separate administration times.

Corticosteroids cause hyperglycemia; adjustment of hypoglycemic agent may be necessary.

Cyclosporine serum concentration is increased; monitor cyclosporine levels and renal function.

CYP2C8/9 inducers: May decrease the levels/effects of glipizide. Example inducers include carbamazepine, phenobarbital, phenytoin, rifampin, rifapentine, and secobarbital.

CYP2C8/9 inhibitors: May increase the levels/effects of glipizide. Example inhibitors include delavirdine, fluconazole, gemfibrozil, ketoconazole, nicardipine, NSAIDs, pioglitazone, and sulfonamides.

Ethanol (large amounts) decreases hypoglycemic effect; avoid concurrent use; rare disulfiram reaction.

H_2 antagonists, antacids, oral sodium bicarbonate may increase the hypoglycemic effect; monitor glucose response.

Rifampin may decrease hypoglycemic effects of glipizide; monitor blood glucose.

Tacrolimus serum concentrations may be increased; monitor tacrolimus serum concentrations and renal function.

Ethanol/Nutrition/Herb Interactions

Ethanol: Caution with ethanol (may cause hypoglycemia or rare disulfiram reaction).

Food: A delayed release of insulin may occur if glipizide is taken with food. Immediate release tablets should be administered 30 minutes before meals to avoid erratic absorption.

Herb/Nutraceutical: Caution with chromium, garlic, gymnema (may cause hypoglycemia).

Dietary Considerations Take immediate release tablets 30 minutes before meals; extended release tablets should be taken with breakfast. Dietary modification based on ADA recommendations is a part of therapy. Decreases blood glucose concentration. Hypoglycemia may occur. Must be able to recognize symptoms of hypoglycemia (palpitations, sweaty palms, lightheadedness).

Dosage Forms

Tablet (Glucotrol®): 5 mg, 10 mg

Tablet, extended release: 5 mg, 10 mg

Glucotrol® XL: 2.5 mg, 5 mg, 10 mg

- ♦ **GlucaGen®** *see* Glucagon *on page 596*
- ♦ **GlucaGen® Diagnostic Kit** *see* Glucagon *on page 596*
- ♦ **GlucaGen® HypoKit™** *see* Glucagon *on page 596*

Glucagon (GLOO ka gon)

Medication Safety Issues

Sound-alike/look-alike issues:

Glucagon may be confused with Glaucon®

U.S. Brand Names GlucaGen®; GlucaGen® Diagnostic Kit; GlucaGen® HypoKit™; Glucagon Diagnostic Kit [DSC]; Glucagon Emergency Kit

Synonyms Glucagon Hydrochloride

Pharmacologic Category Antidote; Diagnostic Agent

Generic Available No

Use Management of hypoglycemia; diagnostic aid in radiologic examinations to temporarily inhibit GI tract movement

Unlabeled/Investigational Use Used with some success as a cardiac stimulant in management of severe cases of beta-adrenergic blocking agent overdosage; treatment of myocardial depression due to calcium channel blocker overdose

Mechanism of Action Stimulates adenylate cyclase to produce increased cyclic AMP, which promotes hepatic glycogenolysis and gluconeogenesis, causing a raise in blood glucose levels

Pharmacodynamics/Kinetics

Onset of action: Peak effect: Blood glucose levels: Parenteral:

I.V.: 5-20 minutes

I.M.: 30 minutes

SubQ: 30-45 minutes
Duration: Hyperglycemia: 60-90 minutes
Metabolism: Primarily hepatic; some inactivation occurring renally and in plasma
Half-life elimination, plasma: 3-10 minutes

Dosage

Hypoglycemia or insulin shock therapy: I.M., I.V., SubQ:

Children <20 kg: 0.5 mg or 20-30 mcg/kg/dose; repeated in 20 minutes as needed

Children ≥20 kg and Adults: 1 mg; may repeat in 20 minutes as needed

Note: If patient fails to respond to glucagon, I.V. dextrose must be given.

Beta-blocker overdose, calcium channel blocker overdose (unlabeled use): Adults: I.V.: 5-10 mg over 1 minutes followed by an infusion of 1-10 mg/hour. The following has also been reported for beta-blocker overdose: 3-10 mg or initially 0.5-5 mg bolus followed by continuous infusion 1-5 mg/hour

Diagnostic aid: Adults: I.M., I.V.: 0.25-2 mg 10 minutes prior to procedure

Stability Prior to reconstitution, store at controlled room temperature of 20°C to 25°C (69°F to 77°F); do not freeze. Reconstitute powder for injection by adding 1 mL of sterile diluent to a vial containing 1 unit of the drug, to provide solutions containing 1 mg of glucagon/mL. Gently roll vial to dissolve. If dose to be administered is <2 mg of the drug, then use only the diluent provided by the manufacturer. If >2 mg, use sterile water for injection. Use immediately after reconstitution. May be kept at 5°C for up to 48 hours if necessary.

Administration I.V.: Bolus may be associated with nausea and vomiting. Continuous infusions may be used in beta-blocker overdose/toxicity.

Monitoring Parameters Blood pressure, blood glucose, heart rate

Anesthesia and Critical Care Concerns/Other Considerations 1 unit = 1 mg

Pregnancy Risk Factor B

Contraindications Hypersensitivity to glucagon or any component of the formulation; insulinoma; pheochromocytoma

Warnings/Precautions Use caution with prolonged fasting, starvation, adrenal insufficiency or chronic hypoglycemia; levels of glucose stores in liver may be decreased. Following response to therapy, oral carbohydrates should be administered to prevent hypoglycemia.

Adverse Reactions Frequency not defined.

Cardiovascular: Hypotension (up to 2 hours after GI procedures), hypertension, tachycardia

Gastrointestinal: Nausea, vomiting (high incidence with rapid administration of high doses)

Miscellaneous: Hypersensitivity reactions, anaphylaxis

Overdosage/Toxicology Symptoms include hypokalemia, nausea and vomiting, inhibition of GI tract motility, decreased blood pressure, tachycardia

Drug Interactions Oral anticoagulant: Hypoprothrombinemic effects may be increased possibly with bleeding; effect seen with glucagon doses of 50 mg administered over 1-2 days

Ethanol/Nutrition/Herb Interactions Glucagon depletes glycogen stores.

Dietary Considerations Administer carbohydrates to patient as soon as possible after response to treatment.

Dosage Forms Injection, powder for reconstitution, as hydrochloride:

GlucaGen®: 1 mg [equivalent to 1 unit; contains lactose 107 mg]

GlucaGen® Diagnostic Kit: 1 mg [equivalent to 1 unit; contains lactose 107 mg; packaged with sterile water]

GlucaGen® HypoKit™: 1 mg [equivalent to 1 unit; contains lactose 107 mg; packaged with prefilled syringe containing sterile water]

Glucagon®: 1 mg [equivalent to 1 unit; contains lactose 49 mg]

Glucagon Diagnostic Kit, Glucagon Emergency Kit: 1 mg [equivalent to 1 unit; contains lactose 49 mg; packaged with diluent syringe containing glycerin 12 mg/mL and water for injection]

References

Mokhlesi B, Leikin JB, Murray P, et al, "Adult Toxicology in Critical Care. Part 11: Specific Poisonings," *Chest*, 2003, 123(3):897-922.

- **Glucagon Diagnostic Kit [DSC]** *see* Glucagon *on page 596*
- **Glucagon Emergency Kit** *see* Glucagon *on page 596*
- **Glucagon Hydrochloride** *see* Glucagon *on page 596*
- **Glucophage®** *see* Metformin *on page 810*
- **Glucophage® XR** *see* Metformin *on page 810*

- **Glucotrol®** *see* GlipiZIDE *on page 594*
- **Glucotrol® XL** *see* GlipiZIDE *on page 594*
- **Glulisine Insulin** *see* Insulin Glulisine *on page 685*
- **Glumetza® (Can)** *see* Metformin *on page 810*
- **Glybenclamide** *see* GlyBURIDE *on page 598*
- **Glybenzcyclamide** *see* GlyBURIDE *on page 598*

GlyBURIDE (GLYE byoor ide)

Medication Safety Issues

Sound-alike/look-alike issues:

GlyBURIDE may be confused with glipiZIDE, Glucotrol®

Diaβeta® may be confused with Diabinese®, Zebeta®

Micronase® may be confused with microK®, miconazole, Micronor®

Related Information

Thiazolidinediones *on page 1577*

Perioperative Management of the Diabetic Patient *on page 1464*

U.S. Brand Names Diaβeta®; Glynase® PresTab®; Micronase®

Canadian Brand Names Albert® Glyburide; Apo-Glyburide®; Diaβeta®; Euglucon®; Gen-Glybe; Novo-Glyburide; Nu-Glyburide; PMS-Glyburide; ratio-Glyburide; Sandoz-Glyburide

Synonyms Diabeta; Glibenclamide; Glybenclamide; Glybenzcyclamide

Pharmacologic Category Antidiabetic Agent, Sulfonylurea

Generic Available Yes

Use Management of type 2 diabetes mellitus (noninsulin dependent, NIDDM)

Unlabeled/Investigational Use Alternative to insulin in women for the treatment of gestational diabetes (11-33 weeks gestation)

Mechanism of Action Stimulates insulin release from the pancreatic beta cells; reduces glucose output from the liver; insulin sensitivity is increased at peripheral target sites

Pharmacodynamics/Kinetics

Onset of action: Serum insulin levels begin to increase 15-60 minutes after a single dose

Duration: ≤24 hours

Protein binding, plasma: >99%

Metabolism: To one moderately active and several inactive metabolites

Half-life elimination: 5-16 hours; may be prolonged with renal or hepatic impairment

Time to peak, serum: Adults: 2-4 hours

Excretion: Feces (50%) and urine (50%) as metabolites

Dosage Oral:

Adults:

Initial: 2.5-5 mg/day, administered with breakfast or the first main meal of the day. In patients who are more sensitive to hypoglycemic drugs, start at 1.25 mg/day.

Increase in increments of no more than 2.5 mg/day at weekly intervals based on the patient's blood glucose response

Maintenance: 1.25-20 mg/day given as single or divided doses; maximum: 20 mg/day

Elderly: Initial: 1.25-2.5 mg/day, increase by 1.25-2.5 mg/day every 1-3 weeks

Micronized tablets (Glynase® PresTab®): Adults:

Initial: 1.5-3 mg/day, administered with breakfast or the first main meal of the day in patients who are more sensitive to hypoglycemic drugs, start at 0.75 mg/day. Increase in increments of no more than 1.5 mg/day in weekly intervals based on the patient's blood glucose response.

Maintenance: 0.75-12 mg/day given as a single dose or in divided doses. Some patients (especially those receiving >6 mg/day) may have a more satisfactory response with twice-daily dosing.

Dosing adjustment/comments in renal impairment: Cl_{cr} <50 mL/minute: **Not recommended**

Dosing adjustment in hepatic impairment: Use conservative initial and maintenance doses and avoid use in severe disease

Administration Administer with meals at the same time each day. Patients who are anorexic or NPO may need to have their dose held to avoid hypoglycemia.

Monitoring Parameters Signs and symptoms of hypoglycemia, fasting blood glucose, hemoglobin A_{1c}

Reference Range Target range: Adults:

Fasting blood glucose: <120 mg/dL

Glycosylated hemoglobin: <7%

Anesthesia and Critical Care Concerns/Other Considerations The possibility of higher doses of sulfonylureas eliciting an increase in cardiovascular events, because of their effects on blocking potassium sensitive ATP channels, has been raised. Longer-term prospective trials of sulfonylurea therapy, such as the UKPDS, do not reveal any increased cardiovascular mortality.

Pregnancy Risk Factor C

Contraindications Hypersensitivity to glyburide, any component of the formulation, or other sulfonamides; type 1 diabetes mellitus (insulin dependent, IDDM), diabetic ketoacidosis with or without coma

Warnings/Precautions Elderly: Rapid and prolonged hypoglycemia (>12 hours) despite hypertonic glucose injections have been reported; age and hepatic and renal impairment are independent risk factors for hypoglycemia; dosage titration should be made at weekly intervals. Use with caution in patients with renal and hepatic impairment, malnourished or debilitated conditions, or adrenal or pituitary insufficiency.

Chemical similarities are present among sulfonamides, sulfonylureas, carbonic anhydrase inhibitors, thiazides, and loop diuretics (except ethacrynic acid). Use in patients with sulfonamide allergy is specifically contraindicated in product labeling, however, a risk of cross-reaction exists in patients with allergy to any of these compounds; avoid use when previous reaction has been severe.

Product labeling states oral hypoglycemic drugs may be associated with an increased cardiovascular mortality as compared to treatment with diet alone or diet plus insulin. Data to support this association are limited, and several studies, including a large prospective trial (UKPDS) have not supported an association.

Adverse Reactions Frequency not defined.

Central nervous system: Headache, dizziness

Dermatologic: Pruritus, rash, urticaria, photosensitivity reaction

Endocrine & metabolic: Hypoglycemia, hyponatremia (SIADH reported with other sulfonylureas)

Gastrointestinal: Nausea, epigastric fullness, heartburn, constipation, diarrhea, anorexia

Genitourinary: Nocturia

Hematologic: Leukopenia, thrombocytopenia, hemolytic anemia, aplastic anemia, bone marrow suppression, agranulocytosis

Hepatic: Cholestatic jaundice, hepatitis

Neuromuscular & skeletal: Arthralgia, paresthesia

Ocular: Blurred vision

Renal: Diuretic effect (minor)

Overdosage/Toxicology Symptoms of overdose include severe hypoglycemia, seizures, cerebral damage, tingling of lips and tongue, nausea, yawning, confusion, agitation, tachycardia, sweating, convulsions, stupor, and coma. Intoxication with sulfonylureas can cause hypoglycemia and is best managed with glucose administration (oral for milder hypoglycemia or by injection in more severe forms).

Drug Interactions **Inhibits** CYP2C8 (weak), 3A4 (weak)

Decreased effect: Thiazides may decrease effectiveness of glyburide

Increased effect: Possible interaction between glyburide and fluoroquinolone antibiotics has been reported resulting in a potentiation of hypoglycemic action of glyburide

Increased toxicity:

- Since this agent is highly protein bound, the toxic potential is increased when given concomitantly with other highly protein bound drugs (ie, phenylbutazone, oral anticoagulants, hydantoins, salicylates, NSAIDs, beta-blockers, sulfonamides) - increase hypoglycemic effect
- Ethanol increases disulfiram reactions
- Phenylbutazone can increase hypoglycemic effects
- Certain drugs tend to produce hyperglycemia and may lead to loss of control (ie, thiazides and other diuretics, corticosteroids, phenothiazines, thyroid products, estrogens, oral contraceptives, phenytoin, nicotinic acid, sympathomimetics, calcium channel blocking drugs, and isoniazid)

(Continued)

GlyBURIDE *(Continued)*

Possible interactions between glyburide and coumarin derivatives have been reported that may either potentiate or weaken the effects of coumarin derivatives

Ethanol/Nutrition/Herb Interactions

Ethanol: Caution with ethanol (may cause hypoglycemia).

Herb/Nutraceutical: Caution with chromium, garlic, gymnema (may cause hypoglycemia).

Dietary Considerations Should be taken with meals at the same time each day. Dietary modification based on ADA recommendations is a part of therapy. Decreases blood glucose concentration. Hypoglycemia may occur. Must be able to recognize symptoms of hypoglycemia (palpitations, sweaty palms, lightheadedness).

Dosage Forms [DSC] = Discontinued product

Tablet (Diaβeta®, Micronase®): 1.25 mg, 2.5 mg, 5 mg

Tablet, micronized: 1.5 mg, 3 mg, 6 mg

Glynase® PresTab®: 1.5 mg [DSC], 3 mg, 6 mg

- **Glyceryl Trinitrate** *see* Nitroglycerin *on page 928*
- **Glycon (Can)** *see* Metformin *on page 810*

Glycopyrrolate (glye koe PYE roe late)

U.S. Brand Names Robinul®; Robinul® Forte

Canadian Brand Names Glycopyrrolate Injection, USP

Synonyms Glycopyrronium Bromide

Pharmacologic Category Anticholinergic Agent

Generic Available Yes: Injection

Use Inhibit salivation and excessive secretions of the respiratory tract preoperatively; reversal of neuromuscular blockade; control of upper airway secretions; adjunct in treatment of peptic ulcer

Mechanism of Action Blocks the action of acetylcholine at parasympathetic sites in smooth muscle, secretory glands, and the CNS

Pharmacodynamics/Kinetics

Onset of action: Oral: 50 minutes; I.M.: 15-30 minutes; I.V.: ~1 minute

Peak effect: Oral: ~1 hour; I.M.: 30-45 minutes

Duration: Vagal effect: 2-3 hours; Inhibition of salivation: Up to 7 hours; Anticholinergic: Oral: 8-12 hours

Absorption: Oral: Poor and erratic

Distribution: V_d: 0.2-0.62 L/kg

Metabolism: Hepatic (minimal)

Bioavailability: ~10%

Half-life elimination: Infants: 22-130 minutes; Children 19-99 minutes; Adults: ~30-75 minutes

Excretion: Urine (as unchanged drug, I.M.: 80%, I.V.: 85%); bile (as unchanged drug)

Dosage

Children:

Reduction of secretions (preanesthetic):

Oral: 40-100 mcg/kg/dose 3-4 times/day

I.M., I.V.: 4-10 mcg/kg/dose every 3-4 hours; maximum: 0.2 mg/dose or 0.8 mg/24 hours

Intraoperative: I.V.: 4 mcg/kg not to exceed 0.1 mg; repeat at 2- to 3-minute intervals as needed

Preoperative: I.M.:

<2 years: 4-9 mcg/kg 30-60 minutes before procedure

>2 years: 4 mcg/kg 30-60 minutes before procedure

Children and Adults: Reverse neuromuscular blockade: I.V.: 0.2 mg for each 1 mg of neostigmine or 5 mg of pyridostigmine administered or 5-15 mcg/kg glycopyrrolate with 25-70 mcg/kg of neostigmine or 0.1-0.3 mg/kg of pyridostigmine (agents usually administered simultaneously, but glycopyrrolate may be administered first if bradycardia is present)

Adults:

Reduction of secretions:

Intraoperative: I.V.: 0.1 mg repeated as needed at 2- to 3-minute intervals

Preoperative: I.M.: 4 mcg/kg 30-60 minutes before procedure

Peptic ulcer:

Oral: 1-2 mg 2-3 times/day

I.M., I.V.: 0.1-0.2 mg 3-4 times/day

Stability Store at 20°C to 25°C (68°F to 77°F).

Administration For I.V. administration, glycopyrrolate may also be administered via the tubing of a running I.V. infusion of a compatible solution; may be administered in the same syringe with neostigmine or pyridostigmine.

Monitoring Parameters Heart rate; anticholinergic effects; bowel sounds

Pregnancy Risk Factor B

Contraindications Hypersensitivity to glycopyrrolate or any component of the formulation; severe ulcerative colitis, toxic megacolon complicating ulcerative colitis, paralytic ileus, obstructive disease of GI tract, intestinal atony in the elderly or debilitated patient; unstable cardiovascular status in acute hemorrhage; narrow-angle glaucoma; acute hemorrhage; tachycardia; obstructive uropathy; myasthenia gravis

Warnings/Precautions Use caution in elderly, patients with autonomic neuropathy, hepatic or renal disease, ulcerative colitis (may precipitate/aggravate toxic megacolon), hyperthyroidism, CAD, CHF, arrhythmias, tachycardia, BPH, or hiatal hernia with reflux. Use of anticholinergics in gastric ulcer treatment may cause a delay in gastric emptying due to antral statis. Caution should be used in individuals demonstrating decreased pigmentation (skin and iris coloration, dark versus light) since there has been some evidence that these individuals have an enhanced sensitivity to the anticholinergic response. May cause drowsiness, eye sensitivity to light, or blurred vision; caution should be used when performing tasks which require mental alertness, such as driving. The risk of heat stroke with this medication may be increased during exercise or hot weather. Infants, patients with Down syndrome, and children with spastic paralysis or brain damage may be hypersensitive to antimuscarine effects. Product packaging may contain latex. Injection contains benzyl alcohol (associated with gasping syndrome in neonates). Not recommended for use in children <12 years of age for the management of peptic ulcer or <16 years for preanesthetic use.

Adverse Reactions Frequency not defined. **Note:** Includes adverse effects which may occur as an extension of the pharmacologic action of anticholinergics (including glycopyrrolate) and adverse effects reported postmarketing with glycopyrrolate.

Cardiovascular: Arrhythmias, cardiac arrest, heart block, hyper-/hypotension, malignant hyperthermia, palpitation, QT_c interval prolongation, tachycardia

Central nervous system: Confusion, dizziness, drowsiness, excitement, headache, insomnia, nervousness, seizures

Dermatologic: Dry skin, pruritus, sensitivity to light increased

Endocrine & metabolic: Lactation suppression

Gastrointestinal: Bloated feeling, constipation, loss of taste, nausea, vomiting, xerostomia

Genitourinary: Impotence, urinary hesitancy, urinary retention

Local: Irritation at injection site

Neuromuscular & skeletal: Weakness

Ocular: Blurred vision, cycloplegia, mydriasis, ocular tension increased, photophobia, sensitivity to light increased

Respiratory: Respiratory depression

Miscellaneous: Anaphylactoid reactions, diaphoresis decreased, hypersensitivity reactions

Overdosage/Toxicology

Symptoms of overdose include blurred vision, urinary retention, tachycardia, and absent bowel sounds. For peripheral adverse effects, a quaternary ammonium anticholinesterase, such as neostigmine methylsulfate, may be given I.V. in increments of 0.25 mg in adults; may repeat every 5-10 minutes (up to a maximum of 2.5 mg) based upon decrease in heart rate and return of bowel sounds. For overdose exhibiting CNS symptoms (eg, excitement, restlessness, convulsions, psychotic behavior), physostigmine 0.5-2 mg I.V. slowly, may be given and repeated as necessary, up to 5 mg. Proportionally smaller doses should be used for pediatric patients. Artificial respiration should be given to individuals experiencing a neuromuscular or curare-like effect which could lead to muscular weakness or possible paralysis. Additional care should be symptomatic and supportive.

Drug Interactions

Anticholinergic agents: Effects of other anticholinergic agents or medications with anticholinergic activity may be increased by glycopyrrolate.

(Continued)

Glycopyrrolate *(Continued)*

Potassium chloride: Severity of potassium chloride-induced gastrointestinal lesions (when potassium is given in a wax matrix formulation, eg, Klor-Con®) may be increased by glycopyrrolate.

Pramlinitide: May enhance the anticholinergic effects of anticholinergics. These effects are specific to the GI tract.

Dosage Forms

Injection, solution (Robinul®): 0.2 mg/mL (1 mL, 2 mL, 5 mL, 20 mL) [contains benzyl alcohol]

Tablet:

Robinul®: 1 mg

Robinul® Forte: 2 mg

- **Glycopyrrolate Injection, USP (Can)** *see* Glycopyrrolate *on page 600*
- **Glycopyrronium Bromide** *see* Glycopyrrolate *on page 600*
- **Glydiazinamide** *see* GlipiZIDE *on page 594*
- **Glynase® PresTab®** *see* GlyBURIDE *on page 598*
- **GMD-Azithromycin (Can)** *see* Azithromycin *on page 149*
- **GMD-Fluconazole (Can)** *see* Fluconazole *on page 530*
- **GMD-Sertraline (Can)** *see* Sertraline *on page 1161*
- **GR38032R** *see* Ondansetron *on page 959*

Granisetron (gra NI se tron)

Medication Safety Issues

Sound-alike/look-alike issues:

Granisetron may be confused with dolasetron, ondansetron, palonosetron

Related Information

Postoperative Nausea and Vomiting *on page 1477*

U.S. Brand Names Kytril®

Canadian Brand Names Kytril®

Synonyms BRL 43694

Pharmacologic Category Antiemetic; Selective 5-HT_3 Receptor Antagonist

Generic Available No

Use Prophylaxis of nausea and vomiting associated with emetogenic chemotherapy and radiation therapy, (including total body irradiation and fractionated abdominal radiation); prophylaxis and treatment of postoperative nausea and vomiting (PONV)

Generally **not** recommended for treatment of existing chemotherapy-induced emesis (CIE) or for prophylaxis of nausea from agents with a low emetogenic potential.

Mechanism of Action Selective 5-HT_3-receptor antagonist, blocking serotonin, both peripherally on vagal nerve terminals and centrally in the chemoreceptor trigger zone

Pharmacodynamics/Kinetics

Duration: Generally up to 24 hours

Absorption: Tablets and oral solution are bioequivalent

Distribution: V_d: 2-4 L/kg; widely throughout body

Protein binding: 65%

Metabolism: Hepatic via N-demethylation, oxidation, and conjugation; some metabolites may have 5-HT_3 antagonist activity

Half-life elimination: Terminal: 5-9 hours

Excretion: Urine (12% as unchanged drug, 48% to 49% as metabolites); feces (34% to 38% as metabolites)

Dosage

Oral: Adults:

Prophylaxis of chemotherapy-related emesis: 2 mg once daily up to 1 hour before chemotherapy or 1 mg twice daily; the first 1 mg dose should be given up to 1 hour before chemotherapy.

Prophylaxis of radiation therapy-associated emesis: 2 mg once daily given 1 hour before radiation therapy.

I.V.:

Children ≥2 years and Adults: Prophylaxis of chemotherapy-related emesis:

Within U.S.: 10 mcg/kg/dose (maximum: 1 mg/dose) given 30 minutes prior to chemotherapy; for some drugs (eg, carboplatin, cyclophosphamide) with a later onset of emetic action, 10 mcg/kg every 12 hours may be necessary

Outside U.S.: 40 mcg/kg/dose (or 3 mg/dose); maximum: 9 mg/24 hours

Breakthrough: Granisetron has not been shown to be effective in terminating nausea or vomiting once it occurs and should not be used for this purpose.

Adults: PONV:

Prevention: 1 mg given undiluted over 30 seconds; administer before induction of anesthesia or immediately before reversal of anesthesia

Treatment: 1 mg given undiluted over 30 seconds

Dosing interval in renal impairment: No dosage adjustment required.

Dosing interval in hepatic impairment: Kinetic studies in patients with hepatic impairment showed that total clearance was approximately halved, however, standard doses were very well tolerated, and dose adjustments are not necessary.

Stability

I.V.: Store at 15°C to 30°C (59°F to 86°F). Stable when mixed in NS or D_5W for 7 days under refrigeration and for 3 days at room temperature. Protect from light. Do not freeze vials.

Oral: Store tablet or oral solution at 15°C to 30°C (59°F to 86°F). Protect from light.

Administration

Oral: Doses should be given up to 1 hour prior to initiation of chemotherapy/radiation

I.V.: Administer I.V. push over 30 seconds or as a 5-10 minute-infusion

Prevention of PONV: Administer before induction of anesthesia or immediately before reversal of anesthesia.

Treatment of PONV: Administer undiluted over 30 seconds.

Pregnancy Risk Factor B

Contraindications Previous hypersensitivity to granisetron, other 5-HT_3 receptor antagonists, or any component of the formulation

Warnings/Precautions Chemotherapy-related emesis: **Granisetron should be used on a scheduled basis, not on an "as needed" (PRN) basis**, since data support the use of this drug in the prevention of nausea and vomiting and not in the rescue of nausea and vomiting. Granisetron should be used only in the first 24-48 hours of receiving chemotherapy or radiation. Data do not support any increased efficacy of granisetron in delayed nausea and vomiting. May be prescribed for patients who are refractory to or have severe adverse reactions to standard antiemetic therapy or young patients (ie, <45 years of age who are more likely to develop extrapyramidal symptoms to high-dose metoclopramide) who are to receive highly emetogenic chemotherapeutic agents. Should not be prescribed for chemotherapeutic agents with a low emetogenic potential (eg, bleomycin, busulfan, etoposide, 5-fluorouracil, vinblastine, vincristine).

Routine prophylaxis for PONV is not recommended. In patients where nausea and vomiting must be avoided postoperatively, administer to all patients even when expected incidence of nausea and vomiting is low. Use caution following abdominal surgery or in chemotherapy-induced nausea and vomiting; may mask progressive ileus or gastric distention. Use caution in patients with liver disease or in pregnancy. Safety and efficacy in children <2 years of age have not been established. Injection contains benzyl alcohol (1 mg/mL) and should not be used in neonates.

Adverse Reactions

>10%:

Central nervous system: Headache (9% to 21%)

Gastrointestinal: Constipation (3% to 18%)

Neuromuscular & skeletal: Weakness (5% to 18%)

1% to 10%:

Cardiovascular: Hypertension (1% to 2%)

Central nervous system: Pain (10%), fever (3% to 9%), dizziness (4% to 5%), insomnia (<2% to 5%), somnolence (1% to 4%), anxiety (2%), agitation (<2%), CNS stimulation (<2%)

Dermatologic: Rash (1%)

Gastrointestinal: Diarrhea (3% to 9%), abdominal pain (4% to 6%), dyspepsia (3% to 6%), taste perversion (2%)

(Continued)

Granisetron *(Continued)*

Hepatic: Liver enzymes increased (5% to 6%)
Renal: Oliguria (2%)
Respiratory: Cough (2%)
Miscellaneous: Infection (3%)

<1% (Limited to important or life-threatening): Agitation, allergic reactions; anaphylaxis (including hypotension, dyspnea, urticaria); angina, arrhythmias, atrial fibrillation, extrapyramidal syndrome, hot flashes, hypotension, hypersensitivity, syncope

Overdosage/Toxicology Overdoses of up to 38.5 mg have been reported without symptoms or with only slight headache. In the event of an overdose, treatment should be symptomatic and supportive.

Drug Interactions Substrate of CYP3A4 (minor)

Apomorphine: Due to reports of profound hypotension during concomitant therapy with other 5-HT3 antagonists, the manufacturer of apomorphine contraindicates its use with granisetron.

Ethanol/Nutrition/Herb Interactions Herb/Nutraceutical: St John's wort may decrease granisetron levels.

Dosage Forms

Injection, solution: 1 mg/mL (1 mL, 4 mL) [contains benzyl alcohol]
Injection, solution [preservative free]: 0.1 mg/mL (1 mL)
Solution, oral: 2 mg/10 mL (30 mL) [contains sodium benzoate; orange flavor]
Tablet: 1 mg

♦ **Granulocyte Colony Stimulating Factor** *see* Filgrastim *on page 525*
♦ **Halcion®** *see* Triazolam *on page 1316*
♦ **Haldol®** *see* Haloperidol *on page 604*
♦ **Haldol® Decanoate** *see* Haloperidol *on page 604*
♦ **Halfprin® [OTC]** *see* Aspirin *on page 129*

Haloperidol (ha loe PER i dole)

Medication Safety Issues

Sound-alike/look-alike issues:
Haloperidol may be confused Halotestin®
Haldol® may be confused with Halcion®, Halenol®, Halog®, Halotestin®, Stadol®

Related Information

Sedative Agents in the Intensive Care Unit *on page 1576*

U.S. Brand Names Haldol®; Haldol® Decanoate

Canadian Brand Names Apo-Haloperidol®; Apo-Haloperidol LA®; Haloperidol Injection, USP; Haloperidol-LA; Haloperidol-LA Omega; Haloperidol Long Acting; Novo-Peridol; Peridol; PMS-Haloperidol LA

Synonyms Haloperidol Decanoate; Haloperidol Lactate

Pharmacologic Category Antipsychotic Agent, Typical

Generic Available Yes

Use Management of schizophrenia; control of tics and vocal utterances of Tourette's disorder in children and adults; severe behavioral problems in children

Unlabeled/Investigational Use Treatment of psychosis; may be used for the emergency sedation of severely-agitated or delirious patients; adjunctive treatment of ethanol dependence; antiemetic

Mechanism of Action Haloperidol is a butyrophenone antipsychotic which blocks postsynaptic mesolimbic dopaminergic D_1 and D_2 receptors in the brain; depresses the release of hypothalamic and hypophyseal hormones; believed to depress the reticular activating system thus affecting basal metabolism, body temperature, wakefulness, vasomotor tone, and emesis

Pharmacodynamics/Kinetics

Onset of action: Sedation: I.V.: ~1 hour
Duration: Decanoate: ~3 weeks
Distribution: Crosses placenta; enters breast milk
Protein binding: 90%
Metabolism: Hepatic to inactive compounds
Bioavailability: Oral: 60%
Half-life elimination: 20 hours
Time to peak, serum: 20 minutes
Excretion: Urine (33% to 40% as metabolites) within 5 days; feces (15%)

Dosage

Children: 3-12 years (15-40 kg): Oral:

Initial: 0.05 mg/kg/day or 0.25-0.5 mg/day given in 2-3 divided doses; increase by 0.25-0.5 mg every 5-7 days; maximum: 0.15 mg/kg/day

Usual maintenance:

Agitation or hyperkinesia: 0.01-0.03 mg/kg/day once daily

Nonpsychotic disorders: 0.05-0.075 mg/kg/day in 2-3 divided doses

Psychotic disorders: 0.05-0.15 mg/kg/day in 2-3 divided doses

Children 6-12 years: Sedation/psychotic disorders: I.M. (as lactate): 1-3 mg/dose every 4-8 hours to a maximum of 0.15 mg/kg/day; change over to oral therapy as soon as able

Adults:

Psychosis:

Oral: 0.5-5 mg 2-3 times/day; usual maximum: 30 mg/day

I.M. (as lactate): 2-5 mg every 4-8 hours as needed

I.M. (as decanoate): Initial: 10-20 times the daily oral dose administered at 4-week intervals

Maintenance dose: 10-15 times initial oral dose; used to stabilize psychiatric symptoms

Delirium in the intensive care unit (unlabeled use, unlabeled route):

I.V.: 2-10 mg; may repeat bolus doses every 20-30 minutes until calm achieved then administer 25% of the maximum dose every 6 hours; monitor ECG and QT_c interval

Intermittent I.V.: 0.03-0.15 mg/kg every 30 minutes to 6 hours

Oral: Agitation: 5-10 mg

Continuous intravenous infusion (100 mg/100 mL D_5W): Rates of 3-25 mg/hour have been used

Rapid tranquilization of severely-agitated patient (unlabeled use): Administer every 30-60 minutes:

Oral: 5-10 mg

I.M.: 5 mg

Average total dose (oral or I.M.) for tranquilization: 10-20 mg

Elderly: Initial: Oral: 0.25-0.5 mg 1-2 times/day; increase dose at 4- to 7-day intervals by 0.25-0.5 mg/day; increase dosing intervals (twice daily, 3 times/day, etc) as necessary to control response or side effects

Hemodialysis/peritoneal dialysis: Supplemental dose is not necessary

Stability

Protect oral dosage forms from light

Haloperidol lactate injection should be stored at controlled room temperature and protected from light, freezing and temperatures >40°C; exposure to light may cause discoloration and the development of a grayish-red precipitate over several weeks

Haloperidol lactate may be administered IVPB or I.V. infusion in D_5W solutions; NS solutions should not be used due to reports of decreased stability and incompatibility

Standardized dose: 0.5-100 mg/50-100 mL D_5W

Stability of standardized solutions is 38 days at room temperature (24°C)

Administration The decanoate injectable formulation should be administered I.M. only, **do not administer decanoate I.V.** Dilute the oral concentrate with water or juice before administration. Avoid skin contact with oral suspension or solution; may cause contact dermatitis.

Monitoring Parameters Vital signs; lipid profile, fasting blood glucose/Hgb A_{1c}; BMI; mental status, abnormal involuntary movement scale (AIMS), extrapyramidal symptoms (EPS)

Reference Range

Therapeutic: 5-20 ng/mL (SI: 10-40 nmol/L) (psychotic disorders - less for Tourette's and mania)

Toxic: >42 ng/mL (SI: >84 nmol/L)

Anesthesia and Critical Care Concerns/Other Considerations

Delirium in the ICU Patient: Set goals for control of delirium. Haloperidol has not been studied in well-controlled trials enrolling ICU patients with acute delirium or agitation. Avoid use in patients with underlying QT prolongation, in those taking medicines that prolong the QT interval, or cause polymorphic ventricular tachycardia. Even when used at recommended doses, cardiac arrhythmias have occurred. Monitor ECG closely for dose-related QT effects. Once the patient has been stable for a few days, taper the dose and reassess the patient. Haloperidol

(Continued)

Haloperidol *(Continued)*

may cause extrapyramidal symptoms. It is the most frequently implicated antipsychotic associated with neuroleptic malignant syndrome.

Pregnancy Risk Factor C

Contraindications Hypersensitivity to haloperidol or any component of the formulation; Parkinson's disease; severe CNS depression; bone marrow suppression; severe cardiac or hepatic disease; coma

Warnings/Precautions Hypotension may occur, particularly with parenteral administration. Decanoate form should never be administered I.V. Avoid in thyrotoxicosis. May be sedating, use with caution in disorders where CNS depression is a feature. Caution in patients with hemodynamic instability, predisposition to seizures, subcortical brain damage, renal or respiratory disease. Esophageal dysmotility and aspiration have been associated with antipsychotic use - use with caution in patients at risk of pneumonia (ie, Alzheimer's disease). Caution in breast cancer or other prolactin-dependent tumors (may elevate prolactin levels). May alter temperature regulation or mask toxicity of other drugs due to antiemetic effects. May alter cardiac conduction - life-threatening arrhythmias have occurred with therapeutic doses of antipsychotics. Adverse effects of decanoate may be prolonged. May cause orthostatic hypotension - use with caution in patients at risk of this effect or those who would tolerate transient hypotensive episodes (cerebrovascular disease, cardiovascular disease, or other medications which may predispose). Some tablets contain tartrazine.

May cause anticholinergic effects (confusion, agitation, constipation, xerostomia, blurred vision, urinary retention). Therefore, they should be used with caution in patients with decreased gastrointestinal motility, urinary retention, BPH, xerostomia, or visual problems. Conditions which also may be exacerbated by cholinergic blockade include narrow-angle glaucoma (screening is recommended) and worsening of myasthenia gravis. Relative to other neuroleptics, haloperidol has a low potency of cholinergic blockade.

May cause extrapyramidal symptoms, including pseudoparkinsonism, acute dystonic reactions, akathisia, and tardive dyskinesia (risk of these reactions is high relative to other neuroleptics). May be associated with neuroleptic malignant syndrome (NMS) or pigmentary retinopathy.

Adverse Reactions Frequency not defined.

Cardiovascular: Hyper-/hypotension, tachycardia, arrhythmia, abnormal T waves with prolonged ventricular repolarization, torsade de pointes (case-control study ~4%)

Central nervous system: Restlessness, anxiety, extrapyramidal reactions, dystonic reactions, pseudoparkinsonian signs and symptoms, tardive dyskinesia, neuroleptic malignant syndrome (NMS), altered central temperature regulation, akathisia, tardive dystonia, insomnia, euphoria, agitation, drowsiness, depression, lethargy, headache, confusion, vertigo, seizure

Dermatologic: Hyperpigmentation, pruritus, rash, contact dermatitis, alopecia, photosensitivity (rare)

Endocrine & metabolic: Amenorrhea, galactorrhea, gynecomastia, sexual dysfunction, lactation, breast engorgement, mastalgia, menstrual irregularities, hyperglycemia, hypoglycemia, hyponatremia

Gastrointestinal: Nausea, vomiting, anorexia, constipation, diarrhea, hypersalivation, dyspepsia, xerostomia

Genitourinary: Urinary retention, priapism

Hematologic: Cholestatic jaundice, obstructive jaundice

Ocular: Blurred vision

Respiratory: Laryngospasm, bronchospasm

Miscellaneous: Heat stroke, diaphoresis

Overdosage/Toxicology Symptoms of overdose include deep sleep, dystonia, agitation, dysrhythmias, and extrapyramidal symptoms. Treatment is supportive and symptomatic.

Drug Interactions **Substrate** of CYP1A2 (minor), 2D6 (major), 3A4 (major); **Inhibits** CYP2D6 (moderate), 3A4 (moderate)

Acetylcholinesterase inhibitors (central): May increase the risk of antipsychotic-related extrapyramidal symptoms; monitor.

Anticholinergics: May inhibit the therapeutic response to haloperidol and excess anticholinergic effects may occur; tardive dyskinesias have also been reported; includes benztropine and trihexyphenidyl

Antihypertensives: Concurrent use of haloperidol with an antihypertensive may produce additive hypotensive effects (particularly orthostasis)

Bromocriptine: Antipsychotics inhibit the ability of bromocriptine to lower serum prolactin concentrations

Chloroquine: Serum concentrations of haloperidol may be increased by chloroquine

CNS depressants: Sedative effects may be additive; monitor for increased effect; includes barbiturates, benzodiazepines, narcotic analgesics, ethanol and other sedative agents

CYP2D6 inhibitors: May increase the levels/effects of haloperidol. Example inhibitors include chlorpromazine, delavirdine, fluoxetine, miconazole, paroxetine, pergolide, quinidine, quinine, ritonavir, and ropinirole.

CYP2D6 substrates: Haloperidol may increase the levels/effects of CYP2D6 substrates. Example substrates include amphetamines, selected beta-blockers, dextromethorphan, fluoxetine, lidocaine, mirtazapine, nefazodone, paroxetine, risperidone, ritonavir, thioridazine, tricyclic antidepressants, and venlafaxine.

CYP2D6 prodrug substrates: Haloperidol may decrease the levels/effects of CYP2D6 prodrug substrates. Example prodrug substrates include codeine, hydrocodone, oxycodone, and tramadol.

CYP3A4 inducers: CYP3A4 inducers may decrease the levels/effects of haloperidol. Example inducers include aminoglutethimide, carbamazepine, nafcillin, nevirapine, phenobarbital, phenytoin, and rifamycins.

CYP3A4 inhibitors: May increase the levels/effects of haloperidol. Example inhibitors include azole antifungals, clarithromycin, diclofenac, doxycycline, erythromycin, imatinib, isoniazid, nefazodone, nicardipine, propofol, protease inhibitors, quinidine, telithromycin, and verapamil.

CYP3A4 substrates: Haloperidol may increase the levels/effects of CYP3A4 substrates. Example substrates include benzodiazepines, calcium channel blockers, cyclosporine, mirtazapine, nateglinide, nefazodone, sildenafil (and other PDE-5 inhibitors), tacrolimus, and venlafaxine. Selected benzodiazepines (midazolam and triazolam), cisapride, ergot alkaloids, selected HMG-CoA reductase inhibitors (lovastatin and simvastatin), and pimozide are generally contraindicated with strong CYP3A4 inhibitors.

Indomethacin: Haloperidol in combination with indomethacin may result in drowsiness, tiredness, and confusion; monitor for adverse effects

Inhalation anesthetics: Haloperidol in combination with certain forms of induction anesthesia may produce peripheral vasodilitation and hypotension

Levodopa: Haloperidol may inhibit the antiparkinsonian effect of levodopa; avoid this combination

Lithium: Haloperidol may produce neurotoxicity with lithium; this is a rare effect

Methyldopa: Effect of haloperidol may be altered; enhanced effects, as well as reduced efficacy have been reported

Metoclopramide: May increase extrapyramidal symptoms (EPS) or risk.

Nefazodone: Haloperidol and nefazodone may produce additive CNS toxicity, including sedation

Propranolol: Serum concentrations of haloperidol may be increased

Quinidine: May increase haloperidol concentrations; monitor for EPS and/or QT_c prolongation

SSRIs: Fluoxetine, fluvoxamine, and paroxetine may inhibit the metabolism of haloperidol resulting in EPS; monitor for EPS

Sulfadoxine-pyrimethamine: May increase fluphenazine concentrations

Tricyclic antidepressants: Concurrent use may produce increased toxicity or altered therapeutic response

Trazodone: Haloperidol and trazodone may produce additive hypotensive effects

Ethanol/Nutrition/Herb Interactions

Ethanol: Avoid ethanol (may increase CNS depression).

Herb/Nutraceutical: Avoid valerian, St John's wort, kava kava, gotu kola (may increase CNS depression).

Dosage Forms [DSC] = Discontinued product. **Note:** Strength expressed as base.

Injection, oil, as decanoate (Haldol® Decanoate): 50 mg/mL (1 mL, 5 mL); 100 mg/mL (1 mL, 5 mL) [contains benzyl alcohol, sesame oil]

Injection, solution, as lactate: 5 mg/mL (1 mL, 10 mL)

Haldol®: 5 mg/mL (1 mL; 10 mL [DSC])

Solution, oral concentrate, as lactate: 2 mg/mL (15 mL, 120 mL)

Tablet: 0.5 mg, 1 mg, 2 mg, 5 mg, 10 mg, 20 mg

(Continued)

Haloperidol *(Continued)*

References

Barton MD, Libonati M, and Cohen PJ, "The Use of Haloperidol for Treatment of Postoperative Nausea and Vomiting - A Double-Blind Placebo-Controlled Trial," *Anesthesiology*, 1975, 42(4):508-12.

Jacobi J, Fraser GL, Coursin DB, et al, "Clinical Practice Guidelines for the Sustained Use of Sedatives and Analgesics in the Critically Ill Adult," *Crit Care Med*, 2002, 30(1):119-41. Available at: http://www.sccm.org/pdf/sedatives.pdf.

Riker RR, Fraser GL, and Cox PM, "Continuous Infusion of Haloperidol Controls Agitation in Critically Ill Patients," *Crit Care Med*, 1994, 22(3):433-40.

♦ **Haloperidol Decanoate** *see* Haloperidol *on page 604*
♦ **Haloperidol Injection, USP (Can)** *see* Haloperidol *on page 604*
♦ **Haloperidol-LA (Can)** *see* Haloperidol *on page 604*
♦ **Haloperidol Lactate** *see* Haloperidol *on page 604*
♦ **Haloperidol-LA Omega (Can)** *see* Haloperidol *on page 604*
♦ **Haloperidol Long Acting (Can)** *see* Haloperidol *on page 604*

Halothane (HA loe thane)

Medication Safety Issues
Sound-alike/look-alike issues:
Halothane may be confused with Halotestin®

Related Information
Anesthesia Considerations for Neurosurgery *on page 1401*
Anesthesia for Patients With Liver Disease *on page 1421*
Inhalational Anesthetics *on page 1528*

Pharmacologic Category General Anesthetic, Inhalation

Generic Available Yes

Use Induction and maintenance of general anesthesia

Pharmacodynamics/Kinetics
Onset of action: 1.5-3 minutes
Duration: Emergence time: Depends on blood concentration when halothane is discontinued
Metabolism: Hepatic (20% to 50%) via CYP, both oxidatively and reductively
Excretion: Exhaled gases within 24 hours

Dosage Minimum alveolar concentration (MAC), the concentration at which 50% of patients do not respond to surgical incision, is 0.74% for halothane. The concentration at which amnesia and loss of awareness occur (MAC - awake) is 0.41%. Surgical levels of anesthesia are maintained with concentrations between 0.5% to 2%; inspired concentrations of up to 3% required for induction of anesthesia. MAC is reduced in the elderly.

Stability Halothane mixed with oxygen or air is not flammable or explosive

Administration Via halothane-specific calibrated vaporizer

Monitoring Parameters Blood pressure, heart rate and rhythm, temperature, oxygen saturation, end-tidal CO_2 and end-tidal halothane concentrations should be monitored prior to and throughout anesthesia.

Pregnancy Risk Factor C

Contraindications Hypersensitivity to halothane or any component of the formulation; known or suspected history of malignant hyperthermia; history of hepatitis after a previous anesthetic

Warnings/Precautions Decrease in blood pressure is dose dependent, due to myocardial depression and blunting of the baroreceptor mediated tachycardic response to hypotension. Sinus bradycardia, wandering pacemaker, and junctional rhythm are not uncommon. Respiration is depressed (increase $PaCO_2$ at 1 MAC to 45 mm Hg with spontaneous ventilation). Hypoxic pulmonary vasoconstriction is depressed which may lead to increased pulmonary shunt. Hypoxemia-induced increase in ventilation is abolished at low halothane concentration. Halothane dilates the cerebral vasculature and may, in certain conditions, increase intracranial pressure. Renal, splenic, and hepatic blood flow are reduced. Halothane induces hepatic microsomal enzymes function. Incidence of halothane-induced hepatitis is 1/10,000 to 1/30,000 anesthetics (less in children); it most often occurs following repeat administration (etiology is likely immune-mediated, mortality is 50%). Halothane is a trigger of malignant hyperthermia. Halothane can produce elevated carbon monoxide levels in the presence of a dry carbon dioxide absorbent within the circle breathing system of an anesthetic machine.

Adverse Reactions Frequency not defined.

Cardiovascular: Myocardial depression, hypotension, bradycardia, reflex tachycardia, ventricular or supraventricular arrhythmias
Central nervous system: Agitation, restlessness
Gastrointestinal: Nausea, vomiting
Respiratory: Respiratory depression/arrest, hypoxemia
Miscellaneous: Shivering

Drug Interactions Substrate of CYP2A6 (minor), 2B6 (minor), 2C9 (minor), 2D6 (minor), 2E1 (major), 3A4 (minor)

Aminophylline: Increased risk of arrhythmias with combined use.
Antihypertensives: Excessive hypotension may occur with combined use.
Benzodiazepines, opioids: Concurrent use of opioids and/or benzodiazepines decreases the MAC of halothane.
CYP2E1 inhibitors: May increase the levels/effects of halothane. Example inhibitors include disulfiram, isoniazid, and miconazole.
Epinephrine: Increased risk of arrhythmias with combined use. Do not exceed 0.1 mg in 10 minutes or 0.3 mg in 1 hour. Avoid concurrent use.
Isoniazid: Increased risk of hepatotoxicity with combined use.
Neuromuscular-blocking agents (nondepolarizing): Halothane may potentiate the action of nondepolarizing, neuromuscular-blocking agents.
Rifampin: Increased risk of hepatotoxicity with combined use.

Dosage Forms [DSC] = Discontinued product

Liquid: 125 mL [DSC], 250 mL

References

Campagna JA, Miller KW, and Forman SA, "Mechanisms of Action of Inhaled Anesthetics," *N Engl J Med*, 2003, 348(21):2110-23.
Eger EI 2nd, Smith NT, Stoelting RK, et al, "Cardiovascular Effects of Halothane in Man," *Anesthesiology*, 1970, 32(5):396-409.
Fee JP and Thompson GH, "Comparative Tolerability Profiles of the Inhaled Anaesthetics," *Drug Saf*, 1997, 16(3):157-70.
"Summary of the National Halothane Study. Possible Association Between Halothane Anesthesia and Postoperative Hepatic Necrosis," *JAMA*, 1966, 197(10):775-88.
Yasuda N, Lockhart SH, Eger EI 2nd, et al, "Kinetics of Desflurane, Isoflurane, and Halothane in Humans," *Anesthesiology*, 1991, 74(3):489-98.

- **Havrix®** *see* Hepatitis A Vaccine *on page 616*
- **Havrix® and Engerix-B®** *see* Hepatitis A Inactivated and Hepatitis B (Recombinant) Vaccine *on page 615*
- **HBIG** *see* Hepatitis B Immune Globulin *on page 618*
- **hBNP** *see* Nesiritide *on page 913*
- **HCTZ (error-prone abbreviation)** *see* Hydrochlorothiazide *on page 634*
- **HDCV** *see* Rabies Virus Vaccine *on page 1101*
- **Helixate® FS** *see* Antihemophilic Factor (Recombinant) *on page 113*
- **Hemorrhoidal HC** *see* Hydrocortisone *on page 639*
- **Hemril®-30** *see* Hydrocortisone *on page 639*
- **HepaGam B™** *see* Hepatitis B Immune Globulin *on page 618*
- **Hepalean® (Can)** *see* Heparin *on page 609*
- **Hepalean® Leo (Can)** *see* Heparin *on page 609*
- **Hepalean®-LOK (Can)** *see* Heparin *on page 609*

Heparin (HEP a rin)

Medication Safety Issues

Sound-alike/look-alike issues:
Heparin may be confused with Hespan®

High alert medication: The Institute for Safe Medication Practices (ISMP) includes this medication among its list of drugs which have a heightened risk of causing significant patient harm when used in error.

Heparin lock flush solution is intended only to maintain patency of I.V. devices and is **not** to be used for anticoagulant therapy.

Note: The 100 unit/mL concentration should not be used in neonates or infants <10 kg, The 10 unit/mL concentration may cause systemic anticoagulation in infants <1 kg who receive frequent flushes.

Related Information

Continuous Renal Replacement Therapy *on page 1447*
Heparin and Low Molecular Weight Heparin (LMWH) *on page 1527*
(Continued)

Heparin *(Continued)*

U.S. Brand Names HepFlush®-10; Hep-Lock®

Canadian Brand Names Hepalean®; Hepalean® Leo; Hepalean®-LOK

Synonyms Heparin Calcium; Heparin Lock Flush; Heparin Sodium

Pharmacologic Category Anticoagulant

Generic Available Yes

Use Prophylaxis and treatment of thromboembolic disorders

Note: Heparin lock flush solution is intended only to maintain patency of I.V. devices and is **not** to be used for anticoagulant therapy.

Unlabeled/Investigational Use Acute MI — combination regimen of heparin (unlabeled dose), tenecteplase (half dose), and abciximab (full dose)

Mechanism of Action Potentiates the action of antithrombin III and thereby inactivates thrombin (as well as activated coagulation factors IX, X, XI, XII, and plasmin) and prevents the conversion of fibrinogen to fibrin; heparin also stimulates release of lipoprotein lipase (lipoprotein lipase hydrolyzes triglycerides to glycerol and free fatty acids)

Pharmacodynamics/Kinetics

Onset of action: Anticoagulation: I.V.: Immediate; SubQ: ~20-30 minutes

Absorption: Oral, rectal, I.M.: Erratic at best from all these routes of administration; SubQ absorption is also erratic, but considered acceptable for prophylactic use

Distribution: Does not cross placenta; does not enter breast milk

Metabolism: Hepatic; may be partially metabolized in the reticuloendothelial system

Half-life elimination: Mean: 1.5 hours; Range: 1-2 hours; affected by obesity, renal function, hepatic function, malignancy, presence of pulmonary embolism, and infections

Excretion: Urine (small amounts as unchanged drug)

Dosage

Children:

Intermittent I.V.: Initial: 50-100 units/kg, then 50-100 units/kg every 4 hours

I.V. infusion: Initial: 50 units/kg, then 15-25 units/kg/hour; increase dose by 2-4 units/kg/hour every 6-8 hours as required

Adults:

Prophylaxis (low-dose heparin): SubQ: 5000 units every 8-12 hours

Intermittent I.V.: Initial: 10,000 units, then 50-70 units/kg (5000-10,000 units) every 4-6 hours

I.V. infusion (weight-based dosing per institutional nomogram recommended):

Acute coronary syndromes: MI: Fibrinolytic therapy:

Full-dose alteplase, reteplase, or tenecteplase with dosing as follows: Concurrent bolus of 60 units/kg (maximum: 4000 units), then 12 units/kg/hour (maximum: 1000 units/hour) as continuous infusion. Check aPTT every 4-6 hours; adjust to target of 1.5-2 times the upper limit of control (50-70 seconds in clinical trials); usual range 10-30 units/kg/hour. Duration of heparin therapy depends on concurrent therapy and the specific patient risks for systemic or venous thromboembolism.

Combination regimen (unlabeled): Half-dose tenecteplase (15-25 mg based on weight) and abciximab 0.25 mg/kg bolus then 0.125 mcg/kg/minute (maximum 10 mcg/minute) for 12 hours with heparin dosing as follows: Concurrent bolus of 40 units/kg (maximum 3000 units), then 7 units/kg/hour (maximum: 800 units/hour) as continuous infusion. Adjust to a aPTT target of 50-70 seconds.

Streptokinase: Heparin use optional depending on concurrent therapy and specific patient risks for systemic or venous thromboembolism (anterior MI, CHF, previous embolus, atrial fibrillation, LV thrombus): If heparin is administered, start when aPTT <2 times the upper limit of control; do not use a bolus, but initiate infusion adjusted to a target aPTT of 1.5-2 times the upper limit of control (50-70 seconds in clinical trials). If heparin is not administered by infusion, 7500-12,500 units SubQ every 12 hours (when aPTT <2 times the upper limit of control) is recommended.

Percutaneous coronary intervention: Heparin bolus and infusion may be administered to an activated clotting time (ACT) of 300-350 seconds if no concurrent GPIIb/IIIa receptor antagonist is administered or 200-250 seconds if a GPIIb/IIIa receptor antagonist is administered.

Treatment of unstable angina (high-risk and some intermediate-risk patients): Initial bolus of 60-70 units/kg (maximum: 5000 units), followed by an initial infusion of 12-15 units/kg/hour (maximum: 1000 units/hour). The American College of Chest Physicians consensus conference has recommended dosage adjustments to correspond to a therapeutic range equivalent to heparin levels of 0.3-0.7 units/mL by antifactor Xa determinations.

Treatment of venous thromboembolism:

DVT/PE: I.V. push: 80 units/kg followed by continuous infusion of 18 units/kg/hour

DVT: SubQ: 17,500 units every 12 hours

Line flushing: When using daily flushes of heparin to maintain patency of single and double lumen central catheters, 10 units/mL is commonly used for younger infants (eg, <10 kg) while 100 units/mL is used for older infants, children, and adults. Capped PVC catheters and peripheral heparin locks require flushing more frequently (eg, every 6-8 hours). Volume of heparin flush is usually similar to volume of catheter (or slightly greater). Additional flushes should be given when stagnant blood is observed in catheter, after catheter is used for drug or blood administration, and after blood withdrawal from catheter.

Addition of heparin (0.5-3 unit/mL) to peripheral and central parenteral nutrition has not been shown to decrease catheter-related thrombosis. The final concentration of heparin used for TPN solutions may need to be decreased to 0.5 units/mL in small infants receiving larger amounts of volume in order to avoid approaching therapeutic amounts. Arterial lines are heparinized with a final concentration of 1 unit/mL.

Using a standard heparin solution (25,000 units/500 mL D_5W), the following infusion rates can be used to achieve the listed doses.

For a dose of:

400 units/hour: Infuse at 8 mL/hour
500 units/hour: Infuse at 10 mL/hour
600 units/hour: Infuse at 12 mL/hour
700 units/hour: Infuse at 14 mL/hour
800 units/hour: Infuse at 16 mL/hour
900 units/hour: Infuse at 18 mL/hour
1000 units/hour: Infuse at 20 mL/hour
1100 units/hour: Infuse at 22 mL/hour
1200 units/hour: Infuse at 24 mL/hour
1300 units/hour: Infuse at 26 mL/hour
1400 units/hour: Infuse at 28 mL/hour
1500 units/hour: Infuse at 30 mL/hour
1600 units/hour: Infuse at 32 mL/hour
1700 units/hour: Infuse at 34 mL/hour
1800 units/hour: Infuse at 36 mL/hour
1900 units/hour: Infuse at 38 mL/hour
2000 units/hour: Infuse at 40 mL/hour

Dosing adjustments in the elderly: Patients >60 years of age may have higher serum levels and clinical response (longer aPTTs) as compared to younger patients receiving similar dosages; lower dosages may be required

Stability

Heparin solutions are colorless to slightly yellow; minor color variations do not affect therapeutic efficacy

Heparin should be stored at controlled room temperature and protected from freezing and temperatures >40°C

Stability at room temperature and refrigeration:

Prepared bag: 24 hours
Premixed bag: After seal is broken 4 days
Out of overwrap stability: 30 days

Standard diluent: 25,000 units/500 mL D_5W (premixed)

Minimum volume: 250 mL D_5W

Administration SubQ: Inject in subcutaneous tissue only (not muscle tissue). Injection sites should be rotated (usually left and right portions of the abdomen, above iliac crest).

Do not administer I.M. due to pain, irritation, and hematoma formation; central venous catheters must be flushed with heparin solution when newly inserted, daily (at the time of tubing change), after blood withdrawal or transfusion, and after an intermittent infusion through an injectable cap. A volume of at least 10 mL

(Continued)

Heparin *(Continued)*

of blood should be removed and discarded from a heparinized line before blood samples are sent for coagulation testing.

Using a standard heparin solution (25,000 units/500 mL D_5W), the following infusion rates can be used to achieve the listed doses.

For a dose of:

400 units/hour: Infuse at 8 mL/hour
500 units/hour: Infuse at 10 mL/hour
600 units/hour: Infuse at 12 mL/hour
700 units/hour: Infuse at 14 mL/hour
800 units/hour: Infuse at 16 mL/hour
900 units/hour: Infuse at 18 mL/hour
1000 units/hour: Infuse at 20 mL/hour
1100 units/hour: Infuse at 22 mL/hour
1200 units/hour: Infuse at 24 mL/hour
1300 units/hour: Infuse at 26 mL/hour
1400 units/hour: Infuse at 28 mL/hour
1500 units/hour: Infuse at 30 mL/hour
1600 units/hour: Infuse at 32 mL/hour
1700 units/hour: Infuse at 34 mL/hour
1800 units/hour: Infuse at 36 mL/hour
1900 units/hour: Infuse at 38 mL/hour
2000 units/hour: Infuse at 40 mL/hour

Monitoring Parameters Platelet counts, hemoglobin, hematocrit, signs of bleeding; aPTT or ACT depending upon indication

For intermittent I.V. injections, aPTT is measured 3.5-4 hours after I.V. injection

Note: Continuous I.V. infusion is preferred over I.V. intermittent injections. For full-dose heparin (ie, nonlow-dose), the dose should be titrated according to aPTT results. For anticoagulation, an aPTT 1.5-2.5 times normal is usually desired. Because of variation among hospitals in the control aPTT values, nomograms should be established at each institution, designed to achieve aPTT values in the target range (eg, for a control aPTT of 30 seconds, the target range [1.5-2.5 times control] would be 45-75 seconds). Measurements should be made prior to heparin therapy, 6 hours after initiation, and 6 hours after any dosage change, and should be used to adjust the heparin infusion until the aPTT exhibits a therapeutic level. When two consecutive aPTT values are therapeutic, the measurements may be made every 24 hours, and if necessary, dose adjustment carried out. In addition, a significant change in the patient's clinical condition (eg, recurrent ischemia, bleeding, hypotension) should prompt an immediate aPTT determination, followed by dose adjustment if necessary. Increase or decrease infusion by 2-4 units/kg/hour dependent upon aPTT.

Heparin infusion dose adjustment:

aPTT >3x control: Decrease infusion rate 50%
aPTT 2-3x control: Decrease infusion rate 25%
aPTT 1.5-2x control: No change
aPTT <1.5x control: Increase rate of infusion 25%; max 2500 units/hour

Reference Range Heparin: 0.3-0.5 unit/mL; aPTT: 1.5-2.5 times **the patient's baseline**

Anesthesia and Critical Care Concerns/Other Considerations In the treatment of unstable angina/non-ST-segment elevation MI, parenteral anticoagulation with unfractionated heparin or low molecular weight heparin is recommended.

Thrombocytopenia: Heparin-associated thrombocytopenia (HAT) commonly occurs within 48-72 hours of initiation. Platelet counts usually fall below 100,000 cells/mm^3 and return to normal within 4 days with continued heparin therapy. Heparin-induced thrombocytopenia (HIT) is a serious, immunoglobulin-mediated reaction with a high risk for thromboembolic events. In HIT, thrombocytopenia usually begins 5-10 days following heparin initiation; HIT can begin within ~10 hours in patients who have received heparin within the previous 100 days (Warkentin T, 2001). Thrombocytopenia can be severe; heparin of all forms must be stopped including flushes and heparin-coated indwelling catheters.

The addition of heparin to parenteral nutrition solutions does not significantly decrease the risk of catheter-related thrombosis (Klerk C, 2003).

Pregnancy Risk Factor C

Contraindications Hypersensitivity to heparin or any component of the formulation; severe thrombocytopenia; uncontrolled active bleeding except when due to DIC; suspected intracranial hemorrhage; not for I.M. use; not for use when appropriate monitoring parameters cannot be obtained

Warnings/Precautions Use cautiously in patients with a documented hypersensitivity reaction and only in life-threatening situations. Hemorrhage is the most common complication. Monitor for signs and symptoms of bleeding. Certain patients are at increased risk of bleeding. Risk factors include bacterial endocarditis; congenital or acquired bleeding disorders; active ulcerative or angiodysplastic GI diseases; severe uncontrolled hypertension; hemorrhagic stroke; or use shortly after brain, spinal, or ophthalmology surgery; patient treated concomitantly with platelet inhibitors; conditions associated with increased bleeding tendencies (hemophilia, vascular purpura); recent GI bleeding; thrombocytopenia or platelet defects; severe liver disease; hypertensive or diabetic retinopathy; or in patients undergoing invasive procedures. A higher incidence of bleeding has been reported in patients >60 years of age, particularly women. They are also more sensitive to the dose.

Patients who develop thrombocytopenia on heparin may be at risk of developing a new thrombus ("White-clot syndrome"). Hypersensitivity reactions can occur. Osteoporosis can occur following long-term use (>6 months). Monitor for hyperkalemia. Discontinue therapy and consider alternatives if platelets are <100,000/mm^3. Patients >60 years of age may require lower doses of heparin.

Some preparations contain benzyl alcohol as a preservative. In neonates, large amounts of benzyl alcohol (>100 mg/kg/day) have been associated with fatal toxicity (gasping syndrome). The use of preservative-free heparin is, therefore, recommended in neonates. Some preparations contain sulfite which may cause allergic reactions.

Heparin does not possess fibrinolytic activity and, therefore, cannot lyse established thrombi; discontinue heparin if hemorrhage occurs; severe hemorrhage or overdosage may require protamine

Adverse Reactions

Cardiovascular: Chest pain, vasospasm (possibly related to thrombosis), hemorrhagic shock

Central nervous system: Fever, headache, chills

Dermatologic: Unexplained bruising, urticaria, alopecia, dysesthesia pedis, purpura, eczema, cutaneous necrosis (following deep SubQ injection), erythematous plaques (case reports)

Endocrine & metabolic: Hyperkalemia (supression of aldosterone), rebound hyperlipidemia on discontinuation

Gastrointestinal: Nausea, vomiting, constipation, hematemesis

Genitourinary: Frequent or persistent erection

Hematologic: Hemorrhage, blood in urine, bleeding from gums, epistaxis, adrenal hemorrhage, ovarian hemorrhage, retroperitoneal hemorrhage, thrombocytopenia (see note)

Hepatic: Elevated liver enzymes (AST/ALT)

Local: Irritation, ulceration, cutaneous necrosis have been rarely reported with deep SubQ injections; I.M. injection (not recommended) is associated with a high incidence of these effects

Neuromuscular & skeletal: Peripheral neuropathy, osteoporosis (chronic therapy effect)

Ocular: Conjunctivitis (allergic reaction)

Respiratory: Hemoptysis, pulmonary hemorrhage, asthma, rhinitis, bronchospasm (case reports)

Miscellaneous: Allergic reactions, anaphylactoid reactions

Note: Thrombocytopenia has been reported to occur at an incidence between 0% and 30%. It is often of no clinical significance. However, immunologically mediated heparin-induced thrombocytopenia has been estimated to occur in 1% to 2% of patients, and is marked by a progressive fall in platelet counts and, in some cases, thromboembolic complications (skin necrosis, pulmonary embolism, gangrene of the extremities, stroke or MI). For recommendations regarding platelet monitoring during heparin therapy, consult "Seventh ACCP Consensus Conference on Antithrombotic and Thrombolytic Therapy."

Overdosage/Toxicology The primary symptom of overdose is bleeding. Antidote is protamine; dose 1 mg neutralizes 1 mg (100 units) of heparin. Discontinue all heparin if evidence of progressive immune thrombocytopenia occurs.

(Continued)

Heparin *(Continued)*

Drug Interactions

Cephalosporins which contain the MTT side chain may increase the risk of hemorrhage.

Drugs which affect platelet function (eg, aspirin, NSAIDs, dipyridamole, ticlopidine, clopidogrel, IIb/IIIa antagonists) may potentiate the risk of hemorrhage.

Nitroglycerin (I.V.) may decrease heparin's anticoagulant effect. This interaction has not been validated in some studies, and may only occur at high nitroglycerin dosages.

Penicillins (parenteral) may prolong bleeding time via inhibition of platelet aggregation, potentially increasing the risk of hemorrhage.

Thrombolytic agents increase the risk of hemorrhage.

Warfarin: Risk of bleeding may be increased during concurrent therapy. Heparin is commonly continued during the initiation of warfarin therapy to assure anticoagulation and to protect against possible transient hypercoagulability.

Other drugs reported to increase heparin's anticoagulant effect include antihistamines, tetracycline, quinine, nicotine, and cardiac glycosides (digoxin).

Ethanol/Nutrition/Herb Interactions

Food: When taking for >6 months, may interfere with calcium absorption.

Herb/Nutraceutical: Avoid cat's claw, dong quai, evening primrose, feverfew, red clover, horse chestnut, garlic, green tea, ginseng, ginkgo (all have additional antiplatelet activity).

Test Interactions Increased thyroxine (S) (competitive protein binding methods); increased PT, increased aPTT, increased bleeding time

Dosage Forms [DSC] = Discontinued product

Infusion, as sodium [premixed in NaCl 0.45%; porcine intestinal mucosa source]: 12,500 units (250 mL); 25,000 units (250 mL, 500 mL)

Infusion, as sodium [preservative free; premixed in D_5W; porcine intestinal mucosa source]: 10,000 units (100 mL) [contains sodium metabisulfite]; 12,500 units (250 mL) [contains sodium metabisulfite]; 20,000 units (500 mL) [contains sodium metabisulfite]; 25,000 units (250 mL, 500 mL) [contains sodium metabisulfite]

Infusion, as sodium [preservative free; premixed in NaCl 0.9%; porcine intestinal mucosa source]: 1000 units (500 mL); 2000 units (1000 mL)

Injection, solution, as sodium [beef lung source; multidose vial]: 1000 units/mL (10 mL, 30 mL); 5000 units/mL (10 mL), 10,000 units/mL (1 mL, 4 mL) [contains benzyl alcohol] [DSC]

Injection, solution, as sodium [lock flush preparation; porcine intestinal mucosa source; multidose vial]: 10 units/mL (1 mL, 10 mL, 30 mL) [contains parabens]; 100 units/mL (1 mL, 5 mL) [contains parabens]

Injection, solution, as sodium [lock flush preparation; porcine intestinal mucosa source; multidose vial]: 10 units/mL (10 mL, 30 mL); 100 units/mL (10 mL, 30 mL) [contains benzyl alcohol]

Hep-Lock®: 10 units/mL (1 mL, 2 mL, 10 mL, 30 mL); 100 units/mL (1 mL, 2 mL, 10 mL, 30 mL) [contains benzyl alcohol]

Injection, solution, as sodium [lock flush preparation; porcine intestinal mucosa source; prefilled syringe]: 10 units/mL (1 mL, 2 mL, 3 mL, 5 mL); 100 units/mL (1 mL, 2 mL, 3 mL, 5 mL) [contains benzyl alcohol]

Injection, solution, as sodium [preservative free; lock flush preparation; porcine intestinal mucosa source; prefilled syringe]: 100 units/mL (5 mL)

Injection, solution, as sodium [preservative free; lock flush preparation; porcine intestinal mucosa source; vial] (HepFlush®-10): 10 units/mL (10 mL)

Injection, solution, as sodium [porcine intestinal mucosa source; multidose vial]: 1000 units/mL (1 mL, 10 mL, 30 mL) [contains benzyl alcohol]; 1000 units/mL (1 mL, 10 mL, 30 mL) [contains methylparabens]; 5000 units/mL (1 mL, 10 mL) [contains benzyl alcohol]; 5000 units/mL (1 mL) [contains methylparabens]; 10,000 units/mL (1 mL, 4 mL) [contains benzyl alcohol]; 10,000 units/mL (1 mL, 5 mL) [contains methylparabens]; 20,000 units/mL (1 mL) [contains methylparabens]

Injection, solution, as sodium [porcine intestinal mucosa source; prefilled syringe]: 5000 units/mL (1 mL) [contains benzyl alcohol]

Injection, solution, as sodium [preservative free; porcine intestinal mucosa source; prefilled syringe]: 10,000 units/mL (0.5 mL)

Injection, solution, as sodium [preservative free; porcine intestinal mucosa source; vial]: 1000 units/mL (2 mL); 2000 units/mL (5 mL); 2500 units/mL (10 mL)

References

Dager WE and White RH, "Pharmacotherapy of Heparin-Induced Thrombocytopenia," *Expert Opin Pharmacother*, 2003, 4(6):919-40.

Klerk CP, Smorenburg SM, and Buller HR, "Thrombosis Prophylaxis in Patient Populations With a Central Venous Catheter: A Systematic Review," *Arch Intern Med*, 2003, 163(16):1913-21.

Verma AK, Levine M, Shalansky SJ, et al, "Frequency of Heparin-Induced Thrombocytopenia in Critical Care Patients," *Pharmacotherapy*, 2003, 23(6):745-53.

Warkentin TE and Kelton JG, "Temporal Aspects of Heparin-Induced Thrombocytopenia," *N Engl J Med*, 2001, 344(17):1286-92.

Warkentin TE, Levine MN, Hirsch J, et al, "Heparin-Induced Thrombocytopenia in Patients Treated With Low-Molecular Weight Heparin or Unfractionated Heparin," *N Engl J Med*, 1995, 332(20):1330-5.

♦ **Heparin Calcium** *see* Heparin *on page 609*
♦ **Heparin Cofactor I** *see* Antithrombin III *on page 115*
♦ **Heparin Lock Flush** *see* Heparin *on page 609*
♦ **Heparin Sodium** *see* Heparin *on page 609*

Hepatitis A Inactivated and Hepatitis B (Recombinant) Vaccine

(hep a TYE tis aye in ak ti VAY ted & hep a TYE tis bee ree KOM be nant vak SEEN)

U.S. Brand Names Twinrix®

Canadian Brand Names Twinrix®

Synonyms Engerix-B® and Havrix®; Havrix® and Engerix-B®; Hepatitis B (Recombinant) and Hepatitis A Inactivated Vaccine

Pharmacologic Category Vaccine

Generic Available No

Use Active immunization against disease caused by hepatitis A virus and hepatitis B virus (all known subtypes) in populations desiring protection against or at high risk of exposure to these viruses.

Populations include travelers to areas of intermediate/high endemicity for **both** HAV and HBV; those at increased risk of HBV infection due to behavioral or occupational factors; patients with chronic liver disease; laboratory workers who handle live HAV and HBV; healthcare workers, police, and other personnel who render first-aid or medical assistance; workers who come in contact with sewage; employees of day care centers and correctional facilities; patients/staff of hemodialysis units; male homosexuals; patients frequently receiving blood products; military personnel; users of injectable illicit drugs; close household contacts of patients with hepatitis A and hepatitis B infection.

Mechanism of Action

Hepatitis A vaccine (Havrix®), an inactivated virus vaccine, offers active immunization against hepatitis A virus infection at an effective immune response rate in up to 99% of subjects.

Recombinant hepatitis B vaccine (Engerix-B®) is a noninfectious subunit viral vaccine. The vaccine is derived from hepatitis B surface antigen (HB_sAg) produced through recombinant DNA techniques from yeast cells. The portion of the hepatitis B gene which codes for HB_sAg is cloned into yeast which is then cultured to produce hepatitis B vaccine.

In immunocompetent people, Twinrix® provides active immunization against hepatitis A virus infection (at an effective immune response rate >99% of subjects) and against hepatitis B virus infection (at an effective immune response rate of 93% to 97%) 30 days after completion of the 3-dose series. This is comparable to using hepatitis A vaccine (Havrix®) and hepatitis B vaccine (Engerix-B®) concomitantly.

Pharmacodynamics/Kinetics

Onset of action: Seroconversion for antibodies against HAV and HBV were detected 1 month after completion of the 3-dose series.

Duration: Patients remained seropositive for at least 4 years during clinical studies.

Dosage I.M.: Adults: Primary immunization: Three doses (1 mL each) given on a 0-, 1-, and 6-month schedule

(Continued)

Hepatitis A Inactivated and Hepatitis B (Recombinant) Vaccine *(Continued)*

Stability Store in refrigerator at 2°C to 8°C (36°F to 46°F); do not freeze (discard if frozen)

Administration I.M.: Shake well prior to use. Do not dilute prior to administration. Administer in the deltoid region; do not administer in the gluteal region (may give suboptimal response). Do not administer at the same site, or using the same syringe, as additional vaccines or immunoglobulins.

For patients at risk of hemorrhage following intramuscular injection, the ACIP recommends "it should be administered intramuscularly if, in the opinion of the physician familiar with the patients bleeding risk, the vaccine can be administered with reasonable safety by this route. If the patient receives antihemophilia or other similar therapy, intramuscular vaccination can be scheduled shortly after such therapy is administered. A fine needle (23 gauge or smaller) can be used for the vaccination and firm pressure applied to the site (without rubbing) for at least 2 minutes. The patient should be instructed concerning the risk of hematoma from the injection."

Pregnancy Risk Factor C

Contraindications Hypersensitivity to hepatitis A vaccine or hepatitis B vaccine, or any component of the formulation

Warnings/Precautions Use caution in patients on anticoagulants, with thrombocytopenia, or bleeding disorders (bleeding may occur following intramuscular injection). Treatment for anaphylactic reactions should be immediately available. Postpone vaccination in moderate to severe acute illness (minor illness is not a contraindication). May not prevent infection if adequate antibody titers are not achieved (including immunosuppressed patients, patients on immunosuppressant therapy). Safety and efficacy in patients <18 years of age have not been established.

See individual agents.

Adverse Reactions All serious adverse reactions must be reported to the U.S. Department of Health and Human Services (DHHS) Vaccine Adverse Event Reporting System (VAERS) 1-800-822-7967.

Incidence of adverse effects of the combination product were similar to those occurring after administration of hepatitis A vaccine and hepatitis B vaccine alone. (Incidence reported is not versus placebo.)

>10%:

Central nervous system: Headache (13% to 22%), fatigue (11% to 14%)

Local: Injection site reaction: Soreness (37% to 41%), redness (9% to 11%)

1% to 10%:

Central nervous system: Fever (2% to 3%)

Gastrointestinal: Diarrhea (4% to 6%), nausea (2% to 4%), vomiting (≤1%)

Local: Injection site reaction: Swelling (4% to 6%), induration

Respiratory: Upper respiratory tract infection

Miscellaneous: Flu-like syndrome

<1% (Limited to important or life-threatening): Also see individual agents: Allergic reactions, anaphylaxis, anaphylactoid reactions, arthralgia, Bell's palsy, bronchospasm, bruising at injection site, diaphoresis, dizziness, dyspnea, encephalopathy, erythema, erythema multiforme, flushing, Guillain-Barré syndrome, liver function test abnormalities, pruritus at injection site, rash, somnolence, Stevens-Johnson syndrome, syncope, urticaria, vertigo, vomiting, weakness

Drug Interactions Immunosuppressant agents: May decrease immune response to vaccine

Dosage Forms Injection, suspension: Inactivated hepatitis A virus 720 ELISA units and hepatitis B surface antigen 20 mcg per mL (1 mL) [prefilled syringe; single-dose vial]

Hepatitis A Vaccine (hep a TYE tis aye vak SEEN)

U.S. Brand Names Havrix®; VAQTA®

Canadian Brand Names Avaxim®; Avaxim®-Pediatric; Havrix®; VAQTA®

Pharmacologic Category Vaccine

Generic Available No

Use

Active immunization against disease caused by hepatitis A virus in populations desiring protection against or at high risk of exposure

Populations at high risk of exposure to hepatitis A virus may include children and adolescents in selected states and regions, travelers to developing countries, household and sexual contacts of persons infected with hepatitis A, child day care employees, patients with chronic liver disease, illicit drug users, male homosexuals, institutional workers (eg, institutions for the mentally and physically handicapped persons, prisons), and healthcare workers who may be exposed to hepatitis A virus (eg, laboratory employees)

Mechanism of Action As an inactivated virus vaccine, hepatitis A vaccine offers active immunization against hepatitis A virus infection at an effective immune response rate in up to 99% of subjects

Pharmacodynamics/Kinetics

Onset of action (protection): 4 weeks after a single dose

Duration: Neutralizing antibodies have persisted for up to 8 years; based on kinetic models, antibodies may be present >20 years

Dosage I.M.:

Havrix®:

- Children 12 months to 18 years: 720 ELISA units (0.5 mL) with a booster dose of 720 ELISA units 6-12 months following primary immunization
- Adults: 1440 ELISA units (1 mL) with a booster 6-12 months following primary immunization

VAQTA®:

- Children 12 months to 18 years: 25 units (0.5 mL) with 25 units (0.5 mL) booster to be given 6-18 months after primary immunization (6-12 months if initial dose was with Havrix®)
- Adults: 50 units (1 mL) with 50 units (1 mL) booster to be given 6-18 months after primary immunization (6-12 months if initial dose was with Havrix®)

Stability Store under refrigeration at 2°C to 8°C (36°F to 46°F); do not freeze

Administration The deltoid muscle is the preferred site for injection. Shake well prior to use. For optimal protection, travelers should receive 1st dose at least 4 weeks prior to departure. For patients at risk of hemorrhage following intramuscular injection, the ACIP recommends "it should be administered intramuscularly if, in the opinion of the physician familiar with the patients bleeding risk, the vaccine can be administered with reasonable safety by this route. If the patient receives antihemophilia or other similar therapy, intramuscular vaccination can be scheduled shortly after such therapy is administered. A fine needle (23 gauge or smaller) can be used for the vaccination and firm pressure applied to the site (without rubbing) for at least 2 minutes. The patient should be instructed concerning the risk of hematoma from the injection."

Monitoring Parameters Liver function tests

Pregnancy Risk Factor C

Contraindications Hypersensitivity to hepatitis A vaccine or any component of the formulation

Warnings/Precautions Use caution in patients on anticoagulants, with thrombocytopenia, or bleeding disorders (bleeding may occur following intramuscular injection). Treatment for anaphylactic reactions should be immediately available. Postpone vaccination with acute infection or febrile illness. May not prevent infection if adequate antibody titers are not achieved (including immunosuppressed patients, patients on immunosuppressant therapy).

Adverse Reactions All serious adverse reactions must be reported to the U.S. Department of Health and Human Services (DHHS) Vaccine Adverse Event Reporting System (VAERS) 1-800-822-7967.

Frequency dependant upon age, product used, and concomitant vaccine administration. In general, injection site reactions were less common in younger children.

>10%:

- Central nervous system: Irritability (11% to 36%), drowsiness (15% to 17%), headache (2% to 16%), fever ≥100.4°F (9% to 11%)
- Gastrointestinal: Anorexia (1% to 19%)
- Local: Injection site: Pain, soreness, tenderness (3% to 56%), erythema (1% to 22%), warmth (<1% to 17%), swelling (1% to 14%)

1% to 10%:

- Central nervous system: Fever ≥102°F (3% to 4%)
- Dermatologic: Rash (≤1% to 5%)
- Endocrine & metabolic: Menstrual disorder (1%)

(Continued)

Hepatitis A Vaccine *(Continued)*

Gastrointestinal: Diarrhea (<1% to 6%), vomiting (<1% to 4%), nausea (2%), abdominal pain (<1% to 2%), anorexia (1%)
Local: Injection site bruising (1% to 2%)
Neuromuscular & skeletal: Weakness/fatigue (4%), myalgia (<1% to 2%), arm pain (1%), back pain (1%), stiffness (1%)
Ocular: Conjunctivitis (1%)
Otic: Otitis media (8%), otitis (2%)
Respiratory: Upper respiratory tract infection (<1% to 10%), rhinorrhea (6%), cough (1% to 5%), pharnyngitis (<1% to 3%), respiratory congestion (2%), nasal congestion (1%), laryngotracheobronchitis (1%)
Miscellaneous: Crying (2%), viral exanthema (1%)

<1% (Limited to importantor life threatening): Allergic reaction, anaphylaxis, angioedema, arthralgia, asthma, bronchial constriction, cerebellar ataxia, CK increased, dermatitis, dizziness, dyspnea, encephalitis, erythema multiforme, eosinophilia, Guillain-Barre syndrome, hepatitis, hyperhydrosis, hypertonic episode, injection site hematoma, injection site itching, injection site rash, insomnia, jaundice, liver function tests increased, lymphadenopathy, multiple sclerosis, myelitis, neuropathy, paresthesia, photophobia, pruritus, seizure, somnolence, syncope, taste disturbance, thrombocytopenia, urine protein increased, vertigo, wheezing

Drug Interactions

Immune globulin: May be administered concomitantly (using separate sites and syringes)

Vaccines: May be administered concomitantly with cholera, diphtheria, MMR II, Japanese encephalitis, poliovirus, rabies, tetanus, typhoid or yellow fever vaccines using separate sites and syringes. May be administered simultaneously with hepatitis B vaccine.

Dosage Forms

Injection, suspension, adult:
Havrix®: Viral antigen 1440 ELISA units/mL (1 mL) [contains trace amounts of neomycin; syringe plunger contains latex rubber; available in prefilled syringe or single-dose vial]
VAQTA®: HAV antigen 50 units/mL (1 mL) [vial stopper and syringe plunger contain latex rubber; available in prefilled syringe or single-dose vial]

Injection, suspension, pediatric (Havrix®): Viral antigen 720 ELISA units/0.5 mL (0.5 mL) [contains trace amounts of neomycin; syringe plunger contains latex rubber; available in prefilled syringe or single-dose vial]

Injection, suspension, pediatric/adolescent (VAQTA®): HAV antigen 25 units/0.5 mL (0.5 mL) [vial stopper and syringe plunger contain latex rubber; available in prefilled syringe or single-dose vial]

Hepatitis B Immune Globulin

(hep a TYE tis bee i MYUN GLOB yoo lin)

U.S. Brand Names BayHep B®; HepaGam B™; Nabi-HB®

Canadian Brand Names BayHep B®; HyperHep B®

Synonyms HBIG

Pharmacologic Category Immune Globulin

Generic Available No

Use Passive prophylactic immunity to hepatitis B following: Acute exposure to blood containing hepatitis B surface antigen (HBsAg); perinatal exposure of infants born to HBsAg-positive mothers; sexual exposure to HBsAg-positive persons; household exposure to persons with acute HBV infection

Note: Hepatitis B immune globulin is not indicated for treatment of active hepatitis B infection and is ineffective in the treatment of chronic active hepatitis B infection.

Unlabeled/Investigational Use

Prevention of hepatitis B virus recurrence after liver transplantation

Mechanism of Action Hepatitis B immune globulin (HBIG) is a nonpyrogenic sterile solution containing immunoglobulin G (IgG) specific to hepatitis B surface antigen (HB_sAg). HBIG differs from immune globulin in the amount of anti-HB_s. Immune globulin is prepared from plasma that is not preselected for anti-HB_s content. HBIG is prepared from plasma preselected for high titer anti-HB_s. In the U.S., HBIG has an anti-HB_s high titer >1:100,000 by IRA.

Pharmacodynamics/Kinetics

Absorption: Slow

Half-life: 17-25 days

Distribution: V_d: 7-15 L

Time to peak, serum: 2-10 days

Dosage I.M.:

Newborns: Hepatitis B: 0.5 mL as soon after birth as possible (within 12 hours); may repeat at 3 months in order for a higher rate of prevention of the carrier state to be achieved; at this time an active vaccination program with the vaccine may begin

Infants <12 months: Household exposure prophylaxis: 0.5 mL (to be administered if mother or primary caregiver has acute HBV infection)

Adults: Postexposure prophylaxis: 0.06 mL/kg as soon as possible after exposure (ie, within 24 hours of needlestick, ocular, or mucosal exposure or within 14 days of sexual exposure); usual dose: 3-5 mL; repeat at 28-30 days after exposure in nonresponders or in patients who refuse vaccination

Note: HBIG may be administered at the same time (but at a different site) or up to 1 month preceding hepatitis B vaccination without impairing the active immune response

I.V. (unlabeled route of administration):

Prevention of hepatitis B virus recurrence after liver transplantation (unlabeled use): Consult institutional protocols; specific protocols may vary among transplant centers. Typical HBIG protocols (Nabi-HB®): 10,000-20,000 units intraoperatively during anhepatic phase, followed by 10,000 units daily for 7 days, then as required to maintain adequate quantitative HB_s antibody levels. Used in combination with nucleoside analog (eg, lamivudine) with anti-HBV activity. Subsequent HBIG doses may be administered at fixed intervals or on an "as needed" basis to maintain goal antibody level. Goal antibody titers and HBIG requirements may differ among patients depending upon viral load pretransplant and the presence of other risk factors for recurrence.

Stability Refrigerate at 2°C to 8°C (36°F to 46°F); do not freeze. Use within 6 hours of entering vial.

Administration I.M. injection only in anterolateral aspect of upper thigh and deltoid muscle of upper arm; to prevent injury from injection, care should be taken when giving to patients with thrombocytopenia or bleeding disorders; has been administered intravenously in hepatitis B-positive liver transplant patients (unlabeled route)

Anesthesia and Critical Care Concerns/Other Considerations Hepatitis B immune globulin has been administered intravenously in hepatitis B-positive liver transplant patients.

Pregnancy Risk Factor C

Contraindications Hypersensitivity to hepatitis B immune globulin or any component of the formulation; severe allergy to gamma globulin or anti-immunoglobulin therapies

Warnings/Precautions Have epinephrine 1:1000 available for anaphylactic reactions. As a product of human plasma, this product may potentially transmit disease; screening of donors, as well as testing and/or inactivation of certain viruses reduces this risk. Use caution in patients with thrombocytopenia or coagulation disorders (I.M. injections may be contraindicated), in patients with isolated IgA deficiency, or in patients with previous systemic hypersensitivity to human immunoglobulins. Not approved for intravenous administration.

Adverse Reactions Frequency not defined.

Central nervous system: Chills, dizziness, fever, headache, lethargy, malaise

Dermatologic: Angioedema, erythema, rash, urticaria

Gastrointestinal: Nausea, vomiting

Genitourinary: Nephrotic syndrome

Local: Muscular stiffness, pain, and tenderness at injection site

Neuromuscular & skeletal: Arthralgia, back pain, myalgia

Miscellaneous: Anaphylaxis, flu-like syndrome

Drug Interactions Live virus vaccines: Interferes with immune response of live virus vaccines; defer live virus vaccine for about 3 months after immune globulin

Note: HBIG may be administered at the same time (but at a different site) or up to 1 month preceding hepatitis B vaccination without impairing the active immune response

Dosage Forms Note: Potency expressed in international units as compared to the WHO standard

(Continued)

Hepatitis B Immune Globulin *(Continued)*

Injection, solution [preservative free]:

BayHepB®: 15%-18% protein (0.5 mL) [neonatal single-dose syringe]; (1 mL) [single-dose syringe or single-dose vial]; (5 mL) [single-dose vial]

Nabi-HB®: 5% (1 mL, 5 mL) [>312 int. units/mL; single-dose vial]

HepaGam B™: 5% (1 mL, 5 mL) [>312 int. units/mL; contains maltose, single-dose vial]

- ♦ **Hepatitis B Inactivated Virus Vaccine (plasma derived)** *see* Hepatitis B Vaccine *on page 620*
- ♦ **Hepatitis B Inactivated Virus Vaccine (recombinant DNA)** *see* Hepatitis B Vaccine *on page 620*
- ♦ **Hepatitis B (Recombinant) and Hepatitis A Inactivated Vaccine** *see* Hepatitis A Inactivated and Hepatitis B (Recombinant) Vaccine *on page 615*

Hepatitis B Vaccine (hep a TYE tis bee vak SEEN)

Medication Safety Issues

Sound-alike/look-alike issues:

Recombivax HB® may be confused with Comvax®

U.S. Brand Names Engerix-B®; Recombivax HB®

Canadian Brand Names Engerix-B®; Recombivax HB®

Synonyms Hepatitis B Inactivated Virus Vaccine (plasma derived); Hepatitis B Inactivated Virus Vaccine (recombinant DNA)

Pharmacologic Category Vaccine

Generic Available No

Use Immunization against infection caused by all known subtypes of hepatitis B virus, in individuals considered at high risk of potential exposure to hepatitis B virus or HB_sAg-positive materials: See table.

Pre-exposure Prophylaxis for Hepatitis B
Healthcare workers[1]
Special patient groups (eg, adolescents, infants born to HB_sAg-positive mothers, children born after 11/21/91, military personnel, etc)
Hemodialysis patients[2] (see dosing recommendations)
Recipients of certain blood products[3]
Lifestyle factors
Homosexual and bisexual men
Intravenous drug abusers
Heterosexually-active persons with multiple sexual partners or recently acquired sexually-transmitted diseases
Environmental factors
Household and sexual contacts of HBV carriers
Prison inmates
Clients and staff of institutions for the mentally handicapped
Residents, immigrants, and refugees from areas with endemic HBV infection
International travelers at increased risk of acquiring HBV infection

[1]The risk of hepatitis B virus (HBV) infection for healthcare workers varies both between hospitals and within hospitals. Hepatitis B vaccination is recommended for all healthcare workers with blood exposure.

[2]Hemodialysis patients often respond poorly to hepatitis B vaccination; higher vaccine doses or increased number of doses are required. A special formulation of one vaccine is now available for such persons (Recombivax HB®, 40 mcg/mL). The anti-Hb_s (antibody to hepatitis B surface antigen) response of such persons should be tested after they are vaccinated, and those who have not responded should be revaccinated with 1-3 additional doses.

Patients with chronic renal disease should be vaccinated as early as possible, ideally before they require hemodialysis. In addition, their anti-HB_s levels should be monitored at 6- to 12-month intervals to assess the need for revaccination.

[3]Patients with hemophilia should be immunized subcutaneously, not intramuscularly.

Mechanism of Action Recombinant hepatitis B vaccine is a noninfectious subunit viral vaccine. The vaccine is derived from hepatitis B surface antigen (HB_sAg) produced through recombinant DNA techniques from yeast cells. The portion of the hepatitis B gene which codes for HB_sAg is cloned into yeast which is then cultured to produce hepatitis B vaccine.

Pharmacodynamics/Kinetics Duration of action: Following a 3-dose series, immunity lasts ~5-7 years

Dosage I.M.:

Immunization regimen: Regimen consists of 3 doses (0, 1, and 6 months): First dose given on the elected date, second dose given 1 month later, third dose given 6 months after the first dose; see table.

Routine Immunization Regimen of Three I.M. Hepatitis B Vaccine Doses

Age	Initial		1 mo		6 mo	
	Recombivax HB® (mL)	Engerix-B® (mL)	Recombivax HB® (mL)	Engerix-B® (mL)	Recombivax HB® (mL)	Engerix-B® (mL)
Birth[1] to 19 y	0.5[2]	0.5[3]	0.5[2]	0.5[3]	0.5[2]	0.5[3]
≥20 y	1[4]	1[5]	1[4]	1[5]	1[4]	1[5]
Dialysis or immunocompromised patients[6]	1[7]	2[8]	1[7]	2[8]	1[7]	2[8]

[1]Infants born of HB_sAg **negative** mothers.

[2]5 mcg/0.5 mL pediatric/adolescent formulation

[3]10 mcg/0.5 mL formulation

[4]10 mcg/mL adult formulation

[5]20 mcg/mL formulation

[6]Revaccinate if anti-HB_s <10 mIU/mL ≥1-2 months after third dose.

[7]40 mcg/mL dialysis formulation

[8]Two 1 mL doses given at different sites using the 40 mcg/2 mL dialysis formulation

Alternative dosing schedule for **Recombivax HB®:** Children 11-15 years (10 mcg/mL adult formulation): First dose of 1 mL given on the elected date, second dose given 4-6 months later

Alternative dosing schedules for **Engerix-B®:**

Children ≤10 years (10 mcg/0.5 mL formulation): High-risk children: 0.5 mL at 0, 1, 2, and 12 months; lower-risk children ages 5-10 who are candidates for an extended administration schedule may receive an alternative regimen of 0.5 mL at 0, 12, and 24 months. If booster dose is needed, revaccinate with 0.5 mL.

Adolescents 11-19 years (20 mcg/mL formulation): 1 mL at 0, 1, and 6 months. High-risk adolescents: 1 mL at 0, 1, 2, and 12 months; lower-risk adolescents 11-16 years who are candidates for an extended administration schedule may receive an alternative regimen of 0.5 mL (using the 10 mcg/0.5 mL) formulation at 0, 12, and 24 months. If booster dose is needed, revaccinate with 20 mcg.

Adults ≥20 years: High-risk adults (20 mcg/mL formulation): 1 mL at 0, 1, 2, and 12 months. If booster dose is needed, revaccinate with 1 mL.

Postexposure prophylaxis: See table.

Postexposure Prophylaxis Recommended Dosage for Infants Born to HB_sAg-Positive Mothers

Treatment	Birth	Within 7 d	1 mo	6 mo
Engerix-B® (pediatric formulation 10 mcg/0.5 mL)[1]	Note[2]	0.5 mL[2]	0.5 mL	0.5 mL
Recombivax HB® (pediatric/adolescent formulation 5 mcg/0.5 mL)	Note[2]	0.5 mL[2]	0.5 mL	0.5 mL
Hepatitis B immune globulin	0.5 mL	—	—	—

[1]An alternate regimen is administration of the vaccine at birth, within 7 days of birth, and 1, 2, and 12 months later.

[2]The first dose may be given at birth at the same time as HBIG, but give in the opposite anterolateral thigh. This may better ensure vaccine absorption.

Stability Refrigerate at 2°C to 8°C (36°F to 46°F). Do not freeze.

Administration It is possible to interchange the vaccines for completion of a series or for booster doses; the antibody produced in response to each type of vaccine is comparable, however, the quantity of the vaccine will vary

(Continued)

Hepatitis B Vaccine *(Continued)*

I.M. injection only; in adults, the deltoid muscle is the preferred site; the anterolateral thigh is the recommended site in infants and young children. Not for gluteal administration. Shake well prior to withdrawal and use.

For patients at risk of hemorrhage following intramuscular injection, the ACIP recommends "it should be administered intramuscularly if, in the opinion of the physician familiar with the patients bleeding risk, the vaccine can be administered with reasonable safety by this route. If the patient receives antihemophilia or other similar therapy, intramuscular vaccination can be scheduled shortly after such therapy is administered. A fine needle (23 gauge or smaller) can be used for the vaccination and firm pressure applied to the site (without rubbing) for at least 2 minutes. The patient should be instructed concerning the risk of hematoma from the injection."

Federal law requires that the date of administration, the vaccine manufacturer, lot number of vaccine, and the administering person's name, title, and address be entered into the patient's permanent medical record.

Pregnancy Risk Factor C

Contraindications Hypersensitivity to yeast, hepatitis B vaccine, or any component of the formulation

Warnings/Precautions Immediate treatment for anaphylactic/anaphylactoid reaction should be available during vaccine use; consider delaying vaccination during acute febrile illness; use caution with decreased cardiopulmonary function; unrecognized hepatitis B infection may be present, immunization may not prevent infection in these patients; patients >65 years may have lower response rates

Adverse Reactions All serious adverse reactions must be reported to the U.S. Department of Health and Human Services (DHHS) Vaccine Adverse Event Reporting System (VAERS) 1-800-822-7967.

Frequency not defined. The most common adverse effects reported with both products included injection site reactions (>10%).

Cardiovascular: Hypotension

Central nervous system: Agitation, chills, dizziness, fatigue, fever (≥37.5°C / 100°F), flushing, headache, insomnia, irritability, lightheadedness, malaise, vertigo

Dermatologic: Angioedema, petechiae, pruritus, rash, urticaria

Gastrointestinal: Abdominal pain, appetite decreased, cramps, diarrhea, dyspepsia, nausea, vomiting

Genitourinary: Dysuria

Local: Injection site reactions: Ecchymosis, erythema, induration, pain, nodule formation, soreness, swelling, tenderness, warmth

Neuromuscular & skeletal: Achiness, arthralgia, back pain, myalgia, neck pain, neck stiffness, paresthesia, shoulder pain, weakness

Otic: Earache

Respiratory: Cough, pharyngitis, rhinitis, upper respiratory tract infection

Miscellaneous: Lymphadenopathy, diaphoresis

Postmarketing and/or case reports: Alopecia, anaphylaxis, arthritis, Bell's palsy, bronchospasm, conjunctivitis, constipation, eczema, encephalitis, erythema nodosum, erythema multiforme, erythrocyte sedimentation rate increased, Guillain-Barré syndrome, herpes zoster, hypoesthesia, keratitis, liver enzyme elevation, migraine, multiple sclerosis, optic neuritis, palpitation, paresis, paresthesia, purpura, seizure, serum-sickness like syndrome (may be delayed days to weeks), Stevens-Johnson syndrome, syncope, tachycardia, thrombocytopenia, transverse myelitis, visual disturbances, vertigo

Drug Interactions

DTaP: Vaccines may be administered together (using separate sites and syringes).

Haemophilus b conjugate vaccine (PedvaxHIB®): Vaccines may be administered together (using separate sites and syringes).

Immunosuppressant medications: The effect of the vaccine may be decreased; consider deferring vaccination for 3 months after immunosuppressant therapy is discontinued.

MMR: Vaccines may be administered together (using separate sites and syringes).

OPV: Vaccines may be administered together.

Dosage Forms Injection, suspension [recombinant DNA]:

Engerix-B®:

Adult: Hepatitis B surface antigen 20 mcg/mL (1 mL) [contains trace amounts of thimerosal]

Pediatric/adolescent: Hepatitis B surface antigen 10 mcg/0.5 mL (0.5 mL) [contains trace amounts of thimerosal]

Recombivax HB®:

Adult [preservative free]: Hepatitis B surface antigen 10 mcg/mL (1 mL, 3 mL)

Dialysis [preservative free]: Hepatitis B surface antigen 40 mcg/mL (1 mL)

Pediatric/adolescent [preservative free]: Hepatitis B surface antigen 5 mcg/0.5 mL (0.5 mL)

- **HepFlush®-10** *see* Heparin *on page 609*
- **Hep-Lock®** *see* Heparin *on page 609*
- **Hepsera™** *see* Adefovir *on page 43*
- **Heptovir® (Can)** *see* Lamivudine *on page 725*
- **HES** *see* Hetastarch *on page 623*
- **Hespan®** *see* Hetastarch *on page 623*

Hetastarch (HET a starch)

Medication Safety Issues

Sound-alike/look-alike issues:

Hespan® may be confused with heparin

U.S. Brand Names Hespan®; Hextend®

Canadian Brand Names Hextend®; Voluven®

Synonyms HES; Hydroxyethyl Starch

Pharmacologic Category Plasma Volume Expander, Colloid

Generic Available Yes: Sodium chloride infusion

Use Blood volume expander used in treatment of hypovolemia

Hespan®: Adjunct in leukapheresis to improve harvesting and increasing the yield of granulocytes by centrifugal means

Unlabeled/Investigational Use Hextend®: Priming fluid in pump oxygenators during cardiopulmonary bypass, and as a plasma volume expander during cardiopulmonary bypass

Mechanism of Action Produces plasma volume expansion by virtue of its highly colloidal starch structure, similar to albumin

Pharmacodynamics/Kinetics

Onset of action: Volume expansion: I.V.: ~30 minutes

Duration: 24-36 hours

Metabolism: Molecules >50,000 daltons require enzymatic degradation by the reticuloendothelial system or amylases in the blood

Excretion: Urine (~40%) within 24 hours; smaller molecular weight molecules readily excreted

Dosage I.V. infusion (requires an infusion pump):

Children: Safety and efficacy have not been established

Plasma volume expansion:

Adults: 500-1000 mL (up to 1500 mL/day) or 20 mL/kg/day (up to 1500 mL/day); larger volumes (15,000 mL/24 hours) have been used safely in small numbers of patients

Leukapheresis: 250-700 mL; **Note:** Citrate anticoagulant is added before use.

Dosing adjustment in renal impairment: Cl_{cr} <10 mL/minute: Initial dose is the same but subsequent doses should be reduced by 20% to 50% of normal

Stability Store at room temperature; do not freeze. Do not use if crystalline precipitate forms or is turbid deep brown. In leukapheresis, admixtures of 500-560 mL of Hespan® with citrate concentrations up to 2.5% are compatible for 24 hours.

Administration Administer I.V. only; infusion pump is required. May administer up to 1.2 g/kg/hour (20 mL/kg/hour). Change I.V. tubing or flush copiously with normal saline before administering blood through the same line. Change I.V. tubing at least every 24 hours. Do not administer Hextend® with blood through the same administration set. Anaphylactoid reactions can occur, have epinephrine and resuscitative equipment available.

Leukapheresis: Mix Hespan® and citrate well. Administer to the input line of the centrifuge apparatus at a ration of 1:8 to 1:13 to venous whole blood.

(Continued)

Hetastarch *(Continued)*

Monitoring Parameters Volume expansion: Blood pressure, heart rate, capillary refill time, CVP, RAP, MAP, urine output; if pulmonary artery catheter in place, monitor PCWP, SVR, and PVR; hemoglobin, hematocrit, cardiac index

Leukapheresis: CBC, total leukocyte and platelet counts, leukocyte differential count, hemoglobin, hematocrit, PT, PTT

Anesthesia and Critical Care Concerns/Other Considerations Hetastarch is a synthetic polymer derived from a waxy starch composed of amylopectin.

Hespan®: 6% hetastarch in 0.9% sodium chloride
- Molecular weight: 450,000
- Sodium: 154 mEq/L
- Chloride: 154 mEq/L

Hextend®: 6% hetastarch in lactated electrolyte injection
- Molecular weight: 670,000
- Sodium: 143 mEq/L
- Chloride: 124 mEq/L
- Calcium: 5 mEq/L
- Potassium: 3 mEq/L
- Magnesium: 0.9 mEq/L
- Lactate: 28 mEq/L
- Dextrose: 0.99 g/L

Both Hextend® and Hespan® will expand the intravascular volume the same as an equal volume of 5% albumin. Hetastarch will increase the intravascular volume up to 24-36 hours. Hetastarch does not have oxygen-carrying capacity and is not a substitute for blood or plasma. Large volumes of Hespan® or Hextend® may interfere with platelet function, prolong PT and PTT times and cause hemodilution, however, clinically Hextend® has not been associated with coagulation abnormalities in doses >20 mL/kg up to a total of 5000 mL.

Hextend®: Formulated with near physiologic levels of sodium, chloride, calcium, potassium, magnesium; may be associated with less electrolyte abnormalities than Hespan®; not to be used for the treatment of lactic acidosis; should not be administered through the same line as blood products; use with caution in patients with congestive heart failure.

Hespan®: Intraoperative use in patients undergoing cardiac surgery with cardiopulmonary bypass may increase bleeding; each 500 mL provides 77 mEq sodium chloride and may cause hyperchloremic metabolic acidosis in large volumes; critically-ill patients receiving hetastarch infusions (goal: PCWP 12-18 mm Hg) had an increase in cardiac index, oxygen delivery and consumption.

Hextend® and Hespan®: May increase serum amylase temporarily without an association with pancreatitis; not eliminated by hemodialysis.

Pregnancy Risk Factor C

Contraindications Hypersensitivity to hydroxyethyl starch or any component of the formulation; severe bleeding disorders, renal failure with oliguria or anuria, or severe congestive heart failure; per the manufacturer, Hextend® is also contraindicated in the treatment of lactic acidosis and in leukapheresis

Warnings/Precautions Anaphylactoid reactions have occurred; use caution in patients allergic to corn (may have cross allergy to hetastarch); use with caution in patients with thrombocytopenia (may interfere with platelet function); large volume may cause drops in hemoglobin concentrations; use with caution in patients at risk from overexpansion of blood volume, including the very young or aged patients, those with CHF or pulmonary edema; volumes >1500 mL may interfere with platelet function and prolong PT and PTT times; use with caution in patients with history of liver disease; note electrolyte content of Hextend® including calcium, lactate, and potassium; use caution in situations where electrolyte and/or acid-base disturbances may be exacerbated (renal impairment, respiratory alkalosis). Safety and efficacy in pediatric patients have not been established, but limited data available.

Adverse Reactions Frequency not defined.

Cardiovascular: Circulatory overload, heart failure, peripheral edema

Central nervous system: Chills, fever, headache, intracranial bleeding

Dermatologic: Itching, pruritus, rash

Endocrine & metabolic: Amylase levels increased, parotid gland enlargement, indirect bilirubin increased, metabolic acidosis

Gastrointestinal: Vomiting

Hematologic: Bleeding, factor VIII:C plasma levels decreased, decreased plasma aggregation decreased, von Willebrand factor decreased, dilutional coagulopathy; prolongation of PT, PTT, clotting time, and bleeding time; thrombocytopenia, anemia, disseminated intravascular coagulopathy (rare), hemolysis (rare)

Neuromuscular & skeletal: Myalgia

Miscellaneous: Anaphylactoid reactions, hypersensitivity, flu-like symptoms (mild)

Overdosage/Toxicology Symptoms of overdose include heart failure, nausea, vomiting, circulatory overload, and bleeding. Treatment is supportive. Hetastarch is not eliminated by hemodialysis.

Dosage Forms

Infusion [premixed in lactated electrolyte injection] (Hextend®): 6% (500 mL)

Infusion, solution [premixed in NaCl 0.9%] (Hespan®): 6% (500 mL)

References

Abbott Laboratories, Hextend® Product Labeling, Revised January, 1999.

Bick RL, "Evaluation of a New Hydroxyethyl Starch Preparation (Hextend®) on Selected Coagulation Parameters," *Clin Appl Thrombosis/Hemostasis*, 1995, 1(3):215-29.

Boldt J, Heesen M, Müller M, et al, "The Effects of Albumin Versus Hydroxyethyl Starch Solution on Cardiorespiratory and Circulatory Variables in Critically Ill Patients," *Anesth Analg*, 1996, 83(2):254-61.

Brutocao D, Bratton SL, Thomas JR, et al, "Comparison of Hetastarch With Albumin for Postoperative Volume Expansion in Children After Cardiopulmonary Bypass," *J Cardiothoracic Vasc Anesth*, 1996, 10(3):348-51.

Gan TJ, Bennett-Guerrero E, Phillips-Bute B, et al "Hextend®, a Physiologically Balanced Plasma Expander for Large Volume Use in Major Surgery: A Randomized Phase III Clinical Trial," *Anesth Analg*, 1999, 88(5):992-8.

Gan TJ, Wright D, Robertson C, et al, "Randomized Comparison of the Coagulation Profile When Hextend® or 5% Albumin is Used for Intraoperative Fluid Resuscitation," *Anesthesiology*, 2001, 95:A193.

Knutson JE, Deering JA, Hall FW, et al, "Does Intraoperative Hetastarch Administration Increase Blood Loss and Transfusion Requirements After Cardiac Surgery?" *Anesth Analg*, 2000, 90(4):801-7.

Wilkes NJ, Woolf RL, Powanda MC, et al, "Hydroxyethyl Starch in Balanced Electrolyte Solution (Hextend®) - Pharmacokinetic and Pharmacodynamic Profiles in Healthy Volunteers," *Anesth Analg*, 2002, 94(3):538-44.

♦ **Hextend®** *see* Hetastarch *on page 623*

♦ **hGH** *see* Human Growth Hormone *on page 625*

♦ **Hibiclens® [OTC]** *see* Chlorhexidine Gluconate *on page 267*

♦ **Hibidil® 1:2000 (Can)** *see* Chlorhexidine Gluconate *on page 267*

♦ **Hibistat® [OTC]** *see* Chlorhexidine Gluconate *on page 267*

♦ **Hirulog** *see* Bivalirudin *on page 178*

♦ **HMR 3647** *see* Telithromycin *on page 1235*

♦ **Humalog®** *see* Insulin Lispro *on page 688*

♦ **Humalog® Mix 25 (Can)** *see* Insulin Lispro Protamine and Insulin Lispro *on page 689*

♦ **Humalog® Mix 50/50™** *see* Insulin Lispro Protamine and Insulin Lispro *on page 689*

♦ **Humalog® Mix 75/25™** *see* Insulin Lispro Protamine and Insulin Lispro *on page 689*

♦ **Human Diploid Cell Cultures Rabies Vaccine** *see* Rabies Virus Vaccine *on page 1101*

Human Growth Hormone (HYU man grothe HOR mone)

Medication Safety Issues

Sound-alike/look-alike issues:

Somatrem may be confused with somatropin

Somatropin may be confused with somatrem, sumatriptan

U.S. Brand Names Genotropin®; Genotropin Miniquick®; Humatrope®; Norditropin®; Norditropin® NordiFlex®; Nutropin®; Nutropin AQ®; Omnitrope™; Saizen®; Serostim®; Tev-Tropin™; Zorbtive™

Canadian Brand Names Humatrope®; Nutropin® AQ; Nutropine®; Saizen®; Serostim®

Synonyms hGH; Human Growth Hormone; Somatrem

Pharmacologic Category Growth Hormone

Generic Available No

(Continued)

Human Growth Hormone *(Continued)*

Use

Children:

Long-term treatment of growth failure due to inadequate endogenous growth hormone secretion (Genotropin®, Humatrope®, Norditropin®, Nutropin®, Nutropin AQ®, Omnitrope™, Saizen®, Tev-Tropin™)

Long-term treatment of short stature associated with Turner syndrome (Genotropin®, Humatrope®, Nutropin®, Nutropin AQ®)

Treatment of Prader-Willi syndrome (Genotropin®)

Treatment of growth failure associated with chronic renal insufficiency (CRI) up until the time of renal transplantation (Nutropin®, Nutropin AQ®)

Long-term treatment of growth failure in children born small for gestational age who fail to manifest catch-up growth by 2 years of age (Genotropin®)

Long-term treatment of idiopathic short stature (nongrowth hormone-deficient short stature) defined by height standard deviation score (SDS) less than or equal to -2.25 and growth rate not likely to attain normal adult height (Humatrope®, Nutropin®, Nutropin AQ®)

Adults:

AIDS-wasting or cachexia with concomitant antiviral therapy (Serostim®)

Replacement of endogenous growth hormone in patients with adult growth hormone deficiency who meet both of the following criteria (Genotropin®, Humatrope®, Norditropin®, Nutropin®, Nutropin AQ®, Omnitrope™, Saizen®):

Biochemical diagnosis of adult growth hormone deficiency by means of a subnormal response to a standard growth hormone stimulation test (peak growth hormone ≤5 mcg/L)

and

Adult-onset: Patients who have adult growth hormone deficiency whether alone or with multiple hormone deficiencies (hypopituitarism) as a result of pituitary disease, hypothalamic disease, surgery, radiation therapy, or trauma

or

Childhood-onset: Patients who were growth hormone deficient during childhood, confirmed as an adult before replacement therapy is initiated

Treatment of short-bowel syndrome (Zorbtive™)

Unlabeled/Investigational Use Investigational: Congestive heart failure; AIDS-wasting/cachexia in children (Serostim®)

Mechanism of Action Somatropin is a purified polypeptide hormones of recombinant DNA origin; somatropin contains the identical sequence of amino acids found in human growth hormone; human growth hormone stimulates growth of linear bone, skeletal muscle, and organs; stimulates erythropoietin which increases red blood cell mass; exerts both insulin-like and diabetogenic effects; enhances the transmucosal transport of water, electrolytes, and nutrients across the gut

Pharmacodynamics/Kinetics

Duration: Maintains supraphysiologic levels for 18-20 hours

Absorption: I.M., SubQ: Well absorbed

Metabolism: Hepatic and renal (~90%)

Half-life elimination: Preparation and route of administration dependent

Excretion: Urine

Dosage

Children (individualize dose):

Growth hormone deficiency:

Genotropin®, Omnitrope™: SubQ: Weekly dosage: 0.16-0.24 mg/kg divided into 6-7 doses

Humatrope®: I.M., SubQ: Weekly dosage: 0.18 mg/kg; maximum replacement dose: 0.3 mg/kg/week; dosing should be divided into equal doses given 3 times/week on alternating days, 6 times/week, or daily

Norditropin®: SubQ: 0.024-0.034 mg/kg/day, 6-7 times/week

Nutropin®, Nutropin® AQ: SubQ: Weekly dosage: 0.3 mg/kg divided into daily doses; pubertal patients: ≤0.7 mg/kg/week divided daily

Tev-Tropin™: SubQ: Up to 0.1 mg/kg administered 3 times/week

Saizen®: I.M., SubQ: 0.06 mg/kg/dose administered 3 times/week

Note: Therapy should be discontinued when patient has reached satisfactory adult height, when epiphyses have fused, or when the patient ceases to respond. Growth of 5 cm/year or more is expected, if growth rate does not exceed 2.5 cm in a 6-month period, double the dose for the next 6 months; if there is still no satisfactory response, discontinue therapy

Chronic renal insufficiency (CRI): Nutropin®, Nutropin® AQ: SubQ: Weekly dosage: 0.35 mg/kg divided into daily injections; continue until the time of renal transplantation

Dosage recommendations in patients treated for CRI who require dialysis:

Hemodialysis: Administer dose at night prior to bedtime or at least 3-4 hours after hemodialysis to prevent hematoma formation from heparin

CCPD: Administer dose in the morning following dialysis

CAPD: Administer dose in the evening at the time of overnight exchange

Turner syndrome:

Genotropin®: SubQ: Weekly dosage: 0.33 mg/kg divided into 6-7 doses

Humatrope®, Nutropin®, Nutropin® AQ: SubQ: Weekly dosage: ≤0.375 mg/kg divided into equal doses 3-7 times per week

Prader-Willi syndrome: Genotropin®: SubQ: Weekly dosage: 0.24 mg/kg divided into 6-7 doses

Small for gestational age: Genotropin®: SubQ: Weekly dosage: 0.48 mg/kg divided into 6-7 doses

Idiopathic short stature:

Humatrope®: SubQ: Weekly dosage: 0.37 mg/kg divided into equal doses 6-7 times per week

Nutropin®, Nutropin AQ®: SubQ: Weekly dosage: Up to 0.3 mg/kg divided into daily doses

AIDS-wasting or cachexia (unlabeled use): Serostim®: SubQ: Limited data; doses of 0.04 mg/kg/day were reported in five children, 6-17 years of age; doses of 0.07 mg/kg/day were reported in six children, 8-14 years of age

Adults:

Growth hormone deficiency: To minimize adverse events in older or overweight patients, reduced dosages may be necessary. During therapy, dosage should be decreased if required by the occurrence of side effects or excessive IGF-I levels.

Norditropin®: SubQ: Initial dose ≤0.004 mg/kg/day; after 6 weeks of therapy, may increase dose to 0.016 mg/kg/day

Nutropin®, Nutropin® AQ: SubQ: ≤0.006 mg/kg/day; dose may be increased according to individual requirements, up to a maximum of 0.025 mg/kg/day in patients <35 years of age, or up to a maximum of 0.0125 mg/kg/day in patients ≥35 years of age

Humatrope®: SubQ: ≤0.006 mg/kg/day; dose may be increased according to individual requirements, up to a maximum of 0.0125 mg/kg/day

Genotropin®, Omnitrope™: SubQ: Weekly dosage: ≤0.04 mg/kg divided into 6-7 doses; dose may be increased at 4- to 8-week intervals according to individual requirements, to a maximum of 0.08 mg/kg/week

Saizen®: SubQ: ≤0.005 mg/kg/day; dose may be increased to not more than 0.01 mg/kg/day after 4 weeks, based on individual requirements.

AIDS-wasting or cachexia:

Serostim®: SubQ: Dose should be given once daily at bedtime; patients who continue to lose weight after 2 weeks should be re-evaluated for opportunistic infections or other clinical events; rotate injection sites to avoid lipodystrophy

Daily dose based on body weight:

<35 kg: 0.1 mg/kg

35-45 kg: 4 mg

45-55 kg: 5 mg

>55 kg: 6 mg

Short-bowel syndrome (Zorbtive™): SubQ: 0.1 mg/kg once daily for 4 weeks (maximum: 8 mg/day)

Fluid retention (moderate) or arthralgias: Treat symptomatically or reduce dose by 50%

Severe toxicity: Discontinue therapy for up to 5 days; when symptoms resolve, restart at 50% of dose. If severe toxicity recurs or does not disappear within 5 days after discontinuation, permanently discontinue treatment.

Elderly: Patients ≥65 years of age may be more sensitive to the action of growth hormone and more prone to adverse effects; in general, dosing should be cautious, beginning at low end of dosing range

(Continued)

Human Growth Hormone *(Continued)*

Dosage adjustment in renal impairment Reports indicate patients with chronic renal failure tend to have decreased clearance; specific dosing suggestions not available

Dosage adjustment in hepatic impairment: Clearance may be reduced in patients with severe hepatic dysfunction; specific dosing suggestions not available

Stability

Genotropin®: Store at 2°C to 8°C (36°F to 46°F); do not freeze, protect from light. Following reconstitution of 5.8 mg and 13.8 mg cartridge, store under refrigeration and use within 21 days.

Miniquick®: Store in refrigerator prior to dispensing, but may be stored ≤25°C (77°F) for up to 3 months after dispensing; once reconstituted, solution must be refrigerated and used within 24 hours; discard unused portion

Omnitrope™: Prior to reconstitution, store under refrigeration at 2°C to 8°C (36°F to 46°F); do not freeze, protect from light. Reconstitute with provided diluent. Swirl gently, do not shake. Following reconstitution with the provided diluents, the 1.5 mg vial may be stored under refrigeration for up to 24 hours and the 5.8 mg vial may be stored under refrigeration for up to 3 weeks. Store vial in carton to protect from light.

Humatrope®:

Vial: Before and after reconstitution, store at 2°C to 8°C (36°F to 46°F), avoid freezing; when reconstituted with bacteriostatic water for injection, use within 14 days; when reconstituted with sterile water for injection, use within 24 hours and discard unused portion

Cartridge: Before and after reconstitution, store at 2°C to 8°C (36°F to 46°F), avoid freezing; following reconstitution, stable for 14 days under refrigeration. Dilute with solution provided with cartridges **ONLY**; do not use diluent provided with vials

Norditropin®: Store at 2°C to 8°C (36°F to 46°F), do not freeze; avoid direct light

Cartridge: Must be used within 4 weeks once inserted into pen

Prefilled pen: Must be used within 4 weeks after initial injection

Nutropin®: Before and after reconstitution, store at 2°C to 8°C (36°F to 46°F), avoid freezing

Vial: Reconstitute with bacteriostatic water for injection; use reconstituted vials within 14 days; when reconstituted with sterile water for injection, use immediately and discard unused portion

AQ formulation: Use within 28 days following initial use

Saizen®: Prior to reconstitution, store at room temperature 15°C to 30°C (59°F to 86°F). Following reconstitution with bacteriostatic water for injection, reconstituted solution should be refrigerated and used within 14 days; when reconstituted with sterile water for injection, use immediately and discard unused portion.

5 mg vial: Reconstitute with 1-3 mL bacteriostatic water for injection or sterile water for injection; gently swirl; do not shake.

8.8 mg vial: Reconstitute with 2-3 mL bacteriostatic water for injection or sterile water for injection; gently swirl; do not shake.

Serostim®: Prior to reconstitution, store at room temperature 15°C to 30°C (59°F to 86°F); reconstitute with sterile water for injection; store reconstituted solution under refrigeration and use within 24 hours, avoid freezing. Do not use if cloudy

Tev-Tropin™: Prior to reconstitution, store at 2°C to 8°C (36°F to 46°F). Reconstitute with 1-5 mL of diluent provided. Gently swirl; do not shake. May use preservative free NS for use in newborns. Following reconstitution with bacteriostatic NS, solution should be refrigerated and used within 14 days. Some cloudiness may occur; do not use if cloudiness persists after warming to room temperature.

Zorbtive™: Store unopened vials and diluent at room temperature of 15°C to 30°C (59°F to 86°F).

8.8 mg vial: Reconstitute with 1-2 mL bacteriostatic water for injection, use within 14 days; store under refrigeration at 2°C to 8°C (36°F to 46°F); avoid freezing

Administration Do not shake; administer SubQ or I.M. (rotate administration sites to avoid tissue atrophy); refer to product labeling; when administering to newborns, reconstitute with sterile water for injection. **Note:** Not all products are approved for I.M. administration.

Norditropin® cartridge must be administered using the corresponding color-coded NordiPen® injection pen.

Monitoring Parameters Growth curve, periodic thyroid function tests, bone age (annually), periodical urine testing for glucose, somatomedin C (IGF-I) levels; funduscopic examinations at initiation of therapy and periodically during treatment; serum phosphorus, alkaline phosphatase and parathyroid hormone. If growth deceleration is observed in children treated for growth hormone deficiency, and not due to other causes, evaluate for presence of antibody formation. Strict blood glucose monitoring in diabetic patients.

Prader-Willi syndrome: Monitor for sleep apnea, respiratory infections, snoring (onset of or increased)

Pregnancy Risk Factor B/C (depending upon manufacturer)

Contraindications Hypersensitivity to growth hormone or any component of the formulation; growth promotion in pediatric patients with closed epiphyses; progression of any underlying intracranial lesion or actively growing intracranial tumor; acute critical illness due to complications following open heart or abdominal surgery; multiple accidental trauma or acute respiratory failure; evidence of active malignancy; use in patients with Prader-Willi syndrome **without** growth hormone deficiency (except Genotropin®) or in patients with Prader-Willi syndrome **with** growth hormone deficiency who are severely obese or have severe respiratory impairment. Saizen® and Norditropin® are contraindicated with proliferative or preproliferative retinopathy.

Warnings/Precautions Use with caution in patients with diabetes or with risk factors for glucose intolerance. Intracranial hypertension has been reported with growth hormone product, funduscopic examinations are recommended. Progression of scoliosis may occur in children experiencing rapid growth. Patients with growth hormone deficiency may develop slipped capital epiphyses more frequently, evaluate any child with new onset of a limp or with complaints of hip or knee pain. Patients with Turner syndrome are at increased risk for otitis media and other ear/hearing disorders, cardiovascular disorders (including stroke, aortic aneurysm, hypertension), and thyroid disease, monitor carefully. Concurrent glucocorticoid therapy may inhibit growth promotion effects; may require dosage adjustment or replacement glucocorticoid therapy in patients with ACTH deficiency. Products may contain benzyl alcohol. When administering to newborns, reconstitute with sterile water or saline for injection. Not for I.V. injection.

Fatalities have been reported in pediatric patients with Prader-Willi syndrome following the use of growth hormone. The reported fatalities occurred in patients with one or more risk factors, including severe obesity, sleep apnea, respiratory impairment, or unidentified respiratory infection; male patients with one or more of these factors may be at greater risk. Treatment interruption is recommended in patients who show signs of upper airway obstruction, including the onset of, or increased, snoring. In addition, evaluation of and/or monitoring for sleep apnea and respiratory infections are recommended.

Adverse Reactions

Growth hormone deficiency: Antigrowth hormone antibodies, carpal tunnel syndrome (rare), eosinophilia, fluid balance disturbances, glucosuria, gynecomastia (rare), Hb A_{1c} elevated, headache, hematoma, hematuria, hyperglycemia (mild), hypertriglyceridemia, hypoglycemia, hypothyroidism, leg pain, leukemia, lipoatrophy, muscle pain, increased growth of pre-existing nevi (rare), pain/ local reactions at the injection site, pancreatitis (rare), peripheral edema, exacerbation of psoriasis, rash, seizure, weakness

Idiopathic short stature: (From ISS NCGS Cohort; all frequencies <1%): Arthralgia, avascular necrosis, bone growth (abnormal), carpal tunnel syndrome, diabetes mellitus, edema, fracture, gynecomastia, injection site reaction, intracranial hypertension, neoplasm (new onset or recurring), scoliosis (new onset or progression), slipped capital femoral epiphysis, tumor (new onset or recurring). Additional adverse effects noted in product literature (Humatrope®; frequency not established in large cohort): Hip pain, hyperlipidemia, hypertension, hypothyroidism, myalgia, otitis media.

Prader-Willi syndrome: Genotropin®: Aggressiveness, arthralgia, edema, hair loss, headache, benign intracranial hypertension, myalgia; fatalities associated with use in this population have been reported

Turner syndrome: Ear disorders, hypothyroidism, increased nevi, joint pain, otitis media, peripheral edema, surgical procedures

Adult growth hormone replacement: Increased ALT, increased AST, arthralgia, back pain, carpal tunnel syndrome, diabetes mellitus, fatigue, flu-like syndrome,

(Continued)

Human Growth Hormone *(Continued)*

gastritis, gastroenteritis, generalized edema, glucose intolerance, gynecomastia (rare), headache, hypertension, hypoesthesia, hypothyroidism, infection (nonviral), insomnia, joint disorder, laryngitis, myalgia, nausea, increased growth of pre-existing nevi, pain, pancreatitis (rare), paresthesia, peripheral edema, pharyngitis, rhinitis, stiffness in extremities, weakness

AIDS wasting or cachexia (limited): Serostim®: Musculoskeletal discomfort (54%), increased tissue turgor (27%), diarrhea (26%), neuropathy (26%), nausea (26%), fatigue (17%), albuminuria (15%), increased diaphoresis (14%), anorexia (12%), anemia (12%), increased AST (12%), insomnia (11%), tachycardia (11%), hyperglycemia (10%), increased ALT (10%)

Postmarketing and/or case reports: Diabetes, diabetic ketoacidosis, glucose intolerance

Short-bowel syndrome: Zorbtive™: Peripheral edema (69% to 81%), edema (facial: 44% to 50%; peripheral 13%), arthralgia (13% to 44%), injection site reaction (19% to 31%), flatulence (25%), abdominal pain (20% to 25%), vomiting (19%), malaise (13%), nausea (13%), diaphoresis increased (13%), rhinitis (7%), dizziness (6%)

Postmarketing and/or case reports: Carpal tunnel syndrome

Small for gestational age: Genotropin®: Mild, transient hyperglycemia; benign intracranial hypertension (rare); central precocious puberty; jaw prominence (rare); aggravation of pre-existing scoliosis (rare); injection site reactions; progression of pigmented nevi

Overdosage/Toxicology Symptoms of acute overdose may include initial hypoglycemia (with subsequent hyperglycemia), fluid retention, headache, nausea, and vomiting. Long-term overdose may result in signs and symptoms of acromegaly.

Drug Interactions

Glucocorticoids: May inhibit growth-promoting effects.

Insulin: Growth hormone may induce insulin resistance in patients with diabetes mellitus; monitor glucose and adjust insulin dose as necessary

Dietary Considerations

Prader-Willi syndrome: All patients should have effective weight control (use is contraindicated in severely-obese patients).

Short-bowel syndrome: Intravenous parenteral nutrition requirements may need reassessment as gastrointestinal absorption improves.

Dosage Forms

Injection, powder for reconstitution [rDNA origin]:

- Genotropin®: 5.8 mg [15 units/mL; delivers 5 mg/mL]; 13.8 mg [36 int units/mL; delivers 12 mg/mL]
- Genotropin Miniquick® [preservative free]: 0.2 mg, 0.4 mg, 0.6 mg, 0.8 mg, 1 mg, 1.2 mg, 1.4 mg, 1.6 mg, 1.8 mg, 2 mg [each strength delivers 0.25 mL]
- Humatrope®: 5 mg [~15 int. units], 6 mg [18 int. units], 12 mg [36 int. units], 24 mg [72 int. units]
- Nutropin®: 5 mg [~15 int. units; packaged with diluent containing benzyl alcohol]; 10 mg [~30 int. units; packaged with diluent containing benzyl alcohol]
- Omnitrope™: 1.5 mg [~4.5 int. units; packaged with preservative free diluent]; 5.8 mg [~17.4 int. units; packaged with diluent containing benzyl alcohol]
- Tev-Tropin™: 5 mg [15 int. units/mL; packaged with diluent containing benzyl alcohol]
- Saizen®: 5 mg [~15 int. units; contains sucrose 34.2 mg; packaged with diluent containing benzyl alcohol]; 8.8 mg [~26.4 int. units; contains sucrose 60.2 mg; packaged with diluent containing benzyl alcohol]
- Serostim®: 4 mg [12 int. units; contains sucrose 27.3 mg]; 5 mg [15 int. units; contains sucrose 34.2 mg]; 6 mg [18 int. units; contains sucrose 41 mg]
- Zorbtive™: 8.8 mg [~26.4 int. units; contains sucrose 60.19 mg; packaged with diluent containing benzyl alcohol]

Injection, solution [rDNA origin]:

- Norditropin®: 5 mg/1.5 mL (1.5 mL); 15 mg/1.5 mL (1.5 mL) [cartridge]
- Norditropin® NordiFlex®: 5 mg/1.5 mL (1.5 mL); 15 mg/1.5 mL (1.5 mL) [prefilled pen]
- Nutropin AQ®: 5 mg/mL (2 mL) [~15 int. units/mL; vial or cartridge]

- ♦ **Humatrope®** *see* Human Growth Hormone *on page 625*
- ♦ **Humulin® 20/80 (Can)** *see* Insulin NPH and Insulin Regular *on page 691*
- ♦ **Humulin® 50/50** *see* Insulin NPH and Insulin Regular *on page 691*

- ♦ **Humulin® 70/30** *see* Insulin NPH and Insulin Regular *on page 691*
- ♦ **Humulin® N** *see* Insulin NPH *on page 690*
- ♦ **Humulin® R** *see* Insulin Regular *on page 693*
- ♦ **Humulin® R (Concentrated) U-500** *see* Insulin Regular *on page 693*

Hyaluronidase (hye al yoor ON i dase)

Medication Safety Issues

Sound-alike/look-alike issues:

Wydase may be confused with Lidex®, Wyamine®

U.S. Brand Names Amphadase™; Hydase™; Hylenex™; Vitrase®

Pharmacologic Category Enzyme

Generic Available No

Use Increase the dispersion and absorption of other drugs; increase rate of absorption of parenteral fluids given by hypodermoclysis; adjunct in subcutaneous urography for improving resorption of radiopaque agents

Unlabeled/Investigational Use Management of drug extravasations

Mechanism of Action Modifies the permeability of connective tissue through hydrolysis of hyaluronic acid, one of the chief components of tissue cement which offers resistance to diffusion of liquids through tissues; hyaluronidase increases both the distribution and absorption of locally injected substances.

Pharmacodynamics/Kinetics

Onset of action: SubQ: Immediate

Duration: 24-48 hours

Dosage Note: A preliminary skin test for hypersensitivity can be performed. ACTH, antihistamines, corticosteroids, estrogens, and salicylates, when used in large doses, may cause tissues to be partly resistant to hyaluronidase. May require larger doses of hyaluronidase for the same effect.

Skin test: Intradermal: 0.02 mL (3 units) of a 150 units/mL solution. Positive reaction consists of a wheal with pseudopods appearing within 5 minutes and persisting for 20-30 minutes with localized itching.

Hypodermoclysis: SubQ: 15 units is added to each 100 mL of I.V. fluid to be administered; 150 units facilitates absorption of >1000 mL of solution

Premature Infants and Neonates: Volume of a single clysis should not exceed 25 mL/kg and the rate of administration should not exceed 2 mL/minute

Children <3 years: Volume of a single clysis should not exceed 200 mL

Children ≥3 years and Adults: Rate and volume of a single clysis should not exceed those used for infusion of I.V. fluids

Urography: Children and Adults: SubQ: 75 units over each scapula followed by injection of contrast medium at the same site; patient should be in the prone position.

Extravasation (unlabeled use): Adults: SubQ: Inject 1 mL of a 150 unit/mL solution (as 5-10 injections of 0.1-0.2 mL) into affected area; doses of 15-250 units have been reported. **Note:** Do not use for extravasation of pressor agents (eg, dopamine, norepinephrine).

Elderly: See Adults dosing. Adjust dose carefully to individual patient.

Stability

Amphadase™, Hydase™, Hylenex™: Store in refrigerator at 2°C to 8°C (35°F to 46°F); do not freeze

Vitrase®: Store unopened vial in refrigerator at 2°C to 8°C (35°F to 46°F). Add 6.2 mL of NaCl to vial (1000 units/mL); further dilute with NaCl before administration. After reconstitution, store at 20°C to 25°C (68°F to 77°F) and use within 6 hours.

For 50 units/mL, draw up 0.05 mL of hyaluronidase reconstituted solution (1000 units/mL) and add 0.95 mL of NaCl.

For 75 units/mL, draw up 0.075 mL of hyaluronidase reconstituted solution and add 0.925 mL of NaCl.

For 150 units/mL, draw up 0.15 mL of hyaluronidase reconstituted solution and add 0.85 mL of NaCl.

For 300 units/mL, draw up 0.3 mL of hyaluronidase reconstituted solution and add 0.7 mL of NaCl.

Administration Do **not** administer I.V.

Pregnancy Risk Factor C

Contraindications Hypersensitivity to hyaluronidase or any component of the formulation

(Continued)

Hyaluronidase *(Continued)*

Warnings/Precautions Do not inject in or around infected or inflamed areas; may spread localized infection. Should not be used for extravasation management of dopamine or alpha agonists or to reduce swelling of bites or stings. Do not administer intravenously. Do not apply directly to the cornea. Discontinue if sensitization occurs.

Adverse Reactions

Frequency not defined:

Cardiovascular: Edema

Local: Injection site reactions

<1%: Allergic reactions, anaphylactic-like reactions (retrobulbar block or I.V. injections), angioedema, urticaria

Overdosage/Toxicology Symptoms of overdose include local edema, urticaria, erythema, chills, nausea, vomiting, dizziness, tachycardia, and hypotension. Treatment is symptom-directed and supportive.

Drug Interactions

Local anesthetics: Hyaluronidase may increase absorption and toxicity of local anesthetics.

Dosage Forms

Injection, powder for reconstitution:

Vitrase®: 6200 units [ovine derived; contains lactose]

Injection, solution:

Amphadase™: 150 units/mL (2 mL) [bovine derived; contains edetate disodium 1 mg, thimerosal ≤0.1 mg]

Injection, solution [preservative free]:

Hydase™: 150 units/mL (2 mL) [bovine derived; contains edetate disodium 1 mg]

Hylenex™: 150 units/mL (1 mL, 2 mL) [recombinant; contains human albumin and edetate disodium]

Vitrase®: 200 units/mL (2 mL) [ovine derived; contains lactulose]

- **hycet™** *see* Hydrocodone and Acetaminophen *on page 636*
- **Hycort™ (Can)** *see* Hydrocortisone *on page 639*
- **Hydase™** *see* Hyaluronidase *on page 631*
- **Hydeltra T.B.A.® (Can)** *see* PrednisoLONE *on page 1046*
- **Hyderm (Can)** *see* Hydrocortisone *on page 639*

HydrALAZINE (hye DRAL a zeen)

Medication Safety Issues

Sound-alike/look-alike issues:

HydrALAZINE may be confused with hydrOXYzine

Related Information

Chronic Renal Failure *on page 1437*

Heart Failure (Systolic) *on page 1607*

Hypertension *on page 1620*

Postoperative Hypertension *on page 1471*

Canadian Brand Names Apo-Hydralazine®; Apresoline®; Novo-Hylazin; Nu-Hydral

Synonyms Apresoline [DSC]; Hydralazine Hydrochloride

Pharmacologic Category Vasodilator

Generic Available Yes

Use Management of moderate to severe hypertension, congestive heart failure, hypertension secondary to pre-eclampsia/eclampsia; treatment of primary pulmonary hypertension

Mechanism of Action Direct vasodilation of arterioles (with little effect on veins) with decreased systemic resistance

Pharmacodynamics/Kinetics

Onset of action: Oral: 20-30 minutes; I.V.: 5-20 minutes

Duration: Oral: Up to 8 hours; I.V.: 1-4 hours; **Note:** May vary depending on acetylator status of patient

Distribution: Crosses placenta; enters breast milk

Protein binding: 85% to 90%

Metabolism: Hepatically acetylated; extensive first-pass effect (oral)

Bioavailability: 30% to 50%; increased with food

Half-life elimination: Normal renal function: 2-8 hours; End-stage renal disease: 7-16 hours

Excretion: Urine (14% as unchanged drug)

Dosage

Children:

Oral: Initial: 0.75-1 mg/kg/day in 2-4 divided doses; increase over 3-4 weeks to maximum of 7.5 mg/kg/day in 2-4 divided doses; maximum daily dose: 200 mg/day

I.M., I.V.: 0.1-0.2 mg/kg/dose (not to exceed 20 mg) every 4-6 hours as needed, up to 1.7-3.5 mg/kg/day in 4-6 divided doses

Adults:

Oral:

Hypertension:

Initial dose: 10 mg 4 times/day for first 2-4 days; increase to 25 mg 4 times/day for the balance of the first week

Increase by 10-25 mg/dose gradually to 50 mg 4 times/day (maximum: 300 mg/day); usual dose range (JNC 7): 25-100 mg/day in 2 divided doses

Congestive heart failure:

Initial dose: 10-25 mg 3-4 times/day

Adjustment: Dosage must be adjusted based on individual response

Target dose: 225-300 mg/day in divided doses; use in combination with isosorbide dinitrate

I.M., I.V.:

Hypertension: Initial: 10-20 mg/dose every 4-6 hours as needed, may increase to 40 mg/dose; change to oral therapy as soon as possible.

Pre-eclampsia/eclampsia: 5 mg/dose then 5-10 mg every 20-30 minutes as needed.

Elderly: Oral: Initial: 10 mg 2-3 times/day; increase by 10-25 mg/day every 2-5 days.

Dosing interval in renal impairment:

Cl_{cr} 10-50 mL/minute: Administer every 8 hours.

Cl_{cr} <10 mL/minute: Administer every 8-16 hours in fast acetylators and every 12-24 hours in slow acetylators.

Hemodialysis: Supplemental dose is not necessary.

Peritoneal dialysis: Supplemental dose is not necessary.

Stability Intact ampuls/vials of hydralazine should not be stored under refrigeration because of possible precipitation or crystallization. Hydralazine should be diluted in NS for IVPB administration due to decreased stability in D_5W. Stability of IVPB solution in NS is 4 days at room temperature.

Administration Inject over 1 minute. Hypotensive effect may be delayed and unpredictable in some patients.

Monitoring Parameters Blood pressure (monitor closely with I.V. use), standing and sitting/supine, heart rate, ANA titer

Anesthesia and Critical Care Concerns/Other Considerations May be combined with isosorbide dinitrate for the treatment of heart failure. It is considered to be safe for the management of blood pressure during pregnancy.

Pregnancy Risk Factor C

Contraindications Hypersensitivity to hydralazine or any component of the formulation; mitral valve rheumatic heart disease

Warnings/Precautions May cause a drug-induced lupus-like syndrome (more likely on larger doses, longer duration). Adjust dose in severe renal dysfunction. Use with caution in CAD (increase in tachycardia may increase myocardial oxygen demand). Use with caution in pulmonary hypertension (may cause hypotension). Patients may be poorly compliant because of frequent dosing.

Monitor blood pressure closely following I.V. administration. Response may be delayed and unpredictable in some patients. Titrate cautiously to response. Hydralazine-induced fluid and sodium retention may require addition or increased dosage of a diuretics.

Adverse Reactions Frequency not defined.

Cardiovascular: Tachycardia, angina pectoris, orthostatic hypotension (rare), dizziness (rare), paradoxical hypertension, peripheral edema, vascular collapse (rare), flushing

Central nervous system: Increased intracranial pressure (I.V., in patient with pre-existing increased intracranial pressure), fever (rare), chills (rare), anxiety*, disorientation*, depression*, coma*

Dermatologic: Rash (rare), urticaria (rare), pruritus (rare)

(Continued)

HydrALAZINE *(Continued)*

Gastrointestinal: Anorexia, nausea, vomiting, diarrhea, constipation, adynamic ileus

Genitourinary: Difficulty in micturition, impotence

Hematologic: Hemolytic anemia (rare), eosinophilia (rare), decreased hemoglobin concentration (rare), reduced erythrocyte count (rare), leukopenia (rare), agranulocytosis (rare), thrombocytopenia (rare)

Neuromuscular & skeletal: Rheumatoid arthritis, muscle cramps, weakness, tremor, peripheral neuritis (rare)

Ocular: Lacrimation, conjunctivitis

Respiratory: Nasal congestion, dyspnea

Miscellaneous: Drug-induced lupus-like syndrome (dose related; fever, arthralgia, splenomegaly, lymphadenopathy, asthenia, myalgia, malaise, pleuritic chest pain, edema, positive ANA, positive LE cells, maculopapular facial rash, positive direct Coombs' test, pericarditis, pericardial tamponade), diaphoresis

*Seen in uremic patients and severe hypertension where rapidly escalating doses may have caused hypotension leading to these effects.

Overdosage/Toxicology Symptoms of overdose include hypotension, tachycardia, and shock. Treatment is supportive and symptomatic.

Drug Interactions **Inhibits** CYP3A4 (weak)

Beta-blockers (metoprolol, propranolol) serum concentrations and pharmacologic effects may be increased. Monitor cardiovascular status.

Propranolol increases hydralazine's serum concentrations. Acebutolol, atenolol, and nadolol (low hepatic clearance or no first-pass metabolism) are unlikely to be affected.

NSAIDs may decrease the hemodynamic effects of hydralazine; avoid use if possible or closely monitor cardiovascular status.

Ethanol/Nutrition/Herb Interactions

Ethanol: Avoid ethanol (may increase CNS depression).

Food: Food enhances bioavailability of hydralazine.

Herb/Nutraceutical: Avoid dong quai if using for hypertension (has estrogenic activity). Avoid ephedra, yohimbe, ginseng (may worsen hypertension). Avoid garlic (may have increased antihypertensive effect).

Dietary Considerations Administer with meals.

Dosage Forms

Injection, solution, as hydrochloride: 20 mg/mL (1 mL)

Tablet, as hydrochloride: 10 mg, 25 mg, 50 mg, 100 mg

References

Erstad BL and Barletta JF, "Treatment of Hypertension in the Perioperative Patient," *Ann Pharmacother*, 2000, 34(1):66-79.

♦ **Hydralazine Hydrochloride** *see* HydrALAZINE *on page 632*

♦ **Hydramine® [OTC]** *see* DiphenhydrAMINE *on page 399*

♦ **Hydrated Chloral** *see* Chloral Hydrate *on page 261*

♦ **Hydrea®** *see* Hydroxyurea *on page 648*

Hydrochlorothiazide (hye droe klor oh THYE a zide)

Medication Safety Issues

Sound-alike/look-alike issues:

Hydrochlorothiazide may be confused with hydrocortisone, hydroflumethiazide

Esidrix may be confused with Lasix®

HCTZ is an error-prone abbreviation (mistaken as hydrocortisone)

Related Information

Heart Failure (Systolic) *on page 1607*

U.S. Brand Names Microzide™

Canadian Brand Names Apo-Hydro®; Novo-Hydrazide; PMS-Hydrochlorothiazide

Synonyms HCTZ (error-prone abbreviation)

Pharmacologic Category Diuretic, Thiazide

Generic Available Yes

Use Management of mild to moderate hypertension; treatment of edema in congestive heart failure and nephrotic syndrome

Unlabeled/Investigational Use Treatment of lithium-induced diabetes insipidus

Mechanism of Action Inhibits sodium reabsorption in the distal tubules causing increased excretion of sodium and water as well as potassium and hydrogen ions

Pharmacodynamics/Kinetics

Onset of action: Diuresis: ~2 hours

Peak effect: 4-6 hours

Duration: 6-12 hours

Absorption: ~50% to 80%

Distribution: 3.6-7.8 L/kg

Protein binding: 68%

Metabolism: Not metabolized

Bioavailability: 50% to 80%

Half-life elimination: 5.6-14.8 hours

Time to peak: 1-2.5 hours

Excretion: Urine (as unchanged drug)

Dosage Oral (effect of drug may be decreased when used every day):

Children (in pediatric patients, chlorothiazide may be preferred over hydrochlorothiazide as there are more dosage formulations [eg, suspension] available):

<6 months: 2-3 mg/kg/day in 2 divided doses

>6 months: 2 mg/kg/day in 2 divided doses

Adults:

Edema: 25-100 mg/day in 1-2 doses; maximum: 200 mg/day

Hypertension: 12.5-50 mg/day; minimal increase in response and more electrolyte disturbances are seen with doses >50 mg/day

Elderly: 12.5-25 mg once daily

Dosing adjustment/comments in renal impairment: Cl_{cr} <10 mL/minute: Avoid use. Usually ineffective with GFR <30 mL/minute. Effective at lower GFR in combination with a loop diuretic.

Administration May be taken with food or milk. Take early in day to avoid nocturia. Take the last dose of multiple doses no later than 6 PM unless instructed otherwise.

Monitoring Parameters Assess weight, I & O reports daily to determine fluid loss; blood pressure, serum electrolytes, BUN, creatinine

Anesthesia and Critical Care Concerns/Other Considerations If given the morning of surgery it may render the patient volume depleted and blood pressure may be labile during general anesthesia.

Thiazide diuretics are effective first-line therapeutic agents in the management of hypertension and have proven to be of benefit in terms of cardiovascular outcome. They may act synergistically to lower blood pressure when combined with an ACE inhibitor or beta-blocker.

Pregnancy Risk Factor B (manufacturer); D (expert analysis)

Contraindications Hypersensitivity to hydrochlorothiazide or any component of the formulation, thiazides, or sulfonamide-derived drugs; anuria; renal decompensation; pregnancy

Warnings/Precautions Avoid in severe renal disease (ineffective). Electrolyte disturbances (hypokalemia, hypochloremic alkalosis, hyponatremia) can occur. Use with caution in severe hepatic dysfunction; hepatic encephalopathy can be caused by electrolyte disturbances. Gout can be precipitate in certain patients with a history of gout, a familial predisposition to gout, or chronic renal failure. Cautious use in diabetics; may see a change in glucose control. Hypersensitivity reactions can occur. Can cause SLE exacerbation or activation. Use with caution in patients with moderate or high cholesterol concentrations. Photosensitization may occur. Correct hypokalemia before initiating therapy.

Chemical similarities are present among sulfonamides, sulfonylureas, carbonic anhydrase inhibitors, thiazides, and loop diuretics (except ethacrynic acid). Use in patients with sulfonamide allergy is specifically contraindicated in product labeling, however, a risk of cross-reaction exists in patients with allergy to any of these compounds; avoid use when previous reaction has been severe.

Adverse Reactions

1% to 10%:

Cardiovascular: Orthostatic hypotension, hypotension

Dermatologic: Photosensitivity

Endocrine & metabolic: Hypokalemia

Gastrointestinal: Anorexia, epigastric distress

<1% (Limited to important or life-threatening): Agranulocytosis, allergic myocarditis, allergic reactions (possibly with life-threatening anaphylactic shock),

(Continued)

Hydrochlorothiazide *(Continued)*

alopecia, aplastic anemia, eosinophilic pneumonitis, erythema multiforme, exfoliative dermatitis, hemolytic anemia, hepatic function impairment, hypercalcemia, interstitial nephritis, leukopenia, pancreatitis, renal failure, respiratory distress, Stevens-Johnson syndrome, thrombocytopenia, toxic epidermal necrolysis

Overdosage/Toxicology Symptoms of overdose include hypermotility, diuresis, lethargy, confusion, and muscle weakness. Treatment is supportive.

Drug Interactions

ACE inhibitors: Increased hypotension if aggressively diuresed with a thiazide diuretic.

Beta-blockers increase hyperglycemic effects in type 2 diabetes mellitus (noninsulin dependent, NIDDM)

Cholestyramine: Hydrochlorothiazide absorption may be decreased.

Colestipol: Hydrochlorothiazide absorption may be decreased.

Cyclosporine and thiazides can increase the risk of gout or renal toxicity; avoid concurrent use.

Digoxin toxicity can be exacerbated if a thiazide induces hypokalemia or hypomagnesemia.

Lithium toxicity can occur by reducing renal excretion of lithium; monitor lithium concentration and adjust as needed.

Neuromuscular blocking agents can prolong blockade; monitor serum potassium and neuromuscular status.

NSAIDs can decrease the efficacy of thiazides reducing the diuretic and antihypertensive effects.

Ethanol/Nutrition/Herb Interactions

Food: Hydrochlorothiazide peak serum levels may be decreased if taken with food. This product may deplete potassium, sodium, and magnesium.

Herb/Nutraceutical: Avoid dong quai if using for hypertension (has estrogenic activity). Dong quai may also cause photosensitization. Avoid ephedra, ginseng, yohimbe (may worsen hypertension). Avoid garlic (may have increased antihypertensive effect).

Test Interactions Increased creatine phosphokinase [CPK] (S), ammonia (B), amylase (S), calcium (S), chloride (S), cholesterol (S), glucose, increased acid (S), decreased chloride (S), magnesium, potassium (S), sodium (S); Tyramine and phentolamine tests, histamine tests for pheochromocytoma

Dosage Forms

Capsule (Microzide™): 12.5 mg

Tablet: 25 mg, 50 mg

Hydrocodone and Acetaminophen

(hye droe KOE done & a seet a MIN oh fen)

Medication Safety Issues

Sound-alike/look-alike issues:

- Lorcet® may be confused with Fioricet®
- Lortab® may be confused with Cortef®, Lorabid®, Luride®
- Vicodin® may be confused with Hycodan®, Hycomine®, Indocin®, Uridon®
- Zydone® may be confused with Vytone®

Related Information

Acute Postoperative Pain *on page 1388*

Chronic Pain Management *on page 1430*

U.S. Brand Names Anexsia®; Bancap HC®; Ceta-Plus®; Co-Gesic®; hycet™; Lorcet® 10/650; Lorcet®-HD [DSC]; Lorcet® Plus; Lortab®; Margesic® H; Maxidone™; Norco®; Stagesic®; Vicodin®; Vicodin® ES; Vicodin® HP; Zydone®

Synonyms Acetaminophen and Hydrocodone

Pharmacologic Category Analgesic Combination (Narcotic)

Restrictions C-III

Generic Available Yes

Use Relief of moderate to severe pain

Mechanism of Action Hydrocodone, as with other narcotic (opiate) analgesics, blocks pain perception in the cerebral cortex by binding to specific receptor molecules (opiate receptors) within the neuronal membranes of synapses. This binding results in a decreased synaptic chemical transmission throughout the CNS thus inhibiting the flow of pain sensations into the higher centers. Mu and kappa are the two subtypes of the opiate receptor which hydrocodone binds to cause analgesia.

Acetaminophen inhibits the synthesis of prostaglandins in the CNS and peripherally blocks pain impulse generation; produces antipyresis from inhibition of hypothalamic heat-regulating center.

Pharmacodynamics/Kinetics

Acetaminophen: See Acetaminophen monograph.

Hydrocodone:

Onset of action: Narcotic analgesic: 10-20 minutes

Duration: 4-8 hours

Distribution: Crosses placenta

Metabolism: Hepatic; O-demethylation; N-demethylation and 6-ketosteroid reduction

Half-life elimination: 3.3-4.4 hours

Excretion: Urine

Dosage Oral (doses should be titrated to appropriate analgesic effect): Analgesic:

Children 2-13 years or <50 kg: Hydrocodone 0.135 mg/kg/dose every 4-6 hours; do not exceed 6 doses/day or the maximum recommended dose of acetaminophen

Children and Adults ≥50 kg: Average starting dose in opioid naive patients: Hydrocodone 5-10 mg 4 times/day; the dosage of acetaminophen should be limited to ≤4 g/day (and possibly less in patients with hepatic impairment or ethanol use).

Dosage ranges (based on specific product labeling): Hydrocodone 2.5-10 mg every 4-6 hours; maximum: 60 mg hydrocodone/day (maximum dose of hydrocodone may be limited by the acetaminophen content of specific product)

Elderly: Doses should be titrated to appropriate analgesic effect; 2.5-5 mg of the hydrocodone component every 4-6 hours. Do not exceed 4 g/day of acetaminophen.

Dosage adjustment in hepatic impairment: Use with caution. Limited, low-dose therapy usually well tolerated in hepatic disease/cirrhosis; however, cases of hepatotoxicity at daily acetaminophen dosages <4 g/day have been reported. Avoid chronic use in hepatic impairment.

Monitoring Parameters Pain relief, respiratory and mental status, blood pressure

Anesthesia and Critical Care Concerns/Other Considerations Doses of agent must be individualized according to degree of pain; commonly used in place of Tylenol® with Codeine; patients on this drug chronically should have liver function monitored secondary to acetaminophen in the product. Keep acetaminophen dose ≤4 g/day. Patients with chronic alcoholism, liver disease, or those who are fasting can develop severe hepatic disease even at therapeutic doses.

Pregnancy Risk Factor C/D (prolonged use or high doses near term)

Contraindications Hypersensitivity to hydrocodone, acetaminophen, or any component of the formulation; CNS depression; severe respiratory depression

Warnings/Precautions Use with caution in patients with hypersensitivity reactions to other phenanthrene derivative opioid agonists (morphine, hydromorphone, levorphanol, oxycodone, oxymorphone); tolerance or drug dependence may result from extended use.

Respiratory depressant effects may be increased with head injuries. Use caution with acute abdominal conditions; clinical course may be obscured. Use caution with thyroid dysfunction, prostatic hyperplasia, hepatic or renal disease, and in the elderly. Causes sedation; caution must be used in performing tasks which require alertness (eg, operating machinery or driving).

Limit acetaminophen to <4 g/day. May cause severe hepatic toxicity in acute overdose; in addition, chronic daily dosing in adults has resulted in liver damage in some patients. Use with caution in patients with alcoholic liver disease; consuming ≥3 alcoholic drinks/day may increase the risk of liver damage. Use caution in patients with known G6PD deficiency.

Adverse Reactions Frequency not defined.

Cardiovascular: Bradycardia, cardiac arrest, circulatory collapse, coma, hypotension

Central nervous system: Anxiety, dizziness, drowsiness, dysphoria, euphoria, fear, lethargy, lightheadedness, malaise, mental clouding, mental impairment, mood changes, physiological dependence, sedation, somnolence, stupor

(Continued)

Hydrocodone and Acetaminophen *(Continued)*

Dermatologic: Pruritus, rash
Endocrine & metabolic: Hypoglycemic coma
Gastrointestinal: Abdominal pain, constipation, gastric distress, heartburn, nausea, peptic ulcer, vomiting
Genitourinary: Ureteral spasm, urinary retention, vesical sphincter spasm
Hematologic: Agranulocytosis, bleeding time prolonged, hemolytic anemia, iron deficiency anemia, occult blood loss, thrombocytopenia
Hepatic: Hepatic necrosis, hepatitis
Neuromuscular & skeletal: Skeletal muscle rigidity
Otic: Hearing impairment or loss (chronic overdose)
Renal: Renal toxicity, renal tubular necrosis
Respiratory: Acute airway obstruction, apnea, dyspnea, respiratory depression (dose related)
Miscellaneous: Allergic reactions, clamminess, diaphoresis

Overdosage/Toxicology Symptoms of overdose include hepatic necrosis, blood dyscrasias, and respiratory depression. Treatment consists of acetylcysteine 140 mg/kg orally (loading) followed by 70 mg/kg every 4 hours for 17 doses; therapy should be initiated based upon laboratory analysis suggesting a high probability for hepatotoxic potential. Naloxone, 2 mg I.V. with repeat administration as necessary up to a total of 10 mg, can also be used to reverse toxic effects of the opiate. Activated charcoal is effective at binding certain chemicals, and this is especially true for acetaminophen.

Drug Interactions

Hydrocodone: **Substrate** of CYP2D6 (major)
Acetaminophen: **Substrate** (minor) of CYP1A2, 2A6, 2C9, 2D6, 2E1, 3A4; **Inhibits** CYP3A4 (weak)
Acetaminophen component: Refer to Acetaminophen monograph.
Hydrocodone component:
- CYP2D6 inhibitors may decrease the effects of hydrocodone. Example inhibitors include chlorpromazine, delavirdine, fluoxetine, miconazole, paroxetine, pergolide, quinidine, quinine, ritonavir, and ropinirole.
- CNS depressants (including antianxiety agents, antihistamines, antipsychotics, narcotics): CNS depression is additive; dose adjustment may be needed
- MAO inhibitors: May see increased effects of MAO inhibitor and hydrocodone.
- Tricyclic antidepressants (TCAs): May see increased effects of TCA and hydrocodone.

Ethanol/Nutrition/Herb Interactions

Ethanol: Avoid ethanol (may increase CNS depression); consuming ≥3 alcoholic drinks/day may increase the risk of liver damage
Herb/Nutraceutical: Avoid valerian, St John's wort, SAMe, kava kava (may increase risk of excessive sedation).

Dosage Forms

Capsule (Bancap HC®, Ceta-Plus®, Margesic® H, Stagesic®): Hydrocodone bitartrate 5 mg and acetaminophen 500 mg
Elixir: Hydrocodone bitartrate 7.5 mg and acetaminophen 500 mg per 15 mL (480 mL)
- Lortab®: Hydrocodone bitartrate 7.5 mg and acetaminophen 500 mg per 15 mL (480 mL) [contains alcohol 7%; tropical fruit punch flavor]

Solution, oral (hycet™): Hydrocodone bitartrate 7.5 mg and acetaminophen 325 mg per 15 mL (480 mL) [contains alcohol 7%; tropical fruit punch flavor]
Tablet:
- Hydrocodone bitartrate 2.5 mg and acetaminophen 500 mg
- Hydrocodone bitartrate 5 mg and acetaminophen 325 mg
- Hydrocodone bitartrate 5 mg and acetaminophen 500 mg
- Hydrocodone bitartrate 7.5 mg and acetaminophen 325 mg
- Hydrocodone bitartrate 7.5 mg and acetaminophen 500 mg
- Hydrocodone bitartrate 7.5 mg and acetaminophen 650 mg
- Hydrocodone bitartrate 7.5 mg and acetaminophen 750 mg
- Hydrocodone bitartrate 10 mg and acetaminophen 325 mg
- Hydrocodone bitartrate 10 mg and acetaminophen 500 mg
- Hydrocodone bitartrate 10 mg and acetaminophen 650 mg
- Hydrocodone bitartrate 10 mg and acetaminophen 660 mg
- Anexsia®:
  - 5/500: Hydrocodone bitartrate 5 mg and acetaminophen 500 mg
  - 7.5/650: Hydrocodone bitartrate 7.5 mg and acetaminophen 650 mg

Co-Gesic® 5/500: Hydrocodone bitartrate 5 mg and acetaminophen 500 mg
Lorcet® 10/650: Hydrocodone bitartrate 10 mg and acetaminophen 650 mg
Lorcet® Plus: Hydrocodone bitartrate 7.5 mg and acetaminophen 650 mg
Lortab®:
  2.5/500: Hydrocodone bitartrate 2.5 mg and acetaminophen 500 mg
  5/500: Hydrocodone bitartrate 5 mg and acetaminophen 500 mg
  7.5/500: Hydrocodone bitartrate 7.5 mg and acetaminophen 500 mg
  10/500: Hydrocodone bitartrate 10 mg and acetaminophen 500 mg
Maxidone™: Hydrocodone bitartrate 10 mg and acetaminophen 750 mg
Norco®:
  Hydrocodone bitartrate 5 mg and acetaminophen 325 mg
  Hydrocodone bitartrate 7.5 mg and acetaminophen 325 mg
  Hydrocodone bitartrate 10 mg and acetaminophen 325 mg
Vicodin®: Hydrocodone bitartrate 5 mg and acetaminophen 500 mg
Vicodin® ES: Hydrocodone bitartrate 7.5 mg and acetaminophen 750 mg
Vicodin® HP: Hydrocodone bitartrate 10 mg and acetaminophen 660 mg
Zydone®:
  Hydrocodone bitartrate 5 mg and acetaminophen 400 mg
  Hydrocodone bitartrate 7.5 mg and acetaminophen 400 mg
  Hydrocodone bitartrate 10 mg and acetaminophen 400 mg

Hydrocortisone (hye droe KOR ti sone)

Medication Safety Issues

Sound-alike/look-alike issues:

- Hydrocortisone may be confused with hydrocodone, hydroxychloroquine, hydrochlorothiazide
- Anusol® may be confused with Anusol-HC®, Aplisol®, Aquasol®
- Anusol-HC® may be confused with Anusol®
- Cortef® may be confused with Lortab®
- Cortizone® may be confused with cortisone
- HCT (occasional abbreviation for hydrocortisone) is an error-prone abbreviation (mistaken as hydrochlorothiazide)
- Hytone® may be confused with Vytone®
- Proctocort® may be confused with ProctoCream®
- ProctoCream® may be confused with Proctocort®

Related Information

Allergic Reactions *on page 1395*
Corticosteroids *on page 1561*
Latex Allergy *on page 1398*
Stress Replacement of Corticosteroids *on page 1494*

U.S. Brand Names Anucort-HC®; Anusol-HC®; Anusol® HC-1 [OTC]; Aquanil™ HC [OTC]; Beta-HC®; Caldecort® [OTC]; Cetacort®; Colocort®; Cortaid® Intensive Therapy [OTC]; Cortaid® Maximum Strength [OTC]; Cortaid® Sensitive Skin [OTC]; Cortef®; Corticool® [OTC]; Cortifoam®; Cortizone®-10 Maximum Strength [OTC]; Cortizone®-10 Plus Maximum Strength [OTC]; Cortizone®-10 Quick Shot [OTC]; Dermarest Dricort® [OTC]; Dermtex® HC [OTC]; EarSol® HC; Encort™; Hemril®-30; HydroZone Plus [OTC]; Hytone®; IvySoothe® [OTC]; Locoid®; Locoid Lipocream®; Nupercainal® Hydrocortisone Cream [OTC]; Nutracort®; Pandel®; Post Peel Healing Balm [OTC]; Preparation H® Hydrocortisone [OTC]; Proctocort®; ProctoCream® HC; Procto-Kit™; Procto-Pak™; Proctosert; Proctosol-HC®; Proctozone-HC™; Sarnol®-HC [OTC]; Solu-Cortef®; Summer's Eve® SpecialCare™ Medicated Anti-Itch Cream [OTC]; Texacort®; Tucks® Anti-Itch [OTC]; Westcort®

Canadian Brand Names Aquacort®; Cortamed®; Cortef®; Cortenema®; Cortifoam™; Emo-Cort®; Hycort™; Hyderm; HydroVal®; Locoid®; Prevex® HC; Sarna® HC; Solu-Cortef®; Westcort®

Synonyms A-hydroCort; Compound F; Cortisol; Hemorrhoidal HC; Hydrocortisone Acetate; Hydrocortisone Butyrate; Hydrocortisone Probutate; Hydrocortisone Sodium Succinate; Hydrocortisone Valerate

Pharmacologic Category Corticosteroid, Rectal; Corticosteroid, Systemic; Corticosteroid, Topical

Generic Available Yes: Excludes acetate foam, butyrate cream and ointment, gel as base, otic drops as base, probutate cream, sodium succinate injection

(Continued)

Hydrocortisone *(Continued)*

Use Management of adrenocortical insufficiency; relief of inflammation of corticosteroid-responsive dermatoses (low and medium potency topical corticosteroid); adjunctive treatment of ulcerative colitis

Mechanism of Action Decreases inflammation by suppression of migration of polymorphonuclear leukocytes and reversal of increased capillary permeability

Pharmacodynamics/Kinetics

Onset of action:

Hydrocortisone acetate: Slow

Hydrocortisone sodium succinate (water soluble): Rapid

Duration: Hydrocortisone acetate: Long

Absorption: Rapid by all routes, except rectally

Metabolism: Hepatic

Half-life elimination: Biologic: 8-12 hours

Excretion: Urine (primarily as 17-hydroxysteroids and 17-ketosteroids)

Dosage Dose should be based on severity of disease and patient response

Acute adrenal insufficiency: I.M., I.V.:

Infants and young Children: Succinate: 1-2 mg/kg/dose bolus, then 25-150 mg/day in divided doses every 6-8 hours

Older Children: Succinate: 1-2 mg/kg bolus then 150-250 mg/day in divided doses every 6-8 hours

Adults: Succinate: 100 mg I.V. bolus, then 300 mg/day in divided doses every 8 hours or as a continuous infusion for 48 hours; once patient is stable change to oral, 50 mg every 8 hours for 6 doses, then taper to 30-50 mg/day in divided doses

Chronic adrenal corticoid insufficiency: Adults: Oral: 20-30 mg/day

Anti-inflammatory or immunosuppressive:

Infants and Children:

Oral: 2.5-10 mg/kg/day **or** 75-300 mg/m^2/day every 6-8 hours

I.M., I.V.: Succinate: 1-5 mg/kg/day **or** 30-150 mg/m^2/day divided every 12-24 hours

Adolescents and Adults: Oral, I.M., I.V.: Succinate: 15-240 mg every 12 hours

Congenital adrenal hyperplasia: Oral: Initial: 10-20 mg/m^2/day in 3 divided doses; a variety of dosing schedules have been used. **Note:** Inconsistencies have occurred with liquid formulations; tablets may provide more reliable levels. Doses must be individualized by monitoring growth, bone age, and hormonal levels. Mineralocorticoid and sodium supplementation may be required based upon electrolyte regulation and plasma renin activity.

Physiologic replacement: Children:

Oral: 0.5-0.75 mg/kg/day **or** 20-25 mg/m^2/day every 8 hours

I.M.: Succinate: 0.25-0.35 mg/kg/day **or** 12-15 mg/m^2/day once daily

Shock: I.M., I.V.: Succinate:

Children: Initial: 50 mg/kg, then repeated in 4 hours and/or every 24 hours as needed

Adolescents and Adults: 500 mg to 2 g every 2-6 hours

Status asthmaticus: Children and Adults: I.V.: Succinate: 1-2 mg/kg/dose every 6 hours for 24 hours, then maintenance of 0.5-1 mg/kg every 6 hours

Adults:

Rheumatic diseases:

Intralesional, intra-articular, soft tissue injection: Acetate:

Large joints: 25 mg (up to 37.5 mg)

Small joints: 10-25 mg

Tendon sheaths: 5-12.5 mg

Soft tissue infiltration: 25-50 mg (up to 75 mg)

Bursae: 25-37.5 mg

Ganglia: 12.5-25 mg

Stress dosing (surgery) in patients known to be adrenally-suppressed or on chronic systemic steroids: I.V.:

Minor stress (ie, inguinal herniorrhaphy): 25 mg/day for 1 day

Moderate stress (ie, joint replacement, cholecystectomy): 50-75 mg/day (25 mg every 8-12 hours) for 1-2 days

Major stress (pancreatoduodenectomy, esophagogastrectomy, cardiac surgery): 100-150 mg/day (50 mg every 8-12 hours) for 2-3 days

Dermatosis: Children >2 years and Adults: Topical: Apply to affected area 2-4 times/day (Buteprate: Apply once or twice daily). Therapy should be discontinued when control is achieved; if no improvement is seen, reassessment of diagnosis may be necessary.

Ulcerative colitis: Adults: Rectal: 10-100 mg 1-2 times/day for 2-3 weeks

Stability Store at controlled room temperature 20°C to 25°C (59°F to 86°F). Hydrocortisone sodium phosphate and hydrocortisone sodium succinate are clear, light yellow solutions which are heat labile.

Sodium succinate: Reconstitute 100 mg vials with bacteriostatic water (not >2 mL). Act-O-Vial (self-contained powder for injection plus diluent) may be reconstituted by pressing the activator to force diluent into the powder compartment. Following gentle agitation, solution may be withdrawn via syringe through a needle inserted into the center of the stopper. May be administered (I.V. or I.M.) without further dilution. After initial reconstitution, hydrocortisone sodium succinate solutions are stable for 3 days at room temperature or under refrigeration when protected from light. Stability of parenteral admixture (Solu-Cortef®) at room temperature (25°C) and at refrigeration temperature (4°C) is concentration-dependent:

Stability of concentration 1 mg/mL: 24 hours

Stability of concentration 2 mg/mL to 60 mg/mL: At least 4 hours

Solutions for I.V. infusion: Reconstituted solutions may be added to an appropriate volume of compatible solution for infusion. Concentration should generally not exceed 1 mg/mL. However, in cases where administration of a small volume of fluid is desirable, 100-3000 mg may be added to 50 mL of D_5W or NS (stability limited to 4 hours).

Administration

Oral: Administer with food or milk to decrease GI upset

Parenteral: Hydrocortisone sodium succinate may be administered by I.M. or I.V. routes

I.V. bolus: Dilute to 50 mg/mL and administer over 30 seconds to several minutes (depending on the dose)

I.V. intermittent infusion: Dilute to 1 mg/mL and administer over 20-30 minutes

Topical: Apply a thin film to clean, dry skin and rub in gently

Monitoring Parameters Blood pressure, weight, serum glucose, and electrolytes

Reference Range Therapeutic: AM: 5-25 mcg/dL (SI: 138-690 nmol/L), PM: 2-9 mcg/dL (SI: 55-248 nmol/L) depending on test, assay

Anesthesia and Critical Care Concerns/Other Considerations Hydrocortisone is a long-acting corticosteroid with minimal sodium-retaining potential.

Neuromuscular Effects: ICU-acquired paresis was recently studied in 5 ICUs (3 medical and 2 surgical ICUs) at 4 French hospitals. All ICU patients without pre-existing neuromuscular disease admitted from March 1999 through June 2000 were evaluated (De Jonghe B, 2002). Each patient had to be mechanically ventilated for ≥7 days and was screened daily for awakening. The first day the patient was considered awake was Study Day 1. Patients with severe muscle weakness on Study Day 7 were considered to have ICU-acquired paresis. Among the 95 patients who were evaluable, about 25% developed ICU-acquired paresis. Independent predictors included: female gender, the number of days with ≥2 organ dysfunction, and administration of corticosteroids. Further studies may be required to verify and characterize the association between the development of ICU-acquired paresis and use of corticosteroids. Concurrent use of a corticosteroid and muscle relaxant appear to increase the risk of certain ICU myopathies; avoid or administer the corticosteroid at the lowest dose possible.

Adrenal Insufficiency: Patients will often have steroid-induced adverse effects on glucose tolerance and lipid profiles. When discontinuing steroid therapy in patients on long-term steroid supplementation, it is important that the steroid therapy be discontinued gradually. Abrupt withdrawal may result in adrenal insufficiency with hypotension and hyperkalemia. Patients on long-term steroid supplementation will require higher corticosteroid doses when subject to stress (ie, trauma, surgery, severe infection). Guidelines for glucocorticoid replacement during various surgical procedures has been published (Salem M, 1994, Coursin DB, 2002).

Septic Shock: A recent randomized, double-blind, placebo controlled trial assessed whether low dose corticosteroid administration could improve 28-day survival in patients with septic shock and relative adrenal insufficiency. Relative adrenal insufficiency was defined as an inappropriate response to corticotropin administration (increase of serum cortisol of ≤9 mcg/dL from baseline). Cortisol

(Continued)

Hydrocortisone *(Continued)*

levels were drawn immediately before corticotropin administration and 30 to 60 minutes afterwards. Three hundred adult septic shock patients requiring mechanical ventilation and vasopressor support were randomized to either hydrocortisone (50 mg IVP every 6 hours) and fludrocortisone (50 mcg tablet daily via nasogastric tube) or matching placebos for 7 days. In patients who did not appropriately respond to corticotropin (nonresponders), there were significantly fewer deaths in the active treatment group. Vasopressor therapy was withdrawn more frequently in this subset of the active treatment group. Adverse events were similar in both groups. Patients who lack adrenal reserve and thus have relative adrenal insufficiency during the stress of septic shock may benefit from physiologic steroid replacement. However, there was a trend for increased mortality in patients who responded to the corticotropin test (increase serum cortisol >9 mcg/dL from baseline). These patients may not benefit from physiologic steroid replacement. Further study is required to better characterize the patient populations who may benefit.

The 2004 Surviving Sepsis Campaign guidelines for steroid use are as follows:
Intravenous corticosteroids (hydrocortisone 200-300 mg/day for 7 days in 3 or 4 divided doses or by continuous infusion) are recommended in patients with septic shock who, despite adequate fluid replacement, require vasopressor therapy to maintain blood pressure (grade C).
Some experts would use a 250 mcg ACTH stimulation test to identify responders (>9 mcg/dL increase in cortisol 30-60 minutes post-ACTH administration) and discontinue therapy in these patients. Clinicians should not wait for ACTH stimulation results to administer corticosteroids (grade E).
Some experts would decrease dosage of steroids after resolution of septic shock (grade E).
Some experts would consider tapering the dose of corticosteroids at the end of therapy (grade E).
Some experts would add fludrocortisone to the regimen (grade E).
Doses of corticosteroids >300 mg of hydrocortisone/day should not be used to treat severe sepsis or septic shock (grade A).
In the absence of shock, corticosteroids should not be administered to treat sepsis. Use of maintenance steroid therapy or stress dose steroids is fine if the patient's history supports it.

Pregnancy Risk Factor C

Contraindications Hypersensitivity to hydrocortisone or any component of the formulation; serious infections, except septic shock or tuberculous meningitis; viral, fungal, or tubercular skin lesions

Warnings/Precautions

Use with caution in patients with hyperthyroidism, cirrhosis, nonspecific ulcerative colitis, hypertension, osteoporosis, thromboembolic tendencies, CHF, convulsive disorders, myasthenia gravis, thrombophlebitis, peptic ulcer, diabetes, glaucoma, cataracts, or tuberculosis. Use caution in hepatic impairment.

May cause HPA axis suppression. Acute adrenal insufficiency may occur with abrupt withdrawal after long-term therapy or with stress; young pediatric patients may be more susceptible to adrenal axis suppression from topical therapy. Avoid use of topical preparations with occlusive dressings or on weeping or exudative lesions.

Because of the risk of adverse effects, systemic corticosteroids should be used cautiously in the elderly, in the smallest possible dose, and for the shortest possible time

Adverse Reactions

Systemic:

>10%:
- Central nervous system: Insomnia, nervousness
- Gastrointestinal: Increased appetite, indigestion

1% to 10%:
- Dermatologic: Hirsutism
- Endocrine & metabolic: Diabetes mellitus
- Neuromuscular & skeletal: Arthralgia
- Ocular: Cataracts
- Respiratory: Epistaxis

<1% (Limited to important or life-threatening): Hypertension, edema, euphoria, headache, delirium, hallucinations, seizure, mood swings, acne, dermatitis, skin atrophy, bruising, hyperpigmentation, hypokalemia, hyperglycemia, Cushing's

syndrome, sodium and water retention, bone growth suppression, amenorrhea, peptic ulcer, abdominal distention, ulcerative esophagitis, pancreatitis, muscle wasting, hypersensitivity reactions, immunosuppression

Topical:

>10%: Dermatologic: Eczema (12.5%)

1% to 10%: Dermatologic: Pruritus (6%), stinging (2%), dry skin (2%)

<1% (Limited to important or life-threatening): Allergic contact dermatitis, burning, dermal atrophy, folliculitis, HPA axis suppression, hypopigmentation; metabolic effects (hyperglycemia, hypokalemia); striae

Overdosage/Toxicology When consumed in high doses for prolonged periods, systemic hypercorticism and adrenal suppression may occur. In those cases, discontinuation of the corticosteroid should be done judiciously.

Drug Interactions Substrate of CYP3A4 (minor); **Induces** CYP3A4 (weak)

Decreased effect:

Insulin decreases hypoglycemic effect

Phenytoin, phenobarbital, ephedrine, and rifampin increase metabolism of hydrocortisone and decrease steroid blood level

Increased toxicity:

Oral anticoagulants change prothrombin time

Potassium-depleting diuretics increase risk of hypokalemia

Cardiac glucosides increase risk of arrhythmias or digitalis toxicity secondary to hypokalemia

Ethanol/Nutrition/Herb Interactions

Ethanol: Avoid ethanol (may enhance gastric mucosal irritation).

Food: Hydrocortisone interferes with calcium absorption.

Herb/Nutraceutical: St John's wort may decrease hydrocortisone levels. Avoid cat's claw, echinacea (have immunostimulant properties).

Dietary Considerations Systemic use of corticosteroids may require a diet with increased potassium, vitamins A, B_6, C, D, folate, calcium, zinc, phosphorus, and decreased sodium. Sodium content of 1 g (sodium succinate injection): 47.5 mg (2.07 mEq)

Dosage Forms [DSC] = Discontinued product

Aerosol, rectal, as acetate (Cortifoam®): 10% (15 g) [90 mg/applicator]

Cream, rectal, as acetate (Nupercainal® Hydrocortisone Cream): 1% (30 g) [strength expressed as base]

Cream, rectal, as base:

Cortizone®-10: 1% (30 g) [contains aloe]

Preparation H® Hydrocortisone: 1% (27 g)

Cream, topical, as acetate: 0.5% (9 g, 30 g, 60 g) [available with aloe]; 1% (30 g, 454 g) [available with aloe]

Cream, topical, as base: 0.5% (30 g); 1% (1.5 g, 30 g, 114 g, 454 g); 2.5% (20 g, 30 g, 454 g)

Anusol-HC®: 2.5% (30 g) [contains benzyl alcohol]

Caldecort®: 1% (30 g) [contains aloe vera gel]

Cortaid® Intensive Therapy: 1% (60 g)

Cortaid® Maximum Strength: 1% (15 g, 30 g, 40 g, 60 g) [contains aloe vera gel and benzyl alcohol]

Cortaid® Sensitive Skin: 0.5% (15 g) [contains aloe vera gel]

Cortizone®-10 Maximum Strength: 1% (15 g, 30 g, 60 g) [contains aloe]

Cortizone®-10 Plus Maximum Strength: 1% (30 g, 60 g) [contains vitamins A, D, E and aloe]

Dermarest® Dricort®: 1% (15 g, 30 g)

HydroZone Plus, Proctocort®, Procto-Pak™: 1% (30 g)

Hytone®: 2.5% (30 g, 60 g)

IvySoothe®: 1% (30 g) [contains aloe]

Post Peel Healing Balm: 1% (23 g)

ProctoCream® HC: 2.5% (30 g) [contains benzyl alcohol]

Procto-Kit™: 1% (30 g) [packaged with applicator tips and finger cots]; 2.5% (30 g) [packaged with applicator tips and finger cots]

Proctosol-HC®, Proctozone-HC™: 2.5% (30 g)

Summer's Eve® SpecialCare™ Medicated Anti-Itch Cream: 1% (30 g)

Cream, topical, as butyrate (Locoid®, Locoid Lipocream®): 0.1% (15 g, 45 g)

Cream, topical, as probutate (Pandel®): 0.1% (15 g, 45 g, 80 g)

Cream, topical, as valerate (Westcort®): 0.2% (15 g, 45 g, 60 g)

Gel, topical, as base (Corticool®): 1% (45 g)

(Continued)

Hydrocortisone *(Continued)*

Injection, powder for reconstitution, as sodium succinate (Solu-Cortef®): 100 mg, 250 mg, 500 mg, 1 g [diluent contains benzyl alcohol; strength expressed as base]
Lotion, topical, as base: 1% (120 mL); 2.5% (60 mL)
  Aquanil™ HC: 1% (120 mL)
  Beta-HC®, Cetacort®, Sarnol®-HC: 1% (60 mL)
  HydroZone Plus: 1% (120 mL)
  Hytone®: 2.5% (60 mL)
  Nutracort®: 1% (60 mL, 120 mL); 2.5% (60 mL, 120 mL)
Ointment, topical, as acetate: 1% (30 g) [strength expressed as base; available with aloe]
  Anusol® HC-1: 1% (21 g) [strength expressed as base]
  Cortaid® Maximum Strength: 1% (15 g, 30 g) [strength expressed as base]
Ointment, topical, as base: 0.5% (30 g); 1% (30 g, 454 g); 2.5% (20 g, 30 g, 454 g)
  Cortizone®-10 Maximum Strength: 1% (30 g, 60 g)
  Hytone®: 2.5% (30 g) [DSC]
Ointment, topical, as butyrate (Locoid®): 0.1% (15 g, 45 g)
Ointment, topical, as valerate (Westcort®): 0.2% (15 g, 45 g, 60 g)
Solution, otic, as base (EarSol® HC): 1% (30 mL) [contains alcohol 44%, benzyl benzoate, yerba santa]
Solution, topical, as base (Texacort®): 2.5% (30 mL) [contains alcohol]
Solution, topical, as butyrate (Locoid®): 0.1% (20 mL, 60 mL) [contains alcohol 50%]
Solution, topical spray, as base:
  Cortaid® Intensive Therapy: 1% (60 mL) [contains alcohol]
  Cortizone®-10 Quick Shot: 1% (44 mL) [contains benzyl alcohol]
  Dermtex® HC: 1% (52 mL) [contains menthol 1%]
Suppository, rectal, as acetate: 25 mg (12s, 24s, 100s)
  Anucort-HC®, Tucks® Anti-Itch: 25 mg (12s, 24s, 100s) [strength expressed as base; Anucort-HC® *renamed* Tucks® Anti-Itch]
  Anusol-HC®, Proctosol-HC®: 25 mg (12s, 24s)
  Encort™: 30 mg (12s)
  Hemril®-30, Proctocort®, Proctosert: 30 mg (12s, 24s)
Suspension, rectal, as base: 100 mg/60 mL (7s)
  Colocort®: 100 mg/60 mL (1s, 7s)
Tablet, as base: 20 mg
  Cortef®: 5 mg, 10 mg, 20 mg

References

Abraham E and Evans T, "Corticosteroids and Septic Shock (editorial)," *JAMA*, 2002, 288(7):886-7.
Annane D, Sebille V, Charpentier C, et al, "Effect of Treatment With Low Doses of Hydrocortisone and Fludrocortisone on Mortality in Patients With Septic Shock," *JAMA*, 2002, 288(7):862-71.
Cooper MS and Stewart PM, "Corticosteroid Insufficiency in Acutely Ill Patients," *N Engl J Med*, 2003, 348(8):727-34.
Coursin DB and Wood KE, "Corticosteroid Supplementation for Adrenal Insufficiency," *JAMA*, 2002, 287(2):236-40.
De Jonghe B, Sharshar T, Lefaucheur JP, et al, "Paresis Acquired in the Intensive Care Unit. A Prospective Multicenter Study," *JAMA*, 2002, 288(22):2859-67.
Dellinger RP, Carlet JM, Masur H, et al, "Surviving Sepsis Campaign Guidelines for Management of Severe Sepsis and Septic Shock," *Crit Care Med*, 2004, 32(3):858-73.
Hotchkiss RS and Karl IE, "The Pathophysiology and Treatment of Sepsis," *N Engl J Med*, 2003, 348(2):138-50.
Salem M, Tainsh RE, Jr, Bromberg J, et al, "Perioperative Glucocorticoid Coverage: A Reassessment 42 Years After Emergence of a Problem," *Ann Surg*, 1994, 219(4):416-25.

- **Hydrocortisone Acetate** *see* Hydrocortisone *on page 639*
- **Hydrocortisone Butyrate** *see* Hydrocortisone *on page 639*
- **Hydrocortisone Probutate** *see* Hydrocortisone *on page 639*
- **Hydrocortisone Sodium Succinate** *see* Hydrocortisone *on page 639*
- **Hydrocortisone Valerate** *see* Hydrocortisone *on page 639*
- **Hydromorph Contin® (Can)** *see* Hydromorphone *on page 644*
- **Hydromorph-IR® (Can)** *see* Hydromorphone *on page 644*

Hydromorphone (hye droe MOR fone)

Medication Safety Issues

Sound-alike/look-alike issues:
  Dilaudid® may be confused with Demerol®, Dilantin®

Hydromorphone may be confused with morphine; significant overdoses have occurred when hydromorphone products have been inadvertently administered instead of morphine sulfate. Commercially available prefilled syringes of both products looks similar and are often stored in close proximity to each other. **Note:** Hydromorphone 1 mg oral is approximately equal to morphine 4 mg oral; hydromorphone 1 mg I.V. is approximately equal to morphine 5 mg I.V.

Dilaudid®, Dilaudid-HP®: Extreme caution should be taken to avoid confusing the highly-concentrated (Dilaudid-HP®) injection with the less-concentrated (Dilaudid®) injectable product.

Related Information

Acute Postoperative Pain *on page 1388*
Anesthesia Considerations for Neurosurgery *on page 1401*
Chronic Pain Management *on page 1430*
Narcotic / Opioid Analgesics *on page 1568*
Opioids *on page 1535*

U.S. Brand Names Dilaudid®; Dilaudid-HP®; Palladone™ *[Withdrawn]*

Canadian Brand Names Dilaudid®; Dilaudid-HP®; Dilaudid-HP-Plus®; Dilaudid® Sterile Powder; Dilaudid-XP®; Hydromorph Contin®; Hydromorph-IR®; Hydromorphone HP; Hydromorphone HP® 10; Hydromorphone HP® 20; Hydromorphone HP® 50; Hydromorphone HP® Forte; Hydromorphone Hydrochloride Injection, USP; PMS-Hydromorphone

Synonyms Dihydromorphinone; Hydromorphone Hydrochloride

Pharmacologic Category Analgesic, Narcotic

Restrictions C-II

Generic Available Yes: Excludes capsule, liquid, powder for injection

Use Management of moderate-to-severe pain

Unlabeled/Investigational Use Antitussive

Mechanism of Action Binds to opiate receptors in the CNS, causing inhibition of ascending pain pathways, altering the perception of and response to pain; causes cough supression by direct central action in the medulla; produces generalized CNS depression

Pharmacodynamics/Kinetics

Onset of action: Analgesic: Immediate release formulations:
- Oral: 15-30 minutes
- Peak effect: Oral: 30-60 minutes

Duration: Immediate release formulations: 4-5 hours
Absorption: I.M.: Variable and delayed; Palladone™: Biphasic
Distribution: V_d: 4 L/kg
Protein binding: ~20%
Metabolism: Hepatic; to inactive metabolites
Bioavailability: 62%
Half-life elimination:
- Immediate release formulations: 1-3 hours
- Palladone™: 18.6 hours

Excretion: Urine (primarily as glucuronide conjugates)

Dosage

Acute pain (moderate to severe): **Note:** These are guidelines and do not represent the maximum doses that may be required in all patients. Doses should be titrated to pain relief/prevention.
- Young Children ≥6 months and <50 kg:
  - Oral: 0.03-0.08 mg/kg/dose every 3-4 hours as needed
  - I.V.: 0.015 mg/kg/dose every 3-6 hours as needed
- Older Children >50 kg and Adults:
  - Oral: Initial: Opiate-naive: 2-4 mg every 3-4 hours as needed; patients with prior opiate exposure may require higher initial doses; usual dosage range: 2-8 mg every 3-4 hours as needed
  - I.V.: Initial: Opiate-naive: 0.2-0.6 mg every 2-3 hours as needed; patients with prior opiate exposure may tolerate higher initial doses
    - **Note:** More frequent dosing may be needed.
    - Mechanically-ventilated patients (based on 70 kg patient): 0.7-2 mg every 1-2 hours as needed; infusion (based on 70 kg patient): 0.5-1 mg/hour
  - Patient-controlled analgesia (PCA): (Opiate-naive: Consider lower end of dosing range)
    - Usual concentration: 0.2 mg/mL
    - Demand dose: Usual: 0.1-0.2 mg; range: 0.05-0.5 mg

(Continued)

Hydromorphone *(Continued)*

Lockout interval: 5-15 minutes
4-hour limit: 4-6 mg

Epidural:
Bolus dose: 1-1.5 mg
Infusion concentration: 0.05-0.075 mg/mL
Infusion rate: 0.04-0.4 mg/hour
Demand dose: 0.15 mg
Lockout interval: 30 minutes

I.M., SubQ: **Note:** I.M. use may result in variable absorption and a lag time to peak effect.
Initial: Opiate-naive: 0.8-1 mg every 4-6 hours as needed; patients with prior opiate exposure may require higher initial doses; usual dosage range: 1-2 mg every 3-6 hours as needed

Rectal: 3 mg every 4-8 hours as needed

Chronic pain: Adults: Oral: **Note:** Patients taking opioids chronically may become tolerant and require doses higher than the usual dosage range to maintain the desired effect. Tolerance can be managed by appropriate dose titration. There is no optimal or maximal dose for hydromorphone in chronic pain. The appropriate dose is one that relieves pain throughout its dosing interval without causing unmanageable side effects.

Controlled release formulation (Hydromorph Contin®, not available in U.S.): 3-30 mg every 12 hours. **Note:** A patient's hydromorphone requirement should be established using prompt release formulations; conversion to long acting products may be considered when chronic, continuous treatment is required. Higher dosages should be reserved for use only in opioid-tolerant patients.

Extended release formulation (Palladone™): For use only in opioid-tolerant patients requiring extended treatment of pain. Initial Palladone™ dose should be calculated using standard conversion estimates based on previous total daily opioid dose, rounding off to the most appropriate strength available. Doses should be administered once every 24 hours. Discontinue all previous around-the-clock opioids when treatment is initiated. Dose may be adjusted every 2 days as needed.

Conversion from transdermal fentanyl to oral Palladone™ (limited clinical experience): Initiate Palladone™ 18 hours after removal of patch; substitute Palladone™ 12 mg/day for each fentanyl 50 mcg/hour patch; monitor closely

Conversion from opioid combination drugs: Initial dose: Palladone™ 12 mg/day in patients receiving around-the-clock fixed combination-opioid analgesics with a total dose greater than or equal to oxycodone 45 mg/day, hydrocodone 45 mg/day, or codeine 300 mg/day

Antitussive (unlabeled use): Oral:
Children 6-12 years: 0.5 mg every 3-4 hours as needed
Children >12 years and Adults: 1 mg every 3-4 hours as needed

Dosing adjustment in hepatic impairment: Should be considered

Stability Store injection and oral dosage forms at 25°C (77°F). Protect tablets from light. A slightly yellowish discoloration has not been associated with a loss of potency; I.V. is **incompatible** when mixed with minocycline, prochlorperazine, sodium bicarbonate, tetracycline, thiopental.

Administration

Parenteral: May be given SubQ or I.M.; vial stopper contains latex
I.V.: For IVP, must be given slowly over 2-3 minutes (rapid IVP has been associated with an increase in side effects, especially respiratory depression and hypotension)

Oral:
Hydromorph Contin®: Capsule should be swallowed whole; do not crush or chew; contents may be sprinkled on soft food and swallowed
Palladone™: Capsule must be swallowed whole; do not break open, crush, chew, dissolve, or sprinkle on food.

Monitoring Parameters Pain relief, respiratory and mental status, blood pressure

Anesthesia and Critical Care Concerns/Other Considerations When developing a therapeutic plan for pain control, scheduled, intermittent opioid dosing or continuous infusion is preferred over the "as needed" regimen. The

2002 ACCM/SCCM guidelines for analgesia (critically-ill adult) recommend fentanyl in patients who need immediate pain relief because of its rapid onset of action; fentanyl or hydromorphone is preferred in patients who are hypotensive or have renal dysfunction. Morphine or hydromorphone is recommended for intermittent, scheduled therapy. Both have a longer duration of action requiring less frequent administration. Hydromorphone does not have any active metabolites, has less protein binding than other opiates and does not cause histamine release. If the patient has required high-dose analgesia or has used for a prolonged period (~7 days), taper dose to prevent withdrawal; monitor for signs and symptoms of withdrawal.

Equianalgesic doses: Morphine 10 mg I.M. = hydromorphone 1.5 mg I.M.

Pregnancy Risk Factor C/D (prolonged use or high doses at term)

Contraindications Hypersensitivity to hydromorphone, any component of the formulation, or other phenanthrene derivative; increased intracranial pressure; acute or severe asthma, severe respiratory depression (in absence of resuscitative equipment or ventilatory support); severe CNS depression; pregnancy (prolonged use or high doses at term)

Palladone™ is also contraindicated with known or suspected paralytic ileus.

Warnings/Precautions Controlled release capsules should only be used when continuous analgesia is required over an extended period of time. Palladone™ should only be used in opioid tolerant patients requiring doses of hydromorphone >12 mg/day (or equianalgesic dose of another opioid) and who have been at that dose for >7 days. Controlled release products are not to be used on an as needed basis. Hydromorphone shares toxic potential of opiate agonists, and precaution of opiate agonist therapy should be observed; use with caution in patients with hypersensitivity to other phenanthrene opiates, respiratory disease, biliary tract disease, acute pancreatitis, or severe liver or renal failure; tolerance or drug dependence may result from extended use. Those at risk for opioid abuse include patients with a history of substance abuse or mental illness.

An opioid-containing analgesic regimen should be tailored to each patient's needs and based upon the type of pain being treated (acute versus chronic), the route of administration, degree of tolerance for opioids (naive versus chronic user), age, weight, and medical condition. The optimal analgesic dose varies widely among patients. Doses should be titrated to pain relief/prevention. I.M. use may result in variable absorption and a lag time to peak effect.

Some dosage forms contain trace amounts of sodium bisulfite which may cause allergic reactions in susceptible individuals.

Adverse Reactions Frequency not defined.

Cardiovascular: Palpitations, hypotension, peripheral vasodilation, tachycardia, bradycardia, flushing of face

Central nervous system: CNS depression, increased intracranial pressure, fatigue, headache, nervousness, restlessness, dizziness, lightheadedness, drowsiness, hallucinations, mental depression, seizure

Dermatologic: Pruritus, rash, urticaria

Endocrine & metabolic: Antidiuretic hormone release

Gastrointestinal: Nausea, vomiting, constipation, stomach cramps, xerostomia, anorexia, biliary tract spasm, paralytic ileus

Genitourinary: Decreased urination, ureteral spasm, urinary tract spasm

Hepatic: LFTs increased, AST increased, ALT increased

Local: Pain at injection site (I.M.)

Neuromuscular & skeletal: Trembling, weakness, myoclonus

Ocular: Miosis

Respiratory: Respiratory depression, dyspnea

Miscellaneous: Histamine release, physical and psychological dependence

Overdosage/Toxicology Symptoms of overdose include CNS depression, respiratory depression, miosis, apnea, pulmonary edema, and convulsions. Along with supportive measures, naloxone, 2 mg I.V. with repeat administration as necessary up to a total of 10 mg, can also be used to reverse toxic effects of the opiate.

Drug Interactions

CNS depressants: Effects with hydromorphone may be additive.

Pegvisomant: Analgesics (narcotic) may diminish the therapeutic effect of pegvisomant; increased pegvisomant doses may be needed.

Phenothiazines: May enhance the hypotensive and CNS depressant effects of hydromorphone.

Selective serotonin reuptake inhibitors (SSRIs): Serotonergic effects may be additive, leading to serotonin syndrome.

(Continued)

Hydromorphone *(Continued)*

Ethanol/Nutrition/Herb Interactions

Ethanol: Avoid ethanol (may increase CNS depression).

Herb/Nutraceutical: Avoid valerian, St John's wort, kava kava, gotu kola (may increase CNS depression).

Test Interactions

Some quinolones may produce a false-positive urine screening result for opiates using commercially-available immunoassay kits. This has been demonstrated most consistently for levofloxacin and ofloxacin, but other quinolones have shown cross-reactivity in certain assay kits. Confirmation of positive opiate screens by more specific methods should be considered.

Dosage Forms [CAN] = Canadian brand name

Capsule, controlled release (Hydromorph Contin®) [CAN]: 3 mg, 6 mg, 12 mg, 18 mg, 24 mg, 30 mg [not available in U.S.]

Capsule, extended release, as hydrochloride (Palladone™): 12 mg, 16 mg, 24 mg, 32 mg *[withdrawn from market]*

Injection, powder for reconstitution, as hydrochloride (Dilaudid-HP®): 250 mg

Injection, solution, as hydrochloride: 1 mg/mL (1 mL); 2 mg/mL (1 mL, 20 mL); 4 mg/mL (1 mL); 10 mg/mL (1 mL, 5 mL, 10 mL)

Dilaudid®: 1 mg/mL (1 mL); 2 mg/mL (1 mL, 20 mL) [20 mL size contains edetate sodium; vial stopper contains latex]; 4 mg/mL (1 mL)

Dilaudid-HP®: 10 mg/mL (1 mL, 5 mL, 50 mL)

Liquid, oral, as hydrochloride (Dilaudid®): 1 mg/mL (480 mL) [may contain trace amounts of sodium bisulfite]

Suppository, rectal, as hydrochloride (Dilaudid®): 3 mg (6s)

Tablet, as hydrochloride (Dilaudid®): 2 mg, 4 mg, 8 mg (8 mg tablets may contain trace amounts of sodium bisulfite)

References

Agency for Health Care Policy and Research, "Acute Pain Management in Infants, Children and Adolescents: Operative and Medical Procedures," *Am Fam Physician*, 1992, 46(2):469-79.

"Clinical Practice Guidelines for the Sustained Use of Sedatives and Analgesics in the Critically Ill Adult. Task Force of the American College of Critical Care Medicine (ACCM) of the Society of Critical Care Medicine (SCCM), American Society of Health-System Pharmacists (ASHP), American College of Chest Physicians," *Am J Health Syst Pharm*, 2002, 59(2):150-78.

Jacobi J, Fraser GL, Coursin DB, et al, "Clinical Practice Guidelines for the Sustained Use of Sedatives and Analgesics in the Critically Ill Adult," *Crit Care Med*, 2002, 30(1):119-41. Available at: http://www.sccm.org/pdf/sedatives.pdf.

Levy MH, "Pharmacologic Treatment of Cancer Pain," *N Engl J Med*, 1996, 335(15):1124-32.

Mokhlesi B, Leikin JB, Murray P, et al, "Adult Toxicology in Critical Care. Part 11: Specific Poisonings," *Chest*, 2003, 123(3):897-922.

Nasraway SA, "Use of Sedative Medications in the Intensive Care Unit," *Sem Resp Crit Care Med*, 2001, 22(2):165-74.

"Principles of Analgesic Use in the Treatment of Acute Pain and Cancer Pain," 5th ed, Glenview, IL: American Pain Society, 2003.

- **Hydromorphone HP (Can)** *see* Hydromorphone *on page 644*
- **Hydromorphone HP® 10 (Can)** *see* Hydromorphone *on page 644*
- **Hydromorphone HP® 20 (Can)** *see* Hydromorphone *on page 644*
- **Hydromorphone HP® 50 (Can)** *see* Hydromorphone *on page 644*
- **Hydromorphone HP® Forte (Can)** *see* Hydromorphone *on page 644*
- **Hydromorphone Hydrochloride** *see* Hydromorphone *on page 644*
- **Hydromorphone Hydrochloride Injection, USP (Can)** *see* Hydromorphone *on page 644*
- **HydroVal® (Can)** *see* Hydrocortisone *on page 639*
- **4-Hydroxybutyrate** *see* Sodium Oxybate *on page 1187*
- **Hydroxycarbamide** *see* Hydroxyurea *on page 648*
- **Hydroxyethyl Starch** *see* Hetastarch *on page 623*

Hydroxyurea (hye droks ee yoor EE a)

Medication Safety Issues

Sound-alike/look-alike issues:

Hydroxyurea may be confused with hydrOXYzine

U.S. Brand Names Droxia®; Hydrea®; Mylocel™

Canadian Brand Names Apo-Hydroxyurea®; Gen-Hydroxyurea; Hydrea®

Synonyms Hydroxycarbamide

Pharmacologic Category Antineoplastic Agent, Antimetabolite

Generic Available Yes: Capsule

Use Treatment of melanoma, refractory chronic myelocytic leukemia (CML), relapsed and refractory metastatic ovarian cancer; radiosensitizing agent in the treatment of squamous cell head and neck cancer (excluding lip cancer); adjunct in the management of sickle cell patients who have had at least three painful crises in the previous 12 months (to reduce frequency of these crises and the need for blood transfusions)

Unlabeled/Investigational Use Treatment of HIV; treatment of psoriasis, treatment of hematologic conditions such as essential thrombocythemia, polycythemia vera, hypereosinophilia, and hyperleukocytosis due to acute leukemia; treatment of uterine, cervix and nonsmall cell lung cancers; radiosensitizing agent in the treatment of primary brain tumors; has shown activity against renal cell cancer and prostate cancer

Mechanism of Action Thought to interfere (unsubstantiated hypothesis) with synthesis of DNA, during the S phase of cell division, without interfering with RNA synthesis; inhibits ribonucleoside diphosphate reductase, preventing conversion of ribonucleotides to deoxyribonucleotides; cell-cycle specific for the S phase and may hold other cells in the G_1 phase of the cell cycle.

Pharmacodynamics/Kinetics

Absorption: Readily (≥80%)

Distribution: Readily crosses blood-brain barrier; distributes into intestine, brain, lung, kidney tissues, effusions and ascites

Metabolism: 60% via hepatic and GI tract

Half-life elimination: 3-4 hours

Time to peak: 1-4 hours

Excretion: Urine (80%, 50% as unchanged drug, 30% as urea); exhaled gases (as CO_2)

Dosage Oral (refer to individual protocols): All dosage should be based on ideal or actual body weight, whichever is less:

Children (unlabeled use):

No FDA-approved dosage regimens have been established; dosages of 1500-3000 mg/m² as a single dose in combination with other agents every 4-6 weeks have been used in the treatment of pediatric astrocytoma, medulloblastoma, and primitive neuroectodermal tumors

CML: Initial: 10-20 mg/kg/day once daily; adjust dose according to hematologic response

Adults: Dose should always be titrated to patient response and WBC counts; usual oral doses range from 10-30 mg/kg/day or 500-3000 mg/day; if WBC count falls to <2500 cells/mm³, or the platelet count to <100,000/mm³, therapy should be stopped for at least 3 days and resumed when values rise toward normal

Solid tumors:

Intermittent therapy: 80 mg/kg as a single dose every third day

Continuous therapy: 20-30 mg/kg/day given as a single dose/day

Concomitant therapy with irradiation: 80 mg/kg as a single dose every third day starting at least 7 days before initiation of irradiation

Resistant chronic myelocytic leukemia: Continuous therapy: 20-30 mg/kg as a single daily dose

HIV (unlabeled use; in combination with antiretroviral agents): 1000-1500 mg daily in a single dose or divided doses

Psoriasis (unlabeled use): 1000-1500 mg/day in a single dose or divided doses

Sickle cell anemia (moderate/severe disease): Initial: 15 mg/kg/day, increased by 5 mg/kg every 12 weeks if blood counts are in an acceptable range until the maximum tolerated dose of 35 mg/kg/day is achieved or the dose that does not produce toxic effects

Acceptable range:

Neutrophils ≥2500 cells/mm³

Platelets ≥95,000/mm³

Hemoglobin >5.3 g/dL, and

Reticulocytes ≥95,000/mm³ if the hemoglobin concentration is <9 g/dL

Toxic range:

Neutrophils <2000 cells/mm³

Platelets <80,000/mm³

Hemoglobin <4.5 g/dL

Reticulocytes <80,000/mm³ if the hemoglobin concentration is <9 g/dL

Monitor for toxicity every 2 weeks; if toxicity occurs, stop treatment until the bone marrow recovers; restart at 2.5 mg/kg/day less than the dose at which toxicity occurs; if no toxicity occurs over the next 12 weeks, then

(Continued)

Hydroxyurea *(Continued)*

the subsequent dose should be increased by 2.5 mg/kg/day; reduced dosage of hydroxyurea alternating with erythropoietin may decrease myelotoxicity and increase levels of fetal hemoglobin in patients who have not been helped by hydroxyurea alone

Dosing adjustment in renal impairment:

Sickle cell anemia: Cl_{cr} <60 mL/minute or ESRD: Reduce initial dose to 7.5 mg/kg; titrate to response/avoidance of toxicity (refer to usual dosing)

Other indications:

Cl_{cr} 10-50 mL/minute: Administer 50% of normal dose

Cl_{cr} <10 mL/minute: Administer 20% of normal dose

Hemodialysis: Administer dose after dialysis on dialysis days; supplemental dose is not necessary. Hydroxyurea is a low molecular weight compound with high aqueous solubility that may be freely dialyzable, however, clinical studies confirming this hypothesis have not been performed.

CAPD effects: Unknown

CAVH effects: Dose for GFR 10-50 mL/minute

Stability Store at room temperature between 15°C and 30°C (59°F and 86°F).

Administration Capsules may be opened and emptied into water (will not dissolve completely); observe proper handling procedures

Monitoring Parameters CBC with differential and platelets, renal function and liver function tests, serum uric acid

Sickle cell disease: Monitor for toxicity every 2 weeks. If toxicity occurs, stop treatment until the bone marrow recovers; restart at 2.5 mg/kg/day less than the dose at which toxicity occurs. If no toxicity occurs over the next 12 weeks, then the subsequent dose should be increased by 2.5 mg/kg/day. Reduced dosage of hydroxyurea alternating with erythropoietin may decrease myelotoxicity and increase levels of fetal hemoglobin in patients who have not been helped by hydroxyurea alone.

Acceptable range: Neutrophils ≥2500 cells/mm^3, platelets ≥95,000/mm^3, hemoglobin >5.3 g/dL, and reticulocytes ≥95,000/mm^3 if the hemoglobin concentration is <9 g/dL

Toxic range: Neutrophils <2000 cells/mm^3, platelets <80,000/mm^3, hemoglobin <4.5 g/dL, and reticulocytes <80,000/mm^3 if the hemoglobin concentration is <9 g/dL

Anesthesia and Critical Care Concerns/Other Considerations If WBC decreases to <2500/mm^3 or platelet count to <100,000/mm^3, interrupt therapy until values rise significantly toward normal. Treat anemia with whole blood replacement; do not interrupt therapy. Almost all patients receiving hydroxyurea in clinical trials needed to have their medication stopped for a time to allow their low blood count to return to acceptable levels.

Myelosuppressive effects:

WBC: Moderate

Platelets: Moderate

Onset: 24-48 hours

Nadir: 10 days

Recovery: 7 days after stopping drug

Pregnancy Risk Factor D

Contraindications Hypersensitivity to hydroxyurea or any component of the formulation; severe anemia; severe bone marrow suppression; WBC <2500/mm^3 or platelet count <100,000/mm^3; pregnancy

Warnings/Precautions Hazardous agent — use appropriate precautions for handling and disposal. Patients with a history of prior cytotoxic chemotherapy and radiation therapy are more likely to experience bone marrow depression. Patients with a history of radiation therapy are also at risk for exacerbation of post irradiation erythema. Megaloblastic erythropoiesis may be seen early in hydroxyurea treatment; plasma iron clearance may be delayed and the rate of utilization of iron by erythrocytes may be delayed. HIV-infected patients treated with hydroxyurea and didanosine (with or without stavudine) are at higher risk for pancreatitis, hepatotoxicity, hepatic failure, and severe peripheral neuropathy. Treatment of myeloproliferative disorders (polycythemia vera and thrombocythemia) with long-term hydroxyurea is associated with secondary leukemia; it is unknown if this is drug-related or disease-related. Cutaneous vasculitic toxicities (vasculitic ulceration and gangrene) have been reported with hydroxyurea treatment, most often in patients with a history of or receiving concurrent interferon therapy;

discontinue hydroxyurea and consider alternate cytoreductive therapy if cutaneous vasculitic toxicity develops. Use caution with renal dysfunction; may require dose reductions. Safety and efficacy in children have not been established.

Adverse Reactions Frequency not defined.

Cardiovascular: Edema

Central nervous system: Chills, disorientation, dizziness, drowsiness (dose-related), fever, hallucinations, headache, malaise, seizure

Dermatologic: Alopecia (rare), cutaneous vasculitic toxicities, dermatomyositis-like skin changes, dry skin, facial erythema, gangrene, hyperpigmentation, maculopapular rash, nail atrophy, nail pigmentation, peripheral erythema, scaling, skin atrophy, skin cancer, vasculitis ulcerations, violet papules

Endocrine & metabolic: Hyperuricemia

Gastrointestinal: Anorexia, constipation, diarrhea, gastrointestinal irritation and mucositis, (potentiated with radiation therapy), nausea, pancreatitis, stomatitis, vomiting

Genitourinary: Dysuria (rare)

Hematologic: Myelosuppression (primarily leukopenia; onset: 24-48 hours; nadir: 10 days; recovery: 7 days after stopping drug; reversal of WBC count occurs rapidly but the platelet count may take 7-10 days to recover); thrombocytopenia and anemia, megaloblastic erythropoiesis, macrocytosis, hemolysis, serum iron decreased, persistent cytopenias, secondary leukemias (long-term use)

Hepatic: Hepatic enzymes increased, hepatotoxicity

Neuromuscular & skeletal: Weakness, peripheral neuropathy

Renal: BUN increased, creatinine increased

Respiratory: Acute diffuse pulmonary infiltrates (rare), dyspnea, pulmonary fibrosis (rare)

Overdosage/Toxicology Symptoms of overdose include myelosuppression, facial swelling, hallucinations, disorientation, soreness, violet erythema, edema on palms and soles, scaling on hands and feet, severe generalized hyperpigmentation of the skin, and stomatitis. Treatment is symptom-directed and supportive.

Drug Interactions

Didanosine: Hydroxyurea may increase risk of didanosine-induced pancreatitis, hepatotoxicity, or neuropathy; concomitant use is not recommended

Dosage Forms

Capsule: 500 mg

Droxia®: 200 mg, 300 mg, 400 mg

Hydrea®: 500 mg

Tablet (Mylocel™): 1000 mg

- **HydroZone Plus [OTC]** *see* Hydrocortisone *on page 639*
- **Hylenex**™ *see* Hyaluronidase *on page 631*
- **Hyoscine Butylbromide** *see* Scopolamine *on page 1152*
- **Hyoscine Hydrobromide** *see* Scopolamine *on page 1152*
- **Hyperal** *see* Total Parenteral Nutrition *on page 1293*
- **Hyperalimentation** *see* Total Parenteral Nutrition *on page 1293*
- **HyperHep B® (Can)** *see* Hepatitis B Immune Globulin *on page 618*
- **Hytone®** *see* Hydrocortisone *on page 639*
- **Hytrin®** *see* Terazosin *on page 1243*
- **Ibidomide Hydrochloride** *see* Labetalol *on page 721*
- **Ibu-200 [OTC]** *see* Ibuprofen *on page 651*

Ibuprofen (eye byoo PROE fen)

Medication Safety Issues

Sound-alike/look-alike issues:

Haltran® may be confused with Halfprin®

Related Information

Acetaminophen and NSAIDS, Dosing Data *on page 1543*

Acute Postoperative Pain *on page 1388*

Anesthesia for Patients With Liver Disease *on page 1421*

Chronic Pain Management *on page 1430*

U.S. Brand Names Advil® [OTC]; Advil® Children's [OTC]; Advil® Infants' [OTC]; Advil® Junior [OTC]; Advil® Migraine [OTC]; ElixSure™ IB [OTC]; Genpril® [OTC]; Ibu-200 [OTC]; I-Prin [OTC]; Midol® Cramp and Body Aches [OTC]; Motrin®; (Continued)

Ibuprofen *(Continued)*

Motrin® Children's [OTC]; Motrin® IB [OTC]; Motrin® Infants' [OTC]; Motrin® Junior Strength [OTC]; NeoProfen®; Proprinal [OTC]; Ultraprin [OTC]

Canadian Brand Names Advil®; Apo-Ibuprofen®; Motrin® (Children's); Motrin® IB; Novo-Profen; Nu-Ibuprofen

Synonyms Ibuprofen Lysine; *p*-Isobutylhydratropic Acid

Pharmacologic Category Nonsteroidal Anti-inflammatory Drug (NSAID), Oral; Nonsteroidal Anti-inflammatory Drug (NSAID), Parenteral

Restrictions A medication guide should be dispensed with each prescription for oral administration. A template for the required MedGuide can be found on the FDA website at: http://www.fda.gov/medwatch/SAFETY/2005/safety05.htm#NSAID

Generic Available Yes: Caplet, suspension, tablet

Use

Oral: Inflammatory diseases and rheumatoid disorders including juvenile rheumatoid arthritis, mild-to-moderate pain, fever, dysmenorrhea

Injection: Ibuprofen lysine is for use in premature infants weighing between 500-1500 g and who are ≤32 weeks gestational age (GA) to induce closure of a clinically-significant patent ductus arteriosus (PDA) when usual treatments are ineffective

Unlabeled/Investigational Use Cystic fibrosis, gout, ankylosing spondylitis, acute migraine headache

Mechanism of Action Inhibits prostaglandin synthesis by decreasing the activity of the enzyme, cyclooxygenase, which results in decreased formation of prostaglandin precursors

Pharmacodynamics/Kinetics

Onset of action: Analgesic: 30-60 minutes; Anti-inflammatory: ≤7 days
- Peak effect: 1-2 weeks

Duration: 4-6 hours

Absorption: Oral: Rapid (85%)

Distribution: Premature infants with ductal closure (highly variable between studies):
- Day 3: 145-349 mL/kg
- Day 5: 72-222 mL/kg

Protein binding: 90% to 99%

Metabolism: Hepatic via oxidation

Half-life elimination:
- Premature infants (highly variable between studies):
  - Day 3: 35-51 hours
  - Day 5: 20-33 hours
- Children 3 months to 10 years: 1.6 ± 0.7 hours
- Adults: 2-4 hours; End-stage renal disease: Unchanged

Time to peak: ~1-2 hours

Excretion: Urine (1% as free drug); some feces

Dosage

I.V.: Infants between 500-1500 g and ≤32 weeks GA: Patent ductus arteriosus: Initial dose: Ibuprofen 10 mg/kg, followed by two doses of 5 mg/kg at 24 and 48 hours. Dose should be based on birth weight.

Oral:

Children:
- Antipyretic: 6 months to 12 years: Temperature <102.5°F (39°C): 5 mg/kg/dose; temperature >102.5°F: 10 mg/kg/dose given every 6-8 hours (maximum daily dose: 40 mg/kg/day)
- Juvenile rheumatoid arthritis: 30-50 mg/kg/24 hours divided every 8 hours; start at lower end of dosing range and titrate upward (maximum: 2.4 g/day)
- Analgesic: 4-10 mg/kg/dose every 6-8 hours
- Cystic fibrosis (unlabeled use): Chronic (>4 years) twice daily dosing adjusted to maintain serum levels of 50-100 mcg/mL has been associated with slowing of disease progression in younger patients with mild lung disease
- OTC labeling (analgesic, antipyretic):
  - Children 6 months to 11 years: See table on next page; use of weight to select dose is preferred; doses may be repeated every 6-8 hours (maximum: 4 doses/day)
  - Children ≥12 years: 200 mg every 4-6 hours as needed (maximum: 1200 mg/24 hours)

Ibuprofen Dosing

Weight (lb)	Age	Dosage (mg)
12-17	6-11 mo	50
18-23	12-23 mo	75
24-35	2-3 y	100
35-47	4-5 y	150
48-59	6-8 y	200
60-71	9-10 y	250
72-95	11 y	300

Adults:

Inflammatory disease: 400-800 mg/dose 3-4 times/day (maximum dose: 3.2 g/day)

Analgesia/pain/fever/dysmenorrhea: 200-400 mg/dose every 4-6 hours (maximum daily dose: 1.2 g, unless directed by physician)

OTC labeling (analgesic, antipyretic): 200 mg every 4-6 hours as needed (maximum: 1200 mg/24 hours)

Dosing adjustment/comments in severe hepatic impairment: Avoid use

Stability Injection: Store at room temperature of 20°C to 25°C (68°F to 77°F); protect from light. Dilute with dextrose or saline to an appropriate volume. Following dilution, administer within 30 minutes of preparation.

Administration

Oral: Administer with food

I.V.: For I.V. administration only; administration via umbilical line has not been evaluated. Infuse over 15 minutes through port closest to insertion site. Avoid extravasation. Do not administer simultaneously via same line with TPN. If needed, interrupt TPN for 15 minutes prior to and after ibuprofen administration, keeping line open with dextrose or saline.

Monitoring Parameters CBC; occult blood loss and periodic liver function tests; monitor response (pain, range of motion, grip strength, mobility, ADL function), inflammation; observe for weight gain, edema; monitor renal function (urine output, serum BUN and creatinine); observe for bleeding, bruising; evaluate gastrointestinal effects (abdominal pain, bleeding, dyspepsia); mental confusion, disorientation; with long-term therapy, periodic ophthalmic exams

Injection: Renal function, signs of infection or bleeding, ECG

Reference Range Plasma concentrations >200 mcg/mL may be associated with severe toxicity

PDA: Minimum effective level: 10-12 mg/L

Anesthesia and Critical Care Concerns/Other Considerations The 2002 ACCM/SCCM guidelines for analgesia (critically-ill adult) suggest that NSAIDs may be used in combination with opioids in select patients for pain management. Concern about adverse events (increased risk of renal dysfunction, altered platelet function and gastrointestinal irritation) limits its use in patients who have other underlying risks for these events.

In short-term use, NSAIDs vary considerably in their effect on blood pressure. When NSAIDs are used in patients with hypertension, appropriate monitoring of blood pressure responses should be completed and the duration of therapy, when possible, kept short. The use of NSAIDs in the treatment of patients with congestive heart failure may be associated with an increased risk for fluid accumulation and edema. May precipitate renal failure in dehydrated patients.

Pregnancy Risk Factor C/D (3rd trimester)

Contraindications Hypersensitivity to ibuprofen, aspirin, other NSAIDs, or any component of the formulation; perioperative pain in the setting of coronary artery bypass surgery (CABG); pregnancy (3rd trimester)

Ibuprofen lysine is contraindicated in preterm infants with untreated proven or suspected infection; congenital heart disease where patency of the PDA is necessary for pulmonary or systemic blood flow; bleeding (especially with active intracranial hemorrhage or GI bleed); thrombocytopenia; coagulation defects; proven or suspected necrotizing enterocolitis (NEC); significant renal dysfunction

Warnings/Precautions **[U.S. Boxed Warning]: NSAIDs are associated with an increased risk of adverse cardiovascular events, including MI, stroke, and new onset or worsening of pre-existing hypertension.** Risk may be

(Continued)

Ibuprofen *(Continued)*

increased with duration of use or pre-existing cardiovascular risk-factors or disease. Carefully evaluate individual cardiovascular risk profiles prior to prescribing. Use caution with fluid retention, CHF or hypertension.

Use of NSAIDs can compromise existing renal function. Renal toxicity can occur in patient with impaired renal function, dehydration, heart failure, liver dysfunction, those taking diuretics and ACEI and the elderly. Rehydrate patient before starting therapy. Monitor renal function closely. Ibuprofen is not recommended for patients with advanced renal disease.

NSAIDs may increase risk of gastrointestinal irritation, ulceration, bleeding, and perforation. These events may occur at any time during therapy and without warning. Use caution with a history of GI disease (bleeding or ulcers), concurrent therapy with aspirin, anticoagulants and/or corticosteroids, smoking, use of alcohol, the elderly or debilitated patients.

Use the lowest effective dose for the shortest duration of time, consistent with individual patient goals, to reduce risk of cardiovascular or GI adverse events. Alternate therapies should be considered for patients at high risk.

NSAIDs may cause serious skin adverse events including exfoliative dermatitis, Stevens-Johnson syndrome (SJS) and toxic epidermal necrolysis (TEN). Anaphylactoid reactions may occur, even without prior exposure; patients with "aspirin triad" (bronchial asthma, aspirin intolerance, rhinitis) may be at increased risk. Do not use in patients who experience bronchospasm, asthma, rhinitis, or urticaria with NSAID or aspirin therapy.

Use with caution in patients with decreased hepatic function. Closely monitor patients with any abnormal LFT. Severe hepatic reactions (eg, fulminant hepatitis, liver failure) have occurred with NSAID use, rarely; discontinue if signs or symptoms of liver disease develop, or if systemic manifestations occur.

The elderly are at increased risk for adverse effects (especially peptic ulceration, CNS effects, renal toxicity) from NSAIDs even at low doses.

Withhold for at least 4-6 half-lives prior to surgical or dental procedures.

Injection: Hold second or third doses if urinary output is <0.6 mL/kg/hour. May alter signs of infection. May inhibit platelet aggregation; monitor for signs of bleeding. May displace bilirubin; use caution when total bilirubin is elevated. Long-term evaluations of neurodevelopment, growth, or diseases associated with prematurity following treatment have not been conducted. A second course of treatment, alternative pharmacologic therapy or surgery may be needed if the ductus arteriosus fails to close or reopens following the initial course of therapy.

OTC labeling: Prior to self-medication, patients should contact health care provider if they have had recurring stomach pain or upset, ulcers, bleeding problems, high blood pressure, heart or kidney disease, other serious medical problems, are currently taking a diuretic, or are ≥60 years of age. Recommended dosages should not be exceeded, due to an increased risk of GI bleeding. Consuming ≥3 alcoholic beverages/day or taking longer than recommended may increase the risk of GI bleeding. When used for self-medication, patients should contact healthcare provider if used for fever lasting >3 days or for pain lasting >10 days in adults or >3 days in children. In children with a sore throat, do not use for >2 days or administer to children <3 years of age unless instructed by healthcare provider. Consult healthcare provider when sore throat pain is severe, persistent, or accompanied by fever, headache, nausea, and/or vomiting. Notify healthcare provider of worsening stomach pain, feeling faint, vomiting of blood or bloody black stools.

Adverse Reactions

Oral:

1% to 10%:

- Cardiovascular: Edema (1% to 3%)
- Central nervous system: Dizziness (3% to 9%), headache (1% to 3%), nervousness (1% to 3%)
- Dermatologic: Itching (1% to 3%), rash (3% to 9%)
- Endocrine & metabolic: Fluid retention (1% to 3%)
- Gastrointestinal: Dyspepsia (1% to 3%), vomiting (1% to 3%), abdominal pain/cramps/distress (1% to 3%), heartburn (3% to 9%), nausea (3% to 9%), diarrhea (1% to 3%), constipation (1% to 3%), flatulence (1% to 3%), epigastric pain (3% to 9%), appetite decreased (1% to 3%)

Otic: Tinnitus (3% to 9%)

<1% (Limited to important or life-threatening): Acute renal failure, agranulocytosis, anaphylaxis, aplastic anemia, azotemia, blurred vision, bone marrow suppression, confusion, creatinine clearance decreased, duodenal ulcer, edema, eosinophilia, epistaxis, erythema multiforme, gastric ulcer, GI bleed, GI hemorrhage, GI ulceration, hallucinations, hearing decreased, hematuria, hematocrit decreased, hemoglobin decreased, hemolytic anemia, hepatitis, hypertension, inhibition of platelet aggregation, jaundice, liver function tests abnormal, leukopenia, melena, neutropenia, pancreatitis, photosensitivity, Stevens-Johnson syndrome, thrombocytopenia, toxic amblyopia, toxic epidermal necrolysis, urticaria, vesiculobullous eruptions, vision changes

Injection:

>10%:

Cardiovascular: Intraventricular hemorrhage (29%; grade 3/4: 15%)
Dermatologic: Skin irritation (16%)
Endocrine & metabolic: Hypocalcemia (12%), hypoglycemia (12%)
Gastrointestinal: GI disorders, non NEC (22%)
Hematologic: Anemia (32%)
Respiratory: Apnea (28%), respiratory infection (19%)
Miscellaneous: Sepsis (43%)

1% to 10%:

Cardiovascular: Edema (4%)
Endocrine & metabolic: Adrenal insufficiency (7%), hypernatremia (7%)
Genitourinary: Urinary tract infection (9%)
Renal: Urea increased (7%), renal impairment (6%), creatinine increased (3%), urine output decreased (3%; small decrease reported on days 2-6 with compensatory increase in output on day 9)
Respiratory: Respiratory failure (10%), atelectasis (4%)

Frequency not defined: Abdominal distension, cardiac failure, cholestasis, convulsions, feeding problems, gastritis, GI reflux, hyperglycemia, hypotension, ileus, infection, inguinal hernia, injection-site reaction, jaundice, neutropenia, tachycardia, thrombocytopenia

Overdosage/Toxicology Symptoms of overdose include apnea, metabolic acidosis, coma, nystagmus, seizures, leukocytosis, and renal failure. Management of NSAID intoxication is supportive and symptomatic. Since many NSAIDs undergo enterohepatic cycling, multiple doses of charcoal may be needed to reduce the potential for delayed toxicities.

Drug Interactions Substrate (minor) of CYP2C9, 2C19; **Inhibits** CYP2C9 (strong)

ACE inhibitors: Antihypertensive effects may be decreased by concurrent therapy with NSAIDs; monitor blood pressure.

Aminoglycosides: NSAIDs may decrease the excretion of aminoglycosides; this is of particular concern in preterm infants.

Angiotensin II antagonists: Antihypertensive effects may be decreased by concurrent therapy with NSAIDs; monitor blood pressure.

Anticoagulants (warfarin, heparin, LMWHs) in combination with NSAIDs can cause increased risk of bleeding.

Antiplatelet drugs (ticlopidine, clopidogrel, aspirin, abciximab, dipyridamole, eptifibatide, tirofiban) can cause an increased risk of bleeding.

Aspirin: Ibuprofen and other COX-1 inhibitors may reduce the cardioprotective effects of aspirin. Avoid giving prior to aspirin therapy or on a regular basis in patients with CAD.

Beta-blockers: NSAIDs may decrease the antihypertensive effect of beta-blockers. Monitor.

Bisphosphonate derivatives: NSAIDs may enhance the adverse/toxic effect of bisphosphonate derivatives. An increased incidence of gastrointestinal ulceration is of concern.

Cholestyramine (and other bile acid sequestrants): May decrease the absorption of NSAIDs. Separate by at least 2 hours.

Corticosteroids: May increase the risk of GI ulceration; avoid concurrent use

Cyclosporine: NSAIDs may increase serum creatinine, potassium, blood pressure, and cyclosporine levels; monitor cyclosporine levels and renal function carefully.

CYP2C9 Substrates: Ibuprofen may increase the levels/effects of CYP2C9 substrates. Example substrates include bosentan, dapsone, fluoxetine, glimepiride, glipizide, losartan, montelukast, nateglinide, paclitaxel, phenytoin, warfarin, and zafirlukast.

(Continued)

Ibuprofen *(Continued)*

Hydralazine's antihypertensive effect is decreased; avoid concurrent use

Lithium levels can be increased; avoid concurrent use if possible or monitor lithium levels and adjust dose. Sulindac may have the least effect. When NSAID is stopped, lithium will need adjustment again.

Loop diuretics efficacy (diuretic and antihypertensive effect) is reduced. Indomethacin reduces this efficacy, however, it may be anticipated with any NSAID.

Methotrexate: Severe bone marrow suppression, aplastic anemia, and GI toxicity have been reported with concomitant NSAID therapy. Avoid use during moderate or high-dose methotrexate (increased and prolonged methotrexate levels). NSAID use during low-dose treatment of rheumatoid arthritis has not been fully evaluated; extreme caution is warranted.

Pemetrexed: NSAIDs may decrease the excretion of pemetrexed.

Probenecid: Probenecid may increase the serum concentration of NSAIDs.

Vancomycin: NSAIDs may decrease the excretion of vancomycin; this is of particular concern in preterm infants.

Warfarin's INRs may be increased by piroxicam. Other NSAIDs may have the same effect depending on dose and duration. Monitor INR closely. Use the lowest dose of NSAIDs possible and for the briefest duration. May alter the anticoagulant effects of warfarin; concurrent use with other antiplatelet agents or anticoagulants may increase risk of bleeding.

Ethanol/Nutrition/Herb Interactions

Ethanol: Avoid ethanol (may enhance gastric mucosal irritation).

Food: Ibuprofen peak serum levels may be decreased if taken with food.

Herb/Nutraceutical: Avoid alfalfa, anise, bilberry, bladderwrack, bromelain, cat's claw, celery, coleus, cordyceps, dong quai, evening primrose, feverfew, fenugreek, garlic, ginger, ginkgo biloba, red clover, horse chestnut, grapeseed, green tea, ginseng, guggul, horse chestnut seed, horseradish, licorice, prickly ash, red clover, reishi, SAMe, sweet clover, turmeric, white willow (all have additional antiplatelet activity).

Dietary Considerations Should be taken with food. Chewable tablets may contain phenylalanine; amount varies by product, consult manufacturers labeling.

Dosage Forms

Caplet: 200 mg [OTC]
- Advil®: 200 mg [contains sodium benzoate]
- Ibu-200, Motrin® IB: 200 mg
- Motrin® Junior Strength: 100 mg

Capsule, liqui-gel:
- Advil®: 200 mg
- Advil® Migraine: 200 mg [solubilized ibuprofen; contains potassium 20 mg]

Gelcap:
- Advil®: 200 mg [contains coconut oil]

Injection, solution, as lysine [preservative free]:
- NeoProfen®: 17.1 mg/mL (2 mL) [equivalent to ibuprofen 10 mg/mL]

Suspension, oral: 100 mg/5 mL (5 mL, 120 mL, 480 mL)
- Advil® Children's: 100 mg/5 mL (60 mL, 120 mL) [contains sodium benzoate; blue raspberry, fruit, and grape flavors]
- ElixSure™ IB: 100 mg/5 mL (120 mL) [berry flavor]
- Motrin® Children's: 100 mg/5 mL (60 mL, 120 mL) [contains sodium benzoate; berry, dye free berry, bubble gum, and grape flavors]

Suspension, oral drops: 40 mg/mL (15 mL)
- Advil® Infants': 40 mg/mL (15 mL) [contains sodium benzoate; fruit and grape flavors]
- Motrin® Infants': 40 mg/mL (15 mL, 30 mL) [contains sodium benzoate; berry and dye-free berry flavors]

Tablet: 200 mg [OTC], 400 mg, 600 mg, 800 mg
- Advil®: 200 mg [contains sodium benzoate]
- Advil® Junior: 100 mg [contains sodium benzoate; coated tablets]
- Genpril®, I-Prin, Midol® Cramp and Body Aches, Motrin® IB, Proprinal, Ultraprin: 200 mg
- Motrin®: 400 mg, 600 mg, 800 mg

Tablet, chewable:
- Advil® Children's: 50 mg [contains phenylalanine 2.1 mg; grape flavors]
- Advil® Junior: 100 mg [contains phenylalanine 4.2 mg; grape flavors]
- Motrin® Children's: 50 mg [contains phenylalanine 1.4 mg; grape and orange flavor]

Motrin® Junior Strength: 100 mg [contains phenylalanine 2.1 mg; grape and orange flavors]

- **Ibuprofen Lysine** *see* Ibuprofen *on page 651*

Ibutilide (i BYOO ti lide)

Related Information

Management of Postoperative Arrhythmias *on page 1451*

U.S. Brand Names Corvert®

Synonyms Ibutilide Fumarate

Pharmacologic Category Antiarrhythmic Agent, Class III

Generic Available No

Use Acute termination of atrial fibrillation or flutter of recent onset; the effectiveness of ibutilide has not been determined in patients with arrhythmias >90 days in duration

Mechanism of Action Exact mechanism of action is unknown; prolongs the action potential in cardiac tissue

Pharmacodynamics/Kinetics

Onset of action: ~90 minutes after start of infusion ($^1/_2$ of conversions to sinus rhythm occur during infusion)

Distribution: V_d: 11 L/kg

Protein binding: 40%

Metabolism: Extensively hepatic; oxidation

Half-life elimination: 2-12 hours (average: 6 hours)

Excretion: Urine (82%, 7% as unchanged drug and metabolites); feces (19%)

Dosage I.V.: Initial:

Adults:

<60 kg: 0.01 mg/kg over 10 minutes

≥60 kg: 1 mg over 10 minutes

If the arrhythmia does not terminate within 10 minutes after the end of the initial infusion, a second infusion of equal strength may be infused over a 10-minute period

Elderly: Dose selection should be cautious, usually starting at the lower end of the dosing range.

Stability Admixtures are chemically and physically stable for 24 hours at room temperature and for 48 hours at refrigerated temperatures

Administration May be administered undiluted or diluted in 50 mL diluent (0.9% NS or D_5W); infuse over 10 minutes

Monitoring Parameters Observe patient with continuous ECG monitoring for at least 4 hours following infusion or until QT_c has returned to baseline; skilled personnel and proper equipment should be available during administration of ibutilide and subsequent monitoring of the patient

Anesthesia and Critical Care Concerns/Other Considerations Ibutilide may lower the energy requirement for direct current cardioversion in atrial fibrillation; effective for termination of postsurgical atrial fibrillation or atrial flutter, but at the risk of precipitating ventricular arrhythmias.

Pregnancy Risk Factor C

Contraindications Hypersensitivity to ibutilide or any component of the formulation; QT_c >440 msec

Warnings/Precautions **[U.S. Boxed Warning]: Potentially fatal arrhythmias (eg, polymorphic ventricular tachycardia) can occur with ibutilide, usually in association with torsade de pointes (QT prolongation).** Studies indicate a 1.7% incidence of arrhythmias in treated patients. The drug should be given in a setting of continuous ECG monitoring and by personnel trained in treating arrhythmias particularly polymorphic ventricular tachycardia. **[U.S. Boxed Warning]: Patients with chronic atrial fibrillation may not be the best candidates for ibutilide since they often revert after conversion and the risks of treatment may not be justified when compared to alternative management.** Dosing adjustments are not required in patients with renal or hepatic dysfunction since a maximum of only two 10-minute infusions are utilized. Drug distribution, rather than administration, is one of the primary mechanisms responsible for termination of the pharmacologic effect. Use caution in elderly patients. Safety and efficacy in children have not been established. Avoid any drug that can prolong QT interval. Correct hyperkalemia and hypomagnesemia before using. Monitor for heart block.

(Continued)

Ibutilide *(Continued)*

Adverse Reactions

1% to 10%:

Cardiovascular: Sustained polymorphic ventricular tachycardia (ie, torsade de pointes) (2%, often requiring cardioversion), nonsustained polymorphic ventricular tachycardia (3%), nonsustained monomorphic ventricular tachycardia (5%), ventricular extrasystoles (5%), nonsustained monomorphic VT (5%), tachycardia/supraventricular tachycardia (3%), hypotension (2%), bundle branch block (2%), AV block (2%), bradycardia (1%), QT segment prolongation, hypertension (1%), palpitation (1%)

Central nervous system: Headache (4%)

Gastrointestinal: Nausea (>1%)

<1% (Limited to important or life-threatening): CHF, erythematous bullous lesions, idioventricular rhythm, nodal arrhythmia, renal failure, supraventricular extrasystoles, sustained monomorphic ventricular tachycardia, syncope (0.3%, not > placebo)

Overdosage/Toxicology Symptoms of overdose include CNS depression, rapid gasping breathing, and convulsions. Arrhythmias occur. Treatment is supportive. Antiarrhythmics are generally avoided.

Drug Interactions

Antiarrhythmics: Class Ia antiarrhythmic drugs (disopyramide, quinidine, and procainamide) and other class III drugs such as amiodarone and sotalol, should not be given concomitantly with ibutilide due to their potential to prolong refractoriness.

Other drugs which may prolong QT interval: Phenothiazines, tricyclic and tetracyclic antidepressants, and cisapride, sparfloxacin, gatifloxacin, moxifloxacin, erythromycin may increase risk of toxicity; avoid concurrent use.

Digoxin: Signs of digoxin toxicity may be masked when coadministered with ibutilide.

Dosage Forms Injection, solution, as fumarate: 0.1 mg/mL (10 mL)

- ♦ **Ibutilide Fumarate** *see* Ibutilide *on page 657*
- ♦ **ICI-182,780** *see* Fulvestrant *on page 571*
- ♦ **IgG4-Kappa Monoclonal Antibody** *see* Natalizumab *on page 904*

Iloprost (EYE loe prost)

U.S. Brand Names Ventavis™

Synonyms Iloprost Tromethamine; Prostacyclin PGI_2

Pharmacologic Category Prostaglandin

Generic Available No

Use Treatment of idiopathic pulmonary arterial hypertension in patients with NYHA Class III or IV symptoms

Mechanism of Action Acutely, iloprost dilates systemic and pulmonary arterial vascular beds. In longer-term use, alters pulmonary vascular resistance and suppresses vascular smooth muscle proliferation. In addition, it is a potent endogenous inhibitor of platelet aggregation.

Pharmacodynamics/Kinetics

Duration: 30-90 minutes

Protein binding: ~60%, primarily to albumin

Metabolism: Hepatic via beta oxidation of the carboxyl side chain; main metabolite, tetranor-iloprost (inactive in animal studies)

Half-life elimination: 20-30 minutes

Dosage Inhalation: Adults: Initial: 2.5 mcg/dose; if tolerated, increase to 5 mcg/dose; administer 6-9 times daily (dosing at intervals ≥2 hours while awake); maintenance dose: 5 mcg/dose; maximum daily dose: 45 mcg

Dosage adjustment in renal impairment: Adjustments are not necessary. Use caution in dialysis patients; may be more susceptible to hypotension.

Dosage adjustment in hepatic impairment: Use caution

Stability Store at 15°C to 30°C (59°F to 86°F)

Administration Do not mix with other medications. For inhalation only via the I-neb® AAD® system or Prodose® ADD® system. Transfer entire contents of ampul into the medication chamber. Only use 1 mL ampul with I-neb® ADD® system. After use, discard remainder of the medicine; not for reuse.

Monitoring Parameters Vital signs at baseline, with initiation and dosage adjustments. Monitor for improvements in pulmonary function, improved exercise tolerance, NYHA Class improvement; side effects

Pregnancy Risk Factor C

Contraindications Hypersensitivity to iloprost or any component of the formulation

Warnings/Precautions Intended for inhalation administration using the I-neb® AAD® system or Prodose® ADD® drug delivery system. Monitor vital signs during initiation. Avoid use in patients with hypotension (systolic BP <85 mm Hg). Use caution with concurrent conditions or medications that may increase risk of syncope. Dosage or therapy adjustment may be required if exertional syncope occurs. If pulmonary edema occurs during administration, discontinue therapy. Use caution in patients with active bleeding or at increased risk of bleeding; potent inhibitor of platelet aggregation. Use caution in dialysis patients and in those with Child Pugh Class B and C hepatic dysfunction. Safety and efficacy have not been established in patients with other concurrent pulmonary diseases (eg, COPD, severe asthma, or acute infections). Safety and efficacy in pediatric patients have not been established.

Adverse Reactions

>10%:

Cardiovascular: Flushing (27%), hypotension (11%)
Central nervous system: Headache (30%)
Gastrointestinal: Nausea (13%)
Neuromuscular & skeletal: Trismus (12%)
Respiratory: Cough increased (39%)
Miscellaneous: Flu-like syndrome (14%), jaw pain (12%)

1% to 10%:

Cardiovascular: Syncope (8%), palpitation (7%)
Central nervous system: Insomnia (8%)
Gastrointestinal: Vomiting (7%)
Hepatic: Alkaline phosphatase increased (6%), GGT increased (6%)
Neuromuscular & skeletal: Back pain (7%), muscle cramps (6%)
Respiratory: Hemoptysis (5%), pneumonia (4%)

<1% (Limited to important or life-threatening): Chest pain, CHF, dyspnea, kidney failure, paradoxical reaction (increased PVR), peripheral edema, supraventricular tachycardia

Overdosage/Toxicology Treatment is symptom-directed and supportive.

Drug Interactions

Anticoagulants and antiplatelet agents: Increased risk of bleeding with concurrent use of iloprost.

Antihypertensives: Hypotensive effects of iloprost may be exacerbated by concurrent use of antihypertensives.

Vasodilators: Hypotensive effects of iloprost may be exacerbated by concurrent use of other vasodilators.

Dosage Forms Solution for oral inhalation [preservative-free]: 10 mcg/mL (1 mL, 2 mL) [ampul]

References

Badesch DB, Abman SH, Ahearn GS, et al, "Medical Therapy for Pulmonary Arterial Hypertension: ACCP Evidence-Based Clinical Practice Guidelines," *Chest*, 2004, 126(1 Suppl):35-62.

Emmel M, Keuth B, and Schickendantz S, "Paradoxical Increase of Pulmonary Vascular Resistance During Testing of Inhaled Iloprost," *Heart*, 2004, 90(1):e2.

Humbert M, Sitbon O, and Simmoneau G, "Treatment of Pulmonary Arterial hypertension," *N Engl J Med*, 2004, 351(14):1425-36.

Olschewski H, Simonneau G, Galie N, et al, "Inhaled Iloprost for Severe Pulmonary Hypertension," *N Engl J Med*, 2002, 347(5):322-9.

♦ **Iloprost Tromethamine** *see* Iloprost *on page 658*

♦ **Imipemide** *see* Imipenem and Cilastatin *on page 659*

Imipenem and Cilastatin (i mi PEN em & sye la STAT in)

Medication Safety Issues

Sound-alike/look-alike issues:

Primaxin® may be confused with Premarin®, Primacor®

(Continued)

Imipenem and Cilastatin *(Continued)*

U.S. Brand Names Primaxin®

Canadian Brand Names Primaxin®; Primaxin® I.V.

Synonyms Imipemide

Pharmacologic Category Antibiotic, Carbapenem

Generic Available No

Use Treatment of respiratory tract, urinary tract, intra-abdominal, gynecologic, bone and joint, skin structure, and polymicrobic infections as well as bacterial septicemia and endocarditis. Antibacterial activity includes resistant gram-negative bacilli (*Pseudomonas aeruginosa* and *Enterobacter* sp), gram-positive bacteria (methicillin-sensitive *Staphylococcus aureus* and *Streptococcus* sp) and anaerobes.

Mechanism of Action Inhibits bacterial cell wall synthesis by binding to one or more of the penicillin binding proteins (PBPs); which in turn inhibits the final transpeptidation step of peptidoglycan synthesis in bacterial cell walls, thus inhibiting cell wall biosynthesis. Bacteria eventually lyse due to ongoing activity of cell wall autolytic enzymes (autolysins and murein hydrolases) while cell wall assembly is arrested. Cilastatin prevents renal metabolism of imipenem by competitive inhibition of dehydropeptidase along the brush border of the renal tubules.

Pharmacodynamics/Kinetics

Absorption: I.M.: Imipenem: 60% to 75%; cilastatin: 95% to 100%

Distribution: Rapidly and widely to most tissues and fluids including sputum, pleural fluid, peritoneal fluid, interstitial fluid, bile, aqueous humor, reproductive organs, and bone; highest concentrations in pleural fluid, interstitial fluid, peritoneal fluid, and reproductive organs; low concentrations in CSF; crosses placenta; enters breast milk

Metabolism: Renally by dehydropeptidase; activity is blocked by cilastatin; cilastatin is partially metabolized renally

Half-life elimination: Both drugs: 60 minutes; prolonged with renal impairment

Excretion: Both drugs: Urine (~70% as unchanged drug)

Dosage

Usual dosage ranges: Note: Dosage based on **imipenem** content:

Neonates: Non-CNS infections: I.V.:

- <1 week: 25 mg/kg every 12 hours
- 1-4 weeks: 25 mg/kg every 8 hours
- 4 weeks to 3 months: 25 mg/kg every 6 hours

Children >3 months: Non-CNS infections: I.V.: 15-25 mg/kg every 6 hours; maximum dosage: Susceptible infections: 2 g/day; moderately-susceptible organisms: 4 g/day

Adults: **Note:** For adults weighing <70 kg, refer to Dosing Adjustment in Renal Impairment:

- I.M.: 500-750 mg every 12 hours
- I.V.: 250-1000 mg every 6-8 hours; maximum: 50 mg/kg/day or 4 g/day, whichever is lower

Indication-specific dosing: Note: Doses based on imipenem content. I.M. administration is not intended for severe or life-threatening infections (eg, septicemia, endocarditis, shock):

Children: I.V.:

Burkholderia mallei (melioidosis): 20 mg/kg every 8 hours for 10 days

Cystic fibrosis: Doses up to 90 mg/kg/day have been used

Adults:

Burkholderia mallei (melioidosis): I.V.: 20 mg/kg every 8 hours for 10 days

Intra-abdominal infections: I.V.: Mild infection: 750 mg every 12 hours; severe: 500 mg every 6 hours

Liver abscess: I.V.: 500 mg every 6 hours for 2-3 weeks, then appropriate oral therapy for a total of 4-6 weeks

Mild infection: Note: Rarely a suitable option in mild infections; normally reserved for moderate-severe cases:

I.M.: 500 mg every 12 hours

I.V.:

Fully-susceptible organisms: 250 mg every 6 hours

Moderately-susceptible organisms: 500 mg every 6 hours

Moderate infection:

I.M.: 750 mg every 12 hours

I.V.:

Fully-susceptible organisms: 500 mg every 6-8 hours

Moderately-susceptible organisms: 500 mg every 6 hours or 1 g every 8 hours

Neutropenic fever, otitis externa, *Pseudomonas* infections: I.V.: 500 mg every 6 hours

Severe infection: I.V.:

Fully-susceptible organisms: 500 mg every 6 hours

Moderately-susceptible organisms: 1 g every 6-8 hours

Maximum daily dose should not exceed 50 mg/kg or 4 g/day, whichever is lower

Urinary tract infection: I.V.:

Uncomplicated: 250 mg every 6 hours

Complicated: 500 mg every 6 hours

Imipenem and Cilastatin Dosage in Renal Impairment

Reduced I.V. Dosage Regimen Based on Creatinine Clearance (mL/minute/1.73 m²) and/or Body Weight <70 kg					
	Body Weight (kg)				
	≥70	60	50	40	30
Total daily dose for normal renal function: 1 g/day					
Cl_{cr} ≥71	250 mg q6h	250 mg q8h	125 mg q6h	125 mg q6h	125 mg q8h
Cl_{cr} 41-70	250 mg q8h	125 mg q6h	125 mg q6h	125 mg q8h	125 mg q8h
Cl_{cr} 21-40	250 mg q12h	250 mg q12h	125 mg q8h	125 mg q12h	125 mg q12h
Cl_{cr} 6-20	250 mg q12h	125 mg q12h	125 mg q12h	125 mg q12h	125 mg q12h
Total daily dose for normal renal function: 1.5 g/day					
Cl_{cr} ≥71	500 mg q8h	250 mg q6h	250 mg q6h	250 mg q8h	125 mg q6h
Cl_{cr} 41-70	250 mg q6h	250 mg q8h	250 mg q8h	125 mg q6h	125 mg q8h
Cl_{cr} 21-40	250 mg q8h	250 mg q8h	250 mg q12h	125 mg q8h	125 mg q8h
Cl_{cr} 6-20	250 mg q12h	250 mg q12h	250 mg q12h	125 mg q12h	125 mg q12h
Total daily dose for normal renal function: 2 g/day					
Cl_{cr} ≥71	500 mg q6h	500 mg q8h	250 mg q6h	250 mg q6h	250 mg q8h
Cl_{cr} 41-70	500 mg q8h	250 mg q6h	250 mg q6h	250 mg q8h	125 mg q6h
Cl_{cr} 21-40	250 mg q6h	250 mg q8h	250 mg q8h	250 mg q12h	125 mg q8h
Cl_{cr} 6-20	250 mg q12h	250 mg q12h	250 mg q12h	250 mg q12h	125 mg q12h
Total daily dose for normal renal function: 3 g/day					
Cl_{cr} ≥71	1000 mg q8h	750 mg q8h	500 mg q6h	500 mg q8h	250 mg q6h
Cl_{cr} 41-70	500 mg q6h	500 mg q8h	500 mg q8h	250 mg q6h	250 mg q8h
Cl_{cr} 21-40	500 mg q8h	500 mg q8h	250 mg q6h	250 mg q8h	250 mg q8h
Cl_{cr} 6-20	500 mg q12h	500 mg q12h	250 mg q12h	250 mg q12h	250 mg q12h
Total daily dose for normal renal function: 4 g/day					
Cl_{cr} ≥71	1000 mg q6h	1000 mg q8h	750 mg q8h	500 mg q6h	500 mg q8h
Cl_{cr} 41-70	750 mg q8h	750 mg q8h	500 mg q6h	500 mg q8h	250 mg q6h
Cl_{cr} 21-40	500 mg q6h	500 mg q8h	500 mg q8h	250 mg q6h	250 mg q8h
Cl_{cr} 6-20	500 mg q12h	500 mg q12h	500 mg q12h	250 mg q12h	250 mg q12h

(Continued)

Imipenem and Cilastatin *(Continued)*

Dosage adjustment in renal impairment: I.V.: **Note:** Adjustments have not been established for I.M. dosing:

Patients with a Cl_{cr} <5 mL/minute/1.73 m^2 should not receive imipenem/cilastatin unless hemodialysis is instituted within 48 hours.

Patients weighing <30 kg with impaired renal function should not receive imipenem/cilastatin.

Hemodialysis: Use the dosing recommendation for patients with a Cl_{cr} 6-20 mL/minute

Peritoneal dialysis: Dose as for Cl_{cr} <10 mL/minute

Continuous arteriovenous or venovenous hemofiltration: Dose as for Cl_{cr} 20-30 mL/minute; monitor for seizure activity; imipenem is well removed by CAVH but cilastatin is not; removes 20 mg of imipenem per liter of filtrate per day

See table on previous page.

Stability Imipenem/cilastatin powder for injection should be stored at <25°C (77°F).

I.M.: Prepare 500 mg vial with 2 mL 1% lidocaine (do not use lidocaine with epinephrine). The I.V. formulation does not form a stable suspension in lidocaine and cannot be used to prepare an I.M dose. The I.M. suspension should be used within 1 hour of reconstitution.

I.V.: Prior to use, dilute dose into 100-250 mL of an appropriate solution. Imipenem is inactivated at acidic or alkaline pH. Final concentration should not exceed 5 mg/mL. The I.M. formulation is not buffered and cannot be used to prepare I.V. solutions. Reconstituted I.V. solutions are stable for 4 hours at room temperature and 24 hours when refrigerated. Do not freeze.

Administration

I.M.: **Note:** I.M. administration is not intended for severe or life-threatening infections (eg, septicemia, endocarditis, shock). Administer by deep injection into a large muscle (gluteal or lateral thigh). **Only the I.M. formulation can be used for I.M. administration.**

I.V.: Do not administer I.V. push. Infuse doses ≤500 mg over 20-30 minutes; infuse doses ≥750 mg over 40-60 minutes. **Only the I.V. formulation can be used for I.V. administration.**

Monitoring Parameters Periodic renal, hepatic, and hematologic function tests; monitor for signs of anaphylaxis during first dose

Pregnancy Risk Factor C

Contraindications Hypersensitivity to imipenem/cilastatin or any component of the formulation

Warnings/Precautions Dosage adjustment required in patients with impaired renal function; prolonged use may result in superinfection; has been associated with CNS adverse effects, including confusional states and seizures; use with caution in patients with a history of seizures or hypersensitivity to beta-lactams (including penicillins and cephalosporins); serious hypersensitivity reactions, including anaphylaxis, have been reported (some without a history of previous allergic reactions to beta-lactams); elderly patients often require lower doses (adjust carefully to renal function); not recommended in pediatric CNS infections. Doses for I.M. administration are mixed with lidocaine, consult information on lidocaine for associated warnings/precautions. Two different imipenem/cilastatin products are available; due to differences in formulation, the I.V. and I.M. preparations **cannot** be interchanged.

Adverse Reactions

1% to 10%:

Gastrointestinal: Nausea/diarrhea/vomiting (1% to 2%)

Local: Phlebitis (3%), pain at I.M. injection site (1%)

<1% (Limited to important or life-threatening): Anaphylaxis, angioneurotic edema, confusion (acute), drug fever, dyspnea, emergence of resistant strains of *P. aeruginosa*, encephalopathy, eosinophilia, erythema multiforme, hallucinations, hemolytic anemia, hemorrhagic colitis, hepatitis, hypersensitivity, hypotension, increased PT, jaundice, leukopenia, neutropenia (including agranulocytosis), pancytopenia, paresthesia, positive Coombs' test, pruritus, pseudomembranous colitis, psychic disturbances, rash, renal failure (acute), seizure, somnolence, Stevens-Johnson syndrome, thrombocytopenia, toxic epidermal necrolysis, urticaria, vertigo

Overdosage/Toxicology Symptoms of overdose include neuromuscular hypersensitivity and seizures. Hemodialysis may be helpful to aid in removal of the drug from blood; otherwise, treatment is supportive or symptom-directed.

Drug Interactions Valproic acid: Imipenem may decrease valproic acid concentrations to subtherapeutic levels; monitor.

Test Interactions Interferes with urinary glucose determination using Clinitest®

Dietary Considerations Sodium content of 500 mg injection:

I.M.: 32 mg (1.4 mEq)

I.V.: 37.5 mg (1.6 mEq)

Dosage Forms

Injection, powder for reconstitution [I.M.]: Imipenem 500 mg and cilastatin 500 mg [contains sodium 32 mg (1.4 mEq)]

Injection, powder for reconstitution [I.V.]: Imipenem 250 mg and cilastatin 250 mg [contains sodium 18.8 mg (0.8 mEq)]; imipenem 500 mg and cilastatin 500 mg [contains sodium 37.5 mg (1.6 mEq)]

References

American Thoracic Society and Infectious Diseases Society of America, "Guidelines for the Management of Adults With Hospital-Acquired, Ventilator-Associated, and Healthcare-Associated Pneumonia," *Am J Respir Crit Care Med*, 2005, 171(4):388-416.

Imipramine (im IP ra meen)

Medication Safety Issues

Sound-alike/look-alike issues:

Imipramine may be confused with amitriptyline, desipramine, Norpramin®

Related Information

Antidepressant Agents *on page 1551*

Chronic Pain Management *on page 1430*

U.S. Brand Names Tofranil®; Tofranil-PM®

Canadian Brand Names Apo-Imipramine®; Novo-Pramine; Tofranil®

Synonyms Imipramine Hydrochloride; Imipramine Pamoate

Pharmacologic Category Antidepressant, Tricyclic (Tertiary Amine)

Restrictions A medication guide concerning the use of antidepressants in children and teenagers can be found on the FDA website at http://www.fda.gov/cder/Offices/ODS/labeling.htm. It should be dispensed to parents or guardians of children and teenagers receiving this medication.

Generic Available Yes: Tablet

Use Treatment of depression; treatment of nocturnal enuresis in children

Unlabeled/Investigational Use Analgesic for certain chronic and neuropathic pain; panic disorder; attention-deficit/hyperactivity disorder (ADHD)

Mechanism of Action Traditionally believed to increase the synaptic concentration of serotonin and/or norepinephrine in the central nervous system by inhibition of their reuptake by the presynaptic neuronal membrane. However, additional receptor effects have been found including desensitization of adenyl cyclase, down regulation of beta-adrenergic receptors, and down regulation of serotonin receptors.

Pharmacodynamics/Kinetics

Onset of action: Peak antidepressant effect: Usually after ≥2 weeks

Absorption: Well absorbed

Distribution: Crosses placenta

Metabolism: Hepatic via CYP to desipramine (active) and other metabolites; significant first-pass effect

Half-life elimination: 6-18 hours

Excretion: Urine (as metabolites)

Dosage Oral:

Children:

Depression (unlabeled use): 1.5 mg/kg/day with dosage increments of 1 mg/kg every 3-4 days to a maximum dose of 5 mg/kg/day in 1-4 divided doses; monitor carefully especially with doses ≥3.5 mg/kg/day

Enuresis: ≥6 years: Initial: 25 mg at bedtime, if inadequate response still seen after 1 week of therapy, increase by 25 mg/day; dose should not exceed 2.5 mg/kg/day or 50 mg at bedtime if 6-12 years of age or 75 mg at bedtime if ≥12 years of age

Adjunct in the treatment of cancer pain (unlabeled use): Initial: 0.2-0.4 mg/kg at bedtime; dose may be increased by 50% every 2-3 days up to 1-3 mg/kg/dose at bedtime

Adolescents: Depression: Initial: 30-40 mg/day; increase gradually; maximum: 100 mg/day in single or divided doses

(Continued)

Imipramine *(Continued)*

Adults: Depression: Initial: 25 mg 3-4 times/day, increase dose gradually, total dose may be given at bedtime; maximum: 300 mg/day

Elderly: Initial: 10-25 mg at bedtime; increase by 10-25 mg every 3 days for inpatients and weekly for outpatients if tolerated; average daily dose to achieve a therapeutic concentration: 100 mg/day; range: 50-150 mg/day

Monitoring Parameters Monitor blood pressure and pulse rate prior to and during initial therapy; ECG in older adults; evaluate mental status; blood levels are useful for therapeutic monitoring

Reference Range Therapeutic: Imipramine and desipramine: 150-250 ng/mL (SI: 530-890 nmol/L); desipramine: 150-300 ng/mL (SI: 560-1125 nmol/L); Toxic: >500 ng/mL (SI: 446-893 nmol/L); utility of serum level monitoring controversial

Pregnancy Risk Factor D

Contraindications Hypersensitivity to imipramine (cross-reactivity with other dibenzodiazepines may occur) or any component of the formulation; concurrent use of MAO inhibitors (within 14 days); in a patient during acute recovery phase of MI; pregnancy

Warnings/Precautions [U.S. Boxed Warning]: Antidepressants increase the risk of suicidal thinking and behavior in children and adolescents with major depressive disorder (MDD) and other depressive disorders; consider risk prior to prescribing. Closely monitor for clinical worsening, suicidality, or unusual changes in behavior; the child's family or caregiver should be instructed to closely observe the patient and communicate condition with healthcare provider. Such observation would generally include at least weekly face-to-face contact with patients or their family members or caregivers during the first 4 weeks of treatment, then every other week visits for the next 4 weeks, then at 12 weeks, and as clinically indicated beyond 12 weeks. Additional contact by telephone may be appropriate between face-to-face visits. Adults treated with antidepressants should be observed similarly for clinical worsening and suicidality, especially during the initial few months of a course of drug therapy, or at times of dose changes, either increases or decreases. A medication guide should be dispensed with each prescription. **Imipramine is FDA approved for the treatment of nocturnal enuresis in children ≥6 years of age.**

The possibility of a suicide attempt is inherent in major depression and may persist until remission occurs. Monitor for worsening of depression or suicidality, especially during initiation of therapy or with dose increases or decreases. Worsening depression and severe abrupt suicidality that are not part of the presenting symptoms may require discontinuation or modification of drug therapy. Use caution in high-risk patients during initiation of therapy. Prescriptions should be written for the smallest quantity consistent with good patient care. The patient's family or caregiver should be alerted to monitor patients for the emergence of suicidality and associated behaviors such as anxiety, agitation, panic attacks, insomnia, irritability, hostility, impulsivity, akathisia, hypomania, and mania; patients should be instructed to notify their healthcare provider if any of these symptoms or worsening depression occur. May worsen psychosis in some patients or precipitate a shift to mania or hypomania in patients with bipolar disorder. Monotherapy in patients with bipolar disorder should be avoided. Patients presenting with depressive symptoms should be screened for bipolar disorder. **Imipramine is not FDA approved for the treatment of bipolar depression.**

May cause sedation, resulting in impaired performance of tasks requiring alertness (eg, operating machinery or driving). Sedative effects may be additive with other CNS depressants and/or ethanol. The degree of sedation is high relative to other antidepressants. May increase the risks associated with electroconvulsive therapy. Consider discontinuing, when possible, prior to elective surgery. Therapy should not be abruptly discontinued in patients receiving high doses for prolonged periods.

May cause orthostatic hypotension (risk is very high relative to other antidepressants) - use with caution in patients at risk of hypotension or in patients where transient hypotensive episodes would be poorly tolerated (cardiovascular disease or cerebrovascular disease). The degree of anticholinergic blockade produced by this agent is high relative to other cyclic antidepressants - use caution in patients with urinary retention, benign prostatic hyperplasia, narrow-angle glaucoma, xerostomia, visual problems, constipation, or history of bowel obstruction.

Use with caution in patients with a history of cardiovascular disease (including previous MI, stroke, tachycardia, or conduction abnormalities). The risk of conduction abnormalities with this agent is high relative to other antidepressants. ECG monitoring is recommended if high dosages are used. Use caution in patients with a previous seizure disorder or condition predisposing to seizures such as brain damage, alcoholism, or concurrent therapy with other drugs which lower the seizure threshold. Use with caution in hyperthyroid patients or those receiving thyroid supplementation. Use with caution in patients with hepatic or renal dysfunction and in elderly patients. Has been associated with photosensitization.

Adverse Reactions Frequency not defined.

Cardiovascular: Orthostatic hypotension, arrhythmia, tachycardia, hypertension, palpitation, MI, heart block, ECG changes, CHF, stroke

Central nervous system: Dizziness, drowsiness, headache, agitation, insomnia, nightmares, hypomania, psychosis, fatigue, confusion, hallucinations, disorientation, delusions, anxiety, restlessness, seizure

Endocrine & metabolic: Gynecomastia, breast enlargement, galactorrhea, increase or decrease in libido, increase or decrease in blood sugar, SIADH

Gastrointestinal: Nausea, unpleasant taste, weight gain/loss, xerostomia, constipation, ileus, stomatitis, abdominal cramps, vomiting, anorexia, epigastric disorders, diarrhea, black tongue

Genitourinary: Urinary retention, impotence

Neuromuscular & skeletal: Weakness, numbness, tingling, paresthesia, incoordination, ataxia, tremor, peripheral neuropathy, extrapyramidal symptoms

Ocular: Blurred vision, disturbances of accommodation, mydriasis

Otic: Tinnitus

Miscellaneous: Diaphoresis

<1% (Limited to important or life-threatening): Agranulocytosis, alopecia, cholestatic jaundice, eosinophilia, increased liver enzymes, itching, petechiae, photosensitivity, purpura, rash, thrombocytopenia, urticaria

Overdosage/Toxicology Symptoms of overdose include confusion, hallucinations, constipation, cyanosis, tachycardia, urinary retention, ventricular tachycardia, and seizures. Following initiation of essential overdose management, toxic symptoms should be treated. Ventricular arrhythmias often respond to concurrent systemic alkalinization (sodium bicarbonate 0.5-2 mEq/kg I.V.) Physostigmine (1-2 mg I.V. slowly for adults) may be indicated to reverse life-threatening cardiac arrhythmias.

Drug Interactions **Substrate** of CYP1A2 (minor), 2B6 (minor), 2C19 (major), 2D6 (major), 3A4 (minor); **Inhibits** CYP1A2 (weak), 2C19 (weak), 2D6 (moderate), 2E1 (weak)

Altretamine: Concurrent use may cause orthostatic hypertension

Amphetamines: TCAs may enhance the effect of amphetamines; monitor for adverse CV effects

Anticholinergics: Combined use with TCAs may produce additive anticholinergic effects

Antihypertensives: TCAs may inhibit the antihypertensive response to bethanidine, clonidine, debrisoquin, guanadrel, guanethidine, guanabenz, guanfacine; monitor BP; consider alternate antihypertensive agent

Beta-agonists: When combined with TCAs may predispose patients to cardiac arrhythmias

Bupropion: May increase the levels of tricyclic antidepressants; based on limited information; monitor response

Carbamazepine: Tricyclic antidepressants may increase carbamazepine levels; monitor

Cholestyramine and colestipol: May bind TCAs and reduce their absorption; monitor for altered response

Clonidine: Abrupt discontinuation of clonidine may cause hypertensive crisis, amitriptyline may enhance the response

CNS depressants: Amitriptyline may be additive with or may potentiate sedation; sedative effects may be additive with TCAs; monitor for increased effect; includes benzodiazepines, barbiturates, antipsychotics, ethanol, and other sedative medications

CYP2C19 inducers: May decrease the levels/effects of imipramine. Example inducers include aminoglutethimide, carbamazepine, phenytoin, and rifampin.

CYP2C19 inhibitors: May increase the levels/effects of imipramine. Example inhibitors include delavirdine, fluconazole, fluvoxamine, gemfibrozil, isoniazid, omeprazole, and ticlopidine.

(Continued)

Imipramine *(Continued)*

CYP2D6 inhibitors: May increase the levels/effects of imipramine. Example inhibitors include chlorpromazine, delavirdine, fluoxetine, miconazole, paroxetine, pergolide, quinidine, quinine, ritonavir, and ropinirole.

Epinephrine (and other direct alpha-agonists): The pressor response to I.V. epinephrine, norepinephrine, and phenylephrine may be enhanced in patients receiving TCAs; this combination is best avoided

Fenfluramine: May increase tricyclic antidepressant levels/effects

Hypoglycemic agents (including insulin): TCAs may enhance the hypoglycemic effects of tolazamide, chlorpropamide, or insulin; monitor for changes in blood glucose levels; reported with chlorpropamide, tolazamide, and insulin

Levodopa: Tricyclic antidepressants may decrease the absorption (bioavailability) of levodopa; rare hypertensive episodes have also been attributed to this combination

Linezolid: Hyperpyrexia, hypertension, tachycardia, confusion, seizures, and **deaths have been reported** with agents which inhibit MAO (serotonin syndrome); this combination should be avoided

Lithium: Concurrent use with a TCA may increase the risk for neurotoxicity

MAO inhibitors: Hyperpyrexia, hypertension, tachycardia, confusion, seizures, and **deaths have been reported** (serotonin syndrome); this combination should be avoided

Methylphenidate: Metabolism of TCAs may be decreased

Phenothiazines: Serum concentrations of some TCAs may be increased; in addition, TCAs may increase concentration of phenothiazines; monitor for altered clinical response

QT_c-prolonging agents: Concurrent use of tricyclic agents with other drugs which may prolong QT_c interval may increase the risk of potentially fatal arrhythmias; includes type Ia and type III antiarrhythmics agents, selected quinolones (sparfloxacin, gatifloxacin, moxifloxacin, grepafloxacin), cisapride, and other agents

Ritonavir: Combined use of high-dose tricyclic antidepressants with ritonavir may cause serotonin syndrome in HIV-positive patients; monitor

Sucralfate: Absorption of tricyclic antidepressants may be reduced with coadministration

Sympathomimetics, indirect-acting: Tricyclic antidepressants may result in a decreased sensitivity to indirect-acting sympathomimetics; includes dopamine and ephedrine; also see interaction with epinephrine (and direct-acting sympathomimetics)

Tramadol: Tramadol's risk of seizures may be increased with TCAs

Valproic acid: May increase serum concentrations/adverse effects of some tricyclic antidepressants

Warfarin (and other oral anticoagulants): TCAs may increase the anticoagulant effect in patients stabilized on warfarin; monitor INR

Ethanol/Nutrition/Herb Interactions

Ethanol: Avoid ethanol (may increase CNS depression).

Food: Grapefruit juice may inhibit the metabolism of some TCAs and clinical toxicity may result.

Herb/Nutraceutical: St John's wort may decrease imipramine levels. Avoid valerian, St John's wort, SAMe, kava kava (may increase risk of serotonin syndrome and/or excessive sedation).

Dosage Forms

Capsule, as pamoate (Tofranil-PM®): 75 mg, 100 mg, 125 mg, 150 mg

Tablet, as hydrochloride (Tofranil®): 10 mg, 25 mg, 50 mg [generic tablets may contain sodium benzoate]

- **Imipramine Hydrochloride** *see* Imipramine *on page 663*
- **Imipramine Pamoate** *see* Imipramine *on page 663*
- **Imitrex®** *see* Sumatriptan *on page 1222*
- **Imitrex® DF (Can)** *see* Sumatriptan *on page 1222*
- **Imitrex® Nasal Spray (Can)** *see* Sumatriptan *on page 1222*

Immune Globulin (Intravenous)

(i MYUN GLOB yoo lin, IN tra VEE nus)

Medication Safety Issues

Sound-alike/look-alike issues:

Gamimune® N may be confused with CytoGam®

U.S. Brand Names Carimune™ NF; Gammagard® Liquid; Gammagard® S/D; Gammar®-P I.V.; Gamunex®; Iveegam EN; Octagam®; Panglobulin® NF; Polygam® S/D

Canadian Brand Names Gamimune® N; Gammagard® Liquid; Gammagard® S/D; Gamunex®; Iveegam Immuno®

Synonyms IVIG

Pharmacologic Category Immune Globulin

Generic Available No

Use

Treatment of primary immunodeficiency syndromes (congenital agammaglobulinemia, severe combined immunodeficiency syndromes [SCIDS], common variable immunodeficiency, X-linked immunodeficiency, Wiskott-Aldrich syndrome); idiopathic thrombocytopenic purpura (ITP); Kawasaki disease (in combination with aspirin)

Prevention of bacterial infection in B-cell chronic lymphocytic leukemia (CLL); pediatric HIV infection; bone marrow transplant (BMT)

Unlabeled/Investigational Use Autoimmune diseases (myasthenia gravis, SLE, bullous pemphigoid, severe rheumatoid arthritis), Guillain-Barré syndrome; used in conjunction with appropriate anti-infective therapy to prevent or modify acute bacterial or viral infections in patients with iatrogenically-induced or disease-associated immunodepression; autoimmune hemolytic anemia or neutropenia, refractory dermatomyositis/polymyositis

Mechanism of Action Replacement therapy for primary and secondary immunodeficiencies; interference with F_c receptors on the cells of the reticuloendothelial system for autoimmune cytopenias and ITP; possible role of contained antiviral-type antibodies

Pharmacodynamics/Kinetics

Onset of action: I.V.: Provides immediate antibody levels

Duration: Immune effect: 3-4 weeks (variable)

Distribution: V_d: 0.09-0.13 L/kg

Intravascular portion (primarily): Healthy subjects: 41% to 57%; Patients with congenital humoral immunodeficiencies: ~70%

Half-life elimination: IgG (variable among patients): Healthy subjects: 14-24 days; Patients with congenital humoral immunodeficiencies: 26-40 days; hypermetabolism associated with fever and infection have coincided with a shortened half-life

Dosage Approved doses and regimens may vary between brands; check manufacturer guidelines. **Note:** Some clinicians dose IVIG on ideal body weight or an adjusted ideal body weight in morbidly obese patients.

Infants and Children: Prevention of gastroenteritis (unlabeled use): Oral: 50 mg/kg/day divided every 6 hours

Children: I.V.:

Pediatric HIV: 400 mg/kg every 28 days

Severe systemic viral and bacterial infections (unlabeled use): 500-1000 mg/kg/week

Children and Adults: I.V.:

Primary immunodeficiency disorders: 200-400 mg/kg every 4 weeks or as per monitored serum IgG concentrations

Gammagard® Liquid, Gamunex®, Octagam®: 300-600 mg/kg every 3-4 weeks; adjusted based on dosage and interval in conjunction with monitored serum IgG concentrations.

B-cell chronic lymphocytic leukemia (CLL): 400 mg/kg/dose every 3 weeks

Idiopathic thrombocytopenic purpura (ITP):

Acute: 400 mg/kg/day for 5 days or 1000 mg/kg/day for 1-2 days

Chronic: 400 mg/kg as needed to maintain platelet count >30,000/mm^3; may increase dose to 800 mg/kg (1000 mg/kg if needed)

Kawasaki disease: Initiate therapy within 10 days of disease onset: 2 g/kg as a single dose administered over 10 hours, or 400 mg/kg/day for 4 days. **Note:** Must be used in combination with aspirin: 80-100 mg/kg/day in 4 divided doses for 14 days; when fever subsides, dose aspirin at 3-5 mg/kg once daily for ≥6-8 weeks

Acquired immunodeficiency syndrome (patients must be symptomatic) (unlabeled use): Various regimens have been used, including:

200-250 mg/kg/dose every 2 weeks

or

400-500 mg/kg/dose every month or every 4 weeks

(Continued)

Immune Globulin (Intravenous) *(Continued)*

Autoimmune hemolytic anemia and neutropenia (unlabeled use): 1000 mg/kg/dose for 2-3 days

Autoimmune diseases (unlabeled use): 400 mg/kg/day for 4 days

Bone marrow transplant: 500 mg/kg beginning on days 7 and 2 pretransplant, then 500 mg/kg/week for 90 days post-transplant

Adjuvant to severe cytomegalovirus infections (unlabeled use): 500 mg/kg/dose every other day for 7 doses

Guillain-Barré syndrome (unlabeled use): Various regimens have been used, including:

400 mg/kg/day for 4 days

or

1000 mg/kg/day for 2 days

or

2000 mg/kg/day for one day

Refractory dermatomyositis (unlabeled use): 2 g/kg/dose every month x 3-4 doses

Refractory polymyositis (unlabeled use): 1 g/kg/day x 2 days every month x 4 doses

Chronic inflammatory demyelinating polyneuropathy (unlabeled use): Various regimens have been used, including:

400 mg/kg/day for 5 doses once each month

or

800 mg/kg/day for 3 doses once each month

or

1000 mg/kg/day for 2 days once each month

Dosing adjustment/comments in renal impairment: Cl_{cr} <10 mL/minute: Avoid use; in patients at risk of renal dysfunction, consider infusion at a rate less than maximum.

Stability Stability and dilution is dependent upon the manufacturer and brand; do not mix with other drugs; do not freeze; do not shake, avoid foaming; discard unused portion:

Carimune™ NF, Panglobulin® NF: Prior to reconstitution, store at or below 30°C (86°F). Reconstitute with NS, D_5W, or SWFI. Following reconstitution, store under refrigeration; use within 24 hours. Do not freeze.

Gammagard® Liquid: May be stored for up to 9 months at room temperature of 25°C (77°F) within 24 months of manufacture date. May be stored for up to 36 months under refrigeration at 2°C to 8°C (36°F to 46°F). May dilute in D_5W only. Do not freeze.

Gammagard® S/D, Polygam® S/D: Store below 25°C (77°F). Reconstitute with SWFI; may store diluted solution under refrigeration for up to 24 hours.

Gammar®-P I.V.: Store below 25°C (77°F). Reconstitute with SWFI.

Gamunex®: May be stored for up to 5 months at room temperature up to 25°C (up to 77°F) within 18 months of manufacture date.

Iveegam EN: Store at 2°C to 8°C (36°F to 46°F). Reconstitute with SWFI; use immediately after reconstitution.

Octagam®: Store at 2°C to 8°C (36°F to 46°F) for 24 months or ≤25°C (77°F) for 18 months.

Polygam® S/D: Store at room temperature at or below 25°C (77°F). Do not freeze.

Administration I.V. infusion over 2-24 hours; for initial treatment, a lower concentration and/or a slower rate of infusion should be used. Administer in separate infusion line from other medications; if using primary line, flush with saline prior administration. Refrigerated product should be warmed to room temperature prior to infusion. Decrease dose, rate and/or concentration of infusion in patients who may be at risk of renal failure. Decreasing the rate or stopping the infusion may help relieve some adverse effects (flushing, changes in pulse rate, changes in blood pressure). Epinephrine should be available during administration.

Monitoring Parameters Renal function, urine output, hemoglobin and hematocrit, infusion-related adverse reactions, anaphylaxis

Pregnancy Risk Factor C

Contraindications Hypersensitivity to immune globulin or any component of the formulation; selective IgA deficiency

Warnings/Precautions [U.S. Boxed Warning]: Acute renal dysfunction (increased serum creatinine, oliguria, acute renal failure) can rarely occur; usually within 7 days of use (more likely with products stabilized with

sucrose); use with caution in the elderly, patients with renal disease, diabetes mellitus, volume depletion, sepsis, paraproteinemia, and nephrotoxic medications due to risk of renal dysfunction. Anaphylactic hypersensitivity reactions can occur, especially in IgA-deficient patients; studies indicate that the currently available products have no discernible risk of transmitting HIV or hepatitis B; aseptic meningitis may occur with high doses (≥2 g/kg). Patients should be adequately hydrated prior to therapy. Use caution in patients with a history of thrombotic events or cardiovascular disease; there is clinical evidence of a possible association between thrombotic events and administration of intravenous immune globulin. For intravenous administration only.

Adverse Reactions Frequency not defined.

Cardiovascular: Flushing of the face, tachycardia, hyper-/hypotension, chest tightness, angioedema, lightheadedness, chest pain, MI, CHF, pulmonary embolism

Central nervous system: Anxiety, chills, dizziness, drowsiness, fatigue, fever, headache, irritability, lethargy, malaise, aseptic meningitis syndrome

Dermatologic: Pruritus, rash, urticaria

Gastrointestinal: Abdominal cramps, diarrhea, nausea, sore throat, vomiting

Hematologic: Autoimmune hemolytic anemia, hematocrit decreased, leukopenia, mild hemolysis

Hepatic: Liver function test increased

Local: Pain or irritation at the infusion site

Neuromuscular & skeletal: Arthralgia, back or hip pain, myalgia, nuchal rigidity

Ocular: Photophobia, painful eye movements

Renal: Acute renal failure, acute tubular necrosis, anuria, BUN increased, creatinine increased, nephrotic syndrome, oliguria, proximal tubular nephropathy, osmotic nephrosis

Respiratory: Cough, dyspnea, wheezing, nasal congestion, pharyngeal pain, rhinorrhea, sinusitis

Miscellaneous: Diaphoresis, hypersensitivity reactions, anaphylaxis

Postmarketing and/or case reports: Abdominal pain, apnea, ARDS, bronchospasm, bullous dermatitis, cardiac arrest, Coombs' test positive, cyanosis, epidermolysis, erythema multiforme, hepatic dysfunction, hypoxemia, leukopenia, loss of consciousness, pancytopenia, pulmonary edema, rigors, seizure, Stevens-Johnson syndrome, thromboembolism, transfusion-related acute lung injury (TRALI), tremor, vascular collapse

Drug Interactions Live virus, vaccines (eg, measles, mumps, rubella): May have impaired response to vaccines; separate administration by at least 3 months.

Test Interactions Octagam® contains maltose. Falsely-elevated blood glucose levels may occur when glucose monitoring devices and test strips utilizing the glucose dehydrogenase pyrroloquinolinequinone (GDH-PQQ) based methods are used. Glucose monitoring devices and test strips which utilize the glucose-specific method are recommended.

Dietary Considerations Octagam® contains sodium 30 mmol/L

Dosage Forms

Injection, powder for reconstitution [preservative free]:

Gammar®-P I.V.: 5 g, 10 g [stabilized with human albumin and sucrose]

Iveegam EN: 5 g [stabilized with glucose]

Injection, powder for reconstitution [preservative free, nanofiltered]:

Carimune™ NF: 3 g, 6 g, 12 g [contains sucrose]

Panglobulin® NF: 6 g, 12 g [contains sucrose]

Injection, powder for reconstitution [preservative free, solvent detergent-treated]:

Gammagard® S/D: 2.5 g, 5 g, 10 g [stabilized with human albumin, glycine, glucose, and polyethylene glycol]

Polygam® S/D: 5 g, 10 g [stabilized with human albumin, glycine, glucose, and polyethylene glycol]

Injection, solution [preservative free; solvent detergent-treated]:

Gammagard® Liquid: 10% [100 mg/mL] (10 mL, 25 mL, 50 mL, 100 mL, 200 mL) [latex free, sucrose free; stabilized with glycine]

Octagam®: 5% [50 mg/mL] (20 mL, 50 mL, 100 mL, 200 mL) [sucrose free; contains sodium 30 mmol/L and maltose]

Injection, solution [preservative free] (Gamunex®): 10% (10 mL, 25 mL, 50 mL, 100 mL, 200 mL) [caprylate/chromatography purified]

- **Immunine® VH (Can)** *see* Factor IX *on page 502*
- **Imogam® Rabies-HT** *see* Rabies Immune Globulin (Human) *on page 1100*
- **Imogam® Rabies Pasteurized (Can)** *see* Rabies Immune Globulin (Human) *on page 1100*

- **Imovax® Rabies** *see* Rabies Virus Vaccine *on page 1101*
- **Imuran®** *see* Azathioprine *on page 148*

Inamrinone (eye NAM ri none)

Medication Safety Issues

Sound-alike/look-alike issues:

Amrinone may be confused with amiloride, amiodarone

Related Information

Heart Failure (Systolic) *on page 1607*

Hemodynamic Support, Intravenous *on page 1566*

Synonyms Amrinone Lactate

Pharmacologic Category Phosphodiesterase Enzyme Inhibitor

Generic Available Yes

Use Infrequently used as a last resort, short-term therapy in patients with intractable heart failure

Mechanism of Action Inhibits myocardial cyclic adenosine monophosphate (cAMP) phosphodiesterase activity and increases cellular levels of cAMP resulting in a positive inotropic effect and increased cardiac output; also possesses systemic and pulmonary vasodilator effects resulting in pre- and afterload reduction; slightly increases atrioventricular conduction

Pharmacodynamics/Kinetics

Onset of action: I.V.: 2-5 minutes

Peak effect: ~10 minutes

Duration (dose dependent): Low dose: ~30 minutes; Higher doses: ~2 hours

Half-life elimination, serum: Adults: Healthy volunteers: 3.6 hours, Congestive heart failure: 5.8 hours

Dosage Dosage is based on clinical response (**Note:** Dose should not exceed 10 mg/kg/24 hours).

Infants, Children, and Adults: 0.75 mg/kg I.V. bolus over 2-3 minutes followed by maintenance infusion of 5-10 mcg/kg/minute; I.V. bolus may need to be repeated in 30 minutes.

Dosing adjustment in renal failure: Cl_{cr} <10 mL/minute: Administer 50% to 75% of dose.

Stability May be administered undiluted for I.V. bolus doses. For continuous infusion: Dilute with 0.45% or 0.9% sodium chloride to final concentration of 1-3 mg/mL; use within 24 hours; do not directly dilute with dextrose-containing solutions, chemical interaction occurs; may be administered I.V. into running dextrose infusions. Furosemide forms a precipitate when injected in I.V. lines containing inamrinone.

Administration May be administered undiluted for I.V. bolus doses. For continuous infusion: Dilute with 0.45% or 0.9% sodium chloride to final concentration of 1-3 mg/mL use within 24 hours.

Monitoring Parameters Cardiac index, stroke volume, systemic vascular resistance, and pulmonary vascular resistance (if Swan-Ganz catheter available); CVP, SBP, DBP, heart rate; platelet count, CBC, liver function and renal function tests

Anesthesia and Critical Care Concerns/Other Considerations To avoid confusion with similarly sounding medication names, the generic name "amrinone" changed to "inamrinone" in July, 2000.

Preliminary pharmacokinetic studies estimate total initial bolus doses of 3-4.5 mg/kg given in divided doses in neonates and infants to obtain serum concentrations similar to therapeutic adult levels; the actual use of these higher doses has been reported in a very small number of infants (n=7). Further studies are needed to define pediatric dosing guidelines.

Although the phosphodiesterase inhibitor drugs may induce short-term improvement in clinical status in patients with intractable heart failure, longer-term studies of these drugs in heart failure have suggested that there is a net increase in mortality.

Pregnancy Risk Factor C

Contraindications Hypersensitivity to inamrinone, any component of the formulation, or bisulfites (contains sodium metabisulfite); patients with severe aortic or pulmonic valvular disease

Warnings/Precautions Due to a slight effect on AV conduction, may increase ventricular response rate in atrial fibrillation/atrial flutter; prior treatment with digoxin is recommended. Monitor liver function. Discontinue therapy if alteration in LFTs and clinical symptoms of hepatotoxicity occur. Observe for arrhythmias in this very high-risk patient population. Not recommended in acute MI treatment. Monitor fluid status closely; patients may require adjustment of diuretic and electrolyte replacement therapy. Can cause thrombocytopenia (dose dependent). Correct hypokalemia before initiating therapy. Increase risk of hospitalization and death with long-term therapy.

Adverse Reactions

1% to 10%:

- Cardiovascular: Arrhythmias (3%, especially in high-risk patients), hypotension (1% to 2%) (may be infusion rate-related)
- Gastrointestinal: Nausea (1% to 2%)
- Hematologic: Thrombocytopenia (may be dose related)

<1% (Limited to important or life-threatening): Chest pain, fever, hepatotoxicity, hypersensitivity (especially with prolonged therapy), vomiting; contains sulfites resulting in allergic reactions in susceptible people

Drug Interactions

Furosemide: A precipitate forms on admixture with inamrinone.

Diuretics may cause significant hypovolemia and decrease filling pressure.

Digitalis: Inotropic effects are additive.

Dosage Forms Injection, solution, as lactate: 5 mg/mL (20 mL) [contains sodium metabisulfite]

- **Inapsine®** *see* Droperidol *on page 432*
- **Inderal®** *see* Propranolol *on page 1077*
- **Inderal® LA** *see* Propranolol *on page 1077*

Indinavir (in DIN a veer)

Medication Safety Issues

Sound-alike/look-alike issues:

Indinavir may be confused with Denavir™

Related Information

Moderate Sedation *on page 1442*

U.S. Brand Names Crixivan®

Canadian Brand Names Crixivan®

Synonyms Indinavir Sulfate

Pharmacologic Category Antiretroviral Agent, Protease Inhibitor

Generic Available No

Use Treatment of HIV infection; should always be used as part of a multidrug regimen (at least three antiretroviral agents)

Mechanism of Action Indinavir is a human immunodeficiency virus protease inhibitor, binding to the protease activity site and inhibiting the activity of this enzyme. HIV protease is an enzyme required for the cleavage of viral polyprotein precursors into individual functional proteins found in infectious HIV. Inhibition prevents cleavage of these polyproteins resulting in the formation of immature noninfectious viral particles.

Pharmacodynamics/Kinetics

Absorption: Administration with a high fat, high calorie diet resulted in a reduction in AUC and in maximum serum concentration (77% and 84% respectively); lighter meal resulted in little or no change in these parameters.

Protein binding, plasma: 60%

Metabolism: Hepatic via CYP3A4; seven metabolites of indinavir identified

Bioavailability: Good

Half-life elimination: 1.8 ± 0.4 hour

Time to peak: 0.8 ± 0.3 hour

Excretion: Urine and feces

Dosage

Children 4-15 years (investigational): 500 mg/m^2 every 8 hours

Adults: Oral:

Unboosted regimen: 800 mg every 8 hours

Ritonavir-boosted regimens:

Ritonavir 100-200 mg twice daily plus indinavir 800 mg twice daily **or**

Ritonavir 400 mg twice daily plus indinavir 400 mg twice daily

(Continued)

Indinavir *(Continued)*

Dosage adjustments for indinavir when administered in combination therapy:

Delavirdine, itraconazole, or ketoconazole: Reduce indinavir dose to 600 mg every 8 hours
Efavirenz: Increase indinavir dose to 1000 mg every 8 hours
Lopinavir and ritonavir (Kaletra™): Indinavir 600 mg twice daily
Nelfinavir: Increase indinavir dose to 1200 mg twice daily
Nevirapine: Increase indinavir dose to 1000 mg every 8 hours
Rifabutin: Reduce rifabutin to ½ the standard dose plus increase indinavir to 1000 mg every 8 hours

Dosage adjustment in hepatic impairment: Mild-moderate impairment due to cirrhosis: 600 mg every 8 hours or with ketoconazole coadministration

Stability Capsules are sensitive to moisture; medication should be stored and used in the original container and the desiccant should remain in the bottle

Administration Drink at least 48 oz of water daily. Administer with water, 1 hour before or 2 hours after a meal. Administer around-the-clock to avoid significant fluctuation in serum levels. May be taken with food when administered in combination with ritonavir.

Monitoring Parameters Monitor viral load, CD4 count, triglycerides, cholesterol, glucose, liver function tests, CBC, urinalysis (severe leukocyturia should be monitored frequently).

Pregnancy Risk Factor C

Contraindications Hypersensitivity to indinavir or any component of the formulation; concurrent use of amiodarone, cisapride, triazolam, midazolam, pimozide, or ergot alkaloids

Warnings/Precautions Because indinavir may cause nephrolithiasis/urolithiasis the drug should be discontinued if signs and symptoms occur; risk is substantially higher in pediatric patients versus adults. Adequate hydration is recommended. May cause tubulointerstitial nephritis (rare); severe asymptomatic leukocyturia may warrant evaluation. Indinavir should not be administered concurrently with lovastatin or simvastatin (caution with atorvastatin and cerivastatin) because of competition for metabolism of these drugs through the CYP3A4 system, and potential serious or life-threatening events. Use caution with other drugs metabolized by this enzyme (particular caution with phosphodiesterase-5 inhibitors, including sildenafil). Avoid concurrent use of St John's wort (may lead to loss of virologic response and/or resistance). Patients with hepatic insufficiency due to cirrhosis should have dose reduction. Warn patients about fat redistribution that can occur. Indinavir has been associated with hemolytic anemia (discontinue if diagnosed), hepatitis, and hyperglycemia (exacerbation or new-onset diabetes). Treatment may result in immune reconstitution syndrome (acute inflammatory response to indolent or residual opportunistic infections). Use caution in patients with hemophilia; spontaneous bleeding has been reported.

Adverse Reactions Protease inhibitors cause dyslipidemia which includes elevated cholesterol and triglycerides and a redistribution of body fat centrally to cause increased abdominal girth, buffalo hump, facial atrophy, and breast enlargement. These agents also cause hyperglycemia (exacerbation or new-onset diabetes).

>10%:
- Gastrointestinal: Nausea (12%)
- Hepatic: Hyperbilirubinemia (14%)
- Renal: Nephrolithiasis/urolithiasis (29%, pediatric patients; 12%, adult patients)

1% to 10%:
- Central nervous system: Headache (6%), insomnia (3%)
- Gastrointestinal: Abdominal pain (9%), diarrhea/vomiting (4% to 5%), taste perversion (3%)
- Neuromuscular & skeletal: Weakness (4%), flank pain (3%)
- Renal: Hematuria

<1% (Limited to important or life-threatening): Acute renal failure, alopecia, anaphylactoid reactions, angina, anorexia, bleeding (spontaneous in patients with hemophilia A or B), crystalluria, decreased hemoglobin, depression, dizziness, dysuria, erythema multiforme, fever, hemolytic anemia, hepatic failure, hepatitis, hyperglycemia, increased serum cholesterol, immune reconstitution syndrome, interstitial nephritis (with medullary calcification and cortical atrophy), leukocyturia (severe and asymptomatic), malaise, MI, new-onset

diabetes, pancreatitis, paresthesia (oral), pruritus, pyelonephritis, somnolence, Stevens-Johnson syndrome, urticaria, vasculitis, xerostomia

Drug Interactions Substrate of CYP2D6 (minor), 3A4 (major); **Inhibits** CYP2C9 (weak), 2C19 (weak), 2D6 (weak), 3A4 (strong)

Amiodarone: Serum levels/toxicity may be increased by indinavir; serious and/or life-threatening reactions may occur; concurrent use is contraindicated.

Anticonvulsants: Phenobarbital, and carbamazepine may decrease serum levels and consequently effectiveness of indinavir.

Benzodiazepines: An increase in midazolam and triazolam serum levels may occur resulting in significant oversedation when administered with indinavir. Concurrent use is contraindicated. Use caution with other benzodiazepines.

Calcium channel blockers: Indinavir may increase the serum concentrations of calcium channel blockers.

Cisapride: Indinavir inhibits the metabolism of cisapride and should not be administered concurrently due to risk of life-threatening cardiac arrhythmias.

CYP3A4 inducers: CYP3A4 inducers may decrease the levels/effects of indinavir. Example inducers include aminoglutethimide, carbamazepine, nafcillin, nevirapine, phenobarbital, phenytoin, and rifamycins. Dosage adjustment may be recommended; see individual agents.

CYP3A4 inhibitors: May increase the levels/effects of indinavir. Example inhibitors include azole antifungals, clarithromycin, diclofenac, doxycycline, erythromycin, imatinib, isoniazid, nefazodone, nicardipine, propofol, protease inhibitors, quinidine, telithromycin, and verapamil.

CYP3A4 substrates: Indinavir may increase the levels/effects of CYP3A4 substrates. Example substrates include benzodiazepines, calcium channel blockers, mirtazapine, nateglinide, nefazodone, and tacrolimus. Selected benzodiazepines (midazolam and triazolam), cisapride, ergot alkaloids, selected HMG-CoA reductase inhibitors (lovastatin and simvastatin), and pimozide are generally contraindicated with strong CYP3A4 inhibitors.

Didanosine: Separate administration of indinavir from buffered formulations by at least 1 hour.

Ergot alkaloids: Serum levels/toxicity may be increased by indinavir; serious and/or life-threatening reactions may occur; concurrent use is contraindicated.

HMG-CoA reductase inhibitors: Indinavir may increase levels of HMG-CoA reductase inhibitors, increasing the risk of myopathy. Lovastatin and simvastatin should not be coadministered with indinavir (per manufacturer). Atorvastatin may be used with careful monitoring, in the lowest dose possible. Fluvastatin and pravastatin may have lowest risk.

Immunosuppressants: Indinavir may increase the serum levels of cyclosporine, sirolimus or tacrolimus.

Itraconazole or ketoconazole: May increase the serum concentrations of indinavir. Dosage adjustment of indinavir is recommended.

Non-nucleoside reverse transcriptase inhibitors: When used with delavirdine, serum levels of indinavir are increased. The serum concentrations of indinavir may be decreased by efavirenz or nevirapine. Dosage adjustment of indinavir may be required for these combinations.

Phosphodiesterase-5 (PDE-5) inhibitors (sildenafil, tadalafil, vardenafil): Serum concentrations/effects may be substantially increased by indinavir. Dosage restriction/limitation is recommended.

Pimozide: Serum levels/toxicity may be increased by indinavir; serious and/or life-threatening reactions may occur; concurrent use is contraindicated.

Protease inhibitors: Serum levels of both nelfinavir and indinavir are increased with concurrent use. Serum concentrations of indinavir may be increased by ritonavir. Serum levels of ritonavir and saquinavir may be increased. Dosage adjustments of both agents may be required during concurrent therapy. Concurrent use of atazanavir may increase the risk of hyperbilirubinemia.

Quinidine: Serum levels/toxicity may be increased by indinavir; serious and/or life-threatening reactions may occur; concurrent use is contraindicated.

Rifabutin: A 200% increase in rifabutin plasma AUC has been observed when coadministered with indinavir. Rifabutin may decrease the serum concentrations of indinavir. Dosage adjustment of both agents required.

Rifampin: Rifampin decreases indinavir's serum concentrations; loss of virologic response and resistance may occur; the two drugs should not be administered together.

St John's wort (*Hypericum perforatum*): Appears to induce CYP3A enzymes and may lead to reduction in trough serum concentrations, which may lead to

(Continued)

Indinavir *(Continued)*

treatment failures. Alternatively, changes may involve P-glycoprotein. The two drugs should not be used together.

Venlafaxine: May decrease indinavir levels/effects; use caution.

Ethanol/Nutrition/Herb Interactions

Food: Indinavir bioavailability may be decreased if taken with food. Meals high in calories, fat, and protein result in a significant decrease in drug levels. Indinavir serum concentrations may be decreased by grapefruit juice.

Herb/Nutraceutical: St John's wort *(Hypericum)* appears to induce CYP3A enzymes and has lead to 57% reductions in indinavir AUCs and 81% reductions in trough serum concentrations, which may lead to treatment failures; should not be used concurrently with indinavir.

Dietary Considerations Should be taken without food but with water 1 hour before or 2 hours after a meal. Administration with lighter meals (eg, dry toast, skim milk, corn flakes) resulted in little/no change in indinavir concentration. If taking with ritonavir, may take with food. Patient should drink at least 48 oz of water daily. May be taken with food when administered in combination with ritonavir.

Dosage Forms Capsule: 100 mg, 200 mg, 333 mg, 400 mg

- **Indinavir Sulfate** *see* Indinavir *on page 671*
- **Indocid® P.D.A. (Can)** *see* Indomethacin *on page 674*
- **Indocin®** *see* Indomethacin *on page 674*
- **Indocin® I.V.** *see* Indomethacin *on page 674*
- **Indocin® SR** *see* Indomethacin *on page 674*
- **Indo-Lemmon (Can)** *see* Indomethacin *on page 674*
- **Indometacin** *see* Indomethacin *on page 674*

Indomethacin (in doe METH a sin)

Medication Safety Issues

Sound-alike/look-alike issues:

Indocin® may be confused with Imodium®, Lincocin®, Minocin®, Vicodin®

Related Information

Chronic Pain Management *on page 1430*

U.S. Brand Names Indocin®; Indocin® I.V.; Indocin® SR

Canadian Brand Names Apo-Indomethacin®; Indocid® P.D.A.; Indocin®; Indo-Lemmon; Indotec; Novo-Methacin; Nu-Indo; Rhodacine®

Synonyms Indometacin; Indomethacin Sodium Trihydrate

Pharmacologic Category Nonsteroidal Anti-inflammatory Drug (NSAID), Oral; Nonsteroidal Anti-inflammatory Drug (NSAID), Parenteral

Restrictions A medication guide should be dispensed with each prescription. A template for the required MedGuide can be found on the FDA website at: http://www.fda.gov/medwatch/SAFETY/2005/safety05.htm#NSAID

Generic Available Yes: Capsule, suspension

Use Acute gouty arthritis, acute bursitis/tendonitis, moderate to severe osteoarthritis, rheumatoid arthritis, ankylosing spondylitis; I.V. form used as alternative to surgery for closure of patent ductus arteriosus in neonates

Mechanism of Action Inhibits prostaglandin synthesis by decreasing the activity of the enzyme, cyclooxygenase, which results in decreased formation of prostaglandin precursors

Pharmacodynamics/Kinetics

Onset of action: ~30 minutes

Duration: 4-6 hours

Absorption: Prompt and extensive

Distribution: V_d: 0.34-1.57 L/kg; crosses blood brain barrier and placenta; enters breast milk

Protein binding: 99%

Metabolism: Hepatic; significant enterohepatic recirculation

Bioavailability: 100%

Half-life elimination: 4.5 hours; prolonged in neonates

Time to peak: Oral: 2 hours

Excretion: Urine (60%, primarily as glucuronide conjugates); feces (33%, primarily as metabolites)

Dosage

Patent ductus arteriosus:

Neonates: I.V.: Initial: 0.2 mg/kg, followed by 2 doses depending on postnatal age (PNA):

PNA **at time of first dose** <48 hours: 0.1 mg/kg at 12- to 24-hour intervals

PNA **at time of first dose** 2-7 days: 0.2 mg/kg at 12- to 24-hour intervals

PNA **at time of first dose** >7 days: 0.25 mg/kg at 12- to 24-hour intervals

In general, may use 12-hour dosing interval if urine output >1 mL/kg/hour after prior dose; use 24-hour dosing interval if urine output is <1 mL/kg/hour but >0.6 mL/kg/hour; doses should be withheld if patient has oliguria (urine output <0.6 mL/kg/hour) or anuria

Inflammatory/rheumatoid disorders: Oral: Use lowest effective dose.

Children >2 years: 1-2 mg/kg/day in 2-4 divided doses; maximum dose: 4 mg/kg/day; not to exceed 150-200 mg/day

Adults: 25-50 mg/dose 2-3 times/day; maximum dose: 200 mg/day; extended release capsule should be given on a 1-2 times/day schedule; maximum dose for sustained release is 150 mg/day. In patients with arthritis and persistent night pain and/or morning stiffness may give the larger portion (up to 100 mg) of the total daily dose at bedtime.

Bursitis/tendonitis: Oral: Adults: Initial dose: 75-150 mg/day in 3-4 divided doses; usual treatment is 7-14 days

Acute gouty arthritis: Oral: Adults: 50 mg 3 times daily until pain is tolerable then reduce dose; usual treatment <3-5 days

Elderly: Refer to Adults dosing; best to start older adults on 25 mg dose given 2-3 times/day

Dosage adjustment in renal impairement: Not recommended in patients with advanced renal disease

Stability I.V.: Store below 30°C (86°F). Protect from light; not stable in alkaline solution; reconstitute just prior to administration; discard any unused portion; do not use preservative-containing diluents for reconstitution

Administration

Oral: Administer with food, milk, or antacids to decrease GI adverse effects; extended release capsules must be swallowed whole, do not crush

I.V.: Administer over 20-30 minutes at a concentration of 0.5-1 mg/mL in preservative-free sterile water for injection or normal saline. Reconstitute I.V. formulation just prior to administration; discard any unused portion; avoid I.V. bolus administration or infusion via an umbilical catheter into vessels near the superior mesenteric artery as these may cause vasoconstriction and can compromise blood flow to the intestines. Do not administer intra-arterially.

Monitoring Parameters Monitor response (pain, range of motion, grip strength, mobility, ADL function), inflammation; observe for weight gain, edema; monitor renal function (serum creatinine, BUN); observe for bleeding, bruising; evaluate gastrointestinal effects (abdominal pain, bleeding, dyspepsia); mental confusion, disorientation, CBC, liver function tests

Anesthesia and Critical Care Concerns/Other Considerations The 2002 ACCM/SCCM guidelines for analgesia (critically-ill adult) suggest that NSAIDs may be used in combination with opioids in select patients for pain management. Concern about adverse events (increased risk of renal dysfunction, altered platelet function and gastrointestinal irritation) limits its use in patients who have other underlying risks for these events.

In short-term use, NSAIDs vary considerably in their effect on blood pressure. When NSAIDs are used in patients with hypertension, appropriate monitoring of blood pressure responses should be completed and the duration of therapy, when possible, kept short. The use of NSAIDs in the treatment of patients with congestive heart failure may be associated with an increased risk for fluid accumulation and edema; may precipitate renal failure in dehydrated patients.

Pregnancy Risk Factor C/D (3rd trimester)

Contraindications Hypersensitivity to indomethacin, aspirin, other NSAIDs, or any component of the formulation; perioperative pain in the setting of coronary artery bypass surgery (CABG); pregnancy (3rd trimester)

Neonates: Necrotizing enterocolitis, impaired renal function, active bleeding, thrombocytopenia, coagulation defects, untreated infection

Warnings/Precautions [U.S. Boxed Warning]: NSAIDs are associated with an increased risk of adverse cardiovascular events, including MI, stroke, and new onset or worsening of pre-existing hypertension. Risk may be increased with duration of use or pre-existing cardiovascular risk-factors or

(Continued)

Indomethacin *(Continued)*

disease. Carefully evaluate individual cardiovascular risk profiles prior to prescribing. Use caution with fluid retention, CHF or hypertension.

Use of NSAIDs can compromise existing renal function. Renal toxicity can occur in patient with impaired renal function, dehydration, heart failure, liver dysfunction, those taking diuretics and ACEI and the elderly. Rehydrate patient before starting therapy. Monitor renal function closely. Indomethacin is not recommended for patients with advanced renal disease.

[U.S. Boxed Warning]: NSAIDs may increase risk of gastrointestinal irritation, ulceration, bleeding, and perforation. These events may occur at any time during therapy and without warning. Use caution with a history of GI disease (bleeding or ulcers), concurrent therapy with aspirin, anticoagulants and/or corticosteroids, smoking, use of alcohol, the elderly or debilitated patients.

Use the lowest effective dose for the shortest duration of time, consistent with individual patient goals, to reduce risk of cardiovascular or GI adverse events. Alternate therapies should be considered for patients at high risk.

NSAIDs may cause serious skin adverse events including exfoliative dermatitis, Stevens-Johnson syndrome (SJS) and toxic epidermal necrolysis (TEN). Anaphylactoid reactions may occur, even without prior exposure; patients with "aspirin triad" (bronchial asthma, aspirin intolerance, rhinitis) may be at increased risk. Do not use in patients who experience bronchospasm, asthma, rhinitis, or urticaria with NSAID or aspirin therapy.

Use with caution in patients with decreased hepatic function. Closely monitor patients with any abnormal LFT. Severe hepatic reactions (eg, fulminant hepatitis, liver failure) have occurred with NSAID use, rarely; discontinue if signs or symptoms of liver disease develop, or if systemic manifestations occur.

Withhold for at least 4-6 half-lives prior to surgical or dental procedures.

Adverse Reactions

>10%: Central nervous system: Headache (12%)

1% to 10%:

Central nervous system: Dizziness (3% to 9%), drowsiness (<1%), fatigue (<3%), vertigo (<3%), depression (<3%), malaise (<3%), somnolence (<3%)

Gastrointestinal: Nausea (3% to 9%), epigastric pain (3% to 9%), abdominal pain/cramps/distress (<3%), heartburn (3% to 9%), indigestion (3% to 9%), constipation (<3%), diarrhea (<3%), dyspepsia (3% to 9%), vomiting

Otic: Tinnitus (<3%)

<1% (Limited to important or life-threatening): Acute respiratory distress, agranulocytosis, allergic rhinitis, anaphylaxis, anemia, angioedema, aplastic anemia, arrhythmia, aseptic meningitis, asthma, bone marrow suppression, bronchospasm, chest pain, cholestatic jaundice, coma, confusion, CHF, cystitis, depersonalization, depression, dilutional hyponatremia (I.V.), diplopia, disseminated intravascular coagulation, dysarthria, dyspnea, ecchymosis, edema, epistaxis, erythema multiforme, erythema nodosum, exfoliative dermatitis, fluid retention, flushing, hair loss, gastric perforation (rare), gastritis, GI bleeding, GI ulceration, gynecomastia, hearing decreased, hematuria, hemolytic anemia, hepatitis (including fatal cases), hot flashes, hyperkalemia, hypersensitivity reactions, hypertension, hypoglycemia (I.V.), interstitial nephritis, involuntary muscle movements, leukopenia, necrotizing fasciitis, nephrotic syndrome, oliguria, paresthesias, parkinson's exacerbation, peptic ulcer, peripheral neuropathy, proctitis, psychosis, pulmonary edema, purpura, syncope, renal insufficiency, renal failure, retinal/macular disturbances, seizure exacerbation, shock, somnolence, Stevens-Johnson syndrome, stomatitis, thrombocytopenia, thrombocytopenic purpura, thrombophlebitis, toxic amblyopia, toxic epidermal necrolysis

Overdosage/Toxicology Symptoms of overdose include drowsiness, lethargy, nausea, vomiting, seizures, paresthesia, headache, dizziness, GI bleeding, cerebral edema, tinnitus, leukocytosis, and renal failure. Management of NSAID intoxication is supportive and symptomatic.

Drug Interactions **Substrate** (minor) of CYP2C9, 2C19; **Inhibits** CYP2C9 (strong), 2C19 (weak)

ACE inhibitors: Antihypertensive effects may be decreased by concurrent therapy with NSAIDs; monitor blood pressure.

Aminoglycosides: NSAIDs may decrease the excretion of aminoglycosides.

Angiotensin II antagonists: Antihypertensive effects may be decreased by concurrent therapy with NSAIDs; monitor blood pressure.

Anticoagulants (warfarin, heparin, LMWHs) in combination with NSAIDs can cause increased risk of bleeding.

Antiplatelet drugs (ticlopidine, clopidogrel, aspirin, abciximab, dipyridamole, eptifibatide, tirofiban) can cause an increased risk of bleeding.

Beta-blockers: NSAIDs may diminish the antihypertensive effects of beta blockers.

Bisphosphonates: NSAIDs may increase the risk of gastrointestinal ulceration.

Cholestyramine (and other bile acid sequestrants): May decrease the absorption of NSAIDs. Separate by at least 2 hours.

Corticosteroids may increase the risk of GI ulceration; avoid concurrent use.

Cyclosporine: NSAIDs may increase serum creatinine, potassium, blood pressure, and cyclosporine levels; monitor cyclosporine levels and renal function carefully.

CYP2C9 Substrates: Indomethacin may increase the levels/effects of CYP2C9 substrates. Example substrates include bosentan, dapsone, fluoxetine, glimepiride, glipizide, losartan, montelukast, nateglinide, paclitaxel, phenytoin, warfarin, and zafirlukast.

Gentamicin and amikacin serum concentrations are increased by indomethacin in premature infants. Results may apply to other aminoglycosides and NSAIDs.

Hydralazine's antihypertensive effect is decreased; avoid concurrent use.

Lithium levels can be increased; avoid concurrent use if possible or monitor lithium levels and adjust dose. Sulindac may have the least effect. When NSAID is stopped, lithium will need adjustment again.

Loop diuretics efficacy (diuretic and antihypertensive effect) is reduced. Indomethacin reduces this efficacy, however, it may be anticipated with any NSAID.

Methotrexate: Severe bone marrow suppression, aplastic anemia, and GI toxicity have been reported with concomitant NSAID therapy. Avoid use during moderate or high-dose methotrexate (increased and prolonged methotrexate levels). NSAID use during low-dose treatment of rheumatoid arthritis has not been fully evaluated; extreme caution is warranted.

Pemetrexed: NSAIDs may decrease the excretion of pemetrexed. Patients with Cl_{cr} 45-79 mL/minute should avoid short acting NSAIDs for 2 days before and 2 days after pemetrexed treatment.

Thiazides antihypertensive effects are decreased; avoid concurrent use.

Tiludronate: Indomethacin may increase serum concentration of tiludronate.

Treprostinil: May enhance the risk of bleeding with concurrent use.

Vancomycin: NSAIDs may decrease the excretion of vancomycin.

Ethanol/Nutrition/Herb Interactions

Ethanol: Avoid ethanol (may enhance gastric mucosal irritation).

Food: Food may decrease the rate but not the extent of absorption. Indomethacin peak serum levels may be delayed if taken with food.

Herb/Nutraceutical: Avoid alfalfa, anise, bilberry, bladderwrack, bromelain, cat's claw, celery, coleus, cordyceps, dong quai, evening primrose, feverfew, fenugreek, garlic, ginger, ginkgo biloba, ginseng, grapeseed, green tea, guggul, horse chestnut seed, horseradish, licorice, prickly ash, red clover, reishi, SAMe, sweet clover, turmeric, white willow (all have additional antiplatelet activity).

Test Interactions False-negative dexamethasone suppression test

Dietary Considerations May cause GI upset; take with food or milk to minimize

Dosage Forms

Capsule (Indocin®): 25 mg, 50 mg

Capsule, sustained release (Indocin® SR): 75 mg

Injection, powder for reconstitution, as sodium trihydrate (Indocin® I.V.): 1 mg

Suspension, oral (Indocin®): 25 mg/5 mL (237 mL) [contains alcohol 1%; pineapple-coconut-mint flavor]

- **Indomethacin Sodium Trihydrate** *see* Indomethacin *on page 674*
- **Indotec (Can)** *see* Indomethacin *on page 674*
- **Infantaire [OTC]** *see* Acetaminophen *on page 26*
- **Infasurf®** *see* Calfactant *on page 218*
- **Inflamase® Mild (Can)** *see* PrednisoLONE *on page 1046*

Infliximab (in FLIKS e mab)

Medication Safety Issues

Sound-alike/look-alike issues:

Remicade® may be confused with Renacidin®, Rituxan®

Infliximab may be confused with rituximab

(Continued)

Infliximab *(Continued)*

U.S. Brand Names Remicade®

Canadian Brand Names Remicade®

Synonyms Infliximab, Recombinant; NSC-728729

Pharmacologic Category Antirheumatic, Disease Modifying; Gastrointestinal Agent, Miscellaneous; Monoclonal Antibody; Tumor Necrosis Factor (TNF) Blocking Agent

Generic Available No

Use

Ankylosing spondylitis: Improving signs and symptoms of disease

Crohn's disease: Induction and maintenance of remission in patients with moderate to severe disease who have an inadequate response to conventional therapy; to reduce the number of draining enterocutaneous and rectovaginal fistulas and to maintain fistula closure

Psoriatic arthritis: Improving signs and symptoms of active arthritis in patients with psoriatic arthritis

Rheumatoid arthritis: Inhibits the progression of structural damage and improves physical function in patients with moderate to severe disease; used with methotrexate

Ulcerative colitis (UC): To reduce signs and symptoms, achieve clinical remission and mucosal healing and eliminate corticosteroid use in moderately to severely active UC inadequately responsive to conventional therapy

Unlabeled/Investigational Use Graft-versus-host disease (GVHD)

Mechanism of Action Infliximab is a chimeric monoclonal antibody that binds to human tumor necrosis factor alpha (TNFα), thereby interfering with endogenous TNFα activity. Biological activities of TNFα include the induction of proinflammatory cytokines (interleukins), enhancement of leukocyte migration, activation of neutrophils and eosinophils, and the induction of acute phase reactants and tissue degrading enzymes. Animal models have shown TNFα expression causes polyarthritis, and infliximab can prevent disease as well as allow diseased joints to heal.

Pharmacodynamics/Kinetics

Onset of action: Crohn's disease: ~2 weeks

Half-life elimination: 8-9.5 days

Dosage I.V.:

Children ≥6 years: Crohn's disease: 5 mg/kg at 0, 2, and 6 weeks, followed by a maintenance dose of 5 mg/kg every 8 weeks

Adults:

Crohn's disease: Induction regimen: 5 mg/kg at 0, 2, and 6 weeks, followed by 5 mg/kg every 8 weeks thereafter; dose may be increased to 10 mg/kg in patients who respond but then lose their response. If no response by week 14, consider discontinuing therapy.

Psoriatic arthritis (with or without methotrexate): 5 mg/kg at 0, 2, and 6 weeks, then every 8 weeks

Rheumatoid arthritis (in combination with methotrexate therapy): 3 mg/kg at 0, 2, and 6 weeks, then every 8 weeks thereafter; doses have ranged from 3-10 mg/kg intravenous infusion repeated at 4- to 8-week intervals

Ankylosing spondylitis: 5 mg/kg at 0, 2, and 6 weeks, followed by 5 mg/kg every 6 weeks thereafter

Ulcerative colitis: 5 mg/kg at 0, 2, and 6 weeks, followed by 5 mg/kg every 8 weeks thereafter

GVHD (unlabeled use): 10 mg/kg weekly for up to 8 weeks (median 4 weeks of treatment)

Dosage adjustment with CHF: Weigh risk versus benefits for individual patient: NYHA Class III or IV: ≤5 mg/kg

Dosage adjustment in renal impairment: No specific adjustment is recommended

Dosage adjustment in hepatic impairment: No specific adjustment is recommended

Stability Store vials at 2°C to 8°C (36°F to 46°F); do not freeze. Reconstitute vials with 10 mL sterile water for injection; swirl vial gently to dissolve powder, do not shake, allow solution to stand for 5 minutes; total dose of reconstituted product should be further diluted to 250 mL of 0.9% sodium chloride injection; infusion of dose should begin within 3 hours of preparation

Administration Infuse over at least 2 hours; do not infuse with other agents; use in-line low protein binding filter (≤1.2 micron)

Monitoring Parameters Improvement of symptoms; signs of infection; LFTs (discontinue if >5 times ULN); place and read PPD before initiation.

Pregnancy Risk Factor B (manufacturer)

Contraindications Hypersensitivity to murine proteins or any component of the formulation; doses >5 mg/kg in patients with moderate or severe congestive heart failure (NYHA Class III/IV)

Warnings/Precautions **[U.S. Boxed Warning]: Opportunistic infections and/or re-activation of latent infections have been associated with infliximab therapy.** Tuberculosis (may be disseminated or extrapulmonary) has been reactivated in patients previously exposed to TB while on infliximab. Most cases have been reported within the first 3-6 months of treatment. Other opportunistic infections (eg, invasive fungal infections, listeriosis, *Pneumocystis*) have occurred during therapy. Patients should be evaluated for latent tuberculosis infection with a tuberculin skin test prior to infliximab therapy. Treatment of latent tuberculosis should be initiated before infliximab is used. The risk/benefit ratio should be weighed in patients who have resided in regions where histoplasmosis is endemic.

Serious infections (including sepsis, pneumonia, and fatal infections) have been reported in patients receiving TNF-blocking agents. Many of the serious infections in patients treated with infliximab have occurred in patients on concomitant immunosuppressive therapy. Caution should be exercised when considering the use of infliximab in patients with a chronic infection or history of recurrent infection. Infliximab should not be given to patients with a clinically important, active infection. Patients who develop a new infection while undergoing treatment with infliximab should be monitored closely. If a patient develops a serious infection or sepsis, infliximab should be discontinued. Rare reactivation of hepatitis B has occurred in chronic virus carriers; evaluate prior to initiation and during treatment.

[U.S. Boxed Warning]: Hepatosplenic T-cell lymphoma has been reported (rarely) in adolescent and young adults with Crohn's disease treated with infliximab and azathioprine or 6-mercaptopurine. The impact of infliximab on the development and course of malignancies is not fully defined, but may be dose dependent. As compared to the general population, an increased risk of lymphoma has been noted in clinical trials; however, rheumatoid arthritis alone has been previously associated with an increased rate of lymphoma.

Severe hepatic reactions have been reported during treatment; discontinue with jaundice or marked increase in liver enzymes. Use caution with heart failure; if a decision is made to use with heart failure, monitor closely and discontinue if exacerbated or new symptoms occur. Use caution with history of hematologic abnormalities; hematologic toxicities (eg, leukopenia, neutropenia, thrombocytopenia, pancytopenia) have been reported; discontinue if significant abnormalities occur. Autoimmune antibodies and a lupus-like syndrome have been reported. If antibodies to double-stranded DNA are confirmed in a patient with lupus-like symptoms, infliximab should be discontinued. Rare cases of optic neuritis and demyelinating disease have been reported; use with caution in patients with pre-existing or recent onset CNS demyelinating disorders, or seizures; discontinue if significant CNS adverse reactions develop.

Medications for the treatment of hypersensitivity reactions should be available for immediate use. Safety and efficacy for use in juvenile rheumatoid arthritis or pediatric ulcerative colitis have not been established.

Adverse Reactions **Although profile is similar, frequency of adverse effects may vary with disease state. Except where noted, percentages reported in adults with rheumatoid arthritis:**

>10%:

- Central nervous system: Headache (18%)
- Gastrointestinal: Nausea (21%), diarrhea (12%), abdominal pain (12%, Crohn's 26%)
- Hepatic: ALT increased (risk increased with concomitant methotrexate)
- Local: Infusion reactions (20%)
- Respiratory: Upper respiratory tract infection (32%), cough (12%), sinusitis (14%), pharyngitis (12%)
- Miscellaneous: Development of antinuclear antibodies (~50%), infection (36%), development of antibodies to double-stranded DNA (17%); Crohn's patients with fistulizing disease: Development of new abscess (15%)

(Continued)

Infliximab *(Continued)*

5% to 10%:

Cardiovascular: Hypertension (7%)
Central nervous system: Fatigue (9%), pain (8%), fever (7%)
Dermatologic: Rash (10%), pruritus (7%)
Gastrointestinal: Dyspepsia (10%)
Genitourinary: Urinary tract infection (8%)
Neuromuscular & skeletal: Arthralgia (8%), back pain (8%)
Respiratory: Bronchitis (10%), rhinitis (8%), dyspnea (6%)
Miscellaneous: Moniliasis (5%)

<5%: Abscess, adult respiratory distress syndrome, allergic reaction, anemia, arrhythmia, basal cell carcinoma, biliary pain, bradycardia, brain infarction, breast cancer, cardiac arrest, cellulitis, cholecystitis, cholelithiasis, circulatory failure, confusion, constipation, dehydration, diaphoresis increased, dizziness, edema, gastrointestinal hemorrhage, heart failure, hemolytic anemia, hepatitis, hypersensitivity reactions, hypotension, ileus, intervertebral disk herniation, intestinal obstruction, intestinal perforation, intestinal stenosis, leukopenia, lymphadenopathy, lymphoma, meningitis, menstrual irregularity, MI, neuritis, pancreatitis, pancytopenia, peripheral neuropathy, peritonitis, pleural effusion, pleurisy, proctalgia, pulmonary edema, pulmonary embolism, renal failure, respiratory insufficiency, seizure, sepsis, serum sickness, suicide attempt, syncope, tachycardia, tendon disorder, thrombocytopenia, thrombophlebitis (deep), ulceration

The following adverse events were reported in children with Crohn's disease and were found more frequently in children than adults:

>10%:

Hepatic: Liver enzymes increased (18%; ≥5 times ULN: 1%)
Hematologic: Anemia (11%)
Miscellaneous: Infections (56%; more common with every 8-week versus every 12-week infusions)

1% to 10%:

Central nervous system: Flushing (9%)
Gastrointestinal: Blood in stool (10%)
Hematologic: Leukopenia (9%), neutropenia (7%)
Respiratory: Respiratory tract allergic reaction (6%), bacterial infection (6%), antibodies to infliximab (3%)
Neuromuscular & skeletal: Bone fracture (7%)

Postmarketing and/or case reports (adults or children): Anaphylactic reactions, angioedema; demyelinating disorders (eg, multiple sclerosis, optic neuritis); drug-induced lupus-like syndrome, Guillain-Barré syndrome, heart failure (worsening), hepatitis B reactivation, hepatosplenic T-cell lymphoma, idiopathic thrombocytopenia purpura, interstitial fibrosis, interstitial pneumonitis, jaundice, latent tuberculosis reactivation, liver failure, liver function tests increased, metallic taste, neuropathy, neutropenia, pericardial effusion, pneumonia, thrombotic thrombocytopenia purpura, transverse myelitis, tuberculosis, urticaria, vasculitis (systemic and cutaneous)

Overdosage/Toxicology Doses of up to 20 mg/kg have been given without toxic effects. In case of overdose, treatment should be symptom-directed and supportive.

Drug Interactions Specific drug interaction studies have not been conducted

Abatacept: Infliximab may enhance the adverse/toxic effects of abatacept; increased risk of serious infection has been reported.

Abciximab: May increase potential for hypersensitivity reaction to infliximab, and may increase risk of thrombocytopenia and/or reduced therapeutic efficacy of infliximab.

Anakinra: Anti-TNF agents may increase the risk of serious infection when used in combination with anakinra. This effect has been observed with etanercept.

Vaccines, live: Concomitant use has not be studied; currently recommended not to administer live vaccines during infliximab therapy

Ethanol/Nutrition/Herb Interactions Herb/Nutraceutical: Echinacea may diminish the therapeutic effect of infliximab.

Dosage Forms

Injection, powder for reconstitution [preservative free]:
Remicade®: 100 mg [contains sucrose and polysorbate 80]

♦ **Infliximab, Recombinant** *see* Infliximab *on page 677*

- **Infumorph®** *see* Morphine Sulfate *on page 867*
- **INH** *see* Isoniazid *on page 703*
- **Inhaled Insulin** *see* Insulin Inhalation *on page 686*
- **Inhibace® (Can)** *see* Cilazapril *on page 277*
- **Innohep®** *see* Tinzaparin *on page 1272*
- **InnoPran XL™** *see* Propranolol *on page 1077*
- **INOmax®** *see* Nitric Oxide *on page 925*
- **Insoluble Prussian Blue** *see* Ferric Hexacyanoferrate *on page 521*
- **Inspra™** *see* Eplerenone *on page 461*

Insulin Aspart (IN soo lin AS part)

Medication Safety Issues

Sound-alike/look-alike issues:

NovoLog® may be confused with Novolin®

NovoLog® Mix 70/30 may be confused with NovoLog®

High alert medication: The Institute for Safe Medication Practices (ISMP) includes this medication among its list of drugs which have a heightened risk of causing significant patient harm when used in error. ***Due to the number of insulin preparations, it is essential to identify/clarify the type of insulin to be used.***

Related Information

Insulin Regular *on page 693*

U.S. Brand Names NovoLog®

Canadian Brand Names NovoRapid®

Synonyms Aspart Insulin

Pharmacologic Category Antidiabetic Agent, Insulin

Generic Available No

Use Treatment of type 1 diabetes mellitus (insulin dependent, IDDM); type 2 diabetes mellitus (noninsulin dependent, NIDDM) to control hyperglycemia

Mechanism of Action Refer to Insulin Regular *on page 693*. Insulin aspart is a rapid-acting insulin analog.

Pharmacodynamics/Kinetics

Onset of action: 0.2-0.5 hours

Duration: 3-5 hours

Time to peak: 1-3 hours

Excretion: Urine

Dosage Refer to Insulin Regular *on page 693*. Insulin aspart is a rapid-acting insulin analog which is normally administered as a a premeal component of the insulin regimen. It is normally used along with a long-acting (basal) form of insulin.

Dosing adjustment in renal impairment: Insulin requirements are reduced due to changes in insulin clearance or metabolism.

Stability Insulin aspart (NovoLog®): Store unopened container in refrigerator; do not use if it has been frozen. If not refrigerated, use within 28 days and protect from heat and light. Once opened (in use), vials may be stored in refrigerator or for up to 28 days at room temperature. Cartridges that are in use should be stored at room temperature and used within 28 days; do not refrigerate. Insulin in reservoir should be replaced every 48 hours. Discard if exposed to temperatures ≥37°C (98.6°F).

Administration

SubQ: Should be administered immediately before a meal (within 5-10 minutes of the start of a meal). Cold injections should be avoided. SubQ administration is usually made into the thighs, arms, buttocks, or abdomen, with sites rotated. When mixing regular insulin with other preparations of insulin, regular insulin should be drawn into syringe first. Can be infused SubQ by external insulin pump; however, when used in an external pump, should not be diluted with other insulins.

I.V.: Insulin aspart may be administered I.V. in selected clinical situations to control hyperglycemia. Appropriate medical supervision is required. May be diluted to a concentration between 0.05 and 1 unit/mL with NS, D_5W, or $D_{10}W$ with 40 mmol/L potassium chloride.

Monitoring Parameters Urine sugar and acetone, serum glucose, electrolytes, Hb A_{1c}, lipid profile; when used intravenously, close monitoring of serum glucose and potassium are required to avoid hypoglycemia and/or hypokalemia

Reference Range Refer to Insulin Regular *on page 693*.

(Continued)

Insulin Aspart *(Continued)*

Pregnancy Risk Factor C

Contraindications Hypersensitivity to any component of the formulation

Warnings/Precautions Refer to Insulin Regular *on page 693.*

In type 1 diabetes mellitus (insulin dependent, IDDM), insulin lispro (Humalog®) and insulin glulisine (Apidra™) should be used in combination with a long-acting insulin. However, in type 2 diabetes mellitus (noninsulin dependent, NIDDM), insulin lispro (Humalog®) may be used without a long-acting insulin when used in combination with a sulfonylurea.

Adverse Reactions Refer to Insulin Regular *on page 693.*

Overdosage/Toxicology Refer to Insulin Regular *on page 693.*

Drug Interactions Refer to Insulin Regular *on page 693.*

Ethanol/Nutrition/Herb Interactions Refer to Insulin Regular *on page 693.*

Dietary Considerations Dietary modification based on ADA recommendations is a key component of therapy.

Dosage Forms Injection, solution (NovoLog®): 100 units/mL (3 mL) [FlexPen® prefilled syringe or PenFill® prefilled cartridge]; (10 mL) [vial]

♦ **Insulin Aspart and Insulin Aspart Protamine** *see* Insulin Aspart Protamine and Insulin Aspart *on page 682*

Insulin Aspart Protamine and Insulin Aspart

(IN soo lin AS part PROE ta meen & IN soo lin AS part)

Medication Safety Issues

Sound-alike/look-alike issues:

NovoLog® Mix 70/30 may be confused with Novolin® 70/30

High alert medication: The Institute for Safe Medication Practices (ISMP) includes this medication among its list of drugs which have a heightened risk of causing significant patient harm when used in error. ***Due to the number of insulin preparations, it is essential to identify/clarify the type of insulin to be used.***

Related Information

Insulin Regular *on page 693*

U.S. Brand Names NovoLog® Mix 70/30

Synonyms Insulin Aspart and Insulin Aspart Protamine

Pharmacologic Category Antidiabetic Agent, Insulin

Generic Available No

Use Treatment of type 1 diabetes mellitus (insulin dependent, IDDM); type 2 diabetes mellitus (noninsulin dependent, NIDDM) to control hyperglycemia

Mechanism of Action Refer to Insulin Regular *on page 693.* Insulin aspart protamine and insulin aspart is a combination insulin product with intermediate-acting characteristics. Normally administered twice daily.

Pharmacodynamics/Kinetics

Onset of action: 0.2 hours

Duration: 18-24 hours

Half-life: 8-9 hours

Time to peak: 1-4 hours

Excretion: Urine

Dosage Refer to Insulin Regular *on page 693.* Fixed ratio insulins (such as insulin aspart protamine and insulin aspart combination) are normally administered in 2 daily doses.

Dosing adjustment in renal impairment: Insulin requirements are reduced due to changes in insulin clearance or metabolism.

Stability NovoLog® Mix 70/30: Store unopened container in refrigerator. Do not use if frozen. If refrigeration is not possible, vial (in use) may be stored at room temperature for up to 28 days. The pen in use should **not** be refrigerated, store below 30°C (86°F) away from direct heat or light; discard after 14 days. If refrigeration is not available, opened vials may be stored unrefrigerated in cool place away from heat and sunlight.

Administration Aspart protamine human suspension and aspart human solution (NovoLog® Mix 70/30): SubQ administration only. Cold injections should be avoided. Should be administered within 15 minutes before a meal. Normally administered twice daily (before breakfast and supper). SubQ administration is usually made into the thighs, arms, buttocks, or abdomen, with sites rotated.

Resuspend immediately prior to use. Gently roll vial or pen in the palms of the hands to resuspend before using. Do not mix or dilute with other insulins.

Pregnancy Risk Factor C

Contraindications Hypersensitivity to any component of the formulation; during episodes of hypoglycemia

Warnings/Precautions Refer to Insulin Regular *on page 693*. Safety and efficacy of this insulin product have not been established in pediatric patients.

In type 1 diabetes mellitus (insulin dependent, IDDM), insulin lispro (Humalog®) and insulin glulisine (Apidra™) should be used in combination with a long-acting insulin. However, in type 2 diabetes mellitus (noninsulin dependent, NIDDM), insulin lispro (Humalog®) may be used without a long-acting insulin when used in combination with a sulfonylurea.

Adverse Reactions Refer to Insulin Regular *on page 693*.

Dosage Forms Injection, suspension (NovoLog® Mix 70/30): Insulin aspart protamine suspension 70% [intermediate acting] and insulin aspart solution 30% [rapid acting]: 100 units/mL (3 mL) [PenFill® prefilled cartridge or FlexPen® prefilled syringe]; (10 mL) [vial]

Insulin Detemir (IN soo lin DE te mir)

Medication Safety Issues

High alert medication: The Institute for Safe Medication Practices (ISMP) includes this medication among its list of drugs which have a heightened risk of causing significant patient harm when used in error. ***Due to the number of insulin preparations, it is essential to identify/clarify the type of insulin to be used.***

Note: Insulin detemir is a clear solution, but it is NOT intended for I.V. or I.M. administration.

Related Information

Insulin Regular *on page 693*

U.S. Brand Names Levemir®

Canadian Brand Names Levemir®

Synonyms Detemir Insulin

Pharmacologic Category Antidiabetic Agent, Insulin

Generic Available No

Use Treatment of type 1 diabetes mellitus (insulin dependent, IDDM); type 2 diabetes mellitus (noninsulin dependent, NIDDM) to control hyperglycemia

Mechanism of Action Refer to Insulin Regular *on page 693*. The product labeling identifies this product as a long-acting insulin analog; however, at lower dosages (<0.6 units/kg) its pharmacodynamic characteristics and dosing are consistent with intermediate insulin forms. In some patients, or at higher dosages, it may have a duration of action approaching 24 hours, which is consistent with a long-acting insulin.

Pharmacodynamics/Kinetics

Onset of action: 3-4 hours

Duration: Dose dependent: 6-23 hours

Note: Duration is dose-dependent. At lower dosages (0.1-0.2 units/kg), mean duration is variable (5.7-12.1 hours). At 0.6 units/kg, the mean duration was 19.9 hours. At high dosages (>0.6 units/kg) the duration is longer and less variable (mean of 22-23 hours).

Bioavailability: 60%

Half-life: 5-7 hours (dose dependent)

Protein binding: >98% (albumin)

Distribution: V_d: 0.1 L/kg

Time to peak: 6-8 hours

Excretion: Urine

Dosage Also refer to Insulin Regular *on page 693*.

Notes: Duration is dose-dependent. Dosage must be carefully titrated (adjustment of dose and timing. Adjustment of concomitant antidiabetic treatment (short-acting insulins or oral antidiabetic agents) may be required. In Canada, insulin detemir is not approved for use in children.

SubQ: Children ≥6 years and Adults: Type 1 or type 2 diabetes:

Basal insulin or basal-bolus: May be substituted on a unit-per-unit basis. Adjust dose to achieve glycemic targets.

(Continued)

Insulin Detemir *(Continued)*

Insulin-naive patients (type 2 diabetes only): 0.1-0.2 units/kg once daily in the evening or 10 units once or twice daily. Adjust dose to achieve glycemic targets. Note: Canadian labeling recommends 10 units once daily (twice daily dosing is not included).

Dosage adjustment in renal impairment: Insulin requirements are reduced due to changes in insulin clearance or metabolism.

Stability Insulin detemir (Levemir®): Store unopened container in refrigerator; do not use if it has been frozen. Once opened (in use), vials may be stored in refrigerator or for up to 42 days at room temperature (below 30°C). Cartridges and prefilled syringes that are in use should be stored at room temperature and used within 42 days; do not refrigerate. Do not store with needle in place. All opened (in-use) vials should be stored away from direct heat and sunlight.

Administration Insulin detemir is a clear solution but it is NOT intended for I.V. or I.M. administration.

Insulin detemir (Levemir®): SubQ administration: Cold injections should be avoided. SubQ administration is usually made into the thighs, arms, buttocks, or abdomen, with sites rotated. Not for infusion pumps. Cannot be diluted or mixed with other insulins.

Once daily: Administer with evening meal or at bedtime.

Twice daily: Administer evening dose with evening meal, at bedtime, or 12 hours following morning dose.

Monitoring Parameters Urine sugar and acetone, serum glucose, electrolytes, Hb A_{1c}, lipid profile

Reference Range Refer to Insulin Regular *on page 693*.

Pregnancy Risk Factor C

Contraindications Hypersensitivity to any component of the formulation

Warnings/Precautions Refer to Insulin Regular *on page 693*. Safety and efficacy not established in children <6 years of age.

Careful adjustment of dosage and timing is required to achieve glycemic targets. Adjustment of other antidiabetic therapy (short-acting or oral antidiabetic agents) may be required. The duration of of action of insulin detemir is dose-dependent and this factor must be considered during dosage adjustment and titration. Insulin detemir is a clear solution, but it is not for intravenous administration.

In type 1 diabetes mellitus (insulin dependent, IDDM), insulin lispro (Humulin®) and insulin glulisine (Apidra™) should be used in combination with a long-acting insulin.

Adverse Reactions Refer to Insulin Regular *on page 693*.

Overdosage/Toxicology Refer to Insulin Regular *on page 693*.

Drug Interactions Refer to Insulin Regular *on page 693*.

Ethanol/Nutrition/Herb Interactions Refer to Insulin Regular *on page 693*.

Dietary Considerations Dietary modification based on ADA recommendations is a key component of therapy.

Dosage Forms Injection, solution (Levemir®): 100 units/mL (3 mL) [Innolet® prefilled syringe, Penfill® prefilled cartridge, or FlexPen® prefilled syringe]; (10 mL) [vial]

References

Plank J, Bodenlenz M, Sinner F, et al, "A Double-Blind, Randomized, Dose-Response Study Investigating the Pharmacodynamic and Pharmacokinetic Properties of the Long-Acting Insulin Analog Detemir," *Diabetes Care*, 2005, 28(5):1107-12.

Insulin Glargine (IN soo lin GLAR jeen)

Medication Safety Issues

Sound-alike/look-alike issues:

Lantus® may be confused with Lente®

Lente® may be confused with Lantus®

High alert medication: The Institute for Safe Medication Practices (ISMP) includes this medication among its list of drugs which have a heightened risk of causing significant patient harm when used in error. ***Due to the number of insulin preparations, it is essential to identify/clarify the type of insulin to be used.***

Related Information

Insulin Regular *on page 693*

U.S. Brand Names Lantus®

Canadian Brand Names Lantus®; Lantus® OptiSet®

Synonyms Glargine Insulin

Pharmacologic Category Antidiabetic Agent, Insulin

Generic Available No

Use Treatment of type 1 diabetes mellitus (insulin dependent, IDDM); type 2 diabetes mellitus (noninsulin dependent, NIDDM) requiring basal (long-acting) insulin to control hyperglycemia

Mechanism of Action Refer to Insulin Regular *on page 693*. Insulin glargine is a long-acting insulin analog.

Pharmacodynamics/Kinetics

Onset of action: 3-4 hours

Duration: 24 hours

Absorption: Slow; forms microprecipitates which allow small amounts to release over time

Metabolism: Partially metabolized in the skin to form teo active metabolites

Time to peak: No pronounced peak

Excretion: Urine

Dosage SubQ: Adults:

Type 1 diabetes: Refer to Insulin Regular *on page 693*.

Type 2 diabetes:

Patient not already on insulin: 10 units once daily, adjusted according to patient response (range in clinical study: 2-100 units/day)

Patient already receiving insulin: In clinical studies, when changing to insulin glargine from once-daily NPH or Ultralente® insulin, the initial dose was not changed; when changing from twice-daily NPH to once-daily insulin glargine, the total daily dose was reduced by 20% and adjusted according to patient response

Dosage adjustment in renal impairment: Insulin requirements are reduced due to changes in insulin clearance or metabolism.

Stability Insulin glargine (Lantus®): Store unopened container in refrigerator; do not use if it has been frozen. If not refrigerated, use within 28 days and protect from heat and light. Once opened (in use), vials may be stored in refrigerator or for up to 28 days at room temperature. Cartridges in use should be stored at room temperature and used within 28 days.

Administration Insulin glargine (Lantus®): SubQ administration: Should be administered once daily, at any time of day, but should be administered at the same time each day. Cold injections should be avoided. SubQ administration is usually made into the thighs, arms, buttocks, or abdomen, with sites rotated. Cannot be diluted or mixed with any other insulin or solution.

Monitoring Parameters Urine sugar and acetone, serum glucose, electrolytes, Hb A_{1c}, lipid profile

Reference Range Refer to Insulin Regular *on page 693* .

Pregnancy Risk Factor C

Contraindications Hypersensitivity to any component of the formulation

Warnings/Precautions Refer to Insulin Regular *on page 693*. Safety and efficacy not established in children <6 years of age.

In type 1 diabetes mellitus (insulin dependent, IDDM), insulin lispro (Humalog®) and insulin glulisine (Apidra™) should be used in combination with a long-acting insulin. However, in type 2 diabetes mellitus (noninsulin dependent, NIDDM), insulin lispro (Humalog®) may be used without a long-acting insulin when used in combination with a sulfonylurea.

Adverse Reactions Refer to Insulin Regular *on page 693*.

Overdosage/Toxicology Refer to Insulin Regular *on page 693*.

Drug Interactions Refer to Insulin Regular *on page 693*.

Ethanol/Nutrition/Herb Interactions Refer to Insulin Regular *on page 693*.

Dosage Forms Injection, solution (Lantus®): 100 units/mL (3 mL) [cartridge]; (10 mL) [vial]

Insulin Glulisine (IN soo lin gloo LIS een)

Medication Safety Issues

High alert medication: The Institute for Safe Medication Practices (ISMP) includes this medication among its list of drugs which have a heightened risk of causing significant patient harm when used in error. ***Due to the number of***

(Continued)

Insulin Glulisine *(Continued)*

insulin preparations, it is essential to identify/clarify the type of insulin to be used.

Related Information

Insulin Regular *on page 693*

U.S. Brand Names Apidra®

Canadian Brand Names Apidra®

Synonyms Glulisine Insulin

Pharmacologic Category Antidiabetic Agent, Insulin

Generic Available No

Use Treatment of type 1 diabetes mellitus (insulin dependent, IDDM); type 2 diabetes mellitus (noninsulin dependent, NIDDM) to control hyperglycemia

Mechanism of Action Refer to Insulin Regular *on page 693*. Insulin glulisine is a rapid-acting insulin analog.

Pharmacodynamics/Kinetics

Onset of action: 0.2-0.5 hours

Duration: 3-4 hours

Time to Peak: 30-90 minutes

Excretion: Urine

Dosage Refer to Insulin Regular *on page 693*.

Dosing adjustment in renal impairment: Insulin requirements are reduced due to changes in insulin clearance or metabolism.

Stability Insulin glulisine (Apidra®): Store unopened vials in refrigerator at 2°C to 8°C (36°F to 46°F); do not freeze. Once opened, may store under refrigeration or at room temperature ≤25°C (77°F); use within 28 days. Stable in infusion pump for up to 48 hours. Discard if exposed to temperatures >37°C (98.6°F).

Administration Insulin glulisine (Apidra®): SubQ administration: Cold injections should be avoided. SubQ administration is usually made into the thighs, arms, buttocks, or abdomen, with sites rotated. Can be infused SubQ by external insulin pump; however, when used in an external pump, should not be diluted or mixed with other insulins.

Monitoring Parameters Urine sugar and acetone, serum glucose, electrolytes, Hb A_{1c}, lipid profile

Reference Range Refer to Insulin Regular *on page 693*.

Pregnancy Risk Factor C

Contraindications Hypersensitivity to any component of the formulation

Warnings/Precautions Refer to Insulin Regular *on page 693*.

In type 1 diabetes mellitus (insulin dependent, IDDM), insulin lispro (Humalog®) and insulin glulisine (Apidra®) should be used in combination with a long-acting insulin. However, in type 2 diabetes mellitus (noninsulin dependent, NIDDM), insulin lispro (Humalog®) may be used without a long-acting insulin when used in combination with a sulfonylurea.

Adverse Reactions Refer to Insulin Regular *on page 693*.

Overdosage/Toxicology Refer to Insulin Regular *on page 693*.

Drug Interactions Refer to Insulin Regular *on page 693*.

Ethanol/Nutrition/Herb Interactions Refer to Insulin Regular *on page 693*.

Dosage Forms

Injection, solution:

Apidra®: 100 units/mL (3 mL [cartridge], 10 mL [vial])

Insulin Inhalation (IN soo lin in ha LAY shun)

Medication Safety Issues

High alert medication: The Institute for Safe Medication Practices (ISMP) includes this medication among its list of drugs which have a heightened risk of causing significant patient harm when used in error. **Due to the number of insulin preparations, it is essential to identify/clarify the type of insulin to be used. The inhalation form of insulin is expressed in milligrams rather than units, potentially leading to confusion. Absolute conversion between doses of inhalation and injection insulin is not possible.**

Related Information

Insulin Regular *on page 693*

U.S. Brand Names Exubera®

Synonyms Inhaled Insulin

Pharmacologic Category Antidiabetic Agent, Insulin

Restrictions A medication guide must be distributed to each patient to whom this medication is dispensed.

Use Treatment of type 1 diabetes mellitus (insulin dependent, IDDM); type 2 diabetes mellitus (noninsulin dependent, NIDDM)

Mechanism of Action Refer to Insulin Regular *on page 693*. Insulin inhalation is a rapid-acting form of human insulin.

Pharmacodynamics/Kinetics

Onset of action: 0.2-0.4 hours

Duration: 6-8 hours

Absorption: Rapid

Bioavailability: Absolute bioavailability not defined (depends on inspiratory flow characteristics); systemic exposure may be up to 2-5 times higher in smokers

Time to peak, plasma: 30-90 minutes

Excretion: Urine

Dosage Inhalation: Children ≥6 years and Adults:

Initial: 0.05 mg/kg (rounded down to nearest whole milligram) 3 times/daily administered within 10 minutes of a meal

Adjustment: Dosage may be increased or decreased based on serum glucose monitoring, meal size, nutrient composition, time of day, and exercise patterns.

Note: A 1 mg blister is approximately equivalent to 3 units of regular insulin, while a 3 mg blister is approximately equivalent to 8 units of regular insulin administered subcutaneously. Patients should combine 1 mg and 3 mg blisters so that the fewest blisters are required to achieve the prescribed dose. Consecutive inhalation of three 1 mg blisters results in significantly higher insulin levels as compared to inhalation of a single 3 mg blister (do not substitute). In a patient stabilized on a dosage which uses 3 mg blisters, if 3 mg blister is temporarily unavailable, inhalation of two 1 mg blisters may be substituted.

Dosing adjustment in renal impairment: Insulin requirements are reduced due to changes in insulin clearance or metabolism.

Stability Insulin inhalation (Exubera®): Store unopened blisters, in-use blisters, and inhaler at controlled room temperature (25°C); excursions permitted to 15°C to 30°C (59°F to 86°F). Do not freeze or refrigerate. Once foil overwrap is opened, blisters should be used within 3 months. Avoid exposure to excess humidity.

Administration Insulin inhalation (Exubera®): Administer no more than 10 minutes before a meal using the Exubera® inhalation device. The Exubera® Release Unit in the inhaler should be changed every 2 weeks; the Exubera® inhaler may be used for 1 year.

Monitoring Parameters Pulmonary function testing at baseline and periodically during therapy; blood glucose, urine sugar and acetone, serum glucose, electrolytes, Hb A_{1c}, lipid profile

Reference Range Refer to Insulin Regular *on page 693*.

Pregnancy Risk Factor C

Contraindications Hypersensitivity to any component of the formulation; smokers or patients who have discontinued smoking for <6 months; poorly-controlled or unstable lung disease

Warnings/Precautions Also refer to Insulin Regular *on page 693*.

Due to increased systemic absorption, the risk of hypoglycemia is greatly increased in patients who smoke or who have stopped smoking for less than 6 months. The effect of passive exposure to smoke has not been fully evaluated but may result in alteration in absorption and/or hypoglycemia. Insulin inhalation should be immediately discontinued in any patient who resumes smoking.

Decreases in pulmonary function have been associated with use. Due the potential impact on pulmonary function, testing should be performed prior to the initiation of inhaled insulin therapy. Not recommended for use in patients with lung disease (asthma, COPD). Monitor closely during periods of intercurrent respiratory illness.

In type 1 diabetes mellitus (insulin dependent, IDDM), rapid-acting insulins including insulin inhalation should be used in combination with a long-acting insulin. However, in type 2 diabetes mellitus (noninsulin dependent, NIDDM), rapid-acting agents may be used without a long-acting insulin when used as monotherapy or combined with an oral antidiabetic agent.

Use caution in renal and/or hepatic impairment.

(Continued)

Insulin Inhalation *(Continued)*

Adverse Reactions Also refer to Insulin Regular *on page 693.*

Cardiovascular: Chest pain (5%; usually mild to moderate)

Dermatologic: Rash (rare)

Endocrine & metabolic: Hypoglycemia

Gastrointestinal: Xerostomia (2%)

Otic: Otitis media (pediatric patients 7%), ear pain (4%), ear disorder (1%)

Respiratory: Respiratory infection (30% to 43%), cough increased (22% to 30%), pharyngitis (10% to 18%), rhinitis (9% to 15%), sinusitis (5% to 10%), dyspnea (4%), sputum increased (3% to 4%), bronchitis (3% to 5%), epistaxis (1%), laryngitis (1%), voice alteration (1%), bronchospasm (rare)

Note: Decreases in pulmonary function (reduced FEV1, DLco) have been associated with use, usually noted in the initial weeks of therapy; declines from baseline of 20% in, respectively, FEV1 and DLco, were reported in 5.1% and 1.5% of patients as compared to 3.6% and 1.3% in comparator-treated patients.

Miscellaneous: Allergic reactions, anaphylaxis (including tachycardia and hypotension), diaphoresis increased

Overdosage/Toxicology Refer to Insulin Regular *on page 693.*

Drug Interactions Refer to Insulin Regular *on page 693.*

Ethanol/Nutrition/Herb Interactions Refer to Insulin Regular *on page 693.*

Dietary Considerations Dietary modification based on ADA recommendations is a key component of therapy.

Dosage Forms

Powder for oral inhalation [prefilled blister pack]: 1 mg (90s) [purchased with or provided with inhaler and 2 release units]; 3 mg (90s) [purchased with or provided with inhaler and 2 release units]

Combination package [prefilled blister pack]: Powder for inhalation: 1 mg (90s); powder for inhalation: 3 mg (90s)

References

Skyler JS, Weinstock RS, and Raskin P, "Use of Inhaled Insulin in a Basal/Bolus Insulin Regimen in Type 1 Diabetic Subjects: A 6-Month, Randomized, Comparative Trial," *Diabetes Care*, 2005, 28(7):1630-5.

Insulin Lispro (IN soo lin LYE sproe)

Medication Safety Issues

Sound-alike/look-alike issues:

Humalog® may be confused with Humulin®, Humira®

High alert medication: The Institute for Safe Medication Practices (ISMP) includes this medication among its list of drugs which have a heightened risk of causing significant patient harm when used in error. ***Due to the number of insulin preparations, it is essential to identify/clarify the type of insulin to be used.***

Related Information

Insulin Regular *on page 693*

U.S. Brand Names Humalog®

Canadian Brand Names Humalog®

Synonyms Lispro Insulin

Pharmacologic Category Antidiabetic Agent, Insulin

Generic Available No

Use Treatment of type 1 diabetes mellitus (insulin dependent, IDDM); type 2 diabetes mellitus (noninsulin dependent, NIDDM) to control hyperglycemia

Note: In type 1 diabetes mellitus (insulin dependent, IDDM), insulin lispro (Humalog®) should be used in combination with a long-acting insulin. However, in type 2 diabetes mellitus (noninsulin dependent, NIDDM), insulin lispro (Humalog®) may be used without a long-acting insulin when used in combination with a sulfonylurea.

Mechanism of Action Refer to Insulin Regular *on page 693.* Insulin lispro is a rapid-acting form of insulin.

Pharmacodynamics/Kinetics

Onset of action: 0.2-0.5 hours

Duration: 3-4 hours

Distribution: 0.26-0.36 L/kg

Bioavailability: 55% to 77%
Time to peak: 30-90 minutes
Excretion: Urine

Dosage Refer to Insulin Regular *on page 693.* Insulin lispro is equipotent to insulin regular, but has a more rapid onset.

Dosing adjustment in renal impairment: Insulin requirements are reduced due to changes in insulin clearance or metabolism.

Stability Insulin lispro (Humalog®): Store unopened container in refrigerator; do not use if it has been frozen. If not refrigerated, use within 28 days and protect from heat and light. Once opened (in use), vials may be stored in refrigerator or for up to 28 days at room temperature. Cartridges/pens should be stored at room temperature and used within 28 days. When used in an external pump, replace insulin in reservoir within 48 hours and cartridges within 7 days; do not expose to temperatures >37°C (98.6°F). If diluted with sterile diluent (available from manufacturer), 1:10 dilutions are stable for 28 days stored at 5°C (41°F) or 14 days stored at 30°C (86°F).

Administration Insulin lispro (Humalog®): SubQ administration: May be administered within 15 minutes before or immediately after a meal. Cold injections should be avoided. SubQ administration is usually made into the thighs, arms, buttocks, or abdomen, with sites rotated. Can be infused SubQ by external insulin pump; however, when used in an external pump, should not be diluted or mixed with other insulins.

Note: May be mixed in the same syringe as Humulin® N or Humulin® U, but Humalog® should be drawn into the syringe first.

Monitoring Parameters Urine sugar and acetone, serum glucose, electrolytes, Hb A_{1c}, lipid profile

Reference Range Refer to Insulin Regular *on page 693.*

Pregnancy Risk Factor B

Contraindications Hypersensitivity to any component of the formulation

Warnings/Precautions Refer to Insulin Regular *on page 693.*

In type 1 diabetes mellitus (insulin dependent, IDDM), insulin lispro (Humalog®) and insulin glulisine (Apidra™) should be used in combination with a long-acting insulin. However, in type 2 diabetes mellitus (noninsulin dependent, NIDDM), insulin lispro (Humalog®) may be used without a long-acting insulin when used in combination with a sulfonylurea.

Adverse Reactions Refer to Insulin Regular *on page 693.*

Overdosage/Toxicology Refer to Insulin Regular *on page 693.*

Drug Interactions Refer to Insulin Regular *on page 693.*

Ethanol/Nutrition/Herb Interactions Refer to Insulin Regular *on page 693.*

Dietary Considerations Dietary modification based on ADA recommendations is a key component of therapy.

Dosage Forms Injection, solution (Humalog®): 100 units/mL (3 mL) [prefilled cartridge or prefilled disposable pen]; (10 mL) [vial]

♦ **Insulin Lispro and Insulin Lispro Protamine** *see* Insulin Lispro Protamine and Insulin Lispro *on page 689*

Insulin Lispro Protamine and Insulin Lispro

(IN soo lin LYE sproe PROE ta meen & IN soo lin LYE sproe)

Medication Safety Issues

Sound-alike/look-alike issues:

Humalog® Mix 75/25™ may be confused with Humulin® 70/30.

High alert medication: The Institute for Safe Medication Practices (ISMP) includes this medication among its list of drugs which have a heightened risk of causing significant patient harm when used in error. ***Due to the number of insulin preparations, it is essential to identify/clarify the type of insulin to be used.***

Related Information

Insulin Regular *on page 693*

U.S. Brand Names Humalog® Mix 50/50™; Humalog® Mix 75/25™

Canadian Brand Names Humalog® Mix 25

Synonyms Insulin Lispro and Insulin Lispro Protamine

Pharmacologic Category Antidiabetic Agent, Insulin

Generic Available No

(Continued)

Insulin Lispro Protamine and Insulin Lispro *(Continued)*

Use Treatment of type 1 diabetes mellitus (insulin dependent, IDDM); type 2 diabetes mellitus (noninsulin dependent, NIDDM) to control hyperglycemia

Mechanism of Action Refer to Insulin Regular *on page 693*. Insulin lispro protamine and insulin lispro is a combination product with a rapid onset, and a duration of action which is similar to intermediate-acting insulin products.

Pharmacodynamics/Kinetics

Onset of action: 0.2-0.5 hours

Duration: 18-24 hours

Time to peak: 2-12 hours

Excretion: Urine

Dosage Refer to Insulin Regular *on page 693*. Fixed ratio insulins (such as insulin lispro protamine and insulin lispro) are normally administered in 2 daily doses.

Dosage adjustment in renal impairment: Insulin requirements are reduced due to changes in insulin clearance or metabolism.

Stability Insulin lispro protamine and insulin lispro (Humalog® Mix): Store unopened container in refrigerator; do not use if it has been frozen. Once opened (in use), vials may be stored in refrigerator or for up to 28 days at room temperature. Pens should be stored at room temperature and used within 10 days. Do not expose to temperatures >37°C (98.6°F).

Administration Insulin lispro protamine and insulin lispro (Humalog® Mix 75/25™): SubQ administration only. Should be administered within 15 minutes before or after a meal. Normally administered twice daily (breakfast and supper). Cold injections should be avoided. SubQ administration is usually made into the thighs, arms, buttocks, or abdomen, with sites rotated. Resuspend immediately prior to use. Gently roll vial or pen in the palms of the hands to resuspend before using. Do not mix or dilute with other insulins.

Pregnancy Risk Factor B

Contraindications Hypersensitivity to any component of the formulation; during episodes of hypoglycemia

Warnings/Precautions Refer to Insulin Regular *on page 693*. Safety and efficacy in children <18 years of age have not been established.

In type 1 diabetes mellitus (insulin dependent, IDDM), insulin lispro (Humalog®) and insulin glulisine (Apidra™) should be used in combination with a long-acting insulin. However, in type 2 diabetes mellitus (noninsulin dependent, NIDDM), insulin lispro (Humalog®) may be used without a long-acting insulin when used in combination with a sulfonylurea.

Adverse Reactions Refer to Insulin Regular *on page 693*.

Drug Interactions Refer to Insulin Regular *on page 693*.

Ethanol/Nutrition/Herb Interactions Refer to Insulin Regular *on page 693*.

Dietary Considerations Dietary modification based on ADA recommendations is a key component of therapy.

Dosage Forms Injection, suspension:

Humalog® Mix 50/50™: Insulin lispro protamine suspension 50% [intermediate acting] and insulin lispro solution 50% [rapid acting]: 100 units/mL (3 mL) [disposable pen]

Humalog® Mix 75/25™: Insulin lispro protamine suspension 75% [intermediate acting] and insulin lispro solution 25% [rapid acting]: 100 units/mL (3 mL) [disposable pen]; (10 mL) [vial]

Insulin NPH (IN soo lin N P H)

Medication Safety Issues

Sound-alike/look-alike issues:

Humulin® may be confused with Humalog®, Humira®

Novolin® may be confused with NovoLog®

High alert medication: The Institute for Safe Medication Practices (ISMP) includes this medication among its list of drugs which have a heightened risk of causing significant patient harm when used in error. ***Due to the number of insulin preparations, it is essential to identify/clarify the type of insulin to be used.***

Related Information

Insulin Regular *on page 693*

U.S. Brand Names Humulin® N; Novolin® N

Canadian Brand Names Humulin® N; Novolin® ge NPH

Synonyms Isophane Insulin; NPH Insulin

Pharmacologic Category Antidiabetic Agent, Insulin

Generic Available No

Use Treatment of type 1 diabetes mellitus (insulin dependent, IDDM); type 2 diabetes mellitus (noninsulin dependent, NIDDM) to control hyperglycemia

Mechanism of Action Refer to Insulin Regular *on page 693*. Insulin NPH is an intermediate-acting form of insulin.

Pharmacodynamics/Kinetics

Onset of action: 1-2 hours

Duration: 18-24 hours

Time to peak: 6-12 hours

Excretion: Urine

Dosage Refer to Insulin Regular *on page 693*. Insulin NPH is usually administered 1-2 times daily.

Dosing adjustment in renal impairment: Insulin requirements are reduced due to changes in insulin clearance or metabolism.

Stability Insulin NPH (Humulin® N, Novolin® N): Store unopened container in refrigerator at 2°C to 8°C (36°F to 46°F); do not freeze. Vial in use may be stored under refrigeration or at room temperature. Humulin® N Pen in use should not be refrigerated; store below 30°C (86°F) away from direct heat or light; discard after 2 weeks.

Administration Insulin NPH (intermediate-acting insulin): SubQ administration: May be administered 1-2 times/day. Cold injections should be avoided. SubQ administration is usually made into the thighs, arms, buttocks, or abdomen, with sites rotated. When mixing regular insulin with other preparations of insulin, regular insulin should be drawn into syringe first. Gently roll vial or pen in the palms of the hands to resuspend before using. Insulin lispro (Humalog®) may be mixed in the same syringe as Humulin® N, but Humalog® should be drawn into the syringe first.

Monitoring Parameters Urine sugar and acetone, serum glucose, electrolytes, Hb A_{1c}, lipid profile

Reference Range Refer to Insulin Regular *on page 693.*

Pregnancy Risk Factor B

Contraindications Hypersensitivity to any component of the formulation

Warnings/Precautions Refer to Insulin Regular *on page 693.*

In type 1 diabetes mellitus (insulin dependent, IDDM), insulin lispro (Humalog®) and insulin glulisine (Apidra™) should be used in combination with a long-acting insulin. However, in type 2 diabetes mellitus (noninsulin dependent, NIDDM), insulin lispro (Humalog®) may be used without a long-acting insulin when used in combination with a sulfonylurea.

Adverse Reactions Refer to Insulin Regular *on page 693.*

Overdosage/Toxicology Refer to Insulin Regular *on page 693.*

Drug Interactions Refer to Insulin Regular *on page 693.*

Ethanol/Nutrition/Herb Interactions Refer to Insulin Regular *on page 693.*

Dietary Considerations Dietary modification based on ADA recommendations is a key component of therapy.

Dosage Forms [CAN] = Canadian brand name

Injection, suspension:

- Humulin® N: 100 units/mL (3 mL) [disposable pen]; (10 mL) [vial]
- Novolin® ge NPH [CAN]: 100 units/mL (3 mL) [NovolinSet® prefilled syringe or PenFill® prefilled cartridge]; 10 mL [vial]
- Novolin® N: 100 units/mL (3 mL) [InnoLet® prefilled syringe or PenFill® prefilled cartridge]; (10 mL) [vial]

Insulin NPH and Insulin Regular

(IN soo lin N P H & IN soo lin REG yoo ler)

Medication Safety Issues

Sound-alike/look-alike issues:

- Humulin® 70/30 may be confused with Humalog® Mix 75/25
- Novolin® 70/30 may be confused with NovoLog® Mix 70/30

High alert medication: The Institute for Safe Medication Practices (ISMP) includes this medication among its list of drugs which have a heightened risk of

(Continued)

Insulin NPH and Insulin Regular *(Continued)*

causing significant patient harm when used in error. ***Due to the number of insulin preparations, it is essential to identify/clarify the type of insulin to be used.***

Related Information

Insulin Regular *on page 693*

U.S. Brand Names Humulin® 50/50; Humulin® 70/30; Novolin® 70/30

Canadian Brand Names Humulin® 20/80; Humulin® 70/30; Novolin® ge 10/90; Novolin® ge 20/80; Novolin® ge 30/70; Novolin® ge 40/60; Novolin® ge 50/50

Synonyms Insulin Regular and Insulin NPH; Isophane Insulin and Regular Insulin; NPH Insulin and Regular Insulin

Pharmacologic Category Antidiabetic Agent, Insulin

Generic Available No

Use Treatment of type 1 diabetes mellitus (insulin dependent, IDDM); type 2 diabetes mellitus (noninsulin dependent, NIDDM) to control hyperglycemia

Mechanism of Action Refer to Insulin Regular *on page 693*. Insulin NPH and insulin regular is a combination insulin product with intermediate-acting characteristics. It may be administered once or twice daily.

Pharmacodynamics/Kinetics

Onset of action: 0.5 hours

Duration: 18-24 hours

Time to peak: 2-12 hours

Excretion: Urine

Dosage Refer to Insulin Regular *on page 693*. Fixed ratio insulins are normally administered in 1-2 daily doses.

Stability Store unopened container in refrigerator. Do not use if it has been frozen. The pen in use should not be refrigerated; store below 30°C (86°F) away from direct heat or light; discard after 10 days. If refrigeration is not available, opened vials may be stored unrefrigerated in cool place away from heat and sunlight.

Administration SubQ administration only. Should be administered ~30 minutes before a meal. Normally administered once or twice daily (before breakfast and supper). Cold injections should be avoided. SubQ administration is usually made into the thighs, arms, buttocks, or abdomen, with sites rotated. Resuspend immediately prior to use. Gently roll vial or pen in the palms of the hands to resuspend before using.

Pregnancy Risk Factor C

Contraindications Hypersensitivity to any component of the formulation; during episodes of hypoglycemia

Warnings/Precautions Refer to Insulin Regular *on page 693*.

In type 1 diabetes mellitus (insulin dependent, IDDM), insulin lispro (Humalog®) and insulin glulisine (Apidra™) should be used in combination with a long-acting insulin. However, in type 2 diabetes mellitus (noninsulin dependent, NIDDM), insulin lispro (Humalog®) may be used without a long-acting insulin when used in combination with a sulfonylurea.

Dosage Forms

Injection, suspension:

Humulin® 50/50: Insulin NPH suspension 50% [intermediate acting] and insulin regular solution 50% [short acting]: 100 units/mL (10 mL) [vial]

Humulin® 70/30: Insulin NPH suspension 70% [intermediate acting] and insulin regular solution 30% [short acting]: 100 units/mL (3 mL) [disposable pen]; (10 mL) [vial]

Novolin® 70/30: Insulin NPH suspension 70% [intermediate acting] and insulin regular solution 30% [short acting]: 100 units/mL (3 mL) [InnoLet® prefilled syringe or PenFill® prefilled cartridge]; (10 mL) [vial]

Additional formulations available in Canada: Injection, suspension:

Humulin® 20/80: Insulin regular solution 20% [short acting] and insulin NPH suspension 80% [intermediate acting]: 100 units/mL (3 mL) [PenFill® prefilled cartridge]

Novolin® ge 10/90: Insulin regular solution 10% [short acting] and insulin NPH suspension 90% [intermediate acting]: 100 units/mL (3 mL) [PenFill® prefilled cartridge]

Novolin® ge 20/80: Insulin regular solution 20% [short acting] and insulin NPH suspension 80% [intermediate acting]: 100 units/mL (3 mL) [PenFill® prefilled cartridge]

Novolin® ge 30/70: Insulin regular solution 30% [short acting] and insulin NPH suspension 70% [intermediate acting]: 100 units/mL (3 mL) [prefilled syringe or PenFill® prefilled cartridge]; (10 mL) [vial]
Novolin® ge 40/60: Insulin regular solution 40% [short acting] and insulin NPH suspension 60% [intermediate acting]: 100 units/mL (3 mL) [PenFill® prefilled cartridge]
Novolin® ge 50/50: Insulin regular solution 50% [short acting] and insulin NPH suspension 50% [intermediate acting]: 100 units/mL (3 mL) [PenFill® prefilled cartridge]

Insulin Regular (IN soo lin REG yoo ler)

Medication Safety Issues

Sound-alike/look-alike issues:

Humulin® may be confused with Humalog®, Humira®
Novolin® may be confused with NovoLog®

High alert medication: The Institute for Safe Medication Practices (ISMP) includes this medication among its list of drugs which have a heightened risk of causing significant patient harm when used in error. ***Due to the number of insulin preparations, it is essential to identify/clarify the type of insulin to be used.***

Concentrated solutions (eg, U-500) should not be available in patient care areas.

Related Information

Insulin Aspart *on page 681*
Insulin Aspart Protamine and Insulin Aspart *on page 682*
Insulin Detemir *on page 683*
Insulin Glargine *on page 684*
Insulin Glulisine *on page 685*
Insulin Inhalation *on page 686*
Insulin Lispro *on page 688*
Insulin Lispro Protamine and Insulin Lispro *on page 689*
Insulin NPH *on page 690*
Insulin NPH and Insulin Regular *on page 691*

U.S. Brand Names Humulin® R; Humulin® R (Concentrated) U-500; Novolin® R

Canadian Brand Names Humulin® R; Novolin® ge Toronto

Synonyms Regular Insulin

Pharmacologic Category Antidiabetic Agent, Insulin; Antidote

Generic Available No

Use Treatment of type 1 diabetes mellitus (insulin dependent, IDDM); type 2 diabetes mellitus (noninsulin dependent, NIDDM) unresponsive to treatment with diet and/or oral hypoglycemics, to control hyperglycemia; adjunct to parenteral nutrition; diabetic ketoacidosis (DKA)

Unlabeled/Investigational Use Hyperkalemia (regular insulin only; use with glucose to shift potassium into cells to lower serum potassium levels)

Mechanism of Action Insulin acts via specific membrane-bound receptors on target tissues to regulate metabolism of carbohydrate, protein, and fats. Insulin facilitates entry of glucose into muscle, adipose, and other tissues via hexose transporters, including GLUT4. Insulin stimulates the cellular uptake of amino acids and increases cellular permeability to several ions, including potassium, magnesium, and phosphate. By activating sodium-potassium ATPases, insulin promotes the intracellular movement of potassium.

Target organs for insulin include the liver, skeletal muscle, and adipose tissue. Within the liver, insulin stimulates hepatic glycogen synthesis through the activation of the enzymes hexokinase, phosphofructokinase, and glycogen synthase as well as the inhibition of glucose-6 phosphatase. Insulin promotes hepatic synthesis of fatty acids, which are released into the circulation as lipoproteins. Skeletal muscle effects of insulin include increased protein synthesis and increased glycogen synthesis. Within adipose tissue, insulin stimulates the processing of circulating lipoproteins to provide free fatty acids, facilitating triglyceride synthesis and storage by adipocytes. Insulin also directly inhibits the hydrolysis of triglycerides.

Normally secreted by the pancreas, insulin products are manufactured for pharmacologic use through recombinant DNA technology using either *E. coli* or *Saccharomyces cerevisiae*. Insulins are categorized based on promptness and duration of effect, including rapid-, short-, intermediate-, and long-acting insulins.
(Continued)

Insulin Regular *(Continued)*

Pharmacodynamics/Kinetics

Onset of action: 0.5 hours

Duration: 6-8 hours (may increase with dose)

Time to peak: 2-4 hours

Excretion: Urine

Dosage SubQ (regular insulin may also be administered I.V.): The number and size of daily doses, time of administration, and diet and exercise require continuous medical supervision. In addition, specific formulations may require distinct administration procedures.

Type 1 Diabetes Mellitus: Children and Adults: **Note:** Multiple daily doses guided by blood glucose monitoring are the standard of diabetes care. Combinations of insulin are commonly used.

Initial dose: 0.2-0.6 units/kg/day in divided doses. Conservative initial doses of 0.2-0.4 units/kg/day are often recommended to avoid the potential for hypoglycemia.

Division of daily insulin requirement: Generally, 50% to 75% of the daily insulin dose is given as an intermediate- or long-acting form of insulin (in 1-2 daily injections). The remaining portion of the 24-hour insulin requirement is divided and administered as a rapid-acting or short-acting form of insulin. These may be given with meals (before or at the time of meals depending on the form of insulin) or at the same time as injections of intermediate forms (some premixed combinations are intended for this purpose).

Adjustment of dose: Dosage must be titrated to achieve glucose control and avoid hypoglycemia. Adjust dose to maintain premeal and bedtime glucose of 80-140 mg/dL (children <5 years: 100-200 mg/dL). Since combinations of agents are frequently used, dosage adjustment must address the individual component of the insulin regimen which most directly influences the blood glucose value in question, based on the known onset and duration of the insulin component.

Usual maintenance range: 0.5-1.2 units/kg/day in divided doses. An estimate of anticipated needs may be based on body weight and/or activity factors as follows:

Adolescents: May require ≤1.5 units/kg/day during growth spurts

Nonobese: 0.4-0.6 units/kg/day

Obese: 0.8-1.2 units/kg/day

Renal failure: Due to alterations in pharmacokinetics of insulin, may require <0.2 units/kg/day

Type 2 Diabetes Mellitus:

Augmentation therapy: Initial dosage of 0.15 (insulin glargine, corresponding to ~10 units) to 0.2 units/kg/day (insulins other than glargine) have been recommended. Dosage must be carefully adjusted.

Note: Administered when residual beta-cell function is present, as a supplemental agent when oral hypoglycemics have not achieved goal glucose control. Twice daily NPH, or an evening dose of NPH, lente, or glargine insulin may be added to oral therapy with metformin or a sulfonylurea. Augmentation to control postprandial glucose may be accomplished with regular, glulisine, aspart, or lispro insulin.

Monotherapy: Initial dose: Highly variable: See Augmentation therapy dosing.

Note: An empirically-defined scheme for dosage estimation based on fasting plasma glucose and degree of obesity has been published with recommended doses ranging from 6-77 units/day (Holman, 1995). In the setting of glucose toxicity (loss of beta-cell sensitivity to glucose concentrations), insulin therapy may be used for short-term management to restore sensitivity of beta-cells; in these cases, the dose may need to be rapidly reduced/withdrawn when sensitivity is re-established.

Diabetic ketoacidosis:

Children <20 years:

I.V.: Regular insulin infused at 0.1 units/kg/hour; continue until acidosis clears, then decrease to 0.05 units/kg/hour until SubQ replacement dosing can be initiated

SubQ, I.M.: If no I.V. infusion access, regular insulin 0.1 units/kg I.M. bolus followed by 0.1 units/kg/hour SubQ or I.M.; continue until acidosis clears, then decrease to 0.05 units/kg/hour until SubQ replacement dosing can be initiated

Adults:

I.V.: Regular insulin 0.15 units/kg initially followed by an infusion of 0.1 units/kg/hour

SubQ, I.M.: Regular insulin 0.4 units/kg given half as I.V. bolus and half as SubQ or I.M., followed by 0.1 units/kg/hour SubQ or I.M.

If serum glucose does not fall by 50-70 mg/dL in the first hour, double insulin dose hourly until glucose falls at an hourly rate of 50-70 mg/dL. Decrease dose to 0.05-0.1 units/kg/hour once serum glucose reaches 250 mg/dL.

Note: Newly-diagnosed patients with IDDM presenting in DKA and patients with blood sugars <800 mg/dL may be relatively "sensitive" to insulin and should receive loading and initial maintenance doses ~50% of those indicated.

Infusion should continue until reversal of acid-base derangement/ketonemia. Serum glucose is not a direct indicator of these abnormalities, and may decrease more rapidly than correction of the range of metabolic abnormalities.

Hyperkalemia (unlabeled use): Children and Adults: I.V.: Administer dextrose at 0.5-1 mL/kg and regular insulin 1 unit for every 4-5 g dextrose given

Dosing adjustment in renal impairment (regular): Insulin requirements are reduced due to changes in insulin clearance or metabolism

Cl_{cr} 10-50 mL/minute: Administer at 75% of normal dose

Cl_{cr} <10 mL/minute: Administer at 25% to 50% of normal dose and monitor glucose closely

Hemodialysis: Because of a large molecular weight (6000 daltons), insulin is not significantly removed by either peritoneal or hemodialysis

Supplemental dose is not necessary

Peritoneal dialysis: Supplemental dose is not necessary

Continuous arteriovenous or venovenous hemofiltration effects: Supplemental dose is not necessary

Stability Insulin, regular (Humulin® R, Novolin® R): Store unopened containers in refrigerator at 2°C to 8°C (36°F to 46°F); do not freeze. Vial in use may be stored under refrigeration or at room temperature; store below 30°C (86°F) away from direct heat or light. Regular insulin should only be used if clear.

Note: Standard diluent for regular insulin: 100 units/100 mL NS; all bags should be prepared fresh; tubing should be flushed 30 minutes prior to administration to allow adsorption as time permits. Can be given as a more diluted solution (eg, 100 units/250 mL 0.45% NS).

Administration

SubQ administration: Cold injections should be avoided. SubQ administration is usually made into the thighs, arms, buttocks, or abdomen, with sites rotated. When mixing regular insulin with other preparations of insulin, regular insulin should be drawn into syringe first. Except for rapid-acting, short-acting, or insulin glargine, gently roll vial or pen in the palms of the hands to resuspend before using. When rapid-acting insulin is mixed with an intermediate- or long-acting insulin, it should be administered within 15 minutes before a meal. Human regular insulin: Should be administered within 30-60 minutes before a meal; may be administered by SubQ, I.M., or I.V. routes.

I.V. administration (requires use of an infusion pump): **Only regular insulin** may be administered I.V.

I.V. infusions: To minimize adsorption problems to I.V. solution bag:

If new tubing is **not** needed: Wait a minimum of 30 minutes between the preparation of the solution and the initiation of the infusion.

If new tubing is needed: After receiving the insulin drip solution, the administration set should be attached to the I.V. container and the line should be flushed with the insulin solution. The nurse should wait 30 minutes, then flush the line again with the insulin solution prior to initiating the infusion.

If insulin is required prior to the availability of the insulin drip, regular insulin should be administered by I.V. push injection.

Because of adsorption, the actual amount of insulin being administered could be substantially less than the apparent amount. Therefore, adjustment of the insulin drip rate should be based on effect and not solely on the apparent insulin dose. Furthermore, the apparent dose should not be used as the basis for determining the subsequent insulin dose upon discontinuing the insulin drip. Dose requires continuous medical supervision.

Monitoring Parameters Urine sugar and acetone, serum glucose, electrolytes, Hb A_{1c}, lipid profile

(Continued)

Insulin Regular *(Continued)*

DKA: Arterial blood gases, CBC with differential, urinalysis, serum glucose (baseline and every hour until reaches 250 mg/dL), BUN, creatinine, electrolytes, anion gap

Hyperkalemia: Serum potassium and glucose must be closely monitored to avoid hypoglycemia and/or hypokalemia.

Reference Range

Therapeutic, serum insulin (fasting): 5-20 μIU/mL (SI: 35-145 pmol/L)

Glucose, fasting:

- Newborns: 60-110 mg/dL
- Adults: 60-110 mg/dL
- Elderly: 100-180 mg/dL

Recommendations for glycemic control, adults with type 1 diabetes:

- Hb A_{1c}: <7%
- Preprandial capillary plasma glucose: 90-130 mg/dL
- Peak postprandial capillary blood glucose: <180 mg/dL
- Blood pressure: <130/80 mm Hg

Criteria for diagnosis of DKA:

- Serum glucose: >250 mg/dL
- Arterial pH: <7.3
- Bicarbonate: <15 mEq/L
- Moderate ketonuria or ketonemia

Anesthesia and Critical Care Concerns/Other Considerations Intensive insulin therapy in critically-ill patients may have beneficial effects on mortality and morbidity.

Surgical Patients: Van den Berghe and colleagues (2001) performed a single-center, prospective, randomized, controlled study in 1548 surgical intensive care patients. Authors compared "conventional" control of blood glucose (180-200 mg/dL) versus "intensive" control of blood glucose (80-110 mg/dL). Primary outcome was ICU mortality. The authors showed an absolute mortality reduction of 3.4% (8.0% vs 4.6%; p: <0.04) in the intensive insulin therapy arm. Intensive insulin therapy also reduced bloodstream infections (7.8% vs 4.2%; p: 0.003), acute renal failure requiring hemodialysis (8.2 vs 4.8%; p: 0.007), and critical-illness polyneuropathy (51.9% vs 28.7%; p: <0.001). Greatest mortality reduction appeared in patients with an ICU stay >5 days, reducing mortality by 9.6% (20.2% vs 10.6%; p: 0.005). Other authors have shown intensive insulin therapy to reduce morbidity and mortality after myocardial infarction and coronary bypass.

Medical Patients: More recently, Van den Berghe (2006) did a similar study in adults admitted to the medical intensive care unit who were assumed to require at least 3 days of ICU care. The primary outcome was hospital mortality. Mortality in the ICU, 90 day mortality, days to wean from mechanical ventilation, days in ICU and hospital, new kidney injury were some of the secondary outcome measurements evaluated. A subgroup analysis was planned for patients staying in the ICU for > 3 days. Twelve hundred patients were randomized to conventional versus intensive blood glucose control. Intensive insulin therapy did not significantly reduce in-hospital mortality (40% conventional treatment group vs 37% intensive treatment group, p = 0.33). Morbidity was significantly reduced in the intensive group by the prevention of newly acquired kidney injury, accelerated weaning from mechanical ventilation and shortened stay in the ICU/hospital. For patients who stayed in the ICU for <3 days, mortality was greater in those receiving intensive insulin therapy. A subset of patients who remained in the ICU for 3 or more days was evaluated and in-hospital mortality was significantly reduced in those who received intensive insulin therapy.

Guidelines: The American College of Endocrinology recommends patients in an intensive care setting maintain serum glucose levels ≤110 mg/dL. In other inpatient units, patients may have preprandial glucoses ≤110 mg/dL and maximal glucose ≤180 mg/dL. The Surviving Sepsis Campaign guidelines recommend maintaining blood glucose <150 mg/dL.

Pregnancy Risk Factor B

Contraindications Hypersensitivity to any component of the formulation

Warnings/Precautions Hypoglycemia is the most common adverse effect of insulin. The timing of hypoglycemia differs among various insulin formulations. Any change of insulin should be made cautiously; changing manufacturers, type, and/or method of manufacture may result in the need for a change of dosage.

Human insulin differs from animal-source insulin. Regular insulin is the only insulin to be used I.V. Hypoglycemia may result from increased work or exercise without eating; use of long-acting insulin preparations (insulin glargine, Ultralente®, insulin U) may delay recovery from hypoglycemia. Use with caution in renal or hepatic impairment.

The general objective of insulin replacement therapy is to approximate the physiologic pattern of insulin secretion. This requires a basal level of insulin throughout the day, supplemented by additional insulin at mealtimes. Since combinations of agents are frequently used, dosage adjustment must address the individual component of the insulin regimen which most directly influences the blood glucose value in question, based on the known onset and duration of the insulin component. The frequency of doses and monitoring must be individualized in consideration of the patient's ability to manage therapy. Diabetic education and nutritional counseling are essential to maximize the effectiveness of therapy.

In type 1 diabetes mellitus (insulin dependent, IDDM), insulin lispro (Humalog®) and insulin glulisine (Apidra™) should be used in combination with a long-acting insulin. However, in type 2 diabetes mellitus (noninsulin dependent, NIDDM), insulin lispro (Humalog®) may be used without a long-acting insulin when used in combination with a sulfonylurea.

Adverse Reactions Frequency not defined.

Cardiovascular: Palpitation, pallor, tachycardia

Central nervous system: Fatigue, headache, hypothermia, loss of consciousness, mental confusion

Dermatologic: Urticaria, redness

Endocrine & metabolic: Hypoglycemia

Gastrointestinal: Hunger, nausea, numbness of mouth

Local: Atrophy or hypertrophy of SubQ fat tissue; edema, itching, pain or warmth at injection site; stinging

Neuromuscular & skeletal: Muscle weakness, paresthesia, tremor

Ocular: Transient presbyopia or blurred vision

Miscellaneous: Anaphylaxis, diaphoresis, local allergy, systemic allergic symptoms

Overdosage/Toxicology Symptoms of overdose include tachycardia, anxiety, hunger, tremor, pallor, headache, motor dysfunction, speech disturbances, sweating, palpitations, coma, and death. Antidote is glucose and glucagon, if necessary.

Drug Interactions Induces CYP1A2 (weak)

Drugs which **DECREASE** hypoglycemic effect of insulin:

Contraceptives (oral), corticosteroids, dextrothyroxine, diltiazem, dobutamine, epinephrine, niacin, smoking, thiazide diuretics, thyroid hormone

Drugs which **INCREASE** hypoglycemic effect of insulin:

Alcohol, alpha-blockers, anabolic steroids, beta-blockers (see "Note", clofibrate, guanethidine, MAO inhibitors, pentamidine, phenylbutazone, salicylates, sulfinpyrazone, tetracyclines. **Note:** Nonselective beta-blockers may delay recovery from hypoglycemic episodes and mask signs/symptoms of hypoglycemia. Cardioselective agents may be alternatives.

Insulin increases the risk of hypoglycemia associated with oral hypoglycemic agents (including sulfonylureas, metformin, pioglitazone, rosiglitazone, and troglitazone).

Ethanol/Nutrition/Herb Interactions

Ethanol: Caution with ethanol (may increase hypoglycemia).

Food: Insulin shifts potassium from extracellular to intracellular space. Decreases potassium serum concentration.

Herb/Nutraceutical: Use caution with chromium, garlic, gymnema (may increase hypoglycemia).

Dietary Considerations Dietary modification based on ADA recommendations is a part of therapy.

Dosage Forms

Injection, solution:

- Humulin® R: 100 units/mL (10 mL) [vial]
- Novolin® R: 100 units/mL (3 mL) [InnoLet® prefilled syringe or PenFill® prefilled cartridge]; (10 mL) [vial]

Injection, solution [concentrate] (Humulin® R U-500): 500 units/mL (20 mL vial)

References

American Diabetes Association, "Standards of Medical Care in Diabetes," *Diabetes Care*, 2005, 28(Suppl 1):4-36.

(Continued)

Insulin Regular *(Continued)*

Antman EM, Anbe SC, Alpert JS, et al, "ACC/AHA Guidelines for the Management of Patients With ST-Elevation Myocardial Infarction - Executive Summary: A Report of the American College of Cardiology/American Heart Association Task Force on Practice Guidelines (Writing Committee to Revise the 1999 Guidelines for the Management of Patients With Acute Myocardial Infarction)," *Circulation*, 2004, 110:588-636. Available at: http://www.circulationaha.org/cgi/content/full/110/5/588. Last accessed October 26, 2004.

Brown G and Dodek P, "Intravenous Insulin Nomogram Improves Blood Glucose Control in the Critically Ill," *Crit Care Med*, 2001, 29(9):1714-9.

Dailey G, "New Strategies for Basal Insulin Treatment in Type 2 Diabetes Mellitus," *Clin Ther*, 2004, 26(6):889-901.

Dellinger RP, Carlet JM, Masur H, et al, "Surviving Sepsis Campaign Guidelines for Management of Severe Sepsis and Septic Shock," *Crit Care Med*, 2004, 32(3):858-73.

Holman RR and Turner RC, "Insulin Therapy in Type II Diabetes," *Diabetes Res Clin Pract*, 1995, (28 Suppl):179-84.

Hopkins DF, Cotton SJ, and Williams G, "Effective Treatment of Insulin-Induced Edema Using Ephedrine," *Diabetes Care*, 1993, 16(7):1026-8.

Joint Commission on Accreditation of Healthcare Organizations, "2005 National Patient Safety Goals," available at http://www.jcaho.org/accredited+organizations/patient+safety/05_npsg_guidelines.

Kitabchi AE, Umpierrez GE, Murphy MB, et al, "Hyperglycemic Crises in Diabetes," *Diabetes Care*, 2004, 27(Suppl 1): 94-102.

Lazar HL, Philippides G, Fitzgerald C, et al, "Glucose-Insulin-Potassium Solutions Enhance Recovery After Urgent Coronary Artery Bypass Grafting," *J Thorac Cardiovasc Surg*, 1997, 113(2):354-60.

Levine DF and Bulstrode C, "Managing Suicidal Insulin Overdose," *Br Med J (Clin Res Ed)*, 1982, 285(6346):974-5.

Malhotra A, "Intensive Insulin in Intensive Care," *N Engl J Med*, 2006, 354(5):516-8.

Malmberg K, "Prospective Randomised Study of Intensive Insulin Treatment on Long Term Survival After Acute Myocardial Infarction in Patients With Diabetes Mellitus. DIGAMI (Diabetes Mellitus, Insulin Glucose Infusion in Acute Myocardial Infarction) Study Group," *BMJ*, 1997, 314(7093):1512-5.

Mokhlesi B, Leikin JB, Murray P, et al, "Adult Toxicology in Critical Care: Part II: Specific Poisonings," *Chest*, 2003, 123(3):897-922.

Morley JE and Perry HM 3d, "The Management of Diabetes Mellitus in Older Individuals," *Drugs*, 1991, 41(4):548-65.

Mueller-Schoop J, "Accidental Intravenous Self-Injection With Insulin Pen," *Lancet*, 1993, 341(8849):894.

Nathan DM, "Insulin Treatment in the Elderly Diabetic Patient," *Clin Geriatr Med*, 1990, 6(4):923-31.

Oiknine R, Bernbaum M, and Mooradian AD, "A Critical Appraisal of the Role of Insulin Analogues in the Management of Diabetes Mellitus," *Drugs*, 2005, 65(3):325-40.

"Proceedings of the American College of Endocrinology Task Force on Inpatient Diabetes and Metabolic Control Consensus Conference, Washington, DC, USA, December 2003," *Endocr Pract*, 2004, (10 Suppl 2):3-108.

Roberge RJ, Martin TG, and Delbridge TR, "Intentional Massive Insulin Overdose: Recognition and Management," *Ann Emerg Med*, 1993, 22(2):228-34.

Silverstein J, Klingensmith G, Copeland K, et al, "Care of Children and Adolescents With Type 1 Diabetes: A Statement of the American Diabetes Association," *Diabetes Care*, 2005, 28(1):186-212.

Simeon PS, Geffner ME, Levin SR, et al, "Continuous Insulin Infusions in Neonates: Pharmacologic Availability of Insulin in Intravenous Solutions," *J Pediatr*, 1994, 124(5 Pt 1):818-20.

Van den Berghe G, Wilmer A, Hermans G, et al, "Intensive Insulin Therapy in the Medical ICU," *N Engl J Med*, 2006, 354(5):449-6.

Van den Berghe G, Wouters P, Weekers F, et al, "Intensive Insulin Therapy in the Critically Ill Patients," *N Engl J Med*, 2001, 345(19):1359-67.

- **Insulin Regular and Insulin NPH** *see* Insulin NPH and Insulin Regular *on page 691*
- **Integrilin®** *see* Eptifibatide *on page 471*
- **Intralipid®** *see* Fat Emulsion *on page 508*
- **Intravenous Fat Emulsion** *see* Fat Emulsion *on page 508*
- **Intrifiban** *see* Eptifibatide *on page 471*
- **Intropin** *see* DOPamine *on page 414*
- **Invanz®** *see* Ertapenem *on page 473*
- **Invirase®** *see* Saquinavir *on page 1149*
- **Iodine** *see* Trace Metals *on page 1296*
- **Iodopen®** *see* Trace Metals *on page 1296*
- **Ionsys™** *see* Fentanyl *on page 514*
- **Iopidine®** *see* Apraclonidine *on page 119*

Ipratropium (i pra TROE pee um)

Medication Safety Issues

Sound-alike/look-alike issues:

Atrovent® may be confused with Alupent®

U.S. Brand Names Atrovent®; Atrovent® HFA

Canadian Brand Names Alti-Ipratropium; Apo-Ipravent®; Atrovent®; Atrovent® HFA; Gen-Ipratropium; Novo-Ipramide; Nu-Ipratropium; PMS-Ipratropium

Synonyms Ipratropium Bromide

Pharmacologic Category Anticholinergic Agent

Generic Available Yes: Excludes solution for oral inhalation

Use Anticholinergic bronchodilator used in bronchospasm associated with COPD, bronchitis, and emphysema; symptomatic relief of rhinorrhea associated with the common cold and allergic and nonallergic rhinitis

Mechanism of Action Blocks the action of acetylcholine at parasympathetic sites in bronchial smooth muscle causing bronchodilation

Pharmacodynamics/Kinetics

Onset of action: Bronchodilation: 1-3 minutes

Peak effect: 1.5-2 hours

Duration: ≤4 hours

Absorption: Negligible

Distribution: Inhalation: 15% of dose reaches lower airways

Dosage

Nebulization:

Infants and Children ≤12 years: 125-250 mcg 3 times/day

Children >12 years and Adults: 500 mcg (one unit-dose vial) 3-4 times/day with doses 6-8 hours apart

Oral inhalation: MDI:

Children 3-12 years: 1-2 inhalations 3 times/day, up to 6 inhalations/24 hours

Children >12 years and Adults: 2 inhalations 4 times/day, up to 12 inhalations/24 hours

Intranasal: Nasal spray:

Symptomatic relief of rhinorrhea associated with the common cold (safety and efficacy of use beyond 4 days in patients with the common cold have not been established):

Children 5-11 years: 0.06%: 2 sprays in each nostril 3 times/day

Children ≥5 years and Adults: 0.06%: 2 sprays in each nostril 3-4 times/day

Symptomatic relief of rhinorrhea associated with allergic/nonallergic rhinitis:

Children ≥6 years and Adults: 0.03%: 2 sprays in each nostril 2-3 times/day

Stability Store at 15°C to 30°C (59°F to 86°F); do not store near heat or open flame.

Administration

Atrovent®: Shake inhaler before each use; rinsing mouth after each use decreases dry mouth side effect

Atrovent® HFA: Prime inhaler by releasing 2 test sprays into the air. If the inhaler has not been used for >3 days, reprime.

Pregnancy Risk Factor B

Contraindications Hypersensitivity to ipratropium, atropine, its derivatives, or any component of the formulation

In addition, Atrovent® inhalation aerosol is contraindicated in patients with hypersensitivity to soya lecithin or related food products (eg, soybean and peanut). **Note:** Other formulations may include these components; refer to product-specific labeling.

Warnings/Precautions Not indicated for the initial treatment of acute episodes of bronchospasm; use with caution in patients with myasthenia gravis, narrow-angle glaucoma, benign prostatic hyperplasia (BPH), or bladder neck obstruction

Adverse Reactions

Inhalation aerosol and inhalation solution:

>10%: Bronchitis (10% to 23%), upper respiratory tract infection (13%)

1% to 10%:

Cardiovascular: Palpitation

Central nervous system: Dizziness (2% to 3%)

Dermatologic: Rash (1%)

Gastrointestinal: Nausea, xerostomia, stomach upset, dry mucous membranes

Renal: Urinary tract infection

Respiratory: Nasal congestion, dyspnea (10%), sputum increased (1%), bronchospasm (2%), pharyngitis (3%), rhinitis (2%), sinusitis (5%)

Miscellaneous: Flu-like syndrome

<1% (Limited to important or life-threatening): Anaphylactic reaction, angioedema, atrial fibrillation, bitter taste, blurred vision, bronchospasm, constipation,

(Continued)

Ipratropium *(Continued)*

eye pain (acute), glaucoma, hypersensitivity reactions, insomnia, laryngospasm, mucosal ulcers, nervousness, palpitations, rash, stomatitis, tachycardia (including supraventricular), tremor, urinary retention, urticaria

Nasal spray: Respiratory: Epistaxis (8%), nasal dryness (5%), nausea (2%)

Overdosage/Toxicology Symptoms of overdose include dry mouth, drying of respiratory secretions, cough, nausea, GI distress, blurred vision or impaired visual accommodation, headache, and nervousness. Acute overdose with ipratropium by inhalation is unlikely since it is so poorly absorbed. However, if poisoning occurs, it can be treated like any other anticholinergic toxicity. An anticholinergic overdose with severe life-threatening symptoms may be treated with physostigmine 1-2 mg SubQ or I.V. slowly.

Drug Interactions Anticholinergics: Concurrent use with ipratropium may increase risk of adverse events.

Dietary Considerations Some dosage forms may contain soya lecithin. Do not use in patients allergic to soya lecithin or related food products such as soybean and peanut.

Dosage Forms [DSC] = Discontinued product

Aerosol for oral inhalation, as bromide (Atrovent®): 18 mcg/actuation (14 g) [contains soya lecithin and chlorofluorocarbons] [DSC]

Aerosol for oral inhalation, as bromide (Atrovent® HFA): 17 mcg/actuation (12.9 g)

Solution for nebulization, as bromide: 0.02% (2.5 mL)

Solution, intranasal, as bromide [spray] (Atrovent®): 0.03% (30 mL); 0.06% (15 mL)

- **Ipratropium Bromide** *see* Ipratropium *on page 698*
- **I-Prin [OTC]** *see* Ibuprofen *on page 651*
- **Iproveratril Hydrochloride** *see* Verapamil *on page 1352*
- **Iquix®** *see* Levofloxacin *on page 746*

Irbesartan (ir be SAR tan)

Medication Safety Issues

Sound-alike/look-alike issues:

Avapro® may be confused with Anaprox®

Related Information

Angiotensin Agents *on page 1544*

U.S. Brand Names Avapro®

Canadian Brand Names Avapro®

Pharmacologic Category Angiotensin II Receptor Blocker

Generic Available No

Use Treatment of hypertension alone or in combination with other antihypertensives; treatment of diabetic nephropathy in patients with type 2 diabetes mellitus (noninsulin dependent, NIDDM) and hypertension

Mechanism of Action Irbesartan is an angiotensin receptor antagonist. Angiotensin II acts as a vasoconstrictor. In addition to causing direct vasoconstriction, angiotensin II also stimulates the release of aldosterone. Once aldosterone is released, sodium as well as water are reabsorbed. The end result is an elevation in blood pressure. Irbesartan binds to the AT1 angiotensin II receptor. This binding prevents angiotensin II from binding to the receptor thereby blocking the vasoconstriction and the aldosterone secreting effects of angiotensin II.

Pharmacodynamics/Kinetics

Onset of action: Peak effect: 1-2 hours

Duration: >24 hours

Distribution: V_d: 53-93 L

Protein binding, plasma: 90%

Metabolism: Hepatic, primarily CYP2C9

Bioavailability: 60% to 80%

Half-life elimination: Terminal: 11-15 hours

Time to peak, serum: 1.5-2 hours

Excretion: Feces (80%); urine (20%)

Dosage Oral:

Hypertension:

Children:

<6 years: Safety and efficacy have not been established.

≥6-12 years: Initial: 75 mg once daily; may be titrated to a maximum of 150 mg once daily

Children ≥13 years and Adults: 150 mg once daily; patients may be titrated to 300 mg once daily

Note: Starting dose in volume-depleted patients should be 75 mg

Nephropathy in patients with type 2 diabetes and hypertension: Adults: Target dose: 300 mg once daily

Dosage adjustment in renal impairment: No dosage adjustment necessary with mild to severe impairment unless the patient is also volume depleted.

Stability Store at room temperature of 15°C to 30°C (59°F to 86°F).

Anesthesia and Critical Care Concerns/Other Considerations The angiotensin II receptor antagonists appear to have similar indications as the ACE inhibitors. In heart failure, the angiotensin II antagonists are especially useful in providing an alternative therapy in those patients who have intractable cough in response to ACE inhibitor therapy. Candesartan has been studied as an alternative therapy in chronic heart failure patients who cannot tolerate an ACE-I (CHARM-Alternative) and as an added therapy in heart failure patients who are maintained on an ACE-I (CHARM-Added). In both studies the combined endpoint of cardiovascular death or heart failure hospitalizations was significantly improved over the placebo treated group. Similar to ACE inhibitors, pre-existing volume depletion caused by diuretic therapy may potentiate hypotension in response to angiotensin II antagonists. Concomitant NSAID therapy may attenuate blood pressure control; use of NSAIDs should be avoided or limited, with monitoring of blood pressure control. In the setting of heart failure, NSAID use may be associated with an increased risk for fluid accumulation and edema.

Pregnancy Risk Factor C/D (2nd and 3rd trimesters)

Contraindications Hypersensitivity to irbesartan or any component of the formulation; hypersensitivity to other A-II receptor antagonists; bilateral renal artery stenosis; pregnancy (2nd and 3rd trimesters)

Warnings/Precautions [U.S. Boxed Warning]: Based on human data, drugs that act on the angiotensin system can cause injury and death to the developing fetus when used in the second and third trimesters. Angiotensin receptor blockers should be discontinued as soon as possible once pregnancy is detected. Avoid use or use smaller doses in patients who are volume depleted; correct depletion first. Deterioration in renal function can occur with initiation. Use with caution in unilateral renal artery stenosis and pre-existing renal insufficiency; significant aortic/mitral stenosis. Safety and efficacy have not been established in pediatric patients <6 years of age.

Adverse Reactions Unless otherwise indicated, percentage of incidence is reported for patients with hypertension.

>10%: Endocrine & metabolic: Hyperkalemia (19%, diabetic nephropathy; rarely seen in HTN)

1% to 10%:

Cardiovascular: Orthostatic hypotension (5%, diabetic nephropathy)

Central nervous system: Fatigue (4%), dizziness (10%, diabetic nephropathy)

Gastrointestinal: Diarrhea (3%), dyspepsia (2%)

Respiratory: Upper respiratory infection (9%), cough (2.8% versus 2.7% in placebo)

<1% (Limited to important or life-threatening): Angina, angioedema, arrhythmia, cardiopulmonary arrest, conjunctivitis, depression, dyspnea, ecchymosis, edema, epistaxis, gout, heart failure, hepatitis, hypotension, jaundice, libido decreased, MI, orthostatic hypotension, paresthesia, sexual dysfunction, stroke, transaminases increased, urticaria. May be associated with worsening of renal function in patients dependent on renin-angiotensin-aldosterone system.

Overdosage/Toxicology Likely manifestations of overdose include hypotension and tachycardia. Treatment is supportive. Not removed by hemodialysis.

Drug Interactions Substrate of CYP2C9 (minor); **Inhibits** CYP2C8 (moderate), 2C9 (moderate), 2D6 (weak), 3A4 (weak)

CYP2C8 Substrates: Irbesartan may increase the levels/effects of CYP2C8 substrates. Example substrates include amiodarone, paclitaxel, pioglitazone, repaglinide, and rosiglitazone.

CYP2C9 Substrates: Irbesartan may increase the levels/effects of CYP2C9 substrates. Example substrates include bosentan, dapsone, fluoxetine, glimepiride, glipizide, losartan, montelukast, nateglinide, paclitaxel, phenytoin, warfarin, and zafirlukast.

Lithium: Risk of toxicity may be increased by irbesartan; monitor lithium levels.

(Continued)

Irbesartan *(Continued)*

NSAIDs: May decrease angiotensin II antagonist efficacy; effect has been seen with losartan, but may occur with other medications in this class; monitor blood pressure

Potassium-sparing diuretics (amiloride, potassium, spironolactone, triamterene): Increased risk of hyperkalemia.

Potassium supplements may increase the risk of hyperkalemia.

Trimethoprim (high dose) may increase the risk of hyperkalemia.

Ethanol/Nutrition/Herb Interactions Herb/Nutraceutical: Avoid dong quai if using for hypertension (has estrogenic activity). Avoid ephedra, yohimbe, ginseng (may worsen hypertension). Avoid garlic (may have increased antihypertensive effect).

Dietary Considerations May be taken with or without food.

Dosage Forms Tablet: 75 mg, 150 mg, 300 mg

♦ **Isoamyl Nitrite** *see* Amyl Nitrite *on page 112*

Isoflurane (eye soe FLURE ane)

Medication Safety Issues

Sound-alike/look-alike issues:

Isoflurane may be confused with enflurane, isoflurophate

Related Information

Anesthesia Considerations for Neurosurgery *on page 1401*

Inhalational Anesthetics *on page 1528*

U.S. Brand Names Forane®; Terrell™

Canadian Brand Names Forane®

Pharmacologic Category General Anesthetic, Inhalation

Generic Available Yes

Use Maintenance of general anesthesia

Pharmacodynamics/Kinetics

Onset of action: 7-10 minutes (pungent odor limits inhalation rate)

Duration: Emergence time: Depends on blood concentration when discontinued

Metabolism: Hepatic (0.2%)

Excretion: Exhaled gases

Dosage Minimum alveolar concentration (MAC), the concentration at which 50% of patients do not respond to surgical incision, is 1.2% for isoflurane. The concentration at which amnesia and loss of awareness occur (MAC - awake) is 0.4%. Surgical levels of anesthesia are achieved with concentrations between 1% to 2.5%. MAC is reduced in the elderly.

Administration Via isoflurane-specific calibrated vaporizer

Monitoring Parameters Blood pressure, heart rate and rhythm, oxygen saturation, end-tidal CO_2 and isoflurane concentrations should be monitored prior to and throughout anesthesia

Anesthesia and Critical Care Concerns/Other Considerations Use of isoflurane for induction of anesthesia is limited by its pungent odor which may cause breath holding or coughing.

Pregnancy Risk Factor C

Contraindications Hypersensitivity to isoflurane or any component of the formulation; known or suspected history of malignant hyperthermia

Warnings/Precautions Decrease in blood pressure is dose dependent due to peripheral vasodilation primarily in skin and muscle; cardiac output is maintained. Isoflurane may produce cardiac steal (due to coronary vasodilation) in patients with hypertension under certain conditions (eg, unusual coronary artery anatomy). Isoflurane may produce reflex tachycardia, but does not alter atrioventricular conduction or sensitize the myocardium to epinephrine-induced arrhythmias. Respiration is depressed as is the normal hyperventilatory response to hypoxia. Hypoxic pulmonary vasoconstriction is depressed which may lead to pulmonary shunt. Isoflurane dilates the cerebral vasculature and may, in certain conditions, increase intracranial pressure. Renal, splenic, and hepatic blood flow are reduced. Isoflurane is a trigger of malignant hyperthermia. Hypoxemia-induced increase in ventilation is abolished at low isoflurane concentration. Isoflurane can produce elevated carbon monoxide levels in the presence of a dry carbon dioxide absorbent within the circle breathing system of an anesthetic machine.

Adverse Reactions Frequency not defined.

Cardiovascular: Hypotension, myocardial depression
Respiratory: Respiratory depression/arrest
Gastrointestinal: Nausea, vomiting
Miscellaneous: Shivering

Drug Interactions **Substrate** of CYP2E1 (major); **Inhibits** CYP2B6 (weak)

Antihypertensives: Excessive hypotension may occur with combined use.

Benzodiazepines, opioids: Concurrent use of opioids and/or benzodiazepines decreases the MAC of isoflurane.

CYP2E1 inhibitors: May increase the levels/effects of isoflurane. Example inhibitors include disulfiram, isoniazid, and miconazole.

Isoniazid: Increased risk of hepatotoxicity with combined use.

Neuromuscular-blocking agents (nondepolarizing): Isoflurane may potentiate the action of nondepolarizing, neuromuscular-blocking agents.

Dosage Forms Liquid, for inhalation: >99.9% (100 mL, 250 mL)

References

Campagna JA, Miller KW, and Forman SA, "Mechanisms of Action of Inhaled Anesthetics," *N Engl J Med*, 2003, 348(21):2110-23.

Ebert TJ and Muzi M, "Sympathetic Hyperactivity During Desflurane Anesthesia in Healthy Volunteers. A Comparison With Isoflurane," *Anesthesiology*, 1993, 79(3):444-53.

Eger EI 2nd, "Isoflurane: A Review," *Anesthesiology*, 1981, 55(5):559-76.

Fee JP and Thompson GH, "Comparative Tolerability Profiles of the Inhaled Anaesthetics," *Drug Saf*, 1997, 16(3):157-70.

Park KW, "Cardiovascular Effects of Inhalational Anesthetics," *Int Anesthesiol Clin*, 2002, 40(1):1-14.

Yasuda N, Lockhart SH, Eger EI 2nd, et al, "Comparison of Kinetics of Sevoflurane and Isoflurane in Humans," *Anesth Analg*, 1991, 72(3):316-24.

Yasuda N, Lockhart SH, Eger EI 2nd, et al, "Kinetics of Desflurane, Isoflurane, and Halothane in Humans," *Anesthesiology*, 1991, 74(3):489-98.

Isoniazid (eye soe NYE a zid)

U.S. Brand Names Nydrazid® [DSC]

Canadian Brand Names Isotamine®; PMS-Isoniazid

Synonyms INH; Isonicotinic Acid Hydrazide

Pharmacologic Category Antitubercular Agent

Generic Available Yes

Use Treatment of susceptible tuberculosis infections; treatment of latent tuberculosis infection (LTBI)

Mechanism of Action Unknown, but may include the inhibition of myocolic acid synthesis resulting in disruption of the bacterial cell wall

Pharmacodynamics/Kinetics

Absorption: Rapid and complete; rate can be slowed with food

Distribution: All body tissues and fluids including CSF; crosses placenta; enters breast milk

Protein binding: 10% to 15%

Metabolism: Hepatic with decay rate determined genetically by acetylation phenotype

Half-life elimination: Fast acetylators: 30-100 minutes; Slow acetylators: 2-5 hours; may be prolonged with hepatic or severe renal impairment

Time to peak, serum: 1-2 hours

Excretion: Urine (75% to 95%); feces; saliva

Dosage Recommendations often change due to resistant strains and newly-developed information; consult *MMWR* for current CDC recommendations:

Oral (injectable is available for patients who are unable to either take or absorb oral therapy):

Infants and Children:

Treatment of latent TB infection (LTBI): 10-20 mg/kg/day in 1-2 divided doses (maximum: 300 mg/day) or 20-40 mg/kg (maximum: 900 mg/dose) twice weekly for 9 months

Treatment of active TB infection:

Daily therapy: 10-15 mg/kg/day in 1-2 divided doses (maximum: 300 mg/day)

Twice weekly directly observed therapy (DOT): 20-30 mg/kg (maximum: 900 mg)

Adults:

Treatment of latent tuberculosis infection (LTBI): 300 mg/day or 900 mg twice weekly for 6-9 months in patients who do not have HIV infection (9 months is optimal, 6 months may be considered to reduce costs of therapy) and 9 months in patients who have HIV infection. Extend to 12 months of therapy if interruptions in treatment occur.

(Continued)

Isoniazid *(Continued)*

Treatment of active TB infection (drug susceptible):

Daily therapy: 5 mg/kg/day given daily (usual dose: 300 mg/day); 10 mg/kg/day in 1-2 divided doses in patients with disseminated disease

Twice weekly directly observed therapy (DOT): 15 mg/kg (maximum: 900 mg); 3 times/week therapy: 15 mg/kg (maximum: 900 mg)

Note: Treatment may be defined by the number of doses administered (eg, "six-month" therapy involves 192 doses of INH and rifampin, and 56 doses of pyrazinamide). Six months is the shortest interval of time over which these doses may be administered, assuming no interruption of therapy.

Note: Concomitant administration of 6-50 mg/day pyridoxine is recommended in malnourished patients or those prone to neuropathy (eg, alcoholics, diabetics)

Dosing adjustment in renal impairment:

Cl_{cr} <10 mL/minute: Administer 50% of normal dose

Hemodialysis: Dialyzable (50% to 100%)

Administer dose postdialysis

Peritoneal dialysis, continuous arteriovenous or venovenous hemofiltration: Dose for Cl_{cr} <10 mL/minute

Dosing adjustment in hepatic impairment: Dose should be reduced in severe hepatic disease

Stability Protect oral dosage forms from light

Administration Should be administered 1 hour before or 2 hours after meals on an empty stomach.

Monitoring Parameters Periodic liver function tests; sputum cultures monthly (until 2 consecutive negative cultures reported); monitoring for prodromal signs of hepatitis

Reference Range Therapeutic: 1-7 mcg/mL (SI: 7-51 μmol/L); Toxic: 20-710 mcg/mL (SI: 146-5176 μmol/L)

Pregnancy Risk Factor C

Contraindications Hypersensitivity to isoniazid or any component of the formulation; acute liver disease; previous history of hepatic damage during isoniazid therapy

Warnings/Precautions Use with caution in patients with renal impairment and chronic liver disease. **[U.S. Boxed Warning]: Severe and sometimes fatal hepatitis may occur or develop even after many months of treatment.** Patients must report any prodromal symptoms of hepatitis, such as fatigue, weakness, malaise, anorexia, nausea, or vomiting. Malnourished patients should receive concomitant pyridoxine therapy. Periodic ophthalmic examinations are recommended even when usual symptoms do not occur; pyridoxine (10-50 mg/day) is recommended in individuals likely to develop peripheral neuropathies.

Adverse Reactions Frequency not defined.

Cardiovascular: Hypertension, palpitation, tachycardia, vasculitis

Central nervous system: Dizziness, encephalopathy, memory impairment, slurred speech, lethargy, fever, depression, psychosis, seizure

Dermatologic: Rash (morbilliform, maculopapular, pruritic, or exfoliative), flushing

Endocrine & metabolic: Hyperglycemia, metabolic acidosis, gynecomastia, pellagra, pyridoxine deficiency

Gastrointestinal: Anorexia, nausea, vomiting, stomach pain

Hematologic: Agranulocytosis, anemia (sideroblastic, hemolytic, or aplastic), thrombocytopenia, eosinophilia, lymphadenopathy

Hepatic: LFTs mildly increased (10% to 20%); hyperbilirubinemia, jaundice, hepatitis (may involve progressive liver damage; risk increases with age; 2.3% in patients >50 years)

Neuromuscular & skeletal: Weakness, peripheral neuropathy (dose-related incidence, 10% to 20% incidence with 10 mg/kg/day), hyper-reflexia, arthralgia, lupus-like syndrome

Ocular: Blurred vision, loss of vision, optic neuritis and atrophy

Overdosage/Toxicology Symptoms of overdose generally occur within 30 minutes to 3 hours, and may include nausea, vomiting, slurred speech, dizziness, blurred vision, metabolic acidosis, hallucinations, stupor, coma, and intractable seizures. Because of high morbidity and mortality rates with isoniazid overdose, patients who are asymptomatic after an overdose should be monitored for 4-6 hours. Pyridoxine has been shown to be effective in the treatment of intoxication, especially when seizures occur. Pyridoxine I.V. is administered on a milligram to milligram dose. If the amount of isoniazid ingested is unknown, 5 g of pyridoxine should be given over 3-5 minutes and may be followed by an additional 5 g in 30 minutes. Treatment is supportive. Forced diuresis and hemodialysis can result in more rapid removal.

Drug Interactions **Substrate** of CYP2E1 (major); **Inhibits** CYP1A2 (weak), 2A6 (moderate), 2C9 (weak), 2C19 (strong), 2D6 (moderate), 2E1 (moderate), 3A4 (strong); **Induces** CYP2E1 (after discontinuation) (weak)

Acetaminophen: Isoniazid may enhance the adverse/toxic effect of acetaminophen.

Antacids: Antacids may decrease the absorption of isoniazid.

Benzodiazepines (metabolized by oxidation): Isoniazid may decrease the metabolism, via CYP isoenzymes, of benzodiazepines (metabolized by oxidation).

Carbamazepine: Isoniazid may decrease the metabolism of carbamazepine.

Cycloserine: Cycloserine may enhance the CNS depressant effect of isoniazid.

CYP2A6 substrates: Isoniazid may increase the levels/effects of CYP2A6 substrates. Example substrates include dexmedetomidine and ifosfamide.

CYP2C19 substrates: Isoniazid may increase the levels/effects of CYP2C19 substrates. Example substrates include citalopram, diazepam, methsuximide, phenytoin, propranolol, and sertraline.

CYP2D6 substrates: Isoniazid may increase the levels/effects of CYP2D6 substrates. Example substrates include amphetamines, selected beta-blockers, dextromethorphan, fluoxetine, lidocaine, mirtazapine, nefazodone, paroxetine, risperidone, ritonavir, thioridazine, tricyclic antidepressants, and venlafaxine.

CYP2D6 prodrug substrates: Isoniazid may decrease the levels/effects of CYP2D6 prodrug substrates. Example prodrug substrates include codeine, hydrocodone, oxycodone, and tramadol.

CYP2E1 substrates: Isoniazid may increase the levels/effects of CYP2E1 substrates. Example substrates include inhalational anesthetics, theophylline, and trimethadione.

CYP3A4 substrates: Isoniazid may increase the levels/effects of CYP3A4 substrates. Example substrates include benzodiazepines, calcium channel blockers, mirtazapine, nateglinide, nefazodone, tacrolimus, and venlafaxine. Selected benzodiazepines (midazolam and triazolam), cisapride, ergot alkaloids, selected HMG-CoA reductase inhibitors (lovastatin and simvastatin), and pimozide are generally contraindicated with strong CYP3A4 inhibitors.

Disulfiram: Isoniazid may enhance the adverse/toxic effect of disulfiram.

Phenytoin: Isoniazid may decrease the metabolism, via CYP isoenzymes, of phenytoin.

Theophylline: Isoniazid may decrease the metabolism, via CYP isoenzymes, of theophylline derivatives.

Valproic Acid: Isoniazid may increase the serum concentration of valproic acid.

Ethanol/Nutrition/Herb Interactions

Ethanol: Avoid ethanol (increases the risk of hepatitis).

Food: Isoniazid serum levels may be decreased if taken with food. Has some ability to inhibit tyramine metabolism; several case reports of mild reactions (flushing, palpitations) after ingestion of cheese with or without wine. Isoniazid decreases folic acid absorption. Isoniazid alters pyridoxine metabolism.

Test Interactions False-positive urinary glucose with Clinitest®

Dietary Considerations Should be taken 1 hour before or 2 hours after meals on an empty stomach; increase dietary intake of folate, niacin, magnesium. No need to restrict tyramine-containing foods.

Dosage Forms [DSC] = Discontinued product

Injection, solution (Nydrazid®): 100 mg/mL (10 mL) [DSC]

Syrup: 50 mg/5 mL (473 mL) [orange flavor]

Tablet: 100 mg, 300 mg

- **Isonicotinic Acid Hydrazide** *see* Isoniazid *on page 703*
- **Isonipecaine Hydrochloride** *see* Meperidine *on page 801*
- **Isophane Insulin** *see* Insulin NPH *on page 690*
- **Isophane Insulin and Regular Insulin** *see* Insulin NPH and Insulin Regular *on page 691*

Isoproterenol (eye soe proe TER e nole)

Medication Safety Issues

Sound-alike/look-alike issues:

Isuprel® may be confused with Disophrol®, Ismelin®, Isordil®

(Continued)

Isoproterenol *(Continued)*

Related Information

Hemodynamic Support, Intravenous *on page 1566*

U.S. Brand Names Isuprel®

Synonyms Isoproterenol Hydrochloride

Pharmacologic Category $Beta_1$- & $Beta_2$-Adrenergic Agonist Agent

Generic Available Yes

Use Ventricular arrhythmias due to AV nodal block; hemodynamically compromised bradyarrhythmias or atropine- and dopamine-resistant bradyarrhythmias (when transcutaneous/venous pacing is not available); temporary use in third-degree AV block until pacemaker insertion

Unlabeled/Investigational Use Pharmacologic overdrive pacing for torsade de pointes; diagnostic aid (vasovagal syncope)

Mechanism of Action Stimulates $beta_1$- and $beta_2$-receptors resulting in relaxation of bronchial, GI, and uterine smooth muscle, increased heart rate and contractility, vasodilation of peripheral vasculature

Pharmacodynamics/Kinetics

Onset of action: Bronchodilation: I.V.: Immediate

Duration: I.V.: 10-15 minutes

Metabolism: Via conjugation in many tissues including hepatic and pulmonary

Half-life elimination: 2.5-5 minutes

Excretion: Urine (primarily as sulfate conjugates)

Dosage I.V.: Cardiac arrhythmias:

Children: Initial: 0.1 mcg/kg/minute (usual effective dose 0.2-2 mcg/kg/minute)

Adults: Initial: 2 mcg/minute; titrate to patient response (2-10 mcg/minute)

Stability Isoproterenol solution should be stored at room temperature; it should not be used if a color or precipitate is present. Exposure to air, light, or increased temperature may cause a pink to brownish pink color to develop. Stability of parenteral admixture at room temperature (25°C) or at refrigeration (4°C) is 24 hours.

Standard diluent: 2 mg/500 mL D_5W; 4 mg/500 mL D_5W

Minimum volume: 1 mg/100 mL D_5W

Incompatible with alkaline solutions, aminophylline and furosemide

Administration I.V. infusion administration requires the use of an infusion pump. To prepare for infusion: 1 mg isoproterenol to 500 mL D_5W, final concentration 2 mcg/mL

Monitoring Parameters ECG, heart rate, respiratory rate, arterial blood gas, arterial blood pressure, CVP; serum glucose, serum potassium, serum magnesium

Anesthesia and Critical Care Concerns/Other Considerations Pharmacologic overdrive pacing with isoproterenol may be helpful in the treatment of torsade de pointes. In patients with recurrent torsade de pointes, treatment consists of correcting underlying cause (eg, electrolyte abnormalities or drug ingestion). Supportive therapy consists of increasing heart rate so as to decrease the QT interval.

Pregnancy Risk Factor C

Contraindications Hypersensitivity to sulfites or isoproterenol, any component of the formulation, or other sympathomimetic amines; angina, pre-existing cardiac arrhythmias (ventricular); tachycardia or AV block caused by cardiac glycoside intoxication

Warnings/Precautions Use with extreme caution; not currently a treatment of choice; use with caution in elderly patients, diabetics, renal or cardiovascular disease, seizure disorder, or hyperthyroidism; excessive or prolonged use may result in decreased effectiveness.

Adverse Reactions Frequency not defined.

Cardiovascular: Premature ventricular beats, bradycardia, hyper-/hypotension, chest pain, palpitation, tachycardia, ventricular arrhythmia, MI size increased

Central nervous system: Headache, nervousness or restlessness

Endocrine & metabolic: Serum glucose increased, serum potassium decreased, hypokalemia

Gastrointestinal: Nausea, vomiting

Respiratory: Dyspnea

Overdosage/Toxicology Symptoms of overdose include tachycardia, tremor, hypertension or hypotension, angina, and seizures. Hypokalemia also may occur.

Cardiac arrest and death may be associated with abuse of beta-agonist bronchodilators. Treatment includes immediate discontinuation and symptomatic and supportive therapies. Cautious use of beta-adrenergic blocking agents may be considered in severe cases.

Drug Interactions Increased toxicity: Sympathomimetic agents may cause headaches and elevate blood pressure; general anesthetics may cause arrhythmias

Ethanol/Nutrition/Herb Interactions Herb/Nutraceutical: Avoid ephedra, yohimbe (may cause CNS stimulation).

Dosage Forms Injection, solution, as hydrochloride: 0.02 mg/mL (10 mL); 0.2 mg/mL (1:5000) (1 mL, 5 mL) [contains sodium metabisulfite]

References

"2005 American Heart Association Guidelines for Cardiopulmonary Resuscitation and Emergency Cardiovascular Care," *Circulation*, 2005, 112(24 Suppl): 130.

Almquist A, Goldenberg IF, Milstein S, et al, "Provocation of Bradycardia and Hypotension by Isoproterenol and Upright Posture in Patients With Unexplained Syncope," *N Engl J Med*, 1989, 320(6):346-51.

Hemstreet MP, Miles MV, and Rutland RO, "Effect of Intravenous Isoproterenol on Theophylline Kinetics," *J Allergy Clin Immunol*, 1982, 69(4):360-4.

Illi A, Sundberg S, Ojala-Karlsson P, et al, "The Effect of Entacapone on the Disposition and Hemodynamic Effects of Intravenous Isoproterenol and Epinephrine," *Clin Pharmacol Ther*, 1995, 58(2):221-7.

Lang CC, Stein CM, Brown RM, et al, "Attenuation of Isoproterenol-Mediated Vasodilatation in Blacks," *N Engl J Med*, 1995, 333(3):155-60.

Rachelefsky GS and Siegel SC, "Asthma in Infants and Children - Treatment of Childhood Asthma: Part II," *J Allergy Clin Immunol*, 1985, 76(3):409-25.

♦ **Isoproterenol Hydrochloride** *see* Isoproterenol *on page 705*
♦ **Isoptin® SR** *see* Verapamil *on page 1352*
♦ **Isopto® Atropine** *see* Atropine *on page 144*
♦ **Isopto® Carbachol** *see* Carbachol *on page 224*
♦ **Isopto® Eserine (Can)** *see* Physostigmine *on page 1026*
♦ **Isopto® Hyoscine** *see* Scopolamine *on page 1152*
♦ **Isotamine® (Can)** *see* Isoniazid *on page 703*
♦ **Istalol™** *see* Timolol *on page 1268*
♦ **Isuprel®** *see* Isoproterenol *on page 705*
♦ **Iveegam EN** *see* Immune Globulin (Intravenous) *on page 666*
♦ **Iveegam Immuno® (Can)** *see* Immune Globulin (Intravenous) *on page 666*
♦ **IVIG** *see* Immune Globulin (Intravenous) *on page 666*
♦ **IvySoothe® [OTC]** *see* Hydrocortisone *on page 639*
♦ **Jantoven™** *see* Warfarin *on page 1362*
♦ **Kadian®** *see* Morphine Sulfate *on page 867*

Kanamycin (kan a MYE sin)

Medication Safety Issues

Sound-alike/look-alike issues:

Kanamycin may be confused with Garamycin®, gentamicin

U.S. Brand Names Kantrex®

Canadian Brand Names Kantrex®

Synonyms Kanamycin Sulfate

Pharmacologic Category Antibiotic, Aminoglycoside

Generic Available No

Use Treatment of serious infections caused by susceptible strains of *E. coli*, *Proteus* species, *Enterobacter aerogenes*, *Klebsiella pneumoniae*, *Serratia marcescens*, and *Acinetobacter* species; second-line treatment of *Mycobacterium tuberculosis*

Mechanism of Action Interferes with protein synthesis in bacterial cell by binding to ribosomal subunit

Pharmacodynamics/Kinetics

Distribution:

Relative diffusion from blood into CSF: Good only with inflammation (exceeds usual MICs)

CSF:blood level ratio: Normal meninges: Nil; Inflamed meninges: 43%

Half-life elimination: 2-4 hours; Anuria: 80 hours; End-stage renal disease: 40-96 hours

Time to peak, serum: I.M.: 1-2 hours (decreased in burn patients)

Excretion: Urine (entire amount)

(Continued)

Kanamycin *(Continued)*

Dosage Note: Dosing should be based on ideal body weight

Children: Infections: I.M., I.V.: 15 mg/kg/day in divided doses every 8-12 hours

Adults:

Infections: I.M., I.V.: 5-7.5 mg/kg/dose in divided doses every 8-12 hours (<15 mg/kg/day)

Intraperitoneal: After contamination in surgery: 500 mg

Irrigating solution: 0.25%; maximum 1.5 g/day (via all administration routes)

Aerosol: 250 mg 2-4 times/day

Dosing adjustment/interval in renal impairment:

Cl_{cr} 50-80 mL/minute: Administer 60% to 90% of dose or administer every 8-12 hours

Cl_{cr} 10-50 mL/minute: Administer 30% to 70% of dose or administer every 12 hours

Cl_{cr} <10 mL/minute: Administer 20% to 30% of dose or administer every 24-48 hours

Stability Store vial at controlled room temperature. Darkening of vials does not indicate loss of potency.

I.V.: Must be further diluted prior to I.V. infusion. For adults, dilute 500 mg in 100-200 mL of appropriate solution or 1 g in 200-400 mL; for pediatric patients, use sufficient amount to infuse solution over 30-60 minutes.

Intraperitoneal: Dilute dose in 20 mL sterile distilled water.

Aerosol: Dilute 250 mg in 3 mL normal saline.

Administration

I.M.: Administer deeply in upper outer quadrant of the gluteal muscle.

I.V.: Infuse over 30-60 minutes.

Some penicillins (eg, carbenicillin, ticarcillin and piperacillin) have been shown to inactivate aminoglycosides *in vitro*. This has been observed to a greater extent with tobramycin and gentamicin, while amikacin has shown greater stability against inactivation. Concurrent use of these agents may pose a risk of reduced antibacterial efficacy *in vivo*, particularly in the setting of profound renal impairment. However, definitive clinical evidence is lacking. If combination penicillin/aminoglycoside therapy is desired in a patient with renal dysfunction, separation of doses (if feasible), and routine monitoring of aminoglycoside levels, CBC, and clinical response should be considered.

Monitoring Parameters Serum creatinine and BUN every 2-3 days; peak and trough concentrations; hearing

Some penicillin derivatives may accelerate the degradation of aminoglycosides*in vitro*. This may be clinically-significant for certain penicillin (ticarcillin, piperacillin, carbenicillin) and aminoglycoside (gentamicin, tobramycin) combination therapy in patients with significant renal impairment. Close monitoring of aminoglycoside levels is warranted.

Reference Range Therapeutic: Peak: 15-30 mcg/mL; Trough: 5-10 mcg/mL; Toxic: Peak: >35 mcg/mL; Trough: >10 mcg/mL

Pregnancy Risk Factor D

Contraindications Hypersensitivity to kanamycin, any component of the formulation, or other aminoglycosides; pregnancy

Warnings/Precautions [U.S. Boxed Warning]: Aminoglycosides may cause neurotoxicity and/or nephrotoxicity; usual risk factors include prexisiting renal impairment, concomitant neuro-/nephrotoxic medications, advanced age and dehydration. Ototoxicity may be directly proportional to the amount of drug given and the duration of treatment; tinnitus or vertigo are indications of vestibular injury and impending hearing loss; renal damage is usually reversible

Not intended for long-term therapy due to toxic hazards associated with extended administration; use caution in pre-existing renal insufficiency, vestibular or cochlear impairment, myasthenia gravis, hypocalcemia, conditions which depress neuromuscular transmission. Dosage modification required in patients with impaired renal function

Adverse Reactions Frequency not defined.

Cardiovascular: Edema

Central nervous system: Neurotoxicity, drowsiness, headache, pseudomotor cerebri

Dermatologic: Skin itching, redness, rash, photosensitivity, erythema

Gastrointestinal: Nausea, vomiting, diarrhea, malabsorption syndrome (with prolonged and high-dose therapy of hepatic coma), anorexia, weight loss, salivation increased, enterocolitis

Hematologic: Granulocytopenia, agranulocytosis, thrombocytopenia
Local: Burning, stinging
Neuromuscular & skeletal: Weakness, tremor, muscle cramps
Otic: Ototoxicity (auditory), ototoxicity (vestibular)
Renal: Nephrotoxicity
Respiratory: Dyspnea

Overdosage/Toxicology Symptoms of overdose include ototoxicity, nephrotoxicity, and neuromuscular toxicity. The treatment of choice following a single acute overdose appears to be the maintenance of good urine output of at least 3 mL/kg/hour. Hemodialysis or peritoneal dialysis may enhance kanamycin elimination; exchange transfusion may also be considered in the newborn infant.

Drug Interactions

Amphotericin B: Concomitant use may lead to nephrotoxicity (reported with gentamicin).
Bisphosphonate derivatives: Concomitant use may lead to hypocalcemia (reported with amikacin and clodronate).
Cisplatin: Concomitant use may lead to increased nephrotoxicity.
Loop diuretics: May increase risk of ototoxicity (reported with ethacrynic acid) and nephrotoxicity.
Neuromuscular-blocking agents: Increase risk of neuromuscular blockade

Test Interactions Some penicillin derivatives may accelerate the degradation of aminoglycosides *in vitro*, leading to a potential underestimation of aminoglycoside serum concentration.

Dosage Forms Injection, solution, as sulfate: 1 g/3 mL (3 mL) [contains sodium bisulfate]

- **Kanamycin Sulfate** *see* Kanamycin *on page 707*
- **Kantrex®** *see* Kanamycin *on page 707*
- **Kayexalate®** *see* Sodium Polystyrene Sulfonate *on page 1193*
- **Kenalog®** *see* Triamcinolone *on page 1311*
- **Kenalog-10®** *see* Triamcinolone *on page 1311*
- **Kenalog-40®** *see* Triamcinolone *on page 1311*
- **Kenalog® in Orabase (Can)** *see* Triamcinolone *on page 1311*
- **Kerlone®** *see* Betaxolol *on page 173*
- **Kerr Insta-Char® [OTC]** *see* Charcoal *on page 259*
- **Ketalar®** *see* Ketamine *on page 709*

Ketamine (KEET a meen)

Medication Safety Issues

Sound-alike/look-alike issues:
Ketalar® may be confused with Kenalog®

Related Information

Acute Postoperative Pain *on page 1388*
Anesthesia Considerations for Neurosurgery *on page 1401*
Chronic Renal Failure *on page 1437*
Intravenous Anesthetic Agents *on page 1531*

U.S. Brand Names Ketalar®

Canadian Brand Names Ketalar®; Ketamine Hydrochloride Injection, USP

Synonyms Ketamine Hydrochloride

Pharmacologic Category General Anesthetic

Restrictions C-III

Generic Available Yes

Use Induction and maintenance of general anesthesia, especially when cardiovascular depression must be avoided (ie, hypotension, hypovolemia, cardiomyopathy, constrictive pericarditis); sedation; analgesia

Mechanism of Action Produces a cataleptic-like state in which the patient is dissociated from the surrounding environment by direct action on the cortex and limbic system. Releases endogenous catecholamines (epinephrine, norepinephrine) which maintain blood pressure and heart rate. Reduces polysynaptic spinal reflexes.

Pharmacodynamics/Kinetics

Onset of action:
I.V.: General anesthesia: 1-2 minutes; Sedation: 1-2 minutes
I.M.: General anesthesia: 3-8 minutes

(Continued)

Ketamine *(Continued)*

Duration: I.V.: 5-15 minutes; I.M.: 12-25 minutes

Metabolism: Hepatic via hydroxylation and N-demethylation; the metabolite norketamine is 25% as potent as parent compound

Half-life elimination: 11-17 minutes; Elimination: 2.5-3.1 hours

Excretion: Clearance: 18 mL/kg/minute

Dosage Used in combination with anticholinergic agents to decrease hypersalivation

Children:

Oral: 6-10 mg/kg for 1 dose (mixed in 0.2-0.3 mL/kg of cola or other beverage) given 30 minutes before the procedure

I.M.: 3-7 mg/kg

I.V.: Range: 0.5-2 mg/kg, use smaller doses (0.5-1 mg/kg) for sedation for minor procedures; usual induction dosage: 1-2 mg/kg

Continuous I.V. infusion: Sedation: 5-20 mcg/kg/minute

Adults:

I.M.: 3-8 mg/kg

I.V.: Range: 1-4.5 mg/kg; usual induction dosage: 1-2 mg/kg

Children and Adults: Maintenance: Supplemental doses of $^1/_3$ to $^1/_2$ of initial dose

Stability Do not mix with barbiturates or diazepam (precipitation may occur).

Administration

Oral: Use 100 mg/mL I.V. solution and mix the appropriate dose in 0.2-0.3 mL/kg of cola or other beverage

Parenteral: I.V.: Do not exceed 0.5 mg/kg/minute or administer faster than 60 seconds; do not exceed final concentration of 2 mg/mL; dilute for I.V. administration with normal saline, sterile water, or D_5W

Monitoring Parameters Cardiovascular effects, heart rate, blood pressure, respiratory rate, transcutaneous O_2 saturation

Anesthesia and Critical Care Concerns/Other Considerations Produces emergence psychosis including auditory and visual hallucinations, restlessness, disorientation, vivid dreams, and irrational behavior in 15% to 30% of patients; pretreatment with a benzodiazepine reduces incidence of psychosis by >50%. Spontaneous involuntary movements, nystagmus, hypertonus, and vocalizations are also commonly seen.

The analgesia outlasts the general anesthetic component. Bronchodilation is beneficial in asthmatic or COPD patients. Laryngeal reflexes may remain intact or may be obtunded. The direct myocardial depressant action of ketamine can be seen in stressed, catecholamine-deficient patients. Ketamine increases cerebral metabolism and cerebral blood flow while producing a noncompetitive block of the neuronal postsynaptic NMDA receptor. It lowers seizure threshold and stimulates salivary secretions (atropine/scopolamine treatment is recommended).

Ketamine increases myocardial oxygen demand secondary to catecholamine release.

Pregnancy Risk Factor D

Contraindications Hypersensitivity to ketamine or any component of the formulation; elevated intracranial pressure; hypertension, aneurysms, thyrotoxicosis, congestive heart failure, angina, psychotic disorders; pregnancy

Warnings/Precautions Use with caution in patients with coronary artery disease, catecholamine depletion, and tachycardia. **[U.S. Boxed Warning]: Postanesthetic emergence reactions which can manifest as vivid dreams, hallucinations, and/or frank delirium occur in 12% of patients; these reactions are less common in patients >65 years of age and when given I.M.** Emergence reactions, confusion, or irrational behavior may occur up to 24 hours postoperatively and may be reduced by pretreatment with a benzodiazepine. May cause dependence (withdrawal symptoms on discontinuation) and tolerance with prolonged use.

Adverse Reactions

>10%:

Cardiovascular: Hypertension, increased cardiac output, paradoxical direct myocardial depression, tachycardia

Central nervous system: Increased intracranial pressure, visual hallucinations, vivid dreams

Neuromuscular & skeletal: Tonic-clonic movements, tremor

Miscellaneous: Emergence reactions, vocalization

1% to 10%:
- Cardiovascular: Bradycardia, hypotension
- Dermatologic: Pain at injection site, skin rash
- Gastrointestinal: Anorexia, nausea, vomiting
- Ocular: Diplopia, nystagmus
- Respiratory: Respiratory depression

<1% (Limited to important or life-threatening): Anaphylaxis, cardiac arrhythmia, cough reflex may be depressed, decreased bronchospasm, fasciculations, hypersalivation, increased airway resistance, increased intraocular pressure, increased metabolic rate, increased skeletal muscle tone, laryngospasm, myocardial depression, respiratory depression or apnea with large doses or rapid infusions

Overdosage/Toxicology

Symptoms of overdose include respiratory depression with excessive dosing or too rapid administration

Supportive care is the treatment of choice; mechanical support of respiration is preferred

Drug Interactions Substrate (major) of CYP2B6, 2C9, 3A4

CYP2B6 inhibitors: May increase the levels/effects of ketamine. Example inhibitors include desipramine, paroxetine, and sertraline.

CYP2C9 Inhibitors may increase the levels/effects of ketamine. Example inhibitors include delavirdine, fluconazole, gemfibrozil, ketoconazole, nicardipine, NSAIDs, sulfonamides and tolbutamide.

CYP3A4 inhibitors: May increase the levels/effects of ketamine. Example inhibitors include azole antifungals, clarithromycin, diclofenac, doxycycline, erythromycin, imatinib, isoniazid, nefazodone, nicardipine, propofol, protease inhibitors, quinidine, telithromycin, and verapamil.

Increased effect: Barbiturates, narcotics, hydroxyzine increase prolonged recovery; nondepolarizing may increase effects

Increased toxicity: Muscle relaxants, thyroid hormones may increase blood pressure and heart rate; halothane may decrease BP

Dosage Forms

Injection, solution: 50 mg/mL (10 mL); 100 mg/mL (5 mL)

Ketalar®: 10 mg/mL (20 mL); 50 mg/mL (10 mL); 100 mg/mL (5 mL)

References

Clements JA and Nimmo WS, "Pharmacokinetics and Analgesic Effect of Ketamine in Man," *Br J Anaesth*, 1981, 53(1):27-30.

Kohrs R and Durieux ME, "Ketamine: Teaching an Old Drug New Tricks," *Anesth Analg*, 1998, 87(5):1186-93.

♦ **Ketamine Hydrochloride** *see* Ketamine *on page 709*

♦ **Ketamine Hydrochloride Injection, USP (Can)** *see* Ketamine *on page 709*

♦ **Ketek®** *see* Telithromycin *on page 1235*

Ketoconazole (kee toe KOE na zole)

Medication Safety Issues

Sound-alike/look-alike issues:

Nizoral® may be confused with Nasarel®, Neoral®, Nitrol®

U.S. Brand Names Nizoral®; Nizoral® A-D [OTC]

Canadian Brand Names Apo-Ketoconazole®; Ketoderm®; Novo-Ketoconazole

Pharmacologic Category Antifungal Agent, Oral; Antifungal Agent, Topical

Generic Available Yes

Use Treatment of susceptible fungal infections, including candidiasis, oral thrush, blastomycosis, histoplasmosis, paracoccidioidomycosis, coccidioidomycosis, chromomycosis, candiduria, chronic mucocutaneous candidiasis, as well as certain recalcitrant cutaneous dermatophytoses; used topically for treatment of tinea corporis, tinea cruris, tinea versicolor, and cutaneous candidiasis, seborrheic dermatitis

Unlabeled/Investigational Use Treatment of prostate cancer (androgen synthesis inhibitor)

Mechanism of Action Alters the permeability of the cell wall by blocking fungal cytochrome P450; inhibits biosynthesis of triglycerides and phospholipids by fungi; inhibits several fungal enzymes that results in a build-up of toxic concentrations of hydrogen peroxide; also inhibits androgen synthesis

Pharmacodynamics/Kinetics

Absorption: Oral: Rapid (~75%); Shampoo: None

(Continued)

Ketoconazole *(Continued)*

Distribution: Well into inflamed joint fluid, saliva, bile, urine, breast milk, sebum, cerumen, feces, tendons, skin and soft tissues, and testes; crosses blood-brain barrier poorly; only negligible amounts reach CSF
Protein binding: 93% to 96%
Metabolism: Partially hepatic via CYP3A4 to inactive compounds
Bioavailability: Decreases as gastric pH increases
Half-life elimination: Biphasic: Initial: 2 hours; Terminal: 8 hours
Time to peak, serum: 1-2 hours
Excretion: Feces (57%); urine (13%)

Dosage

Fungal infections:
Oral:
Children ≥2 years: 3.3-6.6 mg/kg/day as a single dose for 1-2 weeks for candidiasis, for at least 4 weeks in recalcitrant dermatophyte infections, and for up to 6 months for other systemic mycoses
Adults: 200-400 mg/day as a single daily dose for durations as stated above
Shampoo: Apply twice weekly for 4 weeks with at least 3 days between each shampoo
Topical: Rub gently into the affected area once daily to twice daily
Prostate cancer (unlabeled use): Oral: Adults: 400 mg 3 times/day
Dosing adjustment in hepatic impairment: Dose reductions should be considered in patients with severe liver disease
Hemodialysis: Not dialyzable (0% to 5%)

Administration Administer tablets 2 hours prior to antacids to prevent decreased absorption due to the high pH of gastric contents.

Monitoring Parameters Liver function tests

Pregnancy Risk Factor C

Contraindications Hypersensitivity to ketoconazole or any component of the formulation; CNS fungal infections (due to poor CNS penetration); coadministration with ergot derivatives or cisapride is contraindicated due to risk of potentially fatal cardiac arrhythmias

Warnings/Precautions [U.S. Boxed Warning]: Ketoconazole has been associated with hepatotoxicity, including some fatalities; use with caution in patients with impaired hepatic function and perform periodic liver function tests. **[U.S. Boxed Warning]: Concomitant use with cisapride is contraindicated due to the occurrence of ventricular arrythmias.** High doses of ketoconazole may depress adrenocortical function.

Adverse Reactions

Oral:
1% to 10%:
Dermatologic: Pruritus (2%)
Gastrointestinal: Nausea/vomiting (3% to 10%), abdominal pain (1%)
<1% (Limited to important or life-threatening): Bulging fontanelles, chills, depression, diarrhea, dizziness, fever, gynecomastia, headache, hemolytic anemia, hepatotoxicity, impotence, leukopenia, photophobia, somnolence, thrombocytopenia
Cream: Severe irritation, pruritus, stinging (~5%)
Shampoo: Increases in normal hair loss, irritation (<1%), abnormal hair texture, scalp pustules, mild dryness of skin, itching, oiliness/dryness of hair

Overdosage/Toxicology Oral: Symptoms of overdose include dizziness, headache, nausea, vomiting, diarrhea. Overdoses are well tolerated. Treatment includes supportive measures and gastric decontamination.

Drug Interactions Substrate of CYP3A4 (major); **Inhibits** CYP1A2 (strong), 2A6 (moderate), 2B6 (weak), 2C8 (weak), 2C9 (strong), 2C19 (moderate), 2D6 (moderate), 3A4 (strong)

Benzodiazepines: Alprazolam, diazepam, temazepam, triazolam, and midazolam serum concentrations may be increased; consider a benzodiazepine not metabolized by CYP3A4 (such as lorazepam) or another antifungal that is metabolized by CYP3A4. Concurrent use is contraindicated.
Buspirone: Serum concentrations may be increased; monitor for sedation
Busulfan: Serum concentrations may be increased; avoid concurrent use
Calcium channel blockers: Serum concentrations may be increased (applies to those agents metabolized by CYP3A4, including felodipine, nifedipine, and verapamil); consider another agent instead of a calcium channel blocker,

another antifungal, or reduce the dose of the calcium channel blocker; monitor blood pressure

Cisapride: Serum concentration is increased which may lead to malignant arrhythmias; concurrent use is contraindicated

CYP1A2 substrates: Ketoconazole may increase the levels/effects of CYP1A2 substrates. Example substrates include aminophylline, fluvoxamine, mexiletine, mirtazapine, ropinirole, theophylline, and trifluoperazine.

CYP2A6 substrates: Ketoconazole may increase the levels/effects of CYP2A6 substrates. Example substrates include dexmedetomidine and ifosfamide.

CYP2C9 substrates: Ketoconazole may increase the levels/effects of CYP2C9 substrates. Example substrates include bosentan, dapsone, fluoxetine, glimepiride, glipizide, losartan, montelukast, nateglinide, paclitaxel, phenytoin, warfarin, and zafirlukast.

CYP2C19 substrates: Ketoconazole may increase the levels/effects of CYP2C19 substrates. Example substrates include citalopram, diazepam, methsuximide, phenytoin, propranolol, and sertraline.

CYP2D6 substrates: Ketoconazole may increase the levels/effects of CYP2D6 substrates. Example substrates include amphetamines, selected beta-blockers, dextromethorphan, fluoxetine, lidocaine, mirtazapine, nefazodone, paroxetine, risperidone, ritonavir, thioridazine, tricyclic antidepressants, and venlafaxine.

CYP2D6 prodrug substrates: Ketoconazole may decrease the levels/effects of CYP2D6 prodrug substrates. Example prodrug substrates include codeine, hydrocodone, oxycodone, and tramadol.

CYP3A4 inducers: CYP3A4 inducers may decrease the levels/effects of ketoconazole. Example inducers include aminoglutethimide, carbamazepine, nafcillin, nevirapine, phenobarbital, phenytoin, and rifamycins.

CYP3A4 substrates: Ketoconazole may increase the levels/effects of CYP3A4 substrates. Example substrates include benzodiazepines, calcium channel blockers, mirtazapine, nateglinide, nefazodone, tacrolimus, and venlafaxine. Selected benzodiazepines (midazolam and triazolam), cisapride, ergot alkaloids, selected HMG-CoA reductase inhibitors (lovastatin and simvastatin), and pimozide are generally contraindicated with strong CYP3A4 inhibitors.

Didanosine: May decrease absorption of ketoconazole (due to buffering capacity of oral solution); applies only to oral solution formulation of didanosine

Docetaxel: Serum concentrations may be increased; avoid concurrent use

Erythromycin (and clarithromycin): May increase serum concentrations of ketoconazole.

H_2 blockers: May decrease ketoconazole absorption. Ketoconazole depends on gastric acidity for absorption. Avoid concurrent use.

HMG-CoA reductase inhibitors (except pravastatin and fluvastatin): Serum concentrations may be increased. The risk of myopathy/rhabdomyolysis may be increased. Switch to pravastatin/fluvastatin or suspend treatment during course of ketoconazole therapy.

Immunosuppressants: Cyclosporine, sirolimus, and tacrolimus: Serum concentrations may be increased; monitor serum concentrations and renal function

Methylprednisolone: Serum concentrations may be increased; monitor

Nevirapine: May decrease serum concentrations of ketoconazole; monitor

Oral contraceptives: Efficacy may be reduced by ketoconazole (limited data); use barrier birth control method during concurrent use

Phenytoin: Serum concentrations may be increased; monitor phenytoin levels and adjust dose as needed

Protease inhibitors: May increase serum concentrations of ketoconazole. Includes amprenavir, indinavir, nelfinavir, ritonavir, and saquinavir; monitor

Proton pump inhibitors: May decrease ketoconazole absorption. Ketoconazole depends on gastric acidity for absorption. Avoid concurrent use (includes omeprazole, lansoprazole).

Quinidine: Serum levels may be increased; monitor

Rifampin: Rifampin decreases ketoconazole's serum concentration to levels which are no longer effective; avoid concurrent use.

Sildenafil: Serum concentrations may be increased by ketoconazole; consider dosage reduction. A maximum sildenafil dose of 25 mg in 48 hours is recommended with other strong CYP3A4 inhibitors.

Tadalafil: Serum concentrations may be increased by ketoconazole. A maximum tadalafil dose of 10 mg in 72 hours is recommended with strong CYP3A4 inhibitors.

Trimetrexate: Serum concentrations may be increased; monitor

(Continued)

Ketoconazole *(Continued)*

Vardenafil: Serum concentrations may be increased by ketoconazole. If ketoconazole dose is 200 mg/day, limit vardenafil to a maximum of 5 mg/24 hours. If ketoconazole dose is 400 mg/day, limit vardenafil dose to a maximum of 2.5 mg/24 hours.

Warfarin: Anticoagulant effects may be increased; monitor INR and adjust warfarin's dose as needed

Vinca alkaloids: Serum concentrations may be increased; avoid concurrent use

Zolpidem: Serum levels may be increased; monitor

Ethanol/Nutrition/Herb Interactions

Food: Ketoconazole peak serum levels may be prolonged if taken with food.

Herb/Nutraceutical: St John's wort may decrease ketoconazole levels.

Dietary Considerations May be taken with food or milk to decrease GI adverse effects.

Dosage Forms

Cream, topical: 2% (15 g, 30 g, 60 g)

Shampoo, topical (Nizoral® A-D): 1% (6 mL, 120 mL, 210 mL)

Tablet (Nizoral®): 200 mg

- **Ketoderm® (Can)** *see* Ketoconazole *on page 711*

Ketoprofen (kee toe PROE fen)

Medication Safety Issues

Sound-alike/look-alike issues:

Oruvail® may be confused with Clinoril®, Elavil®

Related Information

Acetaminophen and NSAIDS, Dosing Data *on page 1543*

Chronic Pain Management *on page 1430*

U.S. Brand Names Orudis® KT [OTC] [DSC]

Canadian Brand Names Apo-Keto®; Apo-Keto-E®; Apo-Keto SR®; Novo-Keto; Novo-Keto-EC; Nu-Ketoprofen; Nu-Ketoprofen-E; Oruvail®; Rhodis™; Rhodis-EC™; Rhodis SR™

Pharmacologic Category Nonsteroidal Anti-inflammatory Drug (NSAID), Oral

Restrictions A medication guide should be dispensed with each prescription. A template for the required MedGuide can be found on the FDA website at: http://www.fda.gov/medwatch/SAFETY/2005/safety05.htm#NSAID

Generic Available Yes: Capsule

Use Acute and long-term treatment of rheumatoid arthritis and osteoarthritis; primary dysmenorrhea; mild to moderate pain

Mechanism of Action Inhibits prostaglandin synthesis by decreasing the activity of the enzyme, cyclooxygenase, which results in decreased formation of prostaglandin precursors

Pharmacodynamics/Kinetics

Absorption: Almost complete

Protein binding: >99%, primarily albumin

Metabolism: Hepatic via glucuronidation; metabolite can be converted back to parent compound; may have enterohepatic recirculation

Half-life elimination:

Capsule: 2-4 hours; moderate-severe renal impairment: 5-9 hours

Capsule, extended release: ~3-7.5 hours

Time to peak, serum:

Capsule: 0.5-2 hours

Capsule, extended release: 6-7 hours

Excretion: Urine (~80%, primarily as glucuronide conjugates)

Dosage Oral:

Children ≥16 years and Adults:

Rheumatoid arthritis or osteoarthritis (lower doses may be used in small patients or in the elderly, or debilitated):

Capsule: 50-75 mg 3-4 times/day up to a maximum of 300 mg/day

Capsule, extended release: 200 mg once daily

Mild-to-moderate pain: Capsule: 25-50 mg every 6-8 hours up to a maximum of 300 mg/day

OTC labeling: 12.5 mg every 4-6 hours, up to a maximum of 6 tablets/24 hours

Elderly: Initial dose should be decreased in patients >75 years; use caution when dosage changes are made

Dosage adjustment in renal impairment: In general, NSAIDs are not recommended for use in patients with advanced renal disease, but the manufacturer of ketoprofen does provide some guidelines for adjustment in renal dysfunction:

Mild impairment: Maximum dose: 150 mg/day

Severe impairment: Cl_{cr}<25 mL/minute: Maximum dose: 100 mg/day

Dosage adjustment in hepatic impairment and serum albumin <3.5 g/dL: Maximum dose: 100 mg/day

Administration May take with food to reduce GI upset. Do not crush or break extended release capsules.

Anesthesia and Critical Care Concerns/Other Considerations The 2002 ACCM/SCCM guidelines for analgesia (critically-ill adult) suggest that NSAIDs may be used in combination with opioids in select patients for pain management. Concern about adverse events (increased risk of renal dysfunction, altered platelet function and gastrointestinal irritation) limits its use in patients who have other underlying risks for these events.

In short-term use, NSAIDs vary considerably in their effect on blood pressure. When NSAIDs are used in patients with hypertension, appropriate monitoring of blood pressure responses should be completed and the duration of therapy, when possible, kept short. The use of NSAIDs in the treatment of patients with congestive heart failure may be associated with an increased risk for fluid accumulation and edema; may precipitate renal failure in dehydrated patients.

Pregnancy Risk Factor C/D (3rd trimester)

Contraindications Hypersensitivity to ketoprofen, aspirin, other NSAIDs, or any component of the formulation; perioperative pain in the setting of coronary artery bypass surgery (CABG); pregnancy (3rd trimester)

Warnings/Precautions [U.S. Boxed Warning]: NSAIDs are associated with an increased risk of adverse cardiovascular events, including MI, stroke, and new onset or worsening of pre-existing hypertension. Risk may be increased with duration of use or pre-existing cardiovascular risk-factors or disease. Carefully evaluate individual cardiovascular risk profiles prior to prescribing. Use caution with fluid retention, CHF or hypertension.

Use of NSAIDs can compromise existing renal function. Renal toxicity can occur in patient with impaired renal function, dehydration, heart failure, liver dysfunction, those taking diuretics and ACEI and the elderly. Rehydrate patient before starting therapy. Monitor renal function closely. Ketoprofen is not recommended for patients with advanced renal disease.

[U.S. Boxed Warning]: NSAIDs may increase risk of gastrointestinal irritation, ulceration, bleeding, and perforation. These events may occur at any time during therapy and without warning. Use caution with a history of GI disease (bleeding or ulcers), concurrent therapy with aspirin, anticoagulants and/or corticosteroids, smoking, use of alcohol, the elderly or debilitated patients.

Use the lowest effective dose for the shortest duration of time, consistent with individual patient goals, to reduce risk of cardiovascular or GI adverse events. Alternate therapies should be considered for patients at high risk.

NSAIDs may cause serious skin adverse events including exfoliative dermatitis, Stevens-Johnson syndrome (SJS) and toxic epidermal necrolysis (TEN). Anaphylactoid reactions may occur, even without prior exposure; patients with "aspirin triad" (bronchial asthma, aspirin intolerance, rhinitis) may be at increased risk. Do not use in patients who experience bronchospasm, asthma, rhinitis, or urticaria with NSAID or aspirin therapy.

Use with caution in patients with decreased hepatic function. Closely monitor patients with any abnormal LFT. Severe hepatic reactions (eg, fulminant hepatitis, liver failure) have occurred with NSAID use, rarely; discontinue if signs or symptoms of liver disease develop, or if systemic manifestations occur.

Withhold for at least 4-6 half-lives prior to surgical or dental procedures. Safety and efficacy have not been established in pediatric patients.

Adverse Reactions

>10%: Gastrointestinal: Dyspepsia (11%)

1% to 10%:

Central nervous system: Headache (3% to 9%), depression, dizziness (>1%), dreams, insomnia, malaise, nervousness, somnolence

Dermatologic: Rash

(Continued)

Ketoprofen *(Continued)*

Gastrointestinal: Abdominal pain (3% to 9%), constipation (3% to 9%), diarrhea (3% to 9%), flatulence (3% to 9%), nausea (3% to 9%), anorexia (>1%), stomatitis (>1%), vomiting (>1%)

Genitourinary: Urinary tract infection (>1%)

Ocular: Visual disturbances

Otic: Tinnitus

Renal: Renal dysfunction (3% to 9%)

<1% (Limited to important or life-threatening): Agranulocytosis, allergic reaction, allergic rhinitis, alopecia, anaphylaxis, anemia, angioedema, arrhythmia, aseptic meningitis, blurred vision, bone marrow suppression, buccal necrosis, bullous rash, cholestatic hepatitis, confusion, CHF, conjunctivitis, cystitis, diabetes mellitus (aggravated), drowsiness, dry eyes, dysphoria, dyspnea, eczema, epistaxis, erythema multiforme, exfoliative dermatitis, gastritis, gastrointestinal perforation, GI ulceration, gynecomastia, hallucinations, hearing decreased, hemolytic anemia, hepatic dysfunction, hepatitis, hot flashes, hypertension, hyponatremia, impotence, interstitial nephritis, intestinal ulceration, jaundice, leukopenia, microvesicular steatosis, migraine, myocardial infarction, nephrotic syndrome, nightmares, onycholysis, pancreatitis, peptic ulcer, peripheral neuropathy, peripheral vascular disease, photosensitivity, polydipsia, polyuria, purpura, renal failure, retinal hemorrhage, Stevens-Johnson syndrome, tachycardia, taste perversion, thrombocytopenia, toxic amblyopia, toxic epidermal necrolysis, tubulopathy, ulcerative colitis, urticaria

Overdosage/Toxicology Common symptoms of acute NSAID overdose include lethargy, drowsiness, nausea, vomiting and epigastric pain. Respiratory depression, coma, convulsions, GI bleeding, or acute renal failure are rare. Management of NSAID intoxication is supportive and symptomatic; multiple dosing of activated charcoal may be effective.

Drug Interactions Inhibits CYP2C9 (weak)

ACE inhibitors: Antihypertensive effects may be decreased by concurrent therapy with NSAIDs; monitor blood pressure

Aminoglycosides: NSAIDs may decrease the excretion of aminoglycosides.

Angiotensin II antagonists: Antihypertensive effects may be decreased by concurrent therapy with NSAIDs; monitor blood pressure.

Anticoagulants (warfarin, heparin, LMWHs): In combination with NSAIDs can cause increased risk of bleeding.

Antiplatelet agents (ticlopidine, clopidogrel, aspirin, abciximab, dipyridamole, eptifibatide, tirofiban): In combination with NSAIDs can cause an increased risk of bleeding.

Beta-blockers: NSAIDs may decrease the antihypertensive effect of beta-blockers. Monitor.

Bisphosphonates: NSAIDs may increase the risk of gastrointestinal ulceration.

Cholestyramine (and other bile acid sequestrants): May decrease the absorption of NSAIDs. Separate by at least 2 hours.

Corticosteroids: May increase the risk of GI ulceration; avoid concurrent use.

Cyclosporine: NSAIDs may increase serum creatinine, potassium, blood pressure, and cyclosporine levels; monitor cyclosporine levels and renal function carefully.

Hydralazine: Antihypertensive effect is decreased; avoid concurrent use.

Lithium: Lithium levels can be increased; avoid concurrent use if possible or monitor lithium levels and adjust dose. Sulindac may have the least effect. When NSAID is stopped, lithium will need adjustment again.

Loop diuretics: Antihypertensive and diuretic effects may be diminished. Indomethacin reduces this efficacy, however, it may be anticipated with any NSAID.

Methotrexate: Severe bone marrow suppression, aplastic anemia, and GI toxicity have been reported with concomitant NSAID therapy. Avoid use during moderate or high-dose methotrexate (increased and prolonged methotrexate levels). NSAID use during low-dose treatment of rheumatoid arthritis has not been fully evaluated; extreme caution is warranted.

Pemetrexed: NSAIDs may decrease the excretion of pemetrexed. Patients with Cl_{cr} 45-79 mL/minute should avoid long acting NSAIDs for 5 days before and 2 days after pemetrexed treatment.

Probenecid: May increase the serum concentration of ketoprofen.

Thiazides: Antihypertensive effects may be decreased; avoid concurrent use.

Treprostinil: May enhance the risk of bleeding with concurrent use.

Vancomycin: NSAIDs may decrease the excretion of vancomycin.

Ethanol/Nutrition/Herb Interactions

Ethanol: Avoid ethanol (due to GI irritation).

Food: Food slows rate of absorption resulting in delayed and reduced peak serum concentrations.

Herb/Nutraceutical: Avoid alfalfa, anise, bilberry, bladderwrack, bromelain, cat's claw, celery, coleus, cordyceps, dong quai, evening primrose, feverfew, fenugreek, garlic, ginger, ginkgo biloba, red clover, horse chestnut, grapeseed, green tea, ginseng, guggul, horse chestnut seed, horseradish, licorice, prickly ash, red clover, reishi, SAMe, sweet clover, turmeric, white willow (all have additional antiplatelet activity).

Dietary Considerations In order to minimize gastrointestinal effects, ketoprofen can be prescribed to be taken with food or milk.

Dosage Forms [DSC] = Discontinued product

Capsule: 50 mg, 75 mg

Capsule, extended release: 200 mg

Tablet (Orudis® KT): 12.5 mg [contains tartrazine and sodium benzoate] [DSC]

Ketorolac (KEE toe role ak)

Medication Safety Issues

Sound-alike/look-alike issues:

Acular® may be confused with Acthar®, Ocular®

Toradol® may be confused with Foradil®, Inderal®, Tegretol®, Torecan®, tramadol

Related Information

Acetaminophen and NSAIDS, Dosing Data *on page 1543*

Acute Postoperative Pain *on page 1388*

Chronic Pain Management *on page 1430*

U.S. Brand Names Acular®; Acular LS™; Acular® PF; Toradol®

Canadian Brand Names Acular®; Acular LS™; Apo-Ketorolac®; Apo-Ketorolac Injectable®; Ketorolac Tromethamine Injection, USP; Novo-Ketorolac; ratio-Ketorolac; Toradol®; Toradol® IM

Synonyms Ketorolac Tromethamine

Pharmacologic Category Nonsteroidal Anti-inflammatory Drug (NSAID), Ophthalmic; Nonsteroidal Anti-inflammatory Drug (NSAID), Oral; Nonsteroidal Anti-inflammatory Drug (NSAID), Parenteral

Restrictions A medication guide should be dispensed with each prescription. A template for the required MedGuide can be found on the FDA website at: http://www.fda.gov/medwatch/SAFETY/2005/safety05.htm#NSAID

Generic Available Yes: Injection, tablet

Use

Oral, injection: Short-term (≤5 days) management of moderately-severe acute pain requiring analgesia at the opioid level

Ophthalmic: Temporary relief of ocular itching due to seasonal allergic conjunctivitis; postoperative inflammation following cataract extraction; reduction of ocular pain and photophobia following incisional refractive surgery, reduction of ocular pain, burning and stinging following corneal refractive surgery

Mechanism of Action Inhibits prostaglandin synthesis by decreasing the activity of the enzyme, cyclooxygenase, which results in decreased formation of prostaglandin precursors

Pharmacodynamics/Kinetics

Onset of action: Analgesic: I.M.: ~10 minutes

Peak effect: Analgesic: 2-3 hours

Duration: Analgesic: 6-8 hours

Absorption: Oral: Well absorbed

Distribution: Poor penetration into CSF; crosses placenta; enters breast milk

Protein binding: 99%

Metabolism: Hepatic

Half-life elimination: 2-8 hours; prolonged 30% to 50% in elderly

Time to peak, serum: I.M.: 30-60 minutes

Excretion: Urine (61% as unchanged drug)

Dosage

Children 2-16 years: **Do not exceed adult doses**

Single-dose treatment:

I.M.: 1 mg/kg (maximum: 30 mg)

I.V.: 0.5 mg/kg (maximum: 15 mg)

(Continued)

Ketorolac *(Continued)*

Oral (unlabeled): 1 mg/kg as a single dose reported in one study

Multiple-dose treatment (unlabeled): Limited pediatric studies. The maximum combined duration of treatment (for parenteral and oral) is 5 days.

I.V.: Initial dose: 0.5 mg/kg, followed by 0.25-1 mg/kg every 6 hours for up to 48 hours (maximum daily dose: 90 mg)

Oral: 0.25 mg/kg every 6 hours

Adults (pain relief usually begins within 10 minutes with parenteral forms): **Note:** The maximum combined duration of treatment (for parenteral and oral) is 5 days; do not increase dose or frequency; supplement with low-dose opioids if needed for breakthrough pain. For patients <50 kg and/or ≥65 years, see Elderly dosing.

I.M.: 60 mg as a single dose or 30 mg every 6 hours (maximum daily dose: 120 mg)

I.V.: 30 mg as a single dose or 30 mg every 6 hours (maximum daily dose: 120 mg)

Oral: 20 mg, followed by 10 mg every 4-6 hours; do not exceed 40 mg/day; oral dosing is intended to be a continuation of I.M. or I.V. therapy only

Ophthalmic: Children ≥3 years and Adults:

Allergic conjunctivitis (relief of ocular itching) (Acular®): Instill 1 drop (0.25 mg) 4 times/day for seasonal allergic conjunctivitis

Inflammation following cataract extraction (Acular®): Instill 1 drop (0.25 mg) to affected eye(s) 4 times/day beginning 24 hours after surgery; continue for 2 weeks

Pain and photophobia following incisional refractive surgery (Acular® PF): Instill 1 drop (0.25 mg) 4 times/day to affected eye for up to 3 days

Pain following corneal refractive surgery (Acular LS™): Instill 1 drop 4 times/day as needed to affected eye for up to 4 days

Elderly >65 years: Renal insufficiency or weight <50 kg: **Note:** Ketorolac has decreased clearance and increased half-life in the elderly. In addition, the elderly have reported increased incidence of GI bleeding, ulceration, and perforation. The maximum combined duration of treatment (for parenteral and oral) is 5 days.

I.M.: 30 mg as a single dose or 15 mg every 6 hours (maximum daily dose: 60 mg)

I.V.: 15 mg as a single dose or 15 mg every 6 hours (maximum daily dose: 60 mg)

Oral: 10 mg every 4-6 hours; do not exceed 40 mg/day; oral dosing is intended to be a continuation of I.M. or I.V. therapy only

Dosage adjustment in renal impairment: Do not use in patients with advanced renal impairment. Patients with moderately-elevated serum creatinine should use half the recommended dose, not to exceed 60 mg/day I.M./I.V.

Dosage adjustment in hepatic impairment: Use with caution, may cause elevation of liver enzymes

Stability Ketorolac injection and ophthalmic solution should be stored at controlled room temperature and protected from light; injection is clear and has a slight yellow color; precipitation may occur at relatively low pH values. Store tablets at controlled room temperature.

Compatible with NS, D_5W, D_5NS, LR

Incompatible with meperidine, morphine, promethazine, and hydroxyzine

Administration

Oral: May take with food to reduce GI upset

I.M.: Administer slowly and deeply into the muscle. Analgesia begins in 30 minutes and maximum effect within 2 hours

I.V.: Administer I.V. bolus over a minimum of 15 seconds; onset within 30 minutes; peak analgesia within 2 hours

Ophthalmic solution: Contact lenses should be removed before instillation.

Monitoring Parameters Monitor response (pain, range of motion, grip strength, mobility, ADL function), inflammation; observe for weight gain, edema; monitor renal function (serum creatinine, BUN, urine output); observe for bleeding, bruising; evaluate gastrointestinal effects (abdominal pain, bleeding, dyspepsia); mental confusion, disorientation, CBC, liver function tests

Reference Range Serum concentration: Therapeutic: 0.3-5 mcg/mL; Toxic: >5 mcg/mL

Anesthesia and Critical Care Concerns/Other Considerations The 2002 ACCM/SCCM guidelines for analgesia (critically-ill adult) recommend that ketorolac therapy be limited to a maximum of 5 days with close attention to gastrointestinal and renal function. The risk of developing renal dysfunction or gastrointestinal bleeding further increases as treatment extends beyond 5 days.

In short-term use, NSAIDs vary considerably in their effect on blood pressure. When NSAIDs are used in patients with hypertension, appropriate monitoring of blood pressure responses should be completed and the duration of therapy, when possible, kept short. The use of NSAIDs in the treatment of patients with congestive heart failure may be associated with an increased risk for fluid accumulation and edema; may precipitate renal failure in dehydrated patients.

Ketorolac is contraindicated during labor and delivery (may inhibit uterine contractions and adversely affect fetal circulation). Avoid use of ketorolac ophthalmic solution during late pregnancy.

Equivalent dosing: 30 mg provides the analgesia comparable to morphine 12 mg or meperidine 100 mg.

Pregnancy Risk Factor C/D (3rd trimester)

Contraindications Hypersensitivity to ketorolac, aspirin, other NSAIDs, or any component of the formulation; active or history of peptic ulcer disease; recent or history of GI bleeding or perforation; patients with advanced renal disease or risk of renal failure; labor and delivery; nursing mothers; prophylaxis before major surgery; suspected or confirmed cerebrovascular bleeding; hemorrhagic diathesis; concurrent ASA or other NSAIDs; epidural or intrathecal administration; concomitant probenecid; perioperative pain in the setting of coronary artery bypass surgery (CABG); pregnancy (3rd trimester)

Warnings/Precautions

Systemic: Treatment should be started with I.V./I.M. administration then changed to oral only as a continuation of treatment. Total therapy is not to exceed 5 days. Should not be used for minor or chronic pain.

May prolong bleeding time; do not use when hemostasis is critical. Patients should be euvolemic prior to treatment. Low doses of narcotics may be needed for breakthrough pain.

[U.S. Boxed Warning]: NSAIDs are associated with an increased risk of adverse cardiovascular events, including MI, stroke, and new onset or worsening of pre-existing hypertension. Risk may be increased with duration of use or pre-existing cardiovascular risk-factors or disease. Carefully evaluate individual cardiovascular risk profiles prior to prescribing. Use caution with fluid retention, CHF or hypertension.

Use of NSAIDs can compromise existing renal function. Renal toxicity can occur in patient with impaired renal function, dehydration, heart failure, liver dysfunction, those taking diuretics and ACEI and the elderly. Rehydrate patient before starting therapy. Monitor renal function closely. Ketorolac is not recommended for patients with advanced renal disease.

[U.S. Boxed Warning]: NSAIDs may increase risk of gastrointestinal irritation, ulceration, bleeding, and perforation. These events may occur at any time during therapy and without warning. Use caution with a history of GI disease (bleeding or ulcers), concurrent therapy with aspirin, anticoagulants and/or corticosteroids, smoking, use of alcohol, the elderly or debilitated patients.

Use the lowest effective dose for the shortest duration of time, consistent with individual patient goals, to reduce risk of cardiovascular or GI adverse events. Alternate therapies should be considered for patients at high risk.

NSAIDs may cause serious skin adverse events including exfoliative dermatitis, Stevens-Johnson syndrome (SJS) and toxic epidermal necrolysis (TEN). Anaphylactoid reactions may occur, even without prior exposure; patients with "aspirin triad" (bronchial asthma, aspirin intolerance, rhinitis) may be at increased risk. Do not use in patients who experience bronchospasm, asthma, rhinitis, or urticaria with NSAID or aspirin therapy.

Use with caution in patients with decreased hepatic function. Closely monitor patients with any abnormal LFT. Severe hepatic reactions (eg, fulminant hepatitis, liver failure) have occurred with NSAID use, rarely; discontinue if signs or symptoms of liver disease develop, or if systemic manifestations occur.

The elderly are at increased risk for adverse effects (especially peptic ulceration, CNS effects, renal toxicity) from NSAIDs even at low doses.

(Continued)

Ketorolac *(Continued)*

Withhold for at least 4-6 half-lives prior to surgical or dental procedures.

Ophthalmic: May increase bleeding time associated with ocular surgery. Use with caution in patients with known bleeding tendencies or those receiving anticoagulants. Healing time may be slowed or delayed. Corneal thinning, erosion, or ulceration have been reported with topical NSAIDs; discontinue if corneal epithelial breakdown occurs. Use caution with complicated ocular surgery, corneal denervation, corneal epithelial defects, diabetes, rheumatoid arthritis, ocular surface disease, or ocular surgeries repeated within short periods of time; risk of corneal epithelial breakdown may be increased. Use for >24 hours prior to or for >14 days following surgery also increases risk of corneal adverse effects. Do not administer while wearing soft contact lenses. Safety and efficacy in pediatric patients <3 years of age have not been established.

Adverse Reactions

Systemic:

>10%:

Central nervous system: Headache (17%)
Gastrointestinal: Gastrointestinal pain (13%), dyspepsia (12%), nausea (12%)

>1% to 10%:

Cardiovascular: Edema (4%), hypertension
Central nervous system: Dizziness (7%), drowsiness (6%)
Dermatologic: Pruritus, purpura, rash
Gastrointestinal: Diarrhea (7%), constipation, flatulence, gastrointestinal fullness, vomiting, stomatitis
Local: Injection site pain (2%)
Miscellaneous: Diaphoresis

≤1% (Limited to important or life-threatening): Abnormal vision, acute renal failure, anaphylactoid reaction, anaphylaxis, asthma, azotemia, bronchospasm, cholestatic jaundice, convulsions, eosinophilia, epistaxis, esophagitis, extrapyramidal symptoms, GI hemorrhage, GI perforation, hallucinations, hearing loss, hematemesis, hematuria, hepatitis, hypersensitivity reactions, liver failure, Lyell's syndrome, maculopapular rash, nephritis, peptic ulceration, Stevens-Johnson syndrome, tinnitus, toxic epidermal necrolysis, urticaria, vertigo, wound hemorrhage (postoperative)

Ophthalmic solution:

>10%: Ocular: Transient burning/stinging (Acular®: 40%; Acular® PF: 20%)

>1% to 10%:

Central nervous system: Headache
Ocular: Conjunctival hyperemia, corneal infiltrates, iritis, ocular edema, ocular inflammation, ocular irritation, ocular pain, superficial keratitis, superficial ocular infection
Miscellaneous: Allergic reactions

≤1% (Limited to important or life-threatening): Blurred vision corneal ulcer, corneal erosion, corneal perforation, corneal thinning, dry eyes, epithelial breakdown

Overdosage/Toxicology Symptoms of overdose include abdominal pain, peptic ulcers, and metabolic acidosis. Management of NSAID intoxication is supportive and symptomatic. Dialysis is not effective.

Drug Interactions

ACE inhibitors: Antihypertensive effects may be decreased by concurrent therapy with NSAIDs; monitor blood pressure.

Angiotensin II antagonists: Antihypertensive effects may be decreased by concurrent therapy with NSAIDs; monitor blood pressure.

Anticoagulants: Increased risk of bleeding complications with concomitant use; monitor closely.

Antiepileptic drugs (carbamazepine, phenytoin): Sporadic cases of seizures have been reported with concomitant use.

Beta-blockers: NSAIDs may decrease the antihypertensive effect of beta-blockers. Monitor.

Cholestyramine (and other bile acid sequestrants): May decrease the absorption of NSAIDs. Separate by at least 2 hours.

Diuretics: May see decreased effect of diuretics.

Hydralazine's antihypertensive effect may be reduced; monitor.

Lithium: May increase lithium levels; monitor.

Methotrexate: Severe bone marrow suppression, aplastic anemia, and GI toxicity have been reported with concomitant NSAID therapy. Avoid use during moderate or high-dose methotrexate (increased and prolonged methotrexate levels). NSAID use during low-dose treatment of rheumatoid arthritis has not been fully evaluated; extreme caution is warranted.

Nondepolarizing muscle relaxants: Concomitant use has resulted in apnea.

NSAIDs, salicylates: Concomitant use increases NSAID-induced adverse effects; contraindicated.

Probenecid: Probenecid significantly decreases ketorolac clearance, increases ketorolac plasma levels, and doubles the half-life of ketorolac; concomitant use is contraindicated.

Psychoactive drugs (alprazolam, fluoxetine, thiothixene): Hallucinations have been reported with concomitant use.

Ethanol/Nutrition/Herb Interactions

Ethanol: Avoid ethanol (may enhance gastric mucosal irritation).

Food: Oral: High-fat meals may delay time to peak (by ~1 hour) and decrease peak concentrations.

Herb/Neutraceuticals: Avoid alfalfa, anise, bilberry, bladderwrack, bromelain, cat's claw, celery, coleus, cordyceps, dong quai, evening primrose, feverfew, fenugreek, garlic, ginger, ginkgo biloboa, red clover, horse chestnut, grapeseed, green tea, ginseng, guggul, horse chestnut seed, horseradish, licorice, prickly ash, red clover, reishi, SAMe, sweet clover, turmeric, white willow (all have additional antiplatelet activity).

Dietary Considerations Administer tablet with food or milk to decrease gastrointestinal distress.

Dosage Forms [DSC] = Discontinued product

Injection, solution, as tromethamine: 15 mg/mL (1 mL); 30 mg/mL (1 mL, 2 mL, 10 mL) [contains alcohol]

Solution, ophthalmic, as tromethamine:

Acular®: 0.5% (3 mL, 5 mL, 10 mL) [contains benzalkonium chloride]

Acular LS™: 0.4% (5 mL) [contains benzalkonium chloride]

Acular® P.F. [preservative free]: 0.5% (0.4 mL)

Tablet, as tromethamine: 10 mg

Toradol®: 10 mg [DSC]

- **Ketorolac Tromethamine** *see* Ketorolac *on page 717*
- **Ketorolac Tromethamine Injection, USP (Can)** *see* Ketorolac *on page 717*
- **Kidkare Decongestant [OTC]** *see* Pseudoephedrine *on page 1085*
- **Kionex™** *see* Sodium Polystyrene Sulfonate *on page 1193*
- **Klonopin®** *see* Clonazepam *on page 313*
- **Kodet SE [OTC]** *see* Pseudoephedrine *on page 1085*
- **Kogenate® (Can)** *see* Antihemophilic Factor (Recombinant) *on page 113*
- **Kogenate® FS** *see* Antihemophilic Factor (Recombinant) *on page 113*
- **Konakion (Can)** *see* Phytonadione *on page 1027*
- **Kristalose™** *see* Lactulose *on page 724*
- **Kytril®** *see* Granisetron *on page 602*
- **L-749,345** *see* Ertapenem *on page 473*
- **L-M-X™ 4 [OTC]** *see* Lidocaine *on page 755*
- **L-M-X™ 5 [OTC]** *see* Lidocaine *on page 755*
- **L 754030** *see* Aprepitant *on page 121*
- **LA 20304a** *see* Gemifloxacin *on page 587*

Labetalol (la BET a lole)

Medication Safety Issues

Sound-alike/look-alike issues:

Labetalol may be confused with betaxolol, Hexadrol®, lamotrigine

Trandate® may be confused with tramadol, Trendar®, Trental®, Tridrate®

Related Information

Anesthesia for Patients With Liver Disease *on page 1421*

Beta-Blockers *on page 1557*

Hypertension *on page 1620*

Postoperative Hypertension *on page 1471*

(Continued)

Labetalol *(Continued)*

U.S. Brand Names Trandate®

Canadian Brand Names Apo-Labetalol®; Labetalol Hydrochloride Injection, USP; Normodyne®; Trandate®

Synonyms Ibidomide Hydrochloride; Labetalol Hydrochloride

Pharmacologic Category Beta Blocker With Alpha-Blocking Activity

Generic Available Yes

Use Treatment of mild to severe hypertension; I.V. for hypertensive emergencies

Mechanism of Action Blocks alpha-, beta$_1$-, and beta$_2$-adrenergic receptor sites; elevated renins are reduced

Pharmacodynamics/Kinetics

Onset of action: Oral: 20 minutes to 2 hours; I.V.: 2-5 minutes

Peak effect: Oral: 1-4 hours; I.V.: 5-15 minutes

Duration: Oral: 8-24 hours (dose dependent); I.V.: 2-4 hours

Distribution: V_d: Adults: 3-16 L/kg; mean: <9.4 L/kg; moderately lipid soluble, therefore, can enter CNS; crosses placenta; small amounts enter breast milk

Protein binding: 50%

Metabolism: Hepatic, primarily via glucuronide conjugation; extensive first-pass effect

Bioavailability: Oral: 25%; increased with liver disease, elderly, and concurrent cimetidine

Half-life elimination: Normal renal function: 2.5-8 hours

Excretion: Urine (<5% as unchanged drug)

Clearance: Possibly decreased in neonates/infants

Dosage Due to limited documentation of its use, labetalol should be initiated cautiously in pediatric patients with careful dosage adjustment and blood pressure monitoring.

Children:

Oral: Limited information regarding labetalol use in pediatric patients is currently available in literature. Some centers recommend initial oral doses of 4 mg/kg/day in 2 divided doses. Reported oral doses have started at 3 mg/kg/day and 20 mg/kg/day and have increased up to 40 mg/kg/day.

I.V., intermittent bolus doses of 0.3-1 mg/kg/dose have been reported.

For treatment of pediatric hypertensive emergencies, initial continuous infusions of 0.4-1 mg/kg/hour with a maximum of 3 mg/kg/hour have been used. Administration requires the use of an infusion pump.

Adults:

Oral: Initial: 100 mg twice daily, may increase as needed every 2-3 days by 100 mg until desired response is obtained; usual dose: 200-400 mg twice daily; may require up to 2.4 g/day.

Usual dose range (JNC 7): 200-800 mg/day in 2 divided doses

I.V.: 20 mg (0.25 mg/kg for an 80 kg patient) IVP over 2 minutes; may administer 40-80 mg at 10-minute intervals, up to 300 mg total dose.

I.V. infusion: Initial: 2 mg/minute; titrate to response up to 300 mg total dose, if needed. Administration requires the use of an infusion pump.

I.V. infusion (500 mg/250 mL D_5W) rates:

1 mg/minute: 30 mL/hour
2 mg/minute: 60 mL/hour
3 mg/minute: 90 mL/hour
4 mg/minute: 120 mL/hour
5 mg/minute: 150 mL/hour
6 mg/minute: 180 mL/hour

Dialysis: Not removed by hemo- or peritoneal dialysis; supplemental dose is not necessary.

Dosage adjustment in hepatic impairment: Dosage reduction may be necessary.

Stability

Labetalol should be stored at room temperature or under refrigeration and should be protected from light and freezing; the solution is clear to slightly yellow

Stability of parenteral admixture at room temperature (25°C) and refrigeration temperature (4°C): 3 days

Standard diluent: 500 mg/250 mL D_5W

Minimum volume: 250 mL D_5W

Incompatible with sodium bicarbonate, most stable at pH of 2-4; **incompatible** with alkaline solutions

Administration Bolus administered over 2 minutes.

Monitoring Parameters Blood pressure, standing and sitting/supine, pulse, cardiac monitor and blood pressure monitor required for I.V. administration

Anesthesia and Critical Care Concerns/Other Considerations Due to alterations in the beta-adrenergic autonomic nervous system, beta-adrenergic blockade may result in less hemodynamic response in the elderly than seen in younger adults. Despite decreased sensitivity to the chronotropic effects of beta blockade with age, there appears to be an increased myocardial sensitivity to the negative inotropic effect during stress (eg, exercise).

Pregnancy Risk Factor C (manufacturer); D (2nd and 3rd trimesters - expert analysis)

Contraindications Hypersensitivity to labetalol or any component of the formulation; sinus bradycardia; heart block greater than first degree (except in patients with a functioning artificial pacemaker); cardiogenic shock; bronchial asthma; uncompensated cardiac failure; pregnancy (2nd and 3rd trimesters)

Warnings/Precautions Use only with extreme caution in compensated heart failure and monitor for a worsening of the condition. Avoid abrupt discontinuation in patients with a history of CAD; slowly wean while monitoring for signs and symptoms of ischemia. Use caution with concurrent use of beta-blockers and either verapamil or diltiazem; bradycardia or heart block can occur. Avoid concurrent I.V. use of both agents. Patients with bronchospastic disease should not receive beta-blockers. Labetalol may be used with caution in patients with nonallergic bronchospasm (chronic bronchitis, emphysema). Use cautiously in diabetics because it can mask prominent hypoglycemic symptoms. Can mask signs of thyrotoxicosis. Can cause fetal harm when administered in pregnancy. Use cautiously in the hepatically impaired. Use caution when using I.V. labetalol and inhalational anesthetics concurrently (significant myocardial depression).

Adverse Reactions

>10%:

- Central nervous system: Dizziness (1% to 16%)
- Gastrointestinal: Nausea (0% to 19%)

1% to 10%:

- Cardiovascular: Edema (0% to 2%), hypotension (1% to 5%); with IV use, hypotension may occur in up to 58%
- Central nervous system: Fatigue (1% to 10%), paresthesia (1% to 5%), headache (2%), vertigo (2%)
- Dermatologic: Rash (1%), scalp tingling (1% to 5%)
- Gastrointestinal: Vomiting (<1% to 3%), dyspepsia (1% to 4%)
- Genitourinary: Ejaculatory failure (0% to 5%), impotence (1% to 4%)
- Hepatic: Transaminases increased (4%)
- Neuromuscular & skeletal: Weakness (1%)
- Respiratory: Nasal congestion (1% to 6%), dyspnea (2%)
- Miscellaneous: Taste disorder (1%), abnormal vision (1%)

<1% (Limited to important or life-threatening): Alopecia (reversible), anaphylactoid reaction, angioedema, bradycardia, bronchospasm, cholestatic jaundice, CHF, diabetes insipidus, heart block, hepatic necrosis, hepatitis, hypersensitivity, hypotension, Peyronie's disease, positive ANA, pruritus, Raynaud's syndrome, syncope, systemic lupus erythematosus, toxic myopathy, urinary retention, urticaria, ventricular arrhythmia (I.V.)

Other adverse reactions noted with beta-adrenergic blocking agents include mental depression, catatonia, short-term memory loss, emotional lability, intensification of pre-existing AV block, laryngospasm, respiratory distress, agranulocytosis, thrombocytopenic purpura, nonthrombocytopenic purpura, mesenteric artery thrombosis, and ischemic colitis.

Overdosage/Toxicology Symptoms of intoxication include cardiac disturbances, CNS toxicity, bronchospasm, hypoglycemia, and hyperkalemia. The most common cardiac symptoms include hypotension and bradycardia. Atrioventricular block, intraventricular conduction disturbances, cardiogenic shock, and asystole may occur with severe overdose, especially with membrane-depressant drugs (eg, propranolol). CNS effects include convulsions, coma, and respiratory arrest and are commonly seen with propranolol and other membrane-depressant and lipid-soluble drugs. Treatment is symptomatic. Glucagon may be administered to improve cardiac function.

Drug Interactions **Substrate** of CYP2D6 (major); **Inhibits** CYP2D6 (weak)

Alpha-blockers (prazosin, terazosin): Concurrent use of beta-blockers may increase risk of orthostasis.

Cimetidine increases the bioavailability of labetalol.

(Continued)

Labetalol *(Continued)*

CYP2D6 inhibitors: May increase the levels/effects of labetalol. Example inhibitors include chlorpromazine, delavirdine, fluoxetine, miconazole, paroxetine, pergolide, quinidine, quinine, ritonavir, and ropinirole.

Halothane, isoflurane, enflurane (possibly other inhalational anesthetics): Excessive hypotension may occur.

NSAIDs may reduce antihypertensive efficacy of labetalol.

Salicylates may reduce the antihypertensive effects of beta-blockers.

Sulfonylureas: Effects may be decreased by beta-blockers.

Verapamil or diltiazem may have synergistic or additive pharmacological effects when taken concurrently with beta-blockers; avoid concurrent I.V. use.

Ethanol/Nutrition/Herb Interactions

Food: Labetalol serum concentrations may be increased if taken with food.

Herb/Nutraceutical: Avoid dong quai if using for hypertension (has estrogenic activity). Avoid ephedra, yohimbe, ginseng (may worsen hypertension). Avoid natural licorice (causes sodium and water retention and increases potassium loss). Avoid garlic (may have increased antihypertensive effect).

Test Interactions False-positive urine catecholamines, VMA if measured by fluorometric or photometric methods; use HPLC or specific catecholamine radioenzymatic technique

Dosage Forms

Injection, solution, as hydrochloride: 5 mg/mL (4 mL, 20 mL, 40 mL)

Trandate®: 5 mg/mL (20 mL, 40 mL)

Tablet, as hydrochloride: 100 mg, 200 mg, 300 mg

Trandate®: 100 mg, 200 mg [contains sodium benzoate], 300 mg

References

Erstad BL and Barletta JF, "Treatment of Hypertension in the Perioperative Patient," *Ann Pharmacother*, 2000, 34(1):66-79.

Mokhlesi B, Leikin JB, Murray P, et al, "Adult Toxicology in Critical Care. Part 11: Specific Poisonings," *Chest*, 2003, 123(3):897-922.

♦ **Labetalol Hydrochloride** *see* Labetalol *on page 721*

♦ **Labetalol Hydrochloride Injection, USP (Can)** *see* Labetalol *on page 721*

Lactulose (LAK tyoo lose)

Medication Safety Issues

Sound-alike/look-alike issues:

Lactulose may be confused with lactose

U.S. Brand Names Constulose®; Enulose®; Generlac; Kristalose™

Canadian Brand Names Acilac; Apo-Lactulose®; Laxilose; PMS-Lactulose

Pharmacologic Category Ammonium Detoxicant; Laxative, Osmotic

Generic Available Yes

Use Adjunct in the prevention and treatment of portal-systemic encephalopathy; treatment of chronic constipation

Mechanism of Action The bacterial degradation of lactulose resulting in an acidic pH inhibits the diffusion of NH_3 into the blood by causing the conversion of NH_3 to NH_4+; also enhances the diffusion of NH_3 from the blood into the gut where conversion to NH_4+ occurs; produces an osmotic effect in the colon with resultant distention promoting peristalsis

Pharmacodynamics/Kinetics

Absorption: Not appreciable

Metabolism: Via colonic flora to lactic acid and acetic acid; requires colonic flora for drug activation

Excretion: Primarily feces and urine (~3%)

Dosage Diarrhea may indicate overdosage and responds to dose reduction

Prevention of portal systemic encephalopathy (PSE): Oral:

Infants: 2.5-10 mL/day divided 3-4 times/day; adjust dosage to produce 2-3 stools/day

Older Children: Daily dose of 40-90 mL divided 3-4 times/day; if initial dose causes diarrhea, then reduce it immediately; adjust dosage to produce 2-3 stools/day

Constipation: Oral:

Children: 5 g/day (7.5 mL) after breakfast

Adults: 15-30 mL/day increased to 60 mL/day in 1-2 divided doses if necessary

Acute PSE: Adults:

Oral: 20-30 g (30-45 mL) every 1-2 hours to induce rapid laxation; adjust dosage daily to produce 2-3 soft stools; doses of 30-45 mL may be given hourly to cause rapid laxation, then reduce to recommended dose; usual daily dose: 60-100 g (90-150 mL) daily

Rectal administration: 200 g (300 mL) diluted with 700 mL of H_2O or NS; administer rectally via rectal balloon catheter and retain 30-60 minutes every 4-6 hours

Stability Keep solution at room temperature to reduce viscosity; discard solution if cloudy or very dark

Administration Dilute lactulose in water, usually 60-120 mL, prior to administering through a gastric or feeding tube. Syrup formulation has been used in preparation of rectal solution.

Monitoring Parameters Blood pressure, standing/supine; serum potassium, bowel movement patterns, fluid status, serum ammonia

Pregnancy Risk Factor B

Contraindications Hypersensitivity to lactulose or any component of the formulation; galactosemia (or patients requiring a low galactose diet)

Warnings/Precautions Use with caution in patients with diabetes mellitus; monitor periodically for electrolyte imbalance when lactulose is used >6 months or in patients predisposed to electrolyte abnormalities (eg, elderly); patients receiving lactulose and an oral anti-infective agent should be monitored for possible inadequate response to lactulose

Adverse Reactions Frequency not defined: Gastrointestinal: Flatulence, diarrhea (excessive dose), abdominal discomfort, nausea, vomiting, cramping

Overdosage/Toxicology Symptoms of overdose include diarrhea, abdominal pain, hypochloremic alkalosis, dehydration, hypotension, and hypokalemia. Treatment includes supportive care.

Drug Interactions Decreased effect: Oral neomycin, laxatives, antacids

Dietary Considerations Contraindicated in patients on galactose-restricted diet; may be mixed with fruit juice, milk, water, or citrus-flavored carbonated beverages.

Dosage Forms

Crystals for reconstitution (Kristalose™): 10 g/packet (30s), 20 g/packet (30s)

Syrup: 10 g/15 mL (15 mL, 30 mL, 237 mL, 473 mL, 946 mL, 1890 mL)

Constulose®: 10 g/15 mL (240 mL, 960 mL)

Enulose®: 10 g/15 mL (480 mL)

Generlac: 10 g/15 mL (480 mL, 1920 mL)

♦ **L-AmB** *see* Amphotericin B (Liposomal) *on page 100*

♦ **Lamictal®** *see* Lamotrigine *on page 727*

Lamivudine (la MI vyoo deen)

Medication Safety Issues

Sound-alike/look-alike issues:

Lamivudine may be confused with lamotrigine

Epivir® may be confused with Combivir®

U.S. Brand Names Epivir®; Epivir-HBV®

Canadian Brand Names Heptovir®; 3TC®

Synonyms 3TC

Pharmacologic Category Antiretroviral Agent, Reverse Transcriptase Inhibitor (Nucleoside)

Generic Available No

Use

Epivir®: Treatment of HIV infection when antiretroviral therapy is warranted; should always be used as part of a multidrug regimen (at least three antiretroviral agents)

Epivir-HBV®: Treatment of chronic hepatitis B associated with evidence of hepatitis B viral replication and active liver inflammation

Unlabeled/Investigational Use Prevention of HIV following needlesticks (with or without protease inhibitor)

Mechanism of Action Lamivudine is a cytosine analog. After lamivudine is triphosphorylated, the principle mode of action is inhibition of HIV reverse transcription via viral DNA chain termination; inhibits RNA- and DNA-dependent DNA polymerase activities of reverse transcriptase. The monophosphate form of

(Continued)

Lamivudine *(Continued)*

lamivudine is incorporated into the viral DNA by hepatitis B virus polymerase, resulting in DNA chain termination.

Pharmacodynamics/Kinetics

Absorption: Rapid
Distribution: V_d: 1.3 L/kg
Protein binding, plasma: <36%
Metabolism: 5.6% to trans-sulfoxide metabolite
Bioavailability: Absolute; Cp_{max} decreased with food although AUC not significantly affected
- Children: 66%
- Adults: 87%

Half-life elimination: Children: 2 hours; Adults: 5-7 hours
Excretion: Primarily urine (as unchanged drug)

Dosage Note: The formulation and dosage of Epivir-HBV® are not appropriate for patients infected with both HBV and HIV. Use with at least two other antiretroviral agents when treating HIV

Oral:
- Children 3 months to 16 years: HIV: 4 mg/kg twice daily (maximum: 150 mg twice daily)
- Children 2-17 years: Treatment of hepatitis B (Epivir-HBV®): 3 mg/kg once daily (maximum: 100 mg/day)
- Adolescents and Adults: Prevention of HIV following needlesticks (unlabeled use): 150 mg twice daily (with zidovudine with or without a protease inhibitor, depending on risk)
- Adults:
  - HIV: 150 mg twice daily **or** 300 mg once daily
    - <50 kg: 4 mg/kg twice daily (maximum: 150 mg twice daily)
  - Treatment of hepatitis B (Epivir-HBV®): 100 mg/day

Dosing interval in renal impairment in pediatric patients: Insufficient data; however, dose reduction should be considered.

Dosing interval in renal impairment in patients >16 years for HIV:
- Cl_{cr} 30-49 mL/minute: Administer 150 mg once daily
- Cl_{cr} 15-29 mL/minute: Administer 150 mg first dose, then 100 mg once daily
- Cl_{cr} 5-14 mL/minute: Administer 150 mg first dose, then 50 mg once daily
- Cl_{cr} <5 mL/minute: Administer 50 mg first dose, then 25 mg once daily

Dosing interval in renal impairment in adult patients with hepatitis B:
- Cl_{cr} 30-49: Administer 100 mg first dose then 50 mg once daily
- Cl_{cr} 15-29: Administer 100 mg first dose then 25 mg once daily
- Cl_{cr} 5-14: Administer 35 mg first dose then 15 mg once daily
- Cl_{cr} <5: Administer 35 mg first dose then 10 mg once daily

Dialysis: Negligible amounts are removed by 4-hour hemodialysis or peritoneal dialysis. Supplemental dosing is not required.

Stability Store at 2°C to 25°C (68°F to 77°F) tightly closed.

Administration May be taken with or without food. Adjust dosage in renal failure.

Monitoring Parameters Amylase, bilirubin, liver enzymes, hematologic parameters, viral load, and CD4 count; signs and symptoms of pancreatitis

Pregnancy Risk Factor C

Contraindications Hypersensitivity to lamivudine or any component of the formulation

Warnings/Precautions A decreased dosage is recommended in patients with renal dysfunction since AUC, C_{max}, and half-life increased with diminishing renal function; use with extreme caution in children with history of pancreatitis or risk factors for development of pancreatitis. Do not use as monotherapy in treatment of HIV. Treatment of HBV in patients with unrecognized/untreated HIV may lead to rapid HIV resistance. In addition, treatment of HIV in patients with unrecognized/untreated HBV may lead to rapid HBV resistance. **[U.S. Boxed Warning]: Do not use Epivir-HBV® tablets or oral solution for the treatment of HIV.**

[U.S. Boxed Warning]: Lactic acidosis and severe hepatomegaly with steatosis have been reported, including fatal cases. Use caution in hepatic impairment. Pregnancy, obesity, and/or prolonged therapy may increase the risk of lactic acidosis and liver damage.

[U.S. Boxed Warning]: Monitor patients closely for several months following discontinuation of therapy for chronic hepatitis B; clinical exacerbations may occur.

Adverse Reactions (As reported in adults treated for HIV infection)

>10%:

Central nervous system: Headache, fatigue

Gastrointestinal: Nausea, diarrhea, vomiting, pancreatitis (range: 0.5% to 18%; higher percentage in pediatric patients)

Neuromuscular & skeletal: Peripheral neuropathy, paresthesia, musculoskeletal pain

1% to 10%:

Central nervous system: Dizziness, depression, fever, chills, insomnia

Dermatologic: Rash

Gastrointestinal: Anorexia, abdominal pain, heartburn, elevated amylase

Hematologic: Neutropenia

Hepatic: Elevated AST, ALT

Neuromuscular & skeletal: Myalgia, arthralgia

Respiratory: Nasal signs and symptoms, cough

<1% (Limited to important or life-threatening): Alopecia, anaphylaxis, anemia, hepatomegaly, hyperbilirubinemia, hyperglycemia, increased CPK, lactic acidosis, lymphadenopathy, peripheral neuropathy, pruritus, red cell aplasia, rhabdomyolysis, splenomegaly, steatosis, stomatitis, thrombocytopenia, urticaria, weakness

Overdosage/Toxicology Limited information is available, although there have been no clinical signs or symptoms noted, and hematologic tests remained normal in overdose. No antidote is available. Limited (negligible) removal following 4-hour hemodialysis. It is not known if continuous 24-hour hemodialysis would be effective.

Drug Interactions

Ribavirin: Concomitant use of ribavirin and nucleoside analogues may increase the risk of developing lactic acidosis (includes adefovir, didanosine, lamivudine, stavudine, zalcitabine, zidovudine).

Sulfamethoxazole/trimethoprim: Increased AUC and decreased clearance of lamivudine with concomitant use

Trimethoprim (and other drugs excreted by organic cation transport): May increase serum levels/effects of lamivudine.

Zalcitabine: Intracellular phosphorylation of lamivudine and zalcitabine may be inhibited if used together; concomitant use should be avoided.

Zidovudine: Plasma levels of zidovudine are increased by ~39% with concomitant use.

Ethanol/Nutrition/Herb Interactions Food: Food decreases the rate of absorption and C_{max}; however, there is no change in the systemic AUC. Therefore, may be taken with or without food.

Dietary Considerations May be taken with or without food. Each 5 mL of oral solution contains 1 g of sucrose.

Dosage Forms

Solution, oral:

Epivir®: 10 mg/mL (240 mL) [strawberry-banana flavor]

Epivir-HBV®: 5 mg/mL (240 mL) [strawberry-banana flavor]

Tablet:

Epivir®: 150 mg, 300 mg

Epivir-HBV®: 100 mg

Lamotrigine (la MOE tri jeen)

Medication Safety Issues

Sound-alike/look-alike issues:

Lamotrigine may be confused with labetalol, Lamisil®, lamivudine, Lomotil®, ludiomil

Lamictal® may be confused with Lamisil®, Lomotil®, ludiomil

Related Information

Perioperative Management of Patients on Antiseizure Medication *on page 1458*

U.S. Brand Names Lamictal®

Canadian Brand Names Apo-Lamotrigine®; Gen-Lamotrigine; Lamictal®; Novo-Lamotrigine; PMS-Lamotrigine; ratio-Lamotrigine

Synonyms BW-430C; LTG

Pharmacologic Category Anticonvulsant, Miscellaneous

Generic Available No

(Continued)

Lamotrigine *(Continued)*

Use Adjunctive therapy in the treatment of generalized seizures of Lennox-Gastaut syndrome and partial seizures in adults and children ≥2 years of age; conversion to monotherapy in adults with partial seizures who are receiving treatment with valproate or a single enzyme-inducing antiepileptic drug; maintenance treatment of bipolar disorder

Mechanism of Action A triazine derivative which inhibits release of glutamate (an excitatory amino acid) and inhibits voltage-sensitive sodium channels, which stabilizes neuronal membranes. Lamotrigine has weak inhibitory effect on the 5-HT_3 receptor; *in vitro* inhibits dihydrofolate reductase.

Pharmacodynamics/Kinetics

Distribution: V_d: 1.1 L/kg

Protein binding: 55%

Metabolism: Hepatic and renal; metabolized by glucuronic acid conjugation to inactive metabolites

Bioavailability: 98%

Half-life elimination: Adults: 25-33 hours; Concomitant valproic acid therapy: 59-70 hours; Concomitant phenytoin or carbamazepine therapy: 13-14 hours

Time to peak, plasma: 1-4 hours

Excretion: Urine (94%, ~90% as glucuronide conjugates and ~10% unchanged); feces (2%)

Dosage Note: Only whole tablets should be used for dosing, round calculated dose down to the nearest whole tablet: Oral:

Children 2-12 years: Lennox-Gastaut (adjunctive) or partial seizures (adjunctive): **Note:** Children 2-6 years will likely require maintenance doses at the higher end of recommended range:

Patients receiving AED regimens containing valproic acid:

Weeks 1 and 2: 0.15 mg/kg/day in 1-2 divided doses; round dose down to the nearest whole tablet. For patients >6.7 kg and <14 kg, dosing should be 2 mg every other day.

Weeks 3 and 4: 0.3 mg/kg/day in 1-2 divided doses; round dose down to the nearest whole tablet; may use combinations of 2 mg and 5 mg tablets. For patients >6.7 kg and <14 kg, dosing should be 2 mg/day.

Maintenance dose: Titrate dose to effect; after week 4, increase dose every 1-2 weeks by a calculated increment; calculate increment as 0.3 mg/kg/day rounded down to the nearest whole tablet; add this amount to the previously administered daily dose; usual maintenance: 1-5 mg/kg/day in 1-2 divided doses; maximum: 200 mg/day given in 1-2 divided doses

Patients receiving enzyme-inducing AED regimens without valproic acid:

Weeks 1 and 2: 0.6 mg/kg/day in 2 divided doses; round dose down to the nearest whole tablet

Weeks 3 and 4: 1.2 mg/kg/day in 2 divided doses; round dose down to the nearest whole tablet

Maintenance dose: Titrate dose to effect; after week 4, increase dose every 1-2 weeks by a calculated increment; calculate increment as 1.2 mg/kg/day rounded down to the nearest whole tablet; add this amount to the previously administered daily dose; usual maintenance: 5-15 mg/kg/day in 2 divided doses; maximum: 400 mg/day

Children >12 years: Lennox-Gastaut (adjunctive) or partial seizures (adjunctive): Refer to Adults dosing

Children ≥16 years: Conversion from single enzyme-inducing AED regimen to monotherapy: Refer to Adults dosing

Adults:

Lennox-Gastaut (adjunctive) or treatment of partial seizures (adjunctive):

Patients receiving AED regimens containing valproic acid: Initial dose: 25 mg every other day for 2 weeks, then 25 mg every day for 2 weeks. Dose may be increased by 25-50 mg every day for 1-2 weeks in order to achieve maintenance dose. Maintenance dose: 100-400 mg/day in 1-2 divided doses (usual range 100-200 mg/day).

Patients receiving enzyme-inducing AED regimens without valproic acid: Initial dose: 50 mg/day for 2 weeks, then 100 mg in 2 doses for 2 weeks; thereafter, daily dose can be increased by 100 mg every 1-2 weeks to be given in 2 divided doses. Usual maintenance dose: 300-500 mg/day in 2 divided doses; doses as high as 700 mg/day have been reported

Conversion to monotherapy (partial seizures in patients ≥16 years of age):

Adjunctive therapy with valproate: Initiate and titrate as per recommendations to a lamotrigine dose of 200 mg/day. Then taper valproate dose in decrements of not more than 500 mg/day at intervals of one week (or longer) to a valproate dosage of 500 mg/day; this dosage should be maintained for one week. The lamotrigine dosage should then be increased to 300 mg/day while valproate is decreased to 250 mg/day; this dosage should be maintained for one week. Valproate may then be discontinued, while the lamotrigine dose is increased by 100 mg/day at weekly intervals to achieve a lamotrigine maintenance dose of 500 mg/day.

Adjunctive therapy with enzyme-inducing AED: Initiate and titrate as per recommendations to a lamotrigine dose of 500 mg/day. Concomitant enzyme-inducing AED should then be withdrawn by 20% decrements each week over a 4-week period. Patients should be monitored for rash.

Adjunctive therapy with nonenzyme-inducing AED: No specific guidelines available

Bipolar disorder: 25 mg/day for 2 weeks, followed by 50 mg/day for 2 weeks, followed by 100 mg/day for 1 week; thereafter, daily dosage may be increased to 200 mg/day

Patients receiving valproic acid: Initial: 25 mg every other day for 2 weeks, followed by 25 mg/day for 2 weeks, followed by 50 mg/day for 1 week, followed by 100 mg/day (target dose) thereafter. **Note:** If valproate is discontinued, increase daily lamotrigine dose in 50 mg increments at weekly intervals until daily dosage of 200 mg is attained.

Patients receiving enzyme-inducing drugs (eg, carbamazepine): Initial: 50 mg/day for 2 weeks, followed by 100 mg/day (in divided doses) for 2 weeks, followed by 200 mg/day (in divided doses) for 1 week, followed by 300 mg/day (in divided doses) for 1 week. May increase to 400 mg/day (in divided doses) during week 7 and thereafter. **Note:** If carbamazepine (or other enzyme-inducing drug) is discontinued, decrease daily lamotrigine dose in 100 mg increments at weekly intervals until daily dosage of 200 mg is attained.

Discontinuing therapy: Children and Adults: Decrease dose by ~50% per week, over at least 2 weeks unless safety concerns require a more rapid withdrawal.

Restarting therapy after discontinuation: If lamotrigine has been withheld for >5 half-lives, consider restarting according to initial dosing recommendations.

Dosage adjustment in renal impairment: Decreased dosage may be effective in patients with significant renal impairment; use with caution

Dosage adjustment in hepatic impairment:

Child-Pugh Grade B: Reduce initial, escalation, and maintenance doses by 50%

Child-Pugh Grade C: Reduce initial, escalation, and maintenance doses by 75%

Stability Store at 25°C (77°F); excursions are permitted to 15°C to 30°C (59°F to 86°F); protect from light

Administration Doses should be rounded down to the nearest whole tablet. Dispersible tablets may be chewed, dispersed in water, or swallowed whole. To disperse tablets, add to a small amount of liquid (just enough to cover tablet); let sit ~1 minute until dispersed; swirl solution and consume immediately. Do not administer partial amounts of liquid. If tablets are chewed, a small amount of water or diluted fruit juice should be used to aid in swallowing.

Monitoring Parameters Seizure, frequency and duration, serum levels of concurrent anticonvulsants, hypersensitivity reactions, especially rash

Reference Range A therapeutic serum concentration range has not been established for lamotrigine. Dosing should be based on therapeutic response. Lamotrigine plasma concentrations of 0.25-29.1 mcg/mL have been reported in the literature.

Anesthesia and Critical Care Concerns/Other Considerations Low water solubility; less sedating than other antiepileptic drugs. Use gastric lavage with activated charcoal and a cathartic for overdose. Worsens myoclonic seizure activity.

Pregnancy Risk Factor C

Contraindications Hypersensitivity to lamotrigine or any component of the formulation

(Continued)

Lamotrigine *(Continued)*

Warnings/Precautions [U.S. Boxed Warning]: Severe and potentially life-threatening skin rashes requiring hospitalization have been reported (children 0.8%, adults 0.3%); risk may be increased by coadministration with valproic acid, higher than recommended starting doses, and rapid dose titration. The majority of cases occur in the first 8 weeks; however, isolated cases may occur after prolonged treatment. Discontinue at first sign of rash unless rash is clearly not drug related. Use caution in patients with impaired renal, hepatic, or cardiac function. Avoid abrupt cessation, taper over at least 2 weeks if possible. May cause CNS depression, which may impair physical or mental abilities. Patients must be cautioned about performing tasks which require mental alertness (eg, operating machinery or driving). Effects with other sedative drugs or ethanol may be potentiated. Binds to melanin and may accumulate in the eye and other melanin-rich tissues; the clinical significance of this is not known. Safety and efficacy has not been established for use as initial monotherapy, conversion to monotherapy from nonenzyme-inducing antiepileptic drugs (AED) except valproate, or conversion to monotherapy from two or more AEDs. **Use caution in writing and/or interpreting prescriptions/orders; medication dispensing errors have occurred with similar-sounding medications (Lamisil®, ludiomil, lamivudine, labetalol, and Lomotil®).**

Adverse Reactions Percentages reported in adults receiving adjunctive therapy:

>10%:

Central nervous system: Headache (29%), dizziness (38%), ataxia (22%), somnolence (14%)

Gastrointestinal: Nausea (19%)

Ocular: Diplopia (28%), blurred vision (16%)

Respiratory: Rhinitis (14%)

1% to 10%:

Cardiovascular: Peripheral edema

Central nervous system: Depression (4%), anxiety (4%), irritability (3%), confusion, speech disorder (3%), difficulty concentrating (2%), malaise, seizure (includes exacerbations) (2% to 3%), incoordination (6%), insomnia (6%), pain, amnesia, hostility, memory decreased, nervousness, vertigo

Dermatologic: Hypersensitivity rash (10%; serious rash requiring hospitalization - adults 0.3%, children 0.8%), pruritus (3%)

Gastrointestinal: Abdominal pain (5%), vomiting (9%), diarrhea (6%), dyspepsia (5%), xerostomia, constipation (4%), anorexia (2%), tooth disorder (3%)

Genitourinary: Vaginitis (4%), dysmenorrhea (7%), amenorrhea (2%)

Neuromuscular & skeletal: Tremor (4%), arthralgia (2%), neck pain (2%)

Ocular: Nystagmus (2%), visual abnormality

Respiratory: Epistaxis, bronchitis, dyspnea

Miscellaneous: Flu syndrome (7%), fever (6%)

<1% (Limited to important or life-threatening): Acne, acute renal failure, agranulocytosis, allergic reactions, alopecia, anemia, angina, angioedema, aplastic anemia, apnea, atrial fibrillation, back pain, bronchospasm, bruising, chills, depersonalization, disseminated intravascular coagulation (DIC), dysarthria, dysphagia, eosinophilia, erythema multiforme, esophagitis, facial edema, GI hemorrhage, gingival hyperplasia, halitosis, hemolytic anemia, hemorrhage, hepatitis, hot flashes, hypersensitivity reactions (including rhabdomyolysis), hypertension, immunosuppression (progressive), impotence, leukopenia, lupus-like reaction, maculopapular rash, malaise, mania, migraine, movement disorder, multiorgan failure, neutropenia, palpitation, pancreatitis, pancytopenia, paralysis, Parkinson's disease exacerbation, photosensitivity (rare), postural hypotension, rash, red cell aplasia, Stevens-Johnson syndrome, stroke, suicidal ideation, thrombocytopenia, tics, toxic epidermal necrolysis, urticaria, vasculitis, vesiculobullous rash

Overdosage/Toxicology Symptoms of overdose include QRS prolongation, AV block, dizziness, drowsiness, sedation, and ataxia. Enhancement of elimination: Multiple dosing of activated charcoal may be useful.

Drug Interactions

Acetaminophen: May reduce serum concentrations of lamotrigine; mechanism not defined; of clinical concern only with chronic acetaminophen dosing (not single doses).

Carbamazepine: Lamotrigine may increase the epoxide metabolite of carbamazepine resulting in toxicity. Carbamazepine may decrease plasma levels of lamotrigine. Dosage adjustments may be needed when adding or withdrawing agents; monitor.

Oral contraceptives (estrogens): Oral contraceptives may decrease the serum concentration of lamotrigine; monitor. Dosage adjustment of lamotrigine may be required when starting/stopping oral contraceptives.

Phenytoin: May decrease plasma levels of lamotrigine. Dosage adjustments may be needed when adding or withdrawing agents; monitor.

Phenobarbital (barbiturates): May increase the metabolism of lamotrigine. Dosage adjustment may be needed when adding or withdrawing agent; monitor.

SSRIs (sertraline): Toxicity has been reported following the addition of sertraline; limited documentation; monitor.

Valproic acid: Inhibits the clearance of lamotrigine, dosage adjustment required when adding or withdrawing valproic acid. Inhibition appears maximal at valproic acid 250-500 mg/day. The incidence of serious rash may be increased by valproic acid.

Ethanol/Nutrition/Herb Interactions

Ethanol: Avoid ethanol (may increase CNS depression).

Food: Has no effect on absorption.

Herb/Nutraceutical: Avoid evening primrose (seizure threshold decreased).

Dietary Considerations Take without regard to meals; drug may cause GI upset.

Dosage Forms

Tablet: 25 mg, 100 mg, 150 mg, 200 mg [contains lactose]

Tablet, combination package [each unit-dose starter kit contains]:

- Lamictal® (blue kit; for patients taking valproate):
  - Tablet: Lamotrigine 25 mg (35s)
- Lamictal® (green kit; for patients taking carbamazepine, phenytoin, phenobarbital, primidone, or rifampin and **not** taking valproate):
  - Tablet: Lamotrigine 25 mg (84s)
  - Tablet: Lamotrigine 100 mg (14s)
- Lamictal® (orange kit; for patients **not** taking carbamazepine, phenytoin, phenobarbital, primidone, rifampin, or valproate; for use in bipolar patients only):
  - Tablet: Lamotrigine 25 mg (42s)
  - Tablet: Lamotrigine 100 mg (7s)

Tablet, dispersible/chewable: 2 mg, 5 mg, 25 mg [black currant flavor]

♦ **Lanoxicaps®** *see* Digoxin *on page 388*

♦ **Lanoxin®** *see* Digoxin *on page 388*

Lansoprazole (lan SOE pra zole)

Medication Safety Issues

Sound-alike/look-alike issues:

Prevacid® may be confused with Pravachol®, Prevpac®, Prilosec®, Prinivil®

U.S. Brand Names Prevacid®; Prevacid® SoluTab™

Canadian Brand Names Prevacid®

Pharmacologic Category Proton Pump Inhibitor; Substituted Benzimidazole

Generic Available No

Use

Oral: Short-term treatment of active duodenal ulcers; maintenance treatment of healed duodenal ulcers; as part of a multidrug regimen for *H. pylori* eradication to reduce the risk of duodenal ulcer recurrence; short-term treatment of active benign gastric ulcer; treatment of NSAID-associated gastric ulcer; to reduce the risk of NSAID-associated gastric ulcer in patients with a history of gastric ulcer who require an NSAID; short-term treatment of symptomatic GERD; short-term treatment for all grades of erosive esophagitis; to maintain healing of erosive esophagitis; long-term treatment of pathological hypersecretory conditions, including Zollinger-Ellison syndrome

I.V.: Short-term treatment (≤7 days) of erosive esophagitis in adults unable to take oral medications

Unlabeled/Investigational Use Active ulcer bleeding (parenteral formulation)

Mechanism of Action A proton pump inhibitor which decreases acid secretion in gastric parietal cells

(Continued)

Lansoprazole *(Continued)*

Pharmacodynamics/Kinetics

Duration: >1 day

Absorption: Rapid

Protein binding: 97%

Metabolism: Hepatic via CYP2C19 and 3A4, and in parietal cells to two inactive metabolites

Bioavailability: 80%; decreased 50% to 70% if given 30 minutes after food

Half-life elimination: 2 hours; Elderly: 2-3 hours; Hepatic impairment: ≤7 hours

Time to peak, plasma: 1.7 hours

Excretion: Feces (67%); urine (33%)

Dosage

Children 1-11 years: GERD, erosive esophagitis: Oral:

≤30 kg: 15 mg once daily

>30 kg: 30 mg once daily

Note: Doses were increased in some pediatric patients if still symptomatic after 2 or more weeks of treatment (maximum dose: 30 mg twice daily)

Children 12-17 years: Oral:

Nonerosive GERD: 15 mg once daily for up to 8 weeks

Erosive esophagitis: 30 mg once daily for up to 8 weeks

Adults:

Duodenal ulcer: Oral: Short-term treatment: 15 mg once daily for 4 weeks; maintenance therapy: 15 mg once daily

Gastric ulcer: Oral: Short-term treatment: 30 mg once daily for up to 8 weeks

NSAID-associated gastric ulcer (healing): Oral: 30 mg once daily for 8 weeks; controlled studies did not extend past 8 weeks of therapy

NSAID-associated gastric ulcer (to reduce risk): Oral: 15 mg once daily for up to 12 weeks; controlled studies did not extend past 12 weeks of therapy

Symptomatic GERD: Oral: Short-term treatment: 15 mg once daily for up to 8 weeks

Erosive esophagitis:

Oral: Short-term treatment: 30 mg once daily for up to 8 weeks; continued treatment for an additional 8 weeks may be considered for recurrence or for patients that do not heal after the first 8 weeks of therapy; maintenance therapy: 15 mg once daily

I.V.: 30 mg once daily for up to 7 days; patients should be switched to an oral formulation as soon as they can take oral medications

Hypersecretory conditions: Oral: Initial: 60 mg once daily; adjust dose based upon patient response and to reduce acid secretion to <10 mEq/hour (5 mEq/hour in patients with prior gastric surgery); doses of 90 mg twice daily have been used; administer doses >120 mg/day in divided doses

Helicobacter pylori eradication: Oral: Currently accepted recommendations (may differ from product labeling): Dose varies with regimen: 30 mg once daily or 60 mg/day in 2 divided doses; requires combination therapy with antibiotics

Prevention of rebleeding in peptic ulcer bleed (unlabeled use): I.V.: 60 mg, followed by 6 mg/hour infusion for 72 hours

Elderly: No dosage adjustment is needed in elderly patients with normal hepatic function

Dosage adjustment in renal impairment: No dosage adjustment is needed

Dosing adjustment in hepatic impairment: Dose reduction is necessary for severe hepatic impairment

Stability Store at 15°C to 30°C (59°F to 86°F); protect from light and moisture.

Oral suspension: Empty packet into container with 2 tablespoons of water. Do **not** mix with other liquids or food. Stir well and drink immediately.

Powder for injection: Reconstitute with sterile water 5 mL; mix gently until dissolved. Prior to administration, further dilute with 50 mL of NS, LR, or D_5W. After reconstitution, the solution may be stored for up to 1 hour at room temperature prior to final dilution. Following final dilution, solutions mixed with NS or LR are stable at room temperature for 24 hours; solutions mixed with D_5W are stable for 12 hours

Administration

Oral: Administer before food; best if taken before breakfast. The intact granules should not be chewed or crushed; however, in addition to oral suspension, several options are available for those patients unable to swallow capsules:

Capsules may be opened and the intact granules sprinkled on 1 tablespoon of applesauce, Ensure® pudding, cottage cheese, yogurt, or strained pears. The granules should then be swallowed immediately.

Capsules may be opened and emptied into ~60 mL orange juice, apple juice, or tomato juice; mix and swallow immediately. Rinse the glass with additional juice and swallow to assure complete delivery of the dose.

Capsule granules may be mixed with apple, cranberry, grape, orange, pineapple, prune, tomato and V-8® juice and stored for up to 30 minutes.

Delayed release oral suspension granules should be mixed with 2 tablespoonfuls (30 mL) of water; no other liquid should be used. Stir well and drink immediately. Should not be administered through enteral administration tubes.

Orally-disintegrating tablets: Should not be swallowed whole or chewed. Place tablet on tongue; allow to dissolve (with or without water) until particles can be swallowed. Orally-disintegrating tablets may also be administered via an oral syringe: Place the 15 mg tablet in an oral syringe and draw up ~4 mL water, or place the 30 mg tablet in an oral syringe and draw up ~10 mL water. After tablet has dispersed, administer within 15 minutes. Refill the syringe with water (2 mL for the 15 mg tablet; 4 mL for the 30 mg tablet), shake gently, then administer any remaining contents.

I.V.: Administer over 30 minutes. Use of an in-line filter is required. Before and after administration, flush I.V. line with NS, LR, or D_5W. Do not administer with other medications.

Nasogastric tube administration:

Capsule: Capsule can be opened, the granules mixed (not crushed) with 40 mL of apple juice and then injected through the NG tube into the stomach, then flush tube with additional apple juice.

Orally-disintegrating tablet: Nasogastric tube ≥8 French: Place a 15 mg tablet in a syringe and draw up ~4 mL water, or place the 30 mg tablet in a syringe and draw up ~10 mL water. After tablet has dispersed, administer within 15 minutes. Refill the syringe with ~5 mL water, shake gently, and then flush the nasogastric tube.

Monitoring Parameters Patients with Zollinger-Ellison syndrome should be monitored for gastric acid output, which should be maintained at ≤10 mEq/hour during the last hour before the next lansoprazole dose; lab monitoring should include CBC, liver function, renal function, and serum gastrin levels

Anesthesia and Critical Care Concerns/Other Considerations Intravenous omeprazole has been studied in prevention of rebleeding in ulcer patients who are at high risk for rebleeding (endoscopic findings of active bleeding or nonbleeding visible vessel) after successful hemostasis (Lin HJ, 1998; Lau JY, 2000). Lin and his group treated 100 ulcer patients (actively bleeding ulcers or ulcers with nonbleeding visible vessels) endoscopically and then randomized them to cimetidine (300 mg bolus followed by 50 mg/hour infusion) or omeprazole (40 mg bolus, ~7 mg/hour infusion) for 72 hours. Patients were discharged on the oral form of the drug arm they were assigned to. The omeprazole group maintained an intragastric pH >6 for about 84% of the infusion duration, while the cimetidine group maintained their pH >6 only about 50% of the time. Rebleeding occurred significantly more often in the cimetidine group. Lau and his colleagues treated patients with actively bleeding ulcers or ulcers with nonbleeding visible vessels with an epinephrine infusion followed by thermocoagulation. They were then randomized to omeprazole (80 mg bolus followed by a continuous infusion of 8 mg/hour for 72 hours) or placebo. All patients were discharged on oral omeprazole (20 mg/day) for 8 weeks and received *H. pylori* treatment if indicated. The primary goal was to evaluate the rate of rebleeding during the first 30 days after endoscopy. Two hundred and forty patients were enrolled with randomization of 120 into each group. Bleeding recurred in significantly more patients receiving placebo than omeprazole infusion. The authors concluded that after endoscopic therapy, omeprazole reduces the risk of rebleeding in patients with actively bleeding ulcers or ulcers with nonbleeding visible vessels.

Pregnancy Risk Factor B

Contraindications Hypersensitivity to lansoprazole, substituted benzimidazoles (ie, esomeprazole, omeprazole, pantoprazole, rabeprazole), or any component of the formulation

(Continued)

Lansoprazole *(Continued)*

Warnings/Precautions Severe liver dysfunction may require dosage reductions. Symptomatic response does not exclude malignancy. Safety and efficacy have not been established in children <1 year of age.

Adverse Reactions

1% to 10%:

Central nervous system: Headache (children 1-11 years 3%, 12-17 years 7%)

Gastrointestinal: Abdominal pain (children 12-17 years 5%; adults 2%), constipation (children 1-11 years 5%; adults 1%), diarrhea (4%; 4% to 7% at doses of 30-60 mg/day), nausea (children 12-17 years 3%; adults 1%)

<1% (Limited to important or life-threatening): Abnormal vision, agitation, allergic reaction, ALT increased, anaphylactoid reaction, anemia, angina, anxiety, aplastic anemia, arrhythmia, AST increased, chest pain, convulsion, depression, dizziness, dry eyes, dry mouth, erythema multiforme, esophagitis, gastrin levels increased, gastrointestinal disorder, glucocorticoids increased, globulins increased, hemolysis, hemolytic anemia, hepatotoxicity, hyperglycemia, LDH increased, maculopapular rash, pancreatitis, photophobia, rash, RBC abnormal, taste perversion, Stevens-Johnson syndrome, thrombocytopenia, tinnitus, toxic epidermal necrolysis (some fatal), tremor, vertigo, visual field defect, vomiting, WBC abnormal

Overdosage/Toxicology No symptoms of toxicity were observed in animal studies; limited human experience in overdose. Treatment is symptomatic and supportive. Lansoprazole is not removed by hemodialysis.

Drug Interactions **Substrate** of CYP2C9 (minor), 2C19 (major), 3A4 (major); **Inhibits** CYP2C9 (weak), 2C19 (moderate), 2D6 (weak), 3A4 (weak); **Induces** CYP1A2 (weak)

CYP2C19 inducers: May decrease the levels/effects of lansoprazole. Example inducers include aminoglutethimide, carbamazepine, phenytoin, and rifampin.

CYP2C19 substrates: Lansoprazole may increase the levels/effects of CYP2C19 substrates. Example substrates include citalopram, diazepam, methsuximide, phenytoin, propranolol, and sertraline.

CYP3A4 inducers: CYP3A4 inducers may decrease the levels/effects of lansoprazole. Example inducers include aminoglutethimide, carbamazepine, nafcillin, nevirapine, phenobarbital, phenytoin, and rifamycins.

Itraconazole and ketoconazole: Proton pump inhibitors may decrease the absorption of itraconazole and ketoconazole.

Protease inhibitors: Proton pump inhibitors may decrease absorption of some protease inhibitors (atazanavir and indinavir).

Ethanol/Nutrition/Herb Interactions

Ethanol: Avoid ethanol (may cause gastric mucosal irritation).

Food: Lansoprazole serum concentrations may be decreased if taken with food.

Dietary Considerations Should be taken before eating; best if taken before breakfast. Prevacid® SoluTab™ contains phenylalanine 2.5 mg per 15 mg tablet; phenylalanine 5.1 mg per 30 mg tablet.

Dosage Forms

Capsule, delayed release (Prevacid®): 15 mg, 30 mg

Granules, for oral suspension, delayed release (Prevacid®): 15 mg/packet (30s), 30 mg/packet (30s) [strawberry flavor]

Injection, powder for reconstitution (Prevacid®): 30 mg

Tablet, orally disintegrating (Prevacid® SoluTab™): 15 mg [contains phenylalanine 2.5 mg; strawberry flavor]; 30 mg [contains phenylalanine 5.1 mg; strawberry flavor]

References

Allen ME, Kopp BJ, and Erstad BL, "Stress Ulcer Prophylaxis in the Postoperative Period," *Am J Health Syst Pharm*, 2004, 61(6):588-96.

Jung R and MacLaren R, "Proton-Pump Inhibitors for Stress Ulcer Prophylaxis in Critically Ill Patients," *Ann Pharmacother*, 2002, 36(12):1929-37.

Lau JY, Sung JJ, Lee KK, et al, "Effect of Intravenous Omeprazole on Recurrent Bleeding After Endoscopic Treatment of Bleeding Peptic Ulcers," *N Engl J Med*, 2000, 343(5):310-6.

Lin HJ, Lo WC, Lee FY, et al, "A Prospective Randomized Comparative Trial Showing That Omeprazole Prevents Rebleeding in Patients With Bleeding Peptic Ulcer After Successful Endoscopic Therapy," *Arch Intern Med*, 1998, 158(1):54-8.

♦ **Lantus®** *see* Insulin Glargine *on page 684*

♦ **Lantus® OptiSet® (Can)** *see* Insulin Glargine *on page 684*

♦ **Largactil® (Can)** *see* ChlorproMAZINE *on page 273*

♦ **Lasix®** *see* Furosemide *on page 572*

♦ **Lasix® Special (Can)** *see* Furosemide *on page 572*

- **Lavacol® [OTC]** *see* Alcohol (Ethyl) *on page 53*
- **Laxilose (Can)** *see* Lactulose *on page 724*
- **L-Deprenyl** *see* Selegiline *on page 1157*

Lepirudin (leh puh ROO din)

U.S. Brand Names Refludan®

Canadian Brand Names Refludan®

Synonyms Lepirudin (rDNA); Recombinant Hirudin

Pharmacologic Category Anticoagulant, Thrombin Inhibitor

Generic Available No

Use Indicated for anticoagulation in patients with heparin-induced thrombocytopenia (HIT) and associated thromboembolic disease in order to prevent further thromboembolic complications

Unlabeled/Investigational Use Investigational: Prevention or reduction of ischemic complications associated with unstable angina

Mechanism of Action Lepirudin is a highly specific direct inhibitor of thrombin; lepirudin is a recombinant hirudin derived from yeast cells

Pharmacodynamics/Kinetics

Distribution: Two-compartment model; confined to extracellular fluids.

Metabolism: Via release of amino acids via catabolic hydrolysis of parent drug

Half-life elimination: Initial: ~10 minutes: Terminal: Healthy volunteers: 1.3 hours; Marked renal impairment (Cl_{cr} <15 mL/minute and on hemodialysis): ≤2 days

Excretion: Urine (~48%, 35% as unchanged drug and unchanged drug fragments of parent drug); systemic clearance is proportional to glomerular filtration rate or creatinine clearance

Dosage Adults: Maximum dose: Do not exceed 0.21 mg/kg/hour unless an evaluation of coagulation abnormalities limiting response has been completed. **Dosing is weight-based, however, patients weighing >110 kg should not receive doses greater than the recommended dose for a patient weighing 110 kg (44 mg bolus and initial maximal infusion rate of 16.5 mg/hour).**

Heparin-induced thrombocytopenia: Bolus dose: 0.4 mg/kg IVP (over 15-20 seconds), followed by continuous infusion at 0.15 mg/kg/hour; bolus and infusion must be reduced in renal insufficiency

Note: Due to potential renal insufficiency in critical care patients, some clinicians suggest that for isolated HIT (without thromboembolic complications), the initial infusion rate should be 0.1 mg/kg/hour (omit the initial bolus dose unless acute HITTS).

Concomitant use with thrombolytic therapy: Bolus dose: 0.2 mg/kg IVP (over 15-20 seconds), followed by continuous infusion at 0.1 mg/kg/hour

Dosing adjustments during infusions: Monitor first aPTT 4 hours after the start of the infusion. Subsequent determinations of aPTT should be obtained at least once daily during treatment. More frequent monitoring is recommended in renally impaired patients. Any aPTT ratio measurement out of range (1.5-2.5) should be confirmed prior to adjusting dose, unless a clinical need for immediate reaction exists. If the aPTT is below target range, increase infusion by 20%. If the aPTT is in excess of the target range, stop infusion for 2 hours and when re-started the infusion rate should be decreased by 50%. A repeat aPTT should be obtained 4 hours after any dosing change.

Use in patients scheduled for switch to oral anticoagulants: Reduce lepirudin dose gradually to reach aPTT ratio just above 1.5 before starting warfarin therapy; as soon as INR reaches 2.0, lepirudin therapy should be discontinued.

Dosing adjustment in renal impairment: All patients with a creatinine clearance of <60 mL/minute or a serum creatinine of >1.5 mg/dL should receive a reduction in lepirudin dosage; there is only limited information on the therapeutic use of lepirudin in HIT patients with significant renal impairment; the following dosage recommendations are mainly based on single-dose studies in a small number of patients with renal impairment.

Initial: Bolus dose: 0.2 mg/kg IVP (over 15-20 seconds), followed by adjusted infusion based on renal function; refer to the following infusion rate adjustments based on creatinine clearance (mL/minute) and serum creatinine (mg/dL):

Lepirudin infusion rates in patients with renal impairment: See table on next page.

Note: Acute renal failure or hemodialysis: Infusion is to be avoided or stopped. Following the bolus dose, additional bolus doses of 0.1 mg/kg may be administered every other day (only if aPTT falls below lower therapeutic limit).

(Continued)

Lepirudin *(Continued)*

Lepirudin Infusion Rates in Patients With Renal Impairment

Creatinine Clearance (mL/min)	Serum Creatinine (mg/dL)	Adjusted Infusion Rate	
		% of Standard Initial Infusion Rate	mg/kg/h
45-60	1.6-2.0	50%	0.075
30-44	2.1-3.0	30%	0.045
15-29	3.1-6.0	15%	0.0225
<15	>6.0	Avoid or STOP infusion	

Stability

Intact vials should be stored at 2°C to 25°C (36°F to 77°F)

Intravenous bolus: Use a solution with a concentration of 5 mg/mL

Preparation of a lepirudin solution with a concentration of 5 mg/mL: Reconstitute one vial (50 mg) of lepirudin with 1 mL of sterile water for injection or 0.9% sodium chloride injection; the final concentration of 5 mg/mL is obtained by transferring the contents of the vial into a sterile, single-use syringe (of at least 10 mL capacity) and diluting the solution to a total volume of 10 mL using sterile water for injection, 0.9% sodium chloride, or 5% dextrose in water

Intravenous infusion: For continuous intravenous infusion, solutions with concentrations of 0.2 or 0.4 mg/mL may be used

Preparation of a lepirudin solution with a concentration of 0.2 mg/mL or 0.4 mg/mL: Reconstitute 2 vials (50 mg each) of lepirudin with 1 mL each using either sterile water for injection or 0.9% sodium chloride injection; the final concentration of 0.2 mg/mL or 0.4 mg/mL is obtained by transferring the contents of both vials into an infusion bag containing 500 mL or 250 mL of 0.9% sodium chloride injection or 5% dextrose injection

Reconstituted solutions of lepirudin are stable for 24 hours at room temperature

Administration Administer **only** intravenously; administer I.V. bolus over 15-20 seconds

Monitoring Parameters aPTT levels; some clinicians recommend obtaining aPTT levels every 4 hours until steady state is reached (2 consecutive aPTTs in the same range) then daily monitoring.

Reference Range aPTT 1.5 to 2.5 times the control value

Anesthesia and Critical Care Concerns/Other Considerations

Heparin-Induced Thrombocytopenia (HIT): In a case series of 9 patients with HIT, the combination of lepirudin and a GP IIb/IIIa inhibitor was safe and effective during PCI (Pinto DS, 2003). Another case report describes use in patients with HIT during cardiopulmonary bypass (Liu H, 2002). During prolonged treatment (>5 days) in HIT patients, anticoagulant activity should be monitored daily (Eichler P, 2000). Antihirudin antibodies develop frequently and may enhance lepirudin's activity. In this trial, about half of the patients who developed antihirudin antibodies required a 45% (range: 17% to 90%) decrease in dose.

Pregnancy Risk Factor B

Contraindications Hypersensitivity to hirudins or any component of the formulation

Warnings/Precautions Cautiously administer after a thrombolytic episode; risk of intracranial bleeding. Hemorrhage is the most common complication. Monitor for signs and symptoms of bleeding. Certain patients are at increased risk of bleeding. Risk factors include bacterial endocarditis; congenital or acquired bleeding disorders; recent puncture of large vessels or organ biopsy; recent CVA, stroke, intracerebral surgery, or other neuraxial procedure; severe uncontrolled hypertension; renal impairment; recent major surgery; recent major bleeding (intracranial, GI, intraocular, or pulmonary). With renal impairment, relative overdose might occur even with standard dosage regimen. The bolus dose and rate of infusion must be reduced in patients with known or suspected renal insufficiency. Strict monitoring of aPTT is required; formation of antihirudin antibodies can increase the anticoagulant effect of lepirudin. Use cautiously in cirrhosis. Allergic reactions may occur frequently in patients treated concomitantly with streptokinase. Be cautious in re-exposing patients (anaphylaxis has been reported).

Adverse Reactions As with all anticoagulants, bleeding is the most common adverse event associated with lepirudin. Hemorrhage may occur at virtually any site. Risk is dependent on multiple variables.

HIT patients:

>10%: Hematologic: Anemia (12%), bleeding from puncture sites (11%), hematoma (11%)

1% to 10%:

Cardiovascular: Heart failure (3%), pericardial effusion (1%), ventricular fibrillation (1%)

Central nervous system: Fever (7%)

Dermatologic: Eczema (3%), maculopapular rash (4%)

Gastrointestinal: GI bleeding/rectal bleeding (5%)

Genitourinary: Vaginal bleeding (2%)

Hepatic: Transaminases increased (6%)

Renal: Hematuria (4%)

Respiratory: Epistaxis (4%)

<1% (Limited to important or life-threatening): Allergic reactions, anaphylaxis, hemoperitoneum, hemoptysis, injection site reactions, intracranial bleeding, liver bleeding, mouth bleeding, pruritus, pulmonary bleeding, retroperitoneal bleeding, thrombocytopenia, urticaria

Non-HIT populations (including those receiving thrombolytics and/or contrast media):

1% to 10%: Respiratory: Bronchospasm/stridor/dyspnea/cough

<1% (Limited to important or life-threatening): Allergic reactions (unspecified), anaphylactoid reactions, anaphylaxis, angioedema, intracranial bleeding (0.6%), laryngeal edema, thrombocytopenia, tongue edema

Overdosage/Toxicology Risk of bleeding is increased, and therefore management is directed towards control of bleeding.

Drug Interactions

Cephalosporins which contain the MTT side chain may increase the risk of hemorrhage.

Drugs which affect platelet function (eg, aspirin, NSAIDs, dipyridamole, ticlopidine, clopidogrel) may potentiate the risk of hemorrhage.

Penicillins (parenteral) may prolong bleeding time via inhibition of platelet aggregation, potentially increasing the risk of hemorrhage.

Thrombolytic agents increase the risk of hemorrhage.

Warfarin: Risk of bleeding may be increased during concurrent therapy. During the initiation of warfarin therapy, heparin is commonly continued to assure anticoagulation and to protect against possible transient hypercoagulability. It is probable that a similar approach would be used in situations where lepirudin is required.

Ethanol/Nutrition/Herb Interactions Herb/Nutraceutical: Avoid cat's claw, dong quai, evening primrose, feverfew, garlic, ginger, ginkgo, red clover, horse chestnut, green tea, ginseng (all have additional antiplatelet activity)

Dosage Forms Injection, powder for reconstitution: 50 mg

References

Eichler P, Friesen HJ, Lubenow N, et al, "Antihirudin Antibodies in Patients With Heparin-Induced Thrombocytopenia Treated With Lepirudin: Incidence, Effects on aPTT, and Clinical Relevance," *Blood*, 2000, 96(7):2373-8.

Liu H. Fleming NW, and Moore PG, "Anticoagulation for Patients With Heparin-Induced Thrombocytopenia Using Recombinant Hirudin During Cardiopulmonary Bypass," *J Clin Anesth*, 2002, 14(6):452-5.

Lubenow N, Eichler P, Lietz T, et al, "Lepirudin in Patients With Heparin-Induced Thrombocytopenia-Results of the Third Prospective Study (HAT-3) and a Combined Analysis of HAT-1. HAT-2, and HAT-3," *J Thromb Haemost*, 2005, 3(11):2428-36.

Pinto DS, Sperling RT, Tu TM, et al, "Combination Platelet Glycoprotein IIb/IIIa Receptor and Lepirudin Administration During Percutaneous Coronary Intervention in Patients With Heparin-Induced Thrombocytopenia," *Cathet Cardiovasc Intervent*, 2003, 58(1):65-8.

◆ **Lepirudin (rDNA)** *see* Lepirudin *on page 735*

◆ **Lescol®** *see* Fluvastatin *on page 552*

◆ **Lescol® XL** *see* Fluvastatin *on page 552*

Leucovorin (loo koe VOR in)

Medication Safety Issues

Sound-alike/look-alike issues:

Leucovorin may be confused with Leukeran®, Leukine®

Folinic acid may be confused with folic acid

Synonyms Calcium Leucovorin; Citrovorum Factor; Folinic Acid; 5-Formyl Tetrahydrofolate; Leucovorin Calcium

Pharmacologic Category Antidote; Vitamin, Water Soluble

Generic Available Yes

Use Antidote for folic acid antagonists (methotrexate, trimethoprim, pyrimethamine); treatment of megaloblastic anemias when folate is deficient as in infancy, sprue, pregnancy, and nutritional deficiency when oral folate therapy is not possible; in combination with fluorouracil in the treatment of colon cancer

Mechanism of Action A reduced form of folic acid, leucovorin supplies the necessary cofactor blocked by methotrexate, enters the cells via the same active transport system as methotrexate. Stabilizes the binding of 5-dUMP and thymidylate synthetase, enhancing the activity of fluorouracil.

Pharmacodynamics/Kinetics

Onset of action: Oral: ~30 minutes; I.V.: ~5 minutes

Absorption: Oral, I.M.: Rapid and well absorbed

Metabolism: Intestinal mucosa and hepatically to 5-methyl-tetrahydrofolate (5MTHF; active)

Bioavailability: 31% following 200 mg dose; 98% following doses ≤25 mg

Half-life elimination: Leucovorin: 15 minutes; 5MTHF: 33-35 minutes

Excretion: Urine (80% to 90%); feces (5% to 8%)

Dosage Children and Adults:

Treatment of folic acid antagonist overdosage: Oral: 2-15 mg/day for 3 days or until blood counts are normal, **or** 5 mg every 3 days; doses of 6 mg/day are needed for patients with platelet counts <100,000/mm^3

Folate-deficient megaloblastic anemia: I.M.: 1 mg/day

Megaloblastic anemia secondary to congenital deficiency of dihydrofolate reductase: I.M.: 3-6 mg/day

Rescue dose: Initial: I.V.: 10 mg/m^2, then:

Oral, I.M., I.V., SubQ: 10-15 mg/m^2 every 6 hours until methotrexate level <0.05 micromole/L; if methotrexate level remains >5 micromole/L at 48-72 hours after the end of the methotrexate infusion, increase to 20-100 mg/m^2 every 6 hours until methotrexate level <0.05 micromole/L

Investigational: Post I.T. methotrexate: Oral, I.V.: 12 mg/m^2 as a single dose

Stability Store at room temperature; protect from light. Leucovorin should be reconstituted with SWFI, bacteriostatic NS, BWFI, NS, or D_5W; dilute in 100-1000 mL NS, D_5W for infusion. Reconstituted solution is chemically stable for 7 days; reconstitutions with bacteriostatic water for injection, U.S.P., must be used within 7 days. Parenteral admixture is stable for 24 hours stored at room temperature (25°C) and for 4 days when stored under refrigeration (4°C).

Administration Refer to individual protocols. Leucovorin calcium should be administered I.M. or I.V. Leucovorin should not be administered concurrently with methotrexate. It is commonly initiated 24 hours after the start of methotrexate. Toxicity to normal tissues may be irreversible if leucovorin is not initiated by ~40 hours after the start of methotrexate. **Note:** The manufacturer states that leucovorin should not be given intrathecally/intraventricularly; however, it has been given by these routes.

As a rescue after folate antagonists: Leucovorin may be administered by I.V. bolus injection, I.M. injection, or orally. Doses >25 mg should be administered parenterally.

In combination with fluorouracil: When leucovorin is used to modulate fluorouracil activity, the fluorouracil is usually given after, or at the midpoint, of the leucovorin infusion. Leucovorin is usually administered by I.V. bolus injection or short (10-15 minutes) I.V. infusion. Other administration schedules have been used; refer to individual protocols.

Monitoring Parameters Plasma methotrexate concentration as a therapeutic guide to high-dose methotrexate therapy with leucovorin factor rescue. Leucovorin is continued until the plasma methotrexate level <0.05 micromole/L.

With 4- to 6-hour high-dose methotrexate infusions, plasma drug values in excess of 50 and 1 micromole/L at 24 and 48 hours after starting the infusion, respectively, are often predictive of delayed methotrexate clearance

Pregnancy Risk Factor C

Contraindications Hypersensitivity to leucovorin or any component of the formulation; pernicious anemia or vitamin B_{12}-deficient megaloblastic anemias

Adverse Reactions Frequency not defined.

Dermatologic: Rash, pruritus, erythema, urticaria
Hematologic: Thrombocytosis
Respiratory: Wheezing
Miscellaneous: Anaphylactoid reactions

Drug Interactions May decrease efficacy of co-trimoxazole against *Pneumocystis carinii* pneumonitis

Dosage Forms

Injection, powder for reconstitution, as calcium: 50 mg, 100 mg, 200 mg, 350 mg, 500 mg
Injection, solution, as calcium: 10 mg/mL (50 mL)
Tablet, as calcium: 5 mg, 10 mg, 15 mg, 25 mg

♦ **Leucovorin Calcium** *see* Leucovorin *on page 738*

Levalbuterol (leve al BYOO ter ole)

Medication Safety Issues

Sound-alike/look-alike issues:
Xopenex® may be confused with Xanax®

U.S. Brand Names Xopenex®; Xopenex HFA™

Canadian Brand Names Xopenex®

Synonyms Levalbuterol Hydrochloride; Levalbuterol Tartrate; R-albuterol

Pharmacologic Category $Beta_2$-Adrenergic Agonist

Generic Available No

Use Treatment or prevention of bronchospasm in children and adults with reversible obstructive airway disease

Mechanism of Action Relaxes bronchial smooth muscle by action on beta-2 receptors with little effect on heart rate

Pharmacodynamics/Kinetics

Onset of action:
Aerosol: 5.5-10.2 minutes
Peak effect: ~77 minutes
Nebulization: 10-17 minutes (measured as a 15% increase in FEV_1)
Peak effect: 1.5 hours
Duration:
Aerosol: 3-4 hours (up to 6 hours in some patients)
Nebulization: 5-6 hours (up to 8 hours in some patients)
Absorption: A portion of inhaled dose is absorbed to systemic circulation
Half-life elimination: 3.3-4 hours
Time to peak, serum:
Aerosol: 0.5 hours
Nebulization: 0.2 hours

Dosage

Metered-dose inhalation: Aerosol: Children ≥4 years and Adults: 1-2 puffs every 4-6 hours
Nebulization:
Children 6-11 years: 0.31 mg 3 times/day (maximum dose: 0.63 mg 3 times/day)
Children >12 years and Adults: 0.63 mg 3 times/day at intervals of 6-8 hours; dosage may be increased to 1.25 mg 3 times/day with close monitoring for adverse effects. Most patients gain optimal benefit from regular use
Elderly: Only a small number of patients have been studied. Although greater sensitivity of some elderly patients cannot be ruled out, no overall differences in safety or effectiveness were observed. An initial dose of 0.63 mg should be used in all patients >65 years of age.

Stability Aerosol: Store at room temperature of 20°C to 25°C (68°F to 77°F); protect from freezing and direct sunlight. Store with mouthpiece up. Discard after 200 actuations.

Solution for nebulization: Store in protective foil pouch at room temperature of 20°C to 25°C (68°F to 77°F). Protect from light and excessive heat. Vials should

(Continued)

Levalbuterol *(Continued)*

be used within 2 weeks after opening protective pouch. Use within 1 week and protect from light if removed from pouch. Vials of concentrated solution should be used immediately after removing from protective pouch. Concentrated solution should be diluted with 2.5 mL NS prior to use.

Administration Inhalation:

Aerosol: Shake well before use; prime with 4 test sprays prior to first use or if inhaler has not been use of more than 3 days. Clean actuator (mouthpiece) weekly.

Solution for nebulization: Safety and efficacy were established when administered with the following nebulizers: PARI LC Jet™, PARI LC Plus™, as well as the following compressors: PARI Master®, Dura-Neb® 2000, and Dura-Neb® 3000. Concentrated solution should be diluted prior to use.

Monitoring Parameters Asthma symptoms; FEV_1, peak flow, and/or other pulmonary function tests; heart rate, blood pressure, CNS stimulation; arterial blood gases (if condition warrants); serum potassium, serum glucose (in selected patients)

Pregnancy Risk Factor C

Contraindications Hypersensitivity to levalbuterol, albuterol, or any component of the formulation

Warnings/Precautions Optimize anti-inflammatory treatment before initiating maintenance treatment with levalbuterol. Do not use as a component of chronic therapy without an anti-inflammatory agent. Only the mildest form of asthma (Step 1 and/or exercise-induced) would not require concurrent use based upon asthma guidelines. Patient must be instructed to seek medical attention in cases where acute symptoms are not relieved or a previous level of response is diminished. The need to increase frequency of use may indicate deterioration of asthma, and treatment must not be delayed.

Use caution in patients with cardiovascular disease (arrhythmia or hypertension or CHF), convulsive disorders, diabetes, glaucoma, hyperthyroidism, or hypokalemia. Beta agonists may cause elevation in blood pressure, heart rate, and result in CNS stimulation/excitation. $Beta_2$ agonists may increase risk of arrhythmia, increase serum glucose, or decrease serum potassium.

Do not exceed recommended dose; serious adverse events including fatalities, have been associated with excessive use of inhaled sympathomimetics. Rarely, paradoxical bronchospasm may occur with use of inhaled bronchodilating agents; this should be distinguished from inadequate response. Use with caution during labor and delivery. Safety and efficacy have not been established in patients <4 years of age.

Adverse Reactions Immediate hypersensitivity reactions have occurred, including angioedema, oropharyngeal edema, urticaria, rash, and anaphylaxis.

>10%:

Endocrine & metabolic: Serum glucose increased, serum potassium decreased

Respiratory: Viral infection (7% to 12%), rhinitis (3% to 11%)

>2% to <10%:

Central nervous system: Nervousness (3% to 10%), tremor (≤7%), anxiety (3%), dizziness (1% to 3%), migraine (≤3%), pain (1% to 3%)

Cardiovascular: Tachycardia (~3%)

Gastrointestinal: Dyspepsia (1% to 3%)

Neuromuscular & skeletal: Leg cramps (≤3%)

Respiratory: Asthma (9%), pharyngitis (8%), cough (1% to 4%), nasal edema (1% to 3%), sinusitis (1% to 4%)

Miscellaneous: Flu-like syndrome (1% to 4%), accidental injury (≤3%)

<2% (Limited to important or life-threatening): Angina, arrhythmia, atrial fibrillation, extrasystole, headache, hematuria, hyper-/hypotension, hypokalemia, insomnia, oropharyngeal dryness, paresthesia, supraventricular arrhythmia, syncope, tremor, vertigo; immediate hypersensitivity reactions have occurred (including angioedema, oropharyngeal edema, urticaria, rash, and anaphylaxis)

Overdosage/Toxicology Symptoms of overdose include tachycardia, tremor, hypertension, angina, and seizures. Hypokalemia also may occur. Cardiac arrest and death may be associated with abuse of beta-agonist bronchodilators. Treatment includes immediate discontinuation and symptomatic and supportive therapies. Cautious use of beta-adrenergic blocking agents may be considered in severe cases.

Drug Interactions

Anesthetics (inhaled): Cardiac effects of levalbuterol may be potentiated; use with caution.

Beta-blockers (particularly nonselective agents): May block the effect of levalbuterol and also produce severe bronchospasm.

Diuretics (nonpotassium-sparing): ECG changes and/or hypokalemia may result from concomitant use; use caution.

Digoxin: Plasma levels of digoxin may be decreased by 16% to 22%; monitor.

MAO inhibitors: Cardiac effects of levalbuterol may be potentiated; use with extreme caution or within 2 weeks of discontinuing MAO inhibitor.

Sympathomimetics (including amphetamine, dobutamine): Cardiac effects of levalbuterol may be potentiated; use with caution.

Tricyclic antidepressants (TCAs): Cardiac effects of levalbuterol may be potentiated; use with extreme caution or within 2 weeks of discontinuing TCAs

Dosage Forms Note: Strength expressed as base.

Aerosol, oral, as tartrate:

Xopenex HFA™: 45 mcg/actuation (15 g) [200 doses; chlorofluorocarbon free]

Solution for nebulization, as hydrochloride:

Xopenex®: 0.31 mg/3 mL (24s); 0.63 mg/3 mL (24s); 1.25 mg/3 mL (24s)

Solution for nebulization, concentrate, as hydrochloride:

Xopenex®: 1.25 mg/0.5 mL (30s)

- ♦ **Levalbuterol Hydrochloride** *see* Levalbuterol *on page 739*
- ♦ **Levalbuterol Tartrate** *see* Levalbuterol *on page 739*
- ♦ **Levaquin®** *see* Levofloxacin *on page 746*
- ♦ **Levarterenol Bitartrate** *see* Norepinephrine *on page 936*
- ♦ **Levate® (Can)** *see* Amitriptyline *on page 89*
- ♦ **Levemir®** *see* Insulin Detemir *on page 683*
- ♦ **Levitra®** *see* Vardenafil *on page 1339*

Levobupivacaine (LEE voe byoo PIV a kane)

U.S. Brand Names Chirocaine® [DSC]

Canadian Brand Names Chirocaine®

Pharmacologic Category Local Anesthetic

Generic Available No

Use Production of local or regional anesthesia for surgery and obstetrics, and for postoperative pain management

Mechanism of Action Levobupivacaine is the S-enantiomer of bupivacaine. It blocks both the initiation and transmission of nerve impulses by decreasing the neuronal membrane's permeability to sodium ions, which results in inhibition of depolarization with resultant blockade of conduction. Local anesthetics reversibly prevent generation and conduction of electrical impulses in neurons by decreasing the transient increase in permeability to sodium. The differential sensitivity generally depends on the size of the fiber; small fibers are more sensitive than larger fibers and require a longer period for recovery. Sensory pain fibers are usually blocked first, followed by fibers that transmit sensations of temperature, touch, and deep pressure. High concentrations block sympathetic somatic sensory and somatic motor fibers. The spread of anesthesia depends upon the distribution of the solution. This is primarily dependent on the site of administration and volume of drug injected.

Pharmacodynamics/Kinetics

Onset of action: Epidural: 10-14 minutes

Duration (dose dependent): 1-8 hours

Absorption: Dependent on route of administration and dose

Distribution: 67 L

Protein binding, plasma: >97%

Metabolism: Extensively hepatic via CYP3A4 and CYP1A2

Half-life elimination: 1.3 hours

Time to peak: Epidural: 30 minutes

Excretion: Urine (71%) and feces (24%) as metabolites

Dosage Adults: **Note:** Rapid injection of a large volume of local anesthetic solution should be avoided. Fractional (incremental) doses are recommended.

Guidelines (individual response varies): See table on next page.

Maximum dosage: Epidural doses up to 375 mg have been administered incrementally to patients during a surgical procedure.

(Continued)

Levobupivacaine *(Continued)*

	Concentration	Volume	Dose	Motor Block
Surgical Anesthesia				
Epidural for surgery	0.5%-0.75%	10-20 mL	50-150 mg	Moderate to complete
Epidural for C-section	0.5%	20-30 mL	100-150 mg	Moderate to complete
Peripheral nerve	0.25%-0.5%	0.4 mL/kg (30 mL)	1-2 mg/kg (75-150 mg)	Moderate to complete
Ophthalmic	0.75%	5-15 mL	37.5-112.5 mg	Moderate to complete
Local infiltration	0.25%	60 mL	150 mg	Not applicable
Pain Management				
Levobupivacaine can be used epidurally with fentanyl or clonidine; dilutions for epidural administration should be made with preservative free 0.9% saline according to standard hospital procedures for sterility				
Labor analgesia (epidural bolus)	0.25%	10-20 mL	25-50 mg	Minimal to moderate
Postoperative pain (epidural infusion)	0.125%[1]-0.25%	4-10 mL/h	5-25 mg/h	Minimal to moderate

[1]0.125%: Adjunct therapy with fentanyl or clonidine.

Intraoperative block and postoperative pain: 695 mg in 24 hours
Postoperative epidural infusion over 24 hours: 570 mg
Single-fractionated injection for brachial plexus block: 300 mg

Stability

Store at room temperature (20°C to 25°C/68°F to 77°F). Disinfectants containing heavy metals should not be used for mucous membrane disinfection since they have been related to incidents of swelling and edema. Isopropyl or ethyl alcohol is recommended. Stability of solution in vial has been demonstrated following an autoclave cycle at 121°C for 15 minutes.

Not compatible with alkaline pH solutions (pH >8.5). Compatible with 0.9% Sodium Chloride Injection USP, and with saline solutions containing fentanyl, and clonidine. Stable for 24 hours in PVC bags at room temperature when diluted in normal saline. Use preservative free 0.9% sodium chloride in epidural infusion.

Administration Isopropyl or ethyl alcohol are recommended to disinfect the surface of the vial. Disinfectants containing heavy metals should not be used for mucous membrane disinfection since they have been related to incidents of swelling and edema. Prior to administration, it is essential that aspiration for blood or cerebrospinal fluid (where applicable) be performed prior to injecting any local anesthetic, both before the original dosage and at all subsequent doses (to avoid intravascular or intrathecal injection). A negative aspiration does not ensure against intrathecal or intravascular injection. Rapid injection of a large volume of local anesthetic solution should be avoided. Fractional (incremental) doses are recommended. Monitor patient during and after injection for symptoms of CNS or cardiac toxicity.

Monitoring Parameters Monitor the patient during and after injection for symptoms of CNS or cardiac toxicity

Pregnancy Risk Factor B

Contraindications Hypersensitivity to levobupivacaine, any component of the formulation, bupivacaine, or any local anesthetic of the amide type

Warnings/Precautions Unintended intravenous injection may result in cardiac arrest. Use caution when the higher concentration formulations of levobupivacaine are used. Volumes of the high concentration are more likely to produce cardiac toxicity. The 0.75% solution should not be used in obstetrical patients. Use with caution in patients with hypotension, hypovolemia, heart block, hepatic or cardiac impairment.

Local anesthetics should be administered by clinicians familiar with the use of local anesthetic agents and performance of anesthetic procedures, as well as the management of drug-related toxicity and other acute emergencies. Resuscitative equipment and medications should be readily available. Not for use in intravenous regional anesthesia (Bier block) or to produce obstetrical paracervical block anesthesia. Use with caution in patients receiving other local anesthetics or structurally related agents.

Adverse Reactions

>10%:

Cardiovascular: Hypotension (20% to 31%)

Central nervous system: Pain (postoperative) (7% to 18%), fever (7% to 17%)

Gastrointestinal: Nausea (12% to 21%), vomiting (8% to 14%)

Hematologic: Anemia (10% to 12%)

1% to 10%:

Central nervous system: Pain (4% to 8%), headache (5% to 7%), dizziness (5% to 6%), hypoesthesia (3%), somnolence (1%), anxiety (1%), hypothermia (2%)

Cardiovascular: Abnormal ECG (3%), bradycardia (2%), tachycardia (2%), hypertension (1%)

Dermatologic: Pruritus (4% to 9%), purpura (1%)

Endocrine & metabolic: Breast pain - female (1%)

Gastrointestinal: Constipation (3% to 7%), enlarged abdomen (3%), flatulence (2%), abdominal pain (2%), dyspepsia (2%), diarrhea (1%)

Genitourinary: Urinary incontinence (1%), urine flow decreased (1%), urinary tract infection (1%)

Hematologic: Leukocytosis (1%)

Local: Anesthesia (1%)

Neuromuscular & skeletal: Back pain (6%), rigors (3%), paresthesia (2%)

Ocular: Diplopia (3%)

Renal: Albuminuria (3%), hematuria (2%)

Respiratory: Cough (1%)

Miscellaneous: Fetal distress (5% to 10%), delayed delivery (6%), hemorrhage in pregnancy (2%), uterine abnormality (2%), increased wound drainage (1%)

<1% (Limited to important or life-threatening): Apnea, arrhythmia, atrial fibrillation, bronchospasm, cardiac arrest, confusion, dyspnea, generalized spasm, ileus, involuntary muscle contraction, pulmonary edema, skin discoloration, syncope

Overdosage/Toxicology Related to local concentration or due to unintended intrathecal or intravenous injection. Symptoms may include restlessness, anxiety, incoherent speech, lightheadedness, numbness and tingling of the mouth and lips, metallic taste, tinnitus, dizziness, blurred vision, tremors, respiratory arrest, twitching, depression or drowsiness. In addition, cardiac toxicity, including AV block, bradycardia, arrhythmia, and hypotension may occur. Treatment is symptomatic.

Drug Interactions Substrate (minor) of CYP1A2, 3A4

Ethanol/Nutrition/Herb Interactions Herb/Nutraceutical: St John's wort may decrease levobupivacaine levels.

Dosage Forms [DSC] = Discontinued product

Injection, solution [preservative free]: 2.5 mg/mL (10 mL, 30 mL); 5 mg/mL (10 mL, 30 mL); 7.5 mg/mL (10 mL, 30 mL) [DSC]

Levodopa and Carbidopa (lee voe DOE pa & kar bi DOE pa)

U.S. Brand Names Parcopa™; Sinemet®; Sinemet® CR

Canadian Brand Names Apo-Levocarb®; Apo-Levocarb® CR; Endo®-Levodopa/Carbidopa; Novo-Levocarbidopa; Nu-Levocarb; Sinemet®; Sinemet® CR

Synonyms Carbidopa and Levodopa

Pharmacologic Category Anti-Parkinson's Agent, Dopamine Agonist

Generic Available Yes: Excludes orally-disintegrating tablet

Use Idiopathic Parkinson's disease; postencephalitic parkinsonism; symptomatic parkinsonism

Unlabeled/Investigational Use Restless leg syndrome

Mechanism of Action Parkinson's symptoms are due to a lack of striatal dopamine; levodopa circulates in the plasma to the blood-brain-barrier (BBB), where it crosses, to be converted by striatal enzymes to dopamine; carbidopa inhibits the peripheral plasma breakdown of levodopa by inhibiting its decarboxylation, and thereby increases available levodopa at the BBB

Pharmacodynamics/Kinetics

Duration: Variable, 6-12 hours; longer with sustained release forms

See individual agents.

Dosage Oral: Adults:

Parkinson's disease:

Immediate release tablet:

Initial: Carbidopa 25 mg/levodopa 100 mg 3 times/day

(Continued)

Levodopa and Carbidopa *(Continued)*

Dosage adjustment: Alternate tablet strengths may be substituted according to individual carbidopa/levodopa requirements. Increase by 1 tablet every other day as necessary, except when using the carbidopa 25 mg/levodopa 250 mg tablets where increases should be made using ½-1 tablet every 1-2 days. Use of more than 1 dosage strength or dosing 4 times/day may be required (maximum: 8 tablets of any strength/day or 200 mg of carbidopa and 2000 mg of levodopa)

Sustained release tablet:

Initial: Carbidopa 50 mg/levodopa 200 mg 2 times/day, at intervals not <6 hours

Dosage adjustment: May adjust every 3 days; intervals should be between 4-8 hours during the waking day (maximum: 8 tablets/day)

Restless leg syndrome (unlabeled use): Carbidopa 25 mg/levodopa 100 mg given 30-60 minutes before bedtime; may repeat dose once

Elderly: Initial: Carbidopa 25 mg/levodopa 100 mg twice daily, increase as necessary

Stability Store at 20°C to 25°C (68°F to 77°F); excursions are allowed between 15°C to 30°C (59°F to 86°F); protect from light and moisture

Administration Space doses evenly over the waking hours. Give with meals to decrease GI upset. Sustained release product should not be crushed. Orally-disintegrating tablets do not require water; the tablet should disintegrate on the tongue's surface before swallowing.

Monitoring Parameters Blood pressure, standing and sitting/supine; symptoms of parkinsonism, dyskinesias, mental status

Anesthesia and Critical Care Concerns/Other Considerations Consider use of alternative therapies before attempting to use levodopa containing products.

50-100 mg/day of carbidopa is needed to block the peripheral conversion of levodopa to dopamine. "On-off" (a clinical syndrome characterized by sudden periods of drug activity/inactivity), can be managed by giving smaller, more frequent doses of Sinemet® or adding a dopamine agonist or selegiline; when adding a new agent, doses of Sinemet® can usually be decreased. Protein in the diet should be distributed throughout the day to avoid fluctuations in levodopa absorption. Levodopa is the drug of choice when rigidity is the predominant presenting symptom.

Pregnancy Risk Factor C

Contraindications Hypersensitivity to levodopa, carbidopa, or any component of the formulation; narrow-angle glaucoma; use of MAO inhibitors within prior 14 days (however, may be administered concomitantly with the manufacturer's recommended dose of an MAO inhibitor with selectivity for MAO type B); history of melanoma or undiagnosed skin lesions

Warnings/Precautions Use with caution in patients with history of cardiovascular disease (including myocardial infarction and arrhythmias); pulmonary diseases such as asthma, psychosis, wide-angle glaucoma, peptic ulcer disease; as well as in renal, hepatic, or endocrine disease. Sudden discontinuation of levodopa may cause a worsening of Parkinson's disease. Elderly may be more sensitive to CNS effects of levodopa. May cause or exacerbate dyskinesias. May cause orthostatic hypotension; Parkinson's disease patients appear to have an impaired capacity to respond to a postural challenge; use with caution in patients at risk of hypotension (such as those receiving antihypertensive drugs) or where transient hypotensive episodes would be poorly tolerated (cardiovascular disease or cerebrovascular disease). Observe patients closely for development of depression with concomitant suicidal tendencies. Has been associated with a syndrome resembling neuroleptic malignant syndrome on withdrawal or significant dosage reduction after long-term use. Protein in the diet should be distributed throughout the day to avoid fluctuations in levodopa absorption.

Adverse Reactions Frequency not defined.

Cardiovascular: Orthostatic hypotension, arrhythmia, chest pain, hypertension, syncope, palpitation, phlebitis

Central nervous system: Dizziness, anxiety, confusion, nightmares, headache, hallucinations, on-off phenomenon, decreased mental acuity, memory impairment, disorientation, delusions, euphoria, agitation, somnolence, insomnia, gait abnormalities, nervousness, ataxia, EPS, falling, psychosis, peripheral neuropathy, seizure (causal relationship not established)

Dermatologic: Rash, alopecia, malignant melanoma, hypersensitivity (angioedema, urticaria, pruritus, bullous lesions, Henoch-Schönlein purpura)
Endocrine & metabolic: Increased libido
Gastrointestinal: Anorexia, nausea, vomiting, constipation, GI bleeding, duodenal ulcer, diarrhea, dyspepsia, taste alterations, sialorrhea, heartburn
Genitourinary: Discoloration of urine, urinary frequency
Hematologic: Hemolytic anemia, agranulocytosis, thrombocytopenia, leukopenia; decreased hemoglobin and hematocrit; abnormalities in AST and ALT, LDH, bilirubin, BUN, Coombs' test
Neuromuscular & skeletal: Choreiform and involuntary movements, paresthesia, bone pain, shoulder pain, muscle cramps, weakness
Ocular: Blepharospasm, oculogyric crises (may be associated with acute dystonic reactions)
Renal: Difficult urination
Respiratory: Dyspnea, cough
Miscellaneous: Hiccups, discoloration of sweat, diaphoresis (increased)

Overdosage/Toxicology Symptoms of overdose include palpitations, arrhythmias, spasms; may cause hypertension or hypotension. Treatment is supportive. ECG monitoring is warranted. May precipitate a variety of arrhythmias.

Drug Interactions

Antacids: Levodopa absorption may be increased; monitor
Anticholinergics: May reduce the efficacy of levodopa, possibly due to reduced gastrointestinal absorption (also see tricyclic antidepressants); limited evidence of clinical significance; monitor
Antipsychotics: May inhibit the antiparkinsonian effects of levodopa via dopamine receptor blockade; use antipsychotics with low dopamine blockade (clozapine, olanzapine, quetiapine)
Benzodiazepines: May inhibit the antiparkinsonian effects of levodopa; monitor for reduced effect
Clonidine: May reduce the efficacy of levodopa; monitor
Dextromethorphan: Toxic reactions have occurred with dextromethorphan
Furazolidone: May increase the effect/toxicity of levodopa; hypertensive episodes have been reported; monitor
Iron salts: Binds levodopa and reduces its bioavailability; separate doses of iron and levodopa
Linezolid: Due to MAO inhibition (see note on MAO inhibitors), this agent is best avoided
MAO inhibitors: Concurrent use of levodopa with nonselective MAO inhibitors may result in hypertensive reactions via an increased storage and release of dopamine, norepinephrine, or both; use with carbidopa to minimize reactions if combination is necessary, otherwise avoid combination.
L-methionine: May inhibit levodopa's antiparkinsonian effects; monitor for reduced effect
Metoclopramide: May increase the absorption/effect of levodopa; hypertensive episodes have been reported. Levodopa antagonizes metoclopramide's effects on lower esophageal sphincter pressure. Avoid use of metoclopramide for reflux, monitor response to levodopa carefully if used.
Methyldopa: May potentiate the effects of levodopa; levodopa may increase the hypotensive response to methyldopa; monitor
Papaverine: May decrease the efficacy of levodopa; includes other similar agents (ethaverine); monitor
Penicillamine: May increase serum concentrations of levodopa; monitor for increased effect
Phenytoin: May inhibit levodopa's antiparkinsonian effects; monitor for reduced effect
Pyridoxine: May inhibit levodopa's antiparkinsonian effects; monitor for reduced effect (pyridoxine in doses >10-25 mg for levodopa alone, higher doses >200 mg/day may be a problem for levodopa/carbidopa)
Spiramycin: May inhibit levodopa's antiparkinsonian effects; monitor for reduced effect
Tacrine: May inhibit the effects of levodopa via enhanced cholinergic activity; monitor for reduced effect
Tricyclic antidepressants: May decrease the absorption (bioavailability) of levodopa; rare hypertensive episodes have also been attributed to this combination

Ethanol/Nutrition/Herb Interactions

Ethanol: Avoid ethanol (due to CNS depression).
Food: Avoid high protein diets and high intakes of vitamin B_6.
(Continued)

Levodopa and Carbidopa *(Continued)*

Herb/Nutraceutical: Avoid kava kava (may decrease effects). Pyridoxine in doses >10-25 mg (for levodopa alone) or higher doses >200 mg/day (for levodopa/carbidopa) may decrease efficacy.

Test Interactions False-positive reaction for urinary glucose with Clinitest®; false-negative reaction using Clinistix®; false-positive urine ketones with Acetest®, Ketostix®, Labstix®

Dietary Considerations Levodopa peak serum concentrations may be decreased if taken with food. High protein diets (>2 g/kg) may decrease the efficacy of levodopa via competition with amino acids in crossing the blood-brain barrier.

Parcopa™: Contains phenylalanine 3.4 mg per 10/100 mg and 25/100 mg strengths; phenylalanine 8.4 mg in 25/250 mg strength

Dosage Forms

Tablet immediate release (Sinemet®):
- 10/100: Carbidopa 10 mg and levodopa 100 mg
- 25/100: Carbidopa 25 mg and levodopa 100 mg
- 25/250: Carbidopa 25 mg and levodopa 250 mg

Tablet, immediate release, orally disintegrating (Parcopa™):
- 10/100: Carbidopa 10 mg and levodopa 100 mg [contains phenylalanine 3.4 mg/tablet; mint flavor]
- 25/100: Carbidopa 25 mg and levodopa 100 mg [contains phenylalanine 3.4 mg/tablet; mint flavor]
- 25/250: Carbidopa 25 mg and levodopa 250 mg [contains phenylalanine 8.4 mg/tablet; mint flavor]

Tablet, sustained release (Sinemet® CR):
- Carbidopa 25 mg and levodopa 100 mg
- Carbidopa 50 mg and levodopa 200 mg

♦ **Levo-Dromoran®** *see* Levorphanol *on page 750*

Levofloxacin (lee voe FLOKS a sin)

U.S. Brand Names Iquix®; Levaquin®; Quixin™

Canadian Brand Names Levaquin®; Novo-Levofloxacin

Pharmacologic Category Antibiotic, Quinolone

Generic Available No

Use

Systemic: Treatment of mild, moderate, or severe infections caused by susceptible organisms. Includes the treatment of community-acquired pneumonia, including multidrug resistant strains of *S. pneumoniae* (MDRSP); nosocomial pneumonia; chronic bronchitis (acute bacterial exacerbation); acute bacterial sinusitis; urinary tract infection (uncomplicated or complicated), including acute pyelonephritis caused by *E. coli*; prostatitis (chronic bacterial); skin or skin structure infections (uncomplicated or complicated); prevention of inhalational anthrax (postexposure)

Ophthalmic: Treatment of bacterial conjunctivitis caused by susceptible organisms (Quixin™ 0.5% ophthalmic solution); treatment of corneal ulcer caused by susceptible organisms (Iquix® 1.5% ophthalmic solution)

Unlabeled/Investigational Use Diverticulitis, enterocolitis, (*Shigella* sp), gonococcal infections, Legionnaires' disease, peritonitis, PID

Mechanism of Action As the S (-) enantiomer of the fluoroquinolone, ofloxacin, levofloxacin, inhibits DNA-gyrase in susceptible organisms thereby inhibits relaxation of supercoiled DNA and promotes breakage of DNA strands. DNA gyrase (topoisomerase II), is an essential bacterial enzyme that maintains the superhelical structure of DNA and is required for DNA replication and transcription, DNA repair, recombination, and transposition.

Pharmacodynamics/Kinetics

Absorption: Rapid and complete

Distribution: V_d: 1.25 L/kg; CSF concentrations ~15% of serum levels; high concentrations are achieved in prostate, lung, and gynecological tissues, sinus, saliva

Protein binding: 50%

Metabolism: Minimally hepatic

Bioavailability: 99%

Half-life elimination: 6-8 hours

Time to peak, serum: 1-2 hours
Excretion: Primarily urine (as unchanged drug)

Dosage Note: Sequential therapy (intravenous to oral) may be instituted based on prescriber's discretion.

Usual dosage range:
Children ≥1 year: Ophthalmic: 1-2 drops every 2-6 hours
Adults:
Ophthalmic: 1-2 drops every 2-6 hours
Oral, I.V.: 250-500 mg every 24 hours; severe or complicated infections: 750 mg every 24 hours

Indication-specific dosing:
Children ≥1 year and Adults: Ophthalmic:
Conjunctivitis (0.5% ophthalmic solution):
Treatment day 1 and day 2: Instill 1-2 drops into affected eye(s) every 2 hours while awake, up to 8 times/day
Treatment day 3 through day 7: Instill 1-2 drops into affected eye(s) every 4 hours while awake, up to 4 times/day
Children ≥6 years and Adults: Ophthalmic:
Corneal ulceration (1.5% ophthalmic solution): Treatment day 1 through day 3: Instill 1-2 drops into affected eye(s) every 30 minutes to 2 hours while awake and 4-6 hours after retiring.
Adults: Oral, I.V.:
Anthrax (inhalational): 500 mg every 24 hours for 60 days, beginning as soon as possible after exposure
Chronic bronchitis (acute bacterial exacerbation): 500 mg every 24 hours for at least 7 days
Diverticulitis, peritonitis (unlabeled use): 750 mg every 24 hours for 7-10 days; use adjunctive metronidazole therapy
Dysenteric enterocolitis, *Shigella spp.* (unlabeled use): 500 mg every 24 hours for 3-5 days
Gonococcal infection (unlabeled use):
Cervicitis, urethritis: 250 mg for one dose with azithromycin or doxycycline
Disseminated infection: 250 mg I.V. once daily; 24 hours after symptoms improve may change to 500 mg orally every 24 hours to complete total therapy of 7 days
Epididymo-orchitis: 750 mg once daily for 10-14 days
***Legionella* (unlabeled use):** 500 mg every 24 hours for 10-21 days or 750 mg every 24 hours for 5 days
Pelvic inflammatory disease (unlabeled use): 500 mg every 24 hours for 14 days with adjunctive metronidazole
Pneumonia:
Community-acquired: 500 mg every 24 hours for 7-14 days or 750 mg every 24 hours for 5 days (efficacy of 5-day regimen for MDRSP not established)
Nosocomial: 750 mg every 24 hours for 7-14 days
Prostatitis (chronic bacterial): 500 mg every 24 hours for 28 days
Sinusitis (bacterial, acute): 500 mg every 24 hours for 10-14 days or 750 mg every 24 hours for 5 days
Skin and skin structure infections:
Uncomplicated: 500 mg every 24 hours for 7-10 days
Complicated: 750 mg every 24 hours for 7-14 days
Traveler's diarrhea (unlabeled use): 500 mg for one dose
Urinary tract infections:
Uncomplicated: 250 mg once daily for 3 days
Complicated, including pyelonephritis: 250 mg once daily for 10 days

Dosing adjustment in renal impairment:
Chronic bronchitis, acute bacterial sinusitis, uncomplicated skin infection, community-acquired pneumonia, chronic bacterial prostatitis, or inhalational anthrax: Initial: 500 mg, then as follows:
Cl_{cr} 20-49 mL/minute: 250 mg every 24 hours
Cl_{cr} 10-19 mL/minute: 250 mg every 48 hours
Hemodialysis/CAPD: 250 mg every 48 hours
Uncomplicated UTI: No dosage adjustment required
Complicated UTI, acute pyelonephritis: Cl_{cr} 10-19 mL/minute: 250 mg every 48 hours

(Continued)

Levofloxacin *(Continued)*

Complicated skin infection, acute bacterial sinusitis, community-acquired pneumonia, or nosocomial pneumonia: Initial: 750 mg, then as follows:

Cl_{cr} 20-49 mL/minute: 750 mg every 48 hours

Cl_{cr} 10-19 mL/minute: 500 mg every 48 hours

Hemodialysis/CAPD: 500 mg every 48 hours

Stability

Solution for injection:

Vial: Store at room temperature; protect from light. When diluted to 5 mg/mL in a compatible I.V. fluid, solution is stable for 72 hours when stored at room temperature; stable for 14 days when stored under refrigeration. When frozen, stable for 6 months; do not refreeze. Do not thaw in microwave or by bath immersion.

Premixed: Store at ≤25°C (77°F); brief exposure to 40°C (104°F) does not affect product; protect from freezing and light.

Tablet, oral solution: Store at 25°C (77°F); excursions permitted to 15°C to 25°C (59°F to 77°F).

Ophthalmic solution: Store at 15°C to 25°C (59°F to 77°F).

Administration

Oral: Tablets may be administered without regard to meals. Oral solution should be administered 1 hour before or 2 hours after meals.

I.V.: Infuse 250-500 mg I.V. solution over 60 minutes; infuse 750 mg I.V. solution over 90 minutes. Too rapid of infusion can lead to hypotension. Avoid administration through an intravenous line with a solution containing multivalent cations (eg, magnesium, calcium).

Monitoring Parameters Evaluation of organ system functions (renal, hepatic, ophthalmologic, and hematopoietic) is recommended periodically during therapy; the possibility of crystalluria should be assessed; WBC and signs of infection

Pregnancy Risk Factor C

Contraindications Hypersensitivity to levofloxacin, any component of the formulation, or other quinolones

Warnings/Precautions

Systemic: Not recommended in children <18 years of age; CNS stimulation may occur (tremor, restlessness, confusion, and very rarely hallucinations or seizures). Potential for seizures, although very rare, may be increased with concomitant NSAID therapy. Use with caution in individuals at risk of seizures, with known or suspected CNS disorders or renal dysfunction; use caution to avoid possible photosensitivity reactions during and for several days following fluoroquinolone therapy

Rare cases of torsade de pointes have been reported in patients receiving levofloxacin. Risk may be minimized by avoiding use in patients with known prolongation of QT interval, bradycardia, hypokalemia, hypomagnesemia, cardiomyopathy, or in those receiving concurrent therapy with Class Ia or Class III antiarrhythmics.

Severe hypersensitivity reactions, including anaphylaxis, have occurred with quinolone therapy. If an allergic reaction occurs (itching, urticaria, dyspnea or facial edema, loss of consciousness, tingling, cardiovascular collapse), discontinue drug immediately. Prolonged use may result in superinfection; pseudomembranous colitis may occur and should be considered in all patients who present with diarrhea. Tendon inflammation and/or rupture has been reported; risk may be increased with concurrent corticosteroids, particularly in the elderly. Discontinue at first sign of tendon inflammation or pain. Peripheral neuropathies have been linked to levofloxacin use; discontinue if numbness, tingling, or weakness develops. Quinolones may exacerbate myasthenia gravis; use with caution (rare, potentially life-threatening weakness of respiratory muscles may occur).

Ophthalmic solution: For topical use only. Do not inject subconjunctivally or introduce into anterior chamber of the eye. Contact lenses should not be worn during treatment for bacterial conjunctivitis. Safety and efficacy in children <1 year of age (Quixin™) or <6 years of age (Iquix®) have not been established. **Note:** Indications for ophthalmic solutions are product concentration-specific and should not be used interchangeably.

Adverse Reactions

1% to 10%:

Cardiovascular: Chest pain (1%)

Central nervous system: Headache (6%), insomnia (5%), dizziness (2%), fatigue (1%), pain (1%), fever

Dermatologic: Pruritus (1%), rash (1%)

Gastrointestinal: Nausea (7%), diarrhea (5%), abdominal pain (3%), constipation (3%), dyspepsia (2%), vomiting (2%), flatulence (1%)

Genitourinary: Vaginitis (1%)

Hematologic: Lymphopenia (2%)

Ocular (with ophthalmic solution use): Decreased vision (transient), foreign body sensation, transient ocular burning, ocular pain or discomfort, photophobia

Respiratory: Pharyngitis (4%), dyspnea (1%), rhinitis (1%), sinusitis (1%)

<1% (Limited to important or life-threatening):

Systemic: Acute renal failure; allergic reaction (including pneumonitis rash, pneumonitis, and anaphylaxis); agranulocytosis, anaphylactoid reaction, anorexia, anxiety, arrhythmia (including atrial/ventricular tachycardia/fibrillation and torsade de pointes), arthralgia, ascites, bradycardia, bronchospasm, carcinoma, cardiac failure, cerebrovascular disorder, cholecystitis, cholelithiasis, confusion, cnjunctivitis, dehydration, depression, ear disorder, edema, EEG abnormalities, electrolyte abnormality, encephalopathy, eosinophilia, erythema multiforme, gangrene, GI hemorrhage, granulocytopenia, hallucination, heart block, hematoma, hemolytic anemia, hemoptysis, hepatic failure, hyper-/hypotension, infection, INR increased, intestinal obstruction, intracranial hypertension, involuntary muscle contractions, jaundice, leukocytosis, leukopenia, leukorrhea, lymphadenopathy, MI, migraine, multiple organ failure, pancreatitis, paralysis, paresthesia, peripheral neuropathy, phlebitis, photosensitivity (<0.1%), pleural effusion, postural hypotension, prothrombin time increased/decreased, pseudomembraneous colitis, pulmonary edema,pulmonary embolism, purpura, QT_c prolongation, respiratory depression, respiratory disorder, rhabdomyolysis, seizure, skin disorder, somnolence,speech disorder, Stevens-Johnson syndrome, stupor, syncope, taste perversion, tendon rupture, tongue edema, transaminases increased, thrombocythemia, thrombocytopenia, tremor, WBC abnormality

Overdosage/Toxicology

Symptoms of overdose include acute renal failure, seizures

Treatment should include GI decontamination and supportive care; not removed by peritoneal or hemodialysis

Drug Interactions

Corticosteroids: Concurrent use may increase the risk of tendon rupture, particularly in elderly patients (overall incidence rare).

Glyburide: Quinolones may increase the effect of glyburide; monitor

Metal cations (aluminum, calcium, iron, magnesium, and zinc) bind quinolones in the gastrointestinal tract and inhibit absorption. Concurrent administration of most antacids, oral electrolyte supplements, quinapril, sucralfate, some didanosine formulations (chewable/buffered tablets and pediatric powder for oral suspension), and other highly-buffered oral drugs, should be avoided. Levofloxacin should be administered 2 hours before or 2 hours after these agents.

Probenecid: May decrease renal secretion of levofloxacin.

QT_c-prolonging agents: Effects may be additive with levofloxacin. Avoid concurrent use with Class Ia and Class III antiarrhythmics, erythromycin, cisapride, antipsychotics, and cyclic antidepressants.

Warfarin: The hypoprothrombinemic effect of warfarin may be enhanced by some quinolone antibiotics; monitor INR.

Test Interactions Some quinolones may produce a false-positive urine screening result for opiates using commercially-available immunoassay kits. This has been demonstrated most consistently for levofloxacin and ofloxacin, but other quinolones have shown cross-reactivity in certain assay kits. Confirmation of positive opiate screens by more specific methods should be considered.

Dietary Considerations Tablets may be taken without regard to meals. Oral solution should be administered on an empty stomach (1 hour before or 2 hours after a meal).

Dosage Forms

Infusion [premixed in D_5W] (Levaquin®): 250 mg (50 mL); 500 mg (100 mL); 750 mg (150 mL)

Injection, solution [preservative free] (Levaquin®): 25 mg/mL (20 mL, 30 mL)

Solution, ophthalmic:

Iquix®: 1.5% (5 mL)

Quixin™: 0.5% (5 mL) [contains benzalkonium chloride]

(Continued)

Levofloxacin *(Continued)*

Solution, oral (Levaquin®): 25 mg/mL (480 mL) [contains benzyl alcohol]
Tablet (Levaquin®): 250 mg, 500 mg, 750 mg
Levaquin® Leva-Pak: 750 mg (5s)

References

American Thoracic Society and Infectious Diseases Society of America, "Guidelines for the Management of Adults With Hospital-Acquired, Ventilator-Associated, and Healthcare-Associated Pneumonia," *Am J Respir Crit Care Med*, 2005, 171(4):388-416.

♦ **Levophed®** *see* Norepinephrine *on page 936*

Levorphanol (lee VOR fa nole)

Related Information

Chronic Pain Management *on page 1430*
Narcotic / Opioid Analgesics *on page 1568*

U.S. Brand Names Levo-Dromoran®

Synonyms Levorphanol Tartrate; Levorphan Tartrate

Pharmacologic Category Analgesic, Narcotic

Restrictions C-II

Generic Available Yes: Tablet

Use Relief of moderate to severe pain; also used parenterally for preoperative sedation and an adjunct to nitrous oxide/oxygen anesthesia

Mechanism of Action Levorphanol tartrate is a synthetic opioid agonist that is classified as a morphinan derivative. Opioids interact with stereospecific opioid receptors in various parts of the central nervous system and other tissues. Analgesic potency parallels the affinity for these binding sites. These drugs do not alter the threshold or responsiveness to pain, but the perception of pain.

Pharmacodynamics/Kinetics

Onset of action: Oral: 10-60 minutes
Duration: 4-8 hours
Metabolism: Hepatic
Half-life elimination: 11-16 hours
Excretion: Urine (as inactive metabolite)

Dosage Adults: **Note:** These are guidelines and do not represent the maximum doses that may be required in all patients. Doses should be titrated to pain relief/prevention.

Acute pain (moderate to severe):

- Oral: Initial: Opiate-naive: 2 mg every 6-8 hours as needed; patients with prior opiate exposure may require higher initial doses; usual dosage range: 2-4 mg every 6-8 hours as needed
- I.M., SubQ: Initial: Opiate-naive: 1 mg every 6-8 hours as needed; patients with prior opiate exposure may require higher initial doses; usual dosage range: 1-2 mg every 6-8 hours as needed
- Slow I.V.: Initial: Opiate-naive: Up to 1 mg/dose every 3-6 hours as needed; patients with prior opiate exposure may require higher initial doses

Chronic pain: Patients taking opioids chronically may become tolerant and require doses higher than the usual dosage range to maintain the desired effect. Tolerance can be managed by appropriate dose titration. **There is no optimal or maximal dose for levorphanol in chronic pain. The appropriate dose is one that relieves pain throughout its dosing interval without causing unmanageable side effects.**

Premedication: I.M., SubQ: 1-2 mg/dose 60-90 minutes prior to surgery; older or debilitated patients usually require less drug

Dosing adjustment in hepatic disease: Reduction is necessary in patients with liver disease

Stability Store at room temperature, protect from freezing; I.V. is **incompatible** when mixed with aminophylline, barbiturates, heparin, methicillin, phenytoin, sodium bicarbonate

Administration I.V.: Inject 3 mg over 4-5 minutes

Monitoring Parameters Pain relief, respiratory and mental status, blood pressure

Anesthesia and Critical Care Concerns/Other Considerations Acutely, levorphanol 2 mg I.M. produces analgesia comparable to that produced by morphine 10 mg I.M.

Pregnancy Risk Factor B/D (prolonged use or high doses at term)

Contraindications Hypersensitivity to levorphanol or any component of the formulation; pregnancy (prolonged use or high doses at term)

Warnings/Precautions An opioid-containing analgesic regimen should be tailored to each patient's needs and based upon the type of pain being treated (acute versus chronic), the route of administration, degree of tolerance for opioids (naive versus chronic user), age, weight, and medical condition. The optimal analgesic dose varies widely among patients. Doses should be titrated to pain relief/prevention.

Use with caution in patients with hypersensitivity reactions to other phenanthrene derivative opioid agonists (morphine, hydrocodone, hydromorphone, levorphanol, oxycodone, oxymorphone); respiratory diseases including asthma, emphysema, COPD or severe liver or renal insufficiency; some preparations contain sulfites which may cause allergic reactions; tolerance or dependence may result from extended use; dextromethorphan has equivalent antitussive activity but has much lower toxicity in accidental overdose. Elderly may be particularly susceptible to the CNS depressant and constipating effects of narcotics.

Adverse Reactions Frequency not defined.

Cardiovascular: Palpitations, hypotension, bradycardia, peripheral vasodilation, cardiac arrest, shock, tachycardia

Central nervous system: CNS depression, fatigue, drowsiness, dizziness, nervousness, headache, restlessness, anorexia, malaise, confusion, coma, convulsion, insomnia, amnesia, mental depression, hallucinations, paradoxical CNS stimulation, intracranial pressure (increased)

Dermatologic: Pruritus, urticaria, rash

Endocrine & metabolic: Antidiuretic hormone release

Gastrointestinal: Nausea, vomiting, dyspepsia, stomach cramps, xerostomia, constipation, abdominal pain, dry mouth, biliary tract spasm, paralytic ileus

Genitourinary: Decreased urination, urinary tract spasm, urinary retention

Local: Pain at injection site

Neuromuscular & skeletal: Weakness

Ocular: Miosis, diplopia

Respiratory: Respiratory depression, apnea, hypoventilation, cyanosis

Miscellaneous: Histamine release, physical and psychological dependence

Overdosage/Toxicology Symptoms of overdose include CNS depression, respiratory depression, miosis, apnea, pulmonary edema, and convulsions. Naloxone, 2 mg I.V. with repeat administration as necessary up to a total dose of 10 mg, can be used to reverse opiate effects.

Drug Interactions Increased toxicity: CNS depressants increase CNS depression

Ethanol/Nutrition/Herb Interactions

Ethanol: Avoid or limit ethanol (may increase CNS depression). Watch for sedation.

Herb/Nutraceutical: Avoid valerian, St John's wort, kava kava, gotu kola (may increase CNS depression).

Dosage Forms

Injection, solution, as tartrate: 2 mg/mL (1 mL, 10 mL)

Tablet, as tartrate: 2 mg

♦ **Levorphanol Tartrate** *see* Levorphanol *on page 750*

♦ **Levorphan Tartrate** *see* Levorphanol *on page 750*

♦ **Levothroid®** *see* Levothyroxine *on page 751*

Levothyroxine (lee voe thye ROKS een)

Medication Safety Issues

Sound-alike/look-alike issues:

Levothyroxine may be confused with liothyronine

Levoxyl® may be confused with Lanoxin®, Luvox®

Synthroid® may be confused with Symmetrel®

To avoid errors due to misinterpretation of a decimal point, always express dosage in mcg (**not** mg).

U.S. Brand Names Levothroid®; Levoxyl®; Synthroid®; Unithroid®

Canadian Brand Names Eltroxin®; Gen-Levothyroxine; Levothyroxine Sodium; Synthroid®

(Continued)

Levothyroxine *(Continued)*

Synonyms Levothyroxine Sodium; *L*-Thyroxine Sodium; T_4

Pharmacologic Category Thyroid Product

Generic Available Yes

Use Replacement or supplemental therapy in hypothyroidism; pituitary TSH suppression

Mechanism of Action Exact mechanism of action is unknown; however, it is believed the thyroid hormone exerts its many metabolic effects through control of DNA transcription and protein synthesis; involved in normal metabolism, growth, and development; promotes gluconeogenesis, increases utilization and mobilization of glycogen stores, and stimulates protein synthesis, increases basal metabolic rate

Pharmacodynamics/Kinetics

Onset of action: Therapeutic: Oral: 3-5 days; I.V. 6-8 hours

Peak effect: I.V.: ~24 hours

Absorption: Oral: Erratic (40% to 80%); decreases with age

Protein binding: >99%

Metabolism: Hepatic to triiodothyronine (active)

Time to peak, serum: 2-4 hours

Half-life elimination: Euthyroid: 6-7 days; Hypothyroid: 9-10 days; Hyperthyroid: 3-4 days

Excretion: Urine and feces; decreases with age

Dosage Doses should be adjusted based on clinical response and laboratory parameters.

Oral:

Children: Hypothyroidism:

Newborns: Initial: 10-15 mcg/kg/day. Lower doses of 25 mcg/day should be considered in newborns at risk for cardiac failure. Newborns with T_4 levels <5 mcg/dL should be started at 50 mcg/day. Adjust dose at 4- to 6-week intervals.

Infants and Children: Dose based on body weight and age as listed below. Children with severe or chronic hypothyroidism should be started at 25 mcg/day; adjust dose by 25 mcg every 2-4 weeks. In older children, hyperactivity may be decreased by starting with 1/4 of the recommended dose and increasing by 1/4 dose each week until the full replacement dose is reached. Refer to adult dosing once growth and puberty are complete.

0-3 months: 10-15 mcg/kg/day
3-6 months: 8-10 mcg/kg/day
6-12 months: 6-8 mcg/kg/day
1-5 years: 5-6 mcg/kg/day
6-12 years: 4-5 mcg/kg/day
>12 years: 2-3 mcg/kg/day

Adults:

Hypothyroidism: 1.7 mcg/kg/day in otherwise healthy adults <50 years old, children in whom growth and puberty are complete, and older adults who have been recently treated for hyperthyroidism or who have been hypothyroid for only a few months. Titrate dose every 6 weeks. Average starting dose ~100 mcg; usual doses are ≤200 mcg/day; doses ≥300 mcg/day are rare (consider poor compliance, malabsorption, and/or drug interactions). **Note:** For patients >50 years or patients with cardiac disease, refer to Elderly dosing.

Severe hypothyroidism: Initial: 12.5-25 mcg/day; adjust dose by 25 mcg/day every 2-4 weeks as appropriate; **Note:** Oral agents are not recommended for myxedema (see I.V. dosing).

Subclinical hypothyroidism (if treated): 1 mcg/kg/day

TSH suppression:

Well-differentiated thyroid cancer: Highly individualized; Doses >2 mcg/kg/day may be needed to suppress TSH to <0.1 mU/L.

Benign nodules and nontoxic multinodular goiter: Goal TSH suppression: 0.1-0.3 mU/L

Elderly: Hypothyroidism:

>50 years without cardiac disease **or** <50 years with cardiac disease: Initial: 25-50 mcg/day; adjust dose at 6- to 8-week intervals as needed

>50 years with cardiac disease: Initial: 12.5-25 mcg/day; adjust dose by 12.5-25 mcg increments at 4- to 6-week intervals. (**Note:** Many clinicians prefer to adjust at 6- to 8-week intervals.)

Note: Elderly patients may require <1 mcg/kg/day

I.M., I.V.: Children, Adults, Elderly: Hypothyroidism: 50% of the oral dose

I.V.:

Adults: Myxedema coma or stupor: 200-500 mcg, then 100-300 mcg the next day if necessary; smaller doses should be considered in patients with cardiovascular disease

Elderly: Myxedema coma: Refer to Adults dosing; lower doses may be needed

Stability

Tablet: Store at room temperature of 15°C to 30°C (59°F to 86°F). Protect from light and moisture.

Injection: Store at room temperature of 15°C to 30°C (59°F to 86°F). Dilute vials for injection with 5 mL normal saline and shake well; reconstituted solutions should be used immediately and any unused portions discarded. Do not mix I.V. solution with other I.V. infusion solutions.

Administration

Oral: Administer in the morning on an empty stomach, at least 30 minutes before food. Tablets may be crushed and suspended in 1-2 teaspoonfuls of water; suspension should be used immediately. Levoxyl® should be administered with a full glass of water to prevent gagging (due to tablet swelling).

Parenteral: Dilute vial with 5 mL normal saline; use immediately after reconstitution; should not be admixed with other solutions

Monitoring Parameters Thyroid function test (serum thyroxine, thyrotropin concentrations), resin triiodothyronine uptake (rT_3U), free thyroxine index (FTI), T_4, TSH, heart rate, blood pressure, clinical signs of hypo- and hyperthyroidism; TSH is the most reliable guide for evaluating adequacy of thyroid replacement dosage. TSH may be elevated during the first few months of thyroid replacement despite patients being clinically euthyroid. In cases where T_4 remains low and TSH is within normal limits, an evaluation of "free" (unbound) T_4 is needed to evaluate further increase in dosage

Infants: Monitor closely for cardiac overload, arrhythmias, and aspiration from avid suckling

Infants/children: Monitor closely for under/overtreatment. Undertreatment may decrease intellectual development and linear growth, and lead to poor school performance due to impaired concentration and slowed mentation. Overtreatment may adversely affect brain maturation, accelerate bone age (leading to premature closure of the epiphyses and reduced adult height); craniosynostosis has been reported in infants. Treated children may experience a period of catch-up growth. Monitor TSH and total or free T_4 at 2 and 4 weeks after starting treatment; every 1-2 months for first year of life; every 2-3 months during years 1-3; every 3-12 months until growth completed.

Adults: Monitor TSH every 6-8 weeks until normalized; 8-12 weeks after dosage changes; every 6-12 months throughout therapy

Reference Range Pediatrics: Cord T_4 and values in the first few weeks are much higher, falling over the first months and years. ≥10 years: ~5.8-11 mcg/dL (SI: 75-142 nmol/L). Borderline low: ≤4.5-5.7 mcg/dL (SI: 58-73 nmol/L); low: ≤4.4 mcg/dL (SI: 57 nmol/L); results <2.5 mcg/dL (SI: <32 nmol/L) are strong evidence for hypothyroidism.

Approximate adult normal range: 4-12 mcg/dL (SI: 51-154 nmol/L). Borderline high: 11.1-13 mcg/dL (SI: 143-167 nmol/L); high: ≥13.1 mcg/dL (SI: 169 nmol/L). Normal range is increased in women on birth control pills (5.5-12 mcg/dL); normal range in pregnancy: ~5.5-16 mcg/dL (SI: ~71-206 nmol/L). TSH: 0.4-10 (for those ≥80 years) mIU/L; T_4: 4-12 mcg/dL (SI: 51-154 nmol/L); T_3 (RIA) (total T_3): 80-230 ng/dL (SI: 1.2-3.5 nmol/L); T_4 free (free T_4): 0.7-1.8 ng/dL (SI: 9-23 pmol/L).

Anesthesia and Critical Care Concerns/Other Considerations Equivalent doses: The following statement on relative potency of thyroid products is included in a joint statement by American Thyroid Association (ATA), American Association of Clinical Endocrinologists (AACE) and The Endocrine Society (TES): For purposes of conversion, levothyroxine sodium (T_4) 100 mcg is usually considered equivalent to desiccated thyroid 60 mg, thyroglobulin 60 mg, or liothyronine sodium (T_3) 25 mcg. However, these are rough guidelines only and do not obviate the careful re-evaluation of a patient when switching thyroid hormone preparations, including a change from one brand of levothyroxine to another. Joint position statement is available at http://www.thyroid.org/professionals/advocacy/04_12_08_thyroxine.html.

(Continued)

Levothyroxine *(Continued)*

Note: Several medications have effects on thyroid production or conversion. The impact in thyroid replacement has not been specifically evaluated, but patient response should be monitored:

Methimazole: Decreases thyroid hormone secretion, while propylthiouracil decrease thyroid hormone secretion and decreases conversion of T_4 to T_3.

Beta-adrenergic antagonists: Decrease conversion of T_4 to T_3 (dose related, propranolol ≥160 mg/day); patients may be clinically euthyroid.

Iodide, iodine-containing radiographic contrast agents may decrease thyroid hormone secretion; may also increase thyroid hormone secretion, especially in patients with Graves' disease.

Other agents reported to impact on thyroid production/conversion include aminoglutethimide, amiodarone, chloral hydrate, diazepam, ethionamide, interferon-alpha, interleukin-2, lithium, lovastatin (case report), glucocorticoids (dose-related), mercaptopurine, sulfonamides, thiazide diuretics, and tolbutamide.

In addition, a number of medications have been noted to cause transient depression in TSH secretion, which may complicate interpretation of monitoring tests for levothyroxine, including corticosteroids, octreotide, and dopamine. Metoclopramide may increase TSH secretion

Soy protein may interfere with absorption of levothyroxine sodium. An enteral formula without soy protein should be selected and thyroid function monitored during tube feeding.

Pregnancy Risk Factor A

Contraindications Hypersensitivity to levothyroxine sodium or any component of the formulation; recent MI or thyrotoxicosis; uncorrected adrenal insufficiency

Warnings/Precautions [U.S. Boxed Warning]: Ineffective and potentially toxic for weight reduction. High doses may produce serious or even life-threatening toxic effects particularly when used with some anorectic drugs. Use with caution and reduce dosage in patients with angina pectoris or other cardiovascular disease; use cautiously in elderly since they may be more likely to have compromised cardiovascular functions. Patients with adrenal insufficiency, myxedema, diabetes mellitus and insipidus may have symptoms exaggerated or aggravated; thyroid replacement requires periodic assessment of thyroid status. Chronic hypothyroidism predisposes patients to coronary artery disease. Levoxyl® may rapidly swell and disintegrate causing choking or gagging (should be administered with a full glass of water); use caution in patients with dysphagia or other swallowing disorders.

Adverse Reactions Frequency not defined.

Cardiovascular: Angina, arrhythmia, blood pressure increased, cardiac arrest, flushing, heart failure, MI, palpitation, pulse increased, tachycardia

Central nervous system: Anxiety, emotional lability, fatigue, fever, headache, hyperactivity, insomnia, irritability, nervousness, pseudotumor cerebri (children), seizure (rare)

Dermatologic: Alopecia

Endocrine & metabolic: Fertility impaired, menstrual irregularities

Gastrointestinal: Abdominal cramps, appetite increased, diarrhea, vomiting, weight loss

Hepatic: Liver function tests increased

Neuromuscular & skeletal: Bone mineral density decreased, muscle weakness, tremor, slipped capital femoral epiphysis (children)

Respiratory: Dyspnea

Miscellaneous: Diaphoresis, heat intolerance, hypersensitivity (to inactive ingredients, symptoms include urticaria, pruritus, rash, flushing, angioedema, GI symptoms, fever, arthralgia, serum sickness, wheezing)

Levoxyl®: Choking, dysphagia, gagging

Overdosage/Toxicology

Chronic: Chronic overdose may cause hyperthyroidism, weight loss, nervousness, sweating, tachycardia, insomnia, heat intolerance, menstrual irregularities, palpitations, psychosis, and fever. Overtreatment of children may result in premature closure of epiphyses or craniosynostosis (infants). Reduce dose or temporarily discontinue therapy. Hypothalamic-pituitary-thyroid axis will return to normal in 6-8 weeks. Serum T_4 levels do not correlate well with toxicity. Provide general supportive care

Acute: Acute overdose may cause fever, hypoglycemia, CHF, and unrecognized adrenal insufficiency. Acute massive overdose may be life-threatening; treatment should be symptomatic and supportive. Massive overdose may be a require beta-blockers for increased sympathomimetic activity.

Drug Interactions

Aluminum- and magnesium-containing antacids, calcium carbonate, simethicone, or sucralfate: May decrease T_4 absorption; separate dose from levothyroxine by at least 4 hours.

Antidiabetic agents (biguanides, meglitinides, sulfonylureas, thiazolidinediones, insulin): Changes in thyroid function may alter requirements of antidiabetic agent. Monitor closely at initiation of therapy, or when dose is changed or discontinued.

Cholestyramine and colestipol: Decrease T_4 absorption; separate dose from levothyroxine by at least 2 hours.

Digoxin: Digoxin levels may be reduced in hyperthyroidism; therapeutic effect may be reduced. Impact of thyroid replacement should be monitored.

Estrogens: May decrease serum free thyroxine concentrations.

Imatinib: May decrease the effects of thyroid replacement therapy; monitor.

Iron: Decreases T_4 absorption; separate dose from levothyroxine by at least 4 hours.

Kayexalate®: Decreases T_4 absorption; separate dose from levothyroxine by at least 4 hours.

Ketamine: May cause marked hypertension and tachycardia; monitor.

Theophylline, caffeine: Decreased theophylline clearance in hypothyroid patients; monitor during thyroid replacement.

Tricyclic and tetracyclic antidepressants: Therapeutic and toxic effects of levothyroxine and the antidepressant are increased.

Warfarin (and other oral anticoagulants): The hypoprothrombinemic response to warfarin may be altered by a change in thyroid function or replacement. Replacement may dramatically increase response to warfarin. However, initiation of warfarin in a patient stabilized on a dose of levothyroxine does not appear to require a significantly different approach.

Ethanol/Nutrition/Herb Interactions Food: Taking levothyroxine with enteral nutrition may cause reduced bioavailability and may lower serum thyroxine levels leading to signs or symptoms of hypothyroidism. Limit intake of goitrogenic foods (eg, asparagus, cabbage, peas, turnip greens, broccoli, spinach, Brussels sprouts, lettuce, soybeans). Soybean flour (infant formula), cottonseed meal, walnuts, and dietary fiber may decrease absorption of levothyroxine from the GI tract.

Test Interactions Many drugs may have effects on thyroid function tests. Pregnancy, infectious hepatitis, and acute intermittent porphyria may increase TBG concentrations; nephrosis, severe hypoproteinemia, severe liver disease, and acromegaly may decrease TBG concentrations.

Dietary Considerations Should be taken on an empty stomach, at least 30 minutes before food.

Dosage Forms

Injection, powder for reconstitution, as sodium: 0.2 mg, 0.5 mg

Tablet, as sodium: 25 mcg, 50 mcg, 75 mcg, 88 mcg, 100 mcg, 112 mcg, 125 mcg, 150 mcg, 175 mcg, 200 mcg, 300 mcg

- Levothroid®: 25 mcg, 50 mcg, 75 mcg, 88 mcg, 100 mcg, 112 mcg, 125 mcg, 150 mcg, 175 mcg, 200 mcg, 300 mcg
- Levoxyl®, Synthroid®: 25 mcg, 50 mcg, 75 mcg, 88 mcg, 100 mcg, 112 mcg, 125 mcg, 137 mcg, 150 mcg, 175 mcg, 200 mcg, 300 mcg
- Unithroid®: 25 mcg, 50 mcg, 75 mcg, 88 mcg, 100 mcg, 112 mcg, 125 mcg, 150 mcg, 175 mcg, 200 mcg, 300 mcg

♦ **Levothyroxine Sodium (Can)** *see* Levothyroxine *on page 751*

♦ **Levoxyl®** *see* Levothyroxine *on page 751*

♦ **Librium®** *see* Chlordiazepoxide *on page 264*

♦ **LidaMantle®** *see* Lidocaine *on page 755*

Lidocaine (LYE doe kane)

Medication Safety Issues

High alert medication: The Institute for Safe Medication Practices (ISMP) includes this medication (I.V. formulation) among its list of drugs which have a heightened risk of causing significant patient harm when used in error.

(Continued)

Lidocaine *(Continued)*

Transdermal patch may contain conducting metal (eg, aluminum); remove patch prior to MRI.

Related Information

Acute Postoperative Pain *on page 1388*
Anesthesia for Obstetric Patients in Nonobstetric Surgery *on page 1416*
Anesthesia for Patients With Liver Disease *on page 1421*
Antiarrhythmic Drugs *on page 1548*
Chronic Pain Management *on page 1430*
Local Anesthetics *on page 1532*
Management of Postoperative Arrhythmias *on page 1451*

U.S. Brand Names Anestacon®; Band-Aid® Hurt-Free™ Antiseptic Wash [OTC]; Burnamycin [OTC]; Burn Jel [OTC]; Burn-O-Jel [OTC]; LidaMantle®; Lidoderm®; L-M-X™ 4 [OTC]; L-M-X™ 5 [OTC]; LTA® 360; Premjact® [OTC]; Solarcaine® Aloe Extra Burn Relief [OTC]; Topicaine® [OTC]; Xylocaine®; Xylocaine® MPF; Xylocaine® Viscous; Zilactin-L® [OTC]

Canadian Brand Names Betacaine®; Lidodan™; Lidoderm®; Xylocaine®; Xylocard®; Zilactin®

Synonyms Lidocaine Hydrochloride; Lignocaine Hydrochloride

Pharmacologic Category Analgesic, Topical; Antiarrhythmic Agent, Class Ib; Local Anesthetic

Generic Available Yes: Cream, infusion, injection, jelly, lotion, ointment, solution

Use Local anesthetic and acute treatment of ventricular arrhythmias from myocardial infarction, or cardiac manipulation

Rectal: Temporary relief of pain and itching due to anorectal disorders

Topical: Local anesthetic for use in laser, cosmetic, and outpatient surgeries; minor burns, cuts, and abrasions of the skin

Lidoderm® Patch: Relief of allodynia (painful hypersensitivity) and chronic pain in postherpetic neuralgia

Unlabeled/Investigational Use ACLS guidelines (not considered drug of choice): Stable monomorphic VT (preserved ventricular function), polymorphic VT (preserved ventricular function), drug-induced monomorphic VT

Mechanism of Action Class Ib antiarrhythmic; suppresses automaticity of conduction tissue, by increasing electrical stimulation threshold of ventricle, His-Purkinje system, and spontaneous depolarization of the ventricles during diastole by a direct action on the tissues; blocks both the initiation and conduction of nerve impulses by decreasing the neuronal membrane's permeability to sodium ions, which results in inhibition of depolarization with resultant blockade of conduction

Pharmacodynamics/Kinetics

Onset of action: Single bolus dose: 45-90 seconds

Duration: 10-20 minutes

Distribution: V_d: 1.1-2.1 L/kg; alterable by many patient factors; decreased in CHF and liver disease; crosses blood-brain barrier

Protein binding: 60% to 80% to $alpha_1$ acid glycoprotein

Metabolism: 90% hepatic; active metabolites monoethylglycinexylidide (MEGX) and glycinexylidide (GX) can accumulate and may cause CNS toxicity

Half-life elimination: Biphasic: Prolonged with congestive heart failure, liver disease, shock, severe renal disease; Initial: 7-30 minutes; Terminal: Infants, premature: 3.2 hours, Adults: 1.5-2 hours

Dosage

Antiarrhythmic:

Children:

I.V., I.O.: **Note:** For use in pulseless VT or VF, give after defibrillation, CPR, and epinephrine:

Loading dose: 1 mg/kg (maximum 100 mg); follow with continuous infusion; may administer second bolus of 0.5-1 mg/kg if delay between bolus and start of infusion is >15 minutes

Continuous infusion: 20-50 mcg/kg/minute. Use 20 mcg/kg/minute in patients with shock, hepatic disease, cardiac arrest, mild CHF; moderate-to-severe CHF may require ½ loading dose and lower infusion rates to avoid toxicity.

E.T. (loading dose only): 2-10 times the I.V. bolus dose; dilute with NS to a volume of 3-5 mL and follow with several positive-pressure ventilations

Adults:

Ventricular fibrillation or pulseless ventricular tachycardia (after defibrillation, CPR, and vasopressor administration): I.V.: Initial: 1-1.5 mg/kg. Refractory ventricular tachycardia or ventricular fibrillation, a repeat 0.5-0.75 mg/kg bolus may be given every 5-10 minutes after initial dose for a maximum of 3 doses. Total dose should not exceed 3 mg/kg. Follow with continuous infusion (1-4 mg/minute) after return of perfusion. Reappearance of arrhythmia during constant infusion: 0.5 mg/kg bolus and reassessment of infusion.

E.T. (loading dose only): 2-2.5 times the recommended I.V. dose; dilute in 10 mL NS or distilled water. **Note:** Absorption is greater with distilled water, but causes more adverse effects on PaO_2.

Hemodynamically stable VT: 0.5-0.75 mg/kg followed by synchronized cardioversion

Note: Decrease dose in patients with CHF, shock, or hepatic disease.

Anesthesia, topical:

Cream:

LidaMantle®: Skin irritation: Children and Adults: Apply to affected area 2-3 times/day as needed

L-M-X™ 4: Children ≥2 years and Adults: Apply 1/4 inch thick layer to intact skin. Leave on until adequate anesthetic effect is obtained. Remove cream and cleanse area before beginning procedure.

L-M-X™ 5: Relief of anorectal pain and itching: Children ≥12 years and Adults: Rectal: Apply topically to clean, dry area **or** using applicator, insert rectally, up to 6 times/day

Gel, ointment, solution: Adults: Apply to affected area ≤3 times/day as needed (maximum dose: 4.5 mg/kg, not to exceed 300 mg)

Jelly:

Children ≥10 years: Dose varies with age and weight (maximum dose: 4.5 mg/kg)

Adults (maximum dose: 30 mL [600 mg] in any 12-hour period):

Anesthesia of male urethra: 5-30 mL

Anesthesia of female urethra: 3-5 mL

Lubrication of endotracheal tube: Apply a moderate amount to external surface only

Liquid: Cold sores and fever blisters: Children ≥5 years and Adults: Apply to affected area every 6 hours as needed

Patch: Postherpetic neuralgia: Adults: Apply patch to most painful area. Up to 3 patches may be applied in a single application. Patch may remain in place for up to 12 hours in any 24-hour period.

Anesthetic, local injectable: Children and Adults: Varies with procedure, degree of anesthesia needed, vascularity of tissue, duration of anesthesia required, and physical condition of patient; maximum: 4.5 mg/kg/dose; do not repeat within 2 hours.

Dosage adjustment in renal impairment: Not dialyzable (0% to 5%) by hemo- or peritoneal dialysis; supplemental dose is not necessary.

Dosage adjustment in hepatic impairment: Reduce dose in acute hepatitis and decompensated cirrhosis by 50%.

Stability Lidocaine injection is stable at room temperature. Stability of parenteral admixture at room temperature (25°C) is the expiration date on premixed bag; out of overwrap stability is 30 days.

Standard diluent: 2 g/250 mL D_5W

Administration

Intratracheal: Dilute in NS or distilled water. Absorption is greater with distilled water, but causes more adverse effects on PaO_2. Pass catheter beyond tip of tracheal tube, stop compressions, spray drug quickly down tube. Follow immediately with several quick insufflations and continue chest compressions.

I.V.: Use microdrip (60 gtt/mL) or infusion pump to administer an accurate dose

Infusion rates: 2 g/250 mL D_5W (infusion pump should be used):

1 mg/minute: 7.5 mL/hour

2 mg/minute: 15 mL/hour

3 mg/minute: 22.5 mL/hour

4 mg/minute: 30 mL/hour

Buffered lidocaine for injectable local anesthetic: Add 2 mL of sodium bicarbonate 8.4% to 18 mL of lidocaine 1%

Topical:

Gel (Topicaine®): Avoid mucous membranes; remove prior to laser treatment.

Transdermal: Apply to painful area of skin immediately after removal from protective envelope. May be cut to appropriate size. After removal from skin,

(Continued)

Lidocaine *(Continued)*

fold used transdermal systems so the adhesive side sticks to itself. Remove immediately if burning sensation occurs. Wash hands after application.

Reference Range

Therapeutic: 1.5-5.0 mcg/mL (SI: 6-21 μmol/L)
Potentially toxic: >6 mcg/mL (SI: >26 μmol/L)
Toxic: >9 mcg/mL (SI: >38 μmol/L)

Anesthesia and Critical Care Concerns/Other Considerations

Cardiac Arrest: Amiodarone was recently compared to lidocaine (ALIVE trial) in out-of-hospital cardiac arrest victims whose ventricular fibrillation was resistant to 3 defibrillation attempts in addition to epinephrine and a fourth defibrillation attempt (Dorian, 2002). Other inclusion criteria included ventricular fibrillation unrelated to trauma (or with other arrhythmias that converted to ventricular fibrillation) and recurrent ventricular fibrillation after successful initial defibrillation. This was a randomized, double-blind comparison. The primary endpoint was the number of patients who were admitted to the hospital intensive care unit alive. Three hundred and forty-seven patients were enrolled. The initial amiodarone dose was 5 mg/kg and the lidocaine dose was 1.5 mg/kg. If ventricular fibrillation persisted after another shock, then the study drug could be administered again (amiodarone 2.5 mg/kg, lidocaine 1.5 mg/kg). Significantly more amiodarone patients (~23%) were admitted to the hospital alive than lidocaine patients (12%). The majority (>90%) of patients in the ALIVE trial had ventricular fibrillation as the initial arrhythmia. The authors concluded that intravenous amiodarone is superior to lidocaine in the treatment of shock-resistant, out-of-hospital ventricular fibrillation. Lidocaine is not as effective as amiodarone for improving intermediate outcomes, but neither has improved survival until hospital discharge among patients with VF cardiac arrest.

Monitoring: Great care is needed in administration of lidocaine in the elderly and in patients with heart failure, shock, or hepatic disease, as toxic effects of lidocaine may become evident earlier in these patients. The half-life of lidocaine increases after 24-48 hours as the drug inhibits its own hepatic metabolism. The dose should be reduced after 24 hours or blood levels should be monitored. While lidocaine toxicity may elicit seizures, lidocaine may also cause respiratory arrest and cardiac toxicity (eg, sinus arrest, AV block, asystole, and hypotension).

Pregnancy Risk Factor B

Contraindications Hypersensitivity to lidocaine or any component of the formulation; hypersensitivity to another local anesthetic of the amide type; Adam-Stokes syndrome; severe degrees of SA, AV, or intraventricular heart block (except in patients with a functioning artificial pacemaker); premixed injection may contain corn-derived dextrose and its use is contraindicated in patients with allergy to corn-related products

Warnings/Precautions

Intravenous: Constant ECG monitoring is necessary during I.V. administration. Use cautiously in hepatic impairment, any degree of heart block, Wolff-Parkinson-White syndrome, CHF, marked hypoxia, severe respiratory depression, hypovolemia, history of malignant hyperthermia, or shock. Increased ventricular rate may be seen when administered to a patient with atrial fibrillation. Correct any underlying causes of ventricular arrhythmias. Monitor closely for signs and symptoms of CNS toxicity. The elderly may be prone to increased CNS and cardiovascular side effects. Reduce dose in hepatic dysfunction and CHF.

Injectable anesthetic: Follow appropriate administration techniques so as not to administer any intravascularly. Solutions containing antimicrobial preservatives should not be used for epidural or spinal anesthesia. Some solutions contain a bisulfite; avoid in patients who are allergic to bisulfite. Resuscitative equipment, medicine and oxygen should be available in case of emergency. Use products containing epinephrine cautiously in patients with significant vascular disease, compromised blood flow, or during or following general anesthesia (increased risk of arrhythmias). Adjust the dose for the elderly, pediatric, acutely ill, and debilitated patients.

Topical: L-M-X™ 4 cream: Do not leave on large body areas for >2 hours. Observe young children closely to prevent accidental ingestion. Not for use ophthalmic use or for use on mucous membranes.

Transdermal patch: May contain conducting metal (eg, aluminum); remove patch prior to MRI.

Adverse Reactions Effects vary with route of administration. Many effects are dose related.

Frequency not defined.

Cardiovascular: Arrhythmia, bradycardia, arterial spasms, cardiovascular collapse, defibrillator threshold increased, edema, flushing, heart block, hypotension, sinus node supression, vascular insufficiency (periarticular injections)

Central nervous system: Agitation, anxiety, apprehension, coma, confusion, disorientation, dizziness, drowsiness, euphoria, hallucinations, headache, hyperesthesia, hypoesthesia, lethargy, lightheadedness, nervousness, psychosis, seizure, slurred speech, somnolence, unconsciousness

Dermatologic: Angioedema, bruising (transdermal system), contact dermatitis, depigmentation (transdermal system), edema of the skin, itching, petechia (transdermal system), pruritus, rash, urticaria

Gastrointestinal: Metallic taste, nausea, vomiting

Local: Irritation (transdermal system), thrombophlebitis

Neuromuscular & skeletal: Pain exacerbation (transdermal system), paresthesia, transient radicular pain (subarachnoid administration; up to 1.9%), tremor, twitching, weakness

Ocular: Diplopia, visual changes

Otic: Tinnitus

Respiratory: Bronchospasm, dyspnea, respiratory depression or arrest

Miscellaneous: Allergic reactions, anaphylactoid reaction, sensitivity to temperature extremes

Following spinal anesthesia positional headache (3%), shivering (2%) nausea, peripheral nerve symptoms, respiratory inadequacy and double vision (<1%), hypotension, cauda equina syndrome

Postmarketing and/or case reports: ARDS (inhalation), asystole, disorientation, methemoglobinemia, skin reaction

Overdosage/Toxicology Lidocaine has a narrow therapeutic index. Severe toxicity may occur at doses slightly above the therapeutic range, especially in conjunction with other antiarrhythmic drugs. Symptoms of overdose include sedation, confusion, coma, seizures, respiratory arrest, and cardiac toxicity (sinus arrest, AV block, asystole, and hypotension). QRS and QT intervals are usually normal, although they may be prolonged after massive overdose. Other effects include dizziness, paresthesia, tremor, ataxia, and GI disturbance. Treatment is supportive.

Drug Interactions Substrate of CYP1A2 (minor), 2A6 (minor), 2B6 (minor), 2C9 (minor), 2D6 (major), 3A4 (major); **Inhibits** CYP1A2 (strong), 2D6 (moderate), 3A4 (moderate)

Cimetidine increases lidocaine blood levels; monitor levels or use an alternative H_2 antagonist.

CYP1A2 substrates: Lidocaine may increase the levels/effects of CYP1A2 substrates. Example substrates include aminophylline, fluvoxamine, mexiletine, mirtazapine, ropinirole, theophylline, and trifluoperazine.

CYP2D6 inhibitors: May increase the levels/effects of lidocaine. Example inhibitors include chlorpromazine, delavirdine, fluoxetine, miconazole, paroxetine, pergolide, quinidine, quinine, ritonavir, and ropinirole.

CYP2D6 substrates: Lidocaine may increase the levels/effects of CYP2D6 substrates. Example substrates include amphetamines, selected beta-blockers, dextromethorphan, fluoxetine, mirtazapine, nefazodone, paroxetine, risperidone, ritonavir, thioridazine, tricyclic antidepressants, and venlafaxine.

CYP2D6 prodrug substrates: Lidocaine may decrease the levels/effects of CYP2D6 prodrug substrates. Example prodrug substrates include codeine, hydrocodone, oxycodone, and tramadol.

CYP3A4 inducers: CYP3A4 inducers may decrease the levels/effects of lidocaine. Example inducers include aminoglutethimide, carbamazepine, nafcillin, nevirapine, phenobarbital, phenytoin, and rifamycins.

CYP3A4 inhibitors: May increase the levels/effects of lidocaine. Example inhibitors include amiodarone (doses >400 mg/day), azole antifungals, clarithromycin, diclofenac, doxycycline, erythromycin, imatinib, isoniazid, nefazodone, nicardipine, propofol, protease inhibitors, quinidine, telithromycin, and verapamil.

CYP3A4 substrates: Lidocaine may increase the levels/effects of CYP3A4 substrates. Example substrates include benzodiazepines, calcium channel blockers, cyclosporine, mirtazapine, nateglinide, nefazodone, sildenafil (and other PDE-5 inhibitors), tacrolimus, and venlafaxine. Selected benzodiazepines

(Continued)

Lidocaine *(Continued)*

(midazolam and triazolam), cisapride, ergot alkaloids, selected HMG-CoA reductase inhibitors (lovastatin and simvastatin), and pimozide are generally contraindicated with strong CYP3A4 inhibitors.

Propranolol: Increases lidocaine blood levels.

Protease inhibitors (eg, amprenavir, ritonavir): May increase lidocaine blood levels.

Ethanol/Nutrition/Herb Interactions Herb/Nutraceutical: St John's wort may decrease lidocaine levels; avoid concurrent use.

Dietary Considerations Premixed injection may contain corn-derived dextrose and its use is contraindicated in patients with allergy to corn-related products.

Dosage Forms [DSC] = Discontinued product

Cream, rectal (L-M-X™ 5): 5% (15 g) [contains benzyl alcohol; packaged with applicator]; (30 g) [contains benzyl alcohol]

Cream, topical (L-M-X™ 4): 4% (5 g) [contains benzyl alcohol; packaged with Tegaderm™ dressing]; (15 g, 30 g) [contains benzyl alcohol]

Cream, topical, as hydrochloride: 3% (30 g)

LidaMantle®: 3% (30 g, 85 g)

Gel, topical:

Burn-O-Jel: 0.5% (90 g)

Topicaine®: 4% (10 g, 30 g, 113 g) [contains alcohol 35%, benzyl alcohol, aloe vera, and jojoba]

Gel, topical, as hydrochloride:

Burn Jel: 2% (3.5 g, 120 g)

Solarcaine® Aloe Extra Burn Relief: 0.5% (113 g, 226 g) [contains aloe vera gel and tartrazine]

Infusion, as hydrochloride [premixed in D_5W]: 0.4% [4 mg/mL] (250 mL, 500 mL); 0.8% [8 mg/mL] (250 mL, 500 mL)

Injection, solution, as hydrochloride: 0.5% [5 mg/mL] (50 mL); 1% [10 mg/mL] (2 mL, 10 mL, 20 mL, 30 mL, 50 mL); 2% [20 mg/mL] (2 mL, 5 mL, 20 mL, 50 mL)

Xylocaine®: 0.5% [5 mg/mL] (50 mL); 1% [10 mg/mL] (10 mL, 20 mL, 50 mL); 2% [20 mg/mL] (1.8 mL, 10 mL, 20 mL, 50 mL)

Injection, solution, as hydrochloride [preservative free]: 0.5% [5 mg/mL] (50 mL); 1% [10 mg/mL] (2 mL, 5 mL, 30 mL); 1.5% [15 mg/mL] (20 mL); 2% [20 mg/mL] (2 mL, 5 mL, 10 mL); 4% [40 mg/mL] (5 mL)

Xylocaine®: 10% [100 mg/mL] (5 mL) [for ventricular arrhythmias]

Xylocaine® MPF: 0.5% [5 mg/mL] (50 mL); 1% [10 mg/mL] (2 mL, 5 mL, 10 mL, 30 mL); 1.5% [15 mg/mL] (10 mL, 20 mL); 2% [20 mg/mL] (2 mL, 5 mL, 10 mL); 4% [40 mg/mL] (5 mL)

Injection, solution, as hydrochloride [premixed in $D_{7.5}W$, preservative free]: 5% (2 mL)

Xylocaine® MPF: 1.5% (2 mL) [DSC]

Jelly, topical, as hydrochloride: 2% (5 mL, 30 mL)

Anestacon®: 2% (15 mL) [contains benzalkonium chloride]

Xylocaine®: 2% (5 mL, 30 mL)

Liquid, topical (Zilactin®-L): 2.5% (7.5 mL)

Lotion, topical, as hydrochloride (LidaMantle®): 3% (177 mL)

Ointment, topical: 5% (37 g, 50 g)

Solution, topical, as hydrochloride: 4% [40 mg/mL] (50 mL)

Band-Aid® Hurt-Free™ Antiseptic Wash: 2% (180 mL)

LTA® 360: 4% [40 mg/mL] (4 mL) [packaged with cannula for laryngotracheal administration]

Xylocaine®: 4% [40 mg/mL] (50 mL)

Solution, viscous, as hydrochloride: 2% [20 mg/mL] (20 mL, 100 mL)

Xylocaine® Viscous: 2% [20 mg/mL] (100 mL, 450 mL)

Spray, topical:

Burnamycin: 0.5% (60 mL) [contains aloe vera gel and menthol]

Premjact®: 9.6% (13 mL)

Solarcaine® Aloe Extra Burn Relief: 0.5% (127 g) [contains aloe vera]

Transdermal system, topical (Lidoderm®): 5% (30s)

References

"2005 American Heart Association Guidelines for Cardiopulmonary Resuscitation and Emergency Cardiovascular Care," *Circulation*, 2005;112 (Suppl IV):1-211.

Dorian P, Cass D, Schwartz B, et al, "Amiodarone as Compared With Lidocaine for Shock-Resistant Ventricular Fibrillation," *N Engl J Med*, 2002, 346(12):884-90.

Lidocaine and Bupivacaine (LYE doe kane & byoo PIV a kane)

U.S. Brand Names Duocaine™

Synonyms Bupivacaine and Lidocaine; Lidocaine Hydrochloride and Bupivacaine Hydrochloride

Pharmacologic Category Local Anesthetic

Generic Available No

Use Local or regional anesthesia in ophthalmologic surgery by peripheral nerve block techniques such as peribulbar, retrobulbar, and facial blocks; may be used with or without epinephrine

Mechanism of Action Blocks both the initiation and conduction of nerve impulses by decreasing the neuronal membrane's permeability to sodium ions, which results in inhibition of depolarization with resultant blockade of conduction.

Pharmacodynamics/Kinetics Also see individual agents.

Protein binding: Lidocaine: Fraction bound decreases with increased concentration; also dependent upon plasma concentration of alpha$_1$-acid glycoprotein

Metabolism: Lidocaine: Hepatic, forms metabolites; Bupivacaine: hepatic, forms metabolites

Half-life elimination: Lidocaine: I.V.: 1.5-2 hours; Bupivacaine: I.V.: 2.7 hours

Time to peak, plasma: Following peribulbar block: Lidocaine: 20 minutes; Bupivacaine: 21 minutes

Excretion: Urine

Dosage Adults: **Note:** Use lowest effective dose to limit toxic effects. Dosing based on lidocaine 1% and bupivacaine 0.375%

Retrobulbar injection: 2-5 mL; a portion of dose is injected retrobulbarly and remainder may be used to block the facial nerve

Peribulbar block: 6-12 mL

Maximum dose: 0.18 mL/kg or 12 mL; if used with epinephrine, the dose should not exceed 0.28 mL/kg or 20 mL

Dosage adjustment in renal impairment: Lidocaine: Accumulation of metabolites may increase with renal impairment

Dosage adjustment in hepatic impairment:

Lidocaine: Half-life of lidocaine is increased twofold with hepatic impairment

Bupivacaine: Toxicities may be increased with hepatic impairment

Stability Store at 15°C to 25°C (59°F to 77°F)

Pregnancy Risk Factor C

Contraindications Hypersensitivity to lidocaine, bupivacaine, amide-type local anesthetics (etidocaine, mepivacaine, prilocaine, ropivacaine) or any component of the formulation; Stokes-Adams syndrome; Wolff-Parkinson-White syndrome; severe degrees of sinoatrial, atrioventricular, or intraventricular block without artificial pacemaker

Warnings/Precautions Local anesthetics have been associated with rare occurrences of sudden respiratory arrest; convulsions due to systemic toxicity leading to cardiac arrest have also been reported, presumably following unintentional intravascular injection. Resuscitative equipment and medications should be available for immediate use. Repeated doses may lead to significant increases in blood levels due to accumulation of drug and metabolites. Use caution with elderly, debilitated, or acutely ill. Use caution in patients with shock, heart block without functional pacemakers, or hepatic or cardiac dysfunction. Use not intended for spinal anesthesia. Safety and efficacy have not been established in pediatric patients <12 years of age.

Adverse Reactions Frequency not defined; reactions may be dose related or due to unintentional intravascular injection.

Cardiovascular: Bradycardia, cardiac arrest, cardiac output decreased, heart block, hypotension, myocardium depression, ventricular arrhythmia

Central nervous system: Anxiety, chills, convulsions, depression, dizziness, drowsiness, excitation, restlessness

Gastrointestinal: Nausea, vomiting

Neuromuscular & skeletal: Tremors

Ocular: Blurred vision, pupil constriction, permanent injury to extraocular muscle

Otic: Tinnitus

Respiratory: Respiratory arrest

Miscellaneous: Allergic reaction

Following unintentional subarachnoid injection: Backache, cranial nerve palsies, headache, incontinence (fecal or urinary), meningismus, paralysis, paresthesia,

(Continued)

Lidocaine and Bupivacaine *(Continued)*

perineal sensation loss, persistent anesthesia, septic meningitis, sexual function loss, spinal block, urinary retention, weakness

Overdosage/Toxicology See individual agents. Toxicity thresholds of serum concentrations in humans are 6000 ng/mL for lidocaine and 1600 ng/mL for bupivacaine. Cardiovascular effects include cardiac conduction and excitability possibly leading to atrioventricular block, ventricular arrhythmias, and cardiac arrest. Central nervous system effects include stimulation, depression or both.

Drug Interactions Lidocaine: **Substrate** of CYP1A2 (minor), 2A6 (minor), 2B6 (minor), 2C9 (minor), 2D6 (major), 3A4 (major); **Inhibits** CYP1A2 (strong), 2D6 (moderate), 3A4 (moderate)

Also See individual agents.

Epinephrine: May be used to decrease systemic absorption of lidocaine/bupivacaine; if used, see Epinephrine monograph Drug Interactions.

Dosage Forms Injection, solution [preservative free]: Lidocaine hydrochloride 1% and bupivacaine hydrochloride 0.375% (10 mL)

- **Lidocaine Hydrochloride** *see* Lidocaine *on page 755*
- **Lidocaine Hydrochloride and Bupivacaine Hydrochloride** *see* Lidocaine and Bupivacaine *on page 761*
- **Lidodan™ (Can)** *see* Lidocaine *on page 755*
- **Lidoderm®** *see* Lidocaine *on page 755*
- **Lignocaine Hydrochloride** *see* Lidocaine *on page 755*
- **Lin-Buspirone (Can)** *see* BusPIRone *on page 205*

Linezolid (li NE zoh lid)

Medication Safety Issues

Sound-alike/look-alike issues:

Zyvox™ may be confused with Vioxx®, Ziox™, Zosyn®, Zovirax®

U.S. Brand Names Zyvox™

Canadian Brand Names Zyvoxam®

Pharmacologic Category Antibiotic, Oxazolidinone

Generic Available No

Use Treatment of vancomycin-resistant *Enterococcus faecium* (VRE) infections, nosocomial pneumonia caused by *Staphylococcus aureus* including MRSA or *Streptococcus pneumoniae* (including multidrug-resistant strains [MDRSP]), complicated and uncomplicated skin and skin structure infections (including diabetic foot infections without concomitant osteomyelitis), and community-acquired pneumonia caused by susceptible gram-positive organisms

Mechanism of Action Inhibits bacterial protein synthesis by binding to bacterial 23S ribosomal RNA of the 50S subunit. This prevents the formation of a functional 70S initiation complex that is essential for the bacterial translation process. Linezolid is bacteriostatic against enterococci and staphylococci and bactericidal against most strains of streptococci.

Pharmacodynamics/Kinetics

Absorption: Rapid and extensive

Distribution: V_{dss}: Adults: 40-50 L

Protein binding: Adults: 31%

Metabolism: Hepatic via oxidation of the morpholine ring, resulting in two inactive metabolites (aminoethoxyacetic acid, hydroxyethyl glycine); does not involve CYP

Bioavailability: 100%

Half-life elimination: Children ≥1 week (full-term) to 11 years: 1.5-3 hours; Adults: 4-5 hours

Time to peak: Adults: Oral: 1-2 hours

Excretion: Urine (30% as parent drug, 50% as metabolites); feces (9% as metabolites)

Nonrenal clearance: 65%; increased in children ≥1 week to 11 years

Dosage

VRE infections: Oral, I.V.:

Preterm neonates (<34 weeks gestational age): 10 mg/kg every 12 hours; neonates with a suboptimal clinical response can be advanced to 10 mg/kg every 8 hours. By day 7 of life, all neonates should receive 10 mg/kg every 8 hours.

Infants (excluding preterm neonates <1 week) and Children ≤11 years: 10 mg/kg every 8 hours for 14-28 days

Children ≥12 years and Adults: 600 mg every 12 hours for 14-28 days

Nosocomial pneumonia, complicated skin and skin structure infections, community acquired pneumonia including concurrent bacteremia: Oral, I.V.:

Infants (excluding preterm neonates <1 week) and Children ≤11 years: 10 mg/kg every 8 hours for 10-14 days

Children ≥12 years and Adults: 600 mg every 12 hours for 10-14 days

Uncomplicated skin and skin structure infections: Oral:

Infants (excluding preterm neonates <1 week) and Children <5 years: 10 mg/kg every 8 hours for 10-14 days

Children 5-11 years: 10 mg/kg every 12 hours for 10-14 days

Children ≥12-18 years: 600 mg every 12 hours for 10-14 days

Adults: 400 mg every 12 hours for 10-14 days

Elderly: No dosage adjustment required

Dosage adjustment in renal impairment: No adjustment is recommended. The two primary metabolites may accumulate in patients with renal impairment but the clinical significance is unknown. Weigh the risk of accumulation of metabolites versus the benefit of therapy. Both linezolid and the two metabolites are eliminated by dialysis. Linezolid should be given after hemodialysis.

Dosage adjustment in hepatic impairment: No dosage adjustment required for mild to moderate hepatic insufficiency (Child-Pugh Class A or B). Use in severe hepatic insufficiency has not been adequately evaluated.

Stability

Infusion: Store at 25°C (77°F). Protect from light. Keep infusion bags in overwrap until ready for use. Protect infusion bags from freezing.

Oral suspension: Following reconstitution, store at room temperature; use reconstituted suspension within 21 days

Administration

I.V.: Administer intravenous infusion over 30-120 minutes. Do not mix or infuse with other medications. When the same intravenous line is used for sequential infusion of other medications, flush line with D_5W, NS, or LR before and after infusing linezolid. The yellow color of the injection may intensify over time without affecting potency.

Oral suspension: Invert gently to mix prior to administration, do not shake.

Monitoring Parameters Weekly CBC and platelet counts, particularly in patients at increased risk of bleeding, with pre-existing myelosuppression, on concomitant medications that cause bone marrow suppression, in those who require >2 weeks of therapy, or in those with chronic infection who have received previous or concomitant antibiotic therapy; visual function with extended therapy (≥3 months) or in patients with new onset visual symptoms, regardless of therapy length

Anesthesia and Critical Care Concerns/Other Considerations Linezolid has mild MAO inhibitor properties and should be used with caution in patients with cardiovascular disease, particularly those with hypertension. Avoid use with sympathomimetic and dopaminergic agents.

Pregnancy Risk Factor C

Contraindications Hypersensitivity to linezolid or any other component of the formulation

Warnings/Precautions Myelosuppression has been reported and may be dependent on duration of therapy (generally >2 weeks of treatment); use with caution in patients with pre-existing myelosuppression, in patients receiving other drugs which may cause bone marrow suppression, or in chronic infection (previous or concurrent antibiotic therapy). Weekly CBC monitoring is recommended. Discontinue linezolid in patients developing myelosuppression (or in whom myelosuppression worsens during treatment).

Lactic acidosis has been reported with use. Patients who develop recurrent nausea and vomiting, unexplained acidosis, or low bicarbonate levels need immediate evaluation.

Linezolid exhibits mild MAO inhibitor properties and has the potential to have the same interactions as other MAO inhibitors; use with caution in uncontrolled hypertension, pheochromocytoma, carcinoid syndrome, or untreated hyperthyroidism; avoid use with serotonergic agents such as TCAs, venlafaxine, trazodone, sibutramine, meperidine, dextromethorphan, and SSRIs; concomitant use has been associated with the development of serotonin syndrome. Unnecessary use may lead to the development of resistance to linezolid; consider alternatives before initiating outpatient treatment.

(Continued)

Linezolid *(Continued)*

Peripheral and optic neuropathy (with vision loss) has been reported and may occur primarily with extended courses of therapy >28 days; any symptoms of visual change or impairment warrant immediate ophthalmic evaluation and possible discontinuation of therapy.

Due to inconsistent therapeutic concentrations in the CSF, empiric use in pediatric patients with CNS infections is not recommended.

Adverse Reactions Percentages as reported in adults; frequency similar in pediatric patients

>10%:

Central nervous system: Headache (<1% to 11%)
Gastrointestinal: Diarrhea (3% to 11%)

1% to 10%:

Central nervous system: Insomnia (3%), dizziness (0.4% to 2%), fever (2%)
Dermatologic: Rash (2%)
Gastrointestinal: Nausea (3% to 10%), vomiting (1% to 4%), pancreatic enzymes increased (<1% to 4%), constipation (2%), taste alteration (1% to 2%), tongue discoloration (0.2% to 1%), oral moniliasis (0.4% to 1%), pancreatitis
Genitourinary: Vaginal moniliasis (1% to 2%)
Hematologic: Thrombocytopenia (0.3% to 10%), hemoglobin decreased (0.9% to 7%), anemia, leukopenia, neutropenia; **Note:** Myelosuppression (including anemia, leukopenia, pancytopenia, and thrombocytopenia; may be more common in patients receiving linezolid for >2 weeks)
Hepatic: Abnormal LFTs (0.4% to 1%)
Renal: BUN increased (<1% to 2%)
Miscellaneous: Fungal infection (0.1% to 2%), lactate dehydrogenase increased (<1% to 2%)

<1% or frequency not defined (limited to important or life-threatening): Blurred vision, *C. difficile*-related complications, creatinine increased, dyspepsia, hypertension, localized abdominal pain, pruritus, lactic acidosis, peripheral neuropathy, optic neuropathy, serotonin syndrome (with concurrent use of other serotonergic agents)

Overdosage/Toxicology Treatment includes supportive care. Hemodialysis may improve elimination (30% of a dose is removed during a 3-hour hemodialysis session).

Drug Interactions

Adrenergic agents (eg, phenylpropanolamine, pseudoephedrine, sympathomimetic agents, vasopressor or dopaminergic agents) may cause hypertension.
Myelosuppressive medications: Concurrent use may increase risk of myelosuppression with linezolid.
Serotonergic agents (eg, TCAs, venlafaxine, trazodone, sibutramine, meperidine, dextromethorphan, and SSRIs) may cause a serotonin syndrome (eg, hyperpyrexia, cognitive dysfunction) when used concomitantly.
Tramadol: Concurrent use may increase risk of seizures.

Ethanol/Nutrition/Herb Interactions

Ethanol: Avoid ethanol (may contain tyramine, hypertensive crisis may result).
Food: Avoid foods (eg, cheese) and beverages containing tyramine in patients receiving linezolid (hypertensive crisis may result).

Dietary Considerations Take with or without food. Avoid foods with high tyramine content (eg, pickled or fermented foods, cheese, beer and wine). Suspension contains 20 mg phenylalanine per teaspoonful. Sodium content: 0.1 mEq/tablet; 0.4 mEq/5 mL; 1.7 mEq/100 mL infusion; 3.3 mEq/200 mL infusion; 5 mEq/300 mL infusion

Dosage Forms

Infusion [premixed]: 200 mg (100 mL) [contains sodium 1.7 mEq]; 400 mg (200 mL) [contains sodium 3.3 mEq]; 600 mg (300 mL) [contains sodium 5 mEq]
Powder for oral suspension: 20 mg/mL (150 mL) [contains phenylalanine 20 mg/5 mL, sodium benzoate, and sodium 0.4 mEq/5 mL; orange flavor]
Tablet: 600 mg [contains sodium 0.1 mEq/tablet]

References

American Thoracic Society and Infectious Diseases Society of America, "Guidelines for the Management of Adults With Hospital-Acquired, Ventilator-Associated, and Healthcare-Associated Pneumonia," *Am J Respir Crit Care Med*, 2005, 171(4):388-416.

♦ **Lin-Sotalol (Can)** *see* Sotalol *on page 1198*
♦ **Lioresal®** *see* Baclofen *on page 156*

♦ **Liotec (Can)** *see* Baclofen *on page 156*

Liothyronine (lye oh THYE roe neen)

Medication Safety Issues

Sound-alike/look-alike issues:

Liothyronine may be confused with levothyroxine

T3 is an error-prone abbreviation (mistaken as acetaminophen and codeine [ie, Tylenol® #3])

U.S. Brand Names Cytomel®; Triostat®

Canadian Brand Names Cytomel®

Synonyms Liothyronine Sodium; Sodium *L*-Triiodothyronine; T_3 Sodium (error-prone abbreviation)

Pharmacologic Category Thyroid Product

Generic Available No

Use

Oral: Replacement or supplemental therapy in hypothyroidism; management of nontoxic goiter; a diagnostic aid

I.V.: Treatment of myxedema coma/precoma

Mechanism of Action Exact mechanism of action is unknown; however, it is believed the thyroid hormone exerts its many metabolic effects through control of DNA transcription and protein synthesis; involved in normal metabolism, growth, and development; promotes gluconeogenesis, increases utilization and mobilization of glycogen stores, and stimulates protein synthesis, increases basal metabolic rate

Pharmacodynamics/Kinetics

Onset of action: 2-4 hours

Peak response: 2-3 days

Absorption: Oral: Well absorbed (95% in 4 hours)

Half-life elimination: 2.5 days

Excretion: Urine

Dosage Doses should be adjusted based on clinical response and laboratory parameters.

Children: Congenital hypothyroidism: Oral: 5 mcg/day increase by 5 mcg every 3-4 days until the desired response is achieved. Usual maintenance dose: 20 mcg/day for infants, 50 mcg/day for children 1-3 years of age, and adult dose for children >3 years.

Adults:

Hypothyroidism: Oral: 25 mcg/day increase by increments of 12.5-25 mcg/day every 1-2 weeks to a maximum of 100 mcg/day; usual maintenance dose: 25-75 mcg/day.

Patients with cardiovascular disease: Refer to Elderly dosing.

T_3 suppression test: Oral: 75-100 mcg/day for 7 days; use lowest dose for elderly

Myxedema: Oral: Initial: 5 mcg/day; increase in increments of 5-10 mcg/day every 1-2 weeks. When 25 mcg/day is reached, dosage may be increased at intervals of 5-25 mcg/day every 1-2 weeks. Usual maintenance dose: 50-100 mcg/day.

Myxedema coma: I.V.: 25-50 mcg

Patients with known or suspected cardiovascular disease: 10-20 mcg

Note: Normally, at least 4 hours should be allowed between doses to adequately assess therapeutic response and no more than 12 hours should elapse between doses to avoid fluctuations in hormone levels. Oral therapy should be resumed as soon as the clinical situation has been stabilized and the patient is able to take oral medication. If levothyroxine rather than liothyronine sodium is used in initiating oral therapy, the physician should bear in mind that there is a delay of several days in the onset of levothyroxine activity and that I.V. therapy should be discontinued gradually.

Simple (nontoxic) goiter: Oral: Initial: 5 mcg/day; increase by 5-10 mcg every 1-2 weeks; after 25 mcg/day is reached, may increase dose by 12.5-25 mcg. Usual maintenance dose: 75 mcg/day

Elderly: Oral: 5 mcg/day; increase by 5 mcg/day every 2 weeks

Stability Vials must be stored under refrigeration at 2°C to 8°C (36°F to 46°F). Store tablets at 15°C to 30°C (59°F to 86°F).

Administration I.V.: For I.V. use only; **do not administer I.M. or SubQ**

Administer doses at least 4 hours, and no more than 12 hours, apart

(Continued)

Liothyronine *(Continued)*

Resume oral therapy as soon as the clinical situation has been stabilized and the patient is able to take oral medication

When switching to tablets, discontinue the injectable, initiate oral therapy at a low dosage and increase gradually according to response

If **levothyroxine** is used for oral therapy, there is a delay of several days in the onset of activity; therefore, discontinue I.V. therapy gradually

Monitoring Parameters T_3, TSH, heart rate, blood pressure, renal function, clinical signs of hypo- and hyperthyroidism; TSH is the most reliable guide for evaluating adequacy of thyroid replacement dosage. TSH may be elevated during the first few months of thyroid replacement despite patients being clinically euthyroid. In cases where T_4 remains low and TSH is within normal limits, an evaluation of "free" (unbound) T_4 is needed to evaluate further increase in dosage.

Reference Range Free T_3, serum: 250-390 pg/dL; TSH: 0.4 and up to 10 (≥80 years) mIU/L; remains normal in pregnancy

Anesthesia and Critical Care Concerns/Other Considerations Equivalent doses: The following statement on relative potency of thyroid products is included in a joint statement by American Thyroid Association (ATA), American Association of Clinical Endocrinologists (AACE) and The Endocrine Society (TES): For purposes of conversion, levothyroxine sodium (T_4) 100 mcg is usually considered equivalent to desiccated thyroid 60 mg, thyroglobulin 60 mg, or liothyronine sodium (T_3) 25 mcg. However, these are rough guidelines only and do not obviate the careful re-evaluation of a patient when switching thyroid hormone preparations, including a change from one brand of levothyroxine to another. Joint position statement is available at http://www.thyroid.org/professionals/advocacy/04_12_08_thyroxine.html.

Pregnancy Risk Factor A

Contraindications Hypersensitivity to liothyronine sodium or any component of the formulation; undocumented or uncorrected adrenal insufficiency; recent myocardial infarction or thyrotoxicosis; artificial rewarming (injection)

Warnings/Precautions [U.S. Boxed Warning]: Ineffective for weight reduction. High doses may produce serious or even life-threatening toxic effects particularly when used with some anorectic drugs. Use with extreme caution in patients with angina pectoris or other cardiovascular disease (including hypertension) or coronary artery disease; use with caution in elderly patients since they may be more likely to have compromised cardiovascular function. Patients with adrenal insufficiency, myxedema, diabetes mellitus and insipidus may have symptoms exaggerated or aggravated; thyroid replacement requires periodic assessment of thyroid status. Chronic hypothyroidism predisposes patients to coronary artery disease.

Adverse Reactions

1% to 10%: Cardiovascular: Arrhythmia (6%), tachycardia (3%), cardiopulmonary arrest (2%), hypotension (2%), MI (2%)

<1% (Limited to important or life-threatening): Allergic skin reactions, angina, CHF, fever, hypertension, phlebitis, twitching

Overdosage/Toxicology Chronic overdose may cause hyperthyroidism, weight loss, nervousness, sweating, tachycardia, insomnia, heat intolerance, menstrual irregularities, palpitations, psychosis, and fever. Acute overdose may cause fever, hypoglycemia, CHF, unrecognized adrenal insufficiency.

Reduce dose or temporarily discontinue therapy. Normal hypothalamic-pituitary-thyroid axis will return to normal in 6-8 weeks. Serum T_4 levels do not correlate well with toxicity. In massive acute ingestion, reduce GI absorption and give general supportive care. Excessive adrenergic activity (tachycardia) requires propranolol 1-3 mg I.V. over 10 minutes or 80-160 mg orally/day.

Drug Interactions

Aluminum- and magnesium-containing antacids, calcium carbonate, simethicone, or sucralfate: May decrease T_4 absorption; separate dose from thyroid hormones by at least 4 hours.

Antidiabetic agents (biguanides, meglitinides, sulfonylureas, thiazolidinediones, insulin): Changes in thyroid function may alter requirements of antidiabetic agent. Monitor closely at initiation of therapy, or when dose is changed or discontinued.

Cholestyramine and colestipol: Decrease T_4 absorption; separate dose from thyroid hormones by at least 2 hours.

Digoxin: Digoxin levels may be reduced in hyperthyroidism; therapeutic effect may be reduced. Impact of thyroid replacement should be monitored.

Estrogens: May decrease serum free-thyroxine concentrations.

Iron: Decreases T_4 absorption; separate dose from thyroid hormones by at least 4 hours

Kayexalate®: Decreases T_4 absorption; separate dose from thyroid hormones by at least 4 hours

Ketamine: May cause marked hypertension and tachycardia; monitor

Theophylline, caffeine: Decreased theophylline clearance in hypothyroid patients; monitor during thyroid replacement.

Tricyclic and tetracyclic antidepressants: Therapeutic and toxic effects of thyroid hormones and the antidepressant are increased.

Warfarin (and other oral anticoagulants): The hypoprothrombinemic response to warfarin may be altered by a change in thyroid function or replacement. Replacement may dramatically increase response to warfarin. However, initiation of warfarin in a patient stabilized on a dose of thyroid hormones does not appear to require a significantly different approach.

Ethanol/Nutrition/Herb Interactions Food: Limit intake of goitrogenic foods (asparagus, cabbage, peas, turnip greens, broccoli, spinach, Brussels sprouts, lettuce, soybeans)

Dosage Forms

Injection, solution, as sodium (Triostat®): 10 mcg/mL (1 mL) [contains alcohol 6.8%]

Tablet, as sodium (Cytomel®): 5 mcg, 25 mcg, 50 mcg

- ♦ **Liothyronine Sodium** *see* Liothyronine *on page 765*
- ♦ **Lipitor®** *see* Atorvastatin *on page 139*
- ♦ **Liposyn® II (Can)** *see* Fat Emulsion *on page 508*
- ♦ **Liposyn® III** *see* Fat Emulsion *on page 508*
- ♦ **Liquid Antidote** *see* Charcoal *on page 259*

Lisinopril (lyse IN oh pril)

Medication Safety Issues

Sound-alike/look-alike issues:

Lisinopril may be confused with fosinopril, Lioresal®, Risperdal®

Prinivil® may be confused with Plendil®, Pravachol®, Prevacid®, Prilosec®, Proventil®

Zestril® may be confused with Desyrel®, Restoril®, Vistaril®, Zetia™, Zostrix®

Related Information

Angiotensin Agents *on page 1544*

Heart Failure (Systolic) *on page 1607*

U.S. Brand Names Prinivil®; Zestril®

Canadian Brand Names Apo-Lisinopril®; Prinivil®; Zestril®

Pharmacologic Category Angiotensin-Converting Enzyme (ACE) Inhibitor

Generic Available Yes

Use Treatment of hypertension, either alone or in combination with other antihypertensive agents; adjunctive therapy in treatment of CHF (afterload reduction); treatment of acute myocardial infarction within 24 hours in hemodynamically-stable patients to improve survival; treatment of left ventricular dysfunction after myocardial infarction

Mechanism of Action Competitive inhibitor of angiotensin-converting enzyme (ACE); prevents conversion of angiotensin I to angiotensin II, a potent vasoconstrictor; results in lower levels of angiotensin II which causes an increase in plasma renin activity and a reduction in aldosterone secretion; a CNS mechanism may also be involved in hypotensive effect as angiotensin II increases adrenergic outflow from CNS; vasoactive kallikreins may be decreased in conversion to active hormones by ACE inhibitors, thus reducing blood pressure

Pharmacodynamics/Kinetics

Onset of action: 1 hour

Peak effect: Hypotensive: Oral: ~6 hours

Duration: 24 hours

Absorption: Well absorbed; unaffected by food

Protein binding: 25%

Half-life elimination: 11-12 hours

Excretion: Primarily urine (as unchanged drug)

(Continued)

Lisinopril *(Continued)*

Dosage Oral:

Hypertension:

Children ≥6 years: Initial: 0.07 mg/kg once daily (up to 5 mg); increase dose at 1- to 2-week intervals; doses >0.61 mg/kg or >40 mg have not been evaluated.

Adults: Usual dosage range (JNC 7): 10-40 mg/day

Not maintained on diuretic: Initial: 10 mg/day

Maintained on diuretic: Initial: 5 mg/day

Note: Antihypertensive effect may diminish toward the end of the dosing interval especially with doses of 10 mg/day. An increased dose may aid in extending the duration of antihypertensive effect. Doses up to 80 mg/day have been used, but do not appear to give greater effect (Zesteril® Product Information, 12/04).

Elderly: Initial: 2.5-5 mg/day; increase doses 2.5-5 mg/day at 1- to 2-week intervals; maximum daily dose: 40 mg

Patients taking diuretics should have them discontinued 2-3 days prior to initiating lisinopril if possible. Restart diuretic after blood pressure is stable if needed. If diuretic cannot be discontinued prior to therapy, begin with 5 mg with close supervision until stable blood pressure. In patients with hyponatremia (<130 mEq/L), start dose at 2.5 mg/day

Congestive heart failure: Adults: Initial: 2.5-5 mg once daily; then increase by no more than 10 mg increments at intervals no less than 2 weeks to a maximum daily dose of 40 mg. Usual maintenance: 5-40 mg/day as a single dose. Target dose: 20-40 mg once daily (ACC/AHA 2005 Heart Failure Guidelines)

Note: If patient has hyponatremia (serum sodium <130 meq/L) or renal impairment (Cl_{cr} <30 mL/minute or creatinine >3 mg/dL), then initial dose should be 2.5 mg/day

Acute myocardial infarction (within 24 hours in hemodynamically stable patients): Oral: 5 mg immediately, then 5 mg at 24 hours, 10 mg at 48 hours, and 10 mg every day thereafter for 6 weeks. Patients should continue to receive standard treatments such as thrombolytics, aspirin, and beta-blockers.

Dosing adjustment in renal impairment:

Hypertension:

Adults: Initial doses should be modified and upward titration should be cautious, based on response (maximum: 40 mg/day)

Cl_{cr} >30 mL/minute: Initial: 10 mg/day

Cl_{cr} 10-30 mL/minute: Initial: 5 mg/day

Hemodialysis: Initial: 2.5 mg/day; dialyzable (50%)

Children: Use in not recommended in pediatric patients with GFR <30 mL/minute/1.73 m^2

Congestive heart failure: Adults: Cl_{cr} <30 mL/minute or creatinine >3 mg/dL): Initial: 2.5 mg/day

Administration Watch for hypotensive effects within 1-3 hours of first dose or new higher dose.

Monitoring Parameters BUN, serum creatinine, renal function, WBC, and potassium

Anesthesia and Critical Care Concerns/Other Considerations Due to decreases in glomerular filtration (also creatinine clearance) with aging, severe congestive heart failure and renal failure, these patients may experience renal dysfunction with ACE inhibitor administration.

ACE inhibitor therapy may elicit rapid increases in potassium and creatinine, especially when used in patients with bilateral renal artery stenosis. When ACE inhibition is introduced in patients with pre-existing diuretic therapy who are hypovolemic, the ACE inhibitor may induce acute hypotension. Concomitant NSAID therapy may attenuate blood pressure control. Because of the potent teratogenic effects of ACE inhibitors, these drugs should be avoided, if possible, when treating women of childbearing potential not on effective birth control measures.

Pregnancy Risk Factor C (1st trimester)/D (2nd and 3rd trimesters)

Contraindications Hypersensitivity to lisinopril or any component of the formulation; angioedema related to previous treatment with an ACE inhibitor; bilateral renal artery stenosis; pregnancy (2nd and 3rd trimesters)

Warnings/Precautions Anaphylactic reactions can occur. Angioedema can occur at any time during treatment (especially following first dose). It may involve head and neck (potentially affecting the airway) or the intestine (presenting with abdominal pain). Prolonged monitoring may be required especially if tongue, glottis, or larynx are involved as they are associated with airway obstruction. Those with a history of airway surgery in this situation have a higher risk. Careful blood pressure monitoring with first dose (hypotension can occur especially in volume-depleted patients). **[U.S. Boxed Warning]: Based on human data, ACEIs can cause injury and death to the developing fetus when used in the second and third trimesters. ACEIs should be discontinued as soon as possible once pregnancy is detected.** Dosage adjustment needed in renal impairment. Use with caution in hypovolemia; collagen vascular diseases; valvular stenosis (particularly aortic stenosis); hyperkalemia; or before, during, or immediately after anesthesia. Avoid rapid dosage escalation, which may lead to renal insufficiency. Rare toxicities associated with ACE inhibitors include cholestatic jaundice (which may progress to hepatic necrosis) and neutropenia/agranulocytosis with myeloid hyperplasia. If patient has renal impairment then a baseline WBC with differential and serum creatinine should be evaluated and monitored closely during the first 3 months of therapy. Hypersensitivity reactions may be seen during hemodialysis with high-flux dialysis membranes (eg, AN69). Deterioration in renal function can occur with initiation. Use with caution in unilateral renal artery stenosis and pre-existing renal insufficiency. Safety and efficacy have not been established in children <6 years of age.

Adverse Reactions Note: Frequency ranges include data from hypertension and heart failure trials. Higher rates of adverse reactions have generally been noted in patients with CHF. However, the frequency of adverse effects associated with placebo is also increased in this population.

1% to 10%:

- Cardiovascular: Orthostatic effects (1%), hypotension (1% to 4%)
- Central nervous system: Headache (4% to 6%), dizziness (5% to 12%), fatigue (3%)
- Dermatologic: Rash (1% to 2%)
- Endocrine & metabolic: Hyperkalemia (2% to 5%)
- Gastrointestinal: Diarrhea (3% to 4%), nausea (2%), vomiting (1%), abdominal pain (2%)
- Genitourinary: Impotence (1%)
- Hematologic: Decreased hemoglobin (small)
- Neuromuscular & skeletal: Chest pain (3%), weakness (1%)
- Renal: BUN increased (2%); deterioration in renal function (in patients with bilateral renal artery stenosis or hypovolemia); serum creatinine increased (often transient)
- Respiratory: Cough (4% to 9%), upper respiratory infection (2% to 2%)

<1% (Limited to important or life-threatening): Acute renal failure, alopecia, anaphylactoid reactions, angioedema, anuria, arrhythmia, arthralgia, asthma, ataxia, azotemia, bone marrow suppression, bronchospasm, cardiac arrest, decreased libido, gout, hepatic necrosis, hepatitis, hyperkalemia, hyponatremia, increased bilirubin, transaminases increased, infiltrates, jaundice (cholestatic), MI, neutropenia, oliguria, orthostatic hypotension, pancreatitis, paresthesia, pemphigus, peripheral neuropathy, photosensitivity, pleural effusion, pulmonary embolism, Stevens-Johnson syndrome, stroke, systemic lupus erythematosus, thrombocytopenia, TIA, toxic epidermal necrolysis, tremor, urticaria, vasculitis, vertigo, vision loss. In addition, a syndrome which may include fever, myalgia, arthralgia, interstitial nephritis, vasculitis, rash, eosinophilia and positive ANA, and elevated ESR has been reported with ACE inhibitors.

Overdosage/Toxicology Mild hypotension has been the primary toxic effect seen with acute overdose. Bradycardia may also occur; hyperkalemia occurs even with therapeutic doses, especially in patients with renal insufficiency and those taking NSAIDs. Treatment and is symptomatic and supportive.

Drug Interactions

- Allopurinol: Case reports (rare) indicate a possible increased risk of hypersensitivity reactions when combined with lisinopril.
- Alpha$_1$ blockers: Hypotensive effect increased.
- Aspirin: The effects of ACE inhibitors may be blunted by aspirin administration, particularly at higher dosages and/or increase adverse renal effects.
- Diuretics: Hypovolemia due to diuretics may precipitate acute hypotensive events or acute renal failure.
- Insulin: Risk of hypoglycemia may be increased.
- Lithium: Risk of lithium toxicity may be increased; monitor lithium levels, especially the first 4 weeks of therapy.

(Continued)

Lisinopril *(Continued)*

Mercaptopurine: Risk of neutropenia may be increased.

NSAIDs: May attenuate hypertensive efficacy; effect has been seen with captopril and may occur with other ACE inhibitors; monitor blood pressure. May increase adverse renal effects.

Potassium-sparing diuretics (amiloride, spironolactone, triamterene): Increased risk of hyperkalemia.

Potassium supplements may increase the risk of hyperkalemia.

Trimethoprim (high dose) may increase the risk of hyperkalemia.

Ethanol/Nutrition/Herb Interactions Herb/Nutraceutical: Avoid dong quai if using for hypertension (has estrogenic activity). Avoid ephedra, yohimbe, ginseng (may worsen hypertension). Avoid garlic (may have increased antihypertensive effect).

Test Interactions May cause false-positive results in urine acetone determinations using sodium nitroprusside reagent; increased potassium (S); increased serum creatinine/BUN

Dosage Forms [DSC] = Discontinued product

Tablet: 2.5 mg, 5 mg, 10 mg, 20 mg, 30 mg, 40 mg

Prinivil®: 5 mg, 10 mg, 20 mg, 30 mg; 40 mg [DSC]

Zestril®: 2.5 mg, 5 mg, 10 mg, 20 mg, 30 mg, 40 mg

◆ **Lispro Insulin** *see* Insulin Lispro *on page 688*

◆ **Lithane™ (Can)** *see* Lithium *on page 770*

Lithium (LITH ee um)

Medication Safety Issues

Sound-alike/look-alike issues:

Eskalith® may be confused with Estratest®

Lithobid® may be confused with Levbid®, Lithostat®

U.S. Brand Names Eskalith® [DSC]; Eskalith CR®; Lithobid®

Canadian Brand Names Apo-Lithium®; Apo-Lithium® Carbonate SR; Carbolith™; Duralith®; Lithane™; PMS-Lithium Carbonate; PMS-Lithium Citrate

Synonyms Lithium Carbonate; Lithium Citrate

Pharmacologic Category Lithium

Generic Available Yes

Use Management of bipolar disorders; treatment of mania in individuals with bipolar disorder (maintenance treatment prevents or diminishes intensity of subsequent episodes)

Unlabeled/Investigational Use Potential augmenting agent for antidepressants; aggression, post-traumatic stress disorder, conduct disorder in children

Mechanism of Action Alters cation transport across cell membrane in nerve and muscle cells and influences reuptake of serotonin and/or norepinephrine; second messenger systems involving the phosphatidylinositol cycle are inhibited; postsynaptic D2 receptor supersensitivity is inhibited

Pharmacodynamics/Kinetics

Absorption: Rapid and complete

Distribution: V_d: Initial: 0.3-0.4 L/kg; V_{dss}: 0.7-1 L/kg; crosses placenta; enters breast milk at 35% to 50% the concentrations in serum; distribution is complete in 6-10 hours

CSF, liver concentrations: $1/3$ to $1/2$ of serum concentration

Erythrocyte concentration: ~$1/2$ of serum concentration

Heart, lung, kidney, muscle concentrations: Equivalent to serum concentration

Saliva concentration: 2-3 times serum concentration

Thyroid, bone, brain tissue concentrations: Increase 50% over serum concentrations

Protein binding: Not protein bound

Metabolism: Not metabolized

Bioavailability: Not affected by food; Capsule, immediate release tablet: 95% to 100%; Extended release tablet: 60% to 90%; Syrup: 100%

Half-life elimination: 18-24 hours; can increase to more than 36 hours in elderly or with renal impairment

Time to peak, serum: Nonsustained release: ~0.5-2 hours; slow release: 4-12 hours; syrup: 15-60 minutes

Excretion: Urine (90% to 98% as unchanged drug); sweat (4% to 5%); feces (1%)

Clearance: 80% of filtered lithium is reabsorbed in the proximal convoluted tubules; therefore, clearance approximates 20% of GFR or 20-40 mL/minute

Dosage Oral: Monitor serum concentrations and clinical response (efficacy and toxicity) to determine proper dose

Children 6-12 years:
- Bipolar disorder: 15-60 mg/kg/day in 3-4 divided doses; dose not to exceed usual adult dosage
- Conduct disorder (unlabeled use): 15-30 mg/kg/day in 3-4 divided doses; dose not to exceed usual adult dosage

Adults: Bipolar disorder: 900-2400 mg/day in 3-4 divided doses or 900-1800 mg/day (sustained release) in 2 divided doses

Elderly: Bipolar disorder: Initial dose: 300 mg once or twice daily; increase weekly in increments of 300 mg/day, monitoring levels; rarely need >900-1200 mg/day

Dosing adjustment in renal impairment:
- Cl_{cr} 10-50 mL/minute: Administer 50% to 75% of normal dose
- Cl_{cr} <10 mL/minute: Administer 25% to 50% of normal dose

Hemodialysis: Dialyzable (50% to 100%); 4-7 times more efficient than peritoneal dialysis

Administration Administer with meals to decrease GI upset. Slow release tablets must be swallowed whole; do not crush or chew.

Monitoring Parameters Serum lithium every 4-5 days during initial therapy; draw lithium serum concentrations 8-12 hours postdose; renal, thyroid, and cardiovascular function; fluid status; serum electrolytes; CBC with differential, urinalysis; monitor for signs of toxicity; beta-hCG pregnancy test for all females not known to be sterile

Reference Range Levels should be obtained twice weekly until both patient's clinical status and levels are stable then levels may be obtained every 1-3 months

Timing of serum samples: Draw trough just before next dose (8-12 hours after previous dose)

Therapeutic levels:
- Acute mania: 0.6-1.2 mEq/L (SI: 0.6-1.2 mmol/L)
- Protection against future episodes in most patients with bipolar disorder: 0.8-1 mEq/L (SI: 0.8-1.0 mmol/L); a higher rate of relapse is described in subjects who are maintained at <0.4 mEq/L (SI: 0.4 mmol/L)
- Elderly patients can usually be maintained at lower end of therapeutic range (0.6-0.8 mEq/L)

Toxic concentration: >1.5 mEq/L (SI: >2 mmol/L)

Adverse effect levels:
- GI complaints/tremor: 1.5-2 mEq/L
- Confusion/somnolence: 2-2.5 mEq/L
- Seizures/death: >2.5 mEq/L

Pregnancy Risk Factor D

Contraindications Hypersensitivity to lithium or any component of the formulation; avoid use in patients with severe cardiovascular or renal disease, or with severe debilitation, dehydration, or sodium depletion; pregnancy

Warnings/Precautions **[U.S. Boxed Warning]: Lithium toxicity is closely related to serum levels and can occur at therapeutic doses; serum lithium determinations are required to monitor therapy.** Use with caution in patients with thyroid disease, mild-moderate renal impairment, or mild-moderate cardiovascular disease. Use caution in patients receiving medications which alter sodium excretion (eg, diuretics, ACE inhibitors, NSAIDs), or in patients with significant fluid loss (protracted sweating, diarrhea, or prolonged fever); temporary reduction or cessation of therapy may be warranted. Some elderly patients may be extremely sensitive to the effects of lithium, see Dosage and Reference Range. Chronic therapy results in diminished renal concentrating ability (nephrogenic DI); this is usually reversible when lithium is discontinued. Changes in renal function should be monitored, and re-evaluation of treatment may be necessary. Use caution in patients at risk of suicide (suicidal thoughts or behavior).

Morphologic changes with glomerular and interstitial fibrosis and nephron atrophy have been reported in patients on chronic lithium therapy; morphologic changes have also been reported in manic-depressive patients never exposed to lithium. The relationship between morphologic changes and renal function, and the association with lithium therapy, have not been established.

Use with caution in patients receiving neuroleptic medications - a syndrome resembling NMS has been associated with concurrent therapy. Lithium may impair the patient's alertness, affecting the ability to operate machinery or driving

(Continued)

Lithium *(Continued)*

a vehicle. Neuromuscular-blocking agents should be administered with caution; the response may be prolonged.

Higher serum concentrations may be required and tolerated during an acute manic phase; however, the tolerance decreases when symptoms subside. Normal fluid and salt intake must be maintained during therapy.

Safety and efficacy have not been established in children <12 years of age.

Adverse Reactions Frequency not defined.

Cardiovascular: Cardiac arrhythmia, hypotension, sinus node dysfunction, flattened or inverted T waves (reversible), edema, bradycardia, syncope

Central nervous system: Dizziness, vertigo, slurred speech, blackout spells, seizure, sedation, restlessness, confusion, psychomotor retardation, stupor, coma, dystonia, fatigue, lethargy, headache, pseudotumor cerebri, slowed intellectual functioning, tics

Dermatologic: Dry or thinning of hair, folliculitis, alopecia, exacerbation of psoriasis, rash

Endocrine & metabolic: Euthyroid goiter and/or hypothyroidism, hyperthyroidism, hyperglycemia, diabetes insipidus

Gastrointestinal: Polydipsia, anorexia, nausea, vomiting, diarrhea, xerostomia, metallic taste, weight gain, salivary gland swelling, excessive salivation

Genitourinary: Incontinence, polyuria, glycosuria, oliguria, albuminuria

Hematologic: Leukocytosis

Neuromuscular & skeletal: Tremor, muscle hyperirritability, ataxia, choreoathetoid movements, hyperactive deep tendon reflexes, myasthenia gravis (rare)

Ocular: Nystagmus, blurred vision, transient scotoma

Miscellaneous: Coldness and painful discoloration of fingers and toes

Overdosage/Toxicology Symptoms include sedation, confusion, tremors, joint pain, visual changes, seizures, and coma. There is no specific antidote for lithium poisoning. For acute ingestion, following initiation of essential overdose management, discontinue lithium and remove any unabsorbed lithium via gastric lavage (activated charcoal is ineffective as it does not bind lithium). Correct fluid and electrolyte imbalances, provide supportive care. In severe cases, patient should be dialyzed. Hemodialysis is preferred (and more effective) than peritoneal dialysis. The goal is to decrease serum lithium level to <1 mEq/L on a serum sample drawn 6-8 hours after completion of dialysis. Agents that increase the excretion of lithium are of questionable value.

Drug Interactions

ACE inhibitors: May increase the risk of lithium toxicity via sodium depletion; monitor

Angiotensin receptor antagonists (losartan): May reduce the renal clearance of lithium; monitor

Caffeine (xanthine derivatives): May lower lithium serum concentrations by increasing urinary lithium excretion; monitor.

Carbamazepine: Concurrent use of lithium with carbamazepine may increase the risk for neurotoxicity; monitor

Carbonic anhydrase inhibitors: May decrease lithium levels; includes acetazolamide; monitor

Calcium channel blockers (diltiazem and verapamil): May increase the risk for neurotoxicity (ataxia, tremors, nausea, vomiting, diarrhea, and/or tinnitus); monitor; does not appear to involve dihydropyridine class

Chlorpromazine: May lower serum concentrations of both drugs; monitor

COX-2 inhibitors (celecoxib): May increase lithium plasma concentrations (similar to NSAIDs); monitor.

Haloperidol: May increase the risk for neurotoxicity and encephalopathy; a rare encephalopathic syndrome resulting in irreversible brain damage has been reported in a few patients (causal relationship not established); monitor

Iodine salts: May enhance the hypothyroid effects of lithium; monitor

Loop diuretics: May decrease the renal excretion of lithium, leading to toxicity; monitor

MAO inhibitors: Should generally be avoided due to use reports of fatal malignant hyperpyrexia when combined with lithium

Methyldopa: May increase the risk for neurotoxicity; monitor

Metronidazole: May increase lithium toxicity (rare); monitor

Neuromuscular-blocking agents: Lithium may potentiate the response to neuromuscular blockade, resulting in prolonged blockade and possible delayed recovery

NSAIDs: Renal lithium excretion may be decreased leading to increased serum lithium concentrations; sulindac and aspirin may be the exceptions; monitor

Phenothiazines: May increase the risk for neurotoxicity; monitor

Phenytoin: May enhance lithium toxicity; monitor

Selegiline: Risk of severe reactions when combined with MAO inhibitors may be decreased when administered with selective MAO type B inhibitor, particularly at selegiline doses <10 mg/day; however, theoretical risk is still present

SSRIs: May increase the risk for neurotoxicity; monitor; effect noted with fluoxetine, fluvoxamine

Sibutramine: Combined use of lithium with sibutramine may increase the risk of serotonin syndrome; this combination is best avoided

Sodium-containing products: Bicarbonate and/or high sodium intake may reduce serum lithium concentrations via enhanced excretion; monitor. **Note:** Reabsorption of lithium in the proximal convoluted tubule occurs against electrical and concentration gradients that do not distinguish between lithium and sodium. Therefore, lithium clearance may increase or decrease 30% to 50% with sodium load or depletion, respectively. Sodium depletion usually has the greater effect.

Sympathomimetics: Lithium may blunt the pressor response to sympathomimetics (epinephrine, phenylephrine, norepinephrine)

Tetracyclines: May increase lithium levels; monitor

Theophylline: May increase real clearance of lithium, resulting in a decrease in serum lithium concentrations; monitor

Thiazide diuretics: May increase serum lithium concentration via sodium depletion and decreased lithium clearance; a lithium dose reduction of 50% is commonly recommended

Tricyclic antidepressants: May increase the risk for neurotoxicity; monitor

Urea: May lower lithium serum concentrations by increasing urinary excretion; monitor.

Ethanol/Nutrition/Herb Interactions Food: Lithium serum concentrations may be increased if taken with food. Limit caffeine.

Dietary Considerations May be taken with meals to avoid GI upset; have patient drink 2-3 L of water daily.

Dosage Forms

[DSC] = Discontinued product

Capsule, as carbonate: 150 mg, 300 mg, 600 mg

Eskalith®: 300 mg [contains benzyl alcohol] [DSC]

Syrup, as citrate: 300 mg/5 mL (5 mL, 10 mL, 480 mL) [contains alcohol]

Tablet, as carbonate: 300 mg

Tablet, controlled release, as carbonate (Eskalith CR®): 450 mg

Tablet, slow release, as carbonate (Lithobid®): 300 mg

References

Mokhlesi B, Leikin JB, Murray P, et al, "Adult Toxicology in Critical Care. Part 11: Specific Poisonings," *Chest*, 2003, 123(3):897-922.

Szerlip HM, Heeger P, and Feldman GM, "Comparison Between Acetate and Bicarbonate Dialysis for the Treatment of Lithium Intoxication," *Am J Nephrol*, 1992, 12(1-2):116-20.

♦ **Lithium Carbonate** *see* Lithium *on page 770*

♦ **Lithium Citrate** *see* Lithium *on page 770*

♦ **Lithobid®** *see* Lithium *on page 770*

♦ **LMD®** *see* Dextran *on page 372*

♦ **Locoid®** *see* Hydrocortisone *on page 639*

♦ **Locoid Lipocream®** *see* Hydrocortisone *on page 639*

♦ **Lodine® [DSC]** *see* Etodolac *on page 496*

♦ **Lodine® XL [DSC]** *see* Etodolac *on page 496*

♦ **Loniten®** *see* Minoxidil *on page 856*

♦ **Lopressor®** *see* Metoprolol *on page 839*

Lorazepam (lor A ze pam)

Medication Safety Issues

Sound-alike/look-alike issues:

Lorazepam may be confused with alprazolam, clonazepam, diazepam, temazepam

(Continued)

Lorazepam *(Continued)*

Ativan® may be confused with Atarax®, Atgam®, Avitene®

Related Information

Anesthesia Considerations for Neurosurgery *on page 1401*
Anesthesia for Patients With Liver Disease *on page 1421*
Benzodiazepines *on page 1555*
Epilepsy *on page 1604*
Intravenous Anesthetic Agents *on page 1531*
Perioperative Management of Patients on Antiseizure Medication *on page 1458*
Sedative Agents in the Intensive Care Unit *on page 1576*

U.S. Brand Names Ativan®; Lorazepam Intensol®

Canadian Brand Names Apo-Lorazepam®; Ativan®; Lorazepam Injection, USP; Novo-Lorazepam; Nu-Loraz; PMS-Lorazepam; Riva-Lorazepam

Pharmacologic Category Benzodiazepine

Restrictions C-IV

Generic Available Yes

Use

Oral: Management of anxiety disorders or short-term relief of the symptoms of anxiety or anxiety associated with depressive symptoms

I.V.: Status epilepticus, preanesthesia for desired amnesia, antiemetic adjunct

Unlabeled/Investigational Use Ethanol detoxification; insomnia; psychogenic catatonia; partial complex seizures; agitation (I.V.)

Mechanism of Action Binds to stereospecific benzodiazepine receptors on the postsynaptic GABA neuron at several sites within the central nervous system, including the limbic system, reticular formation. Enhancement of the inhibitory effect of GABA on neuronal excitability results by increased neuronal membrane permeability to chloride ions. This shift in chloride ions results in hyperpolarization (a less excitable state) and stabilization.

Pharmacodynamics/Kinetics

Onset of action:
- Hypnosis: I.M.: 20-30 minutes
- Sedation: I.V.: 5-20 minutes
- Anticonvulsant: I.V.: 5 minutes, oral: 30-60 minutes

Duration: 6-8 hours

Absorption: Oral, I.M.: Prompt

Distribution:
- V_d: Neonates: 0.76 L/kg, Adults: 1.3 L/kg; crosses placenta; enters breast milk

Protein binding: 85%; free fraction may be significantly higher in elderly

Metabolism: Hepatic to inactive compounds

Half-life elimination: Neonates: 40.2 hours; Older children: 10.5 hours; Adults: 12.9 hours; Elderly: 15.9 hours; End-stage renal disease: 32-70 hours

Excretion: Urine; feces (minimal)

Dosage

Antiemetic:
- Children 2-15 years: I.V.: 0.05 mg/kg (up to 2 mg/dose) prior to chemotherapy
- Adults: Oral, I.V. (**Note:** May be administered sublingually; not a labeled route): 0.5-2 mg every 4-6 hours as needed

Anxiety and sedation:
- Infants and Children: Oral, I.M., I.V.: Usual: 0.05 mg/kg/dose (range: 0.02-0.09 mg/kg) every 4-8 hours
  - I.V.: May use smaller doses (eg, 0.01-0.03 mg/kg) and repeat every 20 minutes, as needed to titrate to effect
- Adults: Oral: 1-10 mg/day in 2-3 divided doses; usual dose: 2-6 mg/day in divided doses
- Elderly: 0.5-4 mg/day; initial dose not to exceed 2 mg

Insomnia: Adults: Oral: 2-4 mg at bedtime

Preoperative: Adults:
- I.M.: 0.05 mg/kg administered 2 hours before surgery (maximum: 4 mg/dose)
- I.V.: 0.044 mg/kg 15-20 minutes before surgery (usual maximum: 2 mg/dose)

Preprocedural anxiety (dental use): Adults: Oral: 1-2 mg 1 hour before procedure

Operative amnesia: Adults: I.V.: Up to 0.05 mg/kg (maximum: 4 mg/dose)

Sedation (preprocedure): Infants and Children:
- Oral, I.M., I.V.: Usual: 0.05 mg/kg (range: 0.02-0.09 mg/kg);
  - I.V.: May use smaller doses (eg, 0.01-0.03 mg/kg) and repeat every 20 minutes, as needed to titrate to effect

Status epilepticus: I.V.:

Infants and Children: 0.1 mg/kg slow I.V. over 2-5 minutes; do not exceed 4 mg/single dose; may repeat second dose of 0.05 mg/kg slow I.V. in 10-15 minutes if needed

Adolescents: 0.07 mg/kg slow I.V. over 2-5 minutes; maximum: 4 mg/dose; may repeat in 10-15 minutes

Adults: 4 mg/dose slow I.V. over 2-5 minutes; may repeat in 10-15 minutes; usual maximum dose: 8 mg

Rapid tranquilization of agitated patient (administer every 30-60 minutes):

Oral: 1-2 mg

I.M.: 0.5-1 mg

Average total dose for tranquilization: Oral, I.M.: 4-8 mg

Agitation in the ICU patient (unlabeled):

I.V.: 0.02-0.06 mg/kg every 2-6 hours

I.V. infusion: 0.01-0.1 mg/kg/hour

Stability

I.V.: Intact vials should be refrigerated, protected from light; do not use discolored or precipitate-containing solutions. May be stored at room temperature for up to 60 days. Parenteral admixture is stable at room temperature (25°C) for 24 hours. Dilute I.V. dose with equal volume of compatible diluent (D_5W, NS, SWI).

Infusion: Use 2 mg/mL injectable solution to prepare; dilute ≤1 mg/mL and mix in glass bottle; precipitation may develop; can also be administered undiluted via infusion.

Tablet: Store at room temperature.

Administration May be administered by I.M., I.V., or orally

I.M.: Should be administered deep into the muscle mass

I.V.: Do not exceed 2 mg/minute or 0.05 mg/kg over 2-5 minutes; dilute I.V. dose with equal volume of compatible diluent (D_5W, NS, SWI).

Monitoring Parameters Respiratory and cardiovascular status, blood pressure, heart rate, symptoms of anxiety

Reference Range Therapeutic: 50-240 ng/mL (SI: 156-746 nmol/L)

Anesthesia and Critical Care Concerns/Other Considerations Lorazepam 2 mg/mL and 4 mg/mL each contains propylene glycol 830 mg/mL (80% v/v).

Agitation in the ICU Patient: Lorazepam has a slower onset of action than midazolam or diazepam, making it less useful for treatment of acute agitation. The polyethylene glycol and propylene glycol solvents in lorazepam injection can accumulate and lead to reversible acute tubular necrosis, lactic acidosis and hyperosmolar states with prolonged, high-dose infusions. Yaucher (2003) and colleagues recently performed a retrospective review of patients who received lorazepam infusions and developed increases in serum creatinine. Eight patients from the medical-surgical intensive care unit or burn unit were evaluated. Lorazepam infusions ranged from 2-28 mg/hour. The mean cumulative dose of lorazepam was 4305 mg and the mean propylene glycol level determined at the time of peak serum creatinine concentration was 1103 mcg/mL. The duration of lorazepam infusion and magnitude of serum creatinine concentration rise correlated (r: 0.60). Propylene glycol levels strongly correlated with both serum osmolality and osmol gap. These authors suggest that serum osmolality and osmol gap may be useful markers of propylene glycol toxicity. A recent case report described a critically-ill man who developed acute tubular necrosis while receiving a lorazepam infusion and sulfamethoxazole-trimethoprim (Hayman, 2003). The addition of sulfamethoxazole-trimethoprim contributed to the development of propylene glycol toxicity. More recently, a prospective, observational study was performed in a medical intensive care unit evaluating patients receiving high-dose lorazepam (≥10 mg/hour) infusions (Arroliga, 2004). The primary objective was to evaluate the relationship between high-dose lorazepam and serum propylene glycol concentrations. Nine patients met the criteria for entry. Baseline creatinine clearances were between 50-100 mL/minute. Propylene glycol accumulation was observed in these patients receiving high-dose lorazepam infusions for ≥48 hours. A significant correlation between high-dose lorazepam infusion rate and serum propylene glycol concentrations was observed. However, osmol gap was the strongest predictor (r^2: 0.80) of serum propylene glycol concentrations. Study findings suggest that in critically-ill adults with normal renal function, serum propylene glycol concentrations may be predicted by the osmol gap. Based on these findings, propylene glycol accumulation may occur as early as 48 hours when using high-dose lorazepam infusions.

(Continued)

Lorazepam *(Continued)*

More recently, a prospective, observational study was performed in a medical intensive care unit evaluating patients receiving high-dose lorazepam (≥10 mg/hour) infusions (Arroliga, 2004). The primary objective was to evaluate the relationship between high-dose lorazepam and serum propylene glycol concentrations. Nine patients met the criteria for entry. Baseline creatinine clearances were 50-100 mL/minute. Propylene glycol accumulation was observed in these patients receiving high-dose lorazepam infusions for ≥48 hours. A significant correlation between high-dose lorazepam infusion rate and serum propylene glycol concentrations was observed. However, osmol gap was the strongest predictor (R^2 = 0.80) of serum propylene glycol concentrations. Study findings suggest that in critically ill adults with normal renal function, serum propylene glycol concentrations may be predicted by the osmol gap. Based on these findings, propylene glycol accumulation may occur as early as 48 hours when using high-dose lorazepam infusions.

To calculate osmolarity: [2 x sodium (mEq/L)] + [glucose (mg/dL)/18] + [BUN (mg/dL)/2.8]

To calculate osmol gap (normal range: 0-5): (measured osmolality minus calculated osmolarity)

Lorazepam is recommended for the sedation of most patients. Use a defined endpoint in titration of the dose. Use a system to minimize prolonged sedative effects. If patient has received high-dose or >7 days of continuous therapy, consider tapering infusion to prevent withdrawal symptoms.

Status Epilepticus: A randomized, double-blind trial (Treiman, 1998) evaluated the efficacy of four treatments in overt status epilepticus. Treatment arms were designed based upon accepted practices of North American neurologists. The treatments were: 1) lorazepam 0.1 mg/kg, 2) diazepam 0.15 mg/kg followed by phenytoin 18 mg/kg, 3) phenytoin 18 mg/kg alone, and 4) phenobarbital 15 mg/kg. Treatment was considered successful if the seizures were terminated (clinically and by EEG) within 20 minutes of start of therapy without seizure recurrence within 60 minutes from the start of therapy. Patients who failed the first treatment received a second and a third, if necessary. Patients did not receive randomized treatments after the first one, but the treating physician remained blinded. Treatment success: Lorazepam 64.9%, phenobarbital 58.2%, diazepam/phenytoin 55.8%, and phenytoin alone 43.6%. Using an "intention-to-treat" analysis, there was no statistical difference between the groups. Results of subsequent treatments in patients who failed the first therapy indicated that response rate significantly dropped regardless of treatment. Aggregate response rate to the second treatment was 7.0% and third treatment 2.3%.

Pregnancy Risk Factor D

Contraindications Hypersensitivity to lorazepam or any component of the formulation (cross-sensitivity with other benzodiazepines may exist); acute narrow-angle glaucoma; sleep apnea (parenteral); intra-arterial injection of parenteral formulation; severe respiratory insufficiency (except during mechanical ventilation); pregnancy

Warnings/Precautions Use with caution in elderly or debilitated patients, patients with hepatic disease (including alcoholics) or renal impairment. Use with caution in patients with respiratory disease or impaired gag reflex. Initial doses in elderly or debilitated patients should not exceed 2 mg. Prolonged lorazepam use may have a possible relationship to GI disease, including esophageal dilation.

The parenteral formulation of lorazepam contains polyethylene glycol and propylene glycol. Also contains benzyl alcohol - avoid in neonates. Concurrent administration with scopolamine results in an increased risk of hallucinations, sedation, and irrational behavior.

Causes CNS depression (dose-related) resulting in sedation, dizziness, confusion, or ataxia which may impair physical and mental capabilities. Patients must be cautioned about performing tasks which require mental alertness (eg, operating machinery or driving). Use with caution in patients receiving other CNS depressants or psychoactive agents. Effects with other sedative drugs or ethanol may be potentiated. Benzodiazepines have been associated with falls and traumatic injury and should be used with extreme caution in patients who are at risk of these events (especially the elderly).

Lorazepam may cause anterograde amnesia. Paradoxical reactions, including hyperactive or aggressive behavior have been reported with benzodiazepines, particularly in adolescent/pediatric or psychiatric patients. Does not have analgesic, antidepressant, or antipsychotic properties.

Use caution in patients with depression, particularly if suicidal risk may be present. Use with caution in patients with a history of drug dependence. Benzodiazepines have been associated with dependence and acute withdrawal symptoms on discontinuation or reduction in dose. Acute withdrawal, including seizures, may be precipitated after administration of flumazenil to patients receiving long-term benzodiazepine therapy.

As a hypnotic agent, should be used only after evaluation of potential causes of sleep disturbance. Failure of sleep disturbance to resolve after 7-10 days may indicate psychiatric or medical illness. A worsening of insomnia or the emergence of new abnormalities of thought or behavior may represent unrecognized psychiatric or medical illness and requires immediate and careful evaluation.

Adverse Reactions

>10%:

- Central nervous system: Sedation
- Respiratory: Respiratory depression

1% to 10%:

- Cardiovascular: Hypotension
- Central nervous system: Confusion, dizziness, akathisia, unsteadiness, headache, depression, disorientation, amnesia
- Dermatologic: Dermatitis, rash
- Gastrointestinal: Weight gain/loss, nausea, changes in appetite
- Neuromuscular & skeletal: Weakness
- Respiratory: Nasal congestion, hyperventilation, apnea

<1% (Limited to important or life-threatening): Menstrual irregularities, increased salivation, blood dyscrasias, reflex slowing, physical and psychological dependence with prolonged use, polyethylene glycol or propylene glycol poisoning (prolonged I.V. infusion)

Overdosage/Toxicology Symptoms of overdose include confusion, coma, hypoactive reflexes, dyspnea, labored breathing. **Note:** Prolonged infusions have been associated with toxicity from propylene glycol and/or polyethylene glycol. Treatment for benzodiazepine overdose is supportive. Flumazenil has been shown to selectively block the binding of benzodiazepines to CNS receptors, resulting in a reversal of benzodiazepine-induced CNS depression but not respiratory depression

Drug Interactions

CNS depressants: Sedative effects and/or respiratory depression may be additive with CNS depressants; includes ethanol, barbiturates, narcotic analgesics, and other sedative agents; monitor for increased effect

Levodopa: Lorazepam may decrease the antiparkinsonian efficacy of levodopa (limited documentation); monitor

Loxapine: There are rare reports of significant respiratory depression, stupor, and/or hypotension with concomitant use of loxapine and lorazepam; use caution if concomitant administration of loxapine and CNS drugs is required

Scopolamine: May increase the incidence of sedation, hallucinations, and irrational behavior; reported only with parenteral lorazepam

Theophylline: May partially antagonize some of the effects of benzodiazepines; monitor for decreased response; may require higher doses for sedation

Ethanol/Nutrition/Herb Interactions

Ethanol: Avoid or limit ethanol (may increase CNS depression).

Herb/Nutraceutical: Avoid valerian, St John's wort, kava kava, gotu kola (may increase CNS depression).

Dosage Forms

Injection, solution (Ativan®): 2 mg/mL (1 mL, 10 mL); 4 mg/mL (1 mL, 10 mL) [contains benzyl alcohol]

Solution, oral concentrate (Lorazepam Intensol®): 2 mg/mL (30 mL) [alcohol free, dye free]

Tablet (Ativan®): 0.5 mg, 1 mg, 2 mg

References

Alldredge BK, Gelb AM, Isaacs SM, et al, "A Comparison of Lorazepam, Diazepam, and Placebo for the Treatment of Out-of-Hospital Status Epilepticus," *N Engl J Med*, 2001, 345(9):631-7.

Arroliga AC, Shehab N, McCarthy K, et al, "Relationship of Continuous Infusion Lorazepam to Serum Propylene Glycol Concentration in Critically Ill Adults," *Crit Care Med*, 2004, 32(8):1709-14.

Barnes BJ, Gerst C, Smith JR, et al, "Osmol Gap as a Surrogate Marker for Serum Propylene Glycol Concentrations in Patients Receiving Lorazepam for Sedation," *Pharmacotherapy*, 2006, 26(1):23-33.

(Continued)

Lorazepam *(Continued)*

Bleck TP, "Seizures, Stroke, and Other Neurologic Emergencies," *Multidisciplinary Critical Care Review*, Zimmerman JL and Roberts PR, eds, Des Plaines, IL: Society of Critical Care Medicine, 2003, 325-34.

Crawford TO, Mitchell WG, and Snodgrass SR, "Lorazepam in Childhood Status Epilepticus and Serial Seizures: Effectiveness and Tachyphylaxis," *Neurology*, 1987, 37(2):190-5.

Hayman M, Seidl EC, Ali M, et al, "Acute Tubular Necrosis Associated With Propylene Glycol From Concomitant Administration of Intravenous Lorazepam and Trimethoprim-Sulfamethoxazole," *Pharmacotherapy*, 2003, 23(9):1190-4.

Jacobi J, Fraser GL, Coursin DB, et al, "Clinical Practice Guidelines for the Sustained Use of Sedatives and Analgesics in the Critically Ill Adult," *Crit Care Med*, 2002, 30(1):119-41. Available at: http://www.sccm.org/pdf/sedatives.pdf.

Mokhlesi B, Leikin JB, Murray P, et al, "Adult Toxicology in Critical Care. Part 11: Specific Poisonings," *Chest*, 2003, 123(3):897-922.

"New Treatment Strategies in the Treatment of Status Epilepticus," *Mayo Clin Proc*, 2003, 78(4):508-18.

Treiman DM, Meyers PD, Walton NY, et al, "A Comparison of Four Treatments for Generalized Convulsive Status Epilepticus. Veterans Affairs Status Epilepticus Cooperative Study Group," *N Engl J Med*, 1998, 339(12):792-8.

Yaucher NE, Fish JT, Smith HW, et al, "Propylene Glycol-Associated Renal Toxicity From Lorazepam Infusion," *Pharmacotherapy*, 2003, 23(9):1094-9.

- **Lorazepam Injection, USP (Can)** *see* Lorazepam *on page 773*
- **Lorazepam Intensol®** *see* Lorazepam *on page 773*
- **Lorcet® 10/650** *see* Hydrocodone and Acetaminophen *on page 636*
- **Lorcet®-HD [DSC]** *see* Hydrocodone and Acetaminophen *on page 636*
- **Lorcet® Plus** *see* Hydrocodone and Acetaminophen *on page 636*
- **Lortab®** *see* Hydrocodone and Acetaminophen *on page 636*

Losartan (loe SAR tan)

Medication Safety Issues

Sound-alike/look-alike issues:

Losartan may be confused with valsartan

Cozaar® may be confused with Hyzaar®, Zocor®

Related Information

Angiotensin Agents *on page 1544*

U.S. Brand Names Cozaar®

Canadian Brand Names Cozaar®

Synonyms DuP 753; Losartan Potassium; MK594

Pharmacologic Category Angiotensin II Receptor Blocker

Generic Available No

Use Treatment of hypertension (HTN); treatment of diabetic nephropathy in patients with type 2 diabetes mellitus (noninsulin dependent, NIDDM) and a history of hypertension; stroke risk reduction in patients with HTN and left ventricular hypertrophy (LVH)

Mechanism of Action As a selective and competitive, nonpeptide angiotensin II receptor antagonist, losartan blocks the vasoconstrictor and aldosterone-secreting effects of angiotensin II; losartan interacts reversibly at the AT1 and AT2 receptors of many tissues and has slow dissociation kinetics; its affinity for the AT1 receptor is 1000 times greater than the AT2 receptor. Angiotensin II receptor antagonists may induce a more complete inhibition of the renin-angiotensin system than ACE inhibitors, they do not affect the response to bradykinin, and are less likely to be associated with nonrenin-angiotensin effects (eg, cough and angioedema). Losartan increases urinary flow rate and in addition to being natriuretic and kaliuretic, increases excretion of chloride, magnesium, uric acid, calcium, and phosphate.

Pharmacodynamics/Kinetics

Onset of action: 6 hours

Distribution: V_d: Losartan: 34 L; E-3174: 12 L; does not cross blood brain barrier

Protein binding, plasma: High

Metabolism: Hepatic (14%) via CYP2C9 and 3A4 to active metabolite, E-3174 (40 times more potent than losartan); extensive first-pass effect

Bioavailability: 25% to 33%; AUC of E-3174 is four times greater than that of losartan

Half-life elimination: Losartan: 1.5-2 hours; E-3174: 6-9 hours

Time to peak, serum: Losartan: 1 hour; E-3174: 3-4 hours

Excretion: Urine (4% as unchanged drug, 6% as active metabolite)

Clearance: Plasma: Losartan: 600 mL/minute; Active metabolite: 50 mL/minute

Dosage Oral:

Hypertension:

Children 6-16 years: 0.7 mg/kg once daily (maximum: 50 mg/day); adjust dose based on response; doses >1.4 mg/kg (maximum: 100 mg) have not been studied

Adults: Usual starting dose: 50 mg once daily; can be administered once or twice daily with total daily doses ranging from 25-100 mg

Patients receiving diuretics or with intravascular volume depletion: Usual initial dose: 25 mg

Nephropathy in patients with type 2 diabetes and hypertension: Adults: Initial: 50 mg once daily; can be increased to 100 mg once daily based on blood pressure response

Stroke reduction (HTN with LVH): Adults: 50 mg once daily (maximum daily dose: 100 mg); may be used in combination with a thiazide diuretic

Dosing adjustment in renal impairment:

Children: Use is not recommended if Cl_{cr} <30 mL/minute.

Adults: No adjustment necessary.

Dosing adjustment in hepatic impairment: Reduce the initial dose to 25 mg/day; divide dosage intervals into two.

Stability Store at 15°C to 30°C (59°F to 86°F); protect from light

Administration May be administered with or without food.

Monitoring Parameters Supine blood pressure, electrolytes, serum creatinine, BUN, urinalysis, symptomatic hypotension and tachycardia, CBC

Anesthesia and Critical Care Concerns/Other Considerations The angiotensin II receptor antagonists appear to have similar indications as the ACE inhibitors. In heart failure, the angiotensin II antagonists are especially useful in providing an alternative therapy in those patients who have intractable cough in response to ACE inhibitor therapy. Candesartan has been studied as an alternative therapy in chronic heart failure patients who cannot tolerate an ACE-I (CHARM-Alternative) and as an added therapy in heart failure patients who are maintained on an ACE-I (CHARM-Added). In both studies the combined endpoint of cardiovascular death or heart failure hospitalizations was significantly improved over the placebo treated group. Similar to ACE inhibitors, pre-existing volume depletion caused by diuretic therapy may potentiate hypotension in response to angiotensin II antagonists. Concomitant NSAID therapy may attenuate blood pressure control; use of NSAIDs should be avoided or limited, with monitoring of blood pressure control. In the setting of heart failure, NSAID use may be associated with an increased risk for fluid accumulation and edema.

Pregnancy Risk Factor C/D (2nd and 3rd trimesters)

Contraindications Hypersensitivity to losartan or any component of the formulation; hypersensitivity to other A-II receptor antagonists; bilateral renal artery stenosis; pregnancy (2nd and 3rd trimesters)

Warnings/Precautions [U.S. Boxed Warning]: Based on human data, drugs that act on the angiotensin system can cause injury and death to the developing fetus when used in the second and third trimesters. Angiotensin receptor blockers should be discontinued as soon as possible once pregnancy is detected. Avoid use or use a smaller dose in patients who are volume depleted; correct depletion first. Deterioration in renal function can occur with initiation. May cause hyperkalemia; avoid potassium supplementation unless specifically required by healthcare provider. Use with caution in unilateral renal artery stenosis and pre-existing renal insufficiency; significant aortic/mitral stenosis. When used to reduce the risk of stroke in patients with HTN and LVH, may not be effective in the African-American population. Use caution with hepatic dysfunction, dose adjustment may be needed. Safety and efficacy in children <6 years of age have not been established.

Adverse Reactions

>10%:

Cardiovascular: Chest pain (12% diabetic nephropathy)

Central nervous system: Fatigue (14% diabetic nephropathy)

Endocrine: Hypoglycemia (14% diabetic nephropathy)

Gastrointestinal: Diarrhea (2% hypertension to 15% diabetic nephropathy)

Genitourinary: Urinary tract infection (13% diabetic nephropathy)

Hematologic: Anemia (14% diabetic nephropathy)

Neuromuscular & skeletal: Weakness (14% diabetic nephropathy), back pain (2% hypertension to 12% diabetic nephropathy)

Respiratory: Cough (≤3% to 11%; similar to placebo; incidence higher in patients with previous cough related to ACE inhibitor therapy)

(Continued)

Losartan *(Continued)*

1% to 10%:

Cardiovascular: Hypotension (7% diabetic nephropathy), orthostatic hypotension (4% hypertension to 4% diabetic nephropathy), first-dose hypotension (dose related: <1% with 50 mg, 2% with 100 mg)

Central nervous system: Dizziness (4%), hypoesthesia (5% diabetic nephropathy), fever (4% diabetic nephropathy), insomnia (1%)

Dermatology: Cellulitis (7% diabetic nephropathy)

Endocrine: Hyperkalemia (<1% hypertension to 7% diabetic nephropathy)

Gastrointestinal: Gastritis (5% diabetic nephropathy), weight gain (4% diabetic nephropathy), dyspepsia (1% to 4%), abdominal pain (2%), nausea (2%)

Neuromuscular & skeletal: Muscular weakness (7% diabetic nephropathy), knee pain (5% diabetic nephropathy), leg pain (1% to 5%), muscle cramps (1%), myalgia (1%)

Respiratory: Bronchitis (10% diabetic nephropathy), upper respiratory infection (8%), nasal congestion (2%), sinusitis (1% hypertension to 6% diabetic nephropathy)

Miscellaneous: Infection (5% diabetic nephropathy), flu-like syndrome (10% diabetic nephropathy)

>1% but frequency ≤ placebo: Edema, abdominal pain, nausea, headache, pharyngitis

<1% (Limited to important or life-threatening): Acute psychosis with paranoid delusions, ageusia, alopecia, anemia, angina, angioedema, arrhythmia, AV block (second degree), depression, dysgeusia, dyspnea, gout, Henoch-Schönlein purpura, hepatitis, hyperkalemia, hyponatremia, impotence, maculopapular rash, MI, panic disorder, pancreatitis, paresthesia, peripheral neuropathy, photosensitivity, renal impairment (patients dependent on renin-angiotensin-aldosterone system), rhabdomyolysis (rare), stroke, syncope, thrombocytopenia (rare), urticaria, vasculitis, vertigo

Overdosage/Toxicology Hypotension and tachycardia may occur with significant overdose. Treatment should be supportive. Not removed via hemodialysis.

Drug Interactions Substrate (major) of CYP2C9, 3A4; **Inhibits** CYP1A2 (weak), 2C8 (moderate), 2C9 (moderate), 2C19 (weak), 3A4 (weak)

CYP2C9 inducers: May decrease the levels/effects of losartan. Example inducers include carbamazepine, phenobarbital, phenytoin, rifampin, rifapentine, and secobarbital.

CYP2C8 Substrates: Losartan may increase the levels/effects of CYP2C8 substrates. Example substrates include amiodarone, paclitaxel, pioglitazone, repaglinide, and rosiglitazone.

CYP2C9 Substrates: Losartan may increase the levels/effects of CYP2C9 substrates. Example substrates include bosentan, dapsone, fluoxetine, glimepiride, glipizide, montelukast, nateglinide, paclitaxel, phenytoin, warfarin, and zafirlukast.

CYP3A4 inducers: CYP3A4 inducers may decrease the levels/effects of losartan. Example inducers include aminoglutethimide, carbamazepine, nafcillin, nevirapine, phenobarbital, phenytoin, and rifamycins.

Fluconazole: Increases plasma levels of losartan via 2C8/9 inhibition (decreases the plasma levels of the active metabolite). Monitor for increased losartan efficacy.

Lithium: Risk of toxicity may be increased by losartan; monitor lithium levels.

NSAIDs: May decrease angiotensin II antagonist efficacy; effect has been seen with losartan, but may occur with other medications in this class; monitor blood pressure

Potassium-sparing diuretics (amiloride, potassium, spironolactone, triamterene): Increased risk of hyperkalemia.

Potassium supplements may increase the risk of hyperkalemia.

Rifampin may reduce antihypertensive efficacy of losartan.

Trimethoprim (high dose) may increase the risk of hyperkalemia.

Ethanol/Nutrition/Herb Interactions Herb/Nutraceutical: St John's wort may decrease levels. Avoid dong quai if using for hypertension (has estrogenic activity). Avoid ephedra, yohimbe, ginseng (may worsen hypertension). Avoid garlic (may have increased antihypertensive effect).

Dietary Considerations May be taken with or without food.

Dosage Forms Tablet, as potassium: 25 mg, 50 mg, 100 mg

- **Losartan Potassium** *see* Losartan *on page 778*
- **Losec® (Can)** *see* Omeprazole *on page 957*

- **Losec MUPS® (Can)** *see* Omeprazole *on page 957*
- **Lotemax®** *see* Loteprednol *on page 781*
- **Lotensin®** *see* Benazepril *on page 163*

Loteprednol (loe te PRED nol)

U.S. Brand Names Alrex®; Lotemax®

Canadian Brand Names Alrex®; Lotemax®

Synonyms Loteprednol Etabonate

Pharmacologic Category Corticosteroid, Ophthalmic

Generic Available No

Use

Suspension, 0.2% (Alrex®): Temporary relief of signs and symptoms of seasonal allergic conjunctivitis

Suspension, 0.5% (Lotemax®): Inflammatory conditions (treatment of steroid-responsive inflammatory conditions of the palpebral and bulbar conjunctiva, cornea, and anterior segment of the globe such as allergic conjunctivitis, acne rosacea, superficial punctate keratitis, herpes zoster keratitis, iritis, cyclitis, selected infective conjunctivitis, when the inherent hazard of steroid use is accepted to obtain an advisable diminution in edema and inflammation) and treatment of postoperative inflammation following ocular surgery

Mechanism of Action Corticosteroids inhibit the inflammatory response including edema, capillary dilation, leukocyte migration, and scar formation. Loteprednol is highly lipid soluble and penetrates cells readily to induce the production of lipocortins. These proteins modulate the activity of prostaglandins and leukotrienes.

Pharmacodynamics/Kinetics Absorption: None

Dosage Adults: Ophthalmic:

Suspension, 0.2% (Alrex®): Instill 1 drop into affected eye(s) 4 times/day

Suspension, 0.5% (Lotemax®):

Inflammatory conditions: Apply 1-2 drops into the conjunctival sac of the affected eye(s) 4 times/day. During the initial treatment within the first week, the dosing may be increased up to 1 drop every hour. Advise patients not to discontinue therapy prematurely. If signs and symptoms fail to improve after 2 days, re-evaluate the patient.

Postoperative inflammation: Apply 1-2 drops into the conjunctival sac of the operated eye(s) 4 times/day beginning 24 hours after surgery and continuing throughout the first 2 weeks of the postoperative period

Administration Shake well before using

Monitoring Parameters Intraocular pressure (if >10 days)

Pregnancy Risk Factor C

Contraindications Hypersensitivity to loteprednol, other corticosteroids, and any component of the formulation; viral diseases of the cornea and conjunctiva; mycobacterial infection of the eye; fungal diseases of ocular structures

Warnings/Precautions For ophthalmic use only; patients should be re-evaluated if symptoms fail to improve after 2 days. Intraocular pressure should be monitored if this product is used >10 days. Prolonged use may result in glaucoma and injury to the optic nerve. Visual defects in acuity and field of vision may occur. Posterior subcapsular cataracts may form after long-term use. Use with caution in presence of glaucoma (steroids increase intraocular pressure). Perforation may occur with topical steroids in diseases which thin the cornea or sclera. Steroids may mask infection or enhance existing infection. Steroid use may delay healing after cataract surgery.

Adverse Reactions

>10%:

Central nervous system: Headache

Respiratory: Rhinitis, pharyngitis

1% to 10%: Ocular: Abnormal vision/blurring, burning on instillation, chemosis, dry eyes, itching, injection, conjunctivitis/irritation, corneal abnormalities, eyelid erythema, papillae uveitis

<1% (Limited to important or life-threatening): Cataract formation, changes in visual acuity and/or field defects, global perforation in disease which thins cornea or sclera, increased intraocular pressure, secondary ocular infection

Dosage Forms Suspension, ophthalmic, as etabonate:

Alrex®: 0.2% (5 mL, 10 mL) [contains benzalkonium chloride]

Lotemax®: 0.5% (2.5 mL, 5 mL, 10 mL, 15 mL) [contains benzalkonium chloride]

♦ **Loteprednol Etabonate** *see* Loteprednol *on page 781*
♦ **Lotronex®** *see* Alosetron *on page 63*

Lovastatin (LOE va sta tin)

Medication Safety Issues
Sound-alike/look-alike issues:
Lovastatin may be confused with Leustatin®, Livostin®, Lotensin®
Mevacor® may be confused with Mivacron®

Related Information
Hyperlipidemia Management *on page 1614*

U.S. Brand Names Altoprev™; Mevacor®

Canadian Brand Names Apo-Lovastatin®; CO Lovastatin; Gen-Lovastatin; Mevacor®; Novo-Lovastatin; Nu-Lovastatin; PMS-Lovastatin; RAN™-Lovastatin; ratio-Lovastatin; Riva-Lovastatin; Sandoz-Lovastatin

Synonyms Mevinolin; Monacolin K

Pharmacologic Category Antilipemic Agent, HMG-CoA Reductase Inhibitor

Generic Available Yes: Immediate release tablet

Use
Adjunct to dietary therapy to decrease elevated serum total and LDL-cholesterol concentrations in primary hypercholesterolemia
Primary prevention of coronary artery disease (patients without symptomatic disease with average to moderately elevated total and LDL-cholesterol and below average HDL-cholesterol); slow progression of coronary atherosclerosis in patients with coronary heart disease
Adjunct to dietary therapy in adolescent patients (10-17 years of age, females >1 year postmenarche) with heterozygous familial hypercholesterolemia having LDL >189 mg/dL, **or** LDL >160 mg/dL with positive family history of premature cardiovascular disease (CVD), **or** LDL >160 mg/dL with the presence of at least two other CVD risk factors

Mechanism of Action Lovastatin acts by competitively inhibiting 3-hydroxyl-3-methylglutaryl-coenzyme A (HMG-CoA) reductase, the enzyme that catalyzes the rate-limiting step in cholesterol biosynthesis

Pharmacodynamics/Kinetics
Onset of action: LDL-cholesterol reductions: 3 days
Absorption: 30%; increased with extended release tablets when taken in the fasting state
Protein binding: 95%
Metabolism: Hepatic; extensive first-pass effect; hydrolyzed to B-hydroxy acid (active)
Bioavailability: Increased with extended release tablets
Half-life elimination: 1.1-1.7 hours
Time to peak, serum: 2-4 hours
Excretion: Feces (~80% to 85%); urine (10%)

Dosage Oral:
Adolescents 10-17 years: Immediate release tablet:
LDL reduction <20%: Initial: 10 mg/day with evening meal
LDL reduction ≥20%: Initial: 20 mg/day with evening meal
Usual range: 10-40 mg with evening meal, then adjust dose at 4-week intervals
Adults: Initial: 20 mg with evening meal, then adjust at 4-week intervals; maximum dose: 80 mg/day immediate release tablet **or** 60 mg/day extended release tablet

Dosage modification/limits based on concurrent therapy:
Cyclosporine and other immunosuppressant drugs: Initial dose: 10 mg/day with a maximum recommended dose of 20 mg/day
Concurrent therapy with fibrates, danazol, and/or lipid-lowering doses of niacin (>1 g/day): Maximum recommended dose: 20 mg/day. Concurrent use with fibrates should be avoided unless risk to benefit favors use.
Concurrent therapy with amiodarone or verapamil: Maximum recommended dose: 40 mg/day of regular release or 20 mg/day with extended release.

Dosage adjustment in renal impairment: Cl_{cr} <30 mL/minute: Use doses >20 mg/day with caution.

Stability
Tablet, immediate release: Store between 5°C to 30°C (41°F to 86°F); protect from light

Tablet, extended release: Store between 20°C to 25°C (68°F to 77°F); avoid excessive heat and humidity

Administration Administer immediate release tablet with meals. Administer extended release tablet at bedtime; do not crush or chew.

Monitoring Parameters

Obtain baseline LFTs and total cholesterol profile. LFTs should also be assessed prior to upwards dosage adjustment to ≥40 mg daily or when otherwise indicated clinically. Enzyme levels should be followed periodically thereafter as clinically warranted.

Reference Range NCEP classification of pediatric patients with familial history of hypercholesterolemia or premature CVD: Acceptable total cholesterol: <170 mg/dL, LDL: <110 mg/dL

Anesthesia and Critical Care Concerns/Other Considerations Myopathy: Currently-marketed HMG-CoA reductase inhibitors appear to have a similar potential for causing myopathy. Incidence of severe myopathy is about 0.08% to 0.09%. The factors that increase risk include advanced age (especially >80 years), gender (occurs in women more frequently than men), small body frame, frailty, multisystem disease (eg, chronic renal insufficiency especially due to diabetes), multiple medications, **perioperative periods (higher risk when continued during hospitalization for major surgery)**, and drug interactions (use with caution or avoid).

Pregnancy Risk Factor X

Contraindications Hypersensitivity to lovastatin or any component of the formulation; active liver disease; unexplained persistent elevations of serum transaminases; pregnancy; breast-feeding

Warnings/Precautions Liver function tests should be assessed before initiation of therapy in patients with a history of liver disease, prior to upwards dosage adjustment to ≥40 mg daily or when otherwise indicated; enzyme levels should be followed periodically thereafter as clinically warranted. Rhabdomyolysis with or without acute renal failure has occurred. Risk is dose-related and is increased with concurrent use of lipid-lowering agents which may cause rhabdomyolysis (gemfibrozil, fibric acid derivatives, or niacin at doses ≥1 g/day) or during concurrent use with potent CYP3A4 inhibitors. Avoid concurrent use of azole antifungals, macrolide antibiotics, and protease inhibitors. Use caution/limit dose with amiodarone, cyclosporine, danazol, gemfibrozil (or other fibrates), lipid-lowering doses of niacin, or verapamil. Patients should be instructed to report unexplained muscle pain or weakness; lovastatin should be discontinued if myopathy is suspected/confirmed. Temporarily discontinue in any patient experiencing an acute or serious condition predisposing to renal failure secondary to rhabdomyolysis. Use with caution in patients who consume large amounts of ethanol or have a history of liver disease. Safety and efficacy of the immediate release tablet have not been evaluated in prepubertal patients, patients <10 years of age, or doses >40 mg/day in appropriately-selected adolescents; extended release tablets have not been studied in patients <20 years of age.

Adverse Reactions Percentages as reported with immediate release tablets; similar adverse reactions seen with extended release tablets.

>10%: Neuromuscular & skeletal: Increased CPK (>2x normal) (11%)

1% to 10%:

- Central nervous system: Headache (2% to 3%), dizziness (0.5% to 1%)
- Dermatologic: Rash (0.8% to 1%)
- Gastrointestinal: Abdominal pain (2% to 3%), constipation (2% to 4%), diarrhea (2% to 3%), dyspepsia (1% to 2%), flatulence (4% to 5%), nausea (2% to 3%)
- Neuromuscular & skeletal: Myalgia (2% to 3%), weakness (1% to 2%), muscle cramps (0.6% to 1%)
- Ocular: Blurred vision (0.8% to 1%)

<1% (Limited to important or life-threatening): Acid regurgitation, alopecia, arthralgia, chest pain, dermatomyositis, eye irritation, insomnia, leg pain, paresthesia, pruritus, vomiting, xerostomia

Additional class-related events or case reports (not necessarily reported with lovastatin therapy): Alkaline phosphatase increased, alopecia, alteration in taste, anaphylaxis, angioedema, anorexia, anxiety, arthritis, cataracts, chills, cholestatic jaundice, cirrhosis, CPK increased (>10x normal), depression, dryness of skin/mucous membranes, dyspnea, eosinophilia, erectile dysfunction, erythema multiforme, ESR increased, facial paresis, fatty liver, fever, flushing, fulminant hepatic necrosis, GGT increased, gynecomastia, hemolytic anemia, hepatitis, hepatoma, hyperbilirubinemia, hypersensitivity reaction, impaired extraocular muscle movement, impotence, leukopenia, libido

(Continued)

Lovastatin *(Continued)*

decreased, malaise, memory loss, myopathy, nail changes, nodules, ophthalmoplegia, pancreatitis, paresthesia, peripheral nerve palsy, peripheral neuropathy, photosensitivity, polymyalgia rheumatica, positive ANA, pruritus, psychic disturbance, purpura, rash, renal failure (secondary to rhabdomyolysis), rhabdomyolysis, skin discoloration, Stevens-Johnson syndrome, systemic lupus erythematosus-like syndrome, thrombocytopenia, thyroid dysfunction, toxic epidermal necrolysis, transaminases increased, tremor, urticaria, vasculitis, vertigo, vomiting

Overdosage/Toxicology Few adverse events have been reported. Treatment is symptomatic.

Drug Interactions **Substrate** of CYP3A4 (major); **Inhibits** CYP2C9 (weak), 2D6 (weak), 3A4 (weak)

Amiodarone: Inhibits metabolism of lovastatin and may increase lovastatin-induced myopathy and rhabdomyolysis. Concurrent use is not recommended, but if unavoidable, dose of lovastatin should be limited.

Antacids: Plasma concentrations may be decreased when given with magnesium-aluminum hydroxide containing antacids (reported with atorvastatin and pravastatin). Clinical efficacy is not altered, no dosage adjustment is necessary

Azole antifungals: May decrease the metabolism, via CYP isoenzymes, of HMG-CoA reductase inhibitors and may increase risk of lovastatin-induced myopathy and rhabdomyolysis. Avoid concurrent use.

Cholestyramine reduces absorption of several HMG-CoA reductase inhibitors. Separate administration times by at least 4 hours.

Cholestyramine and colestipol (bile acid sequestrants): Cholesterol-lowering effects are additive.

Clofibrate and fenofibrate may increase the risk of myopathy and rhabdomyolysis; limit dose of lovastatin

Cyclosporine: Concurrent use may increase risk of myopathy; limit dose of lovastatin

CYP3A4 inhibitors: May increase the levels/effects of lovastatin. Example inhibitors include azole antifungals, clarithromycin, diclofenac, doxycycline, erythromycin, imatinib, isoniazid, nefazodone, nicardipine, propofol, protease inhibitors, quinidine, telithromycin, and verapamil. Avoid concurrrent use.

Danazol: Concurrent use may increase risk of myopathy; limit dose of lovastatin.

Gemfibrozil: Increased risk of myopathy and rhabdomyolysis; limit dose of lovastatin

Grapefruit juice may inhibit metabolism of lovastatin via CYP3A4; avoid high dietary intakes of grapefruit juice.

Isradipine may decrease lovastatin blood levels.

Macrolide antibiotics: May decrease the metabolism, via CYP isoenzymes, of HMG-CoA reductase inhibitors and may increase risk of lovastatin-induced myopathy and rhabdomyolysis. Avoid concurrent use.

Nefazodone: May decrease the metabolism, via CYP isoenzymes, of HMG-CoA reductase inhibitors and may increase risk of lovastatin-induced myopathy and rhabdomyolysis. Avoid concurrent use.

Niacin (at higher dosages ≥1 g/day) may increase risk of myopathy and rhabdomyolysis; limit dose of lovastatin

Protease inhibitors: Concurrent use increases the risk of myopathy and rhabdomyolysis; concurrent use should be avoided.

Verapamil: Inhibits metabolism of lovastatin and may increase lovastatin-induced myopathy and rhabdomyolysis. Concurrent use is not recommended, but if unavoidable, dose of lovastatin should be limited.

Warfarin effect (hypoprothrombinemic response) may be increased; monitor INR closely when lovastatin is initiated or discontinued.

Ethanol/Nutrition/Herb Interactions

Ethanol: Avoid excessive ethanol consumption (due to potential hepatic effects).

Food: Food **decreases** the bioavailability of lovastatin extended release tablets and **increases** the bioavailability of lovastatin immediate release tablets. Lovastatin serum concentrations may be increased if taken with grapefruit juice; avoid concurrent intake of large quantities (>1 quart/day). Red yeast rice contains an estimated 2.4 mg lovastatin per 600 mg rice.

Herb/Nutraceutical: St John's wort may decrease lovastatin levels.

Test Interactions Altered thyroid function tests

Dietary Considerations Before initiation of therapy, patients should be placed on a standard cholesterol-lowering diet for 6 weeks and the diet should be continued during drug therapy. Avoid intake of large quantities of grapefruit juice (≥1 quart/day); may increase toxicity. Red yeast rice contains an estimated 2.4 mg lovastatin per 600 mg rice.

Dosage Forms

Tablet: 10 mg, 20 mg, 40 mg

Mevacor®: 20 mg, 40 mg

Tablet, extended release (Altoprev™): 10 mg, 20 mg, 40 mg, 60 mg

- ♦ **Lovenox®** *see* Enoxaparin *on page 451*
- ♦ **Lovenox® HP (Can)** *see* Enoxaparin *on page 451*
- ♦ **LTA® 360** *see* Lidocaine *on page 755*
- ♦ **LTG** *see* Lamotrigine *on page 727*
- ♦ ***L*-Thyroxine Sodium** *see* Levothyroxine *on page 751*
- ♦ **Lucidex [OTC]** *see* Caffeine *on page 211*
- ♦ **Luminal® Sodium** *see* Phenobarbital *on page 1008*
- ♦ **Luxiq®** *see* Betamethasone *on page 169*
- ♦ **LY146032** *see* Daptomycin *on page 352*
- ♦ **Macrobid®** *see* Nitrofurantoin *on page 927*
- ♦ **Macrodantin®** *see* Nitrofurantoin *on page 927*

Mafenide (MA fe nide)

U.S. Brand Names Sulfamylon®

Synonyms Mafenide Acetate

Pharmacologic Category Antibiotic, Topical

Generic Available No

Use Adjunct in the treatment of second- and third-degree burns to prevent septicemia caused by susceptible organisms such as *Pseudomonas aeruginosa*

Orphan drug: Prevention of graft loss of meshed autografts on excised burn wounds

Mechanism of Action Interferes with bacterial folic acid synthesis through competitive inhibition of para-aminobenzoic acid

Pharmacodynamics/Kinetics

Absorption: Diffuses through devascularized areas and is rapidly absorbed from burned surface

Metabolism: To para-carboxybenzene sulfonamide, a carbonic anhydrase inhibitor

Time to peak, serum: 2-4 hours

Excretion: Urine (as metabolites)

Dosage Children and Adults: Topical: Apply once or twice daily with a sterile gloved hand; apply to a thickness of approximately 16 mm; the burned area should be covered with cream at all times

Stability

Mafenide 5% topical solution preparation:

Dissolve the 50 g mafenide acetate (Sulfamylon®) packet in 200 mL of either sterile water for irrigation or sterile saline for irrigation (minimum solubility of 50 g of mafenide is in 200 mL of either solution)

Sterilize this solution by pushing through a 0.22 micron filter

Further dissolve this 200 mL of sterile Sulfamylon® solution in 800 mL of the initial diluent (either sterile water for irrigation or normal saline for irrigation)

This solution is stable and sterile for a total of 48 hours at room temperature

Note: Mafenide acetate topical solution CANNOT be mixed with nystatin due to reduced activity of mafenide

Note: Pilot *in vitro* studies: Silvadene® and Furacin® cream combined with nystatin cream were equally effective against the microorganisms as were the individual drugs. However, Sulfamylon® cream combined with nystatin lost its antimicrobial capability (*J Burn Care Rehabil*, 1989, 109:508-11).

Monitoring Parameters Acid base balance

Pregnancy Risk Factor C

Contraindications Hypersensitivity to mafenide, sulfites, or any component of the formulation

Warnings/Precautions Use with caution in patients with renal impairment and in patients with G6PD deficiency; prolonged use may result in superinfection

Adverse Reactions Frequency not defined.

Cardiovascular: Facial edema

Central nervous system: Pain

(Continued)

Mafenide *(Continued)*

Dermatologic: Rash, erythema
Endocrine & metabolic: Hyperchloremia, metabolic acidosis
Hematologic: Porphyria, bone marrow suppression, hemolytic anemia, bleeding
Local: Burning sensation, excoriation
Respiratory: Hyperventilation, tachypnea, dyspnea
Miscellaneous: Hypersensitivity

Drug Interactions No data reported

Dosage Forms

Cream, topical, as acetate: 85 mg/g (60 g, 120 g, 454 g) [contains sodium metabisulfite]
Powder, for topical solution: 5% (5s) [50 g/packet]

♦ **Mafenide Acetate** *see* Mafenide *on page 785*

Magnesium Citrate (mag NEE zhum SIT rate)

Canadian Brand Names Citro-Mag®

Synonyms Citrate of Magnesia

Pharmacologic Category Laxative, Saline; Magnesium Salt

Generic Available Yes

Use Evacuation of bowel prior to certain surgical and diagnostic procedures or overdose situations

Mechanism of Action Promotes bowel evacuation by causing osmotic retention of fluid which distends the colon with increased peristaltic activity

Pharmacodynamics/Kinetics

Absorption: Oral: 15% to 30%
Excretion: Urine

Dosage Cathartic: Oral:

Children:

<6 years: 0.5 mL/kg up to a maximum of 200 mL repeated every 4-6 hours until stools are clear
6-12 years: 100-150 mL

Children ≥12 years and Adults: ½ to 1 full bottle (120-300 mL)

Administration To increase palatability, chill the solution prior to administration.

Reference Range Serum magnesium: 1.5-2.5 mg/dL; slightly different ranges are reported by different laboratories

Pregnancy Risk Factor B

Contraindications Renal failure, appendicitis, abdominal pain, intestinal impaction, obstruction or perforation, diabetes mellitus, complications in gastrointestinal tract, patients with colostomy or ileostomy, ulcerative colitis or diverticulitis

Warnings/Precautions Use with caution in patients with impaired renal function, especially if Cl_{cr} <30 mL/minute (accumulation of magnesium which may lead to magnesium intoxication). Use caution in patients receiving a cardiac glycoside; may increase the AV-blocking effects. Use with caution in patients with lithium administration; use with caution with neuromuscular-blocking agents, and CNS depressants.

Adverse Reactions 1% to 10%:

Cardiovascular: Hypotension
Endocrine & metabolic: Hypermagnesemia
Gastrointestinal: Abdominal cramps, diarrhea, gas formation
Respiratory: Respiratory depression

Overdosage/Toxicology

Serious, potentially life-threatening electrolyte disturbances may occur with long-term use or overdosage due to diarrhea; hypermagnesemia may occur. CNS depression, confusion, hypotension, muscle weakness, blockage of peripheral neuromuscular transmission.

Serum level >4 mEq/L (4.8 mg/dL): Deep tendon reflexes may be depressed

Serum level ≥10 mEq/L (12 mg/dL): Deep tendon reflexes may disappear, respiratory paralysis may occur, heart block may occur

I.V. calcium (5-10 mEq) will reverse respiratory depression or heart block; in extreme cases, peritoneal dialysis or hemodialysis may be required.

Serum level >12 mEq/L may be fatal, serum level ≥10 mEq/L may cause complete heart block

Test Interactions Increased magnesium; decreased protein, decreased calcium (S), decreased potassium (S)

Dietary Considerations Magnesium content of 5 mL: 3.85-4.71 mEq

Dosage Forms

Solution, oral: 290 mg/5 mL (300 mL) [cherry and lemon flavors]
Tablet: 100 mg [as elemental magnesium]

♦ **Magnesium Hydroxide and Aluminum Hydroxide** *see* Aluminum Hydroxide and Magnesium Hydroxide *on page 76*

Magnesium Sulfate (mag NEE zhum SUL fate)

Medication Safety Issues

Sound-alike/look-alike issues:

Magnesium sulfate may be confused with manganese sulfate, morphine sulfate
$MgSO_4$ is an error-prone abbreviation (mistaken as morphine sulfate)

High alert medication: The Institute for Safe Medication Practices (ISMP) includes this medication (I.V. formulation) among its list of drugs which have a heightened risk of causing significant patient harm when used in error.

Synonyms Epsom Salts; $MgSO_4$ (error-prone abbreviation)

Pharmacologic Category Anticonvulsant, Miscellaneous; Electrolyte Supplement, Parenteral; Laxative, Saline; Magnesium Salt

Generic Available Yes

Use Treatment and prevention of hypomagnesemia; seizure prevention in severe pre-eclampsia or eclampsia, pediatric acute nephritis; torsade de pointes; treatment of cardiac arrhythmias (VT/VF) caused by hypomagnesemia; short-term treatment of constipation; soaking aid

Mechanism of Action When taken orally, magnesium promotes bowel evacuation by causing osmotic retention of fluid which distends the colon with increased peristaltic activity; parenterally, magnesium decreases acetylcholine in motor nerve terminals and acts on myocardium by slowing rate of S-A node impulse formation and prolonging conduction time. Magnesium is necessary for the movement of calcium, sodium, and potassium in and out of cells, as well as stabilizing excitable membranes.

Pharmacodynamics/Kinetics

Onset of action: Oral: Cathartic: 1-2 hours; I.M.: 1 hour; I.V.: Immediate
Duration: I.M.: 3-4 hours; I.V.: 30 minutes
Absorption: Oral: Inversely proportional to amount ingested; 40% to 60% under controlled dietary conditions; 15% to 36% at higher doses
Distribution: Bone (50% to 60%); extracellular fluid (1% to 2%)
Protein binding: 30%, to albumin
Excretion: Urine (as magnesium)

Dosage Dose represented as magnesium sulfate unless stated otherwise. **Note:** Serum magnesium is poor reflection of repletional status as the majority of magnesium is intracellular; serum levels may be transiently normal for a few hours after a dose is given, therefore, aim for consistently high normal serum levels in patients with normal renal function for most efficient repletion.

Hypomagnesemia: Note: Treatment depends on severity and clinical status:

Children: I.V., I.O. : 25-50 mg/kg/dose (0.2-0.4 mEq/kg/dose) over 10-20 minutes (faster in torsade); maximum single dose: 2000 mg (16 mEq)

Adults: I.V.:

Severe or smptomatic: 1-2 g over 5-60 minutes
Hypomagnesemia with seizures: 2 g over 10 minutes; calcium administration may also be appropriate

Eclampsia, pre-eclampsia: Adults: I.V.: 4-6 g over 15-20 minutes followed by 2 g/hour

Torsade de pointes: Adults: I.V.:

Pulseless: 1-2 g over 5-20 minutes
With pulse: 1-2 g over 5-60 minutes. **Note:** Slower administration preferable for stable patients.

Cathartic: Oral:

Children:

2-5 years: 2.5-5 g/kg/day in divided doses
6-11 years: 5-10 g/day in divided doses

Children ≥12 years and Adults: 10-30 g/day in divided doses

Parenteral nutrition supplementation (elemental magnesium): I.V.:

Children:

<50 kg: 0.3-0.5 mEq/kg/day
>50 kg: 10-30 mEq/day

(Continued)

Magnesium Sulfate *(Continued)*

Adults: 8-20 mEq/day

Soaking aid: Topical: Adults: Dissolve 2 cupfuls of powder per gallon of warm water

RDA (elemental magnesium):

Children:
- 1-3 years: 80 mg/day
- 4-8 years: 130 mg/day
- 9-13 years: 240 mg/day
- 14-18 years:
  - Female: 360 mg/day
  - Pregnant female: 400 mg/day
  - Male: 410 mg/day

Adults:
- 19-30 years:
  - Female: 310 mg/day
  - Pregnant female: 350 mg/day
  - Male: 400 mg/day
- ≥31 years:
  - Female: 320 mg/day
  - Pregnant female: 360 mg/day
  - Male: 420 mg/day

Dosage adjustment in renal impairment: Cl_{cr} <30 mL/minute: Use with caution; monitor for hypermagnesemia

Stability Prior to use, store at controlled room temperature. Refrigeration of solution may result in precipitation or crystallization.

Administration

Oral: Dissolve powder in ½ glass of water; may add lemon juice to improve taste

Injection: May be administered I.M. or I.V.

I.M.: A 25% or 50% concentration may be used for adults and a 20% solution is recommended for children

I.V.: Magnesium may be administered IVP, IVPB or I.V.; when giving I.V. push, must dilute first and should not be given any faster than 150 mg/minute. Hypotension and asystole may occur with rapid administration.

Maximal rate of infusion: 2 g/hour to avoid hypotension; doses of 4 g/hour have been given in emergencies (eclampsia, seizures); optimally, should add magnesium to I.V. fluids, but bolus doses are also effective

Topical: Dissolve 2 cups of powder per gallon of warm water to use as a soaking aid. To make a compress, dissolve 2 cups of powder per 2 cups of hot water and use a towel to apply as a wet dressing.

Monitoring Parameters Monitor blood pressure when administering magnesium sulfate I.V.; serum magnesium levels should be monitored to avoid overdose; monitor for diarrhea; monitor for arrhythmias, hypotension, respiratory and CNS depression during rapid I.V. administration

Reference Range Serum magnesium: 1.5-2.5 mg/dL; slightly different ranges are reported by different laboratories

Anesthesia and Critical Care Concerns/Other Considerations Hypomagnesemia can hinder the replenishment of intracellular potassium and should be corrected in order to correct hypokalemia.

Pregnancy Risk Factor A/C (manufacturer dependent)

Contraindications Hypersensitivity to any component of the formulation; heart block; myocardial damage

Warnings/Precautions Use with caution in patients with impaired renal function, hepatitis, or Addison's disease (accumulation of magnesium may lead to magnesium intoxication). Monitor serum magnesium level, respiratory rate, deep tendon reflex, renal function when magnesium sulfate is administered parenterally. Use with extreme caution in patients with myasthenia gravis or other neuromuscular disease.

Constipation (self-medication, OTC use): For occasional use only; serious side effects may occur with prolonged use. For use only under the supervision of a healthcare provider in patients with kidney dysfunction, or with a sudden change in bowel habits which persist for >2 weeks. Do not use if abdominal pain, nausea, or vomiting are present.

Adverse Reactions Adverse effects on neuromuscular function may occur at lower levels in patients with neuromuscular disease (eg, myasthenia gravis).

Frequency not defined: Gastrointestinal: Diarrhea (excessive oral doses)

Overdosage/Toxicology Serious, potentially life-threatening electrolyte disturbances may occur with long-term use or overdosage due to diarrhea; hypermagnesemia may occur.

Symptoms of overdose usually present with magnesium serum level >4 mEq/L

Serum magnesium >4 mEq/L: Deep tendon reflexes may be depressed; drowsiness, flushing, headache, lethargy, or nausea may be present

Serum magnesium 6-10 mEq/L: Deep tendon reflexes may disappear; respiratory paralysis may occur; bradycardia, ECG changes, hypocalcemia, hypotension, or somnolence may be present

Serum level 10 mEq/L may be fatal; muscle or respiratory paralysis may be present, complete heart block or cardiac arrest may occur

Calcium chloride 10%: 500-1000 mg can be used to correct arrhythmias; dialysis may be needed for severe hypermagnesemia

Drug Interactions

Calcium channel blockers: Calcium channel blockers may enhance the adverse/toxic effect of magnesium salts. Magnesium salts may enhance the hypotensive effect of calcium channel blockers.

Neuromuscular-blocking agents: Magnesium salts may enhance the neuromuscular-blocking effect of neuromuscular-blocking agents. Only of concern in patients with increased serum magnesium concentrations.

Dietary Considerations Whole grains, legumes and dark-green leafy vegetables are dietary sources of magnesium.

10% elemental magnesium; 8.1 mEq magnesium/g; 4 mmol magnesium/g

500 mg magnesium sulfate = 4.06 mEq magnesium = 49.3 mg elemental magnesium

Dosage Forms

Infusion [premixed in D_5W]: 10 mg/mL (100 mL); 20 mg/mL (500 mL, 1000 mL)

Infusion [premixed in water for injection]: 40 mg/mL (100 mL, 500 mL, 1000 mL); 80 mg/mL (50 mL)

Injection, solution: 125 mg/mL (8 mL); 500 mg/mL (2 mL, 5 mL, 10 mL, 20 mL, 50 mL)

Powder: Magnesium sulfate USP (480 g, 1810 g, 1920 g)

Manganese (MAN ga nees)

Medication Safety Issues

Sound-alike/look-alike issues:

Manganese sulfate may be confused with magnesium sulfate

U.S. Brand Names Mangimin [OTC]

Synonyms Manganese Chloride; Manganese Sulfate

Pharmacologic Category Trace Element, Parenteral

Generic Available Yes

Use Trace element added to total parenteral nutrition (TPN) solution to prevent manganese deficiency; orally as a dietary supplement

Mechanism of Action Cofactor in many enzyme systems, stimulates synthesis of cholesterol and fatty acids in liver, and influences mucopolysaccharide synthesis

Pharmacodynamics/Kinetics

Absorption: Oral: Poor (3% to 4%)

Distribution: Concentrated in mitochondria of pituitary gland, pancreas, liver, kidney, and bone

Excretion: Bile (primarily); urine (negligible)

Dosage

Oral: Adequate intake:

- 0-6 months: 0.003 mg/day
- 7-12 months: 0.6 mg/day
- 1-3 years: 1.2 mg/day
- 4-8 years: 1.5 mg/day
- 9 years to Adults, Male: 1.9-2.3 mg/day
- 9 years to Adults, Female: 1.6-1.8 mg/day
  - Pregnancy: 2 mg/day
  - Lactation: 2.6 mg/day

I.V.:

Children: 2-10 mcg/kg/day usually administered in TPN solutions

(Continued)

Manganese *(Continued)*

Note: Use caution in premature neonates; manganese chloride solution for injection contains aluminum

Adults: 150-800 mcg/day usually administered in TPN solutions

Dosage adjustment in renal impairment: Use caution; manganese chloride solution for injection contains aluminum

Dosage adjustment in hepatic impairment: Use caution; dose may need to be decreased or withheld

Stability Solution for injection: Store at controlled room temperature of 15°C to 30°C (59°F to 86°F); compatible with electrolytes usually present in amino acid/dextrose solution used for TPN solutions.

Administration Solution for injection: Do not administer I.M. or by direct I.V. injection; acidic pH of the solution may cause tissue irritations and it is hypotonic

Monitoring Parameters Periodic manganese plasma level

Reference Range Plasma: 0.6-2 ng/mL

Pregnancy Risk Factor C

Contraindications High manganese levels; severe liver dysfunction or cholestasis (conjugated bilirubin >2 mg/dL) due to reduced biliary excretion

Warnings/Precautions Manganese chloride solution for injection contains aluminum; use caution with impaired renal function and in premature infants. Use caution with hepatic impairment.

Overdosage/Toxicology Acute poisoning due to ingestion of manganese or manganese salts is rare (poor oral absorption). Manganese chloride solution for injection contains aluminum; aluminum doses >4-5 mcg/kg/day are associated with toxicity in patients with renal impairment and in premature neonates. The main symptoms of chronic poisoning, either from injection or usually inhalation of manganese dust or fumes, include extrapyramidal symptoms that can lead to progressive deterioration in the central nervous system.

Dosage Forms

Injection, solution, as chloride [preservative free]: 0.1 mg/mL (10 mL) [contains aluminum ≤100 mcg/mL]

Injection, solution, as sulfate: 0.1 mg/mL (10 mL)

Tablet, as aspartate: 93 mg [equivalent to elemental manganese 25 mg]

Tablet, as gluconate: 5.7 mg [as elemental manganese]; 550 mg [equivalent to elemental manganese 30 mg]; 600 mg [equivalent to elemental manganese 50 mg]

Tablet, chelated: 50 mg [as elemental manganese]

Mangimin: 10 mg [as elemental manganese]

- **Manganese Chloride** *see* Manganese *on page 789*
- **Manganese Sulfate** *see* Manganese *on page 789*
- **Mangimin [OTC]** *see* Manganese *on page 789*

Mannitol (MAN i tole)

Medication Safety Issues

Sound-alike/look-alike issues:

Osmitrol® may be confused with esmolol

U.S. Brand Names Osmitrol®; Resectisol®

Canadian Brand Names Osmitrol®

Synonyms *D*-Mannitol

Pharmacologic Category Diuretic, Osmotic

Generic Available Yes

Use Reduction of increased intracranial pressure associated with cerebral edema; promotion of diuresis in the prevention and/or treatment of oliguria or anuria due to acute renal failure; reduction of increased intraocular pressure; promoting urinary excretion of toxic substances; genitourinary irrigant in transurethral prostatic resection or other transurethral surgical procedures

Mechanism of Action Increases the osmotic pressure of glomerular filtrate, which inhibits tubular reabsorption of water and electrolytes and increases urinary output

Pharmacodynamics/Kinetics

Onset of action: Diuresis: Injection: 1-3 hours; Reduction in intracranial pressure: ~15-30 minutes

Duration: Reduction in intracranial pressure: 1.5-6 hours

Distribution: Remains confined to extracellular space (except in extreme concentrations); does not penetrate the blood-brain barrier (generally, penetration is low)

Metabolism: Minimally hepatic to glycogen

Half-life elimination: 1.1-1.6 hours

Excretion: Primarily urine (as unchanged drug)

Dosage

Children: I.V.:

Test dose (to assess adequate renal function): 200 mg/kg over 3-5 minutes to produce a urine flow of at least 1 mL/kg for 1-3 hours

Initial: 0.25-1 g/kg

Maintenance: 0.25-0.5 g/kg given every 4-6 hours

Adults:

I.V.:

Test dose (to assess adequate renal function): 12.5 g (200 mg/kg) over 3-5 minutes to produce a urine flow of at least 30-50 mL of urine per hour. If urine flow does not increase, a second test dose may be given. If test dose does not produce an acceptable urine output, then need to reassess management.

Initial: 0.5-1 g/kg

Maintenance: 0.25-0.5 g/kg every 4-6 hours; usual daily dose: 20-200 g/24 hours

Intracranial pressure: Cerebral edema: 0.25-1.5 g/kg/dose I.V. as a 15% to 20% solution over ≥30 minutes; maintain serum osmolality 310 to <320 mOsm/kg

Prevention of acute renal failure (oliguria): 50-100 g dose

Treatment of oliguria: 100 g dose

Preoperative for neurosurgery: 1.5-2 g/kg administered 1-1.5 hours prior to surgery

Reduction of intraocular pressure: 1.5-2 g/kg as a 15% to 20% solution; administer over 30 minutes

Topical: Transurethral irrigation: Use urogenital solution as required for irrigation

Elderly: Consider initiation at lower end of dosing range

Dosage adjustment in renal impairment: Contraindicated in severe renal impairment. If test dose does not produce adequate urine output reassess options. Use caution in patients with underlying renal disease.

Dosage adjustment in hepatic impairment: No adjustment required.

Stability Should be stored at room temperature (15°C to 30°C) and protected from freezing; crystallization may occur at low temperatures; do not use solutions that contain crystals, heating in a hot water bath and vigorous shaking may be utilized for resolubilization; cool solutions to body temperature before using

Administration Inspect for crystals prior to administration. If crystals present redissolve by warming solution. Use filter-type administration set; in-line 5-micron filter set should always be used for mannitol infusion with concentrations ≥20%; administer test dose (for oliguria) I.V. push over 3-5 minutes; avoid extravasation; for cerebral edema or elevated ICP, administer over 20-30 minutes; crenation and agglutination of red blood cells may occur if administered with whole blood.

Monitoring Parameters Renal function, daily fluid I & O, serum electrolytes, serum and urine osmolality; for treatment of elevated intracranial pressure, maintain serum osmolality 310 to <320 mOsm/kg

Anesthesia and Critical Care Concerns/Other Considerations Mannitol may autoclave or heat to redissolve crystals.

Mannitol 20% has an approximate osmolarity of 1100 mOsm/L.

Mannitol 25% has an approximate osmolarity of 1375 mOsm/L.

Pregnancy Risk Factor C

Contraindications Hypersensitivity to mannitol or any component or the formulation; severe renal disease (anuria); severe dehydration; active intracranial bleeding except during craniotomy; progressive heart failure, pulmonary congestion, or renal dysfunction after mannitol administration; severe pulmonary edema or congestion

Warnings/Precautions Should not be administered until adequacy of renal function and urine flow is established;use 1-2 test doses to assess renal response. Diuretic effects may mask and intensify underlying dehydration; excessive loss of water and electrolytes may lead to imbalances and aggravate preexisting hyponatremia. May cause renal dysfunction especially with high doses; use caution in patients taking other nephrotoxic agents, with sepsis or preexisting renal disease. (Continued)

Mannitol *(Continued)*

To minimize adverse renal effects, adjust to keep serum osmolality less than 320 mOsm/L. Discontinue if evidence of acute tubular necrosis.

In patients being treated for cerebral edema, mannitol may accumulate in the brain (causing rebound increases in intracranial pressure) if circulating for long periods of time as with continuous infusion; intermittent boluses preferred. Cardiovascular status should also be evaluated; do not administer electrolyte-free mannitol solutions with blood. If hypotension occurs monitor cerebral perfusion pressure to insure adequate.

Adverse Reactions Frequency not defined.

Cardiovascular: Chest pain, CHF, circulatory overload, hyper-/hypotension, tachycardia

Central nervous system: Chills, convulsions, dizziness, headache

Dermatologic: Rash, urticaria

Endocrine & metabolic: Fluid and electrolyte imbalance, dehydration and hypovolemia secondary to rapid diuresis, hyperglycemia, hypernatremia, hyponatremia (dilutional), hyperosmolality-induced hyperkalemia, metabolic acidosis (dilutional), osmolar gap increased, water intoxication

Gastrointestinal: Nausea, vomiting, xerostomia

Genitourinary: Dysuria, polyuria

Local: Pain, thrombophlebitis, tissue necrosis

Ocular: Blurred vision

Renal: Acute renal failure, acute tubular necrosis (>200 g/day; serum osmolality >320 mOsm/L)

Respiratory: Pulmonary edema, rhinitis

Miscellaneous: Allergic reactions

Overdosage/Toxicology Symptoms of overdose include acute renal failure, polyuria, hypotension, cardiovascular collapse, pulmonary edema, hyponatremia, hypokalemia, oliguria, and seizures. Increased electrolyte excretion and fluid overload can occur. Hemodialysis will clear mannitol and reduce osmolality.

Drug Interactions Lithium toxicity (with diuretic-induced hyponatremia)

Dosage Forms

Injection, solution: 5% [50 mg/mL] (1000 mL); 10% [100 mg/mL] (500 mL, 1000 mL); 15% [150 mg/mL] (500 mL); 20% [200 mg/mL] (150 mL, 250 mL, 500 mL); 25% [250 mg/mL] (50 mL)

Osmitrol®: 5% [50 mg/mL] (1000 mL); 10% [100 mg/mL] (500 mL, 1000 mL); 15% [150 mg/mL] (500 mL); 20% [200 mg/mL] (250 mL, 500 mL)

Solution, urogenital (Resectisol®): 5% [50 mg/mL] (2000 mL, 4000 mL)

- **Mapap [OTC]** *see* Acetaminophen *on page 26*
- **Mapap Children's [OTC]** *see* Acetaminophen *on page 26*
- **Mapap Extra Strength [OTC]** *see* Acetaminophen *on page 26*
- **Mapap Infants [OTC]** *see* Acetaminophen *on page 26*
- **Mapezine® (Can)** *see* Carbamazepine *on page 225*
- **Marcaine®** *see* Bupivacaine *on page 196*
- **Marcaine® Spinal** *see* Bupivacaine *on page 196*
- **Margesic® H** *see* Hydrocodone and Acetaminophen *on page 636*
- **Marinol®** *see* Dronabinol *on page 430*
- **3M™ Avagard™ [OTC]** *see* Chlorhexidine Gluconate *on page 267*
- **Mavik®** *see* Trandolapril *on page 1300*
- **Maxalt®** *see* Rizatriptan *on page 1134*
- **Maxalt-MLT®** *see* Rizatriptan *on page 1134*
- **Maxalt RPD™ (Can)** *see* Rizatriptan *on page 1134*
- **Maxidex®** *see* Dexamethasone *on page 366*
- **Maxidone™** *see* Hydrocodone and Acetaminophen *on page 636*
- **Maxipime®** *see* Cefepime *on page 238*
- **Maxivate®** *see* Betamethasone *on page 169*
- **MDL 73,147EF** *see* Dolasetron *on page 412*

Meclofenamate (me kloe fen AM ate)

Related Information

Acetaminophen and NSAIDS, Dosing Data *on page 1543*

Chronic Pain Management *on page 1430*

Canadian Brand Names Meclomen®

Synonyms Meclofenamate Sodium

Pharmacologic Category Nonsteroidal Anti-inflammatory Drug (NSAID), Oral

Restrictions A medication guide should be dispensed with each prescription. A template for the required MedGuide can be found on the FDA website at: http://www.fda.gov/medwatch/SAFETY/2005/safety05.htm#NSAID

Generic Available Yes

Use Treatment of inflammatory disorders, arthritis, mild to moderate pain, dysmenorrhea

Mechanism of Action Inhibits prostaglandin synthesis by decreasing the activity of the enzyme, cyclooxygenase, which results in decreased formation of prostaglandin precursors

Pharmacodynamics/Kinetics

Duration: 2-4 hours

Distribution: Crosses placenta

Protein binding: 99%

Half-life elimination: 2-3.3 hours

Time to peak, serum: 0.5-1.5 hours

Excretion: Primarily urine and feces (as metabolites)

Dosage Children >14 years and Adults: Oral:

Mild to moderate pain: 50 mg every 4-6 hours; increases to 100 mg may be required; maximum dose: 400 mg

Rheumatoid arthritis and osteoarthritis: 50 mg every 4-6 hours; increase, over weeks, to 200-400 mg/day in 3-4 divided doses; do not exceed 400 mg/day; maximal benefit for any dose may not be seen for 2-3 weeks

Anesthesia and Critical Care Concerns/Other Considerations The 2002 ACCM/SCCM guidelines for analgesia (critically-ill adult) suggest that NSAIDs may be used in combination with opioids in select patients for pain management. Concern about adverse events (increased risk of renal dysfunction, altered platelet function and gastrointestinal irritation) limits its use in patients who have other underlying risks for these events.

In short-term use, NSAIDs vary considerably in their effect on blood pressure. When NSAIDs are used in patients with hypertension, appropriate monitoring of blood pressure responses should be completed and the duration of therapy, when possible, kept short. The use of NSAIDs in the treatment of patients with congestive heart failure may be associated with an increased risk for fluid accumulation and edema; may precipitate renal failure in dehydrated patients.

Pregnancy Risk Factor C/D (3rd trimester)

Contraindications Hypersensitivity to meclofenamate, aspirin, other NSAIDs, or any component of the formulation; perioperative pain in the setting of coronary artery bypass surgery (CABG); active GI bleeding, ulcer disease; pregnancy (3rd trimester)

Warnings/Precautions **[U.S. Boxed Warning]: NSAIDs are associated with an increased risk of adverse cardiovascular events, including MI, stroke, and new onset or worsening of pre-existing hypertension.** Risk may be increased with duration of use or pre-existing cardiovascular risk-factors or disease. Carefully evaluate individual cardiovascular risk profiles prior to prescribing. Use caution with fluid retention, CHF or hypertension.

Use of NSAIDs can compromise existing renal function. Renal toxicity can occur in patient with impaired renal function, dehydration, heart failure, liver dysfunction, those taking diuretics and ACEI and the elderly. Rehydrate patient before starting therapy. Monitor renal function closely. Use caution in patients with advanced renal disease.

[U.S. Boxed Warning]: NSAIDs may increase risk of gastrointestinal irritation, ulceration, bleeding, and perforation. These events may occur at any time during therapy and without warning. Use caution with a history of GI disease (bleeding or ulcers), concurrent therapy with aspirin, anticoagulants and/or corticosteroids, smoking, use of alcohol, the elderly or debilitated patients.

Use the lowest effective dose for the shortest duration of time, consistent with individual patient goals, to reduce risk of cardiovascular or GI adverse events. Alternate therapies should be considered for patients at high risk.

(Continued)

Meclofenamate *(Continued)*

NSAIDs may cause serious skin adverse events including exfoliative dermatitis, Stevens-Johnson syndrome (SJS) and toxic epidermal necrolysis (TEN). Anaphylactoid reactions may occur, even without prior exposure; patients with "aspirin triad" (bronchial asthma, aspirin intolerance, rhinitis) may be at increased risk. Do not use in patients who experience bronchospasm, asthma, rhinitis, or urticaria with NSAID or aspirin therapy.

Use with caution in patients with decreased hepatic function. Closely monitor patients with any abnormal LFT. Severe hepatic reactions (eg, fulminant hepatitis, liver failure) have occurred with NSAID use, rarely; discontinue if signs or symptoms of liver disease develop, or if systemic manifestations occur.

The elderly are at increased risk for adverse effects (especially peptic ulceration, CNS effects, renal toxicity) from NSAIDs even at low doses

Withhold for at least 4-6 half-lives prior to surgical or dental procedures. Safety and efficacy have not been established in children <14 years of age.

Adverse Reactions

>10%:

- Central nervous system: Dizziness
- Dermatologic: Skin rash
- Gastrointestinal: Abdominal cramps, heartburn, indigestion, nausea

1% to 10%:

- Central nervous system: Headache, nervousness
- Dermatologic: Itching
- Endocrine & metabolic: Fluid retention
- Gastrointestinal: Vomiting
- Otic: Tinnitus

<1% (Limited to important or life-threatening): Acute renal failure, agranulocytosis, angioedema, arrhythmia, aseptic meningitis, bone marrow suppression, confusion, CHF, dyspnea, erythema multiforme, GI ulceration, hallucinations, hemolytic anemia, hepatitis, leukopenia, mental depression, peripheral neuropathy, somnolence, Stevens-Johnson syndrome, tachycardia, thrombocytopenia, toxic amblyopia, toxic epidermal necrolysis, urticaria

Overdosage/Toxicology

Symptoms of overdose include drowsiness, lethargy, nausea, vomiting, seizures, paresthesia, headache, dizziness, GI bleeding, cerebral edema, cardiac arrest, tinnitus

Management of NSAID intoxication is primarily supportive and symptomatic. Fluid therapy is commonly effective in managing the hypotension that may occur following an acute NSAID overdose, except when this is due to an acute blood loss. Seizures tend to be very short-lived and often do not require drug treatment. Although, recurrent seizures should be treated with I.V. diazepam. Since many of the NSAID undergo enterohepatic cycling, multiple doses of charcoal may be needed to reduce the potential for delayed toxicities.

Drug Interactions

ACE inhibitors: Antihypertensive effects may be decreased by concurrent therapy with NSAIDs; monitor blood pressure.

Angiotensin II antagonists: Antihypertensive effects may be decreased by concurrent therapy with NSAIDs; monitor blood pressure.

Anticoagulants (warfarin, heparin, LMWHs) in combination with NSAIDs can cause increased risk of bleeding.

Antiplatelet drugs (ticlopidine, clopidogrel, aspirin, abciximab, dipyridamole, eptifibatide, tirofiban) can cause an increased risk of bleeding.

Beta-blockers: NSAIDs may decrease the antihypertensive effect of beta-blockers. Monitor.

Cholestyramine (and other bile acid sequestrants): May decrease the absorption of NSAIDs. Separate by at least 2 hours.

Corticosteroids may increase the risk of GI ulceration; avoid concurrent use.

Cyclosporine: NSAIDs may increase serum creatinine, potassium, blood pressure, and cyclosporine levels; monitor cyclosporine levels and renal function carefully.

Gentamicin and amikacin serum concentrations are increased by indomethacin in premature infants. Results may apply to other aminoglycosides and NSAIDs.

Hydralazine's antihypertensive effect is decreased; avoid concurrent use.

Lithium levels can be increased; avoid concurrent use if possible or monitor lithium levels and adjust dose. Sulindac may have the least effect. When NSAID is stopped, lithium will need adjustment again.

Loop diuretics efficacy (diuretic and antihypertensive effect) is reduced. Indomethacin reduces this efficacy, however, it may be anticipated with any NSAID.

Methotrexate: Severe bone marrow suppression, aplastic anemia, and GI toxicity have been reported with concomitant NSAID therapy. Avoid use during moderate or high-dose methotrexate (increased and prolonged methotrexate levels). NSAID use during low-dose treatment of rheumatoid arthritis has not been fully evaluated; extreme caution is warranted.

Thiazides antihypertensive effects are decreased; avoid concurrent use.

Verapamil plasma concentration is decreased by diclofenac; avoid concurrent use.

Warfarin's INRs may be increased by piroxicam. Other NSAIDs may have the same effect depending on dose and duration. Monitor INR closely. Use the lowest dose of NSAIDs possible and for the briefest duration.

Ethanol/Nutrition/Herb Interactions

Ethanol: Avoid ethanol (may enhance gastric mucosal irritation).

Herb/Nutraceutical: Avoid alfalfa, anise, bilberry, bladderwrack, bromelain, cat's claw, celery, coleus, cordyceps, dong quai, evening primrose, feverfew, fenugreek, garlic, ginger, ginkgo biloboa, red clover, horse chestnut, grapeseed, green tea, ginseng, guggul, horse chestnut seed, horseradish, licorice, prickly ash, red clover, reishi, SAMe, sweet clover, turmeric, white willow (all have additional antiplatelet activity).

Test Interactions Increased chloride (S), increased sodium (S)

Dietary Considerations May be taken with food, milk, or antacids.

Dosage Forms Capsule, as sodium: 50 mg, 100 mg

- **Meclofenamate Sodium** *see* Meclofenamate *on page 792*
- **Meclomen® (Can)** *see* Meclofenamate *on page 792*
- **Med-Diltiazem (Can)** *see* Diltiazem *on page 394*
- **Medicinal Carbon** *see* Charcoal *on page 259*
- **Medicinal Charcoal** *see* Charcoal *on page 259*
- **Medicone® [OTC]** *see* Phenylephrine *on page 1015*
- **Medrol®** *see* MethylPREDNISolone *on page 830*
- **Mefenamic-250 (Can)** *see* Mefenamic Acid *on page 795*

Mefenamic Acid (me fe NAM ik AS id)

Medication Safety Issues

Sound-alike/look-alike issues:

Ponstel® may be confused with Pronestyl®

Related Information

Acetaminophen and NSAIDS, Dosing Data *on page 1543*

Chronic Pain Management *on page 1430*

U.S. Brand Names Ponstel®

Canadian Brand Names Apo-Mefenamic®; Dom-Mefenamic Acid; Mefenamic-250; Nu-Mefenamic; PMS-Mefenamic Acid; Ponstan®

Pharmacologic Category Nonsteroidal Anti-inflammatory Drug (NSAID), Oral

Restrictions A medication guide should be dispensed with each prescription. A template for the required MedGuide can be found on the FDA website at: http://www.fda.gov/medwatch/SAFETY/2005/safety05.htm#NSAID

Generic Available No

Use Short-term relief of mild to moderate pain including primary dysmenorrhea

Mechanism of Action Inhibits prostaglandin synthesis by decreasing the activity of the enzyme, cyclooxygenase, which results in decreased formation of prostaglandin precursors

Pharmacodynamics/Kinetics

Onset of action: Peak effect: 2-4 hours

Duration: ≤6 hours

Protein binding: High

Metabolism: Conjugated hepatically

Half-life elimination: 3.5 hours

Excretion: Urine (50%) and feces as unchanged drug and metabolites

Dosage Children >14 years and Adults: Oral: 500 mg to start then 250 mg every 4 hours as needed; maximum therapy: 1 week

Dosing adjustment/comments in renal impairment: Not recommended for use

(Continued)

Mefenamic Acid *(Continued)*

Administration May be administered with food, milk, or antacids.

Anesthesia and Critical Care Concerns/Other Considerations The 2002 ACCM/SCCM guidelines for analgesia (critically-ill adult) suggest that NSAIDs may be used in combination with opioids in select patients for pain management. Concern about adverse events (increased risk of renal dysfunction, altered platelet function and gastrointestinal irritation) limits its use in patients who have other underlying risks for these events.

In short-term use, NSAIDs vary considerably in their effect on blood pressure. When NSAIDs are used in patients with hypertension, appropriate monitoring of blood pressure responses should be completed and the duration of therapy, when possible, kept short. The use of NSAIDs in the treatment of patients with congestive heart failure may be associated with an increased risk for fluid accumulation and edema; may precipitate renal failure in dehydrated patients.

Pregnancy Risk Factor C/D (3rd trimester)

Contraindications Hypersensitivity to mefenamic acid, aspirin, other NSAIDs, or any component of the formulation; perioperative pain in the setting of coronary artery bypass surgery (CABG); active ulceration or chronic inflammation of the GI tract; renal disease; pregnancy (3rd trimester)

Warnings/Precautions [U.S. Boxed Warning]: NSAIDs are associated with an increased risk of adverse cardiovascular events, including MI, stroke, and new onset or worsening of pre-existing hypertension. Risk may be increased with duration of use or pre-existing cardiovascular risk-factors or disease. Carefully evaluate individual cardiovascular risk profiles prior to prescribing. Use caution with fluid retention, CHF or hypertension.

Use of NSAIDs can compromise existing renal function. Renal toxicity can occur in patient with impaired renal function, dehydration, heart failure, liver dysfunction, those taking diuretics and ACEI and the elderly. Rehydrate patient before starting therapy. Monitor renal function closely. Mefenamic acid is not recommended for patients with advanced renal disease.

[U.S. Boxed Warning]: NSAIDs may increase risk of gastrointestinal irritation, ulceration, bleeding, and perforation. These events may occur at any time during therapy and without warning. Use caution with a history of GI disease (bleeding or ulcers), concurrent therapy with aspirin, anticoagulants and/or corticosteroids, smoking, use of alcohol, the elderly or debilitated patients.

Use the lowest effective dose for the shortest duration of time, consistent with individual patient goals, to reduce risk of cardiovascular or GI adverse events. Alternate therapies should be considered for patients at high risk.

NSAIDs may cause serious skin adverse events including exfoliative dermatitis, Stevens-Johnson syndrome (SJS) and toxic epidermal necrolysis (TEN). Anaphylactoid reactions may occur, even without prior exposure; patients with "aspirin triad" (bronchial asthma, aspirin intolerance, rhinitis) may be at increased risk. Do not use in patients who experience bronchospasm, asthma, rhinitis, or urticaria with NSAID or aspirin therapy.

Use with caution in patients with decreased hepatic function. Closely monitor patients with any abnormal LFT. Severe hepatic reactions (eg, fulminant hepatitis, liver failure) have occurred with NSAID use, rarely; discontinue if signs or symptoms of liver disease develop, or if systemic manifestations occur.

The elderly are at increased risk for adverse effects (especially peptic ulceration, CNS effects, renal toxicity) from NSAIDs even at low doses.

Withhold for at least 4-6 half-lives prior to surgical or dental procedures. Safety and efficacy have not been established in children <14 years of age.

Adverse Reactions

1% to 10%:

Central nervous system: Headache, nervousness, dizziness (3% to 9%)
Dermatologic: Itching, rash
Endocrine & metabolic: Fluid retention
Gastrointestinal: Abdominal cramps, heartburn, indigestion, nausea (1% to 10%), vomiting (1% to 10%), diarrhea (1% to 10%), constipation (1% to 10%), abdominal distress/cramping/pain (1% to 10%), dyspepsia (1% to 10%), flatulence (1% to 10%), gastric or duodenal ulcer with bleeding or perforation (1% to 10%), gastritis (1% to 10%)

Hematologic: Bleeding (1% to 10%)
Hepatic: Elevated LFTs (1% to 10%)
Otic: Tinnitus (1% to 10%)
<1%: CHF, hypertension, arrhythmia, tachycardia, confusion, hallucinations, aseptic meningitis, mental depression, drowsiness, insomnia, urticaria, erythema multiforme, toxic epidermal necrolysis, Stevens-Johnson syndrome, angioedema, polydipsia, hot flashes, gastritis, GI ulceration, cystitis, polyuria, agranulocytosis, anemia, hemolytic anemia, bone marrow suppression, leukopenia, thrombocytopenia, hepatitis, peripheral neuropathy, toxic amblyopia, blurred vision, conjunctivitis, dry eyes, decreased hearing, acute renal failure, dyspnea, allergic rhinitis, epistaxis, stomatitis

Overdosage/Toxicology

Symptoms of overdose include CNS stimulation, agitation, seizures

Management of NSAID intoxication is primarily supportive and symptomatic. Fluid therapy is commonly effective in managing the hypotension that may occur following an acute NSAIDs overdose, except when this is due to an acute blood loss. Seizures tend to be very short-lived and often do not require drug treatment. Although, recurrent seizures should be treated with I.V. diazepam. Since many of the NSAID undergo enterohepatic cycling, multiple doses of charcoal may be needed to reduce the potential for delayed toxicities.

Drug Interactions **Substrate** of CYP2C9 (minor); **Inhibits** CYP2C9 (strong)

ACE inhibitors: Antihypertensive effects may be decreased by concurrent therapy with NSAIDs; monitor blood pressure.

Angiotensin II antagonists: Antihypertensive effects may be decreased by concurrent therapy with NSAIDs; monitor blood pressure.

Anticoagulants (warfarin, heparin, LMWHs) in combination with NSAIDs can cause increased risk of bleeding.

Antiplatelet drugs (ticlopidine, clopidogrel, aspirin, abciximab, dipyridamole, eptifibatide, tirofiban) can cause an increased risk of bleeding.

Beta-blockers: NSAIDs may decrease the antihypertensive effect of beta-blockers. Monitor.

Cholestyramine (and other bile acid sequestrants): May decrease the absorption of NSAIDs. Separate by at least 2 hours.

Corticosteroids may increase the risk of GI ulceration; avoid concurrent use.

Cyclosporine: NSAIDs may increase serum creatinine, potassium, blood pressure, and cyclosporine levels; monitor cyclosporine levels and renal function carefully.

CYP2C9 Substrates: Mefenamic acid may increase the levels/effects of CYP2C9 substrates. Example substrates include bosentan, dapsone, fluoxetine, glimepiride, glipizide, losartan, montelukast, nateglinide, paclitaxel, phenytoin, warfarin, and zafirlukast.

Gentamicin and amikacin serum concentrations are increased by indomethacin in premature infants. Results may apply to other aminoglycosides and NSAIDs.

Hydralazine's antihypertensive effect is decreased; avoid concurrent use.

Lithium levels can be increased; avoid concurrent use if possible or monitor lithium levels and adjust dose. Sulindac may have the least effect. When NSAID is stopped, lithium will need adjustment again.

Loop diuretics efficacy (diuretic and antihypertensive effect) is reduced. Indomethacin reduces this efficacy, however, it may be anticipated with any NSAID.

Methotrexate: Severe bone marrow suppression, aplastic anemia, and GI toxicity have been reported with concomitant NSAID therapy. Avoid use during moderate or high-dose methotrexate (increased and prolonged methotrexate levels). NSAID use during low-dose treatment of rheumatoid arthritis has not been fully evaluated; extreme caution is warranted.

Thiazides antihypertensive effects are decreased; avoid concurrent use.

Verapamil plasma concentration is decreased by diclofenac; avoid concurrent use.

Warfarin's INRs may be increased by piroxicam. Other NSAIDs may have the same effect depending on dose and duration. Monitor INR closely. Use the lowest dose of NSAIDs possible and for the briefest duration.

Ethanol/Nutrition/Herb Interactions

Ethanol: Avoid ethanol (may enhance gastric mucosal irritation).

Herb/Nutraceutical: Avoid alfalfa, anise, bilberry, bladderwrack, bromelain, cat's claw, celery, coleus, cordyceps, dong quai, evening primrose, feverfew, fenugreek, garlic, ginger, ginkgo biloboa, red clover, horse chestnut, grapeseed, green tea, ginseng, guggul, horse chestnut seed, horseradish, licorice, prickly

(Continued)

Mefenamic Acid *(Continued)*

ash, red clover, reishi, SAMe, sweet clover, turmeric, white willow (all have additional antiplatelet activity).

Test Interactions Increased chloride (S), increased sodium (S), positive Coombs' [direct], false-positive urinary bilirubin

Dosage Forms Capsule: 250 mg

♦ **Mefoxin®** *see* Cefoxitin *on page 244*

♦ **Mellaril® (Can)** *see* Thioridazine *on page 1259*

Meloxicam (mel OKS i kam)

U.S. Brand Names Mobic®

Canadian Brand Names Apo-Meloxicam®; CO Meloxicam; Gen-Meloxicam; Mobic®; Mobicox®; Novo-Meloxicam; PMS-Meloxicam

Pharmacologic Category Nonsteroidal Anti-inflammatory Drug (NSAID), Oral

Restrictions A medication guide should be dispensed with each prescription. A template for the required MedGuide can be found on the FDA website at: http://www.fda.gov/medwatch/SAFETY/2005/safety05.htm#NSAID

Generic Available No

Use Relief of signs and symptoms of osteoarthritis, rheumatoid arthritis, and juvenile rheumatoid arthritis (JRA)

Mechanism of Action Inhibits prostaglandin synthesis by decreasing the activity of the enzyme, cyclooxygenase, which results in decreased formation of prostaglandin precursors

Pharmacodynamics/Kinetics

Distribution: 10 L

Protein binding: 99.4%

Metabolism: Hepatic via CYP2C9 and CYP3A4 (minor); forms 4 metabolites (inactive)

Bioavailability: 89%

Half-life elimination: Adults: 15-20 hours

Time to peak: Initial: 5-10 hours; Secondary: 12-14 hours

Excretion: Urine and feces (as inactive metabolites)

Dosage Oral:

Children ≥2 years: JRA: 0.125 mg/kg/day; maximum dose: 7.5 mg/day

Adults: Osteoarthritis, rheumatoid arthritis: Initial: 7.5 mg once daily; some patients may receive additional benefit from an increased dose of 15 mg once daily; maximum dose: 15 mg/day

Elderly: Increased concentrations may occur in elderly patients (particularly in females); however, no specific dosage adjustment is recommended

Dosage adjustment in renal impairment:

Mild-to-moderate impairment: No specific dosage recommendations

Significant impairment (Cl_{cr} ≤15 mL/minute): Avoid use

Hemodialysis: Supplemental dose after dialysis not necessary.

Dosage adjustment in hepatic impairment:

Mild (Child-Pugh class A) to moderate (Child-Pugh class B) hepatic dysfunction: No dosage adjustment is necessary

Severe hepatic impairment: Patients with severe hepatic impairment have not been adequately studied

Stability Store at 25°C (77°F)

Monitoring Parameters CBC, periodic liver function, renal function (serum BUN, and creatinine)

Anesthesia and Critical Care Concerns/Other Considerations The 2002 ACCM/SCCM guidelines for analgesia (critically-ill adult) suggest that NSAIDs may be used in combination with opioids in select patients for pain management. Concern about adverse events (increased risk of renal dysfunction, altered platelet function and gastrointestinal irritation) limits its use in patients who have other underlying risks for these events.

In short-term use, NSAIDs vary considerably in their effect on blood pressure. When NSAIDs are used in patients with hypertension, appropriate monitoring of blood pressure responses should be completed and the duration of therapy, when possible, kept short. The use of NSAIDs in the treatment of patients with congestive heart failure may be associated with an increased risk for fluid accumulation and edema; may precipitate renal failure in dehydrated patients.

Pregnancy Risk Factor C/D (3rd trimester)

Contraindications Hypersensitivity to meloxicam, aspirin, other NSAIDs, or any component of the formulation; perioperative pain in the setting of coronary artery bypass surgery (CABG); pregnancy (3rd trimester)

Warnings/Precautions [U.S. Boxed Warning]: NSAIDs are associated with an increased risk of adverse cardiovascular events, including MI, stroke, and new onset or worsening of pre-existing hypertension. Risk may be increased with duration of use or pre-existing cardiovascular risk-factors or disease. Carefully evaluate individual cardiovascular risk profiles prior to prescribing. Use caution with fluid retention, CHF or hypertension.

Use of NSAIDs can compromise existing renal function. Renal toxicity can occur in patient with impaired renal function, dehydration, heart failure, liver dysfunction, those taking diuretics and ACEI and the elderly. Rehydrate patient before starting therapy. Monitor renal function closely. Meloxicam is not recommended for patients with advanced renal disease

[U.S. Boxed Warning]: NSAIDs may increase risk of gastrointestinal irritation, ulceration, bleeding, and perforation. These events may occur at any time during therapy and without warning. Use caution with a history of GI disease (bleeding or ulcers), concurrent therapy with aspirin, anticoagulants and/or corticosteroids, smoking, use of alcohol, the elderly or debilitated patients.

Use the lowest effective dose for the shortest duration of time, consistent with individual patient goals, to reduce risk of cardiovascular or GI adverse events. Alternate therapies should be considered for patients at high risk.

NSAIDs may cause serious skin adverse events including exfoliative dermatitis, Stevens-Johnson syndrome (SJS) and toxic epidermal necrolysis (TEN). Anaphylactoid reactions may occur, even without prior exposure; patients with "aspirin triad" (bronchial asthma, aspirin intolerance, rhinitis) may be at increased risk. Do not use in patients who experience bronchospasm, asthma, rhinitis, or urticaria with NSAID or aspirin therapy.

Use with caution in patients with decreased hepatic function. Closely monitor patients with any abnormal LFT. Severe hepatic reactions (eg, fulminant hepatitis, liver failure) have occurred with NSAID use, rarely; discontinue if signs or symptoms of liver disease develop, or if systemic manifestations occur.

The elderly are at increased risk for adverse effects (especially peptic ulceration, CNS effects, renal toxicity) from NSAIDs even at low doses.

Withhold for at least 4-6 half-lives prior to surgical or dental procedures. Safety and efficacy have not been established in pediatric patients <2 years of age.

Adverse Reactions Percentages reported in adult patients; abdominal pain, diarrhea, headache, pyrexia, and vomiting were reported more commonly in pediatric patients

2% to 10%:

- Cardiovascular: Edema (<1% to 4%)
- Central nervous system: Headache (2% to 8%), dizziness (<1% to 4%), insomnia (<1% to 4%)
- Dermatologic: Pruritus (<1% to 2%), rash (<1% to 3%)
- Gastrointestinal: Diarrhea (3% to 8%), dyspepsia (4% to 9%), nausea (2% to 7%), abdominal pain (2% to 5%), constipation (<1% to 3%), flatulence (<1% to 3%), vomiting (<1% to 3%)
- Hematologic: Anemia (<1% to 4%)
- Neuromuscular & skeletal: Arthralgia (<1% to 5%), back pain (<1% to 3%)
- Respiratory: Upper respiratory infection (2% to 8%), cough (<1% to 2%), pharyngitis (<1% to 3%)
- Miscellaneous: Flu-like symptoms (2% to 6%), falls (3%)

<2% (Limited to important or life-threatening): Agranulocytosis, allergic reaction, anaphylactic reaction, anaphylactoid reaction, angina, angioedema, arrhythmia, bronchospasm, bullous eruption, cardiac failure, colitis, depression, duodenal perforation, duodenal ulcer, erythema multiforme, gastric perforation, gastric ulcer, gastroesophageal reflux, gastrointestinal hemorrhage, hepatic failure, hepatitis, hyper-/hypotension, interstitial nephritis, intestinal perforation, jaundice, MI, pancreatitis, paresthesia, photosensitivity reaction, renal failure, seizure, shock, somnolence, Stevens-Johnson syndrome, syncope, thrombocytopenia, tinnitus, toxic epidermal necrolysis, tremor, ulcerative stomatitis, urticaria, vasculitis, vertigo

(Continued)

Meloxicam *(Continued)*

Overdosage/Toxicology Symptoms of overdose include lethargy, drowsiness, nausea, vomiting, and epigastric pain. Rarely, severe symptoms have been associated with NSAID overdose including apnea, metabolic acidosis, coma, nystagmus, seizures, leukocytosis, and renal failure. Management of NSAID intoxication is supportive and symptomatic. Since meloxicam undergoes enterohepatic cycling, multiple doses of charcoal may be needed to reduce the potential for delayed toxicities. Cholestyramine has been shown to increase meloxicam clearance. Meloxicam is not dialyzable.

Drug Interactions Substrate (minor) of CYP2C9, 3A4; **Inhibits** CYP2C9 (weak)

ACE inhibitors: Antihypertensive effects may be decreased by concurrent therapy with NSAIDs; monitor blood pressure

Angiotensin II antagonists: Antihypertensive effects may be decreased by concurrent therapy with NSAIDs; monitor blood pressure

Anticoagulants (warfarin, heparin, LMWHs) in combination with NSAIDs can cause increased risk of bleeding.

Antiplatelet drugs (ticlopidine, clopidogrel, aspirin, abciximab, dipyridamole, eptifibatide, tirofiban) can cause an increased risk of bleeding.

Aspirin increases serum concentrations (AUC) of meloxicam (in addition to potential for additive adverse effects); concurrent use is not recommended.

Beta-blockers: NSAIDs may decrease the antihypertensive effect of beta-blockers. Monitor.

Cholestyramine (and other bile acid sequestrants): May decrease the absorption of NSAIDs. Separate by at least 2 hours.

Corticosteroids may increase the risk of GI ulceration; avoid concurrent use.

Cyclosporine: NSAIDs may increase serum creatinine, potassium, blood pressure, and cyclosporine levels; monitor cyclosporine levels and renal function carefully.

Hydralazine's antihypertensive effect is decreased; avoid concurrent use.

Lithium levels can be increased; avoid concurrent use if possible or monitor lithium levels and adjust dose. When NSAID is stopped, lithium will need adjustment again.

Loop diuretic's efficacy (diuretic and antihypertensive effect) may be reduced by NSAIDs.

Methotrexate: Severe bone marrow suppression, aplastic anemia, and GI toxicity have been reported with concomitant NSAID therapy. Avoid use during moderate or high-dose methotrexate (increased and prolonged methotrexate levels). NSAID use during low-dose treatment of rheumatoid arthritis has not been fully evaluated; extreme caution is warranted.

Thiazide diuretics: Antihypertensive effects of thiazide diuretics are decreased; avoid concurrent use.

Warfarin INRs may be increased by meloxicam. Monitor INR closely, particularly during initiation or change in dose. May increase risk of bleeding. Use lowest possible dose for shortest duration possible.

Ethanol/Nutrition/Herb Interactions

Ethanol: Avoid ethanol (may enhance gastric mucosal irritation).

Herb/Nutraceutical: Avoid alfalfa, anise, bilberry, bladderwrack, bromelain, cat's claw, celery, coleus, cordyceps, dong quai, evening primrose, feverfew, fenugreek, garlic, ginger, ginkgo biloboa, red clover, horse chestnut, grapeseed, green tea, ginseng, guggul, horse chestnut seed, horseradish, licorice, prickly ash, red clover, reishi, SAMe, sweet clover, turmeric, white willow (all have additional antiplatelet activity).

Dietary Considerations Should be taken with food or milk to minimize gastrointestinal irritation.

Dosage Forms

Suspension: 7.5 mg/5 mL (100 mL) [contains sodium benzoate; raspberry flavor]

Tablet: 7.5 mg, 15 mg

References

Jacobi J, Fraser GL, Coursin DB, et al, "Clinical Practice Guidelines for the Sustained Use of Sedatives and Analgesics in the Critically Ill Adult," *Crit Care Med*, 2002, 30(1):119-41. Available at: http://www.sccm.org/pdf/sedatives.pdf.

Meperidine (me PER i deen)

Medication Safety Issues

Sound-alike/look-alike issues:

Meperidine may be confused with meprobamate

Demerol® may be confused with Demulen®, Desyrel®, dicumarol, Dilaudid®, Dymelor®, Pamelor®

Related Information

Acute Postoperative Pain *on page 1388*
Anesthesia Considerations for Neurosurgery *on page 1401*
Anesthesia for Patients With Liver Disease *on page 1421*
Chronic Pain Management *on page 1430*
Chronic Renal Failure *on page 1437*
Moderate Sedation *on page 1442*
Narcotic / Opioid Analgesics *on page 1568*
Opioids *on page 1535*

U.S. Brand Names Demerol®; Meperitab®

Canadian Brand Names Demerol®

Synonyms Isonipecaine Hydrochloride; Meperidine Hydrochloride; Pethidine Hydrochloride

Pharmacologic Category Analgesic, Narcotic

Restrictions C-II

Generic Available Yes

Use Management of moderate to severe pain; adjunct to anesthesia and preoperative sedation

Unlabeled/Investigational Use

Reduce postoperative shivering; reduce rigors from amphotericin

Mechanism of Action Binds to opiate receptors in the CNS, causing inhibition of ascending pain pathways, altering the perception of and response to pain; produces generalized CNS depression

Pharmacodynamics/Kinetics

Onset of action: Analgesic: Oral, SubQ: 10-15 minutes; I.V.: ~5 minutes

Peak effect: SubQ.: ~1 hour; Oral: 2 hours

Duration: Oral, SubQ.: 2-4 hours

Absorption: I.M.: Erratic and highly variable

Distribution: Crosses placenta; enters breast milk

Protein binding: 65% to 75%

Metabolism: Hepatic; hydrolyzed to meperidinic acid (inactive) or undergoes N-demethylation to normeperidine (active; has $1/2$ the analgesic effect and 2-3 times the CNS effects of meperidine)

Bioavailability: ~50% to 60%; increased with liver disease

Half-life elimination:

Parent drug: Terminal phase: Adults: 2.5-4 hours, Liver disease: 7-11 hours

Normeperidine (active metabolite): 15-30 hours; can accumulate with high doses or with decreased renal function

Excretion: Urine (as metabolites)

Dosage Note: Doses should be titrated to necessary analgesic effect. When changing route of administration, note that oral doses are about half as effective as parenteral dose. Not recommended for chronic pain. These are guidelines and do not represent the maximum doses that may be required in all patients. In patients with normal renal function, doses of ≤600 mg/24 hours and use for ≤48 hours are recommended (American Pain Society, 1999).

Children: Pain: Oral, I.M., I.V., SubQ: 1-1.5 mg/kg/dose every 3-4 hours as needed; 1-2 mg/kg as a single dose preoperative medication may be used; maximum 100 mg/dose (Note: Oral route is not recommended for acute pain.)

Adults: Pain:

Oral: Initial: Opiate-naive: 50 mg every 3-4 hours as needed; usual dosage range: 50-150 mg every 2-4 hours as needed (manufacturers recommendation; oral route is not recommended for acute pain)

I.M., SubQ: Initial: Opiate-naive: 50-75 mg every 3-4 hours as needed; patients with prior opiate exposure may require higher initial doses

Preoperatively: 50-100 mg given 30-90 minutes before the beginning of anesthesia

Slow I.V.: Initial: 5-10 mg every 5 minutes as needed

Patient-controlled analgesia (PCA): Usual concentration: 10 mg/mL

(Continued)

Meperidine *(Continued)*

Initial dose: 10 mg

Demand dose: 1-5 mg (manufacturer recommendations); range 5-25 mg (American Pain Society, 1999).

Lockout interval: 5-10 minutes

Elderly:

Oral: 50 mg every 4 hours

I.M.: 25 mg every 4 hours

Dosing adjustment in renal impairment: Avoid repeated administration of meperidine in renal dysfunction:

Cl_{cr} 10-50 mL/minute: Administer at 75% of normal dose

Cl_{cr} <10 mL/minute: Administer at 50% of normal dose

Dosing adjustment/comments in hepatic disease: Increased narcotic effect in cirrhosis; reduction in dose more important for oral than I.V. route

Stability Meperidine injection should be stored at room temperature and protected from light and freezing; protect oral dosage forms from light

Incompatible with aminophylline, heparin, phenobarbital, phenytoin, and sodium bicarbonate

Administration Meperidine may be administered I.M., SubQ, or I.V.; I.V. push should be administered slowly, use of a 10 mg/mL concentration has been recommended. For continuous I.V. infusions, a more dilute solution (eg, 1 mg/mL) should be used.

Oral: Administer syrup diluted in ½ glass of water; undiluted syrup may exert topical anesthetic effect on mucous membranes

Monitoring Parameters Pain relief, respiratory and mental status, blood pressure; observe patient for excessive sedation, CNS depression, seizures, respiratory depression

Reference Range Therapeutic: 70-500 ng/mL (SI: 283-2020 nmol/L); Toxic: >1000 ng/mL (SI: >4043 nmol/L)

Anesthesia and Critical Care Concerns/Other Considerations The 2002 ACCM/SCCM guidelines for analgesia (critically-ill adult) recommend against using meperidine repetitively. The guidelines recommend fentanyl in patients who need immediate pain relief because of its rapid onset of action; fentanyl or hydromorphone is preferred in patients who are hypotensive or have renal dysfunction. Morphine or hydromorphone is recommended for intermittent, scheduled therapy. Both have a longer duration of action requiring less frequent administration.

Pregnancy Risk Factor C/D (prolonged use or high doses at term)

Contraindications Hypersensitivity to meperidine or any component of the formulation; use with or within 14 days of MAO inhibitors; pregnancy (prolonged use or high doses near term)

Warnings/Precautions Meperidine is not recommended for the management of chronic pain. When used for acute pain (in patients without renal or CNS disease), treatment should be limited to 48 hours and doses should not exceed 600 mg/24 hours. Oral meperidine is not recommended for acute pain management. Normeperidine (an active metabolite and CNS stimulant) may accumulate and precipitate anxiety, tremors, or seizures; risk increases with renal dysfunction and cumulative dose.

Use only with extreme caution (if at all) in patients with head injury or increased intracranial pressure (ICP); potential to elevate ICP may be greatly exaggerated in these patients. Use caution with pulmonary, hepatic, or renal disorders, supraventricular tachycardias, acute abdominal conditions, hypothyroidism, Addison's disease, BPH, or urethral stricture.

An opioid-containing analgesic regimen should be tailored to each patient's needs and based upon the type of pain being treated (acute versus chronic), the route of administration, degree of tolerance for opioids (naive versus chronic user), age, weight, and medical condition. The optimal analgesic dose varies widely among patients. Doses should be titrated to pain relief/prevention.

Some preparations contain sulfites which may cause allergic reaction. Tolerance or drug dependence may result from extended use.

Adverse Reactions Frequency not defined.

Cardiovascular: Hypotension

Central nervous system: Fatigue, drowsiness, dizziness, nervousness, headache, restlessness, malaise, confusion, mental depression, hallucinations, paradoxical CNS stimulation, increased intracranial pressure, seizure (associated with metabolite accumulation), serotonin syndrome

Dermatologic: Rash, urticaria

Gastrointestinal: Nausea, vomiting, constipation, anorexia, stomach cramps, xerostomia, biliary spasm, paralytic ileus, sphincter of Oddi spasm

Genitourinary: Ureteral spasms, decreased urination

Local: Pain at injection site

Neuromuscular & skeletal: Weakness

Respiratory: Dyspnea

Miscellaneous: Histamine release, physical and psychological dependence

Overdosage/Toxicology Symptoms of overdose include CNS depression, respiratory depression, mydriasis, bradycardia, pulmonary edema, chronic tremor, CNS excitability, and seizures. Treatment is symptomatic. Naloxone, 2 mg I.V. with repeat administration as necessary up to a total dose of 10 mg, can be used to reverse opiate effects. Naloxone should not be used to treat meperidine-induced seizures. Naloxone does not reverse the adverse effects of normeperidine.

Drug Interactions

Substrate (minor) of CYP2B6, 2C19, 3A4

Acyclovir: May increase meperidine metabolite concentrations. Use caution.

Barbiturates: May decrease analgesic efficacy and increase sedative and/or respiratory depressive effects of meperidine.

Cimetidine: May increase meperidine metabolite concentrations; use caution.

CNS depressants (including benzodiazepines): May potentiate the sedative and/or respiratory depressive effects of meperidine.

MAO inhibitors: May enhance the serotonergic effect of meperidine, which may cause serotonin syndrome. Concurrent use with or within 14 days of an MAO inhibitor is contraindicated.

Phenothiazines: May potentiate the sedative and/or respiratory depressive effects of meperidine; may increase the incidence of hypotension.

Phenytoin: May decrease the analgesic effects of meperidine

Ritonavir: May increase meperidine metabolite concentrations; use caution.

Serotonin agonists: Serotonin agonists and meperidine may enhance serotonin levels in the brain. Serotonin syndrome may occur.

Serotonin reuptake inhibitors: May potentiate the effects of meperidine, increasing serotonin levels in the brain. Serotonin syndrome may occur.

Sibutramine: May enhance the serotonergic effect of meperidine. Serotonin syndrome may occur.

Tricyclic antidepressants: May potentiate the sedative and/or respiratory depressive effects of meperidine. In addition, potentially may increase the risk of serotonin syndrome.

Ethanol/Nutrition/Herb Interactions

Ethanol: Avoid or limit ethanol (may increase CNS depression). Watch for sedation.

Herb/Nutraceutical: Avoid valerian, St John's wort, kava kava, gotu kola (may increase CNS depression).

Test Interactions Increased amylase (S), increased BSP retention, increased CPK (I.M. injections)

Dosage Forms

Injection, solution, as hydrochloride [ampul]: 25 mg/0.5 mL (0.5 mL); 25 mg/mL (1 mL); 50 mg/mL (1 mL, 1.5 mL, 2 mL); 75 mg/mL (1 mL); 100 mg/mL (1 mL)

Injection, solution, as hydrochloride [prefilled syringe]: 25 mg/mL (1 mL); 50 mg/mL (1 mL); 75 mg/mL (1 mL); 100 mg/mL (1 mL)

Injection, solution, as hydrochloride [for PCA pump]: 10 mg/mL (30 mL, 50 mL, 60 mL)

Injection, solution, as hydrochloride [vial]: 25 mg/mL (1 mL); 50 mg/mL (1 mL, 30 mL); 75 mg/mL (1 mL); 100 mg/mL (1 mL, 20 mL) [may contain sodium metabisulfite]

Syrup, as hydrochloride: 50 mg/5 mL (500 mL) [contains sodium benzoate]

Demerol®: 50 mg/5 mL (480 mL) [contains benzoic acid; banana flavor]

Tablet, as hydrochloride (Demerol®, Meperitab®): 50 mg, 100 mg

References

American Academy of Pediatrics Committee on Drugs, "The Transfer of Drugs and Other Chemicals Into Human Milk," *Pediatrics*, 2001, 108(3):776-89.

Armstrong PJ and Bersten A, "Normeperidine Toxicity," *Anesth Analg*, 1986, 65(5):536-8.

(Continued)

Meperidine *(Continued)*

"Drugs for Pain," *Treat Guidel Med Lett*, 2004, 2(23):47-54.

Jacobi J, Fraser GL, Coursin DB, et al, "Clinical Practice Guidelines for the Sustained Use of Sedatives and Analgesics in the Critically Ill Adult," *Crit Care Med*, 2002, 30(1):119-41. Available at: http://www.sccm.org/pdf/sedatives.pdf.

Mokhlesi B, Leikin JB, Murray P, et al, "Adult Toxicology in Critical Care. Part 11: Specific Poisonings," *Chest*, 2003, 123(3):897-922.

"Principles of Analgesic Use in the Treatment of Acute Pain and Chronic Cancer Pain," 5th ed, Glenview, IL: American Pain Society, 2003.

Stone PA, Macintyre PE, and Jarvis DA, "Norpethidine Toxicity and Patient Controlled Analgesia," *Br J Anaesth*, 1993, 71(5):738-40.

♦ **Meperidine Hydrochloride** *see* Meperidine *on page 801*

♦ **Meperitab®** *see* Meperidine *on page 801*

♦ **Mephyton®** *see* Phytonadione *on page 1027*

Mepivacaine (me PIV a kane)

Medication Safety Issues

Sound-alike/look-alike issues:

Mepivacaine may be confused with bupivacaine

Polocaine® may be confused with prilocaine

Related Information

Acute Postoperative Pain *on page 1388*

Local Anesthetics *on page 1532*

U.S. Brand Names Carbocaine®; Polocaine®; Polocaine® Dental; Polocaine® MPF

Canadian Brand Names Carbocaine®; Polocaine®

Synonyms Mepivacaine Hydrochloride

Pharmacologic Category Local Anesthetic

Generic Available No

Use Local or regional analgesia; anesthesia by local infiltration, peripheral and central neural techniques including epidural and caudal blocks; **not** for use in spinal anesthesia

Mechanism of Action Mepivacaine is an amide local anesthetic similar to lidocaine; like all local anesthetics, mepivacaine acts by preventing the generation and conduction of nerve impulses

Pharmacodynamics/Kinetics

Onset of action (route and dose dependent): Range: 3-20 minutes

Duration (route and dose dependent): 2-2.5 hours

Protein binding: ~75%

Metabolism: Primarily hepatic via N-demethylation, hydroxylation, and glucuronidation

Half-life elimination: Neonates: 8.7-9 hours; Adults: 1.9-3 hours

Excretion: Urine (95% as metabolites)

Dosage

Injectable local anesthetic: Dose varies with procedure, degree of anesthesia needed, vascularity of tissue, duration of anesthesia required, and physical condition of patient. The smallest dose and concentration required to produce the desired effect should be used.

Children: Maximum dose: 5-6 mg/kg; only concentrations <2% should be used in children <3 years or <14 kg (30 lbs)

Adults: Maximum dose: 400 mg; do not exceed 1000 mg/24 hours

Cervical, brachial, intercostal, pudenal nerve block: 5-40 mL of a 1% solution (maximum: 400 mg) **or** 5-20 mL of a 2% solution (maximum: 400 mg). For pudenal block, inject ½ the total dose each side.

Transvaginal block (paracervical plus pudenal): Up to 30 mL (both sides) of a 1% solution (maximum: 300 mg). Inject ½ the total dose each side.

Paracervical block: Up to 20 mL (both sides) of a 1% solution (maximum: 200 mg). Inject ½ the total dose to each side. This is the maximum recommended dose per 90-minute procedure; inject slowly with 5 minutes between sides.

Caudal and epidural block (preservative free solutions only): 15-30 mL of a 1% solution (maximum: 300 mg) **or** 10-25 mL of a 1.5% solution (maximum: 375 mg) **or** 10-20 mL of a 2% solution (maximum: 400 mg)

Infiltration: Up to 40 mL of a 1% solution (maximum: 400 mg)

Therapeutic block (pain management): 1-5 mL of a 1% solution (maximum: 50 mg) **or** 1-5 mL of a 2% solution (maximum: 100 mg)

Dental anesthesia: Adults:

Single site in upper or lower jaw: 54 mg (1.8 mL) as a 3% solution

Infiltration and nerve block of entire oral cavity: 270 mg (9 mL) as a 3% solution. Manufacturer's maximum recommended dose is not more than 400 mg to normal healthy adults.

Stability Store at controlled room temperature of 15°C to 30°C (59°F to 86°F); brief exposure up to 40°C (104°F) does not adversely affect the product. Solutions may be sterilized. Dental solutions should be protected from light.

Administration Before injecting, withdraw syringe plunger to ensure injection is not into vein or artery

Monitoring Parameters Vital signs, state of consciousness; signs of CNS toxicity

Anesthesia and Critical Care Concerns/Other Considerations

Peripheral nerve block, caudal/epidural, therapeutic block: 1% or 2% solution

Transvaginal, paracervical block: 1% solution

Infiltration: 0.5% to 1% solution

Dental procedures: Mepivacaine 3% or mepivacaine 2% solution with levonordefrin

Pregnancy Risk Factor C

Contraindications Hypersensitivity to mepivacaine, other amide-type local anesthetics, or any component of the formulation

Warnings/Precautions Use with caution in patients with cardiac disease, hepatic or renal disease, or hyperthyroidism. Local anesthetics have been associated with rare occurrences of sudden respiratory arrest; convulsions due to systemic toxicity leading to cardiac arrest have been reported presumably due to intravascular injection. A test dose is recommended prior to epidural administration and all reinforcing doses with continuous catheter technique. Do not use solutions containing preservatives for caudal or epidural block. Use caution in debilitated, elderly, or acutely-ill patients; dose reduction may be required.

Adverse Reactions Degree of adverse effects in the CNS and cardiovascular system is directly related to the blood levels of mepivacaine, route of administration, and physical status of the patient. The effects below are more likely to occur after systemic administration rather than infiltration.

Cardiovascular: Bradycardia, cardiac arrest, cardiac output decreased, heart block, hyper-/hypotension, myocardial depression, syncope, tachycardia, ventricular arrhythmias

Central nervous system: Anxiety, chills, convulsions, depression, dizziness, excitation, restlessness, tremors

Dermatologic: Angioneurotic edema, diaphoresis, erythema, pruritus, urticaria

Gastrointestinal: Fecal incontinence, nausea, vomiting

Genitourinary: Incontinence, urinary retention

Neuromuscular & skeletal: Paralysis

Ocular: Blurred vision, pupil constriction

Otic: Tinnitus

Respiratory: Apnea, hypoventilation, sneezing

Miscellaneous: Allergic reaction, anaphylactoid reaction

Overdosage/Toxicology Symptoms of overdose include dizziness, cyanosis, tremor, and bronchial spasm. Treatment is symptomatic and supportive. Termination of anesthesia by pneumatic tourniquet inflation should be attempted when mepivacaine is administered by infiltration or regional injection.

Dosage Forms

Injection, solution, as hydrochloride [contains methylparabens]:

Carbocaine®: 1% (50 mL); 2% (50 mL)

Polocaine®: 1% (50 mL); 2% (50 mL)

Injection, solution, as hydrochloride [preservative free]:

Carbocaine®: 1% (30 mL); 1.5% (30 mL); 2% (20 mL); 3% (1.8 mL) [dental cartridge]

Polocaine® Dental: 3% (1.8 mL) [dental cartridge]

Polocaine® MPF: 1% (30 mL); 1.5% (30 mL); 2% (20 mL)

- **Mepivacaine Hydrochloride** *see* Mepivacaine *on page 804*
- **Mercapturic Acid** *see* Acetylcysteine *on page 35*

Meropenem (mer oh PEN em)

U.S. Brand Names Merrem® I.V.

Canadian Brand Names Merrem®

Pharmacologic Category Antibiotic, Carbapenem

Generic Available No

Use Treatment of intra-abdominal infections (complicated appendicitis and peritonitis); treatment of bacterial meningitis in pediatric patients ≥3 months of age caused by *S. pneumoniae*, *H. influenzae*, and *N. meningitidis*; treatment of complicated skin and skin structure infections caused by susceptible organisms

Unlabeled/Investigational Use Febrile neutropenia, urinary tract infections

Mechanism of Action Inhibits bacterial cell wall synthesis by binding to several of the penicillin-binding proteins, which in turn inhibit the final transpeptidation step of peptidoglycan synthesis in bacterial cell walls, thus inhibiting cell wall biosynthesis; bacteria eventually lyse due to ongoing activity of cell wall autolytic enzymes (autolysins and murein hydrolases) while cell wall assembly is arrested

Pharmacodynamics/Kinetics

Distribution: V_d: Adults: ~0.3 L/kg, Children: 0.4-0.5 L/kg; penetrates well into most body fluids and tissues; CSF concentrations approximate those of the plasma

Protein binding: 2%

Metabolism: Hepatic; metabolized to open beta-lactam form (inactive)

Half-life elimination:

- Normal renal function: 1-1.5 hours
- Cl_{cr} 30-80 mL/minute: 1.9-3.3 hours
- Cl_{cr} 2-30 mL/minute: 3.82-5.7 hours

Time to peak, tissue: 1 hour following infusion

Excretion: Urine (~25% as inactive metabolites)

Dosage

Usual dosage ranges:

Neonates: I.V.:

- Postnatal age 0-7 days: 20 mg/kg/dose every 12 hours
- Postnatal age >7 days:
  - Weight 1200-2000 g: 20 mg/kg/dose every 12 hours
  - Weight >2000 g: 20 mg/kg/dose every 8 hours

Children ≥3 months: I.V.: 60 mg/kg/day divided every 8 hours (maximum dose: 6 g/day)

Adults: I.V.: 1.5-6 g/day divided every 8 hours

Indication-specific dosing:

Children >3 months (<50 kg): I.V.:

- **Febrile neutropenia (unlabeled use):** 20 mg/kg every 8 hours (maximum dose: 1 g every 8 hours)
- **Intra-abdominal infections:** 20 mg/kg every 8 hours (maximum dose: 1 g every 8 hours)
- **Meningitis:** 40 mg/kg every 8 hours (maximum dose: 2 g every 8 hours)
- **Skin and skin structure infections (complicated):** 10 mg/kg every 8 hours (maximum dose: 500 mg every 8 hours)

Children >50 kg and Adults: I.V.:

- ***Burkholderia pseudomallei*** **(melioidosis),** ***Pseudomonas:*** 1 g every 8 hours
- **Cholangitis, intra-abdominal infections, otitis externa, septic lateral sinus thrombosis:** 1 g every 8 hours
- **Febrile neutropenia, pneumonia, other severe infections (unlabeled use):** 1 g every 8 hours
- **Liver abscess:** 1 g every 8 hours for 2-3 weeks, then oral therapy for duration of 4-6 weeks
- **Meningitis:** 2 g every 8 hours
- **Mild-to-moderate infection:** 1.5-3 g/day divided every 8 hours
- **Skin and skin structure infections (complicated):** 500 mg every 8 hours; diabetic foot: 1 g every 8 hours
- **Urinary tract infections, complicated (unlabeled use):** 500 mg to 1 g every 8 hours

Dosing adjustment in renal impairment: Adults:

Cl_{cr} 26-50 mL/minute: Administer recommended dose based on indication every 12 hours

Cl_{cr} 10-25 mL/minute: Administer one-half recommended dose every 12 hours
Cl_{cr} <10 mL/minute: Administer one-half recommended dose every 24 hours
Dialysis: Meropenem and its metabolites are readily dialyzable
Continuous arteriovenous or venovenous hemodiafiltration effects: Dose as Cl_{cr} 10-50 mL/minute

Stability Dry powder should be stored at controlled room temperature 20°C to 25°C (68°F to 77°F). Meropenem infusion vials may be reconstituted with SWFI or a compatible diluent (eg, NS). The 500 mg vials should be reconstituted with 10 mL, and 1 g vials with 20 mL. May be further diluted with compatible solutions for infusion. Consult detailed reference/product labeling for compatibility.

Injection reconstitution: Stability in vial when constituted (up to 50 mg/mL) with:
SWFI: Stable for up to 2 hours at room temperature and for up to 12 hours under refrigeration
Sodium chloride: Stable for up to 2 hours at room temperature or for up to 18 hours under refrigeration.
Dextrose 5% injection: Stable for 1 hour at room temperature or for 8 hours under refrigeration

Infusion admixture (1-20 mg/mL): Solution stability when diluted in NS is 4 hours at room temperature or 24 hours under refrigeration. Stability in D_5W is 1 hour at room temperature and 4 hours under refrigeration.

Administration Administer I.V. infusion over 15-30 minutes; I.V. bolus injection over 3-5 minutes

Monitoring Parameters Monitor for signs of anaphylaxis during first dose

Pregnancy Risk Factor B

Contraindications Hypersensitivity to meropenem, any component of the formulation, or other carbapenems (eg, imipenem); patients who have experienced anaphylactic reactions to other beta-lactams

Warnings/Precautions

Hypersensitivity reactions, including anaphylaxis, have occurred and often require immediate drug discontinuation. Seizures and other CNS adverse reactions have occurred, most commonly in patients with renal impairment and/or underlying neurologic disorders (less frequent than with Primaxin®). Use with caution in renal impairment; dose adjustment is necessary. Thrombocytopenia has been reported in patients with significant renal dysfunction. Pseudomembranous colitis has been associated with meropenem use. Superinfection is possible with long courses of therapy. Safety and efficacy have not been established for children <3 months of age

Adverse Reactions

1% to 10%:
Cardiovascular: Peripheral vascular disorder (<1%)
Central nervous system: Headache (2% to 8%), pain (5%)
Dermatologic: Rash (2% to 3%, includes diaper-area moniliasis in pediatrics), pruritus (1%)
Gastrointestinal: Diarrhea (4% to 5%), nausea/vomiting (1% to 8%), constipation (1% to 7%), oral moniliasis (up to 2% in pediatric patients), glossitis
Hematologic: Anemia (up to 6%)
Local: Inflammation at the injection site (2%), phlebitis/thrombophlebitis (1%), injection site reaction (1%)
Respiratory: Apnea (1%)
Miscellaneous: Sepsis (2%), septic shock (1%)

<1% (Limited to important or life-threatening): Agitation/delirium, agranulocytosis, angioedema, arrhythmia, bilirubin increased, bradycardia, BUN increased, cholestatic creatinine increased, jaundice/jaundice, decreased prothrombin time, dyspepsia, dyspnea, eosinophilia, epistaxis, erythema multiforme, gastrointestinal hemorrhage, hallucinations, hearing loss, heart failure, hemoperitoneum, hepatic failure, hyper-/hypotension, ileus, leukopenia, melena, MI, neutropenia, paresthesia, pleural effusion, pulmonary edema, pulmonary embolism, renal failure, seizure, Stevens-Johnson syndrome, syncope, thrombocytopenia, toxic epidermal necrolysis, urticaria, vaginal moniliasis

Overdosage/Toxicology No cases of acute overdosage are reported which have resulted in symptoms. Accidental overdose is possible with the use of large doses in patients with renal impairment. Supportive therapy is recommended. Meropenem and its metabolite are removable by dialysis.

Drug Interactions

Probenecid: May increase meropenem serum concentrations; use caution.
Valproic acid: Meropenem may decrease valproic acid serum concentrations to subtherapeutic levels; monitor.

(Continued)

Meropenem *(Continued)*

Dietary Considerations 1 g of meropenem contains 90.2 mg of sodium as sodium carbonate (3.92 mEq)

Dosage Forms Injection, powder for reconstitution: 500 mg [contains sodium 45.1 mg as sodium carbonate (1.96 mEq)]; 1 g [contains sodium 90.2 mg as sodium carbonate (3.92 mEq)]

References

American Thoracic Society and Infectious Diseases Society of America, "Guidelines for the Management of Adults With Hospital-Acquired, Ventilator-Associated, and Healthcare-Associated Pneumonia," *Am J Respir Crit Care Med*, 2005, 171(4):388-416.

Tunkel AR, Hartman BJ, Kaplan SL, et al, "Practice Guidelines for the Management of Bacterial Meningitis," *Clin Infect Dis*, 2004, 39(9):1267-84.

Ververs TF, van Dijk A, Vinks SA, et al, "Pharmacokinetics and Dosing Regimen of Meropenem in Critically Ill Patients Receiving Continuous Venovenous Hemofiltration," *Crit Care Med*, 2000, 28(10):3412-6.

♦ **Merrem® (Can)** *see* Meropenem *on page 806*
♦ **Merrem® I.V.** *see* Meropenem *on page 806*
♦ **M-Eslon® (Can)** *see* Morphine Sulfate *on page 867*
♦ **Mestinon®** *see* Pyridostigmine *on page 1087*
♦ **Mestinon®-SR (Can)** *see* Pyridostigmine *on page 1087*
♦ **Mestinon® Timespan®** *see* Pyridostigmine *on page 1087*
♦ **Metacortandralone** *see* PrednisoLONE *on page 1046*
♦ **Metadol™ (Can)** *see* Methadone *on page 813*

Metaproterenol (met a proe TER e nol)

Medication Safety Issues
Sound-alike/look-alike issues:
Metaproterenol may be confused with metipranolol, metoprolol
Alupent® may be confused with Atrovent®

U.S. Brand Names Alupent®

Synonyms Metaproterenol Sulfate; Orciprenaline Sulfate

Pharmacologic Category $Beta_2$-Adrenergic Agonist

Generic Available Yes: Excludes inhaler

Use Bronchodilator in reversible airway obstruction due to asthma or COPD; because of its delayed onset of action (1 hour) and prolonged effect (4 or more hours), this may not be the drug of choice for assessing response to a bronchodilator

Mechanism of Action Relaxes bronchial smooth muscle by action on $beta_2$-receptors with very little effect on heart rate

Pharmacodynamics/Kinetics
Onset of action: Bronchodilation: Oral: ~15 minutes; Inhalation: ~60 seconds
Peak effect: Oral: ~1 hour
Duration: ~1-5 hours

Dosage
Oral:
Children:
<2 years: 0.4 mg/kg/dose given 3-4 times/day; in infants, the dose can be given every 8-12 hours
2-6 years: 1-2.6 mg/kg/day divided every 6 hours
6-9 years: 10 mg/dose 3-4 times/day
Children >9 years and Adults: 20 mg 3-4 times/day
Elderly: Initial: 10 mg 3-4 times/day, increasing as necessary up to 20 mg 3-4 times/day
Inhalation: Children >12 years and Adults: 2-3 inhalations every 3-4 hours, up to 12 inhalations in 24 hours
Nebulizer:
Infants and Children: 0.01-0.02 mL/kg of 5% solution; minimum dose: 0.1 mL; maximum dose: 0.3 mL diluted in 2-3 mL normal saline every 4-6 hours (may be given more frequently according to need)
Adolescents and Adults: 5-20 breaths of full strength 5% metaproterenol **or** 0.2 to 0.3 mL 5% metaproterenol in 2.5-3 mL normal saline until nebulized every 4-6 hours (can be given more frequently according to need)

Stability Store in tight, light-resistant container; do not use if brown solution or contains a precipitate

Administration

Inhalation: Do not use solutions for nebulization if they are brown or contain a precipitate. Shake inhaler well before using.

Oral: Administer around-the-clock to promote less variation in peak and trough serum levels

Monitoring Parameters Assess lung sounds, heart rate, and blood pressure before administration and during peak of medication; observe patient for wheezing after administration, if this occurs, call physician; monitor respiratory rate, arterial or capillary blood gases if applicable; FEV_1, peak flow, and/or other pulmonary function tests; CNS stimulation; serum glucose, serum potassium

Anesthesia and Critical Care Concerns/Other Considerations Hypertension and tachycardia are increased with exogenous sympathomimetics. During endotracheal intubation, $beta_2$-specific agent is more appropriate for perioperative use. Use with caution perioperatively due to $beta_1$ effect of agent.

Pregnancy Risk Factor C

Contraindications Hypersensitivity to metaproterenol or any component of the formulation; pre-existing cardiac arrhythmias associated with tachycardia

Warnings/Precautions Optimize anti-inflammatory treatment before initiating maintenance treatment with metaproterenol. Do not use as a component of chronic therapy without an anti-inflammatory agent. Only the mildest form of asthma (Step 1 and/or exercise-induced) would not require concurrent use based upon asthma guidelines. Patient must be instructed to seek medical attention in cases where acute symptoms are not relieved or a previous level of response is diminished. The need to increase frequency of use may indicate deterioration of asthma, and treatment must not be delayed.

Use caution in patients with cardiovascular disease (arrhythmia or hypertension or CHF), convulsive disorders, diabetes, glaucoma, hyperthyroidism, or hypokalemia. Beta agonists may cause elevation in blood pressure, heart rate, and result in CNS stimulation/excitation. $Beta_2$ agonists may increase risk of arrhythmia, increase serum glucose, or decrease serum potassium.

Do not exceed recommended dose; serious adverse events including fatalities, have been associated with excessive use of inhaled sympathomimetics. Rarely, paradoxical bronchospasm may occur with use of inhaled bronchodilating agents; this should be distinguished from inadequate response. All patients should utilize a spacer device when using a metered-dose inhaler; additionally, a face mask should be used in children <4 years of age.

Metaproterenol has more $beta_1$ activity than $beta_2$-selective agents such as albuterol and, therefore, may no longer be the beta agonist of first choice. Oral use should be avoided due to the increased incidence of adverse effects.

Adverse Reactions

>10%:

- Cardiovascular: Tachycardia (<17%)
- Central nervous system: Nervousness (3% to 14%)
- Endocrine & metabolic: Serum glucose increased, serum potassium decreased
- Neuromuscular & skeletal: Tremor (1% to 33%)

1% to 10%:

- Cardiovascular: Palpitations (<4%)
- Central nervous system: Headache (<4%), dizziness (1% to 4%), insomnia (2%)
- Gastrointestinal: Nausea, vomiting, bad taste, heartburn (≥4%), xerostomia
- Neuromuscular & skeletal: Trembling, muscle cramps, weakness (1%)
- Respiratory: Coughing, pharyngitis (≤4%)
- Miscellaneous: Diaphoresis (increased) (≤4%)

<1% (Limited to important or life-threatening): Angina, chest pain, diarrhea, drowsiness, hypertension, hypokalemia, paradoxical bronchospasm, taste change

Overdosage/Toxicology Symptoms of overdose include tachycardia, tremor, hypertension, angina, and seizures. Hypokalemia also may occur. Cardiac arrest and death may be associated with abuse of beta-agonist bronchodilators. Treatment includes immediate discontinuation and symptomatic and supportive therapies. Cautious use of beta-adrenergic blocking agents may be considered in severe cases.

Drug Interactions

Beta-adrenergic blockers (eg, propranolol) antagonize metaproterenol's effects; avoid concurrent use.

(Continued)

Metaproterenol *(Continued)*

Inhaled ipratropium may increase duration of bronchodilation.
MAO inhibitors may increase side effects; monitor heart rate and blood pressure.
TCAs may increase side effects; monitor heart rate and blood pressure.
Sympathomimetics may increase side effects; monitor heart rate and blood pressure.
Halothane may increase risk of malignant arrhythmias; avoid concurrent use.

Test Interactions Increased potassium (S)

Dosage Forms

Aerosol for oral inhalation, as sulfate (Alupent®): 0.65 mg/inhalation (14 g) [200 doses]
Solution for nebulization, as sulfate [preservative free]: 0.4% [4 mg/mL] (2.5 mL); 0.6% [6 mg/mL] (2.5 mL)
Syrup, as sulfate: 10 mg/5 mL (480 mL) [may contain sodium benzoate]
Tablet, as sulfate: 10 mg, 20 mg

♦ **Metaproterenol Sulfate** *see* Metaproterenol *on page 808*

Metformin (met FOR min)

Medication Safety Issues

Sound-alike/look-alike issues:
Metformin may be confused with metronidazole
Glucophage® may be confused with Glucotrol®, Glutofac®

Related Information

Thiazolidinediones *on page 1577*
Perioperative Management of the Diabetic Patient *on page 1464*

U.S. Brand Names Fortamet™; Glucophage®; Glucophage® XR; Riomet™

Canadian Brand Names Alti-Metformin; Apo-Metformin®; BCI-Metformin; Gen-Metformin; Glucophage®; Glumetza®; Glycon; Novo-Metformin; Nu-Metformin; PMS-Metformin; RAN™-Metformin; Rho®-Metformin; Sandoz-Metformin FC

Synonyms Metformin Hydrochloride

Pharmacologic Category Antidiabetic Agent, Biguanide

Generic Available Yes: Excludes solution

Use Management of type 2 diabetes mellitus (noninsulin dependent, NIDDM) as monotherapy when hyperglycemia cannot be managed on diet alone. May be used concomitantly with a sulfonylurea or insulin to improve glycemic control.

Unlabeled/Investigational Use Treatment of HIV lipodystrophy syndrome

Mechanism of Action Decreases hepatic glucose production, decreasing intestinal absorption of glucose and improves insulin sensitivity (increases peripheral glucose uptake and utilization)

Pharmacodynamics/Kinetics

Onset of action: Within days; maximum effects up to 2 weeks
Distribution: V_d: 654 ± 358 L
Protein binding: Negligible
Bioavailability: Absolute: Fasting: 50% to 60%
Half-life elimination, plasma: 6.2 hours
Excretion: Urine (90% as unchanged drug)

Dosage Note: Allow 1-2 weeks between dose titrations: Generally, clinically significant responses are not seen at doses <1500 mg daily; however, a lower recommended starting dose and gradual increased dosage is recommended to minimize gastrointestinal symptoms

Children 10-16 years: Management of type 2 diabetes mellitus: Oral (500 mg tablet or oral solution): Initial: 500 mg twice daily (given with the morning and evening meals); increases in daily dosage should be made in increments of 500 mg at weekly intervals, given in divided doses, up to a maximum of 2000 mg/day

Adults ≥17 years: Management of type 2 diabetes mellitus: Oral:
Immediate release tablet or oral solution: Initial: 500 mg twice daily (give with the morning and evening meals) **or** 850 mg once daily; increase dosage incrementally.
Incremental dosing recommendations based on dosage form:
500 mg tablet: One tablet/day at weekly intervals
850 mg tablet: One tablet/day every other week
Oral solution: 500 mg twice daily every other week

Doses of up to 2000 mg/day may be given twice daily. If a dose >2000 mg/day is required, it may be better tolerated in three divided doses. Maximum recommended dose 2550 mg/day.

Extended release tablet: Initial: 500 mg once daily (with the evening meal); dosage may be increased by 500 mg weekly; maximum dose: 2000 mg once daily. If glycemic control is not achieved at maximum dose, may divide dose to 1000 mg twice daily. If doses >2000 mg/day are needed, switch to regular release tablets and titrate to maximum dose of 2550 mg/day.

Elderly: The initial and maintenance dosing should be conservative, due to the potential for decreased renal function. Generally, elderly patients should not be titrated to the maximum dose of metformin. Do not use in patients ≥80 years of age unless normal renal function has been established.

Transfer from other antidiabetic agents: No transition period is generally necessary except when transferring from chlorpropamide. When transferring from chlorpropamide, care should be exercised during the first 2 weeks because of the prolonged retention of chlorpropamide in the body, leading to overlapping drug effects and possible hypoglycemia.

Concomitant metformin and oral sulfonylurea therapy: If patients have not responded to 4 weeks of the maximum dose of metformin monotherapy, consider a gradual addition of an oral sulfonylurea, even if prior primary or secondary failure to a sulfonylurea has occurred. Continue metformin at the maximum dose.

Failed sulfonylurea therapy: Patients with prior failure on glyburide may be treated by gradual addition of metformin. Initiate with glyburide 20 mg and metformin 500 mg daily. Metformin dosage may be increased by 500 mg/day at weekly intervals, up to a maximum of 2500 mg/day (dosage of glyburide maintained at 20 mg/day).

Concomitant metformin and insulin therapy: Initial: 500 mg metformin once daily, continue current insulin dose; increase by 500 mg metformin weekly until adequate glycemic control is achieved

Maximum dose: 2500 mg metformin; 2000 mg metformin extended release

Decrease insulin dose 10% to 25% when FPG <120 mg/dL; monitor and make further adjustments as needed

Dosing adjustment/comments in renal impairment: The plasma and blood half-life of metformin is prolonged and the renal clearance is decreased in proportion to the decrease in creatinine clearance. Per the manufacturer, metformin is contraindicated in the presence of renal dysfunction defined as a serum creatinine >1.5 mg/dL in males, or >1.4 mg/dL in females and in patients with abnormal clearance. Clinically, it has been recommended that metformin be avoided in patients with Cl_{cr} <60-70 mL/minute.

Dosing adjustment in hepatic impairment: Avoid metformin; liver disease is a risk factor for the development of lactic acidosis during metformin therapy.

Stability Store tablets and oral solution at 20°C to 25°C (68°F to 77°F).

Administration Extended release dosage form should be swallowed whole; do not crush, break, or chew. Patients who are anorexic or NPO may need to have their dose held to avoid hypoglycemia.

Monitoring Parameters Urine for glucose and ketones, fasting blood glucose, and hemoglobin A_{1c}. Initial and periodic monitoring of hematologic parameters (eg, hemoglobin/hematocrit and red blood cell indices) and renal function should be performed, at least annually. Check vitamin B_{12} and folate if anemia is present.

Reference Range Target range: Adults:

Fasting blood glucose: <120 mg/dL

Glycosylated hemoglobin: <7%

Anesthesia and Critical Care Concerns/Other Considerations While megaloblastic anemia has been rarely seen with metformin, if suspected, vitamin B_{12} deficiency should be excluded. Metformin has a large volume of distribution in liver, kidney, and GI tract where concentration is much larger than in the plasma.

Lactic acidosis is an uncommon side effect in patients without renal or respiratory insufficiency, hepatic failure, or conditions that predispose to hypoxemia. Metformin should be avoided in diabetic patients with heart failure.

Pregnancy Risk Factor B

Contraindications Hypersensitivity to metformin or any component of the formulation; renal disease or renal dysfunction (serum creatinine ≥1.5 mg/dL in males or ≥1.4 mg/dL in females or abnormal creatinine clearance from any cause, including shock, acute myocardial infarction, or septicemia); congestive heart

(Continued)

Metformin *(Continued)*

failure requiring pharmacological management; acute or chronic metabolic acidosis with or without coma (including diabetic ketoacidosis)

Note: Temporarily discontinue in patients undergoing radiologic studies in which intravascular iodinated contrast materials are utilized.

Warnings/Precautions [U.S. Boxed Warning]: Lactic acidosis is a rare, but potentially severe consequence of therapy with metformin. Lactic acidosis should be suspected in any diabetic patient receiving metformin who has evidence of acidosis when evidence of ketoacidosis is lacking. Discontinue metformin in clinical situations predisposing to hypoxemia, including conditions such as cardiovascular collapse, respiratory failure, acute myocardial infarction, acute congestive heart failure, and septicemia.

Metformin is substantially excreted by the kidney. The risk of accumulation and lactic acidosis increases with the degree of impairment of renal function. Patients with renal function below the limit of normal for their age should not receive metformin. In elderly patients, renal function should be monitored regularly; should not be used in any patient ≥80 years of age unless measurement of creatinine clearance verifies normal renal function. Use of concomitant medications that may affect renal function (ie, affect tubular secretion) may also affect metformin disposition. Metformin should be suspended in patients with dehydration and/or prerenal azotemia. Therapy should be suspended for any surgical procedures (resume only after normal intake resumed and normal renal function is verified). Metformin should also be temporarily discontinued for 48 hours in patients undergoing radiologic studies involving the intravascular administration of iodinated contrast materials (potential for acute alteration in renal function).

Avoid use in patients with impaired liver function. Patient must be instructed to avoid excessive acute or chronic ethanol use. Administration of oral antidiabetic drugs has been reported to be associated with increased cardiovascular mortality; metformin does not appear to share this risk. Safety and efficacy of metformin have been established for use in children ≥10 years of age; the extended release preparation is for use in patients ≥17 years of age.

Adverse Reactions

>10%:

- Gastrointestinal: Nausea/vomiting (6% to 25%), diarrhea (10% to 53%), flatulence (12%)
- Neuromuscular & skeletal: Weakness (9%)

1% to 10%:

- Cardiovascular: Chest discomfort, flushing, palpitation
- Central nervous system: Headache (6%), chills, dizziness, lightheadedness
- Dermatologic: Rash
- Endocrine & metabolic: Hypoglycemia
- Gastrointestinal: Indigestion (7%), abdominal discomfort (6%), abdominal distention, abnormal stools, constipation, dyspepsia/ heartburn, taste disorder
- Neuromuscular & skeletal: Myalgia
- Respiratory: Dyspnea, upper respiratory tract infection
- Miscellaneous: Decreased vitamin B_{12} levels (7%), increased diaphoresis, flu-like syndrome, nail disorder

<1% (Limited to important or life-threatening): Lactic acidosis, megaloblastic anemia

Overdosage/Toxicology Hypoglycemia (10% of cases) or lactic acidosis (~32% of cases) may occur. Metformin is dialyzable with a clearance of up to 170 mL/ minute. Hemodialysis may be useful for removal of accumulated drug from patients in whom metformin overdose is suspected. Treatment is supportive.

Drug Interactions

Drugs which tend to produce hyperglycemia (eg, diuretics, corticosteroids, phenothiazines, thyroid products, estrogens, oral contraceptives, phenytoin, nicotinic acid, sympathomimetics, calcium channel blocking drugs, isoniazid) may lead to a loss of glycemic control

Cationic drugs (eg, amiloride, digoxin, morphine, procainamide, quinidine, quinine, ranitidine, triamterene, trimethoprim, and vancomycin) which are eliminated by renal tubular secretion could have the potential for interaction with metformin by competing for common renal tubular transport systems

Cimetidine increases (by 60%) peak metformin plasma and whole blood concentrations

Contrast agents: May increase the risk of metformin-induced lactic acidosis. Discontinue metformin prior to exposure and withhold for 48 hours.

Furosemide increased the metformin plasma and blood C_{max} without altering metformin renal clearance in a single dose study

Ethanol/Nutrition/Herb Interactions

Ethanol: Avoid or limit ethanol (incidence of lactic acidosis may be increased; may cause hypoglycemia).

Food: Food decreases the extent and slightly delays the absorption. May decrease absorption of vitamin B_{12} and/or folic acid.

Herb/Nutraceutical: Caution with chromium, garlic, gymnema (may cause hypoglycemia).

Dietary Considerations Drug may cause GI upset; take with food (to decrease GI upset). Take at the same time each day. Dietary modification based on ADA recommendations is a part of therapy. Monitor for signs and symptoms of vitamin B_{12} and/or folic acid deficiency; supplementation may be required.

Dosage Forms

Solution, oral, as hydrochloride (Riomet™): 100 mg/mL (118 mL, 473 mL) [contains saccharin; cherry flavor]

Tablet, as hydrochloride (Glucophage®): 500 mg, 850 mg, 1000 mg

Tablet, extended release, as hydrochloride: 500 mg

Fortamet™: 500 mg, 1000 mg

Glucophage® XR: 500 mg, 750 mg

◆ **Metformin Hydrochloride** *see* Metformin *on page 810*

Methadone (METH a done)

Medication Safety Issues

Sound-alike/look-alike issues:

Methadone may be confused with Mephyton®, methylphenidate

Related Information

Anesthesia for Patients With Liver Disease *on page 1421*

Chronic Pain Management *on page 1430*

Narcotic / Opioid Analgesics *on page 1568*

U.S. Brand Names Dolophine®; Methadone Diskets®; Methadone Intensol™; Methadose®

Canadian Brand Names Dolophine®; Metadol™; Methadose®

Synonyms Methadone Hydrochloride

Pharmacologic Category Analgesic, Narcotic

Restrictions C-II

When used for treatment of narcotic addiction: May only be dispensed in accordance to guidelines established by the Substance Abuse and Mental Health Services Administration's (SAMHSA) Center for Substance Abuse Treatment (CSAT).

Generic Available Yes

Use Management of severe pain; detoxification and maintenance treatment of narcotic addiction (if used for detoxification and maintenance treatment of narcotic addiction, it must be part of an FDA-approved program)

Mechanism of Action Binds to opiate receptors in the CNS, causing inhibition of ascending pain pathways, altering the perception of and response to pain; produces generalized CNS depression

Pharmacodynamics/Kinetics

Onset of action: Oral: Analgesic: 0.5-1 hour; Parenteral: 10-20 minutes

Peak effect: Parenteral: 1-2 hours

Duration: Oral: 4-8 hours, increases to 22-48 hours with repeated doses

Distribution: V_{dss}: 1-8 L/kg

Protein binding: 85% to 90%

Metabolism: Hepatic; N-demethylation primarily via CYP3A4, CYP2B6, and CYP2C19 to inactive metabolites

Bioavailability: Oral: 36% to 100%

Half-life elimination: 7-59 hours; may be prolonged with alkaline pH, decreased during pregnancy

Excretion: Urine (<10% as unchanged drug); increased with urine pH <6

Dosage Regulations regarding methadone use may vary by state and/or country. Obtain advice from appropriate regulatory agencies and/or consult with pain management/palliative care specialists. **Note:** These are guidelines and do not represent the maximum doses that may be required in all patients. Methadone

(Continued)

Methadone *(Continued)*

accumulates with repeated doses and dosage may need reduction after 3-5 days to prevent CNS depressant effects. Some patients may benefit from every 8-12 hour dosing interval for chronic pain management. Doses should be titrated to appropriate effects.

Children:

Pain (analgesia):

Oral (unlabeled use): Initial: 0.1-0.2 mg/kg 4-8 hours initially for 2-3 doses, then every 6-12 hours as needed. Dosing interval may range from 4-12 hours during initial therapy; decrease in dose or frequency may be required (~ days 2-5) due to accumulation with repeated doses (maximum dose: 5-10 mg)

I.V. (unlabeled use): 0.1 mg/kg every 4-8 hours initially for 2-3 doses, then every 6-12 hours as needed. Dosing interval may range from 4-12 hours during initial therapy; decrease in dose or frequency may be required (~ days 2-5) due to accumulation with repeated doses (maximum dose: 5-8 mg)

Iatrogenic narcotic dependency (unlabeled): Oral: General guidelines: Initial: 0.05-0.1 mg/kg/dose every 6 hours; increase by 0.05 mg/kg/dose until withdrawal symptoms are controlled; after 24-48 hours, the dosing interval can be lengthened to every 12-24 hours; to taper dose, wean by 0.05 mg/kg/day; if withdrawal symptoms recur, taper at a slower rate

Adults:

Pain (analgesia):

Oral: Initial: 5-10 mg; dosing interval may range from 4-12 hours during initial therapy; decrease in dose or frequency may be required (~days 2-5) due to accumulation with repeated doses

Manufacturer's labeling: 2.5-10 mg every 3-4 hours as needed

I.V.: Manufacturers labeling: Initial: 2.5-10 mg every 8-12 hours in opioid-naive patients; titrate slowly to effect; may also be administered by SubQ or I.M. injection

Conversion from oral to parenteral dose: Initial dose: Oral: parenteral: 2:1 ratio

Detoxification: Oral:

Initial: Should not exceed 30 mg; lower doses should be considered in patients with low tolerance at initiation (eg, absence of opioids ≥5 days); an additional 5-10 mg of methadone may be provided if withdrawal symptoms have not been suppressed or if symptoms reappear after 2-4 hours; total daily dose on the first day should not exceed 40 mg, unless the program physician documents in the patient's record that 40 mg did not control opiate abstinence symptoms.

Maintenance: Usual range: 80-120 mg/day (titration should occur cautiously)

Withdrawal: Dose reductions should be <10% of the maintenance dose, every 10-14 days

Detoxification (short-term): Oral:

Initial: Titrate to 40 mg/day in 2 divided doses

Maintenance: Continue 40 mg dose for 2-3 days

Withdrawal: Decrease daily or every other day, keeping withdrawal symptoms tolerable; hospitalized patients may tolerate a 20% reduction/day; ambulatory patients may require a slower reduction

Dosage adjustment during pregnancy: Methadone dose may need to be increased, or the dosing interval decreased; see Pregnancy Implications — use should be reserved for cases where the benefits clearly outweigh the risks

Dosage adjustment in renal impairment: Cl_{cr} <10 mL/minute: Administer 50% to 75% of normal dose

Dosage adjustment in hepatic impairment: Avoid in severe liver disease

Stability

Injection: Store at controlled room temperature of 15°C to 30°C (59°F to 86°F); protect from light

Oral concentrate, oral solution, tablet: Store at controlled room temperature of 15°C to 30°C (59°F to 86°F)

Administration Oral dose for detoxification and maintenance may be administered in fruit juice or water.

Monitoring Parameters Pain relief, respiratory and mental status, blood pressure

Reference Range Therapeutic: 100-400 ng/mL (SI: 0.32-1.29 µmol/L); Toxic: >2 mcg/mL (SI: >6.46 µmol/L)

Anesthesia and Critical Care Concerns/Other Considerations Methadone accumulates with repeated doses and dosage may need to be adjusted downward after 3-5 days to prevent toxic effects. Some patients may benefit from every 8- to 12-hour dosing interval (pain control). Oral dose for detoxification and maintenance may be administered in fruit juice or water.

Pregnancy Risk Factor C/D (prolonged use or high doses at term)

Contraindications Hypersensitivity to methadone or any component of the formulation; respiratory depression (in the absence of resuscitative equipment or in an unmonitored setting); acute bronchial asthma or hypercarbia; pregnancy (prolonged use or high doses near term)

Warnings/Precautions An opioid-containing analgesic regimen should be tailored to each patient's needs and based upon the type of pain being treated (acute versus chronic), the route of administration, degree of tolerance for opioids (naive versus chronic user), age, weight, and medical condition. The optimal analgesic dose varies widely among patients. Doses should be titrated to pain relief/prevention. Patients maintained on stable doses of methadone may need higher and/or more frequent doses in case of acute pain (eg, postoperative pain, physical trauma). Methadone is ineffective for the relief of anxiety.

May prolong the QT interval; use caution in patients at risk for QT prolongation, with medications known to prolong the QT interval, or history of conduction abnormalities. QT interval prolongation and torsade de pointes may be associated with doses >200 mg/day, but have also been observed with lower doses. May cause severe hypotension; use caution with severe volume depletion or other conditions which may compromise maintenance of normal blood pressure. Use caution with cardiovascular disease or patients predisposed to dysrhythmias.

May cause respiratory depression. Use caution in patients with respiratory disease or pre-existing respiratory conditions (eg, severe obesity, asthma, COPD, sleep apnea, CNS depression). Because the respiratory effects last longer than the analgesic effects, slow titration is required. Abrupt cessation may precipitate withdrawal symptoms.

May cause CNS depression, which may impair physical or mental abilities. Patients must be cautioned about performing tasks which require mental alertness (eg, operating machinery or driving). Effects with other sedative drugs or ethanol may be potentiated. Use with caution in patients with depression or suicidal tendencies, or in patients with a history of drug abuse. Tolerance or psychological and physical dependence may occur with prolonged use.

Use with caution in patients with head injury or increased intracranial pressure. May obscure diagnosis or clinical course of patients with acute abdominal conditions. Elderly may be more susceptible to adverse effects (eg, CNS, respiratory, gastrointestinal). Decrease initial dose and use caution in the elderly or debilitated; with hyper/hypothyroidism, prostatic hypertrophy, or urethral stricture; or with severe renal or hepatic failure. Safety and efficacy have not been established in patients <18 years of age. Tablets contain excipients to deter use by injection.

[U.S. Boxed Warning]: When used for treatment of narcotic addiction: May only be dispensed by opiod treatment programs certified by the Substance Abuse and Mental Health Services Administration (SAMHSA) and certified by the designated state authority. Exceptions include inpatient treatment of other conditions and emergency period (not >3 days) while definitive substance abuse treatment is being sought.

Adverse Reactions Frequency not defined. During prolonged administration, adverse effects may decrease over several weeks; however, constipation and sweating may persist.

Cardiovascular: Bradycardia, peripheral vasodilation, cardiac arrest, syncope, faintness, shock, hypotension, edema, arrhythmia, bigeminal rhythms, extrasystoles, tachycardia, torsade de pointes, ventricular fibrillation, ventricular tachycardia, ECG changes, QT interval prolonged, T-wave inversion, cardiomyopathy, flushing, heart failure, palpitation, phlebitis, orthostatic hypotension

Central nervous system: Euphoria, dysphoria, headache, insomnia, agitation, disorientation, drowsiness, dizziness, lightheadedness, sedation, confusion, seizure

Dermatologic: Pruritus, urticaria, rash, hemorrhagic urticaria

Endocrine & metabolic: Libido decreased, hypokalemia, hypomagnesemia, antidiuretic effect, amenorrhea

(Continued)

Methadone *(Continued)*

Gastrointestinal: Nausea, vomiting, constipation, anorexia, stomach cramps, xerostomia, biliary tract spasm, abdominal pain, glossitis, weight gain

Genitourinary: Urinary retention or hesitancy, impotence

Hematologic: Thrombocytopenia (reversible, reported in patients with chronic hepatitis)

Neuromuscular & skeletal: Weakness

Local: I.M./SubQ injection: Pain, erythema, swelling; I.V. injection: pruritus, urticaria, rash, hemorrhagic urticaria (rare)

Ocular: Miosis, visual disturbances

Respiratory: Respiratory depression, respiratory arrest, pulmonary edema

Miscellaneous: Physical and psychological dependence, death, diaphoresis

Overdosage/Toxicology Symptoms include respiratory depression, CNS depression, miosis, hypothermia, circulatory collapse, and convulsions. Treatment includes naloxone 2 mg I.V. (0.01 mg/kg for children), with repeat administration as necessary, up to a total of 10 mg, or as a continuous infusion. Nalmefene may also be used to reverse signs of intoxication. Patient should be monitored for depressant effects of methadone for 36-48 hours and other supportive measures should be employed as needed. Forced diuresis, peritoneal dialysis, hemodialysis, or charcoal hemoperfusion have not been established as beneficial for increasing methadone or metabolite elimination.

Drug Interactions **Substrate** of CYP2C9 (minor), 2C19 (minor), 2D6 (minor), 3A4 (major); **Inhibits** CYP2D6 (moderate), 3A4 (weak)

Agonist/antagonist analgesics (buprenorphine, butorphanol, nalbuphine, pentazocine): May decrease analgesic effect of methadone and precipitate withdrawal symptoms; use is not recommended.

Antiretroviral agents, NNRTI: May decrease levels of methadone, opioid withdrawal syndrome has been reported. Effect reported with efavirenz and nevirapine.

Antiretroviral agents, NRTI: Methadone may increase bioavailability and toxic effects of zidovudine. Methadone may decrease bioavailability of didanosine and stavudine.

Antiretroviral agent, PI: Ritonavir (and combinations) may decrease levels of methadone; withdrawal symptoms have inconsistently been observed, monitor.

CNS depressants (including but not limited to opioid analgesics, general anesthetics, sedatives, hypnotics, ethanol): May cause respiratory depression, hypotension, profound sedation, or coma.

CYP2D6 substrates: Methadone may increase the levels/effects of CYP2D6 substrates. Example substrates include amphetamines, selected beta-blockers, dextromethorphan, fluoxetine, lidocaine, mirtazapine, nefazodone, paroxetine, risperidone, ritonavir, thioridazine, tricyclic antidepressants, and venlafaxine.

CYP2D6 prodrug substrates: Methadone may decrease the levels/effects of CYP2D6 prodrug substrates. Example prodrug substrates include codeine, hydrocodone, oxycodone, and tramadol.

CYP3A4 inducers: CYP3A4 inducers may decrease the levels/effects of methadone. Example inducers include aminoglutethimide, carbamazepine, nafcillin, nevirapine, phenobarbital, phenytoin, and rifamycins.

CYP3A4 inhibitors: May increase the levels/effects of methadone. Example inhibitors include azole antifungals, clarithromycin, diclofenac, doxycycline, erythromycin, imatinib, isoniazid, nefazodone, nicardipine, propofol, protease inhibitors, quinidine, telithromycin, and verapamil.

Desipramine: Levels of desipramine may be increased by methadone.

QT_c interval-prolonging agents (including but may not be limited to amitriptyline, astemizole, bepridil, disopyramide, erythromycin, haloperidol, imipramine, quinidine, pimozide, procainamide, sotalol, and thioridazine): Effect/toxicity increased; use with caution.

Ritonavir: May increase levels/effects of methadone shortly after initiation. May decrease levels/effects of methadone with continued dosing.

Somatostatin: Therapeutic effect of methadone may be decreased; limited documentation; monitor

Zidovudine: serum concentrations may be increased by methadone; monitor

Ethanol/Nutrition/Herb Interactions

Ethanol: Avoid ethanol (may increase CNS effects). Watch for sedation.

Herb/Nutraceutical: Avoid St John's wort (may decrease methadone levels; may increase CNS depression). Avoid valerian, kava kava, gotu kola (may increase

CNS depression). Methadone is metabolized by CYP3A4 in the intestines; avoid concurrent use of grapefruit juice.

Test Interactions

Some quinolones may produce a false-positive urine screening result for opiates using commercially-available immunoassay kits. This has been demonstrated most consistently for levofloxacin and ofloxacin, but other quinolones have shown cross-reactivity in certain assay kits. Confirmation of positive opiate screens by more specific methods should be considered.

Dosage Forms

Injection, solution, as hydrochloride: 10 mg/mL (20 mL)
Solution, oral, as hydrochloride: 5 mg/5 mL (500 mL); 10 mg/5 mL (500 mL) [contains alcohol 8%; citrus flavor]
Solution, oral concentrate, as hydrochloride: 10 mg/mL (946 mL)
 Methadone Intensol™: 10 mg/mL (30 mL)
 Methadose®: 10 mg/mL (1000 mL) [cherry flavor]
 Methadose®: 10 mg/mL (1000 mL) [dye free, sugar free, unflavored]
Tablet, as hydrochloride (Dolophine®, Methadose®): 5 mg, 10 mg
Tablet, dispersible, as hydrochloride:
 Methadose®: 40 mg
 Methadone Diskets®: 40 mg [orange-pineapple flavor]

- ♦ **Methadone Diskets®** *see* Methadone *on page 813*
- ♦ **Methadone Hydrochloride** *see* Methadone *on page 813*
- ♦ **Methadone Intensol™** *see* Methadone *on page 813*
- ♦ **Methadose®** *see* Methadone *on page 813*
- ♦ **Methaminodiazepoxide Hydrochloride** *see* Chlordiazepoxide *on page 264*
- ♦ **Methergine®** *see* Methylergonovine *on page 829*

Methimazole (meth IM a zole)

Medication Safety Issues

Sound-alike/look-alike issues:
 Methimazole may be confused with metolazone

U.S. Brand Names Tapazole®

Canadian Brand Names Dom-Methimazole; PHL-Methimazole; Tapazole®

Synonyms Thiamazole

Pharmacologic Category Antithyroid Agent

Generic Available Yes

Use Palliative treatment of hyperthyroidism, return the hyperthyroid patient to a normal metabolic state prior to thyroidectomy, and to control thyrotoxic crisis that may accompany thyroidectomy. The use of antithyroid thioamides is as effective in elderly as they are in younger adults; however, the expense, potential adverse effects, and inconvenience (compliance, monitoring) make them undesirable. The use of radioiodine due to ease of administration and less concern for long-term side effects and reproduction problems (some older males) makes it a more appropriate therapy.

Mechanism of Action Inhibits the synthesis of thyroid hormones by blocking the oxidation of iodine in the thyroid gland, blocking iodine's ability to combine with tyrosine to form thyroxine and triiodothyronine (T_3), does not inactivate circulating T_4 and T_3

Pharmacodynamics/Kinetics

Onset of action: Antithyroid: Oral: 12-18 hours
Duration: 36-72 hours
Distribution: Concentrated in thyroid gland; crosses placenta; enters breast milk (1:1)
Protein binding, plasma: None
Metabolism: Hepatic
Bioavailability: 80% to 95%
Half-life elimination: 4-13 hours
Excretion: Urine (80%)

Dosage Oral: Administer in 3 equally divided doses at approximately 8-hour intervals

Children: Initial: 0.4 mg/kg/day in 3 divided doses; maintenance: 0.2 mg/kg/day in 3 divided doses up to 30 mg/24 hours maximum
 Alternatively: Initial: 0.5-0.7 mg/kg/day **or** 15-20 mg/m²/day in 3 divided doses
 Maintenance: ¹/₃ to ²/₃ of the initial dose beginning when the patient is euthyroid

(Continued)

Methimazole *(Continued)*

Maximum: 30 mg/24 hours

Adults: Initial: 15 mg/day for mild hyperthyroidism; 30-40 mg/day in moderately severe hyperthyroidism; 60 mg/day in severe hyperthyroidism; maintenance: 5-15 mg/day

Adjust dosage as required to achieve and maintain serum T_3, T_4, and TSH levels in the normal range. An elevated T_3 may be the sole indicator of inadequate treatment. An elevated TSH indicates excessive antithyroid treatment.

Dosing adjustment in renal impairment: Adjustment is not necessary

Stability Protect from light

Monitoring Parameters Monitor for signs of hypothyroidism, hyperthyroidism, T_4, T_3; CBC with differential, liver function (baseline and as needed), serum thyroxine, free thyroxine index

Anesthesia and Critical Care Concerns/Other Considerations Hypothyroidism and congenital defects (rare) may occur. Agranulocytosis, when it occurs, is usually seen during the first several months of therapy and with maintenance doses >40 mg/day.

Pregnancy Risk Factor D

Contraindications Hypersensitivity to methimazole or any component of the formulation; nursing mothers (per manufacturer; however, expert analysis and the AAP state this drug may be used with caution in nursing mothers); pregnancy

Warnings/Precautions Use with extreme caution in patients receiving other drugs known to cause myelosuppression particularly agranulocytosis, patients >40 years of age; avoid doses >40 mg/day (increased myelosuppression); may cause acneiform eruptions or worsen the condition of the thyroid

Adverse Reactions Frequency not defined.

Cardiovascular: Edema

Central nervous system: Headache, vertigo, drowsiness, CNS stimulation, depression

Dermatologic: Skin rash, urticaria, pruritus, erythema nodosum, skin pigmentation, exfoliative dermatitis, alopecia

Endocrine & metabolic: Goiter

Gastrointestinal: Nausea, vomiting, stomach pain, abnormal taste, constipation, weight gain, salivary gland swelling

Hematologic: Leukopenia, agranulocytosis, granulocytopenia, thrombocytopenia, aplastic anemia, hypoprothrombinemia

Hepatic: Cholestatic jaundice, jaundice, hepatitis

Neuromuscular & skeletal: Arthralgia, paresthesia

Renal: Nephrotic syndrome

Miscellaneous: SLE-like syndrome

Overdosage/Toxicology Symptoms of overdose include nausea, vomiting, epigastric distress, headache, fever, arthralgia, pruritus, edema, pancytopenia, and signs of hypothyroidism. Management of overdose is supportive.

Drug Interactions Inhibits CYP1A2 (weak), 2A6 (weak), 2B6 (weak), 2C9 (weak), 2C19 (weak), 2D6 (moderate), 2E1 (weak), 3A4 (weak)

Beta-blockers: Methimazole may decrease beta-blocker clearance due to changes in thyroid function.

Digoxin: Methimazole may increase digoxin levels due to changes in thyroid function.

CYP2D6 substrates: Methimazole may increase the levels/effects of CYP2D6 substrates. Example substrates include amphetamines, selected beta-blockers, dextromethorphan, fluoxetine, lidocaine, mirtazapine, nefazodone, paroxetine, risperidone, ritonavir, thioridazine, tricyclic antidepressants, and venlafaxine.

CYP2D6 prodrug substrates: Methimazole may decrease the levels/effects of CYP2D6 prodrug substrates. Example prodrug substrates include codeine, hydrocodone, oxycodone, and tramadol.

Theophylline: Methimazole may decrease theophylline clearance due to changes in thyroid function.

Warfarin: Anticoagulant effect of warfarin may be decreased.

Dietary Considerations Should be taken consistently in relation to meals every day.

Dosage Forms

Tablet: 5 mg, 10 mg, 20 mg

Tapazole® 5 mg, 10 mg

Methohexital (meth oh HEKS i tal)

Medication Safety Issues
Sound-alike/look-alike issues:
Brevital® may be confused with Brevibloc®

Related Information
Anesthesia Considerations for Neurosurgery *on page 1401*
Anesthesia for Patients With Liver Disease *on page 1421*
Intravenous Anesthetic Agents *on page 1531*

U.S. Brand Names Brevital® Sodium

Canadian Brand Names Brevital®

Synonyms Methohexital Sodium

Pharmacologic Category Barbiturate

Restrictions C-IV

Generic Available No

Use Induction and maintenance of general anesthesia for short procedures

Can be used in pediatric patients ≥1 month of age as follows: For rectal or intramuscular induction of anesthesia prior to the use of other general anesthetic agents, as an adjunct to subpotent inhalational anesthetic agents for short surgical procedures, or for short surgical, diagnostic, or therapeutic procedures associated with minimal painful stimuli

Unlabeled/Investigational Use Wada test

Mechanism of Action Ultra short-acting I.V. barbiturate anesthetic

Pharmacodynamics/Kinetics
Onset of action: I.V.: Immediately
Duration: Single dose: 10-20 minutes

Dosage Doses must be titrated to effect
Manufacturer's recommendations:
Infants <1 month: Safety and efficacy not established
Infants ≥1 month and Children:
I.M.: Induction: 6.6-10 mg/kg of a 5% solution
Rectal: Induction: Usual: 25 mg/kg of a 1% solution
Alternative pediatric dosing:
Children 3-12 years:
I.M.: Preoperative: 5-10 mg/kg/dose
I.V.: Induction: 1-2 mg/kg/dose
Rectal: Preoperative/induction: 20-35 mg/kg/dose; usual: 25 mg/kg/dose; maximum dose: 500 mg/dose; give as 10% aqueous solution
Adults: I.V.:
Induction: 50-120 mg to start; 20-40 mg every 4-7 minutes
Wada test (unlabeled): 3-4 mg over 3 second; following signs of recovery, administer a second dose of 2 mg over 2 seconds

Dosing adjustment/comments in hepatic impairment: Lower dosage and monitor closely

Stability Do not dilute with solutions containing bacteriostatic agents; solutions are alkaline (pH 9.5-11) and **incompatible** with acids (eg, atropine sulfate, succinylcholine, silicone), also **incompatible** with phenol-containing solutions and silicone

Administration Dilute to a maximum concentration of 1% for I.V. use; for Wada testing, a dilution of 1 mg/mL has been reported

Anesthesia and Critical Care Concerns/Other Considerations Methohexital does not possess analgesic properties.

Pregnancy Risk Factor C

Contraindications Hypersensitivity to methohexital or any component of the formulation; porphyria

Warnings/Precautions Use with extreme caution in patients with liver impairment, asthma, cardiovascular instability

Adverse Reactions Frequency not defined.
Cardiovascular: Hypotension, peripheral vascular collapse
Central nervous system: Seizures, headache
Gastrointestinal: Cramping, diarrhea, rectal bleeding, nausea, vomiting, abdominal pain
Hematologic: Hemolytic anemia, thrombophlebitis
Hepatic: Transaminases increased
Local: Pain on I.M. injection
(Continued)

Methohexital *(Continued)*

Neuromuscular & skeletal: Tremor, twitching, rigidity, involuntary muscle movement, radial nerve palsy

Respiratory: Apnea, respiratory depression, laryngospasm, cough, hiccups

Overdosage/Toxicology

Symptoms of overdose include apnea, tachycardia, hypotension

Treatment is primarily supportive with mechanical ventilation if needed

Drug Interactions

Acetaminophen: Barbiturates may enhance the hepatotoxic potential of acetaminophen overdoses

Antiarrhythmics: Barbiturates may increase the metabolism of antiarrhythmics, decreasing their clinical effect; includes disopyramide, propafenone, and quinidine

Anticonvulsants: Barbiturates may increase the metabolism of anticonvulsants; includes ethosuximide, felbamate (possibly), lamotrigine, phenytoin, tiagabine, topiramate, and zonisamide; does not appear to affect gabapentin or levetiracetam

Antineoplastics: Limited evidence suggests that enzyme-inducing anticonvulsant therapy may reduce the effectiveness of some chemotherapy regimens (specifically in ALL); teniposide and methotrexate may be cleared more rapidly in these patients

Antipsychotics: Barbiturates may enhance the metabolism (decrease the efficacy) of antipsychotics; monitor for altered response; dose adjustment may be needed

Beta-blockers: Metabolism of beta-blockers may be increased and clinical effect decreased; atenolol and nadolol are unlikely to interact given their renal elimination

Calcium channel blockers: Barbiturates may enhance the metabolism of calcium channel blockers, decreasing their clinical effect

Chloramphenicol: Barbiturates may increase the metabolism of chloramphenicol and chloramphenicol may inhibit barbiturate metabolism; monitor for altered response

Cimetidine: Barbiturates may enhance the metabolism of cimetidine, decreasing its clinical effect

CNS depressants: Sedative effects and/or respiratory depression with barbiturates may be additive with other CNS depressants; monitor for increased effect; includes ethanol, sedatives, antidepressants, narcotic analgesics, and benzodiazepines

Corticosteroids: Barbiturates may enhance the metabolism of corticosteroids, decreasing their clinical effect

Cyclosporine: Levels may be decreased by barbiturates; monitor

Doxycycline: Barbiturates may enhance the metabolism of doxycycline, decreasing its clinical effect; higher dosages may be required

Estrogens: Barbiturates may increase the metabolism of estrogens and reduce their efficacy

Felbamate may inhibit the metabolism of barbiturates and barbiturates may increase the metabolism of felbamate

Griseofulvin: Barbiturates may impair the absorption of griseofulvin, and griseofulvin metabolism may be increased by barbiturates, decreasing clinical effect

Guanfacine: Effect may be decreased by barbiturates

Immunosuppressants: Barbiturates may enhance the metabolism of immunosuppressants, decreasing its clinical effect; includes both cyclosporine and tacrolimus

Loop diuretics: Metabolism may be increased and clinical effects decreased; established for furosemide, effect with other loop diuretics not established

MAO inhibitors: Metabolism of barbiturates may be inhibited, increasing clinical effect or toxicity of the barbiturates

Methadone: Barbiturates may enhance the metabolism of methadone resulting in methadone withdrawal

Methoxyflurane: Barbiturates may enhance the nephrotoxic effects of methoxyflurane

Oral contraceptives: Barbiturates may enhance the metabolism of oral contraceptives, decreasing their clinical effect; an alternative method of contraception should be considered

Theophylline: Barbiturates may increase metabolism of theophylline derivatives and decrease their clinical effect

Tricyclic antidepressants: Barbiturates may increase metabolism of tricyclic antidepressants and decrease their clinical effect; sedative effects may be additive

Valproic acid: Metabolism of barbiturates may be inhibited by valproic acid; monitor for excessive sedation; a dose reduction may be needed

Warfarin: Barbiturates inhibit the hypoprothrombinemic effects of oral anticoagulants via increased metabolism; this combination should generally be avoided

Dietary Considerations Should not be given to patients with food in stomach because of danger of vomiting during anesthesia.

Dosage Forms Injection, powder for reconstitution, as sodium: 500 mg, 2.5 g, 5 g

♦ **Methohexital Sodium** *see* Methohexital *on page 819*

Methotrexate (meth oh TREKS ate)

Medication Safety Issues

Sound-alike/look-alike issues:

Methotrexate may be confused with metolazone, mitoxantrone

MTX is an error-prone abbreviation (mistaken as mitoxantrone)

High alert medication: The Institute for Safe Medication Practices (ISMP) includes this medication among its list of drugs which have a heightened risk of causing significant patient harm when used in error.

Errors have occurred (resulting in death) when oral methotrexate was administered as "daily" dose instead of the recommended "weekly" dose.

U.S. Brand Names Rheumatrex®; Trexall™

Canadian Brand Names Apo-Methotrexate®; ratio-Methotrexate

Synonyms Amethopterin; Methotrexate Sodium; MTX (error-prone abbreviation); NSC-740

Pharmacologic Category Antineoplastic Agent, Antimetabolite (Antifolate)

Generic Available Yes

Use Treatment of trophoblastic neoplasms; leukemias; psoriasis; rheumatoid arthritis (RA), including polyarticular-course juvenile rheumatoid arthritis (JRA); breast, head and neck, and lung carcinomas; osteosarcoma; soft-tissue sarcomas; carcinoma of gastrointestinal tract, esophagus, testes; lymphomas

Unlabeled/Investigational Use

Treatment and maintenance of remission in Crohn's disease

Mechanism of Action Methotrexate is a folate antimetabolite that inhibits DNA synthesis. Methotrexate irreversibly binds to dihydrofolate reductase, inhibiting the formation of reduced folates, and thymidylate synthetase, resulting in inhibition of purine and thymidylic acid synthesis. Methotrexate is cell cycle specific for the S phase of the cycle.

The MOA in the treatment of rheumatoid arthritis is unknown, but may affect immune function. In psoriasis, methotrexate is thought to target rapidly proliferating epithelial cells in the skin.

In Crohn's disease, it may have immune modulator and anti-inflammatory activity

Pharmacodynamics/Kinetics

Onset of action: Antirheumatic: 3-6 weeks; additional improvement may continue longer than 12 weeks

Absorption: Oral: Rapid; well absorbed at low doses (<30 mg/m^2), incomplete after large doses; I.M.: Complete

Distribution: Penetrates slowly into 3rd space fluids (eg, pleural effusions, ascites), exits slowly from these compartments (slower than from plasma); crosses placenta; small amounts enter breast milk; sustained concentrations retained in kidney and liver

Protein binding: 50%

Metabolism: <10%; degraded by intestinal flora to DAMPA by carboxypeptidase; hepatic aldehyde oxidase converts methotrexate to 7-OH methotrexate; polyglutamates are produced intracellularly and are just as potent as methotrexate; their production is dose- and duration-dependent and they are slowly eliminated by the cell once formed

Half-life elimination: Low dose: 3-10 hours; High dose: 8-12 hours

Time to peak, serum: Oral: 1-2 hours; I.M.: 30-60 minutes

Excretion: Urine (44% to 100%); feces (small amounts)

Dosage Refer to individual protocols.

Note: Doses between 100-500 mg/m^2 **may require** leucovorin rescue. Doses >500 mg/m^2 **require** leucovorin rescue: Oral, I.M., I.V.: Leucovorin 10-15 mg/m^2

(Continued)

Methotrexate *(Continued)*

every 6 hours for 8 or 10 doses, starting 24 hours after the start of methotrexate infusion. Continue until the methotrexate level is ≤0.1 micromolar (10^{-7}M). Some clinicians continue leucovorin until the methotrexate level is <0.05 micromolar (5 x 10^{-8}M) or 0.01 micromolar (10^{-8}M).

If the 48-hour methotrexate level is >1 micromolar (10^{-7}M) or the 72-hour methotrexate level is >0.2 micromolar (2 x 10^{-7}M): I.V., I.M, Oral: Leucovorin 100 mg/m^2 every 6 hours until the methotrexate level is ≤0.1 micromolar (10^{-7}M). Some clinicians continue leucovorin until the methotrexate level is <0.05 micromolar (5 x 10^{-8}M) or 0.01 micromolar (10^{-8}M).

Children:

Dermatomyositis: Oral: 15-20 mg/m^2/week as a single dose once weekly **or** 0.3-1 mg/kg/dose once weekly

Juvenile rheumatoid arthritis: Oral, I.M.: 10 mg/m^2 once weekly, then 5-15 mg/m^2/week as a single dose **or** as 3 divided doses given 12 hours apart

Antineoplastic dosage range:

Oral, I.M.: 7.5-30 mg/m^2/week **or** every 2 weeks

I.V.: 10-18,000 mg/m^2 bolus dosing **or** continuous infusion over 6-42 hours

For dosing schedules, see table.

Methotrexate Dosing Schedules

Dose	Route	Frequency
Conventional		
15-20 mg/m^2	P.O.	Twice weekly
30-50 mg/m^2	P.O., I.V.	Weekly
15 mg/day for 5 days	P.O., I.M.	Every 2-3 weeks
Intermediate		
50-150 mg/m^2*	I.V. push	Every 2-3 weeks
240 mg/m^2*	I.V. infusion	Every 4-7 days
0.5-1 g/m^2**	I.V. infusion	Every 2-3 weeks
High		
1-25 g/m^2*	I.V. infusion	Every 1-3 weeks

*Doses between 100-500 mg/m^2 may require leucovorin rescue in some patients.

**Followed with leucovorin rescue - refer to Leucovorin monograph for details.

Pediatric solid tumors (high-dose): I.V.:

<12 years: 12-25 g/m^2

≥12 years: 8 g/m^2

Acute lymphocytic leukemia (intermediate-dose): I.V.: Loading: 100 mg/m^2 bolus dose, followed by 900 mg/m^2/day infusion over 23-41 hours.

Meningeal leukemia: I.T.: 10-15 mg/m^2 (maximum dose: 15 mg) **or** an age-based dosing regimen; one possible system is:

≤3 months: 3 mg/dose

4-11 months: 6 mg/dose

1 year: 8 mg/dose

2 years: 10 mg/dose

≥3 years: 12 mg/dose

Adults: I.V.: Range is wide from 30-40 mg/m^2/week to 100-12,000 mg/m^2 with leucovorin rescue

Trophoblastic neoplasms:

Oral, I.M.: 15-30 mg/day for 5 days; repeat in 7 days for 3-5 courses

I.V.: 11 mg/m^2 days 1 through 5 every 3 weeks

Head and neck cancer: Oral, I.M., I.V.: 25-50 mg/m^2 once weekly

Mycosis fungoides (cutaneous T-cell lymphoma): Oral, I.M.: Initial (early stages):

5-50 mg once weekly **or**

15-37.5 mg twice weekly

Bladder cancer: I.V.:

30 mg/m^2 day 1 and 8 every 3 weeks **or**

30 mg/m^2 day 1, 15, and 22 every 4 weeks

Breast cancer: I.V.: 30-60 mg/m^2 days 1 and 8 every 3-4 weeks

Gastric cancer: I.V.:1500 mg/m^2 every 4 weeks

Lymphoma, non-Hodgkin's: I.V.:
30 mg/m^2 days 3 and 10 every 3 weeks **or**
120 mg/m^2 day 8 and 15 every 3-4 weeks **or**
200 mg/m^2 day 8 and 15 every 3 weeks **or**
400 mg/m^2 every 4 weeks for 3 cycles **or**
1 g/m^2 every 3 weeks **or**
1.5 g/m^2 every 4 weeks
Sarcoma: I.V.: 8-12 g/m^2 weekly for 2-4 weeks
Rheumatoid arthritis: Oral: 7.5 mg once weekly **or** 2.5 mg every 12 hours for 3 doses/week, not to exceed 20 mg/week
Psoriasis:
Oral: 2.5-5 mg/dose every 12 hours for 3 doses given weekly **or**
Oral, I.M.: 10-25 mg/dose given once weekly
Ectopic pregnancy: I.M., I.V.: 50 mg/m^2 as a single dose
Active Crohn's disease (unlabeled use): Induction of remission: I.M., SubQ: 15-25 mg once weekly; remission maintenance: 15 mg once weekly
Note: Oral dosing has been reported as effective but oral absorption is highly variable. If patient relapses after a switch to oral, may consider returning to injectable.

Elderly: Rheumatoid arthritis/psoriasis: Oral: Initial: 5-7.5 mg/week, not to exceed 20 mg/week
Dosing adjustment in renal impairment:
Cl_{cr} 61-80 mL/minute: Reduce dose to 75% of usual dose
Cl_{cr} 51-60 mL/minute: Reduce dose to 70% of usual dose
Cl_{cr} 10-50 mL/minute: Reduce dose to 30% to 50% of usual dose
Cl_{cr} <10 mL/minute: Avoid use
Hemodialysis: Not dialyzable (0% to 5%); supplemental dose is not necessary
Peritoneal dialysis: Supplemental dose is not necessary
Dosage adjustment in hepatic impairment:
Bilirubin 3.1-5 mg/dL **or** AST >180 units: Administer 75% of usual dose
Bilirubin >5 mg/dL: Do not use

Stability Store tablets and intact vials at room temperature (15°C to 25°C); protect from light. Dilute powder with D_5W or NS to a concentration of ≤25 mg/mL (20 mg and 50 mg vials) and 50 mg/mL (1 g vial). Intrathecal solutions may be reconstituted to 2.5-5 mg/mL with NS, D_5W, lactated Ringer's, or Elliott's B solution. **Use preservative free preparations for intrathecal or high-dose administration.** Further dilution in D_5W or NS is stable for 24 hours at room temperature (21°C to 25°C). Reconstituted solutions with a preservative may be stored under refrigeration for up to 3 months, and up to 4 weeks at room temperature. Intrathecal dilutions are stable at room temperature for 7 days, but it is generally recommended that they be used within 4-8 hours.

Administration Methotrexate may be administered I.M., I.V., or I.T.; I.V. administration may be as slow push, short bolus infusion, or 24- to 42-hour continuous infusion

Specific dosing schemes vary, but high dose should be followed by leucovorin calcium to prevent toxicity; refer to Leucovorin monograph *on page 738*

Monitoring Parameters For prolonged use (especially rheumatoid arthritis, psoriasis) a baseline liver biopsy, repeated at each 1-1.5 g cumulative dose interval, should be performed; WBC and platelet counts every 4 weeks; CBC and creatinine, LFTs every 3-4 months; chest x-ray

Reference Range Therapeutic levels: Variable; Toxic concentration: Variable; therapeutic range is dependent upon therapeutic approach.

High-dose regimens produce drug levels that are between 0.1-1 micromole/L 24-72 hours after drug infusion
Toxic: Low-dose therapy: >0.2 micromole/L; high-dose therapy: >1 micromole/L

Pregnancy Risk Factor X (psoriasis, rheumatoid arthritis)

Contraindications Hypersensitivity to methotrexate or any component of the formulation; severe renal or hepatic impairment; pre-existing profound bone marrow suppression in patients with psoriasis or rheumatoid arthritis, alcoholic liver disease, AIDS, pre-existing blood dyscrasias; pregnancy (in patients with psoriasis or rheumatoid arthritis); breast-feeding

Warnings/Precautions Hazardous agent - use appropriate precautions for handling and disposal. May cause potentially life-threatening pneumonitis (may occur at any time during therapy and at any dosage); monitor closely for pulmonary symptoms, particularly dry, nonproductive cough. Methotrexate may cause photosensitivity and/or severe dermatologic reactions which are not
(Continued)

Methotrexate *(Continued)*

dose-related. Methotrexate has been associated with acute and chronic hepatotoxicity, fibrosis, and cirrhosis. Risk is related to cumulative dose and prolonged exposure. Ethanol abuse, obesity, advanced age, and diabetes may increase the risk of hepatotoxic reactions.

Methotrexate may cause renal failure, gastrointestinal toxicity, or bone marrow depression. Use with caution in patients with renal impairment, peptic ulcer disease, ulcerative colitis, or pre-existing bone marrow suppression. Diarrhea and ulcerative stomatitis may require interruption of therapy; death from hemorrhagic enteritis or intestinal perforation has been reported. Methotrexate penetrates slowly into 3rd space fluids, such as pleural effusions or ascites, and exits slowly from these compartments (slower than from plasma). Dosage reduction may be necessary in patients with renal or hepatic impairment, ascites, and pleural effusion. Toxicity from methotrexate or any immunosuppressive is increased in the elderly.

Severe bone marrow suppression, aplastic anemia, and GI toxicity have occurred during concomitant administration with NSAIDs. Use caution when used with other hepatotoxic agents (azathioprine, retinoids, sulfasalazine). Methotrexate given concomitantly with radiotherapy may increase the risk of soft tissue necrosis and osteonecrosis. Immune suppression may lead to opportunistic infections.

For rheumatoid arthritis and psoriasis, immunosuppressive therapy should only be used when disease is active and less toxic; traditional therapy is ineffective. Discontinue therapy in RA or psoriasis if a significant decrease in hematologic components is noted. Methotrexate formulations and/or diluents containing preservatives should not be used for intrathecal or high-dose therapy. Methotrexate injection may contain benzyl alcohol and should not be used in neonates.

Adverse Reactions Note: Adverse reactions vary by route and dosage. Hematologic and/or gastrointestinal toxicities may be common at dosages used in chemotherapy; these reactions are much less frequent when used at typical dosages for rheumatic diseases.

>10%:

Central nervous system (with I.T. administration or very high-dose therapy):
- Arachnoiditis: Acute reaction manifested as severe headache, nuchal rigidity, vomiting, and fever; may be alleviated by reducing the dose
- Subacute toxicity: 10% of patients treated with 12-15 mg/m^2 of I.T. methotrexate may develop this in the second or third week of therapy; consists of motor paralysis of extremities, cranial nerve palsy, seizure, or coma. This has also been seen in pediatric cases receiving very high-dose I.V. methotrexate.
- Demyelinating encephalopathy: Seen months or years after receiving methotrexate; usually in association with cranial irradiation or other systemic chemotherapy

Dermatologic: Reddening of skin
Endocrine & metabolic: Hyperuricemia, defective oogenesis or spermatogenesis
Gastrointestinal: Ulcerative stomatitis, glossitis, gingivitis, nausea, vomiting, diarrhea, anorexia, intestinal perforation, mucositis (dose dependent; appears in 3-7 days after therapy, resolving within 2 weeks)
Hematologic: Leukopenia, thrombocytopenia
Renal: Renal failure, azotemia, nephropathy
Respiratory: Pharyngitis

1% to 10%:

Cardiovascular: Vasculitis
Central nervous system: Dizziness, malaise, encephalopathy, seizure, fever, chills
Dermatologic: Alopecia, rash, photosensitivity, depigmentation or hyperpigmentation of skin
Endocrine & metabolic: Diabetes
Genitourinary: Cystitis
Hematologic: Hemorrhage
Myelosuppressive: This is the primary dose-limiting factor (along with mucositis) of methotrexate; occurs about 5-7 days after methotrexate therapy, and should resolve within 2 weeks
- WBC: Mild
- Platelets: Moderate

Onset: 7 days
Nadir: 10 days
Recovery: 21 days

Hepatic: Cirrhosis and portal fibrosis have been associated with chronic methotrexate therapy; acute elevation of liver enzymes are common after high-dose methotrexate, and usually resolve within 10 days.

Neuromuscular & skeletal: Arthralgia

Ocular: Blurred vision

Renal: Renal dysfunction: Manifested by an abrupt rise in serum creatinine and BUN and a fall in urine output; more common with high-dose methotrexate, and may be due to precipitation of the drug.

Respiratory: Pneumonitis: Associated with fever, cough, and interstitial pulmonary infiltrates; treatment is to withhold methotrexate during the acute reaction; interstitial pneumonitis has been reported to occur with an incidence of 1% in patients with RA (dose 7.5-15 mg/week)

<1% (Limited to important or life-threatening): Acute neurologic syndrome (at high dosages - symptoms include confusion, hemiparesis, transient blindness, and coma); anaphylaxis, alveolitis, cognitive dysfunction (has been reported at low dosage), decreased resistance to infection, erythema multiforme, hepatic failure, leukoencephalopathy (especially following craniospinal irradiation or repeated high-dose therapy), lymphoproliferative disorders, osteonecrosis and soft tissue necrosis (with radiotherapy), pericarditis, plaque erosions (psoriasis), seizure (more frequent in pediatric patients with ALL), Stevens-Johnson syndrome, thromboembolism

Overdosage/Toxicology Symptoms of overdose include nausea, vomiting, alopecia, melena, and renal failure. Administer leucovorin (see Dosage).

Hydration and alkalinization may be used to prevent precipitation of methotrexate or methotrexate metabolites in the renal tubules. Severe bone marrow toxicity can result from overdose. Generally, neither peritoneal nor hemodialysis have been shown to increase elimination. However, effective clearance of methotrexate has been reported with acute, intermittent hemodialysis using a high-flux dialyzer.

Drug Interactions

Acitretin: May enhance the hepatotoxic effect of methotrexate. Avoid concurrent use.

Cholestyramine: May decrease levels of methotrexate.

Corticosteroids: May decrease uptake of methotrexate into leukemia cells. Administration of these drugs should be separated by 12 hours. Dexamethasone has been reported to not affect methotrexate influx into cells.

Cyclosporine: Concomitant administration with methotrexate may increase levels and toxicity of each.

Cytarabine: Methotrexate, when administered prior to cytarabine, may enhance the efficacy and toxicity of cytarabine. Some combination treatment regimens (eg, hyper-CVAD) have been designed to take advantage of this interaction.

Hepatotoxic agents (azathioprine, retinoids, sulfasalazine) may increase the risk of hepatotoxic reactions

Mercaptopurine: Methotrexate may increase mercaptopurine levels. Dosage adjustment may be required.

NSAIDs: Severe bone marrow suppression, aplastic anemia, and GI toxicity have been reported with concomitant therapy. Should not be used during moderate or high-dose methotrexate due to increased and prolonged methotrexate levels (may increase toxicity); NSAID use during treatment of rheumatoid arthritis has not been fully explored, but continuation of prior regimen has been allowed in some circumstances, with cautious monitoring

Penicillins: May increase methotrexate concentrations (due to a reduction in renal tubular secretion). Primarily a concern with high doses of penicillins and higher dosages of methotrexate.

Probenecid: May increase methotrexate concentrations (due to a reduction in renal tubular secretion). Primarily a concern with higher dosages of methotrexate.

Salicylates: May increase the serum concentration of Methotrexate. Salicylate doses used for prophylaxis of cardiovascular events are not likely to be of concern.

Sulfonamides: May increase methotrexate concentrations (due to a reduction in renal tubular secretion). In addition, sulfonamides may reduce folate levels,

(Continued)

Methotrexate *(Continued)*

increasing the risk/severity of bone marrow suppression. Particularly a concern with higher dosages of methotrexate.

Tetracyclines: May increase methotrexate toxicity; monitor

Theophylline: Methotrexate may increase theophylline levels.

Vaccines (live virus): Concurrent use with methotrexate may result in vaccinia infections.

Ethanol/Nutrition/Herb Interactions

Ethanol: Avoid ethanol (may be associated with increased liver injury).

Food: Methotrexate peak serum levels may be decreased if taken with food. Milk-rich foods may decrease methotrexate absorption. Folate may decrease drug response.

Herb/Nutraceutical: Avoid echinacea (has immunostimulant properties).

Dietary Considerations

Sodium content of 100 mg injection: 20 mg (0.86 mEq)

Sodium content of 100 mg (low sodium) injection: 15 mg (0.65 mEq)

Dosage Forms

Injection, powder for reconstitution [preservative free]: 20 mg, 1 g

Injection, solution: 25 mg/mL (2 mL, 10 mL) [contains benzyl alcohol]

Injection, solution [preservative free]: 25 mg/mL (2 mL, 4 mL, 8 mL, 10 mL)

Tablet: 2.5 mg

Trexall™: 5 mg, 7.5 mg, 10 mg, 15 mg

Tablet, as sodium [dose pack] (Rheumatrex® Dose Pack): 2.5 mg (4 cards with 2, 3, 4, 5, or 6 tablets each)

♦ **Methotrexate Sodium** *see* Methotrexate *on page 821*

Methyldopa (meth il DOE pa)

Medication Safety Issues

Sound-alike/look-alike issues:

Methyldopa may be confused with L-dopa, levodopa

Related Information

Hypertension *on page 1620*

Canadian Brand Names Apo-Methyldopa®; Nu-Medopa

Synonyms Aldomet; Methyldopate Hydrochloride

Pharmacologic Category Alpha-Adrenergic Inhibitor

Generic Available Yes

Use Management of moderate to severe hypertension

Mechanism of Action Stimulation of central alpha-adrenergic receptors by a false transmitter that results in a decreased sympathetic outflow to the heart, kidneys, and peripheral vasculature

Pharmacodynamics/Kinetics

Onset of action: Peak effect: Hypotensive: Oral/parenteral: 3-6 hours

Duration: 12-24 hours

Distribution: Crosses placenta; enters breast milk

Protein binding: <15%

Metabolism: Intestinal and hepatic

Half-life elimination: 75-80 minutes; End-stage renal disease: 6-16 hours

Excretion: Urine (85% as metabolites) within 24 hours

Dosage

Children:

Oral: Initial: 10 mg/kg/day in 2-4 divided doses; increase every 2 days as needed to maximum dose of 65 mg/kg/day; do not exceed 3 g/day.

I.V.: 5-10 mg/kg/dose every 6-8 hours up to a total dose of 65 mg/kg/24 hours or 3 g/24 hours

Adults:

Oral: Initial: 250 mg 2-3 times/day; increase every 2 days as needed (maximum dose: 3 g/day): usual dose range (JNC 7): 250-1000 mg/day in 2 divided doses

I.V.: 250-500 mg every 6-8 hours; maximum dose: 1 g every 6 hours

Dosing interval in renal impairment:

Cl_{cr} >50 mL/minute: Administer every 8 hours.

Cl_{cr} 10-50 mL/minute: Administer every 8-12 hours.

Cl_{cr} <10 mL/minute: Administer every 12-24 hours.

Hemodialysis: Slightly dialyzable (5% to 20%)

Stability Injectable dosage form is most stable at acid to neutral pH; stability of parenteral admixture at room temperature (25°C): 24 hours; stability of parenteral admixture at refrigeration temperature (4°C): 4 days; standard diluent: 250-500 mg/100 mL D_5W

Administration When methyldopa is administered with antihypertensives other than thiazides, limit initial doses to 500 mg/day

Monitoring Parameters Blood pressure, standing and sitting/lying down, CBC, liver enzymes, Coombs' test (direct); blood pressure monitor required during I.V. administration

Anesthesia and Critical Care Concerns/Other Considerations Most effective if used with diuretic. Titrate dose to optimal blood pressure control with minimal side effects. Patients on methyldopa may need less anesthetic agents. Hypotension readily responds to vasopressors because the adrenergic receptors remain sensitive.

It is used in the management of pregnancy-associated hypertension. Although the drug crosses the placenta and may cause hypotension, there is a large body of experience using this drug in the treatment of pregnancy-associated hypertension. Overall, the medication appears to be safe during pregnancy and lactation.

Pregnancy Risk Factor B

Contraindications Hypersensitivity to methyldopa or any component of the formulation; active hepatic disease; liver disorders previously associated with use of methyldopa; on MAO inhibitors; bisulfite allergy if using oral suspension or injectable

Warnings/Precautions May rarely produce hemolytic anemia and liver disorders; positive Coombs' test occurs in 10% to 20% of patients (perform periodic CBCs); sedation usually transient may occur during initial therapy or whenever the dose is increased. Use with caution in patients with previous liver disease or dysfunction, the active metabolites of methyldopa accumulate in uremia. Patients with impaired renal function may respond to smaller doses. Elderly patients may experience syncope (avoid by giving smaller doses). Tolerance may occur usually between the second and third month of therapy. Adding a diuretic or increasing the dosage of methyldopa frequently restores blood pressure control. Because of its CNS effects, methyldopa is not considered a drug of first choice in the elderly. Often considered the drug of choice for treatment of hypertension in pregnancy. Do not use injectable if bisulfite allergy.

Adverse Reactions

>10%: Cardiovascular: Peripheral edema

1% to 10%:

- Central nervous system: Drug fever, mental depression, anxiety, nightmares, drowsiness, headache
- Gastrointestinal: Dry mouth

<1% (Limited to important or life-threatening): Bradycardia (sinus), cholestasis or hepatitis and heptocellular injury, cirrhosis, dyspnea, gynecomastia, hemolytic anemia, hyperprolactinemia, increased liver enzymes, jaundice, leukopenia, orthostatic hypotension, positive Coombs' test, sexual dysfunction, SLE-like syndrome, sodium retention, thrombocytopenia, transient leukopenia or granulocytopenia

Overdosage/Toxicology Symptoms of overdose include hypotension, sedation, bradycardia, dizziness, constipation or diarrhea, flatus, nausea, and vomiting. Treatment is supportive and symptomatic. Can be removed by hemodialysis.

Drug Interactions

Barbiturates and TCAs may reduce response to methyldopa.

Beta-blockers, MAO inhibitors, phenothiazines, and sympathomimetics: Hypertension, sometimes severe, may occur.

Iron supplements can interact and cause a significant **increase** in blood pressure.

Lithium: Methyldopa may increase lithium toxicity; monitor lithium levels.

Tolbutamide, haloperidol, anesthetics, and levodopa effects/toxicity are increased with methyldopa.

Ethanol/Nutrition/Herb Interactions Herb/Nutraceutical: Avoid dong quai if using for hypertension (has estrogenic activity). Avoid ephedra, yohimbe, ginseng (may worsen hypertension). Avoid valerian, St John's wort, kava kava, gotu kola (may increase CNS depression). Avoid natural licorice (causes sodium and water retention and increases potassium loss). Avoid garlic (may have increased antihypertensive effect).

(Continued)

Methyldopa *(Continued)*

Test Interactions Methyldopa interferes with the following laboratory tests: urinary uric acid, serum creatinine (alkaline picrate method), AST (colorimetric method), and urinary catecholamines (falsely high levels)

Dietary Considerations Dietary requirements for vitamin B_{12} and folate may be increased with high doses of methyldopa.

Dosage Forms

Injection, solution, as methyldopate hydrochloride: 50 mg/mL (5 mL) [contains sodium bisulfite]

Tablet: 250 mg, 500 mg

♦ **Methyldopate Hydrochloride** *see* Methyldopa *on page 826*

Methylene Blue (METH i leen bloo)

Medication Safety Issues Due to potential toxicity (hemolytic anemia), do not use methylene blue to color enteral feedings to detect aspiration.

U.S. Brand Names Urolene Blue®

Pharmacologic Category Antidote

Generic Available Yes

Use Antidote for cyanide poisoning and drug-induced methemoglobinemia, indicator dye

Unlabeled/Investigational Use Has been used topically (0.1% solutions) in conjunction with polychromatic light to photoinactivate viruses such as herpes simplex; has been used alone or in combination with vitamin C for the management of chronic urolithiasis

Mechanism of Action Weak germicide in low concentrations, hastens the conversion of methemoglobin to hemoglobin; has opposite effect at high concentrations by converting ferrous ion of reduced hemoglobin to ferric ion to form methemoglobin; in cyanide toxicity, it combines with cyanide to form cyanmethemoglobin preventing the interference of cyanide with the cytochrome system

Pharmacodynamics/Kinetics

Absorption: Oral: 53% to 97%

Excretion: Urine and feces

Dosage

Children: NADPH-methemoglobin reductase deficiency: Oral: 1-1.5 mg/kg/day (maximum: 300 mg/day) given with 5-8 mg/kg/day of ascorbic acid

Children and Adults: Methemoglobinemia: I.V.: 1-2 mg/kg or 25-50 mg/m^2 over several minutes; may be repeated in 1 hour if necessary

Adults: Genitourinary antiseptic: Oral: 65-130 mg 3 times/day with a full glass of water (maximum: 390 mg/day)

Administration Administer I.V. undiluted by direct I.V. injection over several minutes.

Pregnancy Risk Factor C/D (injected intra-amniotically)

Contraindications Hypersensitivity to methylene blue or any component of the formulation; intraspinal injection; renal insufficiency; pregnancy (injected intra-amniotically)

Warnings/Precautions Do not inject SubQ or intrathecally; use with caution in young patients and in patients with G6PD deficiency; continued use can cause profound anemia

Adverse Reactions Frequency not defined.

Cardiovascular: Hypertension, precordial pain

Central nervous system: Dizziness, mental confusion, headache, fever

Dermatologic: Staining of skin

Gastrointestinal: Fecal discoloration (blue-green), nausea, vomiting, abdominal pain

Genitourinary: Discoloration of urine (blue-green), bladder irritation

Hematologic: Anemia

Miscellaneous: Diaphoresis

Overdosage/Toxicology

Symptoms of overdose include nausea, vomiting, precordial pain, hypertension, methemoglobinemia, cyanosis; overdosage has resulted in methemoglobinemia and cyanosis

Treatment is symptomatic and supportive

Dosage Forms

Injection, solution: 10 mg/mL (1 mL, 10 mL)

Tablet (Urolene Blue®): 65 mg

♦ **Methylergometrine Maleate** *see* Methylergonovine *on page 829*

Methylergonovine (meth il er goe NOE veen)

Medication Safety Issues

Sound-alike/look-alike issues:

Methylergonovine and terbutaline parenteral dosage forms look similar. Due to their contrasting indications, use care when administering these agents.

U.S. Brand Names Methergine®

Canadian Brand Names Methergine®

Synonyms Methylergometrine Maleate; Methylergonovine Maleate

Pharmacologic Category Ergot Derivative

Generic Available No

Use Prevention and treatment of postpartum and postabortion hemorrhage caused by uterine atony or subinvolution

Mechanism of Action Similar smooth muscle actions as seen with ergotamine; however, it affects primarily uterine smooth muscles producing sustained contractions and thereby shortens the third stage of labor

Pharmacodynamics/Kinetics

Onset of action: Oxytocic: Oral: 5-10 minutes; I.M.: 2-5 minutes; I.V.: Immediately

Duration: Oral: ~3 hours; I.M.: ~3 hours; I.V.: 45 minutes

Absorption: Rapid

Distribution: V_d: 39-73 L

Rapid; primarily to plasma and extracellular fluid following I.V. administration; tissues

Metabolism: Hepatic

Bioavailability: Oral: 60%; I.M.: 78%

Half-life elimination: Biphasic: Initial: 1-5 minutes; Terminal: 0.5-2 hours

Time to peak, serum: Oral: 0.3-2 hours; I.M.: 0.2-0.6 hours

Excretion: Urine and feces

Dosage Adults:

Oral: 0.2 mg 3-4 times/day for 2-7 days

I.M., I.V.: 0.2 mg after delivery of anterior shoulder, after delivery of placenta, or during puerperium; may be repeated as required at intervals of 2-4 hours

Stability

Ampul: Store under refrigeration at 2°C to 8°C (36°F to 46°F); protect from light

Tablet: Store below 25°C (77°F)

Administration Administer over ≥60 seconds. Should not be routinely administered I.V. because of possibility of inducing sudden hypertension and cerebrovascular accident.

Anesthesia and Critical Care Concerns/Other Considerations This drug should be used extremely carefully because of it's potent vasoconstrictor action. I.V. use may induce sudden hypertension and cerebrovascular accidents. As a last resort, give I.V. slowly over several minutes and monitor blood pressure closely.

Pregnancy Risk Factor C

Contraindications Hypersensitivity to methylergonovine or any component of the formulation; ergot alkaloids are contraindicated with potent inhibitors of CYP3A4 (includes protease inhibitors, azole antifungals, and some macrolide antibiotics); hypertension; toxemia; pregnancy

Warnings/Precautions Use caution in patients with sepsis, obliterative vascular disease, hepatic, or renal involvement, or second stage of labor; administer with extreme caution if using intravenously. Pleural and peritoneal fibrosis have been reported with prolonged daily use. Cardiac valvular fibrosis has also been associated with ergot alkaloids.

Adverse Reactions Frequency not defined.

Cardiovascular: Acute MI, hypertension, temporary chest pain, palpitation

Central nervous system: Hallucinations, dizziness, seizure, headache

Endocrine & metabolic: Water intoxication

Gastrointestinal: Nausea, vomiting, diarrhea, foul taste

Local: Thrombophlebitis

Neuromuscular & skeletal: Leg cramps

Otic: Tinnitus

Renal: Hematuria

(Continued)

Methylergonovine *(Continued)*

Respiratory: Dyspnea, nasal congestion
Miscellaneous: Diaphoresis

Overdosage/Toxicology Symptoms of overdose include prolonged gangrene, numbness in extremities, acute nausea, vomiting, abdominal pain, respiratory depression, hypotension, and seizures. Treatment is symptomatic and supportive.

Drug Interactions Substrate of CYP3A4 (major)

Antifungals, azole derivatives (itraconazole, ketoconazole) increase levels of ergot alkaloids by inhibiting CYP3A4 metabolism, resulting in toxicity; concomitant use is contraindicated.

Antipsychotics: May diminish the effects of methylergonovine (due to dopamine antagonism); these combinations should generally be avoided.

Beta blockers: severe peripheral vasoconstriction has been reported with concomitant use of beta blockers and ergot derivatives. Monitor.

CYP3A4 inhibitors: May increase the levels/effects of methylergonovine. Example inhibitors include azole antifungals, clarithromycin, diclofenac, doxycycline, erythromycin, imatinib, isoniazid, nefazodone, nicardipine, propofol, protease inhibitors, quinidine, telithromycin, and verapamil.

Macrolide antibiotics: Erythromycin, clarithromycin, and troleandomycin may increase levels of ergot alkaloids by inhibiting CYP3A4 metabolism, resulting in toxicity (ischemia, vasospasm); concomitant use is contraindicated.

MAO inhibitors: The serotonergic effects of ergot derivatives may be increased by MAO inhibitors. Monitor for signs and symptoms of serotonin syndrome.

Metoclopramide: May diminish the effects of methylergonovine (due to dopamine antagonism); concurrent therapy should generally be avoided.

Protease inhibitors (ritonavir, amprenavir, atazanavir, indinavir, nelfinavir, and saquinavir) increase blood levels of ergot alkaloids by inhibiting CYP3A4 metabolism, acute ergot toxicity has been reported; concomitant use is contraindicated.

Serotonin agonists: Concurrent use with methylergonovine may increase the risk of serotonin syndrome (includes buspirone, SSRIs, TCAs, nefazodone, sumatriptan, and trazodone).

Sibutramine: May cause serotonin syndrome; concurrent use with ergot alkaloids is contraindicated.

Sumatriptan and other serotonin 5-HT_1 receptor agonists: Prolong vasospastic reactions; do not use sumatriptan or ergot-containing drugs within 24 hours of each other.

Vasoconstrictors: Concomitant use with peripheral vasoconstrictors may cause synergistic elevation of blood pressure; use is contraindicated.

Dosage Forms

Injection, solution, as maleate: 0.2 mg/mL (1 mL)
Tablet, as maleate: 0.2 mg

- **Methylergonovine Maleate** *see* Methylergonovine *on page 829*
- **Methylmorphine** *see* Codeine *on page 325*
- **Methylphytyl Napthoquinone** *see* Phytonadione *on page 1027*

MethylPREDNISolone (meth il pred NIS oh lone)

Medication Safety Issues

Sound-alike/look-alike issues:

MethylPREDNISolone may be confused with medroxyPROGESTERone, predniSONE
Depo-Medrol® may be confused with Solu-Medrol®
Medrol® may be confused with Mebaral®
Solu-Medrol® may be confused with Depo-Medrol®

Related Information

Allergic Reactions *on page 1395*
Contrast Media Reactions, Premedication for Prophylaxis *on page 1602*
Corticosteroids *on page 1561*
Stress Replacement of Corticosteroids *on page 1494*

U.S. Brand Names Depo-Medrol®; Medrol®; Solu-Medrol®

Canadian Brand Names Depo-Medrol®; Medrol®; Methylprednisolone Acetate; Solu-Medrol®

Synonyms 6-α-Methylprednisolone; A-Methapred; Methylprednisolone Acetate; Methylprednisolone Sodium Succinate

Pharmacologic Category Corticosteroid, Systemic

Generic Available Yes: Sodium succinate injection, tablet

Use Primarily as an anti-inflammatory or immunosuppressant agent in the treatment of a variety of diseases including those of hematologic, allergic, inflammatory, neoplastic, and autoimmune origin. Prevention and treatment of graft-versus-host disease following allogeneic bone marrow transplantation.

Mechanism of Action In a tissue-specific manner, corticosteroids regulate gene expression subsequent to binding specific intracellular receptors and translocation into the nucleus. Corticosteroids exert a wide array of physiologic effects including modulation of carbohydrate, protein, and lipid metabolism and maintenance of fluid and electrolyte homeostasis. Moreover cardiovascular, immunologic, musculoskeletal, endocrine, and neurologic physiology are influenced by corticosteroids. Decreases inflammation by suppression of migration of polymorphonuclear leukocytes and reversal of increased capillary permeability.

Pharmacodynamics/Kinetics

Onset of action: Peak effect (route dependent): Oral: 1-2 hours; I.M.: 4-8 days; Intra-articular: 1 week; methylprednisolone sodium succinate is highly soluble and has a rapid effect by I.M. and I.V. routes

Duration (route dependent): Oral: 30-36 hours; I.M.: 1-4 weeks; Intra-articular: 1-5 weeks; methylprednisolone acetate has a low solubility and has a sustained I.M. effect

Distribution: V_d: 0.7-1.5 L/kg

Half-life elimination: 3-3.5 hours; reduced in obese

Excretion: Clearance: Reduced in obese

Dosage Dosing should be based on the lesser of ideal body weight or actual body weight

Only sodium succinate may be given I.V.; methylprednisolone sodium succinate is highly soluble and has a rapid effect by I.M. and I.V. routes. Methylprednisolone acetate has a low solubility and has a sustained I.M. effect.

Children:

Anti-inflammatory or immunosuppressive: Oral, I.M., I.V. (sodium succinate): 0.5-1.7 mg/kg/day **or** 5-25 mg/m²/day in divided doses every 6-12 hours; "Pulse" therapy: 15-30 mg/kg/dose over ≥30 minutes given once daily for 3 days

Status asthmaticus: I.V. (sodium succinate): Loading dose: 2 mg/kg/dose, then 0.5-1 mg/kg/dose every 6 hours for up to 5 days

Acute spinal cord injury: I.V. (sodium succinate): 30 mg/kg over 15 minutes, followed in 45 minutes by a continuous infusion of 5.4 mg/kg/hour for 23 hours

Lupus nephritis: I.V. (sodium succinate): 30 mg/kg over ≥30 minutes every other day for 6 doses

Adults: **Only sodium succinate may be given I.V.;** methylprednisolone sodium succinate is highly soluble and has a rapid effect by I.M. and I.V. routes. Methylprednisolone acetate has a low solubility and has a sustained I.M. effect.

Acute spinal cord injury: I.V. (sodium succinate): 30 mg/kg over 15 minutes, followed in 45 minutes by a continuous infusion of 5.4 mg/kg/hour for 23 hours

Anti-inflammatory or immunosuppressive:

Oral: 2-60 mg/day in 1-4 divided doses to start, followed by gradual reduction in dosage to the lowest possible level consistent with maintaining an adequate clinical response.

I.M. (sodium succinate): 10-80 mg/day once daily

I.M. (acetate): 10-80 mg every 1-2 weeks

I.V. (sodium succinate): 10-40 mg over a period of several minutes and repeated I.V. or I.M. at intervals depending on clinical response; when high dosages are needed, give 30 mg/kg over a period ≥30 minutes and may be repeated every 4-6 hours for 48 hours.

Status asthmaticus: I.V. (sodium succinate): Loading dose: 2 mg/kg/dose, then 0.5-1 mg/kg/dose every 6 hours for up to 5 days

Lupus nephritis: High-dose "pulse" therapy: I.V. (sodium succinate): 1 g/day for 3 days

Aplastic anemia: I.V. (sodium succinate): 1 mg/kg/day or 40 mg/day (whichever dose is higher), for 4 days. After 4 days, change to oral and continue until day 10 or until symptoms of serum sickness resolve, then rapidly reduce over approximately 2 weeks.

(Continued)

MethylPREDNISolone *(Continued)*

Pneumocystis pneumonia in AIDs patients: I.V.: 40-60 mg every 6 hours for 7-10 days

Intra-articular (acetate): Administer every 1-5 weeks.

Large joints: 20-80 mg

Small joints: 4-10 mg

Intralesional (acetate): 20-60 mg every 1-5 weeks

Stability

Intact vials of methylprednisolone sodium succinate should be stored at controlled room temperature

Reconstituted solutions of methylprednisolone sodium succinate should be stored at room temperature (15°C to 30°C) and used within 48 hours

Stability of parenteral admixture at room temperature (25°C) and at refrigeration temperature (4°C): 48 hours

Standard diluent (Solu-Medrol®): 40 mg/50 mL D_5W; 125 mg/50 mL D_5W

Minimum volume (Solu-Medrol®): 50 mL D_5W

Administration

Oral: Administer after meals or with food or milk

Parenteral: Methylprednisolone sodium succinate may be administered I.M. or I.V.; I.V. administration may be IVP over one to several minutes or IVPB or continuous I.V. infusion. **Acetate salt should not be given I.V.**

I.V.: Succinate:

Low dose: ≤1.8 mg/kg or ≤125 mg/dose: I.V. push over 3-15 minutes

Moderate dose: ≥2 mg/kg or 250 mg/dose: I.V. over 15-30 minutes

High dose: 15 mg/kg or ≥500 mg/dose: I.V. over ≥30 minutes

Doses >15 mg/kg or ≥1 g: Administer over 1 hour

Do **not** administer high-dose I.V. push; hypotension, cardiac arrhythmia, and sudden death have been reported in patients given high-dose methylprednisolone I.V. push over <20 minutes; intermittent infusion over 15-60 minutes; maximum concentration: I.V. push 125 mg/mL

Monitoring Parameters Blood pressure, blood glucose, electrolytes

Anesthesia and Critical Care Concerns/Other Considerations

Neuromuscular Effects: ICU-acquired paresis was recently studied in 5 ICUs (3 medical and 2 surgical ICUs) at 4 French hospitals. All ICU patients without pre-existing neuromuscular disease admitted from March 1999 through June 2000 were evaluated (De Jonghe B, 2002). Each patient had to be mechanically ventilated for ≥7 days and was screened daily for awakening. The first day the patient was considered awake was Study Day 1. Patients with severe muscle weakness on Study Day 7 were considered to have ICU-acquired paresis. Among the 95 patients who were evaluable, about 25% developed ICU-acquired paresis. Independent predictors included female gender, the number of days with ≥2 organ dysfunction, and administration of corticosteroids. Further studies may be required to verify and characterize the association between the development of ICU-acquired paresis and use of corticosteroids. Concurrent use of a corticosteroid and muscle relaxant appear to increase the risk of certain ICU myopathies; avoid or administer the corticosteroid at the lowest dose possible.

Adrenal Insufficiency: Patients will often have steroid-induced adverse effects on glucose tolerance and lipid profiles. When discontinuing steroid therapy in patients on long-term steroid supplementation, it is important that the steroid therapy be discontinued gradually. Abrupt withdrawal may result in adrenal insufficiency with hypotension and hyperkalemia. Patients on long-term steroid supplementation will require higher corticosteroid doses when subject to stress (ie, trauma, surgery, severe infection). Guidelines for glucocorticoid replacement during various surgical procedures has been published (Salem M, 1994, Coursin DB, 2002).

Septic Shock: A recent randomized, double-blind, placebo controlled trial assessed whether low dose corticosteroid administration could improve 28-day survival in patients with septic shock and relative adrenal insufficiency. Relative adrenal insufficiency was defined as an inappropriate response to corticotropin administration (increase of serum cortisol of ≤9 mcg/dL from baseline). Cortisol levels were drawn immediately before corticotropin administration and 30 to 60 minutes afterwards. Three hundred adult septic shock patients requiring mechanical ventilation and vasopressor support were randomized to either hydrocortisone (50 mg IVP every 6 hours) and fludrocortisone (50 mcg tablet daily via nasogastric tube) or matching placebos for 7 days. In patients who did not appropriately respond to corticotropin (nonresponders), there were significantly fewer deaths in the active treatment group. Vasopressor therapy was withdrawn more frequently in this subset of the active treatment group. Adverse events were similar in both groups. Patients who lack adrenal reserve and thus have relative adrenal insufficiency during the stress of septic shock may benefit from physiologic steroid replacement. However, there was a trend for increased mortality in patients who responded to the corticotropin test (increase serum cortisol >9 mcg/dL from baseline). These patients may not benefit from physiologic steroid replacement. Further study is required to better characterize the patient populations who may benefit.

Pregnancy Risk Factor C

Contraindications Hypersensitivity to methylprednisolone or any component of the formulation; viral, fungal, or tubercular skin lesions; administration of live virus vaccines; serious infections, except septic shock or tuberculous meningitis. Methylprednisolone formulations containing benzyl alcohol preservative are contraindicated in infants.

Warnings/Precautions Use with caution in patients with hyperthyroidism, cirrhosis, nonspecific ulcerative colitis, hypertension, osteoporosis, thromboembolic tendencies, CHF, convulsive disorders, myasthenia gravis, thrombophlebitis, peptic ulcer, diabetes, glaucoma, cataracts, or tuberculosis. Use caution in hepatic impairment. Because of the risk of adverse effects, systemic corticosteroids should be used cautiously in the elderly, in the smallest possible dose, and for the shortest possible time

Acute adrenal insufficiency may occur with abrupt withdrawal after long-term therapy or with stress; young pediatric patients may be more susceptible to adrenal axis suppression from topical therapy

Adverse Reactions Frequency not defined.

Cardiovascular: Edema, hypertension, arrhythmia

Central nervous system: Insomnia, nervousness, vertigo, seizure, psychoses, pseudotumor cerebri, headache, mood swings, delirium, hallucinations, euphoria

Dermatologic: Hirsutism, acne, skin atrophy, bruising, hyperpigmentation

Endocrine & metabolic: Diabetes mellitus, adrenal suppression, hyperlipidemia, Cushing's syndrome, pituitary-adrenal axis suppression, growth suppression, glucose intolerance, hypokalemia, alkalosis, amenorrhea, sodium and water retention, hyperglycemia

Gastrointestinal: Increased appetite, indigestion, peptic ulcer, nausea, vomiting, abdominal distention, ulcerative esophagitis, pancreatitis

Hematologic: Transient leukocytosis

Neuromuscular & skeletal: Arthralgia, muscle weakness, osteoporosis, fractures

Ocular: Cataracts, glaucoma

Miscellaneous: Infections, hypersensitivity reactions, avascular necrosis, secondary malignancy, intractable hiccups

Overdosage/Toxicology When consumed in high doses for prolonged periods, systemic hypercorticism and adrenal suppression may occur. In these cases, discontinuation should be done judiciously. Arrhythmias and cardiovascular collapse are possible with rapid intravenous infusion of high-dose methylprednisolone. May mask signs and symptoms of infection.

Drug Interactions Substrate of CYP3A4 (minor); **Inhibits** CYP2C8 (weak), 3A4 (weak)

Decreased effect:

- Phenytoin, phenobarbital, rifampin increase clearance of methylprednisolone
- Potassium depleting diuretics enhance potassium depletion

Increased toxicity:

- Skin test antigens, immunizations decrease response and increase potential infections
- Methylprednisolone may increase circulating glucose levels and may need adjustments of insulin or oral hypoglycemics

Ethanol/Nutrition/Herb Interactions

Ethanol: Avoid ethanol (may increase gastric mucosal irritation).

Food: Methylprednisolone interferes with calcium absorption. Limit caffeine.

Herb/Nutraceutical: St John's wort may decrease methylprednisolone levels. Avoid cat's claw, echinacea (have immunostimulant properties).

Test Interactions Interferes with skin tests

(Continued)

MethylPREDNISolone *(Continued)*

Dietary Considerations Should be taken after meals or with food or milk; need diet rich in pyridoxine, vitamin C, vitamin D, folate, calcium, phosphorus, and protein.

Sodium content of 1 g sodium succinate injection: 2.01 mEq; 53 mg of sodium succinate salt is equivalent to 40 mg of methylprednisolone base

Methylprednisolone acetate: Depo-Medrol®

Methylprednisolone sodium succinate: Solu-Medrol®

Dosage Forms

Injection, powder for reconstitution, as sodium succinate: 125 mg [strength expressed as base]

Solu-Medrol®: 40 mg, 125 mg, 500 mg, 1 g, 2 g [packaged with diluent; diluent contains benzyl alcohol; strength expressed as base]

Solu-Medrol®: 500 mg, 1 g

Injection, suspension, as acetate (Depo-Medrol®): 20 mg/mL (5 mL); 40 mg/mL (5 mL); 80 mg/mL (5 mL) [contains benzyl alcohol; strength expressed as base]

Injection, suspension, as acetate [single-dose vial] (Depo-Medrol®): 40 mg/mL (1 mL, 10 mL); 80 mg/mL (1 mL)

Tablet: 4 mg

Medrol®: 2 mg, 4 mg, 8 mg, 16 mg, 32 mg

Tablet, dose-pack: 4 mg (21s)

Medrol® Dosepack™: 4 mg (21s)

References

Abraham E and Evans T, "Corticosteroids and Septic Shock (editorial)," *JAMA*, 2002, 288(7):886-7.

Annane D, Sebille V, Charpentier C, et al, "Effect of Treatment With Low Doses of Hydrocortisone and Fludrocortisone on Mortality in Patients With Septic Shock," *JAMA*, 2002, 288(7):862-71.

Bracken MB, Shepard MJ, Collins WF, et al, "A Randomized, Controlled Trial of Methylprednisolone or Naloxone in the Treatment of Acute Spinal-Cord Injury. Results of the Second National Acute Spinal Cord Injury Study," *N Engl J Med*, 1990, 322(20):1405-11.

Cooper MS and Stewart PM, "Corticosteroid Insufficiency in Acutely Ill Patients," *N Engl J Med*, 2003, 348(8):727-34.

Coursin DB and Wood KE, "Corticosteroid Supplementation for Adrenal Insufficiency," *JAMA*, 2002, 287(2):236-40.

De Jonghe B, Sharshar T, Lefaucheur JP, et al, "Paresis Acquired in the Intensive Care Unit. A Prospective Multicenter Study," *JAMA*, 2002, 288(22):2859-67.

Hotchkiss RS and Karl IE, "The Pathophysiology and Treatment of Sepsis," *N Engl J Med*, 2003, 348(2):138-50.

Salem M, Tainsh RE Jr, Bromberg J, et al, "Perioperative Glucocorticoid Coverage: A Reassessment 42 Years After Emergence of a Problem," *Ann Surg*, 1994, 219(4):416-25.

Steinberg KP, Hudson LD, Goodman RB, et al, "Efficacy and Safety of Corticosteroids for Persistent Acute Respiratory Distress Syndrome. National Heart, Lung and Blood Institute Acute Respiratory Distress Syndrome (ARDS) Clinical Trials Network," *N Engl J Med*, 2006, 354(16):1671-84.

- **6-α-Methylprednisolone** *see* MethylPREDNISolone *on page 830*
- **Methylprednisolone Acetate (Can)** *see* MethylPREDNISolone *on page 830*
- **Methylprednisolone Sodium Succinate** *see* MethylPREDNISolone *on page 830*
- **4-Methylpyrazole** *see* Fomepizole *on page 555*

Metoclopramide (met oh kloe PRA mide)

Medication Safety Issues

Sound-alike/look-alike issues:

Metoclopramide may be confused with metolazone

Reglan® may be confused with Megace®, Regonol®, Renagel®

Related Information

Anesthesia for Obstetric Patients in Nonobstetric Surgery *on page 1416*

Postoperative Nausea and Vomiting *on page 1477*

U.S. Brand Names Reglan®

Canadian Brand Names Apo-Metoclop®; Metoclopramide Hydrochloride Injection; Nu-Metoclopramide

Pharmacologic Category Antiemetic; Gastrointestinal Agent, Prokinetic

Generic Available Yes

Use

Oral: Symptomatic treatment of diabetic gastric stasis; gastroesophageal reflux

I.V., I.M.: Symptomatic treatment of diabetic gastric stasis; postpyloric placement of enteral feeding tubes; prevention and/or treatment of nausea and vomiting associated with chemotherapy, or postsurgery; to stimulate gastric emptying and intestinal transit of barium during radiological examination

Mechanism of Action Blocks dopamine receptors and (when given in higher doses) also blocks serotonin receptors in chemoreceptor trigger zone of the CNS; enhances the response to acetylcholine of tissue in upper GI tract causing enhanced motility and accelerated gastric emptying without stimulating gastric, biliary, or pancreatic secretions; increases lower esophageal sphincter tone

Pharmacodynamics/Kinetics

Onset of action: Oral: 0.5-1 hour; I.V.: 1-3 minutes; I.M.: 10-15 minutes

Duration: Therapeutic: 1-2 hours, regardless of route

Distribution: V_d: 2-4 L/kg

Protein binding: 30%

Bioavailability: Oral: 65% to 95%

Half-life elimination: Normal renal function: 4-6 hours (may be dose dependent)

Time to peak, serum: Oral: 1-2 hours

Excretion: Urine (~85%)

Dosage

Children:

Gastroesophageal reflux (unlabeled use): Oral: 0.1-0.2 mg/kg/dose 4 times/day

Antiemetic (chemotherapy-induced emesis) (unlabeled): I.V.: 1-2 mg/kg 30 minutes before chemotherapy and every 2-4 hours

Postpyloric feeding tube placement: I.V.:

<6 years: 0.1 mg/kg

6-14 years: 2.5-5 mg

>14 years: Refer to Adults dosing.

Adults:

Gastroesophageal reflux: Oral: 10-15 mg/dose up to 4 times/day 30 minutes before meals or food and at bedtime; single doses of 20 mg are occasionally needed for provoking situations. Treatment >12 weeks has not been evaluated.

Diabetic gastric stasis:

Oral: 10 mg 30 minutes before each meal and at bedtime

I.M., I.V. (for severe symptoms): 10 mg over 1-2 minutes; 10 days of I.V. therapy may be necessary for best response

Chemotherapy-induced emesis:

I.V.: 1-2 mg/kg 30 minutes before chemotherapy and repeated every 2 hours for 2 doses, then every 3 hours for 3 doses (manufacturer labeling)

Alternate dosing (with or without diphenhydramine):

Moderate emetic risk chemotherapy: 0.5 mg/kg every 6 hours on days 2-4

Low and minimal risk chemotherapy: 1-2 mg/kg every 3-4 hours

Breakthrough treatment: 1-2 mg/kg every 3-4 hours

Oral (unlabeled use; with or without diphenhydramine):

Moderate emetic risk chemotherapy: 0.5 mg/kg every 6 hours or 20 mg 4 times/day on days 2-4

Low and minimal risk chemotherapy: 20-40 mg every 4-6 hours

Breakthrough treatment: 20-40 mg every 4-6 hours

Postoperative nausea and vomiting: I.M., I.V.: 10-20 mg near end of surgery

Postpyloric feeding tube placement, radiological exam: I.V.: 10 mg

Elderly:

Gastroesophageal reflux: Oral: 5 mg 4 times/day (30 minutes before meals or food and at bedtime); increase dose to 10 mg 4 times/day if no response at lower dose

Gastrointestinal hypomotility:

Oral: Initial: 5 mg 30 minutes before meals and at bedtime; increase if necessary to 10 mg doses

I.V.: Initiate at 5 mg over 1-2 minutes; increase to 10 mg if necessary

Postoperative nausea and vomiting: I.M., I.V.: 5 mg near end of surgery; may repeat dose if necessary

Dosing adjustment in renal impairment: Cl_{cr} <40 mL/minute: Administer at 50% of normal dose

Hemodialysis: Not dialyzable (0% to 5%); supplemental dose is not necessary

Stability

Injection: Store intact vial at controlled room temperature; injection is photosensitive and should be protected from light during storage; parenteral admixtures in D_5W or NS are stable for at least 24 hours, and do not require light protection if used within 24 hours.

Tablet: Store at controlled room temperature.

(Continued)

Metoclopramide *(Continued)*

Administration Injection solution may be given I.M., direct I.V. push, short infusion (15-30 minutes), or continuous infusion; lower doses (≤10 mg) of metoclopramide can be given I.V. push undiluted over 1-2 minutes; higher doses to be given IVPB over at least 15 minutes; continuous SubQ infusion and rectal administration have been reported. **Note:** Rapid I.V. administration may be associated with a transient (but intense) feeling of anxiety and restlessness, followed by drowsiness.

Monitoring Parameters Dystonic reactions; signs of hypoglycemia in patients using insulin and those being treated for gastroparesis; agitation, and onfusion

Anesthesia and Critical Care Concerns/Other Considerations To prevent extrapyramidal symptoms associated with antiemetic dosages, patients may be pretreated with diphenhydramine.

Pregnancy Risk Factor B

Contraindications Hypersensitivity to metoclopramide or any component of the formulation; GI obstruction, perforation or hemorrhage; pheochromocytoma; history of seizures

Warnings/Precautions Use caution with a history of mental illness; has been associated with extrapyramidal symptoms (EPS) and depression. The frequency of EPS is higher in pediatric patients and adults <30 years of age; risk is increased at higher dosages. Extrapyramidal reactions typically occur within the initial 24-48 hours of treatment. Use caution with concurrent use of other drugs associated with EPS. Use caution in the elderly and with Parkinson's disease; may have increased risk of tardive dyskinesia. Use caution in patients with a history of seizures; risk of metoclopramide-associated seizures is increased. Neuroleptic malignant syndrome (NMS) has been reported (rarely) with metoclopramide. Use lowest recommended doses initially; may cause transient increase in serum aldosterone; use caution in patients who are at risk of fluid overload (CHF, cirrhosis). Use caution in patients with hypertension or following surgical anastomosis/closure. Patients with NADH-cytochrome b5 reductase deficiency are at increased risk of methemoglobinemia and/or sulfhemoglobinemia. Abrupt discontinuation may (rarely) result in withdrawal symptoms (dizziness, headache, nervousness). Use caution and adjust dose in renal impairment.

Adverse Reactions Frequency not always defined.

Cardiovascular: AV block, bradycardia, CHF, fluid retention, flushing (following high I.V. doses), hyper-/hypotension, supraventricular tachycardia

Central nervous system: Drowsiness (~10% to 70%; dose related), fatigue (~10%), restlessness (~10%), acute dystonic reactions (<1% to 25%; dose and age related), akathisia, confusion, depression, dizziness, hallucinations (rare), headache, insomnia, neuroleptic malignant syndrome (rare), Parkinsonian-like symptoms, suicidal ideation, seizures, tardive dyskinesia

Dermatologic: Angioneurotic edema (rare), rash, urticaria

Endocrine & metabolic: Amenorrhea, galactorrhea, gynecomastia, impotence

Gastrointestinal: Diarrhea, nausea

Genitourinary: Incontinence, urinary frequency

Hematologic: Agranulocytosis, leukopenia, neutropenia, porphyria

Hepatic: Hepatotoxicity (rare)

Ocular: Visual disturbance

Respiratory: Bronchospasm, laryngeal edema (rare)

Miscellaneous: Allergic reactions, methemoglobinemia, sulfhemoglobinemia

Overdosage/Toxicology Symptoms of overdose include drowsiness, ataxia, extrapyramidal symptoms, seizures, methemoglobinemia (in infants). Disorientation, muscle hypertonia, irritability, and agitation are common. Metoclopramide often causes extrapyramidal symptoms (eg, dystonic reactions) requiring management with diphenhydramine 1-2 mg/kg (adults) up to a maximum of 50-100 mg I.M. or I.V. slow push followed by a maintenance dose (25-50 mg orally every 4-6 hours) for 48-72 hours. When these reactions are unresponsive to diphenhydramine, benztropine mesylate I.V. 1-2 mg (adults) may be effective. These agents are generally effective within 2-5 minutes. Methylene blue is not recommended in patients with G6PD deficiency who experience methemoglobinemia due to metoclopramide.

Drug Interactions Substrate (minor) of CYP1A2, 2D6; **Inhibits** CYP2D6 (weak)

Anticholinergic agents antagonize metoclopramide's actions

Antipsychotic agents: Metoclopramide may increase extrapyramidal symptoms (EPS) or risk when used concurrently.

Cyclosporine: Metoclopramide may increase cyclosporine levels.

Opiate analgesics may increase CNS depression

Ethanol/Nutrition/Herb Interactions Ethanol: Avoid ethanol (may increase CNS depression).

Test Interactions Increased aminotransferase [ALT (SGPT)/AST (SGOT)] (S), increased amylase (S)

Dosage Forms

Injection, solution (Reglan®): 5 mg/mL (2 mL, 10 mL, 30 mL)
Syrup: 5 mg/5 mL (10 mL, 480 mL)
Tablet (Reglan®): 5 mg, 10 mg

♦ **Metoclopramide Hydrochloride Injection (Can)** *see* Metoclopramide *on page 834*

Metolazone (me TOLE a zone)

Medication Safety Issues

Sound-alike/look-alike issues:
Metolazone may be confused with metaxalone, methazolamide, methimazole, methotrexate, metoclopramide, metoprolol, minoxidil
Zaroxolyn® may be confused with Zarontin®

Related Information

Heart Failure (Systolic) *on page 1607*

U.S. Brand Names Zaroxolyn®

Canadian Brand Names Mykrox®; Zaroxolyn®

Pharmacologic Category Diuretic, Thiazide-Related

Generic Available Yes

Use Management of mild to moderate hypertension; treatment of edema in congestive heart failure and nephrotic syndrome, impaired renal function

Mechanism of Action Inhibits sodium reabsorption in the distal tubules causing increased excretion of sodium and water, as well as, potassium and hydrogen ions

Pharmacodynamics/Kinetics

Onset of action: Diuresis: ~60 minutes
Duration: 12-24 hours
Absorption: Incomplete
Distribution: Crosses placenta; enters breast milk
Protein binding: 95%
Metabolism: Undergoes enterohepatic recirculation
Bioavailability: Mykrox® reportedly has highest
Half-life elimination (renal function dependent): 6-20 hours
Excretion: Urine (80% to 95%)

Dosage Adults: Oral:

Edema: 2.5-20 mg/dose every 24 hours (ACC/AHA 2005 Heart Failure Guidelines)
Hypertension (Zaroxolyn®): 2.5-5 mg/dose every 24 hours
Hypertension (Mykrox®): 0.5 mg/day; if response is not adequate, increase dose to maximum of 1 mg/day
Dialysis: Not dialyzable (0% to 5%) via hemo- or peritoneal dialysis; supplemental dose is not necessary

Administration May be taken with food or milk. Take early in day to avoid nocturia. Take the last dose of multiple doses no later than 6 PM unless instructed otherwise.

Monitoring Parameters Serum electrolytes (potassium, sodium, chloride, bicarbonate), renal function, blood pressure (standing, sitting/supine)

Anesthesia and Critical Care Concerns/Other Considerations Metolazone 5 mg is approximately equivalent to hydrochlorothiazide 50 mg; taken the day of surgery may cause hypovolemia and the hypertensive patient undergoing general anesthesia to have labile blood pressure; use with caution prior to surgery or perioperatively

Metolazone is a potent diuretic and is often used in patients refractory to thiazide or loop diuretics. It is important that the patient be closely monitored to avoid profound volume depletion. Also watch for hypomagnesemia.

Pregnancy Risk Factor B (manufacturer); D (expert analysis)

Contraindications Hypersensitivity to metolazone, any component of the formulation, other thiazides, and sulfonamide derivatives; anuria; hepatic coma; pregnancy (expert analysis)

(Continued)

Metolazone *(Continued)*

Warnings/Precautions Electrolyte disturbances (hypokalemia, hypochloremic alkalosis, hyponatremia) can occur. Use with caution in severe hepatic dysfunction; hepatic encephalopathy can be caused by electrolyte disturbances. Gout can be precipitate in certain patients with a history of gout, a familial predisposition to gout, or chronic renal failure. Cautious use in diabetics; may see a change in glucose control. Hypersensitivity reactions can occur. Can cause SLE exacerbation or activation. Use caution in severe renal impairment. Orthostatic hypotension may occur (potentiated by alcohol, barbiturates, narcotics, other antihypertensive drugs). Mykrox® tablets are not interchangeable with Zaroxolyn® tablets. Use with caution in patients with moderate or high cholesterol concentrations. Photosensitization may occur.

Chemical similarities are present among sulfonamides, sulfonylureas, carbonic anhydrase inhibitors, thiazides, and loop diuretics (except ethacrynic acid). Use in patients with thiazide or sulfonamide allergy is specifically contraindicated in product labeling, however, a risk of cross-reaction exists in patients with allergy to any of these compounds; avoid use when previous reaction has been severe.

Adverse Reactions

>10%: Central nervous system: Dizziness

1% to 10%:

- Cardiovascular: Orthostatic hypotension, palpitation, chest pain, cold extremities (rapidly acting), edema (rapidly acting), venous thrombosis (slow acting), syncope (slow acting)
- Central nervous system: Headache, fatigue, lethargy, malaise, lassitude, anxiety, depression, nervousness, "weird" feeling (rapidly acting), chills (slow acting)
- Dermatologic: Rash, pruritus, dry skin (rapidly acting)
- Endocrine & metabolic: Hypokalemia, impotence, reduced libido, excessive volume depletion (slow acting), hemoconcentration (slow acting), acute gouty attach (slow acting)
- Gastrointestinal: Nausea, vomiting, abdominal pain, cramping, bloating, diarrhea or constipation, dry mouth
- Genitourinary: Nocturia
- Neuromuscular & skeletal: Muscle cramps, spasm, weakness
- Ocular: Eye itching (rapidly acting)
- Otic: Tinnitus (rapidly acting)
- Respiratory: Cough (rapidly acting), epistaxis (rapidly acting), sinus congestion (rapidly acting), sore throat (rapidly acting)

<1% (Limited to important or life-threatening): Agranulocytosis, aplastic anemia, cholestasis, cutaneous vasculitis, glycosuria, hepatitis, hypercalcemia, hyperglycemia, leukopenia, pancreatitis, photosensitivity, pruritus, purpura, Stevens-Johnson syndrome, thrombocytopenia, toxic epidermal necrolysis

Overdosage/Toxicology Symptoms of overdose include orthostatic hypotension, dizziness, drowsiness, syncope, hemoconcentration and hemodynamic changes due to plasma volume depletion. Treatment is symptomatic and supportive.

Drug Interactions

ACE inhibitors: Increased hypotension if aggressively diuresed with a thiazide-type diuretic.

Beta-blockers increase hyperglycemic effects in type 2 diabetes mellitus (noninsulin dependent, NIDDM).

Cholestyramine and colestipol may decrease metolazone absorption.

Cyclosporine and thiazide-type compounds can increase the risk of gout or renal toxicity; avoid concurrent use.

Digoxin toxicity can be exacerbated if a diuretic induces hypokalemia or hypomagnesemia.

Lithium toxicity can occur due to a reduced renal excretion of lithium; monitor lithium concentration and adjust as needed.

Loop diuretics (eg, furosemide) may increase the effect of metolazone.

Neuromuscular blocking agents effects may be prolonged; monitor serum potassium and neuromuscular status.

NSAIDs can decrease the efficacy of thiazide-type diuretics.

Ethanol/Nutrition/Herb Interactions Herb/Nutraceutical: Avoid dong quai if using for hypertension (has estrogenic activity). Avoid dong quai, St John's wort (may also cause photosensitization). Avoid ephedra, yohimbe, ginseng (may worsen hypertension). Avoid natural licorice. Avoid garlic (may have increased antihypertensive effect).

Dietary Considerations Should be taken after breakfast; may require potassium supplementation

Dosage Forms Tablet, slow acting: 2.5 mg, 5 mg, 10 mg

Metoprolol (me toe PROE lole)

Medication Safety Issues

Sound-alike/look-alike issues:

Metoprolol may be confused with metaproterenol, metolazone, misoprostol

Toprol-XL® may be confused with Tegretol®, Tegretol®-XR, Topamax®

Related Information

Anesthesia for Patients With Liver Disease *on page 1421*

Antiarrhythmic Drugs *on page 1548*

Beta-Blockers *on page 1557*

Heart Failure (Systolic) *on page 1607*

Management of Postoperative Arrhythmias *on page 1451*

Preoperative Evaluation of the Cardiac Patient for Noncardiac Surgery *on page 1485*

U.S. Brand Names Lopressor®; Toprol-XL®

Canadian Brand Names Apo-Metoprolol®; Betaloc®; Betaloc® Durules®; Lopressor®; Metoprolol Tartrate Injection, USP; Novo-Metoprolol; Nu-Metop; PMS-Metoprolol; Sandoz-Metoprolol; Toprol-XL®

Synonyms Metoprolol Succinate; Metoprolol Tartrate

Pharmacologic Category Beta Blocker, $Beta_1$ Selective

Generic Available Yes: Injection, tablet (nonextended release)

Use Treatment of hypertension and angina pectoris; prevention of myocardial infarction, atrial fibrillation, flutter, symptomatic treatment of hypertrophic subaortic stenosis; to reduce mortality/hospitalization in patients with congestive heart failure (stable NYHA Class II or III) in patients already receiving ACE inhibitors, diuretics, and/or digoxin (sustained-release only)

Unlabeled/Investigational Use Treatment of ventricular arrhythmias, atrial ectopy, migraine prophylaxis, essential tremor, aggressive behavior

Mechanism of Action Selective inhibitor of $beta_1$-adrenergic receptors; competitively blocks $beta_1$-receptors, with little or no effect on $beta_2$-receptors at doses <100 mg; does not exhibit any membrane stabilizing or intrinsic sympathomimetic activity

Pharmacodynamics/Kinetics

Onset of action: Peak effect: Antihypertensive: Oral: 1.5-4 hours

Duration: 10-20 hours

Absorption: 95%

Protein binding: 8%

Metabolism: Extensively hepatic; significant first-pass effect

Bioavailability: Oral: 40% to 50%

Half-life elimination: 3-4 hours; End-stage renal disease: 2.5-4.5 hours

Excretion: Urine (3% to 10% as unchanged drug)

Dosage

Children: Oral: 1-5 mg/kg/24 hours divided twice daily; allow 3 days between dose adjustments

Adults:

Hypertension: Oral: 100-450 mg/day in 2-3 divided doses, begin with 50 mg twice daily and increase doses at weekly intervals to desired effect; usual dosage range (JNC 7): 50-100 mg/day

Extended release: Initial: 25-100 mg/day (maximum: 400 mg/day)

Angina, SVT, MI prophylaxis: Oral: 100-450 mg/day in 2-3 divided doses, begin with 50 mg twice daily and increase doses at weekly intervals to desired effect

Extended release: Initial: 100 mg/day (maximum: 400 mg/day)

Hypertension/ventricular rate control: I.V. (in patients having nonfunctioning GI tract): Initial: 1.25-5 mg every 6-12 hours; titrate initial dose to response. Initially, low doses may be appropriate to establish response; however, up to 15 mg every 3-6 hours has been employed.

Congestive heart failure: Oral (extended release): Initial: 25 mg once daily (reduce to 12.5 mg once daily in NYHA class higher than class II); may double dosage every 2 weeks as tolerated, up to 200 mg/day

(Continued)

Metoprolol *(Continued)*

Myocardial infarction (acute): I.V.: 5 mg every 2 minutes for 3 doses in early treatment of myocardial infarction; thereafter give 50 mg orally every 6 hours 15 minutes after last I.V. dose and continue for 48 hours; then administer a maintenance dose of 100 mg twice daily.

Elderly: Oral: Initial: 25 mg/day; usual range: 25-300 mg/day

Extended release: 25-50 mg/day initially as a single dose; increase at 1- to 2-week intervals.

Hemodialysis: Administer dose posthemodialysis or administer 50 mg supplemental dose; supplemental dose is not necessary following peritoneal dialysis

Dosing adjustment/comments in hepatic disease: Reduced dose probably necessary

Stability

Injection: Do not store above 30°C (86°F); protect from light

Tablet: Store between 15°C to 30°C (59°F to 86°F)

Administration

Oral: Extended release tablets may be divided in half; do not crush or chew.

I.V.: When administered acutely for cardiac treatment, monitor ECG and blood pressure. May administer by rapid infusion (I.V. push) over 1 minute or by slow infusion (ie, 5-10 mg of metoprolol in 50 mL of fluid) over ~30 minutes. Necessary monitoring for surgical patients who are unable to take oral beta-blockers (prolonged ileus) has not been defined. Some institutions require monitoring of baseline and postinfusion heart rate and blood pressure when a patient's response to beta-blockade has not been characterized (ie, the patient's initial dose or following a change in dose). Consult individual institutional policies and procedures.

Monitoring Parameters Acute cardiac treatment: Monitor ECG and blood pressure with I.V. administration; heart rate and blood pressure with oral administration

Anesthesia and Critical Care Concerns/Other Considerations Symptomatic bradycardia may be treated with atropine.

Surgery: Atenolol has also been shown to improve cardiovascular outcomes when used in the perioperative period in patients with underlying cardiovascular disease who are undergoing noncardiac surgery. Bisoprolol in high-risk patients undergoing vascular surgery reduced the perioperative incidence of death from cardiac causes and nonfatal myocardial infarction.

Withdrawal: Beta-blocker therapy should not be withdrawn abruptly, but gradually tapered to avoid acute tachycardia and hypertension.

Pregnancy Risk Factor C (manufacturer); D (2nd and 3rd trimesters - expert analysis)

Contraindications Hypersensitivity to metoprolol or any component of the formulation; sinus bradycardia; heart block greater than first degree (except in patients with a functioning artificial pacemaker); cardiogenic shock; uncompensated cardiac failure; pregnancy (2nd and 3rd trimesters)

Warnings/Precautions Must use care in compensated heart failure and monitor closely for a worsening of the condition (efficacy has not been established for metoprolol). **[U.S. Boxed Warning]: Beta-blocker therapy should not be withdrawn abruptly (particularly in patients with CAD), but gradually tapered to avoid acute tachycardia, hypertension, and/or ischemia.** Beta-blockers may increase the risk of anaphylaxis (in predisposed patients) and blunt response to epinephrine. Use caution in patients with PVD (can aggravate arterial insufficiency). Use caution with concurrent use of beta-blockers and either verapamil or diltiazem; bradycardia or heart block can occur. Avoid concurrent I.V. use of both agents. In general, beta-blockers should be avoided in patients with bronchospastic disease. Metoprolol, with B1 selectivity, should be used cautiously in bronchospastic disease with close monitoring. Use cautiously in diabetics because it can mask prominent hypoglycemic symptoms. Can mask signs of thyrotoxicosis. Can cause fetal harm when administered in pregnancy. Use cautiously in the hepatically impaired. Use care with anesthetic agents which decrease myocardial function. The extended release formulation consists of drug within a nondeformable matrix; following drug release/absorption, the matrix/shell is expelled in the stool. The use of nondeformable products in patients with known stricture/narrowing of the GI tract has been associated with symptoms of obstruction.

Adverse Reactions

>10%:

Central nervous system: Drowsiness, insomnia

Endocrine & metabolic: Decreased sexual ability

1% to 10%:

Cardiovascular: Bradycardia, palpitation, edema, CHF, reduced peripheral circulation

Central nervous system: Mental depression

Gastrointestinal: Diarrhea or constipation, nausea, stomach discomfort

Respiratory: Bronchospasm

Miscellaneous: Cold extremities

<1% (Limited to important or life-threatening): Arrhythmias, arthralgia, chest pain, confusion (especially in the elderly), depression, dyspnea, hallucinations, headache, heart block (second- and third-degree), hepatic dysfunction, hepatitis, jaundice, leukopenia, nervousness, orthostatic hypotension, paresthesia, photosensitivity, thrombocytopenia, vomiting

Overdosage/Toxicology Symptoms of intoxication include cardiac disturbances, CNS toxicity, bronchospasm, hypoglycemia and hyperkalemia. The most common cardiac symptoms include hypotension and bradycardia. Atrioventricular block, intraventricular conduction disturbances, cardiogenic shock, and asystole may occur with severe overdose, especially with membrane-depressant drugs (eg, propranolol). CNS effects include convulsions, coma, and respiratory arrest. Treatment is symptom-directed and supportive.

Drug Interactions **Substrate** of CYP2C19 (minor), 2D6 (major); **Inhibits** CYP2D6 (weak)

Alpha-blockers (prazosin, terazosin): Concurrent use of beta-blockers may increase risk of orthostasis.

AV conduction-slowing agents (digoxin): Effects may be additive with beta-blockers.

Clonidine: Hypertensive crisis after or during withdrawal of either agent.

CYP2D6 inhibitors: May increase the levels/effects of metoprolol. Example inhibitors include chlorpromazine, delavirdine, fluoxetine, miconazole, paroxetine, pergolide, quinidine, quinine, ritonavir, and ropinirole.

Fluoxetine may inhibit the metabolism of metoprolol resulting in cardiac toxicity.

Glucagon: Metoprolol may blunt the hyperglycemic action of glucagon.

Hydralazine may enhance the bioavailability of metoprolol.

Insulin and oral hypoglycemics: Metoprolol may mask tachycardia from hypoglycemia.

Metoprolol reduces antipyrine's clearance by 18%.

NSAIDs (ibuprofen, indomethacin, naproxen, piroxicam) may reduce the antihypertensive effects of beta-blockers.

Oral contraceptives may increase the AUC and C_{max} of metoprolol.

Salicylates may reduce the antihypertensive effects of beta-blockers.

Sulfonylureas: Beta-blockers may alter response to hypoglycemic agents.

Verapamil or diltiazem may have synergistic or additive pharmacological effects when taken concurrently with beta-blockers; avoid concurrent I.V. use.

Ethanol/Nutrition/Herb Interactions

Food: Food increases absorption. Metoprolol serum levels may be increased if taken with food.

Herb/Nutraceutical: Avoid dong quai if using for hypertension (has estrogenic activity). Avoid ephedra, yohimbe, ginseng (may worsen hypertension). Avoid garlic (may have increased antihypertensive effect).

Dietary Considerations Regular tablets should be taken with food. Extended release tablets may be taken without regard to meals.

Dosage Forms

Injection, solution, as tartrate (Lopressor®): 1 mg/mL (5 mL)

Tablet, as tartrate: 25 mg, 50 mg, 100 mg

Lopressor®: 50 mg, 100 mg

Tablet, extended release, as succinate (Toprol-XL®): 25 mg, 50 mg, 100 mg, 200 mg [expressed as mg equivalent to tartrate]

References

Radack K and Deck C, "Beta-Adrenergic Blocker Therapy Does Not Worsen Intermittent Claudication in Subjects With Peripheral Arterial Disease. A Meta-Analysis of Randomized Controlled Trials," *Arch Intern Med*, 1991, 151(9):1769-76.

♦ **Metoprolol Succinate** *see* Metoprolol *on page 839*

♦ **Metoprolol Tartrate** *see* Metoprolol *on page 839*

♦ **Metoprolol Tartrate Injection, USP (Can)** *see* Metoprolol *on page 839*

♦ **MetroCream®** *see* Metronidazole *on page 842*
♦ **MetroGel®** *see* Metronidazole *on page 842*
♦ **MetroGel-Vaginal®** *see* Metronidazole *on page 842*
♦ **MetroLotion®** *see* Metronidazole *on page 842*

Metronidazole (me troe NI da zole)

Medication Safety Issues

Sound-alike/look-alike issues:

Metronidazole may be confused with metformin.

Related Information

Prevention of Wound Infection and Sepsis in Surgical Patients *on page 1588*

Helicobacter pylori Treatment *on page 1613*

U.S. Brand Names Flagyl®; Flagyl ER®; Flagyl® I.V. RTU™; MetroCream®; MetroGel®; MetroGel-Vaginal®; MetroLotion®; Noritate®; Vandazole™

Canadian Brand Names Apo-Metronidazole®; Flagyl®; Florazole® ER; MetroCream®; Metrogel®; Nidagel™; Noritate®; Trikacide

Synonyms Metronidazole Hydrochloride

Pharmacologic Category Amebicide; Antibiotic, Miscellaneous; Antibiotic, Topical; Antiprotozoal, Nitroimidazole

Generic Available Yes: Cream, gel, infusion, tablet

Use Treatment of susceptible anaerobic bacterial and protozoal infections in the following conditions: Amebiasis, symptomatic and asymptomatic trichomoniasis; skin and skin structure infections; CNS infections; intra-abdominal infections (as part of combination regimen); systemic anaerobic infections; treatment of antibiotic-associated pseudomembranous colitis (AAPC), bacterial vaginosis; as part of a multidrug regimen for *H. pylori* eradication to reduce the risk of duodenal ulcer recurrence

Topical: Treatment of inflammatory lesions and erythema of rosacea

Unlabeled/Investigational Use Crohn's disease

Mechanism of Action After diffusing into the organism, interacts with DNA to cause a loss of helical DNA structure and strand breakage resulting in inhibition of protein synthesis and cell death in susceptible organisms

Pharmacodynamics/Kinetics

Absorption: Oral: Well absorbed; Topical: Concentrations achieved systemically after application of 1 g topically are 10 times less than those obtained after a 250 mg oral dose

Distribution: To saliva, bile, seminal fluid, breast milk, bone, liver, and liver abscesses, lung and vaginal secretions; crosses placenta and blood-brain barrier

CSF:blood level ratio: Normal meninges: 16% to 43%; Inflamed meninges: 100%

Protein binding: <20%

Metabolism: Hepatic (30% to 60%)

Half-life elimination: Neonates: 25-75 hours; Others: 6-8 hours, prolonged with hepatic impairment; End-stage renal disease: 21 hours

Time to peak, serum: Oral: Immediate release: 1-2 hours

Excretion: Urine (20% to 40% as unchanged drug); feces (6% to 15%)

Dosage

Infants and Children:

Amebiasis: Oral: 35-50 mg/kg/day in divided doses every 8 hours for 10 days

Trichomoniasis: Oral: 15-30 mg/kg/day in divided doses every 8 hours for 7 days

Anaerobic infections:

Oral: 15-35 mg/kg/day in divided doses every 8 hours

I.V.: 30 mg/kg/day in divided doses every 6 hours

Clostridium difficile (antibiotic-associated colitis): Oral: 20 mg/kg/day divided every 6 hours

Maximum dose: 2 g/day

Adults:

Anaerobic infections (diverticulitis, intra-abdominal, peritonitis, cholangitis, or abscess): Oral, I.V.: 500 mg every 6-8 hours, not to exceed 4 g/day

Acne rosacea: Topical:

0.75%: Apply and rub a thin film twice daily, morning and evening, to entire affected areas after washing. Significant therapeutic results should be noticed within 3 weeks. Clinical studies have demonstrated continuing improvement through 9 weeks of therapy.

1%: Apply thin film to affected area once daily

Amebiasis: Oral: 500-750 mg every 8 hours for 5-10 days

Antibiotic-associated pseudomembranous colitis: Oral: 250-500 mg 3-4 times/day for 10-14 days

Giardiasis: 500 mg twice daily for 5-7 days

Helicobacter pylori eradication: Oral: 250-500 mg with meals and at bedtime for 14 days; requires combination therapy with at least one other antibiotic and an acid-suppressing agent (proton pump inhibitor or H_2 blocker)

Bacterial vaginosis or vaginitis due to *Gardnerella, Mobiluncus*:

Oral: 500 mg twice daily (regular release) or 750 mg once daily (extended release tablet) for 7 days

Vaginal: 1 applicatorful (~37.5 mg metronidazole) intravaginally once or twice daily for 5 days; apply once in morning and evening if using twice daily, if daily, use at bedtime

Trichomoniasis: Oral: 250 mg every 8 hours for 7 days **or** 375 mg twice daily for 7 days **or** 2 g as a single dose

Elderly: Use lower end of dosing recommendations for adults, do not administer as a single dose

Dosing adjustment in renal impairment: Cl_{cr} <10 mL/minute: Administer 50% of dose or every 12 hours

Hemodialysis: Extensively removed by hemodialysis and peritoneal dialysis (50% to 100%); administer dose posthemodialysis

Peritoneal dialysis: Dose as for Cl_{cr} <10 mL/minute

Continuous arteriovenous or venovenous hemofiltration: Administer usual dose

Dosing adjustment/comments in hepatic disease: Unchanged in mild liver disease; reduce dosage in severe liver disease

Stability Metronidazole injection should be stored at 15°C to 30°C and protected from light. Product may be refrigerated but crystals may form; crystals redissolve on warming to room temperature. Prolonged exposure to light will cause a darkening of the product. However, short-term exposure to normal room light does not adversely affect metronidazole stability. Direct sunlight should be avoided. Stability of parenteral admixture at room temperature (25°C): Out of overwrap stability: 30 days.

Standard diluent: 500 mg/100 mL NS

Administration

Oral: May be taken with food to minimize stomach upset. Extended release tablets should be taken on an empty stomach (1 hour before or 2 hours after meals).

Topical: No disulfiram-like reactions have been reported after **topical** application, although metronidazole can be detected in the blood. Apply to clean, dry skin. Cosmetics may be used after application (wait at least 5 minutes after using lotion).

Anesthesia and Critical Care Concerns/Other Considerations Metronidazole may have effects similar to that of disulfiram (Antabuse®). If ethanol is taken during and within 24 hours of the last dose of metronidazole, patients may have severe flushing, headache, nausea, vomiting, or chest and abdominal pain.

Pregnancy Risk Factor B (may be contraindicated in 1st trimester)

Contraindications Hypersensitivity to metronidazole, nitroimidazole derivatives, or any component of the formulation; pregnancy (1st trimester - found to be carcinogenic in rats)

Warnings/Precautions Use with caution in patients with liver impairment due to potential accumulation, blood dyscrasias; history of seizures, CHF, or other sodium retaining states; reduce dosage in patients with severe liver impairment, CNS disease, and severe renal failure (Cl_{cr} <10 mL/minute); if *H. pylori* is not eradicated in patients being treated with metronidazole in a regimen, it should be assumed that metronidazole-resistance has occurred and it should not again be used; seizures and neuropathies have been reported especially with increased doses and chronic treatment; if this occurs, discontinue therapy. **[U.S. Boxed Warning]: Possibly carcinogenic based on animal data.**

Adverse Reactions

Systemic: Frequency not defined:

Cardiovascular: Flattening of the T-wave, flushing

Central nervous system: Ataxia, confusion, coordination impaired, dizziness, fever, headache, insomnia, irritability, seizure, vertigo

(Continued)

Metronidazole *(Continued)*

Dermatologic: Erythematous rash, urticaria
Endocrine & metabolic: Disulfiram-like reaction, dysmenorrhea, libido decreased
Gastrointestinal: Nausea (~12%), anorexia, abdominal cramping, constipation, diarrhea, furry tongue, glossitis, proctitis, stomatitis, unusual/metallic taste, vomiting, xerostomia
Genitourinary: Cystitis, darkened urine (rare), dysuria, incontinence, polyuria, vaginitis
Hematologic: Neutropenia (reversible), thrombocytopenia (reversible, rare)
Neuromuscular & skeletal: Peripheral neuropathy, weakness
Respiratory: Nasal congestion, rhinitis, sinusitis, pharyngitis
Miscellaneous: Flu-like syndrome, moniliasis

Topical: Frequency not defined:
Central nervous system: Headache
Dermatologic: Burning, contact dermatitis, dryness, erythema, irritation, pruritus, rash
Gastrointestinal: Unusual/metallic taste, nausea, constipation
Local: Local allergic reaction
Neuromuscular & skeletal: Tingling/numbness of extremities
Ocular: Eye irritation

Vaginal:
>10%: Genitourinary: Vaginal discharge (12%)
1% to 10%:
Central nervous system: Headache (5%), dizziness (2%)
Gastrointestinal: Gastrointestinal discomfort (7%), nausea and/or vomiting (4%), unusual/metallic taste (2%), diarrhea (1%)
Genitourinary: Vaginitis (10%), vulva/vaginal irritation (9%), pelvic discomfort (3%)
Hematologic: WBC increased (2%)
<1%: Abdominal bloating, abdominal gas, darkened urine, depression, fatigue, itching, rash, thirst, xerostomia

Overdosage/Toxicology Symptoms of overdose include nausea, vomiting, ataxia, seizures, and peripheral neuropathy. Treatment is symptomatic and supportive.

Drug Interactions Inhibits CYP2C9 (weak), 3A4 (moderate)
Cimetidine may increase metronidazole levels.
Cisapride: May inhibit metabolism of cisapride, causing potential arrhythmias; avoid concurrent use
CYP3A4 substrates: Metronidazole may increase the levels/effects of CYP3A4 substrates. Example substrates include benzodiazepines, calcium channel blockers, cyclosporine, mirtazapine, nateglinide, nefazodone, sildenafil (and other PDE-5 inhibitors), tacrolimus, and venlafaxine. Selected benzodiazepines (midazolam and triazolam), cisapride, ergot alkaloids, selected HMG-CoA reductase inhibitors (lovastatin and simvastatin), and pimozide are generally contraindicated with strong CYP3A4 inhibitors.
Ethanol: Ethanol results in disulfiram-like reactions.
Lithium: Metronidazole may increase lithium levels/toxicity; monitor lithium levels.
Phenytoin, phenobarbital may increase metabolism of metronidazole, potentially decreasing its effect.
Warfarin: Metronidazole increases P-T prolongation with warfarin.

Ethanol/Nutrition/Herb Interactions
Ethanol: The manufacturer recommends to avoid all ethanol or any ethanol-containing drugs (may cause disulfiram-like reaction characterized by flushing, headache, nausea, vomiting, sweating or tachycardia).
Food: Peak antibiotic serum concentration lowered and delayed, but total drug absorbed not affected.

Test Interactions May interfere with AST, ALT, triglycerides, glucose, and LDH testing

Dietary Considerations Take on an empty stomach. Drug may cause GI upset; if GI upset occurs, take with food. Extended release tablets should be taken on an empty stomach (1 hour before or 2 hours after meals). Sodium content of 500 mg (I.V.): 322 mg (14 mEq). The manufacturer recommends that ethanol be avoided during treatment and for 3 days after therapy is complete.

Dosage Forms [DSC] = Discontinued product

Capsule (Flagyl®): 375 mg
Cream, topical: 0.75% (45 g)
MetroCream®: 0.75% (45 g) [contains benzyl alcohol]
Noritate®: 1% (60 g)
Gel, topical (MetroGel®): 0.75% (45 g) [DSC], 1% (45 g)
Gel, vaginal (MetroGel-Vaginal®, Vandazole™): 0.75% (70 g)
Infusion (Flagyl® I.V. RTU™) [premixed iso-osmotic sodium chloride solution]: 500 mg (100 mL) [contains sodium 14 mEq]
Lotion, topical (MetroLotion®): 0.75% (60 mL) [contains benzyl alcohol]
Tablet (Flagyl®): 250 mg, 500 mg
Tablet, extended release (Flagyl® ER): 750 mg

References

"Antimicrobial Prophylaxis for Surgery," *Treat Guidel Med Lett*, 2004, 2(20):27-32.

◆ **Metronidazole Hydrochloride** *see* Metronidazole *on page 842*
◆ **Mevacor®** *see* Lovastatin *on page 782*
◆ **Mevinolin** *see* Lovastatin *on page 782*

Mexiletine (MEKS i le teen)

Related Information
Antiarrhythmic Drugs *on page 1548*
Chronic Pain Management *on page 1430*

U.S. Brand Names Mexitil® [DSC]

Canadian Brand Names Novo-Mexiletine

Pharmacologic Category Antiarrhythmic Agent, Class Ib

Generic Available Yes

Use Management of serious ventricular arrhythmias; suppression of PVCs

Unlabeled/Investigational Use Diabetic neuropathy

Mechanism of Action Class IB antiarrhythmic, structurally related to lidocaine, which inhibits inward sodium current, decreases rate of rise of phase 0, increases effective refractory period/action potential duration ratio

Pharmacodynamics/Kinetics
Absorption: Elderly have a slightly slower rate, but extent of absorption is the same as young adults
Distribution: V_d: 5-7 L/kg
Protein binding: 50% to 70%
Metabolism: Hepatic; low first-pass effect
Half-life elimination: Adults: 10-14 hours (average: elderly: 14.4 hours, younger adults: 12 hours); prolonged with hepatic impairment or heart failure
Time to peak: 2-3 hours
Excretion: Urine (10% to 15% as unchanged drug); urinary acidification increases excretion, alkalinization decreases excretion

Dosage Adults: Oral: Initial: 200 mg every 8 hours (may load with 400 mg if necessary); adjust dose every 2-3 days; usual dose: 200-300 mg every 8 hours; maximum dose: 1.2 g/day (some patients respond to every 12-hour dosing). When switching from another antiarrhythmic, initiate a 200 mg dose 6-12 hours after stopping former agents, 3-6 hours after stopping procainamide.
Dosage adjustment in hepatic impairment: Reduce dose to 25% to 30% of usual dose

Administration Administer around-the-clock rather than 3 times/day to promote less variation in peak and trough serum levels; administer with food

Reference Range Therapeutic range: 0.5-2 mcg/mL; potentially toxic: >2 mcg/mL

Anesthesia and Critical Care Concerns/Other Considerations As with other antiarrhythmic agents, mexiletine is also proarrhythmic, particularly in patients with underlying cardiovascular disease and electrolyte abnormalities.

Pregnancy Risk Factor C

Contraindications Hypersensitivity to mexiletine or any component of the formulation; cardiogenic shock; second- or third-degree AV block (except in patients with a functioning artificial pacemaker)

Warnings/Precautions **[U.S. Boxed Warning]: In the Cardiac Arrhythmia Suppression Trial (CAST), recent (>6 days but <2 years ago) myocardial infarction patients with asymptomatic, nonlife-threatening ventricular arrhythmias did not benefit and may have been harmed by attempts to suppress the arrhythmia with flecainide or encainide. An increased mortality or non-fatal cardiac arrest rate (7.7%) was seen in the active**
(Continued)

Mexiletine *(Continued)*

treatment group compared with patients in the placebo group (3%). The applicability of the CAST results to other populations is unknown. Antiarrhythmic agents should be reserved for patients with life-threatening ventricular arrhythmias. Can be proarrhythmic. Electrolyte disturbances alter response; should be corrected before initiating therapy. Use cautiously in patients with first-degree block, pre-existing sinus node dysfunction, intraventricular conduction delays, significant hepatic dysfunction, hypotension, or severe CHF. Alterations in urinary pH may change urinary excretion. Rare hepatic toxicity may occur; may cause acute hepatic injury.

Adverse Reactions

>10%:

Central nervous system: Lightheadedness (11% to 25%), dizziness (20% to 25%), nervousness (5% to 10%), incoordination (10%)

Gastrointestinal: GI distress (41%), nausea/vomiting (40%)

Neuromuscular & skeletal: Trembling, unsteady gait, tremor (13%), ataxia (10% to 20%)

1% to 10%:

Cardiovascular: Chest pain (3% to 8%), premature ventricular contractions (1% to 2%), palpitation (4% to 8%), angina (2%), proarrhythmic (10% to 15% in patients with malignant arrhythmia)

Central nervous system: Confusion, headache, insomnia (5% to 7%), depression (2%)

Dermatologic: Rash (4%)

Gastrointestinal: Constipation or diarrhea (4% to 5%), xerostomia (3%), abdominal pain (1%)

Neuromuscular & skeletal: Weakness (5%), numbness of fingers or toes (2% to 4%), paresthesia (2%), arthralgia (1%)

Ocular: Blurred vision (5% to 7%), nystagmus (6%)

Otic: Tinnitus (2% to 3%)

Respiratory: Dyspnea (3%)

<1% (Limited to important or life-threatening): Agranulocytosis, alopecia, AV block, cardiogenic shock, CHF, dysphagia, exfoliative dermatitis, hallucinations, hepatic necrosis, hepatitis, hypotension, impotence, leukopenia, myelofibrosis, pancreatitis (rare), psychosis, pulmonary fibrosis, seizure, sinus arrest, SLE syndrome, Stevens-Johnson syndrome, syncope, thrombocytopenia, torsade de pointes, upper GI bleeding, urinary retention, urticaria

Overdosage/Toxicology Has a narrow therapeutic index and severe toxicity may occur slightly above the therapeutic range, especially with other antiarrhythmic drugs. Acute ingestion of twice the daily therapeutic dose is potentially life-threatening. Symptoms of overdose include sedation, confusion, coma, seizures, respiratory arrest and cardiac toxicity (sinus arrest, AV block, asystole, and hypotension). The QRS and QT intervals are usually normal, although they may be prolonged after massive overdose. Other effects include dizziness, paresthesia, tremor, ataxia, and GI disturbance. Treatment is symptomatic and supportive.

Drug Interactions Substrate (major) of CYP1A2, 2D6; **Inhibits** CYP1A2 (strong)

CYP1A2 inducers: May decrease the levels/effects of mexiletine. Example inducers include aminoglutethimide, carbamazepine, phenobarbital, and rifampin.

CYP1A2 inhibitors: May increase the levels/effects of mexiletine. Example inhibitors include ciprofloxacin, ketoconazole, norfloxacin, ofloxacin, and rofecoxib.

CYP1A2 substrates: Mexiletine may increase the levels/effects of CYP1A2 substrates. Example substrates include aminophylline, fluvoxamine, mirtazapine, ropinirole, theophylline, and trifluoperazine.

CYP2D6 inhibitors: May increase the levels/effects of mexiletine. Example inhibitors include chlorpromazine, delavirdine, fluoxetine, miconazole, paroxetine, pergolide, quinidine, quinine, ritonavir, and ropinirole.

Fluvoxamine: Clearance of mexiletine was reduced by 38% following coadministration with fluvoxamine. If used concurrently, mexiletine levels should be monitored.

Quinidine may increase mexiletine blood levels.

Theophylline blood levels are increased by mexiletine.

Urinary alkalinizers (antacids, sodium bicarbonate, acetazolamide) may increase mexiletine blood levels.

Ethanol/Nutrition/Herb Interactions Food: Food may decrease the rate, but not the extent of oral absorption; diets which affect urine pH can increase or decrease excretion of mexiletine. Avoid dietary changes that alter urine pH.

Test Interactions Abnormal liver function test, positive ANA, thrombocytopenia

Dosage Forms [DSC] = Discontinued product

Capsule, as hydrochloride: 150 mg, 200 mg, 250 mg

Mexitil®: 150 mg, 200 mg, 250 mg [DSC]

- **Mexitil® [DSC]** *see* Mexiletine *on page 845*
- **$MgSO_4$ (error-prone abbreviation)** *see* Magnesium Sulfate *on page 787*
- **Micardis®** *see* Telmisartan *on page 1237*

Miconazole and Zinc Oxide (mi KON a zole & zink OKS ide)

U.S. Brand Names Vusion™

Synonyms Zinc Oxide and Miconazole Nitrate

Pharmacologic Category Antifungal Agent, Topical

Generic Available No

Use Adjunctive treatment of diaper dermatitis complicated by *Candida albicans* infection

Mechanism of Action

Miconazole inhibits the biosynthesis of ergosterol, damaging the fungal cell wall membrane.

Zinc oxide is a mild astringent with weak antiseptic properties.

Pharmacodynamics/Kinetics Absorption: Topical: Miconazole: Undetectable to 3.8 ng/mL in infants with dermatitis

Dosage Diaper dermatitis: Topical: Children ≥4 weeks: Apply to affected area with each diaper change for 7 days. Treatment should continue for 7 days, even with initial improvement. Do not use for >7 days.

Stability Store at 15°C to 30°C (59°F to 86°F).

Administration Apply thin film to clean, dry skin. Do not rub into skin. Avoid use of scented soaps, shampoos, or lotions in the diaper area. Frequent diaper changes are recommended.

Pregnancy Risk Factor C

Contraindications Hypersensitivity to miconazole, zinc oxide, or any component of the formulation

Warnings/Precautions For use in immunocompetent patients with a candidal infection documented by microscopic evaluation; not intended for prophylactic use. Discontinue in case of irritation or worsening of dermatitis. Safety and efficacy have not been established in children <4 weeks of age, very low-birth-weight infants, incontinent adults, or for duration >7 days. For external use only; not for oral, ophthalmic, or vaginal use.

Dosage Forms Ointment, topical (Vusion™): Miconazole nitrate 0.25% and zinc oxide 15% (30 g)

- **Micronase®** *see* GlyBURIDE *on page 598*
- **Microzide™** *see* Hydrochlorothiazide *on page 634*

Midazolam (MID aye zoe lam)

Medication Safety Issues

Sound-alike/look-alike issues:

Versed may be confused with VePesid®, Vistaril®

Related Information

Anesthesia Considerations for Neurosurgery *on page 1401*
Anesthesia for Patients With Liver Disease *on page 1421*
Benzodiazepines *on page 1555*
Intravenous Anesthetic Agents *on page 1531*
Moderate Sedation *on page 1442*
Sedative Agents in the Intensive Care Unit *on page 1576*

Canadian Brand Names Apo-Midazolam®; Midazolam Injection

Synonyms Midazolam Hydrochloride; Versed

Pharmacologic Category Benzodiazepine

Restrictions C-IV

Generic Available Yes

(Continued)

Midazolam *(Continued)*

Use Preoperative sedation and provides conscious sedation prior to diagnostic or radiographic procedures; ICU sedation (continuous infusion); intravenous anesthesia (induction); intravenous anesthesia (maintenance)

Unlabeled/Investigational Use Anxiety, status epilepticus

Mechanism of Action Binds to stereospecific benzodiazepine receptors on the postsynaptic GABA neuron at several sites within the central nervous system, including the limbic system, reticular formation. Enhancement of the inhibitory effect of GABA on neuronal excitability results by increased neuronal membrane permeability to chloride ions. This shift in chloride ions results in hyperpolarization (a less excitable state) and stabilization.

Pharmacodynamics/Kinetics

Onset of action: I.M.: Sedation: ~15 minutes; I.V.: 1-5 minutes

Peak effect: I.M.: 0.5-1 hour

Duration: I.M.: Up to 6 hours; Mean: 2 hours

Absorption: Oral: Rapid

Distribution: V_d: 0.8-2.5 L/kg; increased with congestive heart failure (CHF) and chronic renal failure

Protein binding: 95%

Metabolism: Extensively hepatic via CYP3A4

Bioavailability: Mean: 45%

Half-life elimination: 1-4 hours; prolonged with cirrhosis, congestive heart failure, obesity, and elderly

Excretion: Urine (as glucuronide conjugated metabolites); feces (~2% to 10%)

Dosage The dose of midazolam needs to be individualized based on the patient's age, underlying diseases, and concurrent medications. Decrease dose (by ~30%) if narcotics or other CNS depressants are administered concomitantly. **Personnel and equipment needed for standard respiratory resuscitation should be immediately available during midazolam administration.**

Children <6 years may require higher doses and closer monitoring than older children; calculate dose on ideal body weight

Conscious sedation for procedures or preoperative sedation:

Oral: 0.25-0.5 mg/kg as a single dose preprocedure, up to a maximum of 20 mg; administer 30-45 minutes prior to procedure. Children <6 years or less cooperative patients may require as much as 1 mg/kg as a single dose; 0.25 mg/kg may suffice for children 6-16 years of age.

Intranasal (not an approved route): 0.2 mg/kg (up to 0.4 mg/kg in some studies), to a maximum of 15 mg; may be administered 30-45 minutes prior to procedure

I.M.: 0.1-0.15 mg/kg 30-60 minutes before surgery or procedure; range 0.05-0.15 mg/kg; doses up to 0.5 mg/kg have been used in more anxious patients; maximum total dose: 10 mg

I.V.:

Infants <6 months: Limited information is available in nonintubated infants; dosing recommendations not clear; infants <6 months are at higher risk for airway obstruction and hypoventilation; titrate dose in small increments to desired effect; monitor carefully

Infants 6 months to Children 5 years: Initial: 0.05-0.1 mg/kg; titrate dose carefully; total dose of 0.6 mg/kg may be required; usual maximum total dose: 6 mg

Children 6-12 years: Initial: 0.025-0.05 mg/kg; titrate dose carefully; total doses of 0.4 mg/kg may be required; usual maximum total dose: 10 mg

Children 12-16 years: Dose as adults; usual maximum total dose: 10 mg

Conscious sedation during mechanical ventilation: Children: Loading dose: 0.05-0.2 mg/kg, followed by initial continuous infusion: 0.06-0.12 mg/kg/hour (1-2 mcg/kg/minute); titrate to the desired effect; usual range: 0.4-6 mcg/kg/minute

Status epilepticus refractory to standard therapy (unlabeled use): Infants >2 months and Children: Loading dose: 0.15 mg/kg followed by a continuous infusion of 1 mcg/kg/minute; titrate dose upward every 5 minutes until clinical seizure activity is controlled; mean infusion rate required in 24 children was 2.3 mcg/kg/minute with a range of 1-18 mcg/kg/minute

Adults:

Preoperative sedation:

I.M.: 0.07-0.08 mg/kg 30-60 minutes prior to surgery/procedure; usual dose: 5 mg; **Note:** Reduce dose in patients with COPD, high-risk patients, patients ≥60 years of age, and patients receiving other narcotics or CNS depressants

I.V.: 0.02-0.04 mg/kg; repeat every 5 minutes as needed to desired effect or up to 0.1-0.2 mg/kg

Intranasal (not an approved route): 0.2 mg/kg (up to 0.4 mg/kg in some studies); administer 30-45 minutes prior to surgery/procedure

Conscious sedation: I.V.: Initial: 0.5-2 mg slow I.V. over at least 2 minutes; slowly titrate to effect by repeating doses every 2-3 minutes if needed; usual total dose: 2.5-5 mg; use decreased doses in elderly

Healthy Adults <60 years: Some patients respond to doses as low as 1 mg; no more than 2.5 mg should be administered over a period of 2 minutes. Additional doses of midazolam may be administered after a 2-minute waiting period and evaluation of sedation after each dose increment. A total dose >5 mg is generally not needed. If narcotics or other CNS depressants are administered concomitantly, the midazolam dose should be reduced by 30%.

Anesthesia: I.V.:

Induction:

Unpremedicated patients: 0.3-0.35 mg/kg (up to 0.6 mg/kg in resistant cases)

Premedicated patients: 0.15-0.35 mg/kg

Maintenance: 0.05-0.3 mg/kg as needed, or continuous infusion 0.25-1.5 mcg/kg/minute

Sedation in mechanically-ventilated patients: I.V. continuous infusion: 100 mg in 250 mL D_5W or NS (if patient is fluid-restricted, may concentrate up to a maximum of 0.5 mg/mL); initial dose: 0.02-0.08 mg/kg (~1 mg to 5 mg in 70 kg adult) initially and either repeated at 5-15 minute intervals until adequate sedation is achieved or continuous infusion rates of 0.04-0.2 mg/kg/hour and titrate to reach desired level of sedation

Elderly: I.V.: Conscious sedation: Initial: 0.5 mg slow I.V.; give no more than 1.5 mg in a 2-minute period; if additional titration is needed, give no more than 1 mg over 2 minutes, waiting another 2 or more minutes to evaluate sedative effect; a total dose of >3.5 mg is rarely necessary

Dosage adjustment in renal impairment:

Hemodialysis: Supplemental dose is not necessary

Peritoneal dialysis: Significant drug removal is unlikely based on physiochemical characteristics

Stability Stable for 24 hours at room temperature/refrigeration; at a final concentration of 0.5 mg/mL, stable for up to 24 hours when diluted with D_5W or NS, or for up to 4 hours when diluted with lactated Ringer's; admixtures do not require protection from light for short-term storage

Administration

Intranasal: Administer using a 1 mL needleless syringe into the nostrils over 15 seconds; use the 5 mg/mL injection; ½ of the dose may be administered to each nostril

Oral: Do not mix with any liquid (such as grapefruit juice) prior to administration

Parenteral:

I.M.: Administer deep I.M. into large muscle.

I.V.: Administer by slow I.V. injection over at least 2-5 minutes at a concentration of 1-5 mg/mL or by I.V. infusion. Continuous infusions should be administered via an infusion pump.

Monitoring Parameters Respiratory and cardiovascular status, blood pressure, blood pressure monitor required during I.V. administration

Anesthesia and Critical Care Concerns/Other Considerations

Agitation in the ICU Patient: Diazepam or midazolam is recommended for rapid sedation of the acutely-agitated patient. Midazolam may accumulate in obesity, in patients with hypoalbuminemia, or renal failure. Concurrent use of CYP3A4 inhibitors may inhibit midazolam's metabolism and prolong its sedative effects. The ACCM/SCCM task force does not recommend midazolam use for ongoing sedation in the practice guidelines for sustained use of sedatives and analgesics in the critically-ill adult. Midazolam is 3-4 times as potent as diazepam. Paradoxical

(Continued)

Midazolam *(Continued)*

reactions associated with midazolam use in children (eg, agitation, restlessness, combativeness) have been successfully treated with flumazenil.

Pregnancy Risk Factor D

Contraindications Hypersensitivity to midazolam or any component of the formulation, including benzyl alcohol (cross-sensitivity with other benzodiazepines may exist); parenteral form is not for intrathecal or epidural injection; narrow-angle glaucoma; concurrent use of potent inhibitors of CYP3A4 (amprenavir, atazanavir, or ritonavir); pregnancy

Warnings/Precautions [U.S. Boxed Warning]: May cause severe respiratory depression, respiratory arrest, or apnea. Use with extreme caution, particularly in noncritical care settings. Appropriate resuscitative equipment and qualified personnel must be available for administration and monitoring. Initial dosing must be cautiously titrated and individualized, particularly in elderly or debilitated patients, patients with hepatic impairment (including alcoholics), or in renal impairment, particularly if other CNS depressants (including opiates) are used concurrently. **[U.S. Boxed Warning]: Initial doses in elderly or debilitated patients should be conservative; as little as 1 mg, but not to exceed 2.5 mg.** Use with caution in patients with respiratory disease or impaired gag reflex. Use during upper airway procedures may increase risk of hypoventilation. Prolonged responses have been noted following extended administration by continuous infusion (possibly due to metabolite accumulation) or in the presence of drugs which inhibit midazolam metabolism.

Causes CNS depression (dose-related) resulting in sedation, dizziness, confusion, or ataxia which may impair physical and mental capabilities. Patients must be cautioned about performing tasks which require mental alertness (eg, operating machinery or driving). A minimum of 1 day should elapse after midazolam administration before attempting these tasks. Use with caution in patients receiving other CNS depressants or psychoactive agents. Effects with other sedative drugs or ethanol may be potentiated. Benzodiazepines have been associated with falls and traumatic injury and should be used with extreme caution in patients who are at risk of these events (especially the elderly).

May cause hypotension - hemodynamic events are more common in pediatric patients or patients with hemodynamic instability. Hypotension and/or respiratory depression may occur more frequently in patients who have received narcotic analgesics. Use with caution in obese patients, chronic renal failure, and CHF. Does not protect against increases in heart rate or blood pressure during intubation. Should not be used in shock, coma, or acute alcohol intoxication. **[U.S. Boxed Warning]: Parenteral form contains benzyl alcohol; avoid rapid injection in neonates or prolonged infusions.** Avoid intra-arterial administration or extravasation of parenteral formulation.

Midazolam causes anterograde amnesia. Paradoxical reactions, including hyperactive or aggressive behavior have been reported with benzodiazepines, particularly in adolescent/pediatric or psychiatric patients. Does not have analgesic, antidepressant, or antipsychotic properties.

Benzodiazepines have been associated with dependence and acute withdrawal symptoms on discontinuation or reduction in dose. Acute withdrawal, including seizures, may be precipitated after administration of flumazenil to patients receiving long-term benzodiazepine therapy.

Adverse Reactions As reported in adults unless otherwise noted:

>10%: Respiratory: Decreased tidal volume and/or respiratory rate decrease, apnea (3% children)

1% to 10%:

- Cardiovascular: Hypotension (3% children)
- Central nervous system: Drowsiness (1%), oversedation, headache (1%), seizure-like activity (1% children)
- Gastrointestinal: Nausea (3%), vomiting (3%)
- Local: Pain and local reactions at injection site (4% I.M., 5% I.V.; severity less than diazepam)
- Ocular: Nystagmus (1% children)
- Respiratory: Cough (1%)
- Miscellaneous: Physical and psychological dependence with prolonged use, hiccups (4%, 1% children), paradoxical reaction (2% children)

<1% (Limited to important or life-threatening): Agitation, amnesia, bigeminy, bronchospasm, emergence delirium, euphoria, hallucinations, laryngospasm, rash

Overdosage/Toxicology Symptoms of overdose include respiratory depression, hypotension, coma, stupor, confusion, and apnea. Treatment for benzodiazepine overdose is supportive. Flumazenil has been shown to selectively block the binding of benzodiazepines to its receptor, resulting in reversal of CNS depression but not always respiratory depression.

Drug Interactions Substrate of CYP2B6 (minor), 3A4 (major); **Inhibits** CYP2C8 (weak), 2C9 (weak), 3A4 (weak)

CNS depressants: Sedative effects and/or respiratory depression may be additive with CNS depressants; includes ethanol, barbiturates, narcotic analgesics, and other sedative agents; monitor for increased effect. **If narcotics or other CNS depressants are administered concomitantly, the midazolam dose should be reduced by 30% if <65 years of age, or by at least 50% if >65 years of age.**

CYP3A4 inducers: CYP3A4 inducers may decrease the levels/effects of midazolam. Example inducers include aminoglutethimide, carbamazepine, nafcillin, nevirapine, phenobarbital, phenytoin, and rifamycins.

CYP3A4 inhibitors: May increase the levels/effects of midazolam. Example inhibitors include azole antifungals, clarithromycin, diclofenac, doxycycline, erythromycin, imatinib, isoniazid, nefazodone, nicardipine, propofol, protease inhibitors, quinidine, telithromycin, and verapamil.

Levodopa: Therapeutic effects may be diminished in some patients following the addition of a benzodiazepine; limited/inconsistent data

Oral contraceptives: May decrease the clearance of some benzodiazepines (those which undergo oxidative metabolism); monitor for increased benzodiazepine effect

Saquinavir: A 56% reduction in clearance and a doubling of midazolam's half-life were seen with concurrent administration with saquinavir.

Theophylline: May partially antagonize some of the effects of benzodiazepines; monitor for decreased response; may require higher doses for sedation

Ethanol/Nutrition/Herb Interactions

Ethanol: Avoid ethanol (may increase CNS depression).

Food: Grapefruit juice may increase serum concentrations of midazolam; avoid concurrent use with oral form.

Herb/Nutraceutical: Avoid concurrent use with St John's wort (may decrease midazolam levels, may increase CNS depression). Avoid concurrent use with valerian, kava kava, gotu kola (may increase CNS depression).

Dietary Considerations Injection: Sodium content of 1 mL: 0.14 mEq

Dosage Forms

Injection, solution: 1 mg/mL (2 mL, 5 mL, 10 mL); 5 mg/mL (1 mL, 2 mL, 5 mL, 10 mL) [contains benzyl alcohol 1%]

Injection, solution [preservative free]: 1 mg/mL (2 mL, 5 mL); 5 mg/mL (1 mL, 2 mL)

Syrup: 2 mg/mL (118 mL) [contains sodium benzoate; cherry flavor]

References

Hughes J, Gill A, Leach HJ, et al, "A Prospective Study of the Adverse Effects of Midazolam on Withdrawal in Critically Ill Children," *Acta Paediatr*, 1994, 83(11):1194-9.

Jacobi J, Fraser GL, Coursin DB, et al, "Clinical Practice Guidelines for the Sustained Use of Sedatives and Analgesics in the Critically Ill Adult," *Crit Care Med*, 2002, 30(1):119-41. Available at: http://www.sccm.org/pdf/sedatives.pdf.

Mokhlesi B, Leikin JB, Murray P, et al, "Adult Toxicology in Critical Care. Part 11: Specific Poisonings," *Chest*, 2003, 123(3):897-922.

Rivera R, Segnini M, Baltodano A, et al, "Midazolam in the Treatment of Status Epilepticus in Children," *Crit Care Med*, 1993, 21(7):991-4.

♦ **Midazolam Hydrochloride** *see* Midazolam *on page 847*

♦ **Midazolam Injection (Can)** *see* Midazolam *on page 847*

♦ **Midol® Cramp and Body Aches [OTC]** *see* Ibuprofen *on page 651*

♦ **Midol® Extended Relief** *see* Naproxen *on page 899*

Milrinone (MIL ri none)

Medication Safety Issues

Sound-alike/look-alike issues:

Primacor® may be confused with Primaxin®

Related Information

Critical Care Infusion Administration Charts *on page 1514*

Hemodynamic Support, Intravenous *on page 1566*

(Continued)

Milrinone *(Continued)*

U.S. Brand Names Primacor®

Canadian Brand Names Milrinone Lactate Injection; Primacor®

Synonyms Milrinone Lactate

Pharmacologic Category Phosphodiesterase Enzyme Inhibitor

Generic Available Yes

Use Short-term I.V. therapy of congestive heart failure; calcium antagonist intoxication

Mechanism of Action Phosphodiesterase inhibitor resulting in vasodilation

Pharmacodynamics/Kinetics

Onset of action: I.V.: 5-15 minutes

Serum level: I.V.: Following a 125 mcg/kg dose, peak plasma concentrations ~1000 ng/mL were observed at 2 minutes postinjection, decreasing to <100 ng/mL in 2 hours

Drug concentration levels:

Therapeutic:

Serum levels of 166 ng/mL, achieved during I.V. infusions of 0.25-1 mcg/kg/minute, were associated with sustained hemodynamic benefit in severe congestive heart failure patients over a 24-hour period

Maximum beneficial effects on cardiac output and pulmonary capillary wedge pressure following I.V. infusion have been associated with plasma milrinone concentrations of 150-250 ng/mL

Toxic: Serum concentrations >250-300 ng/mL have been associated with marked reductions in mean arterial pressure and tachycardia; however, more studies are required to determine the toxic serum levels for milrinone

Distribution: V_{dss}: 0.32 L/kg; Severe congestive heart failure (CHF): V_d: 0.33-0.47 L/kg; not significantly bound to tissues; excretion in breast milk unknown

Protein binding, plasma: ~70%

Metabolism: Hepatic (12%)

Half-life elimination: I.V.: 136 minutes in patients with CHF; patients with severe CHF have a more prolonged half-life, with values ranging from 1.7-2.7 hours. Patients with CHF have a reduction in the systemic clearance of milrinone, resulting in a prolonged elimination half-life. Alternatively, one study reported that 1 month of therapy with milrinone did not change the pharmacokinetic parameters for patients with CHF despite improvement in cardiac function.

Excretion: I.V.: Urine (85% as unchanged drug) within 24 hours; active tubular secretion is a major elimination pathway for milrinone

Clearance: I.V. bolus: 25.9 ± 5.7 L/hour (0.37 L/hour/kg); Severe congestive heart failure: 0.11-0.13 L/hour/kg. The reduction in clearance may be a result of reduced renal function. Creatinine clearance values were ½ those reported for healthy adults in patients with severe congestive heart failure (52 vs 119 mL/minute).

Dosage Adults: I.V.: Loading dose: 50 mcg/kg administered over 10 minutes followed by a maintenance dose titrated according to the hemodynamic and clinical response; see following table:

Maintenance Dosage	Dose Rate (mcg/kg/min)	Total Dose (mg/kg/24 h)
Minimum	0.375	0.59
Standard	0.500	0.77
Maximum	0.750	1.13

Dosing adjustment in renal impairment:

Cl_{cr} 50 mL/minute/1.73 m^2: Administer 0.43 mcg/kg/minute.

Cl_{cr} 40 mL/minute/1.73 m^2: Administer 0.38 mcg/kg/minute.

Cl_{cr} 30 mL/minute/1.73 m^2: Administer 0.33 mcg/kg/minute.

Cl_{cr} 20 mL/minute/1.73 m^2: Administer 0.28 mcg/kg/minute.

Cl_{cr} 10 mL/minute/1.73 m^2: Administer 0.23 mcg/kg/minute.

Cl_{cr} 5 mL/minute/1.73 m^2: Administer 0.2 mcg/kg/minute.

Stability Colorless to pale yellow solution; store at room temperature and protect from light; stable at 0.2 mg/mL in 0.9% sodium chloride or D_5W for 72 hours at room temperature in normal light

Incompatible with furosemide and procainamide; **compatible** with atropine, calcium chloride, digoxin, epinephrine, lidocaine, morphine, propranolol, and sodium bicarbonate

Standard dilution: For a final concentration of 0.2 mg/mL: Dilute Primacor® 1 mg/mL (20 mL) with 80 mL diluent (final volume: 100 mL); may also dilute 1 mg/mL (10 mL) with 40 mL diluent (final volume: 50 mL)

Administration Requires an infusion pump; continuous I.V. infusion; 20 mg/100 mL 0.9% sodium chloride or D_5W (0.2 mg/mL); see table.

Dose (mcg/kg/min)	Rate (mL/kg/h)
0.375	0.11
0.400	0.12
0.500	0.15
0.600	0.18
0.700	0.21
0.750	0.22

Monitoring Parameters Cardiac monitor and blood pressure monitor required; serum potassium

Therapeutic: Patients should be monitored for improvement in the clinical signs and symptoms of congestive heart failure

Toxic: Patients should be monitored for ventricular arrhythmias and exacerbation of anginal symptoms; during I.V. therapy with milrinone, blood pressure and heart rate should be monitored

Anesthesia and Critical Care Concerns/Other Considerations Inotrope of choice for severe congestive heart failure patients taking beta-blockers. Milrinone may be useful for severe CHF patients on beta-blocker who require an intravenous inotrope. If hypotension is a problem, loading doses may be omitted and maintenance infusions initiated. There is some delay in hemodynamic effects, but it is minimal (1-3 hours). Lower maintenance infusions have also been used (0.18-0.25 mcg/kg/minute).

Pregnancy Risk Factor C

Contraindications Hypersensitivity to milrinone, inamrinone, or any component of the formulation; concurrent use of inamrinone

Warnings/Precautions Avoid in severe obstructive aortic or pulmonic valvular disease. It may aggravate outflow tract obstruction in hypertrophic subaortic stenosis. Supraventricular and ventricular arrhythmias have developed in high-risk patients. Monitor closely during the infusion. Ensure that ventricular rate controlled in atrial fibrillation/flutter before initiating. Not recommended for use in acute MI patients. Monitor and correct fluid and electrolyte problems. Adjust dose in renal dysfunction.

Adverse Reactions

>10%: Cardiovascular: Ventricular arrhythmia (ectopy 9%, NSVT 3%, sustained ventricular tachycardia 1%, ventricular fibrillation <1%); life-threatening arrhythmia are infrequent, often associated with underlying factors (eg, pre-existing arrhythmia, electrolyte disturbances, catheter insertion)

1% to 10%:

Cardiovascular: Supraventricular arrhythmia (4%), hypotension

Central nervous system: Headache

<1% (Limited to important or life-threatening): Anaphylaxis, atrial fibrillation, bronchospasm, chest pain, hypokalemia, liver function abnormalities, MI, rash, thrombocytopenia, torsade de pointes, tremor, ventricular fibrillation

Overdosage/Toxicology Treatment is supportive and symptomatic.

Dosage Forms [DSC] = Discontinued product

Infusion [premixed in D_5W] (Primacor®): 200 mcg/mL (100 mL, 200 mL)

Injection, solution: 1 mg/mL (10 mL, 20 mL, 50 mL)

Primacor®: 1 mg/mL (10 mL, 20 mL; 50 mL [DSC])

◆ **Milrinone Lactate** *see* Milrinone *on page 851*
◆ **Milrinone Lactate Injection (Can)** *see* Milrinone *on page 851*
◆ **Minidyne® [OTC]** *see* Povidone-Iodine *on page 1039*
◆ **Minipress®** *see* Prazosin *on page 1044*
◆ **Minirin® (Can)** *see* Desmopressin *on page 363*
◆ **Minitran™** *see* Nitroglycerin *on page 928*

♦ **Minocin®** *see* Minocycline *on page 854*

Minocycline (mi noe SYE kleen)

Medication Safety Issues

Sound-alike/look-alike issues:

Dynacin® may be confused with Dyazide®, Dynabac®, DynaCirc®, Dynapen®

Minocin® may be confused with Indocin®, Lincocin®, Minizide®, Mithracin®, niacin

U.S. Brand Names Dynacin®; Minocin®; myrac™; Solodyn™

Canadian Brand Names Alti-Minocycline; Apo-Minocycline®; Gen-Minocycline; Minocin®; Novo-Minocycline; PMS-Minocycline; Rhoxal-minocycline; Sandoz-Minocycline

Synonyms Minocycline Hydrochloride

Pharmacologic Category Antibiotic, Tetracycline Derivative

Generic Available Yes: Excludes extended release tablet

Use Treatment of susceptible bacterial infections of both gram-negative and gram-positive organisms; treatment of anthrax (inhalational, cutaneous, and gastrointestinal); acne; meningococcal (asymptomatic) carrier state; Rickettsial diseases (including Rocky Mountain spotted fever, Q fever); nongonococcal urethritis, gonorrhea; acute intestinal amebiasis

Mechanism of Action Inhibits bacterial protein synthesis by binding with the 30S and possibly the 50S ribosomal subunit(s) of susceptible bacteria; cell wall synthesis is not affected

Pharmacodynamics/Kinetics

Absorption: Well absorbed

Distribution: Majority deposits for extended periods in fat; crosses placenta; enters breast milk

Protein binding: 70% to 75%

Half-life elimination: 16 hours (range: 11-23 hours)

Time to peak: Capsule, pellet filled: 1-4 hours; Extended release tablet: 3.5-4 hours

Excretion: Urine

Dosage

Usual dosage range:

Children >8 years: Oral: Initial: 4 mg/kg, followed by 2 mg/kg/dose every 12 hours

Adults: Oral: Initial: 200 mg, followed by 100 mg every 12 hours (maximum: 400 mg/day)

Indication-specific dosing:

Children ≥12 years: Inflammatory, non-nodular, moderate-to-severe acne (Solodyn™):

45-59 kg: 45 mg once daily

60-90 kg: 90 mg once daily

91-136 kg: 135 mg once daily

Note: Therapy should be continued for 12 weeks. Higher doses do not confer greater efficacy, and safety of use beyond 12 weeks has not been established.

Adults: Oral:

Acne: 50-100 mg daily

Inflammatory, non-nodular, moderate-to-severe acne (Solodyn™):

45-59 kg: 45 mg once daily

60-90 kg: 90 mg once daily

91-136 kg: 135 mg once daily

Note: Therapy should be continued for 12 weeks. Higher doses do not confer greater efficacy, and safety of use beyond 12 weeks has not been established.

Chlamydial or *Ureaplasma urealyticum* infection, uncomplicated: Urethral, endocervical, or rectal: 100 mg every 12 hours for at least 7 days

Gonococcal infection, uncomplicated (males):

Without urethritis or anorectal infection: Initial: 200 mg, followed by 100 mg every 12 hours for at least 4 days (cultures 2-3 days post-therapy)

Urethritis: 100 mg every 12 hours for 5 days

Meningococcal carrier state: 100 mg every 12 hours for 5 days

***Mycobacterium marinum*:** 100 mg every 12 hours for 6-8 weeks

Nocardiosis, cutaneous (non-CNS): 100 mg every 12 hours

Syphilis: Initial: 200 mg, followed by 100 mg every 12 hours for 10-15 days

Dosage adjustment in renal impairment: Consider decreasing dose or increasing dosing interval; total daily dose should not exceed 200 mg

Stability

Capsule (including pellet-filled), tablet: Store at 20°C to 25°C (68°F to 77°F); protect from light and moisture

Extended release tablet: Store at 15°C to 30°C (59°F to 86°F); protect from light, moisture, and heat

Administration May be taken with food or milk. Administer with adequate fluid to decrease the risk of esophageal irritation and ulceration.

Monitoring Parameters Culture and sensitivity testing prior to initiating therapy; LFTs, BUN, renal function with long-term treatment; if symptomatic for autoimmune disorder, include ANA, CBC

Pregnancy Risk Factor D

Contraindications Hypersensitivity to minocycline, other tetracyclines, or any component of the formulation; pregnancy

Warnings/Precautions May cause tissue hyperpigmentation or permanent tooth discoloration; avoid use during tooth development (children ≤8 years of age) unless other drugs are not likely to be effective or are contraindicated. May be associated with increases in BUN secondary to antianabolic effects; use caution in patients with renal impairment. Hepatotoxicity has been reported; use caution in patients with hepatic insufficiency. Autoimmune syndromes (eg, lupus-like, hepatitis, and vasculitis) have been reported; discontinue if symptoms. CNS effects (lightheadedness, vertigo) may occur; patients must be cautioned about performing tasks which require mental alertness (eg, operating machinery or driving). Has been associated (rarely) with pseudotumor cerebri. May cause photosensitivity; discontinue if skin erythema occurs. May cause overgrowth of nonsusceptible organisms, including fungi; discontinue if superinfection occurs. Avoid use in children ≤8 years of age.

Adverse Reactions Frequency not defined.

Cardiovascular: Myocarditis, pericarditis, vasculitis

Central nervous system: Bulging fontanels, dizziness,f atigue, fever, headache, hypoesthesia, malaise, mood changes, paresthesia, pseudotumor cerebri, sedation, seizure, somnolence, vertigo

Dermatologic: Alopecia, angioedema, erythema multiforme, erythema nodosum, erythematous rash, exfoliative dermatitis, hyperpigmentation of nails, maculopapular rash, photosensitivity, pigmentation of the skin and mucous membranes, pruritus, Stevens-Johnson syndrome, toxic epidermal necrolysis, urticaria

Endocrine & metabolic: Thyroid discoloration, thyroid dysfunction

Gastrointestinal: Anorexia, diarrhea, dyspepsia, dysphagia, enamel hypoplasia, enterocolitis, esophageal ulcerations, esophagitis, glossitis, inflammatory lesions (oral/anogenital), moniliasis, nausea, oral cavity discoloration, pancreatitis, pseudomembranous colitis, stomatitis, tooth discoloration, vomiting, xerostomia

Genitourinary: Balanitis, vulvovaginitis

Hematologic: Agranulocytosis, eosinophilia, hemolytic anemia, leukopenia, neutropenia, pancytopenia, thrombocytopenia

Hepatic: Hepatic cholestasis, hepatic failure, hepatitis, hyperbilirubinemia, jaundice, liver enzyme increases

Neuromuscular & skeletal: Arthralgia, arthritis, bone discoloration, joint stiffness, joint swelling, myalgia

Otic: Hearing loss, tinnitus

Renal: Acute renal failure, BUN increased, interstitial nephritis

Respiratory: Asthma, bronchospasm, cough, dyspnea, pneumonitis, pulmonary infiltrate (with eosinophilia)

Miscellaneous: Anaphylaxis, hypersensitivity, lupus erythematosus, lupus-like syndrome, serum sickness

Overdosage/Toxicology Symptoms of overdose include diabetes insipidus, nausea, anorexia, dizziness, vomiting, and diarrhea. Treatment is symptom-directed and supportive. Not dialyzable (0% to 5%).

Drug Interactions

Calcium-, magnesium-, or aluminum-containing antacids, bile acid sequestrants, bismuth, oral contraceptives, iron, zinc, sodium bicarbonate, penicillins, quinapril: May decrease absorption of tetracyclines.

(Continued)

Minocycline *(Continued)*

Methoxyflurane anesthesia, when concurrent with tetracyclines, may cause fatal nephrotoxicity.

Penicillins: Tetracyclines may reduce bactericidal efficacy of penicillins and cephalosporins.

Retinoic acid derivatives: May increase risk of pseudotumor cerebri.

Typhoid vaccine: Antibacterial agents may decrease the therapeutic efficacy of the live, attenuated typhoid (Ty21a strain) vaccine

Warfarin: Hypoprothrombinemic response may be increased with tetracyclines; monitor INR closely during initiation or discontinuation.

Ethanol/Nutrition/Herb Interactions

Food: Minocycline serum concentrations are not significantly altered if taken with food or dairy products.

Herb/Nutraceutical: Avoid dong quai, St John's wort (may also cause photosensitization).

Test Interactions May cause interference with fluorescence test for urinary catecholamines (false elevations)

Dietary Considerations May be taken with food or milk.

Dosage Forms

Capsule: 50 mg, 75 mg, 100 mg
  Dynacin®: 75 mg, 100 mg

Capsule, pellet filled: 50 mg, 100 mg
  Minocin®: 50 mg, 100 mg

Tablet: 50 mg, 75 mg, 100 mg
  Dynacin®, myrac™: 50 mg, 75 mg, 100 mg

Tablet, extended release:
  Solodyn™: 45 mg, 90 mg, 130 mg

♦ **Minocycline Hydrochloride** *see* Minocycline *on page 854*

♦ **Minox (Can)** *see* Minoxidil *on page 856*

Minoxidil (mi NOKS i dil)

Medication Safety Issues

Sound-alike/look-alike issues:
  Minoxidil may be confused with metolazone, Monopril®
  Loniten® may be confused with clonidine, Lioresal®, Lotensin®

U.S. Brand Names Loniten®; Rogaine® Extra Strength for Men [OTC]; Rogaine® for Men [OTC]; Rogaine® for Women [OTC]

Canadian Brand Names Apo-Gain®; Minox; Rogaine®

Pharmacologic Category Topical Skin Product; Vasodilator

Generic Available Yes

Use Management of severe hypertension (usually in combination with a diuretic and beta-blocker); treatment (topical formulation) of alopecia androgenetica in males and females

Mechanism of Action Produces vasodilation by directly relaxing arteriolar smooth muscle, with little effect on veins; effects may be mediated by cyclic AMP; stimulation of hair growth is secondary to vasodilation, increased cutaneous blood flow and stimulation of resting hair follicles

Pharmacodynamics/Kinetics

Onset of action: Hypotensive: Oral: ~30 minutes
  Peak effect: 2-8 hours

Duration: 2-5 days

Protein binding: None

Metabolism: 88%, primarily via glucuronidation

Bioavailability: Oral: 90%

Half-life elimination: Adults: 3.5-4.2 hours

Excretion: Urine (12% as unchanged drug)

Dosage

Children <12 years: Hypertension: Oral: Initial: 0.1-0.2 mg/kg once daily; maximum: 5 mg/day; increase gradually every 3 days; usual dosage: 0.25-1 mg/kg/day in 1-2 divided doses; maximum: 50 mg/day

Children >12 years and Adults: Hypertension: Oral: Initial: 5 mg once daily, increase gradually every 3 days (maximum: 100 mg/day); usual dose range (JNC 7): 2.5-80 mg/day in 1-2 divided doses

Adults: Alopecia: Topical: Apply twice daily; 4 months of therapy may be necessary for hair growth.

Elderly: Initial: 2.5 mg once daily; increase gradually.

Note: Dosage adjustment is needed when added to concomitant therapy.

Dialysis: Supplemental dose is not necessary via hemo- or peritoneal dialysis.

Stability Store at controlled room temperature of 20°C to 25°C (68°F to 77°F).

Monitoring Parameters Blood pressure, standing and sitting/supine; fluid and electrolyte balance and body weight should be monitored

Anesthesia and Critical Care Concerns/Other Considerations Minoxidil when used in patients with hypertension will not cause regression of left ventricular hypertrophy.

Pregnancy Risk Factor C

Contraindications Hypersensitivity to minoxidil or any component of the formulation; pheochromocytoma; acute MI; dissecting aortic aneurysm

Warnings/Precautions Maximum therapeutic doses of a diuretic and two antihypertensives should be used before this drug is ever added. **[U.S. Boxed Warning]: It can cause pericardial effusion, tamponade, or exacerbate angina pectoris.** Monitor patients who are receiving guanethidine concurrently (orthostasis can be problematic). May need to add a diuretic to minimize fluid gain and a beta-blocker (if no contraindications) to treat tachycardia. Rapid control of blood pressure can lead to syncope, CVA, MI, ischemia. Hypersensitivity reactions occur rarely. Avoid use for a month after acute MI. Inform patients of hair growth patterns before initiating therapy. May take 1-6 months for hypertrichosis to reverse itself after discontinuation of the drug. Use with caution in patients with pulmonary hypertension, significant renal failure, CHF, or ischemic disease. Renal failure and dialysis patients may require a smaller dose.

Adverse Reactions

>10%:

Cardiovascular: CHF, edema, ECG (transient change in T-wave amplitude and direction), tachycardia

Dermatologic: Hypertrichosis (commonly occurs within 1-2 months of therapy)

1% to 10%: Endocrine & metabolic: Fluid and electrolyte imbalance

<1% (Limited to important or life-threatening): Angina, coarsening facial features, leukopenia, pericardial effusion tamponade, rash, Stevens-Johnson syndrome, thrombocytopenia, weight gain

Overdosage/Toxicology

Symptoms of overdose include hypotension, tachycardia, headache, nausea, dizziness, weakness syncope, warm flushed skin and palpitations; lethargy and ataxia may occur in children

Hypotension usually responds to I.V. fluids, Trendelenburg positioning or vasoconstrictor; treatment is primarily supportive and symptomatic

Drug Interactions

Antihypertensives: Effects may be additive.

Guanethidine can cause severe orthostasis; avoid concurrent use - discontinue 1-3 weeks prior to initiating minoxidil.

Ethanol/Nutrition/Herb Interactions Herb/Nutraceutical: Avoid natural licorice (causes sodium and water retention and increases potassium loss).

Dosage Forms [DSC] = Discontinued product

Solution, topical: 2% [20 mg/metered dose] (60 mL); 5% [50 mg/metered dose] (60 mL)

Rogaine® for Men, Rogaine® for Women: 2% [20 mg/metered dose] (60 mL)

Rogaine® Extra Strength for Men: 5% [50 mg/metered dose] (60 mL)

Tablet: 2.5 mg, 10 mg

Loniten®: 2.5 mg [DSC], 10 mg

♦ **Miochol-E®** *see* Acetylcholine *on page 34*

♦ **Miostat®** *see* Carbachol *on page 224*

Misoprostol (mye soe PROST ole)

Medication Safety Issues

Sound-alike/look-alike issues:

Misoprostol may be confused with metoprolol

Cytotec® may be confused with Cytoxan®, Sytobex®

(Continued)

Misoprostol *(Continued)*

U.S. Brand Names Cytotec®

Canadian Brand Names Apo-Misoprostol®; Novo-Misoprostol

Pharmacologic Category Prostaglandin

Generic Available Yes

Use Prevention of NSAID-induced gastric ulcers; medical termination of pregnancy of ≤49 days (in conjunction with mifepristone)

Unlabeled/Investigational Use Cervical ripening and labor induction; NSAID-induced nephropathy; fat malabsorption in cystic fibrosis

Mechanism of Action Misoprostol is a synthetic prostaglandin E_1 analog that replaces the protective prostaglandins consumed with prostaglandin-inhibiting therapies (eg, NSAIDs); has been shown to induce uterine contractions

Pharmacodynamics/Kinetics

Absorption: Rapid

Metabolism: Hepatic; rapidly de-esterified to misoprostol acid (active)

Half-life elimination: Metabolite: 20-40 minutes

Time to peak, serum: Active metabolite: Fasting: 15-30 minutes

Excretion: Urine (64% to 73%) and feces (15%) within 24 hours

Dosage

Oral:

Children 8-16 years: Fat absorption in cystic fibrosis (unlabeled use): 100 mcg 4 times/day

Adults:

Prevention of NSAID-induced gastric ulcers: 200 mcg 4 times/day with food; if not tolerated, may decrease dose to 100 mcg 4 times/day with food or 200 mcg twice daily with food; last dose of the day should be taken at bedtime

Medical termination of pregnancy: Refer to Mifepristone monograph.

Intravaginal: Adults: Labor induction or cervical ripening (unlabeled uses): 25 mcg (1/4 of 100 mcg tablet); may repeat at intervals no more frequent than every 3-6 hours. Do not use in patients with previous cesarean delivery or prior major uterine surgery.

Stability Store at or below 25°C (77°F).

Administration Incidence of diarrhea may be lessened by having patient take dose right after meals. Therapy is usually begun on the second or third day of the next normal menstrual period.

Pregnancy Risk Factor X

Contraindications Hypersensitivity to misoprostol, prostaglandins, or any component of the formulation; pregnancy (when used to reduce NSAID-induced ulcers)

Warnings/Precautions Safety and efficacy have not been established in children <18 years of age; use with caution in patients with renal impairment and the elderly. **[U.S. Boxed Warning]: Not to be used in women of childbearing potential unless woman is capable of complying with effective contraceptive measures;** therapy is normally begun on the second or third day of next normal menstrual period. Uterine perforation and/or rupture have been reported in association with intravaginal use to induce labor or with combined oral/intravaginal use to induce abortion. The manufacturer states that Cytotec® should not be used as a cervical-ripening agent for induction of labor. However, The American College of Obstetricians and Gynecologists (ACOG) continues to support this off-label use.

Adverse Reactions

>10%: Gastrointestinal: Diarrhea, abdominal pain

1% to 10%:

Central nervous system: Headache

Gastrointestinal: Constipation, flatulence, nausea, dyspepsia, vomiting

<1% (Limited to important or life-threatening): Anaphylaxis, anxiety, appetite changes, arrhythmia, arterial thrombosis, bronchospasm, confusion, cramps, depression, drowsiness, edema, fetal or infant death (when used during pregnancy), fever, GI bleeding, GI inflammation, gingivitis, gout, hyper-/hypotension, impotence, loss of libido, MI, neuropathy, neurosis, pulmonary embolism, purpura, rash, reflux, rigors, thrombocytopenia, uterine rupture, weakness, weight changes

Overdosage/Toxicology Symptoms of overdose include sedation, tremor, convulsions, dyspnea, abdominal pain, diarrhea, hypotension, and bradycardia. Treatment is symptom-directed and supportive.

Drug Interactions

Oxytocin: Misoprostol may increase the effect of oxytocin; wait 6-12 hours after misoprostol administration before initiating oxytocin.

Ethanol/Nutrition/Herb Interactions Food: Misoprostol peak serum concentrations may be decreased if taken with food (not clinically significant).

Dietary Considerations Should be taken with food; incidence of diarrhea may be lessened by having patient take dose right after meals.

Dosage Forms Tablet: 100 mcg, 200 mcg

♦ **Mivacron®** *see* Mivacurium *on page 859*

Mivacurium (mye va KYOO ree um)

Medication Safety Issues

Sound-alike/look-alike issues:

Mivacron® may be confused with Mevacor®

High alert medication: The Institute for Safe Medication Practices (ISMP) includes this medication among its list of drugs which have a heightened risk of causing significant patient harm when used in error.

Related Information

Chronic Renal Failure *on page 1437*

Neuromuscular Blocking Agents *on page 1572*

U.S. Brand Names Mivacron®

Canadian Brand Names Mivacron®

Synonyms Mivacurium Chloride

Pharmacologic Category Neuromuscular Blocker Agent, Nondepolarizing

Generic Available No

Use Adjunct to general anesthesia to facilitate endotracheal intubation and to relax skeletal muscles during surgery; to facilitate mechanical ventilation in ICU patients; does not relieve pain or produce sedation

Mechanism of Action Mivacurium is a short-acting, nondepolarizing, neuromuscular-blocking agent. Like other nondepolarizing drugs, mivacurium antagonizes acetylcholine by competitively binding to cholinergic sites on motor endplates in skeletal muscle. This inhibits contractile activity in skeletal muscle leading to muscle paralysis. This effect is reversible with cholinesterase inhibitors such as edrophonium, neostigmine, and physostigmine.

Pharmacodynamics/Kinetics

Onset of action: Neuromuscular blockade (dose dependent): I.V.: 1.5-3 minutes

Duration: Short due to rapid hydrolysis by plasma cholinesterases; clinically effective block may last for 12-20 minutes; spontaneous recovery may be 95% complete in 25-30 minutes; duration shorter in children and may be slightly longer in elderly

Metabolism: Via plasma cholinesterase, inactive metabolites

Half-life elimination: 2 minutes (more active isomers only)

Excretion: Urine (<10%)

Dosage Continuous infusion requires an infusion pump; dose to effect; doses will vary due to interpatient variability; use ideal body weight for obese patients

Children 2-12 years (duration of action is shorter and dosage requirements are higher): 0.2 mg/kg I.V. followed by average infusion rate of 14 mcg/kg/minute (range: 5-31 mcg/kg/minute) upon evidence of spontaneous recovery from initial dose

Adults: Initial: I.V.: 0.15-0.25 mg/kg bolus followed by maintenance doses of 0.1 mg/kg at approximately 15-minute intervals; for prolonged neuromuscular block, initial infusion of 9-10 mcg/kg/minute is used upon evidence of spontaneous recovery from initial dose, usual infusion rate of 6-7 mcg/kg/minute (1-15 mcg/kg/minute) under balanced anesthesia; initial dose after succinylcholine for intubation (balanced anesthesia): Adults: 0.1 mg/kg

Pretreatment/priming: 10% of intubating dose given 3-5 minutes before initial dose

Dosing adjustment in renal impairment: 0.15 mg/kg I.V. bolus; duration of action of blockade: 1.5 times longer in ESRD, may decrease infusion rates by as much as 50%, dependent on degree of renal impairment

Dosing adjustment in hepatic impairment: 0.15 mg/kg I.V. bolus; duration of blockade: 3 times longer in ESLD, may decrease rate of infusion by as much as 50% in ESLD, dependent on the degree of impairment

(Continued)

Mivacurium *(Continued)*

Stability Store at room temperature of 15°C to 25°C (59°F to 77°F); protect from direct ultraviolet light

Administration Children require higher mivacurium infusion rates than adults; during opioid/nitrous oxide/oxygen anesthesia, the infusion rate required to maintain 89% to 99% neuromuscular block averages 14 mcg/kg/minute (range: 5-31). For adults and children, the amount of infusion solution required per hour depends upon the clinical requirements of the patient, the concentration of mivacurium in the infusion solution, and the patient's weight. The contribution of the infusion solution to the fluid requirements of the patient must be considered. See tables.

Infusion Rates for Maintenance of Neuromuscular Block During Opioid/ Nitrous Oxide/Oxygen Anesthesia Using Mivacurium Premixed Infusion (0.5 mg/mL)

Patient Weight (kg)	Drug Delivery Rate (mcg/kg/min)									
	4	5	6	7	8	10	14	16	18	20
	Infusion Delivery Rate (mL/h)									
10	5	6	7	8	10	12	17	19	22	24
15	7	9	11	13	14	18	25	29	32	36
20	10	12	15	17	19	24	34	38	43	48
25	12	15	18	21	24	30	42	48	54	60
35	17	21	26	29	34	42	59	67	76	84
50	24	30	36	42	46	60	84	96	108	120
60	29	36	43	50	58	72	101	115	130	144
70	34	42	50	59	67	84	118	134	151	168
80	39	48	58	67	77	96	134	154	173	192
90	44	54	65	76	86	108	151	173	194	216
100	48	60	72	84	96	120	168	192	216	240

Infusion Rates for Maintenance of Neuromuscular Block During Opioid/Nitrous Oxide/Oxygen Anesthesia Using Mivacurium Injection (2 mg/mL)

Patient Weight (kg)	Drug Delivery Rate (mcg/kg/min)									
	4	5	6	7	8	10	14	16	18	20
	Infusion Delivery Rate (mL/h)									
10	1.2	1.5	1.8	2.1	2.4	3	4.2	4.8	5.4	6
15	1.8	2.3	2.7	3.2	3.6	4.5	6.3	7.2	8.1	9
20	2.4	3	3.6	4.2	4.8	6	8.4	9.5	10.8	12
25	3	3.8	4.5	5.3	6	7.5	10.5	12	13.5	15
35	4.2	5.3	6.3	7.4	8.4	10.5	14.7	16.8	18.9	21
50	6	7.5	9	10.5	12	15	21	24	27	30
60	7.2	9	10.8	12.8	14.4	18	25.2	28.8	32.4	36
70	8.4	10.5	12.6	14.7	16.8	21	29.4	33.6	37.8	42
80	9.6	12	14.4	16.8	19.2	24	33.6	38.4	43.2	48
90	10.8	13.5	16.2	18.9	21.6	27	37.8	43.2	48.6	54
100	12	15	18	21	24	30	42	48	54	60

Anesthesia and Critical Care Concerns/Other Considerations Mivacurium is classified as a short duration neuromuscular-blocking agent; do not mix with barbiturates in same syringe; does not appear to have a cumulative effect on the duration of blockade.

Critically-Ill Adult Patients:

The 2004 Surviving Sepsis Campaign guidelines recommend avoiding use of neuromuscular blockers if at all possible in the septic patient due to the risk of prolonged neuromuscular blockade following discontinuation. If one is required, monitor carefully and observe the following recommendations.

The 2002 ACCM/SCCM/ASHP clinical practice guidelines for sustained neuromuscular blockade in the adult critically-ill patient recommend:

Optimize sedatives and analgesics prior to initiation and monitor and adjust accordingly during course. Neuromuscular blockers do not relieve pain or produce sedation.

Protect patient's eyes from development of keratitis and corneal abrasion by administering ophthalmic ointment and taping eyelids closed or using eye patches. Reposition patient routinely to protect pressure points from breakdown. Address DVT prophylaxis.

Concurrent use of a neuromuscular blocker and corticosteroids appear to increase the risk of certain ICU myopathies; avoid or administer the corticosteroid at the lowest dose possible. Reassess need for neuromuscular blocker daily.

Using daily drug holidays (stopping neuromuscular-blocking agent until patient requires it again) may decrease the incidence of acute quadriplegic myopathy syndrome.

Tachyphylaxis can develop; switch to another neuromuscular blocker (taking into consideration the patient's organ function) if paralysis is still necessary.

Atracurium or cisatracurium is recommended for patients with significant hepatic or renal disease, due to organ-independent Hofmann elimination.

Monitor patients clinically and via "Train of Four" (TOF) testing with a goal of adjusting the degree of blockade to 1-2 twitches or based upon the patient's clinical condition.

Pregnancy Risk Factor C

Contraindications Hypersensitivity to mivacurium chloride, any component of the formulation, or other benzylisoquinolinium agents; use of multidose vials in patients with allergy to benzyl alcohol; pre-existing tachycardia

Warnings/Precautions Ventilation must be supported during neuromuscular blockade; does not counteract bradycardia produced by anesthetics/vagal stimulation; prolonged neuromuscular block may be seen in patients with reduced or atypical plasma cholinesterase activity (eg, pregnancy, liver or kidney disease, infections, peptic ulcer, anemia); patients homozygous for the atypical plasma cholinesterase gene are extremely sensitive to the neuromuscular blocking effect of mivacurium (use extreme caution if at all in those patients); duration prolonged in patients with renal and/or hepatic impairment; reduce initial dosage and inject slowly (over 60 seconds) in patients in whom substantial histamine release would be potentially hazardous; certain clinical conditions may result in potentiation or antagonism of neuromuscular blockade:

Potentiation: Electrolyte abnormalities, severe hyponatremia, severe hypocalcemia, severe hypokalemia, hypermagnesemia, neuromuscular diseases, acidosis, acute intermittent porphyria, renal failure, hepatic failure

Antagonism: Alkalosis, hypercalcemia, demyelinating lesions, peripheral neuropathies, diabetes mellitus

Increased sensitivity in patients with myasthenia gravis, Eaton-Lambert syndrome, resistance in burn patients (>30% of body) for period of 5-70 days postinjury; resistance in patients with muscle trauma, denervation, immobilization, infection. Cross-sensitivity with other neuromuscular-blocking agents may occur; use extreme caution in patients with previous anaphylactic reactions.

Adverse Reactions

>10%: Cardiovascular: Flushing of face

1% to 10%: Cardiovascular: Hypotension

<1% (Limited to important or life-threatening): Acute quadriplegic myopathy syndrome (prolonged use), anaphylactoid reaction, anaphylaxis, bradycardia, bronchospasm, cutaneous erythema, dizziness, endogenous histamine release, hypersensitivity reactions, hypoxemia, injection site reaction, muscle spasms, myositis ossificans (prolonged use), rash, tachycardia, wheezing

Drug Interactions Prolonged neuromuscular blockade: Inhaled anesthetics; local anesthetics; calcium channel blockers; antiarrhythmics (eg, quinidine or procainamide); antibiotics (eg, aminoglycosides, tetracyclines, vancomycin, clindamycin); immunosuppressants (eg, cyclosporine)

Dosage Forms

Injection, solution [preservative free]: 2 mg/mL (5 mL, 10 mL)

Injection, solution: 2 mg/mL (20 mL, 50 mL) [with benzyl alcohol]

References

Cook DR, Freeman JA, Lai AA, et al, "Pharmacokinetics of Mivacurium in Normal Patients and in Those With Hepatic or Renal Failure," *Br J Anaesth*, 1992, 69(6):580-5.

(Continued)

Mivacurium *(Continued)*

Dellinger RP, Carlet JM, Masur H, et al, "Surviving Sepsis Campaign Guidelines for Management of Severe Sepsis and Septic Shock," *Crit Care Med*, 2004, 32(3):858-73.

Moexipril (mo EKS i pril)

Medication Safety Issues

Sound-alike/look-alike issues:

Moexipril may be confused with Monopril®

Related Information

Angiotensin Agents *on page 1544*

Preoperative Evaluation of the Cardiac Patient for Noncardiac Surgery *on page 1485*

U.S. Brand Names Univasc®

Synonyms Moexipril Hydrochloride

Pharmacologic Category Angiotensin-Converting Enzyme (ACE) Inhibitor

Generic Available No

Use Treatment of hypertension, alone or in combination with thiazide diuretics; treatment of left ventricular dysfunction after myocardial infarction

Mechanism of Action Competitive inhibitor of angiotensin-converting enzyme (ACE); prevents conversion of angiotensin I to angiotensin II, a potent vasoconstrictor; results in lower levels of angiotensin II which causes an increase in plasma renin activity and a reduction in aldosterone secretion

Pharmacodynamics/Kinetics

Onset of action: Peak effect: 1-2 hours

Duration: >24 hours

Distribution: V_d (moexiprilat): 180 L

Protein binding, plasma: Moexipril: 90%; Moexiprilat: 50% to 70%

Metabolism: Parent drug: Hepatic and via GI tract to moexiprilat, 1000 times more potent than parent

Bioavailability: Moexiprilat: 13%; reduced with food (AUC decreased by ~40%)

Half-life elimination: Moexipril: 1 hour; Moexiprilat: 2-9 hours

Time to peak: 1.5 hours

Excretion: Feces (50%)

Dosage Adults: Oral: Initial: 7.5 mg once daily (in patients **not** receiving diuretics), 1 hour prior to a meal **or** 3.75 mg once daily (when combined with thiazide diuretics); maintenance dose: 7.5-30 mg/day in 1 or 2 divided doses 1 hour before meals

Dosing adjustment in renal impairment: Cl_{cr} ≤40 mL/minute: Patients may be cautiously placed on 3.75 mg once daily, then upwardly titrated to a maximum of 15 mg/day.

Monitoring Parameters Blood pressure, heart rate, electrolytes, CBC, symptoms of hypotension

Pregnancy Risk Factor C (1st trimester)/D (2nd and 3rd trimesters)

Contraindications Hypersensitivity to moexipril, moexiprilat, or any component of the formulation; hypersensitivity or allergic reactions or angioedema related to previous treatment with an ACE inhibitor; pregnancy (2nd or 3rd trimester)

Warnings/Precautions Anaphylactic reactions can occur. Angioedema can occur at any time during treatment (especially following first dose). It may involve head and neck (potentially affecting the airway) or the intestine (presenting with abdominal pain). Prolonged monitoring may be required especially if tongue, glottis, or larynx are involved as they are associated with airway obstruction.

Those with a history of airway surgery in this situation have a higher risk. Careful blood pressure monitoring with first dose (hypotension can occur especially in volume-depleted patients). **[U.S. Boxed Warning]: Based on human data, ACEIs can cause injury and death to the developing fetus when used in the second and third trimesters. ACEIs should be discontinued as soon as possible once pregnancy is detected.** Dosage adjustment needed in renal impairment. Use with caution in hypovolemia; collagen vascular diseases; valvular stenosis (particularly aortic stenosis); hyperkalemia; or before, during, or immediately after anesthesia. Avoid rapid dosage escalation which may lead to renal insufficiency. Rare toxicities associated with ACE inhibitors include cholestatic jaundice (which may progress to hepatic necrosis) and neutropenia/agranulocytosis with myeloid hyperplasia. If patient has renal impairment then a baseline WBC with differential and serum creatinine should be evaluated and monitored closely during the first 3 months of therapy. Hypersensitivity reactions may be seen during hemodialysis with high-flux dialysis membranes (eg, AN69). Deterioration in renal function can occur with initiation. Use with caution in unilateral renal artery stenosis and pre-existing renal insufficiency.

Adverse Reactions

1% to 10%:

Cardiovascular: Hypotension, peripheral edema
Central nervous system: Headache, dizziness, fatigue
Dermatologic: Alopecia, flushing, rash
Endocrine & metabolic: Hyperkalemia, hyponatremia
Gastrointestinal: Diarrhea, nausea, heartburn
Genitourinary: Polyuria
Neuromuscular & skeletal: Myalgia
Renal: Reversible increases in creatinine or BUN
Respiratory: Cough, pharyngitis, upper respiratory infection, sinusitis

<1% (Limited to important or life-threatening): Alopecia, anemia, angioedema, arrhythmia, bronchospasm, cerebrovascular accident, chest pain, dyspnea, elevated LFTs, eosinophilic pneumonitis, hepatitis, hypercholesterolemia, MI, oliguria, orthostatic hypotension, palpitation, proteinuria, syncope

Overdosage/Toxicology Mild hypotension has been the primary toxic effect seen with acute overdose. Bradycardia may also occur. Hyperkalemia occurs even with therapeutic doses, especially in patients with renal insufficiency and those taking NSAIDs. Treatment is symptom-directed and supportive.

Drug Interactions

ACE inhibitors: Potential for allergic reactions increased with moexipril.
Allopurinol: Potential for allergic reactions increased with moexipril.
$Alpha_1$ blockers: Hypotensive effect increased.
Antacids: May decrease the bioavailability of ACE inhibitors (may be more likely to occur with captopril); separate administration times by 1-2 hours.
Aspirin: The effects of ACE inhibitors may be blunted by aspirin administration, particularly at higher dosages; may increase potential for adverse renal effects.
Diuretics: Hypovolemia due to diuretics may precipitate acute hypotensive events or acute renal failure.
Insulin: Risk of hypoglycemia may be increased.
Lithium: Risk of lithium toxicity may be increased; monitor lithium levels, especially the first 4 weeks of therapy.
Mercaptopurine: Risk of neutropenia may be increased.
NSAIDs: May attenuate hypertensive efficacy; effect has been seen with captopril and may occur with other ACE inhibitors; monitor blood pressure. May increase potential to alter renal function.
Potassium-sparing diuretics (amiloride, potassium, spironolactone, triamterene): Increased risk of hyperkalemia.
Potassium supplements may increase the risk of hyperkalemia.
Probenecid: Blood levels of moexipril are increased (may occur with other ACE inhibitors).
Trimethoprim (high dose) may increase the risk of hyperkalemia.

Ethanol/Nutrition/Herb Interactions

Food: Food may delay and reduce peak serum levels.
Herb/Nutraceutical: Avoid dong quai if using for hypertension (has estrogenic activity). Avoid ephedra, yohimbe, ginseng (may worsen hypertension). Avoid garlic (may have increased antihypertensive effect).

Test Interactions Increases BUN, creatinine, potassium, positive Coombs' [direct]; decreases cholesterol (S); may cause false-positive results in urine acetone determinations using sodium nitroprusside reagent

(Continued)

Moexipril *(Continued)*

Dietary Considerations Administer on an empty stomach.

Dosage Forms Tablet, as hydrochloride [scored]: 7.5 mg, 15 mg

- **Moexipril Hydrochloride** *see* Moexipril *on page 862*
- **Molybdenum** *see* Trace Metals *on page 1296*
- **Molypen®** *see* Trace Metals *on page 1296*
- **Monacolin K** *see* Lovastatin *on page 782*
- **Monocor® (Can)** *see* Bisoprolol *on page 176*
- **Monodox®** *see* Doxycycline *on page 426*
- **Monoethanolamine** *see* Ethanolamine Oleate *on page 494*
- **Mononine®** *see* Factor IX *on page 502*
- **Monopril®** *see* Fosinopril *on page 562*

Montelukast (mon te LOO kast)

Medication Safety Issues

Sound-alike/look-alike issues:

Singulair® may be confused with Sinequan®

U.S. Brand Names Singulair®

Canadian Brand Names Singulair®

Synonyms Montelukast Sodium

Pharmacologic Category Leukotriene-Receptor Antagonist

Generic Available No

Use Prophylaxis and chronic treatment of asthma; relief of symptoms of seasonal allergic rhinitis and perennial allergic rhinitis

Unlabeled/Investigational Use Acute asthma

Mechanism of Action Selective leukotriene receptor antagonist that inhibits the cysteinyl leukotriene receptor. Cysteinyl leukotrienes and leukotriene receptor occupation have been correlated with the pathophysiology of asthma, including airway edema, smooth muscle contraction, and altered cellular activity associated with the inflammatory process, which contribute to the signs and symptoms of asthma.

Pharmacodynamics/Kinetics

Duration: >24 hours

Absorption: Rapid

Distribution: V_d: 8-11 L

Protein binding, plasma: >99%

Metabolism: Extensively hepatic via CYP3A4 and 2C8/9

Bioavailability: Tablet: 10 mg: Mean: 64%; 5 mg: 63% to 73%

Half-life elimination, plasma: Mean: 2.7-5.5 hours

Time to peak, serum: Tablet: 10 mg: 3-4 hours; 5 mg: 2-2.5 hours; 4 mg: 2 hours

Excretion: Feces (86%); urine (<0.2%)

Dosage Oral:

Children:

6-11 months: Asthma (unlabeled use): 4 mg (oral granules) once daily, taken in the evening

6-23 months: Perennial allergic rhinitis: 4 mg (oral granules) once daily

12-23 months: Asthma: 4 mg (oral granules) once daily, taken in the evening

2-5 years: Asthma, seasonal or perennial allergic rhinitis: 4 mg (chewable tablet or oral granules) once daily, taken in the evening

6-14 years: Asthma, seasonal or perennial allergic rhinitis: Chew one 5 mg chewable tablet/day, taken in the evening

Children ≥15 years and Adults:

Asthma, seasonal or perennial allergic rhinitis: 10 mg/day, taken in the evening

Asthma, acute (unlabeled use): 10 mg as a single dose administered with first-line therapy

Dosing adjustment in renal impairment: No adjustment necessary

Dosing adjustment in hepatic impairment: Mild-to-moderate: No adjustment necessary. Patients with severe hepatic disease were **not** studied.

Stability Store at room temperature of 15°C to 30°C (59°F to 86°F); protect from moisture and light

Granules: Use within 15 minutes of opening packet.

Administration When treating asthma, administer dose in the evening. Granules may be administered directly in the mouth or mixed with applesauce, carrots, rice,

ice cream, baby formula, or breast milk; do not add to any other liquids. Administer within 15 minutes of opening packet.

Pregnancy Risk Factor B

Contraindications Hypersensitivity to montelukast or any component of the formulation

Warnings/Precautions Montelukast is not FDA approved for use in the reversal of bronchospasm in acute asthma attacks; some clinicians, however, support its use (Cylly, 2003; Camargo, 2003; Ferreira, 2001). Should not be used as monotherapy for the treatment and management of exercise-induced bronchospasm. Advise patients to have appropriate rescue medication available. Appropriate clinical monitoring and caution are recommended when systemic corticosteroid reduction is considered in patients receiving montelukast. Inform phenylketonuric patients that the chewable tablet contains phenylalanine. Safety and efficacy in children <6 months of age have not been established.

In rare cases, patients on therapy with montelukast may present with systemic eosinophilia, sometimes presenting with clinical features of vasculitis consistent with Churg-Strauss syndrome, a condition which is often treated with systemic corticosteroid therapy. Healthcare providers should be alert to eosinophilia, vasculitic rash, worsening pulmonary symptoms, cardiac complications, and/or neuropathy presenting in their patients. A causal association between montelukast and these underlying conditions has not been established.

Adverse Reactions (As reported in adults)

1% to 10%:

Central nervous system: Dizziness (2%), fatigue (2%), fever (2%)

Dermatologic: Rash (2%)

Gastrointestinal: Abdominal pain (3%), dyspepsia (2%), dental pain (2%), gastroenteritis (2%)

Neuromuscular & skeletal: Weakness (2%)

Respiratory: Cough (3%), nasal congestion (2%), upper respiratory infection (2%)

Miscellaneous: Flu-like symptoms (4%), trauma (1%)

<1% (Limited to important or life-threatening): Agitation, anaphylaxis, angioedema, arthralgia, cholestasis (rare), Churg-Strauss syndrome, eosinophilia, hallucinations, hepatic eosinophilic infiltration (rare); hepatitis (mixed pattern, hepatocellular, and cholestatic); hypoesthesia, insomnia, myalgia, palpitation, pancreatitis, paresthesia, pruritus, seizure, vasculitis

Overdosage/Toxicology No specific antidote

Remove unabsorbed material from the GI tract, employ clinical monitoring and institute supportive therapy if required. Abdominal pain, hyperkinesia, mydriasis, somnolence, and thirst have been reported with acute overdose of ≥150 mg/day.

Drug Interactions Substrate (major) of CYP2C9, 3A4; **Inhibits** CYP2C8 (weak), 2C9 (weak)

CYP2C9 inducers: May decrease the levels/effects of montelukast. Example inducers include carbamazepine, phenobarbital, phenytoin, rifampin, rifapentine, and secobarbital.

CYP3A4 inducers: CYP3A4 inducers may decrease the levels/effects of montelukast. Example inducers include aminoglutethimide, carbamazepine, nafcillin, nevirapine, phenobarbital, phenytoin, and rifamycins.

Ethanol/Nutrition/Herb Interactions Herb/Nutraceutical: St John's wort may decrease montelukast levels.

Dietary Considerations Tablet, chewable: 4 mg strength contains phenylalanine 0.674 mg; 5 mg strength contains phenylalanine 0.842 mg

Dosage Forms

Granules: 4 mg/packet

Tablet: 10 mg

Tablet, chewable: 4 mg [contains phenylalanine 0.674 mg; cherry flavor]; 5 mg [contains phenylalanine 0.842 mg; cherry flavor]

References

Camargo CA Jr, Smithline HA, Malice MP, et al, "A Randomized Controlled Trial of Intravenous Montelukast in Acute Asthma," *Am J Respir Crit Care Med*, 2003, 167(4):528-33.

Cylly A, Kara A, Ozdemir T, et al, "Effects of Oral Montelukast on Airway Function in Acute Asthma," *Respir Med*, 2003, 97(5):533-6.

Ferreira MB, Santos AS, Pregal AL, et al, "Leukotriene Receptor Antagonists (Montelukast) in the Treatment of Asthma Crisis: Preliminary Results of a Double-Blind Placebo Controlled Randomized Study," *Allerg Immunol (Paris)*, 2001, 33(8):315-8.

♦ **Montelukast Sodium** *see* Montelukast *on page 864*

Moricizine (mor I siz een)

Medication Safety Issues

Sound-alike/look-alike issues:

Ethmozine® may be confused with Erythrocin®, erythromycin

Related Information

Antiarrhythmic Drugs *on page 1548*

U.S. Brand Names Ethmozine®

Canadian Brand Names Ethmozine®

Synonyms Moricizine Hydrochloride

Pharmacologic Category Antiarrhythmic Agent, Class I

Generic Available No

Use Treatment of ventricular tachycardia and life-threatening ventricular arrhythmias

Unlabeled/Investigational Use PVCs, complete and nonsustained ventricular tachycardia, atrial arrhythmias

Mechanism of Action Class I antiarrhythmic agent; reduces the fast inward current carried by sodium ions, shortens Phase I and Phase II repolarization, resulting in decreased action potential duration and effective refractory period

Pharmacodynamics/Kinetics

Protein binding, plasma: 95%

Metabolism: Significant first-pass effect; some enterohepatic recycling

Bioavailability: 38%

Half-life elimination: Healthy volunteers: 3-4 hours; Cardiac disease: 6-13 hours

Excretion: Feces (56%); urine (39%)

Dosage Adults: Oral: 200-300 mg every 8 hours, adjust dosage at 150 mg/day at 3-day intervals.

Recommendations for transferring patients from other antiarrhythmic agents to Ethmozine®: See table.

Moricizine

Transferred From	Start Ethmozine®
Encainide, propafenone, tocainide, or mexiletine	8-12 hours after last dose
Flecainide	12-24 hours after last dose
Procainamide	3-6 hours after last dose
Quinidine, disopyramide	6-12 hours after last dose

Dosing interval in renal or hepatic impairment: Start at 600 mg/day or less.

Anesthesia and Critical Care Concerns/Other Considerations This class Ic antiarrhythmic agent was associated with a trend toward increased mortality in the CAST trial and therefore should not be used in patients with cardiovascular disease. Cardiotoxic arrhythmic effects of moricizine and other Class Ic drugs should not be treated using class Ia antiarrhythmics.

Pregnancy Risk Factor B

Contraindications Hypersensitivity to moricizine or any component of the formulation; pre-existing second- or third-degree AV block (except in patients with a functioning artificial pacemaker); right bundle branch block when associated with left hemiblock or bifascicular block (unless functional pacemaker in place); cardiogenic shock

Warnings/Precautions Can be proarrhythmic; watch for new rhythm disturbances or existing arrhythmias that worsen. Use cautiously in CAD, previous history of MI, CHF, and cardiomegaly. **[U.S. Boxed Warning]: The CAST II trial demonstrated a decreased trend in survival for patients receiving moricizine.** Dose-related increases in PR and QRS intervals occur. Use cautiously in patients with pre-existing conduction abnormalities, and significant hepatic impairment. Safety and efficacy have not been established in pediatric patients.

Adverse Reactions

>10%: Central nervous system: Dizziness

1% to 10%:

Cardiovascular: Proarrhythmia, palpitation, cardiac death, ECG abnormalities, CHF

Central nervous system: Headache, fatigue, insomnia

Endocrine & metabolic: Decreased libido
Gastrointestinal: Nausea, diarrhea, ileus
Ocular: Blurred vision, periorbital edema
Respiratory: Dyspnea

<1% (Limited to important or life-threatening): Apnea, cardiac chest pain, hyper-/hypotension, MI, supraventricular arrhythmia, syncope, ventricular tachycardia

Overdosage/Toxicology Has a narrow therapeutic index and severe toxicity may occur slightly above the therapeutic range, especially if combined with other antiarrhythmic drugs. Acute single ingestion of twice the daily therapeutic dose is life-threatening. Symptoms of overdose include increases in PR, QRS, QT intervals and amplitude of the T wave, AV block, bradycardia, hypotension, ventricular arrhythmias (monomorphic or polymorphic ventricular tachycardia), and asystole. Other symptoms include dizziness, blurred vision, headache, and GI upset.

Treatment is symptom-directed and supportive. **Note:** Type Ia antiarrhythmic agents should not be used to treat cardiotoxicity caused by type Ic drugs.

Drug Interactions Substrate of CYP3A4 (major); **Induces** CYP1A2 (weak), 3A4 (weak)

Cimetidine increases moricizine levels by 50%.

CYP3A4 inducers: CYP3A4 inducers may decrease the levels/effects of moricizine. Example inducers include aminoglutethimide, carbamazepine, nafcillin, nevirapine, phenobarbital, phenytoin, and rifamycins.

CYP3A4 inhibitors: May increase the levels/effects of moricizine. Example inhibitors include azole antifungals, clarithromycin, diclofenac, doxycycline, erythromycin, imatinib, isoniazid, nefazodone, nicardipine, propofol, protease inhibitors, quinidine, telithromycin, and verapamil.

Digoxin may result in additive prolongation of the PR interval when combined with moricizine (but not rate of second- and third-degree AV block).

Diltiazem increases moricizine levels resulting in an increased incidence of side effects. Moricizine decreases diltiazem plasma levels and decreases its half-life.

Drugs which may prolong QT interval (including cisapride, erythromycin, phenothiazines, cyclic antidepressants, and some quinolones) are contraindicated with Type Ia antiarrhythmics. Moricizine has some type Ia activity, and caution should be used.

Theophylline levels are decreased by 50% with moricizine due to increased clearance.

Ethanol/Nutrition/Herb Interactions Food: Moricizine peak serum concentrations may be decreased if taken with food.

Dietary Considerations Best if taken on an empty stomach.

Dosage Forms Tablet, as hydrochloride: 200 mg, 250 mg, 300 mg

- ♦ **Moricizine Hydrochloride** *see* Moricizine *on page 866*
- ♦ **Morphine HP® (Can)** *see* Morphine Sulfate *on page 867*
- ♦ **Morphine LP® Epidural (Can)** *see* Morphine Sulfate *on page 867*

Morphine Sulfate (MOR feen SUL fate)

Medication Safety Issues

Sound-alike/look-alike issues:

Morphine may be confused with hydromorphone
Morphine sulfate may be confused with magnesium sulfate
MSO_4 is an error-prone abbreviation (mistaken as magnesium sulfate)
Avinza® may be confused with Evista®, Invanz®
Roxanol™ may be confused with OxyFast®, Roxicet™

Use care when prescribing and/or administering morphine solutions. These products are available in different concentrations. Always prescribe dosage in mg; **not** by volume (mL).

Use caution when selecting a morphine formulation for use in neurologic infusion pumps (eg, Medtronic delivery systems). The product should be appropriately labeled as "preservative-free" and suitable for intraspinal use via continuous infusion. In addition, the product should be formulated in a pH range that is compatible with the device operation specifications.

Related Information

Acute Postoperative Pain *on page 1388*
Anesthesia Considerations for Neurosurgery *on page 1401*
Anesthesia for Patients With Liver Disease *on page 1421*

(Continued)

Morphine Sulfate *(Continued)*

Chronic Pain Management *on page 1430*
Chronic Renal Failure *on page 1437*
Moderate Sedation *on page 1442*
Narcotic / Opioid Analgesics *on page 1568*
Opioids *on page 1535*

U.S. Brand Names Astramorph/PF™; Avinza®; DepoDur™; Duramorph®; Infumorph®; Kadian®; MS Contin®; Oramorph SR®; RMS®; Roxanol™; Roxanol 100™; Roxanol™-T [DSC]

Canadian Brand Names Kadian®; M-Eslon®; Morphine HP®; Morphine LP® Epidural; M.O.S.® 10; M.O.S.® 20; M.O.S.® 30; M.O.S.-SR®; M.O.S.-Sulfate®; MS Contin®; MS-IR®; PMS-Morphine Sulfate SR; ratio-Morphine SR; Statex®; Zomorph®

Synonyms MSO_4 (error-prone abbreviation and should not be used)

Pharmacologic Category Analgesic, Narcotic

Restrictions C-II

Generic Available Yes: Excludes capsule, controlled release tablet, sustained release tablet, extended release liposomal suspension for injection

Use Relief of moderate to severe acute and chronic pain; relief of pain of myocardial infarction; relief of dyspnea of acute left ventricular failure and pulmonary edema; preanesthetic medication

DepoDur™: Epidural (lumbar) single-dose management of surgical pain

Infumorph®: Used in microinfusion devices for intraspinal administration in treatment of intractable chronic pain

Mechanism of Action Binds to opiate receptors in the CNS, causing inhibition of ascending pain pathways, altering the perception of and response to pain; produces generalized CNS depression

Pharmacodynamics/Kinetics

Onset of action: Oral (immediate release): ~30 minutes; I.V.: 5-10 minutes

Duration: Pain relief:

Immediate release formulations: 4 hours

Extended release epidural injection (DepoDur™): >48 hours

Absorption: Variable

Distribution: V_d: 3-4 L/kg; binds to opioid receptors in the CNS and periphery (eg, GI tract)

Protein binding: 30% to 35%

Metabolism: Hepatic via conjugation with glucuronic acid to morphine-3-glucuronide (inactive), morphine-6-glucuronide (active), and in lesser amounts, morphine-3-6-diglucuronide; other minor metabolites include normorphine (active) and the 3-ethereal sulfate

Bioavailability: Oral: 17% to 33% (first-pass effect limits oral bioavailability; oral:parenteral effectiveness reportedly varies from 1:6 in opioid naive patients to 1:3 with chronic use)

Half-life elimination: Adults: 2-4 hours (immediate release forms)

Time to peak, plasma: Kadian®: ~10 hours

Excretion: Urine (primarily as morphine-3-glucuronide, ~2% to 12% excreted unchanged); feces (~7% to 10%). It has been suggested that accumulation of morphine-6-glucuronide might cause toxicity with renal insufficiency. All of the metabolites (ie, morphine-3-glucuronide, morphine-6-glucuronide, and normorphine) have been suggested as possible causes of neurotoxicity (eg, myoclonus).

Dosage Note: These are guidelines and do not represent the doses that may be required in all patients. Doses should be titrated to pain relief/prevention.

Children >6 months and <50 kg: Acute pain (moderate-to-severe):

Oral (prompt release): 0.15-0.3 mg/kg every 3-4 hours as needed

I.M.: 0.1 mg/kg every 3-4 hours as needed

I.V.: 0.05-0.1 mg/kg every 3-4 hours as needed

I.V. infusion: Range: 10-30 mcg/kg/hour

Adolescents >12 years: Sedation/analgesia for procedures: I.V.: 3-4 mg and repeat in 5 minutes if necessary

Adults:

Acute pain (moderate-to-severe):

Oral: Prompt release formulations: Opiate-naive: Initial: 10 mg every 3-4 hours as needed; patients with prior opiate exposure may require higher initial doses: usual dosage range: 10-30 mg every 3-4 hours as needed

I.M., SubQ: **Note:** Repeated SubQ administration causes local tissue irritation, pain, and induration.

Initial: Opiate-naive: 5-10 mg every 3-4 hours as needed; patients with prior opiate exposure may require higher initial doses; usual dosage range: 5-20 mg every 3-4 hours as needed

Rectal: 10-20 mg every 3-4 hours

I.V.: Initial: Opiate-naive: 2.5-5 mg every 3-4 hours; patients with prior opiate exposure may require higher initial doses. **Note:** Repeated doses (up to every 5 minutes if needed) in small increments (eg, 1-4 mg) may be preferred to larger and less frequent doses.

I.V., SubQ continuous infusion: 0.8-10 mg/hour; usual range: Up to 80 mg/hour

Mechanically-ventilated patients (based on 70 kg patient): 0.7-10 mg every 1-2 hours as needed; infusion: 5-35 mg/hour

Patient-controlled analgesia (PCA): (Opiate-naive: Consider lower end of dosing range):

Usual concentration: 1 mg/mL

Demand dose: Usual: 1 mg; range: 0.5-2.5 mg

Lockout interval: 5-10 minutes

Intrathecal (I.T.): **Note:** Administer with extreme caution and in reduced dosage to geriatric or debilitated patients.

Opioid-naive: 0.2-0.25 mg/dose (may provide adequate relief for 24 hours); repeat doses are **not** recommended.

Epidural: **Note:** Administer with extreme caution and in reduced dosage to geriatric or debilitated patients. Vigilant monitoring is particularly important in these patients.

Pain management:

Single-dose (Duramorph®): Initial: 3-5 mg

Infusion:

Bolus dose: 1-6 mg

Infusion rate: 0.1-0.2 mg/hour

Maximum dose: 10 mg/24 hours

Surgical anesthesia: Epidural: Single-dose (extended release, Depo-Dur™): Lumbar epidural only; not recommended in patients <18 years of age:

Cesarean section: 10 mg

Lower abdominal/pelvic surgery: 10-15 mg

Major orthopedic surgery of lower extremity: 15 mg

For Depo-Dur™: To minimize the pharmacokinetic interaction resulting in higher peak serum concentrations of morphine, administer the test dose of the local anesthetic at least 15 minutes prior to Depo-Dur™ administration. Use of Depo-Dur™ with epidural local anesthetics has not been studied. Other medications should not be administered into the epidural space for at least 48 hours after administration of DepoDur™.

Note: Some patients may benefit from a 20 mg dose, however, the incidence of adverse effects may be increased.

Chronic pain: Note: Patients taking opioids chronically may become tolerant and require doses higher than the usual dosage range to maintain the desired effect. Tolerance can be managed by appropriate dose titration. There is no optimal or maximal dose for morphine in chronic pain. The appropriate dose is one that relieves pain throughout its dosing interval without causing unmanageable side effects.

Oral: Controlled-, extended-, or sustained-release formulations: A patient's morphine requirement should be established using prompt-release formulations. Conversion to long-acting products may be considered when chronic, continuous treatment is required. Higher dosages should be reserved for use only in opioid-tolerant patients.

Capsules, extended release (Avinza™): Daily dose administered once daily (for best results, administer at same time each day)

Capsules, sustained release (Kadian®): Daily dose administered once daily or in 2 divided doses daily (every 12 hours)

Tablets, controlled release (MS Contin®), sustained release (Oramorph SR®), or extended release: Daily dose divided and administered every 8 or every 12 hours

Elderly or debilitated patients: Use with caution; may require dose reduction

Dosing adjustment in renal impairment:

Cl_{cr} 10-50 mL/minute: Administer at 75% of normal dose

Cl_{cr} <10 mL/minute: Administer at 50% of normal dose

(Continued)

Morphine Sulfate *(Continued)*

Dosing adjustment/comments in hepatic disease: Unchanged in mild liver disease; substantial extrahepatic metabolism may occur; excessive sedation may occur in cirrhosis

Stability

Capsule, sustained release (Kadian®): Store at controlled room temperature 15°C to 30°C (59°F to 86°F); protect from light and moisture

Suppositories: Store at controlled room temperature 25°C (77°F). Protect from light.

Injection: Store at controlled room temperature. Protect from light. Degradation depends on pH and presence of oxygen; relatively stable in pH ≤4; darkening of solutions indicate degradation. Usual concentration for continuous I.V. infusion: 0.1-1 mg/mL in D_5W.

DepoDur™: Store under refrigeration, 2°C to 8°C (36°F to 46°F); do not freeze. Check freeze indicator before administration; do not administer if bulb is pink or purple. May store at room temperature for up to 7 days. DepoDur™ may be diluted in preservative-free NS to a volume of 5 mL. Gently invert to suspend particles prior to removal from vial. Once vial is opened, use within 4 hours.

Administration

Oral: Do not crush controlled release drug product, swallow whole. Kadian® and Avinza® can be opened and sprinkled on applesauce; do not crush or chew the beads. Contents of Kadian® capsules may be opened and sprinkled over 10 mL water and flushed through prewetted 16F gastrostomy tube; do not administer Kadian® through nasogastric tube. Administration of oral morphine solution with food may increase bioavailability (not observed with Oramorph SR®).

I.V.: When giving morphine I.V. push, it is best to first dilute in 4-5 mL of sterile water, and then to administer slowly (eg, 15 mg over 3-5 minutes)

Epidural: Use preservative-free solutions

Epidural, extended release liposomal suspension (DepoDur™): May be administered undiluted or diluted up to 5 mL total volume in preservative-free NS. Do not use an in-line filter during administration. Not for I.V. or I.M. administration.

Resedation may occur following epidural administration; this may be delayed ≥48 hours in patients receiving extended-release (DepoDur™) injections.

Administration of an epidural test dose (lidocaine 1.5% and epinephrine 1:200,000) may affect the release of morphine from the liposomal preparation. Delaying the dose for an interval of at least 15 minutes following the test dose minimizes this pharmacokinetic interaction. Except for a test dose, other epidural local anesthetics should not be used before or after this product.

Intrathecal: Use preservative-free solutions

Monitoring Parameters Pain relief, respiratory and mental status, blood pressure

Infumorph®: Patients should be observed in a fully-equipped and staffed environment for at least 24 hours following initiation, and as appropriate for the first several days after catheter implantation.

DepoDur™: Patient should be monitored for at least 48 hours following administration.

Reference Range Therapeutic: Surgical anesthesia: 65-80 ng/mL (SI: 227-280 nmol/L); Toxic: 200-5000 ng/mL (SI: 700-17,500 nmol/L)

Anesthesia and Critical Care Concerns/Other Considerations When developing a therapeutic plan for pain control, scheduled, intermittent opioid dosing or continuous infusion is preferred over the "as needed" regimen. The 2002 ACCM/SCCM guidelines for analgesia (critically-ill adult) recommend fentanyl in patients who need immediate pain relief because of its rapid onset of action; fentanyl or hydromorphone is preferred in patients who are hypotensive or have renal dysfunction. Morphine or hydromorphone is recommended for intermittent, scheduled therapy. Both have a longer duration of action requiring less frequent administration. If the patient has required high-dose analgesia or has used for a prolonged period (~7 days), taper dose to prevent withdrawal; monitor for signs and symptoms of withdrawal. Use only preservative-free injections for epidural or intrathecal administration; less adverse effects are associated with epidural compared to intrathecal route of administration.

Pregnancy Risk Factor C/D (prolonged use or high doses at term)

Contraindications Hypersensitivity to morphine sulfate or any component of the formulation; increased intracranial pressure; severe respiratory depression; acute or severe asthma; known or suspected paralytic ileus; sustained release products are not recommended with gastrointestinal obstruction or in acute/postoperative pain; pregnancy (prolonged use or high doses at term)

Warnings/Precautions An opioid-containing analgesic regimen should be tailored to each patient's needs and based upon the type of pain being treated (acute versus chronic), the route of administration, degree of tolerance for opioids (naive versus chronic user), age, weight, and medical condition. The optimal analgesic dose varies widely among patients. Doses should be titrated to pain relief/prevention. When used as an epidural injection, monitor for delayed sedation.

May cause respiratory depression; use with caution in patients (particularly elderly or debilitated) with impaired respiratory function or severe hepatic dysfunction and in patients with hypersensitivity reactions to other phenanthrene derivative opioid agonists (codeine, hydrocodone, hydromorphone, levorphanol, oxycodone, oxymorphone). Some preparations contain sulfites which may cause allergic reactions; infants <3 months of age are more susceptible to respiratory depression, use with caution and generally in reduced doses in this age group. Morphine shares the toxic potential of opiate agonists and usual precautions of opiate agonist therapy should be observed; may cause hypotension in patients with acute myocardial infarction, volume depletion, or concurrent drug therapy which may exaggerate vasodilation. Tolerance or drug dependence may result from extended use. Elderly may be particularly susceptible to the CNS depressant and constipating effects of narcotics.

Extended or sustained-release formulations:

[U.S. Boxed Warning]: Extended or sustained release dosage forms should not be crushed or chewed. Controlled-, extended-, or sustained-release products are not intended for "as needed (PRN)" use. MS Contin® 100 mg or 200 mg tablets are for use only in opioid-tolerant patients requiring >400 mg/day.

[U.S. Boxed Warning]: Avinza®: Do not administer with alcoholic beverages or ethanol-containing products, which may disrupt extended-release characteristic of product.

Injections: Note: Products are designed for administration by specific routes (I.V., intrathecal, epidural). Use caution when prescribing, dispensing, or administering to use formulations only by intended route(s).

[U.S. Boxed Warning]: Duramorph®: Due to the risk of severe and/or sustained cardiopulmonary depressant effects of Duramorph® must be administered in a fully equipped and staffed environment. Naloxone injection should be immediately available. Patient should remain in this environment for at least 24 hours following the initial dose.

Infumorph® solutions are **for use in microinfusion devices only**; not for I.V., I.M., or SubQ administration.

Depo-Dur™: Freezing may adversely affect modified-release mechanism of drug; check freeze indicator within carton prior to administration.

Adverse Reactions Note: Individual patient differences are unpredictable, and percentage may differ in acute pain (surgical) treatment.

Frequency not defined: Flushing, CNS depression, sedation, antidiuretic hormone release, physical and psychological dependence, diaphoresis

>10%:

Cardiovascular: Palpitations, hypotension, bradycardia

Central nervous system: Drowsiness (48%, tolerance usually develops to drowsiness with regular dosing for 1-2 weeks); dizziness (20%), confusion, headache (following epidural or intrathecal use)

Dermatologic: Pruritus (may be secondary to histamine release)

Note: Pruritus may be dose-related, but not confined to the site of administration.

Gastrointestinal: Nausea (28%, tolerance usually develops to nausea and vomiting with chronic use); constipation (40%, tolerance develops very slowly if at all); xerostomia (78%)

Genitourinary: Urinary retention (16%; may be prolonged, up to 20 hours, following epidural or intrathecal use)

Local: Pain at injection site

Neuromuscular & skeletal: Weakness

Miscellaneous: Histamine release

(Continued)

Morphine Sulfate *(Continued)*

1% to 10%:

Cardiovascular: Atrial fibrillation (<3%), chest pain (<3%), edema (<3%), syncope (<3%), tachycardia (<3%)

Central nervous system: Amnesia, anxiety, apathy, ataxia, chills, depression, euphoria, false feeling of well being, fever, headache, hypoesthesia, insomnia, lethargy, malaise, restlessness, seizure, vertigo

Endocrine & metabolic: Hyponatremia (<3%), gynecomastia (<3%)

Gastrointestinal: Anorexia, biliary colic, dyspepsia, dysphagia, GERD, GI irritation, paralytic ileus, vomiting (9%)

Genitourinary: Decreased urination

Hematologic: Anemia (<3%), leukopenia (<3%), thrombocytopenia (<3%)

Neuromuscular & skeletal: Arthralgia, back pain, bone pain, paresthesia, trembling

Ocular: Vision problems

Respiratory: Asthma, atelectasis, dyspnea, hiccups, hypoxia, noncardiogenic pulmonary edema, respiratory depression, rhinitis

Miscellaneous: Diaphoresis, flu-like syndrome, withdrawal syndrome

<1% (Limited to important or life-threatening): Amenorrhea, anaphylaxis, biliary tract spasm, hallucinations, intestinal obstruction, intracranial pressure increased, liver function tests increased, menstrual irregularities, mental depression, miosis, muscle rigidity, myoclonus, oliguria, paradoxical CNS stimulation, peripheral vasodilation, urinary tract spasm, transaminases increased

Overdosage/Toxicology Symptoms of overdose include respiratory depression, miosis, hypotension, bradycardia, apnea, and pulmonary edema. Treatment is symptomatic. Naloxone, 2 mg I.V. with repeat administration as necessary up to a total dose of 10 mg, can be used to reverse opiate effects.

Drug Interactions Substrate of CYP2D6 (minor)

Antipsychotic agents: May increase hypotensive effects of morphine; monitor.

CNS depressants: May increase the effects/toxicity of morphine; monitor.

MAO inhibitors: May increase the effects/toxicity of morphine; some manufacturers recommend avoiding use within 14 days of MAO inhibitors

Pegvisomant: Therapeutic efficacy may be decreased by concomitant opiates, possibly requiring dosage adjustment of pegvisomant.

Rifamycin derivatives: May decrease levels/effects of morphine; monitor.

Selective serotonin reuptake inhibitors (SSRIs) and meperidine: Serotonergic effects may be additive, leading to serotonin syndrome.

Ethanol/Nutrition/Herb Interactions

Ethanol: Avoid ethanol (may increase CNS depression).

Avinza®: Alcoholic beverages or ethanol-containing products may disrupt extended-release formulation resulting in rapid release of entire morphine dose.

Food: Administration of oral morphine solution with food may increase bioavailability (ie, a report of 34% increase in morphine AUC when morphine oral solution followed a high-fat meal). The bioavailability of Oramorph SR® or Kadian® does not appear to be affected by food.

Herb/Nutraceutical: Avoid valerian, St John's wort, kava kava, gotu kola (may increase CNS depression).

Test Interactions

Some quinolones may produce a false-positive urine screening result for opiates using commercially-available immunoassay kits. This has been demonstrated most consistently for levofloxacin and ofloxacin, but other quinolones have shown cross-reactivity in certain assay kits. Confirmation of positive opiate screens by more specific methods should be considered.

Dietary Considerations Morphine may cause GI upset; take with food if GI upset occurs. Be consistent when taking morphine with or without meals.

Dosage Forms [DSC] = Discontinued product

Capsule, extended release (Avinza®): 30 mg, 60 mg, 90 mg, 120 mg

Capsule, sustained release (Kadian®): 20 mg, 30 mg, 50 mg, 60 mg, 100 mg

Infusion [premixed in D_5W]: 1 mg/mL (100 mL, 250 mL)

Injection, extended release liposomal suspension [lumbar epidural injection, preservative free] (DepoDur™): 10 mg/mL (1 mL, 1.5 mL, 2 mL)

Injection, solution: 2 mg/mL (1 mL); 4 mg/mL (1 mL); 5 mg/mL (1 mL); 8 mg/mL (1 mL); 10 mg/mL (1 mL, 10 mL); 15 mg/mL (1 mL, 20 mL); 25 mg/mL (4 mL, 10 mL, 20 mL, 40 mL, 50 mL, 100 mL, 250 mL); 50 mg/mL (20 mL, 40 mL) [some preparations contain sodium metabisulfite]

Injection, solution [epidural, intrathecal, or I.V. infusion; preservative free]:
  Astramorph/PF™: 0.5 mg/mL (2 mL, 10 mL); 1 mg/mL (2 mL, 10 mL)
  Duramorph®: 0.5 mg/mL (10 mL); 1 mg/mL (10 mL)
Injection, solution [epidural or intrathecal infusion via microinfusion device; preservative free] (Infumorph®): 10 mg/mL (20 mL); 25 mg/mL (20 mL)
Injection, solution [I.V. infusion via PCA pump]: 0.5 mg/mL (30 mL); 1 mg/mL (30 mL, 50 mL); 2 mg/mL (30 mL); 5 mg/mL (30 mL, 50 mL)
Injection, solution [preservative free]: 0.5 mg/mL (10 mL); 1 mg/mL (10 mL); 25 mg/mL (4 mL, 10 mL, 20 mL)
Solution, oral: 10 mg/5 mL (5 mL, 10 mL, 100 mL, 500 mL); 20 mg/5 mL (100 mL, 500 mL); 20 mg/mL (30 mL, 120 mL, 240 mL)
  Roxanol™: 20 mg/mL (30 mL, 120 mL)
  Roxanol 100™: 100 mg/5 mL (240 mL) [with calibrated spoon]
  Roxanol™-T: 20 mg/mL (30 mL, 120 mL) [tinted, flavored] [DSC]
Suppository, rectal (RMS®): 5 mg (12s), 10 mg (12s), 20 mg (12s), 30 mg (12s)
Tablet: 15 mg, 30 mg
Tablet, controlled release (MS Contin®): 15 mg, 30 mg, 60 mg, 100 mg, 200 mg
Tablet, extended release: 15 mg, 30 mg, 60 mg, 100 mg, 200 mg
Tablet, sustained release (Oramorph SR®): 15 mg, 30 mg, 60 mg, 100 mg

References

Braunwald E, Antman EM, Beasley JW, et al, "ACC/AHA Guidelines for the Management of Patients With Unstable Angina and Non-ST-Segment Elevation Myocardial Infarction. A Report of the American College of Cardiology/American Heart Association Task Force on Practice Guidelines (Committee on the Management of Patients With Unstable Angina)," *J Am Coll Cardiol*, 2000, 36(3):970-1062.

Golianu B, Krane EJ, Galloway KS, et al, "Pediatric Acute Pain Management," *Pediatr Clin North Am*, 2000, 47(3):559-87.

Jacobi J, Fraser GL, Coursin DB, et al, "Clinical Practice Guidelines for the Sustained Use of Sedatives and Analgesics in the Critically Ill Adult," *Crit Care Med*, 2002, 30(1):119-41. Available at: http://www.sccm.org/pdf/sedatives.pdf.

Mokhlesi B, Leikin JB, Murray P, et al, "Adult Toxicology in Critical Care. Part 11: Specific Poisonings," *Chest*, 2003, 123(3):897-922.

"Principles of Analgesic Use in the Treatment of Acute Pain and Chronic Cancer Pain," 5th ed, Glenview, IL: American Pain Society, 2003.

- **M.O.S.® 10 (Can)** *see* Morphine Sulfate *on page 867*
- **M.O.S.® 20 (Can)** *see* Morphine Sulfate *on page 867*
- **M.O.S.® 30 (Can)** *see* Morphine Sulfate *on page 867*
- **M.O.S.-SR® (Can)** *see* Morphine Sulfate *on page 867*
- **M.O.S.-Sulfate® (Can)** *see* Morphine Sulfate *on page 867*
- **Motrin®** *see* Ibuprofen *on page 651*
- **Motrin® Children's [OTC]** *see* Ibuprofen *on page 651*
- **Motrin® IB [OTC]** *see* Ibuprofen *on page 651*
- **Motrin® Infants' [OTC]** *see* Ibuprofen *on page 651*
- **Motrin® Junior Strength [OTC]** *see* Ibuprofen *on page 651*

Moxifloxacin (moxs i FLOKS a sin)

Medication Safety Issues
Sound-alike/look-alike issues:
  Avelox® may be confused with Avonex®

U.S. Brand Names Avelox®; Avelox® I.V.; Vigamox™

Canadian Brand Names Avelox®; Avelox® I.V.; Vigamox™

Synonyms Moxifloxacin Hydrochloride

Pharmacologic Category Antibiotic, Ophthalmic; Antibiotic, Quinolone

Generic Available No

Use Treatment of mild-to-moderate community-acquired pneumonia, including multidrug-resistant *Streptococcus pneumoniae* (MDRSP); acute bacterial exacerbation of chronic bronchitis; acute bacterial sinusitis; complicated and uncomplicated skin and skin structure infections; complicated intra-abdominal infections; bacterial conjunctivitis (ophthalmic formulation)

Unlabeled/Investigational Use *Legionella*

Mechanism of Action Moxifloxacin is a DNA gyrase inhibitor, and also inhibits topoisomerase IV. DNA gyrase (topoisomerase II) is an essential bacterial enzyme that maintains the superhelical structure of DNA. DNA gyrase is required for DNA replication and transcription, DNA repair, recombination, and transposition; inhibition is bactericidal.

(Continued)

Moxifloxacin *(Continued)*

Pharmacodynamics/Kinetics

Absorption: Well absorbed; not affected by high fat meal or yogurt

Distribution: V_d: 1.7 to 2.7 L/kg; tissue concentrations often exceed plasma concentrations in respiratory tissues, alveolar macrophages, abdominal tissues/fluids, and sinus tissues

Protein binding: 30% to 50%

Metabolism: Hepatic (52% of dose) via glucuronide (14%) and sulfate (38%) conjugation

Bioavailability: 90%

Half-life elimination: Oral: 12 hours; I.V.: 15 hours

Excretion: Approximately 45% of a dose is excreted in feces (25%) and urine (20%) as unchanged drug

Metabolites: Sulfate conjugates in feces, glucuronide conjugates in urine

Dosage

Usual dosage range:

Children ≥1 year and Adults: Ophthalmic: Instill 1 drop into affected eye(s) 3 times/day for 7 days

Adults: Oral, I.V.: 400 mg every 24 hours

Indication-specific dosing:

Children ≥1 year and Adults: Ophthalmic:

Bacterial conjunctivitis: Instill 1 drop into affected eye(s) 3 times/day for 7 days

Adults: Oral, I.V.:

Acute bacterial sinusitis: 400 mg every 24 hours for 10 days

Chronic bronchitis, acute bacterial exacerbation: 400 mg every 24 hours for 5 days

Intra-abdominal infections (complicated): 400 mg every 24 hours for 5-14 days (initiate with I.V.)

Legionella **(unlabeled use):** 400 mg every 24 hours for 10-21 days

Pneumonia, community-acquired (including MDRSP): 400 mg every 24 hours for 7-14 days

Skin and skin structure infections:

Complicated: 400 mg every 24 hours for 7-21 days

Uncomplicated: 400 mg every 24 hours for 7 days

Elderly: No dosage adjustments are required based on age

Dosage adjustment in renal impairment: No dosage adjustment is required, including patients on hemodialysis or CAPD

Dosage adjustment in hepatic impairment: No dosage adjustment is required in mild to moderate hepatic insufficiency (Child-Pugh Class A and B). Not recommended in patients with severe hepatic insufficiency.

Stability Store at 15°C to 30°C (59°F to 86°F). Do not refrigerate infusion solution.

Administration I.V.: Infuse over 60 minutes; do not infuse by rapid or bolus intravenous infusion

Monitoring Parameters WBC, signs of infection

Anesthesia and Critical Care Concerns/Other Considerations Moxifloxacin causes a dose-dependent QT prolongation. Coadministration of moxifloxacin with other drugs that also prolong the QT interval or induce bradycardia (eg, beta-blockers, amiodarone) should be avoided. Careful consideration should be given in the use of moxifloxacin in patients with cardiovascular disease, in those with conduction abnormalities.

Pregnancy Risk Factor C

Contraindications Hypersensitivity to moxifloxacin, other quinolone antibiotics, or any component of the formulation

Warnings/Precautions Use with caution in patients with significant bradycardia or acute myocardial ischemia. Moxifloxacin causes a concentration-dependent QT prolongation. Do not exceed recommended dose or infusion rate. Avoid use with uncorrected hypokalemia, with other drugs that prolong the QT interval or induce bradycardia, or with class IA or III antiarrhythmic agents. Use with caution in individuals at risk of seizures (CNS disorders or concurrent therapy with medications which may lower seizure threshold). Potential for seizures, although very rare, may be increased with concomitant NSAID therapy. Discontinue in patients who experience significant CNS adverse effects (dizziness, hallucinations, suicidal ideation or actions). Not recommended in patients with moderate to severe hepatic insufficiency. Use with caution in diabetes; glucose regulation may be altered. Tendon inflammation and/or rupture have been reported with quinolone antibiotics. Risk may be increased with concurrent corticosteroids, particularly in the elderly. Discontinue at first signs or symptoms of tendon pain.

Severe hypersensitivity reactions, including anaphylaxis, have occurred with quinolone therapy. If an allergic reaction occurs (itching, urticaria, dyspnea or facial edema, loss of consciousness, tingling, cardiovascular collapse) discontinue drug immediately. May cause photosensitivity. Prolonged use may result in superinfection; pseudomembranous colitis may occur and should be considered in all patients who present with diarrhea. Quinolones may exacerbate myasthenia gravis, use with caution (rare, potentially life-threatening weakness of respiratory muscles may occur). Peripheral neuropathy may rarely occur. Safety and efficacy of systemically administered moxifloxacin (oral, intravenous) in patients <18 years of age have not been established.

Ophthalmic: Eye drops should not be injected subconjunctivally or introduced directly into the anterior chamber of the eye. Contact lenses should not be worn during therapy.

Adverse Reactions

Systemic:

3% to 10%: Gastrointestinal: Nausea (6%), diarrhea (5%)

0.1% to 3%:

- Central nervous system: Anxiety, chills, dizziness (2%), headache, insomnia, malaise, nervousness, pain, somnolence, tremor, vertigo
- Dermatologic: Dry skin, pruritus, rash (maculopapular, purpuric, pustular)
- Endocrine & metabolic: Serum chloride increased (≥2%), serum ionized calcium increased (≥2%), serum glucose decreased (≥2%)
- Gastrointestinal: Abdominal pain, amylase increased, amylase decreased (≥2%), anorexia, constipation, dry mouth, dyspepsia, flatulence, glossitis, lactic dehydrogenase increased, stomatitis, taste perversion, vomiting
- Genitourinary: Vaginal moniliasis, vaginitis
- Hematologic: Eosinophilia, leukopenia, prothrombin time prolonged, increased INR, thrombocythemia
  - Increased serum levels of the following (≥2%): MCH, neutrophils, WBC
  - Decreased serum levels of the following (≥2%): Basophils, eosinophils, hemoglobin, RBC, neutrophils
- Hepatic: Bilirubin decreased or increased (≥2%), GGTP increased, liver function test abnormal
- Local: Injection site reaction
- Neuromuscular & skeletal: Arthralgia, myalgia, weakness
- Renal: Serum albumin increased (≥2%)
- Respiratory: Pharyngitis, pneumonia, rhinitis, sinusitis, pO_2 increased (≥2%)
- Miscellaneous: Allergic reaction, infection, diaphoresis, oral moniliasis

Additional reactions with **ophthalmic** preparation: 1% to 6%: Conjunctivitis, dry eye, ocular discomfort, ocular hyperemia, ocular pain, ocular pruritus, subconjunctival hemorrhage, tearing, visual acuity decreased

Overdosage/Toxicology Potential symptoms of overdose may include CNS excitation, seizures, QT prolongation, and arrhythmias (including torsade de pointes). Patients should be monitored by continuous ECG in the event of an overdose. Management is supportive and symptomatic. Hemodialysis only removes ~9% of dose.

Drug Interactions

Corticosteroids: Concurrent use may increase the risk of tendon rupture, particularly in elderly patients (overall incidence rare).

Glyburide: Quinolones may increase the effect of glyburide; monitor

Metal cations (aluminum, calcium, iron, magnesium, and zinc) bind quinolones in the gastrointestinal tract and inhibit absorption. Concurrent administration of most antacids, oral electrolyte supplements, quinapril, sucralfate, some didanosine formulations (chewable/buffered tablets and pediatric powder for oral suspension), and other higly-buffered oral drugs, should be avoided. Moxifloxacin should be administered 4 hours before or 8 hours after these agents. Calcium products do not appear to significantly affect moxifloxacin absorption.

QT_c-prolonging agents: Effects may be additive with moxifloxacin. Avoid concurrent use with Class Ia and Class III antiarrhythmics, erythromycin, cisapride, antipsychotics, and cyclic antidepressants.

Warfarin: The hypoprothrombinemic effect of warfarin may be enhanced by some quinolone antibiotics; monitor INR.

Ethanol/Nutrition/Herb Interactions Food: Absorption is not affected by administration with a high-fat meal or yogurt.

(Continued)

Moxifloxacin *(Continued)*

Test Interactions Some quinolones may produce a false-positive urine screening result for opiates using commercially-available immunoassay kits. This has been demonstrated most consistently for levofloxacin and ofloxacin, but other quinolones have shown cross-reactivity in certain assay kits. Confirmation of positive opiate screens by more specific methods should be considered.

Dietary Considerations May be taken with or without food. Take 4 hours before or 8 hours after multiple vitamins, antacids, or other products containing magnesium, aluminum, iron, or zinc.

Dosage Forms

Infusion [premixed in sodium chloride 0.8%] (Avelox® I.V.): 400 mg (250 mL)
Solution, ophthalmic (Vigamox™): 0.5% (3 mL)
Tablet:
Avelox®: 400 mg
Avelox® ABC Pack [unit-dose pack]: 400 mg (5s)

- ♦ **Moxifloxacin Hydrochloride** *see* Moxifloxacin *on page 873*
- ♦ **4-MP** *see* Fomepizole *on page 555*
- ♦ **MPA** *see* Mycophenolate *on page 877*
- ♦ **MS Contin®** *see* Morphine Sulfate *on page 867*
- ♦ **MS-IR® (Can)** *see* Morphine Sulfate *on page 867*
- ♦ **MSO_4 (error-prone abbreviation and should not be used)** *see* Morphine Sulfate *on page 867*
- ♦ **M.T.E.-4®** *see* Trace Metals *on page 1296*
- ♦ **M.T.E.-5®** *see* Trace Metals *on page 1296*
- ♦ **M.T.E.-6®** *see* Trace Metals *on page 1296*
- ♦ **M.T.E.-7®** *see* Trace Metals *on page 1296*
- ♦ **MTX (error-prone abbreviation)** *see* Methotrexate *on page 821*
- ♦ **Mucomyst® (Can)** *see* Acetylcysteine *on page 35*
- ♦ **Multitrace™-4** *see* Trace Metals *on page 1296*
- ♦ **Multitrace™-4 Neonatal** *see* Trace Metals *on page 1296*
- ♦ **Multitrace™-4 Pediatric** *see* Trace Metals *on page 1296*
- ♦ **Multitrace™-5** *see* Trace Metals *on page 1296*

Mupirocin (myoo PEER oh sin)

Medication Safety Issues

Sound-alike/look-alike issues:
Bactroban® may be confused with bacitracin, baclofen

U.S. Brand Names Bactroban®; Bactroban® Nasal; Centany™

Canadian Brand Names Bactroban®

Synonyms Mupirocin Calcium; Pseudomonic Acid A

Pharmacologic Category Antibiotic, Topical

Generic Available Yes: Topical ointment

Use

Intranasal: Eradication of nasal colonization with MRSA in adult patients and healthcare workers

Topical treatment of impetigo due to *Staphylococcus aureus*, beta-hemolytic *Streptococcus*, and *S. pyogenes*

Unlabeled/Investigational Use Intranasal: Surgical prophylaxis to prevent wound infections

Mechanism of Action Binds to bacterial isoleucyl transfer-RNA synthetase resulting in the inhibition of protein and RNA synthesis

Pharmacodynamics/Kinetics

Absorption: Topical: Penetrates outer layers of skin; systemic absorption minimal through intact skin
Protein binding: 95%
Metabolism: Skin: 3% to monic acid
Half-life elimination: 17-36 minutes
Excretion: Urine

Dosage

Children ≥12 years and Adults: Intranasal: Approximately one-half of the ointment from the single-use tube should be applied into one nostril and the other half into the other nostril twice daily for 5 days

Children ≥3 months and Adults: Topical: Apply small amount to affected area 2-5 times/day for 5-14 days

Stability Do not mix with Aquaphor®, coal tar solution, or salicylic acid

Administration For external use only.

Pregnancy Risk Factor B

Contraindications Hypersensitivity to mupirocin, polyethylene glycol, or any component of the formulation

Warnings/Precautions Potentially toxic amounts of polyethylene glycol contained in the vehicle may be absorbed percutaneously in patients with extensive burns or open wounds; prolonged use may result in over growth of nonsusceptible organisms; for external use only; not for treatment of pressure sores

Adverse Reactions Frequency not defined.

Central nervous system: Dizziness, headache

Dermatologic: Pruritus, rash, erythema, dry skin, cellulitis, dermatitis

Gastrointestinal: Nausea, taste perversion

Local: Burning, stinging, tenderness, edema, pain

Respiratory: Rhinitis, upper respiratory tract infection, pharyngitis, cough

Drug Interactions No data reported

Dosage Forms

Cream, topical, as calcium (Bactroban®): 2% (15 g, 30 g) [contains benzyl alcohol]

Ointment, intranasal, topical, as calcium (Bactroban® Nasal): 2% (1 g) [single-use tube]

Ointment, topical: 2% (0.9 g, 22 g)

Bactroban®: 2% (22 g)

Centany™: 2% (15 g, 30 g)

- **Mupirocin Calcium** *see* Mupirocin *on page 876*
- **Muro 128® [OTC]** *see* Sodium Chloride *on page 1183*
- **Muse®** *see* Alprostadil *on page 68*
- **Muse® Pellet (Can)** *see* Alprostadil *on page 68*
- **Mycinaire™ [OTC]** *see* Sodium Chloride *on page 1183*

Mycophenolate (mye koe FEN oh late)

U.S. Brand Names CellCept®; Myfortic®

Canadian Brand Names CellCept®; Myfortic®

Synonyms MMF; MPA; Mycophenolate Mofetil; Mycophenolate Sodium; Mycophenolic Acid

Pharmacologic Category Immunosuppressant Agent

Generic Available No

Use Prophylaxis of organ rejection concomitantly with cyclosporine and corticosteroids in patients receiving allogenic renal (CellCept®, Myfortic®), cardiac (CellCept®), or hepatic (CellCept®) transplants

Unlabeled/Investigational Use Treatment of rejection in liver transplant patients unable to tolerate tacrolimus or cyclosporine due to neurotoxicity; mild rejection in heart transplant patients; treatment of moderate-severe psoriasis; treatment of proliferative lupus nephritis; treatment of myasthenia gravis

Mechanism of Action MPA exhibits a cytostatic effect on T and B lymphocytes. It is an inhibitor of inosine monophosphate dehydrogenase (IMPDH) which inhibits *de novo* guanosine nucleotide synthesis. T and B lymphocytes are dependent on this pathway for proliferation.

Pharmacodynamics/Kinetics

Onset of action: Peak effect: Correlation of toxicity or efficacy is still being developed, however, one study indicated that 12-hour AUCs >40 mcg/mL/hour were correlated with efficacy and decreased episodes of rejection

T_{max}: Oral: MPA:

CellCept®: 1-1.5 hours

Myfortic®: 1.5-2.5 hours

Absorption: AUC values for MPA are lower in the early post-transplant period versus later (>3 months) post-transplant period. The extent of absorption in pediatrics is similar to that seen in adults, although there was wide variability reported.

Oral: Myfortic®: 93%

Distribution:

CellCept®: MPA: Oral: 4 L/kg; I.V.: 3.6 L/kg

(Continued)

Mycophenolate *(Continued)*

Myfortic®: MPA: Oral: 54 L (at steady state); 112 L (elimination phase)
Protein binding: MPA: 97%, MPAG 82%
Metabolism: Hepatic and via GI tract; CellCept® is completely hydrolyzed in the liver to mycophenolic acid (MPA; active metabolite); enterohepatic recirculation of MPA may occur; MPA is glucuronidated to MPAG (inactive metabolite)
Bioavailability: Oral: CellCept®: 94%; Myfortic®: 72%
Half-life elimination:
CellCept®: MPA: Oral: 18 hours; I.V.: 17 hours
Myfortic®: MPA: Oral: 8-16 hours; MPAG: 13-17 hours
Excretion:
CellCept®: MPA: Urine (<1%), feces (6%); MPAG: Urine (87%)
Myfortic®: MPA: Urine (3%), feces; MPAG: Urine (>60%)

Dosage

Children: Renal transplant: Oral:
CellCept® suspension: 600 mg/m²/dose twice daily; maximum dose: 1 g twice daily
Alternatively, may use solid dosage forms according to BSA as follows:
BSA 1.25-1.5 m²: 750 mg capsule twice daily
BSA >1.5 m²: 1 g capsule or tablet twice daily
Myfortic®: 400 mg/m²/dose twice daily; maximum dose: 720 mg twice daily
BSA <1.19 m²: Use of this formulation is not recommended
BSA 1.19-1.58 m²: 540 mg twice daily (maximum: 1080 mg/day)
BSA >1.58 m²: 720 mg twice daily (maximum: 1440 mg/day)
Adults:
Renal transplant:
CellCept®:
Oral: 1 g twice daily. Doses >2 g/day are not recommended.
I.V.: 1 g twice daily
Myfortic®: Oral: 720 mg twice daily (1440 mg/day)
Cardiac transplantation:
Oral (CellCept®): 1.5 g twice daily
I.V. (CellCept®): 1.5 g twice daily
Hepatic transplantation:
Oral (CellCept®): 1.5 g twice daily
I.V. (CellCept®): 1 g twice daily
Myasthenia gravis (unlabeled use): Oral (CellCept®): 1 g twice daily (range 1-3 g/day)

Dosing adjustment in renal impairment:
Renal transplant: GFR <25 mL/minute in patients outside the immediate post-transplant period:
CellCept®: Doses of >1 g administered twice daily should be avoided; patients should also be carefully observed; no dose adjustments are needed in renal transplant patients experiencing delayed graft function postoperatively
Myfortic®: Cl_{cr} <25 mL/minute: Monitor carefully
Cardiac or liver transplant: No data available; mycophenolate may be used in cardiac or hepatic transplant patients with severe chronic renal impairment if the potential benefit outweighs the potential risk
Hemodialysis: Not removed; supplemental dose is not necessary
Peritoneal dialysis: Supplemental dose is not necessary
Dosage adjustment in hepatic impairment: No dosage adjustment is recommended for renal patients with severe hepatic parenchymal disease; however, it is not currently known whether dosage adjustments are necessary for hepatic disease with other etiologies
Elderly: Dosage is the same as younger patients, however, dosing should be cautious due to possibility of increased hepatic, renal or cardiac dysfunction; elderly patients may be at an increased risk of certain infections, gastrointestinal hemorrhage, and pulmonary edema, as compared to younger patients
Dosing adjustment for toxicity (neutropenia): ANC <1.3 x 10^3/µL: Dosing should be interrupted or the dose reduced, appropriate diagnostic tests performed and patients managed appropriately

Stability

Capsules: Store at room temperature of 15°C to 39°C (59°F to 86°F).
Tablets: Store at room temperature of 15°C to 39°C (59°F to 86°F); protect from light.

Oral suspension: Should be constituted prior to dispensing to the patient and **not** mixed with any other medication. Add 47 mL of water to the bottle and shake well for ~1 minute. Add another 47 mL of water to the bottle and shake well for an additional minute. Final concentration is 200 mg/mL of mycophenolate mofetil.

I.V.: Reconstitute the contents of each vial with 14 mL of 5% dextrose injection; dilute the contents of a vial with 5% dextrose in water to a final concentration of 6 mg mycophenolate mofetil per mL. **Note:** Vial is vacuum-sealed; if a lack of vacuum is noted during preparation, the vial should not be used.

Administration

Oral dosage formulations (tablet, capsule, suspension) should be administered on an empty stomach to avoid variability in MPA absorption. The oral solution may be administered via a nasogastric tube (minimum 8 French, 1.7 mm interior diameter); oral suspension should not be mixed with other medications. Delayed release tablets should not be crushed, cut, or chewed.

Intravenous solutions should be administered over at least 2 hours (either peripheral or central vein); do **not** administer intravenous solution by rapid or bolus injection.

Monitoring Parameters Complete blood count; signs and symptoms of infection

Anesthesia and Critical Care Concerns/Other Considerations Avoid inhalation or direct contact with skin or mucous membranes of the powder in CellCept® capsules. If such contact occurs, wash with soap and water; rinse eyes with plain water. Capsules should not be opened or crushed.

Hypertension may accompany the use of mycophenolate in patients post-transplantation. Furthermore, this drug may also induce increases in cholesterol and potassium, and impair glucose tolerance and phosphate and potassium depletion.

Pregnancy Risk Factor C (manufacturer)

Contraindications Hypersensitivity to mycophenolate mofetil, mycophenolic acid, mycophenolate sodium, or any component of the formulation; intravenous formulation is contraindicated in patients who are allergic to polysorbate 80

Warnings/Precautions Hazardous agent — use appropriate precautions for handling and disposal. Risk for infection and development of lymphoproliferative disorders (particularly of the skin) is increased. Patients should be monitored appropriately, instructed to limit exposure to sunlight/UV light, and given supportive treatment should these conditions occur. Severe neutropenia may occur, requiring interruption of treatment (risk greater from day 31-180 post-transplant). Use caution with active peptic ulcer disease; may be associated with GI bleeding and/or perforation. Use caution in renal impairment as toxicity may be increased; may require dosage adjustment in severe impairment. Patients may be at increased risk of infection.

Because mycophenolate mofetil has demonstrated teratogenic effects in rats and rabbits, tablets should not be crushed, and capsules should not be opened or crushed. Avoid inhalation or direct contact with skin or mucous membranes of the powder contained in the capsules and the powder for oral suspension. Caution should be exercised in the handling and preparation of solutions of intravenous mycophenolate. Avoid skin contact with the intravenous solution and reconstituted suspension. If such contact occurs, wash thoroughly with soap and water, rinse eyes with plain water.

Theoretically, use should be avoided in patients with the rare hereditary deficiency of hypoxanthine-guanine phosphoribosyltransferase (such as Lesch-Nyhan or Kelley-Seegmiller syndrome). Intravenous solutions should be given over at least 2 hours; **never** administer intravenous solution by rapid or bolus injection.

Note: CellCept® and Myfortic® dosage forms should not be used interchangeably due to differences in absorption.

Adverse Reactions As reported in adults following oral dosing of CellCept® alone in renal, cardiac, and hepatic allograft rejection studies. In general, lower doses used in renal rejection patients had less adverse effects than higher doses. Rates of adverse effects were similar for each indication, except for those unique to the specific organ involved. The type of adverse effects observed in pediatric patients was similar to those seen in adults; abdominal pain, anemia, diarrhea, fever, hypertension, infection, pharyngitis, respiratory tract infection, sepsis, and vomiting were seen in higher proportion; lymphoproliferative disorder was the only

(Continued)

Mycophenolate *(Continued)*

type of malignancy observed. Percentages of adverse reactions were similar in studies comparing CellCept® to Myfortic® in patients following renal transplant.

>20%:

Cardiovascular: Hypertension (28% to 77%), hypotension (up to 33%), peripheral edema (27% to 64%), edema (27% to 28%), tachycardia (20% to 22%)

Central nervous system: Pain (31% to 76%), headache (16% to 54%), insomnia (41% to 52%), fever (21% to 52%), dizziness (up to 29%), anxiety (28%)

Dermatologic: Rash (up to 22%)

Endocrine & metabolic: Hyperglycemia (44% to 47%), hypercholesterolemia (41%), hypokalemia (32% to 37%), hypocalcemia (up to 30%), hypomagnesemia (up to 39%), hyperkalemia (up to 22%)

Gastrointestinal: Abdominal pain (25% to 62%), nausea (20% to 54%), diarrhea (31% to 52%), constipation (18% to 41%), vomiting (33% to 34%), anorexia (up to 25%), dyspepsia (22%)

Genitourinary: Urinary tract infection (37%)

Hematologic: Leukopenia (23% to 46%), leukocytosis (22% to 40%), hypochromic anemia (26% to 43%), thrombocytopenia (24% to 36%)

Hepatic: Liver function tests abnormal (up to 25%), ascites (24%)

Neuromuscular & skeletal: Back pain (35% to 47%), weakness (35% to 43%), tremor (24% to 34%), paresthesia (21%)

Renal: BUN increased (up to 35%), creatinine increased (up to 39%)

Respiratory: Dyspnea (31% to 37%), respiratory tract infection (22% to 37%), cough (31%), lung disorder (22% to 30%)

Miscellaneous: Infection (18% to 27%), *Candida* (11% to 22%), herpes simplex (10% to 21%)

3% to <20%:

Cardiovascular: Angina, arrhythmia, arterial thrombosis, atrial fibrillation, atrial flutter, bradycardia, cardiac arrest, cardiac failure, CHF, extrasystole, facial edema, hypervolemia, pallor, palpitation, pericardial effusion, peripheral vascular disorder, postural hypotension, supraventricular extrasystoles, supraventricular tachycardia, syncope, thrombosis, vasodilation, vasospasm, venous pressure increased, ventricular extrasystole, ventricular tachycardia

Central nervous system: Agitation, chills with fever, confusion, convulsion, delirium, depression, emotional lability, hallucinations, hypoesthesia, malaise, nervousness, psychosis, somnolence, thinking abnormal, vertigo

Dermatologic: Acne, alopecia, bruising, cellulitis, hirsutism, petechia, pruritus, skin carcinoma, skin hypertrophy, skin ulcer, vesiculobullous rash

Endocrine & metabolic: Acidosis, Cushing's syndrome, dehydration, diabetes mellitus, gout, hypercalcemia, hyperlipemia, hyperphosphatemia, hyperuricemia, hypochloremia, hypoglycemia, hyponatremia, hypoproteinemia, hypothyroidism, parathyroid disorder, weight gain/loss

Gastrointestinal: Abdomen enlarged, dry mouth, dysphagia, esophagitis, flatulence, gastritis, gastroenteritis, gastrointestinal hemorrhage, gastrointestinal moniliasis, gingivitis, gum hyperplasia, ileus, melena, mouth ulceration, oral moniliasis, stomach disorder, stomatitis

Genitourinary: Impotence, nocturia, pelvic pain, prostatic disorder, scrotal edema, urinary frequency, urinary incontinence, urinary retention, urinary tract disorder

Hematologic: Coagulation disorder, hemorrhage, neutropenia, pancytopenia, polycythemia, prothrombin time increased, thromboplastin increased

Hepatic: Alkaline phosphatase increased, alkalosis, bilirubinemia, cholangitis, cholestatic jaundice, GGT increased, hepatitis, jaundice, liver damage, transaminases increased

Local: Abscess

Neuromuscular & skeletal: Arthralgia, hypertonia, joint disorder, leg cramps, myalgia, myasthenia, neck pain, neuropathy, osteoporosis

Ocular: Amblyopia, cataract, conjunctivitis, eye hemorrhage, lacrimation disorder, vision abnormal

Otic: Deafness, ear disorder, ear pain, tinnitus

Renal: Albuminuria, creatinine increased, dysuria, hematuria, hydronephrosis, kidney failure, kidney tubular necrosis, oliguria

Respiratory: Apnea, asthma, atelectasis, bronchitis, epistaxis, hemoptysis, hiccup, hyperventilation, hypoxia, respiratory acidosis, lung edema, pharyngitis, pleural effusion, pneumonia, pneumothorax, pulmonary hypertension, respiratory moniliasis, rhinitis, sinusitis, sputum increased, voice alteration

Miscellaneous: *Candida* (mucocutaneous 15% to 18%), CMV viremia/syndrome (12% to 14%), CMV tissue invasive disease (6% to 11%), herpes zoster cutaneous disease (4% to 10%), cyst, diaphoresis, flu-like syndrome, fungal dermatitis, healing abnormal, hernia, ileus infection, lactic dehydrogenase increased, peritonitis, pyelonephritis, thirst

Postmarketing and/or case reports: Atypical mycobacterial infection, colitis, infectious endocarditis, interstitial lung disorder, intestinal villous atrophy, meningitis, pancreatitis, pulmonary fibrosis (fatal), tuberculosis

Overdosage/Toxicology There are no reported overdoses with mycophenolate. At plasma concentrations >100 mcg/mL, small amounts of the inactive metabolite MPAG are removed by hemodialysis. Excretion of the active metabolite, MPA, may be increased by using bile acid sequestrants (cholestyramine).

Drug Interactions

Acyclovir and valacyclovir: Levels of both drugs may increase due to competition for tubular secretion; monitor carefully

Antacids (magnesium- and aluminum hydroxide-containing products): Decrease absorption of mycophenolate; do not administer together

Azathioprine: Bone marrow suppression may be caused by both agents; do not administer together

Cholestyramine: Decreases AUC which may lead to decreased efficacy; do not administer together

Ganciclovir and valganciclovir: Levels of both drugs may increase due to competition for tubular secretion; monitor carefully

Oral contraceptives: Progesterone levels are not significantly affected, however, effect on estrogen component varies; although the ovulation-suppression action may not be affected, an additional form of contraception should be used

Probenecid: May increase mycophenolate levels due to inhibition of tubular secretion

Vaccines: Avoid use of live vaccines; vaccinations may be less effective. Influenza vaccine may be of value.

Ethanol/Nutrition/Herb Interactions

Food: Decreases C_{max} of MPA by 40% following CellCept® administration and 33% following Myfortic® use; the extent of absorption is not changed

Herb/Nutraceutical: Avoid cat's claw, echinacea (have immunostimulant properties)

Dietary Considerations Oral dosage formulations should be taken on an empty stomach to avoid variability in MPA absorption. However, in stable renal transplant patients, may be administered with food if necessary. Oral suspension contains 0.56 mg phenylalanine/mL; use caution if administered to patients with phenylketonuria.

Dosage Forms

Capsule, as mofetil (CellCept®): 250 mg

Injection, powder for reconstitution, as mofetil hydrochloride (CellCept®): 500 mg [contains polysorbate 80]

Powder for oral suspension, as mofetil (CellCept®): 200 mg/mL (225 mL) [provides 175 mL suspension following reconstitution; contains phenylalanine 0.56 mg/mL; mixed fruit flavor]

Tablet, as mofetil (CellCept®): 500 mg [may contain ethyl alcohol]

Tablet, delayed release, as mycophenolic acid (Myfortic®): 180 mg, 360 mg [formulated as a sodium salt]

- **Mycophenolate Mofetil** *see* Mycophenolate *on page 877*
- **Mycophenolate Sodium** *see* Mycophenolate *on page 877*
- **Mycophenolic Acid** *see* Mycophenolate *on page 877*
- **Mycostatin®** *see* Nystatin *on page 945*
- **Mydfrin®** *see* Phenylephrine *on page 1015*
- **Mydral™** *see* Tropicamide *on page 1320*
- **Mydriacyl®** *see* Tropicamide *on page 1320*
- **Myfortic®** *see* Mycophenolate *on page 877*
- **Mykrox® (Can)** *see* Metolazone *on page 837*
- **Mylanta™ (Can)** *see* Aluminum Hydroxide and Magnesium Hydroxide *on page 76*
- **Mylocel™** *see* Hydroxyurea *on page 648*
- **Myobloc®** *see* Botulinum Toxin Type B *on page 188*
- **myrac™** *see* Minocycline *on page 854*
- **Nabi-HB®** *see* Hepatitis B Immune Globulin *on page 618*

Nabilone (NA bi lone)

U.S. Brand Names Cesamet™
Canadian Brand Names Cesamet™
Pharmacologic Category Antiemetic
Restrictions C-II
Generic Available No
Use Treatment of refractory nausea and vomiting associated with cancer chemotherapy
Mechanism of Action Not fully characterized; antiemetic activity may be due to effect on cannabinoid receptors (CB1) within the central nervous system.
Pharmacodynamics/Kinetics
Absorption: Rapid and complete
Distribution: ~12.5 L/kg
Metabolism: To several active metabolites by oxidation and stereospecific enzyme reduction; CYP450 enzymes may also be involved
Half-life elimination: Parent compound: 2 hours; Metabolites: 35 hours
Time to peak, serum: Within 2 hours
Excretion: Feces (~60%); renal (~24%)
Dosage Refer to individual protocols. Oral:
Children >4 years (unlabeled use):
<18 kg: 0.5 mg twice daily
18-30 kg: 1 mg twice daily
>30 kg: 1 mg 3 times/day
Adults: 1-2 mg twice daily (maximum: 6 mg divided in 3 doses daily)
Dosage adjustment in renal impairment: No adjustment required.
Stability Store at room temperature between 15°C and 30°C (59°F and 86°F).
Administration Initial dose should be given 1-3 hours before chemotherapy; may be given 2-3 times a day during the entire chemotherapy course and for up to 48 hours after the last dose of chemotherapy; a dose of 1-2 mg the night before chemotherapy may be useful.
Monitoring Parameters Blood pressure, heart rate; signs and symptoms of excessive use, abuse, or misuse
Pregnancy Risk Factor C
Contraindications Hypersensitivity to nabilone, cannabinoids, tetrahydrocannabinol, or any component of the formulation
Warnings/Precautions May affect CNS function; use with caution in the elderly and those with pre-existing CNS depression. May cause additive CNS effects with sedatives, hypnotics, or other psychoactive agents; patients must be cautioned about performing tasks which require mental alertness (eg, operating machinery or driving). Use caution with current or previous history of mental illness; cannabinoid use may reveal symptoms of psychiatric disorders. Psychiatric adverse reactions may persist for up to 3 days after discontinuing treatment. Has potential for abuse and or dependence, use caution in patients with substance abuse history or potential. May cause tachycardia and orthostatic hypotension; use caution with cardiovascular disease. Safety and efficacy in children have not been established.
Adverse Reactions
>10%:
Central nervous system: Dizziness (59%), drowsiness (52% to 66%), vertigo (52% to 59%), euphoria (11% to 38%), ataxia (13% to 14%), depression (14%), concentration decreased (12%), sleep disturbance (11%)
Gastrointestinal: Xerostomia (22% to 36%)
Ocular: Visual disturbance (13%)
1% to 10%:
Cardiovascular: Hypotension (8%)
Central nervous system: Dysphoria (9%), headache (6% to 7%), sedation (3%), depersonalization (2%), disorientation (2%)
Gastrointestinal: Anorexia (8%), nausea (4%), appetite increased (2%)
Neuromuscular & skeletal: Weakness (8%)
<1% (Limited to important or life-threatening) and frequency not reported: Abdominal pain, akathisia, allergic reaction, amblyopia, anemia, anhydrosis, anxiety, apathy, aphthous ulcer, arrhythmia, cerebral vascular accident, chest pain, constipation, cough, diaphoresis, diarrhea, dyspepsia, dyspnea, dystonia, emotional disorder, emotional lability, epistaxis, equilibrium dysfunction, fatigue,

fever, flushing, hallucinations, hot flashes, hyperactivity, hypertension, infection, insomnia, irritation, leukopenia, lightheadedness, malaise, memory disturbance, mood swings, nervousness, neurosis (phobic), numbness, orthostatic hypotension, pain, palpitation, panic disorder, paranoia, paresthesia, perception disturbance, pharyngitis, photophobia, photosensitivity, polyuria, pruritus, psychosis (toxic), pupil dilation, rash, seizure, speech disorder, stupor, syncope, tachycardia, taste perversion, thought disorder, tinnitus, tremor, urination decreased, urinary retention, wheezing, withdrawal

Overdosage/Toxicology Symptoms of overdose include nausea, vomiting, disorientation, CNS/respiratory depression, dysphoria, and euphoria. Although hypertension and hypotension may occur, orthostatic hypotension and tachycardia are most commonly reported. Large overdoses may present with psychotic episodes, hallucinations, anxiety, respiratory depression, and/or coma. Consider overdose in the presence of disturbing psychiatric symptoms. Monitor vital signs, serum electrolytes, and blood gases. Activated charcoal may be used to decrease gastrointestinal absorption. Treatment is otherwise symptom-directed and supportive.

Drug Interactions

Anticholinergic agents (includes antihistamines, atropine, and scopolamine): Tachycardia and drowsiness may be additive.

CNS depressants (includes barbiturates, narcotic analgesics, and other sedative agents): Sedative effects may be additive with CNS depressants; monitor for increased effect.

Naltrexone: Oral cannabinoid effects may be enhanced via opioid receptor blockade.

Opioids: May have cross-tolerance and potentiation.

Sympathomimetic agents (includes amphetamines and cocaine): Hypertension, tachycardia, and cardiotoxicity may be additive.

Tricyclic antidepressants (includes amitriptyline, amoxapine, and desipramine): Tachycardia, hypertension, and drowsiness may be additive.

Ethanol/Nutrition/Herb Interactions Ethanol: Avoid ethanol (may increase CNS depression).

Dosage Forms

Capsule:

Cesamet™: 1 mg

Nabumetone (na BYOO me tone)

Related Information

Chronic Pain Management *on page 1430*

U.S. Brand Names Relafen®

Canadian Brand Names Apo-Nabumetone®; Gen-Nabumetone; Novo-Nabumetone; Relafen™; Rhoxal-nabumetone; Sandoz-Nabumetone

Pharmacologic Category Nonsteroidal Anti-inflammatory Drug (NSAID), Oral

Restrictions A medication guide should be dispensed with each prescription. A template for the required MedGuide can be found on the FDA website at: http://www.fda.gov/medwatch/SAFETY/2005/safety05.htm#NSAID

Generic Available Yes

Use Management of osteoarthritis and rheumatoid arthritis

Unlabeled/Investigational Use Moderate pain

Mechanism of Action Nabumetone is a nonacidic NSAID that is rapidly metabolized after absorption to a major active metabolite, 6-methoxy-2-naphthylacetic acid. As found with previous NSAIDs, nabumetone's active metabolite inhibits the cyclooxygenase enzyme which is indirectly responsible for the production of inflammation and pain during arthritis by way of enhancing the production of endoperoxides and prostaglandins E_2 and I_2 (prostacyclin). The active metabolite of nabumetone is felt to be the compound primarily responsible for therapeutic effect. Comparatively, the parent drug is a poor inhibitor of prostaglandin synthesis.

Pharmacodynamics/Kinetics

Onset of action: Several days

Distribution: Diffusion occurs readily into synovial fluid

V_d: 6MNA: 29-82 L

Protein binding: 6MNA: >99%

(Continued)

Nabumetone *(Continued)*

Metabolism: Prodrug, rapidly metabolized in the liver to an active metabolite [6-methoxy-2-naphthylacetic acid (6MNA)] and inactive metabolites; extensive first-pass effect

Half-life elimination: 6MNA: ~24 hours

Time to peak, serum: 6MNA: Oral: 2.5-4 hours; Synovial fluid: 4-12 hours

Excretion: 6MNA: Urine (80%) and feces (9%)

Dosage Adults: Oral: 1000 mg/day; an additional 500-1000 mg may be needed in some patients to obtain more symptomatic relief; may be administered once or twice daily (maximum dose: 2000 mg/day)

Note: Patients <50 kg are less likely to require doses >1000 mg/day.

Dosage adjustment in renal impairment: In general, NSAIDs are not recommended for use in patients with advanced renal disease, but the manufacturer of nabumetone does provide some guidelines for adjustment in renal dysfunction:

Moderate impairment (Cl_{cr} 30-49 mL/minute): Initial dose: 750 mg/day; maximum dose: 1500 mg/day

Severe impairment (Cl_{cr} <30 mL/minute): Initial dose: 500 mg/day; maximum dose: 1000 mg/day

Monitoring Parameters Patients with renal insufficiency: Baseline renal function followed by repeat test within weeks (to determine if renal function has deteriorated)

Anesthesia and Critical Care Concerns/Other Considerations The 2002 ACCM/SCCM guidelines for analgesia (critically-ill adult) suggest that NSAIDs may be used in combination with opioids in select patients for pain management. Concern about adverse events (increased risk of renal dysfunction, altered platelet function and gastrointestinal irritation) limits its use in patients who have other underlying risks for these events.

In short-term use, NSAIDs vary considerably in their effect on blood pressure. When NSAIDs are used in patients with hypertension, appropriate monitoring of blood pressure responses should be completed and the duration of therapy, when possible, kept short. The use of NSAIDs in the treatment of patients with congestive heart failure may be associated with an increased risk for fluid accumulation and edema; may precipitate renal failure in dehydrated patients.

Pregnancy Risk Factor C/D (3rd trimester)

Contraindications Hypersensitivity to nabumetone, aspirin, other NSAIDs, or any component of the formulation; perioperative pain in the setting of coronary artery bypass surgery (CABG); pregnancy (3rd trimester)

Warnings/Precautions [U.S. Boxed Warning]: NSAIDs are associated with an increased risk of adverse cardiovascular events, including MI, stroke, and new onset or worsening of pre-existing hypertension. Risk may be increased with duration of use or pre-existing cardiovascular risk-factors or disease. Carefully evaluate individual cardiovascular risk profiles prior to prescribing. Use caution with fluid retention, CHF or hypertension.

Use of NSAIDs can compromise existing renal function. Renal toxicity can occur in patient with impaired renal function, dehydration, heart failure, liver dysfunction, those taking diuretics and ACEI and the elderly. Rehydrate patient before starting therapy. Monitor renal function closely. Not recommended for use in patients with advanced renal disease.

[U.S. Boxed Warning]: NSAIDs may increase risk of gastrointestinal irritation, ulceration, bleeding, and perforation. These events may occur at any time during therapy and without warning. Use caution with a history of GI disease (bleeding or ulcers), concurrent therapy with aspirin, anticoagulants and/or corticosteroids, smoking, use of alcohol, the elderly or debilitated patients.

Use the lowest effective dose for the shortest duration of time, consistent with individual patient goals, to reduce risk of cardiovascular or GI adverse events. Alternate therapies should be considered for patients at high risk.

NSAIDs may cause serious skin adverse events including exfoliative dermatitis, Stevens-Johnson syndrome (SJS) and toxic epidermal necrolysis (TEN). Anaphylactoid reactions may occur, even without prior exposure; patients with "aspirin triad" (bronchial asthma, aspirin intolerance, rhinitis) may be at increased risk. Do not use in patients who experience bronchospasm, asthma, rhinitis, or urticaria with NSAID or aspirin therapy.

Use with caution in patients with decreased hepatic function. Closely monitor patients with any abnormal LFT. Severe hepatic reactions (eg, fulminant hepatitis, liver failure) have occurred with NSAID use, rarely; discontinue if signs or symptoms of liver disease develop, or if systemic manifestations occur.

The elderly are at increased risk for adverse effects (especially peptic ulceration, CNS effects, renal toxicity) from NSAIDs even at low doses

Withhold for at least 4-6 half-lives prior to surgical or dental procedures. May cause photosensitivity reactions. Safety and efficacy have not been established in pediatric patients.

Adverse Reactions

>10%: Gastrointestinal: Abdominal pain (12%), diarrhea (14%), dyspepsia (13%)

1% to 10%:

Cardiovascular: Edema (3% to 9%)

Central nervous system: Dizziness (3% to 9%), headache (3% to 9%), fatigue (1% to 3%), insomnia (1% to 3%), nervousness (1% to 3%), somnolence (1% to 3%)

Dermatologic: Pruritus (3% to 9%), rash (3% to 9%)

Gastrointestinal: Constipation (3% to 9%), flatulence (3% to 9%), guaic positive (3% to 9%), nausea (3% to 9%), gastritis (1% to 3%), stomatitis (1% to 3%), vomiting (1% to 3%), xerostomia (1% to 3%)

Otic: Tinnitus

Miscellaneous: Diaphoresis (1% to 3%)

<1% (Limited to important or life-threatening): Abnormal vision, acne, agitation, albuminuria, alopecia, anaphylactoid reaction, anaphylaxis, anemia, angina, angioneurotic edema, anorexia, anxiety, arrhythmia, asthma, azotemia, bilirubinemia duodenitis, bullous eruptions, CHF, chills, confusion, cough, depression, duodenal ulcer, dysphagia, dyspnea, dysuria, eosinophilic pneumonia, eructation, erythema multiforme, fever, gallstones, gastric ulcer, gastroenteritis, gingivitis, GI bleeding, glossitis, granulocytopenia, hematuria, hepatic failure, hyperglycemia, hypersensitivity pneumonitis, hypertension, hyperuricemia, hypokalemia, impotence, interstitial nephritis, interstitial pneumonitis, jaundice, leukopenia, liver function abnormalities, malaise, melena, MI, nephrotic syndrome, nightmares, palpitations, pancreatitis, paresthesia, photosensitivity, pseudoporphyria cutanea tarda, rectal bleeding, renal failure, renal stones, Stevens-Johnson syndrome, syncope, taste disorder, thrombocytopenia, thrombophlebitis, toxic epidermal necrolysis, tremor, urticaria, vasculitis, vertigo, weakness, weight gain/loss

Overdosage/Toxicology Symptoms of overdose include drowsiness, epigastric pain, lethargy, nausea and vomiting. Acute renal failure, coma, hypertension and respiratory depression may also rarely occur. Management of NSAID intoxication is supportive and symptomatic. 6-Methoxy-2-naphthylacetic acid (6MNA) is not dialyzable.

Drug Interactions

ACE inhibitors: Antihypertensive effects may be decreased by concurrent therapy with NSAIDs; monitor blood pressure.

Angiotensin II antagonists: Antihypertensive effects may be decreased by concurrent therapy with NSAIDs; monitor blood pressure.

Anticoagulants (warfarin, heparin, LMWHs) in combination with NSAIDs can cause increased risk of bleeding.

Antiplatelet drugs (ticlopidine, clopidogrel, aspirin, abciximab, dipyridamole, eptifibatide, tirofiban) can cause an increased risk of bleeding.

Beta-blockers: NSAIDs may decrease the antihypertensive effect of beta-blockers. Monitor.

Cholestyramine (and other bile acid sequestrants): May decrease the absorption of NSAIDs. Separate by at least 2 hours.

Corticosteroids may increase the risk of GI ulceration; avoid concurrent use.

Cyclosporine: NSAIDs may increase serum creatinine, potassium, blood pressure, and cyclosporine levels; monitor cyclosporine levels and renal function carefully.

Hydralazine's antihypertensive effect is decreased; avoid concurrent use.

Lithium levels can be increased; avoid concurrent use if possible or monitor lithium levels and adjust dose. Sulindac may have the least effect. When NSAID is stopped, lithium will need adjustment again.

Loop diuretics efficacy (diuretic and antihypertensive effect) is reduced.

Methotrexate: Severe bone marrow suppression, aplastic anemia, and GI toxicity have been reported with concomitant NSAID therapy. Avoid use during

(Continued)

Nabumetone *(Continued)*

moderate or high-dose methotrexate (increased and prolonged methotrexate levels). NSAID use during low-dose treatment of rheumatoid arthritis has not been fully evaluated; extreme caution is warranted.

Thiazides antihypertensive effects are decreased; avoid concurrent use.

Warfarin's INRs may be increased by nabumetone. Monitor INR closely. Use the lowest dose of NSAIDs possible and for the briefest duration.

Ethanol/Nutrition/Herb Interactions

Ethanol: Avoid ethanol (may enhance gastric mucosal irritation).

Food: Nabumetone peak serum concentrations may be increased if taken with food or dairy products.

Herb/Nutraceutical: Avoid alfalfa, anise, bilberry, bladderwrack, bromelain, cat's claw, celery, coleus, cordyceps, dong quai, evening primrose, feverfew, fenugreek, garlic, ginger, ginkgo biloboa, red clover, horse chestnut, grapeseed, green tea, ginseng, guggul, horse chestnut seed, horseradish, licorice, prickly ash, red clover, reishi, SAMe, sweet clover, turmeric, white willow (all have additional antiplatelet activity).

Dosage Forms Tablet: 500 mg, 750 mg

- **NAC** *see* Acetylcysteine *on page 35*
- ***N*-Acetyl-L-cysteine** *see* Acetylcysteine *on page 35*
- ***N*-Acetylcysteine** *see* Acetylcysteine *on page 35*
- **N-Acetyl-P-Aminophenol** *see* Acetaminophen *on page 26*
- **NaCl** *see* Sodium Chloride *on page 1183*

Nadolol (nay DOE lole)

Medication Safety Issues

Sound-alike/look-alike issues:

Nadolol may be confused with Mandol®

Corgard® may be confused with Cognex®

Related Information

Antiarrhythmic Drugs *on page 1548*

Beta-Blockers *on page 1557*

Preoperative Evaluation of the Cardiac Patient for Noncardiac Surgery *on page 1485*

U.S. Brand Names Corgard®

Canadian Brand Names Alti-Nadolol; Apo-Nadol®; Corgard®; Novo-Nadolol

Pharmacologic Category Beta-Adrenergic Blocker, Nonselective

Generic Available Yes

Use Treatment of hypertension and angina pectoris; prophylaxis of migraine headaches

Mechanism of Action Competitively blocks response to $beta_1$- and $beta_2$-adrenergic stimulation; does not exhibit any membrane stabilizing or intrinsic sympathomimetic activity

Pharmacodynamics/Kinetics

Duration: 17-24 hours

Absorption: 30% to 40%

Distribution: Concentration in human breast milk is 4.6 times higher than serum

Protein binding: 28%

Half-life elimination: Adults: 10-24 hours; prolonged with renal impairment; End-stage renal disease: 45 hours

Time to peak, serum: 2-4 hours

Excretion: Urine (as unchanged drug)

Dosage Oral:

Adults: Initial: 40 mg/day, increase dosage gradually by 40-80 mg increments at 3- to 7-day intervals until optimum clinical response is obtained with profound slowing of heart rate; doses up to 160-240 mg/day in angina and 240-320 mg/day in hypertension may be necessary.

Hypertension: Usual dosage range (JNC 7): 40-120 mg once daily

Elderly: Initial: 20 mg/day; increase doses by 20 mg increments at 3- to 7-day intervals; usual dosage range: 20-240 mg/day.

Dosing adjustment in renal impairment:

Cl_{cr} 31-40 mL/minute: Administer every 24-36 hours or administer 50% of normal dose.

Cl_{cr} 10-30 mL/minute: Administer every 24-48 hours or administer 50% of normal dose.

Cl_{cr} <10 mL/minute: Administer every 40-60 hours or administer 25% of normal dose.

Hemodialysis: Moderately dialyzable (20% to 50%); administer dose postdialysis or administer 40 mg supplemental dose.

Peritoneal dialysis: Supplemental dose is not necessary.

Dosing adjustment/comments in hepatic disease: Reduced dose probably necessary.

Anesthesia and Critical Care Concerns/Other Considerations Symptomatic bradycardia may be treated with atropine.

Surgery: Atenolol has also been shown to improve cardiovascular outcomes when used in the perioperative period in patients with underlying cardiovascular disease who are undergoing noncardiac surgery. Bisoprolol in high-risk patients undergoing vascular surgery reduced the perioperative incidence of death from cardiac causes and nonfatal myocardial infarction.

Withdrawal: Beta-blocker therapy should not be withdrawn abruptly, but gradually tapered to avoid acute tachycardia and hypertension.

Pregnancy Risk Factor C

Contraindications Hypersensitivity to nadolol or any component of the formulation; bronchial asthma; sinus bradycardia; sinus node dysfunction; heart block greater than first degree (except in patients with a functioning artificial pacemaker); cardiogenic shock; uncompensated cardiac failure

Warnings/Precautions Administer only with extreme caution in patients with compensated heart failure, monitor for a worsening of the condition. Efficacy in heart failure has not been established for nadolol. **[U.S. Boxed Warning]: Beta-blocker therapy should not be withdrawn abruptly (particularly in patients with CAD), but gradually tapered to avoid acute tachycardia, hypertension, and/or ischemia.** Use caution with concurrent use of beta-blockers and either verapamil or diltiazem; bradycardia or heart block can occur. In general, patients with bronchospastic disease should not receive beta-blockers. Nadolol, if used at all, should be used cautiously in bronchospastic disease with close monitoring. Use cautiously in diabetics because it can mask prominent hypoglycemic symptoms. Can mask signs of thyrotoxicosis. Can cause fetal harm when administered in pregnancy. Use cautiously in the renally impaired (dosage adjustments are required). Use care with anesthetic agents which decrease myocardial function.

Adverse Reactions

>10%:

Central nervous system: Drowsiness, insomnia

Endocrine & metabolic: Decreased sexual ability

1% to 10%:

Cardiovascular: Bradycardia, palpitation, edema, CHF, reduced peripheral circulation

Central nervous system: Mental depression

Gastrointestinal: Diarrhea or constipation, nausea, vomiting, stomach discomfort

Respiratory: Bronchospasm

Miscellaneous: Cold extremities

<1% (Limited to important or life-threatening): Arrhythmias, chest pain, confusion (especially in the elderly), depression, dyspnea, hallucinations, leukopenia, orthostatic hypotension, thrombocytopenia

Overdosage/Toxicology Symptoms of intoxication include cardiac disturbances, CNS toxicity, bronchospasm, hypoglycemia and hyperkalemia. The most common cardiac symptoms include hypotension and bradycardia. Atrioventricular block, intraventricular conduction disturbances, cardiogenic shock, and asystole may occur with severe overdose. CNS effects include convulsions, coma, and respiratory arrest. Treatment is symptom-directed and supportive. Glucagon has been used to reverse cardiac depression.

Drug Interactions

Albuterol (and other $beta_2$ agonists): Effects may be blunted by nonspecific beta-blockers.

Alpha-blockers (prazosin, terazosin): Concurrent use of beta-blockers may increase risk of orthostasis.

Clonidine: Hypertensive crisis after or during withdrawal of either agent.

(Continued)

Nadolol *(Continued)*

Drugs which slow AV conduction (digoxin): Effects may be additive with beta-blockers.

Epinephrine (including local anesthetics with epinephrine): Propranolol may cause hypertension.

Glucagon: Nadolol may blunt the hyperglycemic action of glucagon.

Insulin and oral hypoglycemics: Nadolol may mask symptoms of hypoglycemia.

Nadolol increases antipyrine's half-life.

NSAIDs (ibuprofen, indomethacin, naproxen, piroxicam) may reduce the antihypertensive effects of beta-blockers.

Salicylates may reduce the antihypertensive effects of beta-blockers.

Sulfonylureas: Beta-blockers may alter response to hypoglycemic agents.

Verapamil or diltiazem may have synergistic or additive pharmacological effects when taken concurrently with beta-blockers.

Ethanol/Nutrition/Herb Interactions Herb/Nutraceutical: Avoid dong quai if using for hypertension (has estrogenic activity). Avoid ephedra, garlic, yohimbe, ginseng (may worsen hypertension). Avoid natural licorice (causes sodium and water retention and increases potassium loss).

Dietary Considerations May be taken without regard to meals.

Dosage Forms [DSC] = Discontinued product

Tablet: 20 mg, 40 mg, 80 mg, 120 mg, 160 mg

Corgard®: 20 mg, 40 mg, 80 mg, 120 mg [DSC], 160 mg [DSC]

Nadroparin (nad roe PA rin)

Medication Safety Issues

High alert medication: The Institute for Safe Medication Practices (ISMP) includes this medication among its list of drugs which have a heightened risk of causing significant patient harm when used in error.

Canadian Brand Names Fraxiparine™; Fraxiparine™ Forte

Synonyms Nadroparin Calcium

Pharmacologic Category Low Molecular Weight Heparin

Restrictions Not available in U.S.

Generic Available No

Use Prophylaxis of thromboembolic disorders (particularly deep venous thrombosis and pulmonary embolism) in general and orthopedic surgery; treatment of deep venous thrombosis; prevention of clotting during hemodialysis

Mechanism of Action Nadroparin has high anti-Xa activity, but low anti-IIa activity. The greater ratio of anti-Xa activity has the potential to provide equivalent antithrombic efficacy with reduced hemorrhagic complications.

Pharmacodynamics/Kinetics

Duration: 18 hours

Absorption: SubQ: ≥89%

Time to peak, serum: 3-5 hours

Half-life elimination: 3.5 hours; Renal impairment: 6 hours

Excretion: Urine

Dosage SubQ: Adults:

Prophylaxis of thromboembolic disorders in general surgery: 2850 anti-Xa int. units once daily; begin 2-4 hours before surgery and continue for 7 days

Prophylaxis of thromboembolic disorders in hip replacement: 38 anti-Xa int. units/kg 12 hours before and 12 hours after surgery, **followed by** 38 anti-Xa int. units/kg/day up to and including day 3, **then** 57 anti-Xa int. units/kg/day for up to 10 days total therapy

Treatment of thromboembolic disorders: 171 anti-Xa int. units/kg/day to a maximum of 17,100 int. units; plasma anti-Xa levels should be 1.2-1.8 anti-Xa int. units/mL 3-4 hours postinjection

Patients at increased risk of bleeding: 86 anti-Xa int. units/kg twice daily; plasma anti-Xa levels should be 0.5-1.1 anti-Xa int. units/mL 3-4 hours postinjection

Prevention of clotting during hemodialysis: Single dose of 65 anti-Xa int. units/kg into arterial line at start of each dialysis session; may give additional dose if session lasts longer than 4 hours

Patients at risk of hemorrhage: Administer 50% of dose

Dosage adjustment in renal impairment: Reduced dose recommended

Stability Store between 15°C to 30°C (59°F to 86°F); do not freeze or refrigerate.

Administration SubQ injection into anterolateral abdominal wall with subsequent doses to be administered alternately on right and left side of abdominal wall. The thigh may also be used.

Monitoring Parameters Bleeding complications including stool occult blood tests, hemoglobin, antifactor Xa determinations, platelet counts

Pregnancy Risk Factor B

Contraindications Hypersensitivity to nadroparin or any component of the formulation; acute infective endocarditis; hemorrhage or increased risk of hemorrhage (hemostasis disorder), except for disseminated intravascular coagulation (DIC) not induced by heparin; history of thrombocytopenia with nadroparin; organic lesions likely to bleed (active peptic ulceration); hemorrhagic cerebrovascular event; severe uncontrolled hypertension; diabetic or hemorrhagic retinopathy; injuries to or operations on the CNS, eyes, or ears. Not for I.M. administration.

Warnings/Precautions [U.S. Boxed Warning]: Patients with recent or anticipated neuraxial anesthesia (epidural or spinal anesthesia) are at risk of spinal or epidural hematoma and subsequent paralysis. Consider risk versus benefit prior to neuraxial anesthesia. Risk is increased by concomitant agents which may alter hemostasis, as well as traumatic or repeated epidural or spinal puncture. Patient should be observed closely for bleeding if nadroparin is administered during or immediately following diagnostic lumbar puncture, epidural anesthesia, or spinal anesthesia.

Not to be used interchangeably (unit for unit) with heparin or any other low molecular weight heparins (LMWHs). Use with caution in patients with history of heparin-induced thrombocytopenia. Monitor platelet count closely. Rare thrombocytopenia may occur. Consider discontinuation of nadroparin in any patient developing significant thrombocytopenia. Rare cases of thrombocytopenia with thrombosis have occurred. Use caution in patients with congenital or drug-induced thrombocytopenia or platelet defects.

Monitor patient closely for signs or symptoms of bleeding. Certain patients are at increased risk of bleeding. Risk factors include bacterial endocarditis; congenital or acquired bleeding disorders; active ulcerative or angiodysplastic GI diseases; severe uncontrolled hypertension; hemorrhagic stroke; recent brain, spinal, or ophthalmology surgery; concomitant treatment with platelet inhibitors; recent GI bleeding; thrombocytopenia or platelet defects; severe liver disease; hypertensive or diabetic retinopathy; or in patients undergoing invasive procedures. Use with caution in patients with severe hepatic or renal disease. Safety and efficacy in pediatric patients have not been established.

Heparin can cause hyperkalemia by affecting aldosterone. Similar reactions could occur with LMWHs. Monitor for hyperkalemia. Do not use when abortion is imminent or threatened.

Adverse Reactions Frequency not defined.

Dermatologic: Rash

Endocrine & metabolic: Hypoaldosteronism (causing hyperkalemia and/or hyponatremia)

Hematological: Bleeding, thrombocytopenia

Hepatic: ALT/AST increased

Local: Injection site hematoma, pain at injection site

Neuromuscular & skeletal: Osteopenic effects

Miscellaneous: Allergic reactions

Overdosage/Toxicology The most common symptom is hemorrhage. Platelet count and other coagulation parameters should be monitored. Use of protamine sulfate can be considered in serious cases; a dose of 6 mg (0.6 mL) neutralizes ~0.1 mL of nadroparin or 0.05 mL of nadroparin forte. Do not exceed a rate of 20 mg/minute.

Drug Interactions

Antiplatelet drugs: Drugs which affect platelet function (eg, aspirin, NSAIDs, dipyridamole, ticlopidine, clopidogrel) may increase the risk of hemorrhage.

Thrombolytics (fibrinolytics): Increase risk of hemorrhage.

Warfarin: Risk of bleeding may be increased during concurrent therapy. Nadroparin is commonly continued during the initiation of warfarin therapy to assure anticoagulation and to protect against possible transient hypercoagulability.

Ethanol/Nutrition/Herb Interactions Herb/Nutraceutical: Avoid cat's claw, dong quai, evening primrose, garlic, ginseng (all have anticoagulant or antiplatelet activity).

(Continued)

Nadroparin *(Continued)*

Dosage Forms [CAN] = Canadian brand name

Injection, solution, as calcium:

Fraxiparine™ [CAN]:

9500 anti-Xa int. units/mL (0.2 mL, 0.3 mL, 0.4 mL) [ungraduated prefilled syringe]

9500 anti-Xa int. units/mL (0.6 mL, 0.8 mL, 1 mL) [graduated prefilled syringe]

Fraxiparine™ Forte [CAN]: 19,000 anti-Xa int. units/mL (0.6 mL, 0.8 mL, 1 mL) [graduated prefilled syringe]

♦ **Nadroparin Calcium** *see* Nadroparin *on page 888*

Nafcillin (naf SIL in)

Related Information

Anesthesia for Patients With Liver Disease *on page 1421*

Canadian Brand Names Nallpen®; Unipen®

Synonyms Ethoxynaphthamido Penicillin Sodium; Nafcillin Sodium; Nallpen; Sodium Nafcillin

Pharmacologic Category Antibiotic, Penicillin

Generic Available Yes

Use Treatment of infections such as osteomyelitis, septicemia, endocarditis, and CNS infections caused by susceptible strains of staphylococci species

Mechanism of Action Interferes with bacterial cell wall synthesis during active multiplication, causing cell wall death and resultant bactericidal activity against susceptible bacteria

Pharmacodynamics/Kinetics

Distribution: Widely distributed; CSF penetration is poor but enhanced by meningeal inflammation; crosses placenta

Protein binding: 70% to 90%

Metabolism: Primarily hepatic; undergoes enterohepatic recirculation

Half-life elimination:

Neonates: <3 weeks: 2.2-5.5 hours; 4-9 weeks: 1.2-2.3 hours

Children 3 months to 14 years: 0.75-1.9 hours

Adults: 30 minutes to 1.5 hours with normal renal and hepatic function

Time to peak, serum: I.M.: 30-60 minutes

Excretion: Primarily feces; urine (10% to 30% as unchanged drug)

Dosage

Usual dosage range:

Neonates: I.V.:

<2000 g, <7 days: 50 mg/kg/day divided every 12 hours

>2000 g, <7 days: 50 mg/kg/day divided every 8 hours

<2000 g, >7 days: 75 mg/kg/day divided every 8 hours

>2000 g, >7 days: 75 mg/kg/day divided every 6 hours

Children:

I.M.: 25 mg/kg twice daily

I.V.: 50-200 mg/kg/day in divided doses every 4-6 hours (maximum: 12 g/day)

Adults:

I.M.: 500 mg every 4-6 hours

I.V.: 500-2000 mg every 4-6 hours

Indication-specific dosing:

Neonates:

Arthritis, septic: I.V.:

<2000 g, <7 days: 50 mg/kg/day divided every 12 hours

<2000 g, >7 days: 75 mg/kg/day divided every 8 hours

>2000 g, <7 days: 75 mg/kg/day divided every 8 hours

>2000 g, >7 days: 222 mg/kg/day divided every 6 hours

Children:

Epiglottitis: I.V.: 150-200 mg/kg/day divided in 4 doses

Mild to moderate infections: I.M., I.V.: 50-100 mg/kg/day in divided doses every 6 hours

Severe infections: I.M., I.V.: 100-200 mg/kg/day in divided doses every 4-6 hours (maximum dose: 12 g/day

Toxic epidermal necrolysis: I.V.: 150 mg/kg/day divided every 6 hours for 5-7 days

Adults: I.V.:

Endocarditis: MSSA:

Native valve: 2 g every 4 hours

Prosthetic valve: 1 g every 4 hours with rifampin for 6 weeks with gentamicin for 2 weeks

Tricuspid valve: 2 g every 4 hours with gentamicin for 2 weeks

Joint:

Bursitis, septic: 2 g every 4 hours

Prosthetic: 2 g every 4-6 hours with rifampin for 6 weeks

***Staphylococcus aureus*, methicillin-susceptible infections, including brain abscess, empyema, erysipelas, mastitis, myositis, osteomyelitis, pneumonia, toxic shock, urinary tract (perinephric abscess):** 2 g every 4 hours

Toxic epidermal necrolysis: 2 g every 4 hours

Dosing adjustment in renal impairment: Not necessary

Dosing adjustment in hepatic impairment: In patients with both hepatic and renal impairment, modification of dosage may be necessary; no data available.

Dialysis: Not dialyzable (0% to 5%) via hemodialysis; supplemental dosage not necessary with hemo- or peritoneal dialysis or continuous arteriovenous or venovenous hemofiltration

Stability Reconstituted parenteral solution is stable for 3 days at room temperature and 7 days when refrigerated or 12 weeks when frozen; for I.V. infusion in NS or D_5W, solution is stable for 24 hours at room temperature and 96 hours when refrigerated

Administration

I.M.: Rotate injection sites

I.V.: Vesicant. Administer around-the-clock to promote less variation in peak and trough serum levels; infuse over 30-60 minutes

Extravasation management: Use cold packs. Hyaluronidase: Add 1 mL NS to 150 unit vial to make 150 units/mL of concentration; mix 0.1 mL of above with 0.9 mL NS in 1 mL syringe to make final concentration = 15 units/mL.

Monitoring Parameters Periodic CBC, urinalysis, BUN, serum creatinine, AST and ALT; observe for signs and symptoms of anaphylaxis during first dose

Pregnancy Risk Factor B

Contraindications Hypersensitivity to nafcillin, or any component of the formulation, or penicillins

Warnings/Precautions Extravasation of I.V. infusions should be avoided; modification of dosage is necessary in patients with both severe renal and hepatic impairment; elimination rate will be slow in neonates; use with caution in patients with cephalosporin hypersensitivity

Adverse Reactions Frequency not defined.

Central nervous system: Pain, fever

Dermatologic: Rash

Gastrointestinal: Nausea, diarrhea

Hematologic: Agranulocytosis, bone marrow depression, neutropenia

Local: Pain, swelling, inflammation, phlebitis, skin sloughing, and thrombophlebitis at the injection site; oxacillin (less likely to cause phlebitis) is often preferred in pediatric patients

Renal: Interstitial nephritis (acute)

Miscellaneous: Hypersensitivity reactions

Overdosage/Toxicology Symptoms of penicillin overdose include neuromuscular hypersensitivity (eg, agitation, hallucinations, asterixis, encephalopathy, confusion, and seizures). Electrolyte imbalance may occur if the preparation contains potassium or sodium salts, especially in renal failure. Treatment is supportive or symptom-directed.

Drug Interactions **Induces** CYP3A4 (strong)

Chloramphenicol: May decrease efficacy of nafcillin

Cyclosporine: Levels may be decreased by nafcillin

CYP3A4 substrates: Nafcillin may decrease the levels/effects of CYP3A4 substrates. Example substrates include benzodiazepines, calcium channel blockers, clarithromycin, cyclosporine, erythromycin, estrogens, mirtazapine, nateglinide, nefazodone, nevirapine, protease inhibitors, tacrolimus, and venlafaxine

Methotrexate: Penicillins may increase the exposure to methotrexate during concurrent therapy; monitor.

(Continued)

Nafcillin *(Continued)*

Oral contraceptives: Anecdotal reports suggesting decreased contraceptive efficacy with penicillins have been refuted by more rigorous scientific and clinical data.

Probenecid: May increase levels of penicillins (nafcillin)

Warfarin, oral anticoagulants: Effects of anticoagulants may be decreased

Test Interactions Positive Coombs' test (direct), false-positive urinary and serum proteins; may inactivate aminoglycosides *in vitro*

Dietary Considerations Sodium content of 1 g: 76.6 mg (3.33 mEq)

Dosage Forms

Infusion [premixed iso-osmotic dextrose solution]: 1 g (50 mL); 2 g (100 mL)

Injection, powder for reconstitution, as sodium: 1 g, 2 g, 10 g

♦ **Nafcillin Sodium** *see* Nafcillin *on page 890*

♦ **$NaHCO_3$** *see* Sodium Bicarbonate *on page 1181*

Nalbuphine (NAL byoo feen)

Medication Safety Issues

Sound-alike/look-alike issues:

Nubain® may be confused with Navane®, Nebcin®

Related Information

Anesthesia Considerations for Neurosurgery *on page 1401*

Chronic Pain Management *on page 1430*

Narcotic / Opioid Analgesics *on page 1568*

Opioids *on page 1535*

U.S. Brand Names Nubain®

Synonyms Nalbuphine Hydrochloride

Pharmacologic Category Analgesic, Narcotic

Generic Available Yes

Use Relief of moderate to severe pain; preoperative analgesia, postoperative and surgical anesthesia, and obstetrical analgesia during labor and delivery

Mechanism of Action Agonist of kappa opiate receptors and partial antagonist of mu opiate receptors in the CNS, causing inhibition of ascending pain pathways, altering the perception of and response to pain; produces generalized CNS depression

Pharmacodynamics/Kinetics

Onset of action: Peak effect: SubQ, I.M.: <15 minutes; I.V.: 2-3 minutes

Metabolism: Hepatic

Half-life elimination: 5 hours

Excretion: Feces; urine (~7% as metabolites)

Dosage

Children ≥1 year (unlabeled use): Pain management: I.M., I.V., SubQ: 0.1-0.2 mg/kg every 3-4 hours as needed; maximum: 20 mg/dose and/or 160 mg/day

Adults:

Pain management: I.M., I.V., SubQ: 10 mg/70 kg every 3-6 hours; maximum single dose in nonopioid-tolerant patients: 20 mg; maximum daily dose: 160 mg

Surgical anesthesia supplement: I.V.: Induction: 0.3-3 mg/kg over 10-15 minutes; maintenance doses of 0.25-0.5 mg/kg may be given as required

Dosing adjustment in renal impairment: Use with caution and reduce dose; monitor.

Dosing adjustment in hepatic impairment: Use with caution and reduce dose.

Stability Store at room temperature of 15°C to 30°C (59°F to 86°F); protect from light

Administration Administer I.M., SubQ, or I.V.

Monitoring Parameters Relief of pain, respiratory and mental status, blood pressure

Anesthesia and Critical Care Concerns/Other Considerations Abrupt discontinuation after sustained use (generally >10 days) may cause withdrawal symptoms.

Mixed agonist-antagonist: Incidence of psychomimetic effect is lower than with pentazocine; may precipitate withdrawal in narcotic-dependent patients.

Pregnancy Risk Factor B/D (prolonged use or high doses at term)

Contraindications Hypersensitivity to nalbuphine or any component of the formulation

Warnings/Precautions Use caution in CNS depression. Sedation and psychomotor impairment are likely, and are additive with other CNS depressants or ethanol. May cause respiratory depression. Ambulatory patients must be cautioned about performing tasks which require mental alertness (eg, operating machinery or driving). Use with caution in patients with recent myocardial infarction, biliary tract surgery, head trauma, or increased intracranial pressure. Use caution in patients with decreased hepatic or renal function. May result in tolerance and/or drug dependence with chronic use; use with caution in patients with a history of drug dependence. Abrupt discontinuation following prolonged use may lead to withdrawal symptoms. May precipitate withdrawal symptoms in patients following prolonged therapy with mu opiod agonists. Use with caution in pregnancy (close neonatal monitoring required when used in labor and delivery). Safety and efficacy in pediatric patients (<18 years of age) have not been established.

Adverse Reactions

>10%: Central nervous system: Sedation (36%)

1% to 10%:

Central nervous system: Dizziness (5%), headache (3%)

Gastrointestinal: Nausea/vomiting (6%), xerostomia (4%)

Miscellaneous: Clamminess (9%)

<1% (Limited to important or life-threatening): Abdominal pain, agitation, allergic reaction, anaphylaxis, anaphylactoid reaction, anxiety, asthma, bitter taste, blurred vision, bradycardia, cardiac arrest, confusion, crying, delusion, depersonalization, depression, diaphoresis, dreams (abnormal), dyspepsia, dysphoria, dyspnea, euphoria, faintness, fever, floating sensation, flushing, gastrointestinal cramps, hallucinations, hostility, hypertension, hypotension, injection site reactions (pain, swelling, redness, burning); laryngeal edema, loss of consciousness, nervousness, numbness, pruritus, pulmonary edema, rash, respiratory depression, respiratory distress, restlessness, seizure, sensation of warmth/burning, somnolence, speech disorder, stridor, tachycardia, tingling, tremor, unreality, urinary urgency, urticaria

Overdosage/Toxicology Symptoms of overdose include CNS depression, respiratory depression, miosis, hypotension, and bradycardia. Treatment is symptomatic. Naloxone, 2 mg I.V. with repeat administration as necessary up to a total dose of 10 mg, can be used to reverse opiate effects.

Drug Interactions Increased toxicity: Barbiturate anesthetics may increase CNS depression

Ethanol/Nutrition/Herb Interactions

Ethanol: Avoid ethanol (may increase CNS depression).

Herb/Nutraceutical: Avoid valerian, St John's wort, kava kava, gotu kola (may increase CNS depression).

Dosage Forms [DSC] = Discontinued product

Injection, solution, as hydrochloride: 10 mg/mL (10 mL); 20 mg/mL (10 mL)

Nubain®: 10 mg/mL (10 mL) [DSC]; 20 mg/mL (10 mL)

Injection, solution, as hydrochloride [preservative free]: 10 mg/mL (1 mL); 20 mg/mL (1 mL)

Nubain®: 10 mg/mL (1 mL); 20 mg/mL (1 mL)

♦ **Nalbuphine Hydrochloride** *see* Nalbuphine *on page 892*

♦ **Nalfon®** *see* Fenoprofen *on page 511*

♦ **Nallpen® (Can)** *see* Nafcillin *on page 890*

♦ ***N*-allylnoroxymorphine Hydrochloride** *see* Naloxone *on page 895*

Nalmefene (NAL me feen)

Medication Safety Issues

Sound-alike/look-alike issues:

Revex® may be confused with Nimbex®, ReVia®

Color-coded ampuls denote indication-specific concentrations:

Blue-labeled ampul (for postoperative use) contains 1 mL (100 mcg/mL)

Green-labeled ampul (for overdose management) contains 2 mL (1 mg/mL)

(Continued)

Nalmefene *(Continued)*

U.S. Brand Names Revex®

Synonyms Nalmefene Hydrochloride

Pharmacologic Category Antidote

Generic Available No

Use Complete or partial reversal of opioid drug effects, including respiratory depression induced by natural or synthetic opioids; reversal of postoperative opioid depression; management of known or suspected opioid overdose

Mechanism of Action As a 6-methylene analog of naltrexone, nalmefene acts as a competitive antagonist at opioid receptor sites, preventing or reversing the respiratory depression, sedation, and hypotension induced by opiates; no pharmacologic activity of its own (eg, opioid agonist activity) has been demonstrated

Pharmacodynamics/Kinetics

Onset of action: I.M., SubQ: 5-15 minutes

Distribution: V_d: 8.6 L/kg; rapid

Protein binding: 45%

Metabolism: Hepatic via glucuronide conjugation to metabolites with little or no activity

Bioavailability: I.M., SubQ: 100%

Half-life elimination: 10.8 hours

Time to peak, serum: Serum: I.M.: 2.3 hours; I.V.: <2 minutes; SubQ: 1.5 hours

Excretion: Feces (17%); urine (<5% as unchanged drug)

Clearance: 0.8 L/hour/kg

Dosage I.M., I.V., SubQ:

Reversal of postoperative opioid depression: Blue-labeled product (100 mcg/mL): Titrate to reverse the undesired effects of opioids; initial dose for nonopioid dependent patients: 0.25 mcg/kg followed by 0.25 mcg/kg incremental doses at 2- to 5-minute intervals; after a total dose >1 mcg/kg, further therapeutic response is unlikely

Note: In patients with increased cardiovascular risks, dilute 1:1 in NS or SWFI, and initiate/titrate with 0.1 mcg/kg doses.

Management of known/suspected opioid overdose: Green-labeled product (1 mg/mL): Initial dose: 0.5 mg/70 kg; may repeat with 1 mg/70 kg in 2-5 minutes; further increase beyond a total dose of 1.5 mg/70 kg will not likely result in improved response and may result in cardiovascular stress and precipitated withdrawal syndrome. (If opioid dependency is suspected, administer a challenge dose of 0.1 mg/70 kg; if no withdrawal symptoms are observed in 2 minutes, the recommended doses can be administered.)

Note: If recurrence of respiratory depression is noted, dose may again be titrated to clinical effect using incremental doses.

Note: If I.V. access is lost or not readily obtainable, a single SubQ or I.M. dose of 1 mg may be effective in 5-15 minutes.

Dosing adjustment in renal impairment: Not necessary with single use, however, slow administration (over 60 seconds) of incremental doses is recommended to minimize hypertension and dizziness

Dosing adjustment in hepatic impairment: No adjustment necessary with single use.

Stability Store at controlled room temperature.

Administration Check dosage strength carefully before use to avoid error. Slow administration (over 60 seconds) of incremental doses is recommended to minimize hypertension and dizziness in renal patients. Dilute drug (1:1) with diluent and use smaller doses in patients known to be at increased cardiovascular risk. May be administered via I.M. or SubQ routes if I.V. access is not feasible. A single SubQ or I.M. dose of 1 mg may be effective in 5-15 minutes.

Monitoring Parameters Symptoms of withdrawal; signs/symptoms of respiratory depression; pain

Anesthesia and Critical Care Concerns/Other Considerations Proper steps should be used to prevent use of the incorrect dosage strength. The goal of treatment in the postoperative setting is to achieve reversal of excessive opioid effects without inducing a complete reversal and acute pain. If opioid dependence is suspected, nalmefene should only be used in opioid overdose if the likelihood of overdose is high, based on history or the clinical presentation of respiratory depression with concurrent pupillary constriction present.

Pregnancy Risk Factor B

Contraindications Hypersensitivity to nalmefene, naltrexone, or any component of the formulation

Warnings/Precautions May induce symptoms of acute withdrawal in opioid-dependent patients; recurrence of respiratory depression is possible if the opioid involved is long-acting; observe patients until there is no reasonable risk of recurrent respiratory depression. Safety and efficacy have not been established in children. Avoid abrupt reversal of opioid effects in patients of high cardiovascular risk or who have received potentially cardiotoxic drugs. Pulmonary edema and cardiovascular instability, including ventricular fibrillation, have been reported in association with abrupt reversal with other narcotic antagonists. Animal studies indicate nalmefene may not completely reverse buprenorphine-induced respiratory depression. Use caution with renal impairment.

Adverse Reactions

>10%: Gastrointestinal: Nausea (18%)

1% to 10%:

- Cardiovascular: Tachycardia (5%), hypertension (5%), hypotension (1%), vasodilation (1%)
- Central nervous system: Fever (3%), dizziness (3%), headache (1%), chills (1%)
- Gastrointestinal: Vomiting (9%)
- Miscellaneous: Postoperative pain (4%)

<1% (Limited to important or life-threatening): Agitation, arrhythmia, AST increased, bradycardia, confusion, depression, diarrhea, myoclonus, nervousness, pharyngitis, pruritus, somnolence, tremor, urinary retention, withdrawal syndrome, xerostomia

Overdosage/Toxicology No reported symptoms with significant overdose. Intravenous doses up to 24 mg have been tolerated by healthy volunteers (in the absence of opioid exposure). Large doses of opioids administered to overcome a full blockade of opioid antagonists, however, have resulted in adverse respiratory and circulatory reactions. Treatment is symptom-directed and supportive.

Drug Interactions

Flumazenil: May increase the risk of toxicity with flumazenil. An increased risk of seizures has been associated with flumazenil and nalmefene coadministration

Narcotic analgesics: Decreased effect of narcotic analgesics; may precipitate acute withdrawal reaction in physically dependent patients

Dosage Forms

Injection, solution:

Revex®: 100 mcg/mL (1 mL) [blue label]; 1 mg/mL (2 mL) [green label]

♦ **Nalmefene Hydrochloride** *see* Nalmefene *on page 893*

Naloxone (nal OKS one)

Medication Safety Issues

Sound-alike/look-alike issues:

Naloxone may be confused with naltrexone

Narcan® may be confused with Marcaine®, Norcuron®

Related Information

Chronic Pain Management *on page 1430*

U.S. Brand Names Narcan® [DSC]

Canadian Brand Names Naloxone Hydrochloride Injection®

Synonyms *N*-allylnoroxymorphine Hydrochloride; Naloxone Hydrochloride

Pharmacologic Category Antidote

Generic Available Yes

Use

Complete or partial reversal of opioid depression, including respiratory depression, induced by natural and synthetic opioids, including propoxyphene, methadone, and certain mixed agonist-antagonist analgesics: nalbuphine, pentazocine, and butorphanol

Diagnosis of suspected opioid tolerance or acute opioid overdose

Adjunctive agent to increase blood pressure in the management of septic shock

Unlabeled/Investigational Use PCP and ethanol ingestion

Mechanism of Action Pure opioid antagonist that competes and displaces narcotics at opioid receptor sites

Pharmacodynamics/Kinetics

Onset of action: Endotracheal, I.M., SubQ: 2-5 minutes; I.V.: ~2 minutes

Duration: 20-60 minutes; since shorter than that of most opioids, repeated doses are usually needed

Distribution: Crosses placenta

(Continued)

Naloxone *(Continued)*

Metabolism: Primarily hepatic via glucuronidation
Half-life elimination: Neonates: 1.2-3 hours; Adults: 1-1.5 hours
Excretion: Urine (as metabolites)

Dosage I.M., I.V. (preferred), intratracheal, SubQ:

Postanesthesia narcotic reversal: Infants and Children: 0.01 mg/kg; may repeat every 2-3 minutes, as needed based on response

Opiate intoxication:

Children:

Birth (including premature infants) to 5 years or <20 kg: 0.1 mg/kg; repeat every 2-3 minutes if needed; may need to repeat doses every 20-60 minutes

>5 years or ≥20 kg: 2 mg/dose; if no response, repeat every 2-3 minutes; may need to repeat doses every 20-60 minutes

Children and Adults: Continuous infusion: I.V.: If continuous infusion is required, calculate dosage/hour based on effective intermittent dose used and duration of adequate response seen, titrate dose 0.04-0.16 mg/kg/hour for 2-5 days in children, adult dose typically 0.25-6.25 mg/hour (short-term infusions as high as 2.4 mg/kg/hour have been tolerated in adults during treatment for septic shock); alternatively, continuous infusion utilizes $^2/_3$ of the initial naloxone bolus on an hourly basis; add 10 times this dose to each liter of D_5W and infuse at a rate of 100 mL/hour; $^1/_2$ of the initial bolus dose should be readministered 15 minutes after initiation of the continuous infusion to prevent a drop in naloxone levels; increase infusion rate as needed to assure adequate ventilation

Narcotic overdose: Adults: I.V.: 0.4-2 mg every 2-3 minutes as needed; may need to repeat doses every 20-60 minutes, if no response is observed after 10 mg, question the diagnosis. **Note:** Use 0.1-0.2 mg increments in patients who are opioid dependent and in postoperative patients to avoid large cardiovascular changes.

Stability Store at 25°C (77°F); protect from light; stable in 0.9% sodium chloride and D_5W at 4 mcg/mL for 24 hours; do not mix with alkaline solutions

Administration

Intratracheal: Dilute to 1-2 mL with normal saline
I.V. push: Administer over 30 seconds as undiluted preparation
I.V. continuous infusion: Dilute to 4 mcg/mL in D_5W or normal saline

Monitoring Parameters Respiratory rate, heart rate, blood pressure

Anesthesia and Critical Care Concerns/Other Considerations Naloxone may contain methyl and propylparabens. Proper steps should be used to prevent use of the incorrect dosage strength. the goal of treatment in the postoperative setting is to achieve reversal of excessive opioid effects without inducing a complete reversal and acute pain.

Pregnancy Risk Factor C

Contraindications Hypersensitivity to naloxone or any component of the formulation

Warnings/Precautions Due to an association between naloxone and acute pulmonary edema, use with caution in patients with cardiovascular disease or in patients receiving medications with potential adverse cardiovascular effects (eg, hypotension, pulmonary edema or arrhythmias). Excessive dosages should be avoided after use of opiates in surgery. Abrupt postoperative reversal may result in nausea, vomiting, sweating, tachycardia, hypertension, seizures, and other cardiovascular events (including pulmonary edema and arrhythmias). May precipitate withdrawal symptoms in patients addicted to opiates, including pain, hypertension, sweating, agitation, irritability; in neonates: shrill cry, failure to feed. Recurrence of respiratory depression is possible if the opioid involved is long-acting; observe patients until there is no reasonable risk of recurrent respiratory depression.

Adverse Reactions Frequency not defined.

Cardiovascular: Hyper-/hypotension, tachycardia, ventricular arrhythmia, cardiac arrest
Central nervous system: Irritability, anxiety, narcotic withdrawal, restlessness, seizure
Gastrointestinal: Nausea, vomiting, diarrhea
Neuromuscular & skeletal: Tremulousness
Respiratory: Dyspnea, pulmonary edema, runny nose, sneezing
Miscellaneous: Diaphoresis

Overdosage/Toxicology Naloxone is the drug of choice for respiratory depression that is known or suspected to be caused by overdose of an opiate or opioid. **Caution:** Naloxone's effects are due to its action on narcotic reversal, not due to any direct effect upon opiate receptors. Therefore, adverse events occur secondarily to reversal (withdrawal) of narcotic analgesia and sedation, which can cause severe reactions.

Drug Interactions Narcotic analgesics: Decreased effect of narcotic analgesics; may precipitate acute withdrawal reaction in physically dependent patients

Dosage Forms [DSC] = Discontinued product

Injection, solution, as hydrochloride: 0.4 mg/mL (1 mL, 10 mL)

Narcan®: 0.4 mg/mL (1 mL) [DSC]

References

Boeuf B, Gauvin F, Guerguerian AM, et al, "Therapy of Shock With Naloxone: A Meta-analysis," *Crit Care Med*, 1998, 26(11):1910-6.

Goldfrank L, Weisman RS, Errick JK, et al, "A Dosing Nomogram for Continuous Infusion Intravenous Naloxone," *Ann Emerg Med*, 1986, 15(5):566-70.

Mokhlesi B, Leikin JB, Murray P, et al, "Adult Toxicology in Critical Care. Part 11: Specific Poisonings," *Chest*, 2003, 123(3):897-922.

Tandberg D and Abercrombie D, "Treatment of Heroin Overdose With Endotracheal Naloxone," *Ann Emerg Med*, 1982, 11(8):443-5.

Trujillo MH, Guerrero J, Fragachan C, et al, "Pharmacologic Antidotes in Critical Care Medicine: A Practical Guide for Drug Administration," *Crit Care Med*, 1998, 26(2):377-91.

♦ **Naloxone Hydrochloride** *see* Naloxone *on page 895*

♦ **Naloxone Hydrochloride Injection® (Can)** *see* Naloxone *on page 895*

Naltrexone (nal TREKS one)

Medication Safety Issues

Sound-alike/look-alike issues:

Naltrexone may be confused with naloxone

ReVia® may be confused with Revex®

Related Information

Chronic Pain Management *on page 1430*

U.S. Brand Names Depade®; ReVia®; Vivitrol™

Canadian Brand Names ReVia®

Synonyms Naltrexone Hydrochloride

Pharmacologic Category Antidote

Generic Available Yes: Tablet

Use Treatment of ethanol dependence; blockade of the effects of exogenously administered opioids

Mechanism of Action Naltrexone (a pure opioid antagonist) is a cyclopropyl derivative of oxymorphone similar in structure to naloxone and nalorphine (a morphine derivative); it acts as a competitive antagonist at opioid receptor sites, showing the highest affinity for mu receptors.

Pharmacodynamics/Kinetics

Duration: Oral: 50 mg: 24 hours; 100 mg: 48 hours; 150 mg: 72 hours; I.M.: 4 weeks

Absorption: Oral: Almost complete

Distribution: V_d: 19 L/kg; widely throughout the body but considerable interindividual variation exists

Protein binding: 21%

Metabolism: Noncytochrome-mediated dehydrogenase conversion to 6-β-naltrexol and related minor metabolites; Oral: Extensive first-pass effect

Half-life elimination: Oral: 4 hours; 6-β-naltrexol: 13 hours; I.M.: naltrexone and 6-β-naltrexol: 5-10 days

Time to peak, serum: Oral: ~60 minutes; I.M.: Biphasic: 2 hours (first peak), 2-3 days (second peak)

Excretion: Primarily urine (as metabolites and unchanged drug)

Dosage Adults: Do not give until patient is opioid-free for 7-10 days as determined by urinalysis

Oral: Alcohol dependence, opioid antidote: 25 mg; if no withdrawal signs within 1 hour give another 25 mg; maintenance regimen is flexible, variable and individualized (50 mg/day to 100-150 mg 3 times/week for 12 weeks); up to 800 mg/day has been tolerated in a small number of healthy adults without an adverse effect

I.M.: Alcohol dependence: 380 mg once every 4 weeks

(Continued)

Naltrexone *(Continued)*

Dosage adjustment in renal impairment: Use caution. No adjustment needed in mild impairment. Not adequately studied in moderate-to-severe renal impairment.

Dosage adjustment in hepatic impairment: Use caution. An increase in naltrexone AUC of approximately five- and 10-fold in patients with compensated or decompensated liver cirrhosis respectively, compared with normal liver function has been reported No adjustment required with mild-to-moderate hepatic impairment. Not adequately studied in severe hepatic impairment.

Stability

Injection: Store unopened kit at 2°C to 8°C (36°F to 46°F). Kit may be kept at room temperature of ≤25°C (77°F) for ≤7 days prior to use; do not freeze.

Tablet: Store at 20°C to 25°C (68°F to 77°F).

Administration If there is any question of occult opioid dependence, perform a naloxone challenge test; do not attempt treatment until naloxone challenge is negative.

Oral: To minimize adverse gastrointestinal effects, administer with food or antacids or after meals; advise patient not to self-administer opiates while receiving naltrexone therapy.

I.M.: Vivitrol™: Administer I.M. into the upper outer quadrant of the gluteal area. Injection should alternate between the two buttocks. Do not substitute any components of the dose-pack; administer with needle provided.

Monitoring Parameters For narcotic withdrawal; liver function tests

Anesthesia and Critical Care Concerns/Other Considerations May also be used in detoxification with special guidelines

Pregnancy Risk Factor C

Contraindications Hypersensitivity to naltrexone or any component of the formulation; narcotic dependence or current use of opioid analgesics; acute opioid withdrawal; failure to pass Narcan® challenge or positive urine screen for opioids; acute hepatitis; liver failure

Warnings/Precautions

[U.S. Boxed Warning]: Dose-related hepatocellular injury is possible; the margin of separation between the apparent safe and hepatotoxic doses appears to be only fivefold or less (contraindicated in acute hepatitis or hepatic failure).

May precipitate withdrawal symptoms in patients addicted to opiates, including pain, hypertension, sweating, agitation, irritability; in neonates: shrill cry, failure to feed. Patients should be opiate-free for a minimum of 7-10 days; use naloxone challenge test to confirm. Use with caution in patients with hepatic or renal impairment; not studied in severe hepatic or moderate-to-severe renal impairment..

Patients who had been treated with naltrexone may respond to lower opioid doses than previously used. This could result in potentially life-threatening opioid intoxication. Patients should be aware that they may be more sensitive to lower doses of opioids after naltrexone treatment is discontinued. Use of naltrexone does not eliminate or diminish withdrawal symptoms. Warn patients that attempts to overcome opioid blockade could lead to fatal overdose. Suicidal thoughts and depression have been reported; monitor closely.

Cases of eosinophilic pneumonia have been reported; monitor for hypoxia and dyspnea. Safety and efficacy in children have not been established.

Adverse Reactions Combined reporting of adverse events from oral and injectable formulations:

>10%:

Cardiovascular: Syncope (13%)

Central nervous system: Headache (25%), insomnia (14%), dizziness (13%), anxiety (12%), somnolence (4%), nervousness, fatigue

Gastrointestinal: Nausea (33%), vomiting (14%), appetite decreased (14%), diarrhea (13%), abdominal pain (11%), abdominal cramping

Local: Injection-site reaction (69%)

Neuromuscular & skeletal: Arthralgia (12%), CPK increased (11%)

Respiratory: Upper respiratory tract infection (13%), pharyngitis (11%)

1% to 10%:

Central nervous system: Depression (8%), suicidal thoughts (1%), energy increased, feeling down

Dermatologic: Rash (6%)

Endocrine & metabolic: Polydipsia
Gastrointestinal: Dry mouth (5%)
Genitourinary: Delayed ejaculation, impotency
Hepatic: AST increased (2%)
Neuromuscular & skeletal: Muscle cramps (8%), back pain (6%)

<1% (Limited to important or life-threatening): ALT increased, angina, atrial fibrillation, blood pressure increased, cerebral aneurysm, chest pain, chest tightness, CHF, cholecystitis, cholelithiasis, colitis, COPD, dehydration, delirium, disorientation, DVT, dyspnea, eosinophilic pneumonia, euphoria, GI hemorrhage, hallucinations, hypercholesterolemia, hypersensitivity reaction (includes angioedema and urticaria), hypertension, influenza, ischemic stroke, leukocytosis, lymphadenopathy, MI, narcotic withdrawal, palpitation, paralytic ileus, paranoia, PE, perirectal abscess, pneumonia, pyrexia, rigors, seizures, suicide attempts, tachycardia, thrombocytopenia, tooth abscess, UTI

Overdosage/Toxicology Symptoms of overdose include clonic-tonic convulsions and respiratory failure. Patients receiving up to 800 mg/day for 1 week have shown no toxicity. Seizures and respiratory failure have been seen in animals. Treatment should be symptom-directed and supportive.

Drug Interactions

Narcotic analgesics: Decreased effect of narcotic analgesics; may precipitate acute withdrawal reaction in physically dependent patients; concurrent use is contraindicated

Thioridazine: Lethargy and somnolence have been reported with the combination of naltrexone and thioridazine

Test Interactions May cause cross-reactivity with some opioid immunoassay methods.

Dosage Forms

Injection, powder for suspension [extended-release microspheres]:
Vivitrol™: 380 mg [diluent provided]

Tablet, as hydrochloride: 50 mg
Depade®: 25 mg, 50 mg, 100 mg
ReVia®: 50 mg

References

Mokhlesi B, Leikin JB, Murray P, et al, "Adult Toxicology in Critical Care. Part 11: Specific Poisonings," *Chest*, 2003, 123(3):897-922.

O'Connor PG and Kosten TR, "Rapid and Ultrarapid Opioid Detoxification Techniques," *JAMA*, 1998, 279(3):229-34.

♦ **Naltrexone Hydrochloride** *see* Naltrexone *on page 897*

♦ **Naprelan®** *see* Naproxen *on page 899*

♦ **Naprosyn®** *see* Naproxen *on page 899*

Naproxen (na PROKS en)

Medication Safety Issues

Sound-alike/look-alike issues:
Naproxen may be confused with Natacyn®, Nebcin®
Aleve® may be confused with Alesse®
Anaprox® may be confused with Anaspaz®, Avapro®
Naprelan® may be confused with Naprosyn®
Naprosyn® may be confused with Naprelan®, Natacyn®, Nebcin®

Related Information

Acetaminophen and NSAIDS, Dosing Data *on page 1543*
Acute Postoperative Pain *on page 1388*
Chronic Pain Management *on page 1430*

U.S. Brand Names Aleve® [OTC]; Anaprox®; Anaprox® DS; EC-Naprosyn®; Midol® Extended Relief; Naprelan®; Naprosyn®; Pamprin® Maximum Strength All Day Relief [OTC]

Canadian Brand Names Anaprox®; Anaprox® DS; Apo-Napro-Na®; Apo-Napro-Na DS®; Apo-Naproxen®; Apo-Naproxen SR®; Gen-Naproxen EC; Naprosyn®; Naxen®; Naxen® EC; Novo-Naproc EC; Novo-Naprox; Novo-Naprox Sodium; Novo-Naprox Sodium DS; Novo-Naprox SR; Nu-Naprox; Riva-Naproxen

Synonyms Naproxen Sodium

Pharmacologic Category Nonsteroidal Anti-inflammatory Drug (NSAID), Oral

Restrictions A medication guide should be dispensed with each prescription. A template for the required MedGuide can be found on the FDA website at: http://www.fda.gov/medwatch/SAFETY/2005/safety05.htm#NSAID

(Continued)

Naproxen *(Continued)*

Generic Available Yes

Use Management of ankylosing spondylitis, osteoarthritis, and rheumatoid disorders (including juvenile rheumatoid arthritis); acute gout; mild-to-moderate pain; tendonitis, bursitis; dysmenorrhea; fever

Mechanism of Action Inhibits prostaglandin synthesis by decreasing the activity of the enzyme, cyclooxygenase, which results in decreased formation of prostaglandin precursors

Pharmacodynamics/Kinetics

Onset of action: Analgesic: 1 hour; Anti-inflammatory: ~2 weeks

Peak effect: Anti-inflammatory: 2-4 weeks

Duration: Analgesic: ≤7 hours; Anti-inflammatory: ≤12 hours

Absorption: Almost 100%

Protein binding: >99%; increased free fraction in elderly

Half-life elimination: Normal renal function: 12-17 hours; End-stage renal disease: No change

Time to peak, serum: 1-4 hours

Excretion: Urine (95%)

Dosage Note: Dosage expressed as naproxen base; 200 mg naproxen base is equivalent to 220 mg naproxen sodium.

Oral:

Children >2 years: Juvenile arthritis: 10 mg/kg/day in 2 divided doses

Adults:

Gout, acute: Initial: 750 mg, followed by 250 mg every 8 hours until attack subsides. **Note:** EC-Naprosyn® is not recommended.

Migraine, acute (unlabeled use): Initial: 500-750 mg.; an additional 250-500 mg may be given if needed (maximum: 1250 mg in 24 hours).**Note:** EC-Naprosyn® is not recommended.

Pain (mild-to-moderate), dysmenorrhea, acute tendonitis, bursitis: Initial: 500 mg, then 250 mg every 6-8 hours; maximum: 1250 mg/day naproxen base

Rheumatoid arthritis, osteoarthritis, and ankylosing spondylitis: 500-1000 mg/day in 2 divided doses; may increase to 1.5 g/day of naproxen base for limited time period

OTC labeling: Pain/fever:

Children ≥12 years and Adults ≤65 years: 200 mg naproxen base every 8-12 hours; if needed, may take 400 mg naproxen base for the initial dose; maximum: 600 mg naproxen base/24 hours

Adults >65 years: 200 mg naproxen base every 12 hours

Dosing adjustment in renal impairment: Cl_{cr} <30 mL/minute: use is not recommended

Stability Store oral suspension and tablet at 15°C to 30°C (59°F to 86°F).

Administration Administer with food, milk, or antacids to decrease GI adverse effects

Suspension: Shake suspension well before administration.

Tablet, extended release: Swallow tablet whole; do not break, crush, or chew.

Monitoring Parameters Occult blood loss, periodic liver function test, CBC, BUN, serum creatinine; urine output

Anesthesia and Critical Care Concerns/Other Considerations The 2002 ACCM/SCCM guidelines for analgesia (critically-ill adult) suggest that NSAIDs may be used in combination with opioids in select patients for pain management. Concern about adverse events (increased risk of renal dysfunction, altered platelet function and gastrointestinal irritation) limits its use in patients who have other underlying risks for these events.

In short-term use, NSAIDs vary considerably in their effect on blood pressure. When NSAIDs are used in patients with hypertension, appropriate monitoring of blood pressure responses should be completed and the duration of therapy, when possible, kept short. The use of NSAIDs in the treatment of patients with congestive heart failure may be associated with an increased risk for fluid accumulation and edema; may precipitate renal failure in dehydrated patients.

Pregnancy Risk Factor C/D (3rd trimester)

Contraindications Hypersensitivity to naproxen, aspirin, other NSAIDs, or any component of the formulation; perioperative pain in the setting of coronary artery bypass surgery (CABG); pregnancy (3rd trimester)

Warnings/Precautions

[U.S. Boxed Warning]: NSAIDs are associated with an increased risk of adverse cardiovascular events, including MI, stroke, and new onset or worsening of pre-existing hypertension. Risk may be increased with duration of use or pre-existing cardiovascular risk-factors or disease. Carefully evaluate individual cardiovascular risk profiles prior to prescribing. Use caution with fluid retention, CHF, or hypertension. Use the lowest effective dose for the shortest duration of time, consistent with individual patient goals, to reduce risk of cardiovascular or GI adverse events. Alternate therapies should be considered for patients at high risk.

[U.S. Boxed Warning]: NSAIDs may increase risk of gastrointestinal irritation, ulceration, bleeding, and perforation. These events may occur at any time during therapy and without warning. Use caution with a history of GI disease (bleeding or ulcers), concurrent therapy with aspirin, anticoagulants and/or corticosteroids, smoking, use of alcohol, the elderly or debilitated patients.

Use of NSAIDs can compromise existing renal function. Renal toxicity can occur in patient with impaired renal function, dehydration, heart failure, liver dysfunction, those taking diuretics and ACEI and the elderly. Rehydrate patient before starting therapy. Monitor renal function closely. Naproxen is not recommended for patients with advanced renal disease.

NSAIDs may cause serious skin adverse events including exfoliative dermatitis, Stevens-Johnson Syndrome (SJS) and toxic epidermal necrolysis (TEN). Anaphylactoid reactions may occur, even without prior exposure; patients with "aspirin triad" (bronchial asthma, aspirin intolerance, rhinitis) may be at increased risk. Do not use in patients who experience bronchospasm, asthma, rhinitis, or urticaria with NSAID or aspirin therapy.

Use with caution in patients with decreased hepatic function. Closely monitor patients with any abnormal LFT. Severe hepatic reactions (eg, fulminant hepatitis, liver failure) have occurred with NSAID use, rarely; discontinue if signs or symptoms of liver disease develop, or if systemic manifestations occur.

The elderly are at increased risk for adverse effects (especially peptic ulceration, CNS effects, renal toxicity) from NSAIDs even at low doses.

Withhold for at least 4-6 half-lives prior to surgical or dental procedures. Safety and efficacy have not been established in children <2 years of age.

OTC labeling: Prior to self-medication, patients should contact health care provider if they have had recurring stomach pain or upset, ulcers, bleeding problems, high blood pressure, heart or kidney disease, other serious medical problems, are currently taking a diuretic, or are ≥60 years of age. Recommended dosages should not be exceeded, due to an increased risk of GI bleeding. Consuming ≥3 alcoholic beverages/day or taking longer than recommended may increase the risk of GI bleeding. When used for self-medication, patients should be instructed to contact healthcare provider if used for fever lasting >3 days or for pain lasting >10 days in adults or >3 days in children. Not for self-medication (OTC use) in children <12 years of age.

Adverse Reactions

1% to 10%:

- Cardiovascular: Edema (3% to 9%), palpitations (<3%)
- Central nervous system: Dizziness (3% to 9%), drowsiness (3% to 9%), headache (3% to 9%), lightheadedness (<3%), vertigo (<3%)
- Dermatologic: Pruritus (3% to 9%), skin eruption (3% to 9%), ecchymosis (3% to 9%), purpura (<3%), rash
- Endocrine & metabolic: Fluid retention (3% to 9%)
- Gastrointestinal: Abdominal pain (3% to 9%), constipation (3% to 9%), nausea (3% to 9%), heartburn (3% to 9%), diarrhea (<3%), dyspepsia (<3%), stomatitis (<3%), heartburn (<3%), flatulence, gross bleeding/perforation, indigestion, ulcers, vomiting
- Genitourinary: Abnormal renal function
- Hematologic: Hemolysis (3% to 9%), ecchymosis (3% to 9%), anemia, bleeding time increased
- Hepatic: LFTs increased
- Ocular: Visual disturbances (<3%)
- Otic: Tinnitus (3% to 9%), hearing disturbances (<3%)
- Respiratory: Dyspnea (3% to 9%)
- Miscellaneous: Diaphoresis (<3%), thirst (<3%)

(Continued)

Naproxen *(Continued)*

<1% (Limited to important or life-threatening): Agranulocytosis, alopecia, anaphylactic/anaphylactoid reaction, angioneurotic edema, arrhythmia, aseptic meningitis, asthma, blurred vision, cognitive dysfunction, colitis, coma, confusion, CHF, conjunctivitis, cystitis, depression, dream abnormalities, dysuria, eosinophilia, eosinophilic pneumonitis, erythema multiforme, exfoliative dermatitis, glossitis, granulocytopenia, hallucinations, hematemesis, hepatitis, hyper-/hypoglycemia, hyper-/hypotension, infection, interstitial nephritis, melena, jaundice, leukopenia, liver failure, lymphadenopathy, menstrual disorders, malaise, MI, muscle weakness, myalgia, oliguria, pancreatitis, pancytopenia, paresthesia, photosensitivity, pneumonia, polyuria, proteinuria, pyrexia, rectal bleeding, renal failure, renal papillary necrosis, respiratory depression, sepsis, Stevens-Johnson syndrome, tachycardia, seizure, syncope, thrombocytopenia, toxic epidermal necrolysis ulcerative stomatitis, vasculitis

Overdosage/Toxicology Symptoms of overdose include drowsiness, heartburn, vomiting, CNS depression, leukocytosis, and renal failure. Management is supportive and symptomatic. Seizures tend to be very short-lived and often do not require drug treatment.

Drug Interactions Substrate (minor) of CYP1A2, 2C9

ACE inhibitors: Antihypertensive effects may be decreased by concurrent therapy with NSAIDs; monitor blood pressure.

Angiotensin II antagonists: Antihypertensive effects may be decreased by concurrent therapy with NSAIDs; monitor blood pressure.

Anticoagulants (warfarin, heparin, LMWHs) in combination with NSAIDs can cause increased risk of bleeding.

Antiplatelet drugs (ticlopidine, clopidogrel, aspirin, abciximab, dipyridamole, eptifibatide, tirofiban) can cause an increased risk of bleeding.

Beta-blockers: NSAIDs may decrease the antihypertensive effect of beta-blockers. Monitor.

Cholestyramine (and other bile acid sequestrants): May decrease the absorption of NSAIDs. Separate by at least 2 hours.

Corticosteroids may increase the risk of GI ulceration; avoid concurrent use.

Cyclosporine: NSAIDs may increase serum creatinine, potassium, blood pressure, and cyclosporine levels; monitor cyclosporine levels and renal function carefully.

Hydralazine's antihypertensive effect is decreased; avoid concurrent use.

Lithium levels can be increased; avoid concurrent use if possible or monitor lithium levels and adjust dose. Sulindac may have the least effect. When NSAID is stopped, lithium will need adjustment again.

Loop diuretics efficacy (diuretic and antihypertensive effect) is reduced. Indomethacin reduces this efficacy, however, it may be anticipated with any NSAID.

Methotrexate: Severe bone marrow suppression, aplastic anemia, and GI toxicity have been reported with concomitant NSAID therapy. Avoid use during moderate or high-dose methotrexate (increased and prolonged methotrexate levels). NSAID use during low-dose treatment of rheumatoid arthritis has not been fully evaluated; extreme caution is warranted.

Thiazides antihypertensive effects are decreased; avoid concurrent use.

Warfarin's INRs may be increased by naproxen. Other NSAIDs may have the same effect depending on dose and duration. Monitor INR closely. Use the lowest dose of NSAIDs possible and for the briefest duration.

Ethanol/Nutrition/Herb Interactions

Ethanol: Avoid ethanol (may enhance gastric mucosal irritation).

Food: Naproxen absorption ratelevels may be decreased if taken with food.

Herb/Nutraceutical: Avoid alfalfa, anise, bilberry, bladderwrack, bromelain, cat's claw, celery, coleus, cordyceps, dong quai, evening primrose, feverfew, fenugreek, garlic, ginger, ginkgo biloboa, red clover, horse chestnut, grapeseed, green tea, ginseng, guggul, horse chestnut seed, horseradish, licorice, prickly ash, red clover, reishi, SAMe, sweet clover, turmeric, white willow (all have additional antiplatelet activity).

Test Interactions Naproxen may interfere with 5-HIAA urinary assays; due to an interaction with m-di-nitrobenzene, naproxen should be discontinued 72 hours before adrenal function testing if teh Porter-Silber test is used.

Dietary Considerations Drug may cause GI upset, bleeding, ulceration, perforation; take with food or milk to minimize GI upset.

Dosage Forms

Caplet, as sodium (Aleve®, Midol® Extended Relief, Pamprin® Maximum Strength All Day Relief): 220 mg [equivalent to naproxen 200 mg and sodium 20 mg]

Gelcap, as sodium (Aleve®): 220 mg [equivalent to naproxen 200 mg and sodium 20 mg]

Suspension, oral (Naprosyn®): 125 mg/5 mL (480 mL) [contains sodium 0.3 mEq/mL; orange-pineapple flavor]

Tablet (Naprosyn®): 250 mg, 375 mg, 500 mg

Tablet, as sodium: 220 mg [equivalent to naproxen 200 mg and sodium 20 mg]; 275 mg [equivalent to naproxen 250 mg and sodium 25 mg]; 550 mg [equivalent to naproxen 500 mg and sodium 50 mg]

Aleve®: 220 mg [equivalent to naproxen 200 mg and sodium 20 mg]

Anaprox®: 275 mg [equivalent to naproxen 250 mg and sodium 25 mg]

Anaprox® DS: 550 mg [equivalent to naproxen 500 mg and sodium 50 mg]

Tablet, controlled release, as sodium: 550 mg [equivalent to naproxen 500 mg and sodium 50 mg]

Naprelan®: 421.5 mg [equivalent to naproxen 375 mg and sodium 37.5 mg]; 550 mg [equivalent to naproxen 500 mg and sodium 50 mg]

Tablet, delayed release (EC-Naprosyn®): 375 mg, 500 mg

♦ **Naproxen Sodium** *see* Naproxen *on page 899*

Naratriptan (NAR a trip tan)

Medication Safety Issues

Sound-alike/look-alike issues:

Amerge® may be confused with Altace®, Amaryl®

U.S. Brand Names Amerge®

Canadian Brand Names Amerge®

Synonyms Naratriptan Hydrochloride

Pharmacologic Category Serotonin 5-HT_{1D} Receptor Agonist

Generic Available No

Use Treatment of acute migraine headache with or without aura

Mechanism of Action The therapeutic effect for migraine is due to serotonin agonist activity

Pharmacodynamics/Kinetics

Onset of action: 30 minutes

Absorption: Well absorbed

Protein binding, plasma: 28% to 31%

Metabolism: Hepatic via CYP

Bioavailability: 70%

Time to peak: 2-3 hours

Excretion: Urine

Dosage

Adults: Oral: 1-2.5 mg at the onset of headache; it is recommended to use the lowest possible dose to minimize adverse effects. If headache returns or does not fully resolve, the dose may be repeated after 4 hours; do not exceed 5 mg in 24 hours.

Elderly: Not recommended for use in the elderly

Dosing in renal impairment:

Cl_{cr}: 18-39 mL/minute: Initial: 1 mg; do not exceed 2.5 mg in 24 hours

Cl_{cr}: <15 mL/minute: Do not use

Dosing in hepatic impairment: Contraindicated in patients with severe liver failure; maximum dose: 2.5 mg in 24 hours for patients with mild or moderate liver failure; recommended starting dose: 1 mg

Administration Do **not** crush or chew tablet; swallow whole with water.

Anesthesia and Critical Care Concerns/Other Considerations Naratriptan should not be used in patients with a history of vasospastic disease, Prinzmetal's angina, or any critical vascular disease.

Pregnancy Risk Factor C

Contraindications Hypersensitivity to naratriptan or any component of the formulation; cerebrovascular, peripheral vascular disease (ischemic bowel disease), ischemic heart disease (angina pectoris, history of myocardial infarction, or proven silent ischemia); or in patients with symptoms consistent with ischemic heart disease, coronary artery vasospasm, or Prinzmetal's angina; uncontrolled hypertension or patients who have received within 24 hours another 5-HT agonist (sumatriptan, zolmitriptan) or ergotamine-containing product; patients with known (Continued)

Naratriptan *(Continued)*

risk factors associated with coronary artery disease; patients with severe hepatic or renal disease (Cl_{cr} <15 mL/minute); do not administer naratriptan to patients with hemiplegic or basilar migraine

Warnings/Precautions Use only if there is a clear diagnosis of migraine. May cause vasospastic reactions resulting in colonic, peripheral, or coronary ischemia. Monitor closely, especially after the first dose. Patients who are at risk of CAD (based on risk factor evaluation) but have had a satisfactory cardiovascular evaluation may receive naratriptan, but extreme caution should be used; administration of the first dose in a setting with medical staff and equipment (ie, in a physician's office) is recommended, and ECG monitoring after the first dose should be considered. Periodically re-evaluate risk factors for CAD in patients receiving long-term intermittent treatment. Blood pressure may increase with the administration of naratriptan. If the patient does not respond to the first dose, re-evaluate the diagnosis of migraine before trying a second dose.

Adverse Reactions

1% to 10%:

Central nervous system: Dizziness, drowsiness, malaise/fatigue

Gastrointestinal: Nausea, vomiting

Neuromuscular & skeletal: Paresthesias

Miscellaneous: Pain or pressure in throat or neck

<1% (Limited to important or life-threatening): Allergic reaction, atrial fibrillation, atrial flutter, coronary artery vasospasm, hallucinations, MI, PR prolongation, premature ventricular contractions, QT_c prolongation, seizure, ventricular fibrillation, ventricular tachycardia

Drug Interactions

Decreased effect: Smoking increases the clearance of naratriptan

Increased effect/toxicity: Ergot-containing drugs (dihydroergotamine or methysergide) may cause vasospastic reactions when taken with naratriptan. Avoid concomitant use with ergots; separate dose of naratriptan and ergots by at least 24 hours. Oral contraceptives taken with naratriptan reduced the clearance of naratriptan ~30% which may contribute to adverse effects. Selective serotonin reuptake inhibitors (SSRIs) (eg, fluoxetine, fluvoxamine, paroxetine, sertraline) may cause lack of coordination, hyper-reflexia, or weakness and should be avoided when taking naratriptan.

Dosage Forms Tablet: 1 mg, 2.5 mg

- ♦ **Naratriptan Hydrochloride** *see* Naratriptan *on page 903*
- ♦ **Narcan® [DSC]** *see* Naloxone *on page 895*
- ♦ **Nardil®** *see* Phenelzine *on page 1005*
- ♦ **Naropin®** *see* Ropivacaine *on page 1140*
- ♦ **Nasacort® AQ** *see* Triamcinolone *on page 1311*
- ♦ **NaSal™ [OTC]** *see* Sodium Chloride *on page 1183*
- ♦ **Nasalide® (Can)** *see* Flunisolide *on page 537*
- ♦ **Nasal Moist® [OTC]** *see* Sodium Chloride *on page 1183*
- ♦ **Nasarel®** *see* Flunisolide *on page 537*

Natalizumab (na ta LIZ u mab)

U.S. Brand Names Tysabri®

Synonyms AN100226; Anti-4 Alpha Integrin; IgG4-Kappa Monoclonal Antibody

Pharmacologic Category Monoclonal Antibody, Selective Adhesion-Molecule Inhibitor

Restrictions Patients must be enrolled in the TOUCH Prescribing Program (800-456-2255) to receive natalizumab. Healthcare providers must also register with the program in order to prescribe, dispense or administer natalizumab. A Medication Guide is available (http://www.biogenidec.com/site/TYSABRI-PI-MedGuide.pdf) and should be provided to every patient prior to initiation of therapy.

Generic Available No

Use Treatment of relapsing forms of multiple sclerosis

Unlabeled/Investigational Use Crohn's disease

Mechanism of Action Natalizumab is a monoclonal antibody to the alpha-4 subunit of integrin molecules. These molecules are important to adhesion and migration of cells from the vasculature into inflamed tissue. Natalizumab blocks integrin association with vascular receptors, limiting adhesion and transmigration of leukocytes. Efficacy in specific disorders may be related to reduction in specific inflammatory cell populations in target tissues. In multiple sclerosis, efficacy may be related to blockade of T-lymphocyte migration into the central nervous system; treatment results in a decreased frequency of relapse.

Pharmacodynamics/Kinetics

Distribution: 3.8-7.6 L

Half-life elimination: 7-15 days

Excretion: Clearance: 11-21 mL/hour

Dosage I.V.: Adults:

Multiple sclerosis: 300 mg infused over 1 hour every 4 weeks

Crohn's disease (unlabeled use): 3-6 mg/kg, followed by a second infusion 4 weeks later

Dosage adjustment in renal impairment: No adjustment recommended

Dosage adjustment in hepatic impairment: Not studied

Stability Store concentrated solution under refrigeration between 2°C to 8°C (36°F to 46°F); protect from light; do not shake or freeze. Dilute natalizumab 300 mg in NS 100 mL. Gently invert to mix; do not shake. Following dilution, may store refrigerated for use within up to 8 hours.

Administration Solution may be warmed to room temperature prior to administration. Diluted solution should be infused over 1 hour; do not administer by I.V. bolus or push. Patients should be closely monitored for signs and symptoms of hypersensitivity during the infusion and for at least 1 hour after the infusion is complete. The infusion should be discontinued if a reaction occurs, and treatment of the reaction should be instituted. Following infusion, flush line with NS.

Monitoring Parameters Monitor for hypersensitivity reactions during, and for 1 hour after, infusion.

Signs or symptoms of progressive multifocal leukoencephalopathy (focal neurologic deficits, which may present as hemiparesis, visual field deficits, cognitive impairment, aphasia, ataxia, and/or cranial nerve deficits); baseline and postinfusion gadolinium-enhanced MRIs (at 3 and 6 months after first infusion; every 6 months thereafter); CSF analysis for JC viral DNA. **Note:** Transient and reversible leukocytosis (excluding neutrophils) and mildly reduced hemoglobin may occur with treatment and may require ~4 months for return to baseline values after the last dose.

Pregnancy Risk Factor C

Contraindications Hypersensitivity to natalizumab, murine proteins, or any component of the formulation; pregnancy

Warnings/Precautions [U.S. Boxed Warning]: Increased risk of developing fatal or disabling progressive multifocal leukoencephalopathy (PML); patients must be routinely monitored for signs of PML with baseline and periodic MRI evaluations; access to and provision of therapy requires registration of patients and healthcare providers; concurrent immunomodulator therapy or immunosuppression may be risk factors for the development of PML. Use may be associated with an increased risk of opportunistic infection; concurrent use of antineoplastic, immunosuppressant (including short course corticosteroids) or immunomodulating agents may increase this risk. During clinical studies, ~22% of patients experienced an infusion-related reaction; serious systemic hypersensitivity reactions occurred in <1% of patients. Severe reactions, including anaphylaxis, occur rarely; upon presentation, the infusion should be discontinued immediately. Retreatment is not recommended. Infusion-related reactions may occur more frequently in patients with antibody to natalizumab. Antibody formation (which occurs in about 10% of patients) is associated with a decrease in natalizumab levels and a decrease in the efficacy of natalizumab. Use caution in patients with a history of depression; closely monitor. Safety and efficacy have not been established in chronic progressive multiple sclerosis, for therapy longer than 2 years, or in children (<18 years of age).

Adverse Reactions

>10%:

Central nervous system: Headache (38%), fatigue (27%), depression (19%)

Dermatologic: Rash (12%)

Gastrointestinal: Gastroenteritis (11%), abdominal discomfort (11%)

Genitourinary: Urinary tract infection (21%)

Neuromuscular & skeletal: Arthralgia (19%), extremity pain (16%)

Respiratory: Lower respiratory infection (17%)

Miscellaneous: Infusion-related reaction (24%)

(Continued)

Natalizumab *(Continued)*

1% to 10%:

Cardiovascular: Chest discomfort (5%), peripheral edema (5%)

Central nervous system: Vertigo (6%), syncope (2%), somnolence (2%)

Dermatologic: Dermatitis (7%), pruritus (4%), urticaria (2%)

Endocrine & metabolic: Menstrual irregularities (5%), dysmenorrhea (3%), amenorrhea (2%), ovarian cyst (2%)

Gastrointestinal: Diarrhea (10%), weight changes (2%), cholelithiasis (1%)

Genitourinary: Vaginitis (10%), urinary frequency (9%), urinary incontinence (4%)

Hepatic: Transaminase abnormal (5%)

Local: Bleeding at injection site (3%)

Neuromuscular & skeletal: Muscle cramp (5%), rigors (3%), tremor (3%), joint swelling (2%)

Respiratory: Tonsillitis (7%)

Miscellaneous: Tooth infection (9%), herpes (8%), hypersensitivity reactions (4% to 5%, anaphylaxis/anaphylactoid <1%), serious infection (3%), anaphylaxis (1%), night sweats (1%)

<1% (Limited to important or life-threatening): Appendicitis, opportunistic infections (including progressive multifocal leukoencephalopathy, meningitis, and bronchopulmonary infections), pneumonia, suicidal ideation

Overdosage/Toxicology Safety of doses >300 mg has not been evaluated. Treatment should be symptom-directed and supportive.

Drug Interactions

Immunosuppressive therapy: Concomitant therapy with natalizumab may increase the risk of infection.

Interferon beta-1a: May increase the levels of natalizumab; no dosage adjustment necessary.

Dosage Forms Injection, solution [preservative free]: 300 mg/15 mL (15 mL) [contains polysorbate-80]

References

Ghosh S, Goldin E, Gordon FH, et al, "Natalizumab for Active Crohn's Disease," *N Engl J Med*, 2003, 348(1):24-32.

- **Natrecor®** *see* Nesiritide *on page 913*
- **Natriuretic Peptide** *see* Nesiritide *on page 913*
- **Natural Lung Surfactant** *see* Beractant *on page 168*
- **Naxen® (Can)** *see* Naproxen *on page 899*
- **Naxen® EC (Can)** *see* Naproxen *on page 899*
- **Na-Zone® [OTC]** *see* Sodium Chloride *on page 1183*
- **NebuPent®** *see* Pentamidine *on page 997*

Nelfinavir (nel FIN a veer)

Medication Safety Issues

Sound-alike/look-alike issues:

Nelfinavir may be confused with nevirapine

Viracept® may be confused with Viramune®

U.S. Brand Names Viracept®

Canadian Brand Names Viracept®

Synonyms NFV

Pharmacologic Category Antiretroviral Agent, Protease Inhibitor

Generic Available No

Use In combination with other antiretroviral therapy in the treatment of HIV infection

Mechanism of Action Inhibits the HIV-1 protease; inhibition of the viral protease prevents cleavage of the gag-pol polyprotein resulting in the production of immature, noninfectious virus

Pharmacodynamics/Kinetics

Absorption: Food increases plasma concentration-time curve (AUC) by two- to threefold

Distribution: V_d: 2-7 L/kg

Protein binding: 98%

Metabolism: Hepatic via CYP2C19 and 3A4; major metabolite has activity comparable to parent drug

Half-life elimination: 3.5-5 hours

Time to peak, serum: 2-4 hours

Excretion: Feces (98% to 99%, 78% as metabolites, 22% as unchanged drug); urine (1% to 2%)

Dosage Oral:

Children 2-13 years: 45-55 mg/kg twice daily **or** 25-35 mg/kg 3 times/day (maximum: 2500 mg/day); all doses should be taken with a meal. If tablets are unable to be taken, use oral powder in small amount of water, milk, formula, or dietary supplements; do not use acidic food/juice or store for >6 hours.

Adults: 750 mg 3 times/day with meals or 1250 mg twice daily with meals in combination with other antiretroviral therapies

Dosing adjustment in renal impairment: No adjustment needed

Dosing adjustment in hepatic impairment: Use caution

Stability Store at room temperature of 15°C to 30°C (59°F to 86°F). Oral powder (or dissolved tablets) diluted in nonacidic liquid is stable for 6 hours under refrigeration.

Administration Mix powder or tablets in a small amount of water, milk, formula, soy milk, soy formula, or dietary supplement. Be sure entire contents is consumed to receive full dose. Do not use acidic food/juice to dilute due to bitter taste. One mixed, solution should be used immediately, but may be stored for up to 6 hours if refrigerated.

Monitoring Parameters Liver function tests, viral load, CD4 count, triglycerides, cholesterol, blood glucose, CBC with differential

Pregnancy Risk Factor B

Contraindications Hypersensitivity to nelfinavir or any component of the formulation; concurrent therapy with amiodarone, ergot derivatives, midazolam, pimozide, quinidine, triazolam; additional medications which should not be coadministered (per manufacturer) include lovastatin and simvastatin

Warnings/Precautions Nelfinavir is hepatically metabolized and has multiple drug interactions. A listing of medications that should not be used is available with each bottle and patients should be provided with this information. Use caution with hepatic impairment. Warn patients that redistribution of body fat can occur. New onset diabetes mellitus, exacerbation of diabetes, and hyperglycemia have been reported in HIV-infected patients receiving protease inhibitors. Immune reconstitution syndrome, characterized by an inflammatory response to indolent or residual opportunistic infections, has been reported with nelfinavir; further evaluation and treatment may be required. The oral powder contains phenylalanine; use caution in patients with phenylketonuria.

Adverse Reactions

>10%: Gastrointestinal: Diarrhea

2% to 10%:

Dermatologic: Rash

Gastrointestinal: Nausea, flatulence

Hematologic: Abnormal creatine kinase, hemoglobin, lymphocytes, neutrophils

Hepatic: Abnormal ALT, AST

<2% (Limited to important or life-threatening): Acute iritis, allergic reaction, amylase increased, anemia, anorexia, anxiety, arthralgia, back pain, bilirubinemia, body fat redistribution/accumulation, creatinine phosphokinase increased, dehydration, depression, diaphoresis, dizziness, dyspepsia, dyspnea, epigastric pain, fever, folliculitis, gamma glutamyl transpeptidase increased, gastrointestinal bleeding, headache, hepatitis, hyperkinesia, hyperglycemia, hyperlipemia; hypersensitivity reaction (bronchospasm, rash, edema); hyperuricemia, hypoglycemia, insomnia, jaundice, kidney calculus, lactic dehydrogenase increased, leukopenia, maculopapular rash, metabolic acidosis, myalgia, myasthenia, myopathy, pain, pancreatitis, paresthesia, pruritus, QT_c prolongation, seizure, sexual dysfunction, sleep disorder, somnolence, suicidal ideation, thrombocytopenia, torsade de pointes, urticaria, vomiting, weakness

Overdosage/Toxicology Limited data available; however, unabsorbed drug should be removed via gastric lavage and activated charcoal; significant symptoms beyond gastrointestinal disturbances are likely following acute overdose; hemodialysis will not be effective due to high protein binding of nelfinavir

Drug Interactions Substrate of CYP2C9 (minor), 2C19 (major), 2D6 (minor), 3A4 (major); **Inhibits** CYP1A2 (weak), 2B6 (weak), 2C9 (weak), 2C19 (weak), 2D6 (weak), 3A4 (strong)

Amiodarone: Serum levels/toxicity may be increased by nelfinavir; serious and/or life-threatening reactions may occur; concurrent use is contraindicated.

(Continued)

Nelfinavir *(Continued)*

Anticonvulsants: Phenobarbital, and carbamazepine may decrease serum levels and consequently effectiveness of nelfinavir. Nelfinavir may decrease plasma levels of phenytoin. Consider obtaining nelfinavir levels.

Azithromycin: Serum levels may be increased by azithromycin; monitor

Benzodiazepines: An increase in midazolam and triazolam serum levels may occur resulting in significant oversedation when administered with nelfinavir. Concurrent use is contraindicated. Use caution with other benzodiazepines.

Cisapride: Nelfinavir inhibits the metabolism of cisapride and should, not be administered concurrently due to risk of life-threatening cardiac arrhythmias.

Corticosteroids (eg, fluticasone): Serum concentrations may be increased by nelfinavir, resulting in decreased serum cortisol and HPA axis suppression; monitor.

CYP2C19 inducers: May decrease the levels/effects of nelfinavir. Example inducers include aminoglutethimide, carbamazepine, phenytoin, and rifampin.

CYP3A4 inducers: CYP3A4 inducers may decrease the levels/effects of nelfinavir. Example inducers include aminoglutethimide, carbamazepine, nafcillin, nevirapine, phenobarbital, phenytoin, and rifamycins.

CYP3A4 substrates: Nelfinavir may increase the levels/effects of CYP3A4 substrates. Example substrates include benzodiazepines, calcium channel blockers, mirtazapine, nateglinide, nefazodone, tacrolimus, and venlafaxine. Selected benzodiazepines (midazolam and triazolam), cisapride, ergot alkaloids, selected HMG-CoA reductase inhibitors (lovastatin and simvastatin), and pimozide are generally contraindicated with strong CYP3A4 inhibitors.

Ergot alkaloids: Serum levels/toxicity may be increased by nelfinavir; serious and/or life-threatening reactions may occur; concurrent use is contraindicated.

HMG-CoA reductase inhibitors: Nelfinavir may increase levels of HMG-CoA reductase inhibitors, increasing the risk of myopathy. Lovastatin and simvastatin should not be coadministered with nelfinavir (per manufacturer). Atorvastatin may be used with careful monitoring, in the lowest dose possible. Fluvastatin and pravastatin may have lowest risk.

Immunosuppressants: Nelfinavir may increase the serum levels of cyclosporine, sirolimus or tacrolimus.

Methadone: Serum levels of methadone are decreased by nelfinavir.

Non-nucleoside reverse transcriptase inhibitors: Nevirapine decreases serum levels of nelfinavir. When used with delavirdine, serum levels of nelfinavir are increased and levels of delavirdine are decreased. The safety of these combinations has not been established.

Oral contraceptives: Serum levels of the hormones in oral contraceptives may decrease significantly with administration of nelfinavir. Patients should use alternative methods of contraceptives during nelfinavir therapy. Ethinyl estradiol, norethindrone concentrations are decreased by nelfinavir.

Pimozide: Serum levels/toxicity may be increased by nelfinavir; serious and/or life-threatening reactions may occur; concurrent use is contraindicated.

Protease inhibitors: Serum levels of both nelfinavir and indinavir are increased with concurrent use; nelfinavir increases serum levels of saquinavir; ritonavir increase serum levels of nelfinavir. The safety of these combinations has not been established.

Quinidine: Serum levels/toxicity may be increased by nelfinavir; serious and/or life-threatening reactions may occur; concurrent use is contraindicated.

Rifabutin: A 200% increase in rifabutin plasma AUC has been observed when coadministered with nelfinavir (decrease rifabutin's dose by 50%).

Rifampin: Rifampin decreases nelfinavir's plasma AUC by ~82%; loss of virologic response and resistance may occur; the two drugs should not be administered together.

Sildenafil: Sildenafil serum concentration may be substantially increased (do not exceed single doses of 25 mg in 48 hours).

St John's wort (*Hypericum perforatum*): Appears to induce CYP3A enzymes and may lead to reduction in trough serum concentrations, which may lead to treatment failures. Alternatively, changes may involve P-glycoprotein. The two drugs should not be used together.

Tadalafil: Serum concentrations may be increased by nelfinavir. A maximum tadalafil dose of 10 mg in 72 hours is recommended with strong CYP3A4 inhibitors.

Vardenafil: Serum concentrations may be increased by nelfinavir. Specific dosage adjustment guidelines have not been established. Recommendations for other strong CYP3A4 inhibitors include vardenafil dose not to exceed 2.5 mg in 24 hours.

Ethanol/Nutrition/Herb Interactions

Food: Nelfinavir taken with food increases plasma concentration time curve (AUC) by two- to threefold. Do not administer with acidic food or juice (orange juice, apple juice, or applesauce) since the combination may have a bitter taste.

Herb/Nutraceutical: St John's wort may decrease nelfinavir serum concentrations; avoid concurrent use.

Dietary Considerations Should be taken as scheduled with food. Oral powder contains phenylalanine 11.2 mg/g.

Dosage Forms

Powder, oral: 50 mg/g (144 g) [contains phenylalanine 11.2 mg/g]

Tablet: 250 mg, 625 mg

♦ **Nembutal®** *see* Pentobarbital *on page 999*

♦ **Nembutal® Sodium (Can)** *see* Pentobarbital *on page 999*

♦ **Neo-Fradin™** *see* Neomycin *on page 909*

Neomycin (nee oh MYE sin)

Medication Safety Issues

Sound-alike/look-alike issues:

Myciguent may be confused with Mycitracin®

Related Information

Prevention of Wound Infection and Sepsis in Surgical Patients *on page 1588*

U.S. Brand Names Neo-Fradin™; Neo-Rx

Synonyms Neomycin Sulfate

Pharmacologic Category Ammonium Detoxicant; Antibiotic, Aminoglycoside; Antibiotic, Topical

Generic Available Yes

Use Orally to prepare GI tract for surgery; topically to treat minor skin infections; treatment of diarrhea caused by *E. coli*; adjunct in the treatment of hepatic encephalopathy; bladder irrigation; ocular infections

Mechanism of Action Interferes with bacterial protein synthesis by binding to 30S ribosomal subunits

Pharmacodynamics/Kinetics

Absorption: Oral, percutaneous: Poor (3%)

Distribution: V_d: 0.36 L/kg

Metabolism: Slightly hepatic

Half-life elimination (age and renal function dependent): 3 hours

Time to peak, serum: Oral: 1-4 hours

Excretion: Feces (97% of oral dose as unchanged drug); urine (30% to 50% of absorbed drug as unchanged drug)

Dosage

Children: Oral:

Preoperative intestinal antisepsis: 90 mg/kg/day divided every 4 hours for 2 days; or 25 mg/kg at 1 PM, 2 PM, and 11 PM on the day preceding surgery as an adjunct to mechanical cleansing of the intestine and in combination with erythromycin base

Hepatic encephalopathy: 50-100 mg/kg/day in divided doses every 6-8 hours or 2.5-7 g/m²/day divided every 4-6 hours for 5-6 days not to exceed 12 g/day

Children and Adults: Topical: Topical solutions containing 0.1% to 1% neomycin have been used for irrigation

Adults: Oral:

Preoperative intestinal antisepsis: 1 g each hour for 4 doses then 1 g every 4 hours for 5 doses; or 1 g at 1 PM, 2 PM, and 11 PM on day preceding surgery as an adjunct to mechanical cleansing of the bowel and oral erythromycin; or 6 g/day divided every 4 hours for 2-3 days

Hepatic encephalopathy: 500-2000 mg every 6-8 hours or 4-12 g/day divided every 4-6 hours for 5-6 days

Chronic hepatic insufficiency: 4 g/day for an indefinite period

Monitoring Parameters Renal function tests, audiometry in symptomatic patients

Pregnancy Risk Factor D

Contraindications Hypersensitivity to neomycin or any component of the formulation, or other aminoglycosides; intestinal obstruction

(Continued)

Neomycin *(Continued)*

Warnings/Precautions [U.S. Boxed Warning]: May cause neurotoxicity, nephrotoxicity, and/or neuromuscular blockade and respiratory paralysis; usual risk factors include prexisiting renal impairment, concomitant neuro-/nephrotoxic medications, advanced age and dehydration. The drug's neurotoxicity can result in respiratory paralysis from neuromuscular blockade, especially when the drug is given soon after anesthesia or muscle relaxants. Use with caution in patients with renal impairment, pre-existing hearing impairment, neuromuscular disorders; neomycin is more toxic than other aminoglycosides when given parenterally; **do not administer parenterally**; topical neomycin is a contact sensitizer with sensitivity occurring in 5% to 15% of patients treated with the drug; symptoms include itching, reddening, edema, and failure to heal; **do not use as peritoneal lavage** due to significant systemic adsorption of the drug

Adverse Reactions

Oral:

>10%: Gastrointestinal: Nausea, diarrhea, vomiting, irritation or soreness of the mouth or rectal area

<1% (Limited to important or life-threatening): Dyspnea, eosinophilia, nephrotoxicity, neurotoxicity, ototoxicity (auditory), ototoxicity (vestibular)

Topical: >10%: Dermatologic: Contact dermatitis

Overdosage/Toxicology Symptoms of overdose (rare due to poor oral bioavailability) include ototoxicity, nephrotoxicity, and neuromuscular toxicity. The treatment of choice following a single acute overdose appears to be maintenance of urine output of at least 3 mL/kg/hour during the acute treatment phase. Dialysis is of questionable value in enhancing aminoglycoside elimination. If required, hemodialysis is preferred over peritoneal dialysis in patients with normal renal function. Chelation with penicillin may be of benefit.

Drug Interactions

Decreased effect: May decrease GI absorption of digoxin and methotrexate

Increased effect: Synergistic effects with penicillins

Increased toxicity:

- Oral neomycin may potentiate the effects of oral anticoagulants
- Increased adverse effects with other neurotoxic, ototoxic, or nephrotoxic drugs

Dosage Forms

Powder, micronized, as sulfate [for prescription compounding] (Neo-Rx): (10 g, 100 g)

Solution, oral, as sulfate (Neo-Fradin™): 125 mg/5 mL (60 mL, 480 mL) [contains benzoic acid; cherry flavor]

Tablet, as sulfate: 500 mg

References

"Antimicrobial Prophylaxis for Surgery," *Treat Guidel Med Lett*, 2004, 2(20):27-32.

- **Neomycin Sulfate** *see* Neomycin *on page 909*
- **Neonatal Trace Metals** *see* Trace Metals *on page 1296*
- **NeoProfen®** *see* Ibuprofen *on page 651*
- **Neoral®** *see* CycloSPORINE *on page 337*
- **Neo-Rx** *see* Neomycin *on page 909*

Neostigmine (nee oh STIG meen)

Medication Safety Issues

Sound-alike/look-alike issues:

Prostigmin® may be confused with physostigmine

Related Information

Chronic Renal Failure *on page 1437*

U.S. Brand Names Prostigmin®

Canadian Brand Names Prostigmin®

Synonyms Neostigmine Bromide; Neostigmine Methylsulfate

Pharmacologic Category Acetylcholinesterase Inhibitor

Generic Available Yes: Injection

Use Diagnosis and treatment of myasthenia gravis; prevention and treatment of postoperative bladder distention and urinary retention; reversal of the effects of nondepolarizing neuromuscular-blocking agents after surgery

Mechanism of Action Inhibits destruction of acetylcholine by acetylcholinesterase which facilitates transmission of impulses across myoneural junction

Pharmacodynamics/Kinetics

Onset of action: I.M.: 20-30 minutes; I.V.: 1-20 minutes

Duration: I.M.: 2.5-4 hours; I.V.: 1-2 hours

Absorption: Oral: Poor, <2%

Metabolism: Hepatic

Half-life elimination: Normal renal function: 0.5-2.1 hours; End-stage renal disease: Prolonged

Excretion: Urine (50% as unchanged drug)

Dosage

Myasthenia gravis: Diagnosis: I.M.:

Children: 0.04 mg/kg as a single dose

Adults: 0.02 mg/kg as a single dose

Myasthenia gravis: Treatment:

Children:

Oral: 2 mg/kg/day divided every 3-4 hours

I.M., I.V., SubQ: 0.01-0.04 mg/kg every 2-4 hours

Adults:

Oral: 15 mg/dose every 3-4 hours up to 375 mg/day maximum; interval between doses must be individualized to maximal response

I.M., I.V., SubQ: 0.5-2.5 mg every 1-3 hours up to 10 mg/24 hours maximum

Reversal of nondepolarizing neuromuscular blockade after surgery in conjunction with atropine (must administer atropine several minutes prior to neostigmine): I.V.:

Infants: 0.025-0.1 mg/kg/dose

Children: 0.025-0.08 mg/kg/dose

Adults: 0.5-2.5 mg; total dose not to exceed 5 mg

Bladder atony: Adults: I.M., SubQ:

Prevention: 0.25 mg every 4-6 hours for 2-3 days

Treatment: 0.5-1 mg every 3 hours for 5 doses after bladder has emptied

Dosing adjustment in renal impairment:

Cl_{cr} 10-50 mL/minute: Administer 50% of normal dose

Cl_{cr} <10 mL/minute: Administer 25% of normal dose

Administration May be administered undiluted by slow I.V. injection over several minutes

Anesthesia and Critical Care Concerns/Other Considerations Neostigmine has occasionally been used to improve gastrointestinal motility. Researchers from Amsterdam evaluated a neostigmine infusion (0.4-0.8 mg/hour over 24 hours) in patients with critical illness-related colonic ileus in a randomized, placebo-controlled, double-blind manner (van der Spoel, 2001). Twenty four ICU patients were evaluated and 13 patients initially received neostigmine. Eleven of the patients in the active treatment group passed stools whereas none of the placebo group did. The median time to defecation was 6 hours. None of the patients had the infusion stopped or reduced because of adverse events. Three patients had an increase in saliva and sputum production. No cardiac complications were observed. Three patients developed ischemic colon 7-10 days after treatment. No difference was found in APACHE scores between patients with colonic ischemia and those without, but the median dopamine dose was significantly higher (16 mcg/kg/minute) in patients with ischemia than those without (8 mcg/kg/minute).

Ponec and his associates (1999) studied the use of a single intravenous dose of neostigmine (2 mg over 3-5 minutes) in 21 surgical or medical patients with acute colonic pseudo-obstruction (cecal diameter >10 cm). Patients were randomized to receive neostigmine or placebo and a blinded physician evaluated their responses. Patients received continuous ECG monitoring and atropine was immediately available for treatment of bradycardia. Ten of the 11 patients receiving neostigmine had prompt colonic decompression with a median time to response of 4 minutes. Two that had an initial response to neostigmine required colonic decompression for recurrence of distention. Adverse events included abdominal pain, excessive salivation, and vomiting. In addition, 2 patients had symptomatic bradycardia requiring atropine.

Pregnancy Risk Factor C

Contraindications Hypersensitivity to neostigmine, bromides, or any component of the formulation; GI or GU obstruction

Warnings/Precautions Does **not** antagonize and may prolong the phase I block of depolarizing muscle relaxants (eg, succinylcholine); use with caution in patients with epilepsy, asthma, bradycardia, hyperthyroidism, cardiac arrhythmias, or

(Continued)

Neostigmine *(Continued)*

peptic ulcer; adequate facilities should be available for cardiopulmonary resuscitation when testing and adjusting dose for myasthenia gravis; have atropine and epinephrine ready to treat hypersensitivity reactions; overdosage may result in cholinergic crisis, this must be distinguished from myasthenic crisis; anticholinesterase insensitivity can develop for brief or prolonged periods

Adverse Reactions Frequency not defined.

Cardiovascular: Arrhythmias (especially bradycardia), hypotension, decreased carbon monoxide, tachycardia, AV block, nodal rhythm, nonspecific ECG changes, cardiac arrest, syncope, flushing

Central nervous system: Convulsions, dysarthria, dysphonia, dizziness, loss of consciousness, drowsiness, headache

Dermatologic: Skin rash, thrombophlebitis (I.V.), urticaria

Gastrointestinal: Hyperperistalsis, nausea, vomiting, salivation, diarrhea, stomach cramps, dysphagia, flatulence

Genitourinary: Urinary urgency

Neuromuscular & skeletal: Weakness, fasciculations, muscle cramps, spasms, arthralgia

Ocular: Small pupils, lacrimation

Respiratory: Increased bronchial secretions, laryngospasm, bronchiolar constriction, respiratory muscle paralysis, dyspnea, respiratory depression, respiratory arrest, bronchospasm

Miscellaneous: Diaphoresis (increased), anaphylaxis, allergic reactions

Overdosage/Toxicology Symptoms of overdose include muscle weakness, blurred vision, excessive sweating, tearing and salivation, nausea, vomiting, diarrhea, hypertension, bradycardia, muscle weakness, and paralysis. Atropine sulfate injection should be readily available as an antagonist for the effects of neostigmine.

Drug Interactions

Anticholinergics: Effects may be reduced with cholinesterase inhibitors; atropine antagonizes the muscarinic effects of cholinesterase inhibitors

Beta-blockers without ISA: Activity may increase risk of bradycardia

Calcium channel blockers (diltiazem or verapamil): May increase risk of bradycardia

Cholinergic agonists: Effects may be increased with cholinesterase inhibitors

Corticosteroids: May see increased muscle weakness and decreased response to anticholinesterases shortly after onset of corticosteroid therapy in the treatment of myasthenia gravis. Deterioration in muscle strength, including severe muscular depression, has been documented in patients with myasthenia gravis while receiving corticosteroids and anticholinesterases.

Digoxin: Increased risk of bradycardia with concurrent use

Neuromuscular blockers: Depolarizing neuromuscular blocking agents effects may be increased with cholinesterase inhibitors; nondepolarizing agents are antagonized by cholinesterase inhibitors

Dosage Forms

Injection, solution, as methylsulfate: 0.5 mg/mL (1 mL, 10 mL); 1 mg/mL (10 mL)

Tablet, as bromide: 15 mg

References

Ponec RJ, Saunders MD, and Kimmey MB, "Neostigmine for the Treatment of Acute Colonic Pseudo-Obstruction," *N Engl J Med*, 1999, 341(3):137-41.

van der Spoel JI, Oudemans-van Straaten HM, Stoutenbeek CP, et al, "Neostigmine Resolves Critical Illness-Related Colonic Ileus in Intensive Care Patients With Multiple Organ Failure--A Prospective, Double-Blind, Placebo-Controlled Trial," *Intensive Care Med*, 2001, 27(5):822-7.

♦ **Neostigmine Bromide** *see* Neostigmine *on page 910*

♦ **Neostigmine Methylsulfate** *see* Neostigmine *on page 910*

♦ **Neo-Synephrine® (Can)** *see* Phenylephrine *on page 1015*

♦ **Neo-Synephrine® 12 Hour [OTC]** *see* Oxymetazoline *on page 973*

♦ **Neo-Synephrine® 12 Hour Extra Moisturizing [OTC]** *see* Oxymetazoline *on page 973*

♦ **Neo-Synephrine® Extra Strength [OTC]** *see* Phenylephrine *on page 1015*

♦ **Neo-Synephrine® Mild [OTC]** *see* Phenylephrine *on page 1015*

♦ **Neo-Synephrine® Ophthalmic [DSC]** *see* Phenylephrine *on page 1015*

♦ **Neo-Synephrine® Regular Strength [OTC]** *see* Phenylephrine *on page 1015*

♦ **Neotrace-4®** *see* Trace Metals *on page 1296*

♦ **Nesacaine®** *see* Chloroprocaine *on page 269*

◆ **Nesacaine®-CE (Can)** *see* Chloroprocaine *on page 269*
◆ **Nesacaine®-MPF** *see* Chloroprocaine *on page 269*

Nesiritide (ni SIR i tide)

Medication Safety Issues

High alert medication: The Institute for Safe Medication Practices (ISMP) includes this medication among its list of drugs which have a heightened risk of causing significant patient harm when used in error.

Related Information

Hemodynamic Support, Intravenous *on page 1566*

U.S. Brand Names Natrecor®

Synonyms B-type Natriuretic Peptide (Human); hBNP; Natriuretic Peptide

Pharmacologic Category Natriuretic Peptide, B-Type, Human; Vasodilator

Generic Available No

Use Treatment of acutely decompensated congestive heart failure (CHF) in patients with dyspnea at rest or with minimal activity

Mechanism of Action Binds to guanylate cyclase receptor on vascular smooth muscle and endothelial cells, increasing intracellular cyclic GMP, resulting in smooth muscle cell relaxation. Has been shown to produce dose-dependent reductions in pulmonary capillary wedge pressure (PCWP) and systemic arterial pressure.

Pharmacodynamics/Kinetics

Onset of action: 15 minutes (60% of 3-hour effect achieved)

Duration: >60 minutes (up to several hours) for systolic blood pressure; hemodynamic effects persist longer than serum half-life would predict

Distribution: V_{ss}: 0.19 L/kg

Metabolism: Proteolytic cleavage by vascular endopeptidases and proteolysis following receptor binding and cellular internalization

Half-life elimination: Initial (distribution) 2 minutes; Terminal: 18 minutes

Time to peak: 1 hour

Excretion: Urine

Dosage Adults: I.V.: Initial: 2 mcg/kg (bolus); followed by continuous infusion at 0.01 mcg/kg/minute; **Note:** Should not be initiated at a dosage higher than initial recommended dose. At intervals of ≥3 hours, the dosage may be increased by 0.005 mcg/kg/minute (preceded by a bolus of 1 mcg/kg), up to a maximum of 0.03 mcg/kg/minute. Increases beyond the initial infusion rate should be limited to selected patients and accompanied by hemodynamic monitoring.

Patients experiencing hypotension during the infusion: Infusion should be interrupted. May attempt to restart at a lower dose (reduce initial infusion dose by 30% and omit bolus).

Dosage adjustment in renal impairment: No adjustment required

Stability Vials may be stored at controlled room temperature of 20°C to 25°C (68°F to 77 °F) or under refrigeration at 2°C to 8°C (36°F to 46°F). Following reconstitution, vials are stable under these conditions for up to 24 hours.

Reconstitute 1.5 mg vial with 5 mL of diluent removed from a premixed plastic I.V. bag (compatible with 5% dextrose, 0.9% sodium chloride, 5% dextrose and 0.45% sodium chloride, or 5% dextrose and 0.2% sodium chloride). Do not shake vial to dissolve (roll gently). Withdraw entire contents of vial and add to 250 mL I.V. bag. Resultant concentration of solution approximately 6 mcg/mL.

Administration Do not administer through a heparin-coated catheter (concurrent administration of heparin via a separate catheter is acceptable, per manufacturer).

Prime I.V. tubing with 25 mL of infusion prior to connection with vascular access port and prior to administering bolus or starting the infusion. Withdraw bolus from the prepared infusion bag and administer over 60 seconds. Begin infusion immediately following administration of the bolus. Using a standard 6 mcg/mL concentration, bolus volume in mL = patient weight in kg x 0.33.

Physically incompatible with heparin, insulin, ethacrynate sodium, bumetanide, enalaprilat, hydralazine, and furosemide. Do not administer through the same catheter. Do not administer with any solution containing sodium metabisulfite. Catheter must be flushed between administration of nesiritide and physically incompatible drugs.

Monitoring Parameters Blood pressure, hemodynamic responses (PCWP, RAP, CI)

(Continued)

Nesiritide *(Continued)*

Pregnancy Risk Factor C

Contraindications Hypersensitivity to natriuretic peptide or any component of the formulation; cardiogenic shock (when used as primary therapy); hypotension (systolic blood pressure <90 mm Hg)

Warnings/Precautions May cause hypotension; administer in clinical situations when blood pressure may be closely monitored. Use caution in patients with systolic blood pressure <100 mm Hg (contraindicated if <90 mm Hg); more likely to experience hypotension. Effects may be additive with other agents capable of causing hypotension. Hypotensive effects may last for several hours.

Should not be used in patients with low filling pressures, or in patients with conditions which depend on venous return including significant valvular stenosis, restrictive or obstructive cardiomyopathy, constrictive pericarditis, and pericardial tamponade. May be associated with development of azotemia; use caution in patients with renal impairment or in patients where renal perfusion is dependent on renin-angiotensin-aldosterone system.

Atrial natriuretic peptide (ANP), a related peptide, has been associated with increased vascular permeability and decreased intravascular volume. This has not been observed in clinical trials with nesiritide, however, patients should be monitored for this effect.

Prepared through recombinant technology using *E. coli*; monitor for allergic or anaphylactic reactions. Use caution with prolonged infusions; limited experience for infusions >48 hours. Safety and efficacy in pediatric patients have not been established.

Adverse Reactions Note: Frequencies cited below were recorded in VMAC trial at dosages similar to approved labeling. Higher frequencies have been observed in trials using higher dosages of nesiritide.

>10%:

- Cardiovascular: Hypotension (total: 11%; symptomatic: 4% at recommended dose, up to 17% at higher doses)
- Renal: Increased serum creatinine (28% with >0.5 mg/dL increase over baseline)

1% to 10%:

- Cardiovascular: Ventricular tachycardia (3%)*, ventricular extrasystoles (3%)*, angina (2%)*, bradycardia (1%), tachycardia, atrial fibrillation, AV node conduction abnormalities
- Central nervous system: Headache (8%)*, dizziness (3%)*, insomnia (2%), anxiety (3%), fever, confusion, paresthesia, somnolence, tremor
- Dermatologic: Pruritus, rash
- Gastrointestinal: Nausea (4%)*, abdominal pain (1%)*, vomiting (1%)*
- Hematologic: Anemia
- Local: Injection site reaction
- Neuromuscular & skeletal: Back pain (4%), leg cramps
- Ocular: Amblyopia
- Respiratory: Cough (increased), hemoptysis, apnea
- Miscellaneous: Increased diaphoresis

*Frequency less than or equal to placebo or other standard therapy

Overdosage/Toxicology No data. Symptoms of overdose would be expected to include excessive and/or prolonged hypotension. Treatment is symptomatic and supportive. Drug discontinuation and/or dosage reduction may be required.

Drug Interactions

ACE inhibitors: An increased frequency of symptomatic hypotension was observed with concurrent administration.

Diuretics: Use caution in patients who may have decreased intravascular volume due to diuretic therapy (risk of hypotension and/or renal impairment may be increased). Nesiritide should be avoided in patients with low filling pressures.

Hypotensive agents: Effects on blood pressure are likely to be additive with nesiritide.

Dosage Forms Injection, powder for reconstitution: 1.5 mg

♦ **Neupogen®** *see* Filgrastim *on page 525*
♦ **Neurontin®** *see* Gabapentin *on page 577*
♦ **Neut®** *see* Sodium Bicarbonate *on page 1181*

Nevirapine (ne VYE ra peen)

Medication Safety Issues

Sound-alike/look-alike issues:

Nevirapine may be confused with nelfinavir

Viramune® may be confused with Viracept®

U.S. Brand Names Viramune®

Canadian Brand Names Viramune®

Synonyms NVP

Pharmacologic Category Antiretroviral Agent, Reverse Transcriptase Inhibitor (Non-nucleoside)

Restrictions An FDA-approved medication guide is available at http://www.fda.gov/cder/Offices/ODS/labeling.htm

Generic Available No

Use In combination therapy with other antiretroviral agents for the treatment of HIV-1

Mechanism of Action As a non-nucleoside reverse transcriptase inhibitor, nevirapine has activity against HIV-1 by binding to reverse transcriptase. It consequently blocks the RNA-dependent and DNA-dependent DNA polymerase activities including HIV-1 replication. It does not require intracellular phosphorylation for antiviral activity.

Pharmacodynamics/Kinetics

Absorption: >90%

Distribution: Widely; V_d: 1.2-1.4 L/kg; CSF penetration approximates 40% to 50% of plasma

Protein binding, plasma: 60%

Metabolism: Extensively hepatic via CYP3A4 (hydroxylation to inactive compounds); may undergo enterohepatic recycling

Half-life elimination: Decreases over 2- to 4-week time with chronic dosing due to autoinduction (ie, half-life = 45 hours initially and decreases to 25-30 hours)

Time to peak, serum: 2-4 hours

Excretion: Urine (~81%, primarily as metabolites, <3% as unchanged drug); feces (~10%)

Dosage Oral:

Children 2 months to <8 years: Initial: 4 mg/kg/dose once daily for 14 days; increase dose to 7 mg/kg/dose every 12 hours if no rash or other adverse effects occur; maximum dose: 200 mg/dose every 12 hours

Children ≥8 years: Initial: 4 mg/kg/dose once daily for 14 days; increase dose to 4 mg/kg/dose every 12 hours if no rash or other adverse effects occur; maximum dose: 200 mg/dose every 12 hours

Note: Alternative pediatric dosing (AIDSinfo guidelines): 120-200 mg/m^2 every 12 hours; this dosing has been proposed due to the fact that dosing based on mg/kg may result in an abrupt decrease in dose at the 8th birthday, which may be inappropriate.

Adults: Initial: 200 mg once daily for 14 days; maintenance: 200 mg twice daily (in combination with an additional antiretroviral agent)

Note: If patient experiences a rash during the 14-day lead-in period, dose should not be increased until the rash has resolved. Discontinue if severe rash, or rash with constitutional symptoms, is noted. If therapy is interrupted for >7 days, restart with initial dose for 14 days. Use of prednisone to prevent nevirapine-associated rash is not recommended. Permanently discontinue if symptomatic hepatic events occur.

Prevention of maternal-fetal HIV transmission in women with no prior antiretroviral therapy (AIDS information guidelines):

Mother: 200 mg as a single dose at onset of labor. May be used in combination with zidovudine.

Infant: 2 mg/kg as a single dose at age 48-72 hours. If a maternal dose was given <1 hour prior to delivery, administer a 2 mg/kg dose as soon as possible after birth and repeat at 48-72 hours. May be used in combination with zidovudine.

Dosage adjustment in renal impairment:

Cl_{cr} ≥20 mL/minute: No adjustment required

Hemodialysis: An additional 200 mg dose is recommended following dialysis.

(Continued)

Nevirapine *(Continued)*

Dosage adjustment in hepatic impairment: Use not recommended with moderate-to-severe hepatic impairment. Permanently discontinue if symptomatic hepatic events occur.

Stability Store at room temperature

Administration Oral: May be administered with or without food; may be administered with an antacid or didanosine; shake suspension gently prior to administration

Monitoring Parameters Liver function tests should be monitored at baseline, and intensively during the first 18 weeks of therapy (optimal frequency not established, some practitioners recommend more often than once a month, including prior to dose escalation, and at 2 weeks following dose escalation), then periodically throughout therapy; observe for CNS side effects. Assess/evaluate AST/ALT in any patients with a rash. Permanently discontinue if patient experiences severe rash, constitutional symptoms associated with rash, rash with elevated AST/ALT, or clinical hepatitis, Mild-to-moderate rash without AST/ALT elevation may continue treatment per discretion of prescriber. If mild-to-moderate urticarial rash, do not restart if treatment is interrupted.

Anesthesia and Critical Care Concerns/Other Considerations Nevirapine has a mechanism of action different than nucleoside analogues and protease inhibitors. Potential compliance problems, frequency of administration, and adverse effects should be discussed with patients before initiating therapy to help prevent the emergence of resistance.

Pregnancy Risk Factor C

Contraindications Hypersensitivity to nevirapine or any component of the formulation

Warnings/Precautions [U.S. Boxed Warning]: Severe hepatotoxic reactions may occur (fulminant and cholestatic hepatitis, hepatic necrosis) and, in some cases, have resulted in hepatic failure and death. The greatest risk of these reactions is within the initial 6 weeks of treatment. Patients with a history of chronic hepatitis (B or C) or increased baseline transaminase levels may be at increased risk of hepatotoxic reactions. Female gender and patients with increased $CD4^+$-cell counts may be at substantially greater risk of hepatic events (often associated with rash). Therapy should not be started with elevated $CD4^+$-cell counts unless the benefit of therapy outweighs the risk of serious hepatotoxicity (adult females: $CD4^+$-cell counts >250 cells/mm^3; adult males: $CD4^+$-cell counts >400 cells/mm^3).

[U.S. Boxed Warning]: Severe life-threatening skin reactions (eg, Stevens-Johnson syndrome, toxic epidermal necrolysis, hypersensitivity reactions with rash and organ dysfunction) have occurred; intensive monitoring is required during the initial 18 weeks of therapy to detect potentially life-threatening dermatologic, hypersensitivity, and hepatic reactions. Nevirapine must be initiated with a 14-day lead-in dosing period to decrease the incidence of adverse effects.

If a severe dermatologic or hypersensitivity reaction occurs, or if signs and symptoms of hepatitis occur, nevirapine should be permanently discontinued. These may include a severe rash, or a rash associated with fever, blisters, oral lesions, conjunctivitis, facial edema, muscle or joint aches, general malaise, hepatitis, eosinophilia, granulocytopenia, lymphadenopathy, or renal dysfunction.

Consider alteration of antiretroviral therapies if disease progression occurs while patients are receiving nevirapine. Safety and efficacy have not been established in neonates.

Adverse Reactions Note: Potentially life-threatening nevirapine-associated adverse effects may present with the following symptoms: Abrupt onset of flu-like symptoms, abdominal pain, jaundice, or fever with or without rash; may progress to hepatic failure with encephalopathy. Skin rash is present in ~50% of cases.

Percentages of adverse effects vary by clinical trial:

>10%:

Dermatologic: Rash (grade 1/2: 13%; grade 3/4: 1.5%) is the most common toxicity; occurs most frequently within the first 6 weeks of therapy; women may be at higher risk than men

Hepatic: ALT >250 units/L (5% to 14%); symptomatic hepatic events (4%, range: up to 11%) are more common in women, women with $CD4^+$ cell counts >250 cells/mm^3, and men with $CD4^+$ cell counts >400 cells/mm^3

1% to 10%:

Central nervous system: Headache (1% to 4%), fatigue (up to 5%)

Gastrointestinal: Nausea (<1% to 9%), abdominal pain (<1% to 2%), diarrhea (up to 2%)

Hepatic: AST >250 units/L (4% to 8%); coinfection with hepatitis B or C and/or increased liver function tests at the beginning of therapy are associated with a greater risk of asymptomatic transaminase elevations (ALT or AST >5 times ULN: 6%, range: up to 9%) or symptomatic events occurring ≥6 weeks after beginning treatment

Postmarketing and/or case reports: Allergic reactions, anaphylaxis, anemia, angioedema, arthralgia, blisters, bullous eruptions, conjunctivitis, eosinophilia, facial edema, fever, fulminant and cholestatic hepatitis, granulocytopenia, hepatic failure, hepatic necrosis, hypersensitivity syndrome, jaundice, lymphadenopathy, malaise, neutropenia, oral lesions, paresthesia, redistribution/accumulation of body fat, renal dysfunction, Stevens-Johnson syndrome, somnolence, toxic epidermal necrolysis, ulcerative stomatitis, urticaria, vomiting

Overdosage/Toxicology Edema, erythema nodosum, fatigue, fever, headache, insomnia, nausea, pulmonary infiltrates, rash, vertigo, and weight loss have been reported following large doses.

Drug Interactions Substrate of CYP2B6 (minor), 2D6 (minor), 3A4 (major); **Inhibits** CYP1A2 (weak), 2D6 (weak), 3A4 (weak); **Induces** CYP2B6 (strong), 3A4 (strong)

Antiarrhythmics (includes amiodarone, disopyramide, lidocaine): Serum concentration/effects may be decreased by nevirapine.

Anticonvulsants (includes carbamazepine, clonazepam, ethosuximide): Serum concentration/effects may be decreased by nevirapine.

Calcium channel blockers: Serum concentration may be decreased by nevirapine.

Cimetidine may decrease the metabolism of nevirapine, potentially increasing levels/toxicity.

Clarithromycin: Serum concentration may be decreased by nevirapine; an alternative antimicrobial agent should be considered.

Cyclophosphamide: Serum concentration may be decreased by nevirapine.

CYP2B6 substrates: Nevirapine may decrease the levels/effects of CYP2B6 substrates. Example substrates include bupropion, efavirenz, promethazine, selegiline, and sertraline

CYP3A4 inducers: CYP3A4 inducers may decrease the levels/effects of nevirapine. Example inducers include aminoglutethimide, carbamazepine, nafcillin, nevirapine, phenobarbital, phenytoin, and rifamycins.

CYP3A4 substrates: Nevirapine may decrease the levels/effects of CYP3A4 substrates. Example substrates include benzodiazepines, calcium channel blockers, clarithromycin, cyclosporine, erythromycin, estrogens, mirtazapine, nateglinide, nefazodone, protease inhibitors, tacrolimus, and venlafaxine

Efavirenz: Serum concentration may be decreased by nevirapine; specific adjustments not established

Immunosuppressants: Serum concentration may be decreased by nevirapine.

Ketoconazole: Nevirapine may inhibit ketoconazole absorption. Ketoconazole may inhibit metabolism of nevirapine. Avoid concurrent use.

Methadone: Plasma concentrations may be reduced by nevirapine. Acute withdrawal symptoms have been reported; monitor

Oral contraceptives: Nevirapine may decrease the clinical effect of oral contraceptives; recommend alternative form or additional method of contraception

Prednisone: Concurrent administration of prednisone for the initial 14 days of nevirapine therapy was associated with an increased incidence and severity of rash.

Protease inhibitors: Nevirapine may decrease serum concentrations of some protease inhibitors (AUC of indinavir, lopinavir, nelfinavir, and saquinavir may be decreased - no effect noted with ritonavir), specific dosage adjustments have not been recommended; no adjustment recommended for ritonavir, unless in combination with lopinavir (Kaletra™).

Rifampin, rifabutin: May decrease nevirapine concentrations; rifabutin concentrations may be increased by nevirapine; avoid concurrent use.

St John's wort: Concurrent use may reduce serum concentrations/efficacy of nevirapine. May lead to treatment failure and/or drug resistance. Avoid concurrent use.

Warfarin: Therapeutic effects may be increased; monitor.

(Continued)

Nevirapine *(Continued)*

Ethanol/Nutrition/Herb Interactions Herb/Nutraceutical: Nevirapine serum concentration may be decreased by St John's wort; avoid concurrent use.

Dosage Forms

Suspension, oral: 50 mg/5 mL (240 mL)

Tablet: 200 mg

- ♦ **Nexium®** *see* Esomeprazole *on page 484*
- ♦ **NFV** *see* Nelfinavir *on page 906*
- ♦ **Niastase® (Can)** *see* Factor VIIa (Recombinant) *on page 501*

NiCARdipine (nye KAR de peen)

Medication Safety Issues

Sound-alike/look-alike issues:

NiCARdipine may be confused with niacinamide, NIFEdipine, nimodipine

Cardene® may be confused with Cardizem®, Cardura®, codeine

Related Information

Calcium Channel Blockers *on page 1559*

Critical Care Infusion Administration Charts *on page 1514*

Hypertension *on page 1620*

Postoperative Hypertension *on page 1471*

U.S. Brand Names Cardene®; Cardene® I.V.; Cardene® SR

Synonyms Nicardipine Hydrochloride

Pharmacologic Category Calcium Channel Blocker

Generic Available Yes: Capsule

Use Chronic stable angina (immediate-release product only); management of essential hypertension (immediate and sustained release; parenteral only for short time that oral treatment is not feasible)

Unlabeled/Investigational Use Congestive heart failure

Mechanism of Action Inhibits calcium ion from entering the "slow channels" or select voltage-sensitive areas of vascular smooth muscle and myocardium during depolarization, producing a relaxation of coronary vascular smooth muscle and coronary vasodilation; increases myocardial oxygen delivery in patients with vasospastic angina

Pharmacodynamics/Kinetics

Onset of action: Oral: 0.5-2 hours; I.V.: 10 minutes; Hypotension: ~20 minutes

Duration: ≤8 hours

Absorption: Oral: ~100%

Protein binding: >95%

Metabolism: Hepatic; CYP3A4 substrate (major); extensive first-pass effect (saturable)

Bioavailability: 35%

Half-life elimination: 2-4 hours

Time to peak, serum: 30-120 minutes

Excretion: Urine (60% as metabolites); feces (35%)

Dosage Adults:

Oral:

Immediate release: Initial: 20 mg 3 times/day; usual: 20-40 mg 3 times/day (allow 3 days between dose increases)

Sustained release: Initial: 30 mg twice daily, titrate up to 60 mg twice daily

Note: The total daily dose of immediate-release product may not automatically be equivalent to the daily sustained-release dose; use caution in converting.

I.V. (dilute to 0.1 mg/mL):

Acute hypertension: Initial: 5 mg/hour increased by 2.5 mg/hour every 15 minutes to a maximum of 15 mg/hour; consider reduction to 3 mg/hour after response is achieved. Monitor and titrate to lowest dose necessary to maintain stable blood pressure.

Substitution for oral therapy (approximate equivalents):

20 mg every 8 hours oral, equivalent to 0.5 mg/hour I.V. infusion

30 mg every 8 hours oral, equivalent to 1.2 mg/hour I.V. infusion

40 mg every 8 hours oral, equivalent to 2.2 mg/hour I.V. infusion

Dosing adjustment in renal impairment: Titrate dose beginning with 20 mg 3 times/day (immediate release) or 30 mg twice daily (sustained release).

Specific guidelines for adjustment of I.V. nicardipine are not available, but careful monitoring/adjustment is warranted.

Dosing adjustment in hepatic impairment: Starting dose: 20 mg twice daily (immediate release) with titration. Specific guidelines for adjustment of I.V. nicardipine are not available, but careful monitoring/adjustment is warranted.

Stability Compatible with D_5W, $D_5½NS$, D_5NS, and D_5W with 40 mEq potassium chloride; 0.45% and 0.9% NS; **do not** mix with 5% sodium bicarbonate and lactated Ringer's solution; store at room temperature; protect from light; stable for 24 hours at room temperature

Administration

Oral: The total daily dose of immediate-release product may not automatically be equivalent to the daily sustained-release dose; use caution in converting. Do not chew or crush the sustained release formulation, swallow whole. Do not open or cut capsules.

I.V.: Ampuls must be diluted before use. Administer as a slow continuous infusion.

Anesthesia and Critical Care Concerns/Other Considerations I.V. ampuls must be diluted; dilute each ampul in 240 mL to result in 250 mL of 0.1 mg/mL nicardipine. Nicardipine should be used with caution in patients with heart failure.

Pregnancy Risk Factor C

Contraindications Hypersensitivity to nicardipine or any component of the formulation; advanced aortic stenosis

Warnings/Precautions Blood pressure lowering should be done at a rate appropriate for the patient's condition. Rapid drops in blood pressure can lead to arterial insufficiency. Use with caution in CAD (can cause increase in angina), CHF (can worsen heart failure symptoms), and pheochromocytoma (limited clinical experience). Peripheral infusion sites (for I.V. therapy) should be changed ever 12 hours. Titrate I.V. dose cautiously in patients with CHF, renal, or hepatic dysfunction. Use the I.V. form cautiously in patients with portal hypertension (can cause increase in hepatic pressure gradient). Safety and efficacy have not been demonstrated in pediatric patients. Abrupt withdrawal may cause rebound angina in patients with CAD.

Adverse Reactions

1% to 10%:

Cardiovascular: Flushing (6% to 10%), palpitation (3% to 4%), tachycardia (1% to 3%), peripheral edema (dose related 7% to 8%), increased angina (dose related 5.6%)

Central nervous system: Headache (6% to 8%), dizziness (4% to 7%), somnolence (4% to 6%), paresthesia (1%)

Dermatologic: Rash (1%)

Gastrointestinal: Nausea (2% to 5%), dry mouth (1%)

Neuromuscular & skeletal: Weakness (4% to 6%), myalgia (1%)

<1% (Limited to important or life-threatening): Abnormal ECG, dyspnea, gingival hyperplasia, nervousness, parotitis, sustained tachycardia, syncope

Overdosage/Toxicology The primary cardiac symptoms of calcium blocker overdose include hypotension and bradycardia. Noncardiac symptoms include confusion, stupor, nausea, vomiting, metabolic acidosis, and hyperglycemia. Following initial gastric decontamination, if possible, repeated calcium administration may promptly reverse the depressed cardiac contractility (but not sinus node depression or peripheral vasodilation). Glucagon and epinephrine may treat refractory hypotension. Glucagon and epinephrine also increase the heart rate (outside the U.S., 4-aminopyridine may be available as an antidote). Dialysis and hemoperfusion are not effective in enhancing elimination although repeat-dose activated charcoal may serve as an adjunct with sustained-release preparations.

Drug Interactions Substrate of CYP1A2 (minor), 2C9 (minor), 2D6 (minor), 2E1 (minor), 3A4 (major); **Inhibits** CYP2C9 (strong), 2C19 (moderate), 2D6 (moderate), 3A4 (strong)

Azole antifungals may inhibit the calcium channel blocker's metabolism; avoid this combination. Try an antifungal like terbinafine (if appropriate) or monitor closely for altered effect of the calcium channel blocker.

Calcium may reduce the calcium channel blocker's effects, particularly hypotension.

Cyclosporine's serum concentrations are increased by nicardipine; avoid this combination. Use another calcium channel blocker or monitor cyclosporine trough levels and renal function closely. Tacrolimus may be affected similarly.

(Continued)

NiCARdipine *(Continued)*

CYP2C9 Substrates: Nicardipine may increase the levels/effects of CYP2C9 substrates. Example substrates include bosentan, dapsone, fluoxetine, glimepiride, glipizide, losartan, montelukast, nateglinide, paclitaxel, phenytoin, warfarin, and zafirlukast.

CYP2C19 substrates: Nicardipine may increase the levels/effects of CYP2C19 substrates. Example substrates include citalopram, diazepam, methsuximide, phenytoin, propranolol, and sertraline.

CYP2D6 substrates: Nicardipine may increase the levels/effects of CYP2D6 substrates. Example substrates include amphetamines, selected beta-blockers, dextromethorphan, fluoxetine, lidocaine, mirtazapine, nefazodone, paroxetine, risperidone, ritonavir, thioridazine, tricyclic antidepressants, and venlafaxine.

CYP2D6 prodrug substrates: Nicardipine may decrease the levels/effects of CYP2D6 prodrug substrates. Example prodrug substrates include codeine, hydrocodone, oxycodone, and tramadol.

CYP3A4 inducers: CYP3A4 inducers may decrease the levels/effects of nicardipine. Example inducers include aminoglutethimide, carbamazepine, nafcillin, nevirapine, phenobarbital, phenytoin, and rifamycins.

CYP3A4 inhibitors: May increase the levels/effects of nicardipine. Example inhibitors include azole antifungals, clarithromycin, diclofenac, doxycycline, erythromycin, imatinib, isoniazid, nefazodone, propofol, protease inhibitors, quinidine, telithromycin, and verapamil.

CYP3A4 substrates: Nicardipine may increase the levels/effects of CYP3A4 substrates. Example substrates include benzodiazepines, calcium channel blockers, mirtazapine, nateglinide, nefazodone, tacrolimus, and venlafaxine. Selected benzodiazepines (midazolam and triazolam), cisapride, ergot alkaloids, selected HMG-CoA reductase inhibitors (lovastatin and simvastatin), and pimozide are generally contraindicated with strong CYP3A4 inhibitors.

Metoprolol: Concentration of metoprolol is increased by 25% with concurrent use.

Nafcillin decreases plasma concentration of nicardipine; avoid this combination.

Propranolol: May decrease the metabolism of nicardipine.

Protease inhibitor like amprenavir and ritonavir may increase nicardipine's serum concentration.

Rifampin increases the metabolism of the calcium channel blocker; adjust the dose of the calcium channel blocker to maintain efficacy.

Sildenafil, tadalafil, vardenafil: Blood pressure-lowering effects may be additive; use caution.

Vecuronium: Clearance of vecuronium is decreased by 25% with use of I.V. nicardipine; reduce dose of muscle relaxant.

Ethanol/Nutrition/Herb Interactions

Ethanol: Avoid ethanol (may increase CNS depression).

Food: Nicardipine average peak concentrations may be decreased if taken with food. Serum concentrations/toxicity of nicardipine may be increased by grapefruit juice; avoid concurrent use.

Herb/Nutraceutical: St John's wort may decrease levels. Avoid dong quai if using for hypertension (has estrogenic activity). Avoid ephedra, yohimbe, ginseng (may worsen hypertension). Avoid garlic (may have increased antihypertensive effect).

Dosage Forms

Capsule (Cardene®): 20 mg, 30 mg

Capsule, sustained release (Cardene® SR): 30 mg, 45 mg, 60 mg

Injection, solution (Cardene® IV): 2.5 mg/mL (10 mL)

- **Nicardipine Hydrochloride** *see* NiCARdipine *on page 918*
- **Nidagel™ (Can)** *see* Metronidazole *on page 842*
- **Nifediac™ CC** *see* NIFEdipine *on page 920*
- **Nifedical™ XL** *see* NIFEdipine *on page 920*

NIFEdipine (nye FED i peen)

Medication Safety Issues

Sound-alike/look-alike issues:

NIFEdipine may be confused with niCARdipine, nimodipine, nisoldipine

Procardia XL® may be confused with Cartia® XT

Related Information

Calcium Channel Blockers *on page 1559*

Hypertension *on page 1620*

U.S. Brand Names Adalat® CC; Afeditab™ CR; Nifediac™ CC; Nifedical™ XL; Procardia®; Procardia XL®

Canadian Brand Names Adalat® XL®; Apo-Nifed®; Apo-Nifed PA®; Novo-Nifedin; Nu-Nifed; Procardia®

Pharmacologic Category Calcium Channel Blocker

Generic Available Yes

Use Angina and hypertension (sustained release only), pulmonary hypertension

Mechanism of Action Inhibits calcium ion from entering the "slow channels" or select voltage-sensitive areas of vascular smooth muscle and myocardium during depolarization, producing a relaxation of coronary vascular smooth muscle and coronary vasodilation; increases myocardial oxygen delivery in patients with vasospastic angina

Pharmacodynamics/Kinetics

Onset of action: Immediate release: ~20 minutes

Protein binding (concentration dependent): 92% to 98%

Metabolism: Hepatic to inactive metabolites

Bioavailability: Capsule: 40% to 77%; Sustained release: 65% to 89% relative to immediate release capsules

Half-life elimination: Adults: Healthy: 2-5 hours, Cirrhosis: 7 hours; Elderly: 6.7 hours

Excretion: Urine (as metabolites)

Dosage Oral:

Children: Hypertrophic cardiomyopathy: 0.6-0.9 mg/kg/24 hours in 3-4 divided doses

Adolescents and Adults: (**Note:** When switching from immediate release to sustained release formulations, total daily dose will start the same)

Initial: 30 mg once daily as sustained release formulation, or if indicated, 10 mg 3 times/day as capsules

Usual dose: 10-30 mg 3 times/day as capsules or 30-60 mg once daily as sustained release

Maximum dose: 120-180 mg/day

Increase sustained release at 7- to 14-day intervals

Hemodialysis: Supplemental dose is not necessary.

Peritoneal dialysis effects: Supplemental dose is not necessary.

Dosing adjustment in hepatic impairment: Reduce oral dose by 50% to 60% in patients with cirrhosis.

Administration Extended release tablets should be swallowed whole; do not crush or chew.

Monitoring Parameters Heart rate, blood pressure, signs and symptoms of CHF, peripheral edema

Anesthesia and Critical Care Concerns/Other Considerations Considerable attention has been directed to potential increases in mortality and morbidity when short-acting nifedipine is used in treating hypertension. The rapid reduction in blood pressure may precipitate adverse cardiovascular events. At this time, there is no indication for the use of short-acting calcium channel blocker therapy for angina and hypertension. Nifedipine also has potent negative inotropic effects and can worsen heart failure.

Pregnancy Risk Factor C

Contraindications Hypersensitivity to nifedipine or any component of the formulation; immediate release preparation for treatment of urgent or emergent hypertension; acute MI

Warnings/Precautions **The use of sublingual short-acting nifedipine in hypertensive emergencies and pseudoemergencies is neither safe nor effective and SHOULD BE ABANDONED!** Serious adverse events (cerebrovascular ischemia, syncope, heart block, stroke, sinus arrest, severe hypotension, acute myocardial infarction, ECG changes, and fetal distress) have been reported in relation to such use.

Blood pressure lowering should be done at a rate appropriate for the patient's condition. Rapid drops in blood pressure can lead to arterial insufficiency. Increased angina and/or MI has occurred with initiation or dosage titration of calcium channel blockers. Severe hypotension may occur in patients taking immediate release nifepine concurrently with beta blockers when undergoing CABG with high dose fentanyl anesthesia. When considering surgery with high dose fentanyl, may consider withdrawing nifedipine (>36 hours) before surgery if possible. Use caution in severe aortic stenosis. Use caution in patients with

(Continued)

NIFEdipine *(Continued)*

severe hepatic impairment (may need dosage adjustment). Abrupt withdrawal may cause rebound angina in patients with CAD. Use caution in CHF (may cause worsening of symptoms).

The extended release formulation consists of drug within a nondeformable matrix; following drug release/absorption, the matrix/shell is expelled in the stool. The use of nondeformable products in patients with known stricture/narrowing of the GI tract has been associated with symptoms of obstruction. Avoid grapefruit juice during treatment with nifedipine.

Adverse Reactions

>10%:

Cardiovascular: Flushing (10% to 25%), peripheral edema (dose related 7% to 10%; up to 50%)

Central nervous system: Dizziness/lightheadedness/giddiness (10% to 27%), headache (10% to 23%)

Gastrointestinal: Nausea/heartburn (10% to 11%)

Neuromuscular & skeletal: Weakness (10% to 12%)

≥1% to 10%:

Cardiovascular: Palpitations (≤2% to 7%), transient hypotension (dose related 5%), CHF (2%)

Central nervous system: Nervousness/mood changes (≤2% to 7%), shakiness (≤2%), jitteriness (≤2%), sleep disturbances (≤2%), difficulties in balance (≤2%), fever (≤2%), chills (≤2%)

Dermatologic: Dermatitis (≤2%), pruritus (≤2%), urticaria (≤2%)

Endocrine & metabolic: Sexual difficulties (≤2%)

Gastrointestinal: Diarrhea (≤2%), constipation (≤2%), cramps (≤2%), flatulence (≤2%), gingival hyperplasia (≤10%)

Neuromuscular & skeletal: Muscle cramps/tremor (≤2% to 8%), inflammation (≤2%), joint stiffness (≤2%)

Ocular: Blurred vision (≤2%)

Respiratory: Cough/wheezing (6%), nasal congestion/sore throat (≤2% to 6%), chest congestion (≤2%), dyspnea (≤2%)

Miscellaneous: Diaphoresis (≤2%)

<1% (Limited to important or life-threatening): Agranulocytosis, allergic hepatitis, angina, angioedema, aplastic anemia, arthritis with positive ANA, bezoars (sustained-release preparations), cerebral ischemia, depression, erythema multiforme, erythromelalgia, exfoliative dermatitis, extrapyramidal symptoms, fever, gingival hyperplasia, gynecomastia, leukopenia, memory dysfunction, paranoid syndrome, photosensitivity, purpura, Stevens-Johnson syndrome, syncope, thrombocytopenia, tinnitus, transient blindness

Reported with use of sublingual short-acting nifedipine: Acute MI, cerebrovascular ischemia, ECG changes, fetal distress, heart block, severe hypotension, sinus arrest, stroke, syncope

Overdosage/Toxicology Primary cardiac symptoms of calcium blocker overdose include hypotension and bradycardia. Noncardiac symptoms include confusion, stupor, nausea, vomiting, metabolic acidosis, and hyperglycemia. Following initial gastric decontamination, treat symptomatically.

Drug Interactions **Substrate** of CYP2D6 (minor), 3A4 (major); **Inhibits** CYP1A2 (moderate), 2C9 (weak), 2D6 (weak), 3A4 (weak)

Alpha 1-blockers: May enhance the effects of calcium channel blockers; monitor blood pressure.

Azole antifungals: May inhibit the calcium channel blocker's metabolism; monitor for the toxic effects of calcium channel blocker and adjust accordingly.

Barbiturates: May increase metabolism of calcium channel blocker. Consider therapy modification.

Calcium may reduce the calcium channel blocker's effects.

Calcium channel blocker (nondihydropyridine): May enhance the hypotensive effects of calcium channel blocker (dihydropyridine).

Carbamazepine: May decrease nifedipine serum concentration.

Cimetidine: May increase nifedipine serum concentrations; monitor for toxic effects of calcium channel blocker or choose an alternative H_2 antagonist.

Cisapride: May increase nifedipine's effects; monitor blood pressure.

Cyclosporine: May decrease metabolism of calcium channel blocker (dihydropyridine); monitor for toxic effects of calcium channel blocker.

CYP1A2 substrates: Nifedipine may increase the levels/effects of CYP1A2 substrates. Example substrates include aminophylline, fluvoxamine, mexiletine, mirtazapine, ropinirole, theophylline, and trifluoperazine.

CYP3A4 inducers: CYP3A4 inducers may decrease the levels/effects of nifedipine. Example inducers include aminoglutethimide, carbamazepine, nafcillin, nevirapine, phenobarbital, phenytoin, and rifamycins.

CYP3A4 inhibitors: May increase the levels/effects of nifedipine. Example inhibitors include azole antifungals, clarithromycin, diclofenac, doxycycline, erythromycin, imatinib, isoniazid, nefazodone, nicardipine, propofol, protease inhibitors, quinidine, telithromycin, and verapamil.

Erythromycin: May increase nifedipine serum concentration; monitor blood pressure and adjust if necessary.

Grapefruit juice increases the bioavailability of nifedipine; avoid grapefruit juice.

Magnesium salts: Concurrent use may enhance the adverse/toxic effects of magnesium and enhance the hypotensive effects of the calcium channel blocker.

Nafcillin decreases plasma concentration of nifedipine; avoid this combination.

Neuromuscular-blocking agent (nondepolarizing): Calcium channel blockers may enhance the neuromuscular blocking effect; monitor.

Phenobarbital reduces the plasma concentration of nifedipine. May require much higher dose of nifedipine.

Phenytoin: May decrease nifedipine serum concentration; monitor and adjust if necessary.

Protease inhibitors like amprenavir and ritonavir may increase nifedipine's serum concentration.

Quinidine's serum concentration is reduced and nifedipine's is increased; adjust doses as needed.

Quinupristin/dalfopristin: May increase nifedipine serum concentration; monitor blood pressure and adjust if necessary.

Rifamycin derivatives: Increase the metabolism of the calcium channel blocker; adjust the dose of the calcium channel blocker to maintain efficacy.

Tacrolimus's serum concentrations are increased by nifedipine; monitor tacrolimus trough levels and renal function closely.

Vincristine's half-life is increased by nifedipine; monitor closely for vincristine dose adjustment.

Ethanol/Nutrition/Herb Interactions

Ethanol: Avoid ethanol (may increase CNS depression and may increase the effects of nifedipine). Monitor.

Food: Nifedipine serum levels may be decreased if taken with food. Food may decrease the rate but not the extent of absorption of Procardia XL®. Increased therapeutic and vasodilator side effects, including severe hypotension and myocardial ischemia, may occur if nifedipine is taken by patients ingesting grapefruit.

Herb/Nutraceutical: St John's wort may decrease nifedipine levels. Avoid dong quai if using for hypertension (has estrogenic activity). Avoid ephedra, yohimbe, ginseng (may worsen hypertension). Avoid garlic (may have increased antihypertensive effect).

Dietary Considerations Capsule is rapidly absorbed orally if it is administered without food, but may result in vasodilator side effects; administration with low-fat meals may decrease flushing. Avoid grapefruit juice.

Dosage Forms

Capsule, softgel: 10 mg, 20 mg
  Procardia®: 10 mg
Tablet, extended release: 30 mg, 60 mg, 90 mg
  Adalat® CC, Procardia XL®: 30 mg, 60 mg, 90 mg
  Afeditab™ CR, Nifedical™ XL: 30 mg, 60 mg
  Nifediac™ CC: 30 mg, 60 mg, 90 mg [90 mg tablet contains tartrazine]

♦ **Nilstat (Can)** *see* Nystatin *on page 945*
♦ **Nimbex®** *see* Cisatracurium *on page 294*

Nimodipine (nye MOE di peen)

Medication Safety Issues

Sound-alike/look-alike issues:
  Nimodipine may be confused with niCARdipine, NIFEdipine

(Continued)

Nimodipine *(Continued)*

Nimodipine has inadvertently been administered I.V. when withdrawn from capsules into a syringe for subsequent nasogastric administration. Severe cardiovascular adverse events, including fatalities, have resulted. Employ precautions against such an event.

Related Information

Calcium Channel Blockers *on page 1559*

U.S. Brand Names Nimotop®

Canadian Brand Names Nimotop®

Pharmacologic Category Calcium Channel Blocker

Generic Available No

Use Spasm following subarachnoid hemorrhage from ruptured intracranial aneurysms regardless of the patients neurological condition postictus (Hunt and Hess grades I-V)

Mechanism of Action Nimodipine shares the pharmacology of other calcium channel blockers; animal studies indicate that nimodipine has a greater effect on cerebral arterials than other arterials; this increased specificity may be due to the drug's increased lipophilicity and cerebral distribution as compared to nifedipine; inhibits calcium ion from entering the "slow channels" or select voltage sensitive areas of vascular smooth muscle and myocardium during depolarization

Pharmacodynamics/Kinetics

Protein binding: >95%

Metabolism: Extensively hepatic

Bioavailability: 13%

Half-life elimination: 1-2 hours; prolonged with renal impairment

Time to peak, serum: ~1 hour

Excretion: Urine (50%) and feces (32%) within 4 days

Dosage Note: Capsules and contents are for oral administration **ONLY.**

Adults: Oral: 60 mg every 4 hours for 21 days, start therapy within 96 hours after subarachnoid hemorrhage.

Dialysis: Not removed by hemo- or peritoneal dialysis; supplemental dose is not necessary.

Dosing adjustment in hepatic impairment: Reduce dosage to 30 mg every 4 hours in patients with liver failure.

Administration For oral administration **ONLY.** If the capsules cannot be swallowed, the liquid may be removed by making a hole in each end of the capsule with an 18-gauge needle and extracting the contents into a syringe. If administered via NG tube, follow with a flush of 30 mL NS.

Anesthesia and Critical Care Concerns/Other Considerations Animal studies suggest nimodipine may have a greater effect on cerebral arterioles, possibly due to its lipophilicity which increases cerebral distribution.

Pregnancy Risk Factor C

Contraindications Hypersensitivity to nimodipine or any component of the formulation

Warnings/Precautions May cause reductions in blood pressure. Use caution in hepatic impairment. Intestinal pseudo-obstruction and ileus have been reported during the use of nimodipine. Use caution in patients with decreased GI motility of a history of bowel obstruction. Use caution when treating patients with increased intracranial pressure.

[U.S. Boxed Warning]: Nimodipine has inadvertently been administered I.V. when withdrawn from capsules into a syringe for subsequent nasogastric administration. Severe cardiovascular adverse events, including fatalities, have resulted; precautions should be employed against such an event.

Adverse Reactions

1% to 10%:

Cardiovascular: Reductions in systemic blood pressure (1% to 8%)

Central nervous system: Headache (1% to 4%)

Dermatologic: Rash (1% to 2%)

Gastrointestinal: Diarrhea (2% to 4%), abdominal discomfort (2%)

<1% (Limited to important or life-threatening): Anemia, CHF, deep vein thrombosis, depression, disseminated intravascular coagulation, dyspnea, ECG abnormalities, GI hemorrhage, hemorrhage, hepatitis, jaundice, neurological deterioration, rebound vasospasm, thrombocytopenia, vomiting

Overdosage/Toxicology Primary cardiac symptoms of calcium blocker overdose include hypotension and bradycardia. Noncardiac symptoms include confusion, stupor, nausea, vomiting, metabolic acidosis and hyperglycemia. Treat symptomatically.

Drug Interactions Substrate of CYP3A4 (major)

Antihypertensive agents: Effects may be potentiated by nimodipine.

Azole antifungals may inhibit the calcium channel blocker's metabolism; avoid this combination. Try an antifungal like terbinafine (if appropriate) or monitor closely for altered effect of the calcium channel blocker.

Calcium may reduce the calcium channel blocker's effects, particularly hypotension.

Calcium channel blockers: The effects of other calcium channel blockers may be potentiated by nimodipine.

CYP3A4 inducers: CYP3A4 inducers may decrease the levels/effects of nimodipine. Example inducers include aminoglutethimide, carbamazepine, nafcillin, nevirapine, phenobarbital, phenytoin, and rifamycins.

CYP3A4 inhibitors: May increase the levels/effects of nimodipine. Example inhibitors include azole antifungals, clarithromycin, diclofenac, doxycycline, erythromycin, imatinib, isoniazid, nefazodone, nicardipine, propofol, protease inhibitors, quinidine, telithromycin, and verapamil.

Grapefruit juice increases the bioavailability of nimodipine; monitor for altered nimodipine effects.

Protease inhibitor like amprenavir and ritonavir may increase nimodipine's serum concentration.

Rifampin increases the metabolism of the calcium channel blocker; adjust the dose of the calcium channel blocker to maintain efficacy.

Sildenafil, tadalafil, vardenafil: Blood pressure-lowering effects may be additive; use caution.

Valproic acid increased nimodipine's serum concentration; monitor altered effect of nimodipine.

Ethanol/Nutrition/Herb Interactions

Food: Nimodipine has shown a 1.5-fold increase in bioavailability when taken with grapefruit juice; avoid concurrent use.

Herb/Nutraceutical: St John's wort may decrease levels. Avoid dong quai if using for hypertension (has estrogenic activity). Avoid ephedra, yohimbe, ginseng (may worsen hypertension). Avoid garlic (may have increased antihypertensive effect).

Dosage Forms Capsule, liquid filled: 30 mg

- ♦ **Nimotop®** *see* Nimodipine *on page 923*
- ♦ **Niravam™** *see* Alprazolam *on page 65*
- ♦ **Nitalapram** *see* Citalopram *on page 297*
- ♦ **Nitrek®** *see* Nitroglycerin *on page 928*

Nitric Oxide (NYE trik OKS ide)

U.S. Brand Names INOmax®

Canadian Brand Names INOmax®

Pharmacologic Category Vasodilator, Pulmonary

Generic Available No

Use Treatment of term and near-term (>34 weeks) neonates with hypoxic respiratory failure associated with pulmonary hypertension; used concurrently with ventilatory support and other agents

Unlabeled/Investigational Use Treatment of adult respiratory distress syndrome (ARDS)

Mechanism of Action In neonates with persistent pulmonary hypertension, nitric oxide improves oxygenation. Nitric oxide relaxes vascular smooth muscle by binding to the heme moiety of cytosolic guanylate cyclase, activating guanylate cyclase and increasing intracellular levels of cyclic guanosine 3',5'-monophosphate, which leads to vasodilation. When inhaled, pulmonary vasodilation occurs and an increase in the partial pressure of arterial oxygen results. Dilation of pulmonary vessels in well ventilated lung areas redistributes blood flow away from lung areas where ventilation/perfusion ratios are poor.

Pharmacodynamics/Kinetics

Absorption: Systemic after inhalation

(Continued)

Nitric Oxide *(Continued)*

Metabolism: Nitric oxide combines with hemoglobin that is 60% to 100% oxygenated. Nitric oxide combines with oxyhemoglobin to produce methemoglobin and nitrate. Within the pulmonary system, nitric oxide can combine with oxygen and water to produce nitrogen dioxide and nitrite respectively, which interact with oxyhemoglobin to then produce methemoglobin and nitrate. At 80 ppm the methemoglobin percent is ~5% after 8 hours of administration. Methemoglobin levels >7% were attained only in patients receiving 80 ppm.

Excretion: Urine (as nitrate)

Clearance: Nitrate: At a rate approaching the glomerular filtration rate

Dosage Inhalation: Neonates (up to 14 days old): 20 ppm. Treatment should be maintained up to 14 days or until the underlying oxygen desaturation has resolved and the neonate is ready to be weaned from therapy. In the CINRGI trial, patients whose oxygenation improved had their dose reduced to 5 ppm at the end of 4 hours of treatment. Doses above 20 ppm should not be used because of the risk of methemoglobinemia and elevated NO_2.

Stability Store at 25°C (77°C)

Administration In the ventilated neonate, precise monitoring of inspired nitric oxide and NO_2 should be instituted using a calibrated analysis device with alarms. Sample gas for analysis should be drawn before the Y-piece, proximal to the patient. In addition, oxygen levels should be measured. A backup delivery system should be available in the event of power failure. Do not discontinue abruptly.

Monitoring Parameters Respiratory status including arterial blood gases with close attention to PaO_2, methemoglobin, NO_2 , vital signs, blood sugar, signs and symptoms of infection.

Pregnancy Risk Factor C

Contraindications Hypersensitivity to nitric oxide or any component of the formulation; neonates dependent on right-to-left shunting of blood

Warnings/Precautions Abrupt discontinuation may lead to worsening hypotension, oxygenation, and increasing pulmonary artery pressure (PAP). Worsening oxygenation and increasing PAP may occur in patients who do not respond. Doses above 20 ppm should not be used because of the increased risk of methemoglobinemia and elevated nitrogen dioxide (NO_2) levels. Methemoglobin levels and NO_2 should be monitored.

Adverse Reactions

>10%:

Cardiovascular: Hypotension (13%)

Miscellaneous: Withdrawal syndrome (12%)

1% to 10%:

Dermatologic: Cellulitis (5%)

Endocrine & metabolic: Hyperglycemia (8%)

Genitourinary: Hematuria (8%)

Respiratory: Atelectasis (9% - same as placebo), stridor (5%)

Miscellaneous: Sepsis (7%), infection (6%)

Postmarketing and/or case reports: Headache (environmental exposure, eg, hospital staff); hypoxemia; pulmonary edema (in CREST syndrome patients)

Overdosage/Toxicology Elevations in methemoglobin and nitrogen dioxide may be signs of overdose. Elevated nitrogen dioxide may cause acute lung injury and elevations of methemoglobin reduce the oxygen delivery capacity of the circulation. NO_2 levels >3 ppm or methemoglobin levels >7% were treated by reducing the dose of or discontinuing INOmax®. Methemoglobinemia that does not resolve with dosage reduction or discontinuation of therapy may require intravenous vitamin C, intravenous methylene blue, or blood transfusion, depending on the clinical situation.

Drug Interactions No formal studies have been done. Concurrent use of sodium nitroprusside, nitroglycerin, or prilocaine may result in an increased risk of developing methemoglobinemia. Monitor closely if used. Has been administered with tolazoline, dopamine, dobutamine, steroids, surfactant, and high-frequency ventilation.

Dosage Forms Gas, for inhalation:

100 ppm [nitric oxide 0.01% and nitrogen 99.99%] (353 L) [delivers 344 L], (1963 L) [delivers 1918 L]

800 ppm [nitric oxide 0.08% and nitrogen 99.92%] (353 L) [delivers 344 L], (1963 L) [delivers 1918 L]

References

Davidson D, Barefield ES, Kattwinkel J, et al, "Inhaled Nitric Oxide for the Early Treatment of Persistent Pulmonary Hypertension of the Term Newborn: A Randomized, Double-Masked, Placebo-Controlled, Dose-Response, Multicenter Study: I-NO/PPHN Study Group." *Pediatrics*, 1998, 101(3 Pt 1):325-34.

"Inhaled Nitric Oxide in Full-Term and Nearly Full-term Infants With Hypoxic Respiratory Failure." The Neonatal Inhaled Nitric Oxide Study Group, *N Engl J Med*, 1997, 336(9):597-604.

♦ **Nitro-Bid®** *see* Nitroglycerin *on page 928*

♦ **Nitro-Dur®** *see* Nitroglycerin *on page 928*

Nitrofurantoin (nye troe fyoor AN toyn)

U.S. Brand Names Furadantin®; Macrobid®; Macrodantin®

Canadian Brand Names Apo-Nitrofurantoin®; Macrobid®; Macrodantin®; Novo-Furantoin

Pharmacologic Category Antibiotic, Miscellaneous

Generic Available Yes: Excludes suspension

Use Prevention and treatment of urinary tract infections caused by susceptible gram-negative and some gram-positive organisms; *Pseudomonas*, *Serratia*, and most species of *Proteus* are generally resistant to nitrofurantoin

Mechanism of Action Inhibits several bacterial enzyme systems including acetyl coenzyme A interfering with metabolism and possibly cell wall synthesis

Pharmacodynamics/Kinetics

Absorption: Well absorbed; macrocrystalline form absorbed more slowly due to slower dissolution (causes less GI distress)

Distribution: V_d: 0.8 L/kg; crosses placenta; enters breast milk

Protein binding: 60% to 90%

Metabolism: Body tissues (except plasma) metabolize 60% of drug to inactive metabolites

Bioavailability: Increased with food

Half-life elimination: 20-60 minutes; prolonged with renal impairment

Excretion:

Suspension: Urine (40%) and feces (small amounts) as metabolites and unchanged drug

Macrocrystals: Urine (20% to 25% as unchanged drug)

Dosage Oral:

Children >1 month: 5-7 mg/kg/day in divided doses every 6 hours; maximum: 400 mg/day

UTI prophylaxis (chronic): 1-2 mg/kg/day in divided doses every 12-24 hours; maximum: 100 mg/day

Adults: 50-100 mg/dose every 6 hours

Macrocrystal/monohydrate: 100 mg twice daily

UTI prophylaxis (chronic): 50-100 mg/dose at bedtime

Dosing adjustment in renal impairment: Cl_{cr} <60 mL/minute: Contraindicated

Contraindicated in hemo- and peritoneal dialysis and continuous arteriovenous or venovenous hemofiltration

Stability Store at room temperature 15°C to 30°C (59°F to 86°F).

Administration Administer with meals to slow the rate of absorption and decrease adverse effects; suspension may be mixed with water, milk, fruit juice, or infant formula

Monitoring Parameters Signs of pulmonary reaction, signs of numbness or tingling of the extremities, periodic liver function tests

Pregnancy Risk Factor B (contraindicated at term)

Contraindications Hypersensitivity to nitrofurantoin or any component of the formulation; renal impairment (anuria, oliguria, significantly elevated serum creatinine, or Cl_{cr}< 60 mL/minute); infants <1 month (due to the possibility of hemolytic anemia); pregnancy at term (38-42 weeks gestation), during labor and delivery, or when the onset of labor is imminent

Warnings/Precautions Use with caution in patients with G6PD deficiency or in patients with anemia. Therapeutic concentrations of nitrofurantoin are not attained in urine of patients with Cl_{cr}<60 mL/minute. Use with caution if prolonged therapy is anticipated due to possible pulmonary toxicity. Acute, subacute, or chronic (usually after 6 months of therapy) pulmonary reactions have been observed in patients treated with nitrofurantoin; if these occur, discontinue therapy immediately; monitor closely for malaise, dyspnea, cough, fever, radiologic evidence of diffuse interstitial pneumonitis or fibrosis. Rare, but severe

(Continued)

Nitrofurantoin *(Continued)*

hepatic reactions have been associated with nitrofurantoin (onset may be insidious); discontinue immediately if hepatitis occurs. Has been associated with peripheral neuropathy (rare); risk may be increased by renal impairment, diabetes, vitamin B deficiency, or electrolyte imbalance; use caution.

Adverse Reactions Frequency not defined.

Cardiovascular: Chest pain, cyanosis, ECG changes (associated with pulmonary toxicity)

Central nervous system: Chills, depression, dizziness, drowsiness, fatigue, fever, headache, pseudotumor cerebri, psychotic reaction

Dermatologic: Alopecia, erythema multiforme, exfoliative dermatitis, pruritus, rash, Stevens-Johnson syndrome

Gastrointestinal: Abdominal pain, *C. difficile*-colitis, constipation, diarrhea, dyspepsia, loss of appetite, nausea (most common), pancreatitis, sore throat, vomiting

Hematologic: Agranulocytosis, aplastic anemia, eosinophilia, hemolytic anemia, methemoglobinemia, thrombocytopenia

Hepatic: Cholestasis, hepatitis, hepatic necrosis, transaminases increased, jaundice (cholestatic)

Neuromuscular & skeletal: Arthralgia, numbness, paresthesia, peripheral neuropathy, weakness

Ocular: Amblyopia, nystagmus, optic neuritis (rare)

Respiratory: Cough, dyspnea, pneumonitis, pulmonary fibrosis

Miscellaneous: Hypersensitivity (including acute pulmonary hypersensitivity), lupus-like syndrome

Overdosage/Toxicology Symptoms of overdose include vomiting. Treatment is supportive.

Drug Interactions

Decreased effect: Antacids, especially magnesium salts, decrease absorption of nitrofurantoin; nitrofurantoin may antagonize effects of norfloxacin

Increased toxicity: Probenecid (decreases renal excretion of nitrofurantoin); anticholinergic drugs increase absorption of nitrofurantoin

Ethanol/Nutrition/Herb Interactions

Ethanol: Avoid ethanol (may increase CNS depression).

Food: Nitrofurantoin serum concentrations may be increased if taken with food.

Test Interactions False-positive urine glucose (Benedict's and Fehling's methods); no false positives with enzymatic tests

Dosage Forms

Capsule, macrocrystal: 50 mg, 100 mg

Macrodantin®: 25 mg, 50 mg, 100 mg

Capsule, macrocrystal/monohydrate (Macrobid®): 100 mg

Suspension, oral (Furadantin®): 25 mg/5 mL (470 mL)

Nitroglycerin (nye troe GLI ser in)

Medication Safety Issues

Sound-alike/look-alike issues:

Nitroglycerin may be confused with nitroprusside

Nitro-Bid® may be confused with Nicobid®

Nitroderm may be confused with NicoDerm®

Nitrol® may be confused with Nizoral®

Nitrostat® may be confused with Hyperstat®, Nilstat®, nystatin

Nitroglycerin transdermal patches should be removed prior to defibrillation or MRI study.

Related Information

Critical Care Infusion Administration Charts *on page 1514*

Heart Failure (Systolic) *on page 1607*

Hemodynamic Support, Intravenous *on page 1566*

Hypertension *on page 1620*

Nitrates *on page 1574*

Postoperative Hypertension *on page 1471*

U.S. Brand Names Minitran™; Nitrek®; Nitro-Bid®; Nitro-Dur®; Nitrolingual®; Nitro-Quick®; Nitrostat®; Nitro-Tab®; NitroTime®

Canadian Brand Names Gen-Nitro; Minitran™; Nitro-Dur®; Nitroglycerin Injection, USP; Nitrol®; Nitrostat™; Rho®-Nitro; Transderm-Nitro®; Trinipatch® 0.2; Trinipatch® 0.4; Trinipatch® 0.6

Synonyms Glyceryl Trinitrate; Nitroglycerol; NTG

Pharmacologic Category Vasodilator

Generic Available Yes: Capsule, injection, patch, tablet

Use Treatment of angina pectoris; I.V. for congestive heart failure (especially when associated with acute myocardial infarction); pulmonary hypertension; hypertensive emergencies occurring perioperatively (especially during cardiovascular surgery)

Unlabeled/Investigational Use Esophageal spastic disorders (sublingual)

Mechanism of Action Works by relaxation of smooth muscle, producing a vasodilator effect on the peripheral veins and arteries with more prominent effects on the veins. Primarily reduces cardiac oxygen demand by decreasing preload (left ventricular end-diastolic pressure); may modestly reduce afterload; dilates coronary arteries and improves collateral flow to ischemic regions

Pharmacodynamics/Kinetics

Onset of action: Sublingual tablet: 1-3 minutes; Translingual spray: 2 minutes; Sustained release: 20-45 minutes; Topical: 15-60 minutes; Transdermal: 40-60 minutes; I.V. drip: Immediate

Peak effect: Sublingual tablet: 4-8 minutes; Translingual spray: 4-10 minutes; Sustained release: 45-120 minutes; Topical: 30-120 minutes; Transdermal: 60-180 minutes; I.V. drip: Immediate

Duration: Sublingual tablet: 30-60 minutes; Translingual spray: 30-60 minutes; Sustained release: 4-8 hours; Topical: 2-12 hours; Transdermal: 18-24 hours; I.V. drip: 3-5 minutes

Protein binding: 60%

Metabolism: Extensive first-pass effect

Half-life elimination: 1-4 minutes

Excretion: Urine (as inactive metabolites)

Dosage Note: Hemodynamic and antianginal tolerance often develop within 24-48 hours of continuous nitrate administration. Nitrate-free interval (10-12 hours/day) is recommended to avoid tolerance development; gradually decrease dose in patients receiving NTG for prolonged period to avoid withdrawal reaction.

Children: Pulmonary hypertension: Continuous infusion: Start 0.25-0.5 mcg/kg/minute and titrate by 1 mcg/kg/minute at 20- to 60-minute intervals to desired effect; usual dose: 1-3 mcg/kg/minute; maximum: 5 mcg/kg/minute

Adults:

Oral: 2.5-9 mg 2-4 times/day (up to 26 mg 4 times/day)

I.V.: 5 mcg/minute, increase by 5 mcg/minute every 3-5 minutes to 20 mcg/minute; if no response at 20 mcg/minute increase by 10 mcg/minute every 3-5 minutes, up to 200 mcg/minute

Ointment: 1/2" upon rising and 1/2" 6 hours later; the dose may be doubled and even doubled again as needed

Patch, transdermal: Initial: 0.2-0.4 mg/hour, titrate to doses of 0.4-0.8 mg/hour; tolerance is minimized by using a patch-on period of 12-14 hours and patch-off period of 10-12 hours

Sublingual: 0.2-0.6 mg every 5 minutes for maximum of 3 doses in 15 minutes; may also use prophylactically 5-10 minutes prior to activities which may provoke an attack

Esophageal spastic disorders (unlabeled use): 0.3-0.4 mg 5 minutes before meals

Translingual: 1-2 sprays into mouth under tongue every 3-5 minutes for maximum of 3 doses in 15 minutes, may also be used 5-10 minutes prior to activities which may provoke an attack prophylactically

Hemodialysis: Supplemental dose is not necessary

Peritoneal dialysis: Supplemental dose is not necessary

Elderly: In general, dose selection should be cautious, usually starting at the low end of the dosing range

Stability Doses should be made in glass bottles, Excell® or PAB® containers; adsorption occurs to soft plastic (ie, PVC)

Nitroglycerin diluted in D_5W or NS in glass containers is physically and chemically stable for 48 hours at room temperature and 7 days under refrigeration; in D_5W or NS in Excell®/PAB® containers is physically and chemically stable for 24 hours at room temperature and 14 days under refrigeration

Premixed bottles are stable according to the manufacturer's expiration dating

(Continued)

Nitroglycerin *(Continued)*

Standard diluent: 50 mg/250 mL D_5W; 50 mg/500 mL D_5W

Minimum volume: 100 mg/250 mL D_5W; concentration should not exceed 400 mcg/mL

Store sublingual tablets and ointment in tightly closed containers at 15°C to 30°C. Store spray and transdermal patch at 25°C, excursions permitted to 15°C to 30°C (59°F to 86°F).

Administration

I.V.: I.V. must be prepared in glass bottles; use special sets intended for nitroglycerin. glass I.V. bottles and administration sets provided by manufacturer.

Sublingual: Do not crush sublingual product (tablet). Place under tongue and allow to dissolve.

Translingual spray: Prime prior to first use (5 sprays into the air). If unused for 6 weeks, a single priming spray should be completed. Primimg sprays should be directed away from patient and others. The end of the pump should be covered by the fluid in the bottle.

Monitoring Parameters Blood pressure, heart rate

Anesthesia and Critical Care Concerns/Other Considerations Nitroglycerin 5 mg/mL contains propylene glycol 518 mg/mL (30% v/v).

In the treatment of unstable angina/non-ST-segment elevation MI, nitroglycerin (sublingual tablet or spray), followed by intravenous administration, is recommended for immediate relief of ischemia and associated symptoms. Note that nitrate use may result in significant hypotension in individuals who are volume depleted.

Nitrate use in right ventricular infarction may induce acute hypotension. Nitrate use in severe pericardial effusion may reduce cardiac filling pressure and precipitate cardiac tamponade.

Pregnancy Risk Factor C

Contraindications Hypersensitivity to organic nitrates; hypersensitivity to isosorbide, nitroglycerin, or any component of the formulation; concurrent use with phosphodiesterase-5 (PDE-5) inhibitors (sildenafil, tadalafil, or vardenafil); angle-closure glaucoma (intraocular pressure may be increased); head trauma or cerebral hemorrhage (increase intracranial pressure); severe anemia; allergy to adhesive (transdermal product)

Additional contraindications for I.V. product: Hypotension; uncorrected hypovolemia; inadequate cerebral circulation; constrictive pericarditis; pericardial tamponade

Warnings/Precautions Severe hypotension can occur. Use with caution in volume depletion, hypotension, and right ventricular infarctions. Paradoxical bradycardia and increased angina pectoris can accompany hypotension. Orthostatic hypotension can also occur. Ethanol can accentuate this. Tolerance does develop to nitrates and appropriate dosing is needed to minimize this (drug-free interval). Safety and efficacy have not been established in pediatric patients. Avoid use of long-acting agents in acute MI or CHF; cannot easily reverse. Nitrate may aggravate angina caused by hypertrophic cardiomyopathy. Nitroglycerin transdermal patches should be removed prior to defibrillation or MRI study.

Adverse Reactions

Translingual spray or patch:

>10%: Central nervous system: Headache (patch 63%, spray 50%)

1% to 10%:

Cardiovascular: Hypotension (patch 4%), increased angina (patch 2%), syncope (patch 4%)

Central nervous system: Lightheadedness (patch 6%)

<1% (Limited to important or life-threatening): Allergic reactions, application site irritation (patch), collapse, dizziness, exfoliative dermatitis, methemoglobinemia (rare, overdose), pallor, palpitation, perspiration, rash, restlessness, vertigo, weakness

Topical, sublingual, intravenous: Frequency not defined:

Cardiovascular: Hypotension (infrequent), postural hypotension, crescendo angina (uncommon), rebound hypertension (uncommon), pallor, cardiovascular collapse, tachycardia, shock, flushing, peripheral edema

Central nervous system: Headache (most common), lightheadedness (related to blood pressure changes), syncope (uncommon), dizziness, restlessness

Gastrointestinal: Nausea, vomiting, bowel incontinence, xerostomia

Genitourinary: Urinary incontinence

Hematologic: Methemoglobinemia (rare, overdose)
Neuromuscular & skeletal: Weakness
Ocular: Blurred vision
Miscellaneous: Cold sweat

Overdosage/Toxicology Symptoms of overdose include hypotension, throbbing headache, palpitations, bloody diarrhea, bradycardia, cyanosis, tissue hypoxia, metabolic acidosis, clonic convulsions, circulatory collapse, and methemoglobinemia with extremely large overdoses. Treatment is supportive and symptomatic. Methemoglobinemia should be treated with methylene blue (1-2 mg/kg over 5 minutes). Additional doses may be necessary (0.5-1 mg/kg) based on follow-up methemoglobin levels (obtained after 30 minutes).

Drug Interactions

Alteplase (tissue plasminogen activator) has a lesser effect when used with I.V. nitroglycerin; avoid concurrent use.

Ergot alkaloids may cause an increase in blood pressure and decrease in antianginal effects; avoid concurrent use.

Ethanol can cause hypotension when nitrates are taken 1 hour or more after ethanol ingestion.

Heparin's effect may be reduced by I.V. nitroglycerin. May affect only a minority of patients.

Sildenafil, tadalafil, vardenafil: Significant reduction of systolic and diastolic blood pressure with concurrent use (contraindicated). Do not administer sildenafil, tadalafil, or vardenafil within 24 hours of a nitrate preparation.

Dosage Forms

Capsule, extended release (Nitro-Time®): 2.5 mg, 6.5 mg, 9 mg

Infusion [premixed in D_5W]: 25 mg (250 mL) [0.1 mg/mL]; 50 mg (250 mL) [0.2 mg/mL]; 50 mg (500 mL) [0.1 mg/mL]; 100 mg (250 mL) [0.4 mg/mL]; 200 mg (500 mL) [0.4 mg/mL]

Injection, solution: 5 mg/mL (5 mL, 10 mL) [contains alcohol and propylene glycol]

Ointment, topical (Nitro-Bid®): 2% [20 mg/g] (1 g, 30 g, 60 g)

Solution, translingual spray (Nitrolingual®): 0.4 mg/metered spray (4.9 g) [contains alcohol 20%; 60 metered sprays]; (12 g) [contains alcohol 20%; 200 metered sprays]

Tablet, sublingual (NitroQuick®, Nitrostat®, Nitro-Tab®): 0.3 mg, 0.4 mg, 0.6 mg

Transdermal system [once daily patch]: 0.1 mg/hour (30s); 0.2 mg/hour (30s); 0.4 mg/hour (30s); 0.6 mg/hour (30s)

Minitran™: 0.1 mg/hour (30s); 0.2 mg/hour (30s); 0.4 mg/hour (30s); 0.6 mg/hour (30s)

Nitrek®: 0.2 mg/hour (30s); 0.4 mg/hour (30s); 0.6 mg/hour (30s)

Nitro-Dur®: 0.1 mg/hour (30s); 0.2 mg/hour (30s); 0.3 mg/hour (30s); 0.4 mg/hour (30s); 0.6 mg/hour (30s); 0.8 mg/hour (30s)

References

Erstad BL and Barletta JF, "Treatment of Hypertension in the Perioperative Patient," *Ann Pharmacother*, 2000, 34(1):66-79.

♦ **Nitroglycerin Injection, USP (Can)** *see* Nitroglycerin *on page 928*
♦ **Nitroglycerol** *see* Nitroglycerin *on page 928*
♦ **Nitrol® (Can)** *see* Nitroglycerin *on page 928*
♦ **Nitrolingual®** *see* Nitroglycerin *on page 928*
♦ **Nitropress®** *see* Nitroprusside *on page 931*

Nitroprusside (nye troe PRUS ide)

Medication Safety Issues

Sound-alike/look-alike issues:
Nitroprusside may be confused with nitroglycerin

High alert medication: The Institute for Safe Medication Practices (ISMP) includes this medication among its list of drugs which have a heightened risk of causing significant patient harm when used in error.

Related Information

Chronic Renal Failure *on page 1437*
Critical Care Infusion Administration Charts *on page 1514*
Heart Failure (Systolic) *on page 1607*
Hemodynamic Support, Intravenous *on page 1566*
Hypertension *on page 1620*
(Continued)

Nitroprusside *(Continued)*

U.S. Brand Names Nitropress®

Synonyms Nitroprusside Sodium; Sodium Nitroferricyanide; Sodium Nitroprusside

Pharmacologic Category Vasodilator

Generic Available Yes

Use Management of hypertensive crises; congestive heart failure; used for controlled hypotension to reduce bleeding during surgery

Mechanism of Action Causes peripheral vasodilation by direct action on venous and arteriolar smooth muscle, thus reducing peripheral resistance; will increase cardiac output by decreasing afterload; reduces aortal and left ventricular impedance

Pharmacodynamics/Kinetics

Onset of action: BP reduction <2 minutes

Duration: 1-10 minutes

Metabolism: Nitroprusside is converted to cyanide ions in the bloodstream; decomposes to prussic acid which in the presence of sulfur donor is converted to thiocyanate (hepatic and renal rhodanase systems)

Half-life elimination: Parent drug: <10 minutes; Thiocyanate: 2.7-7 days

Excretion: Urine (as thiocyanate)

Dosage Administration requires the use of an infusion pump. Average dose: 5 mcg/kg/minute.

Children: Pulmonary hypertension: I.V.: Initial: 1 mcg/kg/minute by continuous I.V. infusion; increase in increments of 1 mcg/kg/minute at intervals of 20-60 minutes; titrating to the desired response; usual dose: 3 mcg/kg/minute, rarely need >4 mcg/kg/minute; maximum: 5 mcg/kg/minute.

Adults: I.V. Initial: 0.3-0.5 mcg/kg/minute; increase in increments of 0.5 mcg/kg/minute, titrating to the desired hemodynamic effect or the appearance of headache or nausea; usual dose: 3 mcg/kg/minute; rarely need >4 mcg/kg/minute; maximum: 10 mcg/kg/minute. When administered by prolonged infusion faster than 2 mcg/kg/minute, cyanide is generated faster than an unaided patient can handle.

Stability

Nitroprusside sodium should be reconstituted freshly by diluting 50 mg in 250-1000 mL of D_5W

Use only clear solutions; solutions of nitroprusside exhibit a color described as brownish, brown, brownish-pink, light orange, and straw. Solutions are highly sensitive to light. Exposure to light causes decomposition, resulting in a highly colored solution of orange, dark brown or blue. **A blue color indicates almost complete degradation and breakdown to cyanide.**

Solutions should be wrapped with aluminum foil or other opaque material to protect from light (do as soon as possible)

Stability of parenteral admixture at room temperature (25°C) and at refrigeration temperature (4°C): 24 hours

Administration I.V. infusion only, not for direct injection

Monitoring Parameters Blood pressure, heart rate; monitor for cyanide and thiocyanate toxicity; monitor acid-base status as acidosis can be the earliest sign of cyanide toxicity; monitor thiocyanate levels if requiring prolonged infusion (>3 days) or dose ≥4 mcg/kg/minute or patient has renal dysfunction; monitor cyanide blood levels in patients with decreased hepatic function; cardiac monitor and blood pressure monitor required

Reference Range Monitor thiocyanate levels if requiring prolonged infusion (>4 days) or ≥4 mcg/kg/minute; not to exceed 100 mcg/mL (or 10 mg/dL) plasma thiocyanate

Thiocyanate:

Therapeutic: 6-29 mcg/mL

Toxic: 35-100 mcg/mL

Fatal: >200 mcg/mL

Cyanide: Normal <0.2 mcg/mL; normal (smoker): <0.4 mcg/mL

Toxic: >2 mcg/mL

Potentially lethal: >3 mcg/mL

Anesthesia and Critical Care Concerns/Other Considerations

Elderly patients may have an increased sensitivity to nitroprusside possibly due to a decreased baroreceptor reflex, altered sensitivity to vasodilating effects or a resistance of cardiac adrenergic receptors to stimulation by catecholamines.

Nitroprusside preparations must be wrapped with aluminum foil to protect from light in order to prevent breakdown of the parent drug to cyanide. A bluish tint to the solution indicates breakdown to cyanide. Thiocyanate levels should be monitored if high doses are used for more than 24 hours. Nitroprusside may also be useful for afterload reduction in patients with severe heart failure. Nitroprusside should be avoided in patients with aortic stenosis or coarctation. Nitroprusside should also be used cautiously in patients with acute myocardial infarction, because of hemodynamic effects and possible coronary steal.

Pregnancy Risk Factor C

Contraindications Hypersensitivity to nitroprusside or any component of the formulation; treatment of compensatory hypertension (aortic coarctation, arteriovenous shunting); high output failure; congenital optic atrophy or tobacco amblyopia

Warnings/Precautions **[U.S. Boxed Warning]: Continuous blood pressure monitoring is needed. Except when used briefly or at low (<2 mcg/kg/minute) infusion rates, nitroprusside gives rise to large cyanide quantities. Do not use the maximum dose for more than 10 minutes; if blood pressure not controlled then discontinue infusion. Monitor for cyanide toxicity via acid-base balance and venous oxygen concentration.** Use with extreme caution in patients with elevated intracranial pressure. Use extreme caution in patients with hepatic or renal dysfunction. Use the lowest end of the dosage range with renal impairment. Thiocyanate toxicity occurs in patients with renal impairment or those on prolonged infusions. **[U.S. Boxed Warning]: Should not be administered by direct injection; must be further diluted with 5% dextrose in water.**

Adverse Reactions 1% to 10%:

Cardiovascular: Excessive hypotensive response, palpitation, substernal distress
Central nervous system: Disorientation, psychosis, headache, restlessness
Endocrine & metabolic: Thyroid suppression
Gastrointestinal: Nausea, vomiting
Neuromuscular & skeletal: Weakness, muscle spasm
Otic: Tinnitus
Respiratory: Hypoxia
Miscellaneous: Diaphoresis, thiocyanate toxicity

Overdosage/Toxicology Symptoms of overdose include hypotension, vomiting, hyperventilation, tachycardia, muscular twitching, hypothyroidism, cyanide or thiocyanate toxicity. Thiocyanate toxicity includes psychosis, hyper-reflexia, confusion, weakness, tinnitus, seizures, and coma; cyanide toxicity includes acidosis (decreased HCO_3, decreased pH, increased lactate), increase in mixed venous blood oxygen tension, tachycardia, altered consciousness, coma, convulsions, and almond smell on breath.

Nitroprusside has been shown to release cyanide *in vivo* with hemoglobin. Cyanide toxicity does not usually occur because of the rapid uptake of cyanide by erythrocytes and its eventual incorporation into thiocyanate in the liver. However, high doses, prolonged administration of nitroprusside, or reduced elimination can lead to cyanide poisoning or thiocyanate intoxication. Anemia and liver impairment pose a risk for cyanide accumulation, while renal impairment predisposes thiocyanate accumulation. If toxicity develops, airway support with oxygen therapy is appropriate, followed closely with antidotal therapy of amyl nitrate perles, sodium nitrate 300 mg I.V. for adults (range based on hemoglobin concentration: 6-12 mg/kg for children) and sodium thiosulfate 12.5 g I.V. for adults (range based on hemoglobin concentration: 0.95-1.95 mL/kg of the 25% solution for children); nitrates should not be administered to neonates and small children. Thiocyanate is dialyzable. May be mixed with sodium thiosulfate in I.V. to prevent cyanide toxicity.

Drug Interactions None noted

Dosage Forms Injection, solution, as sodium: 25 mg/mL (2 mL)

References

Erstad BL and Barletta JF, "Treatment of Hypertension in the Perioperative Patient," *Ann Pharmacother*, 2000, 34(1):66-79.

Vesey CJ and Cole PV, "Blood Cyanide and Thiocyanate Concentrations Produced by Long-Term Therapy With Sodium Nitroprusside," *Br J Anaesth*, 1985, 57(2):148-55.

♦ **Nitroprusside Sodium** *see* Nitroprusside *on page 931*
♦ **NitroQuick®** *see* Nitroglycerin *on page 928*
♦ **Nitrostat®** *see* Nitroglycerin *on page 928*
♦ **Nitro-Tab®** *see* Nitroglycerin *on page 928*
♦ **NitroTime®** *see* Nitroglycerin *on page 928*

Nitrous Oxide (NYE trus OKS ide)

Pharmacologic Category Dental Gases; General Anesthetic

Generic Available Yes

Use Produces sedation and analgesia; principal adjunct to inhalation and intravenous general anesthesia

Mechanism of Action General CNS depressant action; may act similarly as inhalant general anesthetics by stabilizing axonal membranes to partially inhibit action potentials leading to sedation; may partially act on opiate receptor systems to cause mild analgesia; central sympathetic stimulating action supports blood pressure, systemic vascular resistance, and cardiac output; it does not depress carbon dioxide drive to breath. Nitrous oxide increases cerebral blood flow and intracranial pressure while decreasing hepatic and renal blood flow; has analgesic action similar to morphine.

Pharmacodynamics/Kinetics

Onset of action: Inhalation: 2-5 minutes

Absorption: Rapid via lungs; blood/gas partition coefficient is 0.47

Metabolism: Body: <0.004%

Excretion: Primarily exhaled gases; skin (minimal amounts)

Dosage Children and Adults:

Surgical: For sedation and analgesia: Concentrations of 25% to 50% nitrous oxide with oxygen. For general anesthesia, concentrations of 40% to 70% via mask or endotracheal tube. Minimal alveolar concentration (MAC), which can be considered the ED_{50} of inhalational anesthetics, is 105%; therefore delivery in a hyperbaric chamber is necessary to use as a complete anesthetic. When administered at 70%, reduces the MAC of other anesthetics by half.

Dental: For sedation and analgesia: Concentrations of 25% to 50% nitrous oxide with oxygen

Anesthesia and Critical Care Concerns/Other Considerations Nitrous oxide's central sympathetic stimulating action supports blood pressure, systemic vascular resistance, and cardiac output. It does not depress carbon dioxide drive to breathe. It increases cerebral blood flow and intracranial pressure while decreasing hepatic and renal blood flow. Nitrous oxide has analgesic action similar to morphine.

Pregnancy Risk Factor No data reported

Contraindications Hypersensitivity to nitrous oxide or any component of the formulation; nitrous oxide should not be administered without oxygen; should not be given to patients after a full meal

Warnings/Precautions Nausea and vomiting occurs postoperatively in ~15% of patients. Prolonged use may produce bone marrow suppression and/or neurologic dysfunction. Oxygen should be briefly administered during emergence from prolonged anesthesia with nitrous oxide to prevent diffusion hypoxia. Patients with vitamin B_{12} deficiency (pernicious anemia) and those with other nutritional deficiencies (alcoholics) are at increased risk of developing neurologic disease and bone marrow suppression with exposure to nitrous oxide. May be addictive.

Adverse Reactions Frequency not defined.

Cardiovascular: Hypotension

Central nervous system: Headache, dizziness, confusion, CNS excitation

Gastrointestinal: Possibly nausea and vomiting

Respiratory: Apnea

Miscellaneous: Personnel exposed to unscavenged nitrous oxide have an increased risk of renal and hepatic diseases and peripheral neuropathy similar to that of vitamin B_{12} deficiency. Female dental personnel who were exposed to unscavenged nitrous oxide for more than 5 hours/week were significantly less fertile than women who were not exposed, or who were exposed to lower levels of scavenged or unscavenged nitrous oxide.

Drug Interactions No data reported

Dosage Forms Supplied in blue cylinders

Nizatidine (ni ZA ti deen)

Medication Safety Issues

Sound-alike/look-alike issues:

Axid® may be confused with Ansaid®

U.S. Brand Names Axid®; Axid® AR [OTC]

Canadian Brand Names Apo-Nizatidine®; Axid®; Gen-Nizatidine; Novo-Nizatidine; Nu-Nizatidine; PMS-Nizatidine

Pharmacologic Category Histamine H_2 Antagonist

Generic Available Yes: Capsule

Use Treatment and maintenance of duodenal ulcer; treatment of benign gastric ulcer; treatment of gastroesophageal reflux disease (GERD); OTC tablet used for the prevention of meal-induced heartburn, acid indigestion, and sour stomach

Unlabeled/Investigational Use Part of a multidrug regimen for *H. pylori* eradication to reduce the risk of duodenal ulcer recurrence

Mechanism of Action Competitive inhibition of histamine at H_2-receptors of the gastric parietal cells resulting in reduced gastric acid secretion, gastric volume and hydrogen ion concentration reduced. In healthy volunteers, nizatidine suppresses gastric acid secretion induced by pentagastrin infusion or food.

Pharmacodynamics/Kinetics

Distribution: V_d: 0.8-1.5 L/kg

Protein binding: 35% to α_1-acid glycoprotein

Metabolism: Partially hepatic; forms metabolites

Bioavailability: >70%

Half-life elimination: 1-2 hours; prolonged with renal impairment

Time to peak, plasma: 0.5-3.0 hours

Excretion: Urine (90%; ~60% as unchanged drug); feces (<6%)

Dosage Oral:

Children:

<12 years: GERD (unlabeled use): 10 mg/kg/day in divided doses given twice daily; may not be as effective in children <12 years

≥12 years:

GERD: Refer to Adults dosing

Meal-induced heartburn, acid indigestion and sour stomach: Refer to Adults dosing

Adults:

Duodenal ulcer:

Treatment of active ulcer: 300 mg at bedtime or 150 mg twice daily

Maintenance of healed ulcer: 150 mg/day at bedtime

Gastric ulcer: 150 mg twice daily or 300 mg at bedtime

GERD: 150 mg twice daily

Meal-induced heartburn, acid indigestion, and sour stomach: 75 mg tablet [OTC] twice daily, 30 to 60 minutes prior to consuming food or beverages

Helicobacter pylori eradication (unlabeled use): 150 mg twice daily; requires combination therapy

Dosing adjustment in renal impairment:

Active treatment:

Cl_{cr} 20-50 mL/minute: 150 mg/day

Cl_{cr} <20 mL/minute: 150 mg every other day

Maintenance treatment:

Cl_{cr} 20-50 mL/minute: 150 mg every other day

Cl_{cr} <20 mL/minute: 150 mg every 3 days

Pregnancy Risk Factor B

Contraindications Hypersensitivity to nizatidine or any component of the formulation; hypersensitivity to other H_2 antagonists (cross-sensitivity has been observed)

Warnings/Precautions Use with caution in children <12 years of age; use with caution in patients with liver and renal impairment; dosage modification required in patients with renal impairment

Adverse Reactions

>10%: Central nervous system: Headache (16%)

1% to 10%:

Central nervous system: Anxiety, dizziness, fever (reported in children), insomnia, irritability (reported in children), somnolence, nervousness

Dermatologic: Pruritus, rash

(Continued)

Nizatidine *(Continued)*

Gastrointestinal: Abdominal pain, anorexia, constipation, diarrhea, dry mouth, flatulence, heartburn, nausea, vomiting

Respiratory: Reported in children: Cough, nasal congestion, nasopharyngitis

<1% (Limited to important or life-threatening): Alkaline phosphatase increased, anaphylaxis, anemia, AST/ALT increased, bronchospasm, confusion, eosinophilia, exfoliative dermatitis, gynecomastia, hepatitis, jaundice, laryngeal edema, serum-sickness like reactions, thrombocytopenia, thrombocytopenic purpura, vasculitis, ventricular tachycardia

Overdosage/Toxicology Symptoms of overdose include muscular tremor, vomiting, and rapid respiration. LD_{50} ~80 mg/kg. Treatment is symptomatic and supportive.

Drug Interactions Inhibits 3A4 (weak)

Antifungal agents (imidazole): Nizatidine may decrease the absorption of itraconazole or ketoconazole.

Ethanol/Nutrition/Herb Interactions

Ethanol: Avoid ethanol (may cause gastric mucosal irritation).

Food: Administration with apple juice may decrease absorption.

Test Interactions False-positive urine protein using Multistix®, gastric acid secretion test, skin tests allergen extracts, serum creatinine and serum transaminase concentrations, urine protein test

Dosage Forms

Capsule (Axid®): 150 mg, 300 mg

Solution, oral (Axid®): 15 mg/mL (120 mL, 480 mL) [bubble gum flavor]

Tablet (Axid® AR): 75 mg

- ♦ **Nizoral®** *see* Ketoconazole *on page 711*
- ♦ **Nizoral® A-D [OTC]** *see* Ketoconazole *on page 711*
- ♦ **No Doz® Maximum Strength [OTC]** *see* Caffeine *on page 211*
- ♦ **Noradrenaline** *see* Norepinephrine *on page 936*
- ♦ **Noradrenaline Acid Tartrate** *see* Norepinephrine *on page 936*
- ♦ **Norco®** *see* Hydrocodone and Acetaminophen *on page 636*
- ♦ **Norcuron® [DSC]** *see* Vecuronium *on page 1345*
- ♦ **Nordeoxyguanosine** *see* Ganciclovir *on page 581*
- ♦ **Norditropin®** *see* Human Growth Hormone *on page 625*
- ♦ **Norditropin® NordiFlex®** *see* Human Growth Hormone *on page 625*

Norepinephrine (nor ep i NEF rin)

Related Information

Allergic Reactions *on page 1395*

Critical Care Infusion Administration Charts *on page 1514*

Hemodynamic Support, Intravenous *on page 1566*

U.S. Brand Names Levophed®

Canadian Brand Names Levophed®

Synonyms Levarterenol Bitartrate; Noradrenaline; Noradrenaline Acid Tartrate; Norepinephrine Bitartrate

Pharmacologic Category Alpha/Beta Agonist

Generic Available Yes

Use Treatment of shock which persists after adequate fluid volume replacement

Mechanism of Action Stimulates $beta_1$-adrenergic receptors and alpha-adrenergic receptors causing increased contractility and heart rate as well as vasoconstriction, thereby increasing systemic blood pressure and coronary blood flow; clinically alpha effects (vasoconstriction) are greater than beta effects (inotropic and chronotropic effects)

Pharmacodynamics/Kinetics

Onset of action: I.V.: Very rapid-acting

Duration: Limited

Metabolism: Via catechol-o-methyltransferase (COMT) and monoamine oxidase (MAO)

Excretion: Urine (84% to 96% as inactive metabolites)

Dosage Administration requires the use of an infusion pump!

Note: Norepinephrine dosage is stated in terms of norepinephrine base and intravenous formulation is norepinephrine bitartrate

Norepinephrine bitartrate 2 mg = Norepinephrine base 1 mg

Continuous I.V. infusion:

Children: Initial: 0.05-0.1 mcg/kg/minute; titrate to desired effect; maximum dose: 1-2 mcg/kg/minute

Adults: Initial: 0.5-1 mcg/minute and titrate to desired response; 8-30 mcg/minute is usual range; range used in clinical trials: 0.01-3 mcg/kg/minute; ACLS dosage range: 0.5-30 mcg/minute

Stability Readily oxidized, protect from light, do not use if brown coloration; dilute with D_5W or D_5NS, but not recommended to dilute in normal saline; not stable with alkaline solutions; stability of parenteral admixture at room temperature (25°C): 24 hours

Administration Administer into large vein to avoid the potential for extravasation; potent drug, must be diluted prior to use; do not administer $NaHCO_3$ through an I.V. line containing norepinephrine.

Anesthesia and Critical Care Concerns/Other Considerations Norepinephrine is effective at increasing arterial blood pressure through vasoconstriction with little change in heart rate or cardiac output. Adequate fluid resuscitation is essential to the success of norepinephrine in raising blood pressure; may successfully increase blood pressure without causing a deterioration in cardiac index or organ function in patients with septic shock. It should be used early and not withheld as a last resort. The 2004 Surviving Sepsis Campaign guidelines suggest that either norephinephrine or dopamine is the first-choice vasopressor agent. Norephinephrine is more potent than dopamine and may be more effective at reversing hypotension in septic shock.

Pregnancy Risk Factor C

Contraindications Hypersensitivity to norepinephrine, bisulfites (contains metabisulfite), or any component of the formulation; hypotension from hypovolemia except as an emergency measure to maintain coronary and cerebral perfusion until volume could be replaced; mesenteric or peripheral vascular thrombosis unless it is a lifesaving procedure; during anesthesia with cyclopropane or halothane anesthesia (risk of ventricular arrhythmias)

Warnings/Precautions Assure adequate circulatory volume to minimize need for vasoconstrictors. Avoid hypertension; monitor blood pressure closely and adjust infusion rate. Avoid extravasation; infuse into a large vein if possible. Avoid infusion into leg veins. Watch I.V. site closely. **[U.S. Boxed Warning]: If extravasation occurs, infiltrate the area with diluted phentolamine (5-10 mg in 10-15 mL of saline) with a fine hypodermic needle. Phentolamine should be administered as soon as possible after extravasation is noted.**

Adverse Reactions Frequency not defined.

Cardiovascular: Bradycardia, arrhythmia, peripheral (digital) ischemia

Central nervous system: Headache (transient), anxiety

Local: Skin necrosis (with extravasation)

Respiratory: Dyspnea, respiratory difficulty

Overdosage/Toxicology Symptoms of overdose include hypertension, sweating, cerebral hemorrhage, and convulsions. Infiltrate the area of extravasation with phentolamine 5-10 mg in 10-15 mL of saline solution; inject a small amount of this dilution into extravasated area; blanching should reverse immediately. Monitor site; if blanching should recur, additional injections of phentolamine may be needed.

Drug Interactions

Beta-blockers (nonselective ones) may increase hypertensive effect; avoid concurrent use.

Cocaine may cause malignant arrhythmias; avoid concurrent use.

Guanethidine can increase the pressor response; be aware of the patient's drug regimen.

MAO inhibitors potentiate hypertension and hypertensive crisis; avoid concurrent use.

Methyldopa can increase the pressor response; be aware of patient's drug regimen.

Reserpine increases the pressor response; be aware of patient's drug regimen.

TCAs increase the pressor response; be aware of patient's drug regimen.

Dosage Forms Injection, solution, as bitartrate: 1 mg/mL (4 mL) [contains sodium metabisulfite]

References

Dellinger RP, Carlet JM, Masur H, et al, "Surviving Sepsis Campaign Guidelines for Management of Severe Sepsis and Septic Shock," *Crit Care Med*, 2004, 32(3):858-73.

Martin C, Papazian L, Perrin G, et al, "Norepinephrine or Dopamine for the Treatment of Hyperdynamic Septic Shock?" *Chest*, 1993, 103(6):1826-31.

- **Norepinephrine Bitartrate** *see* Norepinephrine *on page 936*
- **Noritate®** *see* Metronidazole *on page 842*
- **Normal Human Serum Albumin** *see* Albumin *on page 48*
- **Normal Saline** *see* Sodium Chloride *on page 1183*
- **Normal Serum Albumin (Human)** *see* Albumin *on page 48*
- **Normodyne® (Can)** *see* Labetalol *on page 721*
- **Norpace®** *see* Disopyramide *on page 404*
- **Norpace® CR** *see* Disopyramide *on page 404*
- **Norpramin®** *see* Desipramine *on page 359*
- **Nortemp Children's [OTC]** *see* Acetaminophen *on page 26*

Nortriptyline (nor TRIP ti leen)

Medication Safety Issues

Sound-alike/look-alike issues:

Nortriptyline may be confused with amitriptyline, desipramine, Norpramin®

Aventyl® HCl may be confused with Bentyl®

Pamelor® may be confused with Demerol®, Dymelor®

Related Information

Antidepressant Agents *on page 1551*

Chronic Pain Management *on page 1430*

U.S. Brand Names Pamelor®

Canadian Brand Names Alti-Nortriptyline; Apo-Nortriptyline®; Aventyl®; Gen-Nortriptyline; Norventyl; Novo-Nortriptyline; Nu-Nortriptyline; PMS-Nortriptyline

Synonyms Nortriptyline Hydrochloride

Pharmacologic Category Antidepressant, Tricyclic (Secondary Amine)

Restrictions A medication guide concerning the use of antidepressants in children and teenagers can be found on the FDA website at http://www.fda.gov/cder/Offices/ODS/labeling.htm. It should be dispensed to parents or guardians of children and teenagers receiving this medication.

Generic Available Yes: Excludes solution

Use Treatment of symptoms of depression

Unlabeled/Investigational Use Chronic pain, anxiety disorders, enuresis, attention-deficit/hyperactivity disorder (ADHD); adjunctive therapy for smoking cessation

Mechanism of Action Traditionally believed to increase the synaptic concentration of serotonin and/or norepinephrine in the central nervous system by inhibition of their reuptake by the presynaptic neuronal membrane. However, additional receptor effects have been found including desensitization of adenyl cyclase, down regulation of beta-adrenergic receptors, and down regulation of serotonin receptors.

Pharmacodynamics/Kinetics

Onset of action: Therapeutic: 1-3 weeks

Distribution: V_d: 21 L/kg

Protein binding: 93% to 95%

Metabolism: Primarily hepatic; extensive first-pass effect

Half-life elimination: 28-31 hours

Time to peak, serum: 7-8.5 hours

Excretion: Urine (as metabolites and small amounts of unchanged drug); feces (small amounts)

Dosage Oral:

Nocturnal enuresis: Children (unlabeled use): 10-20 mg/day; titrate to a maximum of 40 mg/day

Depression (unlabeled use): Children: 1-3 mg/kg/day

Depression:

Adults: 25 mg 3-4 times/day up to 150 mg/day

Elderly (**Note:** Nortriptyline is one of the best tolerated TCAs in the elderly)

Initial: 10-25 mg at bedtime

Dosage can be increased by 25 mg every 3 days for inpatients and weekly for outpatients if tolerated

Usual maintenance dose: 75 mg as a single bedtime dose or 2 divided doses; however, lower or higher doses may be required to stay within the therapeutic window

Myofascial pain, neuralgia, burning mouth syndrome (dental use): Initial: 10-25 mg at bedtime; dosage may be increased by 25 mg/day weekly, if tolerated; usual maintenance dose: 75 mg as a single bedtime dose or 2 divided doses

Chronic urticaria, angioedema, nocturnal pruritus (unlabeled use): Adults: Oral: 75 mg/day

Smoking cessation (unlabeled use): Adults: 25-75 mg/day beginning 10-14 days before "quit" day; continue therapy for ≥12 weeks after "quit" day

Dosing adjustment in hepatic impairment: Lower doses and slower titration dependent on individualization of dosage is recommended

Stability Protect from light

Monitoring Parameters Blood pressure and pulse rate (ECG, cardiac monitoring) prior to and during initial therapy in older adults; weight; blood levels are useful for therapeutic monitoring

Reference Range

Plasma levels do not always correlate with clinical effectiveness

Therapeutic: 50-150 ng/mL (SI: 190-570 nmol/L)

Toxic: >500 ng/mL (SI: >1900 nmol/L)

Anesthesia and Critical Care Concerns/Other Considerations Its maximum antidepressant effect may not be seen for ≥2 weeks after initiation of therapy.

Pregnancy Risk Factor D

Contraindications Hypersensitivity to nortriptyline and similar chemical class, or any component of the formulation; use of MAO inhibitors within 14 days; use in a patient during the acute recovery phase of MI; pregnancy

Warnings/Precautions [U.S. Boxed Warning]: Antidepressants increase the risk of suicidal thinking and behavior in children and adolescents with major depressive disorder (MDD) and other depressive disorders; consider risk prior to prescribing. Closely monitor for clinical worsening, suicidality, or unusual changes in behavior; the child's family or caregiver should be instructed to closely observe the patient and communicate condition with healthcare provider. Such observation would generally include at least weekly face-to-face contact with patients or their family members or caregivers during the first 4 weeks of treatment, then every other week visits for the next 4 weeks, then at 12 weeks, and as clinically indicated beyond 12 weeks. Additional contact by telephone may be appropriate between face-to-face visits. Adults treated with antidepressants should be observed similarly for clinical worsening and suicidality, especially during the initial few months of a course of drug therapy, or at times of dose changes, either increases or decreases. A medication guide should be dispensed with each prescription. **Nortriptyline is not FDA approved for use in children.**

The possibility of a suicide attempt is inherent in major depression and may persist until remission occurs. Monitor for worsening of depression or suicidality, especially during initiation of therapy or with dose increases or decreases. Worsening depression and severe abrupt suicidality that are not part of the presenting symptoms may require discontinuation or modification of drug therapy. Use caution in high-risk patients during initiation of therapy. Prescriptions should be written for the smallest quantity consistent with good patient care. The patient's family or caregiver should be alerted to monitor patients for the emergence of suicidality and associated behaviors such as anxiety, agitation, panic attacks, insomnia, irritability, hostility, impulsivity, akathisia, hypomania, and mania; patients should be instructed to notify their healthcare provider if any of these symptoms or worsening depression occur.

May worsen psychosis in some patients or precipitate a shift to mania or hypomania in patients with bipolar disorder. Monotherapy in patients with bipolar disorder should be avoided. Patients presenting with depressive symptoms should be screened for bipolar disorder. **Nortriptyline is not FDA approved for the treatment of bipolar depression.**

May cause sedation, resulting in impaired performance of tasks requiring alertness (eg, operating machinery or driving). Sedative effects may be additive with other CNS depressants and/or ethanol. The degree of sedation is low-moderate relative to other antidepressants. May increase the risks associated with electroconvulsive therapy. Consider discontinuing, when possible, prior to elective surgery. Therapy should not be abruptly discontinued in patients receiving high doses for prolonged periods. May alter glucose regulation - use caution in patients with diabetes.

(Continued)

Nortriptyline *(Continued)*

May cause orthostatic hypotension (risk is low relative to other antidepressants) - use with caution in patients at risk of hypotension or in patients where transient hypotensive episodes would be poorly tolerated (cardiovascular disease or cerebrovascular disease). The degree of anticholinergic blockade produced by this agent is moderate relative to other cyclic antidepressants, however, caution should still be used in patients with urinary retention, benign prostatic hyperplasia, narrow-angle glaucoma, xerostomia, visual problems, constipation, or history of bowel obstruction.

Use with caution in patients with a history of cardiovascular disease (including previous MI, stroke, tachycardia, or conduction abnormalities). The risk conduction abnormalities with this agent is moderate relative to other antidepressants. Use caution in patients with a previous seizure disorder or condition predisposing to seizures such as brain damage, alcoholism, or concurrent therapy with other drugs which lower the seizure threshold. Use with caution in hyperthyroid patients or those receiving thyroid supplementation. Use with caution in patients with hepatic or renal dysfunction and in elderly patients.

Adverse Reactions Frequency not defined.

Cardiovascular: Postural hypotension, arrhythmia, hypertension, heart block, tachycardia, palpitation, MI

Central nervous system: Confusion, delirium, hallucinations, restlessness, insomnia, disorientation, delusions, anxiety, agitation, panic, nightmares, hypomania, exacerbation of psychosis, incoordination, ataxia, extrapyramidal symptoms, seizure

Dermatologic: Alopecia, photosensitivity, rash, petechiae, urticaria, itching

Endocrine & metabolic: Sexual dysfunction, gynecomastia, breast enlargement, galactorrhea, increase or decrease in libido, increase in blood sugar, SIADH

Gastrointestinal: Xerostomia, constipation, vomiting, anorexia, diarrhea, abdominal cramps, black tongue, nausea, unpleasant taste, weight gain/loss

Genitourinary: Urinary retention, delayed micturition, impotence, testicular edema

Hematologic: Rarely agranulocytosis, eosinophilia, purpura, thrombocytopenia

Hepatic: Increased liver enzymes, cholestatic jaundice

Neuromuscular & skeletal: Tremor, numbness, tingling, paresthesia, peripheral neuropathy

Ocular: Blurred vision, eye pain, disturbances in accommodation, mydriasis

Otic: Tinnitus

Miscellaneous: Diaphoresis (excessive), allergic reactions

Overdosage/Toxicology Symptoms of overdose include agitation, confusion, hallucinations, urinary retention, hypothermia, hypotension, seizures, and ventricular tachycardia. Treatment is symptomatic and supportive. Alkalinization by sodium bicarbonate and/or hyperventilation may limit cardiac toxicity.

Drug Interactions **Substrate** of CYP1A2 (minor), 2C19 (minor), 2D6 (major), 3A4 (minor); **Inhibits** CYP2D6 (weak), 2E1 (weak)

Altretamine: Concurrent use may cause orthostatic hypertension

Amphetamines: TCAs may enhance the effect of amphetamines; monitor for adverse CV effects

Anticholinergics: Combined use with TCAs may produce additive anticholinergic effects

Antihypertensives: TCAs may inhibit the antihypertensive response to bethanidine, clonidine, debrisoquin, guanadrel, guanethidine, guanabenz, guanfacine; monitor BP; consider alternate antihypertensive agent

Beta-agonists: When combined with TCAs may predispose patients to cardiac arrhythmias

Bupropion: May increase the levels of tricyclic antidepressants; based on limited information; monitor response

Carbamazepine: Tricyclic antidepressants may increase carbamazepine levels; monitor

Cholestyramine and colestipol: May bind TCAs and reduce their absorption; monitor for altered response

Clonidine: Abrupt discontinuation of clonidine may cause hypertensive crisis, amitriptyline may enhance the response

CNS depressants: Sedative effects may be additive with TCAs; monitor for increased effect; includes benzodiazepines, barbiturates, antipsychotics, ethanol and other sedative medications

CYP2D6 inhibitors: May increase the levels/effects of nortriptyline. Example inhibitors include chlorpromazine, delavirdine, fluoxetine, miconazole, paroxetine, pergolide, quinidine, quinine, ritonavir, and ropinirole.

Epinephrine (and other direct alpha-agonists): Pressor response to I.V. epinephrine, norepinephrine, and phenylephrine may be enhanced in patients receiving TCAs (**Note:** Effect is unlikely with epinephrine or levonordefrin dosages typically administered as infiltration in combination with local anesthetics)

Fenfluramine: May increase tricyclic antidepressant levels/effects

Hypoglycemic agents (including insulin): TCAs may enhance the hypoglycemic effects of tolazamide, chlorpropamide, or insulin; monitor for changes in blood glucose levels; reported with chlorpropamide, tolazamide, and insulin

Levodopa: Tricyclic antidepressants may decrease the absorption (bioavailability) of levodopa; rare hypertensive episodes have also been attributed to this combination

Linezolid: Hyperpyrexia, hypertension, tachycardia, confusion, seizures, and **deaths have been reported** with agents which inhibit MAO (serotonin syndrome); this combination should be avoided

Lithium: Concurrent use with a TCA may increase the risk for neurotoxicity

MAO inhibitors: Hyperpyrexia, hypertension, tachycardia, confusion, seizures, and **deaths have been reported** (serotonin syndrome); this combination should be avoided

Methylphenidate: Metabolism of TCAs may be decreased

Phenothiazines: Serum concentrations of some TCAs may be increased; in addition, TCAs may increase concentration of phenothiazines; monitor for altered clinical response

QT_c-prolonging agents: Concurrent use of tricyclic agents with other drugs which may prolong QT_c interval may increase the risk of potentially fatal arrhythmias; includes type Ia and type III antiarrhythmics agents, selected quinolones (sparfloxacin, gatifloxacin, moxifloxacin, grepafloxacin), cisapride, and other agents

Ritonavir: Combined use of high-dose tricyclic antidepressants with ritonavir may cause serotonin syndrome in HIV-positive patients; monitor

Sucralfate: Absorption of tricyclic antidepressants may be reduced with coadministration

Sympathomimetics, indirect-acting: Tricyclic antidepressants may result in a decreased sensitivity to indirect-acting sympathomimetics; includes dopamine and ephedrine; also see interaction with epinephrine (and direct-acting sympathomimetics)

Tramadol: Tramadol's risk of seizures may be increased with TCAs

Valproic acid: May increase serum concentrations/adverse effects of some tricyclic antidepressants

Warfarin (and other oral anticoagulants): TCAs may increase the anticoagulant effect in patients stabilized on warfarin; monitor INR

Ethanol/Nutrition/Herb Interactions

Ethanol: Avoid ethanol (may increase CNS depression).

Food: Grapefruit juice may inhibit the metabolism of some TCAs and clinical toxicity may result.

Herb/Nutraceutical: Avoid valerian, St John's wort, SAMe, kava kava (may increase risk of serotonin syndrome and/or excessive sedation).

Dosage Forms

Capsule, as hydrochloride: 10 mg, 25 mg, 50 mg, 75 mg

Pamelor®: 10 mg, 25 mg, 50 mg, 75 mg [may contain benzyl alcohol; 50 mg may also contain sodium bisulfite]

Solution, as hydrochloride (Pamelor®): 10 mg/5 mL (473 mL) [contains alcohol 4% and benzoic acid]

- **Nortriptyline Hydrochloride** *see* Nortriptyline *on page 938*
- **Norventyl (Can)** *see* Nortriptyline *on page 938*
- **Norvir®** *see* Ritonavir *on page 1129*
- **Norvir® SEC (Can)** *see* Ritonavir *on page 1129*
- **Novasen (Can)** *see* Aspirin *on page 129*
- **Novo-Alprazol (Can)** *see* Alprazolam *on page 65*
- **Novo-Amiodarone (Can)** *see* Amiodarone *on page 83*
- **Novo-Ampicillin (Can)** *see* Ampicillin *on page 104*
- **Novo-Atenol (Can)** *see* Atenolol *on page 136*
- **Novo-Azathioprine (Can)** *see* Azathioprine *on page 148*
- **Novo-Azithromycin (Can)** *see* Azithromycin *on page 149*

- **NPH Insulin** *see* Insulin NPH *on page 690*
- **NPH Insulin and Regular Insulin** *see* Insulin NPH and Insulin Regular *on page 691*
- **NRS® [OTC]** *see* Oxymetazoline *on page 973*
- **NSC-740** *see* Methotrexate *on page 821*
- **NSC-15200** *see* Gallium Nitrate *on page 580*
- **NSC-26271** *see* Cyclophosphamide *on page 334*
- **NSC-49842** *see* VinBLAStine *on page 1356*
- **NSC-66847** *see* Thalidomide *on page 1250*
- **NSC-125066** *see* Bleomycin *on page 180*
- **NSC-671663** *see* Octreotide *on page 946*
- **NSC-721517** *see* Zoledronic Acid *on page 1377*
- **NSC-724223** *see* Epoetin Alfa *on page 463*
- **NSC-728729** *see* Infliximab *on page 677*
- **NTG** *see* Nitroglycerin *on page 928*
- **Nu-Acyclovir (Can)** *see* Acyclovir *on page 39*
- **Nu-Alprax (Can)** *see* Alprazolam *on page 65*
- **Nu-Ampi (Can)** *see* Ampicillin *on page 104*
- **Nu-Atenol (Can)** *see* Atenolol *on page 136*
- **Nu-Baclo (Can)** *see* Baclofen *on page 156*
- **Nubain®** *see* Nalbuphine *on page 892*
- **Nu-Beclomethasone (Can)** *see* Beclomethasone *on page 161*
- **Nu-Buspirone (Can)** *see* BusPIRone *on page 205*
- **Nu-Capto (Can)** *see* Captopril *on page 221*
- **Nu-Carbamazepine (Can)** *see* Carbamazepine *on page 225*
- **Nu-Cimet (Can)** *see* Cimetidine *on page 281*
- **Nu-Clonazepam (Can)** *see* Clonazepam *on page 313*
- **Nu-Clonidine (Can)** *see* Clonidine *on page 316*
- **Nu-Cotrimox (Can)** *see* Sulfamethoxazole and Trimethoprim *on page 1215*
- **Nu-Desipramine (Can)** *see* Desipramine *on page 359*
- **Nu-Diclo (Can)** *see* Diclofenac *on page 378*
- **Nu-Diclo-SR (Can)** *see* Diclofenac *on page 378*
- **Nu-Diflunisal (Can)** *see* Diflunisal *on page 385*
- **Nu-Diltiaz (Can)** *see* Diltiazem *on page 394*
- **Nu-Diltiaz-CD (Can)** *see* Diltiazem *on page 394*
- **Nu-Divalproex (Can)** *see* Valproic Acid and Derivatives *on page 1329*
- **Nu-Doxycycline (Can)** *see* Doxycycline *on page 426*
- **Nu-Erythromycin-S (Can)** *see* Erythromycin *on page 476*
- **Nu-Famotidine (Can)** *see* Famotidine *on page 506*
- **Nu-Fluoxetine (Can)** *see* Fluoxetine *on page 539*
- **Nu-Flurprofen (Can)** *see* Flurbiprofen *on page 550*
- **Nu-Gabapentin (Can)** *see* Gabapentin *on page 577*
- **Nu-Glyburide (Can)** *see* GlyBURIDE *on page 598*
- **Nu-Hydral (Can)** *see* HydrALAZINE *on page 632*
- **Nu-Ibuprofen (Can)** *see* Ibuprofen *on page 651*
- **Nu-Indo (Can)** *see* Indomethacin *on page 674*
- **Nu-Ipratropium (Can)** *see* Ipratropium *on page 698*
- **Nu-Ketoprofen (Can)** *see* Ketoprofen *on page 714*
- **Nu-Ketoprofen-E (Can)** *see* Ketoprofen *on page 714*
- **Nu-Levocarb (Can)** *see* Levodopa and Carbidopa *on page 743*
- **Nu-Loraz (Can)** *see* Lorazepam *on page 773*
- **Nu-Lovastatin (Can)** *see* Lovastatin *on page 782*
- **Nu-Medopa (Can)** *see* Methyldopa *on page 826*
- **Nu-Mefenamic (Can)** *see* Mefenamic Acid *on page 795*
- **Nu-Metformin (Can)** *see* Metformin *on page 810*
- **Nu-Metoclopramide (Can)** *see* Metoclopramide *on page 834*
- **Nu-Metop (Can)** *see* Metoprolol *on page 839*
- **Numorphan®** *see* Oxymorphone *on page 974*
- **Nu-Naprox (Can)** *see* Naproxen *on page 899*
- **Nu-Nifed (Can)** *see* NIFEdipine *on page 920*

- ♦ **Nu-Nizatidine (Can)** *see* Nizatidine *on page 935*
- ♦ **Nu-Nortriptyline (Can)** *see* Nortriptyline *on page 938*
- ♦ **Nupercainal® Hydrocortisone Cream [OTC]** *see* Hydrocortisone *on page 639*
- ♦ **Nu-Pirox (Can)** *see* Piroxicam *on page 1032*
- ♦ **Nu-Prazo (Can)** *see* Prazosin *on page 1044*
- ♦ **Nu-Prochlor (Can)** *see* Prochlorperazine *on page 1061*
- ♦ **Nu-Propranolol (Can)** *see* Propranolol *on page 1077*
- ♦ **Nu-Ranit (Can)** *see* Ranitidine *on page 1105*
- ♦ **Nuromax®** *see* Doxacurium *on page 416*
- ♦ **Nu-Selegiline (Can)** *see* Selegiline *on page 1157*
- ♦ **Nu-Sertraline (Can)** *see* Sertraline *on page 1161*
- ♦ **Nu-Sotalol (Can)** *see* Sotalol *on page 1198*
- ♦ **Nu-Sucralate (Can)** *see* Sucralfate *on page 1212*
- ♦ **Nu-Sundac (Can)** *see* Sulindac *on page 1219*
- ♦ **Nu-Temazepam (Can)** *see* Temazepam *on page 1239*
- ♦ **Nu-Terazosin (Can)** *see* Terazosin *on page 1243*
- ♦ **Nu-Ticlopidine (Can)** *see* Ticlopidine *on page 1266*
- ♦ **Nu-Timolol (Can)** *see* Timolol *on page 1268*
- ♦ **Nutracort®** *see* Hydrocortisone *on page 639*
- ♦ **Nu-Trazodone (Can)** *see* Trazodone *on page 1306*
- ♦ **Nutropin®** *see* Human Growth Hormone *on page 625*
- ♦ **Nutropin AQ®** *see* Human Growth Hormone *on page 625*
- ♦ **Nutropine® (Can)** *see* Human Growth Hormone *on page 625*
- ♦ **Nu-Verap (Can)** *see* Verapamil *on page 1352*
- ♦ **NVP** *see* Nevirapine *on page 915*
- ♦ **Nyaderm (Can)** *see* Nystatin *on page 945*
- ♦ **Nyamyc™** *see* Nystatin *on page 945*
- ♦ **Nydrazid® [DSC]** *see* Isoniazid *on page 703*

Nystatin (nye STAT in)

Medication Safety Issues

Sound-alike/look-alike issues:

Nystatin may be confused with Nilstat®, Nitrostat®

Nilstat may be confused with Nitrostat®, nystatin

U.S. Brand Names Bio-Statin®; Mycostatin®; Nyamyc™; Nystat-Rx®; Nystop®; Pedi-Dri®

Canadian Brand Names Candistatin®; Nilstat; Nyaderm; PMS-Nystatin

Pharmacologic Category Antifungal Agent, Oral Nonabsorbed; Antifungal Agent, Topical; Antifungal Agent, Vaginal

Generic Available Yes: Cream, ointment, powder, suspension, tablet

Use Treatment of susceptible cutaneous, mucocutaneous, and oral cavity fungal infections normally caused by the *Candida* species

Mechanism of Action Binds to sterols in fungal cell membrane, changing the cell wall permeability allowing for leakage of cellular contents

Pharmacodynamics/Kinetics

Onset of action: Symptomatic relief from candidiasis: 24-72 hours

Absorption: Topical: None through mucous membranes or intact skin; Oral: Poorly absorbed

Excretion: Feces (as unchanged drug)

Dosage

Oral candidiasis:

Suspension (swish and swallow orally):

Premature infants: 100,000 units 4 times/day

Infants: 200,000 units 4 times/day or 100,000 units to each side of mouth 4 times/day

Children and Adults: 400,000-600,000 units 4 times/day

Powder for compounding: Children and Adults: 1/8 teaspoon (500,000 units) to equal approximately 1/2 cup of water; give 4 times/day

Mucocutaneous infections: Children and Adults: Topical: Apply 2-3 times/day to affected areas; very moist topical lesions are treated best with powder

Intestinal infections: Adults: Oral: 500,000-1,000,000 units every 8 hours

(Continued)

Nystatin *(Continued)*

Vaginal infections: Adults: Vaginal tablets: Insert 1 tablet/day at bedtime for 2 weeks

Stability

Vaginal insert: Store in refrigerator; protect from temperature extremes, moisture, and light

Oral tablet, ointment, topical powder, and oral suspension: Store at controlled room temperature of 15°C to 25°C (59°F to 77°F)

Administration Suspension: Shake well before using. Should be swished about the mouth and retained in the mouth for as long as possible (several minutes) before swallowing.

Pregnancy Risk Factor B/C (oral)

Contraindications Hypersensitivity to nystatin or any component of the formulation

Adverse Reactions

Frequency not defined: Dermatologic: Contact dermatitis, Stevens-Johnson syndrome

1% to 10%: Gastrointestinal: Nausea, vomiting, diarrhea, stomach pain

<1% (Limited to important or life-threatening): Hypersensitivity reactions

Overdosage/Toxicology Symptoms of overdose include nausea, vomiting, and diarrhea. Treatment is supportive.

Drug Interactions No data reported

Dosage Forms

Capsule (Bio-Statin®): 500,000 units, 1 million units

Cream: 100,000 units/g (15 g, 30 g)

- Mycostatin®: 100,000 units/g (30 g)

Ointment, topical: 100,000 units/g (15 g, 30 g)

Powder, for prescription compounding: 50 million units (10 g); 150 million units (30 g); 500 million units (100 g); 2 billion units (400 g)

- Nystat-Rx®: 50 million units (10 g); 150 million units (30 g); 500 million units (100 g); 1 billion units (190 g); 2 billion units (350 g)

Powder, topical:

- Mycostatin®: 100,000 units/g (15 g)
- Nyamyc™: 100,000 units/g (15 g, 30 g)
- Nystop®: 100,000 units/g (15 g, 30 g, 60 g)
- Pedi-Dri®: 100,000 units/g (56.7 g)

Suspension, oral: 100,000 units/mL (5 mL, 60 mL, 480 mL)

Tablet: 500,000 units

Tablet, vaginal: 100,000 units (15s) [packaged with applicator]

- **Nystat-Rx®** *see* Nystatin *on page 945*
- **Nystop®** *see* Nystatin *on page 945*
- **Nytol® (Can)** *see* DiphenhydrAMINE *on page 399*
- **Nytol® Extra Strength (Can)** *see* DiphenhydrAMINE *on page 399*
- **Nytol® Quick Caps [OTC]** *see* DiphenhydrAMINE *on page 399*
- **Nytol® Quick Gels [OTC]** *see* DiphenhydrAMINE *on page 399*
- **NāSop™** *see* Phenylephrine *on page 1015*
- **Nōstrilla® [OTC]** *see* Oxymetazoline *on page 973*
- **Ocean® [OTC]** *see* Sodium Chloride *on page 1183*
- **Oceant® for Kids [OTC]** *see* Sodium Chloride *on page 1183*
- **Octagam®** *see* Immune Globulin (Intravenous) *on page 666*
- **Octostim® (Can)** *see* Desmopressin *on page 363*

Octreotide (ok TREE oh tide)

Medication Safety Issues

Sound-alike/look-alike issues:

- Sandostatin® may be confused with Sandimmune®

U.S. Brand Names Sandostatin®; Sandostatin LAR®

Canadian Brand Names Octreotide Acetate Injection; Octreotide Acetate Omega; Sandostatin®; Sandostatin LAR®

Synonyms NSC-671663; Octreotide Acetate

Pharmacologic Category Antidiarrheal; Somatostatin Analog

Generic Available Yes: Solution

Use Control of symptoms in patients with metastatic carcinoid and vasoactive intestinal peptide-secreting tumors (VIPomas); acromegaly

Unlabeled/Investigational Use AIDS-associated secretory diarrhea (including *Cryptosporidiosis*), control of bleeding of esophageal varices, breast cancer, cryptosporidiosis, Cushing's syndrome (ectopic), insulinomas, small bowel fistulas, pancreatic tumors, gastrinoma, postgastrectomy dumping syndrome, chemotherapy-induced diarrhea, graft-versus-host disease (GVHD) induced diarrhea, Zollinger-Ellison syndrome, congenital hyperinsulinism; hypothalamic obesity

Mechanism of Action Mimics natural somatostatin by inhibiting serotonin release, and the secretion of gastrin, VIP, insulin, glucagon, secretin, motilin, and pancreatic polypeptide. Decreases growth hormone and IGF-1 in acromegaly.

Pharmacodynamics/Kinetics

Duration: SubQ: 6-12 hours

Absorption: SubQ: Rapid

Distribution: V_d: 14 L (13-30 L in acromegaly)

Protein binding: 65%, mainly to lipoprotein (41% in acromegaly)

Metabolism: Extensively hepatic

Bioavailability: SubQ: 100%; I.M: 60% to 63% of SubQ dose

Half-life elimination: 1.7-1.9 hours; up to 3.7 hours with cirrhosis

Time to peak, plasma: SubQ: 0.4 hours (0.7 hours acromegaly); I.M.: 1 hour

Excretion: Urine (32%)

Dosage

Infants and Children:

Secretory diarrhea (unlabeled use): I.V., SubQ: Doses of 1-10 mcg/kg every 12 hours have been used in children beginning at the low end of the range and increasing by 0.3 mcg/kg/dose at 3-day intervals. Suppression of growth hormone (animal data) is of concern when used as long-term therapy.

Congenital hyperinsulinism (unlabeled use): SubQ: Doses of 3-40 mcg/kg/day have been used

Adults: SubQ, I.V.: Initial: 50 mcg 2-3 times/day and titrate dose based on patient tolerance, response, and indication

Carcinoid: Initial 2 weeks: 100-600 mcg/day in 2-4 divided doses; usual range 50-1500 mcg/day

VIPomas: Initial 2 weeks: 200-300 mcg/day in 2-4 divided doses; usual range 150-750 mcg/day

Diarrhea (unlabeled use): Initial: I.V.: 50-100 mcg every 8 hours; increase by 100 mcg/dose at 48-hour intervals; maximum dose: 500 mcg every 8 hours

Esophageal varices bleeding (unlabeled use): I.V. bolus: 25-50 mcg followed by continuous I.V. infusion of 25-50 mcg/hour

Acromegaly: Initial: SubQ: 50 mcg 3 times/day; titrate to achieve growth hormone levels <5 ng/mL or IGF-I (somatomedin C) levels <1.9 U/mL in males and <2.2 U/mL in females; usual effective dose 100 mcg 3 times/day; range 300-1500 mcg/day

Note: Should be withdrawn yearly for a 4-week interval (8 weeks for depot injection) in patients who have received irradiation. Resume if levels increase and signs/symptoms recur.

Acromegaly, carcinoid tumors, and VIPomas (depot injection): Patients must be stabilized on subcutaneous octreotide for at least 2 weeks before switching to the long-acting depot: Upon switch: 20 mg I.M. intragluteally every 4 weeks for 2-3 months, then the dose may be modified based upon response. Patients receiving depot injection for carcinoid tumor or VIPoma should continue to receive their SubQ injections for the first 2 weeks at the same dose in order to maintain therapeutic levels.

Dosage adjustment for acromegaly: After 3 months of depot injections the dosage may be continued or modified as follows:

GH ≤2.5 ng/mL, IGF-1 is normal, symptoms controlled: Maintain octreotide LAR® at 20 mg I.M. every 4 weeks

GH >2.5 ng/mL, IGF-1 is elevated, and/or symptoms uncontrolled: Increase octreotide LAR® to 30 mg I.M. every 4 weeks

GH ≤1 ng/mL, IGF-1 is normal, symptoms controlled: Reduce octreotide LAR® to 10 mg I.M. every 4 weeks

Note: Patients not adequately controlled may increase dose to 40 mg every 4 weeks. Dosages >40 mg are not recommended

Dosage adjustment for carcinoid tumors and VIPomas: After 2 months of depot injections the dosage may be continued or modified as follows:

Increase to 30 mg I.M. every 4 weeks if symptoms are inadequately controlled

(Continued)

Octreotide *(Continued)*

Decrease to 10 mg I.M. every 4 weeks, for a trial period, if initially responsive to 20 mg dose

Dosage >30 mg is not recommended

Elderly: Elimination half-life is increased by 46% and clearance is decreased by 26%; dose adjustment may be required.

Dosage adjustment in renal impairment: Severe renal failure requiring dialysis: Clearance is reduced by ~50%; specific dosing guidelines not available

Stability

Solution: Octreotide is a clear solution and should be stored under refrigeration; may be stored at room temperature for up to 14 days when protected from light. Stability of parenteral admixture is stable in NS for 96 hours at room temperature (25°C) and in D_5W for 24 hours.

Suspension: Prior to dilution, store under refrigeration and protect from light; may be at room temperature for 30-60 minutes prior to use; use suspension immediately after preparation.

Administration

Regular injection formulation (do not use if solution contains particles or is discolored): Administer SubQ or I.V.; I.V. administration may be IVP, IVPB, or continuous I.V. infusion:

IVP should be administered undiluted over 3 minutes

IVPB should be administered over 15-30 minutes

Continuous I.V. infusion rates have ranged from 25-50 mcg/hour for the treatment of esophageal variceal bleeding

Depot formulation: Administer I.M. intragluteal (avoid deltoid administration); alternate gluteal injection sites to avoid irritation. Do not administer Sandostatin LAR® intravenously or subcutaneously; must be administered immediately after mixing.

Monitoring Parameters

Acromegaly: Growth hormone, somatomedin C (IGF-1)

Carcinoid: 5-HIAA, plasma serotonin and plasma substance P

VIPomas: Vasoactive intestinal peptide

Chronic therapy: Thyroid function (baseline and periodic), vitamin B_{12} level, blood glucose, cardiac function (heart rate, EKG)

Reference Range Vasoactive intestinal peptide: <75 ng/L; levels vary considerably between laboratories

Pregnancy Risk Factor B

Contraindications Hypersensitivity to octreotide or any component of the formulation

Warnings/Precautions May impair gall bladder function; monitor patients for cholelithiasis. Use with caution in patients with renal impairment. Somatostatin analogs may affect glucose regulation; in type I diabetes, severe hypoglycemia may occur; in type II diabetes or nondiabetic patients, hyperglycemia may occur. Insulin and other hypoglycemic medication requirements may change. Bradycardia, conduction abnormalities, and arrhythmia have been observed in acromegalic patients; use caution with CHF or concomitant medications that alter heart rate or rhythm. May alter absorption of dietary fats; monitor for pancreatitis. Chronic treatment has been associated with abnormal Schillings test; monitor vitamin B_{12} levels. Tumors which secrete growth hormone may increase in size; monitor. Suppresses secretion of TSH; monitor for hypothyroidism.

Adverse Reactions Adverse reactions vary by route of administration. Frequency of cardiac, endocrine, and gastrointestinal adverse reactions were generally higher in acromegalics.

>16%:

Cardiovascular: Sinus bradycardia (19% to 25%), chest pain (16% to 20%)

Central nervous system: Fatigue (1% to 20%), malaise (16% to 20%), dizziness (5% to 20%), headache (6% to 20%), fever (16% to 20%)

Endocrine & metabolic: Hyperglycemia (27%)

Gastrointestinal: Diarrhea (36% to 58%), abdominal discomfort (5% to 61%), flatulence (<10% to 38%), constipation (9% to 21%), nausea (5% to 61%), cholelithiasis (27%; length of therapy dependent), biliary duct dilatation (12%), biliary sludge (24%; length of therapy dependent), loose stools (5% to 61%), vomiting (4% to 21%)

Hematologic: Antibodies to octreotide (up to 25%; no efficacy change)

Local: Injection pain (2% to 50%; dose- and formulation-related)

Neuromuscular & skeletal: Backache (1% to 20%), arthropathy (16% to 20%)

Respiratory: Dyspnea (16% to 20%), upper respiratory infection (16% to 20%)
Miscellaneous: Flu symptoms (1% to 20%)

5% to 15%:

Cardiovascular: Conduction abnormalities (9% to 10%), arrhythmia (3% to 9%), hypertension, palpitations, peripheral edema
Central nervous system: Anxiety, confusion, depression, hypoesthesia, insomnia, vertigo
Dermatologic: Pruritus, rash
Endocrine & metabolic: Hypothyroidism (2% to 12%), goiter (2% to 8%)
Gastrointestinal: Abdominal pain, anorexia, cramping, dehydration, discomfort, hemorrhoids, tenesmus (4% to 6%), dyspepsia (4% to 15%), steatorrhea (4% to 6%), feces discoloration (4% to 6%), weight loss
Genitourinary: UTI
Hematologic: Anemia
Hepatic: Hepatitis
Neuromuscular & skeletal: Arthralgia, leg cramps, myalgia, paresthesia, rigors, weakness
Otic: Ear ache, otitis media
Renal: Renal calculus
Respiratory: Coughing, pharyngitis, rhinitis, sinusitis
Miscellaneous: Allergy, diaphoresis

1% to 4%:

Cardiovascular: Angina, cardiac failure, cerebral vascular disorder, edema, flushing, hematoma, phlebitis, tachycardia
Central nervous system: Abnormal gait, amnesia, dysphonia, hallucinations, nervousness, neuralgia, neuropathy, somnolence, tremor, vertigo
Dermatologic: Acne, alopecia, bruising, cellulitis, urticaria
Endocrine & metabolic: Hypoglycemia (2% to 4%), hypokalemia, hypoproteinemia, gout, cachexia, menstrual irregularities, breast pain, impotence
Gastrointestinal: Colitis, diverticulitis, dysphagia, fat malabsorption, gastritis, gastroenteritis, gingivitis, glossitis, melena, rectal bleeding, stomatitis, taste perversion, xerostomia
Genitourinary: Incontinence
Hematologic: Epistaxis
Hepatic: Ascites, jaundice
Local: Injection hematoma
Neuromuscular & skeletal: Hyperkinesia, hypertonia, joint pain
Ocular: Blurred vision, visual disturbance
Otic: Tinnitus
Renal: Albuminuria, renal abscess
Respiratory: Bronchitis, pleural effusion, pneumonia, pulmonary embolism
Miscellaneous: Bacterial infection, cold symptoms, moniliasis

<1% (Limited to important or life-threatening): Abdomen enlarged, anaphylactic shock, anaphylactoid reaction, aneurysm, aphasia, appendicitis, arthritis, atrial fibrillation, basal cell carcinoma, Bell's palsy, breast carcinoma, burning eyes, cardiac arrest, CHF, CK increased, creatinine increased, deafness, diabetes insipidus, diabetes mellitus, facial edema, fatty liver, galactorrhea, gallbladder polyp, gallstones, GI hemorrhage, glaucoma, gynecomastia, hematuria, hemiparesis, hepatitis, hyperesthesia, hypertensive reaction, hypoadrenalism, intestinal obstruction, intracranial hemorrhage, iron deficiency, ischemia, joint effusion, lactation, leg cramps, LFTs increased, libido decreased, malignant hyperpyrexia, MI, migraine, muscle cramping, nephrolithiasis, orthostatic hypotension, pancreatitis, paranoia, paresis, peptic ulcer, petechiae, pituitary apoplexy, pneumothorax, pulmonary hypertension, pulmonary nodule, Raynaud's syndrome, renal insufficiency, retinal vein thrombosis, rhinorrhea, scotoma, seizure, status asthmaticus, suicide attempt, throat discomfort, thrombocytopenia, thrombophlebitis, thrombosis, vaginitis, visual field defect, wheal/erythema

Overdosage/Toxicology Symptoms of overdose include hypo- or hyperglycemia, blurred vision, dizziness, drowsiness, nausea, flushing, and loss of motor function. Well-tolerated bolus doses up to 1000 mcg have failed to produce adverse effects. Treatment is symptom-directed and supportive.

Drug Interactions

Bromocriptine: Availability of bromocriptine may be increased by octreotide.
Cyclosporine: Case reports of transplant rejection due to reduction of serum cyclosporine levels when cyclosporine was given orally in conjunction with a somatostatin analogue.

(Continued)

Octreotide *(Continued)*

QT_c-prolonging agents: Octreotide may enhance the adverse/toxic effects of other QT_c-prolonging agents. Use with caution; monitor.

Ethanol/Nutrition/Herb Interactions

Herb/Nutraceutical: Avoid hypoglycemic herbs, including alfalfa, aloe, bilberry, bitter melon, burdock, celery, damiana, fenugreek, garcinia, garlic, ginger, ginseng, gymnema, marshmallow, and stinging nettle (may enhance the hypoglycemic effect of octreotide).

Dietary Considerations Schedule injections between meals to decrease GI effects. May alter absorption of dietary fats.

Dosage Forms

Injection, microspheres for suspension, as acetate [depot formulation]:
  Sandostatin LAR®: 10 mg, 20 mg, 30 mg [with diluent and syringe]
Injection, solution, as acetate: 0.05 mg/mL (1 mL); 0.1 mg/mL (1 mL); 0.2 mg/mL (5 mL); 0.5 mg/mL (1 mL); 1 mg/mL (5 mL)
  Sandostatin®: 0.05 mg/mL (1 mL); 0.1 mg/mL (1 mL); 0.2 mg/mL (5 mL); 0.5 mg/mL (1 mL); 1 mg/mL (5 mL)

References

Corley DA, Cello JP, Adkisson W, et al, "Octreotide for Acute Esophageal Variceal Bleeding: A Meta-Analysis," *Gastroentology*, 2001, 120(4):946-54.
Erstad BL, "Octreotide For Acute Variceal Bleeding," *Ann Pharmacother*, 2001, 35(5):618-26.

- **Octreotide Acetate** *see* Octreotide *on page 946*
- **Octreotide Acetate Injection (Can)** *see* Octreotide *on page 946*
- **Octreotide Acetate Omega (Can)** *see* Octreotide *on page 946*
- **Ocufen®** *see* Flurbiprofen *on page 550*
- **Ocuflox®** *see* Ofloxacin *on page 950*

Ofloxacin (oh FLOKS a sin)

Medication Safety Issues

Sound-alike/look-alike issues:
  Floxin® may be confused with Flexeril®
  Ocuflox® may be confused with Ocufen®

Related Information

Prevention of Wound Infection and Sepsis in Surgical Patients *on page 1588*

U.S. Brand Names Floxin®; Ocuflox®

Canadian Brand Names Apo-Oflox®; Apo-Ofloxacin®; Floxin®; Novo-Ofloxacin; Ocuflox®; PMS-Ofloxacin

Synonyms Floxin Otic Singles

Pharmacologic Category Antibiotic, Quinolone

Generic Available Yes: Tablet, ophthalmic solution

Use Quinolone antibiotic for the treatment of acute exacerbations of chronic bronchitis, community-acquired pneumonia, skin and skin structure infections (uncomplicated), urethral and cervical gonorrhea (acute, uncomplicated), urethritis and cervicitis (nongonococcal), mixed infections of the urethra and cervix, pelvic inflammatory disease (acute), cystitis (uncomplicated), urinary tract infections (complicated), prostatitis

Ophthalmic: Treatment of superficial ocular infections involving the conjunctiva or cornea due to strains of susceptible organisms

Otic: Otitis externa, chronic suppurative otitis media, acute otitis media

Unlabeled/Investigational Use Epididymitis (gonorrhea), leprosy, Traveler's diarrhea

Mechanism of Action Ofloxacin is a DNA gyrase inhibitor. DNA gyrase is an essential bacterial enzyme that maintains the superhelical structure of DNA. DNA gyrase is required for DNA replication and transcription, DNA repair, recombination, and transposition; bactericidal

Pharmacodynamics/Kinetics

Absorption: Well absorbed; food causes only minor alterations
Distribution: V_d: 2.4-3.5 L/kg
Protein binding: 20%
Bioavailability: Oral: 98%
Half-life elimination: Biphasic: 5-7.5 hours and 20-25 hours (accounts for <5%); prolonged with renal impairment
Excretion: Primarily urine (as unchanged drug)

Dosage

Usual dosage range:

Children ≥6 months: Otic: 5 drops daily

Children >1 year: Ophthalmic: 1-2 drops every 30 minutes to 4 hours initially, decreasing to every 4-6 hours

Children >12 years: Otic: 10 drops once or twice daily

Adults:

Ophthalmic: 1-2 drops every 30 minutes to 4 hours initially, decreasing to every 4-6 hours

Oral: 200-400 mg every 12 hours

Otic: 10 drops once or twice daily

Indication-specific dosing:

Acute otitis media with tympanostomy tubes: Children 1-12 years: Otic: Instill 5 drops (or the contents of 1 single-dose container) into affected ear(s) twice daily for 10 days

Otitis externa: Children 6 months to 13 years: Otic: Instill 5 drops (or the contents of 1 single-dose container) into affected ear(s) once daily for 7 days

Children >1 year and Adults: Ophthalmic:

Conjunctivitis: Instill 1-2 drops in affected eye(s) every 2-4 hours for the first 2 days, then use 4 times/day for an additional 5 days

Corneal ulcer: Instill 1-2 drops every 30 minutes while awake and every 4-6 hours after retiring for the first 2 days; beginning on day 3, instill 1-2 drops every hour while awake for 4-6 additional days; thereafter, 1-2 drops 4 times/day until clinical cure.

Children >12 years and Adults:

Otitis media, chronic suppurative with perforated tympanic membranes: Otic: Instill 10 drops (or the contents of 2 single-dose containers) into affected ear twice daily for 14 days

Children ≥13 years and Adults:

Otitis externa: Otic: Instill 10 drops (or the contents of 2 single-dose containers) into affected ear(s) once daily for 7 days

Adults: Oral:

Cervicitis/urethritis (nongonococcal) due to *C. trachomatis*, mixed infection of urethra and cervix due to *C. trachomatis* and *N. gonorrhoea*: 300 mg every 12 hours for 7 days

Chronic bronchitis (acute exacerbation), community-acquired pneumonia, skin and skin structure infections (uncomplicated): 400 mg every 12 hours for 10 days

Cystitis (uncomplicated), *E. coli* or *K. pneumoniae*: 200 mg every 12 hours for 3 days or up to 7 days for other organisms

Epididymitis, gonoccocal (unlabeled use): 300 mg twice daily for 10 days

Leprosy (unlabeled use): 400 mg once daily

Pelvic inflammatory disease (acute): 400 mg every 12 hours for 10-14 days

Prostatitis:

Acute: 400 mg for 1 dose, then 300 mg twice daily for 10 days

Chronic: 200 mg every 12 hours for 6 weeks

Traveler's diarrhea (unlabeled use): 300 mg twice daily for 3 days

Urethral and cervical gonorrhea (acute, uncomplicated): 400 mg as a single dose

UTI (complicated): 200 mg every 12 hours for 10 days

Dosing adjustment/interval in renal impairment: Adults: Oral: After a normal initial dose, adjust as follows:

Cl_{cr} 20-50 mL/minute: Administer usual dose every 24 hours

Cl_{cr} <20 mL/minute: Administer half the usual dose every 24 hours

Continuous arteriovenous or venovenous hemodiafiltration effects: Administer 300 mg every 24 hours

Dosing adjustment in hepatic impairment: Severe impairment: Maximum dose: 400 mg/day

Stability

Ophthalmic and otic solution: Store at 15°C to 25°C (59°F to 77°F)

Otic Singles™: Store at 15°C to 30°C (59°F to 86°F); store in pouch to protect from light

Tablet: Store below 30°C (86°F)

Administration

Ophthalmic: For ophthalmic use only; avoid touching tip of applicator to eye or other surfaces.

(Continued)

Ofloxacin *(Continued)*

Oral: Do not take within 2 hours of food or any antacids which contain zinc, magnesium, or aluminum.

Otic: Prior to use, warm solution by holding container in hands for 1-2 minutes. Patient should lie down with affected ear upward and medication instilled. Pump tragus 4 times to ensure penetration of medication. Patient should remain in this position for 5 minutes.

Pregnancy Risk Factor C

Contraindications Hypersensitivity to ofloxacin or other members of the quinolone group such as nalidixic acid, oxolinic acid, cinoxacin, norfloxacin, and ciprofloxacin; hypersensitivity to any component of the formulation

Warnings/Precautions Use with caution in patients with epilepsy or other CNS diseases which could predispose seizures; potential for seizures, although very rare, may be increased with concomitant NSAID therapy. Use with caution in patients with renal or hepatic impairment. Tendon inflammation and/or rupture have been reported with quinolone antibiotics, including ofloxacin. Risk may be increased with concurrent corticosteroids, particularly in the elderly. Discontinue at first sign of tendon inflammation or pain. Peripheral neuropathies have been linked to ofloxacin use; discontinue if numbness, tingling, or weakness develops.

Rare cases of torsade de pointes have been reported in patients receiving ofloxacin and other quinolones. Risk may be minimized by avoiding use in patients with known prolongation of the QT interval, bradycardia, hypokalemia, hypomagnesemia, cardiomyopathy, or in those receiving concurrent therapy with Class Ia or Class III antiarrhythmics.

Severe hypersensitivity reactions, including anaphylaxis, have occurred with quinolone therapy. If an allergic reaction occurs (itching, urticaria, dyspnea, facial edema, loss of consciousness, tingling, cardiovascular collapse), discontinue drug immediately. Prolonged use may result in superinfection; pseudomembranous colitis may occur and should be considered in all patients who present with diarrhea. Quinolones may exacerbate myasthenia gravis, use with caution (rare, potentially life-threatening weakness of respiratory muscles may occur).

Adverse Reactions

Systemic:

1% to 10%:

Cardiovascular: Chest pain (1% to 3%)

Central nervous system: Headache (1% to 9%), insomnia (3% to 7%), dizziness (1% to 5%), fatigue (1% to 3%), somnolence (1% to 3%), sleep disorders (1% to 3%), nervousness (1% to 3%), pyrexia (1% to 3%)

Dermatologic: Rash/pruritus (1% to 3%)

Gastrointestinal: Diarrhea (1% to 4%), vomiting (1% to 4%), GI distress (1% to 3%), abdominal cramps (1% to 3%), flatulence (1% to 3%), abnormal taste (1% to 3%), xerostomia (1% to 3%), decreased appetite (1% to 3%), nausea (3% to 10%), constipation (1% to 3%)

Genitourinary: Vaginitis (1% to 5%), external genital pruritus in women (1% to 3%)

Ocular: Visual disturbances (1% to 3%)

Respiratory: Pharyngitis (1% to 3%)

Miscellaneous: Trunk pain

<1%, postmarketing, and/or case reports (limited to important or life-threatening): Anaphylaxis reactions, anxiety, blurred vision, chills, cognitive change, cough, depression, dream abnormality, ecchymosis, edema, erythema nodosum, euphoria, extremity pain, hallucinations, hearing acuity decreased, hepatic dysfunction, hepatitis, hyper/hypoglycemia, hypertension, interstitial nephritis, lightheadedness, malaise, myasthenia gravis exacerbation, palpitation, paresthesia, peripheral neuropathy, photophobia, photosensitivity, psychotic reactions, rhabdomyolysis, seizure, Stevens-Johnson syndrome, syncope, tendonitis and tendon rupture, thirst, tinnitus, torsade de pointes, Tourette's syndrome, toxic epidermal necrolysis, vasculitis, vasodilation, vertigo, weakness, weight loss

Ophthalmic: Frequency not defined:

Central nervous system: Dizziness

Gastrointestinal: Nausea

Ocular: Blurred vision, burning, chemical conjunctivitis/keratitis, discomfort, dryness, edema, eye pain, foreign body sensation, itching, photophobia, redness, stinging, tearing

Otic:

>10%: Local: Application site reaction (<1% to 17%)

1% to 10%:

Central nervous system: Dizziness (≤1%), vertigo (≤1%)
Dermatologic: Pruritus (1% to 4%), rash (1%)
Gastrointestinal: Taste perversion (7%)
Neuromuscular & skeletal: Paresthesia (1%)

<1% (Limited to important or life-threatening): Diarrhea, fever, headache, hearing loss (transient), hypertension, nausea, otorrhagia, tinnitus, transient neuropsychiatric disturbances, tremor, vomiting, xerostomia

Overdosage/Toxicology Symptoms of overdose include acute renal failure, seizures, nausea, and vomiting. Treatment includes GI decontamination, if possible, and supportive care. Not removed by peritoneal or hemodialysis.

Drug Interactions Inhibits CYP1A2 (strong)

Corticosteroids: Concurrent use may increase the risk of tendon rupture, particularly in elderly patients (overall incidence rare).

CYP1A2 substrates: Ofloxacin may increase the levels/effects of CYP1A2 substrates. Example substrates include aminophylline, fluvoxamine, mexiletine, mirtazapine, ropinirole, and trifluoperazine.

Glyburide: Quinolones may increase the effect of glyburide; monitor.

Metal cations (aluminum, calcium, iron, magnesium, and zinc) bind quinolones in the gastrointestinal tract and inhibit absorption. Concurrent administration of most antacids, oral electrolyte supplements, quinapril, sucralfate, some didanosine formulations (chewable/buffered tablets and pediatric powder for oral suspension), and other highly-buffered oral drugs, should be avoided. Ofloxacin should be administered 2 hours before or 2 hours after these agents.

Probenecid: May decrease renal secretion of ofloxacin.

QT_c-prolonging agents: Effects may be additive with ofloxacin. Avoid concurrent use with Class Ia and Class III antiarrhythmics; use caution with other drugs known to prolong QT_c, including erythromycin, cisapride, antipsychotics, and cyclic antidepressants.

Theophylline: Ofloxacin may increase plasma levels of theophylline. Monitor.

Warfarin: The hypoprothrombinemic effect of warfarin may be enhanced by some quinolone antibiotics; monitor INR.

Ethanol/Nutrition/Herb Interactions

Food: Ofloxacin average peak serum concentrations may be decreased by 20% if taken with food.

Herb/Nutraceutical: Avoid dong quai, St John's wort (may also cause photosensitization).

Test Interactions Some quinolones may produce a false-positive urine screening result for opiates using commercially-available immunoassay kits. This has been demonstrated most consistently for levofloxacin and ofloxacin, but other quinolones have shown cross-reactivity in certain assay kits. Confirmation of positive opiate screens by more specific methods should be considered.

Dosage Forms [DSC] = Discontinued product

Solution, ophthalmic (Ocuflox®): 0.3% (5 mL; 10 mL [DSC]) [contains benzalkonium chloride]

Solution, otic:

Floxin®: 0.3% (5 mL, 10 mL) [contains benzalkonium chloride]

Floxin® Otic Singles™: 0.3% (0.25 mL) [contains benzalkonium chloride; packaged as 2 single-dose containers per pouch, 10 pouches per carton, total net volume 5 mL]

Tablet (Floxin®): 200 mg, 300 mg, 400 mg

Olmesartan (ole me SAR tan)

Related Information

Angiotensin Agents *on page 1544*

U.S. Brand Names Benicar®

Synonyms Olmesartan Medoxomil

Pharmacologic Category Angiotensin II Receptor Blocker

Generic Available No

Use Treatment of hypertension with or without concurrent use of other antihypertensive agents

(Continued)

Olmesartan *(Continued)*

Mechanism of Action As a selective and competitive, nonpeptide angiotensin II receptor antagonist, olmesartan blocks the vasoconstrictor and aldosterone-secreting effects of angiotensin II; olmesartan interacts reversibly at the AT1 and AT2 receptors of many tissues and has slow dissociation kinetics; its affinity for the AT1 receptor is 12,500 times greater than the AT2 receptor. Angiotensin II receptor antagonists may induce a more complete inhibition of the renin-angiotensin system than ACE inhibitors, they do not affect the response to bradykinin, and are less likely to be associated with nonrenin-angiotensin effects (eg, cough and angioedema). Olmesartan increases urinary flow rate and, in addition to being natriuretic and kaliuretic, increases excretion of chloride, magnesium, uric acid, calcium, and phosphate.

Pharmacodynamics/Kinetics

Distribution: 17 L; does not cross the blood-brain barrier (animal studies)

Protein binding: 99%

Metabolism: Olmesartan medoxomil is hydrolyzed in the GI tract to active olmesartan. No further metabolism occurs.

Bioavailability: 26%

Half-life elimination: Terminal: 13 hours

Time to peak: 1-2 hours

Excretion: All as unchanged drug: Feces (50% to 65%); urine (35% to 50%)

Dosage Oral:

Adults: Initial: Usual starting dose is 20 mg once daily; if initial response is inadequate, may be increased to 40 mg once daily after 2 weeks. May administer with other antihypertensive agents if blood pressure inadequately controlled with olmesartan. Consider lower starting dose in patients with possible depletion of intravascular volume (eg, patients receiving diuretics).

Elderly: No dosage adjustment necessary

Dosage adjustment in renal impairment: No specific guidelines for dosage adjustment; patients undergoing hemodialysis have not been studied.

Dosage adjustment in hepatic impairment: No adjustment necessary.

Stability Store at 20°C to 25°C (68°F to 77°F).

Administration May be administered with or without food.

Monitoring Parameters Blood pressure, serum potassium

Anesthesia and Critical Care Concerns/Other Considerations The angiotensin II receptor antagonists appear to have similar indications as the ACE inhibitors. In heart failure, the angiotensin II antagonists are especially useful in providing an alternative therapy in those patients who have intractable cough in response to ACE inhibitor therapy. Candesartan has been studied as an alternative therapy in chronic heart failure patients who cannot tolerate an ACE-I (CHARM-Alternative) and as an added therapy in heart failure patients who are maintained on an ACE-I (CHARM-Added). In both studies the combined endpoint of cardiovascular death or heart failure hospitalizations was significantly improved over the placebo treated group. Similar to ACE inhibitors, pre-existing volume depletion caused by diuretic therapy may potentiate hypotension in response to angiotensin II antagonists. Concomitant NSAID therapy may attenuate blood pressure control; use of NSAIDs should be avoided or limited, with monitoring of blood pressure control. In the setting of heart failure, NSAID use may be associated with an increased risk for fluid accumulation and edema.

Pregnancy Risk Factor C/D (2nd and 3rd trimesters)

Contraindications Hypersensitivity to olmesartan or any component of the formulation; hypersensitivity to other A-II receptor antagonists; bilateral renal artery stenosis; pregnancy (2nd and 3rd trimesters)

Warnings/Precautions [U.S. Boxed Warning]: Based on human data, drugs that act on the angiotensin system can cause injury and death to the developing fetus when used in the second and third trimesters. Angiotensin receptor blockers should be discontinued as soon as possible once pregnancy is detected. Avoid use or use a smaller dose in patients who are volume depleted; correct depletion first. Deterioration in renal function can occur with initiation. Use with caution in unilateral renal artery stenosis and pre-existing renal insufficiency; significant aortic/mitral stenosis. Safety and efficacy in pediatric patients have not been established.

Adverse Reactions

1% to 10%:

Central nervous system: Dizziness (3%), headache

Endocrine & metabolic: Hyperglycemia, hypertriglyceridemia

Gastrointestinal: Diarrhea
Neuromuscular & skeletal: Back pain, CPK increased
Renal: Hematuria
Respiratory: Bronchitis, pharyngitis, rhinitis, sinusitis
Miscellaneous: Flu-like syndrome

<1% (Limited to important or life-threatening): Abdominal pain, acute renal failure, alopecia, angioedema, arthralgia, arthritis, bilirubin increased, chest pain, dyspepsia, facial edema, fatigue, gastroenteritis, hypercholesterolemia, hyperlipidemia, hyperuricemia, insomnia, liver enzymes increased, myalgia, nausea, pain, peripheral edema, pruritus, rash, rhabdomyolysis, serum creatinine increased, skeletal pain, tachycardia, urinary tract infection, urticaria, vertigo, vomiting

Overdosage/Toxicology Hypotension and tachycardia may occur with significant overdose. Bradycardia is possible if vagal stimulation occurs. Treatment should be supportive.

Drug Interactions

Lithium: Risk of toxicity may be increased by olmesartan; monitor lithium levels.
NSAIDs: May decrease angiotensin II antagonist efficacy; effect has been seen with losartan, but may occur with other medications in this class; monitor blood pressure.
Potassium-sparing diuretics (amiloride, potassium, spironolactone, triamterene): Increased risk of hyperkalemia.
Potassium supplements may increase the risk of hyperkalemia.
Trimethoprim (high dose) may increase the risk of hyperkalemia.

Ethanol/Nutrition/Herb Interactions

Food: Does not affect olmesartan bioavailability.
Herb/Nutraceutical: Avoid ephedra, yohimbe, ginseng (may worsen hypertension). Avoid garlic (may have increased antihypertensive effect).

Dietary Considerations May be taken with or without food.

Dosage Forms Tablet, as medoxomil: 5 mg, 20 mg, 40 mg

♦ **Olmesartan Medoxomil** *see* Olmesartan *on page 953*

Omalizumab (oh mah lye ZOO mab)

U.S. Brand Names Xolair®

Canadian Brand Names Xolair®

Synonyms rhuMAb-E25

Pharmacologic Category Monoclonal Antibody, Anti-Asthmatic

Generic Available No

Use Treatment of moderate-to-severe, persistent allergic asthma not adequately controlled with inhaled corticosteroids

Mechanism of Action Omalizumab is an IgG monoclonal antibody (recombinant DNA-derived) which inhibits IgE binding to the high-affinity IgE receptor on mast cells and basophils. By decreasing bound IgE, the activation and release of mediators in the allergic response (early and late phase) is limited. Serum free IgE levels and the number of high-affinity IgE receptors are decreased. Long-term treatment in patients with allergic asthma showed a decrease in asthma exacerbations and corticosteroid usage.

Pharmacodynamics/Kinetics

Absorption: Slow following SubQ injection
Distribution: V_d: 78 ± 32 mL/kg
Metabolism: Hepatic; IgG degradation by reticuloendothelial system and endothelial cells
Bioavailability: 62%
Half-life elimination: 26 days
Time to peak: 7-8 days
Excretion: Primarily via hepatic degradation; intact IgG may be secreted in bile

Dosage SubQ: Children ≥12 years and Adults: Asthma: Dose is based on pretreatment IgE serum levels and body weight. Dosing should not be adjusted based on IgE levels taken during treatment or <1 year following discontinuation of therapy; doses should be adjusted during treatment for significant changes in body weight

IgE ≥30-100 int. units/mL:
30-90 kg: 150 mg every 4 weeks
>90-150 kg: 300 mg every 4 weeks

IgE >100-200 int. units/mL:
30-90 kg: 300 mg every 4 weeks

(Continued)

Omalizumab *(Continued)*

>90-150 kg: 225 mg every 2 weeks
IgE >200-300 int. units/mL:
30-60 kg: 300 mg every 4 weeks
>60-90 kg: 225 mg every 2 weeks
>90-150 kg: 300 mg every 2 weeks
IgE >300-400 int. units/mL:
30-70 kg: 225 mg every 2 weeks
>70-90 kg: 300 mg every 2 weeks
>90 kg: Do not administer dose
IgE >400-500 int. units/mL:
30-70 kg: 300 mg every 2 weeks
>70-90 kg: 375 mg every 2 weeks
>90 kg: Do not administer dose
IgE >500-600 int. units/mL:
30-60 kg: 300 mg every 2 weeks
>60-70 kg: 375 mg every 2 weeks
>70 kg: Do not administer dose
IgE >600-700 int. units/mL:
30-60 kg: 375 mg every 2 weeks
>60 kg: Do not administer dose

Stability Prior to reconstitution, store under refrigeration at 2°C to 8°C (36°F to 46°F); product may be shipped at room temperature. Prepare using SWFI, USP only; add SWFI 1.4 mL to upright vial and swirl gently for 5-10 seconds every 5 minutes until dissolved, may take >20 minutes to dissolve completely. Resulting solution is 150 mg/1.2 mL. Do not use if powder takes >40 minutes to dissolve. Following reconstitution, protect from direct sunlight. May be stored for up to 8 hours if refrigerated or 4 hours if stored at room temperature.

Administration For SubQ injection only; doses >150 mg should divided over more than one site. Injections may take 5-10 seconds to administer.

Monitoring Parameters Baseline IgE; FEV_1, peak flow, and/or other pulmonary function tests

Pregnancy Risk Factor B

Contraindications Hypersensitivity to omalizumab or any component of the formulation; acute bronchospasm, status asthmaticus

Warnings/Precautions For use in patients with a documented reactivity to a perennial aeroallergen and with symptoms uncontrolled using inhaled corticosteroids; not used to control acute asthma symptoms. Dosing is based on pretreatment IgE serum levels and body weight. IgE levels remain elevated up to 1 year following treatment, therefore, levels taken during treatment can not be used as a dosage guide. Corticosteroid therapy should be tapered gradually, do not discontinue abruptly. Anaphylactic reactions have been reported within 2 hours of initial dose; appropriate medications for the treatment of hypersensitivity reactions should be available. Malignant neoplasms have been reported with use in short-term studies; impact of long-term use is not known. Use caution with and monitor patients at risk for parasitic (helminth) infections. Safety and efficacy in children <12 years of age have not been established.

Adverse Reactions

>10%:

Central nervous system: Headache (15%)

Local: Injection-site reaction (45%; placebo 43%; severe 12%). Most reactions occurred within 1 hour, lasted <8 days, and decreased in frequency with additional dosing.

Respiratory: Upper respiratory tract infection (20%), sinusitis (16%), pharyngitis (11%)

Miscellaneous: Viral infection (23%)

1% to 10%:

Central nervous system: Pain (7%), fatigue (3%), dizziness (3%)

Dermatologic: Dermatitis (2%), pruritus (2%)

Neuromuscular & skeletal: Arthralgia (8%), leg pain (4%), arm pain (2%), fracture (2%)

Otic: Earache (2%)

<1% (Limited to important or life-threatening): Alopecia, anaphylaxis, antibody formation to omalizumab, dermatitis, malignancy (0.5%; placebo 0.2%), throat edema, thrombocytopenia, tongue edema, urticaria

Overdosage/Toxicology Limited data; single doses up to 4000 mg and cumulative doses up to 44,000 mg (over 20 weeks) have not been associated with toxicity. Treatment is symptom-directed and supportive.

Test Interactions Total IgE levels are elevated for up to 1 year following treatment. Total serum IgE may be retested after interruption of therapy for 1 year or more.

Dosage Forms

Injection, powder for reconstitution [preservative free]:

Xolair®: 150 mg [contains sucrose 145.5 g]

Omeprazole (oh ME pray zol)

Medication Safety Issues

Sound-alike/look-alike issues:

Prilosec® may be confused with Plendil®, Prevacid®, predniSONE, prilocaine, Prinivil®, Proventil®, Prozac®

U.S. Brand Names Prilosec®; Prilosec OTC™ [OTC]

Canadian Brand Names Apo-Omeprazole®; Losec®; Losec MUPS®

Pharmacologic Category Proton Pump Inhibitor; Substituted Benzimidazole

Generic Available Yes: Delayed release capsule

Use Short-term (4-8 weeks) treatment of active duodenal ulcer disease or active benign gastric ulcer; treatment of heartburn and other symptoms associated with gastroesophageal reflux disease (GERD); short-term (4-8 weeks) treatment of endoscopically-diagnosed erosive esophagitis; maintenance healing of erosive esophagitis; long-term treatment of pathological hypersecretory conditions; as part of a multidrug regimen for *H. pylori* eradication to reduce the risk of duodenal ulcer recurrence

OTC labeling: Short-term treatment of frequent, uncomplicated heartburn occurring ≥2 days/week

Unlabeled/Investigational Use Healing NSAID-induced ulcers; prevention of NSAID-induced ulcers

Mechanism of Action Suppresses gastric basal and stimulated acid secretion by inhibiting the parietal cell H+/K+ ATP pump

Pharmacodynamics/Kinetics

Onset of action: Antisecretory: ~1 hour

Peak effect: 2 hours

Duration: 72 hours

Protein binding: 95%

Metabolism: Extensively hepatic to inactive metabolites

Bioavailability: Oral: 30% to 40%; increased in Asian patients and patients with hepatic dysfunction

Half-life elimination: Delayed release capsule: 0.5-1 hour

Excretion: Urine (77% as metabolites, very small amount as unchanged drug); feces

Dosage Oral:

Children ≥2 years: GERD or other acid-related disorders:

<20 kg: 10 mg once daily

≥20 kg: 20 mg once daily

Adults:

Active duodenal ulcer: 20 mg/day for 4-8 weeks

Gastric ulcers: 40 mg/day for 4-8 weeks

Symptomatic GERD: 20 mg/day for up to 4 weeks

Erosive esophagitis: 20 mg/day for 4-8 weeks; maintenance of healing: 20 mg/day for up to 12 months total therapy (including treatment period of 4-8 weeks)

Helicobacter pylori eradication: Dose varies with regimen: 20 mg once daily **or** 40 mg/day as single dose or in 2 divided doses; requires combination therapy with antibiotics

Pathological hypersecretory conditions: Initial: 60 mg once daily; doses up to 120 mg 3 times/day have been administered; administer daily doses >80 mg in divided doses

Frequent heartburn (OTC labeling): 20 mg/day for 14 days; treatment may be repeated after 4 months if needed

Dosage adjustment in hepatic impairment: Specific guidelines are not available; bioavailability is increased with chronic liver disease

Stability Store at 15°C to 30°C (59°F to 86°F).

(Continued)

Omeprazole *(Continued)*

Administration

Capsule: Should be swallowed whole; do not chew or crush. Best if taken before breakfast. Delayed release capsule may be opened and contents added to applesauce. Administration via NG tube should be in an acidic juice.

Tablet: Should be swallowed whole; do not crush or chew.

Anesthesia and Critical Care Concerns/Other Considerations A 2 mg/mL oral omeprazole solution (Simplified Omeprazole Solution) can be prepared with five omeprazole 20 mg delayed release capsules and 50 mL 8.4% sodium bicarbonate. Empty capsules into beaker. Add sodium bicarbonate solution. Gently stir (about 15 minutes) until a white suspension is formed. Transfer to amber-colored syringe or bottle. Stable for 14 days at room temperature or for 30 days under refrigeration.

DiGiancinto JL, Olsen KM, Bergman KL, et al, "Stability of Suspension Formulations of Lansoprazole and Omeprazole Stored in Amber-Colored Plastic Oral Syringes," *Ann Pharmacother*, 2000, 34:600-5.

Quercia R, Fan C, Liu X, et al, "Stability of Omeprazole in an Extemporaneously Prepared Oral Liquid," *Am J Health Syst Pharm*, 1997, 54:1833-6.

Sharma V, "Comparison of 24-hour Intragastric pH Using Four Liquid Formulations of Lansoprazole and Omeprazole," *Am J Health Syst Pharm*, 1999, 56(Suppl 4):S18-21.

Pregnancy Risk Factor C

Contraindications Hypersensitivity to omeprazole, substituted benzimidazoles (ie, esomeprazole, lansoprazole, pantoprazole, rabeprazole), or any component of the formulation

Warnings/Precautions In long-term (2-year) studies in rats, omeprazole produced a dose-related increase in gastric carcinoid tumors. While available endoscopic evaluations and histologic examinations of biopsy specimens from human stomachs have not detected a risk from short-term exposure to omeprazole, further human data on the effect of sustained hypochlorhydria and hypergastrinemia are needed to rule out the possibility of an increased risk for the development of tumors in humans receiving long-term therapy. Bioavailability may be increased in the elderly, Asian population, and with hepatic dysfunction. Safety and efficacy have not been established in children <2 years of age. When used for self-medication (OTC), do not use for >14 days; treatment should not be repeated more often than every 4 months; OTC and oral suspension are not approved for use in children <18 years of age.

Adverse Reactions

1% to 10%:

Central nervous system: Headache (3% to 7%), dizziness (2%)

Dermatologic: Rash (2%)

Gastrointestinal: Diarrhea (3% to 4%), abdominal pain (2% to 5%), nausea (2% to 4%), vomiting (2% to 3%), flatulence (3%), acid regurgitation (2%), constipation (1% to 2%), taste perversion

Neuromuscular & skeletal: Weakness (1%), back pain (1%)

Respiratory: Upper respiratory infection (2%), cough (1%)

<1% (Limited to important or life-threatening; adverse event occurrence may vary based on formulation): Abdominal swelling, abnormal dreams, aggression, agranulocytosis, alkaline phosphatase increased, allergic reactions, alopecia, anaphylaxis, anemia, angina, angioedema, anorexia, anxiety, apathy, atrophic gastritis, benign gastric polyps, blurred vision, confusion, creatinine increased, depression, diaphoresis, double vision, dry mouth, dry skin, epistaxis, erythema multiforme, esophageal candidiasis, fatigue, fecal discoloration, flatulence, glycosuria, gynecomastia, hallucinations, hematuria, hemifacial dysesthesia, hemolytic anemia, hepatic encephalopathy, hepatic failure, hepatic necrosis, hyperhidrosis, hypertension, hypoglycemia, hyponatremia, insomnia, interstitial nephritis, irritable colon, jaundice, joint pain, leg pain, leukocytosis, leukopenia, liver disease (hepatocellular, cholestatic, mixed), malaise, microscopic pyuria, mucosal atrophy (tongue), muscle cramps, muscle weakness, myalgia, nervousness, neutropenia, ocular irritation, optic neuropathy, pain, palpitation, pancreatitis, pancytopenia, paresthesia, peripheral edema, petechiae, pharyngeal pain, photosensitivity, pneumothorax, proteinuria, pruritus, psychic disturbance, purpura, rash, skin inflammation, somnolence, Stevens-Johnson syndrome, stomatitis, tachycardia, taste perversion, testicular pain, thrombocytopenia, tinnitus, toxic epidermal necrolysis, tremor, urinary frequency, urinary tract infection, urticaria, vertigo, weight gain

Overdosage/Toxicology Limited experience with overdose in humans. Doses up to 2400 mg have been reported. Symptoms include confusion, drowsiness, blurred vision, tachycardia, nausea, flushing, diaphoresis, headache, and dry mouth. Treatment is symptom-directed and supportive. Not dialyzable.

Drug Interactions **Substrate** of CYP2A6 (minor), 2C9 (minor), 2C19 (major), 2D6 (minor), 3A4 (minor); **Inhibits** CYP1A2 (weak), 2C9 (moderate), 2C19 (strong), 2D6 (weak), 3A4 (weak); **Induces** CYP1A2 (weak)

Benzodiazepines metabolized by oxidation (eg, diazepam, midazolam, triazolam): Esomeprazole and omeprazole may increase levels of benzodiazepines metabolized by oxidation.

Carbamazepine: Esomeprazole and omeprazole may increase carbamazepine levels.

Clozapine: Omeprazole may alter the concentrations/effects of clozapine; monitor.

CYP2C9 substrates: Omeprazole may increase the levels/effects of CYP2C9 substrates. Example substrates include amiodarone, fluoxetine, glimepiride, glipizide, nateglinide, phenytoin, pioglitazone, rosiglitazone, sertraline, and warfarin.

CYP2C19 inducers: May decrease the levels/effects of omeprazole. Example inducers include aminoglutethimide, carbamazepine, phenytoin, and rifampin.

CYP2C19 substrates: Omeprazole may increase the levels/effects of CYP2C19 substrates. Example substrates include citalopram, diazepam, methsuximide, phenytoin, propranolol, and sertraline.

Itraconazole and ketoconazole: Proton pump inhibitors may decrease the absorption of itraconazole and ketoconazole.

Methotrexate: Concurrent use with omeprazole may decrease the excretion of methotrexate. **Note:** Antirheumatic doses of methotrexate probably hold minimal risk.

Phenytoin: Elimination of phenytoin may be prolonged; monitor. Phenytoin may decrease omeprazole levels/effects.

Protease inhibitors: Proton pump inhibitors may decrease absorption of some protease inhibitors (atazanavir and indinavir). Avoid concurrent use.

Warfarin: Elimination of warfarin may be prolonged; monitor.

Ethanol/Nutrition/Herb Interactions

Ethanol: Avoid ethanol (may cause gastric mucosal irritation).

Food: Food delays absorption.

Herb/Nutraceutical: St John's wort may decrease omeprazole levels.

Dietary Considerations Should be taken on an empty stomach; best if taken before breakfast.

Dosage Forms

Capsule, delayed release: 10 mg, 20 mg

Prilosec®: 10 mg, 20 mg, 40 mg

Tablet, delayed release:

Prilosec OTC™: 20 mg

References

Allen ME, Kopp BJ, and Erstad BL, "Stress Ulcer Prophylaxis in the Postoperative Period," *Am J Health Syst Pharm*, 2004, 61(6):588-96.

Jung R and MacLaren R, "Proton-Pump Inhibitors for Stress Ulcer Prophylaxis in Critically Ill Patients," *Ann Pharmacother*, 2002, 36(12):1929-37.

Lau JY, Sung JJ, Lee KK, et al, "Effect of Intravenous Omeprazole on Recurrent Bleeding After Endoscopic Treatment of Bleeding Peptic Ulcers," *N Engl J Med*, 2000, 343(5):310-6.

Lin HJ, Lo WC, Lee FY, et al, "A Prospective Randomized Comparative Trial Showing That Omeprazole Prevents Rebleeding in Patients With Bleeding Peptic Ulcer After Successful Endoscopic Therapy," *Arch Intern Med*, 1998, 158(1):54-8.

♦ **Omnitrope™** *see* Human Growth Hormone *on page 625*

Ondansetron (on DAN se tron)

Medication Safety Issues

Sound-alike/look-alike issues:

Ondansetron may be confused with dolasetron, granisetron, palonosetron

Zofran® may be confused with Zantac®, Zosyn®

Related Information

Postoperative Nausea and Vomiting *on page 1477*

(Continued)

Ondansetron *(Continued)*

U.S. Brand Names Zofran®; Zofran® ODT

Canadian Brand Names Zofran®; Zofran® ODT

Synonyms GR38032R; Ondansetron Hydrochloride

Pharmacologic Category Antiemetic; Selective 5-HT_3 Receptor Antagonist

Generic Available No

Use Prevention of nausea and vomiting associated with moderately- to highly-emetogenic cancer chemotherapy [not recommended for treatment of **existing** chemotherapy-induced emesis (CIE)]; radiotherapy in patients receiving total body irradiation or fractions to the abdomen; prevention of postoperative nausea and vomiting (PONV); treatment of PONV if no prophylactic dose received

Unlabeled/Investigational Use Treatment of early-onset alcoholism; hyperemesis gravidarum

Mechanism of Action Selective 5-HT_3-receptor antagonist, blocking serotonin, both peripherally on vagal nerve terminals and centrally in the chemoreceptor trigger zone

Pharmacodynamics/Kinetics

Onset of action: ~30 minutes

Distribution: V_d: Children: 1.7-3.7 L/kg; Adults: 2.2-2.5 L/kg

Protein binding, plasma: 70% to 76%

Metabolism: Extensively hepatic via hydroxylation, followed by glucuronide or sulfate conjugation; CYP1A2, CYP2D6, and CYP3A4 substrate; some demethylation occurs

Bioavailability: Oral: 56% to 71%; Rectal: 58% to 74%

Half-life elimination: Children <15 years: 2-7 hours; Adults: 3-6 hours
- Mild-to-moderate hepatic impairment: Adults: 12 hours
- Severe hepatic impairment (Child-Pugh C): Adults: 20 hours

Time to peak: Oral: ~2 hours

Excretion: Urine (44% to 60% as metabolites, 5% to 10% as unchanged drug); feces (~25%)

Dosage Note: Studies in adults have shown a single daily dose of 8-12 mg I.V. or 8-24 mg orally to be as effective as mg/kg dosing, and should be considered for **all** patients whose mg/kg dose exceeds 8-12 mg I.V.; oral solution and ODT formulations are bioequivalent to corresponding doses of tablet formulation

Children:

I.V.:

Prevention of chemotherapy-induced emesis: 6 months to 18 years: 0.15 mg/kg/dose administered 30 minutes prior to chemotherapy, 4 and 8 hours after the first dose **or** 0.45 mg/kg/day as a single dose

Prevention of postoperative nausea and vomiting: 1 month to 12 years:
- ≤40 kg: 0.1 mg/kg as a single dose
- >40 kg: 4 mg as a single dose

Oral: Prevention of chemotherapy-induced emesis:
- 4-11 years: 4 mg 30 minutes before chemotherapy; repeat 4 and 8 hours after initial dose, then 4 mg every 8 hours for 1-2 days after chemotherapy completed
- ≥12 years: Refer to adult dosing.

Adults:

I.V.:

Prevention of chemotherapy-induced emesis:
- 0.15 mg/kg 3 times/day beginning 30 minutes prior to chemotherapy **or**
- 0.45 mg/kg once daily **or**
- 8-10 mg 1-2 times/day **or**
- 24 mg or 32 mg once daily

Treatment of hyperemesis gravidum (unlabeled use): 8 mg administered over 15 minutes every 12 hours **or** 1 mg/hour infused continuously for up to 24 hours

I.M., I.V.: Postoperative nausea and vomiting: 4 mg as a single dose approximately 30 minutes before the end of anesthesia, or as treatment if vomiting occurs after surgery

Note: Repeat doses given in response to inadequate control of nausea/vomiting from preoperative doses are generally ineffective.

Oral:

Chemotherapy-induced emesis:

Highly-emetogenic agents/single-day therapy: 24 mg given 30 minutes prior to the start of therapy

Moderately-emetogenic agents: 8 mg every 12 hours beginning 30 minutes before chemotherapy, continuously for 1-2 days after chemotherapy completed

Total body irradiation: 8 mg 1-2 hours before daily each fraction of radiotherapy

Single high-dose fraction radiotherapy to abdomen: 8 mg 1-2 hours before irradiation, then 8 mg every 8 hours after first dose for 1-2 days after completion of radiotherapy

Daily fractionated radiotherapy to abdomen: 8 mg 1-2 hours before irradiation, then 8 mg 8 hours after first dose for each day of radiotherapy

Postoperative nausea and vomiting: 16 mg given 1 hour prior to induction of anesthesia

Treatment of hyperemesis gravidum (unlabeled use): 8 mg every 12 hours

Elderly: No dosing adjustment required

Dosage adjustment in renal impairment: No dosing adjustment required

Dosage adjustment in hepatic impairment: Severe liver disease (Child-Pugh C): Maximum daily dose: 8 mg

Stability

Oral solution: Store between 15°C and 30°C (59°F and 86°F); protect from light

Premixed bag: Store between 2°C and 30°C (36°F and 86°F); protect from light

Tablet: Store between 2°C and 30°C (36°F and 86°F)

Vial: Store between 2°C and 30°C (36°F and 86°F); protect from light. Prior to I.V. infusion, dilute in 50 mL D_5W or NS; solution is stable for 48 hours at room temperature. Do not mix injection with alkaline solutions; precipitate may form.

Administration

Oral: Oral dosage forms should be administered 30 minutes prior to chemotherapy; 1-2 hours before radiotherapy; 1 hour prior to the induction of anesthesia

Orally-disintegrating tablets: Do not remove from blister until needed. Peel backing off the blister, do not push tablet through. Using dry hands, place tablet on tongue and allow to dissolve. Swallow with saliva.

I.M.: Should be administered undiluted

I.V.: Give first dose 30 minutes prior to beginning chemotherapy; the I.V. preparation has been successful when administered orally

I.V. injection: Single doses for prevention of postoperative nausea and vomiting may be administered I.V. over 2-5 minutes as undiluted solution

IVPB: Dilute in 50 mL D_5W or NS. Infuse over 15-30 minutes; 24-hour continuous infusions have been reported, but are rarely used

Monitoring Parameters

Closely monitor patients <4 months of age

Pregnancy Risk Factor B

Contraindications Hypersensitivity to ondansetron, other selective 5-HT_3 antagonists, or any component of the formulation

Warnings/Precautions For chemotherapy, ondansetron should be used on a scheduled basis, not on an "as needed" (PRN) basis, since data support the use of this drug only in the prevention of nausea and vomiting (due to antineoplastic therapy) and not in the rescue of nausea and vomiting. Ondansetron should only be used in the first 24-48 hours of chemotherapy. Data do not support any increased efficacy of ondansetron in delayed nausea and vomiting. Does not stimulate gastric or intestinal peristalsis; may mask progressive ileus and/or gastric distension. Orally-disintegrating tablets contain phenylalanine. Safety and efficacy for children <1 month of age have not been established.

Adverse Reactions

Note: Percentages reported in adult patients.

>10%:

Central nervous system: Headache (9% to 27%), malaise/fatigue (9% to 13%)

Gastrointestinal: Constipation (6% to 11%)

1% to 10%:

Central nervous system: Drowsiness (8%), fever (2% to 8%), dizziness (4% to 7%), anxiety (6%), cold sensation (2%)

Dermatologic: Pruritus (2% to 5%), rash (1%)

Gastrointestinal: Diarrhea (2% to 7%)

(Continued)

Ondansetron *(Continued)*

Genitourinary: Gynecological disorder (7%), urinary retention (5%)
Hepatic: ALT/AST increased (1% to 5%)
Local: Injection site reaction (4%; pain, redness, burning)
Neuromuscular & skeletal: Paresthesia (2%)
Respiratory: Hypoxia (9%)

<1% (Limited to important or life-threatening): Anaphylactoid reactions, anaphylaxis, angina, angioedema, arrhythmia, blindness (transient/following infusion), blurred vision (transient/following infusion), bradycardia, bronchospasm, cardiopulmonary arrest, dyspnea, dystonic reaction, ECG changes, electrocardiographic alterations (second degree heart block and ST-segment depression), extrapyramidal symptoms, flushing, grand mal seizure, hiccups, hypersensitivity reaction, hypokalemia, hypotension, laryngeal edema, laryngospasm, oculogyric crisis, palpitation, premature ventricular contractions (PVC), shock, stridor, supraventricular tachycardia, syncope, tachycardia, urticaria, vascular occlusive events, ventricular arrhythmia

Overdosage/Toxicology Sudden transient blindness, severe constipation, hypotension, and vasovagal episode with transient secondary heart block have been reported in some cases of overdose. I.V. doses of up to 252 mg/day have been inadvertently given without adverse effects. There is no specific antidote. Treatment is symptom-directed and supportive.

Drug Interactions Substrate of CYP1A2 (minor), 2C9 (minor), 2D6 (minor), 2E1 (minor), 3A4 (major); **Inhibits** CYP1A2 (weak), 2C9 (weak), 2D6 (weak)

Apomorphine: Due to reports of profound hypotension during concomitant therapy, the manufacturer of apomorphine contraindicates its use with ondansetron.

CYP3A4 inducers: CYP3A4 inducers may decrease the levels/effects of ondansetron. Example inducers include aminoglutethimide, carbamazepine, nafcillin, nevirapine, phenobarbital, phenytoin, and rifamycins. The manufacturer does not recommend dosage adjustment in patients receiving CYP3A4 inducers.

Ethanol/Nutrition/Herb Interactions

Food: Food increases the extent of absorption. The C_{max} and T_{max} do not change much.

Herb/Nutraceutical: St John's wort may decrease ondansetron levels.

Dietary Considerations Take without regard to meals.

Orally-disintegrating tablet contains <0.03 mg phenylalanine

Dosage Forms [DSC] = Discontinued product

Infusion [premixed in D_5W, preservative free]:
Zofran®: 32 mg (50 mL)

Injection, solution:
Zofran®: 2 mg/mL (2 mL, 20 mL)

Solution, oral:
Zofran®: 4 mg/5 mL (50 mL) [contains sodium benzoate; strawberry flavor]

Tablet:
Zofran®: 4 mg; 8 mg; 24 mg [DSC]

Tablet, orally disintegrating:
Zofran® ODT: 4 mg, 8 mg [each strength contains phenylalanine <0.03 mg/tablet; strawberry flavor]

References

Tramer MR, Moore RA, Reynolds DJ, et al, "A Quantitative Systematic Review of Ondansetron in Treatment of Established Postoperative Nausea and Vomiting," *BMJ*, 1997, 314(7087):1088-92.

- ♦ **Ondansetron Hydrochloride** *see* Ondansetron *on page 959*
- ♦ **OPC-13013** *see* Cilostazol *on page 279*
- ♦ **Operand® [OTC]** *see* Povidone-Iodine *on page 1039*
- ♦ **Operand® Chlorhexidine Gluconate [OTC]** *see* Chlorhexidine Gluconate *on page 267*
- ♦ **Ophtho-Tate® (Can)** *see* PrednisoLONE *on page 1046*
- ♦ **Oracea™** *see* Doxycycline *on page 426*
- ♦ **Oracort (Can)** *see* Triamcinolone *on page 1311*
- ♦ **Oramorph SR®** *see* Morphine Sulfate *on page 867*
- ♦ **Oranyl [OTC]** *see* Pseudoephedrine *on page 1085*
- ♦ **Orapred®** *see* PrednisoLONE *on page 1046*
- ♦ **Orapred ODT™** *see* PrednisoLONE *on page 1046*
- ♦ **Orciprenaline Sulfate** *see* Metaproterenol *on page 808*
- ♦ **ORG 946** *see* Rocuronium *on page 1135*

♦ **ORG NC 45** *see* Vecuronium *on page 1345*
♦ **ORO-Clense (Can)** *see* Chlorhexidine Gluconate *on page 267*
♦ **Orudis® KT [OTC] [DSC]** *see* Ketoprofen *on page 714*
♦ **Oruvail® (Can)** *see* Ketoprofen *on page 714*

Oseltamivir (oh sel TAM i vir)

Medication Safety Issues
Sound-alike/look-alike issues:
Tamiflu® may be confused with Thera-Flu®

U.S. Brand Names Tamiflu®

Canadian Brand Names Tamiflu®

Pharmacologic Category Antiviral Agent; Neuraminidase Inhibitor

Generic Available No

Use Treatment of uncomplicated acute illness due to influenza (A or B) infection in children ≥1 year of age and adults who have been symptomatic for no more than 2 days; prophylaxis against influenza (A or B) infection in children ≥1 year of age and adults

Mechanism of Action Oseltamivir, a prodrug, is hydrolyzed to the active form, oseltamivir carboxylate. It is thought to inhibit influenza virus neuraminidase, with the possibility of alteration of virus particle aggregation and release.

Pharmacodynamics/Kinetics
Absorption: Well absorbed
Distribution: V_d: 23-26 L (oseltamivir carboxylate)
Protein binding, plasma: Oseltamivir carboxylate: 3%; Oseltamivir: 42%
Metabolism: Hepatic (90%) to oseltamivir carboxylate; neither the parent drug nor active metabolite has any effect on CYP
Bioavailability: 75% as oseltamivir carboxylate
Half-life elimination: Oseltamivir: 1-3 hours; Oseltamivir carboxylate: 6-10 hours
Excretion: Urine (>90% as oseltamivir carboxylate); feces

Dosage Oral:
Treatment: Initiate treatment within 2 days of onset of symptoms; duration of treatment: 5 days:
Children: 1-12 years:
≤15 kg: 30 mg twice daily
>15 kg to ≤23 kg: 45 mg twice daily
>23 kg to ≤40 kg: 60 mg twice daily
>40 kg: 75 mg twice daily
Adolescents ≥13 years and Adults: 75 mg twice daily
Prophylaxis: Initiate treatment within 2 days of contact with an infected individual; duration of treatment: 10 days
Children: 1-12 years:
≤15 kg: 30 mg twice daily
>15 kg to ≤23 kg: 45 mg twice daily
>23 kg to ≤40 kg: 60 mg twice daily
>40 kg: 75 mg twice daily
Adolescents ≥13 years and Adults: 75 mg once daily. During community outbreaks, dosing is 75 mg once daily. May be used for up to 6 weeks; duration of protection lasts for length of dosing period
Elderly: Refer to Adults dosing.

Dosage adjustment in renal impairment: Adults:
Cl_{cr} 10-30 mL/minute:
Treatment: Reduce dose to 75 mg once daily for 5 days
Prophylaxis: 75 mg every other day or 30 mg once daily
Cl_{cr} <10 mL/minute: Dosing recommendations are not available

Dosage adjustment in hepatic impairment: Dosing recommendations are not available

Stability
Capsules: Store at 25°C (77°F).
Oral suspension: Store powder for suspension at 25°C (77°F). Reconstitute with 23 mL of water (to make 25 mL total suspension). Once reconstituted, store suspension under refrigeration at 2°C to 8°C (36°F to 46°F); do not freeze. Use within 10 days of preparation.

Pregnancy Risk Factor C

(Continued)

Oseltamivir *(Continued)*

Contraindications Hypersensitivity to oseltamivir or any component of the formulation

Warnings/Precautions Oseltamivir is not a substitute for the influenza virus vaccine. Use caution with renal impairment; dosage adjustment is required for creatinine clearance between 10-30 mL/minute. Also consider primary or concomitant bacterial infections. Safety and efficacy for use in hepatic impairment or for treatment or prophylaxis in immunocompromised patients have not been established. Efficacy has not been established if treatment begins >40 hours after the onset of symptoms or in the treatment of patients with chronic cardiac and/or respiratory disease. Rare but severe hypersensitivity reactions (anaphylaxis, severe dermatologic reactions) have been associated with use. Safety and efficacy in children (<1 year of age) have not been established.

Adverse Reactions

>10%: Gastrointestinal: Vomiting (2% to 15%)

1% to 10%: Gastrointestinal: Nausea (3% to 10%), abdominal pain (2% to 5%)

<1% (Limited to important or life-threatening): Allergy, anaphylactic/anaphylactoid reaction, anemia, angina, arrhythmia, confusion, dermatitis, diabetes aggravation, eczema, erythema multiforme, fracture, hepatitis, liver function tests abnormal, peritonsillar abscess, pneumonia, pseudomembranous colitis, pyrexia, rash, seizure, Stevens-Johnson syndrome, swelling of face or tongue, toxic epidermal necrolysis, urticaria

Overdosage/Toxicology Single doses of 1000 mg resulted in nausea and vomiting.

Drug Interactions Influenza virus vaccine nasal spray (fluMist™): Safety and efficacy for use with influenza virus vaccine nasal spray have not been established. Do not administer nasal spray until 48 hours after stopping antiviral; do not administer antiviral for 2 weeks after receiving influenza virus vaccine nasal spray.

Dietary Considerations Take with or without food; take with food to improve tolerance.

Dosage Forms

Capsule, as phosphate: 75 mg

Powder for oral suspension: 12 mg/mL (25 mL) [contains sodium benzoate; tutti-frutti flavor]

◆ **Osmitrol®** *see* Mannitol *on page 790*

◆ **OsmoPrep™** *see* Sodium Phosphates *on page 1189*

◆ **Ostac® (Can)** *see* Clodronate *on page 308*

Oxaprozin (oks a PROE zin)

Medication Safety Issues

Sound-alike/look-alike issues:

Daypro® may be confused with Diupres®

Oxaprozin may be confused with oxazepam

U.S. Brand Names Daypro®

Canadian Brand Names Apo-Oxaprozin®; Daypro®

Pharmacologic Category Nonsteroidal Anti-inflammatory Drug (NSAID), Oral

Restrictions A medication guide should be dispensed with each prescription. A template for the required MedGuide can be found on the FDA website at: http://www.fda.gov/medwatch/SAFETY/2005/safety05.htm#NSAID

Generic Available Yes

Use Acute and long-term use in the management of signs and symptoms of osteoarthritis and rheumatoid arthritis; juvenile rheumatoid arthritis

Mechanism of Action Inhibits prostaglandin synthesis by decreasing the activity of the enzyme, cyclooxygenase, which results in decreased formation of prostaglandin precursors

Pharmacodynamics/Kinetics

Absorption: Almost complete

Protein binding: >99%

Metabolism: Hepatic via oxidation and glucuronidation; no active metabolites

Half-life elimination: 40-50 hours

Time to peak: 2-4 hours

Excretion: Urine (5% unchanged, 65% as metabolites); feces (35% as metabolites)

Dosage Oral (individualize dosage to lowest effective dose to minimize adverse effects):

Children 6-16 years: Juvenile rheumatoid arthritis:

22-31 kg: 600 mg once daily
32-54 kg: 900 mg once daily
≥55 kg: 1200 mg once daily

Adults:

Osteoarthritis: 600-1200 mg once daily; patients should be titrated to lowest dose possible; patients with low body weight should start with 600 mg daily

Rheumatoid arthritis: 1200 mg once daily; a one-time loading dose of up to 1800 mg/day or 26 mg/kg (whichever is lower) may be given

Maximum doses:

Patient <50 kg: Maximum: 1200 mg/day

Patient >50 kg with normal renal/hepatic function and low risk of peptic ulcer: Maximum: 1800 mg or 26 mg/kg (whichever is lower) in divided doses

Dosing adjustment in renal impairment: In general NSAIDs are not recommended for use in patients with advanced renal disease but the manufacturer of oxaprozin does provide some guidelines for adjustment in renal dysfunction.

Severe renal impairment or on dialysis: 600 mg once daily, may increase cautiously to 1200 mg/day with close monitoring

Dosing adjustment in hepatic impairment: Use caution in patients with severe dysfunction

Stability Store at 25°C (77°F); protect from light; keep bottle tightly closed

Monitoring Parameters Monitor CBC; hepatic, renal, and ocular function

Anesthesia and Critical Care Concerns/Other Considerations The 2002 ACCM/SCCM guidelines for analgesia (critically-ill adult) suggest that NSAIDs may be used in combination with opioids in select patients for pain management. Concern about adverse events (increased risk of renal dysfunction, altered platelet function and gastrointestinal irritation) limits its use in patients who have other underlying risks for these events.

In short-term use, NSAIDs vary considerably in their effect on blood pressure. When NSAIDs are used in patients with hypertension, appropriate monitoring of blood pressure responses should be completed and the duration of therapy, when possible, kept short. The use of NSAIDs in the treatment of patients with congestive heart failure may be associated with an increased risk for fluid accumulation and edema; may precipitate renal failure in dehydrated patients.

Pregnancy Risk Factor C/D (3rd trimester)

Contraindications Hypersensitivity to oxaprozin, aspirin, other NSAIDs, or any component of the formulation; perioperative pain in the setting of coronary artery bypass surgery (CABG); pregnancy (3rd trimester)

Warnings/Precautions [U.S. Boxed Warning]: NSAIDs are associated with an increased risk of adverse cardiovascular events, including MI, stroke, and new onset or worsening of pre-existing hypertension. Risk may be increased with duration of use or pre-existing cardiovascular risk-factors or disease. Carefully evaluate individual cardiovascular risk profiles prior to prescribing. Use caution with fluid retention, CHF or hypertension.

Use of NSAIDs can compromise existing renal function. Renal toxicity can occur in patient with impaired renal function, dehydration, heart failure, liver dysfunction, those taking diuretics and ACEI and the elderly. Rehydrate patient before starting therapy. Monitor renal function closely. Oxaprozin is not recommended for patients with advanced renal disease.

[U.S. Boxed Warning]: NSAIDs may increase risk of gastrointestinal irritation, ulceration, bleeding, and perforation. These events may occur at any time during therapy and without warning. Use caution with a history of GI disease (bleeding or ulcers), concurrent therapy with aspirin, anticoagulants and/or corticosteroids, smoking, use of alcohol, the elderly or debilitated patients.

Use the lowest effective dose for the shortest duration of time, consistent with individual patient goals, to reduce risk of cardiovascular or GI adverse events. Alternate therapies should be considered for patients at high risk.

NSAIDs may cause serious skin adverse events including exfoliative dermatitis, Stevens-Johnson syndrome (SJS) and toxic epidermal necrolysis (TEN). Anaphylactoid reactions may occur, even without prior exposure; patients with "aspirin triad" (bronchial asthma, aspirin intolerance, rhinitis) may be at increased risk. Do not use in patients who experience bronchospasm, asthma, rhinitis, or urticaria with NSAID or aspirin therapy.

(Continued)

Oxaprozin *(Continued)*

Use with caution in patients with decreased hepatic function. Closely monitor patients with any abnormal LFT. Severe hepatic reactions (eg, fulminant hepatitis, liver failure) have occurred with NSAID use, rarely; discontinue if signs or symptoms of liver disease develop, or if systemic manifestations occur.

The elderly are at increased risk for adverse effects (especially peptic ulceration, CNS effects, renal toxicity) from NSAIDs even at low doses.

Withhold for at least 4-6 half-lives prior to surgical or dental procedures. May cause mild photosensitivity reactions. Safety and efficacy have not been established in children <6 years of age.

Adverse Reactions

1% to 10%:

Cardiovascular: Edema

Central nervous system: Confusion, depression, dizziness, headache, sedation, sleep disturbance, somnolence

Dermatologic: Pruritus, rash

Gastrointestinal: Abdominal distress, abdominal pain, anorexia, constipation, diarrhea, flatulence, gastrointestinal ulcer, gross bleeding with perforation, heartburn, nausea, vomiting

Hematologic: Anemia, bleeding time increased

Hepatic: Liver enzyme elevation

Otic: Tinnitus

Renal: Dysuria, renal function abnormal, urinary frequency

<1% (Limited to important or life-threatening; effects reported with oxaprozin or other NSAIDs): Acute interstitial nephritis, acute renal failure, agranulocytosis, anaphylaxis, angioedema, asthma, bruising, CHF, erythema multiforme, exfoliative dermatitis, gastritis, gastrointestinal bleeding, hearing decreased, hematemesis, hematuria, hemorrhoidal bleeding, hepatitis, hypersensitivity reaction, hypertension, jaundice, leukopenia, nephrotic syndrome, pancreatitis, peptic ulcer, photosensitivity, rectal bleeding, renal insufficiency, Stevens-Johnson syndrome, toxic epidermal necrolysis, thrombocytopenia

Overdosage/Toxicology Symptoms of overdose include acute renal failure, vomiting, drowsiness, and leukocytes. Management of NSAID intoxication is supportive and symptomatic. Since many NSAIDs undergo enterohepatic cycling, multiple doses of charcoal may be needed to reduce the potential for delayed toxicities.

Drug Interactions

ACE inhibitors: Antihypertensive effects may be decreased by concurrent therapy with NSAIDs; monitor blood pressure. Oxaprozin may decrease serum concentration of enalapril.

Angiotensin II antagonists: Antihypertensive effects may be decreased by concurrent therapy with NSAIDs; monitor blood pressure.

Anticoagulants (warfarin, heparin, LMWHs) in combination with NSAIDs can cause increased risk of bleeding.

Antiplatelet drugs (ticlopidine, clopidogrel, aspirin, abciximab, dipyridamole, eptifibatide, tirofiban) can cause an increased risk of bleeding.

Beta-blockers: NSAIDs may decrease the antihypertensive effect of beta-blockers. Monitor.

Cholestyramine (and other bile acid sequestrants): May decrease the absorption of NSAIDs. Separate by at least 2 hours.

Corticosteroids may increase the risk of GI ulceration; avoid concurrent use.

Cyclosporine: NSAIDs may increase serum creatinine, potassium, blood pressure, and cyclosporine levels; monitor cyclosporine levels and renal function carefully.

Hydralazine's antihypertensive effect is decreased; avoid concurrent use.

Lithium levels can be increased; avoid concurrent use if possible or monitor lithium levels and adjust dose. Sulindac may have the least effect. When NSAID is stopped, lithium will need adjustment again.

Loop diuretics efficacy (diuretic and antihypertensive effect) may be reduced.

Methotrexate: Severe bone marrow suppression, aplastic anemia, and GI toxicity have been reported with concomitant NSAID therapy. Avoid use during moderate or high-dose methotrexate (increased and prolonged methotrexate levels). NSAID use during low-dose treatment of rheumatoid arthritis has not been fully evaluated; extreme caution is warranted.

Thiazides antihypertensive effects are decreased; avoid concurrent use.

Warfarin's INRs may be increased by piroxicam. Other NSAIDs may have the same effect depending on dose and duration. Monitor INR closely. Use the lowest dose of NSAIDs possible and for the briefest duration.

Ethanol/Nutrition/Herb Interactions

Ethanol: Avoid ethanol (may enhance gastric mucosal irritation).

Herb/Nutraceutical: Avoid alfalfa, anise, bilberry, bladderwrack, bromelain, cat's claw, celery, coleus, cordyceps, dong quai, evening primrose, feverfew, fenugreek, garlic, ginger, ginkgo biloboa, red clover, horse chestnut, grapeseed, green tea, ginseng, guggul, horse chestnut seed, horseradish, licorice, prickly ash, red clover, reishi, SAMe, sweet clover, turmeric, white willow (all have additional antiplatelet activity).

Test Interactions False-positive urine immunoassay screening tests for benzodiazepines have been reported and may occur several days after discontinuing oxaprozin.

Dosage Forms Tablet: 600 mg

- **Oxeze® Turbuhaler® (Can)** *see* Formoterol *on page 559*
- **Oxidized Regenerated Cellulose** *see* Cellulose (Oxidized Regenerated) *on page 258*
- **Oxycocet® (Can)** *see* Oxycodone and Acetaminophen *on page 969*
- **Oxycodan® (Can)** *see* Oxycodone and Aspirin *on page 971*

Oxycodone (oks i KOE done)

Medication Safety Issues

Sound-alike/look-alike issues:

Oxycodone may be confused with OxyContin®

OxyContin® may be confused with oxybutynin, oxycodone

OxyFast® may be confused with Roxanol™

Related Information

Acute Postoperative Pain *on page 1388*

Anesthesia Considerations for Neurosurgery *on page 1401*

Chronic Pain Management *on page 1430*

Narcotic / Opioid Analgesics *on page 1568*

U.S. Brand Names OxyContin®; Oxydose™; OxyFast®; OxyIR®; Roxicodone™; Roxicodone™ Intensol™

Canadian Brand Names OxyContin®; Oxy.IR®; Supeudol®

Synonyms Dihydrohydroxycodeinone; Oxycodone Hydrochloride

Pharmacologic Category Analgesic, Narcotic

Restrictions C-II

Generic Available Yes

Use Management of moderate to severe pain, normally used in combination with non-narcotic analgesics

OxyContin® is indicated for around-the-clock management of moderate to severe pain when an analgesic is needed for an extended period of time. **Note:** OxyContin® is not intended for use as an "as needed" analgesic or for immediately-postoperative pain management (should be used postoperatively only if the patient has received it prior to surgery or if severe, persistent pain is anticipated).

Mechanism of Action Binds to opiate receptors in the CNS, causing inhibition of ascending pain pathways, altering the perception of and response to pain; produces generalized CNS depression

Pharmacodynamics/Kinetics

Onset of action: Pain relief: 10-15 minutes

Peak effect: 0.5-1 hour

Duration: 3-6 hours; Controlled release: ≤12 hours

Metabolism: Hepatic

Half-life elimination: 2-3 hours

Excretion: Urine

Dosage Oral:

Immediate release:

Children:

6-12 years: 1.25 mg every 6 hours as needed

>12 years: 2.5 mg every 6 hours as needed

Adults: 5 mg every 6 hours as needed

Controlled release: Adults:

Opioid naive (not currently on opioid): 10 mg every 12 hours

(Continued)

Oxycodone *(Continued)*

Currently on opioid/ASA or acetaminophen or NSAID combination:
1-5 tablets: 10-20 mg every 12 hours
6-9 tablets: 20-30 mg every 12 hours
10-12 tablets: 30-40 mg every 12 hours
May continue the nonopioid as a separate drug.

Currently on opioids: Use standard conversion chart to convert daily dose to oxycodone equivalent. Divide daily dose in 2 (for every 12-hour dosing) and round down to nearest dosage form.

Note: 80 mg or 160 mg tablets are for use **only** in opioid-tolerant patients. Special safety considerations must be addressed when converting to OxyContin® doses ≥160 mg every 12 hours. Dietary caution must be taken when patients are initially titrated to 160 mg tablets.

Dosing adjustment in hepatic impairment: Reduce dosage in patients with severe liver disease

Stability Tablets should be stored at room temperature.

Administration Do not crush controlled-release tablets; 80 mg and 160 mg tablets are for use **only** in opioid-tolerant patients. Do not administer OxyContin® 160 mg tablet with a high-fat meal.

Monitoring Parameters Pain relief, respiratory and mental status, blood pressure

Reference Range Blood level of 5 mg/L associated with fatality

Pregnancy Risk Factor B/D (prolonged use or high doses at term)

Contraindications Hypersensitivity to oxycodone or any component of the formulation; significant respiratory depression; hypercarbia; acute or severe bronchial asthma; OxyContin® is also contraindicated in paralytic ileus (known or suspected); pregnancy (prolonged use or high doses at term)

Warnings/Precautions Use with caution in patients with hypersensitivity reactions to other phenanthrene derivative opioid agonists (morphine, hydrocodone, hydromorphone, levorphanol, oxycodone, oxymorphone), respiratory diseases including asthma, emphysema, or COPD. Use with caution in pancreatitis or biliary tract disease, acute alcoholism (including delirium tremens), adrenocortical insufficiency, CNS depression/coma, kyphoscoliosis (or other skeletal disorder which may alter respiratory function), hypothyroidism (including myxedema), prostatic hyperplasia, urethral stricture, and toxic psychosis.

Use with caution in the elderly, debilitated, severe hepatic or renal function. Hemodynamic effects (hypotension, orthostasis) may be exaggerated in patients with hypovolemia, concurrent vasodilating drugs, or in patients with head injury. Respiratory depressant effects and capacity to elevate CSF pressure may be exaggerated in presence of head injury, other intracranial lesion, or pre-existing intracranial pressure. Some preparations contain sulfites which may cause allergic reactions.

[U.S. Boxed Warning]: Healthcare provider should be alert to problems of abuse, misuse, and diversion. Tolerance or drug dependence may result from extended use.

Controlled-release formulations:

[U.S. Boxed Warnings]: Do NOT crush controlled-release tablets; 80 mg and 160 mg strengths are for use only in opioid-tolerant patients requiring high daily dosages >160 mg (80 mg formulation) or >320 mg (160 mg formulation). OxyContin® is not for use as an "as-needed" analgesic and is suitable only of continuous, around-the-clock management of moderate to severe pain.

Adverse Reactions

>10%:
Central nervous system: Fatigue, drowsiness, dizziness, somnolence
Dermatologic: Pruritus
Gastrointestinal: Nausea, vomiting, constipation
Neuromuscular & skeletal: Weakness

1% to 10%:
Cardiovascular: Postural hypotension
Central nervous system: Nervousness, headache, restlessness, malaise, confusion, anxiety, abnormal dreams, euphoria, thought abnormalities
Dermatologic: Rash
Gastrointestinal: Anorexia, stomach cramps, xerostomia, biliary spasm, abdominal pain, dyspepsia, gastritis

Genitourinary: Ureteral spasms, decreased urination
Local: Pain at injection site
Respiratory: Dyspnea, hiccups
Miscellaneous: Diaphoresis

<1% (Limited to important or life-threatening): Anaphylaxis, anaphylactoid reaction, dysphagia, exfoliative dermatitis, hallucinations, histamine release, hyponatremia, ileus, intracranial pressure increased, mental depression, paradoxical CNS stimulation, paralytic ileus, physical and psychological dependence, SIADH, syncope, urinary retention, urticaria, vasodilation, withdrawal syndrome (may include seizure)

Note: Deaths due to overdose have been reported due to misuse/abuse after crushing the sustained release tablets.

Overdosage/Toxicology Symptoms of toxicity include CNS depression, respiratory depression, and miosis. Naloxone, 2 mg I.V. with repeat administration as necessary up to a total of 10 mg, can also be used to reverse toxic effects of the opiate.

Drug Interactions **Substrate** of CYP2D6 (major)

CNS depressants, MAO inhibitors, general anesthetics, and tricyclic antidepressants: May potentiate the effects of opiate agonists; dextroamphetamine may enhance the analgesic effect of opiate agonists

CYP2D6 inhibitors: May decrease the effects of oxycodone. Example inhibitors include chlorpromazine, delavirdine, fluoxetine, miconazole, paroxetine, pergolide, quinidine, quinine, ritonavir, and ropinirole.

Ethanol/Nutrition/Herb Interactions

Ethanol: Avoid ethanol (may increase CNS depression).

Food: When taken with a high-fat meal, peak concentration is 25% greater following a single OxyContin® 160 mg tablet as compared to two 80 mg tablets.

Herb/Nutraceutical: Avoid valerian, St John's wort, kava kava, gotu kola (may increase CNS depression).

Test Interactions

Some quinolones may produce a false-positive urine screening result for opiates using commercially-available immunoassay kits. This has been demonstrated most consistently for levofloxacin and ofloxacin, but other quinolones have shown cross-reactivity in certain assay kits. Confirmation of positive opiate screens by more specific methods should be considered.

Dietary Considerations Instruct patient to avoid high-fat meals when taking OxyContin® 160 mg tablets.

Dosage Forms

Capsule, immediate release, as hydrochloride (OxyIR®): 5 mg
Solution, oral, as hydrochloride: 5 mg/5 mL (500 mL)
  Roxicodone™: 5 mg/5 mL (5 mL, 500 mL) [contains alcohol]
Solution, oral concentrate, as hydrochloride: 20 mg/mL (30 mL)
  Oxydose™: 20 mg/mL (30 mL) [contains sodium benzoate; berry flavor]
  OxyFast®, Roxicodone™ Intensol™: 20 mg/mL (30 mL) [contains sodium benzoate]
Tablet, as hydrochloride: 5 mg, 15 mg, 30 mg
  Roxicodone™: 5 mg, 15 mg, 30 mg
Tablet, controlled release, as hydrochloride (OxyContin®): 10 mg, 20 mg, 40 mg, 80 mg, 160 mg
Tablet, extended release, as hydrochloride: 10 mg, 20 mg, 40 mg, 80 mg

Oxycodone and Acetaminophen

(oks i KOE done & a seet a MIN oh fen)

Medication Safety Issues

Sound-alike/look-alike issues:
  Percocet® may be confused with Percodan®
  Roxicet™ may be confused with Roxanol™
  Tylox® may be confused with Trimox®, Tylenol®, Wymox®, Xanax®

U.S. Brand Names Endocet®; Percocet®; Roxicet™; Roxicet™ 5/500; Tylox®

Canadian Brand Names Endocet®; Oxycocet®; Percocet®; Percocet®-Demi; PMS-Oxycodone-Acetaminophen

Synonyms Acetaminophen and Oxycodone

Pharmacologic Category Analgesic, Narcotic

Restrictions C-II

Generic Available Yes: Excludes caplet and solution

(Continued)

Oxycodone and Acetaminophen *(Continued)*

Use Management of moderate to severe pain

Mechanism of Action

Oxycodone, as with other narcotic (opiate) analgesics, blocks pain perception in the cerebral cortex by binding to specific receptor molecules (opiate receptors) within the neuronal membranes of synapses. This binding results in a decreased synaptic chemical transmission throughout the CNS thus inhibiting the flow of pain sensations into the higher centers. Mu and kappa are the two subtypes of the opiate receptor to which oxycodone binds to cause analgesia.

Acetaminophen inhibits the synthesis of prostaglandins in the CNS and peripherally blocks pain impulse generation; produces antipyresis from inhibition of hypothalamic heat-regulating center

Pharmacodynamics/Kinetics See individual agents.

Dosage Oral: Doses should be given every 4-6 hours as needed and titrated to appropriate analgesic effects. **Note:** Initial dose is based on the **oxycodone** content; however, the maximum daily dose is based on the **acetaminophen** content.

Children: Maximum acetaminophen dose: Children <45 kg: 90 mg/kg/day; children >45 kg: 4 g/day

Mild to moderate pain: Initial dose, **based on oxycodone content:** 0.05-0.1 mg/kg/dose

Severe pain: Initial dose, **based on oxycodone content:** 0.3 mg/kg/dose

Adults:

Mild to moderate pain: Initial dose, **based on oxycodone content:** 5 mg

Severe pain: Initial dose, **based on oxycodone content:** 15-30 mg. Do not exceed acetaminophen 4 g/day.

Elderly: Doses should be titrated to appropriate analgesic effects: Initial dose, **based on oxycodone content:** 2.5-5 mg every 6 hours. Do not exceed acetaminophen 4 g/day.

Dosage adjustment in hepatic impairment: Dose should be reduced in patients with severe liver disease.

Stability Store at controlled room temperature of 15°C to 30°C (59°F to 86°F). Protect from moisture.

Monitoring Parameters Monitor for pain relief, respiratory and mental status, blood pressure, constipation

Pregnancy Risk Factor C/D (prolonged periods or high doses at term)

Contraindications Hypersensitivity to oxycodone, acetaminophen, or any component of the formulation; severe respiratory depression (in absence of resuscitative equipment or ventilatory support); pregnancy (prolonged periods or high doses at term)

Warnings/Precautions Use with caution in patients with hypersensitivity reactions to other phenanthrene-derivative opioid agonists (morphine, codeine, hydrocodone, hydromorphone, levorphanol, oxymorphone); respiratory diseases including asthma, emphysema, COPD, or severe liver or renal insufficiency, hypothyroidism, Addison's disease, prostatic hypertrophy, or urethral stricture; some preparations contain sulfites which may cause allergic reactions; may be habit-forming

Use with caution in patients with head injury and increased intracranial pressure (respiratory depressant effects increased and may also elevate CSF pressure). May mask diagnosis or clinical course in patients with acute abdominal conditions.

Enhanced analgesia has been seen in elderly patients on therapeutic doses of narcotics; duration of action may be increased in the elderly; the elderly may be particularly susceptible to the CNS depressant and constipating effects of narcotics

Adverse Reactions Frequency not defined (also see individual agents): Allergic reaction, constipation, dizziness, dysphoria, euphoria, lightheadedness, nausea, pruritus, respiratory depression, sedation, skin rash, vomiting

Overdosage/Toxicology See individual agents.

Drug Interactions Also see individual agents.

Oxycodone: **Substrate** of CYP2D6 (major)

Acetaminophen: **Substrate** (minor) of CYP1A2, 2A6, 2C9, 2D6, 2E1, 3A4

Anesthetics, general: May have additive CNS depression; consider lowering dose of one or both agents

Anticholinergics: Concomitant use may lead to paralytic ileus

CNS depressants: May have additive CNS depression; consider lowering dose of one or both agents

CYP2D6 inhibitors: May decrease the effects of oxycodone. Example inhibitors include chlorpromazine, delavirdine, fluoxetine, miconazole, paroxetine, pergolide, quinidine, quinine, ritonavir, and ropinirole.

Phenothiazines: May have additive CNS depression with phenothiazine and other tranquilizers; consider lowering dose of one or both agents

Sedative hypnotics: May have additive CNS depression; consider lowering dose of one or both agents

Ethanol/Nutrition/Herb Interactions Ethanol: May have additive CNS depression. In addition, excessive intake of ethanol may increase the risk of acetaminophen-induced hepatotoxicity. Avoid ethanol or limit to <3 drinks/day.

Dosage Forms

Caplet:

Roxicet™ 5/500: Oxycodone hydrochloride 5 mg and acetaminophen 500 mg

Capsule: 5/500: Oxycodone hydrochloride 5 mg and acetaminophen 500 mg

Tylox®: 5/500: Oxycodone hydrochloride 5 mg and acetaminophen 500 mg [contains sodium benzoate and sodium metabisulfite]

Solution, oral:

Roxicet™: Oxycodone hydrochloride 5 mg and acetaminophen 325 mg per 5 mL (5 mL, 500 mL) [contains alcohol <0.5%]

Tablet: 5/325: Oxycodone hydrochloride 5 mg and acetaminophen 325 mg; 7.5/325: Oxycodone hydrochloride 7.5 mg and acetaminophen 325 mg; 7.5/500: Oxycodone hydrochloride 7.5 mg and acetaminophen 500 mg; 10/325: Oxycodone hydrochloride 10 mg and acetaminophen 325 mg; 10/650: Oxycodone hydrochloride 10 mg and acetaminophen 650 mg

Endocet® 5/325 [scored]: Oxycodone hydrochloride 5 mg and acetaminophen 325 mg

Endocet® 7.5/325: Oxycodone hydrochloride 7.5 mg and acetaminophen 325 mg

Endocet® 7.5/500: Oxycodone hydrochloride 7.5 mg and acetaminophen 500 mg

Endocet® 10/325: Oxycodone hydrochloride 10 mg and acetaminophen 325 mg

Endocet® 10/650: Oxycodone hydrochloride 10 mg and acetaminophen 650 mg

Percocet® 2.5/325: Oxycodone hydrochloride 2.5 mg and acetaminophen 325 mg

Percocet® 5/325 [scored]: Oxycodone hydrochloride 5 mg and acetaminophen 325 mg

Percocet® 7.5/325: Oxycodone hydrochloride 7.5 mg and acetaminophen 325 mg

Percocet® 7.5/500: Oxycodone hydrochloride 7.5 mg and acetaminophen 500 mg

Percocet® 10/325: Oxycodone hydrochloride 10 mg and acetaminophen 325 mg

Percocet® 10/650: Oxycodone hydrochloride 10 mg and acetaminophen 650 mg

Roxicet™ [scored]: Oxycodone hydrochloride 5 mg and acetaminophen 325 mg

Oxycodone and Aspirin (oks i KOE done & AS pir in)

Medication Safety Issues

Sound-alike/look-alike issues:

Percodan® may be confused with Decadron®, Percocet®, Percogesic®, Periactin®

U.S. Brand Names Endodan® [DSC]; Percodan®

Canadian Brand Names Endodan®; Oxycodan®; Percodan®

Synonyms Aspirin and Oxycodone

Pharmacologic Category Analgesic, Narcotic

Restrictions C-II

Generic Available Yes

Use Management of moderate to severe pain

Mechanism of Action

Oxycodone, as with other narcotic (opiate) analgesics, blocks pain perception in the cerebral cortex by binding to specific receptor molecules (opiate receptors) within the neuronal membranes of synapses. This binding results in a decreased synaptic chemical transmission throughout the CNS thus inhibiting

(Continued)

Oxycodone and Aspirin *(Continued)*

the flow of pain sensations into the higher centers. Mu and kappa are the two subtypes of the opiate receptor to which oxycodone binds to cause analgesia.

Aspirin inhibits prostaglandin synthesis by decreasing the activity of the enzyme, cyclooxygenase, which results in decreased formation of prostaglandin precursors, acts on the hypothalamic heat-regulating center to reduce fever, blocks thromboxane synthetase action which prevents formation of the platelet-aggregating substance thromboxane A_2

Pharmacodynamics/Kinetics See individual agents.

Dosage Oral (based on oxycodone combined salts):

Children: Maximum oxycodone: 5 mg/dose; maximum aspirin dose should not exceed 4 g/day. Doses should be given every 6 hours as needed.

Mild-to-moderate pain: Initial dose, **based on oxycodone content:** 0.05-0.1 mg/kg/dose

Severe pain: Initial dose, **based on oxycodone content**: 0.3 mg/kg/dose

Adults: Percodan®: 1 tablet every 6 hours as needed for pain; maximum aspirin dose should not exceed 4 g/day.

Dosing adjustment in hepatic impairment: Dose should be reduced in patients with severe liver disease.

Pregnancy Risk Factor D

Contraindications Hypersensitivity to oxycodone, salicylates, other NSAIDs, or any component of the formulation; patients with the syndrome of asthma, rhinitis, and nasal polyps; inherited or acquired bleeding disorders (including factor VII and factor IX deficiency); do not use in children (<16 years of age) in the presence of viral infections (chickenpox or flu symptoms), with or without fever, due to a potential association with Reye's syndrome; significant respiratory depression; hypercarbia; known or suspected paralytic ileus; acute or severe bronchial asthma; pregnancy (3rd trimester)

Warnings/Precautions Use with caution in patients with hypersensitivity reactions to other phenanthrene derivative opioid agonists (morphine, hydrocodone, hydromorphone, levorphanol, oxycodone, oxymorphone), respiratory diseases including asthma, emphysema, or COPD. Use with caution in pancreatitis or biliary tract disease, acute alcoholism (including delirium tremens), adrenocortical insufficiency, CNS depression/coma, kyphoscoliosis (or other skeletal disorder which may alter respiratory function), hypothyroidism (including myxedema), prostatic hyperplasia, urethral stricture, and toxic psychosis.

Use with caution in the elderly, debilitated, severe hepatic or renal dysfunction. Hemodynamic effects (hypotension, orthostasis) may be exaggerated in patients with dehydration, hypovolemia, concurrent vasodilating drugs, or in patients with head injury. Respiratory depressant effects and capacity to elevate CSF pressure may be exaggerated in presence of head injury, other intracranial lesion, or pre-existing elevation of intracranial pressure. Tolerance or drug dependence may result from extended use. Healthcare provider should be alert to problems of abuse, misuse, and diversion. Taper dose gradually to avoid withdrawal symptoms in physically dependent patients.

Use with caution in patients with platelet and bleeding disorders, erosive gastritis, or peptic ulcer disease. Heavy ethanol use (>3 drinks/day) can increase bleeding risks. Discontinue use if tinnitus or impaired hearing occurs. Patients with sensitivity to tartrazine dyes, nasal polyps and asthma may have an increased risk of salicylate sensitivity. Surgical patients should avoid ASA if possible, for 1-2 weeks prior to surgery, to reduce the risk of excessive bleeding.

Adverse Reactions Note: Also refer to individual agents

Common (frequency not defined):

Central nervous system: Dizziness, drowsiness, lightheadedness, sedation

Dermatologic: Pruritus

Gastrointestinal: Nausea, vomiting, constipation

<1%, postmarketing, and/or case reports (limited to important or life-threatening): Allergic reaction, anaphylaxis, anaphylactoid reaction, angioedema, apnea, asthma, bradycardia, bronchospasm, circulatory depression, confusion, duodenal ulcer, dysphoria, dyspnea, ecchymosis, euphoria, gastric ulcer, gastrointestinal bleeding, hallucination, hemorrhage, hepatitis, hepatotoxicity, hypotension, hypoglycemia, hyperglycemia, ileus, interstitial nephritis, intestinal obstruction, laryngeal edema, metabolic acidosis, pancreatitis, papillary necrosis, paresthesia, purpura, pulmonary edema, proteinuria, rash, renal

failure, respiratory alkalosis, respiratory depression, Reye syndrome, rhabdomyolysis, seizure, shock, thrombocytopenia, tinnitus

Drug Interactions

Oxycodone: **Substrate** of CYP2D6 (major)

Aspirin: **Substrate** of CYP2C9 (minor)

Also see individual agents.

CYP2D6 inhibitors: May decrease the effects of oxycodone. Example inhibitors include chlorpromazine, delavirdine, fluoxetine, miconazole, paroxetine, pergolide, quinidine, quinine, ritonavir, and ropinirole.

Increased effect/toxicity with CNS depressants, TCAs, dextroamphetamine

Test Interactions May cross-react with urine tests for cocaine or marijuana.

Dietary Considerations May be taken with food or water.

Dosage Forms [DSC] = Discontinued product

Tablet: Oxycodone hydrochloride 4.5 mg, oxycodone terephthalate 0.38 mg, and aspirin 325 mg

Endodan® [DSC], Percodan®: Oxycodone hydrochloride 4.5 mg, oxycodone terephthalate 0.38 mg, and aspirin 325 mg

- ♦ **Oxycodone Hydrochloride** *see* Oxycodone *on page 967*
- ♦ **OxyContin®** *see* Oxycodone *on page 967*
- ♦ **Oxydose™** *see* Oxycodone *on page 967*
- ♦ **OxyFast®** *see* Oxycodone *on page 967*
- ♦ **OxyIR®** *see* Oxycodone *on page 967*

Oxymetazoline (oks i met AZ oh leen)

Medication Safety Issues

Sound-alike/look-alike issues:

Oxymetazoline may be confused with oxymetholone

Afrin® may be confused with aspirin

Visine® may be confused with Visken®

U.S. Brand Names Afrin® Extra Moisturizing [OTC]; Afrin® Original [OTC]; Afrin® Severe Congestion [OTC]; Afrin® Sinus [OTC]; Duramist® Plus [OTC]; Duration® [OTC]; Genasal [OTC]; Neo-Synephrine® 12 Hour [OTC]; Neo-Synephrine® 12 Hour Extra Moisturizing [OTC]; Nōstrilla® [OTC]; NRS® [OTC]; Vicks Sinex® 12 Hour [OTC]; Vicks Sinex® 12 Hour Ultrafine Mist [OTC]; Visine® L.R. [OTC]; 4-Way® 12 Hour [OTC]

Canadian Brand Names Claritin® Allergic Decongestant; Dristan® Long Lasting Nasal; Drixoral® Nasal

Synonyms Oxymetazoline Hydrochloride

Pharmacologic Category Adrenergic Agonist Agent; Imidazoline Derivative; Vasoconstrictor

Generic Available Yes: Nasal spray

Use Adjunctive therapy of middle ear infections, associated with acute or chronic rhinitis, the common cold, sinusitis, hay fever, or other allergies

Ophthalmic: Relief of redness of eye due to minor eye irritations

Mechanism of Action Stimulates alpha-adrenergic receptors in the arterioles of the nasal mucosa to produce vasoconstriction

Pharmacodynamics/Kinetics

Onset of action: Intranasal: 5-10 minutes

Duration: 5-6 hours

Dosage

Intranasal (therapy should not exceed 3 days): Children ≥6 years and Adults: 0.05% solution: Instill 2-3 sprays into each nostril twice daily

Ophthalmic: Children ≥6 years and Adults: 0.025% solution: Instill 1-2 drops in affected eye(s) every 6 hours as needed or as directed by healthcare provider

Stability Store at room temperature.

Contraindications Hypersensitivity to oxymetazoline or any component of the formulation

Warnings/Precautions

Nasal: Rebound congestion may occur with extended use (>3 days). Prior to self-medication (OTC use), contact healthcare provider in the presence of hypertension, diabetes, hyperthyroidism, heart disease, coronary artery disease, cerebral arteriosclerosis, or long-standing bronchial asthma.

Ophthalmic: Prior to OTC use, contact healthcare provider in the presence of glaucoma or if needed for >72 hours.

(Continued)

Oxymetazoline *(Continued)*

Adverse Reactions Frequency not defined.

Cardiovascular: Hypertension, palpitation

Local: Transient burning, stinging

Respiratory: Dryness of the nasal mucosa, rebound congestion with prolonged use, sneezing

Drug Interactions Increased toxicity with MAO inhibitors

Dosage Forms

Solution, intranasal, as hydrochloride [spray]: 0.05% (15 mL, 30 mL)

Afrin® Extra Moisturizing: 0.05% (15 mL) [contains benzyl alcohol and glycerin; regular or no drip formula]

Afrin® Original: 0.05% (15 mL, 30 mL) [contains benzalkonium chloride]

Afrin® Original: 0.05% (15 mL) [contains benzyl alcohol and benzalkonium chloride; no drip formula]

Afrin® Severe Congestion: 0.05% (15 mL) [contains benzyl alcohol and menthol; regular or no drip formula]

Afrin® Sinus: 0.05% (15 mL) [contains benzyl alcohol, benzalkonium chloride, camphor, phenol; regular or no drip formula]

Duramist® Plus, Neo-Synephrine® 12 Hour, Nōstrilla®, Vicks Sinex® 12 Hour Ultrafine Mist, Vicks Sinex® 12 Hour, 4-Way® 12 Hour: 0.05% (15 mL) [contains benzalkonium chloride]

Duration®: 0.05% (30 mL) [contains benzalkonium chloride]

Genasal, NRS®: 0.05% (15 mL, 30 mL) [contains benzalkonium chloride]

Neo-Synephrine® 12 Hour Extra Moisturizing: 0.05% (15 mL) [contains glycerin]

Solution, ophthalmic, as hydrochloride (Visine® L.R.): 0.025% (15 mL, 30 mL) [contains benzalkonium chloride]

♦ **Oxymetazoline Hydrochloride** *see* Oxymetazoline *on page 973*

Oxymorphone (oks i MOR fone)

Medication Safety Issues

Sound-alike/look-alike issues:

Oxymorphone may be confused with oxymetholone

Related Information

Chronic Pain Management *on page 1430*

Narcotic / Opioid Analgesics *on page 1568*

U.S. Brand Names Numorphan®

Synonyms Oxymorphone Hydrochloride

Pharmacologic Category Analgesic, Narcotic

Restrictions C-II

Generic Available No

Use Management of moderate to severe pain and preoperatively as a sedative and a supplement to anesthesia

Mechanism of Action Oxymorphone hydrochloride (Numorphan®) is a potent narcotic analgesic with uses similar to those of morphine. The drug is a semisynthetic derivative of morphine (phenanthrene derivative) and is closely related to hydromorphone chemically (Dilaudid®).

Pharmacodynamics/Kinetics

Onset of action: Analgesic: I.V., I.M., SubQ: 5-10 minutes; Rectal: 15-30 minutes

Duration: Analgesic: Parenteral, rectal: 3-4 hours

Metabolism: Hepatic via glucuronidation

Excretion: Urine

Dosage Adults: **Note:** More frequent dosing may be required.

I.M., SubQ: 0.5 mg initially, 1-1.5 mg every 4-6 hours as needed

I.V.: 0.5 mg initially

Rectal: 5 mg every 4-6 hours

Stability Refrigerate suppository

Monitoring Parameters Respiratory rate, heart rate, blood pressure, CNS activity

Anesthesia and Critical Care Concerns/Other Considerations Equivalent dosing: 5 mg rectal suppository = 5 mg morphine I.M.

Pregnancy Risk Factor B/D (prolonged use or high doses at term)

Contraindications Hypersensitivity to oxymorphone or any component of the formulation; increased intracranial pressure; severe respiratory depression; pregnancy (prolonged use or high doses at term)

Warnings/Precautions Some preparations contain sulfites which may cause allergic reactions; infants <3 months of age are more susceptible to respiratory depression, use with caution and generally in reduced doses in this age group; use with caution in patients with impaired respiratory function or severe hepatic dysfunction and in patients with hypersensitivity reactions to other phenanthrene derivative opioid agonists (codeine, hydrocodone, hydromorphone, levorphanol, oxycodone, oxymorphone); tolerance or drug dependence may result from extended use

Adverse Reactions

>10%:

Cardiovascular: Hypotension
Central nervous system: Fatigue, drowsiness, dizziness
Gastrointestinal: Nausea, vomiting, constipation
Neuromuscular & skeletal: Weakness
Miscellaneous: Histamine release

1% to 10%:

Central nervous system: Nervousness, headache, restlessness, malaise, confusion
Gastrointestinal: Anorexia, stomach cramps, xerostomia, biliary spasm
Genitourinary: Decreased urination, ureteral spasms
Local: Pain at injection site
Respiratory: Dyspnea

<1% (Limited to important or life-threatening): Mental depression, hallucinations, paradoxical CNS stimulation, increased intracranial pressure, rash, urticaria, paralytic ileus, histamine release, physical and psychological dependence

Overdosage/Toxicology Symptoms of overdose include respiratory depression, miosis, hypotension, bradycardia, apnea, and pulmonary edema. Treatment of overdose includes maintaining patent airway and establishing an I.V. line. Naloxone, 2 mg I.V., with repeat administration as necessary up to a total of 10 mg, can also be used to reverse toxic effects of the opiate.

Drug Interactions

Decreased effect with phenothiazines
Increased effect/toxicity with CNS depressants, TCAs, dextroamphetamine

Ethanol/Nutrition/Herb Interactions

Ethanol: Avoid ethanol (may increase CNS depression).
Herb/Nutraceutical: Avoid valerian, St John's wort, kava kava, gotu kola (may increase CNS depression).

Test Interactions

Some quinolones may produce a false-positive urine screening result for opiates using commercially-available immunoassay kits. This has been demonstrated most consistently for levofloxacin and ofloxacin, but other quinolones have shown cross-reactivity in certain assay kits. Confirmation of positive opiate screens by more specific methods should be considered.

Dosage Forms

Injection, solution, as hydrochloride: 1 mg (1 mL); 1.5 mg/mL (10 mL)
Suppository, rectal, as hydrochloride: 5 mg

References

Carr DB, Jacox AK, Chapman RC, et al, "Acute Pain Management," Guideline Technical Report, No. 1. Rockville, MD: U.S. Department of Health and Human Services, Public Health Service, Agency for Health Care Policy and Research. AHCPR Publication No. 95-0034. February 1995.

"Drugs for Pain," *Treat Guidel Med Lett*, 2004, 2(23):47-54.

Mokhlesi B, Leikin JB, Murray P, et al, "Adult Toxicology in Critical Care. Part 11: Specific Poisonings," *Chest*, 2003, 123(3):897-922.

"Principles of Analgesic Use in the Treatment of Acute Pain and Chronic Cancer Pain," 5th ed, Glenview, IL: American Pain Society, 2003.

♦ **Oxymorphone Hydrochloride** *see* Oxymorphone *on page 974*

Oxytocin (oks i TOE sin)

Medication Safety Issues

Sound-alike/look-alike issues:
Pitocin® may be confused with Pitressin®

U.S. Brand Names Pitocin®

Canadian Brand Names Pitocin®; Syntocinon®

Synonyms Pit

Pharmacologic Category Oxytocic Agent

Generic Available Yes

(Continued)

Oxytocin *(Continued)*

Use Induction of labor at term; control of postpartum bleeding; adjunctive therapy in management of abortion

Mechanism of Action Produces the rhythmic uterine contractions characteristic to delivery

Pharmacodynamics/Kinetics

Onset of action: Uterine contractions: I.M.: 3-5 minutes; I.V.: ~1 minute

Duration: I.M.: 2-3 hour; I.V.: 1 hour

Metabolism: Rapidly hepatic and via plasma (by oxytocinase) and to a smaller degree the mammary gland

Half-life elimination: 1-5 minutes

Excretion: Urine

Dosage I.V. administration requires the use of an infusion pump. Adults:

Induction of labor: I.V.: 0.5-1 milliunits/minute; gradually increase dose in increments of 1-2 milliunits/minute until desired contraction pattern is established; dose may be decreased after desired frequency of contractions is reached and labor has progressed to 5-6 cm dilation. Infusion rates of 6 milliunits/minute provide oxytocin levels similar to those at spontaneous labor; rates of >9-10 milliunits/minute are rarely required.

Postpartum bleeding:

I.M.: Total dose of 10 units after delivery

I.V.: 10-40 units by I.V. infusion in 1000 mL of intravenous fluid at a rate sufficient to control uterine atony

Adjunctive treatment of abortion: I.V.: 10-20 milliunits/minute; maximum total dose: 30 units/12 hours

Stability Store oxytocin at 2°C to 8°C (36°F to 46°F); protect from freezing. Pitocin® may also be stored at 15°C to 25°C (59°F to 77°F) for up to 30 days.

Reconstitution: I.V.:

Induction or stimulation of labor: Add oxytocin 10 units to NS or LR 1000 mL to yield a solution containing oxytocin 10 milliunits/mL; rotate solution to mix

Postpartum uterine bleeding: Add oxytocin 10-40 units to running I.V. infusion; maximum: 40 units/1000 mL

Adjunctive management of abortion: Add oxytocin 10 units to 500 mL of a physiologic saline solution or D_5W

Administration I.V.: Refer to Stability (reconstitution) for dilution information; an infusion pump is required for administration

Monitoring Parameters Fluid intake and output during administration; fetal monitoring

Pregnancy Risk Factor X

Contraindications Hypersensitivity to oxytocin or any component of the formulation; significant cephalopelvic disproportion; unfavorable fetal positions; fetal distress; hypertonic or hyperactive uterus; contraindicated vaginal delivery (invasive cervical cancer, active genital herpes, prolapse of the cord, cord presentation, total placenta previa, or vasa previa)

Warnings/Precautions [U.S. Boxed Warning]: To be used for medical rather than elective induction of labor. May produce antidiuretic effect (ie, water intoxication and excess uterine contractions); high doses or hypersensitivity to oxytocin may cause uterine hypertonicity, spasm, tetanic contraction, or rupture of the uterus; severe water intoxication with convulsions, coma, and death is associated with a slow oxytocin infusion over 24 hours

Adverse Reactions Frequency not defined.

Fetus or neonate:

Cardiovascular: Arrhythmias (including premature ventricular contractions), bradycardia

Central nervous system: Brain or CNS damage (permanent), neonatal seizure

Hepatic: Neonatal jaundice

Ocular: Neonatal retinal hemorrhage

Miscellaneous: Fetal death, low Apgar score (5 minute)

Mother:

Cardiovascular: Arrhythmias, hypertensive episodes, premature ventricular contractions

Gastrointestinal: Nausea, vomiting

Genitourinary: Pelvic hematoma, postpartum hemorrhage, uterine hypertonicity, tetanic contraction of the uterus, uterine rupture, uterine spasm

Hematologic: Afibrinogenemia (fatal)

Miscellaneous: Anaphylactic reaction, subarachnoid hemorrhage

Overdosage/Toxicology Symptoms of overdose include tetanic uterine contractions, impaired uterine blood flow, amniotic fluid embolism, uterine rupture, SIADH, and seizures. Treatment is symptom-directed and supportive.

Drug Interactions

Dinoprostone, misoprostol: May increase the effect of oxytocin; wait 6-12 hours after dinoprostone or misoprostol administration before initiating oxytocin.

Dosage Forms

Injection, solution: 10 units/mL (1 mL, 10 mL)

Pitocin®: 10 units/mL (1 mL)

- ♦ **Pacerone®** *see* Amiodarone *on page 83*
- ♦ **Pain-A-Lay® [OTC]** *see* Phenol *on page 1012*
- ♦ **Pain Eze [OTC]** *see* Acetaminophen *on page 26*
- ♦ **Palladone™** ***[Withdrawn]*** *see* Hydromorphone *on page 644*

Palonosetron (pal oh NOE se tron)

Medication Safety Issues

Sound-alike/look-alike issues:

Aloxi® may be confused with oxaliplatin

Palonosetron may be confused with dolasetron, granisetron, ondansetron

U.S. Brand Names Aloxi®

Synonyms Palonosetron Hydrochloride; RS-25259; RS-25259-197

Pharmacologic Category Antiemetic; Selective 5-HT_3 Receptor Antagonist

Generic Available No

Use Prevention of acute (within 24 hours) and delayed (2-5 days) chemotherapy-induced nausea and vomiting

Note: Not recommended for treatment of existing chemotherapy-induced emesis (CIE)

Unlabeled/Investigational Use Prevention of postoperative vomiting

Mechanism of Action Selective 5-HT_3 receptor antagonist, blocking serotonin, both peripherally on vagal nerve terminals and centrally in the chemoreceptor trigger zone

Pharmacodynamics/Kinetics

Distribution: V_d: 8.3 ± 2.5 L/kg

Protein binding: 62%

Metabolism: ~50% metabolized via CYP enzymes (and likely other pathways) to relatively inactive metabolites (N-oxide-palonosetron and 6-S-hydroxy-palonosetron); CYP1A2, 2D6, and 3A4 contribute to its metabolism

Half-life elimination: Terminal: 40 hours

Excretion: Urine (80%, 40% as unchanged drug)

Dosage I.V.: Adults:

Chemotherapy-induced nausea and vomiting: 0.25 mg 30 minutes prior to chemotherapy administration, day 1 of each cycle (doses should not be given more than once weekly)

Breakthrough: Palonosetron has not been shown to be effective in terminating nausea or vomiting once it occurs and should not be used for this purpose.

Postoperative vomiting (unlabeled use): 30 mcg/kg (used in hysterectomy, lower doses ineffective; no significant reduction in nausea at any dose)

Elderly: No dosage adjustment necessary

Dosage adjustment in renal/hepatic impairment: No dosage adjustment necessary

Stability Store intact vials at controlled room temperature of 20°C to 25°C (68°F to 77°F); protect from freezing and light. Solutions of 5 mcg/mL and 30 mcg/mL in NS, D_5W, $D_5$1/2NS, and D_5LR injection are stable for 48 hours at room temperature and 14 days under refrigeration.

Administration I.V.: Infuse over 30 seconds; flush I.V. line with NS prior to and following administration.

Pregnancy Risk Factor B

Contraindications Hypersensitivity to palonosetron or any component of the formulation

Warnings/Precautions Use caution in patients allergic to other 5-HT_3 receptor antagonists; cross-reactivity is possible. Caution in patients with congenital QT

(Continued)

Palonosetron *(Continued)*

syndrome or other risk factors for QT prolongation (eg, drugs, electrolyte abnormalities). Not intended for treatment of nausea and vomiting or for chronic continuous therapy. **For chemotherapy, should be used on a scheduled basis, not on an "as needed" (PRN) basis,** since data support the use of this drug only in the prevention of nausea and vomiting (due to antineoplastic therapy) and not in the rescue of nausea and vomiting. Safety and efficacy in pediatric patients (<18 years of age) have not been established.

Adverse Reactions

>10%: Dermatologic: Pruritus (8% to 22%)

1% to 10%:

Cardiovascular: Bradycardia (1%), hypotension (1%), tachycardia (nonsustained) (1%)

Central nervous system: Headache (6% to 9%), anxiety (1% to 5%), dizziness (1%)

Endocrine & metabolic: Hyperkalemia (1%)

Gastrointestinal: Constipation (5% to 10%), diarrhea (1%)

Neuromuscular & skeletal: Weakness (1%)

<1% (Limited to important or life-threatening): ALT increased, AST increased, bilirubin increased, electrolyte fluctuations, extrasystoles, fever, glycosuria, hyperglycemia, hypertension, metabolic acidosis, myocardial ischemia, QT prolongation, sinus arrhythmia, sinus tachycardia, supraventricular extrasystoles, vein distention

Overdosage/Toxicology Dose-ranging studies in humans using doses up to 25 times the recommended dose of 0.25 mg revealed no increase in the incidence of adverse effects compared to lower dose groups. Due to the large volume of distribution, dialysis would not be effective in the event of an overdose. Treatment should be symptom-directed and supportive.

Drug Interactions Substrate (minor) of CYP1A2, 2D6, 3A4

Apomorphine: Due to reports of profound hypotension during concomitant therapy with other 5-HT_3 antagonists, the manufacturer of apomorphine contraindicates its use with palonosetron.

Dosage Forms

Injection, solution:

Aloxi®: 0.05 mg/mL (5 mL) [contains disodium edetate]

♦ **Palonosetron Hydrochloride** *see* Palonosetron *on page 977*

♦ **2-PAM** *see* Pralidoxime *on page 1040*

♦ **Pamelor®** *see* Nortriptyline *on page 938*

Pamidronate (pa mi DROE nate)

Medication Safety Issues

Sound-alike/look-alike issues:

Aredia® may be confused with Adriamycin

U.S. Brand Names Aredia®

Canadian Brand Names Aredia®; Pamidronate Disodium®; Rhoxal-pamidronate

Synonyms Pamidronate Disodium

Pharmacologic Category Antidote; Bisphosphonate Derivative

Generic Available Yes

Use Treatment of hypercalcemia associated with malignancy; treatment of osteolytic bone lesions associated with multiple myeloma or metastatic breast cancer; moderate to severe Paget's disease of bone

Unlabeled/Investigational Use Treatment of pediatric osteoporosis, treatment of osteogenesis imperfecta

Mechanism of Action A bisphosphonate which inhibits bone resorption via actions on osteoclasts or on osteoclast precursors. Does not appear to produce any significant effects on renal tubular calcium handling and is poorly absorbed following oral administration (high oral doses have been reported effective); therefore, I.V. therapy is preferred.

Pharmacodynamics/Kinetics

Onset of action: 24-48 hours

Peak effect: Maximum: 5-7 days

Absorption: Poor; pharmacokinetic studies lacking

Metabolism: Not metabolized

Half-life elimination: 21-35 hours

Excretion: Biphasic; urine (~50% as unchanged drug) within 120 hours

Dosage Drug must be diluted properly before administration and infused intravenously slowly. Due to risk of nephrotoxicity, doses should not exceed 90 mg.

I.V.: Adults:

Hypercalcemia of malignancy:

Moderate cancer-related hypercalcemia (corrected serum calcium: 12-13.5 mg/dL): 60-90 mg, as a single dose

Severe cancer-related hypercalcemia (corrected serum calcium: >13.5 mg/dL): 90 mg, as a single dose

A period of 7 days should elapse before the use of second course; repeat infusions every 2-3 weeks have been suggested, however, could be administered every 2-3 months according to the degree and of severity of hypercalcemia and/or the type of malignancy.

Osteolytic bone lesions with multiple myeloma: 90 mg monthly

Osteolytic bone lesions with metastatic breast cancer: 90 mg repeated every 3-4 weeks

Paget's disease: 30 mg daily for 3 consecutive days

Elderly: Begin at lower end of adult dosing range.

Dosing adjustment in renal impairment: Not recommended in severe renal impairment (patients with bone metastases); safety and efficacy have not been established in patients with serum creatinine >5 mg/dL; studies are limited in multiple myeloma patients with serum creatinine ≥3 mg/dL

Dosing adjustment in renal toxicity: In patients with bone metastases, treatment should be withheld in patients who experience deterioration in renal function (increase of serum creatinine ≥0.5 mg/dL in patients with normal baseline or ≥1.0 mg/dL in patients with abnormal baseline). Resumption of therapy may be considered when serum creatinine returns to within 10% of baseline.

Stability

Powder for injection: Store below 30°C (86°F). Reconstitute by adding 10 mL of SWFI to each vial of lyophilized pamidronate disodium powder; the resulting solution will be 30 mg/10 mL or 90 mg/10 mL. The reconstituted solution is stable for 24 hours stored under refrigeration at 2°C to 8°C (36°F to 46°F).

Solution for injection: Store below 25°C (77°F)

Pamidronate may be further diluted in 250-1000 mL of 0.45% or 0.9% sodium chloride or 5% dextrose. Pamidronate solution for infusion is stable at room temperature for up to 24 hours.

Administration I.V. infusion over 2-24 hours.

Monitoring Parameters Serum calcium, electrolytes, phosphate, magnesium, CBC with differential; monitor for hypocalcemia for at least 2 weeks after therapy; monitor serum creatinine prior to each dose; dental exam and preventative dentistry for patients at risk for osteonecrosis; patients with pre-existing anemia, leukopenia or thrombocytopenia should be closely monitored during the first 2 weeks of treatment

Reference Range Calcium (total): Adults: 9.0-11.0 mg/dL (SI: 2.05-2.54 mmol/L), may slightly decrease with aging; Phosphorus: 2.5-4.5 mg/dL (SI: 0.81-1.45 mmol/L)

Pregnancy Risk Factor D

Contraindications Hypersensitivity to pamidronate, other bisphosphonates, or any component of the formulation; pregnancy

Warnings/Precautions Bisphosphonate therapy has been associated with osteonecrosis, primarily of the jaw; this has been observed mostly in cancer patients, but also in patients with postmenopausal osteoporosis and other diagnoses. Risk factors include a diagnosis of cancer, with concomitant chemotherapy, radiotherapy or corticosteroids; anemia, coagulopathy, infection or pre-existing dental disease. Symptoms included nonhealing extraction socket or an exposed jawbone. There are no data addressing whether discontinuation of therapy reduces the risk of developing osteonecrosis. However, as a precautionary measure, dental exams and preventative dentistry should be performed prior to placing patients with risk factors on chronic bisphosphonate therapy. Invasive dental procedures should be avoided during treatment.

May cause deterioration in renal function. Use caution in patients with renal impairment and avoid in severe renal impairment. Assess serum creatinine prior to each dose; withhold dose in patients with bone metastases who experience deterioration in renal function. Leukopenia has been observed with oral pamidronate and monitoring of white blood cell counts is suggested. Patients with

(Continued)

Pamidronate *(Continued)*

pre-existing anemia, leukopenia, or thrombocytopenia should be closely monitored during the first 2 weeks of treatment.

Vein irritation and thrombophlebitis may occur with infusions. Monitor serum electrolytes, especially in the elderly.

Severe (and occasionally debilitating) bone, joint, and/or muscle pain have been reported infrequently during bisphosphonate treatment. Onset of pain ranged from a single day to several months, with relief in most cases upon discontinuation of the drug. Patients may experience recurrence when rechallenged with the same drug or another bisphosphonate.

Adverse Reactions Percentage of adverse effect varies upon dose and duration of infusion.

>10%:

Central nervous system: Fatigue (12% to 40%), fever (18% to 39%), headache (24% to 27%), anxiety (8% to 18%), insomnia (1% to 25%), pain (13% to 15%)

Endocrine & metabolic: Hypophosphatemia (9% to 18%), hypokalemia (4% to 18%), hypomagnesemia (4% to 12%), hypocalcemia (1% to 12%)

Gastrointestinal: Nausea (4% to 64%), vomiting (4% to 46%), anorexia (1% to 31%), abdominal pain (1% to 24%), dyspepsia (4% to 23%)

Genitourinary: Urinary tract infection (15% to 20%)

Hematologic: Anemia (6% to 48%), leukopenia (4% to 21%)

Local: Infusion site reaction (4% to 18%)

Neuromuscular & skeletal: Weakness (16% to 26%), myalgia (1% to 26%), arthralgia (11% to 15%)

Renal: Serum creatinine increased (19%)

Respiratory: Dyspnea (22% to 35%), cough (25% to 26%), upper respiratory tract infection (3% to 20%), sinusitis (15% to 16%), pleural effusion (3% to 15%)

1% to 10%:

Cardiovascular: Atrial fibrillation (6%), hypertension (6%), syncope (6%), tachycardia (6%), atrial flutter (1%), cardiac failure (1%), edema (1%)

Central nervous system: Somnolence (1% to 6%), psychosis (4%)

Endocrine & metabolic: Hypothyroidism (6%)

Gastrointestinal: Constipation (4% to 6%), gastrointestinal hemorrhage (6%), diarrhea (1%), stomatitis (1%)

Hematologic: Neutropenia (1%), thrombocytopenia (1%)

Neuromuscular & skeletal: Back pain (5%), bone pain (5%)

Renal: Uremia (4%)

Respiratory: Rales (6%), rhinitis (6%)

Miscellaneous: Moniliasis (6%)

<1% (Limited to important or life-threatening): Allergic reaction, anaphylactic shock, angioedema, episcleritis, hypotension, interstitial pneumonitis, iritis, joint and/or muscle pain, malaise, osteonecrosis (primarily jaws), renal deterioration, scleritis, uveitis

Overdosage/Toxicology Symptoms of overdose include hypocalcemia, hypotension, ECG changes, seizures, bleeding, paresthesia, carpopedal spasm, and fever. Treat with I.V. calcium gluconate, and general supportive care; fever and hypotension can be treated with corticosteroids.

Drug Interactions

Aminoglycosides: May lower serum calcium levels with prolonged administration. Concomitant use may have an additive hypocalcemic effect.

Antacids: May decrease the absorption of bisphosphonate derivatives; should be administered at a different time of the day. Antacids containing aluminum, calcium, or magnesium are of specific concern.

Calcium salts: May decrease the absorption of bisphosphonate derivatives. Separate oral dosing in order to minimize risk of interaction.

Iron salts: May decrease the absorption of bisphosphonate derivatives. Only oral iron salts and oral bisphosphonates are of concern.

Magnesium salts: May decrease the absorption of bisphosphonate derivatives. Only oral magnesium salts and oral bisphosphonates are of concern.

Nonsteroidal anti-inflammatory drugs (NSAIDs): May enhance the gastrointestinal adverse/toxic effects (increased incidence of GI ulcers) of bisphosphonate derivatives.

Phosphate supplements: Bisphosphonate derivatives may enhance the hypocalcemic effect of phosphate supplements.

Test Interactions Bisphosphonates may interfere with diagnostic imaging agents such as technetium-99m-diphosphonate in bone scans.

Dosage Forms

Injection, powder for reconstitution, as disodium (Aredia®): 30 mg, 90 mg
Injection, solution: 3 mg/mL (10 mL); 6 mg/mL (10 mL); 9 mg/mL (10 mL)

- **Pamidronate Disodium® (Can)** *see* Pamidronate *on page 978*
- **p-Aminoclonidine** *see* Apraclonidine *on page 119*
- **Pamprin® Maximum Strength All Day Relief [OTC]** *see* Naproxen *on page 899*

Pancuronium (pan kyoo ROE nee um)

Medication Safety Issues

Sound-alike/look-alike issues:

Pancuronium may be confused with pipecuronium

High alert medication: The Institute for Safe Medication Practices (ISMP) includes this medication among its list of drugs which have a heightened risk of causing significant patient harm when used in error.

Related Information

Chronic Renal Failure *on page 1437*
Neuromuscular Blocking Agents *on page 1572*

Canadian Brand Names Pancuronium Bromide®

Synonyms Pancuronium Bromide; Pavulon [DSC]

Pharmacologic Category Neuromuscular Blocker Agent, Nondepolarizing

Generic Available Yes

Use Adjunct to general anesthesia to facilitate endotracheal intubation and to relax skeletal muscles during surgery; to facilitate mechanical ventilation in ICU patients; does not relieve pain or produce sedation

Drug of choice for neuromuscular blockade except in patients with renal failure, hepatic failure, or cardiovascular instability or in situations not suited for pancuronium's long duration of action

Mechanism of Action Blocks neural transmission at the myoneural junction by binding with cholinergic receptor sites

Pharmacodynamics/Kinetics

Onset of effect: Peak effect: I.V.: 2-3 minutes
Duration (dose dependent): 60-100 minutes
Metabolism: Hepatic (30% to 45%); active metabolite 3-hydroxypancuronium ($^1/_3$ to $^1/_2$ the activity of parent drug)
Half-life elimination: 110 minutes
Excretion: Urine (55% to 70% as unchanged drug)

Dosage Administer I.V.; dose to effect; doses will vary due to interpatient variability; use ideal body weight for obese patients

Surgery:

Neonates <1 month:

Test dose: 0.02 mg/kg to measure responsiveness

Initial: 0.03 mg/kg/dose repeated twice at 5- to 10-minute intervals as needed; maintenance: 0.03-0.09 mg/kg/dose every 30 minutes to 4 hours as needed

Infants >1 month, Children, and Adults: Initial: 0.06-0.1 mg/kg or 0.05 mg/kg after initial dose of succinylcholine for intubation; maintenance dose: 0.01 mg/kg 60-100 minutes after initial dose and then 0.01 mg/kg every 25-60 minutes

Pretreatment/priming: 10% of intubating dose given 3-5 minutes before initial dose

ICU: 0.05-0.1 mg/kg bolus followed by 0.8-1.7 mcg/kg/minute once initial recovery from bolus observed or 0.1-0.2 mg/kg every 1-3 hours

Dosing adjustment in renal impairment: Elimination half-life is doubled, plasma clearance is reduced and rate of recovery is sometimes much slower

Cl_{cr} 10-50 mL/minute: Administer 50% of normal dose
Cl_{cr} <10 mL/minute: Do not use

Dosing adjustment/comments in hepatic/biliary tract disease: Elimination half-life is doubled, plasma clearance is reduced, recovery time is prolonged, volume of distribution is increased (50%) and results in a slower onset, higher total initial dosage and prolongation of neuromuscular blockade

(Continued)

Pancuronium *(Continued)*

Stability Refrigerate; however, is stable for up to 6 months at room temperature; I.V. form is **incompatible** when mixed with diazepam at a Y-site injection

Administration May be administered undiluted by rapid I.V. injection

Monitoring Parameters Heart rate, blood pressure, assisted ventilation status; cardiac monitor, blood pressure monitor, and ventilator required

Anesthesia and Critical Care Concerns/Other Considerations Classified as a long duration neuromuscular-blocking agent; neuromuscular blockade will be prolonged in patients with decreased renal function; may produce cumulative effect on duration of blockade; produces tachycardia secondary to vagolytic activity and sympathetic stimulation.

Critically-Ill Adult Patients:

The 2004 Surviving Sepsis Campaign guidelines recommend avoiding use of neuromuscular blockers if at all possible in the septic patient due to the risk of prolonged neuromuscular blockade following discontinuation. If one is required, monitor carefully and observe the following recommendations.

The 2002 ACCM/SCCM/ASHP clinical practice guidelines for sustained neuromuscular blockade in the adult critically-ill patient recommend:

Optimize sedatives and analgesics prior to initiation and monitor and adjust accordingly during course. Neuromuscular blockers do not relieve pain or produce sedation.

Protect patient's eyes from development of keratitis and corneal abrasion by administering ophthalmic ointment and taping eyelids closed or using eye patches. Reposition patient routinely to protect pressure points from breakdown. Address DVT prophylaxis.

Concurrent use of a neuromuscular blocker and corticosteroids appear to increase the risk of certain ICU myopathies; avoid or administer the corticosteroid at the lowest dose possible. Reassess need for neuromuscular blocker daily.

Using daily drug holidays (stopping neuromuscular-blocking agent until patient requires it again) may decrease the incidence of acute quadriplegic myopathy syndrome.

Tachyphylaxis can develop; switch to another neuromuscular blocker (taking into consideration the patient's organ function) if paralysis is still necessary.

Atracurium or cisatracurium is recommended for patients with significant hepatic or renal disease, due to organ-independent Hofmann elimination.

Monitor patients clinically and via "Train of Four" (TOF) testing with a goal of adjusting the degree of blockade to 1-2 twitches or based upon the patient's clinical condition.

Pregnancy Risk Factor C

Contraindications Hypersensitivity to pancuronium, bromide, or any component of the formulation

Warnings/Precautions Ventilation must be supported during neuromuscular blockade; use with caution in patients with renal and/or hepatic impairment (adjust dose appropriately); certain clinical conditions may result in potentiation or antagonism of neuromuscular blockade:

Potentiation: Electrolyte abnormalities, severe hyponatremia, severe hypocalcemia, severe hypokalemia, hypermagnesemia, neuromuscular diseases, acidosis, acute intermittent porphyria, renal failure, hepatic failure

Antagonism: Alkalosis, hypercalcemia, demyelinating lesions, peripheral neuropathies, diabetes mellitus

Increased sensitivity in patients with myasthenia gravis, Eaton-Lambert syndrome; resistance in burn patients (>30% of body) for period of 5-70 days postinjury; resistance in patients with muscle trauma, denervation, immobilization, infection. Cross-sensitivity with other neuromuscular-blocking agents may occur; use extreme caution in patients with previous anaphylactic reactions.

Adverse Reactions Frequency not defined.

Cardiovascular: Elevation in pulse rate, elevated blood pressure and cardiac output, tachycardia, edema, skin flushing, circulatory collapse

Dermatologic: Rash, itching, erythema, burning sensation along the vein

Gastrointestinal: Excessive salivation

Neuromuscular & skeletal: Profound muscle weakness

Respiratory: Wheezing, bronchospasm

Miscellaneous: Hypersensitivity reaction

Postmarketing and/or case reports: Acute quadriplegic myopathy syndrome (prolonged use), myositis ossificans (prolonged use)

Overdosage/Toxicology Symptoms of overdose include apnea, respiratory depression, and cardiovascular collapse. Pyridostigmine, neostigmine, or edrophonium in conjunction with atropine will usually antagonize the action of pancuronium.

Drug Interactions See table.

Potential Drug Interactions

Potentiation	Antagonism
Anesthetics	Calcium
Desflurane, sevoflurane, enflurane and isoflurane > halothane > nitrous oxide-narcotics	Carbamazepine
Antibiotics	Phenytoin
Aminoglycosides, polymyxins, clindamycin, vancomycin	Steroids (chronic administration)
Magnesium sulfate	Theophylline
Antiarrhythmics	Anticholinesterases[1]
Quinidine, procainamide, bretylium, and possibly lidocaine	Neostigmine, pyridostigmine, edrophonium, echothiophate ophthalmic solution
Diuretics	Caffeine
Furosemide, mannitol	Azathioprine
Amphotericin B (secondary to hypokalemia)	
Local anesthetics	
Dantrolene (directly depresses skeletal muscle)	
Beta agonists	
Beta blockers	
Calcium channel blockers	
Ketamine	
Lithium	
Succinylcholine (when administered prior to nondepolarizing NMB agent)	

[1]Can prolong the effects of acetylcholine.

Dosage Forms Injection, solution, as bromide: 1 mg/mL (10 mL); 2 mg/mL (2 mL, 5 mL) [may contain benzyl alcohol]

References

Dellinger RP, Carlet JM, Masur H, et al, "Surviving Sepsis Campaign Guidelines for Management of Severe Sepsis and Septic Shock," *Crit Care Med*, 2004, 32(3):858-73.

Murray MJ, Cowen J, DeBlock H, et al, "Clinical Practice Guidelines for Sustained Neuromuscular Blockade in the Adult Critically Ill Patient. Task Force of the American College of Critical Care Medicine (ACCM) of the Society of Critical Care Medicine (SCCM), American Society of Health-System Pharmacists, American College of Chest Physicians," *Crit Care Med*, 2002, 30(1):142-56; viewable at http://www.sccm.org/pdf/NeuromuscularBlockade.pdf.

♦ **Pancuronium Bromide® (Can)** *see* Pancuronium *on page 981*

♦ **Pandel®** *see* Hydrocortisone *on page 639*

♦ **Panglobulin® NF** *see* Immune Globulin (Intravenous) *on page 666*

♦ **Panto™ IV (Can)** *see* Pantoprazole *on page 983*

♦ **Pantoloc® (Can)** *see* Pantoprazole *on page 983*

Pantoprazole (pan TOE pra zole)

Medication Safety Issues

Sound-alike/look-alike issues:

Protonix® may be confused with Lotronex®, Lovenox®, protamine

Vials containing Protonix® I.V. for injection are not recommended for use with spiked I.V. system adaptors. Nurses and pharmacists have reported breakage of the glass vials during attempts to connect spiked I.V. system adaptors, which may potentially result in injury to healthcare professionals.

U.S. Brand Names Protonix®

Canadian Brand Names Panto™ IV; Pantoloc®; Protonix®

Pharmacologic Category Proton Pump Inhibitor; Substituted Benzimidazole

Generic Available No

(Continued)

Pantoprazole *(Continued)*

Use

Oral: Treatment and maintenance of healing of erosive esophagitis associated with GERD; reduction in relapse rates of daytime and nighttime heartburn symptoms in GERD; hypersecretory disorders associated with Zollinger-Ellison syndrome or other neoplastic disorders

I.V.: Short-term treatment (7-10 days) of patients with gastroesophageal reflux disease (GERD) and a history of erosive esophagitis; hypersecretory disorders associated with Zollinger-Ellison syndrome or other neoplastic disorders

Unlabeled/Investigational Use Peptic ulcer disease, active ulcer bleeding (parenteral formulation); adjunct treatment with antibiotics for *Helicobacter pylori* eradication

Mechanism of Action Suppresses gastric acid secretin by inhibiting the parietal cell H^+/K^+ ATP pump

Pharmacodynamics/Kinetics

Absorption: Well absorbed

Distribution: V_d: 11-24 L

Protein binding: 98%, primarily to albumin

Metabolism: Extensively hepatic; CYP2C19 (demethylation), CYP3A4; no evidence that metabolites have pharmacologic activity

Bioavailability: 77%

Half-life elimination: 1 hour; increased to 3.5-10 hours with CYP2C19 deficiency

Time to peak: Oral: 2.5 hours

Excretion: Urine (71%); feces (18%)

Dosage Adults:

Oral:

Erosive esophagitis associated with GERD:

Treatment: 40 mg once daily for up to 8 weeks; an additional 8 weeks may be used in patients who have not healed after an 8-week course

Maintenance of healing: 40 mg once daily

Note: Lower doses (20 mg once daily) have been used successfully in mild GERD treatment and maintenance of healing

Hypersecretory disorders (including Zollinger-Ellison): Initial: 40 mg twice daily; adjust dose based on patient needs; doses up to 240 mg/day have been administered

Helicobacter pylori eradication (unlabeled use): Doses up to 40 mg twice daily have been used as part of combination therapy

I.V.:

Erosive esophagitis associated with GERD: 40 mg once daily for 7-10 days

Hypersecretory disorders: 80 mg twice daily; adjust dose based on acid output measurements; 160-240 mg/day in divided doses has been used for a limited period (up to 7 days)

Prevention of rebleeding in peptic ulcer bleed (unlabeled use): 80 mg, followed by 8 mg/hour infusion for 72 hours. **Note:** A daily infusion of 40 mg does not raise gastric pH sufficiently to enhance coagulation in active GI bleeds.

Elderly: Dosage adjustment not required

Dosage adjustment in renal impairment: Not required; pantoprazole is not removed by hemodialysis

Dosage adjustment in hepatic impairment: Not required

Stability

Oral: Store tablet at 15°C to 30°C (59°F to 77°F)

I.V.:

EDTA-stabilized formulation: Prior to use: Store at 15°C to 30°C (59°F to 86°F). Protect from light. When reconstituted with 10 mL NS (final concentration 4 mg/mL), solution is stable up to 24 hours at room temperature. If further diluting in 100 mL of D_5W, LR, or NS, dilute within 6 hours of reconstitution. Diluted solution is stable at room temperature for up to 24 hours from the time of initial reconstitution; protection from light not required.

Original formulation (discontinued): Store at 2°C to 8°C (36°F to 46°F); protect from light. When reconstituted with 10 mL NS (final concentration 4 mg/mL), solution is stable up to 2 hours at room temperature; protection from light not required. When diluted in 100 mL D_5W, LR, or NS, may be stored at room temperature for up to 12 hours.

Administration

I.V.: Flush I.V. line before and after administration. Solutions prepared from original formulation must be infused through an inline filter. Solutions prepared from the EDTA-stabilized formulation do not require an in-line filter (per manufacturer).

2-minute infusion: The volume of reconstituted solution (4 mg/mL) to be injected may be administered intravenously over at least 2 minutes.

15-minute infusion: Infuse over 15 minutes at a rate not to exceed 7 mL/minute (3 mg/minute).

Oral: Tablets should be swallowed whole, do not crush or chew. Best if taken before breakfast.

Monitoring Parameters Hypersecretory disorders: Acid output measurements, target level <10 mEq/hour (<5 mEq/hour if prior gastric acid-reducing surgery)

Anesthesia and Critical Care Concerns/Other Considerations Intravenous omeprazole has been studied in prevention of rebleeding in ulcer patients who are at high risk for rebleeding (endoscopic findings of active bleeding or nonbleeding visible vessel) after successful hemostasis (Lin HJ, 1998; Lau JYW, 2000). Lin and his group treated 100 ulcer patients (actively bleeding ulcers or ulcers with nonbleeding visible vessels) endoscopically and then randomized them to cimetidine (300 mg bolus followed by 50 mg/hour infusion) or omeprazole (40 mg bolus, ~7 mg/hour infusion) for 72 hours. Patients were discharged on the oral form of the drug arm they were assigned to. The omeprazole group maintained an intragastric pH >6 for about 84% of the infusion duration, while the cimetidine group maintained their pH >6 only about 50% of the time. Rebleeding occurred significantly more often in the cimetidine group. Lau and his colleagues treated patients with actively bleeding ulcers or ulcers with nonbleeding visible vessels with an epinephrine infusion followed by thermocoagulation. They were then randomized to omeprazole (80 mg bolus followed by a continuous infusion of 8 mg/hour for 72 hours) or placebo. All patients were discharged on oral omeprazole (20 mg/day) for 8 weeks and received *H. pylori* treatment if indicated. The primary goal was to evaluate the rate of rebleeding during the first 30 days after endoscopy. Two hundred and forty patients were enrolled with randomization of 120 into each group. Bleeding recurred in significantly more patients receiving placebo than omeprazole infusion. The authors concluded that after endoscopic therapy, omeprazole reduces the risk of rebleeding in patients with actively bleeding ulcers or ulcers with nonbleeding visible vessels.

Pregnancy Risk Factor B

Contraindications Hypersensitivity to pantoprazole, substituted benzamidazoles (ie, esomeprazole, lansoprazole, omeprazole, rabeprazole), or any component of the formulation

Warnings/Precautions Symptomatic response does not preclude gastric malignancy. Not indicated for maintenance therapy; safety and efficacy for use beyond 16 weeks have not been established. Prolonged treatment (typically >3 years) may lead to vitamin B_{12} malabsorption. Intravenous preparation contains edetate sodium (EDTA); use caution in patients who are risk for zinc deficiency if other EDTA-containing solutions are coadministered. Safety and efficacy in pediatric patients have not been established.

Adverse Reactions

≥1%:

Cardiovascular: Chest pain

Central nervous system: Headache (5% to 9%), insomnia (<1% to 1%), dizziness, migraine, anxiety

Dermatologic: Rash (<1% to 2%)

Endocrine and metabolic: Hyperglycemia (<1% to 1%), hyperlipidemia

Gastrointestinal: Diarrhea (4% to 6%), flatulence (2% to 4%), abdominal pain (1% to 4%), nausea (≤2%), vomiting (≤2%), eructation (≤1%), constipation, dyspepsia, gastroenteritis, rectal disorder

Genitourinary: Urinary frequency, UTI

Hepatic: Liver function abnormal (up to 2%)

Local: Injection site reaction (includes thrombophlebitis and abscess)

Neuromuscular & skeletal: Arthralgia, back pain, hypertonia, neck pain, weakness

Respiratory: Bronchitis, cough, dyspnea, pharyngitis, rhinitis, sinusitis, upper respiratory tract infection

Miscellaneous: Flu syndrome, infection, pain

<1% (Limited to important or life-threatening): Anaphylaxis, angioedema, anterior ischemic optic neuropathy, albuminuria, alkaline phosphatase increased, allergic reaction, anemia, angina pectoris, aphthous stomatitis, arrhythmia, asthma, atrial fibrillation/flutter, bone pain, breast pain, bursitis, cataract, CHF,

(Continued)

Pantoprazole *(Continued)*

cholecystitis, cholelithiasis, CPK increased, colitis, confusion, contact dermatitis, convulsion, creatinine increased, cystitis, deafness, decreased reflexes, dehydration, depression, diabetes mellitus, duodenitis, dysarthria, dysmenorrhea, dysphagia, dysuria, ecchymosis, eczema, ECG abnormality, eosinophilia, epididymitis, erythema multiforme, extraocular palsy, fever, fungal dermatitis, gastrointestinal carcinoma, gastrointestinal hemorrhage, gastrointestinal moniliasis, generalized edema, glaucoma, glycosuria, goiter, gout, hallucinations, hematuria, hemorrhage, hepatic failure, hepatitis, herpes simplex, herpes zoster, hyperkinesia, hyper-/hypotension, hyperuricemia, hypokinesia, impaired urination, impotence, interstitial nephritis, jaundice, kidney calculus, kidney pain, laryngitis, leukocytosis, leukopenia, lichenoid dermatitis, maculopapular rash, mouth ulceration, myalgia, myocardial ischemia, neoplasm, neuralgia, neuritis, optic neuropathy, palpitation, pancreatitis, pancytopenia, paresthesia, pneumonia, pyelonephritis, rhabdomyolysis, rectal hemorrhage, retinal vascular disorder, scrotal edema, skin ulcer, somnolence, Stevens-Johnson syndrome, stomach ulcer, stomatitis, syncope, tachycardia, tenosynovitis, thrombocytopenia, thrombosis, toxic epidermal necrolysis, urethritis, vasodilation, vision abnormal

Overdosage/Toxicology Treatment of an overdose would include appropriate supportive treatment. No adverse events were seen with ingestions of 400 and 600 mg doses. Pantoprazole is not removed by hemodialysis.

Drug Interactions Substrate of CYP2C19 (major), 3A4 (minor); **Inhibits** 2C9 (moderate); **Induces** CYP1A2 (weak), 3A4 (weak)

CYP2C9 Substrates: Pantoprazole may increase the levels/effects of CYP2C9 substrates. Example substrates include bosentan, dapsone, fluoxetine, glimepiride, glipizide, losartan, montelukast, nateglinide, paclitaxel, phenytoin, warfarin, and zafirlukast.

CYP2C19 inducers: May decrease the levels/effects of pantoprazole. Example inducers include aminoglutethimide, carbamazepine, phenytoin, and rifampin.

Iron salts: Oral absorption may be reduced by pantoprazole.

Itraconazole and ketoconazole: Proton pump inhibitors may decrease the absorption of itraconazole and ketoconazole.

Protease inhibitors: Proton pump inhibitors may decrease absorption of some protease inhibitors (atazanavir and indinavir).

Warfarin: Increased anticoagulant effects/INR have been reported with concurrent use (postmarketing case reports); monitor INR closely.

Ethanol/Nutrition/Herb Interactions

Ethanol: Avoid ethanol (may cause gastric mucosal irritation).

Herb/Nutraceutical: Prolonged treatment (typically >3 years) may lead to vitamin B_{12} malabsorption.

Test Interactions False-positive urine screening tests for tetrahydrocannabinol (THC) have been noted in patients receiving proton pump inhibitors, including pantoprazole.

Dietary Considerations

Oral: May be taken with or without food; best if taken before breakfast.

I.V.: Due to EDTA in preparation, zinc supplementation may be needed in patients prone to zinc deficiency.

Dosage Forms [DSC] = Discontinued product; **Note:** Strength expressed as base

Injection, powder for reconstitution, as sodium: 40 mg [original formulation] [DSC]

Injection, powder for reconstitution, as sodium: 40 mg [contains edetate sodium 1 mg]

Tablet, delayed release, as sodium: 20 mg, 40 mg

References

Allen ME, Kopp BJ, and Erstad BL, "Stress Ulcer Prophylaxis in the Postoperative Period," *Am J Health Syst Pharm*, 2004, 61(6):588-96.

Bardhan KD, Dillon J, Axon AT, et al, "Triple Therapy for *Helicobacter pylori* Eradication: A Comparison of Pantoprazole Once Versus Twice Daily," *Aliment Pharmacol Ther*, 2000, 14(1):59-67.

Brunner G, Luna P, Hartmann M, et al, "Optimizing the Intragastric pH as a Supportive Therapy in Upper Gastrointestinal Bleeding," *Yale J Biol Med*, 1996, 69(3):225-231.

Jung R and MacLaren R, "Proton-Pump Inhibitors for Stress Ulcer Prophylaxis in Critically Ill Patients," *Ann Pharmacother*, 2002, 36(12):1929-37.

Lau JY, Sung JJ, Lee KK, et al, "Effect of Intravenous Omeprazole on Recurrent Bleeding After Endoscopic Treatment of Bleeding Peptic Ulcers," *N Engl J Med*, 2000, 343(5):310-6.

Lew EA, Pisegna JR, Starr JA, et al, "Intravenous Pantoprazole Rapidly Controls Gastric Acid Hypersecretion in Patients With Zollinger-Ellison Syndrome," *Gastroenterology*, 2000, 118(4):696-704.

Lin HJ, Lo WC, Lee FY, et al, "A Prospective Randomized Comparative Trial Showing That Omeprazole Prevents Rebleeding in Patients With Bleeding Peptic Ulcer After Successful Endoscopic Therapy," *Arch Intern Med*, 1998, 158(1):54-8.

Morgan D, "Intravenous Proton-Pump Inhibitors in the Critical Care Setting," *Crit Care Med*, 2002, 30(Suppl):369-72.

◆ **Paracetamol** *see* Acetaminophen *on page 26*

◆ **Parcopa™** *see* Levodopa and Carbidopa *on page 743*

Paregoric (par e GOR ik)

Medication Safety Issues

Sound-alike/look-alike issues:

Camphorated tincture of opium is an error-prone synonym (mistaken as opium tincture)

Paregoric may be confused with Percogesic®

Use care when prescribing opium tincture; each mL contains the equivalent of morphine 10 mg; paregoric contains the equivalent of morphine 0.4 mg/mL

Synonyms Camphorated Tincture of Opium (error-prone synonym)

Pharmacologic Category Analgesic, Narcotic

Restrictions C-III

Generic Available Yes

Use Treatment of diarrhea or relief of pain; neonatal opiate withdrawal

Mechanism of Action Increases smooth muscle tone in GI tract, decreases motility and peristalsis, diminishes digestive secretions

Pharmacodynamics/Kinetics In terms of opium:

Metabolism: Hepatic

Excretion: Urine (primarily as morphine glucuronide conjugates and unchanged drug - morphine, codeine, papaverine, etc)

Dosage Oral:

Neonatal opiate withdrawal: 3-6 drops every 3-6 hours as needed, or initially 0.2 mL every 3 hours; increase dosage by approximately 0.05 mL every 3 hours until withdrawal symptoms are controlled; it is rare to exceed 0.7 mL/dose. Stabilize withdrawal symptoms for 3-5 days, then gradually decrease dosage over a 2- to 4-week period.

Children: 0.25-0.5 mL/kg 1-4 times/day

Adults: 5-10 mL 1-4 times/day

Stability Store in light-resistant, tightly closed container

Pregnancy Risk Factor B/D (prolonged use or high doses)

Contraindications Hypersensitivity to opium or any component of the formulation; diarrhea caused by poisoning until the toxic material has been removed; pregnancy (prolonged use or high doses)

Warnings/Precautions Use with caution in patients with respiratory, hepatic or renal dysfunction, severe prostatic hyperplasia, or history of narcotic abuse; opium shares the toxic potential of opiate agonists, and usual precautions of opiate agonist therapy should be observed; some preparations contain sulfites which may cause allergic reactions; infants <3 months of age are more susceptible to respiratory depression, use with caution and generally in reduced doses in this age group; tolerance or drug dependence may result from extended use

Adverse Reactions Frequency not defined.

Cardiovascular: Hypotension, peripheral vasodilation

Central nervous system: Drowsiness, dizziness, insomnia, CNS depression, mental depression, increased intracranial pressure, restlessness, headache, malaise

Gastrointestinal: Constipation, anorexia, stomach cramps, nausea, vomiting, biliary tract spasm

Genitourinary: Ureteral spasms, decreased urination, urinary tract spasm

Hepatic: Increased liver function tests

Neuromuscular & skeletal: Weakness

Ocular: Miosis

Respiratory: Respiratory depression

Miscellaneous: Physical and psychological dependence, histamine release

Overdosage/Toxicology Symptoms of overdose include hypotension, drowsiness, seizures, and respiratory depression. Naloxone, 2 mg I.V. with repeat administration as necessary up to a total of 10 mg, can be used to reverse opiate effects.

(Continued)

Paregoric *(Continued)*

Drug Interactions Increased effect/toxicity with CNS depressants (eg, alcohol, narcotics, benzodiazepines, TCAs, MAO inhibitors, phenothiazine)

Ethanol/Nutrition/Herb Interactions Ethanol: Avoid ethanol (may increase CNS depression).

Dosage Forms Liquid, oral: Morphine equivalent 2 mg/5 mL (473 mL) [equivalent to opium 20 mg powder; contains alcohol 45% and benzoic acid]

- **Parenteral Nutrition** *see* Total Parenteral Nutrition *on page 1293*
- **Pariet® (Can)** *see* Rabeprazole *on page 1099*
- **Pariprazole** *see* Rabeprazole *on page 1099*
- **Parlodel®** *see* Bromocriptine *on page 191*
- **Parnate®** *see* Tranylcypromine *on page 1302*

Paroxetine (pa ROKS e teen)

Medication Safety Issues

Sound-alike/look-alike issues:

Paroxetine may be confused with paclitaxel, pyridoxine

Paxil® may be confused with Doxil®, paclitaxel, Plavix®, Taxol®

Related Information

Antidepressant Agents *on page 1551*

U.S. Brand Names Paxil®; Paxil CR®; Pexeva®

Canadian Brand Names Apo-Paroxetine®; CO Paroxetine; Gen-Paroxetine; Novo-Paroxetine; Paxil®; Paxil CR®; PMS-Paroxetine; ratio-Paroxetine; Rhoxal-paroxetine; Sandoz-Paroxetine

Synonyms Paroxetine Hydrochloride; Paroxetine Mesylate

Pharmacologic Category Antidepressant, Selective Serotonin Reuptake Inhibitor

Restrictions A medication guide concerning the use of antidepressants in children and teenagers can be found on the FDA website at http://www.fda.gov/cder/Offices/ODS/labeling.htm. It should be dispensed to parents or guardians of children and teenagers receiving this medication.

Generic Available Yes: Tablet, as hydrochloride

Use Treatment of depression in adults; treatment of panic disorder with or without agoraphobia; obsessive-compulsive disorder (OCD) in adults; social anxiety disorder (social phobia); generalized anxiety disorder (GAD); post-traumatic stress disorder (PTSD)

Paxil CR®: Treatment of depression; panic disorder; premenstrual dysphoric disorder (PMDD); social anxiety disorder (social phobia)

Unlabeled/Investigational Use May be useful in eating disorders, impulse control disorders, self-injurious behavior; premenstrual disorders, vasomotor symptoms of menopause; treatment of depression and obsessive-compulsive disorder (OCD) in children

Mechanism of Action Paroxetine is a selective serotonin reuptake inhibitor, chemically unrelated to tricyclic, tetracyclic, or other antidepressants; presumably, the inhibition of serotonin reuptake from brain synapse stimulated serotonin activity in the brain

Pharmacodynamics/Kinetics

Absorption: Completely absorbed following oral administration

Distribution: V_d: 8.7 L/kg (3-28 L/kg)

Protein binding: 93% to 95%

Metabolism: Extensively hepatic via CYP enzymes via oxidation and methylation; nonlinear pharmacokinetics may be seen with higher doses and longer duration of therapy. Saturation of CYP2D6 appears to account for the nonlinearity. C_{min} concentrations 70% to 80% greater in the elderly compared to nonelderly patients; clearance is also decreased.

Half-life elimination: 21 hours (3-65 hours)

Time to peak, serum: Immediate release: 5.2 hours; controlled release: 6-10 hours

Excretion: Urine (64%, 2% as unchanged drug); feces (36% primarily via bile)

Dosage Oral:

Children:

Depression (unlabeled use; not recommended by FDA): Initial: 10 mg/day and adjusted upward on an individual basis to 20 mg/day

OCD (unlabeled use): Initial: 10 mg/day and titrate up as necessary to 60 mg/day

Self-injurious behavior (unlabeled use): 20 mg/day

Social phobia (unlabeled use): 2.5-15 mg/day

Adults:

Depression:

Paxil®, Pexeva®: Initial: 20 mg once daily, preferably in the morning; increase if needed by 10 mg/day increments at intervals of at least 1 week; maximum dose: 50 mg/day

Paxil CR®: Initial: 25 mg once daily; increase if needed by 12.5 mg/day increments at intervals of at least 1 week; maximum dose: 62.5 mg/day

GAD (Paxil®): Initial: 20 mg once daily, preferably in the morning; doses of 20-50 mg/day were used in clinical trials, however, no greater benefit was seen with doses >20 mg. If dose is increased, adjust in increments of 10 mg/day at 1-week intervals.

OCD (Paxil®, Pexeva™): Initial: 20 mg once daily, preferably in the morning; increase if needed by 10 mg/day increments at intervals of at least 1 week; recommended dose: 40 mg/day; range: 20-60 mg/day; maximum dose: 60 mg/day

Panic disorder:

Paxil®, Pexeva®: Initial: 10 mg once daily, preferably in the morning; increase if needed by 10 mg/day increments at intervals of at least 1 week; recommended dose: 40 mg/day; range: 10-60 mg/day; maximum dose: 60 mg/day

Paxil CR®: Initial: 12.5 mg once daily; increase if needed by 12.5 mg/day at intervals of at least 1 week; maximum dose: 75 mg/day

PMDD (Paxil CR®): Initial: 12.5 mg once daily in the morning; may be increased to 25 mg/day; dosing changes should occur at intervals of at least 1 week. May be given daily throughout the menstrual cycle or limited to the luteal phase.

PTSD (Paxil®): Initial: 20 mg once daily, preferably in the morning; increase if needed by 10 mg/day increments at intervals of at least 1 week; range: 20-50 mg. Limited data suggest doses of 40 mg/day were not more efficacious than 20 mg/day.

Social anxiety disorder:

Paxil®: Initial: 20 mg once daily, preferably in the morning; recommended dose: 20 mg/day; range: 20-60 mg/day; doses >20 mg may not have additional benefit

Paxil CR®: Initial: 12.5 mg once daily, preferably in the morning; may be increased by 12.5 mg/day at intervals of at least 1 week; maximum dose: 37.5 mg/day

Vasomotor symptoms of menopause (unlabeled use, Paxil CR®): 12.5-25 mg/day

Elderly:

Paxil®, Pexeva®: Initial: 10 mg/day; increase if needed by 10 mg/day increments at intervals of at least 1 week; maximum dose: 40 mg/day

Paxil CR®; Initial: 12.5 mg/day; increase if needed by 12.5 mg/day increments at intervals of at least 1 week; maximum dose: 50 mg/day

Note: Upon discontinuation of paroxetine therapy, gradually taper dose:

Paxil®: 10 mg/day at weekly intervals; when 20 mg/day dose is reached, continue for 1 week before treatment is discontinued. Some patients may need to be titrated to 10 mg/day for 1 week before discontinuation.

Paxil CR®: Patients receiving 37.5 mg/day in clinical trials had their dose decreased by 12.5 mg/day to a dose of 25 mg/day and remained at a dose of 25 mg/day for 1 week before treatment was discontinued.

Dosage adjustment in severe renal/hepatic impairment: Adults:

Cl_{cr} <30 mL/minute: Mean plasma concentration is ~4 times that seen in normal function.

Cl_{cr} 30-60 mL/minute and hepatic dysfunction: Plasma concentration is 2 times that seen in normal function.

Paxil®, Pexeva®: Initial: 10 mg/day; increase if needed by 10 mg/day increments at intervals of at least 1 week; maximum dose: 40 mg/day

Paxil CR®: Initial: 12.5 mg/day; increase if needed by 12.5 mg/day increments at intervals of at least 1 week; maximum dose: 50 mg/day

Stability

Suspension: Store at ≤25°C (≤77°F)

(Continued)

Paroxetine *(Continued)*

Tablet: Store at 15°C to 30°C (59°F to 86°F)

Administration May be administered with or without food. Do not crush, break, or chew controlled release tablets.

Monitoring Parameters Mental status for depression, suicidal ideation (especially at the beginning of therapy or when doses are increased or decreased), anxiety, social functioning, mania, panic attacks; akathisia

Anesthesia and Critical Care Concerns/Other Considerations Paroxetine has properties similar to fluvoxamine maleate. Buspirone (15-60 mg/day) may be useful in treatment of sexual dysfunction during treatment with a selective serotonin reuptake inhibitor.

Pregnancy Risk Factor D

Contraindications Hypersensitivity to paroxetine or any component of the formulation; use of MAO inhibitors or within 14 days; concurrent use with thioridazine or pimozide

Warnings/Precautions

Major psychiatric warnings:

- **[U.S. Boxed Warning]: Antidepressants increase the risk of suicidal thinking and behavior in children and adolescents with major depressive disorder (MDD) and other depressive disorders;** consider risk prior to prescribing. Closely monitor for clinical worsening, suicidality, or unusual changes in behavior; the child's family or caregiver should be instructed to closely observe the patient and communicate condition with healthcare provider. A medication guide concerning the use of antidepressants in children and teenagers should be dispensed with each prescription. **Paroxetine is not FDA approved for use in children.**
- A higher incidence of suicidal behaviors has been observed in young adults receiving paroxetine for both depressive and nondepressive indications.
- The possibility of a suicide attempt is inherent in major depression and may persist until remission occurs. Patients treated with antidepressants (for any indication) should be observed for clinical worsening and suicidality, especially during the initial few months of a course of drug therapy, or at times of dose changes, either increases or decreases. Worsening depression and severe abrupt suicidality that are not part of the presenting symptoms may require discontinuation or modification of drug therapy. Use caution in high-risk patients during initiation of therapy.
- Prescriptions should be written for the smallest quantity consistent with good patient care. The patient's family or caregiver should be alerted to monitor patients for the emergence of suicidality and associated behaviors such as anxiety, agitation, panic attacks, insomnia, irritability, hostility, impulsivity, akathisia, hypomania, and mania; patients should be instructed to notify their healthcare provider if any of these symptoms or worsening depression or psychosis occur.
- May worsen psychosis in some patients or precipitate a shift to mania or hypomania in patients with bipolar disorder. Monotherapy in patients with bipolar disorder should be avoided. Patients presenting with depressive symptoms should be screened for bipolar disorder. **Paroxetine is not FDA approved for the treatment of bipolar depression.**

Key adverse effects:

- Serotonin syndrome: Symptoms of agitation, confusion, hallucinations, hyperreflexia, myoclonus, shivering, and tachycardia may occur with concomitant proserotonergic drugs or agents which reduce paroxetine's metabolism. Concurrent use of serotonin precursors (eg, tryptophan) is not recommended.
- Akathisia: Inability to remain still due to feelings of agitation or restlessness has been observed with paroxetine and other SSRIs. Usually occurs within the first few weeks of therapy.
- Anticholinergic effects: Has low potential for sedation and anticholinergic effects relative to cyclic antidepressants; however among the SSRI class these effects are relatively higher.
- CNS depression: Has a low potential to impair cognitive or motor performance; caution operating hazardous machinery or driving.
- SIADH and hyponatremia: Has been associated with the development of SIADH; hyponatremia has been reported rarely, predominately in the elderly

Concurrent disease:

- Cardiovascular disease: Use caution in patients with cardiovascular disease; paroxetine has not been systemically evaluated in patients with a recent history of MI or unstable heart disease.
- Hepatic impairment: Use caution; clearance is decreased and plasma concentrations are increased; a lower dosage may be needed.
- Narrow-angle glaucoma: Associated with an increased risk of mydriasis in patients with controlled narrow angle glaucoma.
- Platelet aggregation: May impair platelet aggregation, resulting in bleeding.
- Renal impairment: Use caution; clearance is decreased and plasma concentrations are increased; a lower dosage may be needed.
- Seizure disorders: Use caution with a previous seizure disorder or condition predisposing to seizures such as brain damage or alcoholism.
- Sexual dysfunction: May cause or exacerbate sexual dysfunction.

Concurrent drug therapy:

- Agents which lower seizure threshold: Concurrent therapy with other drugs which lower the seizure threshold.
- Anticoagulants/Antiplatelets: Use caution with concomitant use of NSAIDs, ASA, or other drugs that affect coagulation; the risk of bleeding is potentiated.
- CNS depressants: Use caution with concomitant therapy.
- MAO inhibitors: Potential for severe reaction when used with MAO inhibitors; autonomic instability, coma, death, delirium, diaphoresis, hyperthermia, mental status changes/agitation, muscular rigidity, myoclonus, neuroleptic malignant syndrome features, and seizures may occur. Concurrent use with paroxetine is contraindicated.
- Thioridazine and pimozide: Potential for QT_c prolongation and arrhythmia; concurrent use of paroxetine with either of these agents is contraindicated.

Special populations:

- Elderly: Use caution in elderly patients.
- Pregnancy: Avoid use in the first trimester.

Special notes:

- Electroconvulsive therapy: May increase the risks associated with electroconvulsive therapy; consider discontinuing, when possible, prior to ECT treatment.
- Withdrawal syndrome: May cause dysphoric mood, irritability, agitation, dizziness, sensory disturbances, anxiety, confusion, headache, lethargy, emotional lability, insomnia, hypomania, tinnitus, and seizures. Upon discontinuation of paroxetine therapy, gradually taper dose. If intolerable symptoms occur following a decrease in dosage or upon discontinuation of therapy, then resuming the previous dose with a more gradual taper should be considered.

Adverse Reactions Frequency varies by dose and indication. Adverse reactions reported as a composite of all indications.

>10%:

Central nervous system: Somnolence (15% to 24%), insomnia (11% to 24%), headache (17% to 18%), dizziness (6% to 14%)

Endocrine & metabolic: Libido decreased (6% to 15%)

Gastrointestinal: Nausea (19% to 26%), xerostomia (9% to 18%), constipation (5% to 16%), diarrhea (9% to 12%)

Genitourinary: Ejaculatory disturbances (10% to 28%)

Neuromuscular & skeletal: Weakness (12% to 22%), tremor (4% to 11%)

Miscellaneous: Diaphoresis (5% to 14%)

1% to 10%:

Cardiovascular: Vasodilation (2% to 4%), chest pain (3%), palpitations (2% to 3%), hypertension (≥1%), tachycardia (≥1%)

Central nervous system: Nervousness (4% to 9%), anxiety (5%), agitation (3% to 5%), abnormal dreams (3% to 4%), concentration impaired (3% to 4%), yawning (2% to 4%), depersonalization (up to 3%), amnesia (2%), emotional lability (≥1%), vertigo (≥1%), confusion (1%), chills (2%)

Dermatologic: Rash (2% to 3%), pruritus (≥1%)

Endocrine & metabolic: Orgasmic disturbance (2% to 9%), dysmenorrhea (5%)

Gastrointestinal: Anorexia, appetite decreased (5% to 9%), dyspepsia (2% to 5%), flatulence (4%), abdominal pain (4%), appetite increased (2% to 4%), vomiting (2% to 3%), taste perversion (2%), weight gain (≥1%)

Genitourinary: Impotence (2% to 9%), genital disorder (female 2% to 9%), urinary frequency (2% to 3%), urinary tract infection (2%)

(Continued)

Paroxetine *(Continued)*

Neuromuscular & skeletal: Paresthesia (4%), myalgia (2% to 4%), back pain (3%), myoclonus (2% to 3%), myopathy (2%), myasthenia (1%), arthralgia (≥1%)

Ocular: Blurred vision (4%), abnormal vision (2% to 3%)

Otic: Tinnitus (≥1%)

Respiratory: Respiratory disorder (up to 7%), pharyngitis (4%), sinusitis (up to 4%), rhinitis (3%)

Miscellaneous: Infection (5% to 6%)

<1%, postmarketing, and/or case reports (limited to important or life-threatening): Acute renal failure, adrenergic syndrome, akinesia, alkaline phosphatase increased, allergic reaction, anaphylaxis, anemias (various), angina pectoris, angioedema, aphasia, aphthous stomatitis, arrhythmias (atrial and ventricular), arthrosis, asthma, behavioral disturbances (various), bilirubinemia, bleeding time increased, blood dyscrasias, bloody diarrhea, bradycardia, bronchitis, bulimia, BUN increased, bundle branch block, cardiospasm, cataract, cellulitis, cerebral ischemia, cerebrovascular accident, cholelithiasis, colitis, congestive heart failure, creatinine phosphokinase increased, deafness, dehydration, delirium, diabetes mellitus, drug dependence, dyskinesia, dysphagia, dyspnea, dystonia, ecchymosis, eclampsia, electrolyte abnormalities, emphysema, erythema, exfoliative dermatitis, extrapyramidal syndrome, fecal impactions, fungal dermatitis, gamma globulins increased, gastroenteritis, glaucoma, goiter, Guillain-Barré syndrome, hematemesis, hematoma, hemorrhage, hemoptysis, hepatic necrosis, hepatitis, hypercholesteremia, hyper-/hypoglycemia, hyper-/hypothyroidism, hypotension, ileus, jaundice, ketosis, lactic dehydrogenase increased, liver function tests abnormal, low cardiac output, lung fibrosis, lymphadenopathy, meningitis, MI, migraine, myelitis, neuroleptic malignant syndrome, neuropathy, osteoporosis, pancreatitis, peptic ulcer, peritonitis, phlebitis, pneumonia, platelet count abnormalities, pulmonary edema, pulmonary embolus, pulmonary hypertension, seizure, sepsis, serotonin syndrome, syncope, tetany, tongue edema, torsade de pointes, toxic epidermal necrolysis

Overdosage/Toxicology Symptoms of overdose include somnolence, nausea, vomiting, hepatic dysfunction, drowsiness, sinus tachycardia, urinary retention, renal failure (acute), and dilated pupils. Convulsions, status epilepticus, and ventricular arrhythmias (including torsade de pointes) have been reported, as well as serotonin syndrome and manic reaction. There are no specific antidotes, following attempts at decontamination, treatment is supportive and symptom-directed. Forced diuresis, dialysis, and hemoperfusion are unlikely to be beneficial.

Drug Interactions Substrate of CYP2D6 (major); **Inhibits** CYP1A2 (weak), 2B6 (moderate), 2C9 (weak), 2C19 (weak), 2D6 (strong), 3A4 (weak)

Amphetamines: SSRIs may increase the sensitivity to amphetamines, and amphetamines may increase the risk of serotonin syndrome.

Aspirin (and other antiplatelet drugs): Concomitant use of paroxetine and NSAIDs, aspirin, or other drugs affecting coagulation has been associated with an increased risk of bleeding; monitor.

Atomoxetine: Paroxetine may increase the levels/effects; dose reduction of atomoxetine may be required.

Buspirone: Combined use with SSRIs may cause serotonin syndrome.

Carbamazepine: May increase levels/effects of paroxetine; monitor.

Carvedilol: Serum concentrations may be increased; monitor carefully for increased carvedilol effect (hypotension and bradycardia).

Cimetidine: Cimetidine may reduce the first-pass metabolism of paroxetine resulting in elevated paroxetine serum concentrations; consider an alternative H_2antagonist.

Clozapine: May increase serum levels of clozapine; monitor for increased effect/toxicity.

CYP2B6 substrates: Paroxetine may increase the levels/effects of CYP2B6 substrates. Example substrates include bupropion, promethazine, propofol, selegiline, and sertraline.

CYP2D6 inhibitors: May increase the levels/effects of paroxetine. Example inhibitors include chlorpromazine, delavirdine, fluoxetine, miconazole, pergolide, quinidine, quinine, ritonavir, and ropinirole.

CYP2D6 substrates: Paroxetine may increase the levels/effects of CYP2D6 substrates. Example substrates include amphetamines, selected beta-blockers, dextromethorphan, fluoxetine, lidocaine, mirtazapine, nefazodone, risperidone, ritonavir, thioridazine, tricyclic antidepressants, and venlafaxine.

CYP2D6 prodrug substrates: Paroxetine may decrease the levels/effects of CYP2D6 prodrug substrates. Example prodrug substrates include codeine, hydrocodone, oxycodone, and tramadol.

Cyproheptadine: May inhibit the effects of serotonin reuptake inhibitors; monitor for altered antidepressant response; cyproheptadine acts as a serotonin agonist.

Dextromethorphan: Metabolism of dextromethorphan may be inhibited; visual hallucinations occurred; monitor.

Galantamine: Paroxetine may increase levels/effects; monitor.

Haloperidol: Metabolism may be inhibited and cause extrapyramidal symptoms (EPS); monitor patients for EPS if combination is utilized.

HMG-CoA reductase inhibitors: Metabolism may be inhibited by SSRIs; particularly lovastatin and simvastatin resulting in myositis and rhabdomyolysis; paroxetine appears to have weak interaction with CYP3A4, and therefore, appears to have a low risk of this interaction.

Lithium: Patients receiving SSRIs and lithium have developed neurotoxicity; if combination is used; monitor for neurotoxicity.

Loop diuretics: SSRIs may cause hyponatremia; additive hyponatremic effects may be seen with combined use of a loop diuretic (bumetanide, furosemide, torsemide); monitor for hyponatremia.

MAO inhibitors: SSRIs should not be used with nonselective MAO inhibitors (isocarboxazid, phenelzine); fatal reactions have been reported; this combination should be avoided.

Meperidine: Combined use may cause serotonin syndrome; monitor.

Nefazodone and trazodone: May increase the risk of serotonin syndrome with SSRIs; monitor.

NSAIDs: Concomitant use of paroxetine and NSAIDs, aspirin, or other drugs affecting coagulation has been associated with an increased risk of bleeding; monitor.

Phenytoin: Metabolism of phenytoin may be inhibited, resulting in phenytoin toxicity; monitor for toxicity (ataxia, confusion, dizziness, nystagmus, involuntary muscle movement).

Pimozide: Paroxetine may increase the levels/effects; concomitant use contraindicated.

Procyclidine: Paroxetine increases AUC of procyclidine by 35%; this may result in increased anticholinergic effects; procyclidine dose reduction may be necessary.

Risperidone: Paroxetine, a potent CYP2D6 inhibitor, inhibits the metabolism of risperidone (CYP2D6 substrate) resulting in elevated plasma risperidone levels. The clinical implications are unclear, but clinicians should monitor for potential extrapyramidal symptoms (EPS).

Ritonavir: Combined use of paroxetine with ritonavir may cause serotonin syndrome; monitor.

Selegiline: SSRIs have been reported to cause mania or hypertension when combined with selegiline; this combination is best avoided; concurrent use with SSRIs has also been reported to cause serotonin syndrome; as an MAO type B inhibitor, the risk of serotonin syndrome may be less than with nonselective MAO inhibitors.

Serotonergic uptake inhibitors: Combined use with other drugs which inhibit the reuptake may cause serotonin syndrome.

Sibutramine: May increase the risk of serotonin syndrome with SSRIs; avoid coadministration.

Sumatriptan (and other serotonin agonists): Concurrent use may result in toxicity; weakness, hyper-reflexia, and incoordination have been observed with sumatriptan and SSRIs. In addition, concurrent use may theoretically increase the risk of serotonin syndrome; includes sumatriptan, naratriptan, rizatriptan, and zolmitriptan.

Sympathomimetics: May increase the risk of serotonin syndrome with SSRIs.

Theophylline: Paroxetine may elevate serum levels of theophylline; monitor.

Thioridazine: Paroxetine may inhibit the metabolism of thioridazine, resulting in increased plasma levels and increasing the risk of QT_c interval prolongation. Concurrent use is contraindicated.

Tramadol: Combined use may cause serotonin syndrome; monitor.

Tricyclic antidepressants: The metabolism of tricyclic antidepressants (amitriptyline, desipramine, imipramine, nortriptyline) may be inhibited by SSRIs resulting

(Continued)

Paroxetine *(Continued)*

is elevated serum levels; if combination is warranted, a low dose of TCA (10-25 mg/day) should be utilized.

Tryptophan: May increase serotonergic effects; concomitant use not recommended.

Venlafaxine: Combined use with paroxetine may increase the risk of serotonin syndrome.

Warfarin: May alter the hypoprothrombinemic response to warfarin; monitor INR.

Zolpidem: At least one case of acute delirium in association with combined therapy has been reported.

Ethanol/Nutrition/Herb Interactions

Ethanol: Avoid ethanol.

Food: Peak concentration is increased, but bioavailability is not significantly altered by food.

Herb/Nutraceutical: Avoid valerian, St John's wort, SAMe, kava kava.

Dietary Considerations May be taken with or without food.

Dosage Forms Note: Available as paroxetine hydrochloride or mesylate; mg strength refers to paroxetine

Suspension, oral, as hydrochloride (Paxil®): 10 mg/5 mL (250 mL) [orange flavor]

Tablet, as hydrochloride (Paxil®): 10 mg, 20 mg, 30 mg, 40 mg

Tablet, as mesylate (Pexeva®): 10 mg, 20 mg, 30 mg, 40 mg

Tablet, controlled release, as hydrochloride (Paxil CR®): 12.5 mg, 25 mg, 37.5 mg

- **Paroxetine Hydrochloride** *see* Paroxetine *on page 988*
- **Paroxetine Mesylate** *see* Paroxetine *on page 988*
- **Parvolex® (Can)** *see* Acetylcysteine *on page 35*
- **Pavulon [DSC]** *see* Pancuronium *on page 981*
- **Paxil®** *see* Paroxetine *on page 988*
- **Paxil CR®** *see* Paroxetine *on page 988*
- **PCA (error-prone abbreviation)** *see* Procainamide *on page 1056*
- **PCE®** *see* Erythromycin *on page 476*
- **PCEC** *see* Rabies Virus Vaccine *on page 1101*
- **PediaCare® Decongestant Infants [OTC]** *see* Pseudoephedrine *on page 1085*
- **Pediapred®** *see* PrednisoLONE *on page 1046*
- **Pediatric Digoxin CSD (Can)** *see* Digoxin *on page 388*
- **Pediatrix (Can)** *see* Acetaminophen *on page 26*
- **Pedi-Dri®** *see* Nystatin *on page 945*
- **Pedtrace-4®** *see* Trace Metals *on page 1296*

Penicillin G (Parenteral/Aqueous)

(pen i SIL in jee, pa REN ter al, AYE kwee us)

Medication Safety Issues

Sound-alike/look-alike issues:

Penicillin may be confused with penicillamine

Related Information

Prevention of Wound Infection and Sepsis in Surgical Patients *on page 1588*

U.S. Brand Names Pfizerpen®

Canadian Brand Names Pfizerpen®

Synonyms Benzylpenicillin Potassium; Benzylpenicillin Sodium; Crystalline Penicillin; Penicillin G Potassium; Penicillin G Sodium

Pharmacologic Category Antibiotic, Penicillin

Generic Available Yes

Use Active against some gram-positive organisms, generally not *Staphylococcus aureus*; some gram-negative organisms such as *Neisseria gonorrhoeae*, and some anaerobes and spirochetes

Mechanism of Action Interferes with bacterial cell wall synthesis during active multiplication, causing cell wall death and resultant bactericidal activity against susceptible bacteria

Pharmacodynamics/Kinetics

Distribution: Poor penetration across blood-brain barrier, despite inflamed meninges; crosses placenta; enters breast milk

Relative diffusion from blood into CSF: Good only with inflammation (exceeds usual MICs)

CSF:blood level ratio: Normal meninges: <1%; Inflamed meninges: 3% to 5%
Protein binding: 65%
Metabolism: Hepatic (30%) to penicilloic acid
Half-life elimination:
Neonates: <6 days old: 3.2-3.4 hours; 7-13 days old: 1.2-2.2 hours; >14 days old: 0.9-1.9 hours
Children and Adults: Normal renal function: 20-50 minutes
End-stage renal disease: 3.3-5.1 hours
Time to peak, serum: I.M.: ~30 minutes; I.V. ~1 hour
Excretion: Urine

Dosage

Usual dosage range:
Neonates: I.M., I.V.:
<7 days, <2000 g: 25,000-50,000 units/kg every 12 hours
<7 days, >2000 g: 25,000-50,000 units/kg every 8 hours
>7 days, <2000 g: 25,000-50,000 units/kg every 8 hours
>7 days, >2000 g: 25,000-50,000 units/kg every 6 hours
Infants and Children: I.M., I.V.: 250,000 to 400,000 units/kg/day in divided doses every 4-6 hours (maximum dose: 24 million units/day)
Adults: I.M., I.V.: 2-24 million units/day in divided doses every 4 hours depending on sensitivity of the organism and severity of the infection

Indication-specific dosing:
Infants and Children:
Gonococcal:
Disseminated or ophthalmia: I.V.: 100,000 units/kg/day in 2 divided doses (>1 week of age: 4 divided doses)
Meningitis: I.V.: 150,000 units/kg in 2 divided doses (>1 week of age: 4 divided doses)
Mild-to-moderate infections: I.M., I.V.: 25,000-50,000 units/kg/day in 4 divided doses
Severe infections: I.M., I.V.: 250,000-400,000 units/kg/day in divided doses every 4-6 hours (maximum dose: 24 million units/day)
Syphilis (congenital):
Neonates:
≤7 days: 50,000 units/kg I.V. every 12 hours for a total of 10 days
>7 days: 50,000 units/kg I.V. every 8 hours for a total of 10 days
Infants: I.V.: 50,000 units/kg every 4-6 hours for 10 days
Adults:
***Actinomyces* species:** I.V.: 10-20 million units/day divided every 4-6 hours for 4-6 weeks
Anthrax (cutaneous): I.V.: 2 million units every 3 hours for 5-7 days
Clostridium perfringens: I.V.: 24 million units/day divided every 4-6 hours with clindamycin
Corynebacterium diphtheriae: I.V.: 25,000-50,000 units/kg to maximum 1.2 million units every 12 hours, until oral therapy tolerated
Erysipelas: I.V.: 1-2 million units every 4-6 hours
Erysipelothrix: I.V.: 2-4 million units every 4 hours
Fascial space infections: I.V.: 2-4 million units every 4-6 hours with metronidazole
Leptospirosis: I.V.: 1.5 million units every 6 hours for 7 days
Listeria: I.V.: 300,000 units/kg/day every 4 hours
Lyme disease (meningitis): I.V.: 20 million units/day in divided doses
Neurosyphilis: I.M., I.V.: 18-24 million units/day in divided doses every 4 hours (or by continuous infusion) for 10-14 days
Streptococcus:
Brain abscess: I.V.: 20-24 million units/day in divided doses with metronidazole
Endocarditis or osteomyelitis: I.V.: 3-4 million units every 4 hours for at least 4 weeks
Meningitis: I.V.: 3-4 million units every 4 hours for 2-3 weeks
Pregnancy (prophylaxis GBS): I.V.: 5-6 million units x 1 dose, then 2.5-3 million units every 4 hours until delivery
Skin and soft tissue: I.V.: 3-4 million units every 4 hours for 10 days
Toxic shock: I.V.: 24 million units/day in divided doses with clindamycin
Streptococcal pneumonia:
Meningitis: I.V.: 2-4 million units every 2-4 hours
Nonmeningitis: I.V.: 2-3 million units every 4 hours

(Continued)

Penicillin G (Parenteral/Aqueous) *(Continued)*

Whipple's disease: I.V.: 2 million units every 4 hours (with streptomycin) for 10-14 days, followed by oral trimethoprim/sulfamethoxazole or doxycycline for 1 year

Dosing interval in renal impairment:

Cl_{cr} >10 mL/minute: Administer full loading dose followed by 1/2 loading dose given every 4-5 hours

Cl_{cr} <10 mL/minute: Administer full loading dose followed by 1/2 loading dose given every 8-10 hours

Stability

Penicillin G potassium powder for injection should be stored below 86°F (30°C); following reconstitution, solution may be stored for up to 7 days under refrigeration. Premixed bags for infusion should be stored in the freezer (-20°C to -4°F); frozen bags may be thawed at room temperature or in refrigerator. Once thawed, solution is stable for 14 days if stored in refrigerator or for 24 hours when stored at room temperature. Do not re-freeze once thawed.

Penicillin G sodium powder for injection should be stored at controlled room temperature; reconstituted solution may be stored under refrigeration for up to 3 days.

Administration Administer I.M. by deep injection in the upper outer quadrant of the buttock

Monitoring Parameters Observe for signs and symptoms of anaphylaxis during first dose

Anesthesia and Critical Care Concerns/Other Considerations One million units is approximately equal to 625 mg.

Pregnancy Risk Factor B

Contraindications Hypersensitivity to penicillin or any component of the formulation

Warnings/Precautions Avoid intra-arterial administration or injection into or near major peripheral nerves or blood vessels since such injections may cause severe and/or permanent neurovascular damage; use with caution in patients with renal impairment (dosage reduction required), pre-existing seizure disorders, or with a history of hypersensitivity to cephalosporins

Adverse Reactions Frequency not defined.

Central nervous system: Convulsions, confusion, drowsiness, myoclonus, fever

Dermatologic: Rash

Endocrine & metabolic: Electrolyte imbalance

Hematologic: Positive Coombs' reaction, hemolytic anemia

Local: Injection site reaction, thrombophlebitis

Renal: Acute interstitial nephritis

Miscellaneous: Anaphylaxis, hypersensitivity reactions, Jarisch-Herxheimer reaction

Overdosage/Toxicology Symptoms of penicillin overdose include neuromuscular hypersensitivity (eg, agitation, hallucinations, asterixis, encephalopathy, confusion, and seizures). Electrolyte imbalance may occur if the preparation contains potassium or sodium salts, especially in renal failure. Treatment is supportive or symptom-directed.

Drug Interactions

Aminoglycosides: May be synergistic against selected organisms

Methotrexate: Penicillins may increase the exposure to methotrexate during concurrent therapy; monitor.

Oral contraceptives: Anecdotal reports suggesting decreased contraceptive efficacy with penicillins have been refuted by more rigorous scientific and clinical data.

Probenecid, disulfiram: May increase penicillin levels

Tetracyclines: May decrease penicillin effectiveness

Warfarin: Effects of warfarin may be increased

Test Interactions False-positive or negative urinary glucose determination using Clinitest®; positive Coombs' [direct]; false-positive urinary and/or serum proteins

Dietary Considerations

Injection powder for reconstitution as potassium contains sodium 6.8 mg (0.3 mEq) and potassium 65.6 mg (1.68 mEq) per 1 million units

Dosage Forms

Infusion, as potassium [premixed iso-osmotic dextrose solution, frozen]: 1 million units (50 mL), 2 million units (50 mL), 3 million units (50 mL) [contains sodium 1.02 mEq and potassium 1.7 mEq per 1 million units]

Injection, powder for reconstitution, as potassium (Pfizerpen®): 5 million units, 20 million units [contains sodium 6.8 mg (0.3 mEq) and potassium 65.6 mg (1.68 mEq) per 1 million units]

Injection, powder for reconstitution, as sodium: 5 million units [contains sodium 1.68 mEq per 1 million units]

References

Gilbert DN, Moellering RC, Eliopoulos GM, et al, eds, *The Sanford Guide To Antimicrobial Therapy*, 2006, 36th ed, Hyde Park, VT: Antimicrobial Therapy, Inc, 2006, 6-7.

Tunkel AR, Hartman BJ, Kaplan SL, et al, "Practice Guidelines for the Management of Bacterial Meningitis," *Clin Infect Dis*, 2004, 39(9):1267-84.

◆ **Penicillin G Potassium** *see* Penicillin G (Parenteral/Aqueous) *on page 994*

◆ **Penicillin G Sodium** *see* Penicillin G (Parenteral/Aqueous) *on page 994*

◆ **Pennsaid® (Can)** *see* Diclofenac *on page 378*

◆ **Pentahydrate** *see* Sodium Thiosulfate *on page 1195*

◆ **Pentam-300®** *see* Pentamidine *on page 997*

Pentamidine (pen TAM i deen)

U.S. Brand Names NebuPent®; Pentam-300®

Synonyms Pentamidine Isethionate

Pharmacologic Category Antibiotic, Miscellaneous

Generic Available No

Use Treatment and prevention of pneumonia caused by *Pneumocystis carinii* (PCP)

Unlabeled/Investigational Use Treatment of trypanosomiasis and visceral leishmaniasis

Mechanism of Action Interferes with RNA/DNA, phospholipids and protein synthesis, through inhibition of oxidative phosphorylation and/or interference with incorporation of nucleotides and nucleic acids into RNA and DNA, in protozoa

Pharmacodynamics/Kinetics

Absorption: I.M.: Well absorbed; Inhalation: Limited systemic absorption

Half-life elimination: Terminal: 6.4-9.4 hours; may be prolonged with severe renal impairment

Excretion: Urine (33% to 66% as unchanged drug)

Dosage

Children:

Treatment of PCP pneumonia: I.M., I.V. (I.V. preferred): 4 mg/kg/day once daily for 10-14 days

Prevention of PCP pneumonia:

I.M., I.V.: 4 mg/kg monthly or every 2 weeks

Inhalation (aerosolized pentamidine in children ≥5 years): 300 mg/dose given every 3-4 weeks via Respirgard® II inhaler (8 mg/kg dose has also been used in children <5 years)

Treatment of trypanosomiasis (unlabeled use): I.V.: 4 mg/kg/day once daily for 10 days

Adults:

Treatment: I.M., I.V. (I.V. preferred): 4 mg/kg/day once daily for 14-21 days

Prevention: Inhalation: 300 mg every 4 weeks via Respirgard® II nebulizer

Dialysis: Not removed by hemo or peritoneal dialysis or continuous arteriovenous or venovenous hemofiltration; supplemental dosage is not necessary

Dosing adjustment in renal impairment: Adults: I.V.:

Cl_{cr} 10-50 mL/minute: Administer 4 mg/kg every 24-36 hours

Cl_{cr} <10 mL/minute: Administer 4 mg/kg every 48 hours

Stability

Store intact vials at controlled room temperature and protect from light.

Reconstituted vials with SWFI (60-100 mg/mL) are stable for 48 hours at room temperature protected from light. Diluted solutions in 50-250 mL D_5W for infusion (1-2.5 mg/mL) are stable for at least 24 hours at room temperature.

Powder for inhalation should be reconstituted with SWFI (6 mL per 300 mg vial).

Powder for injection may be reconstituted with SWFI or D_5W (SWFI should be used for I.M. injections). **Do not use NS as a diluent.**

(Continued)

Pentamidine *(Continued)*

Administration

I.V.: Infuse slowly over a period of at least 60 minutes or administer deep I.M.
Inhalation: Deliver until nebulizer is gone (30-45 minutes)

Monitoring Parameters Liver function tests, renal function tests, blood glucose, serum potassium and calcium, ECG, blood pressure

Pregnancy Risk Factor C

Contraindications Hypersensitivity to pentamidine isethionate or any component of the formulation (inhalation and injection)

Warnings/Precautions Use with caution in patients with diabetes mellitus, renal or hepatic dysfunction, hyper-/hypotension, leukopenia, thrombocytopenia, asthma, or hypo-/hyperglycemia.

Adverse Reactions

Inhalation:

>10%:

Cardiovascular: Chest pain
Dermatologic: Rash
Respiratory: Wheezing, dyspnea, cough, pharyngitis

1% to 10%: Gastrointestinal: Bitter or metallic taste

<1% (Limited to important or life-threatening): Hypoglycemia, renal insufficiency

Systemic:

>10%:

Cardiovascular: Hypotension
Dermatologic: Rash
Endocrine & metabolic: Hyperglycemia or hypoglycemia
Gastrointestinal: Nausea, vomiting, anorexia, diarrhea
Hematologic: Leukopenia or neutropenia, thrombocytopenia
Hepatic: Elevated LFTs
Renal: Nephrotoxicity

1% to 10%:

Cardiovascular: Cardiac arrhythmia
Gastrointestinal: Pancreatitis, metallic taste
Hematologic: Anemia
Local: Local reactions at injection site

<1% (Limited to important or life-threatening): Arrhythmias

Overdosage/Toxicology Symptoms of overdose include hypotension, hypoglycemia, and cardiac arrhythmias. Treatment is supportive.

Drug Interactions Substrate of CYP2C19 (major); **Inhibits** CYP2C8/9 (weak), 2C19 (weak), 2D6 (weak), 3A4 (weak)

CYP2C19 inducers: May decrease the levels/effects of pentamidine. Example inducers include aminoglutethimide, carbamazepine, phenytoin, and rifampin.

CYP2C19 inhibitors: May increase the levels/effects of pentamidine. Example inhibitors include delavirdine, fluconazole, fluvoxamine, gemfibrozil, isoniazid, omeprazole, and ticlopidine.

QT_c-prolonging agents: Pentamidine may potentiate the effect of other drugs which prolong QT interval (cisapride, sparfloxacin, gatifloxacin, moxifloxacin, pimozide, and type Ia and type III antiarrhythmics).

Ethanol/Nutrition/Herb Interactions Ethanol: Avoid ethanol (may increase CNS depression or aggravate hypoglycemia).

Dosage Forms

Injection, powder for reconstitution, as isethionate (Pentam-300®): 300 mg
Powder for nebulization, as isethionate (NebuPent®): 300 mg

♦ **Pentamidine Isethionate** *see* Pentamidine *on page 997*
♦ **Pentamycetin® (Can)** *see* Chloramphenicol *on page 262*
♦ **Pentaspan®** *see* Pentastarch *on page 998*

Pentastarch (PEN ta starch)

U.S. Brand Names Pentaspan®
Canadian Brand Names Pentaspan®
Pharmacologic Category Blood Modifiers
Generic Available No
Use Orphan drug: Adjunct in leukapheresis to improve harvesting and increase yield of leukocytes by centrifugal means

Dosage 250-700 mL to which citrate anticoagulant has been added is administered by adding to the input line of the centrifugation apparatus at a ratio of 1:8-1:13 to venous whole blood

Dosage Forms Infusion [premixed in NS]: 10% (500 mL)

Pentobarbital (pen toe BAR bi tal)

Medication Safety Issues

Sound-alike/look-alike issues:

Pentobarbital may be confused with phenobarbital

Nembutal® may be confused with Myambutol®

Related Information

Anesthesia Considerations for Neurosurgery *on page 1401*

Epilepsy *on page 1604*

U.S. Brand Names Nembutal®

Canadian Brand Names Nembutal® Sodium

Synonyms Pentobarbital Sodium

Pharmacologic Category Anticonvulsant, Barbiturate; Barbiturate

Restrictions C-II

Generic Available No

Use Sedative/hypnotic; preanesthetic; high-dose barbiturate coma for treatment of increased intracranial pressure or status epilepticus unresponsive to other therapy

Mechanism of Action Short-acting barbiturate with sedative, hypnotic, and anticonvulsant properties. Barbiturates depress the sensory cortex, decrease motor activity, alter cerebellar function, and produce drowsiness, sedation, and hypnosis. In high doses, barbiturates exhibit anticonvulsant activity; barbiturates produce dose-dependent respiratory depression.

Pharmacodynamics/Kinetics

Onset of action: I.M.: 10-15 minutes; I.V.: ~1 minute

Duration: I.V.: 15 minutes

Distribution: V_d: Children: 0.8 L/kg; Adults: 1 L/kg

Protein binding: 35% to 55%

Metabolism: Extensively hepatic via hydroxylation and oxidation pathways

Half-life elimination: Terminal: Children: 25 hours; Adults: Healthy: 22 hours (range: 15-50 hours)

Excretion: Urine (<1% as unchanged drug)

Dosage

Children:

Hypnotic: I.M.: 2-6 mg/kg; maximum: 100 mg/dose

Preoperative/preprocedure sedation: ≥6 months:

Note: Limited information is available for infants <6 months of age.

I.M.: 2-6 mg/kg; maximum: 100 mg/dose

I.V.: 1-3 mg/kg to a maximum of 100 mg until asleep

Conscious sedation prior to a procedure: Children 5-12 years: I.V.: 2 mg/kg 5-10 minutes before procedures, may repeat one time

Adolescents: Conscious sedation: I.V.: 100 mg prior to a procedure

Children and Adults: Barbiturate coma in head injury patients: I.V.: Loading dose: 5-10 mg/kg given slowly over 1-2 hours; monitor blood pressure and respiratory rate; Maintenance infusion: Initial: 1 mg/kg/hour; may increase to 2-3 mg/kg/hour; maintain burst suppression on EEG

Status epilepticus: I.V.: **Note**: Intubation required; monitor hemodynamics

Children: Loading dose: 5-15 mg/kg given slowly over 1-2 hours; maintenance infusion: 0.5-5 mg/kg/hour

Adults: Loading dose: 2-15 mg/kg given slowly over 1-2 hours; maintenance infusion: 0.5-3 mg/kg/hour

Adults:

Hypnotic:

I.M.: 150-200 mg

I.V.: Initial: 100 mg, may repeat every 1-3 minutes up to 200-500 mg total dose

Preoperative sedation: I.M.: 150-200 mg

Dosing adjustment in hepatic impairment: Reduce dosage in patients with severe liver dysfunction

(Continued)

Pentobarbital *(Continued)*

Stability Protect from freezing; aqueous solutions are not stable, commercially available vehicle (containing propylene glycol) is more stable; low pH may cause precipitate; use only clear solution

Administration Pentobarbital may be administered by deep I.M. or slow I.V. injection.

I.M.: No more than 5 mL (250 mg) should be injected at any one site because of possible tissue irritation.

I.V.: I.V. push doses can be given undiluted, but should be administered no faster than 50 mg/minute; parenteral solutions are highly alkaline; avoid extravasation; avoid rapid I.V. administration >50 mg/minute; avoid intra-arterial injection

Monitoring Parameters Respiratory status (for conscious sedation, includes pulse oximetry), cardiovascular status, CNS status; cardiac monitor and blood pressure monitor required

Reference Range

Therapeutic:

Hypnotic: 1-5 mcg/mL (SI: 4-22 μmol/L)

Coma: 10-50 mcg/mL (SI: 88-221 μmol/L)

Toxic: >10 mcg/mL (SI: >44 μmol/L)

Anesthesia and Critical Care Concerns/Other Considerations Pentobarbital 50 mg/mL contains propylene glycol 414.4 mg/mL (40% v/v).

Pentobarbital is one of the standard choices for refractory status epilepticus. Most patients will require systemic and pulmonary arterial catheterization with fluid and vasoactive therapy to maintain blood pressure. High-dose pentobarbital generally produces poikilothermia. Maintenance anticonvulsant treatment may be substantial in order to wean pentobarbital. High doses of barbiturates are potentially immunosuppressive; guard against infection.

Pregnancy Risk Factor D

Contraindications Hypersensitivity to barbiturates or any component of the formulation; marked hepatic impairment; dyspnea or airway obstruction; porphyria; pregnancy

Warnings/Precautions Tolerance to hypnotic effect can occur; do not use for >2 weeks to treat insomnia. Potential for drug dependency exists, abrupt cessation may precipitate withdrawal, including status epilepticus in epileptic patients. Do not administer to patients in acute pain. Use caution in elderly, debilitated, renally impaired, hepatic dysfunction, or pediatric patients. May cause paradoxical responses, including agitation and hyperactivity, particularly in acute pain and pediatric patients. Use with caution in patients with depression or suicidal tendencies, or in patients with a history of drug abuse. Tolerance, psychological and physical dependence may occur with prolonged use.

May cause CNS depression, which may impair physical or mental abilities. Patients must be cautioned about performing tasks which require mental alertness (eg, operating machinery or driving). Effects with other sedative drugs or ethanol may be potentiated. Use of this agent as a hypnotic in the elderly is not recommended due to its long half-life and potential for physical and psychological dependence.

May cause respiratory depression or hypotension, particularly when administered intravenously. Use with caution in hemodynamically unstable patients or patients with respiratory disease. High doses (loading doses of 15-35 mg/kg given over 1-2 hours) have been utilized to induce pentobarbital coma, but these higher doses often cause hypotension requiring vasopressor therapy.

Adverse Reactions Frequency not defined.

Cardiovascular: Bradycardia, hypotension, syncope

Central nervous system: Drowsiness, lethargy, CNS excitation or depression, impaired judgment, "hangover" effect, confusion, somnolence, agitation, hyperkinesia, ataxia, nervousness, headache, insomnia, nightmares, hallucinations, anxiety, dizziness

Dermatologic: Rash, exfoliative dermatitis, Stevens-Johnson syndrome

Gastrointestinal: Nausea, vomiting, constipation

Hematologic: Agranulocytosis, thrombocytopenia, megaloblastic anemia

Local: Pain at injection site, thrombophlebitis with I.V. use

Renal: Oliguria

Respiratory: Laryngospasm, respiratory depression, apnea (especially with rapid I.V. use), hypoventilation

Miscellaneous: Gangrene with inadvertent intra-arterial injection

Overdosage/Toxicology Symptoms of overdose include unsteady gait, slurred speech, confusion, jaundice, hypothermia, hypotension, respiratory depression, and coma. Treat symptomatically. Charcoal hemoperfusion may be beneficial in stage IV coma due to high serum concentration.

Drug Interactions Induces CYP2A6 (strong), 3A4 (strong)

Acetaminophen: Barbiturates may enhance the hepatotoxic potential of acetaminophen overdoses

Antiarrhythmics: Barbiturates may increase the metabolism of antiarrhythmics, decreasing their clinical effect; includes disopyramide, propafenone, and quinidine

Anticonvulsants: Barbiturates may increase the metabolism of anticonvulsants; includes ethosuximide, felbamate (possibly), lamotrigine, phenytoin, tiagabine, topiramate, and zonisamide; does not appear to affect gabapentin or levetiracetam

Antineoplastics: Limited evidence suggests that enzyme-inducing anticonvulsant therapy may reduce the effectiveness of some chemotherapy regimens (specifically in ALL); teniposide and methotrexate may be cleared more rapidly in these patients

Antipsychotics: Barbiturates may enhance the metabolism (decrease the efficacy) of antipsychotics; monitor for altered response; dose adjustment may be needed

Beta-blockers: Metabolism of beta-blockers may be increased and clinical effect decreased; atenolol and nadolol are unlikely to interact given their renal elimination

Calcium channel blockers: Barbiturates may enhance the metabolism of calcium channel blockers, decreasing their clinical effect

Chloramphenicol: Barbiturates may increase the metabolism of chloramphenicol and chloramphenicol may inhibit barbiturate metabolism; monitor for altered response

Cimetidine: Barbiturates may enhance the metabolism of cimetidine, decreasing its clinical effect

CNS depressants: Sedative effects and/or respiratory depression with barbiturates may be additive with other CNS depressants; monitor for increased effect; includes ethanol, sedatives, antidepressants, narcotic analgesics, and benzodiazepines

Corticosteroids: Barbiturates may enhance the metabolism of corticosteroids, decreasing their clinical effect

Cyclosporine: Levels may be decreased by barbiturates; monitor

CYP2A6 substrates: Pentobarbital may decrease the levels/effects of CYP2A6 substrates. Example substrates include ifosfamide and rifampin.

CYP3A4 substrates: Pentobarbital may decrease the levels/effects of CYP3A4 substrates. Example substrates include benzodiazepines, calcium channel blockers, clarithromycin, cyclosporine, erythromycin, estrogens, mirtazapine, nateglinide, nefazodone, nevirapine, protease inhibitors, tacrolimus, and venlafaxine.

Doxycycline: Barbiturates may enhance the metabolism of doxycycline, decreasing its clinical effect; higher dosages may be required

Estrogens: Barbiturates may increase the metabolism of estrogens and reduce their efficacy

Felbamate may inhibit the metabolism of barbiturates and barbiturates may increase the metabolism of felbamate

Griseofulvin: Barbiturates may impair the absorption of griseofulvin, and griseofulvin metabolism may be increased by barbiturates, decreasing clinical effect

Guanfacine: Effect may be decreased by barbiturates

Immunosuppressants: Barbiturates may enhance the metabolism of immunosuppressants, decreasing its clinical effect; includes both cyclosporine and tacrolimus

Loop diuretics: Metabolism may be increased and clinical effects decreased; established for furosemide, effect with other loop diuretics not established

MAO inhibitors: Metabolism of barbiturates may be inhibited, increasing clinical effect or toxicity of the barbiturates

Methadone: Barbiturates may enhance the metabolism of methadone resulting in methadone withdrawal

Methoxyflurane: Barbiturates may enhance the nephrotoxic effects of methoxyflurane

(Continued)

Pentobarbital *(Continued)*

Oral contraceptives: Barbiturates may enhance the metabolism of oral contraceptives, decreasing their clinical effect; an alternative method of contraception should be considered

Theophylline: Barbiturates may increase metabolism of theophylline derivatives and decrease their clinical effect

Tricyclic antidepressants: Barbiturates may increase metabolism of tricyclic antidepressants and decrease their clinical effect; sedative effects may be additive

Valproic acid: Metabolism of barbiturates may be inhibited by valproic acid; monitor for excessive sedation; a dose reduction may be needed

Warfarin: Barbiturates inhibit the hypoprothrombinemic effects of oral anticoagulants via increased metabolism; this combination should generally be avoided

Ethanol/Nutrition/Herb Interactions Ethanol: Avoid ethanol (may increase CNS depression).

Dosage Forms Injection, solution, as sodium: 50 mg/mL (20 mL, 50 mL) [contains alcohol 10% and propylene glycol 40%]

References

Chapman MG, Smith M, and Hirsch NP, "Status Epilepticus," *Anaesthesia*, 2001, 56(7):648-59.

Fischer JH and Raineri DL, "Pentobarbital Anesthesia for Status Epilepticus," *Clin Pharm*, 1987, 6(8):601-2.

Hubbard AM, Markowitz RI, Kimmel B, et al, "Sedation for Pediatric Patients Undergoing CT and MRI," *J Comput Assist Tomogr*, 1992, 16(1):3-6.

Manno EM, "New Management Strategies in the Treatment of Status Epilepticus," *Mayo Clin Proc*, 2003, 78(4):508-18.

- **Pentobarbital Sodium** *see* Pentobarbital *on page 999*
- **Pentothal®** *see* Thiopental *on page 1257*
- **Pepcid®** *see* Famotidine *on page 506*
- **Pepcid® AC [OTC]** *see* Famotidine *on page 506*
- **Pepcid® I.V. (Can)** *see* Famotidine *on page 506*
- **Percocet®** *see* Oxycodone and Acetaminophen *on page 969*
- **Percocet®-Demi (Can)** *see* Oxycodone and Acetaminophen *on page 969*
- **Percodan®** *see* Oxycodone and Aspirin *on page 971*
- **Periactin** *see* Cyproheptadine *on page 344*
- **Peridex®** *see* Chlorhexidine Gluconate *on page 267*
- **Peridol (Can)** *see* Haloperidol *on page 604*

Perindopril Erbumine (per IN doe pril er BYOO meen)

U.S. Brand Names Aceon®

Canadian Brand Names Coversyl®

Pharmacologic Category Angiotensin-Converting Enzyme (ACE) Inhibitor

Generic Available No

Use Treatment of essential hypertension; reduction of cardiovascular mortality or nonfatal myocardial infarction in patients with stable coronary artery disease

Unlabeled/Investigational Use As a class, ACE inhibitors are recommended in the treatment of congestive heart failure with left ventricular dysfunction.

Mechanism of Action Perindopril is a prodrug for perindoprilat, which acts as a competitive inhibitor of angiotensin-converting enzyme (ACE); prevents conversion of angiotensin I to angiotensin II, a potent vasoconstrictor; results in lower levels of angiotensin II which, in turn, causes an increase in plasma renin activity and a reduction in aldosterone secretion

Pharmacodynamics/Kinetics

Onset of action: Peak effect: 1-2 hours

Distribution: Small amounts enter breast milk

Protein binding: Perindopril: 60%; Perindoprilat: 10% to 20%

Metabolism: Hepatically hydrolyzed to active metabolite, perindoprilat (~17% to 20% of a dose) and other inactive metabolites

Bioavailability: Perindopril: 75%; Perindoprilat ~25% (~16% with food)

Half-life elimination: Parent drug: 1.5-3 hours; Metabolite: Effective: 3-10 hours, Terminal: 30-120 hours

Time to peak: Chronic therapy: Perindopril: 1 hour; Perindoprilat: 3-7 hours (maximum perindoprilat serum levels are 2-3 times higher and T_{max} is shorter following chronic therapy); CHF: Perindoprilat: 6 hours

Excretion: Urine (75%, 4% to 12% as unchanged drug)

Dosage Oral:

Adults:

Essential hypertension: Initial: 4 mg/day but may be titrated to response; usual range: 4-8 mg/day (may be given in 2 divided doses); increase at 1- to 2-week intervals (maximum: 16 mg/day)

Concomitant therapy with diuretics: To reduce the risk of hypotension, discontinue diuretic, if possible, 2-3 days prior to initiating perindopril. If unable to stop diuretic, initiate perindopril at 2-4 mg/day and monitor blood pressure closely for the first 2 weeks of therapy, and after any dose adjustment of perindopril or diuretic.

Stable coronary artery disease: Initial: 4 mg once daily for 2 weeks; increase as tolerated to 8 mg once daily.

Congestive heart failure (unlabeled use): Initial: 2 mg once daily; increase at 1- to 2-week intervals; target dose: 8-16 mg once daily (ACC/AHA 2005 Heart Failure Guidelines)

Elderly:

Essential hypertension: >65 years of age: Initial: 4 mg/day; maintenance: 8 mg/day

Stable coronary artery disease: >70 years of age: Initial: 2 mg/day for 1 week; increase as tolerated to 4 mg/day for 1 week; then increase as tolerated to 8 mg/day

Dosing adjustment in renal impairment:

Cl_{cr} >30 mL/minute: Initial: 2 mg/day; maintenance dosing not to exceed 8 mg/day

Cl_{cr} <30 mL/minute: Safety and efficacy not established.

Hemodialysis: Perindopril and its metabolites are dialyzable

Dosing adjustment in hepatic impairment: None needed

Stability Store at room temperature of 20°C to 25°C (68°F to 77°F); protect from moisture

Monitoring Parameters Serum creatinine, electrolytes, and WBC with differential initially and repeated at 2-week intervals for at least 90 days; urinalysis for protein

Pregnancy Risk Factor C (1st trimester) / D (2nd and 3rd trimesters)

Contraindications Hypersensitivity to perindopril or any component of the formulation; angioedema related to previous treatment with an ACE inhibitor; bilateral renal artery stenosis; pregnancy (2nd and 3rd trimesters)

Warnings/Precautions Anaphylactic reactions can occur. Angioedema can occur at any time during treatment (especially following first dose). It may involve head and neck (potentially affecting the airway) or the intestine (presenting with abdominal pain). Prolonged monitoring may be required especially if tongue, glottis, or larynx are involved as they are associated with airway obstruction. Those with a history of airway surgery in this situation have a higher risk. Careful blood pressure monitoring with first dose (hypotension can occur especially in volume- and/or salt-depleted patients); caution in patients receiving hypotensive-inducing anesthesia. **[U.S. Boxed Warning]: Based on human data, ACEIs can cause injury and death to the developing fetus when used in the second and third trimesters. ACEIs should be discontinued as soon as possible once pregnancy is detected.** Dosage adjustment needed in renal impairment. Avoid rapid dosage escalation, which may lead to renal insufficiency. Use with caution in unilateral renal artery stenosis and pre-existing renal insufficiency.

Use with caution in hypovolemia; collagen vascular diseases; valvular stenosis (particularly aortic stenosis); concomitant use with potassium-sparing agents, potassium supplements or salt substitutes not recommended; risk of hyperkalemia may be increased with renal insufficiency. Rare toxicities associated with ACE inhibitors include cholestatic jaundice (which may progress to hepatic necrosis) and neutropenia/agranulocytosis with myeloid hyperplasia. If patient has renal impairment then a baseline WBC with differential and serum creatinine should be evaluated and monitored closely during the first 3 months of therapy. Hypersensitivity reactions may be seen during hemodialysis with high-flux dialysis membranes (eg, AN69). Safety and efficacy in pediatric patients have not been established.

Adverse Reactions

>10%:

Central nervous system: Headache (24%)

Respiratory: Cough (incidence is higher in women, 3:1) (12%)

(Continued)

Perindopril Erbumine *(Continued)*

1% to 10%:

Cardiovascular: Edema (4%), chest pain (2%)), ECG abnormal (2%), palpitation (1%)

Central nervous system: Dizziness (8%, less than placebo), sleep disorders (3%), depression (2%), fever (2%), nervousness (1%), somnolence (1%)

Dermatologic: Rash (2%)

Endocrine & metabolic: Hyperkalemia (1%, less than placebo), triglycerides increased (1%), menstrual disorder (1%)

Gastrointestinal: Nausea (2%), diarrhea (4%), vomiting (2%), dyspepsia (2%), abdominal pain (3%), flatulence (1%)

Genitourinary: Urinary tract infection (3%), sexual dysfunction (male 1%)

Hepatic: Increased ALT (2%)

Neuromuscular & skeletal: Weakness (8%), back pain (6%), lower extremity pain (5%), upper extremity pain (3%), hypertonia (3%), paresthesia (2%), joint pain (1%), myalgia (1%), arthritis (1%), neck pain (1%)

Renal: Proteinuria (2%)

Respiratory: Upper respiratory tract infection (9%), sinusitis (5%), rhinitis (5%), pharyngitis (3%)

Otic: Tinnitus (2%), ear infection (1%)

Miscellaneous: Viral infection (3%), allergy (2%)

Note: Some reactions occurred at an incidence >1% but ≤ placebo.

<1% (Limited to important or life-threatening): Amnesia, anaphylaxis, angioedema, anxiety, dyspnea, erythema, gout, migraine, MI, nephrolithiasis, orthostatic hypotension, pruritus, psychosocial disorder, pulmonary fibrosis, purpura, stroke, syncope, urinary retention, vertigo

Additional adverse effects that have been reported with **ACE inhibitors** include agranulocytosis (especially in patients with renal impairment or collagen vascular disease), neutropenia, anemia, bullous pemphigus, cardiac arrest, eosinophilic pneumonitis, exfoliative dermatitis, hepatic failure, hyponatremia, jaundice, pancreatitis (acute), pancytopenia, thrombocytopenia; decreases in creatinine clearance in some elderly hypertensive patients or those with chronic renal failure, and worsening of renal function in patients with bilateral renal artery stenosis or hypovolemic patients (diuretic therapy). In addition, a syndrome which may include fever, myalgia, arthralgia, interstitial nephritis, vasculitis, rash, eosinophilia and positive ANA, and elevated ESR has been reported with ACE inhibitors.

Overdosage/Toxicology Mild hypotension has been the primary toxic effect seen with acute overdose. Bradycardia may also occur. Hyperkalemia occurs even with therapeutic doses, especially in patients with renal insufficiency and those taking NSAIDs. Treatment is symptom-directed and supportive. Hemodialysis may be beneficial.

Drug Interactions

Allopurinol: ACE inhibitors may increase hypersensitivity reactions to allopurinol; monitor for at least 5 weeks following initiation of allopurinol.

Alpha$_1$ blockers: Hypotensive effect increased.

Aspirin: The effects of ACE inhibitors may be blunted by aspirin administration, particularly at higher dosages and/or increase adverse renal effects.

Cyclosporine: ACE inhibitors may increase nephrotoxicity of cyclosporine; monitor.

Diuretics: Hypovolemia due to diuretics may precipitate acute hypotensive events or acute renal failure.

Insulin: Risk of hypoglycemia may be increased.

Lithium: Risk of lithium toxicity may be increased; monitor lithium levels, especially the first 4 weeks of therapy.

Mercaptopurine: Risk of neutropenia may be increased.

NSAIDs: May attenuate hypertensive efficacy; effect has been seen with captopril and may occur with other ACE inhibitors; monitor blood pressure. May increase risk of renal effects.

Potassium-sparing diuretics (amiloride, eplerenone, spironolactone, triamterene): Increased risk of hyperkalemia.

Potassium supplements may increase the risk of hyperkalemia.

Trimethoprim (high dose) may increase the risk of hyperkalemia.

Ethanol/Nutrition/Herb Interactions

Food: Perindopril active metabolite concentrations may be lowered if taken with food.

Herb/Nutraceutical: Avoid dong quai if using for hypertension (has estrogenic activity). Avoid ephedra, yohimbe, ginseng (may worsen hypertension). Avoid garlic (may have increased antihypertensive effect).

Dosage Forms Tablet: 2 mg, 4 mg, 8 mg

- **PerioChip®** *see* Chlorhexidine Gluconate *on page 267*
- **PerioGard®** *see* Chlorhexidine Gluconate *on page 267*
- **Periostat®** *see* Doxycycline *on page 426*
- **Persantine®** *see* Dipyridamole *on page 402*
- **Pethidine Hydrochloride** *see* Meperidine *on page 801*
- **Pexeva®** *see* Paroxetine *on page 988*
- **Pexicam® (Can)** *see* Piroxicam *on page 1032*
- **Pfizerpen®** *see* Penicillin G (Parenteral/Aqueous) *on page 994*
- **PGE_1** *see* Alprostadil *on page 68*
- **PGI_2** *see* Epoprostenol *on page 467*
- **PGX** *see* Epoprostenol *on page 467*
- **Phenadoz™** *see* Promethazine *on page 1064*
- **Phenaseptic [OTC]** *see* Phenol *on page 1012*

Phenelzine (FEN el zeen)

Medication Safety Issues

Sound-alike/look-alike issues:

Phenelzine may be confused with phenytoin

Nardil® may be confused with Norinyl®

Related Information

Antidepressant Agents *on page 1551*

U.S. Brand Names Nardil®

Canadian Brand Names Nardil®

Synonyms Phenelzine Sulfate

Pharmacologic Category Antidepressant, Monoamine Oxidase Inhibitor

Restrictions A medication guide concerning the use of antidepressants in children and teenagers can be found on the FDA website at http://www.fda.gov/cder/Offices/ODS/labeling.htm. It should be dispensed to parents or guardians of children and teenagers receiving this medication.

Generic Available No

Use Symptomatic treatment of atypical, nonendogenous, or neurotic depression

Unlabeled/Investigational Use Selective mutism

Mechanism of Action Thought to act by increasing endogenous concentrations of norepinephrine, dopamine, and serotonin through inhibition of the enzyme (monoamine oxidase) responsible for the breakdown of these neurotransmitters

Pharmacodynamics/Kinetics

Onset of action: Therapeutic: 2-4 weeks; geriatric patients receiving an average of 55 mg/day developed a mean platelet MAO activity inhibition of about 85%.

Duration: May continue to have a therapeutic effect and interactions 2 weeks after discontinuing therapy

Absorption: Well absorbed

Metabolism: Oxidized via monoamine oxidase (primary pathway) and acetylation (minor pathway)

Half-life elimination: 11 hours

Excretion: Urine (primarily as metabolites and unchanged drug)

Dosage Oral:

Children: Selective mutism (unlabeled use): 30-60 mg/day

Adults: Depression: 15 mg 3 times/day; may increase to 60-90 mg/day during early phase of treatment, then reduce dose for maintenance therapy slowly after maximum benefit is obtained; takes 2-4 weeks for a significant response to occur

Elderly: Depression: Initial: 7.5 mg/day; increase by 7.5-15 mg/day every 3-4 days as tolerated; usual therapeutic dose: 15-60 mg/day in 3-4 divided doses

Stability Protect from light

Monitoring Parameters Blood pressure, heart rate, diet, weight, mood (if depressive symptoms)

(Continued)

Phenelzine *(Continued)*

Anesthesia and Critical Care Concerns/Other Considerations Pyridoxine deficiency has occurred; symptoms include numbness and edema of hands (may respond to supplementation). Avoid food containing tyramine. The MAO inhibitors are usually reserved for patients who do not tolerate or respond to other antidepressants.

Pregnancy Risk Factor C

Contraindications Hypersensitivity to phenelzine or any component of the formulation; uncontrolled hypertension; pheochromocytoma; hepatic disease; congestive heart failure; concurrent use of sympathomimetics (and related compounds), CNS depressants, ethanol, meperidine, bupropion, buspirone, guanethidine, serotonergic drugs (including SSRIs) - do not use within 5 weeks of fluoxetine discontinuation or 2 weeks of other antidepressant discontinuation; general anesthesia, local vasoconstrictors; spinal anesthesia (hypotension may be exaggerated); foods with a high content of tyramine, tryptophan, or dopamine, chocolate, or caffeine (may cause hypertensive crisis)

Warnings/Precautions Safety in children <16 years of age has not been established; use with caution in patients who are hyperactive, hyperexcitable, or who have glaucoma, hyperthyroidism, suicidal tendencies, or diabetes; avoid use of meperidine within 2 weeks of phenelzine use. Hypertensive crisis may occur with tyramine, tryptophan, or dopamine-containing foods. Should not be used in combination with other antidepressants. Hypotensive effects of antihypertensives (beta-blockers, thiazides) may be exaggerated. Use with caution in depressed patients at risk of suicide. May cause orthostatic hypotension - use with caution in patients with hypotension or patients who would not tolerate transient hypotensive episodes (cardiovascular or cerebrovascular disease) - effects may be additive with other agents which cause orthostasis. Has been associated with activation of hypomania and/or mania in bipolar patients. May worsen psychotic symptoms in some patients. Use with caution in patients at risk of seizures, or in patients

Tyramine-Containing Foods

	Cheese/Dairy Products	
American processed Blue Boursault Brick, natural Brie Camembert	Cheddar Emmenthaler Gruyere Mozzarella Parmesan Romano	Roquefort Sour cream Stilton Yogurt
	Meat/Fish	
Beef or chicken liver, other meats, fish (unrefrigerated, fermented) Meats prepared with tenderizer	Fermented sausages (bologna, pepperoni, salami, summer sausage) Game meat	Caviar Dried fish (salted herring) Herring, pickled, spoiled Shrimp paste
	Alcoholic Beverages (Undistilled)	
Beer and ale (imports, some nonalcoholic)	Red wine (especially Chianti)	Sherry
	Fruit/Vegetables	
Avocados (especially overripe) Yeast extracts (Marmite, etc)	Bananas Figs, canned (overripe) Raisins	Soy sauce Miso soup Bean curd
	Foods Containing Other Vasopressors	
Fava beans (overripe) — dopamine	Caffeine (eg, coffee, tea, colas) — caffeine	Chocolate — phenylethylamine Ginseng

receiving other drugs which may lower seizure threshold. Toxic reactions have occurred with dextromethorphan. Discontinue at least 48 hours prior to myelography.

The MAO inhibitors are effective and generally well tolerated by older patients. It is the potential interactions with tyramine or tryptophan-containing foods and other drugs, and their effects on blood pressure that have limited their use. See table for foods containing tyramine on previous page.

Adverse Reactions Frequency not defined.

Cardiovascular: Orthostatic hypotension, edema

Central nervous system: Dizziness, headache, drowsiness, sleep disturbances, fatigue, hyper-reflexia, twitching, ataxia, mania

Dermatologic: Rash, pruritus

Endocrine & metabolic: Decreased sexual ability (anorgasmia, ejaculatory disturbances, impotence), hypernatremia, hypermetabolic syndrome

Gastrointestinal: Xerostomia, constipation, weight gain

Genitourinary: Urinary retention

Hematologic: Leukopenia

Hepatic: Hepatitis

Neuromuscular & skeletal: Weakness, tremor, myoclonus

Ocular: Blurred vision, glaucoma

Miscellaneous: Diaphoresis

Overdosage/Toxicology Symptoms of overdose include tachycardia, palpitations, muscle twitching, seizures, insomnia, restlessness, transient hypertension, hypotension, drowsiness, hyperpyrexia, and coma. Treatment is symptom-directed and supportive.

Drug Interactions

Amphetamines: MAO inhibitors in combination with amphetamines may result in severe hypertensive reaction; concurrent use is contraindicated.

Anorexiants: Concurrent use of anorexiants may result in serotonin syndrome; these combinations are best avoided; includes dexfenfluramine, fenfluramine, or sibutramine

Barbiturates: MAO inhibitors may inhibit the metabolism of barbiturates and prolong their effect

Bupropion: Concurrent use is contraindicated; allow at least 14 days between discontinuing MAO inhibitor and starting bupropion.

Buspirone: May cause hypertension; wait at least 10 days between discontinuing one agent and starting the other.

CNS stimulants: MAO inhibitors in combination with stimulants (methylphenidate) may result in severe hypertensive reaction; concurrent use is contraindicated.

Dextromethorphan: Concurrent use of MAO inhibitors may result in serotonin syndrome; concurrent use is contraindicated.

Disulfiram: MAO inhibitors may produce delirium in patients receiving disulfiram; monitor.

Guanadrel and guanethidine: MAO inhibitors inhibit the antihypertensive response to guanadrel or guanethidine; concurrent use is contraindicated; use an alternative antihypertensive agent.

Hypoglycemic agents: MAO inhibitors may produce hypoglycemia in patients with diabetes; monitor.

Levodopa: MAO inhibitors in combination with levodopa may result in hypertensive reactions; monitor.

Lithium: MAO inhibitors in combination with lithium have resulted in malignant hyperpyrexia; this combination is best avoided.

Meperidine: May cause serotonin syndrome when combined with an MAO inhibitor; concurrent use is contraindicated; avoid use of meperidine within 2 weeks of phenelzine use.

Nefazodone: Concurrent use of MAO inhibitors may result in serotonin syndrome; these combinations are best avoided

Norepinephrine: MAO inhibitors may increase the pressor response of norepinephrine (effect is generally small); monitor

Reserpine: MAO inhibitors in combination with reserpine may result in hypertensive reactions; monitor

Serotonin agonists: Theoretically may increase the risk of serotonin syndrome; includes sumatriptan, naratriptan, rizatriptan, and zolmitriptan

SSRIs: May cause serotonin syndrome when combined with an MAO inhibitor; avoid this combination. Allow 5 weeks between discontinuing fluoxetine and starting an MAO inhibitor; allow at least 10 days after discontinuing MAO inhibitor and starting fluoxetine.

(Continued)

Phenelzine *(Continued)*

Succinylcholine: MAO inhibitors may prolong the muscle relaxation produced by succinylcholine via decreased plasma pseudocholinesterase

Sympathomimetics (indirect-acting): MAO inhibitors in combination with sympathomimetics such as dopamine, metaraminol, phenylephrine, and decongestants (pseudoephedrine) may result in severe hypertensive reaction; concurrent use is contraindicated.

Tramadol: May increase the risk of seizures and serotonin syndrome in patients receiving an MAO inhibitor

Trazodone: Concurrent use of MAO inhibitors may result in serotonin syndrome; these combinations are best avoided

Tricyclic antidepressants: May cause serotonin syndrome when combined with an MAO inhibitor; avoid this combination

Tyramine: Foods (eg, cheese) and beverages (eg, ethanol) containing tyramine, should be avoided in patients receiving an MAO inhibitor; hypertensive crisis may result

Venlafaxine: Concurrent use of MAO inhibitors may result in serotonin syndrome; these combinations are best avoided

Ethanol/Nutrition/Herb Interactions

Ethanol: Avoid ethanol (alcoholic beverages containing tyramine may induce a severe hypertensive response).

Food: Clinically-severe elevated blood pressure may occur if phenelzine is taken with tyramine-containing foods. Avoid foods containing tryptophan, dopamine, chocolate, or caffeine.

Dosage Forms Tablet: 15 mg

♦ **Phenelzine Sulfate** *see* Phenelzine *on page 1005*

♦ **Phenergan®** *see* Promethazine *on page 1064*

Phenobarbital (fee noe BAR bi tal)

Medication Safety Issues

Sound-alike/look-alike issues:

Phenobarbital may be confused with pentobarbital

Luminal® may be confused with Tuinal®

Related Information

Anesthesia Considerations for Neurosurgery *on page 1401*

Anesthesia for Patients With Liver Disease *on page 1421*

Epilepsy *on page 1604*

Perioperative Management of Patients on Antiseizure Medication *on page 1458*

U.S. Brand Names Luminal® Sodium

Canadian Brand Names PMS-Phenobarbital

Synonyms Phenobarbital Sodium; Phenobarbitone; Phenylethylmalonylurea

Pharmacologic Category Anticonvulsant, Barbiturate; Barbiturate

Restrictions C-IV

Generic Available Yes

Use Management of generalized tonic-clonic (grand mal) and partial seizures; sedative

Unlabeled/Investigational Use Febrile seizures in children; may also be used for prevention and treatment of neonatal hyperbilirubinemia and lowering of bilirubin in chronic cholestasis; neonatal seizures; management of sedative/hypnotic withdrawal

Mechanism of Action Short-acting barbiturate with sedative, hypnotic, and anticonvulsant properties. Barbiturates depress the sensory cortex, decrease motor activity, alter cerebellar function, and produce drowsiness, sedation, and hypnosis. In high doses, barbiturates exhibit anticonvulsant activity; barbiturates produce dose-dependent respiratory depression.

Pharmacodynamics/Kinetics

Onset of action: Oral: Hypnosis: 20-60 minutes; I.V.: ~5 minutes

Peak effect: I.V.: ~30 minutes

Duration: Oral: 6-10 hours; I.V.: 4-10 hours

Absorption: Oral: 70% to 90%

Protein binding: 20% to 45%; decreased in neonates

Metabolism: Hepatic via hydroxylation and glucuronide conjugation

Half-life elimination: Neonates: 45-500 hours; Infants: 20-133 hours; Children: 37-73 hours; Adults: 53-140 hours

Time to peak, serum: Oral: 1-6 hours

Excretion: Urine (20% to 50% as unchanged drug)

Dosage

Children:

Sedation: Oral: 2 mg/kg 3 times/day

Hypnotic: I.M., I.V., SubQ: 3-5 mg/kg at bedtime

Preoperative sedation: Oral, I.M., I.V.: 1-3 mg/kg 1-1.5 hours before procedure

Adults:

Sedation: Oral, I.M.: 30-120 mg/day in 2-3 divided doses

Hypnotic: Oral, I.M., I.V., SubQ: 100-320 mg at bedtime

Preoperative sedation: I.M.: 100-200 mg 1-1.5 hours before procedure

Anticonvulsant: Status epilepticus: **Loading dose:** I.V.:

Infants and Children: 10-20 mg/kg in a single or divided dose; in select patients may administer additional 5 mg/kg/dose every 15-30 minutes until seizure is controlled or a total dose of 40 mg/kg is reached

Adults: 300-800 mg initially followed by 120-240 mg/dose at 20-minute intervals until seizures are controlled or a total dose of 1-2 g

Anticonvulsant maintenance dose: Oral, I.V.:

Infants: 5-8 mg/kg/day in 1-2 divided doses

Children:

1-5 years: 6-8 mg/kg/day in 1-2 divided doses

5-12 years: 4-6 mg/kg/day in 1-2 divided doses

Children >12 years and Adults: 1-3 mg/kg/day in divided doses or 50-100 mg 2-3 times/day

Sedative/hypnotic withdrawal (unlabeled use): Initial daily requirement is determined by substituting phenobarbital 30 mg for every 100 mg pentobarbital used during tolerance testing; then daily requirement is decreased by 10% of initial dose

Dosing interval in renal impairment: Cl_{cr} <10 mL/minute: Administer every 12-16 hours

Hemodialysis: Moderately dialyzable (20% to 50%)

Dosing adjustment/comments in hepatic disease: Increased side effects may occur in severe liver disease; monitor plasma levels and adjust dose accordingly

Stability Protect elixir from light; not stable in aqueous solutions; use only clear solutions; do not add to acidic solutions, precipitation may occur; I.V. form is **incompatible** with benzquinamide (in syringe), cephalothin, chlorpromazine, hydralazine, hydrocortisone, hydroxyzine, insulin, levorphanol, meperidine, methadone, morphine, norepinephrine, pentazocine, prochlorperazine, promazine, promethazine, ranitidine (in syringe), vancomycin

Administration Avoid rapid I.V. administration >50 mg/minute; avoid intra-arterial injection; parenteral solutions are highly alkaline; avoid extravasation

Monitoring Parameters Phenobarbital serum concentrations, mental status, CBC, LFTs, seizure activity

Reference Range

Therapeutic:

Infants and children: 15-30 mcg/mL (SI: 65-129 μmol/L)

Adults: 20-40 mcg/mL (SI: 86-172 μmol/L)

Toxic: >40 mcg/mL (SI: >172 μmol/L)

Toxic concentration: Slowness, ataxia, nystagmus: 35-80 mcg/mL (SI: 150-344 μmol/L)

Coma with reflexes: 65-117 mcg/mL (SI: 279-502 μmol/L)

Coma without reflexes: >100 mcg/mL (SI: >430 μmol/L)

Anesthesia and Critical Care Concerns/Other Considerations Phenobarbital 65 mg/mL and 130 mg/mL each contains propylene glycol 702.4 mg/mL (67.8% v/v).

Status Epilepticus: A randomized, double-blind trial evaluated the efficacy of four treatments in overt status epilepticus. Treatment arms were designed based upon accepted practices of North American neurologists. The treatments were: 1) lorazepam 0.1 mg/kg, 2) diazepam 0.15 mg/kg followed by phenytoin 18 mg/kg, 3) phenytoin 18 mg/kg alone, and 4) phenobarbital 15 mg/kg. Treatment was considered successful if the seizures were terminated (clinically and by EEG) within 20 minutes of start of therapy without seizure recurrence within 60 minutes from the start of therapy. Patients who failed the first

(Continued)

Phenobarbital *(Continued)*

treatment received a second and a third, if necessary. Patients did not receive randomized treatments after the first one but the treating physician remained blinded. Treatment success: Lorazepam 64.9%, phenobarbital 58.2%, diazepam/phenytoin 55.8%, and phenytoin alone 43.6%. Using an "intention-to-treat" analysis, there was no statistical difference between the groups. Results of subsequent treatments in patients who failed the first therapy indicated that response rate significantly dropped regardless of treatment. Aggregate response rate to the second treatment was 7.0% and third treatment 2.3%.

Pregnancy Risk Factor D

Contraindications Hypersensitivity to barbiturates or any component of the formulation; marked hepatic impairment; dyspnea or airway obstruction; porphyria; pregnancy

Warnings/Precautions Potential for drug dependency exists, abrupt cessation may precipitate withdrawal, including status epilepticus in epileptic patients. Do not administer to patients in acute pain. Use caution in elderly, debilitated, renally or hepatic dysfunction, and pediatric patients. May cause paradoxical responses, including agitation and hyperactivity, particularly in acute pain and pediatric patients. Use with caution in patients with depression or suicidal tendencies, or in patients with a history of drug abuse. Tolerance, psychological and physical dependence may occur with prolonged use. May cause CNS depression, which may impair physical or mental abilities. Patients must cautioned about performing tasks which require mental alertness (eg, operating machinery or driving). Effects with other sedative drugs or ethanol may be potentiated. May cause respiratory depression or hypotension, particularly when administered intravenously. Use with caution in hemodynamically unstable patients (hypovolemic shock, CHF) or patients with respiratory disease. Due to its long half-life and risk of dependence, phenobarbital is not recommended as a sedative in the elderly. Use has been associated with cognitive deficits in children. Use with caution in patients with hypoadrenalism.

Adverse Reactions Frequency not defined.

Cardiovascular: Bradycardia, hypotension, syncope

Central nervous system: Drowsiness, lethargy, CNS excitation or depression, impaired judgment, "hangover" effect, confusion, somnolence, agitation, hyperkinesia, ataxia, nervousness, headache, insomnia, nightmares, hallucinations, anxiety, dizziness

Dermatologic: Rash, exfoliative dermatitis, Stevens-Johnson syndrome

Gastrointestinal: Nausea, vomiting, constipation

Hematologic: Agranulocytosis, thrombocytopenia, megaloblastic anemia

Local: Pain at injection site, thrombophlebitis with I.V. use

Renal: Oliguria

Respiratory: Laryngospasm, respiratory depression, apnea (especially with rapid I.V. use), hypoventilation

Miscellaneous: Gangrene with inadvertent intra-arterial injection

Overdosage/Toxicology Symptoms of overdose include unsteady gait, slurred speech, confusion, jaundice, hypothermia, hypotension, respiratory depression, and coma. In severe overdose, charcoal hemoperfusion may accelerate removal. Treatment is symptom-directed and supportive.

Drug Interactions **Substrate** of CYP2C9 (minor), 2C19 (major), 2E1 (minor); **Induces** CYP1A2 (strong), 2A6 (strong), 2B6 (strong), 2C8 (strong), 2C9 (strong), 3A4 (strong)

Acetaminophen: Barbiturates may enhance the hepatotoxic potential of acetaminophen overdoses

Antiarrhythmics: Barbiturates may increase the metabolism of antiarrhythmics, decreasing their clinical effect; includes disopyramide, propafenone, and quinidine

Anticonvulsants: Barbiturates may increase the metabolism of anticonvulsants; includes ethosuximide, felbamate (possibly), lamotrigine, phenytoin, tiagabine, topiramate, and zonisamide; does not appear to affect gabapentin or levetiracetam

Antineoplastics: Limited evidence suggests that enzyme-inducing anticonvulsant therapy may reduce the effectiveness of some chemotherapy regimens (specifically in ALL); teniposide and methotrexate may be cleared more rapidly in these patients

Antipsychotics: Barbiturates may enhance the metabolism (decrease the efficacy) of antipsychotics; monitor for altered response; dose adjustment may be needed

Beta-blockers: Metabolism of beta-blockers may be increased and clinical effect decreased; atenolol and nadolol are unlikely to interact given their renal elimination

Calcium channel blockers: Barbiturates may enhance the metabolism of calcium channel blockers, decreasing their clinical effect

Chloramphenicol: Barbiturates may increase the metabolism of chloramphenicol and chloramphenicol may inhibit barbiturate metabolism; monitor for altered response

Cimetidine: Barbiturates may enhance the metabolism of cimetidine, decreasing its clinical effect

CNS depressants: Sedative effects and/or respiratory depression with barbiturates may be additive with other CNS depressants; monitor for increased effect; includes ethanol, sedatives, antidepressants, narcotic analgesics, and benzodiazepines

Corticosteroids: Barbiturates may enhance the metabolism of corticosteroids, decreasing their clinical effect

Cyclosporine: Levels may be decreased by barbiturates; monitor

CYP1A2 substrates: Phenobarbital may decrease the levels/effects of CYP1A2 substrates. Example substrates include aminophylline, estrogens, fluvoxamine, mirtazapine, ropinirole, and theophylline.

CYP2A6 substrates: Phenobarbital may decrease the levels/effects of CYP2A6 substrates. Example substrates include ifosfamide and rifampin.

CYP2B6 substrates: Phenobarbital may decrease the levels/effects of CYP2B6 substrates. Example substrates include bupropion, efavirenz, promethazine, selegiline, and sertraline.

CYP2C8 Substrates: Phenobarbital may decrease the levels/effects of CYP2C8 substrates. Example substrates include amiodarone, paclitaxel, pioglitazone, repaglinide, and rosiglitazone.

CYP2C9 Substrates: Phenobarbital may decrease the levels/effects of CYP2C9 substrates. Example substrates include bosentan, celecoxib, dapsone, fluoxetine, glimepiride, glipizide, losartan, montelukast, nateglinide, paclitaxel, phenytoin, sulfonamides, trimethoprim, warfarin, and zafirlukast.

CYP2C19 inducers: May decrease the levels/effects of phenobarbital. Example inducers include aminoglutethimide, carbamazepine, phenytoin, and rifampin.

CYP2C19 inhibitors: May increase the levels/effects of phenobarbital. Example inhibitors include delavirdine, fluconazole, fluvoxamine, gemfibrozil, isoniazid, omeprazole, and ticlopidine.

CYP3A4 substrates: Phenobarbital may decrease the levels/effects of CYP3A4 substrates. Example substrates include benzodiazepines, calcium channel blockers, clarithromycin, cyclosporine, erythromycin, estrogens, mirtazapine, nateglinide, nefazodone, nevirapine, protease inhibitors, tacrolimus, and venlafaxine.

Doxycycline: Barbiturates may enhance the metabolism of doxycycline, decreasing its clinical effect; higher dosages may be required

Estrogens: Barbiturates may increase the metabolism of estrogens and reduce their efficacy

Felbamate may inhibit the metabolism of barbiturates and barbiturates may increase the metabolism of felbamate

Griseofulvin: Barbiturates may impair the absorption of griseofulvin, and griseofulvin metabolism may be increased by barbiturates, decreasing clinical effect

Guanfacine: Effect may be decreased by barbiturates

Immunosuppressants: Barbiturates may enhance the metabolism of immunosuppressants, decreasing its clinical effect; includes both cyclosporine and tacrolimus

Loop diuretics: Metabolism may be increased and clinical effects decreased; established for furosemide, effect with other loop diuretics not established

MAO inhibitors: Metabolism of barbiturates may be inhibited, increasing clinical effect or toxicity of the barbiturates

Methadone: Barbiturates may enhance the metabolism of methadone resulting in methadone withdrawal

Methoxyflurane: Barbiturates may enhance the nephrotoxic effects of methoxyflurane

(Continued)

Phenobarbital *(Continued)*

Oral contraceptives: Barbiturates may enhance the metabolism of oral contraceptives, decreasing their clinical effect; an alternative method of contraception should be considered

Theophylline: Barbiturates may increase metabolism of theophylline derivatives and decrease their clinical effect

Tricyclic antidepressants: Barbiturates may increase metabolism of tricyclic antidepressants and decrease their clinical effect; sedative effects may be additive

Valproic acid: Metabolism of barbiturates may be inhibited by valproic acid; monitor for excessive sedation; a dose reduction may be needed

Warfarin: Barbiturates inhibit the hypoprothrombinemic effects of oral anticoagulants via increased metabolism; this combination should generally be avoided

Ethanol/Nutrition/Herb Interactions

Ethanol: Avoid ethanol (may increase CNS depression).

Food: May cause decrease in vitamin D and calcium.

Herb/Nutraceutical: Avoid evening primrose (seizure threshold decreased). Avoid valerian, St John's wort, kava kava, gotu kola (may increase CNS depression).

Test Interactions Assay interference of LDH

Dietary Considerations Vitamin D: Loss in vitamin D due to malabsorption; increase intake of foods rich in vitamin D. Supplementation of vitamin D and/or calcium may be necessary. Sodium content of injection (65 mg, 1 mL): 6 mg (0.3 mEq).

Dosage Forms

Elixir: 20 mg/5 mL (473 mL) [contains alcohol]

Injection, solution, as sodium: 65 mg/mL (1 mL); 130 mg/mL (1 mL) [contains alcohol and propylene glycol]

Luminal® Sodium: 60 mg/mL (1 mL); 130 mg/mL (1 mL) [contains alcohol 10% and propylene glycol]

Tablet: 15 mg, 30 mg, 32 mg, 60 mg, 65 mg, 100 mg

- **Phenobarbital Sodium** *see* Phenobarbital *on page 1008*
- **Phenobarbitone** *see* Phenobarbital *on page 1008*

Phenol (FEE nol)

Medication Safety Issues

Sound-alike/look-alike issues:

Cēpastat® may be confused with Capastat®

U.S. Brand Names Castellani Paint Modified [OTC]; Cepastat® [OTC]; Cepastat® Extra Strength [OTC]; Cheracol® [OTC]; Chloraseptic® Gargle [OTC]; Chloraseptic® Mouth Pain [OTC]; Chloraseptic® Rinse [OTC]; Chloraseptic® Spray [OTC]; Chloraseptic® Spray for Kids [OTC]; Pain-A-Lay® [OTC]; Phenaseptic [OTC]; Phenol EZ® [OTC]; Ulcerease® [OTC]

Canadian Brand Names P & S™ Liquid Phenol

Synonyms Carbolic Acid

Pharmacologic Category Anesthetic, Topical

Generic Available Yes: Oral spray

Use Relief of sore throat pain, mouth, gum, and throat irritations; antiseptic; topical anesthetic

Dosage Oral:

Sore throat:

Children 2-12 years:

Chloraseptic®: Three sprays onto throat or affected area; may repeat every 2 hours

Chloraseptic® for Kids: Five sprays onto throat or affected area; may repeat every 2 hours

Children >3 year (Ulcerease®): Refer to adult dosing.

Children 6-12 years:

Cēpastat®: Up to 1 lozenge every 2 hours as needed (maximum: 18 lozenges/24 hours)

Cēpastat® Extra Strength: Up to 1 lozenge every 2 hours as needed (maximum: 10 lozenges/24 hours)

Pain-A-Lay® Gargle: Using gauze pad, apply 10 mL to affected area, or gargle or swish for 15 seconds, then expectorate

Children ≥12 years and Adults:
Cēpastat® Extra Strength, Cēpastat®: Up to 2 lozenges every 2 hours as needed
Cheracol®, Pain-A-Lay® Spray: Spray directly in throat; rinse for 15 seconds then expectorate; may repeat every 2 hours
Chloraseptic®: Five sprays onto throat or affected area; may repeat every 2 hours
Chloraseptic® Gargle, Chloraseptic® Mouth Pain, Pain-A-Lay® Gargle, Ulcerease®: Gargle or swish for 15 seconds, then expectorate; may repeat every 2 hours

Topical: Antiseptic: Adults: Castellani Paint Modified: Apply small amount to affected area 1-3 times/day

Stability Store at <86°F (30°C); protect from humidity

Administration

Oral: Allow to lozenge dissolve slowly in mouth. Spray should be allowed to remain in mouth for ~15 seconds, then expectorate.

Topical: Castellani Paint Modified: May stain skin and clothing; apply to clean area

Warnings/Precautions

When used for self-medication (OTC) for sore throat: Not for use >7 days or if pain, redness, or irritation continues. If sore throat is severe, not for use >2 days or if followed by fever, headache, rash, nausea, or vomiting. Oral gargles and sprays should not be swallowed.

When used for self-medication (OTC) as a topical antiseptic: Do not use in eyes, or apply to large areas of the body, deep or puncture wounds, animal bites or burns. Do not use for >7 days; do not bandage affected area.

Dosage Forms

Lozenge, oral:
Cēpastat®: 14.5 mg (18s) [sugar free; contains menthol; cherry flavor]
Cēpastat® Extra Strength: 29 mg (18s) [sugar free; contains menthol; eucalyptus flavor]

Solution, oral: 1.4% (180 mL) [spray]
Cheracol® [spray]: Phenol 1.4% (180 mL) [alcohol and sugar free; contains tartrazine]
Chloraseptic® [gargle]: 1.4% (296 mL) [alcohol and sugar free; cool mint flavor]
Chloraseptic® Mouth Pain [rinse]: 1.4% (240 mL) [cinnamon flavor]
Chloraseptic® [spray]: 1.4% (20 mL, 30 mL) [alcohol and sugar free; cherry flavor]; (180 mL) [alcohol and sugar free; cherry, cool mint, and menthol flavors]
Chloraseptic® for Kids [spray]: 0.5% (177 mL) [grape flavor]
Pain-A-Lay® [gargle]: 1.4% (240 mL, 540 mL) [contains tartrazine]
Pain-A-Lay® [spray]: 1.4% (180 mL) [contains tartrazine]
Phenaseptic [spray]: 1.4% (180 mL) [cherry flavor]
Ulcerease® [gargle]: 0.6% (180 mL) [alcohol, dye, and sugar free; contains glycerin]

Solution, topical:
Castellani Paint Modified: Phenol 1.5% (30 mL) [contains alcohol 13%, acetone, basic fuchsin, resorcinol]
Castellani Paint Modified [colorless]: Phenol 1.5% (30 mL) [contains alcohol 13%, acetone, and resorcinol]

Swabs, topical (Phenol EZ®): 89% (30s) [~0.2 mL]

♦ **Phenol EZ® [OTC]** *see* Phenol *on page 1012*

Phentolamine (fen TOLE a meen)

Medication Safety Issues

Sound-alike/look-alike issues:
Phentolamine may be confused with phentermine, Ventolin®

Related Information

Hypertension *on page 1620*

Canadian Brand Names Regitine®; Rogitine®

Synonyms Phentolamine Mesylate; Regitine [DSC]

Pharmacologic Category Alpha$_1$ Blocker

Generic Available Yes

Use Diagnosis of pheochromocytoma and treatment of hypertension associated with pheochromocytoma or other forms of hypertension caused by excess
(Continued)

Phentolamine *(Continued)*

sympathomimetic amines; as treatment of dermal necrosis after extravasation of drugs with alpha-adrenergic effects (norepinephrine, dopamine, epinephrine)

Unlabeled/Investigational Use Treatment of pralidoxime-induced hypertension

Mechanism of Action Competitively blocks alpha-adrenergic receptors to produce brief antagonism of circulating epinephrine and norepinephrine to reduce hypertension caused by alpha effects of these catecholamines; also has a positive inotropic and chronotropic effect on the heart

Pharmacodynamics/Kinetics

Onset of action: I.M.: 15-20 minutes; I.V.: Immediate
Duration: I.M.: 30-45 minutes; I.V.: 15-30 minutes
Metabolism: Hepatic
Half-life elimination: 19 minutes
Excretion: Urine (10% as unchanged drug)

Dosage

Treatment of alpha-adrenergic drug extravasation: SubQ:
- Children: 0.1-0.2 mg/kg diluted in 10 mL 0.9% sodium chloride infiltrated into area of extravasation within 12 hours
- Adults: Infiltrate area with small amount of solution made by diluting 5-10 mg in 10 mL 0.9% sodium chloride within 12 hours of extravasation; do not exceed 0.1-0.2 mg/kg or 5 mg total
- If dose is effective, normal skin color should return to the blanched area within 1 hour

Diagnosis of pheochromocytoma: I.M., I.V.:
- Children: 0.05-0.1 mg/kg/dose, maximum single dose: 5 mg
- Adults: 5 mg

Surgery for pheochromocytoma: Hypertension: I.M., I.V.:
- Children: 0.05-0.1 mg/kg/dose given 1-2 hours before procedure; repeat as needed every 2-4 hours until hypertension is controlled; maximum single dose: 5 mg
- Adults: 5 mg given 1-2 hours before procedure and repeated as needed every 2-4 hours

Hypertensive crisis: Adults: 5-20 mg

Treatment of pralidoxime-induced hypertension (unlabeled use): I.V.:
- Children: 1 mg
- Adults and Elderly: 5 mg

Stability Reconstituted solution is stable for 48 hours at room temperature and 1 week when refrigerated

Administration Infiltrate the area of dopamine extravasation with multiple small injections using only 27- or 30-gauge needles and changing the needle between each skin entry; take care not to cause so much swelling of the extremity or digit that a compartment syndrome occurs. If infiltration is severe, may also need to consult vascular surgeon

Monitoring Parameters Blood pressure, heart rate; area of infiltration; monitor patient for orthostasis; assist with ambulation

Pregnancy Risk Factor C

Contraindications Hypersensitivity to phentolamine or any component of the formulation; renal impairment; coronary or cerebral arteriosclerosis; concurrent use with phosphodiesterase-5 (PDE-5) inhibitors including sildenafil (>25 mg), tadalafil, or vardenafil

Warnings/Precautions Myocardial infarction, cerebrovascular spasm and cerebrovascular occlusion have occurred following administration. Use with caution in patients with gastritis or peptic ulcer, tachycardia, or a history of cardiac arrhythmias.

Adverse Reactions Frequency not defined.

Cardiovascular: Hypotension, tachycardia, arrhythmia, flushing, orthostatic hypotension
Central nervous system: Dizziness
Gastrointestinal: Nausea, vomiting, diarrhea
Neuromuscular & skeletal: Weakness
Respiratory: Nasal congestion
Postmarketing and/or case reports: Pulmonary hypertension

Overdosage/Toxicology Symptoms of overdose include tachycardia, shock, vomiting, and dizziness. If fluid replacement is inadequate to treat hypotension, only alpha-adrenergic vasopressors such as norepinephrine should be used. Mixed agents such as epinephrine may cause more hypotension.

Drug Interactions

Epinephrine, ephedrine: Effects may be decreased.

Ethanol: Increased toxicity (disulfiram reaction).

Sildenafil, tadalafil, vardenafil: Blood pressure-lowering effects are additive. Use of tadalafil or vardenafil is contraindicated by the manufacturer. Use sildenafil with extreme caution (dose ≤25 mg).

Test Interactions Increased LFTs rarely

Dosage Forms Injection, powder for reconstitution, as mesylate: 5 mg

◆ **Phentolamine Mesylate** *see* Phentolamine *on page 1013*

Phenylephrine (fen il EF rin)

Medication Safety Issues

Sound-alike/look-alike issues:

Mydfrin® may be confused with Midrin®

Related Information

Critical Care Infusion Administration Charts *on page 1514*

Hemodynamic Support, Intravenous *on page 1566*

U.S. Brand Names AH-chew® D [OTC] [DSC]; AK-Dilate®; Altafrin; Anu-Med [OTC]; Formulation R™ [OTC]; Medicone® [OTC]; Mydfrin®; NāSop™; Neo-Synephrine® Extra Strength [OTC]; Neo-Synephrine® Mild [OTC]; Neo-Synephrine® Ophthalmic [DSC]; Neo-Synephrine® Regular Strength [OTC]; Rectacaine [OTC]; Relief® [OTC]; Rhinall [OTC]; Sudafed PE™ [OTC]; Tronolane® Suppository [OTC]; Vicks® Sinex® Nasal Spray [OTC]; Vicks® Sinex® UltraFine Mist [OTC]

Canadian Brand Names Dionephrine®; Mydfrin®; Neo-Synephrine®

Synonyms Phenylephrine Hydrochloride; Phenylephrine Tannate

Pharmacologic Category Alpha/Beta Agonist; Ophthalmic Agent, Antiglaucoma; Ophthalmic Agent, Mydriatic

Generic Available Yes: Excludes cream, suspension, tablet

Use Treatment of hypotension, vascular failure in shock; as a vasoconstrictor in regional analgesia; as a mydriatic in ophthalmic procedures and treatment of wide-angle glaucoma; supraventricular tachycardia

For OTC use as symptomatic relief of nasal and nasopharyngeal mucosal congestion, treatment of hemorrhoids, relief of redness of the eye due to irritation

Mechanism of Action Potent, direct-acting alpha-adrenergic stimulator with weak beta-adrenergic activity; causes vasoconstriction of the arterioles of the nasal mucosa and conjunctiva; activates the dilator muscle of the pupil to cause contraction; produces vasoconstriction of arterioles in the body; produces systemic arterial vasoconstriction

Pharmacodynamics/Kinetics

Onset of action: I.M., SubQ: 10-15 minutes; I.V.: Immediate; Ophthalmic: 10-15 minutes

Duration: I.M.: 0.5-2 hours; I.V.: 15-30 minutes; SubQ: 1 hour; Ophthalmic: Maximal mydriasis: 1 hour, recover time: 3-6 hours

Metabolism: Hepatic, via intestinal monoamine oxidase to phenolic conjugates

Excretion: Urine (90%)

Dosage

Hemorrhoids: Children ≥12 years and Adults: Rectal:

Cream/ointment: Apply to clean dry area, up to 4 times/day; may be used externally or inserted rectally using applicator.

Suppository: Insert 1 suppository rectally, up to 4 times/day

Hypotension/shock:

Children:

I.V. bolus: 5-20 mcg/kg/dose every 10-15 minutes as needed

I.V. infusion: 0.1-0.5 mcg/kg/minute

Adults:

I.V. bolus: 0.1-0.5 mg/dose every 10-15 minutes as needed (initial dose should not exceed 0.5 mg)

I.V. infusion: Initial dose: 100-180 mcg/minute; when blood pressure is stabilized, maintenance rate: 40-60 mcg/minute; rates up to 360 mcg/minute have been reported; dosing range: 0.4-9.1 mcg/kg/minute

(Continued)

Phenylephrine *(Continued)*

Nasal decongestant:

Children:

2-6 years:

Intranasal: Instill 1 drop every 2-4 hours of 0.125% solution as needed. (**Note:** Therapy should not exceed 3 continuous days.)

Oral: Tannate salt (NāSop™ suspension): 1.87-3.75 mg every 12 hours

6-12 years:

Intranasal: Instill 1-2 sprays or instill 1-2 drops every 4 hours of 0.25% solution as needed. (**Note:** Therapy should not exceed 3 continuous days.)

Oral:

Hydrochloride salt: 10 mg every 4 hours

Tannate salt (NāSop™ suspension): 3.75-7.5 mg every 12 hours

Children >12 years and Adults:

Intranasal: Instill 1-2 sprays or instill 1-2 drops every 4 hours of 0.25% to 0.5% solution as needed; 1% solution may be used in adult in cases of extreme nasal congestion; do not use nasal solutions more than 3 days

Oral:

Hydrochloride salt: 10-20 mg every 4 hours

Tannate salt (NāSop™ suspension): 7.5-15 mg every 12 hours

Ocular procedures:

Infants <1 year: Instill 1 drop of 2.5% 15-30 minutes before procedures

Children and Adults: Instill 1 drop of 2.5% or 10% solution, may repeat in 10-60 minutes as needed

Ophthalmic irritation (OTC formulation for relief of eye redness): Adults: Instill 1-2 drops 0.12% solution into affected eye, up to 4 times/day; do not use for >72 hours

Paroxysmal supraventricular tachycardia: I.V.:

Children: 5-10 mcg/kg/dose over 20-30 seconds

Adults: 0.25-0.5 mg/dose over 20-30 seconds

Stability

Solution for injection: Store vials at controlled room temperature of 15°C to 30°C (59°F to 86°F); protect from light. Do not use solution if brown or contains a precipitate.

I.V. infusion: May dilute 10 mg in 500 mL NS or D_5W.

I.V. injection: Dilute with SWFI to a concentration of 1 mg/mL.

Ophthalmic solution:

0.12%: Store at controlled room temperature. Protect from light and excessive heat.

2.5% and 10%: Refer to product labeling. Some products are labeled to store at room temperature, others should be stored under refrigeration at 2°C to 8°C (36°F to 46°F); do not use solution if brown or contains a precipitate.

Administration

I.V.: May cause necrosis or sloughing tissue if extravasation occurs during I.V. administration or SubQ administration.

Extravasation management: Use phentolamine as antidote; mix 5 mg with 9 mL of NS. Inject a small amount of this dilution into extravasated area. Blanching should reverse immediately. Monitor site. If blanching should recur, additional injections of phentolamine may be needed.

Oral: NāSop™: Place tablet on tongue and allow to dissolve

Monitoring Parameters Blood pressure, pulse; excitability, irritability, anxiety

Anesthesia and Critical Care Concerns/Other Considerations Phenylephrine allows for close titration of blood pressure and may be used in patients with hypotension or shock due to peripheral vasodilation; can increase blood pressure in fluid-resuscitated septic shock patients; does not impair cardiac or renal function. May be a good choice when tachyarrhythmias limit use of other vasopressors, although experience in patients with septic shock is limited. An increase in oxygen delivery and consumption may occur in >15% of patients according to one study (Flancbaum, 1997).

Extravasation Management: Antidote for peripheral ischemia caused by phenylephrine extravasation: To prevent sloughing and necrosis in ischemic areas, the area should be infiltrated as soon as possible with 5-10 mg of Regitine® (phentolamine), an adrenergic blocking agent, diluted in 10-15 mL of saline. A syringe with a fine hypodermic needle should be used, and the solution liberally infiltrated throughout the ischemic area. Sympathetic blockade with phentolamine causes immediate and conspicuous local hyperemic changes if the area is infiltrated within 12 hours. Therefore, phentolamine should be given as soon as possible after the extravasation is noted, as phentolamine may be ineffective if given >12 hours after extravasation.

Pregnancy Risk Factor C

Contraindications Hypersensitivity to phenylephrine or any component of the formulation; hypertension; ventricular tachycardia

Oral: Use with or within 14 days of MAO inhibitor therapy

Ophthalmic: Narrow-angle glaucoma

Warnings/Precautions Some products contain sulfites which may cause allergic reactions in susceptible individuals.

Intravenous: Use with caution in the elderly, patients with hyperthyroidism, bradycardia, partial heart block, myocardial disease, or severe CAD. Not a substitute for volume replacement. Avoid hypertension; monitor blood pressure closely and adjust infusion rate. Infuse into a large vein if possible. Watch I.V. site closely. Avoid extravasation.

Nasal, oral, rectal: Use caution with hyperthyroidism, diabetes mellitus, cardiovascular disease, ischemic heart disease, increased intraocular pressure, prostatic hyperplasia or in the elderly. Rebound congestion may occur when nasal products are discontinued after chronic use. When used for self-medication (OTC), notify healthcare provider if symptoms do not improve within 7 days (oral, rectal) or 3 days (nasal), are accompanied by fever (oral), or if bleeding occurs (rectal).

Ophthalmic: Use caution with or within 21 days of MAO inhibitor therapy. When used for self-medication (OTC), notify healthcare provider in case of vision changes, continued redness, or if symptoms worsen or do not improve within 3 days.

Adverse Reactions Frequency not defined.

Cardiovascular: Reflex bradycardia, excitability, restlessness, arrhythmia (rare), precordial pain or discomfort, pallor, hypertension, severe peripheral and visceral vasoconstriction, decreased cardiac output

Central nervous system: Headache, anxiety, dizziness, tremor, paresthesia, restlessness

Endocrine & metabolic: Metabolic acidosis

Local: I.V.: Extravasation which may lead to necrosis and sloughing of surrounding tissue, blanching of skin

Neuromuscular & skeletal: Pilomotor response, weakness

Renal: Decreased renal perfusion, reduced urine output

Respiratory: Respiratory distress

Overdosage/Toxicology Symptoms of overdose include vomiting, hypertension, palpitations, paresthesia, and ventricular extrasystoles. Treatment is supportive. In extreme cases, I.V. phentolamine may be used.

Drug Interactions

Beta-blockers (nonselective) may increase hypertensive effect; avoid concurrent use.

MAO inhibitors: May potentiate hypertension and hypertensive crisis; avoid concurrent use.

Methyldopa can increase the pressor response; be aware of patient's drug regimen.

Tricyclic antidepressants: May enhance the vasopressor effect phenylephrine; avoid concurrent use.

Ethanol/Nutrition/Herb Interactions Herb/Nutraceutical: Avoid ephedra, yohimbe (may cause CNS stimulation).

Dietary Considerations NāSop™ contains phenylalanine 4 mg/tablet.

Dosage Forms [DSC] = Discontinued product

Cream, rectal, as hydrochloride (Formulation R™): 0.25% (54 g) [contains sodium benzoate]

Injection, solution, as hydrochloride: 1% [10 mg/mL] (1 mL, 5 mL) [may contain sodium metabisulfite]

Neo-Synephrine®: 1% (1 mL) [contains sodium metabisulfite]

Ointment, rectal, as hydrochloride:

Formulation R™: 0.25% (30 g, 60 g) [contains benzoic acid]

Rectacaine: 0.25% (30 g) [contains shark liver oil]

(Continued)

Phenylephrine *(Continued)*

Solution, intranasal drops, as hydrochloride:
- Neo-Synephrine® Extra Strength: 1% (15 mL) [contains benzalkonium chloride]
- Neo-Synephrine® Regular Strength: 0.5% (15 mL) [contains benzalkonium chloride]
- Rhinall: 0.25% (30 mL) [contains benzalkonium chloride and sodium bisulfite]

Solution, intranasal spray, as hydrochloride:
- Neo-Synephrine® Extra Strength: 1% (15 mL) [contains benzalkonium chloride]
- Neo-Synephrine® Mild: 0.25% (15 mL) [contains benzalkonium chloride]
- Neo-Synephrine® Regular Strength: 0.5% (15 mL) [contains benzalkonium chloride]
- Rhinall: 0.25% (40 mL) [contains benzalkonium chloride and sodium bisulfite]
- Vicks® Sinex®, Vicks® Sinex® UltraFine Mist: 0.5% (15 mL) [contains benzalkonium chloride]

Solution, ophthalmic, as hydrochloride: 2.5% (1 mL, 2 mL, 3 mL, 5 mL, 15 mL) [may contain sodium bisulfite]
- AK-Dilate®: 2.5% (2 mL, 15 mL); 10% (5 mL)
- Altrafrin: 0.12% (15 mL) [OTC]; 2.5% (5 mL, 15 mL) [RX; contains benzalkonium chloride]; 10% (5 mL) [RX; contains benzalkonium chloride]
- Mydfrin®: 2.5% (3 mL, 5 mL) [contains sodium bisulfite]
- Neo-Synephrine®: 2.5% (15 mL); 10% (5 mL) [contains benzalkonium chloride] [DSC]
- Neo-Synephrine® Viscous: 10% (5 mL) [contains benzalkonium chloride] [DSC]

Suppository, rectal, as hydrochloride: 0.25% (12s)
- Anu-Med, Tronolane®: 0.25% (12s)
- Medicone®: 0.25% (18s, 24s)
- Rectacaine: 0.25% (12s) [contains shark liver oil]

Suspension, oral, as tannate (NāSop™): 7.5 mg/5 mL (120 mL) [orange flavor]

Tablet, as hydrochloride (Sudafed PE™): 10 mg

Tablet, chewable, as hydrochloride:
- AH-chew® D: 10 mg [DSC]

Tablet, orally dissolving, as hydrochloride (NāSop™): 10 mg [contains phenylalanine 4 mg/tablet; bubble gum flavor]

References

Bonfiglio MF, Dasta JF, Gregory JS, et al, "High-Dose Phenylephrine Infusion in the Hemodynamic Support of Septic Shock," *DICP*, 1990, 24(10):936-9.

Flancbaum L, Dick M, Dasta J, et al, "A Dose-Response Study of Phenylephrine in Critically Ill, Septic Surgical Patients," *Eur J Clin Pharmacol*, 1997, 51(6):461-5.

Gregory JS, Bonfiglio MF, Dasta JF, et al, "Experience With Phenylephrine as a Component of the Pharmacologic Support of Septic Shock," *Crit Care Med*, 1991, 19(11):1395-400.

"Task Force of the American College of Critical Care Medicine and Society of Critical Care Medicine. Practice Parameters for Hemodynamic Support of Sepsis in Adult Patients," *Crit Care Med*, 1999, 27(3):639-60. Available at: http://www.sccm.org/pdf/Hemodynamic%20Support.pdf.

- ♦ **Phenylephrine Hydrochloride** *see* Phenylephrine *on page 1015*
- ♦ **Phenylephrine Tannate** *see* Phenylephrine *on page 1015*
- ♦ **Phenylethylmalonylurea** *see* Phenobarbital *on page 1008*
- ♦ **Phenytek™** *see* Phenytoin *on page 1018*

Phenytoin (FEN i toyn)

Medication Safety Issues

Sound-alike/look-alike issues:
- Phenytoin may be confused with phenelzine, phentermine
- Dilantin® may be confused with Dilaudid®, diltiazem, Dipentum®

Related Information

Anesthesia for Patients With Liver Disease *on page 1421*
Chronic Pain Management *on page 1430*
Chronic Renal Failure *on page 1437*
Epilepsy *on page 1604*
Perioperative Management of Patients on Antiseizure Medication *on page 1458*

U.S. Brand Names Dilantin®; Phenytek™

Canadian Brand Names Dilantin®

Synonyms Diphenylhydantoin; DPH; Phenytoin Sodium; Phenytoin Sodium, Extended; Phenytoin Sodium, Prompt

Pharmacologic Category Antiarrhythmic Agent, Class Ib; Anticonvulsant, Hydantoin

Generic Available Yes: Excludes chewable tablet

Use Management of generalized tonic-clonic (grand mal), complex partial seizures; prevention of seizures following head trauma/neurosurgery

Unlabeled/Investigational Use Ventricular arrhythmias, including those associated with digitalis intoxication, prolonged QT interval and surgical repair of congenital heart diseases in children; epidermolysis bullosa

Mechanism of Action Stabilizes neuronal membranes and decreases seizure activity by increasing efflux or decreasing influx of sodium ions across cell membranes in the motor cortex during generation of nerve impulses; prolongs effective refractory period and suppresses ventricular pacemaker automaticity, shortens action potential in the heart

Pharmacodynamics/Kinetics

Onset of action: I.V.: ~0.5-1 hour

Absorption: Oral: Slow

Distribution: V_d:

- Neonates: Premature: 1-1.2 L/kg; Full-term: 0.8-0.9 L/kg
- Infants: 0.7-0.8 L/kg
- Children: 0.7 L/kg
- Adults: 0.6-0.7 L/kg

Protein binding:

- Neonates: ≥80% (≤20% free)
- Infants: ≥85% (≤15% free)
- Adults: 90% to 95%
- Others: Decreased protein binding
  - **Disease states resulting in a decrease in serum albumin concentration**: Burns, hepatic cirrhosis, nephrotic syndrome, pregnancy, cystic fibrosis
  - **Disease states resulting in an apparent decrease in affinity of phenytoin for serum albumin**: Renal failure, jaundice (severe), other drugs (displacers), hyperbilirubinemia (total bilirubin >15 mg/dL), Cl_{cr} <25 mL/minute (unbound fraction is increased two- to threefold in uremia)

Metabolism: Follows dose-dependent capacity-limited (Michaelis-Menten) pharmacokinetics with increased V_{max} in infants >6 months of age and children versus adults; major metabolite (via oxidation), HPPA, undergoes enterohepatic recirculation

Bioavailability: Form dependent

Half-life elimination: Oral: 22 hours (range: 7-42 hours)

Time to peak, serum (form dependent): Oral: Extended-release capsule: 4-12 hours; Immediate release preparation: 2-3 hours

Excretion: Urine (<5% as unchanged drug); as glucuronides

- Clearance: Highly variable, dependent upon intrinsic hepatic function and dose administered; increased clearance and decreased serum concentrations with febrile illness

Dosage

Status epilepticus: I.V.:

- Infants and Children: Loading dose: 15-20 mg/kg in a single or divided dose; maintenance dose: Initial: 5 mg/kg/day in 2 divided doses; usual doses:
  - 6 months to 3 years: 8-10 mg/kg/day
  - 4-6 years: 7.5-9 mg/kg/day
  - 7-9 years: 7-8 mg/kg/day
  - 10-16 years: 6-7 mg/kg/day, some patients may require every 8 hours dosing
- Adults: Loading dose: Manufacturer recommends 10-15 mg/kg, however, 15-25 mg/kg has been used clinically; maintenance dose: 300 mg/day or 5-6 mg/kg/day in 3 divided doses or 1-2 divided doses using extended release

Anticonvulsant: Children and Adults: Oral:

- Loading dose: 15-20 mg/kg; based on phenytoin serum concentrations and recent dosing history; administer oral loading dose in 3 divided doses given every 2-4 hours to decrease GI adverse effects and to ensure complete oral absorption; maintenance dose: same as I.V.
- Neurosurgery (prophylactic): 100-200 mg at approximately 4-hour intervals during surgery and during the immediate postoperative period

Dosing adjustment/comments in renal impairment or hepatic disease: Safe in usual doses in mild liver disease; clearance may be substantially reduced in cirrhosis and plasma level monitoring with dose adjustment advisable. Free phenytoin levels should be monitored closely.

Stability

Capsule, tablet: Store below 30°C (86°F); protect from light and moisture

(Continued)

Phenytoin *(Continued)*

Oral suspension: Store at room temperature of 20°C to 25°C (68°F to 77°F); protect from freezing and light.

Solution for injection: Store at room temperature of 15°C to 30°C (59°F to 86°F); use only clear solutions free of precipitate and haziness, slightly yellow solutions may be used. Precipitation may occur if solution is refrigerated and may dissolve at room temperature.

Further dilution of the solution for I.V. infusion is controversial and no consensus exists as to the optimal concentration and length of stability. Stability is concentration and pH dependent. Based on limited clinical consensus, NS or LR are recommended diluents; dilutions of 1-10 mg/mL have been used and should be administered as soon as possible after preparation (some recommend to discard if not used within 4 hours). Do not refrigerate.

I.V. form is highly **incompatible** with many drugs and solutions. Mixing with other medications is not recommended.

Administration

Oral: Suspension: Shake well prior to use. Absorption is impaired when phenytoin suspension is given concurrently to patients who are receiving continuous nasogastric feedings. A method to resolve this interaction is to divide the daily dose of phenytoin and withhold the administration of nutritional supplements for 1-2 hours before and after each phenytoin dose.

I.M.: Although approved for I.M. use, I.M. administration is not recommended due to erratic absorption and pain on injection. Fosphenytoin may be considered.

I.V.: Vesicant. Fosphenytoin may be considered for loading in patients who are in status epilepticus, hemodynamically unstable, or develop hypotension/bradycardia with I.V. administration of phenytoin. Phenytoin may be administered by IVP or IVPB administration. The maximum rate of I.V. administration is 50 mg/minute. Highly sensitive patients (eg, elderly, patients with pre-existing cardiovascular conditions) should receive phenytoin more slowly (eg, 20 mg/minute). An in-line 0.22-5 micron filter is recommended for IVPB solutions due to the high potential for precipitation of the solution. Avoid extravasation. Following I.V. administration, NS should be injected through the same needle or I.V. catheter to prevent irritation.

pH: 10.0-12.3

SubQ: SubQ administration is not recommended because of the possibility of local tissue damage.

Monitoring Parameters Blood pressure, vital signs (with I.V. use), plasma phenytoin level, CBC, liver function tests

Reference Range Timing of serum samples: Because it is slowly absorbed, peak blood levels may occur 4-8 hours after ingestion of an oral dose. The serum half-life varies with the dosage and the drug follows Michaelis-Menten kinetics. The average adult half-life is about 24 hours. Steady-state concentrations are reached in 5-10 days.

Children and Adults: Toxicity is measured clinically, and some patients require levels outside the suggested therapeutic range

Therapeutic range:

Total phenytoin: 10-20 mcg/mL (children and adults), 8-15 mcg/mL (neonates)

Concentrations of 5-10 mcg/mL may be therapeutic for some patients but concentrations <5 mcg/mL are not likely to be effective

50% of patients show decreased frequency of seizures at concentrations >10 mcg/mL

86% of patients show decreased frequency of seizures at concentrations >15 mcg/mL

Add another anticonvulsant if satisfactory therapeutic response is not achieved with a phenytoin concentration of 20 mcg/mL

Free phenytoin: 1-2.5 mcg/mL

Toxic: >30 mcg/mL (SI: <120-200 µmol/L)

Lethal: >100 mcg/mL (SI: >400 µmol/L)

When to draw levels: This is dependent on the disease state being treated and the clinical condition of the patient

Key points:

Slow absorption of extended capsules and prolonged half-life minimize fluctuations between peak and trough concentrations, timing of sampling not crucial

Trough concentrations are generally recommended for routine monitoring. Daily levels are not necessary and may result in incorrect dosage adjustments. If it is determined essential to monitor free phenytoin concentrations, concomitant monitoring of total phenytoin concentrations is not necessary and expensive.

After a loading dose: Draw level within 48-96 hours

Rapid achievement: Draw within 2-3 days of therapy initiation to ensure that the patient's metabolism is not remarkably different from that which would be predicted by average literature-derived pharmacokinetic parameters; early levels should be used cautiously in design of new dosing regimens

Second concentration: Draw within 6-7 days with subsequent doses of phenytoin adjusted accordingly

If plasma concentrations have not changed over a 3- to 5-day period, monitoring interval may be increased to once weekly in the acute clinical setting

In stable patients requiring long-term therapy, generally monitor levels at 3- to 12-month intervals

Adjustment of serum concentration: See tables.

Adjustment of Serum Concentration in Patients With Low Serum Albumin

Measured Total Phenytoin Concentration (mcg/mL)	Patient's Serum Albumin (g/dL)			
	3.5	3	2.5	2
	Adjusted Total Phenytoin Concentration (mcg/mL)[1]			
5	6	7	8	10
10	13	14	17	20
15	19	21	25	30

[1]Adjusted concentration = measured total concentration divided by [(0.2 x albumin) + 0.1].

Adjustment of Serum Concentration in Patients With Renal Failure (Cl_{cr} ≤10 mL/min)

Measured Total Phenytoin Concentration (mcg/mL)	Patient's Serum Albumin (g/dL)				
	4	3.5	3	2.5	2
	Adjusted Total Phenytoin Concentration (mcg/mL)[1]				
5	10	11	13	14	17
10	20	22	25	29	33
15	30	33	38	43	50

[1]Adjusted concentration = measured total concentration divided by [(0.1 x albumin) + 0.1].

Anesthesia and Critical Care Concerns/Other Considerations Because phenytoin induces the metabolism of many drugs, it may alter their effective blood concentration.

The vehicle which contains propylene glycol, ethanol, and sodium hydroxide, may cause hypotension, bradycardia, arrhythmias, or asystole refractory to defibrillation. Phenytoin 50 mg/mL contains propylene glycol 414.4 mg/mL (40% v/v).

Patients on chronic phenytoin therapy require larger and more frequent doses of nondepolarizing muscle relaxants to attain the same degree of muscle relaxation. This is probably due to increased levels of alpha$_1$-acid glycoprotein released by the liver (which bind free phenytoin) during hepatic enzyme induction.

Rapid intravenous administration may cause hypotension. Infuse at a rate no greater than 50 mg/minute in adults and 25 mg/minute in the elderly.

Status Epilepticus: A randomized, double-blind trial (Treiman D, 1998) evaluated the efficacy of four treatments in overt status epilepticus. Treatment arms were designed based upon accepted practices of North American neurologists. The treatments were: 1) lorazepam 0.1 mg/kg, 2) diazepam 0.15 mg/kg followed by phenytoin 18 mg/kg, 3) phenytoin 18 mg/kg alone, and 4) phenobarbital 15 mg/kg. Treatment was considered successful if the seizures were terminated (clinically and by EEG) within 20 minutes of start of therapy without seizure recurrence within 60 minutes from the start of therapy. Patients who failed the first treatment received a second and a third, if necessary. Patients did not receive randomized treatments after the first one but the treating physician remained

(Continued)

Phenytoin *(Continued)*

blinded. Treatment success: Lorazepam 64.9%, phenobarbital 58.2%, diazepam/phenytoin 55.8%, and phenytoin alone 43.6%. Using an intention to treat analysis, there was no statistical difference between the groups. Results of subsequent treatments in patients who failed the first therapy indicated that response rate significantly dropped regardless of treatment. Aggregate response rate to the second treatment was 7.0% and third treatment 2.3%.

Pregnancy Risk Factor D

Contraindications Hypersensitivity to phenytoin, other hydantoins, or any component of the formulation; pregnancy

Warnings/Precautions May increase frequency of petit mal seizures; I.V. form may cause hypotension, skin necrosis at I.V. site; avoid I.V. administration in small veins; use with caution in patients with porphyria; discontinue if rash or lymphadenopathy occurs; use with caution in patients with hepatic dysfunction, sinus bradycardia, SA block, or AV block; use with caution in elderly or debilitated patients, or in any condition associated with low serum albumin levels, which will increase the free fraction of phenytoin in the serum and, therefore, the pharmacologic response. Sedation, confusional states, or cerebellar dysfunction (loss of motor coordination) may occur at higher total serum concentrations, or at lower total serum concentrations when the free fraction of phenytoin is increased. Abrupt withdrawal may precipitate status epilepticus.

Adverse Reactions I.V. effects: Hypotension, bradycardia, cardiac arrhythmia, cardiovascular collapse (especially with rapid I.V. use), venous irritation and pain, thrombophlebitis

Effects not related to plasma phenytoin concentrations: Hypertrichosis, gingival hypertrophy, thickening of facial features, carbohydrate intolerance, folic acid deficiency, peripheral neuropathy, vitamin D deficiency, osteomalacia, systemic lupus erythematosus

Concentration-related effects: Nystagmus, blurred vision, diplopia, ataxia, slurred speech, dizziness, drowsiness, lethargy, coma, rash, fever, nausea, vomiting, gum tenderness, confusion, mood changes, folic acid depletion, osteomalacia, hyperglycemia

Related to elevated concentrations:

>20 mcg/mL: Far lateral nystagmus

>30 mcg/mL: 45° lateral gaze nystagmus and ataxia

>40 mcg/mL: Decreased mentation

>100 mcg/mL: Death

Cardiovascular: Hypotension, bradycardia, cardiac arrhythmia, cardiovascular collapse

Central nervous system: Psychiatric changes, slurred speech, dizziness, drowsiness, headache, insomnia

Dermatologic: Rash

Gastrointestinal: Constipation, nausea, vomiting, gingival hyperplasia, enlargement of lips

Hematologic: Leukopenia, thrombocytopenia, agranulocytosis

Hepatic: Hepatitis

Local: Thrombophlebitis

Neuromuscular & skeletal: Tremor, peripheral neuropathy, paresthesia

Ocular: Diplopia, nystagmus, blurred vision

Rarely seen effects: Blood dyscrasias, coarsening of facial features, dyskinesias, hepatitis, hypertrichosis, lymphadenopathy, lymphoma, pseudolymphoma, SLE-like syndrome, Stevens-Johnson syndrome, venous irritation and pain

Overdosage/Toxicology Symptoms of overdose include unsteady gait, slurred speech, confusion, nausea, hypothermia, fever, hypotension, respiratory depression, coma. Treatment is symptomatic.

Drug Interactions Substrate of CYP2C9 (major), 2C19 (major), 3A4 (minor); **Induces** CYP2B6 (strong), 2C8 (strong), 2C9 (strong), 2C19 (strong), 3A4 (strong)

Acetaminophen: Phenytoin may enhance the hepatotoxic potential of acetaminophen overdoses

Acetazolamide: Concurrent use with phenytoin may result in an increased risk of osteomalacia

Acyclovir: May decrease phenytoin serum levels; limited documentation; monitor

Allopurinol: May increase phenytoin serum concentrations; monitor

Antacids: May decrease absorption of phenytoin; separate oral doses by several hours

Antiarrhythmics: Phenytoin may increase the metabolism of antiarrhythmics, decreasing their clinical effect; includes disopyramide, propafenone, and quinidine; amiodarone also may increase phenytoin concentrations (see CYP inhibitors)

Anticonvulsants: Phenytoin may increase the metabolism of anticonvulsants; includes barbiturates, carbamazepine, ethosuximide, felbamate, lamotrigine, tiagabine, topiramate, and zonisamide; does not appear to affect gabapentin or levetiracetam; felbamate and gabapentin may increase phenytoin levels; monitor

Antineoplastics: Several chemotherapeutic agents have been associated with a decrease in serum phenytoin levels; includes cisplatin, bleomycin, carmustine, methotrexate, and vinblastine; monitor phenytoin serum levels. Limited evidence also suggest that enzyme-inducing anticonvulsant therapy may reduce the effectiveness of some chemotherapy regimens (specifically in ALL). Teniposide and methotrexate may be cleared more rapidly in these patients.

Antipsychotics: Phenytoin may enhance the metabolism (decrease the efficacy) of antipsychotics; monitor for altered response; dose adjustment may be needed; also see note on clozapine

Benzodiazepines: Phenytoin may decrease the serum concentrations of some benzodiazepines; monitor for decreased benzodiazepine effect

Beta-blockers: Metabolism of beta-blockers may be increased and clinical effect decreased; atenolol and nadolol are unlikely to interact given their renal elimination

Calcium channel blockers: Phenytoin may enhance the metabolism of calcium channel blockers, decreasing their clinical effect; calcium channel blockers (diltiazem, nifedipine) have been reported to increase phenytoin levels (case report); monitor.

Capecitabine: May increase the serum concentrations of phenytoin; monitor

Chloramphenicol: Phenytoin may increase the metabolism of chloramphenicol and chloramphenicol may inhibit phenytoin metabolism; monitor for altered response

Cimetidine: May increase the serum concentrations of phenytoin; monitor.

Ciprofloxacin: May decrease serum phenytoin concentrations; monitor.

Clozapine: Phenytoin may decrease levels/effects of clozapine; monitor.

CNS depressants: Sedative effects may be additive with other CNS depressants; monitor for increased effect; includes ethanol, barbiturates, sedatives, antidepressants, narcotic analgesics, and benzodiazepines

Corticosteroids: Phenytoin may increase the metabolism of corticosteroids, decreasing their clinical effect; also see dexamethasone

Cyclosporine and tacrolimus: Levels may be decreased by phenytoin; monitor

CYP2B6 substrates: Phenytoin may decrease the levels/effects of CYP2B6 substrates. Example substrates include bupropion, efavirenz, promethazine, selegiline, and sertraline.

CYP2C9 inducers: May decrease the levels/effects of phenytoin. Example inducers include carbamazepine, phenobarbital, rifampin, rifapentine, and secobarbital.

CYP2C9 Inhibitors may increase the levels/effects of phenytoin. Example inhibitors include delavirdine, fluconazole, gemfibrozil, ketoconazole, nicardipine, NSAIDs, sulfonamides and tolbutamide.

CYP2C8 Substrates: Phenytoin may decrease the levels/effects of CYP2C8 substrates. Example substrates include amiodarone, paclitaxel, pioglitazone, repaglinide, and rosiglitazone.

CYP2C9 Substrates: Phenytoin may decrease the levels/effects of CYP2C9 substrates. Example substrates include bosentan, celecoxib, dapsone, fluoxetine, glimepiride, glipizide, losartan, montelukast, nateglinide, paclitaxel, sulfonamides, trimethoprim, warfarin, and zafirlukast.

CYP2C19 inducers: May decrease the levels/effects of phenytoin. Example inducers include aminoglutethimide, carbamazepine, phenytoin, and rifampin.

CYP2C19 inhibitors: May increase the levels/effects of phenytoin. Example inhibitors include delavirdine, fluconazole, fluvoxamine, gemfibrozil, isoniazid, omeprazole, and ticlopidine.

CYP2C19 substrates: Phenytoin may decrease the levels/effects of CYP2C19 substrates. Example substrates include citalopram, diazepam, methsuximide, propranolol, proton pump inhibitors, sertraline, and voriconazole.

CYP3A4 substrates: Phenytoin may decrease the levels/effects of CYP3A4 substrates. Example substrates include benzodiazepines, calcium channel blockers, clarithromycin, cyclosporine, erythromycin, estrogens, mirtazapine,

(Continued)

Phenytoin *(Continued)*

nateglinide, nefazodone, nevirapine, protease inhibitors, tacrolimus, and venlafaxine.

Digoxin: Effects and/or levels of digitalis glycosides may be decreased by phenytoin

Disulfiram: May increase serum phenytoin concentrations; monitor

Dopamine: Phenytoin (I.V.) may increase the effect of dopamine (enhanced hypotension)

Doxycycline: Phenytoin may enhance the metabolism of doxycycline, decreasing its clinical effect; higher dosages may be required

Estrogens: Phenytoin may increase the metabolism of estrogens, decreasing their clinical effect; monitor

Folic acid: Replacement of folic acid has been reported to increase the metabolism of phenytoin, decreasing its serum concentrations and/or increasing seizures

HMG-CoA reductase inhibitors: Phenytoin may increase the metabolism of these agents, reducing their clinical effect; monitor

Itraconazole: Phenytoin may decrease the effect of itraconazole

Levodopa: Phenytoin may inhibit the anti-Parkinson effect of levodopa

Lithium: Concurrent use of phenytoin and lithium has resulted in lithium intoxication

Methadone: Phenytoin may enhance the metabolism of methadone resulting in methadone withdrawal

Methylphenidate: May increase serum phenytoin concentrations; monitor

Metronidazole: May increase the serum concentrations of phenytoin; monitor.

Neuromuscular-blocking agents: Duration of effect may be decreased by phenytoin

Omeprazole: May increase serum phenytoin concentrations; monitor

Oral contraceptives: Phenytoin may enhance the metabolism of oral contraceptives, decreasing their clinical effect; an alternative method of contraception should be considered

Primidone: Phenytoin enhances the conversion of primidone to phenobarbital resulting in elevated phenobarbital serum concentrations

Quetiapine: Serum concentrations may be substantially reduced by phenytoin, potentially resulting in a loss of efficacy; limited documentation; monitor

SSRIs: May increase phenytoin serum concentrations; fluoxetine and fluvoxamine are known to inhibit metabolism via CYP enzymes; sertraline and paroxetine have also been shown to increase concentrations in some patients; monitor

Sucralfate: May reduce the GI absorption of phenytoin; monitor

Theophylline: Phenytoin may increase metabolism of theophylline derivatives and decrease their clinical effect; theophylline may also increase phenytoin concentrations

Thyroid hormones (including levothyroxine): Phenytoin may alter the metabolism of thyroid hormones, reducing its effect; there is limited documentation of this interaction, but monitoring should be considered

Ticlopidine: May increase serum phenytoin concentrations and/or toxicity; monitor

Tricyclic antidepressants: Phenytoin may increase metabolism of tricyclic antidepressants and decrease their clinical effect; sedative effects may be additive; tricyclics may also increase phenytoin concentrations

Topiramate: Phenytoin may decrease serum levels of topiramate; topiramate may increase the effect of phenytoin

Trazodone: Serum levels of phenytoin may be increased; limited documentation; monitor

Trimethoprim: May increase serum phenytoin concentrations; monitor

Valproic acid (and sulfisoxazole): May displace phenytoin from binding sites; valproic acid may increase, decrease, or have no effect on phenytoin serum concentrations

Vigabatrin: May reduce phenytoin serum concentrations; monitor

Warfarin: Phenytoin transiently increased the hypothrombinemia response to warfarin initially; this is followed by an inhibition of the hypoprothrombinemic response

Ethanol/Nutrition/Herb Interactions

Ethanol:

Acute use: Avoid or limit ethanol (inhibits metabolism of phenytoin). Watch for sedation.

Chronic use: Avoid or limit ethanol (stimulates metabolism of phenytoin).

Food: Phenytoin serum concentrations may be altered if taken with food. If taken with enteral nutrition, phenytoin serum concentrations may be decreased. Tube feedings decrease bioavailability; hold tube feedings 2 hours before and 2 hours after phenytoin administration. May decrease calcium, folic acid, and vitamin D levels.

Herb/Nutraceutical: Avoid evening primrose (seizure threshold decreased). Avoid valerian, St John's wort, kava kava, gotu kola (may increase CNS depression).

Dietary Considerations

Folic acid: Phenytoin may decrease mucosal uptake of folic acid; to avoid folic acid deficiency and megaloblastic anemia, some clinicians recommend giving patients on anticonvulsants prophylactic doses of folic acid and cyanocobalamin. However, folate supplementation may increase seizures in some patients (dose dependent). Discuss with healthcare provider prior to using any supplements.

Calcium: Hypocalcemia has been reported in patients taking prolonged high-dose therapy with an anticonvulsant. Some clinicians have given an additional 4000 units/week of vitamin D (especially in those receiving poor nutrition and getting no sun exposure) to prevent hypocalcemia.

Vitamin D: Phenytoin interferes with vitamin D metabolism and osteomalacia may result; may need to supplement with vitamin D

Tube feedings: Tube feedings decrease phenytoin absorption. To avoid decreased serum levels with continuous NG feeds, hold feedings for 2 hours prior to and 2 hours after phenytoin administration, if possible. There is a variety of opinions on how to administer phenytoin with enteral feedings. Be **consistent** throughout therapy.

Sodium content of 1 g injection: 88 mg (3.8 mEq)

Dosage Forms

Capsule, extended release, as sodium: 100 mg

Dilantin®: 30 mg [contains sodium benzoate], 100 mg

Phenytek™: 200 mg, 300 mg

Capsule, prompt release, as sodium: 100 mg

Injection, solution, as sodium: 50 mg/mL (2 mL, 5 mL) [contains alcohol and propylene glycol]

Suspension, oral: 125 mg/5 mL (240 mL)

Dilantin®: 125 mg/5 mL (240 mL) [contains alcohol <0.6%, sodium benzoate; orange vanilla flavor]

Tablet, chewable:

Dilantin®: 50 mg

References

Black J, Hannaman T, and Malone C, "The Relationship of Serum Albumin Level to Phenytoin Toxicity," *J Clin Pharmacol*, 1987, 27(3):249-50.

Bleck TP, "Seizures, Stroke, and Other Neurologic Emergencies," *Multidisciplinary Critical Care Review*, Zimmerman JL and Roberts PR, eds, Des Plaines, IL: Society of Critical Care Medicine, 2003, 325-34.

Chapman MG, Smith M, and Hirsch NP, "Status Epilepticus," *Anaesthesia*, 56(7):648-59.

Manno EM, "New Management Strategies in the Treatment of Status Epilepticus," *Mayo Clin Proc*, 2003, 78(4):508-18.

Mansur LI, Murrow RW, Garrelts JC, et al, "Rebound of Plasma Free Phenytoin Concentration Following Plasmapheresis in a Patient With Thrombotic Thrombocytopenic Purpura," *Ann Pharmacother*, 1995, 29(6):592-5.

Treiman DM, Meyers PD, Walton NY, et al, "A Comparison of Four Treatments for Generalized Convulsive Status Epilepticus. Veterans Affairs Status Epilepticus Cooperative Study Group," *N Engl J Med*, 1998, 339(12):792-8.

♦ **Phenytoin Sodium** *see* Phenytoin *on page 1018*

♦ **Phenytoin Sodium, Extended** *see* Phenytoin *on page 1018*

♦ **Phenytoin Sodium, Prompt** *see* Phenytoin *on page 1018*

♦ **PHL-Citalopram (Can)** *see* Citalopram *on page 297*

♦ **PHL-Methimazole (Can)** *see* Methimazole *on page 817*

♦ **PHL-Sumatriptan (Can)** *see* Sumatriptan *on page 1222*

♦ **PHL-Topiramate (Can)** *see* Topiramate *on page 1287*

♦ **Phoxal-timolol (Can)** *see* Timolol *on page 1268*

♦ **Phylloquinone** *see* Phytonadione *on page 1027*

Physostigmine (fye zoe STIG meen)

Medication Safety Issues

Sound-alike/look-alike issues:

Physostigmine may be confused with Prostigmin®, pyridostigmine

Canadian Brand Names Eserine®; Isopto® Eserine

Synonyms Eserine Salicylate; Physostigmine Salicylate; Physostigmine Sulfate

Pharmacologic Category Acetylcholinesterase Inhibitor

Generic Available Yes

Use Reverse toxic CNS effects caused by anticholinergic drugs

Mechanism of Action Inhibits destruction of acetylcholine by acetylcholinesterase which facilitates transmission of impulses across myoneural junction and prolongs the central and peripheral effects of acetylcholine

Pharmacodynamics/Kinetics

Onset of action: ~5 minutes

Duration: 0.5-5 hours

Absorption: I.M., SubQ: Readily absorbed

Distribution: Crosses blood-brain barrier readily and reverses both central and peripheral anticholinergic effects

Metabolism: Hepatic and via hydrolysis by cholinesterases

Half-life elimination: 15-40 minutes

Dosage

Children: Anticholinergic drug overdose: Reserve for life-threatening situations only: I.V.: 0.01-0.03 mg/kg/dose (maximum: 0.5 mg/minute); may repeat after 5-10 minutes to a maximum total dose of 2 mg or until response occurs or adverse cholinergic effects occur

Adults: Anticholinergic drug overdose:

I.M., I.V., SubQ: 0.5-2 mg to start, repeat every 20 minutes until response occurs or adverse effect occurs

Repeat 1-4 mg every 30-60 minutes as life-threatening signs (arrhythmias, seizures, deep coma) recur; maximum I.V. rate: 1 mg/minute

Stability Do not use solution if cloudy or dark brown

Administration Injection: Infuse slowly I.V. at a maximum rate of 0.5 mg/minute in children or 1 mg/minute in adults. Too rapid administration (I.V. rate not to exceed 1 mg/minute) can cause bradycardia, hypersalivation leading to respiratory difficulties and seizures.

Monitoring Parameters Heart rate, respiratory rate

Anesthesia and Critical Care Concerns/Other Considerations Cholinergic effects of physostigmine include bradycardia and bradydysrhythmias.

Pregnancy Risk Factor C

Contraindications Hypersensitivity to physostigmine or any component of the formulation; GI or GU obstruction; physostigmine therapy of drug intoxications should be used with extreme caution in patients with asthma, gangrene, severe cardiovascular disease, or mechanical obstruction of the GI tract or urogenital tract. In these patients, physostigmine should be used only to treat life-threatening conditions.

Warnings/Precautions Use with caution in patients with epilepsy, asthma, diabetes, gangrene, cardiovascular disease, bradycardia. Discontinue if excessive salivation or emesis, frequent urination or diarrhea occur. Reduce dosage if excessive sweating or nausea occurs. Administer I.V. slowly or at a controlled rate not faster than 1 mg/minute. Due to the possibility of hypersensitivity or overdose/cholinergic crisis, atropine should be readily available; not intended as a first-line agent for anticholinergic toxicity or Parkinson's disease.

Adverse Reactions Frequency not defined.

Cardiovascular: Palpitations, bradycardia

Central nervous system: Restlessness, nervousness, hallucinations, seizure

Gastrointestinal: Nausea, salivation, diarrhea, stomach pain

Genitourinary: Frequent urge to urinate

Neuromuscular & skeletal: Muscle twitching

Ocular: Lacrimation, miosis

Respiratory: Dyspnea, bronchospasm, respiratory paralysis, pulmonary edema

Miscellaneous: Diaphoresis

Overdosage/Toxicology Symptoms of overdose include muscle weakness, blurred vision, excessive sweating, tearing and salivation, nausea, vomiting, bronchospasm, and seizures. If physostigmine is used in excess or in the absence of an anticholinergic overdose, patients may manifest signs of cholinergic toxicity. At this point, an anticholinergic agent (eg, atropine 0.015-0.05 mg/kg) may be necessary.

Drug Interactions Increased toxicity: Bethanechol, methacholine, succinylcholine may increase neuromuscular blockade with systemic administration

Test Interactions Increased aminotransferase [ALT (SGPT)/AST (SGOT)] (S), increased amylase (S)

Dosage Forms Injection, solution, as salicylate: 1 mg/mL (2 mL) [contains benzyl alcohol and sodium metabisulfite]

- **Physostigmine Salicylate** *see* Physostigmine *on page 1026*
- **Physostigmine Sulfate** *see* Physostigmine *on page 1026*
- **Phytomenadione** *see* Phytonadione *on page 1027*

Phytonadione (fye toe na DYE one)

Medication Safety Issues

Sound-alike/look-alike issues:

Mephyton® may be confused with melphalan, methadone

Management of Elevated INR

INR	Symptom	Action
Above therapeutic range to <5	No significant bleeding	Lower or hold the next dose and monitor frequently; when INR approaches desired range, may resume dosing with a lower dose if INR was significantly above therapeutic range.
≥5 and <9	No significant bleeding	Omit the next 1or 2 doses; monitor INR and resume with a lower dose when the INR approaches the desired range. Alternatively, if there are other risk factors for bleeding, omit the next dose and give vitamin K_1 orally ≤5 mg; resume with a lower dose when the INR approaches the desired range. If rapid reversal is required for surgery, then given vitamin K_1 orally 2-4 mg and hold warfarin. Expect a response within 24 hours; another 1-2 mg may be given orally if needed.
≥9	No significant bleeding	Hold warfarin, give vitamin K_1 orally 5-10 mg, expect the INR to be reduced within 24-48 hours; monitor INR and administer additional vitamin K if necessary. Resume warfarin at lower doses when INR is in the desired range.
Any INR elevation	Serious bleeding	Hold warfarin, give vitamin K_1 (10 mg by slow I.V. infusion), and supplement with fresh plasma transfusion or prothrombin complex concentrate (Factor X complex); recombinant factor VIIa is an alternative to prothrombin complex concentrate. Vitamin K_1 injection can be repeated every 12 hours.
Any INR elevation	Life-threatening bleeding	Hold warfarin, give prothrombin complex concentrate, supplemented with vitamin K_1 (10 mg by slow I.V. infusion); repeat if necessary. Recombinant factor VIIa is an alternative to prothrombin complex concentrate.

Note: Use of high doses of vitamin K_1 (10-15 mg) may cause resistance to warfarin for up to a week. Heparin or low molecular weight heparin can be given until the patient becomes respon sive to warfarin.

Reference: Ansell J, Hirsh J, Poller L et al. "The Pharmacology and Management of the Vitamin K Antagonists," *Chest*, 2004, 126 (3 Suppl):204-33.

(Continued)

Phytonadione *(Continued)*

U.S. Brand Names Mephyton®

Canadian Brand Names AquaMEPHYTON®; Konakion; Mephyton®

Synonyms Methylphytyl Napthoquinone; Phylloquinone; Phytomenadione; Vitamin K_1

Pharmacologic Category Vitamin, Fat Soluble

Generic Available Yes: Injection

Use Prevention and treatment of hypoprothrombinemia caused by coumarin derivative-induced or other drug-induced vitamin K deficiency, hypoprothrombinemia caused by malabsorption or inability to synthesize vitamin K; hemorrhagic disease of the newborn

Mechanism of Action Promotes liver synthesis of clotting factors (II, VII, IX, X); however, the exact mechanism as to this stimulation is unknown. Menadiol is a water soluble form of vitamin K; phytonadione has a more rapid and prolonged effect than menadione; menadiol sodium diphosphate (K_4) is half as potent as menadione (K_3).

Pharmacodynamics/Kinetics

Onset of action: Increased coagulation factors: Oral: 6-10 hours; I.V.: 1-2 hours

Peak effect: INR values return to normal: Oral: 24-48 hours; I.V.: 12-14 hours

Absorption: Oral: From intestines in presence of bile; SubQ: Variable

Metabolism: Rapidly hepatic

Excretion: Urine and feces

Dosage

Adequate intake:

Children:

1-3 years: 30 mcg/day

4-8 years: 55 mcg/day

9-13 years: 60 mcg/day

14-18 years: 75 mcg/day

Adults: Males: 120 mcg/day; Females: 90 mcg/day

Hemorrhagic disease of the newborn:

Prophylaxis: I.M.: 0.5-1 mg within 1 hour of birth

Treatment: I.M., SubQ: 1 mg/dose/day; higher doses may be necessary if mother has been receiving oral anticoagulants

Hypoprothrombinemia due to drugs (other than coumarin derivatives) or factors limiting absorption or synthesis: Adults: Oral, SubQ, I.M., I.V.: Initial: 2.5-25 mg (rarely up to 50 mg)

Vitamin K deficiency secondary to coumarin derivative: Adults: See table on previous page.

Stability

Injection: Store at 15°C to 30°C (59°F to 86°F). Dilute in preservative-free NS, D_5W, or D_5NS.

Note: Store Hospira product at 20°C to 25°C (68°F to 77°F).

Oral: Store tablets at 15°C to 30°C (59°F to 86°F); protect from light.

Administration I.V. administration: Infuse slowly; rate of infusion should not exceed 1 mg/minute. The injectable route should be used only if the oral route is not feasible or there is a greater urgency to reverse anticoagulation.

Oral: The parenteral preparation has been administered orally to neonates.

Monitoring Parameters PT, INR

Pregnancy Risk Factor C

Contraindications Hypersensitivity to phytonadione or any component of the formulation

Warnings/Precautions

Allergic reactions (injectable): [U.S. Boxed Warning]: Severe reactions resembling hypersensitivity (eg, anaphylaxis) reactions have occurred rarely during or immediately after I.V. administration (even with proper dilution and rate of administration). Allergic reactions have also occurred with I.M. and SubQ injections.

Route: Oral administration is the safest and requires the presence of bile salts for absorption. In obstructive jaundice or with biliary fistulas, concurrent administration of bile salts would be necessary for proper absorption. Manufacturers recommend the SubQ route over other parenteral routes, however, SubQ is less predictable when compared to the oral route, and efficacy may be delayed. The American College of Chest Physicians recommends the I.V. route in patients with serious or life-threatening bleeding secondary to use of vitamin K antagonists such as warfarin. The I.V. route should be restricted to emergency situations only where oral phytonadione cannot be used. Efficacy (eg, control of bleeding, decrease in INR) is delayed regardless of route of administration; patient management may require other treatments in the interim.

Reversing anticoagulant induced hypoprothrombinemia: Administer a dose that will quickly lower the INR into a safe range without causing resistance to warfarin. High phytonadione doses may lead to warfarin resistance for at least one week.

Newborns: Use caution in newborns, especially premature infants; hemolysis, jaundice, and hyperbilirubinemia have been reported with larger than recommended doses. Some dosage forms contain benzyl alcohol which has been associated with "gasping syndrome" in premature infants.

Hypoprothrombinemia caused by liver disease: If initial doses do not reverse coagulopathy, then higher doses are unlikely to have any effect. **Note:** Ineffective in hereditary hypoprothrombinemia.

Renal dysfunction: Use caution with renal dysfunction (including premature infants). Injectable products may contain aluminum; may result in toxic levels following prolonged administration.

Adverse Reactions Parenteral administration: Frequency not defined.

Cardiovascular: Cyanosis, flushing, hypotension
Central nervous system: Dizziness
Dermatologic: Scleroderma-like lesions
Endocrine & metabolic: Hyperbilirubinemia (newborn; greater than recommended doses)
Gastrointestinal: Abnormal taste
Local: Injection site reactions
Respiratory: Dyspnea
Miscellaneous: Anaphylactoid reactions, diaphoresis, hypersensitivity reactions

Drug Interactions

Coumarin derivatives: Phytonadione may diminish the anticoagulant effect; monitor INR.

Orlistat: Phytonadione (oral) may not be properly absorbed when administered concurrently; separate doses by at least 2 hours.

Dosage Forms

Injection, aqueous colloidal: 2 mg/mL (0.5 mL); 10 mg/mL (1 mL) [contains benzyl alcohol]

Tablet: 5 mg

References

Martinez-Abad M, Delgado F, Palop V, et al, "Vitamin K_1 and Anaphylactic Shock," *DICP*, 1991, 25(7-8):871-2.

Piperacillin and Tazobactam Sodium

(pi PER a sil in & ta zoe BAK tam SOW dee um)

Medication Safety Issues

Sound-alike/look-alike issues:

Zosyn® may be confused with Zofran®, Zyvox™

U.S. Brand Names Zosyn®

Canadian Brand Names Tazocin®

Synonyms Piperacillin Sodium and Tazobactam Sodium

Pharmacologic Category Antibiotic, Penicillin

Generic Available No

Use Treatment of moderate-to-severe infections caused by susceptible organisms, including infections of the lower respiratory tract (community-acquired pneumonia, nosocomial pneumonia); urinary tract; uncomplicated and complicated skin and skin structures; gynecologic (endometritis, pelvic inflammatory disease); bone and joint infections; intra-abdominal infections (appendicitis with rupture/abscess, peritonitis); and septicemia. Tazobactam expands activity of piperacillin to include beta-lactamase producing strains of *S. aureus*, *H. influenzae*, *Bacteroides*, and other gram-negative bacteria.

Mechanism of Action Inhibits bacterial cell wall synthesis by binding to one or more of the penicillin binding proteins (PBPs); which in turn inhibits the final transpeptidation step of peptidoglycan synthesis in bacterial cell walls, thus inhibiting cell wall biosynthesis. Bacteria eventually lyse due to ongoing activity of cell wall autolytic enzymes (autolysins and murein hydrolases) while cell wall assembly is arrested. Tazobactam inhibits many beta-lactamases, including

(Continued)

Piperacillin and Tazobactam Sodium *(Continued)*

staphylococcal penicillinase and Richmond and Sykes types II, III, IV, and V, including extended spectrum enzymes; it has only limited activity against class I beta-lactamases other than class Ic types.

Pharmacodynamics/Kinetics Both AUC and peak concentrations are dose proportional; hepatic impairment does not affect kinetics

Distribution: Well into lungs, intestinal mucosa, skin, muscle, uterus, ovary, prostate, gallbladder, and bile; penetration into CSF is low in subject with noninflamed meninges

Protein binding: Piperacillin and tazobactam: ~30%

Metabolism:

- Piperacillin: 6% to 9% to desethyl metabolite (weak activity)
- Tazobactam: ~26% to inactive metabolite

Half-life elimination: Piperacillin and tazobactam: 0.7-1.2 hours

Time to peak, plasma: Immediately following infusion of 30 minutes

Excretion: Clearance of both piperacillin and tazobactam are directly proportional to renal function

- Piperacillin: Urine (68% as unchanged drug); feces (10% to 20%)
- Tazobactam: Urine (80% as inactive metabolite)

Dosage

Usual dosage range:

Children ≥6 months and ≤50 kg (unlabeled use): I.V.: 240-450 mg of piperacillin component/kg/day in divided doses every 4-6 hours for severe infections

Children ≥12 years and Adults: I.V.: 2.25-4.5 g every 6-8 hours (maximum 18 g (piperacillin)/day)

Indication-specific dosing:

Children ≥6 months and ≤50 kg (unlabeled use):

Cystic fibrosis, pseudomonal infections: 300-450 mg of piperacillin component/kg/day in divided doses every 6-8 hours have been used

Children ≥12 years and Adults:

Diverticulitis, intra-abdominal abscess, peritonitis: I.V.: 4.5 g every 8 hours or 3.375 g every 6 hours

Moderate infections: I.M.: 2.25 g every 6-8 hours; treatment should be continued for ≥7-10 days depending on severity of disease (**Note:** I.M. route not FDA-approved)

Pneumonia (nosocomial): I.V.: 4.5 g every 6 hours for 7-14 days (when used empirically, combination with an aminoglycoside is recommended; consider discontinuation of aminoglycoside if *P. aeruginosa* is not isolated)

Severe infections: I.V.: 4.5 g every 8 hours or 3.375 g every 6 hours for 7-10 days

Dosing interval in renal impairment:

Cl_{cr} 20-40 mL/minute: Administer 2.25 g every 6 hours (3.375 g every 6 hours for nosocomial pneumonia)

Cl_{cr} <20 mL/minute: Administer 2.25 g every 8 hours (2.25 g every 6 hours for nosocomial pneumonia)

Hemodialysis/CAPD: Administer 2.25 g every 12 hours (every 8 hours for nosocomial pneumonia) with an additional dose of 0.75 g after each dialysis

Continuous arteriovenous or venovenous hemodiafiltration effects: Dose as for Cl_{cr} 10-50 mL/minute

Stability

Vials: Store at controlled room temperature of 20°C to 25°C (68°F to 77°F). Use single-dose vials immediately after reconstitution (discard unused portions after 24 hours at room temperature and 48 hours if refrigerated). Reconstitute with 5 mL of diluent per 1 g of piperacillin and then further dilute. After reconstitution, vials or solution are stable in NS or D_5W for 24 hours at room temperature and 48 hours (vials) or 7 days (solution) when refrigerated.

Premixed solution: Store frozen at -20°C (-4°F). Thawed solution is stable for 24 hours at room temperature or 14 days under refrigeration; do not refreeze.

Administration Administer by I.V. infusion over 30 minutes

Some penicillins (eg, carbenicillin, ticarcillin and piperacillin) have been shown to inactivate aminoglycosides *in vitro*. This has been observed to a greater extent with tobramycin and gentamicin, while amikacin has shown greater stability against inactivation. Concurrent use of these agents may pose a risk of reduced antibacterial efficacy *in vivo*, particularly in the setting of profound renal impairment. However, definitive clinical evidence is lacking. If combination penicillin/

aminoglycoside therapy is desired in a patient with renal dysfunction, separation of doses (if feasible), and routine monitoring of aminoglycoside levels, CBC, and clinical response should be considered.

Monitoring Parameters Creatinine, BUN, CBC with differential, PT, PTT; signs of bleeding; monitor for signs of anaphylaxis during first dose

Pregnancy Risk Factor B

Contraindications Hypersensitivity to penicillins, beta-lactamase inhibitors, or any component of the formulation

Warnings/Precautions Bleeding disorders have been observed, particularly in patients with renal impairment; discontinue if thrombocytopenia or bleeding occurs. Due to sodium load and to the adverse effects of high serum concentrations of penicillins, dosage modification is required in patients with impaired or underdeveloped renal function; use with caution in patients with seizures or in patients with history of beta-lactam allergy; associated with an increased incidence of rash and fever in cystic fibrosis patients. Prolonged use may result in superinfection, including pseudomembranous colitis. Safety and efficacy have not been established in children.

Adverse Reactions

>10%: Gastrointestinal: Diarrhea (11%)

>1% to 10%:

Cardiovascular: Hypertension (2%), chest pain, edema

Central nervous system: Insomnia (7%), headache (7% to 8%), agitation (2%), fever (2%), pain (2%), anxiety, dizziness

Dermatologic: Rash (4%), pruritus (3%)

Gastrointestinal: Constipation (7% to 8%), nausea (7%), vomiting (3%), dyspepsia (3%), stool changes (2%), abdominal pain

Hepatic: Transaminases increased

Respiratory: Dyspnea, rhinitis

Miscellaneous: Moniliasis (2%)

≤1%, postmarketing, and/or case reports: Agranulocytosis, anaphylaxis/anaphylactoid reaction, anemia, arrhythmia, arthralgia, atrial fibrillation, back pain, bradycardia, bronchospasm, candidiasis, cardiac arrest, cardiac failure, circulatory failure, cholestatic jaundice, confusion, convulsions, coughing, depression, diaphoresis, dysuria, epistaxis, erythema multiforme, flatulence, flushing, gastritis, genital pruritus, hallucination, hematuria, hemolytic anemia, hemorrhage, hepatitis, hiccough, hypoglycemia, hypotension, ileus, incontinence, injection site reaction, interstitial nephritis, leukorrhea, malaise, melena, mesenteric embolism, myalgia, myocardial infarction, oliguria, pancytopenia, pharyngitis, phlebitis, photophobia, pseudomembranous colitis, pulmonary edema, pulmonary embolism, purpura, renal failure, retention, rigors, seizure, Stevens-Johnson syndrome, syncope, tachycardia (supraventricular and ventricular), taste perversion, thirst, thrombocytosis, tinnitus, toxic epidermal necrolysis, tremor, ulcerative stomatitis, vaginitis, ventricular fibrillation, vertigo

Overdosage/Toxicology Symptoms of penicillin overdose include neuromuscular hypersensitivity (eg, agitation, hallucinations, asterixis, encephalopathy, confusion, and seizures). Electrolyte imbalance may occur if the preparation contains potassium or sodium salts, especially in renal dysfunction. Hemodialysis may be helpful to aid in removal of the drug from blood; otherwise, treatment is supportive or symptom-directed.

Drug Interactions

Aminoglycosides: May be synergistic against selected organisms; physical inactivation of aminoglycosides in the presence of high concentrations of piperacillin and potential toxicity in patients with mild to moderate renal dysfunction

Heparin: Concomitant use with high-dose parenteral penicillins may result in increased risk of bleeding

Methotrexate: Penicillins may increase the exposure to methotrexate during concurrent therapy; monitor.

Neuromuscular blockers: May increase duration of blockade

Oral contraceptives: Anecdotal reports suggesting decreased contraceptive efficacy with penicillins have been refuted by more rigorous scientific and clinical data.

Probenecid: May increase levels of penicillins (piperacillin)

Tetracyclines: May decrease effectiveness of penicillins (piperacillin)

Warfarin: Effects of warfarin may be increased

Test Interactions Positive Coombs' [direct] test; false positive reaction for urine glucose using copper-reduction method (Clinitest®); may result in false positive results with the Platelia® *Aspergillus* enzyme immunoassay (EIA)

(Continued)

Piperacillin and Tazobactam Sodium *(Continued)*

Some penicillin derivatives may accelerate the degradation of aminoglycosides *in vitro*, leading to a potential underestimation of aminoglycoside serum concentration.

Dietary Considerations

Infusion, premixed: 2.25 g contains sodium 5.58 mEq (128 mg); 3.375 g contains sodium 8.38 mEq (192 mg); 4.5 g contains sodium 11.17 mEq (256 mg)

Injection, powder for reconstitution: 2.25 g contains sodium 5.58 mEq (128 mg); 3.375 g contains sodium 8.38 mEq (192 mg); 4.5 g contains sodium 11.17 mEq (256 mg); 40.5 g contains sodium 100.4 mEq (2304 mg, bulk pharmacy vial)

Dosage Forms Note: 8:1 ratio of piperacillin sodium/tazobactam sodium

Infusion [premixed iso-osmotic solution, frozen]:

- 2.25 g: Piperacillin 2 g and tazobactam 0.25 g (50 mL) [contains sodium 5.58 mEq (128 mg) and EDTA]
- 3.375 g: Piperacillin 3 g and tazobactam 0.375 g (50 mL) [contains sodium 8.38 mEq (192 mg) and EDTA]
- 4.5 g: Piperacillin 4 g and tazobactam 0.5 g (50 mL) [contains sodium 11.17 mEq (256 mg) and EDTA]

Injection, powder for reconstitution:

- 2.25 g: Piperacillin 2 g and tazobactam 0.25 g [contains sodium 5.58 mEq (128 mg) and EDTA]
- 3.375 g: Piperacillin 3 g and tazobactam 0.375 g [contains sodium 8.38 mEq (192 mg) and EDTA]
- 4.5 g: Piperacillin 4 g and tazobactam 0.5 g [contains sodium 11.17 mEq (256 mg) and EDTA]
- 40.5 g: Piperacillin 36 g and tazobactam 4.5 g [contains sodium 100.4 mEq (2304 mg) and EDTA; bulk pharmacy vial]

References

American Thoracic Society and Infectious Diseases Society of America, "Guidelines for the Management of Adults With Hospital-Acquired, Ventilator-Associated, and Healthcare-Associated Pneumonia," *Am J Respir Crit Care Med*, 2005, 171(4):388-416.

♦ **Piperacillin Sodium and Tazobactam Sodium** *see* Piperacillin and Tazobactam Sodium *on page 1029*

Piroxicam (peer OKS i kam)

Related Information

Chronic Pain Management *on page 1430*

U.S. Brand Names Feldene®

Canadian Brand Names Apo-Piroxicam®; Gen-Piroxicam; Novo-Pirocam; Nu-Pirox; Pexicam®

Pharmacologic Category Nonsteroidal Anti-inflammatory Drug (NSAID), Oral

Restrictions A medication guide should be dispensed with each prescription. A template for the required MedGuide can be found on the FDA website at: http://www.fda.gov/medwatch/SAFETY/2005/safety05.htm#NSAID

Generic Available Yes

Use Symptomatic treatment of acute and chronic rheumatoid arthritis and osteoarthritis

Unlabeled/Investigational Use Ankylosing spondylitis

Mechanism of Action Inhibits prostaglandin synthesis, acts on the hypothalamus heat-regulating center to reduce fever, blocks prostaglandin synthetase action which prevents formation of the platelet-aggregating substance thromboxane A_2; decreases pain receptor sensitivity. Other proposed mechanisms of action for salicylate anti-inflammatory action are lysosomal stabilization, kinin and leukotriene production, alteration of chemotactic factors, and inhibition of neutrophil activation. This latter mechanism may be the most significant pharmacologic action to reduce inflammation.

Pharmacodynamics/Kinetics

Onset of action: Analgesic: ~1 hour

Peak effect: 3-5 hours

Protein binding: 99%

Metabolism: Hepatic

Half-life elimination: 45-50 hours

Excretion: Primarily urine and feces (small amounts) as unchanged drug (5%) and metabolites

Dosage Oral:

Children (unlabeled use): 0.2-0.3 mg/kg/day once daily; maximum dose: 15 mg/day

Adults: 10-20 mg/day once daily; although associated with increase in GI adverse effects, doses >20 mg/day have been used (ie, 30-40 mg/day)

Dosing adjustment in renal impairment: Not recommended in patients with advanced renal disease

Dosing adjustment in hepatic impairment: Reduction of dosage is necessary

Monitoring Parameters Occult blood loss, hemoglobin, hematocrit, and periodic renal and hepatic function tests; periodic ophthalmologic exams with chronic use

Anesthesia and Critical Care Concerns/Other Considerations The 2002 ACCM/SCCM guidelines for analgesia (critically-ill adult) suggest that NSAIDs may be used in combination with opioids in select patients for pain management. Concern about adverse events (increased risk of renal dysfunction, altered platelet function and gastrointestinal irritation) limits its use in patients who have other underlying risks for these events.

In short-term use, NSAIDs vary considerably in their effect on blood pressure. When NSAIDs are used in patients with hypertension, appropriate monitoring of blood pressure responses should be completed and the duration of therapy, when possible, kept short. The use of NSAIDs in the treatment of patients with congestive heart failure may be associated with an increased risk for fluid accumulation and edema; may precipitate renal failure in dehydrated patients.

Pregnancy Risk Factor C/D (3rd trimester)

Contraindications Hypersensitivity to piroxicam, aspirin, other NSAIDs or any component of the formulation; perioperative pain in the setting of coronary artery bypass surgery (CABG); pregnancy (3rd trimester or near term)

Warnings/Precautions [U.S. Boxed Warning]: NSAIDs are associated with an increased risk of adverse cardiovascular events, including MI, stroke, and new onset or worsening of pre-existing hypertension. Risk may be increased with duration of use or pre-existing cardiovascular risk-factors or disease. Carefully evaluate individual cardiovascular risk profiles prior to prescribing. Use caution with fluid retention, CHF or hypertension.

Use of NSAIDs can compromise existing renal function. Renal toxicity can occur in patient with impaired renal function, dehydration, heart failure, liver dysfunction, those taking diuretics and ACEI and the elderly. Rehydrate patient before starting therapy. Monitor renal function closely. Not recommended for use in patients with advanced renal disease.

[U.S. Boxed Warning]: NSAIDs may increase risk of gastrointestinal irritation, ulceration, bleeding, and perforation. These events may occur at any time during therapy and without warning. Use caution with a history of GI disease (bleeding or ulcers), concurrent therapy with aspirin, anticoagulants and/or corticosteroids, smoking, use of alcohol, the elderly or debilitated patients.

Use the lowest effective dose for the shortest duration of time, consistent with individual patient goals, to reduce risk of cardiovascular or GI adverse events. Alternate therapies should be considered for patients at high risk.

NSAIDs may cause serious skin adverse events including exfoliative dermatitis, Stevens-Johnson syndrome (SJS) and toxic epidermal necrolysis (TEN). Anaphylactoid reactions may occur, even without prior exposure; patients with "aspirin triad" (bronchial asthma, aspirin intolerance, rhinitis) may be at increased risk. Do not use in patients who experience bronchospasm, asthma, rhinitis, or urticaria with NSAID or aspirin therapy. A serum sickness-like reaction can rarely occur; watch for arthralgias, pruritus, fever, fatigue, and rash.

Use with caution in patients with decreased hepatic function. Closely monitor patients with any abnormal LFT. Severe hepatic reactions (eg, fulminant hepatitis, liver failure) have occurred with NSAID use, rarely; discontinue if signs or symptoms of liver disease develop, or if systemic manifestations occur.

The elderly are at increased risk for adverse effects (especially peptic ulceration, CNS effects, renal toxicity) from NSAIDs even at low doses

Withhold for at least 4-6 half-lives prior to surgical or dental procedures.

Adverse Reactions

>10%:

Central nervous system: Dizziness
Dermatologic: Rash
Gastrointestinal: Abdominal cramps, heartburn, indigestion, nausea

(Continued)

Piroxicam *(Continued)*

1% to 10%:

Central nervous system: Headache, nervousness
Dermatologic: Itching
Endocrine & metabolic: Fluid retention
Gastrointestinal: Vomiting
Otic: Tinnitus

<1%: Acute renal failure, agranulocytosis, allergic rhinitis, anemia, angioedema, arrhythmia, aseptic meningitis, blurred vision, bone marrow suppression, confusion, CHF, conjunctivitis, cystitis, decreased hearing, drowsiness, dry eyes, dyspnea, epistaxis, erythema multiforme, gastritis, GI ulceration, hallucinations, hemolytic anemia, hepatitis, hot flashes, hypertension, insomnia, leukopenia, mental depression, peripheral neuropathy, photosensitivity, polydipsia, polyuria, Stevens-Johnson syndrome, tachycardia, thrombocytopenia, toxic amblyopia, toxic epidermal necrolysis, urticaria

Overdosage/Toxicology Symptoms of overdose include nausea, epigastric distress, CNS depression, leukocytosis, and renal failure. Management of NSAID intoxication is supportive and symptomatic. Multiple doses of activated charcoal may interrupt enterohepatic recycling of some NSAIDs.

Drug Interactions Substrate of CYP2C9 (minor); **Inhibits** CYP2C9 (strong)

ACE inhibitors: Antihypertensive effects may be decreased by concurrent therapy with NSAIDs; monitor blood pressure.

Angiotensin II antagonists: Antihypertensive effects may be decreased by concurrent therapy with NSAIDs; monitor blood pressure.

Anticoagulants (warfarin, heparin, LMWHs) in combination with NSAIDs can cause increased risk of bleeding.

Antiplatelet drugs (ticlopidine, clopidogrel, aspirin, abciximab, dipyridamole, eptifibatide, tirofiban) can cause an increased risk of bleeding.

Beta-blockers: NSAIDs may decrease the antihypertensive effect of beta-blockers. Monitor.

Cholestyramine (and other bile acid sequestrants): May decrease the absorption of NSAIDs. Separate by at least 2 hours.

Corticosteroids may increase the risk of GI ulceration; avoid concurrent use.

Cyclosporine: NSAIDs may increase serum creatinine, potassium, blood pressure, and cyclosporine levels; monitor cyclosporine levels and renal function carefully.

CYP2C9 Substrates: Piroxicam may increase the levels/effects of CYP2C9 substrates. Example substrates include bosentan, dapsone, fluoxetine, glimepiride, glipizide, losartan, montelukast, nateglinide, paclitaxel, phenytoin, warfarin, and zafirlukast.

Hydralazine's antihypertensive effect is decreased; avoid concurrent use.

Lithium levels can be increased; avoid concurrent use if possible or monitor lithium levels and adjust dose.

Loop diuretics efficacy (diuretic and antihypertensive effect) is reduced. Indomethacin reduces this efficacy, however, it may be anticipated with any NSAID.

Methotrexate: Severe bone marrow suppression, aplastic anemia, and GI toxicity have been reported with concomitant NSAID therapy. Avoid use during moderate or high-dose methotrexate (increased and prolonged methotrexate levels). NSAID use during low-dose treatment of rheumatoid arthritis has not been fully evaluated; extreme caution is warranted.

Thiazides antihypertensive effects are decreased; avoid concurrent use.

Warfarin's INRs may be increased by piroxicam. Other NSAIDs may have the same effect depending on dose and duration. Monitor INR closely. Use the lowest dose of NSAIDs possible and for the briefest duration.

Ethanol/Nutrition/Herb Interactions

Ethanol: Avoid ethanol (may enhance gastric mucosal irritation).

Food: Onset of effect may be delayed if piroxicam is taken with food.

Herb/Nutraceutical: Avoid alfalfa, anise, bilberry, bladderwrack, bromelain, cat's claw, celery, coleus, cordyceps, dong quai, evening primrose, feverfew, fenugreek, garlic, ginger, ginkgo biloboa, red clover, horse chestnut, grapeseed, green tea, ginseng, guggul, horse chestnut seed, horseradish, licorice, prickly ash, red clover, reishi, SAMe, sweet clover, turmeric, white willow (all have additional antiplatelet activity).

Test Interactions Increased chloride (S), increased sodium (S), increased bleeding time

Dietary Considerations May be taken with food to decrease GI adverse effect.

Dosage Forms Capsule: 10 mg, 20 mg

- ♦ **PMS-Oxycodone-Acetaminophen (Can)** *see* Oxycodone and Acetaminophen *on page 969*
- ♦ **PMS-Paroxetine (Can)** *see* Paroxetine *on page 988*
- ♦ **PMS-Phenobarbital (Can)** *see* Phenobarbital *on page 1008*
- ♦ **PMS-Pravastatin (Can)** *see* Pravastatin *on page 1042*
- ♦ **PMS-Pseudoephedrine (Can)** *see* Pseudoephedrine *on page 1085*
- ♦ **PMS-Ranitidine (Can)** *see* Ranitidine *on page 1105*
- ♦ **PMS-Salbutamol (Can)** *see* Albuterol *on page 50*
- ♦ **PMS-Sertraline (Can)** *see* Sertraline *on page 1161*
- ♦ **PMS-Simvastatin (Can)** *see* Simvastatin *on page 1174*
- ♦ **PMS-Sodium Polystyrene Sulfonate (Can)** *see* Sodium Polystyrene Sulfonate *on page 1193*
- ♦ **PMS-Sotalol (Can)** *see* Sotalol *on page 1198*
- ♦ **PMS-Sucralate (Can)** *see* Sucralfate *on page 1212*
- ♦ **PMS-Sumatriptan (Can)** *see* Sumatriptan *on page 1222*
- ♦ **PMS-Temazepam (Can)** *see* Temazepam *on page 1239*
- ♦ **PMS-Terazosin (Can)** *see* Terazosin *on page 1243*
- ♦ **PMS-Theophylline (Can)** *see* Theophylline *on page 1253*
- ♦ **PMS-Timolol (Can)** *see* Timolol *on page 1268*
- ♦ **PMS-Tobramycin (Can)** *see* Tobramycin *on page 1278*
- ♦ **PMS-Topiramate (Can)** *see* Topiramate *on page 1287*
- ♦ **PMS-Trazodone (Can)** *see* Trazodone *on page 1306*
- ♦ **PMS-Valproic Acid (Can)** *see* Valproic Acid and Derivatives *on page 1329*
- ♦ **PMS-Valproic Acid E.C. (Can)** *see* Valproic Acid and Derivatives *on page 1329*
- ♦ **PN** *see* Total Parenteral Nutrition *on page 1293*
- ♦ **Polocaine®** *see* Mepivacaine *on page 804*
- ♦ **Polocaine® Dental** *see* Mepivacaine *on page 804*
- ♦ **Polocaine® MPF** *see* Mepivacaine *on page 804*
- ♦ **Polygam® S/D** *see* Immune Globulin (Intravenous) *on page 666*

Polymyxin B (pol i MIKS in bee)

U.S. Brand Names Poly-Rx

Synonyms Polymyxin B Sulfate

Pharmacologic Category Antibiotic, Irrigation; Antibiotic, Miscellaneous

Generic Available Yes

Use Treatment of acute infections caused by susceptible strains of *Pseudomonas aeruginosa*; used occasionally for gut decontamination; parenteral use of polymyxin B has mainly been replaced by less toxic antibiotics, reserved for life-threatening infections caused by organisms resistant to the preferred drugs (eg, pseudomonal meningitis - intrathecal administration)

Mechanism of Action Binds to phospholipids, alters permeability, and damages the bacterial cytoplasmic membrane permitting leakage of intracellular constituents

Pharmacodynamics/Kinetics

Absorption: Well absorbed from peritoneum; minimal from GI tract (except in neonates) from mucous membranes or intact skin

Distribution: Minimal into CSF; does not cross placenta

Half-life elimination: 4.5-6 hours; prolonged with renal impairment

Time to peak, serum: I.M.: ~2 hours

Excretion: Urine (>60% primarily as unchanged drug)

Dosage

Otic (in combination with other drugs): 1-2 drops, 3-4 times/day; should be used sparingly to avoid accumulation of excess debris

Infants <2 years:

I.M.: Up to 40,000 units/kg/day divided every 6 hours (not routinely recommended due to pain at injection sites)

I.V.: Up to 40,000 units/kg/day divided every 12 hours

Intrathecal: 20,000 units/day for 3-4 days, then 25,000 units every other day for at least 2 weeks after CSF cultures are negative and CSF (glucose) has returned to within normal limits

Children ≥2 years and Adults:

I.M.: 25,000-30,000 units/kg/day divided every 4-6 hours (not routinely recommended due to pain at injection sites)

I.V.: 15,000-25,000 units/kg/day divided every 12 hours

Intrathecal: 50,000 units/day for 3-4 days, then every other day for at least 2 weeks after CSF cultures are negative and CSF (glucose) has returned to within normal limits

Total daily dose should not exceed 2,000,000 units/day

Bladder irrigation: Continuous irrigant or rinse in the urinary bladder for up to 10 days using 20 mg (equal to 200,000 units) added to 1 L of normal saline; usually no more than 1 L of irrigant is used per day unless urine flow rate is high; administration rate is adjusted to patient's urine output

Topical irrigation or topical solution: 500,000 units/L of normal saline; topical irrigation should not exceed 2 million units/day in adults

Gut sterilization: Oral: 15,000-25,000 units/kg/day in divided doses every 6 hours

Clostridium difficile enteritis: Oral: 25,000 units every 6 hours for 10 days

Ophthalmic: A concentration of 0.1% to 0.25% is administered as 1-3 drops every hour, then increasing the interval as response indicates to 1-2 drops 4-6 times/day

Dosing adjustment/interval in renal impairment:

Cl_{cr} 20-50 mL/minute: Administer 75% to 100% of normal dose every 12 hours

Cl_{cr} 5-20 mL/minute: Administer 50% of normal dose every 12 hours

Cl_{cr} <5 mL/minute: Administer 15% of normal dose every 12 hours

Stability Prior to reconstitution, store at room temperature of 15°C to 30°C (59°F to 86°F); protect from light. After reconstitution, store under refrigeration at 2°C to 8°C (36°F to 46°F); discard any unused solution after 72 hours. **Incompatible** with strong acids/alkalies, calcium, magnesium, cephalothin, cefazolin, chloramphenicol, heparin, penicillins.

Administration Dissolve 500,000 units in 300-500 mL D_5W for continuous I.V. drip; dissolve 500,000 units in 2 mL water for injection, saline, or 1% procaine solution for I.M. injection; dissolve 500,000 units in 10 mL physiologic solution for intrathecal administration

Extravasation management: Monitor I.V. site closely; extravasation may cause serious injury with possible necrosis and tissue sloughing. Rotate infusion site frequently.

Monitoring Parameters Neurologic symptoms and signs of superinfection; renal function (decreasing urine output and increasing BUN may require discontinuance of therapy)

Reference Range Serum concentrations >5 mcg/mL are toxic in adults

Pregnancy Risk Factor B (per expert opinion)

Contraindications Hypersensitivity to polymyxin B or any component of the formulation; concurrent use of neuromuscular blockers

Warnings/Precautions **[U.S. Boxed Warning]: May cause neurotoxicity, nephrotoxicity, and/or neuromuscular blockade and respiratory paralysis;** usual risk factors include prexisiting renal impairment, concomitant neuro-/nephrotoxic medications, advanced age and dehydration. Use with caution in patients with impaired renal function (modify dosage); polymyxin B-induced nephrotoxicity may be manifested by albuminuria, cellular casts, and azotemia. Discontinue therapy with decreasing urinary output and increasing BUN; neurotoxic reactions are usually associated with high serum levels, often in patients with renal dysfunction. Avoid concurrent or sequential use of other nephrotoxic and neurotoxic drugs (eg, aminoglycosides). The drug's neurotoxicity can result in respiratory paralysis from neuromuscular blockade, especially when the drug is given soon after anesthesia or muscle relaxants. Polymyxin B sulfate is most toxic when given parenterally; avoid parenteral use whenever possible. **[U.S. Boxed Warnings]: Safety in pregnant women not established; intramuscular/intrathecal administration only to hospitalized patinets.**

Adverse Reactions Frequency not defined (limited to important or life-threatening):

Central nervous system: Neurotoxicity (irritability, drowsiness, ataxia, perioral paresthesia, numbness of the extremities, and blurred vision); dizziness

Neuromuscular & skeletal: Neuromuscular blockade

Renal: Nephrotoxicity

Respiratory: Respiratory arrest

(Continued)

Polymyxin B *(Continued)*

Overdosage/Toxicology Symptoms of overdose include respiratory paralysis, ototoxicity, and nephrotoxicity. Supportive care is indicated as treatment.

Drug Interactions Polymyxin may increase/prolong effect of neuromuscular blocking agents; aminoglycosides may increase polymyxin's risk of respiratory paralysis and renal dysfunction

Dosage Forms

Injection, powder for reconstitution: 500,000 units

Powder [for prescription compounding] (Poly-Rx): 100 million units (13 g)

- ♦ **Polymyxin B Sulfate** *see* Polymyxin B *on page 1036*
- ♦ **Poly-Rx** *see* Polymyxin B *on page 1036*
- ♦ **Polyvinylpyrrolidone with Iodine** *see* Povidone-Iodine *on page 1039*
- ♦ **Ponstan® (Can)** *see* Mefenamic Acid *on page 795*
- ♦ **Ponstel®** *see* Mefenamic Acid *on page 795*
- ♦ **Pontocaine®** *see* Tetracaine *on page 1248*
- ♦ **Pontocaine® Niphanoid®** *see* Tetracaine *on page 1248*

Poractant Alfa (por AKT ant AL fa)

U.S. Brand Names Curosurf®

Canadian Brand Names Curosurf®

Pharmacologic Category Lung Surfactant

Generic Available No

Use Orphan drug: Treatment and prevention of respiratory distress syndrome (RDS) in premature infants

Mechanism of Action Endogenous pulmonary surfactant reduces surface tension at the air-liquid interface of the alveoli during ventilation and stabilizes the alveoli against collapse at resting transpulmonary pressures. A deficiency of pulmonary surfactant in preterm infants results in respiratory distress syndrome characterized by poor lung expansion, inadequate gas exchange, and atelectasis. Poractant alpha compensates for the surfactant deficiency and restores surface activity to the infant's lungs. It reduces mortality and pneumothoraces associated with RDS.

Pharmacodynamics/Kinetics Information limited to animal models. No human information about pharmacokinetics exists.

Dosage Intratracheal use **only**: Premature infant with RDS: Initial dose is 2.5 mL/kg of birth weight. Up to 2 subsequent doses of 1.25 mL/kg birth weight can be administered at 12-hour intervals if needed in infants who continue to require mechanical ventilation and supplemental oxygen.

Stability Store under refrigeration at defined temperature of 2°C to 8°C (36°F to 46°F). Unopened, unused vials that have been warmed to room temperature can be returned to refrigerator storage within 24 hours for future use. Do not warm and then refrigerate more than once. Protect from light. Do not shake.

Administration Take from refrigerator and warm to room temperature. Inspect for discoloration. The color should be white to creamy white. Gently turn the vial upside down to get a uniform suspension. Do not shake. Slowly withdraw the entire contents into a 3 mL or 5 mL plastic syringe through a large gauge needle (≥20 gauge). Attach the catheter to the syringe. Fill the catheter with poractant alfa. Discard the excess through the catheter so that only the total dose to be given remains in the syringe.

Before administering, assure proper placement and patency of the endotracheal tube. The endotracheal tube may be suctioned before administering the poractant alpha. The drug is administered intratracheally through a 5-French end-hole catheter cut to a standard length of 8 cm **or** through a secondary lumen of a dual-lumen endotracheal tube (without interrupting mechanical ventilation). Up to 2 repeated doses may be administered, using the same technique at 12-hour intervals.

Administration using a 5-French end-hole catheter: The infant should be stable before proceeding with dosing. The infant's ventilator settings should be changed to a rate of 40-60 breaths/minute, inspiratory time 0.5 seconds, and supplemental oxygen to maintain SaO_2 of 92%. Keep the head and body of the infant in alignment without inclination. Briefly disconnect the endotracheal tube from the ventilator, insert the 5-French catheter. This catheter is inserted into the infant's endotracheal tube with the tip positioned distally in the endotracheal tube.

The catheter tip should not extend beyond the distal tip of the endotracheal tube. Each dose should be administered in two aliquots with each aliquot administered into one of the two main bronchi by positioning the infant with either the right or left side dependent.

Insert the first aliquot (1.25 mL/kg birth weight) and position the infant so that either the right or left side is dependent for the aliquot. Remove the catheter and manually ventilate the infant with 100% oxygen at a rate of 40-60 breaths/minute for 1 minute. When the infant is stable, reposition the infant such that the other side is dependent and administer the remaining aliquot using the same technique. Remove the catheter without flushing. Do not suction the airways for 1 hour after instillation unless signs of significant airway obstruction occur. Resume ventilator management and clinical care.

Administration using the secondary lumen of a dual-lumen endotracheal tube: Administration as a single dose over 1 minute (without interrupting mechanical ventilation); transient increases in F_1O_2, ventilatory rate, or peak inspiratory pressure (PIP) may be required.

Monitoring Parameters Arterial blood gases, ventilator measurement assessment

Contraindications No known contraindications

Warnings/Precautions Marked improvement in oxygenation may occur within minutes of administration, therefore, may require frequent clinical and laboratory assessment so adjustments to oxygen delivery and ventilation settings can be made. Should only be used by those who are experts in care of the premature infant. Stop administration if bradycardia, hypotension, endotracheal tube blockage, or oxygen desaturation occur. May reinstitute after the patient is stable. Correct acidosis, hypotension, anemia, hypoglycemia, and hypothermia before use. Do not use with experimental therapies for RDS.

Adverse Reactions Frequency not defined.

Cardiovascular: Bradycardia, hypotension

Gastrointestinal: Endotracheal tube blockage

Respiratory: Oxygen desaturation

Overdosage/Toxicology There have been no reports. However, in the event of an accidental overdose in which the patient has suffered clinical effects, aspirate as much of the suspension from the lungs as possible and manage with supportive treatment, with emphasis on fluid and electrolyte balance.

Dosage Forms Suspension for intratracheal instillation [preservative free; porcine derived]: 80 mg/mL (1.5 mL, 3 mL)

♦ **Post Peel Healing Balm [OTC]** *see* Hydrocortisone *on page 639*

♦ **Povidine™ [OTC]** *see* Povidone-Iodine *on page 1039*

Povidone-Iodine (POE vi done EYE oh dyne)

Medication Safety Issues

Sound-alike/look-alike issues:

Betadine® may be confused with Betagan®, betaine

U.S. Brand Names Betadine® [OTC]; Betadine® Ophthalmic; Minidyne® [OTC]; Operand® [OTC]; Povidine™ [OTC]; Summer's Eve® Medicated Douche [OTC]; Vagi-Gard® [OTC]

Canadian Brand Names Betadine®; Proviodine

Synonyms Polyvinylpyrrolidone with Iodine; PVP-I

Pharmacologic Category Antiseptic, Ophthalmic; Antiseptic, Topical; Antiseptic, Vaginal; Topical Skin Product

Generic Available Yes

Use External antiseptic with broad microbicidal spectrum for the prevention or treatment of topical infections associated with surgery, burns, minor cuts/scrapes; relief of minor vaginal irritation

Mechanism of Action Povidone-iodine is known to be a powerful broad spectrum germicidal agent effective against a wide range of bacteria, viruses, fungi, protozoa, and spores.

Pharmacodynamics/Kinetics Absorption: Topical: Absorbed systemically as iodine; amount depends upon concentration, route of administration, characteristics of skin

(Continued)

Povidone-Iodine *(Continued)*

Dosage

Antiseptic: Apply topically to affected area as needed. Ophthalmic solution may be used to irrigate the eye or applied to area around the eye such as skin, eyelashes, or lid margins.

Surgical scrub: Topical: Apply solution to wet skin or hands, scrub for ~5 minutes, rinse; refer to product labeling for specific procedure-related instructions.

Vaginal irritation: Douche: Insert 0.3% solution vaginally once daily for 5-7 days

Pregnancy Risk Factor C (ophthalmic)

Contraindications Hypersensitivity to iodine or any component of the formulation

Warnings/Precautions Use caution in patients with thyroid disorders. Toxicity may occur following application of large or prolonged quantities; use caution with renal dysfunction, burns, pediatric patients. When used for self-medication (OTC use) do not apply to deep puncture wounds or serious burns; discontinue in case of redness, swelling, irritation or pain; do not use for longer than 1 week.

Adverse Reactions Frequency not defined.

Local: Edema, irritation, pruritus, rash

Drug Interactions No data reported

Dosage Forms [DSC] = Discontinued product

Gel, topical (Operand®): 10% (120 g)
Liquid, topical: 10% (30 mL)
Ointment, topical: 10% (1 g, 30 g)
  Betadine®: 10% (0.9 g, 3.7 g, 30 g) [DSC]
  Povidine™: 10% (30 g)
Pad [prep pads]: 10% (200s)
  Betadine® SwabAids: 10% (100s)
Scrub brush [solution impregnated]: 7.5% (30s)
Solution, ophthalmic (Betadine®): 5% (50 mL)
Solution, perineal (Operand®): 10% (240 mL) [concentrate]
Solution, topical: 10% (240 mL, 480 mL, 3840 mL)
  Betadine®: 10% (15 mL, 120 mL, 240 mL, 480 mL, 960 mL, 3840 mL)
  Minidyne®: 10% (15 mL)
  Operand®: 10% (60 mL, 120 mL, 240 mL, 480 mL, 960 mL, 3840 mL)
Solution, topical scrub:
  Betadine® Surgical Scrub: 7.5% (120 mL, 480 mL, 960 mL, 3840 mL)
  Betadine® Skin Cleanser: 7.5% (120 mL)
  Operand®: 7.5% (60 mL, 120 mL, 240 mL, 480 mL, 960 mL, 3840 mL)
Solution, topical spray:
  Betadine®: 5% (90 mL) [CFC free; contains dry natural rubber]
  Operand®: 10% (59 mL)
Solution, vaginal douche:
  Operand®: 10% (240 mL) [concentrate]
  Summer's Eve® Medicated Douche: 0.3% (135 mL)
  Vagi-Gard®: 10% (180 mL, 240 mL) [concentrate]
Solution, whirlpool (Operand®): 10% (3840 mL) [concentrate]
Swab [prep-swab ampul]: 10% (0.65 mL)
Swabsticks: 10% (25s, 50s)
  Betadine®: 10% (50s, 150s, 200s)
Swabsticks [gel saturated]: 10% (50s)
Swabsticks, topical scrub: 7.5% (25s, 50s)

Pralidoxime (pra li DOKS eem)

Medication Safety Issues

Sound-alike/look-alike issues:
  Pralidoxime may be confused with pramoxine, pyridoxine
  Protopam® may be confused with Proloprim®, protamine, Protropin®

U.S. Brand Names Protopam®

Canadian Brand Names Protopam®

Synonyms 2-PAM; Pralidoxime Chloride; 2-Pyridine Aldoxime Methochloride

Pharmacologic Category Antidote

Generic Available No

Use Reverse muscle paralysis caused by toxic exposure to organophosphate anticholinesterase pesticides and chemicals; control of overdose of anticholinesterase medications used to treat myasthenia gravis (ambenonium, neostigmine, pyridostigmine)

Unlabeled/Investigational Use Treatment of nerve agent toxicity (chemical warfare) in combination with atropine

Mechanism of Action Reactivates cholinesterase that had been inactivated by phosphorylation due to exposure to organophosphate pesticides by displacing the enzyme from its receptor sites; removes the phosphoryl group from the active site of the inactivated enzyme

Pharmacodynamics/Kinetics

Protein binding: None

Metabolism: Hepatic

Half-life elimination: 74-77 minutes

Time to peak, serum: I.V.: 5-15 minutes

Excretion: Urine (80% to 90% as metabolites and unchanged drug)

Dosage

Organic phosphorus poisoning (use in conjunction with atropine; atropine effects should be established before pralidoxime is administered): I.V. (may be given I.M. or SubQ if I.V. is not feasible):

Children: 20-50 mg/kg/dose; repeat in 1-2 hours if muscle weakness has not been relieved, then at 8- to 12-hour intervals if cholinergic signs recur

Adults: 1-2 g; repeat in 1 hour if muscle weakness has not been relieved, then at 8- to 12-hour intervals if cholinergic signs recur. When the poison has been ingested, continued absorption from the lower bowel may require additional doses; patients should be titrated as long as signs of poisoning recur; dosing may need repeated every 3-8 hours.

Treatment of acetylcholinesterase inhibitor toxicity: Adults: I.V.: Initial: 1-2 g followed by increments of 250 mg every 5 minutes until response is observed

Nerve agent toxicity management (unlabeled use): **Note:** Atropine is a component of the management of nerve agent toxicity; consult atropine monograph for specific route and dose. To be effective, pralidoxime must be administered within minutes to a few hours following exposure (depending on the nerve agent).

Infants and Children:

Prehospital ("in the field"): Mild-to-moderate symptoms: I.M.: 15 mg/kg; severe symptoms: 25 mg/kg

Hospital/emergency department: Mild-to-severe symptoms: I.V.: 15 mg/kg (up to 1 g)

Adults:

Prehospital ("in the field"): Mild-to-moderate symptoms: I.M.: 600 mg; severe symptoms: 1800 mg

Hospital/emergency department: Mild-to-severe symptoms: I.V.: 15 mg/kg (up to 1 g)

Frail patients, elderly:

Prehospital ("in the field"): Mild-to-moderate symptoms: I.M.: 10 mg/kg; severe symptoms: 25 mg/kg

Hospital/emergency department: Mild-to-severe symptoms: I.V.: 5-10 mg/kg

Elderly: Refer to Adults dosing; dosing should be cautious, considering possibility of decreased hepatic, renal, or cardiac function

Dosing adjustment in renal impairment: Dose should be reduced

Stability Store at controlled room temperature of 20°C to 25°C (68°F to 77°F). For I.V. administration, dilute 1 g with 20 mL SWI; solution should be further diluted and administered as 1-2 g in 100 mL NS. If not practical or in cases of fluid overload, may prepare as a 5% solution.

Administration I.V.: Infuse over 15-30 minutes at a rate not to exceed 200 mg/minute; may administer I.M. or SubQ if I.V. is not accessible. If a more concentrated 5% solution is used, infuse over at least 5 minutes.

Monitoring Parameters Heart rate, respiratory rate, blood pressure, continuous ECG; cardiac monitor and blood pressure monitor required for I.V. administration

Reference Range Minimum therapeutic concentration: 4 mcg/mL

Anesthesia and Critical Care Concerns/Other Considerations Use I.V. phentolamine for treatment of pralidoxime-induced hypertension (children: 1 mg; adults: 5 mg).

Pregnancy Risk Factor C

(Continued)

Pralidoxime *(Continued)*

Contraindications Hypersensitivity to pralidoxime or any component of the formulation; poisonings due to phosphorus, inorganic phosphates, or organic phosphates without anticholinesterase activity; poisonings due to pesticides or carbamate class (may increase toxicity of carbaryl)

Warnings/Precautions Use with caution in patients with myasthenia gravis; dosage modification required in patients with impaired renal function; use with caution in patients receiving theophylline, succinylcholine, phenothiazines, respiratory depressants (eg, narcotics, barbiturates).

Adverse Reactions Frequency not defined.

Cardiovascular: Tachycardia, hypertension
Central nervous system: Dizziness, headache, drowsiness
Dermatologic: Rash
Gastrointestinal: Nausea
Hepatic: Transient increases in ALT, AST
Local: Pain at injection site after I.M. administration
Neuromuscular & skeletal: Muscle rigidity, weakness
Ocular: Accommodation impaired, blurred vision, diplopia
Renal: Renal function decreased
Respiratory: Hyperventilation, laryngospasm

Overdosage/Toxicology Symptoms of overdose include blurred vision, nausea, tachycardia, and dizziness. Treatment is supportive.

Drug Interactions

Decreased effect: Atropine, although often used concurrently with pralidoxime to offset muscarinic stimulation, these effects can occur earlier than anticipated

Increased effect: Barbiturates (potentiated)

Increased toxicity: Use with aminophylline, morphine, theophylline, and succinylcholine is contraindicated; use with reserpine and phenothiazines should be avoided in patients with organophosphate poisoning

Dosage Forms Injection, powder for reconstitution, as chloride: 1 g

References

"Medical Management Guidelines (MMGs) for Nerve Agents: Tabun (GA); Sarin (GB); Soman (GD); and VX," available at www.atsdr.cdc.gov/MHMI/mmg166.html.

◆ **Pralidoxime Chloride** *see* Pralidoxime *on page 1040*

◆ **Pravachol®** *see* Pravastatin *on page 1042*

◆ **PravASA (Can)** *see* Aspirin and Pravastatin *on page 135*

Pravastatin (PRA va stat in)

Medication Safety Issues

Sound-alike/look-alike issues:

Pravachol® may be confused with Prevacid®, Prinivil®, propranolol

Related Information

Hyperlipidemia Management *on page 1614*

U.S. Brand Names Pravachol®

Canadian Brand Names Apo-Pravastatin®; CO Pravastatin; Novo-Pravastatin; PMS-Pravastatin; Pravachol®; ratio-Pravastatin; Sandoz-Pravastatin

Synonyms Pravastatin Sodium

Pharmacologic Category Antilipemic Agent, HMG-CoA Reductase Inhibitor

Generic Available No

Use Use with dietary therapy for the following:

Primary prevention of coronary events: In hypercholesterolemic patients without established coronary heart disease to reduce cardiovascular morbidity (myocardial infarction, coronary revascularization procedures) and mortality.

Secondary prevention of cardiovascular events in patients with established coronary heart disease: To slow the progression of coronary atherosclerosis; to reduce cardiovascular morbidity (myocardial infarction, coronary vascular procedures) and to reduce mortality; to reduce the risk of stroke and transient ischemic attacks

Hyperlipidemias: Reduce elevations in total cholesterol, LDL-C, apolipoprotein B, and triglycerides (elevations of 1 or more components are present in Fredrickson type IIa, IIb, III, and IV hyperlipidemias)

Heterozygous familial hypercholesterolemia (HeFH): In pediatric patients, 8-18 years of age, with HeFH having LDL-C ≥190 mg/dL **or** LDL ≥160 mg/dL with positive family history of premature cardiovascular disease (CVD) or 2 or more CVD risk factors in the pediatric patient

Mechanism of Action Pravastatin is a competitive inhibitor of 3-hydroxy-3-methylglutaryl coenzyme A (HMG-CoA) reductase, which is the rate-limiting enzyme involved in *de novo* cholesterol synthesis.

Pharmacodynamics/Kinetics

Onset of action: Several days

Peak effect: 4 weeks

Absorption: Rapidly absorbed; average absorption 34%

Protein binding: 50%

Metabolism: Hepatic to at least two metabolites

Bioavailability: 17%

Half-life elimination: ~2-3 hours

Time to peak, serum: 1-1.5 hours

Excretion: Feces (70%); urine (≤20%, 8% as unchanged drug)

Dosage Oral: **Note:** Doses should be individualized according to the baseline LDL-cholesterol levels, the recommended goal of therapy, and patient response; adjustments should be made at intervals of 4 weeks or more; doses may need adjusted based on concomitant medications

Children: HeFH:

8-13 years: 20 mg/day

14-18 years: 40 mg/day

Dosage adjustment for pravastatin based on concomitant immunosuppressants (ie, cyclosporine): Refer to Adults dosing section

Adults: Hyperlipidemias, primary prevention of coronary events, secondary prevention of cardiovascular events: Initial: 40 mg once daily; titrate dosage to response; usual range: 10-80 mg; (maximum dose: 80 mg once daily)

Dosage adjustment for pravastatin based on concomitant immunosuppressants (ie, cyclosporine): Initial: 10 mg/day, titrate with caution (maximum dose: 20 mg/day)

Elderly: No specific dosage recommendations. Clearance is reduced in the elderly, resulting in an increase in AUC between 25% to 50%. However, substantial accumulation is not expected.

Dosing adjustment in renal impairment: Initial: 10 mg/day

Dosing adjustment in hepatic impairment: Initial: 10 mg/day

Stability Store at 25°C (77°F); excursions permitted to 15°C to 30°C (59°F to 86°F). Protect from moisture and light.

Administration May be taken without regard to meals.

Monitoring Parameters Obtain baseline LFTs and total cholesterol profile; creatine phosphokinase due to possibility of myopathy. Repeat LFTs prior to elevation of dose. May be measured when clinically indicated and/or periodically thereafter.

Anesthesia and Critical Care Concerns/Other Considerations Myopathy: Currently-marketed HMG-CoA reductase inhibitors appear to have a similar potential for causing myopathy. Incidence of severe myopathy is about 0.08% to 0.09%. The factors that increase risk include advanced age (especially >80 years), gender (occurs in women more frequently than men), small body frame, frailty, multisystem disease (eg, chronic renal insufficiency especially due to diabetes), multiple medications, **perioperative periods (higher risk when continued during hospitalization for major surgery)**, and drug interactions (use with caution or avoid).

Pregnancy Risk Factor X

Contraindications Hypersensitivity to pravastatin or any component of the formulation; active liver disease; unexplained persistent elevations of serum transaminases; pregnancy; breast-feeding

Warnings/Precautions Secondary causes of hyperlipidemia should be ruled out prior to therapy. Liver function must be monitored by periodic laboratory assessment. Rhabdomyolysis with acute renal failure has occurred. Risk may be increased with concurrent use of other drugs which may cause rhabdomyolysis (including gemfibrozil, fibric acid derivatives, or niacin at doses ≥1 g/day). Temporarily discontinue in any patient experiencing an acute or serious condition predisposing to renal failure secondary to rhabdomyolysis. Use caution in patients with previous liver disease or heavy ethanol use. Treatment in patients <8 years of age is not recommended.

Adverse Reactions As reported in short-term trials; safety and tolerability with long-term use were similar to placebo

(Continued)

Pravastatin *(Continued)*

1% to 10%:

Cardiovascular: Chest pain (4%)

Central nervous system: Headache (2% to 6%), fatigue (4%), dizziness (1% to 3%)

Dermatologic: Rash (4%)

Gastrointestinal: Nausea/vomiting (7%), diarrhea (6%), heartburn (3%)

Hepatic: Transaminases increased (>3x normal on two occasions - 1%)

Neuromuscular & skeletal: Myalgia (2%)

Respiratory: Cough (3%)

Miscellaneous: Influenza (2%)

<1% (Limited to important or life-threatening): Allergy, lens opacity, libido change, memory impairment, muscle weakness, neuropathy, paresthesia, taste disturbance, tremor, vertigo

Postmarketing and/or case reports: Anaphylaxis, angioedema, cholestatic jaundice, cirrhosis, cranial nerve dysfunction, dermatomyositis, erythema multiforme, ESR increase, fulminant hepatic necrosis, gynecomastia, hemolytic anemia, hepatitis, hepatoma, lupus erythematosus-like syndrome, myopathy, pancreatitis, peripheral nerve palsy, polymyalgia rheumatica, positive ANA, purpura, rhabdomyolysis, Stevens-Johnson syndrome, vasculitis

Additional class-related events or case reports (not necessarily reported with pravastatin therapy): Angioedema, cataracts, depression, dyspnea, eosinophilia, erectile dysfunction, facial paresis, hypersensitivity reaction, impaired extraocular muscle movement, impotence, leukopenia, malaise, memory loss, ophthalmoplegia, paresthesia, peripheral neuropathy, photosensitivity, psychic disturbance, skin discoloration, thrombocytopenia, thyroid dysfunction, toxic epidermal necrolysis, transaminases increased, vomiting

Overdosage/Toxicology Treatment is symptomatic.

Drug Interactions Substrate of CYP3A4 (minor); **Inhibits** CYP2C9 (weak), 2D6 (weak), 3A4 (weak)

Cholestyramine: Reduces pravastatin absorption; separate administration times by at least 4 hours.

Clofibrate and fenofibrate: May increase the risk of myopathy and rhabdomyolysis.

Colestipol: Reduces pravastatin absorption; separate administration by 1 hour.

Cyclosporine: Concurrent use may increase the risk of myopathy and rhabdomyolysis.

Gemfibrozil: Increased risk of myopathy and rhabdomyolysis.

Imidazole antifungals (itraconazole, ketoconazole): May modestly increase pravastatin concentrations (AUC).

Niacin: May increase the risk of myopathy and rhabdomyolysis.

P-glycoprotein inhibitors (eg, amiodarone, cyclosporine, ketoconazole): May increase pravastatin concentrations.

Ethanol/Nutrition/Herb Interactions

Ethanol: Consumption of large amounts of ethanol may increase the risk of liver damage with HMG-CoA reductase inhibitors.

Food: Red yeast rice contains an estimated 2.4 mg lovastatin per 600 mg rice.

Herb/Nutraceutical: St John's wort may decrease pravastatin levels.

Dietary Considerations May be taken without regard to meals. Before initiation of therapy, patients should be placed on a standard cholesterol-lowering diet for 6 weeks and the diet should be continued during drug therapy. Red yeast rice contains an estimated 2.4 mg lovastatin per 600 mg rice.

Dosage Forms Tablet, as sodium: 10 mg, 20 mg, 40 mg, 80 mg

- **Pravastatin and Aspirin** *see* Aspirin and Pravastatin *on page 135*
- **Pravastatin Sodium** *see* Pravastatin *on page 1042*
- **Pravigard™ PAC [DSC]** *see* Aspirin and Pravastatin *on page 135*

Prazosin (PRA zoe sin)

Medication Safety Issues

Sound-alike/look-alike issues:

Prazosin may be confused with prazepam, predniSONE

U.S. Brand Names Minipress®

Canadian Brand Names Apo-Prazo®; Minipress™; Novo-Prazin; Nu-Prazo

Synonyms Furazosin; Prazosin Hydrochloride

Pharmacologic Category $Alpha_1$ Blocker

Generic Available Yes

Use Treatment of hypertension

Unlabeled/Investigational Use Benign prostatic hyperplasia; Raynaud's syndrome

Mechanism of Action Competitively inhibits postsynaptic alpha-adrenergic receptors which results in vasodilation of veins and arterioles and a decrease in total peripheral resistance and blood pressure

Pharmacodynamics/Kinetics

Onset of action: BP reduction: ~2 hours
- Maximum decrease: 2-4 hours

Duration: 10-24 hours

Distribution: Hypertensive adults: V_d: 0.5 L/kg

Protein binding: 92% to 97%

Metabolism: Extensively hepatic

Bioavailability: 43% to 82%

Half-life elimination: 2-4 hours; prolonged with congestive heart failure

Excretion: Urine (6% to 10% as unchanged drug)

Dosage Oral:

Children: Initial: 5 mcg/kg/dose (to assess hypotensive effects); usual dosing interval: every 6 hours; increase dosage gradually up to maximum of 25 mcg/kg/dose every 6 hours

Adults:
- Hypertension: Initial: 1 mg/dose 2-3 times/day; usual maintenance dose: 3-15 mg/day in divided doses 2-4 times/day; maximum daily dose: 20 mg
- Hypertensive urgency: 10-20 mg once, may repeat in 30 minutes
- Raynaud's (unlabeled use): 0.5-3 mg twice daily
- Benign prostatic hyperplasia (unlabeled use): 2 mg twice daily

Stability Store in airtight container; protect from light

Monitoring Parameters Blood pressure, standing and sitting/supine

Anesthesia and Critical Care Concerns/Other Considerations $Alpha_1$ blockers do not affect renal blood flow or glomerular filtration. Orthostatic hypotension, compared to newer alpha-blockers, is more of a concern.

Pregnancy Risk Factor C

Contraindications Hypersensitivity to quinazolines (doxazosin, prazosin, terazosin) or any component of the formulation; concurrent use with phosphodiesterase-5 (PDE-5) inhibitors including sildenafil (>25 mg), tadalafil, or vardenafil

Warnings/Precautions May cause significant orthostatic hypotension and syncope, especially with first dose. Risk is increased at doses >1 mg, hypovolemia, or in patients receiving concurrent beta-blocker therapy. Anticipate a similar effect if therapy is interrupted for a few days, if dosage is rapidly increased, or if another antihypertensive drug is introduced.

Adverse Reactions

>10%: Central nervous system: Dizziness (10%)

1% to 10%:
- Cardiovascular: Palpitations (5%), edema, orthostatic hypotension, syncope (1%)
- Central nervous system: Headache (8%), drowsiness (8%), vertigo, depression, nervousness
- Dermatologic: Rash (1% to 4%)
- Endocrine & metabolic: Decreased energy (7%)
- Gastrointestinal: Nausea (5%), vomiting, diarrhea, constipation
- Genitourinary: Urinary frequency (1% to 5%)
- Neuromuscular & skeletal: Weakness (7%)
- Ocular: Blurred vision, reddened sclera, xerostomia
- Respiratory: Dyspnea, epistaxis, nasal congestion

<1% (Limited to important or life-threatening): Allergic reaction, alopecia, angina, cataplexy, cataracts (both development and disappearance have been reported), hallucinations, impotence, leukopenia, lichen planus, MI, narcolepsy (worsened), pancreatitis, paresthesia, pigmentary mottling and serous retinopathy, priapism, pruritus, systemic lupus erythematosus, tinnitus, urticaria, vasculitis

(Continued)

Prazosin *(Continued)*

Overdosage/Toxicology Symptoms of overdose include hypotension and drowsiness. Treatment is otherwise supportive and symptomatic.

Drug Interactions

ACE inhibitors: Hypotensive effect may be increased.
Beta-blockers: Hypotensive effect may be increased.
Calcium channel blockers: Hypotensive effect may be increased.
NSAIDs may reduce antihypertensive efficacy.
Sildenafil, tadalafil, vardenafil: Blood pressure-lowering effects are additive. Use of tadalafil or vardenafil is contraindicated by the manufacturer. Use sildenafil with extreme caution (dose ≤25 mg).
Tricyclic antidepressants (TCAs) and low-potency antipsychotics: May increase risk of orthostasis.

Ethanol/Nutrition/Herb Interactions

Ethanol: Avoid ethanol (may increase vasodilation).
Food: Food has variable effects on absorption.
Herb/Nutraceutical: Avoid dong quai if using for hypertension (has estrogenic activity). Avoid ephedra, yohimbe, ginseng (may worsen hypertension). Avoid saw palmetto (due to limited experience with this combination). Avoid garlic (may have increased antihypertensive effect).

Test Interactions Increased urinary VMA 17%, norepinephrine metabolite 42%

Dosage Forms Capsule, as hydrochloride: 1 mg, 2 mg, 5 mg

- **Prazosin Hydrochloride** *see* Prazosin *on page 1044*
- **Precedex™** *see* Dexmedetomidine *on page 370*
- **Pred Forte®** *see* PrednisoLONE *on page 1046*
- **Pred Mild®** *see* PrednisoLONE *on page 1046*

PrednisoLONE (pred NISS oh lone)

Medication Safety Issues

Sound-alike/look-alike issues:
PrednisoLONE may be confused with predniSONE
Pediapred® may be confused with Pediazole®

Related Information

Corticosteroids *on page 1561*
Stress Replacement of Corticosteroids *on page 1494*

U.S. Brand Names AK-Pred®; Bubbli-Pred™ [DSC]; Econopred® Plus; Orapred®; Orapred ODT™; Pediapred®; Pred Forte®; Pred Mild®; Prelone®

Canadian Brand Names Diopred®; Hydeltra T.B.A.®; Inflamase® Mild; Novo-Prednisolone; Ophtho-Tate®; Pediapred®; Pred Forte®; Pred Mild®; Sab-Prenase

Synonyms Deltahydrocortisone; Metacortandralone; Prednisolone Acetate; Prednisolone Acetate, Ophthalmic; Prednisolone Sodium Phosphate; Prednisolone Sodium Phosphate, Ophthalmic

Pharmacologic Category Corticosteroid, Ophthalmic; Corticosteroid, Systemic

Generic Available Yes

Use Treatment of palpebral and bulbar conjunctivitis; corneal injury from chemical, radiation, thermal burns, or foreign body penetration; endocrine disorders, rheumatic disorders, collagen diseases, dermatologic diseases, allergic states, ophthalmic diseases, respiratory diseases, hematologic disorders, neoplastic diseases, edematous states, and gastrointestinal diseases; resolution of acute exacerbations of multiple sclerosis; management of fulminating or disseminated tuberculosis and trichinosis; acute or chronic solid organ rejection

Mechanism of Action Decreases inflammation by suppression of migration of polymorphonuclear leukocytes and reversal of increased capillary permeability; suppresses the immune system by reducing activity and volume of the lymphatic system

Pharmacodynamics/Kinetics

Duration: 18-36 hours
Protein binding (concentration dependent): 65% to 91%; decreased in elderly
Metabolism: Primarily hepatic, but also metabolized in most tissues, to inactive compounds
Half-life elimination: 3.6 hours; End-stage renal disease: 3-5 hours
Excretion: Primarily urine (as glucuronides, sulfates, and unconjugated metabolites)

Dosage Dose depends upon condition being treated and response of patient; dosage for infants and children should be based on severity of the disease and response of the patient rather than on strict adherence to dosage indicated by age, weight, or body surface area. Consider alternate day therapy for long-term therapy. Discontinuation of long-term therapy requires gradual withdrawal by tapering the dose. Patients undergoing unusual stress while receiving corticosteroids, should receive increased doses prior to, during, and after the stressful situation.

Children: Oral:

Acute asthma: 1-2 mg/kg/day in divided doses 1-2 times/day for 3-5 days

Anti-inflammatory or immunosuppressive dose: 0.1-2 mg/kg/day in divided doses 1-4 times/day

Nephrotic syndrome:

Initial (first 3 episodes): 2 mg/kg/day **or** 60 mg/m²/day (maximum: 80 mg/day) in divided doses 3-4 times/day until urine is protein free for 3 consecutive days (maximum: 28 days); followed by 1-1.5 mg/kg/dose **or** 40 mg/m²/dose given every other day for 4 weeks

Maintenance (long-term maintenance dose for frequent relapses): 0.5-1 mg/kg/dose given every other day for 3-6 months

Adults: Oral:

Usual range: 5-60 mg/day

Multiple sclerosis: 200 mg/day for 1 week followed by 80 mg every other day for 1 month

Rheumatoid arthritis: Initial: 5-7.5 mg/day; adjust dose as necessary

Ophthalmic suspension/solution: Conjunctivitis, corneal injury: Children and Adults: Instill 1-2 drops into conjunctival sac every hour during day, every 2 hours at night until favorable response is obtained, then use 1 drop every 4 hours.

Elderly: Use lowest effective dose

Dosing adjustment in hyperthyroidism: Prednisolone dose may need to be increased to achieve adequate therapeutic effects

Hemodialysis: Slightly dialyzable (5% to 20%); administer dose posthemodialysis

Peritoneal dialysis: Supplemental dose is not necessary

Stability Store Orapred ODT™ at 20°C to 25°C (68°F to 77°F) in blister pack; protect from moisture

Administration Administer oral formulation with food or milk to decrease GI effects.

Orapred ODT™: Do not break or use partial tablet. Remove tablet from blister pack just prior to use. May swallow whole or allow to dissolve on tongue.

Monitoring Parameters Blood pressure; blood glucose, electrolytes; intraocular pressure (use >6 weeks); bone mineral density

Anesthesia and Critical Care Concerns/Other Considerations

Neuromuscular Effects: ICU-acquired paresis was recently studied in 5 ICUs (3 medical and 2 surgical ICUs) at 4 French hospitals. All ICU patients without pre-existing neuromuscular disease admitted from March 1999 through June 2000 were evaluated (De Jonghe B, 2002). Each patient had to be mechanically ventilated for ≥7 days and was screened daily for awakening. The first day the patient was considered awake was Study Day 1. Patients with severe muscle weakness on Study Day 7 were considered to have ICU-acquired paresis. Among the 95 patients who were evaluable, about 25% developed ICU-acquired paresis. Independent predictors included: female gender, the number of days with ≥2 organ dysfunction, and administration of corticosteroids. Further studies may be required to verify and characterize the association between the development of ICU-acquired paresis and use of corticosteroids. Concurrent use of a corticosteroid and muscle relaxant appear to increase the risk of certain ICU myopathies; avoid or administer the corticosteroid at the lowest dose possible.

Adrenal Insufficiency: Patients will often have steroid-induced adverse effects on glucose tolerance and lipid profiles. When discontinuing steroid therapy in patients on long-term steroid supplementation, it is important that the steroid therapy be discontinued gradually. Abrupt withdrawal may result in adrenal insufficiency with hypotension and hyperkalemia. Patients on long-term steroid supplementation will require higher corticosteroid doses when subject to stress (ie, trauma, surgery, severe infection). Guidelines for glucocorticoid replacement during various surgical procedures has been published (Salem M, 1994, Coursin DB, 2002).

(Continued)

PrednisoLONE *(Continued)*

Septic Shock: A recent randomized, double-blind, placebo controlled trial assessed whether low dose corticosteroid administration could improve 28-day survival in patients with septic shock and relative adrenal insufficiency. Relative adrenal insufficiency was defined as an inappropriate response to corticotropin administration (increase of serum cortisol of ≤9 mcg/dL from baseline). Cortisol levels were drawn immediately before corticotropin administration and 30 to 60 minutes afterwards. Three hundred adult septic shock patients requiring mechanical ventilation and vasopressor support were randomized to either hydrocortisone (50 mg IVP every 6 hours) and fludrocortisone (50 mcg tablet daily via nasogastric tube) or matching placebos for 7 days. In patients who did not appropriately respond to corticotropin (nonresponders), there were significantly fewer deaths in the active treatment group. Vasopressor therapy was withdrawn more frequently in this subset of the active treatment group. Adverse events were similar in both groups. Patients who lack adrenal reserve and thus have relative adrenal insufficiency during the stress of septic shock may benefit from physiologic steroid replacement. However, there was a trend for increased mortality in patients who responded to the corticotropin test (increase serum cortisol >9 mcg/dL from baseline). These patients may not benefit from physiologic steroid replacement. Further study is required to better characterize the patient populations who may benefit.

Pregnancy Risk Factor C

Contraindications Hypersensitivity to prednisolone or any component of the formulation; acute superficial herpes simplex keratitis; live or attenuated virus vaccines (with immunosuppressive doses of corticosteroids); systemic fungal infections; varicella

Warnings/Precautions Use with caution in patients with cirrhosis, nonspecific ulcerative colitis, hypertension, osteoporosis, thromboembolic tendencies, CHF, convulsive disorders, myasthenia gravis, thrombophlebitis, peptic ulcer, diabetes, or tuberculosis; acute adrenal insufficiency may occur with abrupt withdrawal after long-term therapy or with stress; young pediatric patients may be more susceptible to adrenal axis suppression from topical therapy. Changes in thyroid status may necessitate dosage adjustments; metabolic clearance of corticosteroids increases in hyperthyroid patients and decreases in hypothyroid ones.

Prolonged use of corticosteroids may result in glaucoma; damage to the optic nerve (not indicated for treatment of optic neuritis), defects in visual acuity and fields of vision, and posterior subcapsular cataract formation may occur. Prolonged use of corticosteroids may also increase the incidence of secondary infection, mask acute infection (including fungal infections) or prolong or exacerbate viral infections. Exposure to chickenpox should be avoided; corticosteroids should not be used to treat ocular herpes simplex. Use following cataract surgery may delay healing or increase the incidence of bleb formation.

Corticosteroids should not be used for cerebral malaria. Because of the risk of adverse effects, systemic corticosteroids should be used cautiously in the elderly, in the smallest possible dose, and for the shortest possible time.

Adverse Reactions Frequency not defined.

Ophthalmic formulation:

Endocrine & metabolic: Hypercorticoidism (rare)

Ocular: Conjunctival hyperemia, conjunctivitis, corneal ulcers, delayed wound healing, glaucoma, intraocular pressure increased, keratitis, loss of accommodation, optic nerve damage, mydriasis, posterior subcapsular cataract formation, ptosis, secondary ocular infection

Oral formulation:

Cardiovascular: Cardiomyopathy, CHF, edema, facial edema, hypertension

Central nervous system: Convulsions, headache, insomnia, malaise, nervousness, pseudotumor cerebri, psychic disorders, vertigo

Dermatologic: Bruising, facial erythema, hirsutism, petechiae, skin test reaction suppression, thin fragile skin, urticaria

Endocrine & metabolic: Carbohydrate tolerance decreased, Cushing's syndrome, diabetes mellitus, growth suppression, hyperglycemia, hypernatremia, hypokalemia, hypokalemic alkalosis, menstrual irregularities, negative nitrogen balance, pituitary adrenal axis suppression

Gastrointestinal: Abdominal distention, increased appetite, indigestion, nausea, pancreatitis, peptic ulcer, ulcerative esophagitis, weight gain

Hepatic: LFTs increased (usually reversible)

Neuromuscular & skeletal: Arthralgia, aseptic necrosis (humeral/femoral heads), fractures, muscle mass decreased, muscle weakness, osteoporosis, steroid myopathy, tendon rupture, weakness

Ocular: Cataracts, exophthalmus, eyelid edema, glaucoma, intraocular pressure increased, irritation

Respiratory: Epistaxis

Miscellaneous: Diaphoresis increased, impaired wound healing

Overdosage/Toxicology When consumed in high doses for prolonged periods, systemic hypercorticism and adrenal suppression may occur, in those cases discontinuation of the corticosteroid should be done judiciously. Treatment should be symptom-directed and supportive.

Drug Interactions Substrate of CYP3A4 (minor); **Inhibits** CYP3A4 (weak)

Aminoglutethimide: May reduce the serum levels/effects of prednisolone; likely via induction of microsomal isoenzymes.

Antacids: May increase the absorption of corticosteroids; separate administration by ≥2 hours.

Aprepitant: May increase effects of systemic corticosteroids.

Azole antifungals: May increase the serum levels of corticosteroids; monitor.

Barbiturates: May decrease prednisolone levels; monitor.

Bile acid sequestrants: May decrease the absorption of corticosteroids (oral).

Calcium channel blockers (nondihydropyridine): May increase the serum levels of corticosteroids; monitor.

Cyclosporine: Corticosteroids may increase the serum levels of cyclosporine. In addition, cyclosporine may increase levels of corticosteroids; monitor.

Estrogens: May increase the serum levels of corticosteroids; monitor.

Fluoroquinolones: Concurrent use may increase the risk of tendon rupture, particularly in elderly patients (overall incidence rare).

Isoniazid: Serum concentrations may be decreased by corticosteroids.

Ketoconazole: May decrease metabolism of certain corticosteroids leading to increased levels (up to 60%) and increased risk of adverse effects; monitor.

Macrolide antibiotics: May decrease the metabolism of corticosteroids.

Neuromuscular-blocking agents: Concurrent use with corticosteroids may increase the risk of myopathy.

Nonsteroidal anti-inflammatory drugs (NSAIDs), ophthalmic: Concurrent use with ophthalmic corticosteroids may lead to delayed healing.

Potassium-depleting agents (eg, diuretics, amphotericin B): Concurrent use increases risk of hypokalemia (especially if digitalized); monitor.

Primidone: May increase the metabolism of corticosteroids.

Rifampin: May decrease serum levels/effects of prednisolone; monitor.

Salicylates: Salicylates may increase the gastrointestinal adverse effects of corticosteroids.

Skin tests: Corticosteroids may suppress reactions to skin tests.

Vaccines (dead organisms): Immunosuppressants may diminish the effect of these vaccines.

Vaccines (live organisms): Immunosuppressants may enhance the adverse/toxic effects of these vaccines.

Ethanol/Nutrition/Herb Interactions

Ethanol: Avoid ethanol (may increase gastric mucosal irritation).

Food: Prednisolone interferes with calcium absorption. Limit caffeine.

Herb/Nutraceutical: St John's wort may decrease prednisolone levels. Avoid cat's claw, echinacea (have immunostimulant properties).

Test Interactions Response to skin tests

Dietary Considerations Should be taken after meals or with food or milk to decrease GI effects; increase dietary intake of pyridoxine, vitamin C, vitamin D, folate, calcium, and phosphorus.

Dosage Forms [DSC] = Discontinued product

Solution, ophthalmic, as sodium phosphate: 1% (5 mL, 10 mL, 15 mL) [contains benzalkonium chloride]

AK-Pred®: 1% (5 mL, 15 mL) [contains benzalkonium chloride]

Solution, oral, as sodium phosphate: Prednisolone base 5 mg/5 mL (120 mL)

Bubbli-Pred™: Prednisolone base 5 mg/5 mL (120 mL) [bubble gum flavor] [DSC]

Orapred®: 20 mg/5 mL (240 mL) [equivalent to prednisolone base 15 mg/5 mL; dye free; contains alcohol 2%, sodium benzoate; grape flavor]

Pediapred®: 6.7 mg/5 mL (120 mL) [equivalent to prednisolone base 5 mg/5 mL; dye free; raspberry flavor]

(Continued)

PrednisoLONE *(Continued)*

Suspension, ophthalmic, as acetate: 1% (5 mL, 10 mL, 15 mL) [contains benzalkonium chloride]
Econopred® Plus: 1% (5 mL, 10 mL) [contains benzalkonium chloride]
Pred Forte®: 1% (1 mL, 5 mL, 10 mL, 15 mL) [contains benzalkonium chloride and sodium bisulfite]
Pred Mild®: 0.12% (5 mL, 10 mL) [contains benzalkonium chloride and sodium bisulfite]
Syrup, as base: 5 mg/5 mL (120 mL); 15 mg/5 mL (240 mL, 480 mL)
Prelone®: 15 mg/5 mL (240 mL, 480 mL) [contains alcohol 5%, benzoic acid; cherry flavor]
Tablet, as base: 5 mg
Tablet, orally disintegrating, as base:
Orapred ODT™: 10 mg, 15 mg, 30 mg [grape flavor]

References

Abraham E and Evans T, "Corticosteroids and Septic Shock (editorial)," *JAMA*, 2002, 288(7):886-7.
Annane D, Sebille V, Charpentier C, et al, "Effect of Treatment With Low Doses of Hydrocortisone and Fludrocortisone on Mortality in Patients With Septic Shock," *JAMA*, 2002, 288(7):862-71.
Cooper MS and Stewart PM, "Corticosteroid Insufficiency in Acutely Ill Patients," *N Engl J Med*, 2003, 348(8):727-34.
Coursin DB and Wood KE, "Corticosteroid Supplementation for Adrenal Insufficiency," *JAMA*, 2002, 287(2):236-40.
De Jonghe B, Sharshar T, Lefaucheur JP, et al, "Paresis Acquired in the Intensive Care Unit. A Prospective Multicenter Study," *JAMA*, 2002, 288(22):2859-67.
Hotchkiss RS and Karl IE, "The Pathophysiology and Treatment of Sepsis," *N Engl J Med*, 2003, 348(2):138-50.
Salem M, Tainsh RE, Jr, Bromberg J, et al, "Perioperative Glucocorticoid Coverage: A Reassessment 42 Years After Emergence of a Problem," *Ann Surg*, 1994, 219(4):416-25.

- **Prednisolone Acetate** *see* PrednisoLONE *on page 1046*
- **Prednisolone Acetate, Ophthalmic** *see* PrednisoLONE *on page 1046*
- **Prednisolone Sodium Phosphate** *see* PrednisoLONE *on page 1046*
- **Prednisolone Sodium Phosphate, Ophthalmic** *see* PrednisoLONE *on page 1046*

PredniSONE (PRED ni sone)

Medication Safety Issues
Sound-alike/look-alike issues:
PredniSONE may be confused with methylPREDNISolone, Pramosone®, prazosin, prednisoLONE, Prilosec®, primidone, promethazine

Related Information
Contrast Media Reactions, Premedication for Prophylaxis *on page 1602*
Corticosteroids *on page 1561*
Stress Replacement of Corticosteroids *on page 1494*

U.S. Brand Names Prednisone Intensol™; Sterapred®; Sterapred® DS

Canadian Brand Names Apo-Prednisone®; Novo-Prednisone; Winpred™

Synonyms Deltacortisone; Deltadehydrocortisone

Pharmacologic Category Corticosteroid, Systemic

Generic Available Yes

Use Treatment of a variety of diseases including adrenocortical insufficiency, hypercalcemia, rheumatic, and collagen disorders; dermatologic, ocular, respiratory, gastrointestinal, and neoplastic diseases; organ transplantation and a variety of diseases including those of hematologic, allergic, inflammatory, and autoimmune in origin; not available in injectable form, prednisolone must be used

Unlabeled/Investigational Use Investigational: Prevention of postherpetic neuralgia and relief of acute pain in the early stages

Mechanism of Action Decreases inflammation by suppression of migration of polymorphonuclear leukocytes and reversal of increased capillary permeability; suppresses the immune system by reducing activity and volume of the lymphatic system; suppresses adrenal function at high doses. Antitumor effects may be related to inhibition of glucose transport, phosphorylation, or induction of cell death in immature lymphocytes. Antiemetic effects are thought to occur due to blockade of cerebral innervation of the emetic center via inhibition of prostaglandin synthesis.

Pharmacodynamics/Kinetics Refer to PrednisoLONE *on page 1046* for complete information.

Protein binding (concentration dependent): 65% to 91%

Metabolism: Hepatically converted from prednisone (inactive) to prednisolone (active); may be impaired with hepatic dysfunction

Half-life elimination: Normal renal function: 2.5-3.5 hours

Dosage Oral: Dose depends upon condition being treated and response of patient; dosage for infants and children should be based on severity of the disease and response of the patient rather than on strict adherence to dosage indicated by age, weight, or body surface area. Consider alternate day therapy for long-term therapy. Discontinuation of long-term therapy requires gradual withdrawal by tapering the dose.

Children:

Anti-inflammatory or immunosuppressive dose: 0.05-2 mg/kg/day divided 1-4 times/day

Acute asthma: 1-2 mg/kg/day in divided doses 1-2 times/day for 3-5 days

Alternatively (for 3- to 5-day "burst"):

<1 year: 10 mg every 12 hours

1-4 years: 20 mg every 12 hours

5-13 years: 30 mg every 12 hours

>13 years: 40 mg every 12 hours

Asthma long-term therapy (alternative dosing by age):

<1 year: 10 mg every other day

1-4 years: 20 mg every other day

5-13 years: 30 mg every other day

>13 years: 40 mg every other day

Nephrotic syndrome:

Initial (first 3 episodes): 2 mg/kg/day **or** 60 mg/m^2/day (maximum: 80 mg/day) in divided doses 3-4 times/day until urine is protein free for 3 consecutive days (maximum: 28 days); followed by 1-1.5 mg/kg/dose **or** 40 mg/m^2/dose given every other day for 4 weeks

Maintenance dose (long-term maintenance dose for frequent relapses): 0.5-1 mg/kg/dose given every other day for 3-6 months

Children and Adults: Physiologic replacement: 4-5 mg/m^2/day

Children ≥5 years and Adults: Asthma:

Moderate persistent: Inhaled corticosteroid (medium dose) or inhaled corticosteroid (low-medium dose) with a long-acting bronchodilator

Severe persistent: Inhaled corticosteroid (high dose) and corticosteroid tablets or syrup long term: 2 mg/kg/day, generally not to exceed 60 mg/day

Adults:

Immunosuppression/chemotherapy adjunct: Range: 5-60 mg/day in divided doses 1-4 times/day

Allergic reaction (contact dermatitis):

Day 1: 30 mg divided as 10 mg before breakfast, 5 mg at lunch, 5 mg at dinner, 10 mg at bedtime

Day 2: 5 mg at breakfast, 5 mg at lunch, 5 mg at dinner, 10 mg at bedtime

Day 3: 5 mg 4 times/day (with meals and at bedtime)

Day 4: 5 mg 3 times/day (breakfast, lunch, bedtime)

Day 5: 5 mg 2 times/day (breakfast, bedtime)

Day 6: 5 mg before breakfast

Pneumocystis carinii pneumonia (PCP):

40 mg twice daily for 5 days **followed by**

40 mg once daily for 5 days **followed by**

20 mg once daily for 11 days or until antimicrobial regimen is completed

Thyrotoxicosis: Oral: 60 mg/day

Chemotherapy (refer to individual protocols): Oral: Range: 20 mg/day to 100 mg/m^2/day

Rheumatoid arthritis: Oral: Use lowest possible daily dose (often ≤7.5 mg/day)

Idiopathic thrombocytopenia purpura (ITP): Oral: 60 mg daily for 4-6 weeks, gradually tapered over several weeks

Systemic lupus erythematosus (SLE): Oral:

Acute: 1-2 mg/kg/day in 2-3 divided doses

Maintenance: Reduce to lowest possible dose, usually <1 mg/kg/day as single dose (morning)

Elderly: Use the lowest effective dose

Dosing adjustment in hepatic impairment: Prednisone is inactive and must be metabolized by the liver to prednisolone. This conversion may be impaired in patients with liver disease, however, prednisolone levels are observed to be higher in patients with severe liver failure than in normal patients. Therefore,

(Continued)

PredniSONE *(Continued)*

compensation for the inadequate conversion of prednisone to prednisolone occurs.

Dosing adjustment in hyperthyroidism: Prednisone dose may need to be increased to achieve adequate therapeutic effects

Hemodialysis: Supplemental dose is not necessary

Peritoneal dialysis: Supplemental dose is not necessary

Administration Administer with meals to decrease gastrointestinal upset

Monitoring Parameters Blood pressure, blood glucose, electrolytes

Anesthesia and Critical Care Concerns/Other Considerations

Neuromuscular Effects: ICU-acquired paresis was recently studied in 5 ICUs (3 medical and 2 surgical ICUs) at 4 French hospitals. All ICU patients without pre-existing neuromuscular disease admitted from March 1999 through June 2000 were evaluated (De Jonghe B, 2002). Each patient had to be mechanically ventilated for ≥7 days and was screened daily for awakening. The first day the patient was considered awake was Study Day 1. Patients with severe muscle weakness on Study Day 7 were considered to have ICU-acquired paresis. Among the 95 patients who were evaluable, about 25% developed ICU-acquired paresis. Independent predictors included: female gender, the number of days with ≥2 organ dysfunction, and administration of corticosteroids. Further studies may be required to verify and characterize the association between the development of ICU-acquired paresis and use of corticosteroids. Concurrent use of a corticosteroid and muscle relaxant appear to increase the risk of certain ICU myopathies; avoid or administer the corticosteroid at the lowest dose possible.

Adrenal Insufficiency: Patients will often have steroid-induced adverse effects on glucose tolerance and lipid profiles. When discontinuing steroid therapy in patients on long-term steroid supplementation, it is important that the steroid therapy be discontinued gradually. Abrupt withdrawal may result in adrenal insufficiency with hypotension and hyperkalemia. Patients on long-term steroid supplementation will require higher corticosteroid doses when subject to stress (ie, trauma, surgery, severe infection). Guidelines for glucocorticoid replacement during various surgical procedures has been published (Salem M, 1994, Coursin DB, 2002).

Septic Shock: A recent randomized, double-blind, placebo controlled trial assessed whether low dose corticosteroid administration could improve 28-day survival in patients with septic shock and relative adrenal insufficiency. Relative adrenal insufficiency was defined as an inappropriate response to corticotropin administration (increase of serum cortisol of ≤9 mcg/dL from baseline). Cortisol levels were drawn immediately before corticotropin administration and 30 to 60 minutes afterwards. Three hundred adult septic shock patients requiring mechanical ventilation and vasopressor support were randomized to either hydrocortisone (50 mg IVP every 6 hours) and fludrocortisone (50 mcg tablet daily via nasogastric tube) or matching placebos for 7 days. In patients who did not appropriately respond to corticotropin (nonresponders), there were significantly fewer deaths in the active treatment group. Vasopressor therapy was withdrawn more frequently in this subset of the active treatment group. Adverse events were similar in both groups. Patients who lack adrenal reserve and thus have relative adrenal insufficiency during the stress of septic shock may benefit from physiologic steroid replacement. However, there was a trend for increased mortality in patients who responded to the corticotropin test (increase serum cortisol >9 mcg/dL from baseline). These patients may not benefit from physiologic steroid replacement. Further study is required to better characterize the patient populations who may benefit.

Pregnancy Risk Factor B

Contraindications Hypersensitivity to prednisone or any component of the formulation; serious infections, except tuberculous meningitis; systemic fungal infections; varicella

Warnings/Precautions Withdraw therapy with gradual tapering of dose, may retard bone growth. Use with caution in patients with hypothyroidism, cirrhosis, CHF, ulcerative colitis, thromboembolic disorders, and patients at increased risk for peptic ulcer disease. Corticosteroids should be used with caution in patients with diabetes, hypertension, osteoporosis, glaucoma, cataracts, or tuberculosis. Use caution in hepatic impairment. Because of the risk of adverse effects, systemic corticosteroids should be used cautiously in the elderly, in the smallest possible dose, and for the shortest possible time.

Adverse Reactions

>10%:

Central nervous system: Insomnia, nervousness

Gastrointestinal: Increased appetite, indigestion

1% to 10%:

Central nervous system: Dizziness or lightheadedness, headache

Dermatologic: Hirsutism, hypopigmentation

Endocrine & metabolic: Diabetes mellitus, glucose intolerance, hyperglycemia

Neuromuscular & skeletal: Arthralgia

Ocular: Cataracts, glaucoma

Respiratory: Epistaxis

Miscellaneous: Diaphoresis

<1% (Limited to important or life-threatening): Cushing's syndrome, edema, fractures, hallucinations, hypertension, muscle-wasting, osteoporosis, pancreatitis, pituitary-adrenal axis suppression, seizure

Overdosage/Toxicology When consumed in high doses for prolonged periods, systemic hypercorticism and adrenal suppression may occur. In those cases, discontinuation of the corticosteroid should be done judiciously.

Drug Interactions Substrate of CYP3A4 (minor); **Induces** CYP2C19 (weak), 3A4 (weak)

Decreased effect:

Barbiturates, phenytoin, rifampin decrease corticosteroid effectiveness

Decreases salicylates

Decreases vaccines

Decreases toxoids effectiveness

Increased effect/toxicity: NSAIDs: Concurrent use of prednisone may increase the risk of GI ulceration

Ethanol/Nutrition/Herb Interactions

Ethanol: Avoid ethanol (may increase gastric mucosal irritation)

Food: Prednisone interferes with calcium absorption, Limit caffeine.

Herb/Nutraceutical: St John's wort may decrease prednisone levels. Avoid cat's claw, echinacea (have immunostimulant properties).

Test Interactions Response to skin tests

Dietary Considerations Should be taken after meals or with food or milk; increase dietary intake of pyridoxine, vitamin C, vitamin D, folate, calcium, and phosphorus.

Dosage Forms

Solution, oral: 1 mg/mL (5 mL, 120 mL, 500 mL) [contains alcohol 5%, sodium benzoate; vanilla flavor]

Solution, oral concentrate (Prednisone Intensol™): 5 mg/mL (30 mL) [contains alcohol 30%]

Tablet: 1 mg, 2.5 mg, 5 mg, 10 mg, 20 mg, 50 mg

Sterapred®: 5 mg [supplied as 21 tablet 6-day unit-dose package or 48 tablet 12-day unit-dose package]

Sterapred® DS: 10 mg [supplied as 21 tablet 6-day unit-dose package or 48 tablet 12-day unit-dose package]

References

Abraham E and Evans T, "Corticosteroids and Septic Shock (editorial)," *JAMA*, 2002, 288(7):886-7.

Annane D, Sebille V, Charpentier C, et al, "Effect of Treatment With Low Doses of Hydrocortisone and Fludrocortisone on Mortality in Patients With Septic Shock," *JAMA*, 2002, 288(7):862-71.

Cooper MS and Stewart PM, "Corticosteroid Insufficiency in Acutely Ill Patients," *N Engl J Med*, 2003, 348(8):727-34.

Coursin DB and Wood KE, "Corticosteroid Supplementation for Adrenal Insufficiency," *JAMA*, 2002, 287(2):236-40.

De Jonghe B, Sharshar T, Lefaucheur JP, et al, "Paresis Acquired in the Intensive Care Unit. A Prospective Multicenter Study," *JAMA*, 2002, 288(22):2859-67.

Hotchkiss RS and Karl IE, "The Pathophysiology and Treatment of Sepsis," *N Engl J Med*, 2003, 348(2):138-50.

Salem M, Tainsh RE, Jr, Bromberg J, et al, "Perioperative Glucocorticoid Coverage: A Reassessment 42 Years After Emergence of a Problem," *Ann Surg*, 1994, 219(4):416-25.

♦ **Prednisone Intensol™** *see* PredniSONE *on page 1050*

♦ **Prelone®** *see* PrednisoLONE *on page 1046*

♦ **Premarin®** *see* Estrogens (Conjugated/Equine) *on page 488*

♦ **Premjact® [OTC]** *see* Lidocaine *on page 755*

♦ **Preparation H® Hydrocortisone [OTC]** *see* Hydrocortisone *on page 639*

♦ **Pressyn® (Can)** *see* Vasopressin *on page 1342*

♦ **Pressyn® AR (Can)** *see* Vasopressin *on page 1342*

♦ **Pretz® [OTC]** *see* Sodium Chloride *on page 1183*

- **Pretz-D® [OTC]** *see* Ephedrine *on page 455*
- **Prevacid®** *see* Lansoprazole *on page 731*
- **Prevacid® SoluTab™** *see* Lansoprazole *on page 731*
- **Prevex® B (Can)** *see* Betamethasone *on page 169*
- **Prevex® HC (Can)** *see* Hydrocortisone *on page 639*

Prilocaine (PRIL oh kane)

Medication Safety Issues

Sound-alike/look-alike issues:

Prilocaine may be confused with Polocaine®, Prilosec®

Related Information

Local Anesthetics *on page 1532*

U.S. Brand Names Citanest® Plain

Canadian Brand Names Citanest® Plain

Pharmacologic Category Local Anesthetic

Generic Available No

Mechanism of Action Local anesthetics bind selectively to the intracellular surface of sodium channels to block influx of sodium into the axon. As a result, depolarization necessary for action potential propagation and subsequent nerve function is prevented. The block at the sodium channel is reversible. When drug diffuses away from the axon, sodium channel function is restored and nerve propagation returns.

Pharmacodynamics/Kinetics

Onset of action: Infiltration: ~2 minutes; Inferior alveolar nerve block: ~3 minutes

Duration: Infiltration: Complete anesthesia for procedures lasting 20 minutes; Inferior alveolar nerve block: ~2.5 hours

Distribution: V_d: 0.7-4.4 L/kg; crosses blood-brain barrier

Protein binding: 55%

Metabolism: Hepatic and renal

Half-life elimination: 10-150 minutes; prolonged with hepatic or renal impairment

Dosage

Children <10 years: Doses >40 mg (1 mL) as a 4% solution per procedure rarely needed

Children >10 years and Adults: Dental anesthesia, infiltration, or conduction block: Initial: 40-80 mg (1-2 mL) as a 4% solution; up to a maximum of 400 mg (10 mL) as a 4% solution within a 2-hour period. Manufacturer's maximum recommended dose is not more than 600 mg to normal healthy adults. The effective anesthetic dose varies with procedure, intensity of anesthesia needed, duration of anesthesia required and physical condition of the patient. Always use the lowest effective dose along with careful aspiration.

Note: Adult and children doses of prilocaine hydrochloride cited from USP Dispensing Information (USP DI), 17th ed, The United States Pharmacopeial Convention, Inc, Rockville, MD, 1997, 139.

Anesthesia and Critical Care Concerns/Other Considerations Addition of sodium bicarbonate to local anesthetic solution can increase onset and potency. Only preservative-free solutions should be used for epidural administration. The metabolite *o*-toluidine can cause methemoglobinemia when large doses of prilocaine >600 mg are administered.

Pregnancy Risk Factor B

Contraindications Hypersensitivity to local anesthetics of the amide type or any component of the formulation

Warnings/Precautions Aspirate the syringe after tissue penetration and before injection to minimize chance of direct vascular injection

Adverse Reactions

1% to 10%: Cardiovascular: Hypotension

<1% (Limited to important or life-threatening): Anaphylactoid reaction, aseptic meningitis resulting in paralysis, chills, CNS stimulation followed by CNS depression, miosis, nausea, skin discoloration, tinnitus, vomiting

Drug Interactions No data reported

Dosage Forms Injection, solution: Prilocaine hydrochloride 4% (1.8 mL) [prefilled cartridge]

- **Prilosec®** *see* Omeprazole *on page 957*
- **Prilosec OTC™ [OTC]** *see* Omeprazole *on page 957*
- **Primacor®** *see* Milrinone *on page 851*

- **Primatene® Mist [OTC]** *see* Epinephrine *on page 457*
- **Primaxin®** *see* Imipenem and Cilastatin *on page 659*
- **Primaxin® I.V. (Can)** *see* Imipenem and Cilastatin *on page 659*
- **Principen®** *see* Ampicillin *on page 104*
- **Prinivil®** *see* Lisinopril *on page 767*
- **Pristinamycin** *see* Quinupristin and Dalfopristin *on page 1097*

Probenecid (proe BEN e sid)

Medication Safety Issues

Sound-alike/look-alike issues:

Probenecid may be confused with Procanbid®

Canadian Brand Names Benuryl™

Synonyms Benemid [DSC]

Pharmacologic Category Uricosuric Agent

Generic Available Yes

Use Prevention of hyperuricemia associated with gout or gouty arthritis; prolongation and elevation of beta-lactam plasma levels

Mechanism of Action Competitively inhibits the reabsorption of uric acid at the proximal convoluted tubule, thereby promoting its excretion and reducing serum uric acid levels; increases plasma levels of weak organic acids (penicillins, cephalosporins, or other beta-lactam antibiotics) by competitively inhibiting their renal tubular secretion

Pharmacodynamics/Kinetics

Onset of action: Effect on penicillin levels: 2 hours

Absorption: Rapid and complete

Metabolism: Hepatic

Half-life elimination (dose dependent): Normal renal function: 6-12 hours

Time to peak, serum: 2-4 hours

Excretion: Urine

Dosage Oral:

Children:

<2 years: Contraindicated

2-14 years: Prolong penicillin serum levels: Initial: 25 mg/kg, then 40 mg/kg/day given 4 times/day (maximum: 500 mg/dose)

Gonorrhea: >45 kg: Refer to adult guidelines

Adults:

Hyperuricemia with gout: 250 mg twice daily for one week; increase to 250-500 mg/day; may increase by 500 mg/month, if needed, to maximum of 2-3 g/day (dosages may be increased by 500 mg every 6 months if serum urate concentrations are controlled)

Prolong penicillin serum levels: 500 mg 4 times/day

Gonorrhea: CDC guidelines (alternative regimen): Probenecid 1 g orally with cefoxitin 2 g I.M.

Pelvic inflammatory disease: CDC guidelines: Cefoxitin 2 g I.M. plus probenecid 1 g orally as a single dose

Neurosyphilis: CDC guidelines (alternative regimen): Procaine penicillin 2.4 million units/day I.M. plus probenecid 500 mg 4 times/day; both administered for 10-14 days

Dosing adjustment in renal impairment: Cl_{cr} <30 mL/minute: Avoid use

Administration Administer with food or antacids to minimize GI effects

Monitoring Parameters Uric acid, renal function, CBC

Contraindications Hypersensitivity to probenecid or any component of the formulation; high-dose aspirin therapy; blood dyscrasias; uric acid kidney stones; children <2 years of age

Warnings/Precautions Use with caution in patients with peptic ulcer. Salicylates may diminish the therapeutic effect of probenecid. This effect may be more pronounced with high, chronic doses, however, the manufacturer recommends the use of an alternative analgesic even in place of small doses of aspirin. Use of probenecid with penicillin in patients with renal insufficiency is not recommended. Probenecid monotherapy may not be effective in patients with a creatinine clearance <30 mL/minute. May cause exacerbation of acute gouty attack

Adverse Reactions Frequency not defined.

Cardiovascular: Flushing

Central nervous system: Dizziness, fever, headache

(Continued)

Probenecid *(Continued)*

Dermatologic: Alopecia, dermatitis, pruritus, rash
Gastrointestinal: Anorexia, nausea, vomiting, sore gums
Genitourinary: Hematuria, polyuria
Hematologic: Anemia, aplastic anemia, hemolytic anemia, leukopenia
Hepatic: Hepatic necrosis
Neuromuscular & skeletal: Costovertebral pain, gouty arthritis (acute)
Renal: Nephrotic syndrome, renal colic
Miscellaneous: Anaphylaxis, hypersensitivity

Drug Interactions **Inhibits** CYP2C19 (weak)

Carbapenems (ertapenem, imipenem, meropenem): Probenecid may decrease the excretion of carbapenem antibiotics..

Cephalosporins: Probenecid may decrease the excretion of cephalosporin antibiotics. This effect is used advantageously in selected cases to increase serum antibiotic concentrations.

Dapsone: Probenecid may decrease the excretion of dapsone.

Methotrexate: Probenecid may decrease the excretion of methotrexate; concomitant use should be avoided. If used concomitantly, the methotrexate dosage will likely need reduced. Monitor for evidence of methotrexate toxicity.

Nonsteroidal anti-inflammatory agents: Probenecid may increase the serum concentration of NSAIDs. The manufacturer of ketorolac contraindicates concomitant use.

Penicillins: Probenecid may decrease the excretion of penicillin antibiotics. This effect is used advantageously in selected cases to increase serum antibiotic concentrations.

Salicylates: Salicylates may diminish the therapeutic effect of probenecid.

Thiopental: Probenecid may enhance the therapeutic effect of thiopental.

Zidovudine: Probenecid may decrease the metabolism of zidovudine.

Test Interactions False-positive glucosuria with Clinitest®, a falsely high determination of theophylline has occurred and the renal excretion of phenolsulfonphthalein 17-ketosteroids and bromsulfophthalein (BSP) may be inhibited

Dietary Considerations Drug may cause GI upset; take with food if GI upset. Drink plenty of fluids.

Dosage Forms Tablet: 500 mg

Procainamide (proe kane A mide)

Medication Safety Issues

Sound-alike/look-alike issues:
Procanbid® may be confused with probenecid
Pronestyl® may be confused with Ponstel®

PCA is an error-prone abbreviation (mistaken as patient controlled analgesia)

Related Information

Antiarrhythmic Drugs *on page 1548*
Chronic Renal Failure *on page 1437*
Management of Postoperative Arrhythmias *on page 1451*

U.S. Brand Names Procanbid®

Canadian Brand Names Apo-Procainamide®; Procainamide Hydrochloride Injection, USP; Procan® SR; Pronestyl®-SR

Synonyms PCA (error-prone abbreviation); Procainamide Hydrochloride; Procaine Amide Hydrochloride

Pharmacologic Category Antiarrhythmic Agent, Class Ia

Generic Available Yes

Use Treatment of ventricular tachycardia (VT), premature ventricular contractions, paroxysmal atrial tachycardia (PSVT), and atrial fibrillation (AF); prevent recurrence of ventricular tachycardia, paroxysmal supraventricular tachycardia, atrial fibrillation or flutter

Unlabeled/Investigational Use ACLS guidelines:

Stable monomorphic VT (EF >40%, no CHF)
Stable wide complex tachycardia, likely VT (EF >40%, no CHF, patient stable)
Atrial fibrillation or flutter, including pre-excitation syndrome (EF >40%, no CHF)
AV reentrant, narrow complex tachycardia (eg, reentrant SVT) [preserved ventricular function]

PALS guidelines: Tachycardia with pulses and poor perfusion (possible VT)

Mechanism of Action Decreases myocardial excitability and conduction velocity and may depress myocardial contractility, by increasing the electrical stimulation threshold of ventricle, His-Purkinje system and through direct cardiac effects

Pharmacodynamics/Kinetics

Onset of action: I.M. 10-30 minutes

Distribution: V_d: Children: 2.2 L/kg; Adults: 2 L/kg; Congestive heart failure or shock: Decreased V_d

Protein binding: 15% to 20%

Metabolism: Hepatic via acetylation to produce N-acetyl procainamide (NAPA) (active metabolite)

Bioavailability: Oral: 75% to 95%

Half-life elimination:

- Procainamide (hepatic acetylator, phenotype, cardiac and renal function dependent):
  - Children: 1.7 hours; Adults: 2.5-4.7 hours; Anephric: 11 hours
- NAPA (dependent upon renal function):
  - Children: 6 hours; Adults: 6-8 hours; Anephric: 42 hours

Time to peak, serum: Capsule: 45 minutes to 2.5 hours; I.M.: 15-60 minutes

Excretion: Urine (25% as NAPA)

Dosage Must be titrated to patient's response

Children:

- Oral: 15-50 mg/kg/24 hours divided every 3-6 hours
- I.M.: 50 mg/kg/24 hours divided into doses of 1/8 to 1/4 every 3-6 hours in divided doses until oral therapy is possible
- I.V. (infusion requires use of an infusion pump):
  - Load: 3-6 mg/kg/dose over 5 minutes not to exceed 100 mg/dose; may repeat every 5-10 minutes to maximum of 15 mg/kg/load
  - Maintenance as continuous I.V. infusion: 20-80 mcg/kg/minute; maximum: 2 g/24 hours
  - Possible VT (pulses and poor perfusion) [PALS 2005 Guidelines]: I.V.; I.O.: 15 mg/kg over 30-60 minutes

Adults:

- Oral: Usual dose: 50 mg/kg/24 hours: maximum: 5 g/24 hours (**Note:** Twice-daily dosing approved for Procanbid®.)
  - Immediate release formulation: 250-500 mg/dose every 3-6 hours
  - Extended release formulation: 500 mg to 1 g every 6 hours; Procanbid®: 1000-2500 mg every 12 hours
- I.M.: 0.5-1 g every 4-8 hours until oral therapy is possible
- I.V. (infusion requires use of an infusion pump):
  - Loading dose: 15-18 mg/kg administered as slow infusion over 25-30 minutes **or** 100-200 mg/dose repeated every 5 minutes as needed to a total dose of 1 g. Reduce loading dose to 12 mg/kg in severe renal or cardiac impairment.
  - Maintenance dose: 1-4 mg/minute by continuous infusion. Maintenance infusions should be reduced by one-third in patients with moderate renal or cardiac impairment and by two-thirds in patients with severe renal or cardiac impairment.
  - ACLS guidelines: Infuse 20 mg/minute until arrhythmia is controlled, hypotension occurs, QRS complex widens by 50% of its original width, or total of 17 mg/kg is given.

Dosing interval in renal impairment:

- Oral:
  - Cl_{cr} 10-50 mL/minute: Administer every 6-12 hours.
  - Cl_{cr} <10 mL/minute: Administer every 8-24 hours.
- I.V.:
  - Loading dose: Reduce dose to 12 mg/kg in severe renal impairment.
  - Maintenance infusion: Reduce dose by one-third in patients with mild renal impairment. Reduce dose by two-thirds in patients with severe renal impairment.
- Dialysis:
  - Procainamide: Moderately hemodialyzable (20% to 50%): 200 mg supplemental dose posthemodialysis is recommended.
  - N-acetylprocainamide: Not dialyzable (0% to 5%)
  - Procainamide/N-acetylprocainamide: Not peritoneal dialyzable (0% to 5%)
  - Procainamide/N-acetylprocainamide: Replace by blood level during continuous arteriovenous or venovenous hemofiltration

Dosing adjustment in hepatic impairment: Reduce dose by 50%.

(Continued)

Procainamide *(Continued)*

Stability Procainamide may be stored at room temperature up to 27°C; however, refrigeration retards oxidation, which causes color formation. The solution is initially colorless but may turn slightly yellow on standing. Injection of air into the vial causes the solution to darken. Solutions darker than a light amber should be discarded.

Minimum volume: 1 g/250 mL NS/D_5W
Stability of admixture at room temperature in D_5W or NS: 24 hours

Some information indicates that procainamide may be subject to greater decomposition in D_5W unless the admixture is refrigerated or the pH is adjusted. Procainamide is believed to form an association complex with dextrose - the bioavailability of procainamide in this complex is not known and the complex formation is reversible.

Administration

Oral: Do **not** crush or chew extended release drug products.

Must dilute prior to I.V. administration; maximum rate: 50 mg/minute; administer around-the-clock rather than 4 times/day to promote less variation in peak and trough serum levels.

Infusion rate: **2 g/250 mL** (I.V. infusion requires use of an infusion pump):
- 1 mg/minute: 7.5 mL/hour
- 2 mg/minute: 15 mL/hour
- 3 mg/minute: 22.5 mL/hour
- 4 mg/minute: 30 mL/hour
- 5 mg/minute: 37.5 mL/hour
- 6 mg/minute: 45 mL/hour

Monitoring Parameters ECG, blood pressure, CBC with differential, platelet count; cardiac monitor and blood pressure monitor required during I.V. administration; blood levels in patients with renal failure or receiving constant infusion >3 mg/minute for longer than 24 hours

Reference Range

Timing of serum samples: Draw trough just before next oral dose; draw 6-12 hours after I.V. infusion has started; half-life is 2.5-5 hours

Therapeutic levels: Procainamide: 4-10 mcg/mL; NAPA 15-25 mcg/mL; Combined: 10-30 mcg/mL

Toxic concentration: Procainamide: >10-12 mcg/mL

Anesthesia and Critical Care Concerns/Other Considerations In patients with pre-existing cardiovascular disease, the incidence of proarrhythmia and mortality may be increased with Class Ia antiarrhythmic agents.

Procainamide may be used to pharmacologically convert atrial fibrillation to normal sinus rhythm. In this setting, it is important that AV nodal conduction be controlled (eg, digoxin, beta-blocker, calcium channel blocker) prior to cardioversion to inhibit procainamide-induced increases in ventricular response. Patients should be monitored (ECG and BP) in a controlled setting when initiating therapy.

Pregnancy Risk Factor C

Contraindications Hypersensitivity to procaine, other ester-type local anesthetics, or any component of the formulation; complete heart block (except in patients with a functioning artificial pacemaker); second-degree AV block (without a functional pacemaker); various types of hemiblock (without a functional pacemaker); SLE; torsade de pointes; concurrent cisapride use; QT prolongation

Warnings/Precautions Monitor and adjust dose to prevent QT_c prolongation. Watch for proarrhythmic effects. May precipitate or exacerbate CHF. Reduce dosage in renal impairment. May increase ventricular response rate in patients with atrial fibrillation or flutter; control AV conduction before initiating. Correct hypokalemia before initiating therapy. Hypokalemia may worsen toxicity. Use caution in digoxin-induced toxicity (can further depress AV conduction). Reduce dose if first-degree heart block occurs. Use caution with concurrent use of other antiarrhythmics. Avoid use in myasthenia gravis (may worsen condition). Hypersensitivity reactions can occur. Some tablets contain tartrazine; injection may contain bisulfite (allergens).

Potentially fatal blood dyscrasias have occurred with therapeutic doses; close monitoring is recommended during the first 3 months of therapy.

[U.S. Boxed Warning]: Long-term administration leads to the development of a positive antinuclear antibody (ANA) test in 50% of patients which may result in a drug-induced lupus erythematosus-like syndrome (in 20% to 30%

of patients); discontinue procainamide with SLE symptoms and choose an alternative agent

Adverse Reactions

>1%:

Cardiovascular: Hypotension (I.V., up to 5%)

Dermatologic: Rash

Gastrointestinal: Diarrhea (3% to 4%), nausea, vomiting, taste disorder, GI complaints (3% to 4%)

<1% (Limited to important or life-threatening): Agranulocytosis, angioneurotic edema, aplastic anemia, arrhythmia (proarrhythmic effect, new or worsened), bone marrow suppression, cerebellar ataxia, cholestasis, demyelinating polyradiculoneuropathy, depressed myocardial contractility, depression, disorientation, drug fever, granulomatous hepatitis, hallucinations, hemolytic anemia, hepatic failure, hypoplastic anemia, leukopenia, mania, myasthenia gravis (worsened), myocarditis, myopathy, neuromuscular blockade, neutropenia, pancreatitis, pancytopenia, paradoxical increase in ventricular rate in atrial fibrillation/flutter, pericarditis, peripheral neuropathy, pleural effusion, positive ANA, positive Coombs' test, pruritus, pseudo-obstruction, psychosis, pulmonary embolism, QT prolongation (excessive), rash, respiratory failure due to myopathy, second-degree heart block, SLE-like syndrome, thrombocytopenia (0.5%), torsade de pointes, tremor, urticaria, vasculitis, ventricular arrhythmia

Overdosage/Toxicology Procainamide has a low toxic:therapeutic ratio and may easily produce fatal intoxication (acute toxic dose: 5 g in adults). Symptoms of overdose include sinus bradycardia, sinus node arrest or asystole, P-R, QRS, or QT interval prolongation, torsade de pointes (polymorphous ventricular tachycardia), and depressed myocardial contractility, which along with alpha-adrenergic or ganglionic blockade, may result in hypotension and pulmonary edema. Other effects are seizures, coma, and respiratory arrest. Treatment is symptomatic and effects usually respond to conventional therapies. **Note:** Do not use other Type 1A or 1C antiarrhythmic agents to treat ventricular tachycardia. Sodium bicarbonate may treat wide QRS intervals or hypotension. Markedly impaired conduction or high degree AV block, unresponsive to bicarbonate, indicates consideration of a pacemaker.

Drug Interactions Substrate of CYP2D6 (major)

Amiodarone increases procainamide and NAPA blood levels; consider reducing procainamide dosage by 25% with concurrent use.

Cimetidine increases procainamide and NAPA blood concentrations; monitor blood levels closely or use an alternative H_2 antagonist.

Cisapride and procainamide may increase the risk of malignant arrhythmia; concurrent use is contraindicated.

CYP2D6 inhibitors: May increase the levels/effects of procainamide. Example inhibitors include chlorpromazine, delavirdine, fluoxetine, miconazole, paroxetine, pergolide, quinidine, quinine, ritonavir, and ropinirole.

Neuromuscular blocking agents: Procainamide may potentiate neuromuscular blockade.

Ofloxacin may increase procainamide levels due to an inhibition of renal secretion; monitor levels for procainamide closely.

QT_c-prolonging agents (eg, amiodarone, amitriptyline, bepridil, disopyramide, erythromycin, haloperidol, imipramine, pimozide, quinidine, sotalol, and thioridazine): Effects/toxicity may be increased; use with caution.

Sparfloxacin, gatifloxacin, and moxifloxacin may result in additional prolongation of the QT interval; concurrent use is contraindicated.

Trimethoprim increases procainamide and NAPA blood levels; closely monitor levels.

Ethanol/Nutrition/Herb Interactions

Ethanol: Avoid ethanol (acute ethanol administration reduces procainamide serum concentrations).

Herb/Nutraceutical: Avoid ephedra (may worsen arrhythmia).

Dietary Considerations Should be taken with water on an empty stomach.

Dosage Forms

Capsule, as hydrochloride: 250 mg, 500 mg

Injection, solution, as hydrochloride: 100 mg/mL (10 mL); 500 mg/mL (2 mL) [contains sodium metabisulfite]

Tablet, extended release, as hydrochloride: 500 mg, 750 mg, 1000 mg

Procanbid®: 500 mg, 1000 mg

(Continued)

Procainamide *(Continued)*

References

"2005 American Heart Association Guidelines for Cardiopulmonary Resuscitation and Emergency Cardiovascular Care," *Circulation*, 2005, 112(24 Suppl): 1-211.

Coyle JD and Lima JJ, "Procainamide" in *Applied Pharmacokinetics: Principles of Therapeutic Drug Monitoring*, 3rd Ed. Evans WE, Schentag JJ, and Jusko W (eds). Applied Therapeutics, Inc: Spokane, WA, 1992, 22-1-33.

♦ **Procainamide Hydrochloride** *see* Procainamide *on page 1056*

♦ **Procainamide Hydrochloride Injection, USP (Can)** *see* Procainamide *on page 1056*

Procaine (PROE kane)

Related Information

Local Anesthetics *on page 1532*

U.S. Brand Names Novocain®

Synonyms Procaine Hydrochloride

Pharmacologic Category Local Anesthetic

Generic Available No

Use Produces spinal anesthesia and epidural and peripheral nerve block by injection and infiltration methods

Mechanism of Action Blocks both the initiation and conduction of nerve impulses by decreasing the neuronal membrane's permeability to sodium ions, which results in inhibition of depolarization with resultant blockade of conduction

Pharmacodynamics/Kinetics

Onset of action: 2-5 minutes

Duration (patient, type of block, concentration, and method of anesthesia dependent); 0.5-1.5 hours

Metabolism: Rapidly hydrolyzed by plasma enzymes to para-aminobenzoic acid and diethylaminoethanol (80% conjugated before elimination)

Half-life elimination: 7.7 minutes

Excretion: Urine (as metabolites and some unchanged drug)

Dosage Dose varies with procedure, desired depth, and duration of anesthesia, desired muscle relaxation, vascularity of tissues, physical condition, and age of patient

Administration Prior to instillation of anesthetic agent, withdraw plunger to ensure needle is not in artery or vein; resuscitative equipment should be available when local anesthetics are administered

Pregnancy Risk Factor C

Contraindications Hypersensitivity to procaine, PABA, parabens, other ester local anesthetics, or any component of the formulation

Warnings/Precautions Patients with cardiac diseases, hyperthyroidism, or other endocrine diseases may be more susceptible to toxic effects of local anesthetics; some preparations contain metabisulfite

Adverse Reactions

1% to 10%: Local: Burning sensation at site of injection, tissue irritation, pain at injection site

<1% (Limited to important or life-threatening): Aseptic meningitis resulting in paralysis, chills, CNS stimulation followed by CNS depression

Overdosage/Toxicology Treatment is symptomatic and supportive. Termination of anesthesia by pneumatic tourniquet inflation should be attempted when procaine is administered by infiltration or regional injection.

Drug Interactions

Decreased effect of sulfonamides with the PABA metabolite of procaine, chloroprocaine, and tetracaine

Decreased/increased effect of vasopressors, ergot alkaloids, and MAO inhibitors on blood pressure when using anesthetic solutions with a vasoconstrictor

Dosage Forms Injection, solution, as hydrochloride: 1% [10 mg/mL] (2 mL) [contains sodium bisulfite]; 10% (2 mL) [contains sodium bisulfite]

♦ **Procaine Amide Hydrochloride** *see* Procainamide *on page 1056*

♦ **Procaine Hydrochloride** *see* Procaine *on page 1060*

♦ **Procanbid®** *see* Procainamide *on page 1056*

♦ **Procan® SR (Can)** *see* Procainamide *on page 1056*

♦ **Procardia®** *see* NIFEdipine *on page 920*

♦ **Procardia XL®** *see* NIFEdipine *on page 920*

Prochlorperazine (proe klor PER a zeen)

Medication Safety Issues

Sound-alike/look-alike issues:

Prochlorperazine may be confused with chlorproMAZINE

Compazine® may be confused with Copaxone®, Coumadin®

CPZ (occasional abbreviation for Compazine®) is an error-prone abbreviation (mistaken as chlorpromazine)

Related Information

Postoperative Nausea and Vomiting *on page 1477*

U.S. Brand Names Compro™

Canadian Brand Names Apo-Prochlorperazine®; Compazine®; Nu-Prochlor; Stemetil®

Synonyms Chlormeprazine; Compazine; Prochlorperazine Edisylate; Prochlorperazine Maleate

Pharmacologic Category Antiemetic; Antipsychotic Agent, Typical, Phenothiazine

Generic Available Yes: Injection, tablet, suppository

Use Management of nausea and vomiting; psychotic disorders including schizophrenia; anxiety

Unlabeled/Investigational Use Behavioral syndromes in dementia

Mechanism of Action Prochlorperazine is a piperazine phenothiazine antipsychotic which blocks postsynaptic mesolimbic dopaminergic D_1 and D_2 receptors in the brain, including the chemoreceptor trigger zone; exhibits a strong alpha-adrenergic and anticholinergic blocking effect and depresses the release of hypothalamic and hypophyseal hormones; believed to depress the reticular activating system, thus affecting basal metabolism, body temperature, wakefulness, vasomotor tone and emesis

Pharmacodynamics/Kinetics

Onset of action: Oral: 30-40 minutes; I.M.: 10-20 minutes; Rectal: ~60 minutes

Peak antiemetic effect: I.V.: 30-60 minutes

Duration: Rectal: 12 hours; Oral: 3-4 hours; I.M., I.V.: Adults: 4-6 hours; I.M.: Children: 12 hours

Distribution: V_d: 1400-1548 L; crosses placenta; enters breast milk

Metabolism: Primarily hepatic; N-desmethyl prochlorperazine (major active metabolite)

Bioavailability: Oral: 12.5%

Half-life elimination: Oral: 3-5 hours; I.V.: ~7 hours

Dosage

Antiemetic: Children (therapy >1 day usually not required): **Note:** Not recommended for use in children <9 kg or <2 years:

Oral, rectal: >9 kg: 0.4 mg/kg/24 hours in 3-4 divided doses; **or**

9-13 kg: 2.5 mg every 12-24 hours as needed; maximum: 7.5 mg/day

13.1-17 kg: 2.5 mg every 8-12 hours as needed; maximum: 10 mg/day

17.1-37 kg: 2.5 mg every 8 hours or 5 mg every 12 hours as needed; maximum: 15 mg/day

I.M.: 0.13 mg/kg/dose; change to oral as soon as possible

Antiemetic: Adults:

Oral (tablet): 5-10 mg 3-4 times/day; usual maximum: 40 mg/day; larger doses may rarely be required

I.M. (deep): 5-10 mg every 3-4 hours; usual maximum: 40 mg/day

I.V.: 2.5-10 mg; maximum 10 mg/dose or 40 mg/day; may repeat dose every 3-4 hours as needed

Rectal: 25 mg twice daily

Surgical nausea/vomiting: Adults: **Note:** Should not exceed 40 mg/day

I.M.: 5-10 mg 1-2 hours before induction or to control symptoms during or after surgery; may repeat once if necessary

I.V. (administer slow IVP <5 mg/minute): 5-10 mg 15-30 minutes before induction or to control symptoms during or after surgery; may repeat once if necessary

Rectal (unlabeled use): 25 mg

(Continued)

Prochlorperazine *(Continued)*

Antipsychotic:

Children 2-12 years (not recommended in children <9 kg or <2 years):

Oral, rectal: 2.5 mg 2-3 times/day; do not give more than 10 mg the first day; increase dosage as needed to maximum daily dose of 20 mg for 2-5 years and 25 mg for 6-12 years

I.M.: 0.13 mg/kg/dose; change to oral as soon as possible

Adults:

Oral: 5-10 mg 3-4 times/day; titrate dose slowly every 2-3 days; doses up to 150 mg/day may be required in some patients for treatment of severe disturbances

I.M.: Initial: 10-20 mg; if necessary repeat initial dose every 1-4 hours to gain control; more than 3-4 doses are rarely needed. If parenteral administration is still required; give 10-20 mg every 4-6 hours; change to oral as soon as possible.

Nonpsychotic anxiety: Oral (tablet): Adults: Usual dose: 15-20 mg/day in divided doses; do not give doses >20 mg/day or for longer than 12 weeks

Elderly: Behavioral symptoms associated with dementia (unlabeled use): Initial: 2.5-5 mg 1-2 times/day; increase dose at 4- to 7-day intervals by 2.5-5 mg/day; increase dosing intervals (twice daily, 3 times/day, etc) as necessary to control response or side effects; maximum daily dose should probably not exceed 75 mg in elderly; gradual increases (titration) may prevent some side effects or decrease their severity

Stability

Injection: Store at <30°C (<86°F); do not freeze; protect from light. Clear or slightly yellow solutions may be used.

I.V. infusion: Injection may be diluted in 50-100 mL NS or D_5W.

Suppository, tablet: Store at 15°C to 30°C (59°F to 86°F); protect from light.

Administration May be administered orally, I.M., or I.V.

I.M.: Inject by deep IM into outer quadrant of buttocks.

I.V.: Doses should be given as a short (~30 minute) infusion to avoid orthostatic hypotension; administer at ≤5 mg/minute

Monitoring Parameters Vital signs; lipid profile, fasting blood glucose/Hgb A_{1c}; BMI; mental status, abnormal involuntary movement scale (AIMS); periodic ophthalmic exams (if chronically used); extrapyramidal symptoms (EPS)

Anesthesia and Critical Care Concerns/Other Considerations Prochlorperazine is not recommended as an antipsychotic due to inferior efficacy compared to other phenothiazines. Prochlorperazine has a faster onset of action and causes less sedation than promethazine. When compared with ondansetron (4 mg I.V.), prochlorperazine (10 mg I.M.) administered at the end of surgery more effectively reduced postoperative nausea and the need for rescue antiemetics in patients undergoing total hip or knee replacement. In patients undergoing tympanoplasty, prophylactic prochlorperazine (0.02 mg/kg I.M.) administered at the end of surgery was as effective as ondansetron (0.06 mg/kg I.V.) for reducing PONY.

Contraindications Hypersensitivity to prochlorperazine or any component of the formulation (cross-reactivity between phenothiazines may occur); severe CNS depression; coma; pediatric surgery; Reye's syndrome; should not be used in children <2 years of age or <9 kg

Warnings/Precautions May be sedating; use with caution in disorders where CNS depression is a feature. May obscure intestinal obstruction or brain tumor. May impair physical or mental abilities; patients must be cautioned about performing tasks which require mental alertness (eg, operating machinery or driving). Effects with other sedative drugs or ethanol may be potentiated. Use with caution in Parkinson's disease; hemodynamic instability; bone marrow suppression; predisposition to seizures; subcortical brain damage; and in severe cardiac, hepatic, renal or respiratory disease. Caution in breast cancer or other prolactin-dependent tumors (may elevate prolactin levels). May alter temperature regulation or mask toxicity of other drugs. Use caution with exposure to heat. May alter cardiac conduction; life-threatening arrhythmias have occurred with therapeutic doses of phenothiazines. May cause orthostatic hypotension; use with caution in patients at risk of hypotension or where transient hypotensive episodes would be poorly tolerated (cardiovascular disease or cerebrovascular disease). Hypotension may occur following administration, particularly when parenteral form is used or in high dosages.

Phenothiazines may cause anticholinergic effects (eg, constipation, xerostomia, blurred vision, urinary retention); therefore, they should be used with caution in patients with decreased gastrointestinal motility, urinary retention, BPH, xerostomia, or visual problems. Conditions which also may be exacerbated by cholinergic blockade include narrow-angle glaucoma (screening is recommended) and worsening of myasthenia gravis. May cause extrapyramidal symptoms, including pseudoparkinsonism, acute dystonic reactions, akathisia, and tardive dyskinesia (TD). Use caution in the the elderly; incidence of TD may be increased. Children with acute illness or dehydration are more susceptible to neuromuscular reactions (eg, dystonias); use cautiously. May be associated with neuroleptic malignant syndrome (NMS).

Adverse Reactions Reported with prochlorperazine or other phenothiazines. Frequency not defined

Cardiovascular: Cardiac arrest, hypotension, peripheral edema, Q-wave distortions, T-wave distortions

Central nervous system: Agitation, catatonia, cerebral edema, cough reflex suppressed, dizziness, drowsiness, fever (mild — I.M.), headache, hyperactivity, hyperpyrexia, impairment of temperature regulation, insomnia, neuroleptic malignant syndrome (NMS), paradoxical excitement, restlessness, seizure

Dermatologic: Angioedema, contact dermatitis, discoloration of skin (blue-gray), epithelial keratopathy, erythema, eczema, exfoliative dermatitis (injectable), itching, photosensitivity, rash, skin pigmentation, urticaria

Endocrine & metabolic: Amenorrhea, breast enlargement, galactorrhea, gynecomastia, glucosuria, hyperglycemia, hypoglycemia, lactation, libido (changes in), menstrual irregularity, SIADH

Gastrointestinal: Appetite increased, atonic colon, constipation, ileus, nausea, weight gain, xerostomia

Genitourinary: Ejaculating dysfunction, ejaculatory disturbances, impotence, incontinence, polyuria, priapism, urinary retention, urination difficulty

Hematologic: Agranulocytosis, aplastic anemia, eosinophilia, hemolytic anemia, leukopenia, pancytopenia, thrombocytopenic purpura

Hepatic: Biliary stasis, cholestatic jaundice, hepatotoxicity

Neuromuscular & skeletal: Dystonias (torticollis, opisthotonos, carpopedal spasm, trismus, oculogyric crisis, protusion of tongue); extrapyramidal symptoms (pseudoparkinsonism, akathisia, dystonias, tardive dyskinesia); SLE-like syndrome, tremor

Ocular: blurred vision, cornea and lens changes, lenticular/corneal deposits, miosis, mydriasis, pigmentary retinopathy

Respiratory: Asthma, laryngeal edema, nasal congestion

Miscellaneous: Allergic reactions, diaphoresis

Overdosage/Toxicology Symptoms of overdose include deep sleep, coma, extrapyramidal symptoms, abnormal involuntary muscle movements, seizures, and hypotension. Treatment is symptom-directed and supportive. Do not induce emesis because of risk of aspiration if acute dystonic reaction occurred. Extrapyramidal symptoms may be treated with an anticholinergic such as diphenydramine or benzetropine. Treat hypotension with norephinephrine or phenylephrine. Phenothiazines are not dialyzable.

Drug Interactions

Acetylcholinesterase inhibitors (central): May increase the risk of antipsychotic-related extrapyramidal symptoms; monitor.

Alpha-/Beta- agonists: May enhance the arrhythmogenic effect of phenothiazines.

Analgesics (narcotic): Phenothiazines may enhance the hypotensive effect of narcotic analgesics.

Antacids: May decrease the absorption of phenothiazines; monitor.

Antidepressants (serotonin reuptake inhibitors/antagonist): Concurrent use may produce increased hypotension.

Anticholinergics: May inhibit the therapeutic response to phenothiazines and excess anticholinergic effects may occur; includes benztropine, trihexyphenidyl, biperiden, and drugs with significant anticholinergic activity (TCAs, antihistamines, disopyramide)

Antihistamines: May enhance the arrhythmogenic effect of phenothiazines.

Antimalarial agents: May increase phenothiazine concentrations.

Antiparkinson's Agents (dopamine agonists such as levodopa): Phenothiazines may inhibit the antiparkinsonian effect of levodopa; avoid this combination.

Attapulgite: May decrease absorption of phenothiazines.

(Continued)

Prochlorperazine *(Continued)*

Beta blockers: Serum concentrations of phenothiazines may be increased; phenothiazines may increase hypotensive effects of beta blockers.

CNS depressants: Sedative effects may be additive with phenothiazines; monitor for increased effect; includes barbiturates, benzodiazepines, narcotic analgesics, ethanol and other sedative agents.

Epinephrine: Chlorpromazine (and possibly other low potency antipsychotics) may diminish the pressor effects of epinephrine.

False Neurotransmitters (guanadrel, methyldopa): Antihypertensive effects may be inhibited by phenothiazines.

Lithium: Phenothiazines may produce neurotoxicity with lithium; this is a rare effect Phenytoin: Concurrent use may increase CNS depression.

Polypeptide antibiotics: Rare cases of respiratory paralysis have been reported with concurrent use of phenothiazines.

Pramlintide: May enhance the anticholinergic effects of phenothiazines.

QT_c-prolonging agents: Effects on QT_c interval may be additive with phenothiazines, increasing the risk of malignant arrhythmias; includes type Ia antiarrhythmics, TCAs, and some quinolone antibiotics (sparfloxacin, moxifloxacin, and gatifloxacin).

Ethanol/Nutrition/Herb Interactions

Ethanol: Avoid ethanol (may increase CNS depression).

Food: Limit caffeine.

Herb/Nutraceutical: Avoid dong quai, St John's wort (may also cause photosensitization). Avoid kava kava, gotu kola, valerian, St John's wort (may increase CNS depression).

Test Interactions False-positives for phenylketonuria, pregnancy, urinary amylase, uroporphyrins, urobilinogen

Dietary Considerations Increase dietary intake of riboflavin; should be administered with food or water. Rectal suppositories may contain coconut and palm oil.

Dosage Forms

Injection, solution, as edisylate: 5 mg/mL (2 mL, 10 mL) [contains benzyl alcohol]

Suppository, rectal: 2.5 mg (12s), 5 mg (12s), 25 mg (12s) [may contain coconut and palm oil]

Compro™: 25 mg (12s) [contains coconut and palm oils]

Tablet, as maleate: 5 mg, 10 mg

- **Prochlorperazine Edisylate** *see* Prochlorperazine *on page 1061*
- **Prochlorperazine Maleate** *see* Prochlorperazine *on page 1061*
- **Procrit®** *see* Epoetin Alfa *on page 463*
- **Proctocort®** *see* Hydrocortisone *on page 639*
- **ProctoCream® HC** *see* Hydrocortisone *on page 639*
- **Procto-Kit™** *see* Hydrocortisone *on page 639*
- **Procto-Pak™** *see* Hydrocortisone *on page 639*
- **Proctosert** *see* Hydrocortisone *on page 639*
- **Proctosol-HC®** *see* Hydrocortisone *on page 639*
- **Proctozone-HC™** *see* Hydrocortisone *on page 639*
- **Procytox® (Can)** *see* Cyclophosphamide *on page 334*
- **Profilnine® SD** *see* Factor IX Complex (Human) *on page 504*
- **Prograf®** *see* Tacrolimus *on page 1225*
- **Prolixin® [DSC]** *see* Fluphenazine *on page 545*
- **Prolixin Decanoate®** *see* Fluphenazine *on page 545*

Promethazine (proe METH a zeen)

Medication Safety Issues

Sound-alike/look-alike issues:

Promethazine may be confused with chlorproMAZINE, predniSONE, promazine

Phenergan® may be confused with Phenaphen®, Phrenilin®, Theragran®

Related Information

Postoperative Nausea and Vomiting *on page 1477*

U.S. Brand Names Phenadoz™; Phenergan®; Promethegan™

Canadian Brand Names Phenergan®

Synonyms Promethazine Hydrochloride

Pharmacologic Category Antiemetic; Antihistamine; Phenothiazine Derivative; Sedative

Generic Available Yes

Use Symptomatic treatment of various allergic conditions; antiemetic; motion sickness; sedative; postoperative pain (adjunctive therapy); anesthetic (adjunctive therapy); anaphylactic reactions (adjunctive therapy)

Mechanism of Action Blocks postsynaptic mesolimbic dopaminergic receptors in the brain; exhibits a strong alpha-adrenergic blocking effect and depresses the release of hypothalamic and hypophyseal hormones; competes with histamine for the H_1-receptor; reduces stimuli to the brainstem reticular system

Pharmacodynamics/Kinetics

Onset of action: I.M.: ~20 minutes; I.V.: 3-5 minutes

Peak effect: C_{max}: 9.04 ng/mL (suppository); 19.3 ng/mL (syrup)

Duration: 2-6 hours

Absorption:

I.M.: Bioavailability may be greater than with oral or rectal administration

Oral: Rapid and complete; large first pass effect limits systemic bioavailability

Distribution: V_d: 171 L

Protein binding: 93%

Metabolism: Hepatic; primarily oxidation; forms metabolites

Half-life elimination: 9-16 hours

Time to maximum serum concentration: 4.4 hours (syrup); 6.7-8.6 hours (suppositories)

Excretion: Primarily urine and feces (as inactive metabolites)

Dosage

Children ≥2 years:

Allergic conditions: Oral, rectal: 0.1 mg/kg/dose (maximum: 12.5 mg) every 6 hours during the day and 0.5 mg/kg/dose (maximum: 25 mg) at bedtime as needed

Antiemetic: Oral, I.M., I.V., rectal: 0.25-1 mg/kg 4-6 times/day as needed (maximum: 25 mg/dose)

Motion sickness: Oral, rectal: 0.5 mg/kg/dose 30 minutes to 1 hour before departure, then every 12 hours as needed (maximum dose: 25 mg twice daily)

Sedation: Oral, I.M., I.V., rectal: 0.5-1 mg/kg/dose every 6 hours as needed (maximum: 50 mg/dose)

Adults:

Allergic conditions (including allergic reactions to blood or plasma):

Oral, rectal: 25 mg at bedtime **or** 12.5 mg before meals and at bedtime (range: 6.25-12.5 mg 3 times/day)

I.M., I.V.: 25 mg, may repeat in 2 hours when necessary; switch to oral route as soon as feasible

Antiemetic: Oral, I.M., I.V., rectal: 12.5-25 mg every 4-6 hours as needed

Motion sickness: Oral, rectal: 25 mg 30-60 minutes before departure, then every 12 hours as needed

Sedation: Oral, I.M., I.V., rectal: 12.5-50 mg/dose

Stability

Injection: Prior to dilution, store at room temperature; protect from light. Solutions in NS or D_5W are stable for 24 hours at room temperature.

Suppositories: Store refrigerated at 2°C to 8°C (36°F to 46°F)

Tablets: Store at room temperature; protect from light

Administration Formulations available for oral, rectal, I.M./I.V.; not for SubQ or intra-arterial administration. Administer I.M. into deep muscle (preferred route of administration). I.V. administration is **not** the preferred route. Solution for injection should be administered in a maximum concentration of 25 mg/mL and infused at a rate ≤25 mg/minute. Administration via functioning I.V. infusion is preferred.

Monitoring Parameters Relief of symptoms, mental status

Pregnancy Risk Factor C

Contraindications Hypersensitivity to promethazine or any component of the formulation (cross-reactivity between phenothiazines may occur); coma; treatment of lower respiratory tract symptoms, including asthma; children <2 years of age

(Continued)

Promethazine *(Continued)*

Warnings/Precautions Not for SubQ or intra-arterial administration. Injection may contain sodium metabisulfite (may cause allergic reaction). May be sedating; use with caution in disorders where CNS depression is a feature. May impair physical or mental abilities; patients must be cautioned about performing tasks which require mental alertness (eg, operating machinery or driving). Use with caution in Parkinson's disease; hemodynamic instability; bone marrow suppression; subcortical brain damage; and in severe cardiac, hepatic, renal, or respiratory disease. Avoid use in Reye's syndrome. **[U.S. Boxed Warning]: Respiratory fatalities have been reported in children <2 years of age. In children ≥2 years, use the lowest possible dose; other drugs with respiratory depressant effects should be avoided.** May lower seizure threshold; use caution in persons with seizure disorders or in persons using narcotics or local anesthetics which may also affect seizure threshold. May alter temperature regulation or mask toxicity of other drugs due to antiemetic effects. May alter cardiac conduction (life-threatening arrhythmias have occurred with therapeutic doses of phenothiazines). May cause orthostatic hypotension; use with caution in patients at risk of hypotension or where transient hypotensive episodes would be poorly tolerated (cardiovascular disease or cerebrovascular disease).

Phenothiazines may cause anticholinergic effects (constipation, xerostomia, blurred vision, urinary retention); therefore, they should be used with caution in patients with decreased gastrointestinal motility, urinary retention, BPH, xerostomia, or visual problems. Conditions which also may be exacerbated by cholinergic blockade include narrow-angle glaucoma (screening is recommended) and worsening of myasthenia gravis. May cause extrapyramidal symptoms, including pseudoparkinsonism, acute dystonic reactions, akathisia, and tardive dyskinesia. May be associated with neuroleptic malignant syndrome (NMS).

Adverse Reactions

Cardiovascular: Bradycardia, hypertension, nonspecific QT changes, postural hypotension, tachycardia

Central nervous system: Akathisia, catatonic states, confusion, delirium, disorientation, dizziness, drowsiness, dystonias, euphoria, excitation, extrapyramidal symptoms, fatigue, hallucinations, hysteria, insomnia, lassitude, nervousness, neuroleptic malignant syndrome, nightmares, pseudoparkinsonism, sedation, seizure, somnolence, tardive dyskinesia

Dermatologic: Angioneurotic edema, dermatitis, photosensitivity, skin pigmentation (slate gray), urticaria

Endocrine & metabolic: Amenorrhea, breast engorgement, gynecomastia, hyper-/hypoglycemia, lactation

Gastrointestinal: Constipation, nausea, vomiting, xerostomia

Genitourinary: Ejaculatory disorder, impotence, urinary retention

Hematologic: Agranulocytosis, aplastic anemia, eosinophilia, hemolytic anemia, leukopenia, thrombocytopenia, thrombocytopenic purpura

Hepatic: Jaundice

Neuromuscular & skeletal: Incoordination, tremor

Ocular: Blurred vision, corneal and lenticular changes, diplopia, epithelial keratopathy, pigmentary retinopathy

Otic: Tinnitus

Respiratory: Apnea, asthma, nasal congestion, respiratory depression

Overdosage/Toxicology Symptoms of overdose include CNS depression, respiratory depression, possible CNS stimulation, dry mouth, fixed and dilated pupils, and hypotension. Treatment is symptom-directed and supportive. Epinephrine should not be used. Hemodialysis: Not dialyzable (0% to 5%)

Drug Interactions **Substrate** (major) of CYP2B6, 2D6; **Inhibits** CYP2D6 (weak)

Aluminum salts: May decrease the absorption of phenothiazines; monitor

Amphetamines: Efficacy may be diminished by antipsychotics; in addition, amphetamines may increase psychotic symptoms; avoid concurrent use

Anticholinergics: May inhibit the therapeutic response to phenothiazines and excess anticholinergic effects may occur; includes benztropine, trihexyphenidyl, biperiden, and drugs with significant anticholinergic activity (TCAs, antihistamines, disopyramide)

Antihypertensives: Concurrent use of phenothiazines with an antihypertensive may produce additive hypotensive effects (particularly orthostasis)

Bromocriptine: Phenothiazines inhibit the ability of bromocriptine to lower serum prolactin concentrations

CNS depressants: Sedative effects may be additive with phenothiazines; monitor for increased effect; includes barbiturates, benzodiazepines, narcotic analgesics, ethanol, and other sedative agents

CYP2B6 inducers: May decrease the levels/effects of promethazine. Example inducers include carbamazepine, nevirapine, phenobarbital, phenytoin, and rifampin.

CYP2B6 inhibitors: May increase the levels/effects of promethazine. Example inhibitors include desipramine, paroxetine, and sertraline.

CYP2D6 inhibitors: May increase the levels/effects of promethazine. Example inhibitors include chlorpromazine, delavirdine, fluoxetine, miconazole, paroxetine, pergolide, quinidine, quinine, ritonavir, and ropinirole.

Epinephrine: Promethazine may diminish the pressor effects of epinephrine.

Guanethidine and guanadrel: Antihypertensive effects may be inhibited by phenothiazines

Levodopa: Phenothiazines may inhibit the antiparkinsonian effect of levodopa; avoid this combination

Lithium: Phenothiazines may produce neurotoxicity with lithium; this is a rare effect

Propranolol: Serum concentrations of phenothiazines may be increased; propranolol also increases phenothiazine concentrations

Polypeptide antibiotics: Rare cases of respiratory paralysis have been reported with concurrent use of phenothiazines

QT_c-prolonging agents: Effects on QT_c interval may be additive with phenothiazines, increasing the risk of malignant arrhythmias; includes type Ia antiarrhythmics, TCAs, and some quinolone antibiotics (sparfloxacin, moxifloxacin, and gatifloxacin)

Sulfadoxine-pyrimethamine: May increase phenothiazine concentrations

Tricyclic antidepressants: Concurrent use may produce increased toxicity or altered therapeutic response

Trazodone: Phenothiazines and trazodone may produce additive hypotensive effects

Valproic acid: Serum levels may be increased by phenothiazines

Ethanol/Nutrition/Herb Interactions

Ethanol: Avoid ethanol (may increase CNS depression).

Herb/Nutraceutical: Avoid valerian, St John's wort, kava kava, gotu kola (may increase CNS depression).

Test Interactions Alters the flare response in intradermal allergen tests; hCG-based pregnancy tests may result in false-negatives or false-positives; increased serum glucose may be seen with glucose tolerance tests

Dietary Considerations Increase dietary intake of riboflavin.

Dosage Forms [DSC] = Discontinued product

Injection, solution, as hydrochloride: 25 mg/mL (1 mL); 50 mg/mL (1 mL)
  Phenergan®: 25 mg/mL (1 mL); 50 mg/mL (1 mL) [contains sodium metabisulfite]

Suppository, rectal, as hydrochloride: 12.5 mg, 25 mg, 50 mg
  Phenadoz™: 12.5 mg, 25 mg
  Phenergan®: 25 mg, 50 mg [DSC]
  Promethegan™: 12.5 mg, 25 mg, 50 mg

Syrup, as hydrochloride: 6.25 mg/5 mL (120 mL, 480 mL) [contains alcohol]

Tablet, as hydrochloride: 12.5 mg, 25 mg, 50 mg
  Phenergan®: 25 mg [DSC]

References

Blanc VF, Ruest P, Milot J, et al, "Antiemetic Prophylaxis With Promethazine or Droperidol in Paediatric Outpatient Strabismus Surgery," *Can J Anaesth*, 1991, 38(1):54-60.

♦ **Promethazine Hydrochloride** *see* Promethazine *on page 1064*

♦ **Promethegan**™ *see* Promethazine *on page 1064*

♦ **Pronap-100**® *see* Propoxyphene and Acetaminophen *on page 1076*

♦ **Pronestyl®-SR (Can)** *see* Procainamide *on page 1056*

♦ **Propaderm® (Can)** *see* Beclomethasone *on page 161*

Propafenone (proe pa FEEN one)

Related Information

Antiarrhythmic Drugs *on page 1548*

(Continued)

Propafenone *(Continued)*

U.S. Brand Names Rythmol®; Rythmol® SR

Canadian Brand Names Apo-Propafenone®; Rythmol® Gen-Propafenone

Synonyms Propafenone Hydrochloride

Pharmacologic Category Antiarrhythmic Agent, Class Ic

Generic Available Yes: Tablet

Use Treatment of life-threatening ventricular arrhythmias

Rythmol® SR: Maintenance of normal sinus rhythm in patients with symptomatic atrial fibrillation

Unlabeled/Investigational Use Supraventricular tachycardias, including those patients with Wolff-Parkinson-White syndrome

Mechanism of Action Propafenone is a class 1c antiarrhythmic agent which possesses local anesthetic properties, blocks the fast inward sodium current, and slows the rate of increase of the action potential. Prolongs conduction and refractoriness in all areas of the myocardium, with a slightly more pronounced effect on intraventricular conduction; it prolongs effective refractory period, reduces spontaneous automaticity and exhibits some beta-blockade activity.

Pharmacodynamics/Kinetics

Absorption: Well absorbed

Metabolism: Hepatic; two genetically determined metabolism groups exist: fast or slow metabolizers; 10% of Caucasians are slow metabolizers; exhibits nonlinear pharmacokinetics; when dose is increased from 300-900 mg/day, serum concentrations increase tenfold; this nonlinearity is thought to be due to saturable first-pass effect

Bioavailability: 150 mg: 3.4%; 300 mg: 10.6%

Half-life elimination: Single dose (100-300 mg): 2-8 hours; Chronic dosing: 10-32 hours

Time to peak: 150 mg dose: 2 hours, 300 mg dose: 3 hours

Dosage Oral: Adults: **Note:** Patients who exhibit significant widening of QRS complex or second- or third-degree AV block may need dose reduction.

Immediate release tablet: Initial: 150 mg every 8 hours, increase at 3- to 4-day intervals up to 300 mg every 8 hours.

Extended release capsule: Initial: 225 mg every 12 hours; dosage increase may be made at a minimum of 5-day intervals; may increase to 325 mg every 12 hours; if further increase is necessary, may increase to 425 mg every 12 hours

Dosing adjustment in hepatic impairment: Reduction is necessary; however, specific guidelines are not available.

Stability Store at 25°C (77°F); excursions permitted to 15°C to 30°C (59°F to 86°F).

Administration Capsules should be swallowed whole; do not crush or chew.

Monitoring Parameters ECG, blood pressure, pulse (particularly at initiation of therapy)

Anesthesia and Critical Care Concerns/Other Considerations As with other class 1c agents, avoid use in patients with cardiovascular disease.

Pregnancy Risk Factor C

Contraindications Hypersensitivity to propafenone or any component of the formulation; sinoatrial, AV, and intraventricular disorders of impulse generation and/or conduction (except in patients with a functioning artificial pacemaker); sinus bradycardia; cardiogenic shock; uncompensated cardiac failure; hypotension; bronchospastic disorders; uncorrected electrolyte abnormalities; concurrent use of ritonavir (see Drug Interactions)

Warnings/Precautions Monitor for proarrhythmic events. May prolong QT_c interval; use caution with other QT_c-prolonging drugs. **[U.S. Boxed Warning]: In the Cardiac Arrhythmia Suppression Trial (CAST), recent (>6 days but <2 years ago) myocardial infarction patients with asymptomatic, nonlife-threatening ventricular arrhythmias did not benefit and may have been harmed by attempts to suppress the arrhythmia with flecainide or encainide. An increased mortality or nonfatal cardiac arrest rate (7.7%) was seen in the active treatment group compared with patients in the placebo group (3%). The applicability of the CAST results to other populations is unknown. Antiarrhythmic agents should be reserved for patients with life-threatening ventricular arrhythmias.** Can cause or unmask a variety of conduction disturbances. May alter pacing and sensing thresholds of artificial pacemakers. Patients with bronchospastic disease should generally not receive this drug. Monitor for worsening CHF if patient has underlying condition. Administer cautiously in significant hepatic dysfunction.

Adverse Reactions

1% to 10%:

Cardiovascular: New or worsened arrhythmia (proarrhythmic effect) (2% to 10%), angina (2% to 5%), CHF (1% to 4%), ventricular tachycardia (1% to 3%), palpitation (1% to 3%), AV block (first-degree) (1% to 3%), syncope (1% to 2%), increased QRS interval (1% to 2%), chest pain (1% to 2%), PVCs (1% to 2%), bradycardia (1% to 2%), edema (0% to 1%), bundle branch block (0% to 1%), atrial fibrillation (1%), hypotension (0% to 1%), intraventricular conduction delay (0% to 1%)

Central nervous system: Dizziness (4% to 15%), fatigue (2% to 6%), headache (2% to 5%), ataxia (0% to 2%), insomnia (0% to 2%), anxiety (1% to 2%), drowsiness (1%)

Dermatologic: Rash (1% to 3%)

Gastrointestinal: Nausea/vomiting (2% to 11%), unusual taste (3% to 23%), constipation (2% to 7%), dyspepsia (1% to 3%), diarrhea (1% to 3%), xerostomia (1% to 2%), anorexia (1% to 2%), abdominal pain (1% to 2%), flatulence (0% to 1%)

Neuromuscular & skeletal: Tremor (0% to 1%), arthralgia (0% to 1%), weakness (1% to 2%)

Ocular: Blurred vision (1% to 6%)

Respiratory: Dyspnea (2% to 5%)

Miscellaneous: Diaphoresis (1%)

<1% (Limited to important or life-threatening): Agranulocytosis, alopecia, amnesia, anemia, apnea, AV block (second or third degree), AV dissociation, cardiac arrest, cholestasis (0.1%), coma, confusion, CHF, depression, granulocytopenia, hepatitis (0.03%), hyperglycemia, impotence, increased bleeding time, leukopenia, lupus erythematosus, mania, memory loss, nephrotic syndrome, paresthesia, peripheral neuropathy, pruritus, psychosis, purpura, renal failure, seizure (0.3%), SIADH, sinus node dysfunction, thrombocytopenia, tinnitus, vertigo

Overdosage/Toxicology Propafenone has a narrow therapeutic index and severe toxicity may occur slightly above the therapeutic range, especially if combined with other antiarrhythmic drugs. Acute single ingestion of twice the daily therapeutic dose is life-threatening. Symptoms of overdose include increased P-R, QRS, or QT intervals and amplitude of the T wave, AV block, bradycardia, hypotension, ventricular arrhythmias (monomorphic or polymorphic ventricular tachycardia), and asystole. Other symptoms include dizziness, blurred vision, headache, and GI upset. Treatment is supportive. **Note:** Class 1A antiarrhythmic agents should not be used to treat cardiotoxicity caused by Class 1C drugs. Sodium bicarbonate may reverse QRS prolongation, bradycardia, and hypotension. Ventricular pacing may be needed.

Drug Interactions **Substrate** of CYP1A2 (minor), 2D6 (major), 3A4 (minor); **Inhibits** CYP1A2 (weak), 2D6 (weak)

Cimetidine: May increase propafenone levels.

CYP2D6 inhibitors: May increase the levels/effects of propafenone. Example inhibitors include chlorpromazine, delavirdine, fluoxetine, miconazole, paroxetine, pergolide, quinidine, quinine, ritonavir, and ropinirole.

Digoxin: Propafenone may increase digoxin levels; monitor for toxicity.

Metoprolol: Propafenone may increase metoprolol levels.

Phenobarbital: May decrease propafenone levels.

Propranolol: Propafenone may increase propranolol levels.

QT_c-prolonging agents: Effects may be additive with propafenone. Use caution with Class Ia and Class III antiarrhythmics, erythromycin, cisapride, antipsychotics, and cyclic antidepressants.

Quinidine: May increase propafenone levels.

Rifampin: May decrease propafenone levels.

Ritonavir: May increase propafenone levels; concurrent use is contraindicated.

Theophylline: Propafenone may increase theophylline levels.

Warfarin: Propafenone may increase warfarin levels/effects. Monitor INR closely.

Ethanol/Nutrition/Herb Interactions

Food: Propafenone serum concentrations may be increased if taken with food.

Herb/Nutraceutical: St John's wort may decrease propafenone levels. Avoid ephedra (may worsen arrhythmia).

Dietary Considerations

Capsule: May be taken without regard to food.

(Continued)

Propafenone *(Continued)*

Rythmol® SR capsules contain soy lecithin.

Tablet: Should be taken at the same time in relation to meals each day, either always with meals or always between meals.

Dosage Forms

Capsule, extended release, as hydrochloride (Rythmol® SR): 225 mg, 325 mg, 425 mg [contains soy lecithin]

Tablet, as hydrochloride (Rythmol®): 150 mg, 225 mg, 300 mg

- **Propafenone Hydrochloride** *see* Propafenone *on page 1067*
- **Proplex® T** *see* Factor IX Complex (Human) *on page 504*

Propofol (PROE po fole)

Medication Safety Issues

Sound-alike/look-alike issues:

Diprivan® may be confused with Diflucan®, Ditropan®

Related Information

Anesthesia Considerations for Neurosurgery *on page 1401*
Critical Care Infusion Administration Charts *on page 1514*
Epilepsy *on page 1604*
Intravenous Anesthetic Agents *on page 1531*
Sedative Agents in the Intensive Care Unit *on page 1576*

U.S. Brand Names Diprivan®

Canadian Brand Names Diprivan®

Pharmacologic Category General Anesthetic

Generic Available Yes

Use Induction of anesthesia for inpatient or outpatient surgery in patients ≥3 years of age; maintenance of anesthesia for inpatient or outpatient surgery in patients >2 months of age; in adults, for the induction and maintenance of monitored anesthesia care sedation during diagnostic procedures; treatment of agitation in intubated, mechanically-ventilated ICU patients

Unlabeled/Investigational Use Postoperative antiemetic; refractory delirium tremens (case reports); conscious sedation

Mechanism of Action Propofol is a hindered phenolic compound with intravenous general anesthetic properties. The drug is unrelated to any of the currently used barbiturate, opioid, benzodiazepine, arylcyclohexylamine, or imidazole intravenous anesthetic agents.

Pharmacodynamics/Kinetics

Onset of action: Anesthetic: Bolus infusion (dose dependent): 9-51 seconds (average 30 seconds)

Duration (dose and rate dependent): 3-10 minutes

Distribution: V_d: 2-10 L/kg; highly lipophilic

Protein binding: 97% to 99%

Metabolism: Hepatic to water-soluble sulfate and glucuronide conjugates

Half-life elimination: Biphasic: Initial: 40 minutes; Terminal: 4-7 hours (up to 1-3 days)

Excretion: Urine (~88% as metabolites, 40% as glucuronide metabolite); feces (<2%)

Clearance: 20-30 mL/kg/minute; total body clearance exceeds liver blood flow

Dosage Dosage must be individualized based on total body weight and titrated to the desired clinical effect; wait at least 3-5 minutes between dosage adjustments to clinically assess drug effects; smaller doses are required when used with narcotics; the following are general dosing guidelines:

General anesthesia:

Induction: I.V.:

Children 3-16 years, ASA I or II: 2.5-3.5 mg/kg over 20-30 seconds; use a lower dose for children ASA III or IV

Adults, ASA I or II, <55 years: 2-2.5 mg/kg (~40 mg every 10 seconds until onset of induction)

Elderly, debilitated, hypovolemic, or ASA III or IV: 1-1.5 mg/kg (~20 mg every 10 seconds until onset of induction)

Cardiac anesthesia: 0.5-1.5 mg/kg (~20 mg every 10 seconds until onset of induction)

Neurosurgical patients: 1-2 mg/kg (~20 mg every 10 seconds until onset of induction)

Maintenance: I.V. infusion:

Children 2 months to 16 years, ASA I or II: Initial: 200-300 mcg/kg/minute; decrease dose after 30 minutes if clinical signs of light anesthesia are absent; usual infusion rate: 125-150 mcg/kg/minute (range: 125-300 mcg/kg/minute; 7.5-18 mg/kg/hour); children ≤5 years may require larger infusion rates compared to older children

Adults, ASA I or II, <55 years: Initial: 150-200 mcg/kg/minute for 10-15 minutes; decrease by 30% to 50% during first 30 minutes of maintenance; usual infusion rate: 100-200 mcg/kg/minute (6-12 mg/kg/hour)

Elderly, debilitated, hypovolemic, ASA III or IV: 50-100 mcg/kg/minute (3-6 mg/kg/ hour)

Cardiac anesthesia:

Low-dose propofol with primary opioid: 50-100 mcg/kg/minute (see manufacturer's labeling)

Primary propofol with secondary opioid: 100-150 mcg/kg/minute

Neurosurgical patients: 100-200 mcg/kg/minute (6-12 mg/kg/hour)

Maintenance: I.V. intermittent bolus: Adults, ASA I or II, <55 years: 20-50 mg increments as needed

Monitored anesthesia care sedation:

Initiation:

Adults, ASA I or II, <55 years: Slow I.V. infusion: 100-150 mcg/kg/minute for 3-5 minutes **or** slow injection: 0.5 mg/kg over 3-5 minutes

Elderly, debilitated, neurosurgical, or ASA III or IV patients: Use similar doses to healthy adults; avoid rapid I.V. boluses

Maintenance:

Adults, ASA I or II, <55 years: I.V. infusion using variable rates (preferred over intermittent boluses): 25-75 mcg/kg/minute **or** incremental bolus doses: 10 mg or 20 mg

Elderly, debilitated, neurosurgical, or ASA III or IV patients: Use 80% of healthy adult dose; **do not** use rapid bolus doses (single or repeated)

ICU sedation in intubated mechanically-ventilated patients: Avoid rapid bolus injection; individualize dose and titrate to response Continuous infusion: Initial: 0.3 mg/kg/hour (5 mcg/kg/min); increase by 0.3-0.6 mg/kg/hour (5-10 mcg/kg/min) every 5-10 minutes until desired sedation level is achieved; usual maintenance: 0.3-4.8 mg/kg/hour (5-80 mcg/kg/min) or higher; reduce dose by 80% in elderly, debilitated, and ASA III or IV patients; reduce dose after adequate sedation established and adjust to response (ie, evaluate frequently to use minimum dose for sedation). Some clinicians recommend daily interruption of infusion to perform clinical evaluation.

Stability Store at room temperature 4°C to 22°C (40°F to 72°F), refrigeration is not recommended; protect from light. If transferred to a syringe or other container prior to administration, use within 6 hours. If used directly from vial/prefilled syringe, use within 12 hours. Shake well before use. Do not use if there is evidence of separation of phases of emulsion.

Does not need to be diluted; however, propofol may be further diluted in 5% dextrose in water to a concentration of 2 mg/mL and is stable for 8 hours at room temperature.

Y-site administration compatible with D_5LR, D_5W, lactated Ringer's, lidocaine, 5% dextrose and 0.45% sodium chloride, 5% dextrose and 0.2% sodium chloride. Do not mix with other therapeutic agents.

Administration To reduce pain associated with injection, use larger veins of forearm or antecubital fossa; lidocaine I.V. (1 mL of a 1% solution) may also be used prior to administration. Do not use filter with <5 micron for administration. Tubing and any unused portions of propofol vials should be discarded after 12 hours. Strict aseptic technique must be maintained in handling although a preservative has been added. Do not administer through the same I.V. catheter with blood or plasma. The American College of Critical Care Medicine recommends the use of a central vein for administration in an ICU setting.

Monitoring Parameters Cardiac monitor, blood pressure monitor required; serum triglyceride levels should be obtained prior to initiation of therapy (ICU setting) and every 3-7 days thereafter; daily sedation levels using standardized scale. Monitor vital signs (blood pressure, heart rate) during infusion. Unexplained tachycardia should prompt evaluation of metabolic status (including consideration of acid-base status). In patients at risk for renal impairment, urinalysis and urine sediment should be monitored prior to treatment and every other day of sedation.

(Continued)

Propofol *(Continued)*

Diprivan®: Monitor zinc levels in patients predisposed to deficiency (burns, diarrhea, major sepsis) or after 5 days of treatment.

Anesthesia and Critical Care Concerns/Other Considerations On March 26, 2001, a specific warning was issued concerning the use of propofol in pediatric ICU patients. In the opinion of the FDA, a clinical trial evaluating the use of propofol as a sedative agent in this population was associated with a higher number of deaths as compared to standard sedative agents. The warning reminded healthcare professionals that propofol is not approved in the U.S. for sedation in pediatric ICU patients. There have been several case reports of propofol infusion syndrome in critically-ill adults. Clinical features include circulatory collapse, metabolic acidosis, rhabdomyolysis, hepatomegaly, and hyperkalemia. Preservatives (eg, EDTA or sodium metabisulfite) have been added to some products.

Propofol is a negative inotrope and chronotrope.

Bradycardia may respond to atropine.

Very long-term infusions can result in some tolerance; taper propofol infusions to prevent withdrawal. Caution should be exercised when using high doses (>5 mg/kg/hour) and for long-term (>48 hours).

Pregnancy Risk Factor B

Contraindications Hypersensitivity to propofol or any component of the formulation; propofol is also contraindicated when general anesthesia or sedation is contraindicated

Warnings/Precautions Use requires careful patient monitoring, should only be used by experienced personnel who are not actively engaged in the procedure or surgery. If used in a nonintubated and/or nonmechanically-ventilated patient, qualified personnel and appropriate equipment for rapid institution of respiratory and/or cardiovascular support must be immediately available.

Use a slower rate of induction and avoid rapid bolus administration in the elderly, debilitated, or ASA III/IV patients. Use with caution in patients who are hypotensive, hypovolemic, hemodynamically unstable, or have abnormally low vascular tone (eg, sepsis). Use caution in patients with severe cardiac disease (ejection fraction <50%) or respiratory disease; may have more profound adverse cardiovascular responses to propofol. Use caution in patients with a history of epilepsy or seizures; risk of seizure during recovery phase. Use caution in patients with increased intracranial pressure or impaired cerebral circulation - substantial decreases in mean arterial pressure and subsequent decreases in cerebral perfusion pressure may occur.

Use caution in patients with hyperlipidemia as evidenced by increased serum triglyceride levels or serum turbidity. Transient local pain may occur during I.V. injection; perioperative myoclonia has occurred. Not recommended for use in obstetrics, including cesarean section deliveries. Safety and efficacy in pediatric intensive care unit patients have not been established. Several deaths associated with severe metabolic acidosis have been reported in pediatric ICU patients on long-term propofol infusion. Concurrent use of fentanyl and propofol in pediatric patients may result in bradycardia.

Abrupt discontinuation prior to weaning or daily wake up assessments should be avoided. Abrupt discontinuation can result in rapid awakening, anxiety, agitation, and resistance to mechanical ventilation; titrate the infusion rate so the patient awakens slowly. Propofol does not have analgesic properties; pain should be treated with analgesic agents, propofol must be titrated separately from the analgesic agent. Propofol emulsion contains soybean oil, egg phosphatide, and glycerol; some formulations also contain sulfites. Some products may contain benzyl alcohol; benzyl alcohol has been associated with the "gasping syndrome" in neonates and low-birth-weight infants.

Adverse Reactions

>10%:

Cardiovascular: Hypotension (children 17%, adults 3% to 26%)

Central nervous system: Dystonic or choreiform movement (children 17%)

Local: Injection site burning, stinging, or pain (children 10%, adults 18%)

Respiratory: Apnea, lasting 30-60 seconds (children 10%, adults 24%); apnea, lasting >60 seconds (children 5%, adults 12%)

1% to 10%:

Cardiovascular: Hypertension (children 8%), arrhythmia, bradycardia, cardiac output decreased, tachycardia

Central nervous system: Movement (adults)

Dermatologic: Pruritus (children 2%), rash (children 5%)

Endocrine & metabolic: Hyperlipidemia, hypertriglyceridemia

Respiratory: Respiratory acidosis during weaning

<1% (Limited to important or life-threatening): Agitation, amblyopia, anaphylaxis, anaphylactoid reaction, anticholinergic syndrome, asystole, atrial arrhythmia, bigeminy, cardiac arrest, chills, cough, dizziness, delirium; discoloration (green - urine, hair, or nailbeds); dystonia; extremity pain, fever, flushing, hemorrhage, hypersalivation, hypertonia, hypomagnesemia, hypoxia, laryngospasm, leukocytosis, lung function decreased, metabolic acidosis (not associated with "propofol infusion syndrome"), myalgia, nausea, paresthesia, perioperative myoclonia (rarely including convulsions and opisthotonos), phlebitis, postoperative pancreatitis, postoperative unconsciousness with or without increase in muscle tone, premature atrial contractions, premature ventricular contractions, pulmonary edema, rhabdomyolysis, serum triglycerides increased, somnolence, syncope, thrombosis, urine cloudy, vision abnormality, wheezing.

Infusion site reactions include pain, swelling, blisters and/or tissue necrosis following accidental extravasation. **Note:** A "propofol infusion syndrome" has been described in patients receiving high-dose, prolonged infusion; symptoms include severe, sporadic metabolic acidosis and/or lactic acidosis which may be associated with tachycardia, myocardial dysfunction, and/or rhabdomyolysis.

Overdosage/Toxicology

Symptoms of overdose include hypotension, bradycardia, and cardiovascular collapse.

Treatment is symptomatic and supportive. Hypotension usually responds to I.V. fluids and/or Trendelenburg positioning. Parenteral inotropes may be needed. Bradycardia may respond to atropine.

Drug Interactions Substrate of CYP1A2 (minor), 2A6 (minor), 2B6 (major), 2C9 (major), 2C19 (minor), 2D6 (minor), 2E1 (minor), 3A4 (minor); **Inhibits** CYP1A2 (moderate), 2C9 (weak), 2C19 (moderate), 2D6 (weak), 2E1 (weak), 3A4 (strong)

CNS depressants: Additive CNS depression and respiratory depression may necessitate dosage reduction when used with anesthetics, benzodiazepines, opiates, ethanol, phenothiazines.

CYP1A2 substrates: Propofol may increase the levels/effects of CYP1A2 substrates. Example substrates include aminophylline, fluvoxamine, mexiletine, mirtazapine, ropinirole, theophylline, and trifluoperazine.

CYP2B6 inhibitors: May increase the levels/effects of propofol. Example inhibitors include desipramine, paroxetine, and sertraline.

CYP2C9 Inhibitors may increase the levels/effects of propofol. Example inhibitors include delavirdine, fluconazole, gemfibrozil, ketoconazole, nicardipine, NSAIDs, sulfonamides and tolbutamide.

CYP2C19 substrates: Propofol may increase the levels/effects of CYP2C19 substrates. Example substrates include citalopram, diazepam, methsuximide, phenytoin, propranolol, and sertraline.

CYP3A4 substrates: Propofol may increase the levels/effects of CYP3A4 substrates. Example substrates include benzodiazepines, calcium channel blockers, mirtazapine, nateglinide, nefazodone, tacrolimus, and venlafaxine. Selected benzodiazepines (midazolam and triazolam), cisapride, ergot alkaloids, selected HMG-CoA reductase inhibitors (lovastatin and simvastatin), and pimozide are generally contraindicated with strong CYP3A4 inhibitors.

Narcotics: Concomitant use may lead to increased sedative or anesthetic effects of propofol, more pronounced decreases in systolic, diastolic, and mean arterial pressures and cardiac output. Lower doses of propofol may be needed. In addition, fentanyl may cause serious bradycardia when used with propofol in pediatric patients.

Vecuronium: Propofol may potentiate the neuromuscular blockade of vecuronium.

Ethanol/Nutrition/Herb Interactions Food: EDTA, an ingredient of propofol emulsion, may lead to decreased zinc levels in patients on prolonged therapy (>5 days) or those predisposed to deficiency (burns, diarrhea, and/or major sepsis).

Test Interactions Decreased cholesterol (S); increased porphyrin (U); decreased cortisol (S), but does not appear to inhibit adrenal responsiveness to ACTH

Dietary Considerations Propofol is formulated in an oil-in-water emulsion. If on parenteral nutrition, may need to adjust the amount of lipid infused. Propofol

(Continued)

Propofol *(Continued)*

emulsion contains 1.1 kcal/mL. Soybean fat emulsion is used as a vehicle for propofol. Formulations also contain egg phosphatide and glycerol.

Dosage Forms

Injection, emulsion: 10 mg/mL (20 mL, 50 mL, 100 mL) [contains egg lecithin, and soybean oil; may contain either benzyl alcohol or sodium metabisulfite]

Diprivan®: 10 mg/mL (20 mL, 50 mL, 100 mL) [contains egg lecithin, soybean oil, and disodium edetate]

References

Burow BK, Johnson ME, and Packer DL, "Metabolic Acidosis Associated With Propofol in the Absence of Other Causative Factors," *Anesthesiology*, 2004, 101(1):239-41.

Cawley MJ, Guse TM, Laroia A, et al, "Propofol Withdrawal Syndrome in an Adult Patient With Thermal Injury," *Pharmacotherapy*, 2003, 23(7):933-9.

Ernest D and French C, "Propofol Infusion Syndrome - Report of an Adult Fatality," *Anaesth Intensive Care*, 2003, 31(3):316-9.

Funston JS and Prough DS, "Two Reports of Propofol Anesthesia Associated With Metabolic Acidosis in Adults," *Anesthesiology*, 2004, 101(1):6-8.

Jacobi J, Fraser GL, Coursin DB, et al, "Clinical Practice Guidelines for the Sustained Use of Sedatives and Analgesics in the Critically Ill Adult," *Crit Care Med*, 2002, 30(1):119-41. Available at: http://www.sccm.org/pdf/sedatives.pdf.

Kang TM, "Propofol Infusion Syndrome in Critically Ill Patients," *Ann Pharmacother*, 2002, 36(9):1453-6.

McCowan C and Marik P, "Refractory Delirium Tremens Treated With Propofol: A Case Series," *Crit Care Med*, 2000, 28(6):1781-4.

Salengros JC, Velghe-Lenelle CE, Bollens R, et al, "Lactic Acidosis During Propofol-Remifentanil Anesthesia in an Adult," *Anesthesiology*, 2004, 101(1):241-3.

Short TG and Young Y, "Toxicity of Intravenous Anaesthetics," *Best Pract Res Clin Anaesthesiol*, 2003, 17(1):77-89.

Propoxyphene (proe POKS i feen)

Medication Safety Issues

Sound-alike/look-alike issues:

Propoxyphene may be confused with proparacaine

Darvon® may be confused with Devrom®, Diovan®

Darvon-N® may be confused with Darvocet-N®

Related Information

Acute Postoperative Pain *on page 1388*

Chronic Pain Management *on page 1430*

Narcotic / Opioid Analgesics *on page 1568*

U.S. Brand Names Darvon®; Darvon-N®

Canadian Brand Names Darvon-N®; 642® Tablet

Synonyms Dextropropoxyphene; Propoxyphene Hydrochloride; Propoxyphene Napsylate

Pharmacologic Category Analgesic, Narcotic

Restrictions C-IV

Generic Available Yes: Capsule

Use Management of mild to moderate pain

Mechanism of Action Propoxyphene is a weak narcotic analgesic which acts through binding to opiate receptors to inhibit ascending pain pathways. Propoxyphene, as with other narcotic (opiate) analgesics, blocks pain perception in the cerebral cortex by binding to specific receptor molecules (opiate receptors) within the neuronal membranes of synapses. This binding results in a decreased synaptic chemical transmission throughout the CNS thus inhibiting the flow of pain sensations into the higher centers. Mu and kappa are the two subtypes of the opiate receptor which propoxyphene binds to cause analgesia.

Pharmacodynamics/Kinetics

Onset of action: 0.5-1 hour

Duration: 4-6 hours

Metabolism: Hepatic to active metabolite (norpropoxyphene) and inactive metabolites; first-pass effect

Half-life elimination: Adults: Parent drug: 6-12 hours; Norpropoxyphene: 30-36 hours

Excretion: Urine (primarily as metabolites)

Dosage Oral:

Children: Doses for children are not well established; doses of the hydrochloride of 2-3 mg/kg/d divided every 6 hours have been used

Adults:

Hydrochloride: 65 mg every 3-4 hours as needed for pain; maximum: 390 mg/day

Napsylate: 100 mg every 4 hours as needed for pain; maximum: 600 mg/day

Elderly:

Hydrochloride: 65 mg every 4-6 hours as needed for pain

Napsylate: 100 mg every 4-6 hours as needed for pain

Dosing adjustment in renal impairment: Serum concentrations of propoxyphene may be increased or elimination may be delayed. Avoid use in Cl_{cr} <10 mL/minute. Specific dosing recommendations not available for less severe impairment.

Not dialyzable (0% to 5%)

Dosing adjustment in hepatic impairment: Serum concentrations of propoxyphene may be increased or elimination may be delayed; specific dosing recommendations not available.

Stability Store at controlled room temperature of 15°C to 30°C (59°F to 86°F).

Administration Should be administered with glass of water on an empty stomach. Food may decrease rate of absorption, but may slightly increase bioavailability.

Monitoring Parameters Pain relief, respiratory and mental status, blood pressure

Reference Range

Therapeutic: Ranges published vary between laboratories and may not correlate with clinical effect

Therapeutic concentration: 0.1-0.4 mcg/mL (SI: 0.3-1.2 µmol/L)

Toxic: >0.5 mcg/mL (SI: >1.5 µmol/L)

Anesthesia and Critical Care Concerns/Other Considerations Equivalent dosing: 100 mg of napsylate = 65 mg of hydrochloride

Pregnancy Risk Factor C/D (prolonged use)

Contraindications Hypersensitivity to propoxyphene or any component of the formulation

Warnings/Precautions [U.S. Boxed Warning]: When given in excessive doses, either alone or in combination with other CNS depressants (including alcohol), propoxyphene is a major cause of drug-related deaths; recommended dosage must not be exceeded and alcohol intake should be limited. Avoid use in severely depressed or suicidal patients. Should not be prescribed in patients who are addiction prone or suicidal. Use caution in patients taking CNS depressant medications or antidepressants, and in patients who use alcohol in excess.

Use caution in patients dependent on opiates, substitution may result in acute opiate withdrawal symptoms. Tolerance or drug dependence may result from extended use. Propoxyphene should be used with caution in patients with renal or hepatic dysfunction or in the elderly; consider dosing adjustment.

Adverse Reactions Frequency not defined.

Cardiovascular: Hypotension, bundle branch block

Central nervous system: Dizziness, lightheadedness, sedation, paradoxical excitement and insomnia, fatigue, drowsiness, mental depression, hallucinations, paradoxical CNS stimulation, increased intracranial pressure, nervousness, headache, restlessness, malaise, confusion, dysphoria, vertigo

Dermatologic: Rash, urticaria

Endocrine & metabolic: Hypoglycemia, urinary 17-OHCS decreased

Gastrointestinal: Anorexia, stomach cramps, xerostomia, biliary spasm, nausea, vomiting, constipation, paralytic ileus, abdominal pain

Genitourinary: Urination decreased, ureteral spasms

Hepatic: LFTs increased, jaundice

Neuromuscular & skeletal: Weakness

Ocular: Visual disturbances

Respiratory: Dyspnea

Miscellaneous: Psychologic and physical dependence with prolonged use, histamine release, hypersensitivity reaction

Overdosage/Toxicology Symptoms of overdose include CNS disturbances, respiratory depression, hypotension, pulmonary edema, and seizures. Naloxone, 2 mg I.V. with repeat administration as necessary up to a total of 10 mg, can also be used to reverse toxic effects of the opiate. Charcoal is very effective (>95%) at binding propoxyphene.

Drug Interactions Inhibits CYP2C9 (weak), 2D6 (weak), 3A4 (weak)

Decreased effect with charcoal, cigarette smoking

(Continued)

Propoxyphene *(Continued)*

Increased toxicity: CNS depressants may potentiate pharmacologic effects; propoxyphene may inhibit the metabolism and increase the serum concentrations of carbamazepine, phenobarbital, MAO inhibitors, tricyclic antidepressants, and warfarin

Ethanol/Nutrition/Herb Interactions

Ethanol: Avoid or limit ethanol (may increase CNS depression). Watch for sedation.

Food: May decrease rate of absorption, but may slightly increase bioavailability.

Test Interactions False-positive methadone test

Dietary Considerations May administer with food if gastrointestinal distress occurs.

Dosage Forms

Capsule, as hydrochloride (Darvon®): 65 mg

Tablet, as napsylate (Darvon-N®): 100 mg

Propoxyphene and Acetaminophen

(proe POKS i feen & a seet a MIN oh fen)

Medication Safety Issues

Sound-alike/look-alike issues:

Darvocet-N® may be confused with Darvon-N®

U.S. Brand Names Balacet 325™; Darvocet A500™; Darvocet-N® 50; Darvocet-N® 100; Pronap-100®

Canadian Brand Names Darvocet-N® 50; Darvocet-N® 100

Synonyms Acetaminophen and Propoxyphene; Propoxyphene Hydrochloride and Acetaminophen; Propoxyphene Napsylate and Acetaminophen

Pharmacologic Category Analgesic Combination (Narcotic)

Restrictions C-IV

Generic Available Yes

Use Management of mild to moderate pain

Mechanism of Action

Propoxyphene is a weak narcotic analgesic which acts through binding to opiate receptors to inhibit ascending pain pathways

Propoxyphene, as with other narcotic (opiate) analgesics, blocks pain perception in the cerebral cortex by binding to specific receptor molecules (opiate receptors) within the neuronal membranes of synapses. This binding results in a decreased synaptic chemical transmission throughout the CNS thus inhibiting the flow of pain sensations into the higher centers. Mu and kappa are the two subtypes of the opiate receptor to which propoxyphene binds to cause analgesia.

Acetaminophen inhibits the synthesis of prostaglandins in the CNS and peripherally blocks pain impulse generation; produces antipyresis from inhibition of hypothalamic heat-regulating center

Pharmacodynamics/Kinetics See individual agents.

Dosage Oral: Adults:

Darvocet A500™, Darvocet-N® 100: 1 tablet every 4 hours as needed; maximum: 600 mg propoxyphene napsylate/day

Darvocet-N® 50: 1-2 tablets every 4 hours as needed; maximum: 600 mg propoxyphene napsylate/day

Note: Dosage of acetaminophen should not exceed 4 g/day (6 tablets of Darvocet-N® 100); possibly less in patients with ethanol

Elderly: Refer to Adults dosing

Dosing adjustment in renal/hepatic impairment: Serum concentrations of propoxyphene may be increased or elimination may be delayed; specific dosing recommendations not available.

Stability Store at controlled room temperature.

Administration Should be administered with water on an empty stomach.

Pregnancy Risk Factor C

Contraindications Hypersensitivity to propoxyphene, acetaminophen, or any component of the formulation

Warnings/Precautions **[U.S. Boxed Warning]: When given in excessive doses, either alone or in combination with other CNS depressants (including alcohol), propoxyphene is a major cause of drug-related deaths; recommended dosage must not be exceeded and alcohol intake should be**

limited. Avoid use in severely depressed or suicidal patients. Should not be prescribed in patients who are addiction prone or suicidal. Use caution in patients taking CNS depressant medications or antidepressants, and in patients who use alcohol in excess.

Use caution in patients dependent on opiates, substitution may result in acute opiate withdrawal symptoms. Tolerance or drug dependence may result from extended use. Propoxyphene should be used with caution in patients with renal or hepatic dysfunction or in the elderly; consider dosing adjustment.

Propoxyphene should be used with caution in patients with renal or hepatic dysfunction or in the elderly; consider dosing adjustment. Acetaminophen should be used with caution in patients with liver disease; consuming ≥3 alcoholic drinks/day may increase risk of liver damage. Use caution in patients with known G6PD deficiency. Safety and efficacy of this combination have not been established in pediatric patients.

Adverse Reactions See individual agents.

Drug Interactions

Propoxyphene: **Inhibits** CYP2C9 (weak), 2D6 (weak), 3A4 (weak)

Acetaminophen: **Substrate** (minor) of CYP1A2, 2A6, 2C9, 2D6, 2E1, 3A4; **Inhibits** CYP3A4 (weak)

Also see individual agents.

Ethanol/Nutrition/Herb Interactions

Based on **propoxyphene** component:

Ethanol: Avoid or limit ethanol (may increase CNS depression). Watch for sedation.

Food: May decrease rate of absorption, but may slightly increase bioavailability.

Based on **acetaminophen** component:

Ethanol: Excessive intake of ethanol may increase the risk of acetaminophen-induced hepatotoxicity. Avoid ethanol or limit to <3 drinks/day.

Food: Rate of absorption may be decreased when given with food.

Herb/Nutraceutical: St John's wort may decrease acetaminophen levels.

Dietary Considerations May be taken with food if gastrointestinal distress occurs.

Dosage Forms

Tablet: Propoxyphene hydrochloride 65 mg and acetaminophen 650 mg, propoxyphene napsylate 100 mg, and acetaminophen 650 mg

Balacet 325™: Propoxyphene napsylate 100 mg and acetaminophen 325 mg

Darvocet A500™: Propoxyphene napsylate 100 mg and acetaminophen 500 mg [contains lactose]

Darvocet-N® 50: Propoxyphene napsylate 50 mg and acetaminophen 325 mg

Darvocet-N® 100, Pronap-100®: Propoxyphene napsylate 100 mg and acetaminophen 650 mg

- **Propoxyphene Hydrochloride** *see* Propoxyphene *on page 1074*
- **Propoxyphene Hydrochloride and Acetaminophen** *see* Propoxyphene and Acetaminophen *on page 1076*
- **Propoxyphene Napsylate** *see* Propoxyphene *on page 1074*
- **Propoxyphene Napsylate and Acetaminophen** *see* Propoxyphene and Acetaminophen *on page 1076*

Propranolol (proe PRAN oh lole)

Medication Safety Issues

Sound-alike/look-alike issues:

Propranolol may be confused with Pravachol®, Propulsid®

Inderal® may be confused with Adderall®, Enduron®, Enduronyl®, Imdur®, Imuran®, Inderide®, Isordil®, Toradol®

Inderal® 40 may be confused with Enduronyl® Forte

Related Information

Anesthesia for Patients With Liver Disease *on page 1421*

Antiarrhythmic Drugs *on page 1548*

Beta-Blockers *on page 1557*

Preoperative Evaluation of the Cardiac Patient for Noncardiac Surgery *on page 1485*

U.S. Brand Names Inderal®; Inderal® LA; InnoPran XL™

Canadian Brand Names Apo-Propranolol®; Inderal®; Inderal®-LA; Novo-Pranol; Nu-Propranolol; Propranolol Hydrochloride Injection, USP

(Continued)

Propranolol *(Continued)*

Synonyms Propranolol Hydrochloride

Pharmacologic Category Antiarrhythmic Agent, Class II; Beta-Adrenergic Blocker, Nonselective

Generic Available Yes: Excludes capsule

Use Management of hypertension; angina pectoris; pheochromocytoma; essential tremor; tetralogy of Fallot cyanotic spells; arrhythmias (such as atrial fibrillation and flutter, AV nodal re-entrant tachycardias, and catecholamine-induced arrhythmias); prevention of myocardial infarction; migraine headache; symptomatic treatment of hypertrophic subaortic stenosis

Unlabeled/Investigational Use Tremor due to Parkinson's disease; ethanol withdrawal; aggressive behavior; antipsychotic-induced akathisia; prevention of bleeding esophageal varices; anxiety; schizophrenia; acute panic; gastric bleeding in portal hypertension; thyrotoxicosis

Mechanism of Action Nonselective beta-adrenergic blocker (class II antiarrhythmic); competitively blocks response to $beta_1$- and $beta_2$-adrenergic stimulation which results in decreases in heart rate, myocardial contractility, blood pressure, and myocardial oxygen demand

Pharmacodynamics/Kinetics

Onset of action: Beta-blockade: Oral: 1-2 hours

Duration: ~6 hours

Distribution: V_d: 3.9 L/kg in adults; crosses placenta; small amounts enter breast milk

Protein binding: Newborns: 68%; Adults: 93%

Metabolism: Hepatic to active and inactive compounds; extensive first-pass effect

Bioavailability: 30% to 40%; may be increased in Down syndrome

Half-life elimination: Neonates and Infants: Possible increased half-life; Children: 3.9-6.4 hours; Adults: 4-6 hours

Excretion: Urine (96% to 99%)

Dosage

Akathisia: Oral: Adults: 30-120 mg/day in 2-3 divided doses

Angina: Oral: Adults: 80-320 mg/day in doses divided 2-4 times/day

Long-acting formulation: Initial: 80 mg once daily; maximum dose: 320 mg once daily

Essential tremor: Oral: Adults: 20-40 mg twice daily initially; maintenance doses: usually 120-320 mg/day

Hypertension:

Oral:

Children: Initial: 0.5-1 mg/kg/day in divided doses every 6-12 hours; increase gradually every 5-7 days; maximum: 16 mg/kg/24 hours

Adults: Initial: 40 mg twice daily; increase dosage every 3-7 days; usual dose: ≤320 mg divided in 2-3 doses/day; maximum daily dose: 640 mg; usual dosage range (JNC 7): 40-160 mg/day in 2 divided doses

Long-acting formulation: Initial: 80 mg once daily; usual maintenance: 120-160 mg once daily; maximum daily dose: 640 mg; usual dosage range (JNC 7): 60-180 mg/day once daily

I.V.: Children: 0.01-0.05 mg/kg over 1 hour; maximum dose: 10 mg

Hypertrophic subaortic stenosis: Oral: Adults: 20-40 mg 3-4 times/day

Long-acting formulation: 80-160 mg once daily

Migraine headache prophylaxis: Oral:

Children: Initial: 2-4 mg/kg/day **or**

≤35 kg: 10-20 mg 3 times/day

>35 kg: 20-40 mg 3 times/day

Adults: Initial: 80 mg/day divided every 6-8 hours; increase by 20-40 mg/dose every 3-4 weeks to a maximum of 160-240 mg/day given in divided doses every 6-8 hours; if satisfactory response not achieved within 6 weeks of starting therapy, drug should be withdrawn gradually over several weeks

Long-acting formulation: Initial: 80 mg once daily; effective dose range: 160-240 mg once daily

Myocardial infarction prophylaxis: Oral: Adults: 180-240 mg/day in 3-4 divided doses

Pheochromocytoma: Oral: Adults: 30-60 mg/day in divided doses

Tachyarrhythmias:

Oral:

Children: Initial: 0.5-1 mg/kg/day in divided doses every 6-8 hours; titrate dosage upward every 3-7 days; usual dose: 2-6 mg/kg/day; higher doses may be needed; do not exceed 16 mg/kg/day or 60 mg/day

Adults: 10-30 mg/dose every 6-8 hours

Elderly: Initial: 10 mg twice daily; increase dosage every 3-7 days; usual dosage range: 10-320 mg given in 2 divided doses

I.V.:

Children: 0.01-0.1 mg/kg/dose slow IVP over 10 minutes; maximum dose: 1 mg for infants; 3 mg for children

Adults (in patients having nonfunctional GI tract): 1 mg/dose slow IVP; repeat every 5 minutes up to a total of 5 mg; titrate initial dose to desired response

Tetralogy spells: Children:

Oral: Palliation: Initial: 1 mg/kg/day every 6 hours; if ineffective, may increase dose after 1 week by 1 mg/kg/day to a maximum of 5 mg/kg/day; if patient becomes refractory, may increase slowly to a maximum of 10-15 mg/kg/day. Allow 24 hours between dosing changes.

I.V.: 0.01-0.2 mg/kg/dose infused over 10 minutes; maximum initial dose: 1 mg

Thyrotoxicosis:

Oral:

Children: 2 mg/kg/day, divided every 6-8 hours, titrate to effective dose

Adolescents and Adults: Oral: 10-40 mg/dose every 6 hours

I.V.: Adults: 1-3 mg/dose slow IVP as a single dose

Dosing adjustment/comments in renal impairment:

Not dialyzable (0% to 5%); supplemental dose is not necessary.

Peritoneal dialysis effects: Supplemental dose is not necessary.

Dosing adjustment/comments in hepatic disease: Marked slowing of heart rate may occur in cirrhosis with conventional doses; low initial dose and regular heart rate monitoring

Stability **Compatible** in saline, **incompatible** with HCO_3^-; protect injection from light; solutions have maximum stability at pH of 3 and decompose rapidly in alkaline pH; propranolol is stable for 24 hours at room temperature in D_5W or NS

Administration I.V. dose is much smaller than oral dose. When administered acutely for cardiac treatment, monitor ECG and blood pressure. May administer by rapid infusion (I.V. push) at a rate of 1 mg/minute or by slow infusion over ~30 minutes. Necessary monitoring for surgical patients who are unable to take oral beta-blockers (prolonged ileus) has not been defined. Some institutions require monitoring of baseline and postinfusion heart rate and blood pressure when a patient's response to beta-blockade has not been characterized (ie, the patient's initial dose or following a change in dose). Consult individual institutional policies and procedures. Do not crush long-acting oral forms.

Monitoring Parameters

Acute cardiac treatment: Monitor ECG and blood pressure with I.V. administration; heart rate and blood pressure with oral administration

Reference Range Therapeutic: 50-100 ng/mL (SI: 190-390 nmol/L) at end of dose interval

Anesthesia and Critical Care Concerns/Other Considerations Propranolol is not indicated for hypertensive emergencies. It is not significantly removed by hemodialysis.

Myocardial Infarction: Beta-blockers, in general without intrinsic sympathomimetic activity (ISA), have been shown to decrease morbidity and mortality when initiated in the acute treatment of myocardial infarction and continued long-term. In this setting, therapy should be avoided in patients with hypotension, cardiogenic shock, or heart block.

Surgery: Atenolol has also been shown to improve cardiovascular outcomes when used in the perioperative period in patients with underlying cardiovascular disease who are undergoing noncardiac surgery. Bisoprolol in high-risk patients undergoing vascular surgery reduced the perioperative incidence of death from cardiac causes and nonfatal myocardial infarction.

Atrial Fibrillation: Beta-blocker therapy provides effective rate control in patients with atrial fibrillation.

Withdrawal: Beta-blocker therapy should not be withdrawn abruptly, but gradually tapered over 2 weeks to avoid acute tachycardia and hypertension.

(Continued)

Propranolol *(Continued)*

Pregnancy Risk Factor C (manufacturer); D (2nd and 3rd trimesters - expert analysis)

Contraindications Hypersensitivity to propranolol, beta-blockers, or any component of the formulation; uncompensated congestive heart failure (unless the failure is due to tachyarrhythmias being treated with propranolol), cardiogenic shock, bradycardia or heart block (2nd or 3rd degree), pulmonary edema, severe hyperactive airway disease (asthma or COPD), Raynaud's disease; pregnancy (2nd and 3rd trimesters)

Warnings/Precautions Administer cautiously in compensated heart failure and monitor for a worsening of the condition (efficacy of propranolol in CHF has not been demonstrated). **[U.S. Boxed Warning]: Beta-blocker therapy should not be withdrawn abruptly (particularly in patients with CAD), but gradually tapered (over 2 weeks) to avoid acute tachycardia, hypertension, and/or ischemia.** Use caution in patient with PVD. Use caution with concurrent use of beta-blockers and either verapamil or diltiazem; bradycardia or heart block can occur. Avoid concurrent I.V. use of both agents. Use cautiously in diabetics because it can mask prominent hypoglycemic symptoms. Can mask signs of thyrotoxicosis. Can cause fetal harm when administered in pregnancy. Use cautiously in hepatic dysfunction (dosage adjustment required). Use care with anesthetic agents which decrease myocardial function. Not indicated for hypertensive emergencies.

Adverse Reactions Frequency not defined.

Cardiovascular: Bradycardia, CHF, reduced peripheral circulation, chest pain, hypotension, impaired myocardial contractility, worsening of AV conduction disturbance, cardiogenic shock, Raynaud's syndrome, mesenteric thrombosis (rare), syncope

Central nervous system: Mental depression, lightheadedness, amnesia, emotional lability, confusion, hallucinations, dizziness, insomnia, fatigue, vivid dreams, lethargy, cold extremities, vertigo, cognitive dysfunction, psychosis, hypersomnolence

Dermatologic: Alopecia, contact dermatitis, eczematous eruptions, erythema multiforme, exfoliative dermatitis, hyperkeratosis, nail changes, pruritus, psoriasiform eruptions, rash, ulcerative lichenoid, urticaria, Stevens-Johnson syndrome, toxic epidermal necrolysis

Endocrine & metabolic: Hypoglycemia, hyperglycemia, hyperlipidemia, hyperkalemia

Gastrointestinal: Diarrhea, nausea, vomiting, stomach discomfort, constipation, anorexia

Genitourinary: Impotence, proteinuria (rare), oliguria (rare), interstitial nephritis (rare), Peyronie's disease

Hematologic: Agranulocytosis, thrombocytopenia, thrombocytopenic purpura

Neuromuscular & skeletal: Weakness, carpal tunnel syndrome (rare), paresthesia, myotonus, polyarthritis, arthropathy

Ocular: Hyperemia of the conjunctiva, decreased tear production, decreased visual acuity, mydriasis

Respiratory: Wheezing, pharyngitis, bronchospasm, pulmonary edema, respiratory distress, laryngospasm

Miscellaneous: Lupus-like syndrome (rare), anaphylactic/anaphylactoid allergic reaction

Overdosage/Toxicology Symptoms of intoxication include cardiac disturbances, CNS toxicity, bronchospasm, hypoglycemia, and hyperkalemia. The most common cardiac symptoms include hypotension and bradycardia. Atrioventricular block, intraventricular conduction disturbances, cardiogenic shock, and asystole may occur with severe overdose, especially with membrane-depressant drugs (eg, propranolol). CNS effects include convulsions and coma. Respiratory arrest is commonly seen with propranolol and other membrane-depressant and lipid-soluble drugs. Treatment is symptom-directed and supportive.

Drug Interactions Substrate of CYP1A2 (major), 2C19 (minor), 2D6 (major), 3A4 (minor); **Inhibits** CYP1A2 (weak), 2D6 (weak)

Albuterol (and other $beta_2$ agonists): Effects may be blunted by nonspecific beta-blockers.

Alpha-blockers (prazosin, terazosin): Concurrent use of beta-blockers may increase risk of orthostasis.

Aluminum hydroxide: Absorption of propranolol may be decreased.

Cholestyramine, colestipol: Plasma levels of propranolol may be decreased.

Cimetidine increases the plasma concentration of propranolol and its pharmacodynamic effects may be increased.

Clonidine: Hypertensive crisis after or during withdrawal of either agent

CYP1A2 inducers: May decrease the levels/effects of propranolol. Example inducers include aminoglutethimide, carbamazepine, phenobarbital, and rifampin.

CYP1A2 inhibitors: May increase the levels/effects of propranolol. Example inhibitors include ciprofloxacin, fluvoxamine, ketoconazole, norfloxacin, ofloxacin, and rofecoxib.

CYP2D6 inhibitors: May increase the levels/effects of propranolol. Example inhibitors include chlorpromazine, delavirdine, fluoxetine, miconazole, paroxetine, pergolide, quinidine, quinine, ritonavir, and ropinirole.

Diazepam: Metabolism of diazepam may be inhibited; concentrations of diazepam and metabolites may be increased.

Drugs which slow AV conduction (digoxin): Effects may be additive with beta-blockers.

Epinephrine (including local anesthetics with epinephrine): Propranolol may cause hypertension.

Flecainide: Pharmacological activity of both agents may be increased when used concurrently.

Fluoxetine may inhibit the metabolism of propranolol, resulting in cardiac toxicity.

Glucagon: Propranolol may blunt hyperglycemic action.

Haloperidol: Hypotensive effects may be potentiated.

Hydralazine: The bioavailability propranolol (rapid release) and hydralazine may be enhanced with concurrent dosing.

Insulin: Propranolol inhibits recovery and may cause hypertension and bradycardia following insulin-induced hypoglycemia; also masks the tachycardia that usually accompanies insulin-induced hypoglycemia.

Lidocaine: Metabolism of lidocaine may be decreased.

NSAIDs (ibuprofen, indomethacin, naproxen, piroxicam) may reduce the antihypertensive effects of beta-blockers.

Phenothiazines (chlorpromazine, phenothiazine): Plasma levels of propranolol and phenothiazine may both be increased.

Propafenone: May increase the concentrations/effects of propranolol.

Quinidine: May increase plasma levels of propranolol by decreasing metabolism.

Rifampin: May decrease plasma levels of propranolol by increasing metabolism.

Salicylates may reduce the antihypertensive effects of beta-blockers

Serotonin 5-HT_{1D} receptor agonists (such as rizatriptan, zolmitriptan): Propranolol may increase bioavailability of serotonin 5-HT_{1D} receptor agonists.

Sulfonylureas: Beta-blockers may alter response to hypoglycemic agents.

Theophylline: Theophylline clearance may be decreased by propranolol.

Verapamil or diltiazem may have synergistic or additive pharmacological effects when taken concurrently with beta-blockers; avoid concurrent I.V. use of both.

Warfarin: Propranolol may increase bioavailability of warfarin and PT may be increased.

Ethanol/Nutrition/Herb Interactions

Ethanol: Ethanol may decrease plasma levels of propranolol by increasing metabolism.

Food: Propranolol serum levels may be increased if taken with food. Protein-rich foods may increase bioavailability; a change in diet from high carbohydrate/low protein to low carbohydrate/high protein may result in increased oral clearance.

Cigarette: Smoking may decrease plasma levels of propranolol by increasing metabolism.

Herb/Nutraceutical: Avoid dong quai if using for hypertension (has estrogenic activity). Avoid ephedra, yohimbe, ginseng (may worsen hypertension or arrhythmia). Avoid natural licorice (causes sodium and water retention and increases potassium loss). Avoid garlic (may have increased antihypertensive effect).

Dietary Considerations Tablets should be taken on an empty stomach; capsules may be taken with or without food, but should always be taken consistently (with food or on an empty stomach)

Dosage Forms

Capsule, extended release, as hydrochloride (InnoPran XL™): 80 mg, 120 mg

Capsule, sustained release, as hydrochloride (Inderal® LA): 60 mg, 80 mg, 120 mg, 160 mg

Injection, solution, as hydrochloride (Inderal®): 1 mg/mL (1 mL)

(Continued)

Propranolol *(Continued)*

Solution, oral, as hydrochloride: 4 mg/mL (5 mL, 500 mL); 8 mg/mL (500 mL) [strawberry-mint flavor; contains alcohol 0.6%]

Tablet, as hydrochloride (Inderal®): 10 mg, 20 mg, 40 mg, 60 mg, 80 mg

References

Radack K and Deck C, "Beta-Adrenergic Blocker Therapy Does Not Worsen Intermittent Claudication in Subjects With Peripheral Arterial Disease. A Meta-Analysis of Randomized Controlled Trials," *Arch Intern Med*, 1991, 151(9):1769-76.

- **Propranolol Hydrochloride** *see* Propranolol *on page 1077*
- **Propranolol Hydrochloride Injection, USP (Can)** *see* Propranolol *on page 1077*
- **Proprinal [OTC]** *see* Ibuprofen *on page 651*
- **Propulsid®** *see* Cisapride *on page 291*
- **2-Propylpentanoic Acid** *see* Valproic Acid and Derivatives *on page 1329*

Propylthiouracil (proe pil thye oh YOOR a sil)

Medication Safety Issues

Sound-alike/look-alike issues:

Propylthiouracil may be confused with Purinethol®

PTU is an error-prone abbreviation (mistaken as mercaptopurine [Purinethol®; 6-MP])

Canadian Brand Names Propyl-Thyracil®

Synonyms PTU (error-prone abbreviation)

Pharmacologic Category Antithyroid Agent

Generic Available Yes

Use Palliative treatment of hyperthyroidism as an adjunct to ameliorate hyperthyroidism in preparation for surgical treatment or radioactive iodine therapy; management of thyrotoxic crisis

Mechanism of Action Inhibits the synthesis of thyroid hormones by blocking the oxidation of iodine in the thyroid gland; blocks synthesis of thyroxine and triiodothyronine

Pharmacodynamics/Kinetics

Onset of action: Therapeutic: 24-36 hours

Peak effect: Remission: 4 months of continued therapy

Duration: 2-3 hours

Distribution: Concentrated in the thyroid gland

Protein binding: 75% to 80%

Metabolism: Hepatic

Bioavailability: 80% to 95%

Half-life elimination: 1.5-5 hours; End-stage renal disease: 8.5 hours

Time to peak, serum: ~1 hour

Excretion: Urine (35%)

Dosage Oral: Administer in 3 equally divided doses at approximately 8-hour intervals. Adjust dosage to maintain T_3, T_4, and TSH levels in normal range; elevated T_3 may be sole indicator of inadequate treatment. Elevated TSH indicates excessive antithyroid treatment.

Children: Initial: 5-7 mg/kg/day **or** 150-200 mg/m²/day in divided doses every 8 hours

or

6-10 years: 50-150 mg/day

>10 years: 150-300 mg/day

Maintenance: Determined by patient response **or** 1/3 to 2/3 of the initial dose in divided doses every 8-12 hours. This usually begins after 2 months on an effective initial dose.

Adults: Initial: 300 mg/day in divided doses every 8 hours. In patients with severe hyperthyroidism, very large goiters, or both, the initial dosage is usually 450 mg/day; an occasional patient will require 600-900 mg/day; maintenance: 100-150 mg/day in divided doses every 8-12 hours

Elderly: Use lower dose recommendations; Initial: 150-300 mg/day

Withdrawal of therapy: Therapy should be withdrawn gradually with evaluation of the patient every 4-6 weeks for the first 3 months then every 3 months for the first year after discontinuation of therapy to detect any reoccurrence of a hyperthyroid state.

Dosing adjustment in renal impairment: Adjustment is not necessary

Monitoring Parameters CBC with differential, prothrombin time, liver function tests, thyroid function tests (TSH, T_3, T_4); periodic blood counts are recommended chronic therapy

Reference Range Normal laboratory values:

Total T_4: 5-12 mcg/dL

Serum T_3: 90-185 ng/dL

Free thyroxine index (FT_4 I): 6-10.5

TSH: 0.5-4.0 microunits/mL

Anesthesia and Critical Care Concerns/Other Considerations Agranulocytosis, when it occurs, is usually seen during the first several months of therapy.

The use of antithyroid thioamides is as effective in elderly as in younger adults; however, the expense, potential adverse effects, and inconvenience (compliance, monitoring) make them undesirable. The use of radioiodine, due to ease of administration and less concern for long-term side effects and reproduction problems, makes it a more appropriate therapy.

Pregnancy Risk Factor D

Contraindications Hypersensitivity to propylthiouracil or any component of the formulation; pregnancy

Warnings/Precautions Use with caution in patients >40 years of age because PTU may cause hypoprothrombinemia and bleeding; use with extreme caution in patients receiving other drugs known to cause agranulocytosis; may cause agranulocytosis, thyroid hyperplasia, thyroid carcinoma (usage >1 year). Discontinue in the presence of agranulocytosis, aplastic anemia, ANCA-positive vasculitis, hepatitis, unexplained fever, or exfoliative dermatitis. Safety and efficacy have not been established in children <6 years of age.

Adverse Reactions Frequency not defined.

Cardiovascular: Edema, cutaneous vasculitis, leukocytoclastic vasculitis, ANCA-positive vasculitis

Central nervous system: Fever, drowsiness, vertigo, headache, drug fever, dizziness, neuritis

Dermatologic: Skin rash, urticaria, pruritus, exfoliative dermatitis, alopecia, erythema nodosum

Endocrine & metabolic: Goiter, weight gain, swollen salivary glands

Gastrointestinal: Nausea, vomiting, loss of taste perception, stomach pain, constipation

Hematologic: Leukopenia, agranulocytosis, thrombocytopenia, bleeding, aplastic anemia

Hepatic: Cholestatic jaundice, hepatitis

Neuromuscular & skeletal: Arthralgia, paresthesia

Renal: Nephritis, glomerulonephritis, acute renal failure

Respiratory: Interstitial pneumonitis, alveolar hemorrhage

Miscellaneous: SLE-like syndrome

Overdosage/Toxicology Symptoms of overdose include nausea, vomiting, epigastric pain, headache, fever, arthralgia, pruritus, edema, pancytopenia, epigastric distress, headache, fever, CNS stimulation, or depression. Treatment is supportive. Monitor bone marrow response. Forced diuresis, dialysis, and charcoal hemoperfusion have been used to enhance elimination.

Drug Interactions

Anticoagulants: Anticoagulants may be potentiated by antivitamin-K effect of propylthiouracil. Oral anticoagulant activity is increased only until metabolic effect stabilizes.

Correction of hyperthyroidism may alter disposition of beta-blockers, digoxin, and theophylline, necessitating a dose reduction of these agents.

Ethanol/Nutrition/Herb Interactions Food: Propylthiouracil serum levels may be altered if taken with food.

Dietary Considerations Administer at the same time in relation to meals each day, either always with meals or always between meals.

Dosage Forms Tablet: 50 mg

- **Propyl-Thyracil® (Can)** *see* Propylthiouracil *on page 1082*
- **2-Propylvaleric Acid** *see* Valproic Acid and Derivatives *on page 1329*
- **Proquin® XR** *see* Ciprofloxacin *on page 285*
- **ProSom®** *see* Estazolam *on page 487*
- **Prostacyclin** *see* Epoprostenol *on page 467*
- **Prostacyclin PGI_2** *see* Iloprost *on page 658*
- **Prostaglandin E_1** *see* Alprostadil *on page 68*

- **Prostigmin®** *see* Neostigmine *on page 910*
- **Prostin® VR (Can)** *see* Alprostadil *on page 68*
- **Prostin VR Pediatric®** *see* Alprostadil *on page 68*

Protamine Sulfate (PROE ta meen SUL fate)

Medication Safety Issues

Sound-alike/look-alike issues:

Protamine may be confused with ProAmatine®, protamine, Protopam®, Protropin®

Pharmacologic Category Antidote

Generic Available Yes

Use Treatment of heparin overdosage; neutralize heparin during surgery or dialysis procedures

Unlabeled/Investigational Use Treatment of low molecular weight heparin (LMWH) overdose

Mechanism of Action Combines with strongly acidic heparin to form a stable complex (salt) neutralizing the anticoagulant activity of both drugs

Pharmacodynamics/Kinetics Onset of action: I.V.: Heparin neutralization: ~5 minutes

Dosage

Heparin neutralization: I.V.: Protamine dosage is determined by the dosage of heparin; 1 mg of protamine neutralizes 90 USP units of heparin (lung) and 115 USP units of heparin (intestinal); maximum dose: 50 mg

Heparin overdosage, following intravenous administration: I.V.: Since blood heparin concentrations decrease rapidly **after** administration, adjust the protamine dosage depending upon the duration of time since heparin administration as follows: See table.

Time Elapsed	Dose of Protamine (mg) to Neutralize 100 units of Heparin
Immediate	1-1.5
30-60 min	0.5-0.75
>2 h	0.25-0.375

Heparin overdosage, following SubQ injection: I.V.: 1-1.5 mg protamine per 100 units heparin; this may be done by a portion of the dose (eg, 25-50 mg) given slowly I.V. followed by the remaining portion as a continuous infusion over 8-16 hours (the expected absorption time of the SubQ heparin dose)

LMWH overdose (unlabeled use): **Note:** Antifactor Xa activity never completely neutralized (maximum: ~60% to 75%)

Enoxaparin: 1 mg protamine for each mg of enoxaparin; if PTT prolonged 2-4 hours after first dose, consider additional dose of 0.5 mg for each mg of enoxaparin.

Dalteparin or tinzaparin: 1 mg protamine for each 100 anti-Xa int. units of dalteparin or tinzaparin; if PTT prolonged 2-4 hours after first dose, consider additional dose of 0.5 mg for each 100 anti-Xa int. units of dalteparin or tinzaparin.

Note: Excessive protamine doses may worsen bleeding potential.

Stability Refrigerate, avoid freezing; remains stable for at least 2 weeks at room temperature; **incompatible** with cephalosporins and penicillins; preservative-free formulation does not require refrigeration. Reconstitute vial with 5 mL sterile water; if using protamine in neonates, reconstitute with preservative-free sterile water for injection; resulting solution equals 10 mg/mL.

Administration For I.V. use only; **incompatible** with cephalosporins and penicillins; administer slow IVP (50 mg over 10 minutes); rapid I.V. infusion causes hypotension; resulting solution equals 10 mg/mL; inject without further dilution over 1-3 minutes; maximum of 50 mg in any 10-minute period

Monitoring Parameters Coagulation test, aPTT or ACT, cardiac monitor and blood pressure monitor required during administration

Anesthesia and Critical Care Concerns/Other Considerations Monitor vital signs closely during protamine therapy because of possible hypotension during administration.

Anaphylaxis or hypersensitivity responses with acute hypotension to protamine may present with its use, especially in patients with allergies to fish, previous exposure to protamine (through previous use of protamine or protamine-containing insulin), infertile or vasectomized males.

Protamine's reversal of LMWHs is not as complete or predictable as with heparin. Protamine neutralizes the antithrombin activity of LMWHs, but the cationic protein neutralizes the antifactor Xa activity incompletely. A recent case illustrates a failure to reverse enoxaparin (Makris M, 2000). Protamine will not reverse the effects of thrombin inhibitors such as lepirudin, bivalirudin, or argatroban.

Pregnancy Risk Factor C

Contraindications Hypersensitivity to protamine or any component of the formulation

Warnings/Precautions May not be totally effective in some patients following cardiac surgery despite adequate doses; may cause hypersensitivity reaction in patients with a history of allergy to fish (have epinephrine 1:1000 available) and in patients sensitized to protamine (via protamine zinc insulin); too rapid administration can cause severe hypotensive and anaphylactoid-like reactions. Heparin rebound associated with anticoagulation and bleeding has been reported to occur occasionally; symptoms typically occur 8-9 hours after protamine administration, but may occur as long as 18 hours later.

Adverse Reactions Frequency not defined.

Cardiovascular: Sudden fall in blood pressure, bradycardia, flushing, hypotension
Central nervous system: Lassitude
Gastrointestinal: Nausea, vomiting
Hematologic: Hemorrhage
Respiratory: Dyspnea, pulmonary hypertension
Miscellaneous: Hypersensitivity reactions

Overdosage/Toxicology Symptoms of overdose include hypertension. May cause hemorrhage. Doses exceeding 100 mg may cause paradoxical anticoagulation.

Dosage Forms Injection, solution, as sulfate [preservative free]: 10 mg/mL (5 mL, 25 mL)

References

Aren C, "Heparin and Protamine Therapy," *Semin Thorac Cardiovasc Surg*, 1990, 2(4):364-72.
Horrow JC, "Protamine: A Review of Its Toxicity," *Anesth Analg*, 1985, 64(3):348-61.
Jaques LB, "Protamine - Antagonist to Heparin," *Can Med Assoc J*, 1973, 108(10):1291-7.
Kondo NI, Maddi R, Ewenstein BM, et al, "Anticoagulation and Hemostasis in Cardiac Surgical Patients," *J Card Surg*, 1994, 9(4):443-61.
Lindblad B, "Protamine Sulfate: A Review of Its Effects - Hypersensitivity and Toxicity," *Eur J Vasc Surg*, 1989, 3(3):195-201.
Makris M, Hough RE, and Kitchen S, et al, "Poor Reversal of Low Molecular Weight Heparin by Protamine," *Br J Haematol*, 2000, 108(4): 884-5.
Michelson AD, Bovill E, Monagle P, et al, "Antithrombic Therapy in Children," *Chest*, 1998, 114(5 Suppl):748-69.
Mokhlesi B, Leikin JB, Murray P, et al, "Adult Toxicology in Critical Care. Part 11: Specific Poisonings," *Chest*, 2003, 123(3):897-922.
Wakefield TW and Stanley JC, "Intraoperative Heparin Anticoagulation and Its Reversal," *Semin Vasc Surg*, 1996, 9(4):296-302.

♦ **Protein C (Activated), Human, Recombinant** *see* Drotrecogin Alfa *on page 434*
♦ **Prothrombin Complex Concentrate** *see* Factor IX Complex (Human) *on page 504*
♦ **Protonix®** *see* Pantoprazole *on page 983*
♦ **Protopam®** *see* Pralidoxime *on page 1040*
♦ **Protopic®** *see* Tacrolimus *on page 1225*
♦ **Proventil®** *see* Albuterol *on page 50*
♦ **Proventil® HFA** *see* Albuterol *on page 50*
♦ **Proviodine (Can)** *see* Povidone-Iodine *on page 1039*
♦ **Prozac®** *see* Fluoxetine *on page 539*
♦ **Prozac® Weekly™** *see* Fluoxetine *on page 539*
♦ **Prudoxin™** *see* Doxepin *on page 422*
♦ **Prussian Blue** *see* Ferric Hexacyanoferrate *on page 521*

Pseudoephedrine (soo doe e FED rin)

Medication Safety Issues

Sound-alike/look-alike issues:
Dimetapp® may be confused with Dermatop®, Dimetabs®, Dimetane®
Sudafed® may be confused with Sufenta®

(Continued)

Pseudoephedrine *(Continued)*

U.S. Brand Names Biofed [OTC]; Contact® Cold [OTC]; Dimetapp® 12-Hour Non-Drowsy Extentabs® [OTC]; Dimetapp® Decongestant Infant [OTC]; Elix-Sure™ Congestion [OTC]; Genaphed® [OTC]; Kidkare Decongestant [OTC]; Kodet SE [OTC]; Oranyl [OTC]; PediaCare® Decongestant Infants [OTC]; Silfedrine Children's [OTC]; Simply Stuffy™ [OTC]; Sudafed® [OTC]; Sudafed® 12 Hour [OTC]; Sudafed® 24 Hour [OTC]; Sudafed® Children's [OTC]; Sudodrin [OTC]; SudoGest [OTC]; Sudo-Tab® [OTC]

Canadian Brand Names Balminil Decongestant; Benylin® D for Infants; Contac® Cold 12 Hour Relief Non Drowsy; Drixoral® ND; Eltor®; PMS-Pseudoephedrine; Pseudofrin; Robidrine®; Sudafed® Decongestant

Synonyms *d*-Isoephedrine Hydrochloride; Pseudoephedrine Hydrochloride; Pseudoephedrine Sulfate

Pharmacologic Category Alpha/Beta Agonist

Generic Available Yes: Liquid, syrup, tablet

Use Temporary symptomatic relief of nasal congestion due to common cold, upper respiratory allergies, and sinusitis; also promotes nasal or sinus drainage

Mechanism of Action Directly stimulates alpha-adrenergic receptors of respiratory mucosa causing vasoconstriction; directly stimulates beta-adrenergic receptors causing bronchial relaxation, increased heart rate and contractility

Pharmacodynamics/Kinetics

Onset of action: Decongestant: Oral: 15-30 minutes

Duration: Immediate release tablet: 4-6 hours; Extended release: ≤12 hours

Absorption: Rapid

Metabolism: Partially hepatic

Half-life elimination: 9-16 hours

Excretion: Urine (70% to 90% as unchanged drug, 1% to 6% as active norpseudoephedrine); dependent on urine pH and flow rate; alkaline urine decreases renal elimination of pseudoephedrine

Dosage Oral: General dosing guidelines:

Children:

- <2 years: 4 mg/kg/day in divided doses every 6 hours
- 2-5 years: 15 mg every 4-6 hours; maximum: 60 mg/24 hours
- 6-12 years: 30 mg every 4-6 hours; maximum: 120 mg/24 hours

Adults: 30-60 mg every 4-6 hours, sustained release: 120 mg every 12 hours; maximum: 240 mg/24 hours

Dosing adjustment in renal impairment: Reduce dose

Administration Do not crush extended release drug product, swallow whole.

Pregnancy Risk Factor C

Contraindications Hypersensitivity to pseudoephedrine or any component of the formulation; with or within 14 days of MAO inhibitor therapy

Warnings/Precautions Use with caution in patients >60 years of age; administer with caution to patients with hypertension, hyperthyroidism, diabetes mellitus, cardiovascular disease, ischemic heart disease, increased intraocular pressure, or prostatic hyperplasia. Elderly patients are more likely to experience adverse reactions to sympathomimetics. Overdosage may cause hallucinations, seizures, CNS depression, and death. When used for self-medication (OTC), notify healthcare provider if symptoms do not improve within 7 days or are accompanied by fever.

Adverse Reactions Frequency not defined.

Cardiovascular: Tachycardia, palpitation, arrhythmia

Central nervous system: Nervousness, transient stimulation, insomnia, excitability, dizziness, drowsiness, convulsions, hallucinations, headache

Gastrointestinal: Nausea, vomiting

Genitourinary: Dysuria

Neuromuscular & skeletal: Weakness, tremor

Respiratory: Dyspnea

Miscellaneous: Diaphoresis

Overdosage/Toxicology Symptoms of overdose include seizures, nausea, vomiting, cardiac arrhythmias, hypertension, agitation, hallucinations, and death. There is no specific antidote for pseudoephedrine intoxication. Treatment is primarily supportive.

Drug Interactions

Decreased effect of methyldopa, reserpine

Increased toxicity: MAO inhibitors may increase blood pressure effects of pseudoephedrine; propranolol, sympathomimetic agents may increase toxicity

Ethanol/Nutrition/Herb Interactions

Food: Onset of effect may be delayed if pseudoephedrine is taken with food.

Herb/Nutraceutical: Avoid ephedra, yohimbe (may cause hypertension).

Test Interactions Interferes with urine detection of amphetamine (false-positive)

Dietary Considerations Should be taken with water or milk to decrease GI distress.

Dosage Forms

Caplet, extended release, as hydrochloride (Contact® Cold, Sudafed® 12 Hour): 120 mg

Liquid, as hydrochloride: 30 mg/5 mL (120 mL, 480 mL)

- Silfedrine Children's: 15 mg/5 mL (120 mL, 480 mL) [alcohol and sugar free; grape flavor]
- Simply Stuffy™: 15 mg/5 mL (120 mL) [alcohol free; contains sodium benzoate; cherry berry flavor]
- Sudafed® Children's: 15 mg/5 mL (120 mL) [alcohol and sugar free; contains sodium benzoate; grape flavor]

Liquid, oral drops, as hydrochloride:

- Dimetapp® Decongestant Infant Drops: 7.5 mg/0.8 mL (15 mL) [alcohol free; contains sodium benzoate; grape flavor]
- Kidkare Decongestant: 7.5 mg/0.8 mL (30 mL) [alcohol free; contains benzoic acid and sodium benzoate; cherry flavor]
- PediaCare® Decongestant: 7.5 mg/0.8 mL (15 mL) [alcohol free, dye free; contains benzoic acid, sodium benzoate; fruit flavor]

Syrup, as hydrochloride:

- Biofed: 30 mg/5 mL (120 mL, 240 mL, 480 mL, 3840 mL) [alcohol free; contains sodium benzoate]
- ElixSure™ Congestion: 15 mg/5 mL (120 mL) [grape bubble gum flavor]

Tablet, as hydrochloride: 30 mg, 60 mg

- Genaphed®, Kodet SE, Oranyl, Sudafed®, Sudodrin, Sudo-Tab®: 30 mg
- SudoGest: 30 mg, 60 mg

Tablet, chewable, as hydrochloride (Sudafed® Children's): 15 mg [sugar free; contains phenylalanine 0.78 mg/tablet; orange flavor]

Tablet, extended release, as hydrochloride:

- Dimetapp® 12-Hour Non-Drowsy Extentabs®: 120 mg
- Sudafed® 24 Hour: 240 mg

- ♦ **Pseudoephedrine Hydrochloride** *see* Pseudoephedrine *on page 1085*
- ♦ **Pseudoephedrine Sulfate** *see* Pseudoephedrine *on page 1085*
- ♦ **Pseudofrin (Can)** *see* Pseudoephedrine *on page 1085*
- ♦ **Pseudomonic Acid A** *see* Mupirocin *on page 876*
- ♦ **P & S™ Liquid Phenol (Can)** *see* Phenol *on page 1012*
- ♦ **P.T.E.-4®** *see* Trace Metals *on page 1296*
- ♦ **P.T.E.-5®** *see* Trace Metals *on page 1296*
- ♦ **PTU (error-prone abbreviation)** *see* Propylthiouracil *on page 1082*
- ♦ **Pulmophylline (Can)** *see* Theophylline *on page 1253*
- ♦ **Purified Chick Embryo Cell** *see* Rabies Virus Vaccine *on page 1101*
- ♦ **PVP-I** *see* Povidone-Iodine *on page 1039*
- ♦ **2-Pyridine Aldoxime Methochloride** *see* Pralidoxime *on page 1040*

Pyridostigmine (peer id oh STIG meen)

Medication Safety Issues

Sound-alike/look-alike issues:

- Pyridostigmine may be confused with physostigmine
- Mestinon® may be confused with Metatensin®
- Regonol® may be confused with Reglan®, Renagel®

Related Information

Chronic Renal Failure *on page 1437*

U.S. Brand Names Mestinon®; Mestinon® Timespan®; Regonol®

Canadian Brand Names Mestinon®; Mestinon®-SR

Synonyms Pyridostigmine Bromide

Pharmacologic Category Acetylcholinesterase Inhibitor

Generic Available Yes: Tablet

(Continued)

Pyridostigmine *(Continued)*

Use Symptomatic treatment of myasthenia gravis; antidote for nondepolarizing neuromuscular blockers

Military use: Pretreatment for Soman nerve gas exposure

Mechanism of Action Inhibits destruction of acetylcholine by acetylcholinesterase which facilitates transmission of impulses across myoneural junction

Pharmacodynamics/Kinetics

Onset of action: Oral, I.M.: 15-30 minutes; I.V. injection: 2-5 minutes

Duration: Oral: Up to 6-8 hours (due to slow absorption); I.V.: 2-3 hours

Absorption: Oral: Very poor

Distribution: 19 ± 12 L

Metabolism: Hepatic

Bioavailability: 10% to 20%

Half-life elimination: 1-2 hours; Renal failure: ≤6 hours

Excretion: Urine (80% to 90% as unchanged drug)

Dosage

Myasthenia gravis:

Oral:

Children: 7 mg/kg/24 hours divided into 5-6 doses

Adults: Highly individualized dosing ranges: 60-1500 mg/day, usually 600 mg/day divided into 5-6 doses, spaced to provide maximum relief

Sustained release formulation: Highly individualized dosing ranges: 180-540 mg once or twice daily (doses separated by at least 6 hours); **Note:** Most clinicians reserve sustained release dosage form for bedtime dose only.

I.M., slow I.V. push:

Children: 0.05-0.15 mg/kg/dose

Adults: To supplement oral dosage pre- and postoperatively during labor and postpartum, during myasthenic crisis, or when oral therapy is impractical: ~1/30th of oral dose; observe patient closely for cholinergic reactions

or

I.V. infusion: Initial: 2 mg/hour with gradual titration in increments of 0.5-1 mg/hour, up to a maximum rate of 4 mg/hour

Pretreatment for Soman nerve gas exposure (military use): Oral: Adults: 30 mg every 8 hours beginning several hours prior to exposure; discontinue at first sign of nerve agent exposure, then begin atropine and pralidoxime

Reversal of nondepolarizing muscle relaxants: **Note:** Atropine sulfate (0.6-1.2 mg) I.V. immediately prior to pyridostigmine to minimize side effects: I.V.:

Children: Dosing range: 0.1-0.25 mg/kg/dose*

Adults: 0.1-0.25 mg/kg/dose; 10-20 mg is usually sufficient*

*Full recovery usually occurs ≤15 minutes, but ≥30 minutes may be required

Dosage adjustment in renal dysfunction: Lower dosages may be required due to prolonged elimination; no specific recommendations have been published

Stability

Injection: Protect from light.

Tablet:

30 mg: Store under refrigeration at 2°C to 8°C (36°F to 46°F) and protect from light; stable at room temperature for up to 3 months

Mestinon®: Store at 25°C (77°F); protect from moisture

Administration Do **not** crush sustained release tablet.

Monitoring Parameters Observe for cholinergic reactions, particularly when administered I.V.

Anesthesia and Critical Care Concerns/Other Considerations Atropine or glycopyrrolate must be administered in combination with pyridostigmine. Large parenteral doses should be accompanied by parenteral atropine. Ephedrine sulfate and potassium chloride have been used orally (in adult patients) to improve response. Extended release products are preferred for use **only** at bedtime for patients who are very weak upon arising.

Pregnancy Risk Factor B

Contraindications Hypersensitivity to pyridostigmine, bromides, or any component of the formulation; GI or GU obstruction

Warnings/Precautions Use with caution in patients with epilepsy, asthma, bradycardia, hyperthyroidism, cardiac arrhythmias, or peptic ulcer; adequate facilities should be available for cardiopulmonary resuscitation when testing and adjusting dose for myasthenia gravis; have atropine and epinephrine ready to treat hypersensitivity reactions; overdosage may result in cholinergic crisis, this must be distinguished from myasthenic crisis; anticholinesterase insensitivity can develop for brief or prolonged periods. Safety and efficacy in pediatric patients have not been established.

Regonol® injection contains 1% benzyl alcohol as the preservative (not intended for use in newborns).

Adverse Reactions Frequency not defined.

Cardiovascular: Arrhythmias (especially bradycardia), hypotension, decreased carbon monoxide, tachycardia, AV block, nodal rhythm, nonspecific ECG changes, cardiac arrest, syncope, flushing

Central nervous system: Convulsions, dysarthria, dysphonia, dizziness, loss of consciousness, drowsiness, headache

Dermatologic: Skin rash, thrombophlebitis (I.V.), urticaria

Gastrointestinal: Hyperperistalsis, nausea, vomiting, salivation, diarrhea, stomach cramps, dysphagia, flatulence, abdominal pain

Genitourinary: Urinary urgency

Neuromuscular & skeletal: Weakness, fasciculations, muscle cramps, spasms, arthralgia, myalgia

Ocular: Small pupils, lacrimation, amblyopia

Respiratory: Increased bronchial secretions, laryngospasm, bronchiolar constriction, respiratory muscle paralysis, dyspnea, respiratory depression, respiratory arrest, bronchospasm

Miscellaneous: Diaphoresis (increased), anaphylaxis, allergic reactions

Overdosage/Toxicology Symptoms of overdose include muscle weakness, blurred vision, excessive sweating, tearing and salivation, nausea, vomiting, diarrhea, hypertension, bradycardia, and paralysis. Atropine is the treatment of choice for intoxications manifesting significant muscarinic symptoms. Atropine I.V. 2-4 mg every 3-60 minutes should be repeated to control symptoms and then continued as needed for 1-2 days following acute ingestion. Monitor cardiac function and support ventilation.

Drug Interactions

Aminoglycosides (gentamicin, kanamycin, neomycin, streptomycin): Use of high parenteral doses may intensify/prolong neuromuscular blockade, or lead to resistance of neuromuscular blockade reversal, especially if used with other nondepolarizing neuromuscular-blocking drugs.

Antibiotics (bacitracin, colistin, polymyxin B, sodium colistimethate, tetracycline): Use of high parenteral doses may intensify/prolong neuromuscular blockade, or lead to resistance of neuromuscular blockade reversal, especially if used with other nondepolarizing neuromuscular-blocking drugs.

Beta blockers: Pyridostigmine and beta-blockers may both cause bradycardia and hypotension, effect may be additive; monitor.

Depolarizing neuromuscular-blocking agents (succinylcholine): Increased neuromuscular blocking effect with concomitant use.

Edrophonium: Increased toxicity with concomitant use.

Magnesium: Patients with elevated serum magnesium concentrations may experience enhanced neuromuscular blockage with blocking agents. The reversing effect of pyridostigmine may be compensated.

Quinidine: Recurrent paralysis may occur when quinidine is administered with nondepolarizing neuromuscular-blocking drugs. This may complicate attempts to reverse blockade with pyridostigmine.

Quinolone antibiotics (ciprofloxacin, norfloxacin): Case reports suggest these drugs may exhibit neuromuscular-blocking effects (especially in some patients with myasthenia gravis); monitor.

Test Interactions Increased aminotransferase [ALT (SGPT)/AST (SGOT)] (S), increased amylase (S)

Dosage Forms

Injection, solution, as bromide:

Mestinon®: 5 mg/mL (2 mL)

Regonol®: 5 mg/mL (2 mL) [contains benzyl alcohol]

Syrup, as bromide (Mestinon®): 60 mg/5 mL (480 mL) [raspberry flavor; contains alcohol 5%, sodium benzoate]

Tablet, as bromide (Mestinon®): 60 mg

Tablet, sustained release, as bromide (Mestinon® Timespan®): 180 mg

References

Saltis LM, Martin BR, Traeger SM, et al, "Continuous Infusion of Pyridostigmine in the Management of Myasthenic Crisis," *Crit Care Med*,1993, 21(6):938-40.

◆ **Pyridostigmine Bromide** *see* Pyridostigmine *on page 1087*

Pyridoxine (peer i DOKS een)

Medication Safety Issues

Sound-alike/look-alike issues:

Pyridoxine may be confused with paroxetine, pralidoxime, Pyridium®

U.S. Brand Names Aminoxin® [OTC]

Synonyms Pyridoxine Hydrochloride; Vitamin B_6

Pharmacologic Category Vitamin, Water Soluble

Generic Available Yes

Use Prevention and treatment of vitamin B_6 deficiency, pyridoxine-dependent seizures in infants; adjunct to treatment of acute toxicity from isoniazid, cycloserine, or hydrazine overdose

Mechanism of Action Precursor to pyridoxal, which functions in the metabolism of proteins, carbohydrates, and fats; pyridoxal also aids in the release of liver and muscle-stored glycogen and in the synthesis of GABA (within the central nervous system) and heme

Pharmacodynamics/Kinetics

Absorption: Enteral, parenteral: Well absorbed

Metabolism: Via 4-pyridoxic acid (active form) and other metabolites

Half-life elimination: 15-20 days

Excretion: Urine

Dosage

Recommended daily allowance (RDA):

- Children:
  - 1-3 years: 0.9 mg
  - 4-6 years: 1.3 mg
  - 7-10 years: 1.6 mg
- Adults:
  - Male: 1.7-2.0 mg
  - Female: 1.4-1.6 mg

Pyridoxine-dependent Infants:

- Oral: 2-100 mg/day
- I.M., I.V., SubQ: 10-100 mg

Dietary deficiency: Oral:

- Children: 5-25 mg/24 hours for 3 weeks, then 1.5-2.5 mg/day in multiple vitamin product
- Adults: 10-20 mg/day for 3 weeks

Drug-induced neuritis (eg, isoniazid, hydralazine, penicillamine, cycloserine): Oral:

- Children:
  - Treatment: 10-50 mg/24 hours
  - Prophylaxis: 1-2 mg/kg/24 hours
- Adults:
  - Treatment: 100-200 mg/24 hours
  - Prophylaxis: 25-100 mg/24 hours

Treatment of seizures and/or coma from acute isoniazid toxicity, a dose of pyridoxine hydrochloride equal to the amount of INH ingested can be given I.M./I.V. in divided doses together with other anticonvulsants; if the amount INH ingested is not known, administer 5 g I.V. pyridoxine

Treatment of acute hydrazine toxicity, a pyridoxine dose of 25 mg/kg in divided doses I.M./I.V. has been used

Stability Protect from light

Administration Burning may occur at the injection site after I.M. or SubQ administration; seizures have occurred following I.V. administration of very large doses

Reference Range Over 50 ng/mL (SI: 243 nmol/L) (varies considerably with method). A broad range is ~25-80 ng/mL (SI: 122-389 nmol/L). HPLC method for pyridoxal phosphate has normal range of 3.5-18 ng/mL (SI: 17-88 nmol/L).

Pregnancy Risk Factor A/C (dose exceeding RDA recommendation)

Contraindications Hypersensitivity to pyridoxine or any component of the formulation

Warnings/Precautions Dependence and withdrawal may occur with doses >200 mg/day

Adverse Reactions Frequency not defined.

Central nervous system: Headache, seizure (following very large I.V. doses), sensory neuropathy
Endocrine & metabolic: Decreased serum folic acid secretions
Gastrointestinal: Nausea
Hepatic: Increased AST
Neuromuscular & skeletal: Paresthesia
Miscellaneous: Allergic reactions

Overdosage/Toxicology Symptoms of overdose include ataxia and sensory neuropathy with doses of 50 mg to 2 g daily over prolonged periods.

Drug Interactions Decreased serum levels of levodopa, phenobarbital, and phenytoin

Test Interactions Urobilinogen

Dosage Forms
Capsule, as hydrochloride: 250 mg
Injection, solution, as hydrochloride: 100 mg/mL (1 mL)
Tablet, as hydrochloride: 25 mg, 50 mg, 100 mg, 200 mg, 250 mg, 500 mg
Tablet, enteric coated, as hydrochloride (Aminoxin®): 20 mg

References

Mokhlesi B, Leikin JB, Murray P, et al, "Adult Toxicology in Critical Care: Part II: Specific Poisonings," *Chest*, 2003, 123(3):897-922.

- **Pyridoxine Hydrochloride** *see* Pyridoxine *on page 1090*
- **Q-Dryl [OTC]** *see* DiphenhydrAMINE *on page 399*
- **Quelicin®** *see* Succinylcholine *on page 1210*
- **Quenalin [OTC]** *see* DiphenhydrAMINE *on page 399*
- **Quibron®-T** *see* Theophylline *on page 1253*
- **Quibron®-T/SR** *see* Theophylline *on page 1253*
- **Quinalbarbitone Sodium** *see* Secobarbital *on page 1154*

Quinapril (KWIN a pril)

Medication Safety Issues
Sound-alike/look-alike issues:
Accupril® may be confused with Accolate®, Accutane®, AcipHex®, Monopril®

Related Information
Angiotensin Agents *on page 1544*
Heart Failure (Systolic) *on page 1607*
Preoperative Evaluation of the Cardiac Patient for Noncardiac Surgery *on page 1485*

U.S. Brand Names Accupril®

Canadian Brand Names Accupril®

Synonyms Quinapril Hydrochloride

Pharmacologic Category Angiotensin-Converting Enzyme (ACE) Inhibitor

Generic Available Yes

Use Management of hypertension; treatment of congestive heart failure

Unlabeled/Investigational Use Treatment of left ventricular dysfunction after myocardial infarction

Mechanism of Action Competitive inhibitor of angiotensin-converting enzyme (ACE); prevents conversion of angiotensin I to angiotensin II, a potent vasoconstrictor; results in lower levels of angiotensin II which causes an increase in plasma renin activity and a reduction in aldosterone secretion; a CNS mechanism may also be involved in hypotensive effect as angiotensin II increases adrenergic outflow from CNS; vasoactive kallikreins may be decreased in conversion to active hormones by ACE inhibitors, thus reducing blood pressure

Pharmacodynamics/Kinetics
Onset of action: 1 hour
Duration: 24 hours
Absorption: Quinapril: ≥60%
Protein binding: Quinapril: 97%; Quinaprilat: 97%
Metabolism: Rapidly hydrolyzed to quinaprilat, the active metabolite
Half-life elimination: Quinapril: 0.8 hours; Quinaprilat: 3 hours; increases as Cl_{cr} decreases
Time to peak, serum: Quinapril: 1 hour; Quinaprilat: ~2 hours
Excretion: Urine (50% to 60% primarily as quinaprilat)
(Continued)

Quinapril *(Continued)*

Dosage

Adults: Oral:

Hypertension: Initial: 10-20 mg once daily, adjust according to blood pressure response at peak and trough blood levels; initial dose may be reduced to 5 mg in patients receiving diuretic therapy if the diuretic is continued; usual dose range (JNC 7): 10-40 mg once daily

Congestive heart failure or post-MI: Initial: 5 mg once or twice daily, titrated at weekly intervals to 20-40 mg daily in 2 divided doses; target dose (heart failure): 20 mg twice daily (ACC/AHA 2005 Heart Failure Guidelines)

Elderly: Initial: 2.5-5 mg/day; increase dosage at increments of 2.5-5 mg at 1- to 2-week intervals.

Dosing adjustment in renal impairment: Lower initial doses should be used; after initial dose (if tolerated), administer initial dose twice daily; may be increased at weekly intervals to optimal response:

Hypertension: Initial:

Cl_{cr} >60 mL/minute: Administer 10 mg/day

Cl_{cr} 30-60 mL/minute: Administer 5 mg/day

Cl_{cr} 10-30 mL/minute: Administer 2.5 mg/day

Congestive heart failure: Initial:

Cl_{cr} >30 mL/minute: Administer 5 mg/day

Cl_{cr} 10-30 mL/minute: Administer 2.5 mg/day

Dosing comments in hepatic impairment: In patients with alcoholic cirrhosis, hydrolysis of quinapril to quinaprilat is impaired; however, the subsequent elimination of quinaprilat is unaltered.

Stability Store at room temperature; unstable in aqueous solutions; to prepare solution for oral administration, mix prior to administration and use within 10 minutes

Anesthesia and Critical Care Concerns/Other Considerations ACE inhibitors decrease morbidity and mortality in patients with asymptomatic and symptomatic left ventricular dysfunction. ACE inhibitors are also indicated in patients postmyocardial infarction in whom left ventricular ejection fraction is <40%.

ACE inhibitor therapy may elicit rapid increases in potassium and creatinine, especially when used in patients with bilateral renal artery stenosis. When ACE inhibition is introduced in patients with pre-existing diuretic therapy who are hypovolemic, the ACE inhibitor may induce acute hypotension. To prevent this, discontinue diuretics 2-3 days prior to initiating quinapril; may restart diuretics if blood pressure is not controlled by quinapril alone. Because of the potent teratogenic effects of ACE inhibitors, these drugs should be avoided, if possible, when treating women of childbearing potential not on effective birth control measures.

Pregnancy Risk Factor C (1st trimester)/D (2nd and 3rd trimesters)

Contraindications Hypersensitivity to quinapril or any component of the formulation; angioedema related to previous treatment with an ACE inhibitor; bilateral renal artery stenosis; patients with idiopathic or hereditary angioedema; pregnancy (2nd and 3rd trimesters)

Warnings/Precautions Anaphylactic reactions can occur. Angioedema can occur at any time during treatment (especially following first dose). It may involve head and neck (potentially affecting the airway) or the intestine (presenting with abdominal pain). Prolonged monitoring may be required especially if tongue, glottis, or larynx are involved as they are associated with airway obstruction. Those with a history of airway surgery in this situation have a higher risk. Careful blood pressure monitoring with first dose (hypotension can occur especially in volume-depleted patients). **[U.S. Boxed Warning]: Based on human data, ACEIs can cause injury and death to the developing fetus when used in the second and third trimesters. ACEIs should be discontinued as soon as possible once pregnancy is detected.** Dosage adjustment needed in renal impairment. Use with caution in hypovolemia; collagen vascular diseases; valvular stenosis (particularly aortic stenosis); hyperkalemia; or before, during, or immediately after anesthesia. Avoid rapid dosage escalation, which may lead to renal insufficiency. Rare toxicities associated with ACE inhibitors include cholestatic jaundice (which may progress to hepatic necrosis) and neutropenia/agranulocytosis with myeloid hyperplasia. If patient has renal impairment, a baseline WBC with differential and serum creatinine should be evaluated and monitored closely during the first 3 months of therapy.

Hypersensitivity reactions may be seen during hemodialysis with high-flux dialysis membranes (eg, AN69). Patients receiving ACE inhibitors have experienced rare life-threatening anaphylactoid reactions during desensitization. Rare hepatic reactions, progressing from cholestatic jaundice to hepatic necrosis, have been reported with ACE inhibitors. Discontinue if marked elevation of hepatic transaminases or jaundice occurs.

Use with caution in unilateral renal artery stenosis and pre-existing renal insufficiency. Deterioration in renal function can occur with initiation.

Adverse Reactions Note: Frequency ranges include data from hypertension and heart failure trials. Higher rates of adverse reactions have generally been noted in patients with CHF. However, the frequency of adverse effects associated with placebo is also increased in this population.

1% to 10%:

Cardiovascular: Hypotension (3%), chest pain (2%), first-dose hypotension (up to 3%)

Central nervous system: Dizziness (4% to 8%), headache (2% to 6%), fatigue (3%)

Dermatologic: Rash (1%)

Endocrine & metabolic: Hyperkalemia (2%)

Gastrointestinal: Vomiting/nausea (1% to 2%), diarrhea (1.7%)

Neuromuscular & skeletal: Myalgias (2% to 5%), back pain (1%)

Renal: Increased BUN/serum creatinine (2%, transient elevations may occur with a higher frequency), worsening of renal function (in patients with bilateral renal artery stenosis or hypovolemia)

Respiratory: Upper respiratory symptoms, cough (2% to 4%; up to 13% in some studies), dyspnea (2%)

<1% (Limited to important or life-threatening): Acute renal failure, agranulocytosis, alopecia, amblyopia, anaphylactoid reaction, angina, angioedema, arrhythmia, arthralgia, depression, dermatopolymyositis, edema, eosinophilic pneumonitis, exfoliative dermatitis, hemolytic anemia, hepatitis, hyperkalemia, hypertensive crisis, impotence, insomnia, MI, orthostatic hypotension, pancreatitis, paresthesia, pemphigus, photosensitivity, pruritus, shock, somnolence, stroke, syncope, thrombocytopenia, vertigo

A syndrome which may include fever, myalgia, arthralgia, interstitial nephritis, vasculitis, rash, eosinophilia and positive ANA, and elevated ESR has been reported with ACE inhibitors. In addition, pancreatitis, hepatic necrosis, neutropenia, and/or agranulocytosis (particularly in patients with collagen-vascular disease or renal impairment) have been associated with many ACE inhibitors.

Overdosage/Toxicology Mild hypotension has been the primary toxic effect seen with acute overdose. Bradycardia may also occur. Hyperkalemia occurs even with therapeutic doses, especially in patients with renal insufficiency and those taking NSAIDs. Treatment is symptom-directed and supportive.

Drug Interactions

Alpha$_1$ blockers: Hypotensive effect increased.

Aspirin: The effects of ACE inhibitors may be blunted by aspirin administration, particularly at higher dosages and/or increase adverse renal effects.

Diuretics: Hypovolemia due to diuretics may precipitate acute hypotensive events or acute renal failure.

Insulin: Risk of hypoglycemia may be increased.

Lithium: Risk of lithium toxicity may be increased; monitor lithium levels, especially the first 4 weeks of therapy.

Mercaptopurine: Risk of neutropenia may be increased.

NSAIDs: May attenuate hypertensive efficacy; effect has been seen with captopril and may occur with other ACE inhibitors; monitor blood pressure. May increase risk of adverse renal effects.

Potassium-sparing diuretics (amiloride, spironolactone, triamterene): Increased risk of hyperkalemia.

Potassium supplements may increase the risk of hyperkalemia.

Quinolones: Absorption may be decreased by quinapril; separate administration by at least 2-4 hours.

Tetracyclines: Absorption may be reduced by quinapril; separate administration by at least 2-4 hours.

Trimethoprim (high dose) may increase the risk of hyperkalemia.

Ethanol/Nutrition/Herb Interactions Herb/Nutraceutical: Avoid dong quai if using for hypertension (has estrogenic activity). Avoid ephedra, yohimbe, ginseng

(Continued)

Quinapril *(Continued)*

(may worsen hypertension). Avoid garlic (may have increased antihypertensive effect).

Dosage Forms Tablet, as hydrochloride: 5 mg, 10 mg, 20 mg, 40 mg

- **Quinapril Hydrochloride** *see* Quinapril *on page 1091*
- **Quinate® (Can)** *see* Quinidine *on page 1094*

Quinidine (KWIN i deen)

Medication Safety Issues

Sound-alike/look-alike issues:

Quinidine may be confused with clonidine, quinine, Quinora®

Related Information

Antiarrhythmic Drugs *on page 1548*

Canadian Brand Names Apo-Quin-G®; Apo-Quinidine®; BioQuin® Durules™; Novo-Quinidin; Quinate®

Synonyms Quinidine Gluconate; Quinidine Polygalacturonate; Quinidine Sulfate

Pharmacologic Category Antiarrhythmic Agent, Class Ia

Generic Available Yes

Use Prophylaxis after cardioversion of atrial fibrillation and/or flutter to maintain normal sinus rhythm; prevent recurrence of paroxysmal supraventricular tachycardia, paroxysmal AV junctional rhythm, paroxysmal ventricular tachycardia, paroxysmal atrial fibrillation, and atrial or ventricular premature contractions; has activity against *Plasmodium falciparum* malaria

Mechanism of Action Class 1a antiarrhythmic agent; depresses phase O of the action potential; decreases myocardial excitability and conduction velocity, and myocardial contractility by decreasing sodium influx during depolarization and potassium efflux in repolarization; also reduces calcium transport across cell membrane

Pharmacodynamics/Kinetics

Distribution: V_d: Adults: 2-3.5 L/kg, decreased with congestive heart failure, malaria; increased with cirrhosis; crosses placenta; enters breast milk

Protein binding:

Newborns: 60% to 70%; decreased protein binding with cyanotic congenital heart disease, cirrhosis, or acute myocardial infarction

Adults: 80% to 90%

Metabolism: Extensively hepatic (50% to 90%) to inactive compounds

Bioavailability: Sulfate: 80%; Gluconate: 70%

Half-life elimination, plasma: Children: 2.5-6.7 hours; Adults: 6-8 hours; prolonged with elderly, cirrhosis, and congestive heart failure

Excretion: Urine (15% to 25% as unchanged drug)

Dosage Dosage expressed in terms of the salt: 267 mg of quinidine gluconate = 200 mg of quinidine sulfate.

Children: Test dose for idiosyncratic reaction (sulfate, oral or gluconate, I.M.): 2 mg/kg or 60 mg/m^2

Oral (quinidine sulfate): 15-60 mg/kg/day in 4-5 divided doses or 6 mg/kg every 4-6 hours; usual 30 mg/kg/day or 900 mg/m^2/day given in 5 daily doses

I.V. **not** recommended (quinidine gluconate): 2-10 mg/kg/dose given at a rate ≤10 mg/minute every 3-6 hours as needed

Adults: Test dose: Oral, I.M.: 200 mg administered several hours before full dosage (to determine possibility of idiosyncratic reaction)

Oral (for malaria):

Sulfate: 100-600 mg/dose every 4-6 hours; begin at 200 mg/dose and titrate to desired effect (maximum daily dose: 3-4 g)

Gluconate: 324-972 mg every 8-12 hours

I.M.: 400 mg/dose every 2-6 hours; initial dose: 600 mg (gluconate)

I.V.: 200-400 mg/dose diluted and given at a rate ≤10 mg/minute; may require as much as 500-750 mg

Dosing adjustment in renal impairment: Cl_{cr} <10 mL/minute: Administer 75% of normal dose.

Hemodialysis: Slightly hemodialyzable (5% to 20%); 200 mg supplemental dose posthemodialysis is recommended.

Peritoneal dialysis: Not dialyzable (0% to 5%)

Dosing adjustment/comments in hepatic impairment: Larger loading dose may be indicated, reduce maintenance doses by 50% and monitor serum levels closely.

Stability Do not use discolored parenteral solution.

Administration Administer around-the-clock to promote less variation in peak and trough serum levels

Oral: Do not crush, chew, or break sustained release dosage forms.

Parenteral: When injecting I.M., aspirate carefully to avoid injection into a vessel; maximum I.V. infusion rate: 10 mg/minute

Monitoring Parameters Cardiac monitor required during I.V. administration; CBC, liver and renal function tests, should be routinely performed during long-term administration

Reference Range Therapeutic: 2-5 mcg/mL (SI: 6.2-15.4 μmol/L). Patient dependent therapeutic response occurs at levels of 3-6 mcg/mL (SI: 9.2-18.5 μmol/L). Optimal therapeutic level is method dependent; >6 mcg/mL (SI: >18 μmol/L).

Pregnancy Risk Factor C

Contraindications Hypersensitivity to quinidine or any component of the formulation; thrombocytopenia; thrombocytopenic purpura; myasthenia gravis; heart block greater than first degree; idioventricular conduction delays (except in patients with a functioning artificial pacemaker); those adversely affected by anticholinergic activity; concurrent use of quinolone antibiotics which prolong QT interval, cisapride, amprenavir, or ritonavir

Warnings/Precautions Monitor and adjust dose to prevent QT_c prolongation. Watch for proarrhythmic effects. Correct hypokalemia before initiating therapy. Hypokalemia may worsen toxicity. **[U.S. Boxed Warning]: Antiarrhythmic drugs have not been shown to enhance survival in nonlife-threatening ventricular arrhythmias and may increase mortality; the risk is greatest with structural heart disease. Quinidine may increase mortality in treatment of atrial fibrillation/flutter.** May precipitate or exacerbate CHF. Reduce dosage in hepatic impairment. Use may cause digoxin-induced toxicity (adjust digoxin's dose). Use caution with concurrent use of other antiarrhythmics. Hypersensitivity reactions can occur. Can unmask sick sinus syndrome (causes bradycardia). Has been associated with severe hepatotoxic reactions, including granulomatous hepatitis. Hemolysis may occur in patients with G6PD (glucose-6-phosphate dehydrogenase) deficiency. Different salt products are not interchangeable.

Adverse Reactions

Frequency not defined: Hypotension, syncope

>10%:

- Cardiovascular: QT_c prolongation (modest prolongation is common, however, excessive prolongation is rare and indicates toxicity)
- Central nervous system: Lightheadedness (15%)
- Gastrointestinal: Diarrhea (35%), upper GI distress, bitter taste, diarrhea, anorexia, nausea, vomiting, stomach cramping (22%)

1% to 10%:

- Cardiovascular: Angina (6%), palpitation (7%), new or worsened arrhythmia (proarrhythmic effect)
- Central nervous system: Syncope (1% to 8%), headache (7%), fatigue (7%), sleep disturbance (3%), tremor (2%), nervousness (2%), incoordination (1%)
- Dermatologic: Rash (5%)
- Neuromuscular & skeletal: Weakness (5%)
- Ocular: Blurred vision
- Otic: Tinnitus
- Respiratory: Wheezing

<1% (Limited to important or life-threatening): Abnormal pigmentation, acute psychotic reactions, agranulocytosis, angioedema, arthralgia, bronchospasm, cerebral hypoperfusion (possibly resulting in ataxia, apprehension, and seizure), cholestasis, confusion, delirium, depression, drug-induced lupus-like syndrome, eczematous dermatitis, esophagitis, exacerbated bradycardia (in sick sinus syndrome), exfoliative rash, fever, flushing, granulomatous hepatitis, hallucinations, heart block, hemolytic anemia, hepatotoxic reaction (rare), impaired hearing, increased CPK, lichen planus, livedo reticularis, lymphadenopathy, melanin pigmentation of the hard palate, myalgia, mydriasis, nephropathy, optic neuritis, pancytopenia, paradoxical increase in ventricular rate during atrial fibrillation/flutter, photosensitivity, pneumonitis, pruritus, psoriaform rash, QT_c prolongation (excessive), respiratory depression, sicca syndrome, tachycardia, thrombocytopenia, thrombocytopenic purpura, torsade de pointes,

(Continued)

Quinidine *(Continued)*

urticaria, uveitis, vascular collapse, vasculitis, ventricular fibrillation, ventricular tachycardia, vertigo, visual field loss

Note: Cinchonism, a syndrome which may include tinnitus, high-frequency hearing loss, deafness, vertigo, blurred vision, diplopia, photophobia, headache, confusion, and delirium has been associated with quinidine use. Usually associated with chronic toxicity, this syndrome has also been described after brief exposure to a moderate dose in sensitive patients. Vomiting and diarrhea may also occur as isolated reactions to therapeutic quinidine levels.

Overdosage/Toxicology Has a low toxic:therapeutic ratio and may easily produce fatal intoxication (acute toxic dose: 1 g in adults). Symptoms of overdose include sinus bradycardia, sinus node arrest or asystole, P-R, QRS, or QT interval prolongation, torsade de pointes (polymorphous ventricular tachycardia), and depressed myocardial contractility, which along with alpha-adrenergic or ganglionic blockade, may result in hypotension and pulmonary edema. Other effects are anticholinergic (dry mouth, dilated pupils, and delirium) as well as seizures, coma, and respiratory arrest. Treatment is symptomatic and effects usually respond to conventional therapies. **Note:** Do not use other Class 1A or 1C antiarrhythmic agents to treat ventricular tachycardia. Sodium bicarbonate may treat wide QRS intervals or hypotension. Markedly impaired conduction or high degree AV block, unresponsive to bicarbonate, indicates consideration of a pacemaker.

Drug Interactions **Substrate** of CYP2C9 (minor), 2E1 (minor), 3A4 (major); **Inhibits** CYP2C9 (weak), 2D6 (strong), 3A4 (strong)

Amiloride may cause prolonged ventricular conduction leading to arrhythmias.

Amiodarone may increase quinidine blood levels; monitor quinidine levels.

Cimetidine: Increase quinidine blood levels; closely monitor levels or use an alternative H_2 antagonist.

Cisapride and quinidine may increase risk of malignant arrhythmias; concurrent use is contraindicated.

Codeine: Analgesic efficacy may be reduced.

CYP2D6 substrates: Quinidine may increase the levels/effects of CYP2D6 substrates. Example substrates include amphetamines, selected beta-blockers, dextromethorphan, fluoxetine, lidocaine, mirtazapine, nefazodone, paroxetine, risperidone, ritonavir, thioridazine, tricyclic antidepressants, and venlafaxine.

CYP2D6 prodrug substrates: Quinidine may decrease the levels/effects of CYP2D6 prodrug substrates. Example prodrug substrates include codeine, hydrocodone, oxycodone, and tramadol.

CYP3A4 inducers: CYP3A4 inducers may decrease the levels/effects of quinidine. Example inducers include aminoglutethimide, carbamazepine, nafcillin, nevirapine, phenobarbital, phenytoin, and rifamycins.

CYP3A4 inhibitors: May increase the levels/effects of quinidine. Example inhibitors include azole antifungals, clarithromycin, diclofenac, doxycycline, erythromycin, imatinib, isoniazid, nefazodone, nicardipine, propofol, protease inhibitors, telithromycin, and verapamil.

CYP3A4 substrates: Quinidine may increase the levels/effects of CYP3A4 substrates. Example substrates include benzodiazepines, calcium channel blockers, mirtazapine, nateglinide, nefazodone, tacrolimus, and venlafaxine. Selected benzodiazepines (midazolam and triazolam), cisapride, ergot alkaloids, selected HMG-CoA reductase inhibitors (lovastatin and simvastatin), and pimozide are generally contraindicated with strong CYP3A4 inhibitors.

Digoxin blood levels may be increased. Monitor digoxin blood levels.

Metoprolol: Increased metoprolol blood levels.

Mexiletine blood levels may be increased.

Nifedipine blood levels may be increased by quinidine; nifedipine may decrease quinidine blood levels.

Propafenone blood levels may be increased.

Propranolol blood levels may be increased.

QT_c-prolonging agents (eg, amiodarone, amitriptyline, bepridil, disopyramide, erythromycin, haloperidol, imipramine, pimozide, procainamide, sotalol, thioridazine): Effects may be additive; use with caution.

Ritonavir, nelfinavir and amprenavir may increase quinidine levels and toxicity; concurrent use is contraindicated.

Sparfloxacin, gatifloxacin, and moxifloxacin may result in additional prolongation of the QT interval; concurrent use is contraindicated.

Timolol blood levels may be increased.

Urinary alkalinizers (antacids, sodium bicarbonate, acetazolamide) increase quinidine blood levels.

Verapamil and diltiazem increase quinidine blood levels.

Warfarin effects may be increased by quinidine; monitor INR closely during addition or withdrawal of quinidine.

Ethanol/Nutrition/Herb Interactions

Food: Dietary salt intake may alter the rate and extent of quinidine absorption. A decrease in dietary salt may lead to an increase in quinidine serum concentrations. Avoid changes in dietary salt intake. Quinidine serum levels may be increased if taken with food. Food has a variable effect on absorption of sustained release formulation. The rate of absorption of quinidine may be decreased following the ingestion of grapefruit juice. In addition, CYP3A4 metabolism of quinidine may be reduced by grapefruit juice. Grapefruit juice should be avoided. Excessive intake of fruit juices or vitamin C may decrease urine pH and result in increased clearance of quinidine with decreased serum concentration. Alkaline foods may result in increased quinidine serum concentrations.

Herb/Nutraceutical: St John's wort may decrease quinidine levels. Avoid ephedra (may worsen arrhythmia).

Dietary Considerations Administer with food or milk to decrease gastrointestinal irritation. Avoid changes in dietary salt intake.

Dosage Forms

Injection, solution, as gluconate: 80 mg/mL (10 mL) [equivalent to quinidine base 50 mg/mL]

Tablet, as sulfate: 200 mg, 300 mg

Tablet, extended release, as gluconate: 324 mg [equivalent to quinidine base 202 mg]

Tablet, extended release, as sulfate: 300 mg [equivalent to quinidine base 249 mg]

♦ **Quinidine Gluconate** *see* Quinidine *on page 1094*
♦ **Quinidine Polygalacturonate** *see* Quinidine *on page 1094*
♦ **Quinidine Sulfate** *see* Quinidine *on page 1094*

Quinupristin and Dalfopristin (kwi NYOO pris tin & dal FOE pris tin)

U.S. Brand Names Synercid®

Canadian Brand Names Synercid®

Synonyms Pristinamycin; RP-59500

Pharmacologic Category Antibiotic, Streptogramin

Generic Available No

Use Treatment of serious or life-threatening infections associated with vancomycin-resistant *Enterococcus faecium* bacteremia; treatment of complicated skin and skin structure infections caused by methcillin-susceptible *Staphylococcus aureus* or *Streptococcus pyogenes*

Has been studied in the treatment of a variety of infections caused by *Enterococcus faecium* (not *E. fecalis*) including vancomycin-resistant strains. May also be effective in the treatment of serious infections caused by *Staphylococcus* species including those resistant to methicillin.

Mechanism of Action Quinupristin/dalfopristin inhibits bacterial protein synthesis by binding to different sites on the 50S bacterial ribosomal subunit thereby inhibiting protein synthesis

Pharmacodynamics/Kinetics

Distribution: Quinupristin: 0.45 L/kg; Dalfopristin: 0.24 L/kg

Protein binding: Moderate

Metabolism: To active metabolites via nonenzymatic reactions

Half-life elimination: Quinupristin: 0.85 hour; Dalfopristin: 0.7 hour (mean elimination half-lives, including metabolites: 3 and 1 hours, respectively)

Excretion: Feces (75% to 77% as unchanged drug and metabolites); urine (15% to 19%)

Dosage I.V.:

Children (limited information): Dosages similar to adult dosing have been used in the treatment of complicated skin/soft tissue infections and infections caused by vancomycin-resistant *Enterococcus faecium*

(Continued)

Quinupristin and Dalfopristin *(Continued)*

CNS shunt infection due to vancomycin-resistant *Enterococcus faecium*: 7.5 mg/kg/dose every 8 hours; concurrent intrathecal doses of 1-2 mg/day have been administered for up to 68 days

Adults:

Vancomycin-resistant *Enterococcus faecium*: 7.5 mg/kg every 8 hours

Complicated skin and skin structure infection: 7.5 mg/kg every 12 hours

Dosage adjustment in renal impairment: No adjustment required in renal failure, hemodialysis, or peritoneal dialysis

Dosage adjustment in hepatic impairment: Pharmacokinetic data suggest dosage adjustment may be necessary; however, specific recommendations have not been proposed

Elderly: No dosage adjustment is required

Stability Store unopened vials under refrigeration (2°C to 8°C/36°F to 46°F). Reconstitute single dose vial with 5 mL of 5% dextrose in water or sterile water for injection. Swirl gently to dissolve, do not shake (to limit foam formation). The reconstituted solution should be diluted within 30 minutes. Stability of the diluted solution prior to the infusion is established as 5 hours at room temperature or 54 hours if refrigerated at 2°C to 8°C. Reconstituted solution should be added to at least 250 mL of 5% dextrose in water for peripheral administration (increase to 500 mL or 750 mL if necessary to limit venous irritation). An infusion volume of 100 mL may be used for central line infusions. Do not freeze solution.

Administration Line should be flushed with 5% dextrose in water prior to and following administration. Incompatible with saline. Infusion should be completed over 60 minutes (toxicity may be increased with shorter infusion). Compatible (Y-site injection) with aztreonam, ciprofloxacin, haloperidol, metoclopramide or potassium chloride when admixed in 5% dextrose in water. Also compatible (Y-site injection) with fluconazole (used as undiluted solution). If severe venous irritation occurs following peripheral administration of quinupristin/dalfopristin diluted in 250 mL 5% dextrose in water, consideration should be given to increasing the infusion volume to 500 mL or 750 mL, changing the infusion site, or infusing by a peripherally inserted central catheter (PICC) or a central venous catheter.

Pregnancy Risk Factor B

Contraindications Hypersensitivity to quinupristin, dalfopristin, pristinamycin, or virginiamycin, or any component of the formulation

Warnings/Precautions May cause pain and phlebitis when infused through a peripheral line (not relieved by hydrocortisone or diphenhydramine). Superinfection may occur. As with many antibiotics, antibiotic-associated colitis and pseudomembranous colitis may occur. May cause arthralgias, myalgias, and hyperbilirubinemia. May inhibit the metabolism of many drugs metabolized by CYP3A4. Concurrent therapy with cisapride (which may prolong QT_c interval and lead to arrhythmias) should be avoided.

Adverse Reactions

>10%:

Hepatic: Hyperbilirubinemia (3% to 35%)

Local: Inflammation at infusion site (38% to 42%), local pain (40% to 44%), local edema (17% to 18%), infusion site reaction (12% to 13%)

Neuromuscular & skeletal: Arthralgia (up to 47%), myalgia (up to 47%)

1% to 10%:

Central nervous system: Pain (2% to 3%), headache (2%)

Dermatologic: Pruritus (2%), rash (3%)

Endocrine & metabolic: Hyperglycemia (1%)

Gastrointestinal: Nausea (3% to 5%), diarrhea (3%), vomiting (3% to 4%)

Hematologic: Anemia (3%)

Hepatic: GGT increased (2%), LDH increased (3%)

Local: Thrombophlebitis (2%)

Neuromuscular & skeletal: CPK increased (2%)

<1% (Limited to important or life-threatening): Allergic reaction, anaphylactoid reaction, angina, apnea, arrhythmia, cardiac arrest, coagulation disorder, dysautonomia, dyspnea, encephalopathy, gout, hematuria, hemolytic anemia, hepatitis, hyperkalemia, hypotension, maculopapular rash, mesenteric artery occlusion, myasthenia, neuropathy, pancreatitis, pancytopenia, paraplegia, paresthesia, pericarditis, pleural effusion, pseudomembranous colitis, respiratory distress, seizure, shock, stomatitis, syncope, thrombocytopenia, urticaria

Overdosage/Toxicology Symptoms may include dyspnea, emesis, tremors and ataxia. Treatment is supportive. Not removed by hemodialysis or peritoneal dialysis.

Drug Interactions Quinupristin: **Inhibits** CYP3A4 (weak)

Cisapride: The manufacturer states that quinupristin/dalfopristin may increase cisapride concentrations and cause QT_c prolongation, and recommends to avoid concurrent use with cisapride.

Cyclosporine: Quinupristin/dalfopristin may increase cyclosporine concentrations; monitor.

Dosage Forms Injection, powder for reconstitution:

500 mg: Quinupristin 150 mg and dalfopristin 350 mg
600 mg: Quinupristin 180 mg and dalfopristin 420 mg

- **Quixin™** *see* Levofloxacin *on page 746*
- **QVAR®** *see* Beclomethasone *on page 161*
- **RabAvert®** *see* Rabies Virus Vaccine *on page 1101*

Rabeprazole (ra BE pray zole)

Medication Safety Issues

Sound-alike/look-alike issues:

AcipHex® may be confused with Acephen®, Accupril®, Aricept®
Rabeprazole may be confused with aripiprazole

U.S. Brand Names AcipHex®

Canadian Brand Names AcipHex®; Pariet®

Synonyms Pariprazole

Pharmacologic Category Proton Pump Inhibitor; Substituted Benzimidazole

Generic Available No

Use Short-term (4-8 weeks) treatment and maintenance of erosive or ulcerative gastroesophageal reflux disease (GERD); symptomatic GERD; short-term (up to 4 weeks) treatment of duodenal ulcers; long-term treatment of pathological hypersecretory conditions, including Zollinger-Ellison syndrome; *H. pylori* eradication (in combination with amoxicillin and clarithromycin)

Unlabeled/Investigational Use Maintenance of duodenal ulcer

Mechanism of Action Potent proton pump inhibitor; suppresses gastric acid secretion by inhibiting the parietal cell H+/K+ ATP pump

Pharmacodynamics/Kinetics

Onset of action: 1 hour
Duration: 24 hours
Absorption: Oral: Well absorbed within 1 hour
Distribution: 96.3%
Protein binding, serum: 94.8% to 97.5%
Metabolism: Hepatic via CYP3A and 2C19 to inactive metabolites
Bioavailability: Oral: 52%
Half-life elimination (dose dependent): 0.85-2 hours
Time to peak, plasma: 2-5 hours
Excretion: Urine (90% primarily as thioether carboxylic acid); remainder in feces

Dosage Oral: Adults >18 years and Elderly:

GERD: 20 mg once daily for 4-8 weeks; maintenance: 20 mg once daily

Duodenal ulcer: 20 mg/day before breakfast for 4 weeks

H. pylori eradication: 20 mg twice daily for 7 days; to be administered with amoxicillin 1000 mg and clarithromycin 500 mg, also given twice daily for 7 days.

Hypersecretory conditions: 60 mg once daily; dose may need to be adjusted as necessary. Doses as high as 100 mg once daily and 60 mg twice daily have been used.

Dosage adjustment in renal impairment: No dosage adjustment required

Dosage adjustment in hepatic impairment:

Mild to moderate: Elimination decreased; no dosage adjustment required
Severe: Use caution

Stability Rapidly degraded in acid conditions.

Administration May be administered with or without food; best if taken before breakfast. Do not crush, split, or chew tablet. May be administered with an antacid.

Pregnancy Risk Factor B

(Continued)

Rabeprazole *(Continued)*

Contraindications Hypersensitivity to rabeprazole, substituted benzimidazoles (ie, esomeprazole, lansoprazole, omeprazole, pantoprazole), or any component of the formulation

Warnings/Precautions Use caution in severe hepatic impairment; relief of symptoms with rabeprazole does not preclude the presence of a gastric malignancy

Adverse Reactions

1% to 10%: Central nervous system: Headache (2.4%)

<1% (Limited to important or life-threatening): Anaphylaxis, agranulocytosis, allergic reactions, alopecia, amnesia, angina, angioedema, apnea, asthma, bradycardia, bundle branch block, cholecystitis, coma, delirium, depression, dysphagia, dyspnea, erythema multiforme, extrapyramidal reaction, gout, hemolytic anemia, interstitial pneumonia, jaundice, leukopenia, MI, neuralgia, neuropathy, pancreatitis, pancytopenia, paresthesia, photosensitivity, pulmonary embolus, QT prolongation, rash, renal calculus, retinal degeneration, rhabdomyolysis, seizure, strabismus, syncope, tachycardia, thrombocytopenia, toxic epidermal necrolysis, Stevens-Johnson syndrome, ventricular tachycardia, vertigo

Overdosage/Toxicology No experience with large overdose; rabeprazole is not dialyzable. Treatment of overdosage should be symptomatic and supportive.

Drug Interactions Substrate (major) of CYP2C19, 3A4; **Inhibits** CYP2C8 (moderate), 2C19 (moderate), 2DC (weak), 3A4 (weak)

CYP2C8 Substrates: Rabeprazole may increase the levels/effects of CYP2C8 substrates. Example substrates include amiodarone, paclitaxel, pioglitazone, repaglinide, and rosiglitazone.

CYP2C19 inducers: May decrease the levels/effects of rabeprazole. Example inducers include aminoglutethimide, carbamazepine, phenytoin, and rifampin.

CYP2C19 substrates: Rabeprazole may increase the levels/effects of CYP2C19 substrates. Example substrates include citalopram, diazepam, methsuximide, phenytoin, propranolol, and sertraline.

CYP3A4 inducers: CYP3A4 inducers may decrease the levels/effects of rabeprazole. Example inducers include aminoglutethimide, carbamazepine, nafcillin, nevirapine, phenobarbital, phenytoin, and rifamycins.

Itraconazole and ketoconazole: Proton pump inhibitors may decrease the absorption of itraconazole and ketoconazole; concurrent use is contraindicated.

Protease inhibitors: Proton pump inhibitors may decrease absorption of some protease inhibitors (atazanavir and indinavir).

Ethanol/Nutrition/Herb Interactions

Ethanol: Avoid ethanol (may cause gastric mucosal irritation).

Food: High-fat meals may delay absorption, but C_{max} and AUC are not altered.

Dietary Considerations May be taken with or without food; best if taken before breakfast.

Dosage Forms Tablet, delayed release, enteric coated, as sodium: 20 mg

---

Rabies Immune Globulin (Human)

(RAY beez i MYUN GLOB yoo lin, HYU man)

U.S. Brand Names BayRab®; Imogam® Rabies-HT

Canadian Brand Names BayRab™; Imogam® Rabies Pasteurized

Synonyms RIG

Pharmacologic Category Immune Globulin

Generic Available No

Use Part of postexposure prophylaxis of persons with rabies exposure who lack a history of pre-exposure or postexposure prophylaxis with rabies vaccine or a recently documented neutralizing antibody response to previous rabies vaccination; although it is preferable to administer RIG with the first dose of vaccine, it can be given up to 8 days after vaccination

Mechanism of Action Rabies immune globulin is a solution of globulins dried from the plasma or serum of selected adult human donors who have been immunized with rabies vaccine and have developed high titers of rabies antibody. It generally contains 10% to 18% of protein of which not less than 80% is monomeric immunoglobulin G.

Dosage Children and Adults: I.M.: 20 units/kg in a single dose (RIG should always be administered as part of rabies vaccine (HDCV)) regimen (as soon as possible after the first dose of vaccine, up to 8 days); infiltrate ½ of the dose locally around the wound; administer the remainder I.M.

Note: Persons known to have an adequate titer or who have been completely immunized with rabies vaccine should not receive RIG, only booster doses of HDCV

Stability Refrigerate

Administration Intramuscular injection only; injection should be made into the gluteal muscle

Pregnancy Risk Factor C

Contraindications Hypersensitivity to thimerosal or any component of the formulation

Warnings/Precautions Have epinephrine 1:1000 available for anaphylactic reactions. As a product of human plasma, this product may potentially transmit disease; screening of donors, as well as testing and/or inactivation of certain viruses reduces this risk. Use caution in patients with thrombocytopenia or coagulation disorders (I.M. injections may be contraindicated), in patients with isolated IgA deficiency, or in patients with previous systemic hypersensitivity to human immunoglobulins. Not for intravenous administration.

Adverse Reactions

1% to 10%:

Central nervous system: Fever (mild)

Local: Soreness at injection site

<1% (Limited to important or life-threatening): Anaphylactic shock, angioedema, soreness of muscles, stiffness, urticaria

Drug Interactions Decreased effect: Live virus vaccines (eg, MMR, rabies) may have delayed or diminished antibody response with immune globulin administration; should not be administered within 3 months unless antibody titers dictate as appropriate

Dosage Forms Injection, solution:

BayRab®: 150 int. units/mL (2 mL, 10 mL) [solvent/detergent treated]

Imogam® Rabies-HT: 150 int. units/mL (2 mL, 10 mL) [heat treated]

Rabies Virus Vaccine (RAY beez VYE rus vak SEEN)

U.S. Brand Names Imovax® Rabies; RabAvert®

Canadian Brand Names Imovax® Rabies; RabAvert®

Synonyms HDCV; Human Diploid Cell Cultures Rabies Vaccine; PCEC; Purified Chick Embryo Cell

Pharmacologic Category Vaccine

Generic Available No

Use Pre-exposure immunization: Vaccinate persons with greater than usual risk due to occupation or avocation including veterinarians, rangers, animal handlers, certain laboratory workers, and persons living in or visiting countries for longer than 1 month where rabies is a constant threat.

Postexposure prophylaxis: If a bite from a carrier animal is unprovoked, if it is not captured and rabies is present in that species and area, administer rabies immune globulin (RIG) and the vaccine as indicated

Mechanism of Action Rabies vaccine is an inactivated virus vaccine which promotes immunity by inducing an active immune response. The production of specific antibodies requires about 7-10 days to develop. Rabies immune globulin or antirabies serum, equine (ARS) is given in conjunction with rabies vaccine to provide immune protection until an antibody response can occur.

Pharmacodynamics/Kinetics

Onset of action: I.M.: Rabies antibody: ~7-10 days

Peak effect: ~30-60 days

Duration: ≥1 year

Dosage

Pre-exposure prophylaxis: 1 mL I.M. on days 0, 7, and 21 to 28. **Note:** Prolonging the interval between doses does not interfere with immunity achieved after the concluding dose of the basic series.

Postexposure prophylaxis: All postexposure treatment should begin with immediate cleansing of the wound with soap and water

Persons not previously immunized as above: I.M.: 5 doses (1 mL each) on days 0, 3, 7, 14, 28. In addition, patients should receive rabies immune globulin 20 units/kg body weight, half infiltrated at bite site if possible, remainder I.M.)

(Continued)

Rabies Virus Vaccine *(Continued)*

Persons who have previously received postexposure prophylaxis with rabies vaccine, received a recommended I.M. pre-exposure series of rabies vaccine or have a previously documented rabies antibody titer considered adequate: 1 mL of either vaccine I.M. only on days 0 and 3; do not administer RIG

Booster (for occupational or other continuing risk): 1 mL I.M. every 2-5 years or based on antibody titers

Stability Store under refrigeration at 2°C to 8°C (36°F to 46°F); protect from light; do not freeze

Administration For I.M. administration only; this rabies vaccine product must not be administered intradermally; in adults and children, administer I.M. injections in the deltoid muscle, not the gluteal; for younger children, use the outer aspect of the thigh.

For patients at risk of hemorrhage following intramuscular injection, the ACIP recommends "it should be administered intramuscularly if, in the opinion of the physician familiar with the patients bleeding risk, the vaccine can be administered with reasonable safety by this route. If the patient receives antihemophilia or other similar therapy, intramuscular vaccination can be scheduled shortly after such therapy is administered. A fine needle (23 gauge or smaller) can be used for the vaccination and firm pressure applied to the site (without rubbing) for at least 2 minutes. The patient should be instructed concerning the risk of hematoma from the injection."

Monitoring Parameters Serum rabies antibody every 6 months to 2 years in patients at high risk for exposure

Reference Range Antibody titers ≥115 as determined by rapid fluorescent-focus inhibition test are indicative of adequate response; collect titers on day 28 postexposure

Pregnancy Risk Factor C

Contraindications Hypersensitivity to any component of the formulation; developing febrile illness (during pre-exposure therapy only); life-threatening allergic reactions to rabies vaccine or any components of the formulation (however, carefully consider a patient's risk of rabies before continuing therapy)

Warnings/Precautions Report serious reactions to the State Health Department or the manufacturer/distributor, an immune complex reaction is possible 2-21 days following booster doses of HDCV; hypersensitivity reactions may be treated with antihistamines or epinephrine, if severe. Immune response may be decreased in immunosuppressed patients. Imovax® Rabies contains albumin and neomycin. RabAvert® contains amphotericin B, bovine gelatin, chicken protein, chlortetracycline, and neomycin. For I. M. administration only.

Adverse Reactions **All serious adverse reactions must be reported to the U.S. Department of Health and Human Services (DHHS) Vaccine Adverse Event Reporting System (VAERS) 1-800-822-7967.**

Frequency not defined.

Cardiovascular: Edema

Central nervous system: Dizziness, malaise, encephalomyelitis, transverse myelitis, fever, pain, headache, neuroparalytic reactions

Gastrointestinal: Nausea, abdominal pain

Local: Local discomfort, pain at injection site, itching, erythema, swelling or pain

Neuromuscular & skeletal: Myalgia

Postmarketing and/or case reports: Anaphylaxis, encephalitis, Guillain-Barré syndrome, meningitis, transient paralysis, urticaria pigmentosa

Drug Interactions Decreased effect with immunosuppressive agents, corticosteroids, antimalarial drugs (ie, chloroquine); persons on these drugs should receive RIG (3 doses/1 mL each) by the I.M. route

Dosage Forms Injection, powder for reconstitution:

Imovax® Rabies: 2.5 int. units [HDCV; grown in human diploid cell culture; contains albumin <100 mg, neomycin <150 mcg]

RabAvert®: 2.5 int. units [PCEC; grown in chicken fibroblasts; contains amphotericin <2 ng, chlortetracycline <20 ng, and neomycin <1 mcg]

◆ **Racepinephrine** *see* Epinephrine *on page 457*
◆ **Radiogardase™** *see* Ferric Hexacyanoferrate *on page 521*
◆ **rAHF** *see* Antihemophilic Factor (Recombinant) *on page 113*
◆ **R-albuterol** *see* Levalbuterol *on page 739*

Ramipril (ra MI pril)

Medication Safety Issues

Sound-alike/look-alike issues:

Ramipril may be confused with enalapril, Monopril®

Altace® may be confused with alteplase, Amaryl®, Amerge®, Artane®

Related Information

Angiotensin Agents *on page 1544*

Heart Failure (Systolic) *on page 1607*

Preoperative Evaluation of the Cardiac Patient for Noncardiac Surgery *on page 1485*

U.S. Brand Names Altace®

Canadian Brand Names Altace®

Pharmacologic Category Angiotensin-Converting Enzyme (ACE) Inhibitor

Generic Available No

Use Treatment of hypertension, alone or in combination with thiazide diuretics; treatment of left ventricular dysfunction after myocardial infarction; to reduce risk of heart attack, stroke, and death in patients at increased risk for these problems

Unlabeled/Investigational Use Treatment of heart failure

Mechanism of Action Ramipril is an ACE inhibitor which prevents the formation of angiotensin II from angiotensin I and exhibits pharmacologic effects that are similar to captopril. Ramipril must undergo enzymatic saponification by esterases in the liver to its biologically active metabolite, ramiprilat. The pharmacodynamic effects of ramipril result from the high-affinity, competitive, reversible binding of ramiprilat to angiotensin-converting enzyme thus preventing the formation of the potent vasoconstrictor angiotensin II. This isomerized enzyme-inhibitor complex has a slow rate of dissociation, which results in high potency and a long duration of action; a CNS mechanism may also be involved in the hypotensive effect as angiotensin II increases adrenergic outflow from CNS; vasoactive kallikreins may be decreased in conversion to active hormones by ACE inhibitors, thus reducing blood pressure

Pharmacodynamics/Kinetics

Onset of action: 1-2 hours

Duration: 24 hours

Absorption: Well absorbed (50% to 60%)

Distribution: Plasma levels decline in a triphasic fashion; rapid decline is a distribution phase to peripheral compartment, plasma protein and tissue ACE (half-life 2-4 hours); 2nd phase is an apparent elimination phase representing the clearance of free ramiprilat (half-life: 9-18 hours); and final phase is the terminal elimination phase representing the equilibrium phase between tissue binding and dissociation

Metabolism: Hepatic to the active form, ramiprilat

Half-life elimination: Ramiprilat: Effective: 13-17 hours; Terminal: >50 hours

Time to peak, serum: ~1 hour

Excretion: Urine (60%) and feces (40%) as parent drug and metabolites

Dosage Adults: Oral:

Hypertension: 2.5-5 mg once daily, maximum: 20 mg/day

Reduction in risk of MI, stroke, and death from cardiovascular causes: Initial: 2.5 mg once daily for 1 week, then 5 mg once daily for the next 3 weeks, then increase as tolerated to 10 mg once daily (may be given as divided dose)

Heart failure postmyocardial infarction: Initial: 2.5 mg twice daily titrated upward, if possible, to 5 mg twice daily.

Heart failure (unlabeled use): Initial: 1.25-2.5 mg once daily; target dose: 10 mg once daily (ACC/AHA 2005 Heart Failure Guidelines)

Note: The dose of any concomitant diuretic should be reduced. If the diuretic cannot be discontinued, initiate therapy with 1.25 mg. After the initial dose, the patient should be monitored carefully until blood pressure has stabilized.

Dosing adjustment in renal impairment:

Cl_{cr} <40 mL/minute: Administer 25% of normal dose.

Renal failure and hypertension: Administer 1.25 mg once daily, titrated upward as possible.

Renal failure and heart failure: Administer 1.25 mg once daily, increasing to 1.25 mg twice daily up to 2.5 mg twice daily as tolerated.

Stability Store at controlled room temperature.

Administration Capsule is usually swallowed whole, but may be may be mixed in water, apple juice, or applesauce.

(Continued)

Ramipril *(Continued)*

Anesthesia and Critical Care Concerns/Other Considerations A recently completed trial (HOPE), examining the use of ramipril (at a dose of between 2.5-10 mg daily) in patients at high risk for cardiovascular events but who did not have heart failure, documented a significant improvement in cardiovascular outcome in the treated group.

ACE inhibitors decrease morbidity and mortality in patients with asymptomatic and symptomatic left ventricular dysfunction. ACE inhibitors are also indicated in patients postmyocardial infarction in whom left ventricular ejection fraction is <40%.

ACE inhibitor therapy may elicit rapid increases in potassium and creatinine, especially when used in patients with bilateral renal artery stenosis. When ACE inhibition is introduced in patients with pre-existing diuretic therapy who are hypovolemic, the ACE inhibitor may induce acute hypotension. Because of the potent teratogenic effects of ACE inhibitors, these drugs should be avoided, if possible, when treating women of childbearing potential not on effective birth control measures.

Pregnancy Risk Factor C (1st trimester)/D (2nd and 3rd trimesters)

Contraindications Hypersensitivity to ramipril or any component of the formulation; prior hypersensitivity (including angioedema) to ACE inhibitors; bilateral renal artery stenosis; pregnancy (2nd and 3rd trimesters)

Warnings/Precautions Anaphylactic or anaphylactoid reactions can occur. Angioedema can occur at any time during treatment (especially following first dose). It may involve head and neck (potentially affecting the airway) or the intestine (presenting with abdominal pain). Prolonged monitoring may be required especially if tongue, glottis, or larynx are involved as they are associated with airway obstruction. Those with a history of airway surgery in this situation have a higher risk. Careful blood pressure monitoring with first dose (hypotension can occur especially in volume-depleted patients). **[U.S. Boxed Warning]: Based on human data, ACEIs can cause injury and death to the developing fetus when used in the second and third trimesters. ACEIs should be discontinued as soon as possible once pregnancy is detected.** Dosage adjustment needed in renal impairment. Use with caution in hypovolemia; collagen vascular diseases; valvular stenosis (particularly aortic stenosis); hyperkalemia; or before, during, or immediately after anesthesia. Avoid rapid dosage escalation, which may lead to renal insufficiency. Rare toxicities associated with ACE inhibitors include cholestatic jaundice (which may progress to hepatic necrosis) and neutropenia/agranulocytosis with myeloid hyperplasia. If patient has renal impairment then a baseline WBC with differential and serum creatinine should be evaluated and monitored closely during the first 3 months of therapy. Hypersensitivity reactions may be seen during hemodialysis with high-flux dialysis membranes (eg, AN69). Use with caution in unilateral renal artery stenosis and pre-existing renal insufficiency.

Adverse Reactions Note: Frequency ranges include data from hypertension and heart failure trials. Higher rates of adverse reactions have generally been noted in patients with CHF. However, the frequency of adverse effects associated with placebo is also increased in this population.

>10%: Respiratory: Cough (increased) (7% to 12%)

1% to 10%:

- Cardiovascular: Hypotension (11%), angina (3%), postural hypotension (2%), syncope (2%)
- Central nervous system: Headache (1% to 5%), dizziness (2% to 4%), fatigue (2%), vertigo (2%)
- Endocrine & metabolic: Hyperkalemia (1% to 10%)
- Gastrointestinal: Nausea/vomiting (1% to 2%)
- Neuromuscular & skeletal: Chest pain (noncardiac) (1%)
- Renal: Renal dysfunction (1%), elevation in serum creatinine (1% to 2%), increased BUN (<1% to 3%); transient elevations of creatinine and/or BUN may occur more frequently
- Respiratory: Cough (estimated 1% to 10%)

<1% (Limited to important or life-threatening): Agitation, agranulocytosis, amnesia, anaphylactoid reaction, angina, angioedema, arrhythmia, bone marrow depression, convulsions, depression, dysphagia, dyspnea, edema, eosinophilia, erythema multiforme, hearing loss, hemolytic anemia, hepatitis, hypersensitivity reactions (urticaria, rash, fever), impotence, insomnia, myalgia,

MI, neuropathy, onycholysis, pancreatitis, pancytopenia, paresthesia, pemphigoid, pemphigus, photosensitivity, proteinuria, somnolence, Stevens-Johnson syndrome, symptomatic hypotension, syncope, thrombocytopenia, toxic epidermal necrolysis, vertigo

Worsening of renal function may occur in patients with bilateral renal artery stenosis or in hypovolemia. In addition, a syndrome which may include fever, myalgia, arthralgia, interstitial nephritis, vasculitis, rash, eosinophilia and positive ANA, and elevated ESR has been reported with ACE inhibitors. Risk of pancreatitis and/or agranulocytosis may be increased in patients with collagen vascular disease or renal impairment.

Overdosage/Toxicology Mild hypotension has been the primary toxic effect seen with acute overdose. Bradycardia may also occur. Hyperkalemia occurs even with therapeutic doses, especially in patients with renal insufficiency and those taking NSAIDs. Treatment is symptom-directed and supportive.

Drug Interactions

Alpha$_1$ blockers: Hypotensive effect increased.

Aspirin: The effects of ACE inhibitors may be blunted by aspirin administration, particularly at higher dosages and/or increase adverse renal effects.

Diuretics: Hypovolemia due to diuretics may precipitate acute hypotensive events or acute renal failure.

Insulin: Risk of hypoglycemia may be increased.

Lithium: Risk of lithium toxicity may be increased; monitor lithium levels, especially the first 4 weeks of therapy.

Mercaptopurine: Risk of neutropenia may be increased.

NSAIDs: May attenuate hypertensive efficacy; effect has been seen with captopril and may occur with other ACE inhibitors; monitor blood pressure. May increase risk of adverse renal effects or hyperkalemia.

Potassium-sparing diuretics (amiloride, spironolactone, triamterene): Increased risk of hyperkalemia.

Potassium supplements may increase the risk of hyperkalemia.

Trimethoprim (high dose) may increase the risk of hyperkalemia.

Ethanol/Nutrition/Herb Interactions Herb/Nutraceutical: Avoid dong quai if using for hypertension (has estrogenic activity). Avoid ephedra, yohimbe, ginseng (may worsen hypertension). Avoid garlic (may have increased antihypertensive effect).

Test Interactions Increases BUN, creatinine, potassium, positive Coombs' [direct]; decreases cholesterol (S); may cause false-positive results in urine acetone determinations using sodium nitroprusside reagent

Dosage Forms Capsule: 1.25 mg, 2.5 mg, 5 mg, 10 mg

♦ **RAN™-Carvedilol (Can)** *see* Carvedilol *on page 231*

♦ **RAN™-Ciprofloxacin (Can)** *see* Ciprofloxacin *on page 285*

♦ **RAN™-Citalopram (Can)** *see* Citalopram *on page 297*

Ranitidine (ra NI ti deen)

Medication Safety Issues

Sound-alike/look-alike issues:

Ranitidine may be confused with amantadine, rimantadine

Zantac® may be confused with Xanax®, Zarontin®, Zofran®, Zyrtec®

Related Information

Anesthesia for Patients With Liver Disease *on page 1421*

U.S. Brand Names Zantac®; Zantac 75® [OTC]; Zantac 150™ [OTC]; Zantac® EFFERdose®

Canadian Brand Names Alti-Ranitidine; Apo-Ranitidine®; BCI-Ranitidine; CO Ranitidine; Gen-Ranidine; Novo-Ranidine; Nu-Ranit; PMS-Ranitidine; Ranitidine Injection, USP; Rhoxal-ranitidine; Sandoz-Ranitidine; Zantac®; Zantac 75®

Synonyms Ranitidine Hydrochloride

Pharmacologic Category Histamine H_2 Antagonist

Generic Available Yes: Excludes effervescent tablet

Use

Zantac®: Short-term and maintenance therapy of duodenal ulcer, gastric ulcer, gastroesophageal reflux, active benign ulcer, erosive esophagitis, and pathological hypersecretory conditions; as part of a multidrug regimen for *H. pylori* eradication to reduce the risk of duodenal ulcer recurrence

(Continued)

Ranitidine *(Continued)*

Zantac® 75 [OTC]: Relief of heartburn, acid indigestion, and sour stomach

Unlabeled/Investigational Use Recurrent postoperative ulcer, upper GI bleeding, prevention of acid-aspiration pneumonitis during surgery, and prevention of stress-induced ulcers

Mechanism of Action Competitive inhibition of histamine at H_2-receptors of the gastric parietal cells, which inhibits gastric acid secretion, gastric volume, and hydrogen ion concentration are reduced. Does not affect pepsin secretion, pentagastrin-stimulated intrinsic factor secretion, or serum gastrin.

Pharmacodynamics/Kinetics

Absorption: Oral: 50%

Distribution: Normal renal function: V_d: 1.7 L/kg; Cl_{cr} 25-35 mL/minute: 1.76 L/kg minimally penetrates the blood-brain barrier; enters breast milk

Protein binding: 15%

Metabolism: Hepatic to N-oxide, S-oxide, and N-desmethyl metabolites

Bioavailability: Oral: 48%

Half-life elimination:

- Oral: Normal renal function: 2.5-3 hours; Cl_{cr} 25-35 mL/minute: 4.8 hours
- I.V.: Normal renal function: 2-2.5 hours

Time to peak, serum: Oral: 2-3 hours; I.M.: ≤15 minutes

Excretion: Urine: Oral: 30%, I.V.: 70% (as unchanged drug); feces (as metabolites)

Dosage

Children 1 month to 16 years:

- Duodenal and gastric ulcer:
  - Oral:
    - Treatment: 2-4 mg/kg/day divided twice daily; maximum treatment dose: 300 mg/day
    - Maintenance: 2-4 mg/kg once daily; maximum maintenance dose: 150 mg/day
  - I.V.: 2-4 mg/kg/day divided every 6-8 hours; maximum: 150 mg/day
- GERD and erosive esophagitis:
  - Oral: 5-10 mg/kg/day divided twice daily; maximum: GERD: 300 mg/day, erosive esophagitis: 600 mg/day
  - I.V.: 2-4 mg/kg/day divided every 6-8 hours; maximum: 150 mg/day **or as an alternative**
    - Continuous infusion: Initial: 1 mg/kg/dose for one dose followed by infusion of 0.08-0.17 mg/kg/hour or 2-4 mg/kg/day

Children ≥12 years: Prevention of heartburn: Oral: Zantac® 75 [OTC]: 75 mg 30-60 minutes before eating food or drinking beverages which cause heartburn; maximum: 150 mg/24 hours; do not use for more than 14 days

Adults:

- Duodenal ulcer: Oral: Treatment: 150 mg twice daily, or 300 mg once daily after the evening meal or at bedtime; maintenance: 150 mg once daily at bedtime
- *Helicobacter pylori* eradication: 150 mg twice daily; requires combination therapy
- Pathological hypersecretory conditions:
  - Oral: 150 mg twice daily; adjust dose or frequency as clinically indicated; doses of up to 6 g/day have been used
  - I.V.: Continuous infusion for Zollinger-Ellison: 1 mg/kg/hour; measure gastric acid output at 4 hours, if >10 mEq or if patient is symptomatic, increase dose in increments of 0.5 mg/kg/hour; doses of up to 2.5 mg/kg/hour have been used
- Gastric ulcer, benign: Oral: 150 mg twice daily; maintenance: 150 mg once daily at bedtime
- Erosive esophagitis: Oral: Treatment: 150 mg 4 times/day; maintenance: 150 mg twice daily
- Prevention of heartburn: Oral: Zantac® 75 [OTC]: 75 mg 30-60 minutes before eating food or drinking beverages which cause heartburn; maximum: 150 mg in 24 hours; do not use for more than 14 days
- Patients not able to take oral medication:
  - I.M.: 50 mg every 6-8 hours
  - I.V.: Intermittent bolus or infusion: 50 mg every 6-8 hours
  - Continuous I.V. infusion: 6.25 mg/hour

Elderly: Ulcer healing rates and incidence of adverse effects are similar in the elderly, when compared to younger patients; dosing adjustments not necessary based on age alone

Dosing adjustment in renal impairment: Adults: Cl_{cr} <50 mL/minute:

Oral: 150 mg every 24 hours; adjust dose cautiously if needed

I.V.: 50 mg every 18-24 hours; adjust dose cautiously if needed

Hemodialysis: Adjust dosing schedule so that dose coincides with the end of hemodialysis

Dosing adjustment/comments in hepatic disease: Patients with hepatic impairment may have minor changes in ranitidine half-life, distribution, clearance, and bioavailability; dosing adjustments not necessary, monitor

Stability

Injection: Vials: Store between 4°C to 30°C (39°F to 86°F); protect from light; solution is a clear, colorless to yellow solution; slight darkening does not affect potency

Premixed bag: Store between 2°C to 25°C (36°F to 77°F); protect from light

EFFERdose® formulations: Store between 2°C to 30°C (36°F to 86°F)

Syrup: Store between 4°C to 25°C (39°F to 77°F); protect from light

Tablet: Store in dry place, between 15°C to 30°C (59°F to 86°F); protect from light

Vials can be mixed with NS or D_5W; solutions are stable for 48 hours at room temperature

Intermittent bolus injection: Dilute to maximum of 2.5 mg/mL

Intermittent infusion: Dilute to maximum of 0.5 mg/mL

Do not add other medications to premixed bag

Administration

Ranitidine injection may be administered I.M. or I.V.:

I.M.: Injection is administered undiluted

I.V.: Must be diluted; may be administered IVP or IVPB or continuous I.V. infusion

IVP: Ranitidine (usually 50 mg) should be diluted to a total of 20 mL with NS or D_5W and administered over at least 5 minutes

IVPB: Administer over 15-20 minutes

Continuous I.V. infusion: Administer at 6.25 mg/hour and titrate dosage based on gastric pH by continuous infusion over 24 hours

EFFERdose®: Should not be chewed, swallowed whole, or dissolved on tongue:

25 mg tablet: Dissolve in at least 5 mL (1 teaspoonful) of water; wait until completely dissolved before administering

150 mg tablet: Dissolve each dose in 6-8 ounces of water before drinking

Monitoring Parameters AST, ALT, serum creatinine; when used to prevent stress-related GI bleeding, measure the intragastric pH and try to maintain pH >4; signs and symptoms of peptic ulcer disease, occult blood with GI bleeding, monitor renal function to correct dose; monitor for side effects

Anesthesia and Critical Care Concerns/Other Considerations Ranitidine causes fewer CNS adverse reactions and drug interactions compared to cimetidine.

Pregnancy Risk Factor B

Contraindications Hypersensitivity to ranitidine or any component of the formulation

Warnings/Precautions Use with caution in patients with hepatic impairment; use with caution in renal impairment, dosage modification required; avoid use in patients with history of acute porphyria (may precipitate attacks); long-term therapy may be associated with vitamin B_{12} deficiency; EFFERdose® formulations contain phenylalanine; safety and efficacy have not been established for pediatric patients <1 month of age

Adverse Reactions Frequency not defined (limited to important or life-threatening):

Cardiovascular: Arrhythmias, vasculitis

Central nervous system: Dizziness, hallucinations, headache, mental confusion, somnolence, vertigo

Dermatologic: Erythema multiforme, rash

Gastrointestinal: Pancreatitis

Hematologic: Acquired hemolytic anemia, agranulocytosis, aplastic anemia, granulocytopenia, leukopenia, pancytopenia, thrombocytopenia

Hepatic: Hepatic failure

Miscellaneous: Anaphylaxis, hypersensitivity reactions

(Continued)

Ranitidine *(Continued)*

Overdosage/Toxicology Symptoms of overdose include abnormal gait, hypotension, and adverse effects seen with normal use. Treatment is primarily symptomatic and supportive.

Drug Interactions Substrate (minor) of CYP1A2, 2C19, 2D6; **Inhibits** CYP1A2 (weak), 2D6 (weak)

Propantheline: Slight delay and increase in peak ranitidine levels

Triazolam: Ranitidine increases bioavailability of triazolam (10% to 30%), possibly by reducing gastric acidity

Warfarin: May increase or decrease prothrombin time when used concomitantly; monitor

Ethanol/Nutrition/Herb Interactions

Ethanol: Avoid ethanol (may cause gastric mucosal irritation).

Food: Does not interfere with absorption of ranitidine.

Test Interactions False-positive urine protein using Multistix®, gastric acid secretion test, skin test allergen extracts, serum creatinine, urine protein test

Dietary Considerations Oral dosage forms may be taken with or without food.

Zantac® EFFERdose®:

Effervescent tablet 25 mg contains sodium 1.33 mEq/tablet and phenylalanine 2.81 mg/tablet

Effervescent tablet 150 mg contains sodium 7.96 mEq/tablet and phenylalanine 16.84 mg/tablet

Dosage Forms

Capsule, as hydrochloride: 150 mg, 300 mg

Infusion, as hydrochloride [premixed in NaCl 0.45%; preservative free] (Zantac®): 50 mg (50 mL)

Injection, solution, as hydrochloride: 25 mg/mL (2 mL, 6 mL)

Zantac®: 25 mg/mL (2 mL, 6 mL, 40 mL) [contains phenol 0.5% as preservative]

Syrup, as hydrochloride: 15 mg/mL (10 mL) [contains alcohol 7.5%; peppermint flavor]

Zantac®: 15 mg/mL (473 mL) [contains alcohol 7.5%; peppermint flavor]

Tablet, as hydrochloride: 75 mg [OTC], 150 mg, 300 mg

Zantac®: 150 mg, 300 mg

Zantac 75®: 75 mg

Zantac 150™: 150 mg

Tablet, effervescent, as hydrochloride (Zantac® EFFERdose®): 25 mg [contains sodium 1.33 mEq/tablet, phenylalanine 2.81 mg/tablet, and sodium benzoate]; 150 mg [contains sodium 7.96 mEq/tablet, phenylalanine 16.84 mg/tablet, and sodium benzoate]

References

Allen ME, Kopp BJ, and Erstad BL, "Stress Ulcer Prophylaxis in the Postoperative Period," *Am J Health Syst Pharm*, 2004, 61(6):588-96.

"ASHP Therapeutic Guidelines on Stress Ulcer Prophylaxis. ASHP Commission on Therapeutics and Approved by the ASHP Board of Directors on November 14, 1998," *Am J Health Syst Pharm*, 1999, 56(4):347-79.

Cook D, Guyatt G, Marshall J, et al, "A Comparison of Sucralfate and Ranitidine for the Prevention of Upper Gastrointestinal Bleeding in Patients Requiring Mechanical Ventilation. Canadian Critical Care Trials Group," *N Engl J Med*, 1998, 338(12):791-7.

Lopez-Herce J, Albajara L, Codoceo R, et al, "Ranitidine Prophylaxis in Acute Gastric Mucosal Damage in Critically Ill Pediatric Patients," *Crit Care Med*, 1988, 16(6):591-93.

Morris DL, Markham SJ, Beechey A, et al, "Ranitidine-Bolus or Infusion Prophylaxis for Stress Ulcer," *Crit Care Med*, 1988, 16(3):229-32.

◆ **Ranitidine Hydrochloride** *see* Ranitidine *on page 1105*
◆ **Ranitidine Injection, USP (Can)** *see* Ranitidine *on page 1105*
◆ **RAN™-Lovastatin (Can)** *see* Lovastatin *on page 782*
◆ **RAN™-Metformin (Can)** *see* Metformin *on page 810*
◆ **Rapamune®** *see* Sirolimus *on page 1177*
◆ **Raphon [OTC]** *see* Epinephrine *on page 457*
◆ **ratio-Acyclovir (Can)** *see* Acyclovir *on page 39*
◆ **ratio-Azithromycin (Can)** *see* Azithromycin *on page 149*
◆ **ratio-Benzydamine (Can)** *see* Benzydamine *on page 167*
◆ **ratio-Carvedilol (Can)** *see* Carvedilol *on page 231*
◆ **ratio-Cefuroxime (Can)** *see* Cefuroxime *on page 253*
◆ **ratio-Ciprofloxacin (Can)** *see* Ciprofloxacin *on page 285*
◆ **ratio-Citalopram (Can)** *see* Citalopram *on page 297*
◆ **ratio-Clarithromycin (Can)** *see* Clarithromycin *on page 300*

Remifentanil (rem i FEN ta nil)

Medication Safety Issues

Sound-alike/look-alike issues:

Remifentanil may be confused with alfentanil

Related Information

Anesthesia Considerations for Neurosurgery *on page 1401*

Chronic Renal Failure *on page 1437*

Narcotic / Opioid Analgesics *on page 1568*

Substance Abuse and Anesthesia *on page 1496*

U.S. Brand Names Ultiva®

Canadian Brand Names Ultiva®

Synonyms GI87084B

Pharmacologic Category Analgesic, Narcotic

Restrictions C-II

(Continued)

Remifentanil *(Continued)*

Generic Available No

Use Analgesic for use during the induction and maintenance of general anesthesia; for continued analgesia into the immediate postoperative period; analgesic component of monitored anesthesia

Unlabeled/Investigational Use Management of pain in mechanically-ventilated patients

Mechanism of Action Binds with stereospecific mu-opioid receptors at many sites within the CNS, increases pain threshold, alters pain reception, inhibits ascending pain pathways

Pharmacodynamics/Kinetics

Onset of action: I.V.: 1-3 minutes

Distribution: V_d: 100 mL/kg; increased in children

Protein binding: ~70% (primarily alpha$_1$ acid glycoprotein)

Metabolism: Rapid via blood and tissue esterases

Half-life elimination (dose dependent): Terminal: 10-20 minutes; effective: 3-10 minutes

Excretion: Urine

Dosage I.V. continuous infusion: Dose should be based on ideal body weight (IBW) in obese patients (>30% over IBW).

Children birth to 2 months: Maintenance of anesthesia with nitrous oxide (70%): 0.4 mcg/kg/minute (range: 0.4-1 mcg/kg/minute); supplemental bolus dose of 1 mcg/kg may be administered, smaller bolus dose may be required with potent inhalation agents, potent neuraxial anesthesia, significant comorbidities, significant fluid shifts, or without atropine pretreatment. Clearance in neonates is highly variable; dose should be carefully titrated.

Children 1-12 years: Maintenance of anesthesia with halothane, sevoflurane or isoflurane: 0.25 mcg/kg/minute (range 0.05-1.3 mcg/kg/minute); supplemental bolus dose of 1 mcg/kg may be administered every 2-5 minutes. Consider increasing concomitant anesthetics with infusion rate >1 mcg/kg/minute. Infusion rate can be titrated upward in increments up to 50% or titrated downward in decrements of 25% to 50%. May titrate every 2-5 minutes.

Adults:

Induction of anesthesia: 0.5-1 mcg/kg/minute; if endotracheal intubation is to occur in <8 minutes, an initial dose of 1 mcg/kg may be given over 30-60 seconds

Coronary bypass surgery: 1 mcg/kg/minute

Maintenance of anesthesia: **Note:** Supplemental bolus dose of 1 mcg/kg may be administered every 2-5 minutes. Consider increasing concomitant anesthetics with infusion rate >1 mcg/kg/minute. Infusion rate can be titrated upward in increments of 25% to 100% or downward in decrements of 25% to 50%. May titrate every 2-5 minutes.

With nitrous oxide (66%): 0.4 mcg/kg/minute (range: 0.1-2 mcg/kg/minute)

With isoflurane: 0.25 mcg/kg/minute (range: 0.05-2 mcg/kg/minute)

With propofol: 0.25 mcg/kg/minute (range: 0.05-2 mcg/kg/minute)

Coronary bypass surgery: 1 mcg/kg/minute (range: 0.125-4 mcg/kg/minute); supplemental dose: 0.5-1 mcg/kg

Continuation as an analgesic in immediate postoperative period: 0.1 mcg/kg/minute (range: 0.025-0.2 mcg/kg/minute). Infusion rate may be adjusted every 5 minutes in increments of 0.025 mcg/kg/minute. Bolus doses are not recommended. Infusion rates >0.2 mcg/kg/minute are associated with respiratory depression.

Coronary bypass surgery, continuation as an analgesic into the ICU: 1 mcg/kg/minute (range: 0.05-1 mcg/kg/minute)

Analgesic component of monitored anesthesia care: **Note:** Supplemental oxygen is recommended:

Single I.V. dose given 90 seconds prior to local anesthetic:

Remifentanil alone: 1 mcg/kg over 30-60 seconds

With midazolam: 0.5 mcg/kg over 30-60 seconds

Continuous infusion beginning 5 minutes prior to local anesthetic:

Remifentanil alone: 0.1 mcg/kg minute

With midazolam: 0.05 mcg/kg/minute

Continuous infusion given after local anesthetic:

Remifentanil alone: 0.05 mcg/kg/minute (range: 0.025-0.2 mcg/kg/minute)

With midazolam: 0.025 mcg/kg/minute (range: 0.025-0.2 mcg/kg/minute)

Note: Following local or anesthetic block, infusion rate should be decreased to 0.05 mcg/kg/minute; rate adjustments of 0.025 mcg/kg/minute may be done at 5-minute intervals

Mechanically-ventilated patients: Acute pain (moderate-to-severe) (unlabeled use): 0.6-15 mcg/kg/hour

Elderly: Elderly patients have an increased sensitivity to effect of remifentanil, doses should be decreased by 1/2 and titrated

Stability Prior to reconstitution, store at 2°C to 25°C (36°F to 77°F). Prepare solution by adding 1 mL of diluent per 1 mg of remifentanil. Shake well. Further dilute to a final concentration of 20, 25, 50, or 250 mcg/mL. Stable for 24 hours at room temperature after reconstitution and further dilution to concentrations of 20-250 mcg/mL (4 hours if diluted with LR).

Administration An infusion device should be used to administer continuous infusions. During the maintenance of general anesthesia, I.V. boluses may be administered over 30-60 seconds. Injections should be given into I.V. tubing close to the venous cannula; tubing should be cleared after treatment to prevent residual effects when other fluids are administered through the same I.V. line.

Monitoring Parameters Respiratory and cardiovascular status, blood pressure, heart rate

Anesthesia and Critical Care Concerns/Other Considerations Ultra short-acting narcotic that is unique compared to other short-acting narcotics. This agent is not considered suitable as the sole agent for induction; remifentanil should be used in combination with other induction agents; bolus doses are not recommended for sedation cases and in treatment of postoperative pain due to risk of respiratory depression and muscle rigidity; due to remifentanil's short duration of action, when postoperative pain is anticipated, discontinuation of an infusion of remifentanil should be preceded by an adequate postoperative analgesic (ie, fentanyl, morphine).

Elderly patients have an increased sensitivity to effect of remifentanil, doses should be decreased by 1/2 and titrated.

Pregnancy Risk Factor C

Contraindications Not for intrathecal or epidural administration, due to the presence of glycine in the formulation; hypersensitivity to remifentanil, fentanyl, or fentanyl analogs, or any component of the formulation

Warnings/Precautions Remifentanil is not recommended as the sole agent in general anesthesia, because the loss of consciousness cannot be assured and due to the high incidence of apnea, hypotension, tachycardia and muscle rigidity; it should be administered by individuals specifically trained in the use of anesthetic agents and should not be used in diagnostic or therapeutic procedures outside the monitored anesthesia setting; resuscitative and intubation equipment should be readily available.

Interruption of an infusion will result in offset of effects within 5-10 minutes; the discontinuation of remifentanil infusion should be preceded by the establishment of adequate postoperative analgesia orders, especially for patients in whom postoperative pain is anticipated. Use caution in the morbidly obese.

Adverse Reactions

>10%: Gastrointestinal: Nausea, vomiting

1% to 10%:

Cardiovascular: Hypotension (dose dependent), bradycardia (dose dependent), tachycardia, hypertension

Central nervous system: Dizziness, headache, agitation, fever

Dermatologic: Pruritus

Neuromuscular & skeletal: Muscle rigidity (dose dependent)

Ocular: Visual disturbances

Respiratory: Respiratory depression, apnea, hypoxia

Miscellaneous: Shivering, postoperative pain

<1% (Limited to important or life-threatening): Anaphylactic/anaphylactoid reactions, anemia, anxiety, arrhythmia, asystole, bronchospasm, confusion, constipation, CPK-MB increased, diarrhea, dysphagia, electrolyte disorders, hallucinations, heart block, pleural effusion, prolonged emergence from anesthesia, pulmonary edema, syncope, thrombocytopenia, xerostomia

Overdosage/Toxicology

Symptoms of overdose include apnea, chest wall rigidity, seizures, hypoxemia, hypotension and bradycardia

(Continued)

Remifentanil *(Continued)*

Support of patient's airway, establish an I.V. line, administer intravenous fluids and administer naloxone 2 mg I.V. (0.01 mg/kg for children) with repeat administration as needed up to a total of 10 mg; glycopyrrolate or atropine may be useful for the treatment of bradycardia or hypotension

Drug Interactions

Anesthetics: Synergistic with other anesthetics, may need to decrease thiopental, propofol, isoflurane and midazolam by up to 75%

CNS depressants: Increased effect of CNS depressants

Dosage Forms Injection, powder for reconstitution: 1 mg, 2 mg, 5 mg [contains glycine 15 mg]

References

Carr DB, Jacox AK, Chapman RC, et al, "Acute Pain Management," Guideline Technical Report, No. 1. Rockville, MD: U.S. Department of Health and Human Services, Public Health Service, Agency for Health Care Policy and Research. AHCPR Publication No. 95-0034. February 1995.

"Clinical Practice Guidelines for the Sustained Use of Sedatives and Analgesics in the Critically Ill Adult. Task Force of the American College of Critical Care Medicine (ACCM) of the Society of Critical Care Medicine (SCCM), American Society of Health-System Pharmacists (ASHP), American College of Chest Physicians," *Am J Health Syst Pharm*, 2002, 59(2):150-78.

Hogue CW, Bowdle TA, O'Leary C, et al, "A Multicenter Evaluation of Total Intravenous Anesthesia With Remifentanil and Propofol for Elective Inpatient Surgery," *Anesth Analg*, 1996, 83(2):279-85.

Jacobi J, Fraser GL, Coursin DB, et al, "Clinical Practice Guidelines for the Sustained Use of Sedatives and Analgesics in the Critically Ill Adult," *Crit Care Med*, 2002, 30(1):119-41. Available at: http://www.sccm.org/pdf/sedatives.pdf.

Mokhlesi B, Leikin JB, Murray P, et al, "Adult Toxicology in Critical Care. Part 11: Specific Poisonings," *Chest*, 2003, 123(3):897-922.

"Principles of Analgesic Use in the Treatment of Acute Pain and Chronic Cancer Pain," 5th ed, Glenview, IL: American Pain Society, 2003.

Warner DS, Hindman BJ, Todd MM, et al, "Intracranial Pressure and Hemodynamic Effects of Remifentanil Versus Alfentanil in Patients Undergoing Supratentorial Craniotomy," *Anesth Analg*, 1996, 83(2):348-53.

Westmoreland CL, Hoke JF, Sebel PS, et al, "Pharmacokinetics of Remifentanil (GI87084B) and Its Major Metabolite (GI90291) in Patients Undergoing Elective Inpatient Surgery," *Anesthesiology*, 1993, 79(5):893-903.

♦ **Remodulin®** *see* Treprostinil *on page 1309*

♦ **ReoPro®** *see* Abciximab *on page 23*

♦ **Resectisol®** *see* Mannitol *on page 790*

Reserpine (re SER peen)

Medication Safety Issues

Sound-alike/look-alike issues:

Reserpine may be confused with Risperdal®, risperidone

Pharmacologic Category Central Monoamine-Depleting Agent; Rauwolfia Alkaloid

Generic Available Yes

Use Management of mild-to-moderate hypertension; treatment of agitated psychotic states (schizophrenia)

Unlabeled/Investigational Use Management of tardive dyskinesia

Mechanism of Action Reduces blood pressure via depletion of sympathetic biogenic amines (norepinephrine and dopamine); this also commonly results in sedative effects

Pharmacodynamics/Kinetics

Onset of action: Antihypertensive: 3-6 days

Duration: 2-6 weeks

Absorption: ~40%

Distribution: Crosses placenta; enters breast milk

Protein binding: 96%

Metabolism: Extensively hepatic (>90%)

Half-life elimination: 50-100 hours

Excretion: Feces (30% to 60%); urine (10%)

Dosage Note: When used for management of hypertension, full antihypertensive effects may take as long as 3 weeks.

Oral:

Children: Hypertension: 0.01-0.02 mg/kg/24 hours divided every 12 hours; maximum dose: 0.25 mg/day (not recommended in children)

Adults:

Hypertension:

Manufacturer's labeling: Initial: 0.5 mg/day for 1-2 weeks; maintenance: 0.1-0.25 mg/day

Note: Clinically, the need for a "loading" period (as recommended by the manufacturer) is not well supported, and alternative dosing is preferred.

Alternative dosing (unlabeled): Initial: 0.1 mg once daily; adjust as necessary based on response.

Usual dose range (JNC 7): 0.05-0.25 mg once daily; 0.1 mg every other day may be given to achieve 0.05 mg once daily

Schizophrenia (labeled use) or tardive dyskinesia (unlabeled use): Dosing recommendations vary; initial dose recommendations generally range from 0.05-0.25 mg (although manufacturer recommends 0.5 mg once daily initially in schizophrenia). May be increased in increments of 0.1-0.25 mg; maximum dose in tardive dyskinesia: 5 mg/day.

Elderly: Initial: 0.05 mg once daily, increasing by 0.05 mg every week as necessary

Dosing adjustment in renal impairment: Cl_{cr} <10 mL/minute: Avoid use

Dialysis: Not removed by hemo or peritoneal dialysis; supplemental dose is not necessary

Stability Protect oral dosage forms from light

Monitoring Parameters Blood pressure, standing and sitting/supine

Anesthesia and Critical Care Concerns/Other Considerations Currently, reserpine is used only infrequently for treatment of hypertension. Nasal congestion, sedation, depression, and activation of peptic ulcer are important adverse effects.

Pregnancy Risk Factor C

Contraindications Hypersensitivity to reserpine or any component of the formulation; active peptic ulcer disease, ulcerative colitis; history of mental depression (especially with suicidal tendencies); patients receiving electroconvulsive therapy (ECT)

Warnings/Precautions Use with caution in patients with impaired renal function, inflammatory bowel disease, asthma, Parkinson's disease, gallstones, or history of peptic ulcer disease, and the elderly. At high doses, significant mental depression, anxiety, or psychosis may occur (uncommon at dosages <0.25 mg/day). May cause orthostatic hypotension; use with caution in patients at risk of hypotension or in patients where transient hypotensive episodes would be poorly tolerated (cardiovascular disease or cerebrovascular disease). Avoid concurrent use of MAO inhibitors and/or drugs with MAO-inhibiting properties. Some products may contain tartrazine.

Adverse Reactions Frequency not defined.

Cardiovascular: Peripheral edema, arrhythmia, bradycardia, chest pain, PVC, hypotension, syncope

Central nervous system: Dizziness, headache, nightmares, nervousness, drowsiness, fatigue, mental depression, parkinsonism, dull sensorium, paradoxical anxiety

Dermatologic: Rash, pruritus, flushing of skin, purpura

Endocrine & metabolic: Gynecomastia, weight gain

Gastrointestinal: Anorexia, diarrhea, dry mouth, nausea, vomiting, increased salivation, increased gastric acid secretion

Genitourinary: Impotence, decreased libido

Hematologic: Thrombocytopenia purpura

Neuromuscular & skeletal: Muscle ache

Ocular: Blurred vision, optic atrophy

Respiratory: Nasal congestion, dyspnea, epistaxis

Overdosage/Toxicology Symptoms of overdose include hypotension, bradycardia, CNS depression, sedation, coma, hypothermia, miosis, tremor, diarrhea, and vomiting. Treatment is symptom-directed and supportive. Anticholinergic agents may be useful in reducing parkinsonian effects and bradycardia.

Drug Interactions

Antihypertensives: Hypotensive effects may be increased.

CNS depressants, ethanol: Additive CNS effects may occur.

Digitalis glycosides: Concomitant administration may predispose some patients to cardiac arrhythmias.

MAO inhibitors: Reserpine may cause hypertensive reactions; concurrent use is not recommended. Theoretically, risk is decreased if reserpine is initiated several days prior to MAO inhibitors.

(Continued)

Reserpine *(Continued)*

Quinidine, procainamide: Reserpine may increase the risk of cardiac arrhythmias effects.

Sympathomimetics: The effects of direct-acting sympathomimetics (eg, epinephrine, norepinephrine) may be modestly increased/prolonged. However, the effects of indirect-acting sympathomimetics (amphetamines, dopamine) may be blocked by reserpine.

Ethanol/Nutrition/Herb Interactions

Ethanol: Avoid ethanol (may increase CNS depression).

Herb/Nutraceutical: Avoid dong quai if using for hypertension (has estrogenic activity). Avoid ephedra, yohimbe (may worsen hypertension). Avoid valerian, St John's wort, kava kava, gotu kola (may increase CNS depression). Avoid garlic (may have increased antihypertensive effect).

Dosage Forms Tablet: 0.1 mg, 0.25 mg

♦ **Restasis®** *see* CycloSPORINE *on page 337*

♦ **Restoril®** *see* Temazepam *on page 1239*

♦ **Retavase®** *see* Reteplase *on page 1114*

Reteplase (RE ta plase)

Medication Safety Issues

High alert medication: The Institute for Safe Medication Practices (ISMP) includes this medication (I.V.) among its list of drugs which have a heightened risk of causing significant patient harm when used in error.

U.S. Brand Names Retavase®

Canadian Brand Names Retavase®

Synonyms Recombinant Plasminogen Activator; r-PA

Pharmacologic Category Thrombolytic Agent

Generic Available No

Use Management of acute myocardial infarction (AMI); improvement of ventricular function; reduction of the incidence of CHF and the reduction of mortality following AMI

Mechanism of Action Reteplase is a nonglycosylated form of tPA produced by recombinant DNA technology using *E. coli*; it initiates local fibrinolysis by binding to fibrin in a thrombus (clot) and converts entrapped plasminogen to plasmin

Pharmacodynamics/Kinetics

Onset of action: Thrombolysis: 30-90 minutes

Half-life elimination: 13-16 minutes

Excretion: Feces and urine

Clearance: Plasma: 250-450 mL/minute

Dosage

Children: Not recommended

Adults: 10 units I.V. over 2 minutes, followed by a second dose 30 minutes later of 10 units I.V. over 2 minutes

Withhold second dose if serious bleeding or anaphylaxis occurs

Stability Dosage kits should be stored at 2°C to 25°C (36°F to 77°F) and remain sealed until use in order to protect from light

Administration Reteplase should be reconstituted using the diluent, syringe, needle and dispensing pin provided with each kit and the each reconstituted dose should be administered I.V. over 2 minutes; no other medication should be added to the injection solution

Monitoring Parameters Monitor for signs of bleeding (hematuria, GI bleeding, gingival bleeding)

Pregnancy Risk Factor C

Contraindications Hypersensitivity to reteplase or any component of the formulation; active internal bleeding; history of cerebrovascular accident; recent intracranial or intraspinal surgery or trauma; intracranial neoplasm, arteriovenous malformations, or aneurysm; known bleeding diathesis; severe uncontrolled hypertension

Warnings/Precautions Concurrent heparin anticoagulation can contribute to bleeding; careful attention to all potential bleeding sites. I.M. injections and nonessential handling of the patient should be avoided. Venipunctures should be performed carefully and only when necessary. If arterial puncture is necessary, use an upper extremity vessel that can be manually compressed. If serious bleeding occurs then the infusion of anistreplase and heparin should be stopped.

For the following conditions the risk of bleeding is higher with use of reteplase and should be weighed against the benefits of therapy: recent major surgery (eg, CABG, obstetrical delivery, organ biopsy, previous puncture of noncompressible vessels), cerebrovascular disease, recent gastrointestinal or genitourinary bleeding, recent trauma including CPR, hypertension (systolic BP >180 mm Hg and/or diastolic BP >110 mm Hg), high likelihood of left heart thrombus (eg, mitral stenosis with atrial fibrillation), acute pericarditis, subacute bacterial endocarditis, hemostatic defects including ones caused by severe renal or hepatic dysfunction, significant hepatic dysfunction, pregnancy, diabetic hemorrhagic retinopathy or other hemorrhagic ophthalmic conditions, septic thrombophlebitis or occluded AV cannula at seriously infected site, advanced age (eg, >75 years), patients receiving oral anticoagulants, any other condition in which bleeding constitutes a significant hazard or would be particularly difficult to manage because of location.

Coronary thrombolysis may result in reperfusion arrhythmias. Follow standard MI management. Rare anaphylactic reactions can occur. Safety and efficacy in pediatric patients have not been established.

Adverse Reactions Bleeding is the most frequent adverse effect associated with reteplase. Heparin and aspirin have been administered concurrently with reteplase in clinical trials. The incidence of adverse events is a reflection of these combined therapies, and are comparable with comparison thrombolytics.

>10%: Local: Injection site bleeding (4.6% to 48.6%)

1% to 10%:
- Gastrointestinal: Bleeding (1.8% to 9.0%)
- Genitourinary: Bleeding (0.9% to 9.5%)
- Hematologic: Anemia (0.9% to 2.6%)

<1% (Limited to important or life-threatening): Allergic/anaphylactoid reactions, cholesterol embolization, intracranial hemorrhage (0.8%)

Other adverse effects noted are frequently associated with MI (and therefore may or may not be attributable to Retavase®) and include arrhythmia, arrest, cardiac reinfarction, cardiogenic shock, embolism, hypotension, pericarditis, pulmonary edema, tamponade, thrombosis

Overdosage/Toxicology Symptoms of overdose include increased incidence of intracranial bleeding. Treatment is supportive.

Drug Interactions

Aminocaproic acid (antifibrinolytic agent) may decrease effectiveness.

Drugs which affect platelet function (eg, NSAIDs, dipyridamole, ticlopidine, clopidogrel, IIb/IIIa antagonists) may potentiate the risk of hemorrhage; use with caution.

Heparin and aspirin: Use with aspirin and heparin may increase bleeding. However, aspirin and heparin were used concomitantly with reteplase in the majority of patients in clinical studies.

Warfarin or oral anticoagulants: Risk of bleeding may be increased during concurrent therapy.

Dosage Forms Injection, powder for reconstitution [preservative free]: 10.4 units [equivalent to reteplase 18.1 mg; contains sucrose and polysorbate 80; packaged with sterile water for injection]

References

Antman EM, Anbe SC, Alpert JS, et al, "ACC/AHA Guidelines for the Management of Patients With ST-Elevation Myocardial Infarction - Executive Summary: A Report of the American College of Cardiology/American Heart Association Task Force on Practice Guidelines (Writing Committee to Revise the 1999 Guidelines for the Management of Patients With Acute Myocardial Infarction)," *Circulation*, 2004, 110:588-636. Available at: http://www.circulationaha.org/cgi/content/full/110/5/588. Last accessed August 26, 2004.

Ryan TJ, Anderson JK, Antman EM, et al, "ACC/AHA Guidelines for the Management of Patients With Acute Myocardial Infarction: A Report of the American College of Cardiology/American Heart Association Task Force on Practice Guidelines (Committee on Management of Acute Myocardial Infarction)," *J Am Coll Cardiol*, 1996, 28:1328-428.

Topol EJ, GUSTO V Investigators, "Reperfusion Therapy for Acute Myocardial Infarction With Fibrinolytic Therapy or Combination Reduced Fibrinolytic Therapy and Platelet Glycoprotein IIb/IIIa Inhibition: The GUSTO V Randomized Trial," *Lancet*, 2001, 357:1905-14.

- **Retrovir®** *see* Zidovudine *on page 1371*
- **Revatio™** *see* Sildenafil *on page 1169*
- **Reversol®** *see* Edrophonium *on page 439*
- **Revex®** *see* Nalmefene *on page 893*
- **ReVia®** *see* Naltrexone *on page 897*

- **rFVIIa** *see* Factor VIIa (Recombinant) *on page 501*
- **Rheumatrex®** *see* Methotrexate *on page 821*
- **Rhinalar® (Can)** *see* Flunisolide *on page 537*
- **Rhinall [OTC]** *see* Phenylephrine *on page 1015*
- **Rho®-Clonazepam (Can)** *see* Clonazepam *on page 313*
- **Rhodacine® (Can)** *see* Indomethacin *on page 674*
- **Rhodis™ (Can)** *see* Ketoprofen *on page 714*
- **Rhodis-EC™ (Can)** *see* Ketoprofen *on page 714*
- **Rhodis SR™ (Can)** *see* Ketoprofen *on page 714*
- **Rho®-Metformin (Can)** *see* Metformin *on page 810*
- **Rho®-Nitro (Can)** *see* Nitroglycerin *on page 928*
- **Rho®-Sotalol (Can)** *see* Sotalol *on page 1198*
- **Rhoxal-amiodarone (Can)** *see* Amiodarone *on page 83*
- **Rhoxal-atenolol (Can)** *see* Atenolol *on page 136*
- **Rhoxal-ciprofloxacin (Can)** *see* Ciprofloxacin *on page 285*
- **Rhoxal-citalopram (Can)** *see* Citalopram *on page 297*
- **Rhoxal-cyclosporine (Can)** *see* CycloSPORINE *on page 337*
- **Rhoxal-diltiazem CD (Can)** *see* Diltiazem *on page 394*
- **Rhoxal-diltiazem SR (Can)** *see* Diltiazem *on page 394*
- **Rhoxal-diltiazem T (Can)** *see* Diltiazem *on page 394*
- **Rhoxal-fluoxetine (Can)** *see* Fluoxetine *on page 539*
- **Rhoxal-minocycline (Can)** *see* Minocycline *on page 854*
- **Rhoxal-nabumetone (Can)** *see* Nabumetone *on page 883*
- **Rhoxal-pamidronate (Can)** *see* Pamidronate *on page 978*
- **Rhoxal-paroxetine (Can)** *see* Paroxetine *on page 988*
- **Rhoxal-ranitidine (Can)** *see* Ranitidine *on page 1105*
- **Rhoxal-salbutamol (Can)** *see* Albuterol *on page 50*
- **Rhoxal-sertraline (Can)** *see* Sertraline *on page 1161*
- **Rhoxal-sumatriptan (Can)** *see* Sumatriptan *on page 1222*
- **Rhoxal-ticlopidine (Can)** *see* Ticlopidine *on page 1266*
- **Rhoxal-topiramate (Can)** *see* Topiramate *on page 1287*
- **Rhoxal-valproic (Can)** *see* Valproic Acid and Derivatives *on page 1329*
- ***r*HuEPO-α** *see* Epoetin Alfa *on page 463*
- **rhuMAb-E25** *see* Omalizumab *on page 955*
- **Ribasphere™** *see* Ribavirin *on page 1116*

Ribavirin (rye ba VYE rin)

Medication Safety Issues

Sound-alike/look-alike issues:

Ribavirin may be confused with riboflavin

U.S. Brand Names Copegus®; Rebetol®; Ribasphere™; Virazole®

Canadian Brand Names Virazole®

Synonyms RTCA; Tribavirin

Pharmacologic Category Antiviral Agent

Restrictions An FDA-approved medication guide is available at http://www.fda.gov/cder/Offices/ODS/labeling.htm; distribute to each patient to whom this medication is dispensed for the treatment of hepatitis C.

Generic Available Yes: Capsule, tablet

Use

Inhalation: Treatment of patients with respiratory syncytial virus (RSV) infections; specially indicated for treatment of severe lower respiratory tract RSV infections in patients with an underlying compromising condition (prematurity, bronchopulmonary dysplasia and other chronic lung conditions, congenital heart disease, immunodeficiency, immunosuppression), and recent transplant recipients

Oral capsule:

In combination with interferon alfa-2b (Intron® A) injection for the treatment of chronic hepatitis C in patients with compensated liver disease who have relapsed after alpha interferon therapy or were previously untreated with alpha interferons

In combination with peginterferon alfa-2b (PEG-Intron®) injection for the treatment of chronic hepatitis C in patients with compensated liver disease who were previously untreated with alpha interferons

Oral solution: In combination with interferon alfa 2b (Intron® A) injection for the treatment of chronic hepatitis C in patients ≥3 years of age with compensated liver disease who were previously untreated with alpha interferons or patients ≥18 years of age who have relapsed after alpha interferon therapy

Oral tablet: In combination with peginterferon alfa-2a (Pegasys®) injection for the treatment of chronic hepatitis C in patients with compensated liver disease who were previously untreated with alpha interferons (includes patients with histological evidence of cirrhosis [Child-Pugh class A] and patients with clinically-stable HIV disease)

Unlabeled/Investigational Use Used in other viral infections including influenza A and B and adenovirus

Mechanism of Action Inhibits replication of RNA and DNA viruses; inhibits influenza virus RNA polymerase activity and inhibits the initiation and elongation of RNA fragments resulting in inhibition of viral protein synthesis

Pharmacodynamics/Kinetics

Absorption: Inhalation: Systemic; dependent upon respiratory factors and method of drug delivery; maximal absorption occurs with the use of aerosol generator via endotracheal tube; highest concentrations in respiratory tract and erythrocytes

Distribution: Oral capsule: Single dose: V_d 2825 L; distribution significantly prolonged in the erythrocyte (16-40 days), which can be used as a marker for intracellular metabolism

Protein binding: Oral: None

Metabolism: Hepatically and intracellularly (forms active metabolites); may be necessary for drug action

Bioavailability: Oral: 64%

Half-life elimination, plasma:

Children: Inhalation: 6.5-11 hours

Adults: Oral:

Capsule, single dose (Rebetol®, Ribasphere™): 24 hours in healthy adults, 44 hours with chronic hepatitis C infection (increases to ~298 hours at steady state)

Tablet, single dose (Copegus®): 120-170 hours

Time to peak, serum: Inhalation: At end of inhalation period; Oral capsule: Multiple doses: 3 hours; Tablet: 2 hours

Excretion: Inhalation: Urine (40% as unchanged drug and metabolites); Oral capsule: Urine (61%), feces (12%)

Dosage

Aerosol inhalation: Infants and children: Use with Viratek® small particle aerosol generator (SPAG-2) at a concentration of 20 mg/mL (6 g reconstituted with 300 mL of sterile water without preservatives). Continuous aerosol administration: 12-18 hours/day for 3 days, up to 7 days in length

Oral capsule or solution: Children ≥3 years: Chronic hepatitis C (in combination with interferon alfa-2b):

Rebetol®: Oral: **Note:** Oral solution should be used in children 3-5 years of age, children ≤25 kg, or those unable to swallow capsules.

Capsule/solution: 15 mg/kg/day in 2 divided doses (morning and evening)

Capsule dosing recommendations:

25-36 kg: 400 mg/day (200 mg morning and evening)

37-49 kg: 600 mg/day (200 mg in the morning and two 200 mg capsules in the evening)

50-61 kg: 800 mg/day (two 200 mg capsules morning and evening)

>61 kg: Refer to Adults dosing

Note: Duration of therapy is 48 weeks in pediatric patients with genotype 1 and 24 weeks in patients with genotype 2,3. Discontinue treatment in any patient if HCV-RNA is not below the limit of detection of the assay after 24 weeks of therapy.

Note: Also refer to Interferon Alfa-2b/Ribavirin combination pack monograph.

Oral capsule (Rebetol®, Ribasphere™): Adults:

Chronic hepatitis C (in combination with interferon alfa-2b):

≤75 kg: 400 mg in the morning, then 600 mg in the evening

>75 kg: 600 mg in the morning, then 600 mg in the evening

(Continued)

Ribavirin *(Continued)*

Note: If HCV-RNA is undetectable at 24 weeks, duration of therapy is 48 weeks. In patients who relapse following interferon therapy, duration of dual therapy is 24 weeks.

Note: Also refer to Interferon Alfa-2b/Ribavirin combination pack monograph.

Chronic hepatitis C (in combination with peginterferon alfa-2b): 400 mg twice daily; duration of therapy is 1 year; after 24 weeks of treatment, if serum HCV-RNA is not below the limit of detection of the assay, consider discontinuation.

Oral tablet (Copegus®, in combination with peginterferon alfa-2b): Adults: Chronic hepatitis C:

Monoinfection, genotype 1,4:

<75kg: 1000 mg/day in 2 divided doses for 48 weeks

≥75kg: 1200 mg/day in 2 divided doses for 48 weeks

Monoinfection, genotype 2,3: 800 mg/day in 2 divided doses for 24 weeks

Coinfection with HIV: 800 mg/day in 2 divided doses for 48 weeks

Note: Also refer to Peginterferon Alfa-2a monograph.

Dosage adjustment in renal impairment: Cl_{cr} <50 mL/minute: Oral route is contraindicated

Dosage adjustment for toxicity: Oral: Capsule, solution, tablet:

Patient **without** cardiac history:

Hemoglobin <10 g/dL:

Children: 7.5 mg/kg/day

Adults: Decrease dose to 600 mg/day

Hemoglobin <8.5 g/dL: Children and Adults: Permanently discontinue treatment

Patient **with** cardiac history:

Hemoglobin has decreased ≥2 g/dL during any 4-week period of treatment:

Children: 7.5 mg/kg/day

Adults: Decrease dose to 600 mg/day

Hemoglobin <12 g/dL after 4 weeks of reduced dose: Children and Adults: Permanently discontinue treatment

Stability

Inhalation: Store vials in a dry place at 15°C to 25°C (59°F to 78°F). Do not use any water containing an antimicrobial agent to reconstitute drug; reconstituted solution is stable for 24 hours at room temperature. Should not be mixed with other aerosolized medication.

Oral: Store at 15°C to 30°C (59°F to 86°F). Solution may also be refrigerated at 2°C to 8°C (36°F to 46°F).

Administration

Inhalation: Ribavirin should be administered in well-ventilated rooms (at least 6 air changes/hour). In mechanically-ventilated patients, ribavirin can potentially be deposited in the ventilator delivery system depending on temperature, humidity, and electrostatic forces; this deposition can lead to malfunction or obstruction of the expiratory valve, resulting in inadvertently high positive end-expiratory pressures. The use of one-way valves in the inspiratory lines, a breathing circuit filter in the expiratory line, and frequent monitoring and filter replacement have been effective in preventing these problems. Solutions in SPAG-2 unit should be discarded at least every 24 hours and when the liquid level is low before adding newly reconstituted solution. Should not be mixed with other aerosolized medication.

Oral: Administer concurrently with interferon alfa injection. Capsule should not be opened, crushed, chewed, or broken. Capsules are not for use in children <5 years of age. Use oral solution for children 3-5 years, those ≤25 kg, or those who cannot swallow capsules.

Capsule, in combination with interferon alfa-2b: May be administered with or without food, but always in a consistent manner in regard to food intake.

Capsule, in combination with peginterferon alfa 2b: Administer with food.

Solution, in combination with interferon alfa-2b: May be administered with or without food, but always in a consistent manner in regard to food intake.

Tablet: Should be administered with food.

Monitoring Parameters

Inhalation: Respiratory function, hemoglobin, reticulocyte count, CBC, I & O

Oral: CBC with differential (pretreatment, 2- and 4 weeks after initiation); pretreatment and monthly pregnancy test for women of childbearing age; LFTs, TSH,

HCV-RNA after 24 weeks of therapy; ECG in patients with pre-existing cardiac disease

Pregnancy Risk Factor X

Contraindications Hypersensitivity to ribavirin or any component of the formulation; women of childbearing age who will not use contraception reliably; pregnancy

Additional contraindications for oral formulation: Male partners of pregnant women; Cl_{cr}< 50 mL/minute; hemoglobinopathies (eg, thalassemia major, sickle cell anemia); as monotherapy for treatment of chronic hepatitis C; patients with autoimmune hepatitis, anemia, severe heart disease

Refer to individual monographs for Interferon Alfa-2b (Intron® A) and Peginterferon Alfa-2a (Pegasys®) for additional contraindication information.

Warnings/Precautions [U.S. Boxed Warning]: Negative pregnancy test is required before initiation and monthly thereafter. Avoid pregnancy in female patients and female partners of male patients, during therapy, and for at least 6 months after treatment; two forms of contraception should be used. Elderly patients are more susceptible to adverse effects; use caution. Safety and efficacy have not been established in patients who have failed other alpha interferon therapy, received organ transplants, or been coinfected with hepatitis B or HIV (Copegus® may be used in HIV coinfected patients unless CD4+ cell count is <100 cells/microL). **[U.S. Boxed Warning]: Monotherapy not effective for chronic hepatitis C infection.** Safety and efficacy have not been established in patients <3 years of age.

Inhalation: **[U.S. Boxed Warning]: Use with caution in patients requiring assisted ventilation because precipitation of the drug in the respiratory equipment may interfere with safe and effective patient ventilation; sudden deterioration of respiratory function has been observed;** monitor carefully in patients with COPD and asthma for deterioration of respiratory function. Ribavirin is potentially mutagenic, tumor-promoting, and gonadotoxic. Although anemia has not been reported with inhalation therapy, consider monitoring for anemia 1-2 weeks post-treatment. Pregnant healthcare workers may consider unnecessary occupational exposure; ribavirin has been detected in healthcare workers' urine. Healthcare professionals or family members who are pregnant (or may become pregnant) should be counseled about potential risks of exposure and counseled about risk reduction strategies.

Oral: Severe psychiatric events have occurred including depression and suicidal behavior during combination therapy. Avoid use in patients with a psychiatric history; discontinue if severe psychiatric symptoms occur. **[U.S. Boxed Warning]: Hemolytic anemia is a significant toxicity; usually occurring within 1-2 weeks.** Assess cardiac disease before initiation. Anemia may worsen underlying cardiac disease; use caution. If any deterioration in cardiovascular status occurs, discontinue therapy. Use caution in pulmonary disease; pulmonary symptoms have been associated with administration. Discontinue therapy in suspected/confirmed pancreatitis or if hepatic decompensation occurs. Use caution in patients with sarcoidosis (exacerbation reported).

Hemolytic anemia (hemoglobin <10 g/dL) was observed in up to 10% of treated patients in clinical trials when alfa interferons were combined with ribavirin; anemia occurred within 1-2 weeks of initiation of therapy.

Adverse Reactions

Inhalation:

1% to 10%:

Central nervous system: Fatigue, headache, insomnia

Gastrointestinal: Nausea, anorexia

Hematologic: Anemia

<1%: Hypotension, cardiac arrest, digitalis toxicity, conjunctivitis, mild bronchospasm, worsening of respiratory function, apnea

Note: Incidence of adverse effects (approximate) in healthcare workers: Headache (51%); conjunctivitis (32%); rhinitis, nausea, rash, dizziness, pharyngitis, and lacrimation (10% to 20%)

Oral (all adverse reactions are documented while receiving combination therapy with interferon alpha-2b or interferon alpha-2a; percentages as reported in adults):

>10%:

Central nervous system: Fatigue (60% to 70%)*, headache (43% to 66%)*, fever (32% to 46%)*, insomnia (26% to 41%), depression (20% to 36%)*,

(Continued)

Ribavirin *(Continued)*

irritability (23% to 32%), dizziness (14% to 26%), impaired concentration (10% to 14%)*, emotional lability (7% to 12%)*

Dermatologic: Alopecia (27% to 36%), pruritus (13% to 29%), dry skin (13% to 24%), rash (5% to 28%), dermatitis (up to 16%)

Gastrointestinal: Nausea (33% to 47%), anorexia (21% to 32%), weight decrease (10% to 29%), diarrhea (10% to 22%), dyspepsia (8% to 16%), vomiting (9% to 14%)*, abdominal pain (8% to 13%), xerostomia (up to 12%), RUQ pain (up to 12%)

Hematologic: Neutropenia (8% to 27%; 40% with HIV coinfection), hemoglobin decreased (25% to 36%), hyperbilirubinemia (24% to 34%), anemia (11% to 17%), lymphopenia (12% to 14%), absolute neutrophil count <0.5 x 10^9/L (5% to 11%), thrombocytopenia (<1% to 14%), hemolytic anemia (10% to 13%), WBC decreased

Neuromuscular & skeletal: Myalgia (40% to 64%)*, rigors (40% to 48%), arthralgia (22% to 34%)*, musculoskeletal pain (19% to 28%)

Respiratory: Dyspnea (13% to 26%), cough (7% to 23%), pharyngitis (up to 13%), sinusitis (up to 12%)*, nasal congestion

Miscellaneous: Flu-like syndrome (13% to 18%)*, viral infection (up to 12%), diaphoresis increased (up to 11%)

*Similar to interferon alone

1% to 10%:

Cardiovascular: Chest pain (5% to 9%)*, flushing (up to 4%)

Central nervous system: Mood alteration (up to 6%; 9% with HIV coinfection), memory impairment (up to 6%), malaise (up to 6%), nervousness (~5%)*

Dermatologic: Eczema (4% to 5%)

Endocrine & metabolic: Hypothyroidism (up to 5%)

Gastrointestinal: Taste perversion (4% to 9%), constipation (up to 5%)

Genitourinary: Menstrual disorder (up to 7%)

Hepatic: Hepatomegaly (up to 4%)

Neuromuscular & skeletal: Weakness (9% to 10%), back pain (5%)

Ocular: Conjunctivitis (up to 6%), blurred vision (up to 5%)

Respiratory: Rhinitis (up to 8%), exertional dyspnea (up to 7%)

Miscellaneous: Fungal infection (up to 6%)

*Similar to interferon alone

<1% (Limited to important or life-threatening): Aggression, angina, anxiety, aplastic anemia, arrhythmia; autoimmune disorders (systemic lupus erythematosus, rheumatoid arthritis, sarcoidosis); cerebreal hemorrhage, cholangitis, colitis, coma, diabetes mellitus, fatty liver, gastrointestinal bleeding, gout, hepatic dysfunction, hyper-/hypothyroidism, myositis, pancreatitis, peptic ulcer, peripheral neuropathy, psychosis, pulmonary dysfunction, pulmonary embolism, suicidal ideation, suicide, thrombotic thrombocytopenic purpura, thyroid function test abnormalities

Note: Incidence of anorexia, headache, fever, suicidal ideation, and vomiting are higher in children.

Overdosage/Toxicology Treatment is symptom-directed and supportive. Not effectively removed by hemodialysis.

Drug Interactions

Antiretroviral (nucleoside): Concomitant use of ribavirin and nucleoside analogues may increase the risk of developing lactic acidosis (includes adefovir, didanosine, lamivudine, stavudine, zalcitabine, zidovudine). Concurrent use with didanosine has been noted to increase the risk of pancreatitis, peripheral neuropathy in addition to lactic acidosis. Suspend therapy if signs/symptoms of toxicity are present.

Interferons (alfa): Concurrent therapy may increase the risk of hemolytic anemia.

Lamivudine, stavudine: Antagonistic *in vitro*; use with caution (per manufacturer)

Zidovudine: Antagonistic *in vitro*; use with caution (per manufacturer). Concurrent therapy with ribavirin/interferon alfa-2a may cause increased risk of severe anemia and/or severe neutropenia.

Ethanol/Nutrition/Herb Interactions Food: Oral: High-fat meal increases the AUC and C_{max}.

Dietary Considerations When used in combination with interferon alfa-2b, capsules and solution may be taken with or without food, but always in a consistent manner in regard to food intake (ie, always take with food or always take on an empty stomach). When used in combination with peginterferon alfa 2b, capsules should be taken with food. Tablets should be taken with food.

Dosage Forms

Capsule (Rebetol®, Ribasphere™): 200 mg

Powder for aerosol (Virazole®): 6 g

Powder for solution, inhalation [for aerosol administration] (Virazole®): 6 g [reconstituted product provides 20 mg/mL]

Tablet (Copegus®): 200 mg

◆ **Rifadin®** *see* Rifampin *on page 1121*

◆ **Rifampicin** *see* Rifampin *on page 1121*

Rifampin (RIF am pin)

Medication Safety Issues

Sound-alike/look-alike issues:

Rifampin may be confused with rifabutin, Rifamate®, rifapentine, rifaximin

Rifadin® may be confused with Ritalin®

U.S. Brand Names Rifadin®

Canadian Brand Names Rifadin®; Rofact™

Synonyms Rifampicin

Pharmacologic Category Antibiotic, Miscellaneous; Antitubercular Agent

Generic Available Yes

Use Management of active tuberculosis in combination with other agents; elimination of meningococci from the nasopharynx in asymptomatic carriers

Unlabeled/Investigational Use Prophylaxis of *Haemophilus influenzae* type b infection; *Legionella* pneumonia; used in combination with other anti-infectives in the treatment of staphylococcal infections; treatment of *M. leprae* infections

Mechanism of Action Inhibits bacterial RNA synthesis by binding to the beta subunit of DNA-dependent RNA polymerase, blocking RNA transcription

Pharmacodynamics/Kinetics

Duration: ≤24 hours

Absorption: Oral: Well absorbed; food may delay or slightly reduce peak

Distribution: Highly lipophilic; crosses blood-brain barrier well

Relative diffusion from blood into CSF: Adequate with or without inflammation (exceeds usual MICs)

CSF:blood level ratio: Inflamed meninges: 25%

Protein binding: 80%

Metabolism: Hepatic; undergoes enterohepatic recirculation

Half-life elimination: 3-4 hours; prolonged with hepatic impairment; End-stage renal disease: 1.8-11 hours

Time to peak, serum: Oral: 2-4 hours

Excretion: Feces (60% to 65%) and urine (~30%) as unchanged drug

Dosage Oral (I.V. infusion dose is the same as for the oral route):

Tuberculosis therapy (drug susceptible): Note: A four-drug regimen (isoniazid, rifampin, pyrazinamide, and ethambutol) is preferred for the initial, empiric treatment of TB. When the drug susceptibility results are available, the regimen should be altered as appropriate.

Infants and Children <12 years:

Daily therapy: 10-20 mg/kg/day usually as a single dose (maximum: 600 mg/day)

Twice weekly directly observed therapy (DOT): 10-20 mg/kg (maximum: 600 mg)

Adults:

Daily therapy: 10 mg/kg/day (maximum: 600 mg/day)

Twice weekly directly observed therapy (DOT): 10 mg/kg (maximum: 600 mg); 3 times/week: 10 mg/kg (maximum: 600 mg)

Latent tuberculosis infection (LTBI): As an alternative to isoniazid:

Children: 10-20 mg/kg/day (maximum: 600 mg/day) for 6 months

Adults: 10 mg/kg/day (maximum: 600 mg/day) for 4 months. **Note:** Combination with pyrazinamide should not generally be offered (*MMWR*, Aug 8, 2003).

H. influenzae **prophylaxis (unlabeled use):**

Infants and Children: 20 mg/kg/day every 24 hours for 4 days, not to exceed 600 mg/dose

Adults: 600 mg every 24 hours for 4 days

Leprosy (unlabeled use): Adults:

Multibacillary: 600 mg once monthly for 24 months in combination with ofloxacin and minocycline

Paucibacillary: 600 mg once monthly for 6 months in combination with dapsone

(Continued)

Rifampin *(Continued)*

Single lesion: 600 mg as a single dose in combination with ofloxacin 400 mg and minocycline 100 mg

Meningococcal meningitis prophylaxis:

Infants <1 month: 10 mg/kg/day in divided doses every 12 hours for 2 days

Infants ≥1 month and Children: 20 mg/kg/day in divided doses every 12 hours for 2 days (maximum: 600 mg/dose)

Meningitis *(Pneumococcus* or *Staphylococcus):* I.V.: Adults: 600 mg once daily

Adults: 600 mg every 12 hours for 2 days

Nasal carriers of *Staphylococcus aureus* (unlabeled use):

Children: 15 mg/kg/day divided every 12 hours for 5-10 days in combination with other antibiotics

Adults: 600 mg/day for 5-10 days in combination with other antibiotics

Synergy for *Staphylococcus aureus* infections (unlabeled use): Adults: 300-600 mg twice daily with other antibiotics

Dosing adjustment in hepatic impairment: Dose reductions may be necessary to reduce hepatotoxicity

Hemodialysis or peritoneal dialysis: Plasma rifampin concentrations are not significantly affected by hemodialysis or peritoneal dialysis.

Stability Rifampin powder is reddish brown. Intact vials should be stored at room temperature and protected from excessive heat and light. Reconstitute powder for injection with SWFI; prior to injection, dilute in appropriate volume of compatible diluent (eg, 100 mL D_5W). Reconstituted vials are stable for 24 hours at room temperature

Stability of parenteral admixture at room temperature (25°C) is 4 hours for D_5W and 24 hours for NS

Administration

I.V.: Administer I.V. preparation once daily by slow I.V. infusion over 30 minutes to 3 hours at a final concentration not to exceed 6 mg/mL.

Oral: Administer on an empty stomach (ie, 1 hour prior to, or 2 hours after meals or antacids) to increase total absorption. The compounded oral suspension must be shaken well before using. May mix contents of capsule with applesauce or jelly.

Monitoring Parameters Periodic (baseline and every 2-4 weeks during therapy) monitoring of liver function (AST, ALT, bilirubin), CBC; hepatic status and mental status, sputum culture, chest x-ray 2-3 months into treatment

Anesthesia and Critical Care Concerns/Other Considerations Rifampin causes body secretions to turn orange and may stain contact lenses.

Pregnancy Risk Factor C

Contraindications Hypersensitivity to rifampin, any rifamycins, or any component of the formulation; concurrent use of amprenavir, saquinavir/ritonavir (possibly other protease inhibitors)

Warnings/Precautions Use with caution and modify dosage in patients with liver impairment; observe for hyperbilirubinemia; discontinue therapy if this in conjunction with clinical symptoms or any signs of significant hepatocellular damage develop; since rifampin has enzyme-inducing properties, porphyria exacerbation is possible; use with caution in patients with porphyria; do not use for meningococcal disease, only for short-term treatment of asymptomatic carrier states. Use with caution in patients receiving concurrent medications associated with hepatotoxicity (particularly with pyrazinamide), or in patients with a history of alcoholism (even if ethanol consumption is discontinued during therapy).

Monitor for compliance and effects including hypersensitivity, thrombocytopenia in patients on intermittent therapy; urine, feces, saliva, sweat, tears, and CSF may be discolored to red/orange; do not administer I.V. form via I.M. or SubQ routes; restart infusion at another site if extravasation occurs; remove soft contact lenses during therapy since permanent staining may occur; regimens of 600 mg once or twice weekly have been associated with a high incidence of adverse reactions including a flu-like syndrome.

Adverse Reactions

Frequency not defined:

Cardiovascular: Edema, flushing

Central nervous system: Ataxia, behavioral changes, concentration impaired, confusion, dizziness, drowsiness, fatigue, fever, headache, numbness, psychosis

Dermatologic: Pemphigoid reaction, pruritus, urticaria
Endocrine & metabolic: Adrenal insufficiency, menstrual disorders
Hematologic: Agranulocytosis (rare), DIC, eosinophilia, hemoglobin decreased, hemolysis, hemolytic anemia, leukopenia, thrombocytopenia (especially with high-dose therapy)
Hepatic: Hepatitis (rare), jaundice
Neuromuscular & skeletal: Myalgia, osteomalacia, weakness
Ocular: Exudative conjunctivitis, visual changes
Renal: Acute renal failure, BUN increased, hemoglobinuria, hematuria, interstitial nephritis, uric acid increased
Miscellaneous: Flu-like syndrome

1% to 10%:
Dermatologic: Rash (1% to 5%)
Gastrointestinal (1% to 2%): Anorexia, cramps, diarrhea, epigastric distress, flatulence, heartburn, nausea, pseudomembranous colitis, pancreatitis vomiting
Hepatic: LFTs increased (up to 14%)

Overdosage/Toxicology Symptoms of overdose include nausea, vomiting, hepatotoxicity, lethargy, discoloration of bodily fluids, skin, and/or feces, and CNS depression. Treatment is supportive. Plasma rifampin concentrations are not significantly affected by hemodialysis or peritoneal dialysis.

Drug Interactions **Induces** CYP1A2 (strong), 2A6 (strong), 2B6 (strong), 2C8 (strong), 2C9 (strong), 2C19 (strong), 3A4 (strong)

Acetaminophen: Rifampin may increase the metabolism of acetaminophen.
Alfentanil: Rifamycin derivatives may increase the metabolism, via CYP isoenzymes, of alfentanil.
Amiodarone: Rifamycin derivatives may increase the metabolism, via CYP isoenzymes, of amiodarone
Angiotensin II receptor blockers (irbesartan, losartan): Rifamycin derivatives may increase the metabolism, via CYP isoenzymes, of angiotensin II receptor blockers.
Antiemetics (5-HT_3 antagonists): Rifamycin derivatives may increase the metabolism, via CYP isoenzymes, of antiemetics (5-HT_3 antagonists).
Antifungal Agents (imidazole): Rifamycin derivatives may increase the metabolism, via CYP isoenzymes, of antifungal agents (imidazole).
Aprepitant: Rifamycin derivatives may increase the metabolism, via CYP isoenzymes, of aprepitant.
Barbiturates: Rifamycin derivatives may increase the metabolism, via CYP isoenzymes, of barbiturates.
Benzodiazepines (metabolized by oxidation): Rifamycin derivatives may increase the metabolism, via CYP isoenzymes, of benzodiazepines (metabolized by oxidation).
Beta-blockers: Rifamycin derivatives may increase the metabolism, via CYP isoenzymes, of beta-blockers.
Buspirone: Rifamycin derivatives may increase the metabolism, via CYP isoenzymes, of buspirone.
Calcium channel blockers: Rifamycin derivatives may increase the metabolism, via CYP isoenzymes, of calcium channel blockers.
Chloramphenicol: Rifampin may increase the metabolism, via CYP isoenzymes, of chloramphenicol.
Clopidogrel: Rifamycin derivatives may enhance the therapeutic effect of Clopidogrel.
Corticosteroids (systemic): Rifamycin derivatives may increase the metabolism, via CYP isoenzymes, of corticosteroids (systemic).
Cyclosporine: Rifamycin derivatives may increase the metabolism, via CYP isoenzymes, of cyclosporine.
CYP1A2 substrates: Rifampin may decrease the levels/effects of CYP1A2 substrates. Example substrates include aminophylline, estrogens, fluvoxamine, mirtazapine, ropinirole, and theophylline.
CYP2A6 substrates: Rifampin may decrease the levels/effects of CYP2A6 substrates (eg, ifosfamide).
CYP2B6 substrates: Rifampin may decrease the levels/effects of CYP2B6 substrates. Example substrates include bupropion, efavirenz, promethazine, selegiline, and sertraline.
CYP2C8 substrates: Rifampin may decrease the levels/effects of CYP2C8 substrates. Example substrates include amiodarone, paclitaxel, pioglitazone, repaglinide, and rosiglitazone.

(Continued)

Rifampin *(Continued)*

CYP2C9 substrates: Rifampin may decrease the levels/effects of CYP2C9 substrates. Example substrates include bosentan, celecoxib, dapsone, fluoxetine, glimepiride, glipizide, losartan, montelukast, nateglinide, paclitaxel, phenytoin, sulfonamides, trimethoprim, warfarin, and zafirlukast.

CYP2C19 substrates: Rifampin may decrease the levels/effects of CYP2C19 substrates. Example substrates include citalopram, diazepam, methsuximide, phenytoin, propranolol, proton pump inhibitors, sertraline, and voriconazole.

CYP3A4 substrates: Rifampin may decrease the levels/effects of CYP3A4 substrates. Example substrates include benzodiazepines, calcium channel blockers, clarithromycin, cyclosporine, erythromycin, estrogens, mirtazapine, nateglinide, nefazodone, nevirapine, protease inhibitors, tacrolimus, and venlafaxine.

Dapsone: Rifamycin derivatives may increase the metabolism, via CYP isoenzymes, of dapsone.

Disopyramide: Rifamycin derivatives may increase the metabolism, via CYP isoenzymes, of disopyramide.

Estrogens (oral contraceptives): Rifamycin derivatives may decrease the serum concentration of oral contraceptive (estrogens); contraceptive failure is possible.

Fexofenadine: Rifampin may decrease the serum concentration of fexofenadine.

Fluconazole: Rifamycin derivatives may increase the metabolism, via CYP isoenzymes, of fluconazole.

Fusidic Acid: Rifampin may decrease the excretion of fusidic acid.

Gefitinib: Rifamycin derivatives may increase the metabolism, via CYP isoenzymes, of gefitinib.

HMG-CoA reductase inhibitors: Rifamycin derivatives may increase the metabolism, via CYP isoenzymes, of HMG-CoA reductase inhibitors.

Isoniazid: Rifamycin derivatives may enhance the hepatotoxic effect of isoniazid; however, this is a frequently employed combination regimen.

Macrolide antibiotics: Macrolide antibiotics may decrease the metabolism, via CYP isoenzymes, of rifamycin derivatives.

Methadone: Rifamycin derivatives may increase the metabolism, via CYP isoenzymes, of methadone.

Morphine: Rifamycin derivatives may decrease the serum concentration of morphine sulfate.

Phenytoin: Rifamycin derivatives may increase the metabolism, via CYP isoenzymes, of phenytoin.

Progestins (contraceptives): Rifamycin derivatives may decrease the serum concentration of contraceptive (progestins); contraceptive failure is possible.

Propafenone: Rifamycin derivatives may increase the metabolism, via CYP isoenzymes, of propafenone.

Protease inhibitors: Rifamycin derivatives may increase the metabolism, via CYP isoenzymes, of protease inhibitors. Concurrent use with saquinavir/ritonavir increases risk of hepatotoxicity. Rifampin administration should be avoided.

Pyrazinamide: Pyrazinamide may enhance the hepatotoxic effect of rifampin.

Quinidine: Rifamycin derivatives may increase the metabolism, via CYP isoenzymes, of quinidine.

Repaglinide: Rifamycin derivatives may increase the metabolism, via CYP isoenzymes, of repaglinide.

Reverse transcriptase inhibitors (non-nucleoside): Rifamycin derivatives may increase the metabolism, via CYP isoenzymes, of reverse transcriptase inhibitors (non-nucleoside).

Sulfonylureas: Rifampin may increase the metabolism, via CYP isoenzymes, of sulfonylureas.

Tacrolimus: Rifamycin derivatives may increase the metabolism, via CYP isoenzymes, of tacrolimus.

Tamoxifen: Rifamycin derivatives may increase the metabolism, via CYP isoenzymes, of tamoxifen.

Terbinafine: Rifamycin derivatives may increase the metabolism of terbinafine.

Tocainide: Rifamycin derivatives may increase the metabolism, via CYP isoenzymes, of tocainide.

Tricyclic antidepressants: Rifamycin derivatives may increase the metabolism, via CYP isoenzymes, of tricyclic antidepressants.

Warfarin: Rifamycin derivatives may increase the metabolism, via CYP isoenzymes, of warfarin.

Zaleplon: Rifamycin derivatives may increase the metabolism, via CYP isoenzymes, of zaleplon.
Zidovudine: Rifamycin derivatives may increase the metabolism, via CYP isoenzymes, of zidovudine.
Zolpidem: Rifamycin derivatives may increase the metabolism, via CYP isoenzymes, of zolpidem.

Ethanol/Nutrition/Herb Interactions

Ethanol: Avoid ethanol (may increase risk of hepatotoxicity).
Food: Food decreases the extent of absorption; rifampin concentrations may be decreased if taken with food.
Herb/Nutraceutical: St John's wort may decrease rifampin levels.

Test Interactions Positive Coombs' reaction [direct], rifampin inhibits standard assay's ability to measure serum folate and B_{12}; transient increase in LFTs and decreased biliary excretion of contrast media

Dietary Considerations Rifampin should be taken on an empty stomach.

Dosage Forms

Capsule: 150 mg, 300 mg
Injection, powder for reconstitution: 600 mg

References

Tunkel AR, Hartman BJ, Kaplan SL, et al, "Practice Guidelines for the Management of Bacterial Meningitis," *Clin Infect Dis*, 2004, 39(9):1267-84.

- **RIG** *see* Rabies Immune Globulin (Human) *on page 1100*
- **Riomet™** *see* Metformin *on page 810*
- **Risperdal®** *see* Risperidone *on page 1125*
- **Risperdal® M-Tab®** *see* Risperidone *on page 1125*
- **Risperdal® Consta™** *see* Risperidone *on page 1125*

Risperidone (ris PER i done)

Medication Safety Issues

Sound-alike/look-alike issues:
Risperidone may be confused with reserpine
Risperdal® may be confused with lisinopril, reserpine

U.S. Brand Names Risperdal®; Risperdal® Consta™; Risperdal® M-Tab®

Canadian Brand Names Risperdal®; Risperdal® Consta™; Risperdal® M-Tab®

Synonyms Risperdal M-Tab®

Pharmacologic Category Antipsychotic Agent, Atypical

Generic Available No

Use Treatment of schizophrenia; treatment of acute mania or mixed episodes associated with bipolar I disorder (as monotherapy or in combination with lithium or valproate)

Unlabeled/Investigational Use Behavioral symptoms associated with dementia in elderly; treatment of Tourette's disorder; treatment of pervasive developmental disorder and autism in children and adolescents

Mechanism of Action Risperidone is a benzisoxazole atypical antipsychotic with mixed serotonin-dopamine antagonist activity that binds to 5-HT_2-receptors in the CNS and in the periphery with a very high affinity; binds to dopamine-D_2 receptors with less affinity. The binding affinity to the dopamine-D_2 receptor is 20 times lower than the 5-HT_2 affinity. The addition of serotonin antagonism to dopamine antagonism (classic neuroleptic mechanism) is thought to improve negative symptoms of psychoses and reduce the incidence of extrapyramidal side effects. $Alpha_1$, $alpha_2$ adrenergic, and histaminergic receptors are also antagonized with high affinity. Risperidone has low to moderate affinity for 5-HT_{1C}, 5-HT_{1D}, and 5-HT_{1A} receptors, weak affinity for D_1 and no affinity for muscarinics or $beta_1$ and $beta_2$ receptors

Pharmacodynamics/Kinetics

Absorption:
Oral: Rapid and well absorbed; food does not affect rate or extent
Injection: <1% absorbed initially; main release occurs at ~3 weeks and is maintained from 4-6 weeks

Distribution: V_d: 1-2 L/kg
Protein binding, plasma: Risperidone 90%; 9-hydroxyrisperidone: 77%
Metabolism: Extensively hepatic via CYP2D6 to 9-hydroxyrisperidone (similar pharmacological activity as risperidone); *N*-dealkylation is a second minor pathway

(Continued)

Risperidone *(Continued)*

Bioavailability: Solution: 70%; Tablet: 66%; orally-disintegrating tablets and oral solution are bioequivalent to tablets

Half-life elimination: Active moiety (risperidone and its active metabolite 9-hydroxyrisperidone)

Oral: 20 hours (mean)

Extensive metabolizers: Risperidone: 3 hours; 9-hydroxyrisperidone: 21 hours

Poor metabolizers: Risperidone: 20 hours; 9-hydroxyrisperidone: 30 hours

Injection: 3-6 days; related to microsphere erosion and subsequent absorption of risperidone

Time to peak, plasma: Oral: Risperidone: Within 1 hour; 9-hydroxyrisperidone: Extensive metabolizers: 3 hours; Poor metabolizers: 17 hours

Excretion: Urine (70%); feces (15%)

Dosage

Oral:

Children and Adolescents:

Pervasive developmental disorder (unlabeled use): Initial: 0.25 mg twice daily; titrate up 0.25 mg/day every 5-7 days; optimal dose range: 0.75-3 mg/day

Autism (unlabeled use): Initial: 0.25 mg at bedtime; titrate to 1 mg/day (0.1 mg/kg/day)

Schizophrenia (unlabeled use): Initial: 0.5 mg once or twice daily; titrate as necessary up to 2-6 mg/day

Bipolar disorder (unlabeled use): Initial: 0.5 mg; titrate to 0.5-3 mg/day

Tourette's disorder (unlabeled use): Initial: 0.5 mg; titrate to 2-4 mg/day

Adults:

Schizophrenia:

Initial: 1 mg twice daily; may be increased by 2 mg/day to a target dose of 6 mg/day; usual range: 4-8 mg/day; may be given as a single daily dose once maintenance dose is achieved; daily dosages >6 mg do not appear to confer any additional benefit, and the incidence of extrapyramidal symptoms is higher than with lower doses. Further dose adjustments should be made in increments/decrements of 1-2 mg/day on a weekly basis. Dose range studied in clinical trials: 4-16 mg/day.

Maintenance: Target dose: 4 mg once daily (range 2-8 mg/day)

Bipolar mania:

Initial: 2-3 mg once daily; if needed, adjust dose by 1 mg/day in intervals ≥24 hours; dosing range: 1-6 mg/day

Maintenance: No dosing recommendation available for treatment >3 weeks duration.

Elderly: A starting dose of 0.5 mg twice daily, and titration should progress slowly in increments of no more than 0.5 mg twice daily; increases to dosages >1.5 mg twice daily should occur at intervals of ≥1 week.

Additional monitoring of renal function and orthostatic blood pressure may be warranted. If once-a-day dosing in the elderly or debilitated patient is considered, a twice daily regimen should be used to titrate to the target dose, and this dose should be maintained for 2-3 days prior to attempts to switch to a once-daily regimen.

I.M.: Adults: Schizophrenia (Risperdal® Consta™): 25 mg every 2 weeks; some patients may benefit from larger doses; maximum dose not to exceed 50 mg every 2 weeks. Dosage adjustments should not be made more frequently than every 4 weeks.

Note: Oral risperidone (or other antipsychotic) should be administered with the initial injection of Risperdal® Consta™ and continued for 3 weeks (then discontinued) to maintain adequate therapeutic plasma concentrations prior to main release phase of risperidone from injection site. When switching from depot administration to a short-acting formulation, administer short-acting agent in place of the next regularly-scheduled depot injection.

Dosing adjustment in renal impairment: Oral: Starting dose of 0.5 mg twice daily; clearance of the active moiety is decreased by 60% in patients with moderate to severe renal disease compared to healthy subjects.

Dosing adjustment in hepatic impairment: Oral: Starting dose of 0.5 mg twice daily; the mean free fraction of risperidone in plasma was increased by 35% compared to healthy subjects.

Stability

Injection: Risperdal® Consta™: Store in refrigerator at 2°C to 8°C (36°F to 46°F) and protect from light. May be stored at room temperature of 25°C (77°F) for up to 7 days prior to administration. Bring to room temperature prior to reconstitution. Reconstitute with provided diluent only. Shake vigorously to mix; will form thick, milky suspension. Following reconstitution, store at room temperature and use within 6 hours. If suspension settles prior to use, shake vigorously to resuspend.

Oral solution, tablet: Store at 15°C to 25°C (59°F to 77°F). Protect from light and moisture. Keep orally disintegrating tablets sealed in foil pouch until ready to use.

Administration

Oral: Oral solution can be mixed with water, coffee, orange juice, or low-fat milk, but is **not compatible** with cola or tea. May be administered with or without food.

Risperdal® M-Tabs™ should not be removed from blister pack until administered. Using dry hands, place immediately on tongue. Tablet will dissolve within seconds, and may be swallowed with or without liquid. Do not split or chew.

I.M.: Risperdal® Consta™ should be administered into the upper outer quadrant of the gluteal area. Injection should alternate between the two buttocks. Do not combine two different dosage strengths into one single administration. Do not substitute any components of the dose-pack; administer with needle provided.

Monitoring Parameters Vital signs; fasting lipid profile and fasting blood glucose/Hgb A_{1c} (prior to treatment, at 3 months, then annually); BMI, personal/family history of obesity, waist circumference; blood pressure; mental status, abnormal involuntary movement scale (AIMS), extrapyramidal symptoms; orthostatic blood pressure changes for 3-5 days after starting or increasing dose. Weight should be assessed prior to treatment, at 4 weeks, 8 weeks, 12 weeks, and then at quarterly intervals. Consider titrating to a different antipsychotic agent for a weight gain ≥5% of the initial weight.

Anesthesia and Critical Care Concerns/Other Considerations Risperidone may cause orthostatic hypotension and tachycardia but to a degree which may be less than is seen with other agents (eg, phenothiazines: chlorpromazine, thioridazine). Risperidone may also prolong the QT interval. For these reasons, patient's with cardiovascular disease should be monitored closely while on therapy.

Temazepam (30 mg) can be used to treat risperidone-induced insomnia.

Pregnancy Risk Factor C

Contraindications Hypersensitivity to risperidone or any component of the formulation

Warnings/Precautions [U.S. Boxed Warning]: Elderly patients with dementia-related behavioral disorders treated with atypical antipsychotics are at an increased risk of cerebrovascular adverse events and death compared to placebo; risk may be increased with dehydration (increased risk of death observed with concurrent furosemide). Risperidone is not approved for the treatment of dementia-related psychosis.

Low to moderately sedating, use with caution in disorders where CNS depression is a feature. Use with caution in Parkinson's disease. Caution in patients with hemodynamic instability; bone marrow suppression; predisposition to seizures; subcortical brain damage; severe cardiac, hepatic, or respiratory disease. Use with caution in renal or hepatic dysfunction; dose reduction recommended. Esophageal dysmotility and aspiration have been associated with antipsychotic use; use with caution in patients at risk of aspiration pneumonia (ie, Alzheimer's disease). Caution in breast cancer or other prolactin-dependent tumors (elevates prolactin levels). May alter temperature regulation or mask toxicity of other drugs due to antiemetic effects.

May cause orthostasis. Use with caution in patients with cardiovascular diseases (eg, heart failure, history of myocardial infarction or ischemia, cerebrovascular disease, conduction abnormalities). Use caution in patients receiving medications for hypertension (orthostatic effects may be exacerbated) or in patients with hypovolemia or dehydration. May alter cardiac conduction (low risk relative to other neuroleptics); life-threatening arrhythmias have occurred with therapeutic doses of neuroleptics.

(Continued)

Risperidone *(Continued)*

May cause anticholinergic effects (confusion, agitation, constipation, xerostomia, blurred vision, urinary retention); therefore, they should be used with caution in patients with decreased gastrointestinal motility, urinary retention, BPH, xerostomia, or visual problems. Conditions which also may be exacerbated by cholinergic blockade include narrow-angle glaucoma (screening is recommended) and worsening of myasthenia gravis. Relative to other neuroleptics, risperidone has a low potency of cholinergic blockade.

May cause extrapyramidal symptoms, including pseudoparkinsonism, acute dystonic reactions, akathisia, and tardive dyskinesia (risk of these reactions is low relative to other neuroleptics, and is dose dependent). Risk of neuroleptic malignant syndrome (NMS) may be increased in patients with Parkinson's disease or Lewy Body Dementia; monitor for symptoms of confusion, obtundation, postural instability and extrapyramidal symptoms. May cause hyperglycemia; in some cases may be extreme and associated with ketoacidosis, hyperosmolar coma, or death. Use with caution in patients with diabetes or other disorders of glucose regulation; monitor for worsening of glucose control.

The possibility of a suicide attempt is inherent in psychotic illness or bipolar disorder; use caution in high-risk patients during initiation of therapy. Prescriptions should be written for the smallest quantity consistent with good patient care. Safety and efficacy in children have not been established.

Adverse Reactions

Unless otherwise noted, frequency of adverse effects is reported for the oral formulation.

>10%:

Central nervous system: Extrapyramidal symptoms (17% to 34%; dose dependent), somnolence (3% to 28%), insomnia (13% to 26%), agitation (8% to 26%), anxiety (4% to 20%), headache (12% to 14%), dizziness (4% to 11%)

Gastrointestinal: Weight gain (>5% to 18%), constipation (7% to 13%), dyspepsia (5% to 11%), nausea (4% to 11%)

1% to 10%:

Cardiovascular: Tachycardia (3% to 5%), hypertension (3%), chest pain (2% to 3%), hypotension (2% — especially orthostatic)

Central nervous system: Mania (8%), pseudoparkinsonism (6%), dreaming increased (≥5%), sleep prolonged (≥5%) fatigue (4%), fever (2% to 3%), aggressiveness (1% to 3%), hypoesthesia (2%), tardive dyskinesia, neuroleptic malignant syndrome, altered central temperature regulation, nervousness, hallucination, restlessness

Dermatologic: Rash (2% to 5%), dry skin (2% to 4%), acne (2%), pruritus (2%), seborrhea (up to 1%)

Endocrine & metabolic: Sexual dysfunction (≥5%), menorrhagia (≥5%), galactorrhea, gynecomastia

Gastrointestinal: Xerostomia (≥5%), vomiting (5% to 7%), diarrhea (≥5%), salivation increased (2% to 5%), abdominal pain (1% to 4%), toothache (up to 2%), GI upset, anorexia

Genitourinary: Micturition disturbances (≥5%)

Hematologic: Anemia (≥1% I.M. injection)

Hepatic: Transaminases increased (≥1% I.M. injection)

Neuromuscular & skeletal: Myalgia (5%), arthralgia (2% to 3%), skeletal pain (2%), back pain (up to 2%)

Ocular: Abnormal vision (1% to 6%), accommodation disturbances (≥5%)

Respiratory: Rhinitis (3% to 10%), sinusitis (1% to 4%), upper respiratory infection (3%), cough (2% to 3%), pharyngitis (2% to 3%), dyspnea (up to 1%)

Miscellaneous: Injury (up to 2%)

≤1% (Limited to important or life-threatening): Allergic reaction, amenorrhea, amnesia, anaphylactic reaction, anemias (oral formulations), angina pectoris, angioedema, antidiuretic hormone disorder, aphasia, apnea, ascites, aspiration, asthma, atrial fibrillation, AV block, bronchospasm, cachexia, catatonic reaction, cerebrovascular accident, cerebrovascular disorder, cholecystitis, cholelithiasis, cholestatic hepatitis, cholinergic syndrome, coma, confusion, creatine phosphokinase increase, dehydration, delirium, depression, diabetes mellitus, diabetic ketoacidosis, diverticulitis, dysphagia, esophagitis, esophageal dysmotility, fecal incontinence, flu-like symptoms, flushing, gastroenteritis, hematemesis, hematuria, hemorrhage, hepatic failure, hepatocellular damage, hyper-/hypoglycemia, hyperphosphatemia, hypertriglyceridemia, hyperuricemia, hypokalemia, hyponatremia, hypoproteinemia, flu-like symptoms, intestinal obstruction, jaundice, leukocytosis, leukopenia, leukorrhea, liver enzymes increased (oral formulations), lymphadenopathy, mastitis, menstrual irregularities, migraine, myocardial infarction, myocarditis, palpitation, pancreatitis, Pelger-Huët anomaly, photosensitivity (rare), pituitary adenomas, pneumonia, premature atrial contractions, priapism, pulmonary embolism, purpura, QT_c prolongation, RBC disorders, renal insufficiency, rigors, sarcoidosis, skin exfoliation, skin ulceration, ST depression, stomatitis, stridor, stroke, superficial phlebitis, synostosis, T wave inversions, thirst, thrombocytopenia, thrombophlebitis, thrombotic thrombocytopenic purpura, tinnitus, tongue discoloration, tongue edema, tongue paralysis, torticollis, transient ischemic attack, urinary incontinence, urinary retention, urticaria, ventricular extrasystoles, ventricular tachycardia, withdrawal syndrome, xerophthalmia

Overdosage/Toxicology Symptoms of overdose include drowsiness, sedation, tachycardia, hypotension, extrapyramidal symptoms (EPS), torsade de pointes, prolonged QT interval, seizures, and cardiopulmonary arrest. Treatment should be symptom-directed and supportive. Gastric decontamination and cardiac monitoring should be initiated. Consider risk of aspiration. Avoid antiarrhythmic therapy known to prolong the QT interval. Avoid vasopressors which may worsen hypotensive effects.

Drug Interactions Substrate of CYP2D6 (major), 3A4 (minor); **Inhibits** CYP2D6 (weak), 3A4 (weak)

Acetylcholinesterase inhibitors (central): May increase the risk of antipsychotic-related extrapyramidal symptoms; monitor.

Carbamazepine: Plasma concentrations of risperidone and 9-hydroxyrisperidone were decreased by ~50% with concomitant use. The dose of risperidone may need to be titrated accordingly when carbamazepine is added or discontinued.

Clozapine: Decreases clearance of risperidone, increasing its serum concentrations

CNS depressants: May increase adverse effects/toxicity of other CNS depressants.

CYP2D6 inhibitors: May increase the levels/effects of risperidone. Example inhibitors include chlorpromazine, delavirdine, fluoxetine, miconazole, paroxetine, pergolide, quinidine, quinine, ritonavir, and ropinirole.

Lithium: May increase the neurotoxic effects (eg, EPS) of risperidone; monitor.

Pramlintide: May enhance the anticholinergic effect of risperidone. These effects are specific to the GI tract.

SSRIs: May increase the levels/effects of risperidone; monitor.

Verapamil: May increase the levels and effects of risperidone.

Ethanol/Nutrition/Herb Interactions

Ethanol: Avoid ethanol (may increase CNS depression).

Herb/Nutraceutical: Avoid kava kava, gotu kola, valerian, St John's wort (may increase CNS depression).

Dietary Considerations May be taken with or without food. Risperdal® M-Tabs™ contain phenylalanine.

Dosage Forms

Injection, microspheres for reconstitution, extended release (Risperdal® Consta™): 25 mg, 37.5 mg, 50 mg [supplied in a dose-pack containing vial with active ingredient in microsphere formulation, prefilled syringe with diluent, needle-free vial access device, and safety needle]

Solution, oral: 1 mg/mL (30 mL) [contains benzoic acid]

Tablet: 0.25 mg, 0.5 mg, 1 mg, 2 mg, 3 mg, 4 mg

Tablet, orally disintegrating (Risperdal® M-Tabs™): 0.5 mg [contains phenylalanine 0.42 mg]; 3 mg [contains phenylalanine 0.63 mg]; 4 mg [contains phenylalanine 0.84 mg]

Ritonavir (ri TOE na veer)

Medication Safety Issues

Sound-alike/look-alike issues:

Ritonavir may be confused with Retrovir®

Norvir® may be confused with Norvasc®

Related Information

Moderate Sedation *on page 1442*

(Continued)

Ritonavir *(Continued)*

U.S. Brand Names Norvir®

Canadian Brand Names Norvir®; Norvir® SEC

Pharmacologic Category Antiretroviral Agent, Protease Inhibitor

Generic Available No

Use Treatment of HIV infection; should always be used as part of a multidrug regimen (at least three antiretroviral agents); may be used as a pharmacokinetic "booster" for other protease inhibitors

Mechanism of Action Ritonavir inhibits HIV protease and renders the enzyme incapable of processing of polyprotein precursor which leads to production of noninfectious immature HIV particles

Pharmacodynamics/Kinetics

Absorption: Variable; increased with food

Distribution: High concentrations in serum and lymph nodes

Protein binding: 98% to 99%

Metabolism: Hepatic via CYP3A4 and 2D6; five metabolites, low concentration of an active metabolite achieved in plasma (oxidative)

Half-life elimination: 3-5 hours

Time to peak, plasma: 2 hours (fasted); 4 hours (nonfasted)

Excretion: Urine (~11%); feces (~86%)

Dosage Treatment of HIV infection: Oral:

Children >1 month: 350-400 mg/m^2 twice daily (maximum dose: 600 mg twice daily). Initiate dose at 250 mg/m^2 twice daily; titrate dose upward every 2-3 days by 50 mg/m^2 twice daily.

Adults: 600 mg twice daily; dose escalation tends to avoid nausea that many patients experience upon initiation of full dosing. Escalate the dose as follows: 300 mg twice daily for 1 day, 400 mg twice daily for 2 days, 500 mg twice daily for 1 day, then 600 mg twice daily. Ritonavir may be better tolerated when used in combination with other antiretrovirals by initiating the drug alone and subsequently adding the second agent within 2 weeks.

Pharmacokinetic "booster" in combination with other protease inhibitors: 100-400 mg/day

Refer to individual monographs; specific dosage recommendations often require adjustment of both agents.

Note: Dosage adjustments for ritonavir when administered in combination therapy:

Amprenavir: Adjustments necessary for each agent:

Amprenavir 1200 mg with ritonavir 200 mg once daily **or**

Amprenavir 600 mg with ritonavir 100 mg twice daily

Amprenavir plus efavirenz (3-drug regimen): Amprenavir 1200 mg twice daily plus ritonavir 200 mg twice daily plus efavirenz at standard dose

Indinavir: Adjustments necessary for both agents:

Indinavir 800 mg twice daily plus ritonavir 100-200 mg twice daily **or**

Indinavir 400 mg twice daily plus ritonavir 400 mg twice daily

Nelfinavir: Ritonavir 400 mg twice daily

Rifabutin: Decrease rifabutin dose to 150 mg every other day

Saquinavir: Ritonavir 400 mg twice daily

Dosing adjustment in renal impairment: None necessary

Dosing adjustment in hepatic impairment: No adjustment required in mild or moderate impairment; however, careful monitoring is required in moderate hepatic impairment (levels may be decreased); caution advised with severe impairment (no data available)

Stability

Capsule: Store under refrigeration at 2°C to 8°C (36°F to 46°F); may be left out at room temperature of <25°C (<77°F) if used within 30 days. Protect from light. Avoid exposure to excessive heat.

Solution: Store at room temperature at 20°C to 25°C (68°F to 77°F). Do not refrigerate.

Administration Administer with food. Liquid formulations usually have an unpleasant taste. Consider mixing it with chocolate milk or a liquid nutritional supplement. Whenever possible, administer oral solution with calibrated dosing syringe.

Monitoring Parameters Triglycerides, cholesterol, CBC, LFTs, CPK, uric acid, basic HIV monitoring, viral load, CD4 count, glucose, serum amylase and lipase

Anesthesia and Critical Care Concerns/Other Considerations Potential compliance problems, frequency of administration, and adverse effects should be discussed with patients before initiating therapy to help prevent the emergence of resistance.

Pregnancy Risk Factor B

Contraindications Hypersensitivity to ritonavir or any component of the formulation; concurrent alfuzosin, amiodarone, cisapride, dihydroergotamine, ergonovine, ergotamine, flecainide, methylergonovine, midazolam, pimozide, propafenone, quinidine, triazolam, and voriconazole (when ritonavir ≥800 mg/day)

Warnings/Precautions [U.S. Boxed Warning]: Ritonavir may interact with many medications, resulting in potentially serious and/or life-threatening adverse events; careful review is required. A listing of medications that should not be used is available with each bottle and patients should be provided with this information. Avoid concurrent use with lovastatin, simvastatin, and St John's wort; atorvastatin should be used at the lowest possible dose, while fluvastatin or pravastatin may be safer alternatives. Cushing's syndrome and adrenal suppression have been reported in patients receiving concomitant ritonavir and fluticasone; avoid concurrent use unless benefit outweighs risk. Dosage adjustment is required for combination therapy with amprenavir and ritonavir; in addition, the risk of hyperlipidemia may be increased during concurrent therapy. Cardiac and neurological events have been reported with concurrent use of disopyramide, mexiletine, nefazodone, fluoxetine or beta blockers. Pancreatitis has been observed; use with caution in patients with increased triglycerides; monitor serum lipase and amylase.

Use with caution in patients with hemophilia A or B; increased bleeding during protease inhibitor therapy has been reported. Changes in glucose tolerance, hyperglycemia, exacerbation of diabetes, DKA, and new-onset diabetes mellitus have been reported in patients receiving protease inhibitors. May be associated with fat redistribution (buffalo hump, increased abdominal girth, breast engorgement, facial atrophy, and dyslipidemia). Immune reconstitution syndrome may develop resulting in the occurrence of an inflammatory response to an indolent or residual opportunistic infection; further evaluation and treatment may be required. May cause hepatitis or exacerbate pre-existing hepatic dysfunction; use with caution in patients with hepatitis B or C and in hepatic disease. Safety and efficacy have not been established in children <1 month of age.

Adverse Reactions Protease inhibitors cause dyslipidemia which includes elevated cholesterol and triglycerides and a redistribution of body fat centrally to cause increased abdominal girth, buffalo hump, facial atrophy, and breast enlargement. These agents also cause hyperglycemia. Percentages as reported in adults:

>10%:

- Endocrine & metabolic: Hypercholesterolemia (>240 mg/dL: 37% to 45%), triglycerides increased (>800 mg/dL: 17% to 34%; >1500 mg/dL: 1% to 13%)
- Gastrointestinal: Nausea (26% to 30%), diarrhea (15% to 23%), vomiting (14% to 17%), taste perversion (7% to 11%)
- Hematologic: WBCs decreased
- Hepatic: GGT increased (5% to 20%)
- Neuromuscular & skeletal: Weakness (10% to 15%), creatine phosphokinase increased (9% to 12%)

2% to 10%:

- Cardiovascular: Syncope (<1% to 2%), vasodilation (2%)
- Central nervous system: Fever (4% to 5%), dizziness (3% to 4%), insomnia (2% to 3%), somnolence (2% to 3%), anxiety (2%),
- Dermatologic: Rash
- Endocrine & metabolic: Uric acid increased (up to 4%)
- Gastrointestinal: Abdominal pain (6% to 8%), anorexia (2% to 8%), dyspepsia (up to 6%), local throat irritation (2% to 3%)
- Hematologic: Eosinophilia, neutropenia, neutrophilia
- Hepatic: LFTs increased (6% to 10%)
- Neuromuscular & skeletal: Paresthesia (3% to 7%), arthralgia (up to 2%), myalgia (2%)
- Respiratory: Pharyngitis
- Miscellaneous: Circumoral paresthesia, diaphoresis (2% to 3%)

<2% (Limited to important or life-threatening): Acute myeloblastic leukemia, adrenal cortex insufficiency, allergic reaction, amnesia, anemia, aphasia, asthma, bleeding increased (in patients with hemophilia A or B), cachexia, cardiovascular disorder, cerebral ischemia, cerebral venous thrombosis, chest pain, cholestatic jaundice, coma, convulsion, Cushing's syndrome, dehydration,

(Continued)

Ritonavir *(Continued)*

dementia, depersonalization, diabetes mellitus, dyspnea, esophageal ulcer, gastroenteritis, gastrointestinal hemorrhage, hallucinations, hepatic coma, hepatitis, hepatomegaly, hypercholesteremia, hyper-/hypotension, hypothermia, hypoventilation, ileus, interstitial pneumonia, kidney failure, larynx edema, leukopenia, lymphadenopathy, lymphocytosis, manic reaction, MI, myeloproliferative disorder, neuropathy, palpitation, pancreatitis, paralysis, postural hypotension, pseudomembranous colitis, rectal hemorrhage, redistribution of body fat, skin melanoma, subdural hematoma, tachycardia, thrombocytopenia, tongue edema, ulcerative colitis

Overdosage/Toxicology Human experience is limited; there is no specific antidote for overdose with ritonavir. Oral solution contains 43% ethanol by volume, potentially causing significant ethanol-related toxicity in younger patients. Dialysis is unlikely to be beneficial in significant removal of the drug. Charcoal or gastric lavage may be useful to remove unabsorbed drug.

Drug Interactions Substrate of CYP1A2 (minor), 2B6 (minor), 2D6 (major), 3A4 (major); **Inhibits** CYP2C8 (strong), 2C9 (weak), 2C19 (weak), 2D6 (strong), 2E1 (weak), 3A4 (strong); **Induces** CYP1A2 (weak), 2C8 (weak), 2C9 (weak), 3A4 (weak)

Alfuzosin: Serum concentrations may be increased by ritonavir; concurrent use is contraindicated.

Amprenavir: The serum concentrations of ritonavir may be increased by amprenavir. In addition, the risk of cholesterol/triglyceride elevations may be increased. Specific dosing has been recommended for both agents.

Analgesics (eg, tramadol, meperidine, propoxyphene): Serum levels of parent drug or metabolite may be increased by ritonavir.

Antiarrhythmics (eg, disopyramide, mexiletine, lidocaine): Toxicity may be greatly increased; concurrent use of ritonavir is contraindicated with amiodarone, flecainide, propafenone, and quinidine.

Anticonvulsants: Ritonavir may increase levels (carbamazepine, ethosuximide) or decrease levels (lamotrigine, divalproex, phenytoin); monitor.

Antidepressants (eg, bupropion, trazodone, nefazodone, fluoxetine, and possibly other SSRIs): Ritonavir may increase the levels/effects of these agents.

Antipsychotics (clozapine, perphenazine, risperidone, thioridazine): Serum concentrations may be increased by ritonavir. Avoid use with thioridazine.

Benzodiazepines (clorazepate, diazepam, estazolam, flurazepam midazolam, triazolam) toxicity may be increased; concurrent use of midazolam and triazolam is specifically contraindicated.

Beta-blockers: Serum concentrations/effects may be increased by ritonavir.

Calcium channel blockers: Serum concentrations/effects may be increased by ritonavir.

Cimetidine: May increase the levels/effects of ritonavir; monitor.

Cisapride toxicity (arrhythmia) may be increased by ritonavir; concurrent use is contraindicated.

Clarithromycin serum concentrations are increased by ritonavir; dosage adjustment required (based on Cl_{cr}).

CYP2C8 substrates: Ritonavir may increase the levels/effects of CYP2C89 substrates. Example substrates include amiodarone, paclitaxel, pioglitazone, repaglinide, and rosiglitazone.

CYP2D6 substrates: Ritonavir may increase the levels/effects of CYP2D6 substrates. Example substrates include amphetamines, selected beta-blockers, dextromethorphan, fluoxetine, lidocaine, mirtazapine, nefazodone, paroxetine, risperidone, thioridazine, tricyclic antidepressants, and venlafaxine.

CYP2D6 prodrug substrates: Ritonavir may decrease the levels/effects of CYP2D6 prodrug substrates. Example prodrug substrates include codeine, hydrocodone, oxycodone, and tramadol.

CYP3A4 inducers: CYP3A4 inducers may decrease the levels/effects of ritonavir. Example inducers include aminoglutethimide, carbamazepine, nafcillin, nevirapine, phenobarbital, phenytoin, and rifamycins.

CYP3A4 substrates: Ritonavir may increase the levels/effects of CYP3A4 substrates. Example substrates include benzodiazepines, calcium channel blockers, mirtazapine, nateglinide, nefazodone, tacrolimus, and venlafaxine. Selected benzodiazepines (midazolam and triazolam), cisapride, ergot alkaloids, and pimozide are generally contraindicated with strong CYP3A4 inhibitors.

Delavirdine: Ritonavir may increase the levels/toxicity of delavirdine.

Desipramine (and possibly other TCAs at high doses) serum levels may be increased by ritonavir in HIV-positive patients, requiring dosage adjustment; monitor.

Didanosine: Administration should be separated by 2.5 hours to avoid formulation incompatibility.

Digoxin: Serum concentrations may be increased by ritonavir; monitor.

Disulfiram: May cause disulfiram reaction (oral solution contains 43% ethanol)

Eplerenone: Ritonavir may increase the levels/effects of eplerenone; monitor.

Ergot alkaloids (dihydroergotamine, ergotamine, ergonovine, methylergonovine) toxicity (peripheral ischemia, vasospasm) is increased by ritonavir; concurrent use is contraindicated.

Estrogen (oral or transdermal contraceptives): Effects may be decreased (not well characterized). Use alternative contraceptive measures.

Fentanyl: Ritonavir may increase the levels/effects; monitor.

HMG-CoA reductase inhibitors (atorvastatin, cerivastatin, lovastatin, simvastatin) serum concentrations may be increased by ritonavir, increasing the risk of myopathy/rhabdomyolysis. Lovastatin or simvastatin should not be used with ritonavir. Use lowest possible dose of atorvastatin. Fluvastatin and pravastatin may be safer alternatives.

Immunosuppressants (cyclosporine, sirolimus, tacrolimus): Serum levels/effects may be increased by ritonavir; monitor.

Indinavir serum concentrations are increased by ritonavir.

Inhaled corticosteroids (eg, budesonide, fluticasone): Serum concentrations may be increased by ritonavir, resulting in decreased serum cortisol, HPA axis suppression; concurrent use is not recommended.

Itraconazole, ketoconazole serum concentrations are increased by ritonavir. Limit ketoconazole dose to ≤200 mg/day.

Meperidine: Serum concentrations of metabolite (normeperidine) are increased by ritonavir, which may increase the risk of CNS toxicity.

Methadone: Serum concentrations may be decreased by ritonavir; dose adjustment of methadone may be necessary.

Metronidazole: May cause disulfiram reaction (oral solution contains 43% ethanol).

Pimozide toxicity is significantly increased by ritonavir; concurrent use is contraindicated.

Rifabutin and rifabutin metabolite serum concentrations may be increased by ritonavir; reduce rifabutin dose to 150 mg every other day.

Rifampin: May decrease levels/effects of ritonavir; alternative antimycobacterial agent recommended.

Saquinavir: Serum concentrations are increased by ritonavir; dosage of both agents should be adjusted.

Sildenafil: Serum concentrations may be increased by ritonavir; when used concurrently, do not exceed a maximum sildenafil dose of 25 mg in a 48-hour period.

Tadalafil: Serum concentrations may be increased by ritonavir. A maximum tadalafil dose of 10 mg in 72 hours is recommended with strong CYP3A4 inhibitors.

Theophylline: Serum concentrations may be decreased by ritonavir.

Trazodone: Serum concentrations/effects may be increased by ritonavir; use caution and reduce trazodone dose.

Vardenafil: Serum concentrations may be increased by ritonavir; do not exceed vardenafil dose of 2.5 mg in 72 hours.

Voriconazole: Serum levels are reduced by ritonavir. Concurrent use is contraindicated with ritonavir dose ≥800 mg/day. Concomitant use not recommended with lower doses of ritonavir unless benefit outweighs risk.

Zolpidem: Serum levels/effects may be increased by ritonavir; monitor.

Ethanol/Nutrition/Herb Interactions

Food: Food enhances absorption.

Herb/Nutraceutical: St John's wort may decrease ritonavir serum levels. Avoid use.

Dietary Considerations Should be taken with food. Oral solution contains 43% ethanol by volume.

Dosage Forms

Capsule: 100 mg [contains ethanol and polyoxyl 35 castor oil]

Solution: 80 mg/mL (240 mL) [contains ethanol and polyoxyl 35 castor oil; peppermint and caramel flavor]

♦ **Riva-Atenolol (Can)** *see* Atenolol *on page 136*

- ◆ **Riva-Diclofenac (Can)** *see* Diclofenac *on page 378*
- ◆ **Riva-Diclofenac-K (Can)** *see* Diclofenac *on page 378*
- ◆ **Riva-Famotidine (Can)** *see* Famotidine *on page 506*
- ◆ **Riva-Fluconazole (Can)** *see* Fluconazole *on page 530*
- ◆ **Riva-Fosinopril (Can)** *see* Fosinopril *on page 562*
- ◆ **Riva-Lorazepam (Can)** *see* Lorazepam *on page 773*
- ◆ **Riva-Lovastatin (Can)** *see* Lovastatin *on page 782*
- ◆ **Riva-Naproxen (Can)** *see* Naproxen *on page 899*
- ◆ **Rivanase AQ (Can)** *see* Beclomethasone *on page 161*
- ◆ **Riva-Simvastatin (Can)** *see* Simvastatin *on page 1174*
- ◆ **Riva-Sotalol (Can)** *see* Sotalol *on page 1198*
- ◆ **Riva-Sumatriptan (Can)** *see* Sumatriptan *on page 1222*
- ◆ **Riva-Verapamil SR (Can)** *see* Verapamil *on page 1352*
- ◆ **Rivotril® (Can)** *see* Clonazepam *on page 313*

Rizatriptan (rye za TRIP tan)

U.S. Brand Names Maxalt®; Maxalt-MLT®

Canadian Brand Names Maxalt™; Maxalt RPD™

Synonyms MK462

Pharmacologic Category Serotonin 5-HT_{1D} Receptor Agonist

Generic Available No

Use Acute treatment of migraine with or without aura

Mechanism of Action Selective agonist for serotonin (5-HT_{1D} receptor) in cranial arteries to cause vasoconstriction and reduce sterile inflammation associated with antidromic neuronal transmission correlating with relief of migraine

Pharmacodynamics/Kinetics

Onset of action: ~30 minutes

Duration: 14-16 hours

Protein binding: 14%

Metabolism: Via monoamine oxidase-A; first-pass effect

Bioavailability: 40% to 50%

Half-life elimination: 2-3 hours

Time to peak: 1-1.5 hours

Excretion: Urine (82%, 8% to 16% as unchanged drug); feces (12%)

Dosage Note: In patients with risk factors for coronary artery disease, following adequate evaluation to establish the absence of coronary artery disease, the initial dose should be administered in a setting where response may be evaluated (physician's office or similarly staffed setting). ECG monitoring may be considered.

Oral: 5-10 mg, repeat after 2 hours if significant relief is not attained; maximum: 30 mg in a 24-hour period (use 5 mg dose in patients receiving propranolol with a maximum of 15 mg in 24 hours)

Note: For orally-disintegrating tablets (Maxalt-MLT®): Patient should be instructed to place tablet on tongue and allow to dissolve. Dissolved tablet will be swallowed with saliva.

Stability Store in blister pack until administration.

Monitoring Parameters Headache severity, signs/symptoms suggestive of angina; consider monitoring blood pressure, heart rate, and/or ECG with first dose in patients with likelihood of unrecognized coronary disease, such as patients with significant hypertension, hypercholesterolemia, obese patients, diabetics, smokers with other risk factors or strong family history of coronary artery disease

Anesthesia and Critical Care Concerns/Other Considerations Rizatriptan should not be used in patients with a history of vasospastic disease, Prinzmetal's angina, or any critical vascular disease.

Pregnancy Risk Factor C

Contraindications Hypersensitivity to rizatriptan or any component of the formulation; documented ischemic heart disease or Prinzmetal's angina; uncontrolled hypertension; basilar or hemiplegic migraine; during or within 2 weeks of MAO inhibitors; during or within 24 hours of treatment with another 5-HT_1 agonist, or an ergot-containing or ergot-type medication (eg, methysergide, dihydroergotamine)

Warnings/Precautions Use only in patients with a clear diagnosis of migraine. May cause vasospastic reactions resulting in colonic, peripheral, or coronary ischemia. Use with caution in elderly or patients with hepatic or renal impairment (including dialysis patients), history of hypersensitivity to sumatriptan or adverse effects from sumatriptan, and in patients at risk of coronary artery disease (as predicted by presence of risk factors) unless cardiovascular evaluation provides evidence that the patient is free of cardiovascular disease. In patients with risk factors for coronary artery disease, following adequate evaluation to establish the absence of coronary artery disease, the initial dose should be administered in a setting where response may be evaluated (physician's office or similarly staffed setting). ECG monitoring may be considered. Do not use with ergotamines. May increase blood pressure transiently; may cause coronary vasospasm (less than sumatriptan); avoid in patients with signs/symptoms suggestive of reduced arterial flow (ischemic bowel, Raynaud's) which could be exacerbated by vasospasm.

Patients who experience sensations of chest pain/pressure/tightness or symptoms suggestive of angina following dosing should be evaluated for coronary artery disease or Prinzmetal's angina before receiving additional doses.

Reconsider diagnosis of migraine if no response to initial dose. Long-term effects on vision have not been evaluated.

Adverse Reactions

1% to 10%:

- Cardiovascular: Systolic/diastolic blood pressure increases (5-10 mm Hg), chest pain (5%), palpitation
- Central nervous system: Dizziness, drowsiness, fatigue (13% to 30%, dose related)
- Dermatologic: Skin flushing
- Endocrine & metabolic: Mild increase in growth hormone, hot flashes
- Gastrointestinal: Nausea, abdominal pain, dry mouth (<5%)
- Respiratory: Dyspnea

<1% (Limited to important or life-threatening): Akinesia, angina, angioedema, arrhythmia, bradycardia, bradykinesia, decreased mental activity, myalgia, myocardial ischemia, MI, neck pain/stiffness, neurological/psychiatric abnormalities, pruritus, stroke, syncope, tachycardia, tinnitus, toxic epidermal necrolysis, wheezing

Drug Interactions Use within 24 hours of another selective 5-HT_1 agonist or ergot-containing drug should be avoided due to possible additive vasoconstriction

MAO inhibitors and nonselective MAO inhibitors increase concentration of rizatriptan

Propranolol: Plasma concentration of rizatriptan increased 70%

SSRIs: Rarely, concurrent use results in weakness and incoordination; monitor closely

Ethanol/Nutrition/Herb Interactions Food: Food delays absorption.

Dietary Considerations Orally-disintegrating tablet contains phenylalanine (1.05 mg per 5 mg tablet, 2.10 mg per 10 mg tablet).

Dosage Forms

Tablet, as benzoate (Maxalt®): 5 mg, 10 mg

Tablet, orally disintegrating, as benzoate (Maxalt-MLT®): 5 mg [contains phenylalanine 1.05 mg/tablet; peppermint flavor]; 10 mg [contains phenylalanine 2.1 mg/tablet; peppermint flavor]

- ♦ **RMS®** *see* Morphine Sulfate *on page 867*
- ♦ **Robidrine® (Can)** *see* Pseudoephedrine *on page 1085*
- ♦ **Robinul®** *see* Glycopyrrolate *on page 600*
- ♦ **Robinul® Forte** *see* Glycopyrrolate *on page 600*
- ♦ **Rocephin®** *see* Ceftriaxone *on page 250*

Rocuronium (roe kyoor OH nee um)

Medication Safety Issues

Sound-alike/look-alike issues:

Zemuron® may be confused with Remeron®

High alert medication: The Institute for Safe Medication Practices (ISMP) includes this medication among its list of drugs which have a heightened risk of causing significant patient harm when used in error.

Related Information

Chronic Renal Failure *on page 1437*

Neuromuscular Blocking Agents *on page 1572*

(Continued)

Rocuronium *(Continued)*

U.S. Brand Names Zemuron®

Canadian Brand Names Zemuron®

Synonyms ORG 946; Rocuronium Bromide

Pharmacologic Category Neuromuscular Blocker Agent, Nondepolarizing

Generic Available No

Use Adjunct to general anesthesia to facilitate both rapid sequence and routine endotracheal intubation and to relax skeletal muscles during surgery; to facilitate mechanical ventilation in ICU patients; does not relieve pain or produce sedation

Mechanism of Action Blocks acetylcholine from binding to receptors on motor endplate inhibiting depolarization

Pharmacodynamics/Kinetics

Onset of action: Good intubation conditions in 1-2 minutes; maximum neuromuscular blockade within 4 minutes

Duration: ~30 minutes (with standard doses, increases with higher doses)

Metabolism: Minimally hepatic; 17-desacetylrocuronium (5% to 10% activity of parent drug)

Half-life elimination: 60-70 minutes

Excretion: Feces (50%); urine (30%)

Dosage Administer I.V.; dose to effect; doses will vary due to interpatient variability; use ideal body weight for obese patients

Children:

Initial: 0.6 mg/kg under halothane anesthesia produce excellent to good intubating conditions within 1 minute and will provide a median time of 41 minutes of clinical relaxation in children 3 months to 1 year of age, and 27 minutes in children 1-12 years

Maintenance: 0.075-0.125 mg/kg administered upon return of T_1 to 25% of control provides clinical relaxation for 7-10 minutes

Adults:

Tracheal intubation: I.V.:

Initial: 0.6 mg/kg is expected to provide approximately 31 minutes of clinical relaxation under opioid/nitrous oxide/oxygen anesthesia with neuromuscular block sufficient for intubation attained in 1-2 minutes; lower doses (0.45 mg/kg) may be used to provide 22 minutes of clinical relaxation with median time to neuromuscular block of 1-3 minutes; maximum blockade is achieved in <4 minutes

Maximum: 0.9-1.2 mg/kg may be given during surgery under opioid/nitrous oxide/oxygen anesthesia without adverse cardiovascular effects and is expected to provide 58-67 minutes of clinical relaxation; neuromuscular blockade sufficient for intubation is achieved in <2 minutes with maximum blockade in <3 minutes

Maintenance: 0.1, 0.15, and 0.2 mg/kg administered at 25% recovery of control T_1 (defined as 3 twitches of train-of-four) provides a median of 12, 17, and 24 minutes of clinical duration under anesthesia

Rapid sequence intubation: 0.6-1.2 mg/kg in appropriately premedicated and anesthetized patients with excellent or good intubating conditions within 2 minutes

Continuous infusion: Initial: 0.01-0.012 mg/kg/minute only after early evidence of spontaneous recovery of neuromuscular function is evident; infusion rates have ranged from 4-16 mcg/kg/minute

ICU: 10 mcg/kg/minute; adjust dose to maintain appropriate degree of neuromuscular blockade (eg, 1 or 2 twitches on train-of-four)

Dosing adjustment in hepatic impairment: Reductions are necessary in patients with liver disease

Stability Store under refrigeration (2°C to 8°C), do not freeze; when stored at room temperature, it is stable for 30 days; unlike vecuronium, it is stable in 0.9% sodium chloride and 5% dextrose in water, this mixture should be used within 24 hours of preparation

Administration Administer I.V. only; may be administered undiluted as a bolus injection or via a continuous infusion using an infusion pump

Monitoring Parameters Peripheral nerve stimulator measuring twitch response, heart rate, blood pressure, assisted ventilation status

Anesthesia and Critical Care Concerns/Other Considerations Classified as an intermediate duration neuromuscular-blocking agent; do not mix in same syringe with barbiturates.

Critically-Ill Adult Patients:

The 2004 Surviving Sepsis Campaign guidelines recommend avoiding use of neuromuscular blockers if at all possible in the septic patient due to the risk of prolonged neuromuscular blockade following discontinuation. If one is required, monitor carefully and observe the following recommendations.

The 2002 ACCM/SCCM/ASHP clinical practice guidelines for sustained neuromuscular blockade in the adult critically-ill patient recommend:

Optimize sedatives and analgesics prior to initiation and monitor and adjust accordingly during course. Neuromuscular blockers do not relieve pain or produce sedation.

Protect patient's eyes from development of keratitis and corneal abrasion by administering ophthalmic ointment and taping eyelids closed or using eye patches. Reposition patient routinely to protect pressure points from breakdown. Address DVT prophylaxis.

Concurrent use of a neuromuscular blocker and corticosteroids appear to increase the risk of certain ICU myopathies; avoid or administer the corticosteroid at the lowest dose possible. Reassess need for neuromuscular blocker daily.

Using daily drug holidays (stopping neuromuscular-blocking agent until patient requires it again) may decrease the incidence of acute quadriplegic myopathy syndrome.

Tachyphylaxis can develop; switch to another neuromuscular blocker (taking into consideration the patient's organ function) if paralysis is still necessary.

Atracurium or cisatracurium is recommended for patients with significant hepatic or renal disease, due to organ-independent Hofmann elimination.

Monitor patients clinically and via "Train of Four" (TOF) testing with a goal of adjusting the degree of blockade to 1-2 twitches on based upon the patient's clinical condition.

Pregnancy Risk Factor C

Contraindications Hypersensitivity to rocuronium or any component of the formulation

Warnings/Precautions Use with caution in patients with valvular heart disease, pulmonary disease, hepatic impairment; ventilation must be supported during neuromuscular blockade; certain clinical conditions may result in potentiation or antagonism of neuromuscular blockade:

Potentiation: Electrolyte abnormalities, severe hyponatremia, severe hypocalcemia, severe hypokalemia, hypermagnesemia, neuromuscular diseases, acidosis, acute intermittent porphyria, renal failure, hepatic failure

Antagonism: Alkalosis, hypercalcemia, demyelinating lesions, peripheral neuropathies, diabetes mellitus

Increased sensitivity in patients with myasthenia gravis, Eaton-Lambert syndrome; resistance in burn patients (>30% of body) for period of 5-70 days postinjury; resistance in patients with muscle trauma, denervation, immobilization, infection. Cross-sensitivity with other neuromuscular-blocking agents may occur; use extreme caution in patients with previous anaphylactic reactions.

Adverse Reactions

>1%: Cardiovascular: Transient hypotension and hypertension

<1% (Limited to important or life-threatening): Abnormal ECG, acute quadriplegic myopathy syndrome (prolonged use), anaphylaxis, arrhythmia, bronchospasm, edema, hiccups, injection site pruritus, myositis ossificans (prolonged use), nausea, rash, rhonchi, shock, tachycardia, vomiting, wheezing

Overdosage/Toxicology

Symptoms of overdose include prolonged skeletal muscle block, muscle weakness and apnea

Treatment is maintenance of a patent airway and controlled ventilation until recovery of normal neuromuscular block is observed, further recovery may be facilitated by administering an anticholinesterase agent (eg, neostigmine, edrophonium, or pyridostigmine) with atropine, to antagonize the skeletal muscle relaxation; support of the cardiovascular system with fluids and pressors may be necessary

Drug Interactions

Decreased effect: Chronic carbamazepine or phenytoin can shorten the duration of neuromuscular blockade; phenylephrine can severely inhibit neuromuscular blockade

Increased effect: Infusion requirements are reduced 35% to 40% during anesthesia with enflurane or isoflurane

(Continued)

Rocuronium *(Continued)*

Increased toxicity: Aminoglycosides, vancomycin, tetracyclines, bacitracin

Dosage Forms Injection, solution, as bromide: 10 mg/mL (5 mL, 10 mL)

References

Bartkowski RR, Witkowski TA, Azad S, et al, "Rocuronium Onset of Action: A Comparison With Atracurium and Vecuronium," *Anesth Analg*, 1993, 77(3):574-8.

Dellinger RP, Carlet JM, Masur H, et al, "Surviving Sepsis Campaign Guidelines for Management of Severe Sepsis and Septic Shock," *Crit Care Med*, 2004, 32(3):858-73.

Khuenl-Brady KS, Sparr H, Puhringer F, et al, "Rocuronium Bromide in the ICU: Dose Finding and Pharmacokinetics," *Eur J Anaesthesiol Suppl*, 1995, 11:79-80.

Murray MJ, Cowen J, DeBlock H, et al, "Clinical Practice Guidelines for Sustained Neuromuscular Blockade in the Adult Critically Ill Patient. Task Force of the American College of Critical Care Medicine (ACCM) of the Society of Critical Care Medicine (SCCM), American Society of Health-System Pharmacists, American College of Chest Physicians," *Crit Care Med*, 2002, 30(1):142-56. Available at: http://www.sccm.org/pdf/NeuromuscularBlockade.pdf. Accessed August 6, 2003.

Puhringer FK, Khuenl-Brady KS, and Mitterschiffthaler G, "Rocuronium Bromide: Time-Course of Action in Underweight, Normal Weight, Overweight and Obese Patients," *Eur J Anaesthesiol Suppl*, 1995, 11:107-10.

♦ **Rocuronium Bromide** *see* Rocuronium *on page 1135*

♦ **Rofact™ (Can)** *see* Rifampin *on page 1121*

Rofecoxib (roe fe COX ib)

Medication Safety Issues

Sound-alike/look-alike issues:

Vioxx® may be confused with Zyvox™

Related Information

Acetaminophen and NSAIDS, Dosing Data *on page 1543*

U.S. Brand Names Vioxx® [DSC]

Pharmacologic Category Nonsteroidal Anti-inflammatory Drug (NSAID), COX-2 Selective

Generic Available No

Use Relief of the signs and symptoms of osteoarthritis, rheumatoid arthritis, and juvenile rheumatoid arthritis (JRA); management of acute pain; treatment of primary dysmenorrhea; treatment of migraine attacks

Mechanism of Action Inhibits prostaglandin synthesis by decreasing the activity of the enzyme, cyclooxygenase-2 (COX-2), which results in decreased formation of prostaglandin precursors. Rofecoxib does not inhibit cyclooxygenase-1 (COX-1) at therapeutic concentrations.

Pharmacodynamics/Kinetics

Onset of action: 45 minutes

Duration: Up to >24 hours

Distribution: V_{dss} (apparent): 86-91 L

Protein binding: 87%

Metabolism: Hepatic (99%); minor metabolism via CYP2C8/9 isoenzyme; metabolites inactive

Bioavailability: 93%

Half-life elimination: 17 hours

Time to peak: 2-3 hours

Excretion: Urine (72% as metabolites, <1% as unchanged drug); feces (14% as unchanged drug)

Dosage Oral:

Children 2-17 years and ≥10 kg: JRA: 0.6 mg/kg/day (maximum: 25 mg/day)

Adults:

Osteoarthritis: 12.5 mg once daily; may be increased to a maximum of 25 mg once daily

Acute pain and management of dysmenorrhea: 50 mg once daily as needed (use for longer than 5 days has not been studied)

Migraine attack: 25 mg once daily, as needed; may be increased to a maximum of 50 mg once daily

Rheumatoid arthritis: 25 mg once daily

Dosing comment in renal impairment: Use in advanced renal disease is not recommended

Dosing adjustment in hepatic impairment: Moderate hepatic dysfunction (Child-Pugh score 7-9): Maximum dose: 12.5 mg/day

Monitoring Parameters Signs and symptoms of gastrointestinal bleeding

Anesthesia and Critical Care Concerns/Other Considerations Does not inhibit platelets or prolong bleeding.

Pregnancy Risk Factor C/D (3rd trimester)

Contraindications Hypersensitivity to rofecoxib or any component of the formulation, aspirin, or other NSAIDs; patients with "aspirin triad" (bronchial asthma, aspirin intolerance, rhinitis); pregnancy (3rd trimester)

Warnings/Precautions Gastrointestinal irritation, ulceration, bleeding, and perforation may occur with NSAIDs (rofecoxib has been associated with rates of these events which are lower than naproxen, a nonselective NSAID); use the lowest effective dose for the shortest duration possible to decrease risk. Use with caution in patients with a history of GI disease (bleeding or ulcers), decreased renal function, hepatic disease, CHF, hypertension, or asthma. Edema, GI irritation, and/or hypertension occur at an increased frequency with chronic use of 50 mg/day. Use with caution in patients with ischemic heart disease; antiplatelet therapies should be considered (rofecoxib is not a substitute for antiplatelet agents). Anaphylactoid reactions may occur, even with no prior exposure to rofecoxib. Safety and efficacy in pediatric patients <2 years of age and <10 kg, and in cluster headaches have not been established.

Adverse Reactions

2% to 10%:

- Cardiovascular: Peripheral edema (4%), hypertension (up to 10%)
- Central nervous system: Headache (5%), dizziness (3%)
- Gastrointestinal: Diarrhea (7%), nausea (5%), heartburn (4%), epigastric discomfort (4%), dyspepsia (4%), abdominal pain (3%); dry socket (postdental extraction alveolitis 2%)
- Genitourinary: Urinary tract infection (3%)
- Neuromuscular & skeletal: Back pain (3%), weakness (2%)
- Respiratory: Upper respiratory infection (9%), bronchitis (2%), sinusitis (3%)
- Miscellaneous: Flu-like syndrome (3%)

0.1% to 2%:

- Cardiovascular: Chest pain, upper extremity edema, atrial fibrillation, bradycardia, arrhythmia, palpitation, tachycardia, venous insufficiency, fluid retention
- Central nervous system: Anxiety, depression, decreased mental acuity, hypoesthesia, insomnia, neuropathy, migraine, paresthesia, somnolence, vertigo, fever, pain
- Dermatologic: Alopecia, atopic dermatitis, basal cell carcinoma, contact dermatitis, pruritus, rash, erythema, urticaria, dry skin
- Endocrine & metabolic: Weight gain, hypercholesteremia
- Gastrointestinal: Reflux, abdominal distension, abdominal tenderness, constipation, dry mouth, esophagitis, flatulence, gastritis, gastroenteritis, hematochezia, hemorrhoids, oral ulceration, dental caries, aphthous stomatitis
- Genitourinary: Breast mass, cystitis, dysuria, menopausal disorder, nocturia, urinary retention, vaginitis, pelvic pain
- Hematologic: Hematoma
- Hepatic: Transaminases increased >3 times ULN (1%)
- Neuromuscular & skeletal: Muscle spasm, sciatica, arthralgia, bursitis, cartilage trauma, joint swelling, muscle cramps, muscle weakness, myalgia, tendonitis, traumatic arthropathy, fracture (wrist)
- Ocular: Blurred vision, conjunctivitis
- Otic: Otic pain, otitis media, tinnitus
- Respiratory: Asthma, cough, dyspnea, pneumonia, respiratory infection, pulmonary congestion, rhinitis, epistaxis, laryngitis, dry throat, pharyngitis, tonsillitis, diaphragmatic hernia
- Miscellaneous: Allergy, fungal infection, insect bite reaction, syncope, viral syndrome, herpes simplex, herpes zoster, increased diaphoresis

<2% (Limited to important or life-threatening): Allergy, alopecia, angina, arrhythmia, asthma, atopic dermatitis, atrial fibrillation, blurred vision, decreased mental acuity, depression, dyspnea, esophageal reflux, esophagitis, fluid retention, gastritis, hematochezia, hematoma, hemorrhoids, muscle cramps, neuropathy, paresthesia, pruritus, rash, somnolence, syncope, tendonitis, tinnitus, transaminases increased (>3 times ULN), urinary retention, urticaria, venous insufficiency, vertigo

<0.1% (Limited to important or life-threatening): Agranulocytosis, aplastic anemia, breast cancer, cholecystitis, colitis, colonic neoplasm, CHF, deep vein thrombosis, duodenal ulcer, gastrointestinal bleeding, hallucinations, intestinal

(Continued)

Rofecoxib *(Continued)*

obstruction, lymphoma, MI, pancreatitis, pancytopenia, photosensitivity reaction, prostatic cancer, Stevens-Johnson syndrome, stroke, toxic epidermal necrolysis, transient ischemic attack, unstable angina, urolithiasis

Overdosage/Toxicology Symptoms may include epigastric pain, drowsiness, lethargy, nausea, and vomiting. Gastrointestinal bleeding may occur. Rare manifestations include hypertension, respiratory depression, coma, and acute renal failure. Treatment is symptomatic and supportive. Hemodialysis does not remove rofecoxib.

Drug Interactions **Substrate** of CYP2C9 (minor); **Inhibits** CYP1A2 (weak); **Induces** CYP3A4 (weak)

ACE inhibitors: Antihypertensive effects may be reduced by rofecoxib.

Aspirin: Rofecoxib may be used with low-dose aspirin, however, rates of gastrointestinal bleeding may be increased with coadministration.

Cimetidine increases AUC of rofecoxib by 23%.

Diuretics: Thiazide diuretics, loop diuretics: Effects may be diminished by rofecoxib.

Lithium: Serum concentrations/toxicity may be increased by rofecoxib; monitor.

Methotrexate: Severe bone marrow suppression, aplastic anemia, and GI toxicity have been reported with concomitant NSAID therapy. Selective COX-2 inhibitors appear to have a lower risk of this toxicity, however, caution is warranted.

Rifampin reduces the serum concentration of rofecoxib by ~50%; consider using initial dose of 25 mg/day for osteoarthritis.

Theophylline: Serum concentrations may be increased during therapy with rofecoxib; monitor.

Warfarin: Rofecoxib may increase the INR in patients receiving warfarin and may increase the risk of bleeding complications. However, rofecoxib does not appear to inhibit platelet aggregation.

Ethanol/Nutrition/Herb Interactions

Ethanol: Avoid ethanol (may increase gastric mucosal irritation)

Food: Time to peak concentrations are delayed when taken with a high-fat meal, however, peak concentration and AUC are unchanged.

Dietary Considerations May be taken without regard to meals.

Dosage Forms [DSC] = Discontinued product

Suspension, oral [DSC]: 12.5 mg/5 mL (150 mL); 25 mg/5 mL (150 mL) [strawberry flavor]

Tablet [DSC]: 12.5 mg, 25 mg, 50 mg

♦ **Rogaine® (Can)** *see* Minoxidil *on page 856*
♦ **Rogaine® Extra Strength for Men [OTC]** *see* Minoxidil *on page 856*
♦ **Rogaine® for Men [OTC]** *see* Minoxidil *on page 856*
♦ **Rogaine® for Women [OTC]** *see* Minoxidil *on page 856*
♦ **Rogitine® (Can)** *see* Phentolamine *on page 1013*
♦ **Romazicon®** *see* Flumazenil *on page 534*
♦ **Romycin®** *see* Erythromycin *on page 476*

Ropivacaine (roe PIV a kane)

Medication Safety Issues

Sound-alike/look-alike issues:

Ropivacaine may be confused with bupivacaine, ropinirole

Related Information

Acute Postoperative Pain *on page 1388*
Local Anesthetics *on page 1532*

U.S. Brand Names Naropin®

Canadian Brand Names Naropin®

Synonyms Ropivacaine Hydrochloride

Pharmacologic Category Local Anesthetic

Generic Available No

Use Local anesthetic for use in surgery, postoperative pain management, and obstetrical procedures when local or regional anesthesia is needed

Mechanism of Action Blocks both the initiation and conduction of nerve impulses by decreasing the neuronal membrane's permeability to sodium ions, which results in inhibition of depolarization with resultant blockade of conduction

Pharmacodynamics/Kinetics

Onset of action: Anesthesia (route dependent): 3-15 minutes

Duration (dose and route dependent): 3-15 hours

Metabolism: Hepatic

Half-life elimination: Epidural: 5-7 hours; I.V.: 2.4 hours

Excretion: Urine (86% as metabolites)

Dosage Dose varies with procedure, onset and depth of anesthesia desired, vascularity of tissues, duration of anesthesia, and condition of patient: Adults:

Surgical anesthesia:

- Lumbar epidural: 15-30 mL of 0.5% to 1% solution
- Lumbar epidural block for cesarean section:
  - 20-30 mL dose of 0.5% solution
  - 15-20 mL dose of 0.75% solution
- Thoracic epidural block: 5-15 mL dose of 0.5% to 0.75% solution
- Major nerve block:
  - 35-50 mL dose of 0.5% solution (175-250 mg)
  - 10-40 mL dose of 0.75% solution (75-300 mg)
- Field block: 1-40 mL dose of 0.5% solution (5-200 mg)

Labor pain management: Lumbar epidural: Initial: 10-20 mL 0.2% solution; continuous infusion dose: 6-14 mL/hour of 0.2% solution with incremental injections of 10-15 mL/hour of 0.2% solution

Postoperative pain management:

- Lumbar or thoracic epidural: Continuous infusion dose: 6-14 mL/hour of 0.2% solution
- Infiltration/minor nerve block:
  - 1-100 mL dose of 0.2% solution
  - 1-40 mL dose of 0.5% solution

Stability Epidural infusions can be used ≤24 hours.

Administration Administered via local infiltration, epidural block and epidural infusion, or intermittent bolus

Anesthesia and Critical Care Concerns/Other Considerations Addition of sodium bicarbonate to local anesthetic solution will increase onset and potency. Only preservative-free solutions should be used for epidural and spinal administration. Although ropivacaine is chemically related to bupivacaine, it is not a racemic mixture (made up of the S-form enantiomer only) and, is less toxic than bupivacaine.

Pregnancy Risk Factor B

Contraindications Hypersensitivity to amide-type local anesthetics (eg, bupivacaine, mepivacaine, lidocaine) or any component of the formulation; septicemia, severe hypotension and for spinal anesthesia, in the presence of complete heart block

Warnings/Precautions Use with caution in patients with liver disease, cardiovascular disease, neurological or psychiatric disorders; it is not recommended for use in emergency situations where rapid administration is necessary

Adverse Reactions

>5% (dose and route related):

- Cardiovascular: Hypotension, bradycardia
- Central nervous system: Headache
- Dermatologic: Pruritus
- Gastrointestinal: Nausea, vomiting
- Hematologic: Anemia
- Neuromuscular & skeletal: Back pain, paresthesia

1% to 5% (dose related):

- Cardiovascular: Hypertension, tachycardia
- Central nervous system: Dizziness, anxiety, lightheadedness
- Endocrine & metabolic: Hypokalemia
- Genitourinary: Urinary retention
- Neuromuscular & skeletal: Hypoesthesia, rigors, circumoral paresthesia
- Otic: Tinnitus
- Renal: Oliguria
- Respiratory: Dyspnea
- Miscellaneous: Shivering

<1% (Limited to important or life-threatening): Angioedema, apnea (usually associated with epidural block in head/neck region), bronchospasm, cardiac arrest, cardiovascular collapse, dyskinesia, hallucinations, hyperthermia, myocardial depression, MI, rash, seizure, syncope, tinnitus, ventricular arrhythmia

(Continued)

Ropivacaine *(Continued)*

Overdosage/Toxicology Treatment is primarily symptomatic and supportive. Termination of anesthesia by pneumatic tourniquet inflation should be attempted when the agent is administered by infiltration or regional injection. Seizures commonly respond to diazepam, while hypotension responds to I.V. fluids and Trendelenburg positioning. Bradyarrhythmias (when the heart rate is <60) can be treated with I.V. or SubQ atropine 15 mcg/kg. With the development of metabolic acidosis, I.V. sodium bicarbonate 0.5-2 mEq/kg and ventilatory assistance should be instituted. Methemoglobinemia should be treated with methylene blue 1-2 mg/kg in a 1% sterile aqueous solution I.V. push over 4-6 minutes repeated up to a total dose of 7 mg/kg.

Drug Interactions Substrate of CYP1A2 (major), 2B6 (minor), 2D6 (minor), 3A4 (minor; may be major in cases of 1A2 inhibition/deficiency)

Amiodarone (and other class III antiarrhythmics): Cardiac effects during concomitant therapy may be additive. In addition, amiodarone may decrease th metabolism of ropivacaine. Monitor.

Ciprofloxacin: May increase ropivacaine levels/effects; monitor.

CYP1A2 inhibitors: May increase the levels/effects of ropivacaine. Example inhibitors include ketoconazole, norfloxacin, ofloxacin, and rofecoxib.

Fluvoxamine: May increase ropivacaine levels/effects; monitor.

Dosage Forms

Infusion, as hydrochloride: 2 mg/mL (100 mL, 200 mL)

Injection, solution, as hydrochloride [preservative free]: 2 mg/mL (10 mL, 20 mL); 5 mg/mL (20 mL, 30 mL); 7.5 mg/mL (20 mL); 10 mg/mL (10 mL, 20 mL)

References

Alahuhta S, Rasanen J, Jouppila P, et al, "The Effects of Epidural Ropivacaine and Bupivacaine for Cesarean Section on Uteroplacental and Fetal Circulation," *Anesthesiology*, 1995, 83(1):23-32.

Datta S, Camann W, Bader A, et al, "Clinical Effects and Maternal and Fetal Plasma Concentrations of Epidural Ropivacaine Versus Bupivacaine for Cesarean Section," *Anesthesiology*, 1995, 82(6):1346-52.

McClure JH, "Ropivacaine," *Br J Anaesth*, 1996, 76(2):300-7.

Scott DB, Lee A, Fagan D, et al, "Acute Toxicity of Ropivacaine Compared With That of Bupivacaine," *Anesth Analg*, 1989, 69(5):563-9.

Wood MB and Rubin AP, "A Comparison of Epidural 1% Ropivacaine and 0.75% Bupivacaine for Lower Abdominal Gynecologic Surgery," *Anesth Analg*, 1993, 76(6):1274-8.

Zaric D, Axelsson K, Nydahl P, et al, "Sensory and Motor Blockade During Epidural Analgesia With 1%, 0.75%, and 0.5% Ropivacaine - A Double-Blind Study," *Anesth Analg*, 1991, 72(4):509-15.

♦ **Ropivacaine Hydrochloride** *see* Ropivacaine *on page 1140*

Rosuvastatin (roe SOO va sta tin)

Related Information

Hyperlipidemia Management *on page 1614*

U.S. Brand Names Crestor®

Canadian Brand Names Crestor®

Synonyms Rosuvastatin Calcium

Pharmacologic Category Antilipemic Agent, HMG-CoA Reductase Inhibitor

Generic Available No

Use Used with dietary therapy for hyperlipidemias to reduce elevations in total cholesterol (TC), LDL-C, apolipoprotein B, and triglycerides (TG) in patients with primary hypercholesterolemia (elevations of 1 or more components are present in Fredrickson type IIa, IIb, and IV hyperlipidemias); treatment of homozygous familial hypercholesterolemia (FH)

Mechanism of Action Inhibitor of 3-hydroxy-3-methylglutaryl coenzyme A (HMG-CoA) reductase, the rate-limiting enzyme in cholesterol synthesis (reduces the production of mevalonic acid from HMG-CoA); this then results in a compensatory increase in the expression of LDL receptors on hepatocyte membranes and a stimulation of LDL catabolism

Pharmacodynamics/Kinetics

Onset: Within 1 week; maximal at 4 weeks

Distribution: V_d: 134 L

Protein binding: 90%

Metabolism: Hepatic (10%), via CYP2C9 (1 active metabolite identified)

Bioavailability: 20% (high first-pass extraction by liver)

Asian patients have been noted to have increased bioavailability.

Half-life elimination: 19 hours

Time to peak, plasma: 3-5 hours

Excretion: Feces (90%), primarily as unchanged drug

Dosage Adults: Oral:

Heterozygous familial and nonfamilial hypercholesterolemia; mixed dyslipidemia:

Initial dose:

General dosing: 10 mg once daily (20 mg in patients with severe hypercholesterolemia)

Conservative dosing: Patients requiring less aggressive treatment or predisposed to myopathy (including patients of Asian descent): 5 mg once daily

Titration: After 2 weeks, may be increased by 5-10 mg once daily; dosing range: 5-40 mg/day (maximum dose: 40 mg once daily)

Note: The 40 mg dose should be reserved for patients who have not achieved goal cholesterol levels on a dose of 20 mg/day, including patients switched from another HMG-CoA reductase inhibitor.

Homozygous FH: Initial: 20 mg once daily (maximum dose: 40 mg/day)

Dosage adjustment with concomitant medications:

Cyclosporine: Rosuvastatin dose should not exceed 5 mg/day

Gemfibrozil: Rosuvastatin dose should not exceed 10 mg/day

Dosage adjustment for persistent, unexplained proteinuria while on 40 mg/day: Reduce dose and evaluate causes

Dosage adjustment in renal impairment:

Mild-to-moderate impairment: No dosage adjustment required.

Cl_{cr} <30 mL/minute/1.73 m^2: Initial: 5 mg/day; do not exceed 10 mg once daily

Stability Store between 20°C and 25°C (68°F to 77°F); protect from moisture

Administration May be administered with or without food.

Monitoring Parameters Total cholesterol, LDL, and HDL cholesterol; liver function tests should be determined at baseline (prior to initiation), 3 months following initiation, and 3 months after any increase in dose; baseline CPK (recheck CPK in any patient with symptoms suggestive of myopathy)

Anesthesia and Critical Care Concerns/Other Considerations Myopathy: Currently-marketed HMG-CoA reductase inhibitors appear to have a similar potential for causing myopathy. Incidence of severe myopathy is about 0.08% to 0.09%. The factors that increase risk include advanced age (especially >80 years), gender (occurs in women more frequently than men), small body frame, frailty, multisystem disease (eg, chronic renal insufficiency especially due to diabetes), multiple medications, **perioperative periods (higher risk when continued during hospitalization for major surgery)**, and drug interactions (use with caution or avoid).

Pregnancy Risk Factor X

Contraindications Hypersensitivity to rosuvastatin or any component of the formulation; active liver disease; unexplained persistent elevations of serum transaminases (>3 times ULN); pregnancy; breast-feeding

Warnings/Precautions Secondary causes of hyperlipidemia should be ruled out prior to therapy. Liver function must be monitored by periodic laboratory assessment. Use with caution in patients who consume large amounts of ethanol or have a history of liver disease. Rhabdomyolysis with acute renal failure has occurred. Discontinue in any patient in which CPK levels are markedly elevated (>10 times ULN) or if myopathy is suspected/diagnosed. An increased incidence of rosuvastatin-associated myopathy has been reported during concomitant therapy with fibric acid derivatives, niacin, cyclosporine, and in certain subgroups of the Asian population. Risk is also elevated at higher dosages of rosuvastatin. Patients should be instructed to report unexplained muscle pain, tenderness, or weakness, particularly if associated with fever and/or malaise. Use caution in patients predisposed to myopathy (eg, renal failure, advanced age, inadequately treated hypothyroidism). Temporarily withhold in patients experiencing an acute or serious condition predisposing to renal failure secondary to rhabdomyolysis (sepsis, hypotension, major surgery, trauma, severe metabolic or endocrine or electrolyte disorders, uncontrolled seizures). Safety and efficacy have not been established in children (limited experience with homozygous FH in patients >8 years of age).

Adverse Reactions

1% to 10%:

Cardiovascular: Chest pain, hypertension, peripheral edema, palpitation

Central nervous system: Headache (6%), depression, dizziness, insomnia, pain, anxiety, neuralgia, vertigo

Dermatologic: Rash

Gastrointestinal: Pharyngitis (9%), diarrhea, dyspepsia, nausea, abdominal pain, constipation, gastroenteritis, vomiting

(Continued)

Rosuvastatin *(Continued)*

Hematologic: Anemia, bruising

Neuromuscular & skeletal: Myalgia (3%), weakness, back pain, arthritis, arthralgia, hypertonia, paresthesia

Respiratory: Bronchitis, rhinitis, sinusitis, cough

Miscellaneous: Flu-like syndrome

<1% (Limited to important or life-threatening): Arrhythmia, angioedema, hematuria (microscopic), hepatitis, hypersensitivity reactions, jaundice, kidney failure, myasthenia, myositis, myopathy, pancreatitis, photosensitivity, proteinuria (dose related), rhabdomyolysis, syncope

Adverse reactions reported with other HMG-CoA reductase inhibitors include a hypersensitivity syndrome (symptoms may include anaphylaxis, angioedema, arthralgia, erythema multiforme, eosinophilia, hemolytic anemia, lupus syndrome, photosensitivity, polymyalgia rheumatica, positive ANA, purpura, Stevens-Johnson syndrome, toxic epidermal necrolysis, urticaria, vasculitis)

Overdosage/Toxicology No specific experience in overdose. Treatment is supportive. Rosuvastatin is not removed by hemodialysis. CNS vascular lesions and corneal opacities have been reported following high-dose, long-term exposure to HMG-CoA reductase inhibitors in animal studies. The relationship to human exposures has not been established.

Drug Interactions Substrate (minor) of CYP2C9, 3A4

Antacids: Plasma concentrations may be decreased when given with magnesium/aluminum hydroxide-containing antacids. Antacids should be administered at least 2 hours after rosuvastatin.

Cholestyramine and colestipol (bile acid sequestrants): Reduce absorption of several HMG-CoA reductase inhibitors; separate administration times by at least 4 hours. Cholesterol-lowering effects are additive.

Clofibrate and fenofibrate may increase the risk of myopathy and rhabdomyolysis with HMG-CoA reductase inhibitors. Effects on lipid levels may be additive.

Cyclosporine: May increase serum concentrations of rosuvastatin (up to 10 times usual concentrations). Limit dose to 5 mg/day.

Gemfibrozil: Serum concentrations of rosuvastatin may be increased (doubled) during concurrent administration; combination should be avoided. Limit dose to 10 mg/day.

Hormonal contraceptives: Rosuvastatin increases serum concentrations of ethinyl estradiol and norgestrel.

Niacin: May increase the risk of myopathy and rhabdomyolysis with HMG-CoA reductase inhibitors.

Warfarin: Effects may be increased by rosuvastatin. Monitor.

Ethanol/Nutrition/Herb Interactions Ethanol: Avoid excessive ethanol consumption (due to potential hepatic effects).

Food: Red yeast rice contains an estimated 2.4 mg lovastatin per 600 mg rice.

Dietary Considerations May be taken with or without food. Red yeast rice contains an estimated 2.4 mg lovastatin per 600 mg rice.

Dosage Forms Tablet, as calcium: 5 mg, 10 mg, 20 mg, 40 mg

- ♦ **Rosuvastatin Calcium** *see* Rosuvastatin *on page 1142*
- ♦ **Roxanol™** *see* Morphine Sulfate *on page 867*
- ♦ **Roxanol 100™** *see* Morphine Sulfate *on page 867*
- ♦ **Roxanol™-T [DSC]** *see* Morphine Sulfate *on page 867*
- ♦ **Roxicet™** *see* Oxycodone and Acetaminophen *on page 969*
- ♦ **Roxicet™ 5/500** *see* Oxycodone and Acetaminophen *on page 969*
- ♦ **Roxicodone™** *see* Oxycodone *on page 967*
- ♦ **Roxicodone™ Intensol™** *see* Oxycodone *on page 967*
- ♦ **RP-59500** *see* Quinupristin and Dalfopristin *on page 1097*
- ♦ **r-PA** *see* Reteplase *on page 1114*
- ♦ **rPDGF-BB** *see* Becaplermin *on page 160*
- ♦ **RS-25259** *see* Palonosetron *on page 977*
- ♦ **RS-25259-197** *see* Palonosetron *on page 977*
- ♦ **RTCA** *see* Ribavirin *on page 1116*
- ♦ **Rulox [OTC]** *see* Aluminum Hydroxide and Magnesium Hydroxide *on page 76*
- ♦ **Rulox No. 1 [DSC]** *see* Aluminum Hydroxide and Magnesium Hydroxide *on page 76*
- ♦ **Rylosol (Can)** *see* Sotalol *on page 1198*
- ♦ **Rythmodan® (Can)** *see* Disopyramide *on page 404*

- **Rythmodan®-LA (Can)** *see* Disopyramide *on page 404*
- **Rythmol®** *see* Propafenone *on page 1067*
- **Rythmol® Gen-Propafenone (Can)** *see* Propafenone *on page 1067*
- **Rythmol® SR** *see* Propafenone *on page 1067*
- **S2® [OTC]** *see* Epinephrine *on page 457*
- **SAB-Gentamicin (Can)** *see* Gentamicin *on page 589*
- **Sab-Prenase (Can)** *see* PrednisoLONE *on page 1046*
- **Saizen®** *see* Human Growth Hormone *on page 625*
- **Salbu-2 (Can)** *see* Albuterol *on page 50*
- **Salbu-4 (Can)** *see* Albuterol *on page 50*
- **Salbutamol** *see* Albuterol *on page 50*
- **Salflex® (Can)** *see* Salsalate *on page 1147*
- **Salicylsalicylic Acid** *see* Salsalate *on page 1147*
- **SalineX® [OTC]** *see* Sodium Chloride *on page 1183*

Salmeterol (sal ME te role)

Medication Safety Issues

Sound-alike/look-alike issues:

Salmeterol may be confused with Salbutamol

Serevent® may be confused with Serentil®

U.S. Brand Names Serevent® Diskus®

Canadian Brand Names Serevent®

Synonyms Salmeterol Xinafoate

Pharmacologic Category $Beta_2$-Adrenergic Agonist

Restrictions An FDA-approved medication guide is available at http://www.fda.gov/cder/Offices/ODS/labeling.htm; distribute to each patient to whom this medication is dispensed.

Generic Available No

Use Maintenance treatment of asthma and in prevention of bronchospasm with reversible obstructive airway disease, including patients with symptoms of nocturnal asthma; prevention of exercise-induced bronchospasm; maintenance treatment of bronchospasm associated with COPD

Mechanism of Action Relaxes bronchial smooth muscle by selective action on $beta_2$-receptors with little effect on heart rate; because salmeterol acts locally in the lung, therapeutic effect is not predicted by plasma levels

Pharmacodynamics/Kinetics

Onset of action: Asthma: 30-48 minutes, COPD: 2 hours

Peak effect: 2-4 hours, COPD: 3.27-4.75 hours

Duration: 12 hours

Protein binding: 96%

Metabolism: Hepatically hydroxylated

Half-life elimination: 5.5 hours

Excretion: Feces (60%), urine (25%)

Dosage Inhalation, powder (Serevent® Diskus®):

Asthma, maintenance and prevention: Children ≥4 years and Adults: One inhalation (50 mcg) twice daily (~12 hours apart); maximum: 1 inhalation twice daily

Exercise-induced asthma, prevention: Children ≥4 years and Adults: One inhalation (50 mcg) at least 30 minutes prior to exercise; additional doses should not be used for 12 hours; should not be used in individuals already receiving salmeterol twice daily

COPD (maintenance treatment of associated bronchospasm): Adults: One inhalation (50 mcg) twice daily (~12 hours apart); maximum: 1 inhalation twice daily

Stability Inhalation powder: Store at controlled room temperature 20°C to 25°C (68°F to 77°F) in a dry place away from direct heat or sunlight. Stable for 6 weeks after removal from foil pouch.

Administration Inhalation: **Not** to be used for the relief of acute attacks. Not for use with a spacer device. Administer with Diskus® in a level, horizontal position. Do not wash mouthpiece; Diskus® should be kept dry.

Monitoring Parameters FEV_1, peak flow, and/or other pulmonary function tests; blood pressure, heart rate; CNS stimulation; serum glucose, serum potassium. Monitor for increased use of short-acting $beta_2$-agonist inhalers; may be marker of a deteriorating asthma condition.

Pregnancy Risk Factor C

(Continued)

Salmeterol *(Continued)*

Contraindications Hypersensitivity to salmeterol, adrenergic amines, or any component of the formulation; need for acute bronchodilation

Warnings/Precautions

Asthma treatment: [U.S. Boxed Warning]: Long-acting $beta_2$ agonists may increase the risk of asthma-related deaths. In a large, randomized clinical trial (SMART, 2006), salmeterol was associated with a small, but statistically significant increase in asthma-related deaths (when added to usual asthma therapy); risk may be greater in African-American patients versus Caucasians. Should only be used as adjuvant therapy in patients not adequately controlled on inhaled corticosteroids or whose disease requires two maintenance therapies. Salmeterol is not meant to relieve acute asthmatic symptoms, should not be initiated in patients with significantly worsening or acutely deteriorating asthma, and is not a substitute for inhaled or oral corticosteroids. Short-acting $beta_2$ agonist should be used for acute symptoms and symptoms occurring between treatments. Corticosteroids should not be stopped or reduced when salmeterol is initiated. During the initiation of salmeterol watch for signs of worsening asthma.

Concurrent diseases: Use caution in patients with cardiovascular disease (eg, arrhythmia, hypertension, or CHF), seizure disorders, diabetes, glaucoma, hyperthyroidism, hepatic impairment, or hypokalemia. Beta agonists may cause elevation in blood pressure, heart rate, and result in CNS stimulation/excitation. $Beta_2$ agonists may increase risk of arrhythmia, increase serum glucose, or decrease serum potassium.

Adverse events: Salmeterol should not be used more than twice daily; do not exceed recommended dose; do not use with other long-acting $beta_2$ agonists; serious adverse events including fatalities, have been associated with excessive use of inhaled sympathomimetics. Rarely, paradoxical bronchospasm may occur with use of inhaled bronchodilating agents; this should be distinguished from inadequate response. Powder for oral inhalation contains lactose; very rare anaphylactic reactions have been reported in patients with severe milk protein allergy.

Safety and efficacy have not been established in children <4 years of age.

Adverse Reactions

>10%:

Central nervous system: Headache (13% to 17%)
Neuromuscular & skeletal: Pain (1% to 12%)

1% to 10%:

Cardiovascular: Hypertension (4%), edema (1% to <3%)
Central nervous system: Dizziness (4%), sleep disturbance (1% to 3%), fever (1% to 3%), anxiety (1% to <3%), migraine (1% to <3%)
Dermatologic: Rash (1% to 4%), contact dermatitis (1% to 3%), eczema (1% to 3%), urticaria (3%), photodermatitis (1% to 2%)
Endocrine & metabolic: Hyperglycemia (1% to <3%)
Gastrointestinal: Nausea (1% to 3%), dyspepsia (1% to <3%), dental pain (1% to <3%), infections (1% to <3%), oropharyngeal candidiasis (1% to <3%), xerostomia (1% to <3%)
Neuromuscular & skeletal: Muscular cramps/spasm (3%), paresthesia (1% to 3%), arthralgia (1% to <3%), muscular stiffness, rigidity (1% to <3%)
Ocular: Keratitis/conjunctivitis (1% to <3%)
Respiratory: Tracheitis/bronchitis (7%), pharyngitis (up to 6%), cough (5%), influenza (5%), infection (5%), sinusitis (4% to 5%), rhinitis (4% to 5%), nasal congestion (4%), asthma (3% to 4%)

<1% (Limited to important or life-threatening): Anaphylaxis, anaphylactic reaction (severe milk protein allergy), angioedema; arrhythmia (atrial fibrillation, supraventricular tachycardia, extrasystoles); bronchospasm, choking, hypersensitivity reaction, laryngeal spasm, paradoxical bronchospasm, stridor, tachycardia, tremor

Overdosage/Toxicology Symptoms of overdose include tachycardia, tremor, hypertension, angina, and seizures. Hypokalemia also may occur. Cardiac arrest and death may be associated with abuse of beta-agonist bronchodilators. Treatment includes immediate discontinuation and symptomatic and supportive therapies. Cautious use of beta-adrenergic blocking agents may be considered in severe cases.

Drug Interactions Substrate of CYP3A4 (major)

Atomoxetine: May enhance the tachycardia effect of $beta_2$-agonists.

Beta$_2$-agonists: May diminish the bradycardia effect of beta-blockers (beta$_1$ selective).
Beta-blockers (nonselective): May diminish the bronchodilator effect of beta$_2$-agonists.
CYP3A4 inhibitors: May increase the levels/effects of salmeterol. Example inhibitors include amprenavir, atazanavir, clarithromycin, delavirdine, diclofenac, fosamprenavir, imatinib, indinavir, isoniazid, itraconazole, ketoconazole, miconazole, nefazodone, nelfinavir, nicardipine, propofol, quinidine, ritonavir, and telithromycin.
Sympathomimetics: May enhance the adverse/toxic effect of salmeterol.

Dietary Considerations Powder for oral inhalation contains lactose; very rare anaphylactic reactions have been reported in patients with severe milk protein allergy.

Dosage Forms Powder for oral inhalation: 50 mcg (28s, 60s) [delivers 50 mcg/inhalation; contains lactose]

- **Salmeterol Xinafoate** *see* Salmeterol *on page 1145*

Salsalate (SAL sa late)

Medication Safety Issues
Sound-alike/look-alike issues:
Salsalate may be confused with sucralfate, sulfasalazine

Related Information
Chronic Pain Management *on page 1430*

U.S. Brand Names Amigesic®

Canadian Brand Names Amigesic®; Salflex®

Synonyms Disalicylic Acid; Salicylsalicylic Acid

Pharmacologic Category Salicylate

Generic Available Yes

Use Treatment of minor pain or fever; arthritis

Mechanism of Action Inhibits prostaglandin synthesis, acts on the hypothalamus heat-regulating center to reduce fever, blocks prostaglandin synthetase action which prevents formation of the platelet-aggregating substance thromboxane A_2

Pharmacodynamics/Kinetics
Onset of action: Therapeutic: 3-4 days of continuous dosing
Absorption: Complete from small intestine
Metabolism: Hepatically hydrolyzed to two moles of salicylic acid (active)
Half-life elimination: 7-8 hours
Excretion: Primarily urine

Dosage Adults: Oral: 3 g/day in 2-3 divided doses
Dosing comments in renal impairment: In patients with end-stage renal disease undergoing hemodialysis: 750 mg twice daily with an additional 500 mg after dialysis

Anesthesia and Critical Care Concerns/Other Considerations Salsalate does not appear to inhibit platelet aggregation.

Pregnancy Risk Factor C/D (3rd trimester)

Contraindications Hypersensitivity to salsalate or any component of the formulation; GI ulcer or bleeding; pregnancy (3rd trimester)

Warnings/Precautions Use with caution in patients with platelet and bleeding disorders, renal dysfunction, erosive gastritis, or peptic ulcer disease, dehydration, previous nonreaction does not guarantee future safe taking of medication; do not use aspirin in children <16 years of age for chickenpox or flu symptoms due to the association with Reye's syndrome

Adverse Reactions
>10%: Gastrointestinal: Nausea, heartburn, stomach pain, dyspepsia
1% to 10%:
Central nervous system: Drowsiness
Dermatologic: Rash
Gastrointestinal: Gastrointestinal ulceration
Hematologic: Hemolytic anemia
Neuromuscular & skeletal: Weakness
Respiratory: Dyspnea
Miscellaneous: Anaphylactic shock
(Continued)

Salsalate *(Continued)*

<1% (Limited to important or life-threatening): Bronchospasm, does not appear to inhibit platelet aggregation, hepatotoxicity, impaired renal function, iron-deficiency anemia, leukopenia, occult bleeding, thrombocytopenia

Overdosage/Toxicology Symptoms of overdose include respiratory alkalosis, hyperpnea, tachypnea, tinnitus, headache, hyperpyrexia, metabolic acidosis, hypoglycemia, and coma. Nomograms, such as the "Done" nomogram, can be very helpful for estimating the severity of aspirin poisoning and for directing treatment using serum salicylate levels. Treatment can also be based upon symptomatology.

Drug Interactions

Decreased effect with urinary alkalinizers, antacids, corticosteroids; decreased effect of uricosurics, spironolactone; ACE inhibitor effects may be decreased by concurrent therapy with NSAIDs

Increased effect/toxicity of oral anticoagulants, hypoglycemics, methotrexate

Ethanol/Nutrition/Herb Interactions

Ethanol: Avoid ethanol (may enhance gastric mucosal irritation).

Food: Salsalate peak serum levels may be delayed if taken with food.

Herb/Nutraceutical: Avoid cat's claw, dong quai, evening primrose, feverfew, garlic, ginger, ginkgo, red clover, horse chestnut, green tea, ginseng (all have additional antiplatelet activity).

Test Interactions False-negative results for glucose oxidase urinary glucose tests (Clinistix®); false-positives using the cupric sulfate method (Clinitest®); also, interferes with Gerhardt test, VMA determination; 5-HIAA, xylose tolerance test and T_3 and T_4

Dietary Considerations May be taken with food to decrease GI distress.

Dosage Forms

Tablet: 500 mg, 750 mg

Amigesic®: 500 mg, 750 mg

- ♦ **Salt** *see* Sodium Chloride *on page 1183*
- ♦ **Salt Poor Albumin** *see* Albumin *on page 48*
- ♦ **Sal-Tropine™** *see* Atropine *on page 144*
- ♦ **Sandimmune®** *see* CycloSPORINE *on page 337*
- ♦ **Sandimmune® I.V. (Can)** *see* CycloSPORINE *on page 337*
- ♦ **Sandostatin®** *see* Octreotide *on page 946*
- ♦ **Sandostatin LAR®** *see* Octreotide *on page 946*
- ♦ **Sandoz-Amiodarone (Can)** *see* Amiodarone *on page 83*
- ♦ **Sandoz-Atenolol (Can)** *see* Atenolol *on page 136*
- ♦ **Sandoz-Azithromycin (Can)** *see* Azithromycin *on page 149*
- ♦ **Sandoz-Betaxolol (Can)** *see* Betaxolol *on page 173*
- ♦ **Sandoz-Bisoprolol (Can)** *see* Bisoprolol *on page 176*
- ♦ **Sandoz-Ciprofloxacin (Can)** *see* Ciprofloxacin *on page 285*
- ♦ **Sandoz-Citalopram (Can)** *see* Citalopram *on page 297*
- ♦ **Sandoz-Clonazepam (Can)** *see* Clonazepam *on page 313*
- ♦ **Sandoz-Cyclosporine (Can)** *see* CycloSPORINE *on page 337*
- ♦ **Sandoz-Diltiazem CD (Can)** *see* Diltiazem *on page 394*
- ♦ **Sandoz-Diltiazem T (Can)** *see* Diltiazem *on page 394*
- ♦ **Sandoz-Fluoxetine (Can)** *see* Fluoxetine *on page 539*
- ♦ **Sandoz-Glyburide (Can)** *see* GlyBURIDE *on page 598*
- ♦ **Sandoz-Lovastatin (Can)** *see* Lovastatin *on page 782*
- ♦ **Sandoz-Metformin FC (Can)** *see* Metformin *on page 810*
- ♦ **Sandoz-Metoprolol (Can)** *see* Metoprolol *on page 839*
- ♦ **Sandoz-Minocycline (Can)** *see* Minocycline *on page 854*
- ♦ **Sandoz-Nabumetone (Can)** *see* Nabumetone *on page 883*
- ♦ **Sandoz-Paroxetine (Can)** *see* Paroxetine *on page 988*
- ♦ **Sandoz-Pravastatin (Can)** *see* Pravastatin *on page 1042*
- ♦ **Sandoz-Ranitidine (Can)** *see* Ranitidine *on page 1105*
- ♦ **Sandoz-Sertraline (Can)** *see* Sertraline *on page 1161*
- ♦ **Sandoz-Simvastatin (Can)** *see* Simvastatin *on page 1174*
- ♦ **Sandoz-Sumatriptan (Can)** *see* Sumatriptan *on page 1222*
- ♦ **Sandoz-Ticlopidine (Can)** *see* Ticlopidine *on page 1266*

♦ **Sandoz-Timolol (Can)** *see* Timolol *on page 1268*
♦ **Sandoz-Tobramycin (Can)** *see* Tobramycin *on page 1278*
♦ **Sandoz-Topiramate (Can)** *see* Topiramate *on page 1287*
♦ **Sandoz-Valproic (Can)** *see* Valproic Acid and Derivatives *on page 1329*
♦ **Sans Acne® (Can)** *see* Erythromycin *on page 476*

Saquinavir (sa KWIN a veer)

Medication Safety Issues
Sound-alike/look-alike issues:
Saquinavir may be confused with Sinequan®
Fortovase® may be confused with Invirase®
Invirase® may be confused with Fortovase®

Related Information
Moderate Sedation *on page 1442*

U.S. Brand Names Fortovase® [DSC]; Invirase®

Canadian Brand Names Fortovase®; Invirase®

Synonyms Saquinavir Mesylate

Pharmacologic Category Antiretroviral Agent, Protease Inhibitor

Generic Available No

Use Treatment of HIV infection; used in combination with at least two other antiretroviral agents

Mechanism of Action As an inhibitor of HIV protease, saquinavir prevents the cleavage of viral polyprotein precursors which are needed to generate functional proteins in and maturation of HIV-infected cells

Pharmacodynamics/Kinetics
Absorption: Poor; increased with high fat meal; Fortovase® has improved absorption over Invirase®
Distribution: V_d: 700 L; does not distribute into CSF
Protein binding, plasma: ~98%
Metabolism: Extensively hepatic via CYP3A4; extensive first-pass effect
Bioavailability: Invirase®: ~4%; Fortovase®: 12% to 15%
Excretion: Feces (81% to 88%), urine (1% to 3%) within 5 days

Dosage Oral: Children ≥16 years and Adults: **Note:** Fortovase® and Invirase® are not bioequivalent and should not be used interchangeably; only Fortovase® should be used to initiate therapy:
Unboosted regimen: Fortovase®: 1200 mg (six 200 mg capsules) 3 times/day or 1600 mg twice daily within 2 hours after a meal in combination with a nucleoside analog
Note: Saquinavir hard-gel capsules (Invirase®) should not be used in "unboosted regimens."
Ritonavir-boosted regimens:
Fortovase®: 1000 mg (five 200 mg capsules) twice daily in combination with ritonavir 100 mg twice daily
Invirase®: 1000 mg (five 200 mg capsules or two 500 mg tablets) twice daily given in combination with ritonavir 100 mg twice daily. This combination should be given together and within 2 hours after a full meal in combination with a nucleoside analog.
Dosage adjustments of Fortovase® when administered in combination therapy:
Delavirdine: Fortovase® 800 mg 3 times/day
Lopinavir and ritonavir (Kaletra™): Fortovase® or Invirase® 1000 mg twice daily
Nelfinavir: Fortovase®: 1200 mg twice daily
Elderly: Clinical studies did not include sufficient numbers of patients ≥65 years of age; use caution due to increased frequency of organ dysfunction

Stability
Fortovase®: Store in refrigerator. Stable for 3 months when stored at room temperature.
Invirase®: Store at room temperature.

Administration Take saquinavir within 2 hours after a full meal. Avoid direct sunlight when taking saquinavir. When used with ritonavir, saquinavir and ritonavir should be administered at the same time.

Monitoring Parameters Monitor viral load, CD4 count, triglycerides, cholesterol, glucose
(Continued)

Saquinavir *(Continued)*

Anesthesia and Critical Care Concerns/Other Considerations Potential compliance problems, frequency of administration, and adverse effects should be discussed with patients before initiating therapy to help prevent the emergence of resistance.

Pregnancy Risk Factor B

Contraindications Hypersensitivity to saquinavir or any component of the formulation; exposure to direct sunlight without sunscreen or protective clothing; severe hepatic impairment; coadministration with amiodarone, bepridil, cisapride, flecainide, midazolam, pimozide, propafenone, quinidine, rifampin, triazolam, or ergot derivatives

Warnings/Precautions Use caution in patients with hepatic insufficiency. May exacerbate pre-existing hepatic dysfunction; use with caution in patients with hepatitis B or C and in cirrhosis. May be associated with fat redistribution (buffalo hump, increased abdominal girth, breast engorgement, facial atrophy). Use caution in hemophilia. May increase cholesterol and/or triglycerides; hypertriglyceridemia may increase risk of pancreatitis.

Saquinavir interacts with multiple medications (including herbal products) when given concurrently; refer to Drug Interactions. **[U.S. Boxed Warning]: Fortovase® and Invirase® are not bioequivalent and should not be used interchangeably; only Fortovase® should be used to initiate therapy.** Fortovase® is recommended when saquinavir will be given as the sole protease inhibitor; Invirase® may be used only if combined with ritonavir. Safety and efficacy have not been established in children <16 years of age.

Adverse Reactions Protease inhibitors cause dyslipidemia which includes elevated cholesterol and triglycerides and a redistribution of body fat centrally to cause increased abdominal girth, buffalo hump, facial atrophy, and breast enlargement. These agents also cause hyperglycemia.

10%: Gastrointestinal: Diarrhea, nausea

1% to 10%:

- Cardiovascular: Chest pain
- Central nervous system: Anxiety, depression, fatigue, headache, insomnia, pain
- Dermatologic: Rash, verruca
- Endocrine & metabolic: Hyperglycemia, hypoglycemia, hyperkalemia, libido disorder, serum amylase increased
- Gastrointestinal: Abdominal discomfort, abdominal pain, appetite decreased, buccal mucosa ulceration, constipation, dyspepsia, flatulence, taste alteration, vomiting
- Hepatic: AST increased, ALT increased, bilirubin increased
- Neuromuscular & skeletal: Paresthesia, weakness, CPK increased
- Renal: Creatinine kinase increased

<1% (Limited to important or life-threatening): Acute myeloblastic leukemia, alkaline phosphatase increased, allergic reaction, ascites, ataxia, bullous skin eruption, calcium increased, cholangitis, chronic liver disease exacerbation, confusion, hemoglobin decreased, hemolytic anemia, hepatitis, hypokalemia, jaundice, LFTs increased, neuropathy, pain, pancreatitis, polyarthritis, portal hypertension, seizure, serum phosphate decreased, Stevens-Johnson syndrome, syncope, thrombocytopenia, thrombophlebitis, triglycerides increased, upper quadrant abdominal pain

Drug Interactions Substrate of CYP2D6 (minor), 3A4 (major); **Inhibits** CYP2C9 (weak), 2C19 (weak), 2D6 (weak), 3A4 (moderate)

Antiarrhythmics: Serum levels/toxicity may be increased by saquinavir; serious and/or life-threatening reactions may occur. Concurrent use with amiodarone, bepridil, flecainide, propafenone, or quinidine is contraindicated. Use caution with systemic lidocaine.

Anticonvulsants: Saquinavir serum concentrations may be decreased by carbamazepine, phenobarbital, or phenytoin; use with caution.

Azole antifungals (itraconazole, ketoconazole): Serum concentrations of saquinavir may be increased. Dose adjustment was not needed at the study dose when used for a limited time (ketoconazole 400 mg once daily and Fortovase® 1200 mg 3 times daily).

Benzodiazepines: An increase in midazolam and triazolam serum levels may occur resulting in significant over sedation when administered with saquinavir.

Concurrent use is contraindicated. A decreased dose may be considered when used with alprazolam, clorazepate, diazepam, or flurazepam.

Calcium channel blockers: Use with caution; serum concentrations of calcium channel blockers may be increased.

Cisapride: Saquinavir inhibits the metabolism of cisapride and should not be administered concurrently due to risk of life-threatening cardiac arrhythmias.

Clarithromycin: Serum concentrations of saquinavir and clarithromycin may both be increased. Dose adjustment not was not needed at the study dose when used for 7 days (clarithromycin 500 mg twice daily and Fortovase® 1200 mg 3 times/day); dosage adjustment of clarithromycin is recommended in patients with renal impairment.

Corticosteroids: Dexamethasone may decrease serum concentrations of saquinavir; use with caution.

CYP3A4 inducers: CYP3A4 inducers may decrease the levels/effects of saquinavir. Example inducers include aminoglutethimide, carbamazepine, nafcillin, nevirapine, phenobarbital, phenytoin, and rifamycins.

CYP3A4 substrates: Saquinavir may increase the levels/effects of CYP3A4 substrates. Example substrates include benzodiazepines, calcium channel blockers, cyclosporine, mirtazapine, nateglinide, nefazodone, sildenafil (and other PDE-5 inhibitors), tacrolimus, and venlafaxine. Selected benzodiazepines (midazolam and triazolam), cisapride, ergot alkaloids, selected HMG-CoA reductase inhibitors (lovastatin and simvastatin), and pimozide are generally contraindicated with strong CYP3A4 inhibitors.

Ergot alkaloids (dihydroergotamine, ergonovine, ergotamine and methylergonovine): Serum levels/toxicity may be increased by saquinavir; serious and/or life-threatening reactions may occur; concurrent use is contraindicated.

HMG-CoA reductase inhibitors: Saquinavir increased serum concentrations of simvastatin, lovastatin, and atorvastatin; risk of myopathy/rhabdomyolysis may be increased. Avoid use with simvastatin and lovastatin. Use caution with atorvastatin and cerivastatin (fluvastatin, pravastatin, and rosuvastatin are not appreciably metabolized by CYP3A4).

Immunosuppressants: Saquinavir may increase the serum levels of cyclosporine, sirolimus, or tacrolimus.

Methadone: Serum concentrations of methadone may be decreased; an increased dose may be needed when administered with saquinavir

Non-nucleoside reverse transcriptase inhibitors: Saquinavir serum concentrations may be increased by delavirdine. Serum levels of saquinavir and efavirenz may be decreased with concurrent use; saquinavir should not be used as the sole protease inhibitor with efavirenz or nevirapine.

Oral contraceptives: Serum levels of the hormones in oral contraceptives may decrease significantly with administration of saquinavir. Patients should use alternative methods of contraceptives during saquinavir therapy.

PDE-5 inhibitors: Serum concentrations may be increased by saquinavir; dosing adjustment is required. Limit sildenafil dose to 25 mg/48 hours. The maximum dose of tadalafil is 10 mg/72 hours. Vardenafil dosing should not exceed 2.5 mg/24 hours.

Pimozide: Serum levels/toxicity may be increased by saquinavir; serious and/or life-threatening reactions may occur; concurrent use is contraindicated.

Protease inhibitors: Atazanavir, indinavir, and ritonavir may increase serum levels of saquinavir. Serum levels of saquinavir and nelfinavir may be increased with concurrent use. Lopinavir/ritonavir (combination product) may increase serum levels of saquinavir. Refer to Dosage section. Dosage adjustment recommendations with atazanavir have not been established.

Rifabutin: Serum concentrations of saquinavir are decreased and levels of rifabutin are increased. Saquinavir should not be used as the sole protease inhibitor when given with rifabutin.

Rifampin: Serum concentrations of saquinavir are markedly decreased. Risk of hepatotoxicity is increased with concurrent use of ritonavir-boosted saquinavir therapy. Concurrent use is contraindicated.

Tricyclic antidepressants: Serum concentrations of amitriptyline and imipramine may be increased; monitor.

Warfarin: Serum concentrations of warfarin may be affected; monitor.

Ethanol/Nutrition/Herb Interactions

Food: A high-fat meal maximizes bioavailability. Saquinavir levels may increase if taken with grapefruit juice.

(Continued)

Saquinavir *(Continued)*

Herb/Nutraceutical: Saquinavir serum concentrations may be decreased by St John's wort; avoid concurrent use. Garlic capsules may decrease saquinavir serum concentrations; avoid use if saquinavir is the only protease inhibitor.

Dietary Considerations Administer within 2 hours of a meal. Invirase® capsules contain lactose 63.3 mg/capsule (not expected to induce symptoms of intolerance).

Dosage Forms Note: Strength expressed as base; [DSC] = Discontinued product

Capsule, as mesylate:
  Invirase®: 200 mg [contains lactose 63.3 mg/capsule]

Capsule, soft gelatin, as base:
  Fortovase®: 200 mg [DSC]

Tablet, as mesylate:
  Invirase®: 500 mg

- **Saquinavir Mesylate** *see* Saquinavir *on page 1149*
- **Sarafem®** *see* Fluoxetine *on page 539*
- **Sarna® HC (Can)** *see* Hydrocortisone *on page 639*
- **Sarnol®-HC [OTC]** *see* Hydrocortisone *on page 639*
- **SB-265805** *see* Gemifloxacin *on page 587*
- **Scopace™** *see* Scopolamine *on page 1152*

Scopolamine (skoe POL a meen)

Medication Safety Issues

Transdermal patch may contain conducting metal (eg, aluminum); remove patch prior to MRI.

Related Information

Cycloplegic Mydriatics *on page 1564*

U.S. Brand Names Isopto® Hyoscine; Scopace™; Transderm Scōp®

Canadian Brand Names Buscopan®; Transderm-V®

Synonyms Hyoscine Butylbromide; Hyoscine Hydrobromide; Scopolamine Butylbromide; Scopolamine Hydrobromide

Pharmacologic Category Anticholinergic Agent

Generic Available Yes: Injection

Use

Scopolamine hydrobromide:

Injection: Preoperative medication to produce amnesia, sedation, and decrease salivary and respiratory secretions

Ophthalmic: Produce cycloplegia and mydriasis; treatment of iridocyclitis

Oral: Symptomatic treatment of postencephalitic parkinsonism and paralysis agitans; inhibits excessive motility and hypertonus of the genitourinary or gastrointestinal tract in such conditions as the irritable colon syndrome, mild dysentery, diverticulitis, pylorospasm, and cardiospasm

Transdermal: Prevention of nausea/vomiting associated with anesthesia or opiate analgesia; prevention of motion sickness

Scopolamine butylbromide:

Oral/injection: Treatment of smooth muscle spasm of the genitourinary or gastrointestinal tract; injection may also be used to prior to radiological/diagnostic procedures to prevent spasm

Mechanism of Action Blocks the action of acetylcholine at parasympathetic sites in smooth muscle, secretory glands and the CNS; increases cardiac output, dries secretions, antagonizes histamine and serotonin

Pharmacodynamics/Kinetics

Onset of action: Oral, I.M.: 0.5-1 hour; I.V.: 10 minutes
  Peak effect: 20-60 minutes; may take 3-7 days for full recovery; transdermal: 24 hours

Duration: Oral, I.M.: 4-6 hours; I.V.: 2 hours

Absorption: Tertiary salts (hydrobromide) are well absorbed; quaternary salts (butylbromide) are poorly absorbed (local concentrations in the GI tract following oral dosing may be high)

Metabolism: Hepatic

Half-life elimination: 4.8 hours

Excretion: Urine (as metabolites)

Dosage Note: Scopolamine (hyoscine) hydrobromide should not be interchanged with scopolamine butylbromide formulations. Dosages are not equivalent.

Scopolamine hydrobromide:

Preoperative:

Children: I.M., SubQ: 6 mcg/kg/dose (maximum: 0.3 mg/dose) every 6-8 hours

Adults:

I.M., I.V., SubQ: 0.3-0.65 mg; may be repeated every 4-6 hours

Transdermal patch: Apply 2.5 cm^2 patch to hairless area behind ear the night before surgery or 1 hour prior to cesarean section (the patch should be applied no sooner than 1 hour before surgery for best results and removed 24 hours after surgery)

Motion sickness: Transdermal: Adults: Apply 1 disc behind the ear at least 4 hours prior to exposure and every 3 days as needed; effective if applied as soon as 2-3 hours before anticipated need, best if 12 hours before

Refraction: Ophthalmic:

Children: Instill 1 drop of 0.25% to eye(s) twice daily for 2 days before procedure

Adults: Instill 1-2 drops of 0.25% to eye(s) 1 hour before procedure

Iridocyclitis: Ophthalmic:

Children: Instill 1 drop of 0.25% to eye(s) up to 3 times/day

Adults: Instill 1-2 drops of 0.25% to eye(s) up to 4 times/day

Parkinsonism, spasticity, motion sickness: Oral: 0.4-0.8 mg as a range; the dosage may be cautiously increased in parkinsonism and spastic states.

Scopolamine butylbromide:

Gastrointestinal/genitourinary spasm (Buscopan® [CAN]; not available in the U.S.): Adults:

Oral: 10-20 mg daily (1-2 tablets); maximum: 6 tablets/day

I.M., I.V., SubQ: 10-20 mg; maximum: 100 mg/day. Intramuscular injections should be administered 10-15 minutes prior to radiological/diagnostic procedures

Stability Store tablets and/or injection at room temperature of 15°C to 30°C. Protect injection from light.

Hydrobromide injection: Avoid acid solutions, hydrolysis occurs at pH <3.

Butylbromide injection: Stable in D_5W, NS, $D_{10}W$, and LR for up to 8 hours

Administration

I.V.:

Hydrobromide: Dilute with an equal volume of sterile water and administer by direct I.V.; inject over 2-3 minutes

Butylbromide: No dilution is necessary prior to injection; inject at a rate of 1 mL/minute

Transdermal: Topical disc is programmed to deliver *in vivo* 1 mg over 3 days. Once applied, do not remove the patch for 3 full days. Apply to hairless area of skin behind the ear. Wash hands before and after applying the disc to avoid drug contact with eyes.

Anesthesia and Critical Care Concerns/Other Considerations In administering scopolamine, it is important to recognize that lower doses (0.1 mg) may have vagal mimetic effects (ie, increase vagal tone causing paradoxical bradycardia). It is likely that the vagal tonic effects of scopolamine are mediated by blockade of muscarinic receptors at the level of the brain. Disc is programmed to deliver *in vivo* 1 mg over 3 days.

Pregnancy Risk Factor C

Contraindications Hypersensitivity to scopolamine or any component of the formulation; narrow-angle glaucoma; acute hemorrhage; paralytic ileus, GI or GU obstruction; thyrotoxicosis; tachycardia secondary to cardiac insufficiency; myasthenia gravis

Warnings/Precautions Use with caution with hepatic or renal impairment since adverse CNS effects occur more often in these patients; use with caution in infants and children since they may be more susceptible to adverse effects of scopolamine; use with caution in patients with GI obstruction, prostatic hyperplasia (nonobstructive), or urinary retention. Discontinue if patient reports unusual visual disturbances or pain within the eye. Use caution in hiatal hernia, reflux esophagitis, and ulcerative colitis. Scopolamine (hyoscine) hydrobromide should not be interchanged with scopolamine butylbromide formulations; dosages are not equivalent. Transdermal patch may contain conducting metal (eg, aluminum); remove patch prior to MRI.

Adverse Reactions Frequency not defined.

(Continued)

Scopolamine *(Continued)*

Ophthalmic: Note: Systemic adverse effects have been reported following ophthalmic administration.

Cardiovascular: Vascular congestion, edema
Central nervous system: Drowsiness
Dermatologic: Eczematoid dermatitis
Ocular: Blurred vision, photophobia, local irritation, increased intraocular pressure, follicular conjunctivitis, exudate
Respiratory: Congestion

Systemic:

Cardiovascular: Orthostatic hypotension, ventricular fibrillation, tachycardia, palpitation
Central nervous system: Confusion, drowsiness, headache, loss of memory, ataxia, fatigue
Dermatologic: Dry skin, increased sensitivity to light, rash
Endocrine & metabolic: Decreased flow of breast milk
Gastrointestinal: Constipation, xerostomia, dry throat, dysphagia, bloated feeling, nausea, vomiting
Genitourinary: Dysuria
Local: Irritation at injection site
Neuromuscular & skeletal: Weakness
Ocular: Increased intraocular pain, blurred vision
Respiratory: Dry nose
Miscellaneous: Diaphoresis (decreased)
<1% (Limited to important or life-threatening): Anaphylactoid reaction, anaphylaxis, hallucinations, restlessness, retinal pigmentation

Overdosage/Toxicology Symptoms of overdose include dilated pupils, flushed skin, tachycardia, hypertension, and ECG abnormalities. CNS manifestations resemble acute psychosis. CNS depression, circulatory collapse, respiratory failure, and death can occur. For a scopolamine overdose with severe life-threatening symptoms, physostigmine 1-2 mg SubQ or I.V. slowly should be given to reverse toxic effects.

Drug Interactions

Anticholinergic agents: Adverse anticholinergic effects may be additive with other anticholinergic agents (includes tricyclic antidepressants, antihistamines, and phenothiazines).
CNS depressants: Sedative effects may be additive with scopolamine; use caution.

Ethanol/Nutrition/Herb Interactions Ethanol: Avoid ethanol (may increase CNS depression).

Dosage Forms [CAN] = Canadian brand name

Injection, solution, as hydrobromide: 0.4 mg/mL (1 mL)
Injection, solution, as hyoscine-N-butylbromide (Buscopan® [CAN]): 20 mg/mL [not available in U.S.]
Solution, ophthalmic, as hydrobromide (Isopto® Hyoscine): 0.25% (5 mL, 15 mL) [contains benzalkonium chloride]
Tablet, as hyoscine-N-butylbromide (Buscopan® [CAN]): 10 mg [not available in U.S.]
Tablet, soluble, as hydrobromide (Scopace™): 0.4 mg
Transdermal system (Transderm Scōp®): 1.5 mg (4s, 10s, 24s) [releases ~1 mg over 72 hours]

♦ **Scopolamine Butylbromide** *see* Scopolamine *on page 1152*
♦ **Scopolamine Hydrobromide** *see* Scopolamine *on page 1152*

Secobarbital (see koe BAR bi tal)

Medication Safety Issues

Sound-alike/look-alike issues:
Seconal® may be confused with Sectral®

Related Information

Anesthesia Considerations for Neurosurgery *on page 1401*

U.S. Brand Names Seconal®

Synonyms Quinalbarbitone Sodium; Secobarbital Sodium

Pharmacologic Category Barbiturate

Restrictions C-II

Generic Available No

Use Preanesthetic agent; short-term treatment of insomnia

Mechanism of Action Depresses CNS activity by binding to barbiturate site at GABA-receptor complex enhancing GABA activity, depressing reticular activity system; higher doses may be gabamimetic

Pharmacodynamics/Kinetics

Onset of hypnosis: 15-30 minutes

Duration: 3-4 hours with 100 mg dose

Distribution: 1.5 L/kg; crosses the placenta; appears in breast milk

Protein binding: 45% to 60%

Metabolism: Hepatic, by microsomal enzyme system

Half-life elimination: 15-40 hours, mean: 28 hours

Time to peak, serum: Within 2-4 hours

Excretion: Urine (as inactive metabolites, small amounts as unchanged drug)

Dosage Oral:

Children:

Preoperative sedation: 2-6 mg/kg (maximum dose: 100 mg/dose) 1-2 hours before procedure

Sedation: 6 mg/kg/day divided every 8 hours

Adults:

Hypnotic: Usual: 100 mg/dose at bedtime; range 100-200 mg/dose

Preoperative sedation: 100-300 mg 1-2 hours before procedure

Monitoring Parameters Blood pressure, heart rate, respiratory rate, CNS status

Pregnancy Risk Factor D

Contraindications Hypersensitivity to barbiturates or any component of the formulation; marked hepatic impairment; dyspnea or airway obstruction; porphyria; pregnancy

Warnings/Precautions Should be used only after evaluation of potential causes of sleep disturbance. Failure of sleep disturbance to resolve after 7-10 days may indicate psychiatric or medical illness. Potential for drug dependency exists, abrupt cessation may precipitate withdrawal, including status epilepticus in epileptic patients. Do not administer to patients in acute pain. Use caution in elderly, debilitated, renally impaired, or pediatric patients. May cause paradoxical responses, including agitation and hyperactivity, particularly in acute pain and pediatric patients. Use with caution in patients with depression or suicidal tendencies, or in patients with a history of drug abuse. Tolerance, psychological and physical dependence may occur with prolonged use. Use with caution in patients with hepatic function impairment. May cause CNS depression, which may impair physical or mental abilities. Patients must cautioned about performing tasks which require mental alertness (eg, operating machinery or driving). Effects with other sedative drugs or ethanol may be potentiated. May cause respiratory depression or hypotension, Use with caution in hemodynamically unstable patients or patients with respiratory disease.

Adverse Reactions Frequency not defined.

Cardiovascular: Hypotension

Central nervous system: Dizziness, lightheadedness, "hangover" effect, drowsiness, CNS depression, fever, confusion, mental depression, unusual excitement, nervousness, faint feeling, headache, insomnia, nightmares, hallucinations

Dermatologic: Exfoliative dermatitis, rash, Stevens-Johnson syndrome

Gastrointestinal: Nausea, vomiting, constipation

Hematologic: Agranulocytosis, megaloblastic anemia, thrombocytopenia, thrombophlebitis, urticaria apnea

Local: Pain at injection site

Respiratory: Respiratory depression, laryngospasm

Overdosage/Toxicology Symptoms of overdose include unsteady gait, slurred speech, confusion, jaundice, hypothermia, fever, hypotension, respiratory depression, and coma. Charcoal hemoperfusion or hemodialysis may be useful, especially in the presence of very high serum barbiturate levels when the patient is in shock, coma, or renal failure. Forced alkaline diuresis is of no value in the treatment of intoxications with short-acting barbiturates.

Drug Interactions Induces CYP2A6 (strong), 2C8 (strong), 2C9 (strong)

Acetaminophen: Barbiturates may enhance the hepatotoxic potential of acetaminophen overdoses

(Continued)

Secobarbital *(Continued)*

Antiarrhythmics: Barbiturates may increase the metabolism of antiarrhythmics, decreasing their clinical effect; includes disopyramide, propafenone, and quinidine

Anticonvulsants: Barbiturates may increase the metabolism of anticonvulsants; includes ethosuximide, felbamate (possibly), lamotrigine, phenytoin, tiagabine, topiramate, and zonisamide; does not appear to affect gabapentin or levetiracetam

Antineoplastics: Limited evidence suggests that enzyme-inducing anticonvulsant therapy may reduce the effectiveness of some chemotherapy regimens (specifically in ALL); teniposide and methotrexate may be cleared more rapidly in these patients

Antipsychotics: Barbiturates may enhance the metabolism (decrease the efficacy) of antipsychotics; monitor for altered response; dose adjustment may be needed

Beta-blockers: Metabolism of beta-blockers may be increased and clinical effect decreased; atenolol and nadolol are unlikely to interact given their renal elimination

Calcium channel blockers: Barbiturates may enhance the metabolism of calcium channel blockers, decreasing their clinical effect

Chloramphenicol: Barbiturates may increase the metabolism of chloramphenicol and chloramphenicol may inhibit barbiturate metabolism; monitor for altered response

Cimetidine: Barbiturates may enhance the metabolism of cimetidine, decreasing its clinical effect

CNS depressants: Sedative effects and/or respiratory depression with barbiturates may be additive with other CNS depressants; monitor for increased effect; includes ethanol, sedatives, antidepressants, narcotic analgesics, and benzodiazepines

Corticosteroids: Barbiturates may enhance the metabolism of corticosteroids, decreasing their clinical effect

Cyclosporine: Levels may be decreased by barbiturates; monitor

CYP2A6 substrates: Secobarbital may decrease the levels/effects of CYP2A6 substrates. Example substrates include ifosfamide and rifampin.

CYP2C8 Substrates: Secobarbital may decrease the levels/effects of CYP2C8 substrates. Example substrates include amiodarone, paclitaxel, pioglitazone, repaglinide, and rosiglitazone.

CYP2C9 Substrates: Secobarbital may decrease the levels/effects of CYP2C9 substrates. Example substrates include bosentan, celecoxib, dapsone, fluoxetine, glimepiride, glipizide, losartan, montelukast, nateglinide, paclitaxel, phenytoin, sulfonamides, trimethoprim, warfarin, and zafirlukast.

Doxycycline: Barbiturates may enhance the metabolism of doxycycline, decreasing its clinical effect; higher dosages may be required

Estrogens: Barbiturates may increase the metabolism of estrogens and reduce their efficacy

Felbamate may inhibit the metabolism of barbiturates and barbiturates may increase the metabolism of felbamate

Griseofulvin: Barbiturates may impair the absorption of griseofulvin, and griseofulvin metabolism may be increased by barbiturates, decreasing clinical effect

Guanfacine: Effect may be decreased by barbiturates

Immunosuppressants: Barbiturates may enhance the metabolism of immunosuppressants, decreasing its clinical effect; includes both cyclosporine and tacrolimus

Loop diuretics: Metabolism may be increased and clinical effects decreased; established for furosemide, effect with other loop diuretics not established

MAO inhibitors: Metabolism of barbiturates may be inhibited, increasing clinical effect or toxicity of the barbiturates

Methadone: Barbiturates may enhance the metabolism of methadone resulting in methadone withdrawal

Methoxyflurane: Barbiturates may enhance the nephrotoxic effects of methoxyflurane

Oral contraceptives: Barbiturates may enhance the metabolism of oral contraceptives, decreasing their clinical effect; an alternative method of contraception should be considered

Theophylline: Barbiturates may increase metabolism of theophylline derivatives and decrease their clinical effect

Tricyclic antidepressants: Barbiturates may increase metabolism of tricyclic antidepressants and decrease their clinical effect; sedative effects may be additive

Valproic acid: Metabolism of barbiturates may be inhibited by valproic acid; monitor for excessive sedation; a dose reduction may be needed

Warfarin: Barbiturates inhibit the hypoprothrombinemic effects of oral anticoagulants via increased metabolism; this combination should generally be avoided

Ethanol/Nutrition/Herb Interactions

Ethanol: Avoid ethanol (may increase CNS depression).

Herb/Nutraceutical: Avoid valerian, St John's wort, kava kava, gotu kola (may increase CNS depression).

Dosage Forms Capsule, as sodium: 100 mg

♦ **Secobarbital Sodium** *see* Secobarbital *on page 1154*

♦ **Seconal®** *see* Secobarbital *on page 1154*

Selegiline (se LE ji leen)

Medication Safety Issues

Sound-alike/look-alike issues:

Selegiline may be confused with Salagen®, Serentil®, sertraline, Serzone®, Stelazine®

Eldepryl® may be confused with Elavil®, enalapril

U.S. Brand Names Eldepryl®; Emsam®

Canadian Brand Names Apo-Selegiline®; Gen-Selegiline; Novo-Selegiline; Nu-Selegiline

Synonyms Deprenyl; L-Deprenyl; Selegiline Hydrochloride

Pharmacologic Category Anti-Parkinson's Agent, MAO Type B Inhibitor; Antidepressant, Monoamine Oxidase Inhibitor

Generic Available Yes: Excludes transdermal system

Use Adjunct in the management of parkinsonian patients in which levodopa/carbidopa therapy is deteriorating; treatment of major depressive disorder

Unlabeled/Investigational Use Early Parkinson's disease; attention-deficit/hyperactivity disorder (ADHD); negative symptoms of schizophrenia; extrapyramidal symptoms; Alzheimer's disease (studies have shown some improvement in behavioral and cognitive performance)

Mechanism of Action Potent, irreversible inhibitor of monoamine oxidase (MAO). When administered orally, the lower plasma concentrations achieved (due to an extensive first-pass effect) confer selective inhibition of MAO type B, which plays a major role in the metabolism of dopamine; selegiline may also increase dopaminergic activity by interfering with dopamine reuptake at the synapse. When administered transdermally, selegiline achieves higher blood levels and effectively inhibits both MAO-A and MAO-B, which blocks catabolism of other centrally-active biogenic amine neurotransmitters.

Pharmacodynamics/Kinetics

Onset of action: Therapeutic: Oral: Within 1 hour

Duration: Oral: 24-72 hours

Absorption: Transdermal: 25% to 30% (of total selegiline content) over 24 hours

Half-life elimination: 18-25 hours

Protein binding: ~90%

Metabolism: Hepatic via CYP2D6, 2C9, and 3A4/5 to N-desmethylselegiline, methamphetamine and amphetamine

Excretion: Urine; feces

Dosage

Oral:

Children and Adolescents: ADHD (unlabeled use): 5-15 mg/day

Adults: Parkinson's disease: 5 mg twice daily with breakfast and lunch or 10 mg in the morning

Elderly: Parkinson's disease: Initial: 5 mg in the morning, may increase to a total of 10 mg/day

Transdermal (Emsam®): Depression:

Adults: Initial: 6 mg/24 hours once daily; may titrate based on clinical response in increments of 3 mg/day every 2 weeks up to a maximum of 12 mg/24 hours

Elderly: 6 mg/24 hours

Dosage adjustment in renal impairment: No adjustment necessary.

Dosage adjustment in hepatic impairment: No adjustment necessary in mild-moderate hepatic impairment.

(Continued)

Selegiline *(Continued)*

Stability

Tablet, capsule: Store at controlled room temperature 15°C to 30°C (59°F to 86°F).

Transdermal: Store at 20°C to 25°C (68°F to 77°F).

Administration Topical: Transdermal (Emsam®): Apply to clean, dry, intact skin to the upper torso (below the neck and above the waist), upper thigh, or outer surface of the upper arm. Avoid exposure of application site to external heat source, which may increase the amount of drug absorbed. Apply at the same time each day and rotate application sites. Wash hands with soap and water after handling. Avoid touching the sticky side of the patch.

Monitoring Parameters Blood pressure; symptoms of parkinsonism; general mood and behavior (increased anxiety, presence of mania or agitation, or suicidal ideation/tendencies)

Anesthesia and Critical Care Concerns/Other Considerations When adding selegiline to levodopa/carbidopa, the dose of the latter can usually be decreased. Studies are investigating the use of selegiline in early Parkinson's disease to slow the progression of the disease. With doses >10 mg/day, selegiline loses MAO type "B" specificity.

Pregnancy Risk Factor C

Contraindications Hypersensitivity to selegiline or any component of the formulation

Oral: Additional contraindication: Concomitant use of meperidine

Transdermal: Additional contraindications: Pheochromocytoma; concomitant use of meperidine, bupropion, selective or dual serotonin reuptake inhibitors (including SSRIs and SNRIs), tricyclic antidepressants, buspirone, tramadol, propoxyphene, methadone, dextromethorphan, St. John's Wort, mirtazapine, cyclobenzaprine, oral selegiline and other MAO inhibitors; sympathomimetic amines (eg, pseudoephedrine), carbamazepine, and oxcarbazepine; elective surgery requiring general anesthesia, local anesthesia containing sympathomimetic vasoconstrictors

Warnings/Precautions

Oral: MAO-B selective inhibition should not pose a problem with tyramine-containing products as long as the typical oral doses are employed, however, rare reactions have been reported. Increased risk of nonselective MAO inhibition occurs with oral doses >10 mg/day. Use of oral selgiline with tricyclic antidepressants and SSRIs has also been associated with rare reactions and should generally be avoided. Addition to levodopa therapy may result in exacerbation of levodopa adverse effects, requiring a reduction in levodopa dosage.

Transdermal: Nonselective MAO inhibition occurs with transdermal delivery and is necessary for antidepressant efficacy. Hypertensive crisis as a result of ingesting tyramine-rich foods is always a concern with nonselective MAO inhibition. Although transdermal delivery minimizes inhibition of MAO-A in the gut, there is limited data with higher transdermal doses; dietary restrictions are recommended with doses >6 mg/24hours. Monitor for worsening of depression, suicidality and/or associated behaviors such as anxiety, agitation, panic attacks, insomnia, irritability, hostility, impulsivity, hypomania, and mania; worsening depression and severe abrupt suicidality that are not part of the presenting symptoms may require discontinuation or modification of drug therapy. Use caution in high-risk patients during initiation of therapy; prescriptions should be written for the smallest quantity. The patient's family or caregiver should be alerted to monitor patients for the emergence of suicidality and associated behaviors such as anxiety, agitation, panic attacks, insomnia, irritability, hostility, impulsivity, akathisia, hypomania, and mania; patients should be instructed to notify their healthcare provider if any of these symptoms or worsening depression occur.

Transdermal selegiline may worsen psychosis in some patients or precipitate a shift to mania or hypomania in patients with bipolar disorder. Monotherapy in patients with bipolar disorder should be avoided. Patients presenting with depressive symptoms should be screened for bipolar disorder. Selegiline is not FDA approved for the treatment of bipolar depression. **[U.S. Boxed Warning]: Antidepressants increase the risk of suicidal thinking and behavior in children and adolescents with major depressive disorder (MDD) and other depressive disorders. Selegiline is not FDA approved for use in children.**

Should not be used in combination with other antidepressants. Do not use within 5 weeks of fluoxetine discontinuation or 1 week of other antidepressant discontinuation. Wait 2 weeks after discontinuing transdermal selegiline before initiating therapy with buspirone or any other contraindicated drug. May cause orthostatic hypotension - use with caution in patients with hypotension or patients who would not tolerate transient hypotensive episodes (cardiovascular or cerebrovascular disease) - effects may be additive with other agents which cause orthostasis. Discontinue at least 10 days prior to elective surgery.

Medication should not be stopped abruptly; taper off as rapidly as possible. Safety and efficacy in pediatric patients have not been established.

Adverse Reactions Unless otherwise noted, the percentage of adverse events is reported for the transdermal patch:

> 10%:

Central nervous system: Headache (18%), insomnia (12%)

Local: Application site reaction (24%)

1% to 10%:

Cardiovascular: Hypotension (including postural 3% to 10%), chest pain (≥1%), hypertension (≥1%), peripheral edema (≥1%)

Central nervous system: Dizziness (7% oral), hallucinations (3% oral), confusion (3% oral), headache (2%) oral), agitation (≥1%), amnesia (≥1%), thinking abnormal (≥1%)

Dermatologic: Rash (4%), bruising (≥1%), pruritus (≥1%), acne (≥1%)

Endocrine and metabolic: Sexual side effects (≤1%), weight loss (5%)

Gastrointestinal: Nausea (10% oral), diarrhea (9%), xerostomia (8%), abdominal pain (4% oral), dyspepsia (4%), constipation (≥1%), flatulence (≥1%), anorexia (≥1%), gastroenteritis (≥1%), taste perversion (≥1%), vomiting (≥1%)

Genitourinary: Dysmenorrhea (≥1%), metrorrhagia (≥1%), UTI (≥1%), urinary frequency (≥1%)

Neuromuscular & skeletal: Myalgia (≥1%), neck pain (≥1%), paresthesia (≥1%)

Otic: Tinnitus (≥1%)

Respiratory: Pharyngitis (3%), sinusitis (3%), cough (≥1%), bronchitis (≥1%)

Miscellaneous: Diaphoresis (≥1%)

Oral and/or transdermal patch: <1% or frequency not defined (limited to important or life-threatening): Abnormal liver function tests, alkaline phosphatase increased, appetite increased, arrhythmia, asthma, ataxia, atrial fibrillation, bacterial infection, behavior/mood changes, bilirubinemia, bradycardia, bradykinesia, breast neoplasm (female), breast pain, chorea, circumoral paresthesia, colitis, confusion, dehydration, delusions, dental caries, depersonalization, depression, dysphagia, dyspnea, emotional lability, epistaxis, eructation, euphoria, face edema, fever, fungal infection, gastritis, generalized spasm, glossitis, hallucinations, heat stroke, hematuria (female), hernia, hostility, hypercholesterolmia, hyperesthesia, hyperglycemia, hyperkinesias, hypertonia, hypoglycemic reaction, hyponatremia, kidney calculus (female), lactate dehydrogenase increased, laryngismus, leukocytosis, leukopenia, libido increased, loss of balance, lymphadenopathy, maculopapular rash, manic reaction, melena, migraine, moniliasis, myasthenia, myocardial infarct, myoclonus, neoplasia, neurosis, osteoporosis, otitis external, palpitation, paranoid reaction, parasitic infection, parosmia, pelvic pain, periodontal abscess, peripheral vascular disorder, pneumonia, polyuria (female), prostatic hyperplasia, rectal hemorrhage, salivation increased, skin hypertrophy, skin benign neoplasm, suicide attempt, syncope, tachycardia, tenosynovitis, tongue edema, tremor, twitching, urinary retention, urinary urgency (male and female), urination impaired (male), urticaria, vaginal hemorrhage, vaginal moniliasis, vaginitis, vasodilatation, vertigo, vesiculobullous rash, viral infection, visual field defect

Overdosage/Toxicology Symptoms of overdose include tachycardia, palpitations, muscle twitching, and seizures. Both hypertension or hypotension can occur with intoxication. While treating hypertension, care is warranted to avoid sudden drops in blood pressure, since this may worsen MAO inhibitor toxicity. Cardiac arrhythmias are best treated with phenytoin or procainamide. Treatment is generally symptom-directed and supportive.

Drug Interactions Substrate of CYP1A2 (minor), 2A6 (minor), 2B6 (major), 2C9 (major), 2D6 (minor), 3A4 (minor); **Inhibits** CYP1A2 (weak), 2A6 (weak), 2C9 (weak), 2C19 (weak), 2D6 (weak), 2E1 (weak), 3A4 (weak)

Note: Many drug interactions involving selegiline are theoretical, primarily based on interactions with nonspecific MAO inhibitors; at oral doses <10 mg/day, the

(Continued)

Selegiline *(Continued)*

risk of these interactions with selegiline may be very low. Transdermal selegiline results in higher plasma levels and nonselective MAO inhibition.

Amphetamines: MAO inhibitors in combination with amphetamines may result in severe hypertensive reaction or serotonin syndrome; these combinations are best avoided (contraindicated with transdermal selegiline).

Anorexiants: Concurrent use of selegiline (high dose) in combination with CNS stimulants or anorexiants may result in serotonin syndrome; these combinations are best avoided; includes dexfenfluramine, fenfluramine, or sibutramine

Atomoxetine: MAO inhibitors may increase the toxicity of atomoxetine; avoid concomitant use.

Barbiturates: MAO inhibitors may inhibit the metabolism of barbiturates and prolong their effect

Bupropion: MAO inhibitors may increase the toxicity of bupropion; avoid concomitant use.

Buspirone: Concomitant use with selegiline may cause increased blood pressure; avoid combination.

Carbamazepine: May increase levels/effects of selegiline; concomitant use of transdermal selegiline is contraindicated.

CNS stimulants: MAO inhibitors in combination with stimulants (methylphenidate) may result in serotonin syndrome; these combinations are best avoided (contraindicated with transdermal selegiline).

COMT inhibitors (eg, entacapone, tolcapone): May increase to toxicity of MAO inhibitors; avoid concomitant use.

CYP2B6 inducers: May decrease the levels/effects of selegiline. Example inducers include carbamazepine, nevirapine, phenobarbital, phenytoin, and rifampin.

CYP2B6 inhibitors: May increase the levels/effects of selegiline. Example inhibitors include desipramine, paroxetine, and sertraline.

CYP2C9 inducers: May decrease the levels/effects of selegiline. Example inducers include phenobarbital, phenytoin, rifampin, rifapentine, and secobarbital.

CYP2C9 inhibitors: May increase the levels/effects of selegiline. Example inhibitors include delavirdine, fluconazole, gemfibrozil, ketoconazole, nicardipine, NSAIDs, sulfonamides, and tolbutamide.

Dextromethorphan: Concurrent use of selegiline (high dose) may result in serotonin syndrome; these combinations are best avoided (contraindicated with transdermal selegiline).

Disulfiram: MAO inhibitors may produce delirium in patients receiving disulfiram; monitor.

Guanadrel and guanethidine: MAO inhibitors inhibit the antihypertensive response to guanadrel or guanethidine; use an alternative antihypertensive agent.

Hypoglycemic agents: MAO inhibitors may produce hypoglycemia in patients with diabetes; monitor.

Levodopa: MAO inhibitors in combination with levodopa may result in hypertensive reactions; monitor.

Lithium: MAO inhibitors in combination with lithium have resulted in malignant hyperpyrexia; this combination is best avoided.

Meperidine: Use with selegiline (high dose) may result in serotonin syndrome; concurrent use contraindicated.

Methadone: Comcomitant use with an MAO inhibitor may increase the risk of serotonin syndrome (contraindicated with transdermal selegiline).

Mirtazapine, nefazodone: Concurrent use of selegiline (high dose) may result in serotonin syndrome; these combinations are best avoided (contraindicated with transdermal selegiline).

Norepinephrine: MAO inhibitors may increase the pressor response of norepinephrine (effect is generally small); monitor (contraindicated with transdermal selegiline).

Oral contraceptives: Increased selegiline levels have been noted with concurrent administration; monitor

Propoxyphene: Comcomitant use with an MAO inhibitor may increase the risk of serotonin syndrome (contraindicated with transdermal selegiline).

Reserpine: MAO inhibitors in combination with reserpine may result in hypertensive reactions; monitor.

Sibutramine: May cause serotonin syndrome when combined with an MAO inhibitor; avoid this combination.

SSRIs/SNRIs: Concurrent use of selegiline with a selective serotonin or serotonin/norepinephrine reuptake inhibitor may result in mania or hypertension. It is generally best to avoid these combinations (contraindicated with transdermal selegiline).

St John's wort: May cause serotonin syndrome when combined with an MAO inhibitor; avoid this combination.

Sympathomimetics (indirect-acting): MAO inhibitors in combination with sympathomimetics such as dopamine, metaraminol, phenylephrine, and decongestants (pseudoephedrine) may result in severe hypertensive reaction; these combinations are best avoided (contraindicated with transdermal selegiline).

Tramadol: May increase the risk of seizures and serotonin syndrome in patients receiving an MAO inhibitor (contraindicated with transdermal selegiline).

Trazodone: Concurrent use of selegiline (high dose) may result in serotonin syndrome; these combinations are best avoided.

Tricyclic antidepressants: May cause serotonin syndrome when combined with an MAO inhibitor; avoid this combination (contraindicated with transdermal selegiline).

Venlafaxine: Concurrent use of selegiline (high dose) may result in serotonin syndrome; these combinations are best avoided (contraindicated with transdermal selegiline).

Ethanol/Nutrition/Herb Interactions

Ethanol: Avoid ethanol. Avoid beverages containing tyramine (hearty red wine and beer).

Food: Selegiline (>10 mg/day) may cause sudden and severe high blood pressure when taken with food high in tyramine (cheeses, sour cream, yogurt, pickled herring, chicken liver, canned figs, raisins, bananas, avocados, soy sauce, broad bean pods, yeast extracts, meats prepared with tenderizers, and many foods aged to improve flavor). Diet restriction of tyramine-rich foods are not necessary for lowest (6 mg) transdermal dose. Small amounts of caffeine may produce irregular heartbeat or high blood pressure and can interact with this medication for up to 2 weeks after stopping its use.

Herb/Nutraceutical: Avoid valerian, St John's wort, SAMe, kava kava (may increase risk of serotonin syndrome and/or excessive sedation).

Dietary Considerations Emsam® 9 mg/24 hours or 12 mg/24 hours: Avoid tyramine-rich foods or beverages beginning the first day of treatment or for 2 weeks after discontinuation or dose reduction to 6 mg/24 hours.

Dosage Forms

Capsule, as hydrochloride (Eldepryl®): 5 mg

Tablet, as hydrochloride: 5 mg

Transdermal system [once-daily patch] (Emsam®): 6 mg/24 hours (30s) [20 cm^2, total selegiline 20 mg]; 9 mg/24 hours (30s) [30 cm^2, total selegiline 30 mg]; 12 mg/24 hours (30s) [40 cm^2, total selegiline 40 mg]

♦ **Selegiline Hydrochloride** *see* Selegiline *on page 1157*
♦ **Selenium** *see* Trace Metals *on page 1296*
♦ **Selepen®** *see* Trace Metals *on page 1296*
♦ **Sensorcaine®** *see* Bupivacaine *on page 196*
♦ **Sensorcaine®-MPF** *see* Bupivacaine *on page 196*
♦ **Septra®** *see* Sulfamethoxazole and Trimethoprim *on page 1215*
♦ **Septra® DS** *see* Sulfamethoxazole and Trimethoprim *on page 1215*
♦ **Septra® Injection (Can)** *see* Sulfamethoxazole and Trimethoprim *on page 1215*
♦ **Serevent® (Can)** *see* Salmeterol *on page 1145*
♦ **Serevent® Diskus®** *see* Salmeterol *on page 1145*
♦ **Serostim®** *see* Human Growth Hormone *on page 625*

Sertraline (SER tra leen)

Medication Safety Issues

Sound-alike/look-alike issues:

Sertraline may be confused with selegiline, Serentil®

Zoloft® may be confused with Zocor®

Related Information

Antidepressant Agents *on page 1551*

(Continued)

Sertraline *(Continued)*

U.S. Brand Names Zoloft®

Canadian Brand Names Apo-Sertraline®; Gen-Sertraline; GMD-Sertraline; Novo-Sertraline; Nu-Sertraline; PMS-Sertraline; ratio-Sertraline; Rhoxal-sertraline; Sandoz-Sertraline; Zoloft®

Synonyms Sertraline Hydrochloride

Pharmacologic Category Antidepressant, Selective Serotonin Reuptake Inhibitor

Restrictions A medication guide concerning the use of antidepressants in children and teenagers can be found on the FDA website at http://www.fda.gov/cder/Offices/ODS/labeling.htm. It should be dispensed to parents or guardians of children and teenagers receiving this medication.

Generic Available No

Use Treatment of major depression; obsessive-compulsive disorder (OCD); panic disorder; post-traumatic stress disorder (PTSD); premenstrual dysphoric disorder (PMDD); social anxiety disorder

Unlabeled/Investigational Use Eating disorders; generalized anxiety disorder (GAD); impulse control disorders

Mechanism of Action Antidepressant with selective inhibitory effects on presynaptic serotonin (5-HT) reuptake and only very weak effects on norepinephrine and dopamine neuronal uptake. *In vitro* studies demonstrate no significant affinity for adrenergic, cholinergic, GABA, dopaminergic, histaminergic, serotonergic, or benzodiazepine receptors.

Pharmacodynamics/Kinetics

Absorption: Slow

Protein binding: 98%

Metabolism: Hepatic; extensive first-pass metabolism

Bioavailability: 88%

Half-life elimination: Parent drug: 26 hours; Metabolite N-desmethylsertraline: 66 hours (range: 62-104 hours)

Time to peak, plasma: 4.5-8.4 hours

Excretion: Urine and feces

Dosage Oral:

Children and Adolescents: OCD:

6-12 years: Initial: 25 mg once daily

13-17 years: Initial: 50 mg once daily

Note: May increase daily dose, at intervals of not less than 1 week, to a maximum of 200 mg/day. If somnolence is noted, give at bedtime.

Adults:

Depression/OCD: Oral: Initial: 50 mg/day (see "Note" above)

Panic disorder, PTSD, social anxiety disorder: Initial: 25 mg once daily; increase to 50 mg once daily after 1 week (see "Note" above)

PMDD: 50 mg/day either daily throughout menstrual cycle **or** limited to the luteal phase of menstrual cycle, depending on physician assessment. Patients not responding to 50 mg/day may benefit from dose increases (50 mg increments per menstrual cycle) up to 150 mg/day when dosing throughout menstrual cycle **or** up to 100 mg day when dosing during luteal phase only. If a 100 mg/day dose has been established with luteal phase dosing, a 50 mg/day titration step for 3 days should be utilized at the beginning of each luteal phase dosing period.

Elderly: Depression/OCD: Start treatment with 25 mg/day in the morning and increase by 25 mg/day increments every 2-3 days if tolerated to 50-100 mg/day; additional increases may be necessary; maximum dose: 200 mg/day

Dosage adjustment/comment in renal impairment: Multiple-dose pharmacokinetics are unaffected by renal impairment.

Hemodialysis: Not removed by hemodialysis

Dosage adjustment/comment in hepatic impairment: Sertraline is extensively metabolized by the liver; caution should be used in patients with hepatic impairment; a lower dose or less frequent dosing should be used.

Stability Tablets and oral solution should be stored at controlled room temperature of 15°C to 30°C (59°F to 86°F).

Administration Oral concentrate: Must be diluted before use. Immediately before administration, use the dropper provided to measure the required amount of concentrate; mix with 4 ounces ($^1/_2$ cup) of water, ginger ale, lemon/lime soda, lemonade, or orange juice **only**. Do not mix with any other liquids than these. The dose should be taken immediately after mixing; do not mix in advance. A slight haze may appear after mixing; this is normal. **Note:** Use with caution in patients with latex sensitivity; dropper dispenser contains dry natural rubber.

Monitoring Parameters Monitor nutritional intake and weight; mental status for depression, suicidal ideation, anxiety, social functioning, mania, panic attacks; akathisia; growth in pediatric patients

Anesthesia and Critical Care Concerns/Other Considerations Buspirone (15-60 mg/day) may be useful in treatment of sexual dysfunction during treatment with a selective serotonin reuptake inhibitor; may exacerbate tics in Tourette's syndrome.

Pregnancy Risk Factor C

Contraindications Hypersensitivity to sertraline or any component of the formulation; use of MAO inhibitors within 14 days; concurrent use of pimozide; concurrent use of sertraline oral concentrate with disulfiram

Warnings/Precautions

Major psychiatric warnings:

- **[U.S. Boxed Warning]: Antidepressants increase the risk of suicidal thinking and behavior in children and adolescents with major depressive disorder (MDD) and other depressive disorders;** consider risk prior to prescribing. Closely monitor for clinical worsening, suicidality, or unusual changes in behavior; the child's family or caregiver should be instructed to closely observe the patient and communicate condition with healthcare provider. A medication guide concerning the use of antidepressants in children and teenagers should be dispensed with each prescription. **Sertraline is not FDA approved for use in children with major depressive disorder (MDD). However, it is approved for the treatment of obsessive-compulsive disorder (OCD) in children ≥6 years of age.**
- The possibility of a suicide attempt is inherent in major depression and may persist until remission occurs. Patients treated with antidepressants should be observed for clinical worsening and suicidality, especially during the initial few months of a course of drug therapy, or at times of dose changes, either increases or decreases. Worsening depression and severe abrupt suicidality that are not part of the presenting symptoms may require discontinuation or modification of drug therapy. Use caution in high-risk patients during initiation of therapy.
- Prescriptions should be written for the smallest quantity consistent with good patient care. The patient's family or caregiver should be alerted to monitor patients for the emergence of suicidality and associated behaviors such as anxiety, agitation, panic attacks, insomnia, irritability, hostility, impulsivity, akathisia, hypomania, and mania; patients should be instructed to notify their healthcare provider if any of these symptoms or worsening depression or psychosis occur.
- May worsen psychosis in some patients or precipitate a shift to mania or hypomania in patients with bipolar disorder. Monotherapy in patients with bipolar disorder should be avoided. Patients presenting with depressive symptoms should be screened for bipolar disorder. **Sertraline is not FDA approved for the treatment of bipolar depression.**

Key adverse effects:

- Anticholinergic effects: Relatively devoid of these side effects
- CNS depression: Has a low potential to impair cognitive or motor performance; caution operating hazardous machinery or driving.
- SIADH and hyponatremia: Has been associated with the development of SIADH; hyponatremia has been reported rarely, predominately in the elderly

Concurrent disease:

- Hepatic impairment: Use caution; clearance is decreased and plasma concentrations are increased; a lower dosage may be needed.
- Other concurrent illness: Use caution in patients with certain concomitant systemic illness; due to limited experience.
- Platelet aggregation: May impair platelet aggregation, resulting in bleeding.
- Renal impairment: Use caution; clearance is decreased and plasma concentrations are increased; a lower dosage may be needed.
- Seizure disorders: Use caution with a previous seizure disorder or condition predisposing to seizures such as brain damage or alcoholism.
- Sexual dysfunction: May cause or exacerbate sexual dysfunction.
- Uric acid nephropathy: Use caution in patients at risk of uric acid nephropathy; sertraline acts as a mild uricosuric.

(Continued)

Sertraline *(Continued)*

- Weight loss: May cause weight loss. Use caution in patients where weight loss is undesirable.

Concurrent drug therapy:

- Agents which lower seizure threshold: Concurrent therapy with other drugs which lower the seizure threshold.
- Anticoagulants/Antiplatelets: Use caution with concomitant use of NSAIDs, ASA, or other drugs that affect coagulation; the risk of bleeding is potentiated.
- CNS depressants: Use caution with concomitant therapy.
- MAO inhibitors: Potential for severe reaction when used with MAO inhibitors; autonomic instability, coma, death, delirium, diaphoresis, hyperthermia, mental status changes/agitation, muscular rigidity, myoclonus, neuroleptic malignant syndrome features, and seizures may occur.

Special populations:

- Elderly: Use caution in elderly patients.
- Latex sensitivity: Use oral concentrate formulation with caution in patients with latex sensitivity; dropper dispenser contains dry, natural rubber.
- Pediatrics: Monitor growth in pediatric patients.

Special notes:

- Electroconvulsive therapy: May increase the risks associated with electroconvulsive therapy; consider discontinuing, when possible, prior to ECT treatment.
- Withdrawal syndrome: May cause dysphoric mood, irritability, agitation, dizziness, sensory disturbances, anxiety, confusion, headache, lethargy, emotional lability, insomnia, hypomania, tinnitus, and seizures. Upon discontinuation of sertraline therapy, gradually taper dose. If intolerable symptoms occur following a decrease in dosage or upon discontinuation of therapy, then resuming the previous dose with a more gradual taper should be considered.

Adverse Reactions

>10%:

Central nervous system: Insomnia, somnolence, dizziness, headache, fatigue
Gastrointestinal: Xerostomia, diarrhea, nausea
Genitourinary: Ejaculatory disturbances

1% to 10%:

Cardiovascular: Palpitations
Central nervous system: Agitation, anxiety, nervousness
Dermatologic: Rash
Endocrine & metabolic: Decreased libido
Gastrointestinal: Constipation, anorexia, dyspepsia, flatulence, vomiting, weight gain
Genitourinary: Micturition disorders
Neuromuscular & skeletal: Tremors, paresthesia
Ocular: Visual difficulty, abnormal vision
Otic: Tinnitus
Miscellaneous: Diaphoresis (increased)

<1% (Limited to important or life-threatening): Acute renal failure, agranulocytosis, allergic reaction, angioedema, aplastic anemia, atrial arrhythmia, AV block, blindness, dystonia, extrapyramidal symptoms, gum hyperplasia, gynecomastia, hallucinations, hepatic failure, hypothyroidism, jaundice, lupus-like syndrome, neuroleptic malignant syndrome, oculogyric crisis, optic neuritis, pancreatitis (rare), photosensitivity, priapism, psychosis, pulmonary hypertension, QT_c prolongation, serotonin syndrome, serum sickness, SIADH, Stevens-Johnson syndrome (and other severe dermatologic reactions), thrombocytopenia, vasculitis, ventricular tachycardia (including torsade de pointes)

Additional adverse reactions reported in pediatric patients (frequency >2%): Aggressiveness, epistaxis, hyperkinesia, purpura, sinusitis, urinary incontinence

Overdosage/Toxicology Among 634 patients who overdosed on sertraline alone, 8 resulted in a fatal outcome. Symptoms of overdose include somnolence, vomiting, tachycardia, nausea, dizziness, agitation, and tremor. Treatment is symptomatic and supportive.

Drug Interactions Substrate of CYP2B6 (minor), 2C9 (minor), 2C19 (major), 2D6 (major), 3A4 (minor); **Inhibits** CYP1A2 (weak), 2B6 (moderate), 2C8 (weak), 2C9 (weak), 2C19 (moderate), 2D6 (moderate), 3A4 (moderate)

Amphetamines: SSRIs may increase the sensitivity to amphetamines, and amphetamines may increase the risk of serotonin syndrome

Benzodiazepines: Sertraline may inhibit the metabolism of alprazolam and diazepam resulting in elevated serum levels; monitor for increased sedation and psychomotor impairment

Buspirone: Sertraline inhibits the reuptake of serotonin; combined use with a serotonin agonist (buspirone) may cause serotonin syndrome

Carbamazepine: Sertraline may inhibit the metabolism of carbamazepine resulting in increased carbamazepine levels and toxicity; monitor for altered carbamazepine response

Cimetidine: Concurrent use resulted in an increase in sertraline's AUC, C_{max}, and half-life; monitor.

Clozapine: Sertraline may increase serum levels of clozapine; monitor for increased effect/toxicity

Cyclosporine: Sertraline may increase serum levels of cyclosporine (and possibly tacrolimus); monitor

CYP2B6 substrates: Sertraline may increase the levels/effects of CYP2B6 substrates. Example substrates include bupropion, promethazine, propofol, and selegiline.

CYP2C19 inducers: May decrease the levels/effects of sertraline. Example inducers include aminoglutethimide, carbamazepine, phenytoin, and rifampin.

CYP2C19 inhibitors: May increase the levels/effects of sertraline. Example inhibitors include delavirdine, fluconazole, fluvoxamine, gemfibrozil, isoniazid, omeprazole, and ticlopidine.

CYP2C19 substrates: Sertraline may increase the levels/effects of CYP2C19 substrates. Example substrates include citalopram, diazepam, methsuximide, phenytoin, and propranolol.

CYP2D6 inhibitors: May increase the levels/effects of sertraline. Example inhibitors include chlorpromazine, delavirdine, fluoxetine, miconazole, paroxetine, pergolide, quinidine, quinine, ritonavir, and ropinirole.

CYP2D6 substrates: Sertraline may increase the levels/effects of CYP2D6 substrates. Example substrates include amphetamines, selected beta-blockers, dextromethorphan, fluoxetine, lidocaine, mirtazapine, nefazodone, paroxetine, risperidone, ritonavir, thioridazine, tricyclic antidepressants, and venlafaxine.

CYP2D6 prodrug substrates: Sertraline may decrease the levels/effects of CYP2D6 prodrug substrates. Example prodrug substrates include codeine, hydrocodone, oxycodone, and tramadol.

CYP3A4 substrates: Sertraline may increase the levels/effects of CYP3A4 substrates. Example substrates include benzodiazepines, calcium channel blockers, cyclosporine, mirtazapine, nateglinide, nefazodone, sildenafil (and other PDE-5 inhibitors), tacrolimus, and venlafaxine. Selected benzodiazepines (midazolam and triazolam), cisapride, ergot alkaloids, selected HMG-CoA reductase inhibitors (lovastatin and simvastatin), and pimozide are generally contraindicated with strong CYP3A4 inhibitors.

Cyproheptadine: May inhibit the effects of serotonin reuptake inhibitors (fluoxetine); monitor for altered antidepressant response; cyproheptadine acts as a serotonin agonist

Dextromethorphan: Some SSRIs inhibit the metabolism of dextromethorphan; visual hallucinations occurred; monitor for serotonin syndrome

Erythromycin: Serotonin syndrome has been reported when added to sertraline; limited documentation

Haloperidol: Serum concentrations may be increased by sertraline (small increase); monitor

HMG-CoA reductase inhibitors: Sertraline may inhibit the metabolism of lovastatin and simvastatin (metabolized by CYP3A4) resulting in myositis and rhabdomyolysis; although its inhibition is weak, these combinations are best avoided

Lamotrigine: Toxicity has been reported following the addition of sertraline; monitor

Lithium: Patients receiving SSRIs and lithium have developed neurotoxicity; if combination is used, monitor for neurotoxicity

Loop diuretics: Sertraline may cause hyponatremia; additive hyponatremic effects may be seen with combined use of a loop diuretic (bumetanide, furosemide, torsemide); monitor for hyponatremia

MAO inhibitors: Sertraline should not be used with nonselective MAO inhibitors (isocarboxazid, phenelzine); fatal reactions have been reported; this combination is contraindicated.

Meperidine: Concurrent use may result in serotonin syndrome; these combinations are best avoided

Nefazodone: May increase the risk of serotonin syndrome

(Continued)

Sertraline *(Continued)*

NSAIDs: Concomitant use of sertraline and NSAIDs, aspirin, or other drugs affecting coagulation has been associated with an increased risk of bleeding; monitor.

Phenothiazines: Sertraline may inhibit metabolism of thioridazine or mesoridazine, potentially leading to malignant ventricular arrhythmias. Avoid concurrent use. Wait at least 5 weeks after discontinuing sertraline prior to starting thioridazine.

Phenytoin: Sertraline inhibits the metabolism of phenytoin and may result in phenytoin toxicity; monitor for phenytoin toxicity (ataxia, confusion, dizziness, nystagmus, involuntary muscle movement)

Pimozide: Sertraline may increase serum levels of pimozide. Concurrent use is contraindicated.

Ritonavir: Combined use of sertraline with ritonavir may cause serotonin syndrome in HIV-positive patients; monitor

Selegiline: SSRIs have been reported to cause mania or hypertension when combined with selegiline; this combination is best avoided. Concurrent use with SSRIs has been reported to cause serotonin syndrome. As an MAO type B inhibitor, the risk of serotonin syndrome may be less than with nonselective MAO inhibitors.

Sibutramine: May increase the risk of serotonin syndrome with SSRIs; monitor.

SSRIs: Combined use with other drugs which inhibit the reuptake may cause serotonin syndrome

Sumatriptan (and other serotonin agonists): Concurrent use may result in toxicity; weakness, hyper-reflexia, and incoordination have been observed with sumatriptan and SSRIs. In addition, concurrent use may theoretically increase the risk of serotonin syndrome; includes sumatriptan, naratriptan, rizatriptan, and zolmitriptan.

Sympathomimetics: May increase the risk of serotonin syndrome with SSRIs

Tolbutamide: Sertraline may decrease the metabolism of tolbutamide; monitor for changes in glucose control.

Tramadol: Sertraline combined with tramadol (serotonergic effects) may cause serotonin syndrome; monitor

Trazodone: Sertraline may inhibit the metabolism of trazodone resulting in increased toxicity; monitor

Tricyclic antidepressants: Sertraline may inhibit the metabolism of tricyclic antidepressants (amitriptyline, desipramine, imipramine, nortriptyline) resulting is elevated serum levels; if combination is warranted, a low dose of TCA (10-25 mg/day) should be utilized

Tryptophan: Sertraline may inhibit the reuptake of serotonin; combination with tryptophan, a serotonin precursor, may cause agitation and restlessness; this combination is best avoided

Venlafaxine: Sertraline may increase the risk of serotonin syndrome

Warfarin: Sertraline may alter the hypoprothrombinemic response to warfarin; monitor

Zolpidem: Onset of hypnosis may be shortened in patients receiving sertraline; monitor

Ethanol/Nutrition/Herb Interactions

Ethanol: Avoid ethanol (may increase CNS depression).

Food: Sertraline average peak serum levels may be increased if taken with food.

Herb/Nutraceutical: Avoid valerian, St John's wort, kava kava, gotu kola (may increase CNS depression).

Dosage Forms Note: Available as sertraline hydrochloride; mg strength refers to sertraline

Solution, oral concentrate: 20 mg/mL (60 mL) [contains alcohol 12%]

Tablet: 25 mg, 50 mg, 100 mg

♦ **Sertraline Hydrochloride** *see* Sertraline *on page 1161*

Sevoflurane (see voe FLOO rane)

Medication Safety Issues

Sound-alike/look-alike issues:

Ultane® may be confused with Ultram®

Related Information

Anesthesia Considerations for Neurosurgery *on page 1401*

Chronic Renal Failure *on page 1437*

Inhalational Anesthetics *on page 1528*

U.S. Brand Names Ultane®

Canadian Brand Names Sevorane™

Pharmacologic Category General Anesthetic, Inhalation

Generic Available No

Use Induction and maintenance of general anesthesia

Mechanism of Action Inhaled anesthetics alter activity of neuronal ion channels particularly the fast synaptic neurotransmitter receptors (nicotinic acetylcholine, GABA, and glutamate receptors). Limited effects on sympathetic stimulation including cardiovascular system. Seroflurane does not cause respiratory irritation or circulatory stimulation. May depress myocardial contractility, decrease blood pressure through a decrease in systemic vascular resistance and decrease sympathetic nervous activity.

Pharmacodynamics/Kinetics Sevoflurane has a low blood/gas partition coefficient and therefore is associated with a rapid onset of anesthesia and recovery

Onset of action: Time to induction: Within 2 minutes

Duration: Emergence time: Depends on blood concentration when sevoflurane is discontinued. The rate of change of anesthetic concentration in the lung is rapid with sevoflurane because of its low blood gas solubility (0.63). The 90% decrement time (time required for anesthetic concentration in vessel-rich tissues to decrease by 90%) for sevoflurane is short when the duration of anesthesia is <2 hours but increases dramatically as the duration of administration is lengthened.

Metabolism: 3% to 5% hepatic via CYP2E1

Excretion: Exhaled gases

Dosage Minimum alveolar concentration (MAC), the concentration that abolishes movement in response to a noxious stimulus (surgical incision) in 50% of patients, is 2.6% (25 years of age) for sevoflurane. Surgical levels of anesthesia are generally achieved with concentrations from 0.5% to 3%; the concentration at which amnesia and loss of awareness occur is 0.6%.

Minimum alveolar concentrations (MAC) values for surgical levels of anesthesia:

- 0 to 1 month old full-term neonates: Sevoflurane in oxygen: 3.3%
- 1 to <6 months: Sevoflurane in oxygen: 3%
- 6 months to <3 years:
  - Sevoflurane in oxygen: 2.8%
  - Sevoflurane in 60% N_20/40% oxygen: 2%
- 3-12 years: Sevoflurane in oxygen: 2.5%
- 25 years:
  - Sevoflurane in oxygen: 2.6%
  - Sevoflurane in 65% N_20/35% oxygen: 1.4%
- 40 years:
  - Sevoflurane in oxygen: 2.1%
  - Sevoflurane in 65% N_20/35% oxygen: 1.1%
- 60 years:
  - Sevoflurane in oxygen: 1.7%
  - Sevoflurane in 65% N_20/35% oxygen: 0.9%
- 80 years:
  - Sevoflurane in oxygen: 1.4%
  - Sevoflurane in 65% N_20/35% oxygen: 0.7%

Dosage adjustment in renal impairment: Use with caution in renal insufficiency.

Dosage adjustment in hepatic impairment: Use with caution in patients with underlying hepatic conditions.

Stability Store at 15°C to 30°C (59°F to 86°F).

Administration Via sevoflurane-specific calibrated vaporizers; use cautiously in low-flow or closed-circuit systems since sevoflurane is unstable and potentially toxic breakdown products have been liberated.

Monitoring Parameters Blood pressure, temperature, heart rate and rhythm, oxygen saturation, end-tidal CO_2 and end-tidal sevoflurane concentrations should be monitored prior to and throughout anesthesia; temperature of CO_2 absorbent canister

Anesthesia and Critical Care Concerns/Other Considerations When sevoflurane is used in conjunction with desiccated CO_2, isolated reports of fire or extreme heat in the respiratory circuit of anesthesia machines have been reported. Steps that might reduce the risk of these events include: Replace CO_2
(Continued)

Sevoflurane *(Continued)*

absorbent if it has not been used for an extended period of time, shut off anesthesia machine at the end of clinical use or after any case when a subsequent extended period of nonuse is expected, turn off all vaporizers when not in use, verify the integrity of new CO_2 absorbents prior to use, monitor the temperature of the CO_2 absorbent canisters, and monitor the correlation between sevoflurane vaporizer setting and the inspired concentration.

Pregnancy Risk Factor B

Contraindications Previous hypersensitivity to sevoflurane, other halogenated anesthetics, or any component of the formulation; known or suspected susceptibility to malignant hyperthermia

Warnings/Precautions Reaction of sevoflurane with CO_2 absorbents that become desiccated within circle breathing equipment can lead to formation of formaldehyde (causing respiratory irritation) and carbon monoxide; maintain fresh absorbent as per manufacturer guidelines regardless of state of colorimetric indicator. Exothermic reaction of sevoflurane with desiccated CO_2 absorbents has been reported to generate extreme heat, smoke and/or fire within breathing circuit. This reaction also leads to formation of a fluorinated byproduct, compound A, which has been reported to cause nephrotoxicity (eg, proteinuria, glycosuria) in animal studies. Compound A-induced renal toxicity is dose- and exposure time-dependent; minimize exposure risk by not exceeding 2 MAC hours and fresh flow rates <2 L/minute (low fresh gas flow rates maximize rebreathing of the anesthetic).

Causes dose-dependent respiratory depression and blunted ventilatory response to hypoxia and hypercapnia. Hypoxic pulmonary vasoconstriction is blunted which may lead to increased pulmonary shunt. May dilate the cerebral vasculature and increase intracranial pressure. Use cautiously in patients with risk of elevation in intracranial pressure. May cause malignant hyperthermia. Use cautiously in patients with renal dysfunction. Use with caution in patients at risk for seizures; seizures have been reported in children and young adults. Monitor for emergence agitation or delirium. Postoperative hepatitis or hepatic dysfunction with or without jaundice has rarely been reported. Safety in patients with severe hepatic dysfunction has not been determined.

Adverse Reactions

>10%:

Cardiovascular: Hypotension (4% to 11% dose dependent)
Central nervous system: Agitation (7% to 15%)
Gastrointestinal: Nausea (25%), vomiting (18%)
Respiratory: Cough increased (5% to 11%)

1% to 10%:

Cardiovascular: Bradycardia (5%), tachycardia (2% to 6%), hypertension (2%)
Central nervous system: Somnolence (8%), dizziness (4%), hypothermia (1%), headache (1%), fever (1%), emergence delirium
Gastrointestinal: Salivation (2% to 4%)
Respiratory: Laryngospasm (2% to 8%), airway obstruction (8%), breath-holding (2% to 5%), apnea (2%)
Miscellaneous: Shivering (6%)

<1% (Limited to important or life-threatening): Acidosis, albuminuria, alkaline phosphatase increased, allergic reactions, ALT/AST increased, amblyopia, anaphylactic/anaphylactoid reaction, arrhythmia, asthenia, atrial arrhythmia, atrial fibrillation, bigeminy, bilirubinemia, bronchospasm, BUN increased, complete AV block, confusion, conjunctivitis, creatinine increased, crying, dry mouth, dyspnea, fluorosis, glycosuria, hemorrhage, hepatic dysfunction, hepatitis, hiccup, hyperglycemia, hypertonia, hyper-/hypoventilation, hypophosphatemia, hypoxia, insomnia, inverted T wave, jaundice, leukocytosis, LDH increased, liver enzymes increased, malignant hyperthermia, nervousness, oliguria, pain, pharyngitis, pruritus, rash, second degree AV block, seizure, sputum, ST depression, stridor, supraventricular extrasystoles, syncope, taste perversion, thrombocytopenia, urinary retention, ventricular extrasystoles, wheezing

Drug Interactions Substrate of CYP2A6 (minor), 2B6 (minor), 2E1 (major), 3A4 (minor)

Aminoglycosides: Concomitant use may increase risk of nephrotoxicity.
Antihypertensives: Excessive hypotension may occur with combined use.
Benzodiazepines: Concurrent use may decrease the MAC of sevoflurane.

CYP2E1 inhibitors: May increase the levels/effects of sevoflurane. Example inhibitors include disulfiram, isoniazid, and miconazole.

Neuromuscular-blocking agents (nondepolarizing): Sevoflurane may potentiate the action of nondepolarizing, neuromuscular-blocking agents.

Nitrous oxide: Concurrent use may reduce the anesthetic requirement of sevoflurane.

Opioids: Concurrent use may decrease the MAC of sevoflurane.

Dosage Forms Liquid for inhalation: 100% (250 mL)

References

Campagna JA, Miller KW, and Forman SA, "Mechanisms of Action of Inhaled Anesthetics," *N Engl J Med*, 2003, 348(21):2110-23.

Doi M and Ikeda K, "Airway Irritation Produced by Volatile Anaesthetics During Brief Inhalation: Comparison of Halothane, Enflurane, Isoflurane and Sevoflurane," *Can J Anaesth*, 1993, 40(2):122-6.

FDA/CDER resources page, Food and Drug Administration Website, available at: http://www.fda.gov/medwatch/SAFETY/2003/Ultane_deardoc.pdf, last

Frink EJ Jr, Ghantous H, Malan TP, et al, "Plasma Inorganic Fluoride With Sevoflurane Anesthesia: Correlation With Indices of Hepatic and Renal Function," *Anesth Analg*, 1992, 74(2):231-5.

Jones RM, "Desflurane and Sevoflurane: Inhalation Anaesthetics for This Decade?" *Br J Anaesth*, 1990, 65(4):527-36.

Katoh T, Suguro Y, Nakajima R, et al, "Blood Concentrations of Sevoflurane and Isoflurane on Recovery From Anaesthesia," *Br J Anaesth*, 1992, 69(3):259-62.

Smith I, Ding Y, and White PF, "Comparison of Induction, Maintenance, and Recovery Characteristics of Sevoflurane-N20 and Propofol-Sevoflurane-N(2)O With Propofol-Isoflurane-N(2)O Anesthesia," *Anesth Analg*, 1992, 74(2):253-9.

Strum DP and Eger EI 2d, "Partition Coefficients for Sevoflurane in Human Blood, Saline, and Olive Oil," *Anesth Analg*, 1987, 66(7):654-6.

Yasuda N, Lockhart SH, Eger EI 2nd, et al, "Comparison of Kinetics of Sevoflurane and Isoflurane in Humans," *Anesth Analg*, 1991, 72(3):316-24.

- **Sevorane™ (Can)** *see* Sevoflurane *on page 1166*
- **Siladryl® Allergy [OTC]** *see* DiphenhydrAMINE *on page 399*
- **Siladryl® DAS [OTC]** *see* DiphenhydrAMINE *on page 399*
- **Silapap® Children's [OTC]** *see* Acetaminophen *on page 26*
- **Silapap® Infants [OTC]** *see* Acetaminophen *on page 26*

Sildenafil (sil DEN a fil)

Medication Safety Issues

Sound-alike/look-alike issues:

Viagra® may be confused with Allegra®, Vaniqa™

U.S. Brand Names Revatio™; Viagra®

Canadian Brand Names Viagra®

Synonyms UK92480

Pharmacologic Category Phosphodiesterase-5 Enzyme Inhibitor

Generic Available No

Use Treatment of erectile dysfunction; treatment of pulmonary arterial hypertension

Unlabeled/Investigational Use Psychotropic-induced sexual dysfunction; pulmonary arterial hypertension in children

Mechanism of Action

Erectile dysfunction: Does not directly cause penile erections, but affects the response to sexual stimulation. The physiologic mechanism of erection of the penis involves release of nitric oxide (NO) in the corpus cavernosum during sexual stimulation. NO then activates the enzyme guanylate cyclase, which results in increased levels of cyclic guanosine monophosphate (cGMP), producing smooth muscle relaxation and inflow of blood to the corpus cavernosum. Sildenafil enhances the effect of NO by inhibiting phosphodiesterase type 5 (PDE-5), which is responsible for degradation of cGMP in the corpus cavernosum; when sexual stimulation causes local release of NO, inhibition of PDE-5 by sildenafil causes increased levels of cGMP in the corpus cavernosum, resulting in smooth muscle relaxation and inflow of blood to the corpus cavernosum; at recommended doses, it has no effect in the absence of sexual stimulation.

Pulmonary arterial hypertension (PAH): Inhibits phosphodiesterase type 5 (PDE-5) in smooth muscle of pulmonary vasculature where PDE-5 is responsible for the degradation of cyclic guanosine monophosphate (cGMP). Increased cGMP concentration results in pulmonary vasculature relaxation; vasodilation in the pulmonary bed and the systemic circulation (to a lesser degree) may occur.

(Continued)

Sildenafil *(Continued)*

Pharmacodynamics/Kinetics

Onset of action: ~60 minutes
Duration: 2-4 hours
Absorption: Rapid; slower with a high-fat meal
Distribution: V_{dss}: 105 L
Protein binding, plasma: ~96%
Metabolism: Hepatic via CYP3A4 (major) and CYP2C9 (minor route)
Bioavailability: 40%
Half-life elimination: 4 hours
Time to peak: 30-120 minutes; delayed by 60 minutes with a high-fat meal
Excretion: Feces (80%); urine (13%)

Dosage Adults: Oral:

Erectile dysfunction (Viagra®): For most patients, the recommended dose is 50 mg taken as needed, approximately 1 hour before sexual activity. However, sildenafil may be taken anywhere from 30 minutes to 4 hours before sexual activity. Based on effectiveness and tolerance, the dose may be increased to a maximum recommended dose of 100 mg or decreased to 25 mg. The maximum recommended dosing frequency is once daily.

Pulmonary arterial hypertension (Revatio™): 20 mg 3 times/day, taken 4-6 hours apart

Dosage adjustment for patients >65 years of age: Hepatic impairment (cirrhosis), severe renal impairment (creatinine clearance <30 mL/minute): Higher plasma levels have been associated which may result in increase in efficacy and adverse effects; Viagra®: Starting dose of 25 mg should be considered

Dosage considerations for patients taking alpha blockers: Viagra®: Doses of 50 or 100 mg, should not be taken within 4 hours of an alpha blocker; doses of 25 mg may be given at any time

Dosage adjustment for concomitant use of potent CYP34A inhibitors:

Revatio™:
Erythromycin, saquinavir: No dosage adjustment
Itraconazole, ketoconazole, ritonavir: Not recommended

Viagra®:
Erythromycin, itraconazole, ketoconazole, saquinavir: Starting dose of 25 mg should be considered
Ritonavir: Maximum: 25 mg every 48 hours

Stability Store tablets at controlled room temperature of 15°C to 30°C (59°F to 86°F).

Administration

Revatio™: Administer tablets at least 4-6 hours apart
Viagra®: Administer orally ~1 hour before sexual activity (may be used anytime from 4 hours to 30 minutes before).

Anesthesia and Critical Care Concerns/Other Considerations

Use of sildenafil is contraindicated in patients currently taking nitrate preparations. Cardiovascular effects of sildenafil may be potentially hazardous in patients with:

- active coronary ischemia (not on nitrates)
- congestive heart failure and with low blood pressure and low volume status
- complicated, multidrug antihypertensive regimens
- potential for drug-drug interactions that may prolong sildenafil half-life (eg, drugs that predominantly inhibit CYP3A4, such as HMG-CoA reductase inhibitors, protease inhibitors, certain macrolide antibiotics, imidazole antibiotics)

Pregnancy Risk Factor B

Contraindications Hypersensitivity to sildenafil or any component of the formulation; concurrent use of organic nitrates (nitroglycerin) in any form (potentiates the hypotensive effects)

Warnings/Precautions Decreases in blood pressure may occur due to vasodilator effects; use caution in patients with resting hypotension (BP <90/50), hypertension (BP >170/110), fluid depletion, severe left ventricular outflow obstruction, autonomic dysfunction,or taking alpha-blockers. Not recommended for use with pulmonary veno-occlusive disease.

Use caution in patients with cardiovascular disease, including cardiac failure, unstable angina, or a recent history (within the last 6 months) of myocardial infarction, stroke, or life-threatening arrhythmia. Use caution in patients receiving concurrent bosentan.

There is a degree of cardiac risk associated with sexual activity; therefore, physicians may wish to consider the cardiovascular status of their patients prior to initiating any treatment for erectile dysfunction. Sildenafil should be used with caution in patients with anatomical deformation of the penis (angulation, cavernosal fibrosis, or Peyronie's disease), or in patients who have conditions which may predispose them to priapism (sickle cell anemia, multiple myeloma, leukemia).

Rare cases of nonarteritic ischemic optic neuropathy (NAION) have been reported; risk may be increased with history of vision loss. Other risk factors for NAION include low cup-to-disc ratio ("crowded disc"), coronary artery disease, diabetes, hypertension, hyperlipidemia, smoking, and age >50 years.

The safety and efficacy of sildenafil with other treatments for erectile dysfunction have not been established; use is not recommended. May cause dose-related impairment of color discrimination. Use caution in patients with retinitis pigmentosa; a minority have generic disorders of retinal phosphodiesterases (no safety information available). Safety and efficacy in pediatric patients have not been established.

Adverse Reactions Based upon normal doses. (Adverse effects such as flushing, diarrhea, myalgia, and visual disturbances may be increased with doses >100 mg/24 hours.)

>10%:
- Central nervous system: Headache (16% to 46%)
- Gastrointestinal: Dyspepsia (7% to 17%)

1% to 10%:
- Cardiovascular: Flushing (10%)
- Central nervous system: Dizziness, insomnia, pyrexia
- Dermatologic: Erythema, rash
- Gastrointestinal: Diarrhea (3% to 9%), gastritis
- Genitourinary: Urinary tract infection
- Hematologic: Anemia, leukopenia
- Hepatic: LFTs increased
- Neuromuscular & skeletal: Myalgia, paresthesia
- Ocular: Abnormal vision (color changes, blurred or increased sensitivity to light 3%; up to 11% with doses >100 mg)
- Respiratory: Dyspnea exacerbated, epistaxis, nasal congestion, rhinitis, sinusitis

<2% (Limited to important or life-threatening): Abnormal dreams, allergic reaction, anemia, angina pectoris, anorgasmia, asthma, AV block, cardiac arrest, cardiomyopathy, cataract, cerebrovascular hemorrhage, cystitis, depression, dysphagia, hearing decreased, hemorrhage, cerebral thrombosis, colitis, dyspnea, edema, epistaxis, exfoliative dermatitis, eye hemorrhage, gout, heart failure, hematuria, hyper-/hypoglycemia, hypernatremia, hyper-/hypotension, hyperuricemia, intraocular pressure increased, leukopenia, migraine, myocardial ischemia, MI, myasthenia, mydriasis, neuralgia, nonarteritic ischemic optic neuropathy (NAION), palpitation, photosensitivity, postural hypotension, priapism, pulmonary hemorrhage, rectal hemorrhage, retinal vascular disease or bleeding, seizure, shock, stomatitis, syncope, tachycardia, tendon rupture, TIA, urinary incontinence, ventricular arrhythmia, vertigo, visual field loss, vitreous detachment/traction, vomiting

Overdosage/Toxicology In studies with healthy volunteers of single doses up to 800 mg, adverse events were similar to those seen at lower doses but incidence rates were increased. Dialysis not likely to be beneficial due to protein binding.

Drug Interactions Substrate of CYP2C9 (minor), 3A4 (major); **Inhibits** CYP1A2 (weak), 2C9 (weak), 2C19 (weak), 2D6 (weak), 2E1 (weak), 3A4 (weak)

Azole antifungals: May increase the serum concentrations of sildenafil; reduce starting dose to 25 mg.

Alpha-blockers (doxazosin): Concomitant use may lead to symptomatic hypotension in some patients. Sildenafil in doses >25 mg should not be given within 4 hours of administering an alpha-blocker.

Bosentan: May decrease serum concentration and effect of sildenafil.

CYP3A4 inhibitors: May increase the levels/effects of sildenafil. Example inhibitors include azole antifungals, clarithromycin, diclofenac, doxycycline, erythromycin, imatinib, isoniazid, nefazodone, nicardipine, propofol, protease inhibitors, quinidine, telithromycin, and verapamil.

(Continued)

Sildenafil *(Continued)*

Macrolide antibiotics: May increase serum concentrations of sildenafil; reduce starting dose of Viagra® to 25 mg if used with clarithromycin, erythromycin, telithromycin, or troleandomycin. No adjustments with Revatio™ are required.

Nitroglycerin (other nitrates): Concurrent use with sildenafil is contraindicated due to the potential for severe, potentially fatal, hypotensive responses.

Protease inhibitors: May increase the serum concentrations of sildenafil; reduce dose of Viagra® to 25 mg/24 hours; use of Revatio™ is not recommended.

Ethanol/Nutrition/Herb Interactions

Food: Amount and rate of absorption of sildenafil is reduced when taken with a high-fat meal. Serum concentrations/toxicity may be increased with grapefruit juice; avoid concurrent use.

Herb/Nutraceutical: St John's wort may decrease sildenafil levels.

Dosage Forms Tablet:

Revatio™: 20 mg

Viagra®: 25 mg, 50 mg, 100 mg

References

Badesch DB, Abman SH, Ahearn GS, et al, "Medical Therapy for Pulmonary Arterial Hypertension: ACCP Evidence-Based Clinical Practice Guidelines," *Chest*, 2004, 126(1 Suppl):35-62.

Humbert M, Sitbon O, and Simmoneau G, "Treatment of Pulmonary Arterial hypertension," *N Engl J Med*, 2004, 351(14):1425-36.

Jackson G and Chambers J, "Sildenafil for Primary Pulmonary Hypertension: Short and Long-Term Symptomatic Benefit," *Int J Clin Pract*, 2002 56(5):397-8.

Prasad S, Wilkinson J, and Gatzoulis MA, "Sildenafil in Primary Pulmonary Hypertension," *N Engl J Med*, 2000, 343(18):1342.

Watanabe H, Ohashi K, Takeuchi K, et al, "Sildenafil for Primary and Secondary Pulmonary Hypertension," *Clin Pharmacol Ther*, 2002, 71(5):398-402.

♦ **Silfedrine Children's [OTC]** *see* Pseudoephedrine *on page 1085*

♦ **Silphen® [OTC]** *see* DiphenhydrAMINE *on page 399*

♦ **Silvadene®** *see* Silver Sulfadiazine *on page 1173*

Silver Nitrate (SIL ver NYE trate)

Synonyms $AgNO_3$

Pharmacologic Category Antibiotic, Topical; Cauterizing Agent, Topical; Topical Skin Product, Antibacterial

Generic Available Yes

Use Cauterization of wounds and sluggish ulcers, removal of granulation tissue and warts; aseptic prophylaxis of burns

Mechanism of Action Free silver ions precipitate bacterial proteins by combining with chloride in tissue forming silver chloride; coagulates cellular protein to form an eschar; silver ions or salts or colloidal silver preparations can inhibit the growth of both gram-positive and gram-negative bacteria. This germicidal action is attributed to the precipitation of bacterial proteins by liberated silver ions. Silver nitrate coagulates cellular protein to form an eschar, and this mode of action is the postulated mechanism for control of benign hematuria, rhinitis, and recurrent pneumothorax.

Pharmacodynamics/Kinetics

Absorption: Because silver ions readily combine with protein, there is minimal GI and cutaneous absorption of the 0.5% and 1% preparations

Excretion: Highest amounts of silver noted on autopsy have been in kidneys, excretion in urine is minimal

Dosage Children and Adults:

Sticks: Apply to mucous membranes and other moist skin surfaces only on area to be treated 2-3 times/week for 2-3 weeks

Topical solution: Apply a cotton applicator dipped in solution on the affected area 2-3 times/week for 2-3 weeks

Stability Must be stored in a dry place. Store in a tight, light-resistant container. Exposure to light causes silver to oxidize and turn brown, dipping in water causes oxidized film to readily dissolve.

Administration Applicators are **not** for ophthalmic use.

Monitoring Parameters With prolonged use, monitor methemoglobin levels

Pregnancy Risk Factor C

Contraindications Hypersensitivity to silver nitrate or any component of the formulation; not for use on broken skin, cuts, or wounds

Warnings/Precautions Do not use applicator sticks on the eyes. Prolonged use may result in skin discoloration.

Adverse Reactions Frequency not defined.

Dermatologic: Burning and skin irritation, staining of the skin
Endocrine & metabolic: Hyponatremia
Hematologic: Methemoglobinemia

Overdosage/Toxicology Symptoms of overdose include pain and burning of the mouth, salivation, vomiting, diarrhea, shock, coma, convulsions, and death; blackening of skin and mucous membranes. Absorbed nitrate can cause methemoglobinemia. Fatal dose is as low as 2 g; administer sodium chloride in water (10 g/L) to cause precipitation of silver.

Dosage Forms

Applicator sticks, topical: Silver nitrate 75% and potassium nitrate 25% (6", 12", 18")
Solution, topical: 10% (30 mL); 25% (30 mL); 50% (30 mL)

Silver Sulfadiazine (SIL ver sul fa DYE a zeen)

U.S. Brand Names Silvadene®; SSD®; SSD® AF; Thermazene®

Canadian Brand Names Flamazine®

Pharmacologic Category Antibiotic, Topical

Generic Available Yes

Use Prevention and treatment of infection in second and third degree burns

Mechanism of Action Acts upon the bacterial cell wall and cell membrane. Bactericidal for many gram-negative and gram-positive bacteria and is effective against yeast. Active against *Pseudomonas aeruginosa*, *Pseudomonas maltophilia*, *Enterobacter* species, *Klebsiella* species, *Serratia* species, *Escherichia coli*, *Proteus mirabilis*, *Morganella morganii*, *Providencia rettgeri*, *Proteus vulgaris*, *Providencia* species, *Citrobacter* species, *Acinetobacter calcoaceticus*, *Staphylococcus aureus*, *Staphylococcus epidermidis*, *Enterococcus* species, *Candida albicans*, *Corynebacterium diphtheriae*, and *Clostridium perfringens*

Pharmacodynamics/Kinetics

Absorption: Significant percutaneous absorption of silver sulfadiazine can occur especially when applied to extensive burns
Half-life elimination: 10 hours; prolonged with renal impairment
Time to peak, serum: 3-11 days of continuous therapy
Excretion: Urine (~50% as unchanged drug)

Dosage Children and Adults: Topical: Apply once or twice daily with a sterile-gloved hand; apply to a thickness of 1/16"; burned area should be covered with cream at all times

Stability Silvadene® cream will occasionally darken either in the jar or after application to the skin. This color change results from a light catalyzed reaction which is a common characteristic of all silver salts. A similar analogy is the oxidation of silverware. The product of this color change reaction is silver oxide which ranges in color from gray to black. Silver oxide has rarely been associated with permanent skin discoloration. Additionally, the antimicrobial activity of the product is not substantially diminished because the color change reaction involves such a small amount of the active drug and is largely a surface phenomenon.

Administration Apply with a sterile-gloved hand. Apply to a thickness 1/16". Burned area should be covered with cream at all times.

Monitoring Parameters Serum electrolytes, urinalysis, renal function tests, CBC in patients with extensive burns on long-term treatment

Pregnancy Risk Factor B

Contraindications Hypersensitivity to silver sulfadiazine or any component of the formulation; premature infants or neonates <2 months of age (sulfonamides may displace bilirubin and cause kernicterus); pregnancy (approaching or at term)

Warnings/Precautions Use with caution in patients with G6PD deficiency, renal impairment, or history of allergy to other sulfonamides; sulfadiazine may accumulate in patients with impaired hepatic or renal function; fungal superinfection may occur; use of analgesic might be needed before application; systemic absorption is significant and adverse reactions may occur

Adverse Reactions Frequency not defined.

Dermatologic: Itching, rash, erythema multiforme, discoloration of skin, photosensitivity
Hematologic: Hemolytic anemia, leukopenia, agranulocytosis, aplastic anemia
Hepatic: Hepatitis
(Continued)

Silver Sulfadiazine *(Continued)*

Renal: Interstitial nephritis
Miscellaneous: Allergic reactions may be related to sulfa component

Drug Interactions Decreased effect: Topical proteolytic enzymes are inactivated

Dosage Forms

Cream, topical: 1% (25 g, 50 mg, 85 g, 400 g)
Silvadene®, Thermazene®: 1% (20 g, 50 g, 85 g, 400 g, 1000 g)
SSD®: 1% (25 g, 50 g, 85 g, 400 g)
SSD® AF: 1% (50 g, 400 g)

- ♦ **Simply Saline® [OTC]** *see* Sodium Chloride *on page 1183*
- ♦ **Simply Saline® Baby [OTC]** *see* Sodium Chloride *on page 1183*
- ♦ **Simply Saline® Nasal Moist® [OTC]** *see* Sodium Chloride *on page 1183*
- ♦ **Simply Sleep® [OTC]** *see* DiphenhydrAMINE *on page 399*
- ♦ **Simply Stuffy™ [OTC]** *see* Pseudoephedrine *on page 1085*
- ♦ **Simulect®** *see* Basiliximab *on page 158*

Simvastatin (SIM va stat in)

Medication Safety Issues

Sound-alike/look-alike issues:
Zocor® may be confused with Cozaar®, Yocon®, Zoloft®

Related Information

Hyperlipidemia Management *on page 1614*

U.S. Brand Names Zocor®

Canadian Brand Names Apo-Simvastatin®; BCI-Simvastatin; CO Simvastatin; Gen-Simvastatin; Novo-Simvastatin; PMS-Simvastatin; ratio-Simvastatin; Riva-Simvastatin; Sandoz-Simvastatin; Taro-Simvastatin; Zocor®

Pharmacologic Category Antilipemic Agent, HMG-CoA Reductase Inhibitor

Generic Available No

Use Used with dietary therapy for the following:

Secondary prevention of cardiovascular events in hypercholesterolemic patients with established coronary heart disease (CHD) or at high risk for CHD: To reduce cardiovascular morbidity (myocardial infarction, coronary revascularization procedures) and mortality; to reduce the risk of stroke and transient ischemic attacks

Hyperlipidemias: To reduce elevations in total cholesterol, LDL-C, apolipoprotein B, and triglycerides in patients with primary hypercholesterolemia (elevations of 1 or more components are present in Fredrickson type IIa, IIb, III, and IV hyperlipidemias); treatment of homozygous familial hypercholesterolemia

Heterozygous familial hypercholesterolemia (HeFH): In adolescent patients (10-17 years of age, females >1 year postmenarche) with HeFH having LDL-C ≥190 mg/dL **or** LDL ≥160 mg/dL with positive family history of premature cardiovascular disease (CVD), or 2 or more CVD risk factors in the adolescent patient

Mechanism of Action Simvastatin is a methylated derivative of lovastatin that acts by competitively inhibiting 3-hydroxy-3-methylglutaryl-coenzyme A (HMG-CoA) reductase, the enzyme that catalyzes the rate-limiting step in cholesterol biosynthesis

Pharmacodynamics/Kinetics

Onset of action: >3 days
Peak effect: 2 weeks
Absorption: 85%
Protein binding: ~95%
Metabolism: Hepatic via CYP3A4; extensive first-pass effect
Bioavailability: <5%
Half-life elimination: Unknown
Time to peak: 1.3-2.4 hours
Excretion: Feces (60%); urine (13%)

Dosage Oral: **Note:** Doses should be individualized according to the baseline LDL-cholesterol levels, the recommended goal of therapy, and the patient's response; adjustments should be made at intervals of 4 weeks or more; doses may need adjusted based on concomitant medications

Children 10-17 years (females >1 year postmenarche): HeFH: 10 mg once daily in the evening; range: 10-40 mg/day (maximum: 40 mg/day)

Dosage adjustment for simvastatin with concomitant cyclosporine, danazol, fibrates, niacin, amiodarone, or verapamil: Refer to drug-specific dosing in Adults dosing section

Adults:

Homozygous familial hypercholesterolemia: 40 mg once daily in the evening **or** 80 mg/day (given as 20 mg, 20 mg, and 40 mg evening dose)

Prevention of cardiovascular events, hyperlipidemias: 20-40 mg once daily in the evening; range: 5-80 mg/day

Patients requiring only moderate reduction of LDL-cholesterol may be started at 10 mg once daily

Patients requiring reduction of >45% in low-density lipoprotein (LDL) cholesterol may be started at 40 mg once daily in the evening

Patients with CHD or at high risk for CHD: Dosing should be started at 40 mg once daily in the evening; simvastatin may be started simultaneously with diet

Dosage adjustment with concomitant medications:

Cyclosporine or danazol (patient must first demonstrate tolerance to simvastatin ≥5 mg once daily): Initial: 5 mg simvastatin, should **not** exceed 10 mg/day

Fibrates or niacin: Simvastatin dose should **not** exceed 10 mg/day

Amiodarone or verapamil: Simvastatin dose should **not** exceed 20 mg/day

Dosing adjustment/comments in renal impairment: Because simvastatin does not undergo significant renal excretion, modification of dose should not be necessary in patients with mild to moderate renal insufficiency.

Severe renal impairment: Cl_{cr} <10 mL/minute: Initial: 5 mg/day with close monitoring.

Stability Tablets should be stored in tightly-closed containers at temperatures between 5°C to 30°C (41°F to 86°F).

Administration May be taken without regard to meals.

Monitoring Parameters Creatine phosphokinase levels due to possibility of myopathy; serum cholesterol (total and fractionated)

Obtain liver function tests prior to initiation, dose, and thereafter when clinically indicated. Patients titrated to the 80 mg dose should be tested prior to initiation and 3 months after initiating the 80 mg dose. Thereafter, periodic monitoring (ie, semiannually) is recommended for the first year of treatment. Patients with elevated transaminase levels should have a second (confirmatory) test and frequent monitoring until values normalize. Discontinue if increase in ALT/AST is persistently >3 times ULN.

Anesthesia and Critical Care Concerns/Other Considerations Myopathy: Currently-marketed HMG-CoA reductase inhibitors appear to have a similar potential for causing myopathy. Incidence of severe myopathy is about 0.08% to 0.09%. The factors that increase risk include advanced age (especially >80 years), gender (occurs in women more frequently than men), small body frame, frailty, multisystem disease (eg, chronic renal insufficiency especially due to diabetes), multiple medications, **perioperative periods (higher risk when continued during hospitalization for major surgery)**, and drug interactions (use with caution or avoid).

Pregnancy Risk Factor X

Contraindications Hypersensitivity to simvastatin or any component of the formulation; acute liver disease; unexplained persistent elevations of serum transaminases; pregnancy; breast-feeding

Warnings/Precautions Secondary causes of hyperlipidemia should be ruled out prior to therapy. Liver function must be monitored by laboratory assessment. Rhabdomyolysis with acute renal failure has occurred. Risk is dose-related and is increased with concurrent use of lipid-lowering agents which may cause rhabdomyolysis (gemfibrozil, fibric acid derivatives, or niacin at doses ≥1 g/day), during concurrent use with danazol or strong CYP3A4 inhibitors (including amiodarone, clarithromycin, cyclosporine, erythromycin, telithromycin, itraconazole, ketoconazole, nefazodone, grapefruit juice in large quantities, verapamil, or protease inhibitors such as indinavir, nelfinavir, or ritonavir). Weigh the risk versus benefit when combining any of these drugs with simvastatin. Do not initiate simvastatin-containing treatment in a patient with pre-existing therapy of cyclosporine or danazol, unless the patient has previously demonstrated tolerance to ≥5 mg/day simvastatin. Temporarily discontinue in any patient experiencing an acute or serious major medical or surgical condition which may increase the risk of rhabdomyolysis. Discontinue temporarily for elective surgical procedures. Use caution

(Continued)

Simvastatin *(Continued)*

in patients with renal insufficiency. Use with caution in patients who consume large amounts of ethanol or have a history of liver disease. Safety and efficacy have not been established in patients <10 years or in premenarcheal girls.

Adverse Reactions

1% to 10%:

Gastrointestinal: Constipation (2%), dyspepsia (1%), flatulence (2%)

Neuromuscular & skeletal: CPK elevation (>3x normal on one or more occasions - 5%)

Respiratory: Upper respiratory infection (2%)

<1% (Limited to important or life-threatening): Depression, lichen planus, photosensitivity, thrombocytopenia, vertigo

Additional class-related events: Alopecia, anaphylaxis, angioedema, anxiety, cataracts, cholestatic jaundice, depression, dermatomyositis, dyspnea, eosinophilia, erythema multiforme, facial paresis, fulminant hepatic necrosis, gynecomastia, hemolytic anemia, hepatitis, hypersensitivity reaction, impotence, leukopenia, myopathy, ophthalmoplegia, pancreatitis, paresthesia, peripheral nerve palsy, peripheral neuropathy, photosensitivity, polymyalgia rheumatica, psychic disturbance, rash, renal failure (secondary to rhabdomyolysis), rhabdomyolysis, Stevens-Johnson syndrome, systemic lupus erythematosus-like syndrome, thrombocytopenia, thyroid dysfunction, toxic epidermal necrolysis, urticaria, vasculitis, vertigo

Overdosage/Toxicology Very few adverse events. Treatment is symptomatic.

Drug Interactions Substrate of CYP3A4 (major); **Inhibits** CYP2C8 (weak), 2C9 (weak), 2D6 (weak)

Amiodarone may increase the risk of myopathy and rhabdomyolysis; dose of simvastatin should not exceed 20 mg/day.

Antacids: Plasma concentrations may be decreased when given with magnesium-aluminum hydroxide containing antacids (reported with atorvastatin and pravastatin). Clinical efficacy is not altered, no dosage adjustment is necessary

Cholestyramine reduces absorption of several HMG-CoA reductase inhibitors. Separate administration times by at least 4 hours.

Cholestyramine and colestipol (bile acid sequestrants): Cholesterol-lowering effects are additive.

Clofibrate and fenofibrate may increase the risk of myopathy and rhabdomyolysis; dose of simvastatin should not exceed 10 mg/day

Cyclosporine: Concurrent use may increase the risk of myopathy and rhabdomyolysis; dose of simvastatin should not exceed 10 mg/day

CYP3A4 inhibitors: May increase the levels/effects of simvastatin. Example inhibitors include azole antifungals, clarithromycin, diclofenac, doxycycline, erythromycin, imatinib, isoniazid, nefazodone, nicardipine, propofol, protease inhibitors, quinidine, telithromycin, and verapamil.

Danazol: May increase risk of myopathy and rhabdomyolysis; dose of simvastatin should not exceed 10 mg/day.

Gemfibrozil: Increased risk of myopathy and rhabdomyolysis; dose of simvastatin should not exceed 10 mg/day.

Grapefruit juice may inhibit metabolism of simvastatin via CYP3A4; avoid high dietary intakes of grapefruit juice.

Niacin (≥1 g/day): Concurrent use may increase the risk of myopathy and rhabdomyolysis; dose of simvastatin should not exceed 10 mg/day.

Verapamil may increase the risk of myopathy and rhabdomyolysis; dose of simvastatin should not exceed 20 mg/day.

Warfarin effects (hypoprothrombinemic response) may be increased; monitor INR closely when simvastatin is initiated or discontinued.

Ethanol/Nutrition/Herb Interactions

Ethanol: Avoid excessive ethanol consumption (due to potential hepatic effects).

Food: Simvastatin serum concentration may be increased when taken with grapefruit juice; avoid concurrent intake of large quantities (>1 quart/day). Red yeast rice contains an estimated 2.4 mg lovastatin per 600 mg rice.

Herb/Nutraceutical: St John's wort may decrease simvastatin levels.

Dietary Considerations Red yeast rice contains an estimated 2.4 mg lovastatin per 600 mg rice.

Dosage Forms Tablet: 5 mg, 10 mg, 20 mg, 40 mg, 80 mg

♦ **Sinemet®** *see* Levodopa and Carbidopa *on page 743*

♦ **Sinemet® CR** *see* Levodopa and Carbidopa *on page 743*

◆ **Sinequan® [DSC]** *see* Doxepin *on page 422*
◆ **Singulair®** *see* Montelukast *on page 864*

Sirolimus (sir OH li mus)

U.S. Brand Names Rapamune®

Canadian Brand Names Rapamune®

Pharmacologic Category Immunosuppressant Agent

Generic Available No

Use Prophylaxis of organ rejection in patients receiving renal transplants, in combination with corticosteroids and cyclosporine (cyclosporine may be withdrawn in low-to-moderate immunological risk patients after 2-4 months, in conjunction with an increase in sirolimus dosage)

Unlabeled/Investigational Use Investigational: Immunosuppression in other forms of solid organ transplantation and peripheral stem cell/bone marrow transplantation

Mechanism of Action Sirolimus inhibits T-lymphocyte activation and proliferation in response to antigenic and cytokine stimulation. Its mechanism differs from other immunosuppressants. It inhibits acute rejection of allografts and prolongs graft survival.

Pharmacodynamics/Kinetics

Absorption: Rapid

Distribution: 12 L/kg (range: 4-20 L/kg)

Protein binding: 92%, primarily to albumin

Metabolism: Extensively hepatic via CYP3A4; P-glycoprotein-mediated efflux into gut lumen

Bioavailability: Oral solution: 14%; Oral tablet: 18%

Half-life elimination: Mean: 62 hours

Time to peak: 1-2hours

Excretion: Feces (91%); urine (2%)

Dosage

Oral:

Combination therapy with cyclosporine: For *de novo* transplant recipients, a loading dose of 3 times the daily maintenance dose should be administered on day 1 of dosing. Doses should be taken 4 hours after cyclosporine, and should be taken consistently either with or without food.

Children ≥13 years and Adults: Dosing by body weight:

<40 kg: Loading dose: Loading dose: 3 mg/m^2 on day 1, followed by a maintenance dosing of 1 mg/m^2/day

≥40 kg: Loading dose: 6 mg on day 1; maintenance: 2 mg/day

Maintenance therapy after withdrawal of cyclosporine:

Following 2-4 months of combined therapy, withdrawal of cyclosporine may be considered in low-to-moderate risk patients. Cyclosporine withdrawal in not recommended in high immunological risk patients. Cyclosporine should be discontinued over 4-8 weeks, and a necessary increase in the dosage of sirolimus (up to fourfold) should be anticipated due to removal of metabolic inhibition by cyclosporine and to maintain adequate immunosuppressive effects.

Sirolimus dosages should be adjusted to maintain trough concentrations of 12-24 ng/mL. Dosage should be adjusted at intervals of 7-14 days to account for the long half-life of sirolimus. Considerable increases in dosage may require an additional loading dose, calculated as the difference between the target concentration and the current concentration, multiplied by a factor of 3. Loading doses >40 mg may be administered over two days. Serum concentrations should not be used as the sole basis for dosage adjustment (monitor clinical signs/symptoms, tissue biopsy, and laboratory parameters).

Dosage adjustment in renal impairment: No dosage adjustment is necessary in renal impairment

Dosage adjustment in hepatic impairment: Reduce maintenance dose by approximately 33% in hepatic impairment. Loading dose is unchanged.

Stability

Oral solution: Protect from light and store under refrigeration, 2°C to 8°C (36°F to 46°F). A slight haze may develop in refrigerated solutions, but the quality of the product is not affected. After opening, solution should be used in 1 month. If necessary, may be stored at temperatures up to 25°C (77°F) for several days after opening (up to 24 hours for pouches and not >15 days for bottles). Product

(Continued)

Sirolimus *(Continued)*

may be stored in amber syringe for a maximum of 24 hours (at room temperature or refrigerated). Solution should be used immediately following dilution.

Tablet: Store at room temperature of 20°C to 25°C (68°F to 77°F); protect from light

Administration The solution should be mixed with at least 2 ounces of water or orange juice. No other liquids should be used for dilution. Patient should drink diluted solution immediately. The cup should then be refilled with an additional 4 ounces of water or orange juice, stirred vigorously, and the patient should drink the contents at once. Sirolimus should be taken 4 hours after cyclosporine oral solution (modified) or cyclosporine capsules (modified)

Monitoring Parameters Monitor sirolimus levels in pediatric patients, patients ≥13 years of age weighing <40 kg, patients with hepatic impairment, or on concurrent potent inhibitors or inducers of CYP3A4, and/or if cyclosporine dosing is markedly reduced or discontinued. Also monitor serum cholesterol and triglycerides, blood pressure, and serum creatinine. Serum drug concentrations should be determined 3-4 days after loading doses; however, these concentrations should not be used as the sole basis for dosage adjustment, especially during withdrawal of cyclosporine (monitor clinical signs/symptoms, tissue biopsy, and laboratory parameters).

Reference Range Serum trough concentrations:

Concomitant cyclosporine: 5-15 ng/mL

After cyclosporine withdrawal: 12-24 ng/mL

Note: Differences in sensitivity and specificity exist between methods of detection (eg, immunoassay vs. HPLC); target range may vary based on assay conditions

Pregnancy Risk Factor C

Contraindications Hypersensitivity to sirolimus or any component of the formulation

Warnings/Precautions **[U.S. Boxed Warning]: Immunosuppressive agents, including sirolimus, increase the risk of infection and may be associated with the development of lymphoma.** May increase serum lipids (cholesterol and triglycerides). Use with caution in patients with hyperlipidemia. May increase serum creatinine and decrease GFR. Use caution in patients with renal impairment, or when used concurrently with medications which may alter renal function. Monitor renal function closely when combined with cyclosporine; consider dosage adjustment or discontinue in patients with increasing serum creatinine. Has been associated with an increased risk of lymphocele. Cases of interstitial lung disease (eg, pneumonitis, bronchiolitis obliterans organizing pneumonia, pulmonary fibrosis) have been observed; risk may be increased with higher trough levels. Avoid concurrent use of strong CYP3A4 inhibitors or strong inducers of either CYP3A4 or P-glycoprotein. Concurrent use with a calcineurin inhibitor (cyclosporine, tacrolimus) may increase the risk of calcineurin inhibitor-induced hemolytic uremic syndrome/thrombotic thrombocytopenic purpura/thrombotic microangiopathy (HUS/TTP/TMA). Anaphylactic reactions, angioedema and hypersensitivity vasculitis have been reported. May increase sensitivity to UV light; use appropriate sun protection.

Sirolimus is not recommended for use in liver transplant patients; studies indicate an association with an increase risk of hepatic artery thrombosis and graft failure in these patients. Cases of bronchial anastomotic dehiscence have been reported in lung transplant patients when sirolimus was used as part of an immunosuppressive regimen; most of these reactions were fatal. Use in patients with lung transplants is not recommended. Safety and efficacy of cyclosporine withdrawal in high-risk patients is not currently recommended. Safety and efficacy in children <13 years of age, or in adolescent patients <18 years of age considered at high immunological risk, have not been established.

Adverse Reactions Incidence of many adverse effects is dose related

>20%:

Cardiovascular: Hypertension (39% to 49%), peripheral edema (54% to 64%), edema (16% to 24%), chest pain (16% to 24%)

Central nervous system: Fever (23% to 34%), headache (23% to 34%), pain (24% to 33%), insomnia (13% to 22%)

Dermatologic: Acne (20% to 31%)

Endocrine & metabolic: Hypercholesterolemia (38% to 46%), hypophosphatemia (15% to 23%), hyperlipidemia (38% to 57%), hypokalemia (11% to 21%)

Gastrointestinal: Abdominal pain (28% to 36%), nausea (25% to 36%), vomiting (19% to 25%), diarrhea (25% to 42%), constipation (28% to 38%), dyspepsia (17% to 25%), weight gain (8% to 21%)
Genitourinary: Urinary tract infection (20% to 33%)
Hematologic: Anemia (23% to 37%), thrombocytopenia (13% to 40%)
Neuromuscular & skeletal: Arthralgia (25% to 31%), weakness (22% to 40%), back pain (16% to 26%), tremor (21% to 31%)
Renal: Increased serum creatinine (35% to 40%)
Respiratory: Dyspnea (22% to 30%), upper respiratory infection (20% to 26%), pharyngitis (16% to 21%)

3% to 20% (Limited to important or life-threatening):
Cardiovascular: Atrial fibrillation, CHF, postural hypotension, syncope, thrombosis, venous thromboembolism
Central nervous system: Anxiety, confusion, depression, emotional lability, neuropathy, somnolence
Dermatologic: Hirsutism, pruritus, skin hypertrophy, rash (10% to 20%)
Endocrine & metabolic: Cushing's syndrome, diabetes mellitus, hypercalcemia, hyperglycemia, hyperphosphatemia, hypocalcemia, hypoglycemia, hypomagnesemia, hyponatremia, hyperkalemia (12% to 17%)
Gastrointestinal: Esophagitis, gastritis, gingival hyperplasia, ileus
Genitourinary: Impotence
Hematologic: TTP, hemolytic-uremic syndrome, hemorrhage, leukopenia (9% to 15%)
Hepatic: Transaminases increased, ascites
Neuromuscular & skeletal: Increased CPK, bone necrosis, tetany, paresthesia
Otic: Deafness
Renal: Acute tubular necrosis, nephropathy (toxic), urinary retention
Respiratory: Asthma, pulmonary edema, pleural effusion
Miscellaneous: Flu-like syndrome, infection, peritonitis, sepsis

Postmarketing and/or case reports: Anaphylactoid reaction, anaphylaxis, anastomotic disruption, angioedema, fascial dehiscence, hepatic necrosis, hypersensitivity vasculitis; interstitial lung disease (pneumonitis, pulmonary fibrosis, and bronchiolitis obliterans organizing pneumonia) with no identified infectious etiology, lymphedema, neutropenia, pancytopenia. In liver transplant patients (not an approved use), an increase in hepatic artery thrombosis and graft failure were noted in clinical trials. In lung transplant patients (not an approved use), bronchial anastomotic dehiscence has been reported. Calcineurin inhibitor-induced hemolytic uremic syndrome/thrombotic thrombocytopenic purpura/thrombotic microangiopathy (HUS/TTP/TMA) have been reported (with concurrent cyclosporine or tacrolimus).

Overdosage/Toxicology Experience with overdosage has been limited. Dose-limiting toxicities include immune suppression. Reported symptoms of overdose include atrial fibrillation. Treatment is supportive, dialysis is not likely to facilitate removal.

Drug Interactions **Substrate** of CYP3A4 (major); **Inhibits** CYP3A4 (weak)

Antifungal agents, imidazoles (itraconazole, ketoconazole, voriconazole): May increase the levels/effects of sirolimus. Concurrent use is not recommended.

Calcineurin inhibitors (cyclosporine, tacrolimus): Concurrent therapy may increase the risk of HUS/TTP/TMA.

Clarithromycin: May increase serum concentrations of sirolimus. Concurrent use not recommended.

Cyclosporine capsules (modified) or cyclosporine oral solution (modified) increase C_{max} and AUC of sirolimus during concurrent therapy, and cyclosporine clearance may be reduced during concurrent therapy. Sirolimus should be taken 4 hours after cyclosporine oral solution (modified) and/or cyclosporine capsules (modified).

CYP3A4 inducers: CYP3A4 inducers may decrease the levels/effects of sirolimus. Example inducers include aminoglutethimide, carbamazepine, nafcillin, nevirapine, phenobarbital, phenytoin, and rifamycins. Concurrent use is not recommended.

CYP3A4 inhibitors: May increase the levels/effects of sirolimus. Example inhibitors include azole antifungals, clarithromycin, diclofenac, doxycycline, erythromycin, imatinib, isoniazid, nefazodone, nicardipine, propofol, protease inhibitors, quinidine, telithromycin, and verapamil. Concurrent use is not recommended.

Diltiazem may increase serum concentrations of sirolimus; monitor. Verapamil and nicardipine may share this effect.

(Continued)

Sirolimus *(Continued)*

Erythromycin: May increase serum concentrations of sirolimus. Concurrent use is not recommended.

P-gp inducers: May decrease serum concentrations of sirolimus.

Rifampin: May decrease serum concentrations of sirolimus. Concurrent use is not recommended.

Vaccines: Vaccination may be less effective and use of live vaccines should be avoided during sirolimus therapy.

Voriconazole: Sirolimus serum concentrations may be increased; concurrent use is contraindicated.

Ethanol/Nutrition/Herb Interactions

Food: Do not administer with grapefruit juice; may decrease clearance of sirolimus. Ingestion with high-fat meals decreases peak concentrations but increases AUC by 35%. Sirolimus should be taken consistently either with or without food to minimize variability.

Herb/Nutraceutical: St John's wort may decrease sirolimus levels; avoid concurrent use. Avoid cat's claw, echinacea (have immunostimulant properties; consider therapy modifications).

Dietary Considerations Take consistently, with or without food, to minimize variability of absorption.

Dosage Forms

Solution, oral [bottle]: 1 mg/mL (60 mL) [contains ethanol 1.5% to 2.5%; packaged with oral syringes and a carrying case]

Tablet: 1 mg, 2 mg

♦ **SK** *see* Streptokinase *on page 1207*
♦ **Sleep-ettes D [OTC]** *see* DiphenhydrAMINE *on page 399*
♦ **Sleepinal® [OTC]** *see* DiphenhydrAMINE *on page 399*
♦ **SMZ-TMP** *see* Sulfamethoxazole and Trimethoprim *on page 1215*
♦ **Sodium 4-Hydroxybutyrate** *see* Sodium Oxybate *on page 1187*
♦ **Sodium *L*-Triiodothyronine** *see* Liothyronine *on page 765*

Sodium Acetate (SOW dee um AS e tate)

Pharmacologic Category Electrolyte Supplement, Parenteral

Generic Available Yes

Use Sodium source in large volume I.V. fluids to prevent or correct hyponatremia in patients with restricted intake; used to counter acidosis through conversion to bicarbonate

Dosage Sodium acetate is metabolized to bicarbonate on an equimolar basis outside the liver; administer in large volume I.V. fluids as a sodium source. Refer to Sodium Bicarbonate monograph.

Maintenance electrolyte requirements of sodium in parenteral nutrition solutions:

Daily requirements: 3-4 mEq/kg/24 hours or 25-40 mEq/1000 kcal/24 hours

Maximum: 100-150 mEq/24 hours

Stability Protect from light, heat, and from freezing; **incompatible** with acids, acidic salts, alkaloid salts, calcium salts, catecholamines, atropine

Administration Must be diluted prior to I.V. administration; infusion hypertonic solutions (>154 mEq/L) via a central line; maximum rate of administration: 1 mEq/kg/hour

Pregnancy Risk Factor C

Contraindications Alkalosis, hypocalcemia, low sodium diets, edema, cirrhosis

Warnings/Precautions Avoid extravasation, use with caution in patients with hepatic failure

Adverse Reactions 1% to 10%:

Cardiovascular: Thrombosis, hypervolemia

Dermatologic: Chemical cellulitis at injection site (extravasation)

Endocrine & metabolic: Hypernatremia, dilution of serum electrolytes, overhydration, hypokalemia, metabolic alkalosis, hypocalcemia

Gastrointestinal: Gastric distension, flatulence

Local: Phlebitis

Respiratory: Pulmonary edema

Miscellaneous: Congestive conditions

Dietary Considerations Sodium and acetate content of 1 g: 7.3 mEq

Dosage Forms Injection, solution: 2 mEq/mL (20 mL, 50 mL, 100 mL); 4 mEq/mL (50 mL, 100 mL)

- **Sodium Acid Carbonate** *see* Sodium Bicarbonate *on page 1181*
- **Sodium Benzoate and Caffeine** *see* Caffeine *on page 211*

Sodium Bicarbonate (SOW dee um bye KAR bun ate)

Related Information

Allergic Reactions *on page 1395*

U.S. Brand Names Brioschi® [OTC]; Neut®

Synonyms Baking Soda; $NaHCO_3$; Sodium Acid Carbonate; Sodium Hydrogen Carbonate

Pharmacologic Category Alkalinizing Agent; Antacid; Electrolyte Supplement, Oral; Electrolyte Supplement, Parenteral

Generic Available Yes

Use Management of metabolic acidosis; gastric hyperacidity; as an alkalinization agent for the urine; treatment of hyperkalemia; management of overdose of certain drugs, including tricyclic antidepressants and aspirin

Mechanism of Action Dissociates to provide bicarbonate ion which neutralizes hydrogen ion concentration and raises blood and urinary pH

Pharmacodynamics/Kinetics

Onset of action: Oral: Rapid; I.V.: 15 minutes

Duration: Oral: 8-10 minutes; I.V.: 1-2 hours

Absorption: Oral: Well absorbed

Excretion: Urine (<1%)

Dosage

Cardiac arrest: **Routine use of $NaHCO_3$ is not recommended and should be given only after adequate alveolar ventilation has been established and effective cardiac compressions are provided**

Infants and Children: I.V.: 0.5-1 mEq/kg/dose repeated every 10 minutes or as indicated by arterial blood gases; rate of infusion should not exceed 10 mEq/minute; neonates and children <2 years of age should receive 4.2% (0.5 mEq/mL) solution

Adults: I.V.: Initial: 1 mEq/kg/dose one time; maintenance: 0.5 mEq/kg/dose every 10 minutes or as indicated by arterial blood gases

Metabolic acidosis: Infants, Children, and Adults: Dosage should be based on the following formula if blood gases and pH measurements are available:

HCO_3^- (mEq) = 0.3 x weight (kg) x base deficit (mEq/L)

Administer ½ dose initially, then remaining ½ dose over the next 24 hours; monitor pH, serum HCO_3^-, and clinical status

Note: If acid-base status is not available: Dose for older Children and Adults: 2-5 mEq/kg I.V. infusion over 4-8 hours; subsequent doses should be based on patient's acid-base status

Chronic renal failure: Oral: Initiate when plasma HCO_3^- <15 mEq/L

Children: 1-3 mEq/kg/day

Adults: Start with 20-36 mEq/day in divided doses, titrate to bicarbonate level of 18-20 mEq/L

Hyperkalemia: Adults: I.V.: 1 mEq/kg over 5 minutes

Renal tubular acidosis: Oral:

Distal:

Children: 2-3 mEq/kg/day

Adults: 0.5-2 mEq/kg/day in 4-5 divided doses

Proximal: Children and Adults: Initial: 5-10 mEq/kg/day; maintenance: Increase as required to maintain serum bicarbonate in the normal range

Urine alkalinization: Oral:

Children: 1-10 mEq (84-840 mg)/kg/day in divided doses every 4-6 hours; dose should be titrated to desired urinary pH

Adults: Initial: 48 mEq (4 g), then 12-24 mEq (1-2 g) every 4 hours; dose should be titrated to desired urinary pH; doses up to 16 g/day (200 mEq) in patients <60 years and 8 g (100 mEq) in patients >60 years

Antacid: Adults: Oral: 325 mg to 2 g 1-4 times/day

Stability Store injection at room temperature; protect from heat and from freezing; use only clear solutions; Advise patient of milk-alkali syndrome if use is long-term; observe for extravasation when giving I.V.; **incompatible** with acids, acidic salts, alkaloid salts, atropine, calcium salts, catecholamines

(Continued)

Sodium Bicarbonate *(Continued)*

Administration For I.V. administration to infants, use the 0.5 mEq/mL solution or dilute the 1 mEq/mL solution 1:1 with **sterile water**; for direct I.V. infusion in emergencies, administer slowly (maximum rate in infants: 10 mEq/minute); for infusion, dilute to a maximum concentration of 0.5 mEq/mL in dextrose solution and infuse over 2 hours (maximum rate of administration: 1 mEq/kg/hour)

Anesthesia and Critical Care Concerns/Other Considerations The use of bicarbonate for the treatment of lactic acidosis has not been proven useful. Increased pCO_2 after bicarbonate administration may result in an acute decrease in intracellular pH. Bicarbonate does not improve any hemodynamic parameters resulting in improved cardiovascular function. Many clinicians do not use bicarbonate in the treatment of lactic acidosis regardless of the patient's pH level.

Pregnancy Risk Factor C

Contraindications Alkalosis, hypernatremia, severe pulmonary edema, hypocalcemia, unknown abdominal pain

Warnings/Precautions Rapid administration in neonates and children <2 years of age has led to hypernatremia, decreased CSF pressure and intracranial hemorrhage. **Use of I.V. $NaHCO_3$ should be reserved for documented metabolic acidosis and for hyperkalemia-induced cardiac arrest.** Routine use in cardiac arrest is not recommended. Avoid extravasation, tissue necrosis can occur due to the hypertonicity of $NaHCO_3$. May cause sodium retention especially if renal function is impaired; not to be used in treatment of peptic ulcer; use with caution in patients with CHF, edema, cirrhosis, or renal failure. Not the antacid of choice for the elderly because of sodium content and potential for systemic alkalosis.

Adverse Reactions Frequency not defined.

Cardiovascular: Cerebral hemorrhage, CHF (aggravated), edema

Central nervous system: Tetany

Gastrointestinal: Belching, flatulence (with oral), gastric distension

Endocrine & metabolic: Hypernatremia, hyperosmolality, hypocalcemia, hypokalemia, increased affinity of hemoglobin for oxygen-reduced pH in myocardial tissue necrosis when extravasated, intracranial acidosis, metabolic alkalosis, milk-alkali syndrome (especially with renal dysfunction)

Respiratory: Pulmonary edema

Overdosage/Toxicology Symptoms of overdose include hypocalcemia, hypokalemia, hypernatremia, and seizures. Treatment is symptom-directed and supportive.

Drug Interactions

Decreased effect/levels of lithium, chlorpropamide, methotrexate, tetracyclines, and salicylates due to urinary alkalinization

Increased toxicity/levels of amphetamines, anorexiants, mecamylamine, ephedrine, pseudoephedrine, flecainide, quinidine, quinine due to urinary alkalinization

Ethanol/Nutrition/Herb Interactions Herb/Nutraceutical: Concurrent doses with iron may decrease iron absorption.

Dietary Considerations Oral product should be administered 1-3 hours after meals.

Sodium content:

Injection: 50 mL, 8.4% = 1150 mg = 50 mEq; each mL of 8.4% $NaHCO_3$ contains 23 mg sodium; 1 mEq $NaHCO_3$ = 84 mg

Granules: 2.69 g packet or capful = 770 mg sodium

Powder: 30 mEq sodium per ½ teaspoon

Dosage Forms

Granules, effervescent (Brioschi®): 2.69 g/packet (6 g) [unit-dose packets; contains sodium 770 mg/packet; lemon flavor]; 2.69 g/capful (120 g, 240 g) [contains sodium 770 mg/capful; lemon flavor]

Infusion [premixed in sterile water]: 5% (500 mL)

Injection, solution:

4.2% [42 mg/mL = 5 mEq/10 mL] (10 mL)

7.5% [75 mg/mL = 8.92 mEq/10 mL] (50 mL)

8.4% [84 mg/mL = 10 mEq/10 mL] (10 mL, 50 mL)

Neut®: 4% [40 mg/mL = 2.4 mEq/5 mL] (5 mL)

Powder: Sodium bicarbonate USP (120 g, 480 g) [contains sodium 30 mEq per ½ teaspoon]

Tablet: 325 mg [3.8 mEq]; 650 mg [7.6 mEq]

References

Forsythe SM and Schmidt GA, "Sodium Bicarbonate for the Treatment of Lactic Acidosis," *Chest*, 2000, 117(1):260-7.
Mokhlesi B, Leikin JB, Murray P, et al, "Adult Toxicology in Critical Care: Part II: Specific Poisonings," *Chest*, 2003, 123(3):897-922.

Sodium Chloride (SOW dee um KLOR ide)

Medication Safety Issues

Per JCAHO recommendations, concentrated electrolyte solutions (eg, NaCl >0.9%) should not be available in patient care areas.

High alert medication: The Institute for Safe Medication Practices (ISMP) includes this medication (I.V. formulation) among its list of drugs which have a heightened risk of causing significant patient harm when used in error.

U.S. Brand Names Altachlore [OTC]; Altamist [OTC]; Ayr® Baby Saline [OTC]; Ayr® Saline [OTC]; Ayr® Saline No-Drip [OTC]; Breathe Right® Saline [OTC]; Broncho Saline® [OTC]; Deep Sea [OTC]; Entsol® [OTC]; Muro 128® [OTC]; Mycinaire™ [OTC]; NaSal™ [OTC]; Nasal Moist® [OTC]; Na-Zone® [OTC]; Ocean® [OTC]; Oceant® for Kids [OTC]; Pretz® [OTC]; SalineX® [OTC]; Simply Saline® [OTC]; Simply Saline® Baby [OTC]; Simply Saline® Nasal Moist® [OTC]; Syrex; 4-Way® Saline Moisturizing Mist [OTC]; Wound Wash Saline™ [OTC]

Synonyms NaCl; Normal Saline; Salt

Pharmacologic Category Electrolyte Supplement, Parenteral; Lubricant, Ocular; Sodium Salt

Generic Available Yes

Use

Parenteral: Restores sodium ion in patients with restricted oral intake (especially hyponatremia states or low salt syndrome). In general, parenteral saline uses:

- Bacteriostatic sodium chloride: Dilution or dissolving drugs for I.M., I.V., or SubQ injections
- Concentrated sodium chloride: Additive for parenteral fluid therapy
- Hypertonic sodium chloride: For severe hyponatremia and hypochloremia
- Hypotonic sodium chloride: Hydrating solution
- Normal saline: Restores water/sodium losses
- Pharmaceutical aid/diluent for infusion of compatible drug additives

Ophthalmic: Reduces corneal edema

Inhalation: Restores moisture to pulmonary system; loosens and thins congestion caused by colds or allergies; diluent for bronchodilator solutions that require dilution before inhalation

Intranasal: Restores moisture to nasal membranes

Irrigation: Wound cleansing, irrigation, and flushing

Unlabeled/Investigational Use Traumatic brain injury (hypertonic sodium chloride)

Mechanism of Action Principal extracellular cation; functions in fluid and electrolyte balance, osmotic pressure control, and water distribution

Pharmacodynamics/Kinetics

Absorption: Oral, I.V.: Rapid

Distribution: Widely distributed

Excretion: Primarily urine; also sweat, tears, saliva

Dosage

Children: I.V.: Hypertonic solutions (>0.9%) should only be used for the initial treatment of acute serious symptomatic hyponatremia; maintenance: 3-4 mEq/kg/day; maximum: 100-150 mEq/day; dosage varies widely depending on clinical condition

Replacement: Determined by laboratory determinations mEq

Sodium deficiency (mEq/kg) = [% dehydration (L/kg)/100 x 70 (mEq/L)] + [0.6 (L/kg) x (140 - serum sodium) (mEq/L)]

Children ≥2 years and Adults:

Intranasal: 2-3 sprays in each nostril as needed

Irrigation: Spray affected area

Children and Adults: Inhalation: Bronchodilator diluent: 1-3 sprays (1-3 mL) to dilute bronchodilator solution in nebulizer prior to administration

Adults:

GU irrigant: 1-3 L/day by intermittent irrigation

Replacement I.V.: Determined by laboratory determinations mEq

Sodium deficiency (mEq/kg) = [% dehydration (L/kg)/100 x 70 (mEq/L)] + [0.6 (L/kg) x (140 - serum sodium) (mEq/L)]

(Continued)

Sodium Chloride *(Continued)*

To correct acute, serious hyponatremia: mEq sodium = [desired sodium (mEq/L) - actual sodium (mEq/L)] x [0.6 x wt (kg)]; for acute correction use 125 mEq/L as the desired serum sodium; acutely correct serum sodium in 5 mEq/L/dose increments; more gradual correction in increments of 10 mEq/L/day is indicated in the asymptomatic patient

Chloride maintenance electrolyte requirement in parenteral nutrition: 2-4 mEq/kg/24 hours or 25-40 mEq/1000 kcals/24 hours; maximum: 100-150 mEq/24 hours

Sodium maintenance electrolyte requirement in parenteral nutrition: 3-4 mEq/kg/24 hours or 25-40 mEq/1000 kcals/24 hours; maximum: 100-150 mEq/24 hours.

Approximate Deficits of Water and Electrolytes in Moderately Severe Dehydration[1]

Condition	Water (mL/kg)	Sodium (mEq/kg)
Fasting and thirsting	100-120	5-7
Diarrhea		
isonatremic	100-120	8-10
hypernatremic	100-120	2-4
hyponatremic	100-120	10-12
Pyloric stenosis	100-120	8-10
Diabetic acidosis	100-120	9-10

[1]A **negative** deficit indicates total body **excess** prior to treatment.

Adapted from Behrman RE, Kleigman RM, Nelson WE, et al, eds, *Nelson Textbook of Pediatrics*, 14th ed, WB Saunders Co, 1992.

Ophthalmic:

Ointment: Apply once daily or more often

Solution: Instill 1-2 drops into affected eye(s) every 3-4 hours

Stability Store injection at room temperature; protect from heat and from freezing; use only clear solutions

Monitoring Parameters Serum sodium, potassium, chloride, and bicarbonate levels; I & O, weight

Reference Range Serum/plasma sodium levels:

Neonates:

Full-term: 133-142 mEq/L

Premature: 132-140 mEq/L

Children ≥2 months to Adults: 135-145 mEq/L

Anesthesia and Critical Care Concerns/Other Considerations An Australian/New Zealand group recently published results from their evaluation of resuscitation fluid (4% albumin versus normal saline) in a heterogeneous intensive care population (Finfer, 2004). They conducted this multicenter, randomized, double-blind trial to compare the effects of resuscitation fluid on mortality from any cause during the 28-day period after randomization. Patients were eligible for inclusion if the treating clinician judged that fluid resuscitation was required for intravascular fluid depletion as supported by one of the following criteria:

Heart rate >90 bpm

Systolic BP <100 mm Hg

Mean arterial BP <75 mm Hg

Decrease of 40 mm Hg in systolic or mean arterial BP (as compared with baseline)

CVP <10 mm Hg

PCWP <12 mm Hg

Respiratory variation in systolic or mean BP >5 mm Hg

Capillary refill time >1 second

Urine output <0.5 mL/kg for 1 hour

Patients were excluded for a variety of reasons, including ICU transfer following cardiac or liver transplantation surgery, or burn treatment. Almost 7000 patients were randomized; 3497 to albumin and 3500 to saline. Baseline characteristics were similar between the groups, except CVP pressure was slightly higher in the albumin group (9.0 in albumin versus 8.6 in saline). There was no significant mortality difference between groups (726 deaths in albumin group; 729 deaths in saline group). There were no significant differences in secondary endpoints (length of stay in the ICU or hospital, days of mechanical ventilation, and days of renal replacement therapy). Similar outcomes resulted from use of either fluid for resuscitation in this patient population.

The 2004 Surviving Sepsis Campaign guidelines recommend that during the first 6 hours of resuscitation, the goals of sepsis-induced hypoperfusion should include central venous pressure 8-12 mm Hg, mean arterial pressure >65 mm Hg, urine output >0.5 mL/kg/hour, central venous or mixed venous oxygen saturation >70%.

Pregnancy Risk Factor C

Contraindications Hypersensitivity to sodium chloride or any component of the formulation; hypertonic uterus, hypernatremia, fluid retention

Warnings/Precautions Use with caution in patients with CHF, renal insufficiency, liver cirrhosis, hypertension, edema; sodium toxicity is almost exclusively related to how fast a sodium deficit is corrected; both rate and magnitude are extremely important; do not use bacteriostatic sodium chloride in newborns since benzyl alcohol preservatives have been associated with toxicity. Wound Wash Saline™ is for single-patient use only.

Adverse Reactions Frequency not defined.

Cardiovascular: Congestive conditions

Endocrine & metabolic: Extravasation, hypervolemia, hypernatremia, dilution of serum electrolytes, overhydration, hypokalemia

Local: Thrombosis, phlebitis, extravasation

Respiratory: Pulmonary edema

Overdosage/Toxicology

Symptoms of overdose include nausea, vomiting, diarrhea, abdominal cramps, hypocalcemia, hypokalemia, hypernatremia

Hypernatremia is resolved through the use of diuretics and free water replacement

Drug Interactions Decreased levels of lithium

Dosage Forms

Gel, intranasal:
- Ayr® Saline No-Drip: 0.5% (22 mL) [spray gel; contains benzalkonium chloride, benzyl alcohol and soybean oil]
- Ayr® Saline: 0.5% (14 g) [contains soybean oil]
- Entsol®: 3% (20 g) [contains aloe, benzalkonium chloride, and vitamin E]
- Simply Saline® Nasal Moist®: 0.65% (30 g)

Injection, solution [preservative free]: 0.9% (2 mL, 5 mL, 10 mL, 20 mL, 100 mL)

Injection, solution [preservative free, prefilled I.V. flush syringe]: 0.9% (2 mL, 2.5 mL, 3 mL, 5 mL, 10 mL)

Injection, solution: 0.45% (25 mL, 50 mL, 100 mL, 250 mL, 500 mL, 1000 mL); 0.9% (3 mL, 5 mL, 10 mL, 20 mL, 25 mL, 30 mL, 50 mL, 100 mL, 150 mL, 250 mL, 500 mL, 1000 mL); 3% (500 mL); 5% (500 mL)
- Syrex: 0.9% (2.5 mL, 5 mL, 10 mL) [prefilled syringe]

Injection, solution [bacteriostatic]: 0.9% (10 mL, 20 mL, 30 mL) [contains benzyl alcohol]

Injection, solution [concentrate]: 14.6% (2.5 mEq/mL) (20 mL, 40 mL); 23.4% (4 mEq/mL) (30 mL, 100 mL, 200 mL, 250 mL)

Ointment, ophthalmic: 5% (3.5 g)
- Altachlore, Muro 128®: 5% (3.5 g)

Powder for nasal solution (Entsol®): 3% (10.5 g)

Solution for inhalation: 0.45% (3 mL, 5 mL); 0.9% (3 mL, 5 mL, 15 mL); 3% (15 mL); 10% (15 mL)
- Broncho® Saline: 0.9% (90 mL, 240 mL) [for dilution of bronchodilator solutions]

Solution, intranasal: 0.65% (45 mL)
- Altamist: 0.65% (60 mL) [spray; contains benzalkonium chloride]
- Ayr® Baby Saline: 0.65% (30 mL) [spray/drops; contains benzalkonium chloride]
- Ayr® Saline: 0.65% (50 mL) [drops; contains benzalkonium chloride]
- Ayr® Saline: 0.65% (50 mL) [mist, contains benzalkonium chloride]
- Breathe Right® Saline: 0.65% (44 mL) [spray; contains benzalkonium chloride]
- Deep Sea: 0.65% (45 mL) [spray; contains benzalkonium chloride]
- Entsol® Mist: 3% (30 mL) [spray; contains benzalkonium chloride]
- Entsol® [preservative free]: 3% (100 mL) [spray]
- Entsol® [preservative free]: 3% (240 mL) [nasal wash]

(Continued)

Sodium Chloride *(Continued)*

Mycinaire™: 0.65% (30 mL) [mist; contains benzalkonium chloride]
Na-Zone®: 0.65% (60 mL) [spray; contains benzalkonium chloride]
NaSal™: 0.65% (15 mL) [drops; contains benzalkonium chloride], (30 mL) [spray; contains benzalkonium chloride]
Nasal Moist®: 0.65% (45 mL) [spray]
Ocean®: 0.65% (45 mL) [mist/spray/drops; contains benzalkonium chloride]; (473 mL) [refill bottle; contains benzalkonium chloride]
Ocean® for Kids: 0.65% (37.5 mL) [drops/spray/stream; contains benzalkonium chloride]
Pretz®: 0.75% (50 mL) [spray; contains benzalkonium chloride and yerba santa]; (240 mL) [irrigation; contains benzalkonium chloride and yerba santa]; (960 mL) [refill bottle; contains benzalkonium chloride and yerba santa]
SalineX®: 0.4% (15 mL) [drops]; (50 mL) [spray]
Simply Saline®: 0.9% (44 mL, 90 mL) [mist]
Simply Saline® Baby: 0.9% (45 mL) [mist]
4-Way® Saline Moisturizing Mist: 0.74% (30 mL) [alcohol free; contains benzalkonium chloride, eucalyptol, and menthol]

Solution for irrigation: 0.45% (1500 mL, 2000 mL); 0.9% (250 mL, 500 mL, 1000 mL, 1500 mL, 2000 mL, 3000 mL, 4000 mL, 5000 mL)
Wound Wash Saline™: 0.9% (90 mL, 210 mL)

Solution, ophthalmic: 5% (15 mL)
Altachlore: 5% (15 mL, 30 mL)
Muro 128®: 2% (15 mL); 5% (15 mL, 30 mL)

References

Cooper DJ, Myles PS, McDermott FT, et al, "Prehospital Hypertonic Saline Resuscitation of Patients With Hypotension and Severe Traumatic Brain Injury: A Randomized Controlled Trial," *JAMA*, 2004, 291(11):1350-7.

Dellinger RP, Carlet JM, Masur H, et al, "Surviving Sepsis Campaign Guidelines for Management of Severe Sepsis and Septic Shock," *Crit Care Med*, 2004, 32(3):858-73.

Doyle JA, Davis DP, and Hoyt DB, "The Use of Hypertonic Saline in the Treatment of Traumatic Brain Injury," *J Trauma*, 2001, 50(2):367-83.

Finfer S, Bellomo R, Boyce N, et al, "A Comparison of Albumin and Saline for Fluid Resuscitation in the Intensive Care Unit. SAFE Study Investigators," *N Engl J Med*, 2004, 350(22):2247-56.

♦ **Sodium Etidronate** *see* Etidronate Disodium *on page 495*

♦ **Sodium Fusidate** *see* Fusidic Acid *on page 575*

♦ **Sodium Hydrogen Carbonate** *see* Sodium Bicarbonate *on page 1181*

Sodium Hypochlorite Solution

(SOW dee um hye poe KLOR ite soe LOO shun)

U.S. Brand Names Dakin's Solution; Di-Dak-Sol

Synonyms Modified Dakin's Solution

Pharmacologic Category Disinfectant, Antibacterial (Topical)

Generic Available No

Use Treatment of athlete's foot (0.5%); wound irrigation (0.5%); disinfection of utensils and equipment (5%)

Dosage Topical irrigation

Stability Use prepared solution within 7 days.

Administration For external use only; do **not** ingest.

Pregnancy Risk Factor C

Contraindications Hypersensitivity to any component of the formulation

Warnings/Precautions For external use only; avoid eye or mucous membrane contact; do not use on open wounds

Adverse Reactions Frequency not defined.

Dermatologic: Irritating to skin
Hematologic: Dissolves blood clots, delays clotting

Dosage Forms Solution, topical:

Dakin's: 0.25% (480 mL); 0.5% (480 mL, 3840 mL)
Di-Dak-Sol: 0.0125% (480 mL)

♦ **Sodium Hyposulfate** *see* Sodium Thiosulfate *on page 1195*

Sodium Lactate (SOW dee um LAK tate)

Pharmacologic Category Alkalinizing Agent, Parenteral

Generic Available Yes

Use Source of bicarbonate for prevention and treatment of mild to moderate metabolic acidosis

Dosage Dosage depends on degree of acidosis

Administration The rate of I.V. infusion should not exceed 300 mL/hour of the 1/6 molar injection

Pregnancy Risk Factor A

Dosage Forms Injection, solution: 560 mg/mL [sodium 5 mEq and lactate 5 mEq per mL] (10 mL)

- ♦ **Sodium Nafcillin** *see* Nafcillin *on page 890*
- ♦ **Sodium Nitroferricyanide** *see* Nitroprusside *on page 931*
- ♦ **Sodium Nitroprusside** *see* Nitroprusside *on page 931*

Sodium Oxybate (SOW dee um ox i BATE)

U.S. Brand Names Xyrem®

Canadian Brand Names Xyrem®

Synonyms Gamma Hydroxybutyric Acid; GHB; 4-Hydroxybutyrate; Sodium 4-Hydroxybutyrate

Pharmacologic Category Central Nervous System Depressant

Restrictions C-I (illicit use); C-III (medical use)

Sodium oxybate oral solution will be available only to prescribers enrolled in the Xyrem® Patient Success Program® and dispensed to the patient through the designated centralized pharmacy (1-866-997-3688). Prior to dispensing the first prescription, prescribers will be sent educational materials to be reviewed with the patient and enrollment forms for the postmarketing surveillance program. Patients must be seen at least every 3 months; prescriptions can be written for a maximum of 3 months (the first prescription may only be written for a 1-month supply).

An FDA-approved medication guide is available at http://www.fda.gov/cder/Offices/ODS/labeling.htm; distribute to each patient to whom this medication is dispensed.

Generic Available No

Use Treatment of cataplexy and daytime sleepiness in patients with narcolepsy

Mechanism of Action Sodium oxybate is derived from gamma aminobutyric acid (GABA) and acts as an inhibitory chemical transmitter in the brain. May function through specific receptors for gamma hydroxybutyrate (GHB) and GABA (B).

Pharmacodynamics/Kinetics

Absorption: Rapid

Distribution: 190-384 mL/kg

Protein binding: <1%

Metabolism: Primarily via the Krebs cycle to form water and carbon dioxide; secondarily via beta oxidation; significant first-pass effect; no active metabolites; metabolic pathways are saturable

Bioavailability: 25%

Half-life elimination: 30-60 minutes

Time to peak: 30-75 minutes

Excretion: Primarily pulmonary (as carbon dioxide); urine (<5% unchanged drug)

Dosage Oral:

Children ≥16 years and Adults: Narcolepsy: Initial: 4.5 g/day, in 2 equal doses; first dose to be given at bedtime after the patient is in bed, and second dose to be given 2.5-4 hours later. Dose may be increased or adjusted in 2-week intervals; average dose: 6-9 g/day (maximum: 9 g/day)

Elderly: Safety and efficacy have not been studied in patients >65 years.

Dosage adjustment in renal impairment: Adjustment not necessary; consider sodium content

Dosage adjustment in hepatic impairment: Decrease starting dose to half and titrate doses carefully in patients with liver dysfunction. Elimination half-life significantly longer in patients with Child's class C liver dysfunction.

Stability Store at controlled room temperature of 15°C to 30°C (59°F to 86°F) in the original bottle and in a safe and secure place (may need to be locked up). Prepare both doses prior to bedtime and place safely near bed, out of reach of pets and children. Each dose should be diluted with 2 ounces of water in the child-resistant dosing cups. Once diluted, solutions should be used within 24 hours.

(Continued)

Sodium Oxybate *(Continued)*

Administration Take on an empty stomach; separate last meal (or food) and first dose by several hours; try to take at similar time each day. Doses should be administered while patient is sitting up in bed. Both doses should be prepared prior to bedtime. The first dose is taken at bedtime and the second dose is taken 2.5-4 hours later; an alarm clock may need to be set for the second dose. After taking the dose, patient is to lie down and remain in bed.

Monitoring Parameters

Signs and symptoms of depression, drug abuse

Pregnancy Risk Factor B

Contraindications Hypersensitivity to sodium oxybate or any component of the formulation; ethanol and other CNS depressants; semialdehyde dehydrogenase deficiency

Warnings/Precautions [U.S. Boxed Warning]: Sodium oxybate is a CNS depressant with abuse potential; it should not be used with ethanol or other CNS depressants. Seizures, respiratory depression, decreases in level of consciousness, coma, and death have been reported when used for nonprescription purposes. Due to the rapid onset of CNS depressant effects, doses should be administered only at bedtime and while the patient is sitting up in bed. May impair respiratory drive; use caution with compromised respiratory function. Most patients (~80%) in clinical trials were also treated with stimulants; therefore, an independent assessment of the effects of sodium oxybate is lacking. May cause confusion, psychosis, paranoia, hallucinations, agitation, and depression; use caution with history of depression or suicide attempt. May cause sleepwalking, urinary, and/or fecal incontinence. Use caution with hepatic dysfunction. Contains significant amounts of sodium; use caution with heart failure, hypertension, or compromised renal function.

Patients should be instructed not to engage in hazardous activities requiring mental alertness for at least 6 hours after taking this medication and that CNS effects may carryover to the next day. Tolerance to sodium oxybate, or withdrawal following its discontinuation, have not been clearly defined in controlled clinical trials, but have been reported at larger doses used for illicit purposes. Safety and efficacy have not been established in patients <16 years of age.

[U.S. Boxed Warning]: Sodium oxybate oral solution will be available only to prescribers enrolled in the Xyrem® Patient Success Program® and dispensed to the patient through the designated centralized pharmacy (1-866-997-3688).

Adverse Reactions

>10%:

- Central nervous system: Dizziness (8% to 37%), headache (9% to 37%), pain (9% to 20%), somnolence (1% to 14%), confusion (3% to 17%), sleep disorder (6% to 14%)
- Gastrointestinal: Nausea (8% to 40%), vomiting (2% to 23%), abdominal pain (3% to 11%)
- Genitourinary: Urinary incontinence (<1% to 14%, usually nocturnal), enuresis (3% to 17%), cystitis, metrorrhagia, urinary frequency
- Miscellaneous: Diaphoresis (3% to 11%)

1% to 10%:

- Cardiovascular: Hypertension (6%), chest pain, edema
- Central nervous system: Disorientation (up to 9%), inebriation (up to 9%), concentration decreased (3% to 9%), dream abnormality (3% to 9%), sleepwalking (4% to 7%), depression (3% to 6%), amnesia (3% to 6%), anxiety (3% to 6%), thinking abnormality (3% to 6%), lethargy (up to 6%), insomnia (5%), agitation, ataxia, chills, fatigue, malaise, memory impairment, nervousness, pyrexia, seizure, stupor, tremor, vertigo
- Dermatologic: Hyperhidrosis (3% to 6%), pruritus, rash
- Endocrine & metabolic: Dysmenorrhea (3% to 6%)
- Gastrointestinal: Dyspepsia (6% to 9%), diarrhea (6% to 8%), abdominal pain (6%), nausea and vomiting (6%), anorexia, constipation, tooth ache, weight gain
- Hepatic: Alkaline phosphatase increased, hypercholesteremia, hypocalcemia
- Neuromuscular & skeletal: Hypoesthesia (6%), weakness (6% to 8%), myasthenia (3% to 6%), pain (3% to 6%), arthritis, leg cramps, myalgia
- Ocular: Amblyopia (6%), blurred vision (6%)
- Otic: Tinnitus (6%), ear pain

Renal: Albuminuria, hematuria

Respiratory: Pharyngitis (6% to 8%), rhinitis (8%), nasopharyngitis (3% to 8%), infection (3% to 6%), bronchitis, cough, dyspnea

Miscellaneous: Infection (3% to 6%), viral infection (3% to 9%), allergic reaction, flu-like syndrome

<1% (Limited to important or life-threatening): Abdominal distension, accident, acne, affect lability, akathisia, ALT/AST increased, allergic reaction, alopecia, anemia, apathy, apnea, arthritis, asthma, bilirubinemia, bronchitis, bruising, coma, conjunctivitis, contusion, contact dermatitis, creatinine increased, dehydration, depersonalization, dysgeusia, dysphagia, edema, epistaxis, eructation, euphoria, eye irritation, eye pain, eye redness, eye swelling, fall, fecal incontinence, flatulence, fracture, gastroinesophageal reflux disease, gait abnormal, hangover, hematuria, hiccups, hypersensitivity, hyperuricemia, hyperglycemia, hypernatremia, hypertonia, hypotension, infection, injury, keratoconjunctivitis sicca, laceration, leukocytosis, leukopenia, libido decreased, lymphadenopathy, mental impairment, migraine, miosis, mouth ulceration, myoclonus, neck rigidity, neuralgia, night sweats, paralysis, paranoia, polyarthritis, polycythemia, positive ANA test, proteinuria, psychomotor activity, restless leg syndrome, rosacea, salivary hypersecretion, sinusitis, snoring, stomatitis, suicidal behavior/thoughts, suicidal attempts, syncope, tachycardia, taste loss, tendonitis, thirst, urinary urgency, urticaria

Overdosage/Toxicology Signs and symptoms of overdose may be dependent upon dose ingested, time since ingestion, coingestion of CNS depressants, and the fed or fasted state. Signs and symptoms may include depressed consciousness (may fluctuate rapidly between confusion, agitation, combativeness, ataxia, coma); emesis; diaphoresis; headache; impaired psychomotor skills; blurred vision; myoclonus; tonic-clonic seizures; apnea; Cheyne-Stokes respiration; bradycardia; hypothermia; and muscular hypotonia (with tendon reflexes intact). Pupillary reactivity to light is maintained and no typical pupillary changes have been described. Treatment should be symptom-directed and supportive. Atropine may be given for bradycardia.

Drug Interactions CNS depressants: CNS depressant effects are potentiated; concomitant use with sodium oxybate is contraindicated.

Ethanol/Nutrition/Herb Interactions

Ethanol: Avoid ethanol (increases CNS depression).

Food: High-fat meal decreases bioavailability, delays absorption, and decreases peak serum level.

Herb/Nutraceutical: Avoid any products that may cause CNS depression (eg, kava kava or valerian).

Dietary Considerations Take on an empty stomach; separate last meal (or food) and first dose by several hours; try to take at similar time each day.

Contains sodium 0.5 g per 3 g dose or 1.6 g per 9 g dose.

Dosage Forms Solution, oral: 500 mg/mL (180 mL) [supplied in a kit containing two dosing cups and measuring device]

Sodium Phosphates (SOW dee um FOS fates)

Medication Safety Issues

Enemas and oral solution are available in pediatric and adult sizes; prescribe by "volume" not by "bottle."

U.S. Brand Names Fleet® Accu-Prep® [OTC]; Fleet® Enema [OTC]; Fleet® Phospho-Soda® [OTC]; OsmoPrep™; Visicol®

Canadian Brand Names Fleet Enema®; Fleet® Phospho-Soda® Oral Laxative

Pharmacologic Category Cathartic; Electrolyte Supplement, Oral; Electrolyte Supplement, Parenteral; Laxative, Bowel Evacuant

Generic Available Yes: Enema, injection

Use

Oral, rectal: Short-term treatment of constipation and to evacuate the colon for rectal and bowel exams

I.V.: Source of phosphate in large volume I.V. fluids and parenteral nutrition; treatment and prevention of hypophosphatemia

Mechanism of Action As a laxative, exerts osmotic effect in the small intestine by drawing water into the lumen of the gut, producing distention and promoting peristalsis and evacuation of the bowel; phosphorous participates in bone deposition, calcium metabolism, utilization of B complex vitamins, and as a buffer in acid-base equilibrium

(Continued)

Sodium Phosphates *(Continued)*

Pharmacodynamics/Kinetics

Onset of action: Cathartic: 3-6 hours; Rectal: 2-5 minutes
Absorption: Oral: ~1% to 20%

Dosage

Normal requirements elemental phosphorus: Oral:
- 0-6 months: Adequate intake: 100 mg/day
- 6-12 months: Adequate intake: 275 mg/day
- 1-3 years: RDA: 460 mg
- 4-8 years: RDA: 500 mg
- 9-18 years: RDA: 1250 mg
- ≥19 years: RDA: 700 mg

Hypophosphatemia: It is difficult to provide concrete guidelines for the treatment of severe hypophosphatemia because the extent of total body deficits and response to therapy are difficult to predict. Aggressive doses of phosphate may result in a transient serum elevation followed by redistribution into intracellular compartments or bone tissue. Intermittent I.V. infusion should be reserved for severe depletion situations (<1 mg/dL in adults); large doses of oral phosphate may cause diarrhea and intestinal absorption may be unreliable. I.V. solutions should be infused slowly. Use caution when mixing with calcium and magnesium, precipitate may form. The following dosages are empiric guidelines. **Note:** 1 mmol phosphate = 31 mg phosphorus; 1 mg phosphorus = 0.032 mmol phosphate

Hypophosphatemia treatment: Doses listed as mmol of phosphate:
- Intermittent I.V. infusion: Acute repletion or replacement:
  - Children:
    - Low dose: 0.08 mmol/kg over 6 hours; use if losses are recent and uncomplicated
    - Intermediate dose: 0.16-0.24 mmol/kg over 4-6 hours; use if serum phosphorus level 0.5-1 mg/dL
    - High dose: 0.36 mmol/kg over 6 hours; use if serum phosphorus <0.5 mg/dL
  - Adults: Varying dosages: 0.15-0.3 mmol/kg/dose over 12 hours; may repeat as needed to achieve desired serum level **or**
    - 15 mmol/dose over 2 hours; use if serum phosphorus <2 mg/dL **or**
    - Low dose: 0.16 mmol/kg over 4-6 hours; use if serum phosphorus level 2.3-3 mg/dL
    - Intermediate dose: 0.32 mmol/kg over 4-6 hours; use if serum phosphorus level 1.6-2.2 mg/dL
    - High dose: 0.64 mmol/kg over 8-12 hours; use if serum phosphorus <1.5 mg/dL
- Oral: Adults: 0.5-1 g elemental phosphorus 2-3 times/day may be used when serum phosphorus level is 1-2.5 mg/dL

Maintenance: Doses listed as mmol of phosphate:
- Children:
  - Oral: 2-3 mmol/kg/day in divided doses
  - I.V.: 0.5-1.5 mmol/kg/day
- Adults:
  - Oral: 50-150 mmol/day in divided doses
  - I.V.: 50-70 mmol/day

Laxative (Fleet®): Rectal:
- Children 2-<5 years: One-half contents of one 2.25 oz pediatric enema
- Children 5-12 years: Contents of one 2.25 oz pediatric enema, may repeat
- Children ≥12 years and Adults: Contents of one 4.5 oz enema as a single dose, may repeat

Laxative (Fleet® Phospho-Soda®): Oral: Take on an empty stomach; dilute dose with 8 ounces cool water, then follow dose with 8 ounces water; **do not repeat dose within 24 hours**
- Children 5-9 years: 7.5 mL as a single dose; maximum daily dose: 7.5 mL
- Children 10-12 years: 15 mL as a single dose; maximum daily dose: 15 mL
- Children ≥12 years and Adults: 15 mL as a single dose; maximum daily dose: 45 mL

Bowel cleansing prior to colonoscopy: Adults: **Note:** Each dose should be taken with a minimum of 8 ounces of clear liquids. Do not repeat treatment within 7 days. Do not use additional agents, especially sodium phosphate products.

Fleet® Phospho-Soda®: Oral: Prior to procedure (timing of doses determined by prescriber): One dose is equal to 45 mL (2 doses are recommended): Each dose is diluted as follows:

Mix 45 mL with 120 mL clear liquid; drink, then follow with at least 240 mL of clear liquid; **or**

Mix 15 mL with 240 mL clear liquid; drink, then follow with 240 mL clear liquid; repeat every 10 minutes for a total of 45 mL

Visicol™: Oral: Adults: A total of 40 tablets divided as follows:

Evening before colonoscopy: 3 tablets every 15 minutes for 6 doses, then 2 additional tablets in 15 minutes (total of 20 tablets)

3-5 hours prior to colonoscopy: 3 tablets every 15 minutes for 6 doses, then 2 additional tablets in 15 minutes (total of 20 tablets)

OsmoPrep™: A total of 32 tablets divided as follows:

Evening before colonoscopy: 4 tablets every 15 minutes for 5 doses (total of 20 tablets)

3-5 hours prior to colonoscopy: 4 tablets every 15 minutes for 3 doses (total of 12 tablets)

Dosage adjustment in renal impairment: Use with caution; ionized inorganic phosphate is excreted by the kidneys; oral solution is contraindicated in patients with kidney disease

Dosage adjustment in hepatic impairment: Not expected to be metabolized in the liver

Elderly: Use with caution due to increased risk of renal impairment in the elderly

Stability Store at 15°C to 30°C (59°F to 86°F).

Administration

Intermittent I.V. infusion: Dilute at a maximum concentration of 0.12 mmol/mL and infuse over 4-6 hours; maximum rate of infusion: 0.06 mmol/kg/hour

Bowel cleansing: Have patient drink ~8 ounces of water with each dose of sodium phosphate (total of 2 quarts/64 ounces); have patient rehydrate before and after colonoscopy

Monitoring Parameters

I.V.: Serum calcium and phosphate levels; renal function

Oral: Bowel cleansing: Baseline and post-procedure labs (electrolytes, calcium, phosphate, BUN, creatinine) in patients at risk for acute renal nephropathy, seizure, or who have a history of electrolyte abnormality; ECG in patients with risks for prolonged QT or arrhythmias

Pregnancy Risk Factor C

Contraindications Hypersensitivity to sodium phosphate salts or any component of the formulation; congestive heart failure, hyperparathyroidism, ascites

Enema: Imperforate anus

Intravenous preparation: Diseases with hyperphosphatemia, hypocalcemia, or hypernatremia

Oral preparation: Acute colitis, acute phosphate nephropathy (biopsy proven), bowel obstruction, bowel perforation, congenital megacolon, gastric retention, hypomotility syndromes, ileus, pseudo-obstruction, severe chronic constipation, toxic megacolon, unstable angina

Warnings/Precautions Use with caution in patients with impaired renal dysfunction, pre-existing electrolyte imbalances, risk of electrolyte disturbance (hypocalcemia, hyperphosphatemia, hypernatremia) or serious adverse event secondary to one of the above, dehydration, chronic inflammatory bowel disease, gastric bypass or stapling surgery.

Acute phosphate nephropathy may rarely occur during use as a bowel cleanser. Risk factors for acute phosphate nephropathy may include increased age (>62 years of age), renal dysfunction or dehydration, use of medicines that affect renal perfusion or function (eg, ACE inhibitors, angiotensin receptor blockers, diuretics, NSAIDs). Other preventive measures may include avoid excessive doses and concurrent use of other laxatives containing sodium phosphate; encourage patients to drink sufficient quantities of clear fluids during bowel cleansing (eg, electrolyte rehydration solution); obtain baseline and post-procedure labs in patients at risk; consider hospitalization and intravenous hydration during bowel cleansing for patients unable to hydrate themselves.

Use caution in inflammatory bowel disease; may induce colonic aphthous ulceration. Use with caution in patients with a history of seizures, those at higher risk of seizures or on medication that lowers seizure threshold, patients withdrawing

(Continued)

Sodium Phosphates *(Continued)*

from alcohol or benzodiazepines, patients with hyponatremia. Use caution in patients with or at risk for arrhythmias (eg, cardiomyopathy, prolonged QT interval, history of uncontrolled arrhythmias, recent MI). Prolongation of the QT interval has been reported (associated with hypokalemia, hypocalcemia); use caution with concurrent use of other QT prolonging medications. If using as a bowel evacuant, correct electrolyte abnormalities before administration. Inadequate fluid intake may lead to excessive fluid loss and hypovolemia. Use with caution in debilitated patients; consider each patient's ability to hydrate properly. Use with caution in geriatric patients. Laxatives and purgatives have the potential for abuse by bulimia nervosa patients. Other oral medications may not be well absorbed when given during bowel evacuation because of rapid intestinal peristalsis. Enemas and oral solution are available in pediatric and adult sizes; prescribe by "volume" not by "bottle." Safety and efficacy of tablets in children have not been established.

Visicol®: Use caution with history of swallowing difficulties or esophageal narrowing. Tablet particles may be seen in the stool.

Adverse Reactions Frequency not defined.

Cardiovascular: Edema, hypotension

Central nervous system: Dizziness, headache

Endocrine & metabolic: Calcium phosphate precipitation, hypernatremia, hyperphosphatemia, hypocalcemia

Gastrointestinal: Abdominal bloating, abdominal pain, diarrhea, mucosal bleeding, nausea, superficial mucosal ulcerations, vomiting

Renal: Acute renal failure

Postmarketing and/or case reports: Atrial fibrillation following severe vomiting (tablet formulation); nephrocalcinosis (oral solution)

Overdosage/Toxicology Overdose may lead to cardiac arrhythmias, severe electrolyte disturbances, including hyperphosphatemia, hypocalcemia, hypernatremia or hypokalemia. Treat symptomatically.

Drug Interactions

ACE inhibitors or angiotensin-receptor antagonists: May increase the risk of electrolyte disorders or nephrocalcinosis when oral phosphates solution is used as a bowel evacuant. Use caution.

Antacids: Do not give with magnesium- and aluminum-containing antacids which can bind with phosphate.

Bisphosphonates: Increased risk of hypoglycemia with concurrent use.

Diuretics: May increase the risk of electrolyte disorders or nephrocalcinosis when oral phosphates solution is used as a bowel evacuant. Use caution.

Sucralfate: Do not give with sucralfate which can bind with phosphate.

Oral preparations: May affect absorption of other medications due to rapid intestinal peristalsis and watery diarrhea caused by agent

Intravenous preparation: Use caution with thiazide diuretics, may lead to renal damage

Dietary Considerations Should be taken on an empty stomach with water; a clear liquid diet should be used for 12 hours prior to tablet administration.

Oral solution contains 556 mg (24.17 mEq) sodium/ 5 mL; 20.6 mmol phosphate/ 5 mL

Oral tablet contains 312 mg (13.6 mEq) sodium/tablet; 336 mg (10.8 mmol phosphate) elemental phosphorus/tablet

Whole cow's milk: 0.29 mmol/mL phosphate; 0.025 mEq/mL sodium; 0.035 mEq/mL potassium

Dosage Forms

Kit (Fleet® Accu-Prep®):

Solution, oral (Fleet® Phosph-Soda®): Monobasic sodium phosphate monohydrate 2.4 g and dibasic sodium phosphate heptahydrate 0.9 g per 5 mL (15 mL) [contains sodium benzoate; kit contains six 15 mL unit-dose containers (equal to two 45 mL doses)]

Pads, anorectal (Fleet® Relief™): Pramoxine hydrochloride 1% and glycerin 12% (4s)

Injection, solution [preservative free]: Phosphorus 3 mmol and sodium 4 mEq per mL (5 mL, 15 mL, 50 mL)

Solution, oral (Fleet® Phospho-Soda®): Monobasic sodium phosphate monohydrate 2.4 g and dibasic sodium phosphate heptahydrate 0.9 g per 5 mL (45 mL,

90 mL) [contains sodium benzoate; contains 20.6 mmol phosphate/5 mL; unflavored or ginger-lemon flavor]

Solution, rectal [enema]: Monobasic sodium phosphate 19 g and dibasic sodium phosphate 7 g per 118 mL delivered dose (135 mL)

Fleet® Enema: Monobasic sodium phosphate 19 g and dibasic sodium phosphate 7 g per 118 mL delivered dose (135 mL)

Fleet® Enema for Children: Monobasic sodium phosphate 9.5 g and dibasic sodium phosphate 3.5 g per 59 mL delivered dose (68 mL)

Tablet, oral:

OsmoPrep™: Sodium phosphate monobasic monohydrate 1.102 g and sodium phosphate dibasic anhydrous 0.398 g [sodium phosphate 1.5 g per tablet; gluten free]

Visicol®: Sodium phosphate monobasic monohydrate 1.102 g and sodium phosphate dibasic anhydrous 0.398 g [sodium phosphate 1.5 g per tablet]

References

Clark CL, Sacks GS, Dickerson RN, et al, "Treatment of Hypophosphatemia in Patients Receiving Specialized Nutrition Support Using a Graduated Dosing Scheme: Results From a Prospective Clinical Trial," *Crit Care Med*, 1995, 23(9):1504-11.

Dickerson R, "Treating Hypophosphatemia," *Hosp Pharm*, 1985, 20:920-24.

Lentz RD, Brown BM, and Kjellstrand CM, "Treatment of Severe Hypophosphatemia," *Ann Intern Med*, 1978, 89(6):941-4.

Lloyd CW and Johnson CE, "Management of Hypophosphatemia," *Clin Pharm*, 1988, 7(2):123-8.

Rosen GH, Boullata JI, O'Rangers EA, et al, "Intravenous Phosphate Repletion Regimen for Critically Ill Patients With Moderate Hypophosphatemia," *Crit Care Med*, 1995, 23(7):1204-10.

Sodium Polystyrene Sulfonate

(SOW dee um pol ee STYE reen SUL fon ate)

Medication Safety Issues

Sound-alike/look-alike issues:

Kayexalate® may be confused with Kaopectate®

Always prescribe either one-time doses or as a specific number of doses (eg, 15 g q6h x 2 doses). Scheduled doses with no dosage limit could be given for days leading to dangerous hypokalemia.

U.S. Brand Names Kayexalate®; Kionex™; SPS®

Canadian Brand Names Kayexalate®; PMS-Sodium Polystyrene Sulfonate

Pharmacologic Category Antidote

Generic Available Yes

Use Treatment of hyperkalemia

Mechanism of Action Removes potassium by exchanging sodium ions for potassium ions in the intestine before the resin is passed from the body

Pharmacodynamics/Kinetics

Onset of action: 2-24 hours

Absorption: None

Excretion: Completely feces (primarily as potassium polystyrene sulfonate)

Dosage

Children:

Oral: 1 g/kg/dose every 6 hours

Rectal: 1 g/kg/dose every 2-6 hours (In small children and infants, employ lower doses by using the practical exchange ratio of 1 mEq K^+/g of resin as the basis for calculation)

Adults: Hyperkalemia:

Oral: 15 g (60 mL) 1-4 times/day

Rectal: 30-50 g every 6 hours

Stability Store prepared suspensions at 15°C to 30°C (59°F to 86°F); store repackaged product in refrigerator and use within 14 days; freshly prepared suspensions should be used within 24 hours; do not heat resin suspension

Administration

Oral: Administer oral (or NG) as ~25% sorbitol solution; never mix in orange juice. Chilling the oral mixture will increase palatability.

Rectal: Enema route is less effective than oral administration. Administer cleansing enema first. Retain enema in colon for at least 30-60 minutes and for several hours, if possible. Enema should be followed by irrigation with normal saline to prevent necrosis.

Monitoring Parameters Exchange capacity is 1 mEq/g *in vivo*, and *in vitro* capacity is 3.1 mEq/g, therefore, a wide range of exchange capacity exists such

(Continued)

Sodium Polystyrene Sulfonate *(Continued)*

that close monitoring of serum electrolytes (potassium, sodium, calcium, magnesium) is necessary; ECG

Reference Range Serum potassium: Adults: 3.5-5.2 mEq/L

Anesthesia and Critical Care Concerns/Other Considerations While sodium polystyrene sulfonate can be used in the treatment of hyperkalemia, if hyperkalemia is associated with ECG changes, more emergent therapy needs to be used (ie, glucose-insulin or calcium). Sodium polystyrene sulfonate should be used with caution in patients with severe heart failure, hypertension, or renal failure. While rectal administration of sodium polystyrene sulfonate achieves a more rapid action, oral administration results in a more sustained potassium reduction.

Pregnancy Risk Factor C

Contraindications Hypersensitivity to sodium polystyrene sulfonate or any component of the formulation; hypernatremia, hypokalemia, obstructive bowel disease

Warnings/Precautions Use with caution in patients with severe CHF, hypertension, edema, or renal failure; avoid using the commercially available liquid product in neonates due to the preservative content; large oral doses may cause fecal impaction (especially in elderly); enema will reduce the serum potassium faster than oral administration, but the oral route will result in a greater reduction over several hours.

Adverse Reactions Frequency not defined.

Endocrine & metabolic: Hypernatremia, hypokalemia, hypocalcemia, hypomagnesemia

Gastrointestinal: Anorexia, colonic necrosis (rare), constipation, fecal impaction, intestinal obstruction (due to concretions in association with aluminum hydroxide), nausea, vomiting

Overdosage/Toxicology Symptoms of overdose include hypokalemia including cardiac dysrhythmias, confusion, irritability, ECG changes, muscle weakness, and GI effects. Treatment is supportive, limited to management of fluid and electrolytes.

Drug Interactions Systemic alkalosis and seizure has occurred after cation-exchange resins were administered with nonabsorbable cation-donating antacids and laxatives (eg, magnesium hydroxide, aluminum carbonate). Digitalis toxicity may occur with hypokalemia.

Dietary Considerations Do **not** mix in orange juice. Sodium content of 1 g: 31 mg (1.3 mEq).

Dosage Forms

Powder for suspension, oral/rectal:

Kayexalate®: 15 g/4 level teaspoons (480 g) [contains sodium 100 mg (4.1 mEq)/g]

Kionex™: 15 g/4 level teaspoons (454 g) [contains sodium 100 mg (4.1 mEq)/g]

Suspension, oral/rectal: 15 g/60 mL (60 mL, 120 mL, 200 mL, 500 mL) [contains sodium 1500 mg (65 mEq)/60 mL, sorbitol, and alcohol 0.1%; cherry/caramel flavor]

SPS®: 15 g/60 mL (60 mL, 120 mL, 480 mL) [contains alcohol 0.3%, sodium 1500 mg (65 mEq)/60 mL, and sorbitol; cherry flavor]

Sodium Tetradecyl (SOW dee um tetra DEK il)

U.S. Brand Names Sotradecol®

Canadian Brand Names Trombovar®

Synonyms Sodium Tetradecyl Sulfate

Pharmacologic Category Sclerosing Agent

Generic Available No

Use Treatment of small, uncomplicated varicose veins of the lower extremities

Mechanism of Action Acts by irritation of the vein intimal endothelium and causes thrombosis formation leading to occlusion of the injected vein

Dosage I.V.: Test dose: 0.5 mL given several hours prior to administration of larger dose; 0.5-2 mL (preferred maximum: 1 mL) in each vein, maximum: 10 mL per treatment session; 3% solution reserved for large varices

Stability Store at controlled room temperature.

Administration Inject slowly.

Monitoring Parameters Monitor for DVT or PE (up to 4 weeks after injection)

Pregnancy Risk Factor C

Contraindications Hypersensitivity to sodium tetradecyl or any component of the formulation; arterial disease, acute thrombophlebitis; valvular or deep vein incompetence, phlebitis migrans, cellulitis, acute infections; bedridden patients; patients with uncontrolled systemic disease such as diabetes, toxic hyperthyroidism, tuberculosis, asthma, neoplasm, sepsis, blood dyscrasias, and acute respiratory or skin diseases; huge superficial veins with wide open communications to deeper veins; allergic conditions; varicosities caused by abdominal and pelvic tumors (unless tumor has been removed)

Warnings/Precautions Use caution with Buerger's disease or peripheral arteriosclerosis. Avoid extravasation. Observe for hypersensitivity/anaphylactic reaction; emergency resuscitation equipment should be available. Valvular and venous competency should be evaluated prior to use.

Adverse Reactions Frequency not defined.

Central nervous system: Headache

Dermatologic: Discoloration at site of injection, sloughing and tissue necrosis following extravasation

Gastrointestinal: Nausea, vomiting

Local: Pain, itching, or ulceration at injection site

Miscellaneous: Allergic reaction (including hives, asthma, hay fever); anaphylactic shock

Dosage Forms Injection, as sulfate: 1% [10 mg/mL] (2 mL) [contains benzyl alcohol]; 3% [30 mg/mL] (2 mL) [contains benzyl alcohol]

♦ **Sodium Tetradecyl Sulfate** *see* Sodium Tetradecyl *on page 1194*

Sodium Thiosulfate (SOW dee um thye oh SUL fate)

U.S. Brand Names Versiclear™

Synonyms Disodium Thiosulfate Pentahydrate; Pentahydrate; Sodium Hyposulfate; Sodium Thiosulphate; Thiosulfuric Acid Disodium Salt

Pharmacologic Category Antidote

Generic Available Yes: Injection

Use

Parenteral: Used alone or with sodium nitrite or amyl nitrite in cyanide poisoning; reduce the risk of nephrotoxicity associated with cisplatin therapy

Topical: Treatment of tinea versicolor

Unlabeled/Investigational Use Management of I.V. extravasation

Mechanism of Action

Cyanide toxicity: Increases the rate of detoxification of cyanide by the enzyme rhodanese by providing an extra sulfur

Cisplatin toxicity: Complexes with cisplatin to form a compound that is nontoxic to either normal or cancerous cells

Pharmacodynamics/Kinetics

Absorption: Oral: Poor

Distribution: Extracellular fluid

Half-life elimination: 0.65 hour

Excretion: Urine (28.5% as unchanged drug)

Variation of Sodium Nitrite and Sodium Thiosulfate Dose With Hemoglobin Concentration[1]

Hemoglobin (g/dL)	Initial Dose Sodium Nitrite (mg/kg)	Initial Dose Sodium Nitrite 3% (mL/kg)	Initial Dose Sodium Thiosulfate 25% (mL/kg)
7	5.8	0.19	0.95
8	6.6	0.22	1.10
9	7.5	0.25	1.25
10	8.3	0.27	1.35
11	9.1	0.30	1.50
12	10.0	0.33	1.65
13	10.8	0.36	1.80
14	11.6	0.39	1.95

[1]Adapted from Berlin DM Jr, "The Treatment of Cyanide Poisoning in Children," *Pediatrics*, 1970, 46:793.

(Continued)

Sodium Thiosulfate *(Continued)*

Dosage

Cyanide and nitroprusside antidote: I.V.:

Children <25 kg: 50 mg/kg after receiving 4.5-10 mg/kg sodium nitrite; a half dose of each may be repeated if necessary

Children >25 kg and Adults: 12.5 g after 300 mg of sodium nitrite; a half dose of each may be repeated if necessary

Cyanide poisoning: I.V.: Dose should be based on determination as with nitrite, at rate of 2.5-5 mL/minute to maximum of 50 mL.

Variation of sodium nitrite and sodium thiosulfate dose, based on hemoglobin concentration: See table on previous page.

Cisplatin rescue should be given before or during cisplatin administration: I.V. infusion (in sterile water): 12 g/m^2 over 6 hours or 9 g/m^2 I.V. push followed by 1.2 g/m^2 continuous infusion for 6 hours

Tinea versicolor: Children and Adults: Topical: 20% to 25% solution: Apply a thin layer to affected areas twice daily

Drug extravasation (unlabeled use): Children and Adults: SubQ:

2% solution: Infiltrate SubQ into the affected area

1/6 M (~4%) solution: 5-10 mL infused through I.V. line and SubQ into the affected area

Administration

I.V.: Inject slowly, over at least 10 minutes; rapid administration may cause hypotension.

Topical: Do not apply to or near eyes.

Monitoring Parameters Monitor for signs of thiocyanate toxicity

Pregnancy Risk Factor C

Contraindications Hypersensitivity to sodium thiosulfate or any component of the formulation

Warnings/Precautions Safety in pregnancy has not been established; discontinue topical use if irritation or sensitivity occurs; rapid I.V. infusion has caused transient hypotension and ECG changes in dogs; can increase risk of thiocyanate intoxication

Adverse Reactions

1% to 10%:

Cardiovascular: Hypotension

Central nervous system: Coma, CNS depression secondary to thiocyanate intoxication, psychosis, confusion

Dermatologic: Contact dermatitis, local irritation

Neuromuscular & skeletal: Weakness

Otic: Tinnitus

<1% (Limited to important or life-threatening): Gastrointestinal: Diarrhea (following large oral doses)

Dosage Forms

Injection, solution [preservative free]: 100 mg/mL (10 mL); 250 mg/mL (50 mL)

Lotion: Sodium thiosulfate 25% and salicylic acid 1% (120 mL) [contains isopropyl alcohol 10%]

♦ **Sodium Thiosulphate** *see* Sodium Thiosulfate *on page 1195*
♦ **Solaraze®** *see* Diclofenac *on page 378*
♦ **Solarcaine® Aloe Extra Burn Relief [OTC]** *see* Lidocaine *on page 755*

Solifenacin (sol i FEN a sin)

U.S. Brand Names VESIcare®

Synonyms Solifenacin Succinate

Pharmacologic Category Anticholinergic Agent

Generic Available No

Use Treatment of overactive bladder with symptoms of urinary frequency, urgency, or urge incontinence

Mechanism of Action Inhibits muscarinic receptors resulting in decreased urinary bladder contraction, increased residual urine volume, and decreased detrusor muscle pressure.

Pharmacodynamics/Kinetics

Distribution: V_d: 600 L

Protein binding: 98% bound to alpha$_1$-acid glycoprotein

Metabolism: Extensively hepatic; via N-oxidation and 4 R-hydroxylation, forms one active and three inactive metabolites; primary pathway for elimination is via CYP3A4 route
Bioavailability: 90%
Half-life elimination: 45-68 hours following chronic dosing
Time to peak, plasma: 3-8 hours
Excretion: Urine 69% (<15% as unchanged drug); feces 23%

Dosage Oral:
Children: Use is not recommended.
Adults: 5 mg/day; if tolerated, may increase to 10 mg/day
Dosage adjustment in renal impairment: Use with caution in reduced renal function
Cl_{cr} <30 mL/minute: 5 mg/day
Dosage adjustment in hepatic impairment: Use with caution in reduced hepatic function
Moderate: 5 mg/day
Severe: Not recommended

Stability Store at room temperature between 15°C to 30°C (59°F to 86°F).

Administration Swallow tablet whole; may take with liquids, without regard to food.

Monitoring Parameters Anticholinergic effects (eg, fixed and dilated pupils, blurred vision, tremors or dry skin)

Pregnancy Risk Factor C

Contraindications Hypersensitivity to solifenacin or any component of the formulation; urinary retention; gastric retention; uncontrolled narrow-angle glaucoma.

Warnings/Precautions Use with caution in patients with bladder outflow obstruction, gastrointestinal obstructive disorders, and decreased gastrointestinal motility. Use with caution in patients with controlled (treated) narrow-angle glaucoma. Dosage adjustment is required for patients with renal or hepatic impairment. Patients on potent CYP3A4 inhibitors require lower dose. Safety and efficacy in pediatric patients have not been established.

Adverse Reactions Adverse reactions are dose related.
>10%: Gastrointestinal: Xerostomia (11% to 28%), constipation (5% to 13%)
1% to 10%:
Cardiovascular: Edema (up to 1%), hypertension (up to 1%)
Central nervous system: Dizziness (2%), fatigue (1% to 2%), depression (up to 1%)
Gastrointestinal: Nausea (2% to 3%), dyspepsia (1% to 4%), upper abdominal pain (1% to 2%), vomiting (up to 1%)
Genitourinary: Urinary tract infection (3% to 5%), urinary retention (up to 1%)
Ocular: Blurred vision (4% to 5%), dry eyes (up to 2%)
Respiratory: Cough (up to 1%), pharyngitis (up to 1%)
Miscellaneous: Influenza (1% to 2%)
<1% (Limited to important or life-threatening): Angioneurotic edema, gastrointestinal obstruction

Overdosage/Toxicology Overdosage can potentially result in severe central anticholinergic effects. Treatment should include gastric lavage and supportive measures.

Drug Interactions Substrate of CYP3A4 (major)
CYP3A4 inducers: May decrease the levels/effects of solifenacin. Example inducers include aminoglutethimide, carbamazepine, nafcillin, nevirapine, phenobarbital, and phenytoin.
CYP3A4 inhibitors: May increase the levels/effects of solifenacin. Example inhibitors include azole antifungals, clarithromycin, diclofenac, doxycycline, erythromycin, imatinib, isoniazid, nefazodone, nicardipine, propofol, protease inhibitors, quinidine, telithromycin, and verapamil. Solifenacin dose should not exceed 5 mg/day; monitor.
Ketoconazole: May increase serum concentrations of solifenacin. Solifenacin dose should not exceed 5 mg/day; monitor.

Ethanol/Nutrition/Herb Interactions
Food: Grapefruit juice may increase the serum level effects of solifenacin.
Herb/Nutraceutical: St John's wort (*Hypericum*) may decrease the levels/effects of solifenacin.

Dosage Forms Tablet: 5 mg, 10 mg

- **Solifenacin Succinate** *see* Solifenacin *on page 1196*
- **Solodyn™** *see* Minocycline *on page 854*

♦ **Solu-Cortef®** *see* Hydrocortisone *on page 639*
♦ **Solu-Medrol®** *see* MethylPREDNISolone *on page 830*
♦ **Somatrem** *see* Human Growth Hormone *on page 625*
♦ **Sominex® [OTC]** *see* DiphenhydrAMINE *on page 399*
♦ **Sominex® Maximum Strength [OTC]** *see* DiphenhydrAMINE *on page 399*
♦ **Somnote™** *see* Chloral Hydrate *on page 261*
♦ **Som Pam (Can)** *see* Flurazepam *on page 548*
♦ **Sorine®** *see* Sotalol *on page 1198*
♦ **Sotacor® (Can)** *see* Sotalol *on page 1198*

Sotalol (SOE ta lole)

Medication Safety Issues

Sound-alike/look-alike issues:

Sotalol may be confused with Stadol®

Betapace® may be confused with Betapace AF®

Betapace AF® may be confused with Betapace®

Related Information

Antiarrhythmic Drugs *on page 1548*

Beta-Blockers *on page 1557*

Preoperative Evaluation of the Cardiac Patient for Noncardiac Surgery *on page 1485*

U.S. Brand Names Betapace®; Betapace AF®; Sorine®

Canadian Brand Names Alti-Sotalol; Apo-Sotalol®; Betapace AF®; CO Sotalol; Gen-Sotalol; Lin-Sotalol; Novo-Sotalol; Nu-Sotalol; PMS-Sotalol; Rho®-Sotalol; Riva-Sotalol; Rylosol; Sotacor®

Synonyms Sotalol Hydrochloride

Pharmacologic Category Antiarrhythmic Agent, Class II; Antiarrhythmic Agent, Class III; Beta-Adrenergic Blocker, Nonselective

Generic Available Yes

Use Treatment of documented ventricular arrhythmias (ie, sustained ventricular tachycardia), that in the judgment of the physician are life-threatening; maintenance of normal sinus rhythm in patients with symptomatic atrial fibrillation and atrial flutter who are currently in sinus rhythm. Manufacturer states substitutions should not be made for Betapace AF® since Betapace AF® is distributed with a patient package insert specific for atrial fibrillation/flutter.

Mechanism of Action

Beta-blocker which contains both beta-adrenoreceptor-blocking (Vaughan Williams Class II) and cardiac action potential duration prolongation (Vaughan Williams Class III) properties

Class II effects: Increased sinus cycle length, slowed heart rate, decreased AV nodal conduction, and increased AV nodal refractoriness

Class III effects: Prolongation of the atrial and ventricular monophasic action potentials, and effective refractory prolongation of atrial muscle, ventricular muscle, and atrioventricular accessory pathways in both the antegrade and retrograde directions

Sotalol is a racemic mixture of *d*- and *l*-sotalol; both isomers have similar Class III antiarrhythmic effects while the *l*-isomer is responsible for virtually all of the beta-blocking activity

Sotalol has both $beta_1$- and $beta_2$-receptor blocking activity

The beta-blocking effect of sotalol is a noncardioselective [half maximal at about 80 mg/day and maximal at doses of 320-640 mg/day]. Significant beta-blockade occurs at oral doses as low as 25 mg/day.

The Class III effects are seen only at oral doses ≥160 mg/day

Pharmacodynamics/Kinetics

Onset of action: Rapid, 1-2 hours

Peak effect: 2.5-4 hours

Duration: 8-16 hours

Absorption: Decreased 20% to 30% by meals compared to fasting

Distribution: Low lipid solubility; enters milk of laboratory animals and is reported to be present in human milk

Protein binding: None

Metabolism: None

Bioavailability: 90% to 100%

Half-life elimination: 12 hours; Children: 9.5 hours; terminal half-life decreases with age <2 years (may by ≥1 week in neonates)

Excretion: Urine (as unchanged drug)

Dosage Sotalol should be initiated and doses increased in a hospital with facilities for cardiac rhythm monitoring and assessment. Proarrhythmic events can occur after initiation of therapy and with each upward dosage adjustment.

Children: Oral: The safety and efficacy of sotalol in children have not been established

Note: Dosing per manufacturer, based on pediatric pharmacokinetic data; wait at least 36 hours between dosage adjustments to allow monitoring of QT intervals

≤2 years: Dosage should be adjusted (decreased) by plotting of the child's age on a logarithmic scale; see graph or refer to manufacturer's package labeling.

Sotalol Age Factor Nomogram for Patients ≤2 Years of Age

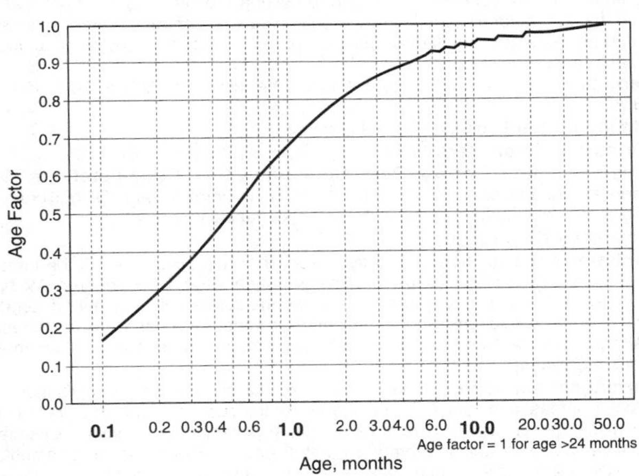

Adapted from U.S. Food and Drug Administration. http://www.fda.gov/cder/foi/label/2001/2115s3lbl.PDF

>2 years: Initial: 90 mg/m²/day in 3 divided doses; may be incrementally increased to a maximum of 180 mg/m²/day

Adults: Oral:

Ventricular arrhythmias (Betapace®, Sorine®):

Initial: 80 mg twice daily

Dose may be increased gradually to 240-320 mg/day; allow 3 days between dosing increments in order to attain steady-state plasma concentrations and to allow monitoring of QT intervals

Most patients respond to a total daily dose of 160-320 mg/day in 2-3 divided doses.

Some patients, with life-threatening refractory ventricular arrhythmias, may require doses as high as 480-640 mg/day; however, these doses should only be prescribed when the potential benefit outweighs the increased of adverse events.

Atrial fibrillation or atrial flutter (Betapace AF®): Initial: 80 mg twice daily

If the initial dose does not reduce the frequency of relapses of atrial fibrillation/flutter and is tolerated without excessive QT prolongation (not >520 msec) after 3 days, the dose may be increased to 120 mg twice daily. This may be further increased to 160 mg twice daily if response is inadequate and QT prolongation is not excessive.

(Continued)

Sotalol *(Continued)*

Elderly: Age does not significantly alter the pharmacokinetics of sotalol, but impaired renal function in elderly patients can increase the terminal half-life, resulting in increased drug accumulation

Dosage adjustment in renal impairment: Adults: Impaired renal function can increase the terminal half-life, resulting in increased drug accumulation. Sotalol (Betapace AF®) is contraindicated per the manufacturer for treatment of atrial fibrillation/flutter in patients with a Cl_{cr} <40 mL/minute.

Ventricular arrhythmias (Betapace®, Sorine®):

- Cl_{cr} >60 mL/minute: Administer every 12 hours
- Cl_{cr} 30-60 mL/minute: Administer every 24 hours
- Cl_{cr} 10-30 mL/minute: Administer every 36-48 hours
- Cl_{cr} <10 mL/minute: Individualize dose

Atrial fibrillation/flutter (Betapace AF®):

- Cl_{cr} >60 mL/minute: Administer every 12 hours
- Cl_{cr} 40-60 mL/minute: Administer every 24 hours
- Cl_{cr} <40 mL/minute: Use is contraindicated

Dialysis: Hemodialysis would be expected to reduce sotalol plasma concentrations because sotalol is not bound to plasma proteins and does not undergo extensive metabolism; administer dose postdialysis or administer supplemental 80 mg dose; peritoneal dialysis does not remove sotalol; supplemental dose is not necessary

Stability Store at 25°C (77°F); excursions permitted to 15°C to 30°C (59°F to 86°F)

Administration Food may decrease adsorption

Monitoring Parameters Serum magnesium, potassium, ECG

Anesthesia and Critical Care Concerns/Other Considerations Withdrawal: Beta-blocker therapy should not be withdrawn abruptly, but gradually tapered to avoid acute tachycardia and hypertension.

Pregnancy Risk Factor B

Contraindications Hypersensitivity to sotalol or any component of the formulation; bronchial asthma; sinus bradycardia; second- and third-degree AV block (unless a functioning pacemaker is present); congenital or acquired long QT syndromes; cardiogenic shock; uncontrolled congestive heart failure. Betapace AF® is contraindicated in patients with significantly reduced renal filtration (Cl_{cr} <40 mL/minute).

Warnings/Precautions Manufacturer recommends initiation (or reinitiation) and doses increased in a hospital setting with continuous monitoring and staff familiar with the recognition and treatment of life-threatening arrhythmias. Dosage of sotalol should be adjusted gradually with 3 days between dosing increments to achieve steady-state concentrations, and to allow time to monitor QT intervals. Some experts will initiate therapy on an outpatient basis in a patient without heart disease or bradycardia, who has a baseline uncorrected QT interval <450 msec, and normal serum potassium and magnesium levels; close EKG monitoring during this time is necessary. ACC/AHA guidelines for management of atrial fibrillation also recommend that for outpatient initiation the patient not have risk factors predisposing to drug-induced ventricular proarrhythmia. Creatinine clearance must be calculated prior to dosing. Use cautiously in the renally-impaired (dosage adjustment required).

Monitor and adjust dose to prevent QT_c prolongation. Concurrent use with other QT_c-prolonging drugs (including Class I and Class III antiarrhythmics) is generally not recommended; withhold for 3 half-lives. Watch for proarrhythmic effects. Correct electrolyte imbalances before initiating (especially hypokalemia and hyperkalemia). Consider pre-existing conditions such as sick sinus syndrome before initiating. Conduction abnormalities can occur particularly sinus bradycardia. Use cautiously within the first 2 weeks post-MI (experience limited). Administer cautiously in compensated heart failure and monitor for a worsening of the condition. Use caution in patients with PVD (can aggravate arterial insufficiency). Beta-blocker therapy should not be withdrawn abruptly (particularly in patients with CAD), but gradually tapered to avoid acute tachycardia, hypertension, and/or ischemia. Use caution with concurrent use of beta-blockers and either verapamil or diltiazem; bradycardia or heart block can occur. Use cautiously in diabetics because it can mask prominent hypoglycemic symptoms. Can mask signs of thyrotoxicosis. Use care with anesthetic agents which decrease myocardial function.

[U.S. Boxed Warning]: Betapace® should not be substituted for Betapace® AF; Betapace® AF is distributed with an educational insert specifically for patients with atrial fibrillation/flutter.

Adverse Reactions

>10%:

- Cardiovascular: Bradycardia (16%), chest pain (16%), palpitation (14%)
- Central nervous system: Fatigue (20%), dizziness (20%), lightheadedness (12%)
- Neuromuscular & skeletal: Weakness (13%)
- Respiratory: Dyspnea (21%)

1% to 10%:

- Cardiovascular: CHF (5%), peripheral vascular disorders (3%), edema (8%), abnormal ECG (7%), hypotension (6%), proarrhythmia (5% in ventricular arrhythmia patients; less than 1% in atrial fibrillation/flutter), syncope (5%)
- Central nervous system: Mental confusion (6%), anxiety (4%), headache (8%), sleep problems (8%), depression (4%)
- Dermatologic: Itching/rash (5%)
- Endocrine & metabolic: Sexual ability decreased (3%)
- Gastrointestinal: Diarrhea (7%), nausea/vomiting (10%), stomach discomfort (3% to 6%), flatulence (2%)
- Genitourinary: Impotence (2%)
- Hematologic: Bleeding (2%)
- Neuromuscular & skeletal: Paresthesia (4%), extremity pain (7%), back pain (3%)
- Ocular: Visual problems (5%)
- Respiratory: Upper respiratory problems (5% to 8%), asthma (2%)

<1% (Limited to important or life-threatening): Alopecia, bronchiolitis obliterans with organized pneumonia (BOOP), cold extremities, diaphoresis, eosinophilia, leukocytoclastic vasculitis, leukopenia, paralysis, phlebitis, photosensitivity reaction, pruritus, pulmonary edema, Raynaud's phenomenon, red crusted skin, retroperitoneal fibrosis, serum transaminases increased, skin necrosis after extravasation, thrombocytopenia, vertigo

Overdosage/Toxicology Symptoms of intoxication include cardiac disturbances, CNS toxicity, bronchospasm, hypoglycemia and hyperkalemia. The most common cardiac symptoms include hypotension and bradycardia; atrioventricular block, intraventricular conduction disturbances, cardiogenic shock, and asystole may occur with severe overdose, especially with membrane-depressant drugs (eg, propranolol); CNS effects include convulsions, coma, and respiratory arrest is commonly seen with propranolol and other membrane-depressant and lipid-soluble drugs.

Treatment includes symptomatic treatment of seizures, hypotension, hyperkalemia and hypoglycemia. Bradycardia and hypotension resistant to atropine, isoproterenol or pacing may respond to glucagon. Wide QRS defects caused by the membrane-depressant poisoning may respond to hypertonic sodium bicarbonate. Repeat-dose charcoal, hemoperfusion, or hemodialysis may be helpful in removal of only those beta-blockers with a small V_d, long half-life, or low intrinsic clearance (acebutolol, atenolol, nadolol, sotalol).

Drug Interactions

Amiodarone: May cause additive effects on QT_c prolongation as well as decreased heart rate, and has been associated with cardiac arrest in patients receiving beta-blockers.

Antacids (aluminum/magnesium) decrease sotalol blood levels; separate administration by 2 hours.

Antiarrhythmics: Concurrent use of Class Ia or Class III antiarrhythmics may result in additive QT_c prolongation; concurrent use is not recommended.

$Beta_2$ agonists: Effects may be diminished by concurrent sotalol; use caution.

Beta-blockers: Due to shared pharmacological effects, heart rate reductions may be additive; concurrent use is not recommended.

Calcium channel blockers: Concurrent use may lead to additive effects on AV conduction, ventricular contractility, and/or hypotension; use caution.

Cisapride: Concurrent use with sotalol increases malignant arrhythmias; contraindicated.

Clonidine: Sotalol may cause rebound hypertension after discontinuation of clonidine.

(Continued)

Sotalol *(Continued)*

QT_c-prolonging drugs: Concurrent use may result in additive QT_c prolongation, potentially increasing the risk of malignant arrhythmias. Use of cisapride, mesoridazine, thioridazine, and pimozide with other QT_c-prolonging agents is contraindicated. Concurrent use of sotalol with Class I and Class III antiarrhythmics is not recommended; withhold for 3 half-lives. Use caution with other QT_c-prolonging agents (including bepridil, erythromycin, clarithromycin), fluoroquinolones (including sparfloxacin, gatifloxacin, and moxifloxacin), haloperidol, and TCAs.

Phenothiazines (mesoridazine and thioridazine): Concurrent use may result in additive QT_c prolongation, potentially increasing the risk of malignant arrhythmias; contraindicated.

Pimozide: Concurrent use may result in additive QT_c prolongation, potentially increasing the risk of malignant arrhythmias; contraindicated.

Ethanol/Nutrition/Herb Interactions

Food: Sotalol peak serum concentrations may be decreased if taken with food.

Herb/Nutraceutical: Avoid ephedra (may worsen arrhythmia).

Dietary Considerations Administer on an empty stomach.

Dosage Forms

Tablet, as hydrochloride: 80 mg, 80 mg [AF], 120 mg, 120 mg [AF], 160 mg, 160 mg [AF], 240 mg

Betapace® [light blue]: 80 mg, 120 mg, 160 mg, 240 mg

Betapace AF® [white]: 80 mg, 120 mg, 160 mg

Sorine® [white]: 80 mg, 120 mg, 160 mg, 240 mg

- ♦ **Sotalol Hydrochloride** *see* Sotalol *on page 1198*
- ♦ **Sotradecol®** *see* Sodium Tetradecyl *on page 1194*
- ♦ **SPA** *see* Albumin *on page 48*
- ♦ **SPD417** *see* Carbamazepine *on page 225*

Spirapril (SPYE ra pril)

Related Information

Angiotensin Agents *on page 1544*

Preoperative Evaluation of the Cardiac Patient for Noncardiac Surgery *on page 1485*

Pharmacologic Category Angiotensin-Converting Enzyme (ACE) Inhibitor

Restrictions Not available in U.S.

Generic Available No

Use Management of mild to severe hypertension; treatment of left ventricular dysfunction after myocardial infarction

Mechanism of Action ACE inhibitor; inhibits renin-angiotensin system

Pharmacodynamics/Kinetics

Absorption: 53% to 60%; delayed by high fat meals

Half-life elimination, serum: 1-2 hours

Dosage Adults: Oral: 12-48 mg once daily

Pregnancy Risk Factor C (1st trimester); D (2nd and 3rd trimesters)

Contraindications Hypersensitivity to spirapril or any component of the formulation; angioedema or other sensitivity to any ACE inhibitor; bilateral renal artery stenosis; pregnancy (2nd and 3rd trimesters)

Warnings/Precautions Anaphylactic reactions can occur. Angioedema can occur at any time during treatment (especially following first dose). It may involve head and neck (potentially affecting the airway) or the intestine (presenting with abdominal pain). Prolonged monitoring may be required especially if tongue, glottis, or larynx are involved as they are associated with airway obstruction. Those with a history of airway surgery in this situation have a higher risk. Careful blood pressure monitoring with first dose (hypotension can occur especially in volume-depleted patients). Dosage adjustment needed in renal impairment. Use with caution in hypovolemia; collagen vascular diseases; valvular stenosis (particularly aortic stenosis); hyperkalemia; or before, during, or immediately after anesthesia. Avoid rapid dosage escalation which may lead to renal insufficiency. Rare toxicities associated with ACE inhibitors include cholestatic jaundice (which may progress to hepatic necrosis) and neutropenia/agranulocytosis with myeloid hyperplasia. If patient has renal impairment then a baseline WBC with differential and serum creatinine should be evaluated and monitored closely during the first 3 months of therapy. Hypersensitivity reactions may be seen during hemodialysis with high-flux dialysis membranes (eg, AN69). Deterioration in renal function can occur with initiation. Use with caution in unilateral renal artery stenosis and pre-existing renal insufficiency.

Adverse Reactions Frequency not defined.

Cardiovascular: Hypotension (orthostatic), angioedema

Central nervous system: Headache, dizziness, migraine headache (exacerbation of), hypoesthesia

Dermatologic: Skin rash

Gastrointestinal: Nausea, diarrhea, vomiting

Neuromuscular & skeletal: Back pain

Ocular: Conjunctivitis

Respiratory: Cough

Drug Interactions

Alpha$_1$ blockers: Hypotensive effect increased.

Aspirin: May decrease ACE inhibitor efficacy and/or increase risk of renal effects.

Diuretics: Hypovolemia due to diuretics may precipitate acute hypotensive events or acute renal failure.

Insulin: Risk of hypoglycemia may be increased.

Lithium: Risk of lithium toxicity may be increased; monitor lithium levels, especially the first 4 weeks of therapy.

Mercaptopurine: Risk of neutropenia may be increased.

NSAIDs: May attenuate hypertensive efficacy; effect has been seen with captopril and may occur with other ACE inhibitors; monitor blood pressure. May increase risk of renal effects.

Potassium-sparing diuretics (amiloride, potassium, spironolactone, triamterene): Increased risk of hyperkalemia.

Potassium supplements may increase the risk of hyperkalemia.

Trimethoprim (high dose) may increase the risk of hyperkalemia.

Dosage Forms Tablet: 3 mg, 6 mg, 12 mg, 24 mg

♦ **Spiriva®** *see* Tiotropium *on page 1274*

Spironolactone (speer on oh LAK tone)

Medication Safety Issues

Sound-alike/look-alike issues:

Aldactone® may be confused with Aldactazide®

Related Information

Heart Failure (Systolic) *on page 1607*

U.S. Brand Names Aldactone®

Canadian Brand Names Aldactone®; Novo-Spiroton

Pharmacologic Category Diuretic, Potassium-Sparing; Selective Aldosterone Blocker

Generic Available Yes

Use Management of edema associated with excessive aldosterone excretion; hypertension; congestive heart failure; primary hyperaldosteronism; hypokalemia; cirrhosis of liver accompanied by edema or ascites

Unlabeled/Investigational Use Female acne (adjunctive therapy); hirsutism; hypertension (pediatric); diuretic (pediatric)

Mechanism of Action Competes with aldosterone for receptor sites in the distal renal tubules, increasing sodium chloride and water excretion while conserving potassium and hydrogen ions; may block the effect of aldosterone on arteriolar smooth muscle as well

Pharmacodynamics/Kinetics

Duration of action: 2-3 days

Protein binding: 91% to 98%

Metabolism: Hepatic to multiple metabolites, including canrenone (active)

Half-life elimination: 78-84 minutes

Time to peak, serum: 1-3 hours (primarily as the active metabolite)

Excretion: Urine and feces

Dosage To reduce delay in onset of effect, a loading dose of 2 or 3 times the daily dose may be administered on the first day of therapy. Oral:

Children:

Diuretic, hypertension (unlabeled use): Children 1-17 years: Initial: 1 mg/kg/day divided every 12-24 hours (maximum dose: 3.3 mg/kg/day, up to 100 mg/day)

Diagnosis of primary aldosteronism (unlabeled use): 125-375 mg/m^2/day in divided doses

(Continued)

Spironolactone *(Continued)*

Adults:

Edema, hypokalemia: 25-200 mg/day in 1-2 divided doses

Hypertension (JNC 7): 25-50 mg/day in 1-2 divided doses

Diagnosis of primary aldosteronism: 100-400 mg/day in 1-2 divided doses

Acne in women (unlabeled use): 25-200 mg once daily

Hirsutism in women (unlabeled use): 50-200 mg/day in 1-2 divided doses

CHF, severe (with ACE inhibitor and a loop diuretic ± digoxin): 12.5-25 mg/day; maximum daily dose: 50 mg (higher doses may occasionallly be used). In the RALES trial, 25 mg every other day was the lowest maintenance dose possible.

Note: If potassium >5.4 mEq/L, consider dosage reduction.

Elderly: Initial: 25-50 mg/day in 1-2 divided doses, increasing by 25-50 mg every 5 days as needed.

Dosing interval in renal impairment:

Cl_{cr} 10-50 mL/minute: Administer every 12-24 hours.

Cl_{cr} <10 mL/minute: Avoid use.

Stability Protect from light

Monitoring Parameters Blood pressure, serum electrolytes (potassium, sodium), renal function, I & O ratios and daily weight throughout therapy

CHF: Potassium levels and renal function should be checked in 3 days and 1 week after initiation, then every 2-4 weeks for 3-12 months, then every 3-6 months.

Anesthesia and Critical Care Concerns/Other Considerations In severe heart failure, spironolactone (25 mg/day), when combined with maximal standard therapy, resulted in a striking improvement in cardiovascular outcome (*N Engl J Med*, 1999, 341:709-17).

Potassium levels should be monitored in patients on an aldosterone blocker, particularly in those who have underlying renal impairment or concurrent ACE inhibitor therapy.

Pregnancy Risk Factor C/D in pregnancy-induced hypertension (per expert analysis)

Contraindications Hypersensitivity to spironolactone or any component of the formulation; anuria; acute renal insufficiency; significant impairment of renal excretory function; hyperkalemia; pregnancy (pregnancy-induced hypertension - per expert analysis)

Warnings/Precautions Avoid potassium supplements, potassium-containing salt substitutes, a diet rich in potassium, or other drugs that can cause hyperkalemia. Monitor for fluid and electrolyte imbalances. Gynecomastia is related to dose and duration of therapy. Diuretic therapy should be carefully used in severe hepatic dysfunction; electrolyte and fluid shifts can cause or exacerbate encephalopathy. Discontinue use prior to adrenal vein catheterization. When evaluating a heart failure patient for spironolactone treatment, creatinine should be ≤2.5 mg/dL in men or ≤2 mg/dL in women and potassium <5 mEq/L. **[U.S. Boxed Warning]: Shown to be a tumorigen in chronic toxicity animal studies. Avoid unnecessary use.**

Adverse Reactions Incidence of adverse events is not always reported (mean daily dose 26 mg).

Cardiovascular: Edema (2%, placebo 2%)

Central nervous system: Disorders (23%, placebo 21%) which may include drowsiness, lethargy, headache, mental confusion, drug fever, ataxia, fatigue

Dermatologic: Maculopapular, erythematous cutaneous eruptions, urticaria, hirsutism, eosinophilia

Endocrine & metabolic: Gynecomastia (men 9%; placebo 1%), breast pain (men 2%; placebo 0.1%), serious hyperkalemia (2%, placebo 1%), hyponatremia, dehydration, hyperchloremic metabolic acidosis (in decompensated hepatic cirrhosis), impotence, menstrual irregularities, amenorrhea, postmenopausal bleeding

Gastrointestinal: Disorders (29%, placebo 29%) which may include anorexia, nausea, cramping, diarrhea, gastric bleeding, ulceration, gastritis, vomiting

Hematologic: Agranulocytosis

Hepatic: Cholestatic/hepatocellular toxicity

Renal: Increased BUN concentration

Miscellaneous: Deepening of the voice, anaphylactic reaction, breast cancer

Overdosage/Toxicology Symptoms of overdose include drowsiness, confusion, clinical signs of dehydration and electrolyte imbalance, and hyperkalemia. Ingestion of large amounts of potassium-sparing diuretics may result in life-threatening hyperkalemia. This can be treated with I.V. glucose, with concurrent regular insulin. Sodium bicarbonate may also be used as a temporary measure. If needed, Kayexalate® oral or rectal solutions in sorbitol may also be used.

Drug Interactions

ACE inhibitors can cause hyperkalemia, especially in patients with renal impairment, potassium-rich diets, or on other drugs causing hyperkalemia; avoid concurrent use or monitor closely.

Cholestyramine can cause hyperchloremic acidosis in cirrhotic patients; avoid concurrent use.

Digoxin's positive inotropic effect may be reduced; serum levels of digoxin may increase.

Mitotane loses its effect; avoid concurrent use.

Potassium supplements may increase potassium retention and cause hyperkalemia; avoid concurrent use.

Salicylates and NSAIDs may interfere with the natriuretic action of spironolactone.

Ethanol/Nutrition/Herb Interactions

Food: Food increases absorption.

Herb/Nutraceutical: Avoid natural licorice (due to mineralocorticoid activity)

Test Interactions May cause false elevation in serum digoxin concentrations measured by RIA

Dietary Considerations Should be taken with food to decrease gastrointestinal irritation and to increase absorption. Excessive potassium intake (eg, salt substitutes, low-salt foods, bananas, nuts) should be avoided.

Dosage Forms Tablet: 25 mg, 50 mg, 100 mg

- **SPS®** *see* Sodium Polystyrene Sulfonate *on page 1193*
- **SSD®** *see* Silver Sulfadiazine *on page 1173*
- **SSD® AF** *see* Silver Sulfadiazine *on page 1173*
- **Stadol®** *see* Butorphanol *on page 208*
- **Stagesic®** *see* Hydrocodone and Acetaminophen *on page 636*
- **Statex® (Can)** *see* Morphine Sulfate *on page 867*
- **Staticin® [DSC]** *see* Erythromycin *on page 476*

Stavudine (STAV yoo deen)

Medication Safety Issues

Sound-alike/look-alike issues:

Zerit® may be confused with Ziac®

U.S. Brand Names Zerit®

Canadian Brand Names Zerit®

Synonyms d4T

Pharmacologic Category Antiretroviral Agent, Reverse Transcriptase Inhibitor (Nucleoside)

Generic Available No

Use Treatment of HIV infection in combination with other antiretroviral agents

Mechanism of Action Stavudine is a thymidine analog which interferes with HIV viral DNA dependent DNA polymerase resulting in inhibition of viral replication; nucleoside reverse transcriptase inhibitor

Pharmacodynamics/Kinetics

Distribution: V_d: 0.5 L/kg

Bioavailability: 86.4%

Metabolism: Undergoes intracellular phosphorylation to an active metabolite

Half-life elimination: 1-1.6 hours

Time to peak, serum: 1 hour

Excretion: Urine (40% as unchanged drug)

Dosage Oral:

Newborns (Birth to 13 days): 0.5 mg/kg every 12 hours

Children:

>14 days and <30 kg: 1 mg/kg every 12 hours

≥30 kg: Refer to Adults dosing

Adults:

≥60 kg: 40 mg every 12 hours

<60 kg: 30 mg every 12 hours

(Continued)

Stavudine *(Continued)*

Dosing adjustment for toxicity: If symptoms of peripheral neuropathy occur, discontinue until symptoms resolve. Treatment may then be resumed at 50% the recommended dose. If symptoms recur at lower dose, permanent discontinuation should be considered.

Dosing adjustment in renal impairment:

Children: Specific recommendations not available. Reduction in dose or increase in dosing interval should be considered.

Adults:

Cl_{cr} >50 mL/minute:
- ≥60 kg: 40 mg every 12 hours
- <60 kg: 30 mg every 12 hours

Cl_{cr} 26-50 mL/minute:
- ≥60 kg: 20 mg every 12 hours
- <60 kg: 15 mg every 12 hours

Cl_{cr} 10-25 mL/minute, hemodialysis (administer dose after hemodialysis on day of dialysis):
- ≥60 kg: 20 mg every 24 hours
- <60 kg: 15 mg every 24 hours

Elderly: Older patients should be closely monitored for signs and symptoms of peripheral neuropathy; dosage should be carefully adjusted to renal function

Stability Capsules and powder for reconstitution may be stored at room temperature. Reconstituted oral solution should be refrigerated and is stable for 30 days.

Administration May be administered without regard to meals. Oral solution should be shaken vigorously prior to use.

Monitoring Parameters Monitor liver function tests and signs and symptoms of peripheral neuropathy; monitor viral load and CD4 count

Pregnancy Risk Factor C

Contraindications Hypersensitivity to stavudine or any component of the formulation

Warnings/Precautions Use with caution in patients who demonstrate previous hypersensitivity to zidovudine, didanosine, zalcitabine, pre-existing bone marrow suppression, renal insufficiency, or peripheral neuropathy. Peripheral neuropathy may be the dose-limiting side effect. Zidovudine should not be used in combination with stavudine. **[U.S. Boxed Warning]: Lactic acidosis and severe hepatomegaly with steatosis have been reported with stavudine use, including fatal cases.** Risk may be increased in obesity, prolonged nucleoside exposure, or in female patients. Suspend therapy in patients with suspected lactic acidosis; consider discontinuation of stavudine if lactic acidosis is confirmed. Pregnant women may be at increased risk of lactic acidosis and liver damage. Severe motor weakness (resembling Guillain-Barré syndrome) has also been reported (including fatal cases, usually in association with lactic acidosis); manufacturer recommends discontinuation if motor weakness develops (with or without lactic acidosis). **[U.S. Boxed Warning]: Pancreatitis (including some fatal cases) has occurred during combination therapy (didanosine with or without hydroxyurea).** Risk increased when used in combination regimen with didanosine and hydroxyurea. Suspend therapy with agents toxic to the pancreas (including stavudine, didanosine, or hydroxyurea) in patients with suspected pancreatitis.

Adverse Reactions All adverse reactions reported below were similar to comparative agent, zidovudine, except for peripheral neuropathy, which was greater for stavudine. Selected adverse events reported as monotherapy or in combination therapy include:

>10%:
- Central nervous system: Headache
- Dermatologic: Rash
- Gastrointestinal: Nausea, vomiting, diarrhea
- Hepatic: Transaminases increased
- Neuromuscular & skeletal: Peripheral neuropathy
- Miscellaneous: Amylase increased

1% to 10%: Hepatic: Bilirubin increased

Postmarketing and/or case reports: Abdominal pain, allergic reaction, anemia, anorexia, chills, fever, hepatitis, hepatomegaly, hepatic failure, hepatic steatosis, insomnia, lactic acidosis, leukopenia, motor weakness (severe), myalgia, pancreatitis, redistribution/accumulation of body fat, thrombocytopenia

Overdosage/Toxicology Acute toxicity was not reported following administration of 12-24 times the recommended dose in adults. Peripheral neuropathy and hepatic toxicity have been reported following chronic overdose. Stavudine may be removed by hemodialysis.

Drug Interactions

Didanosine: Risk of pancreatitis may be increased with concurrent use. Cases of fatal lactic acidosis have been reported with this combination when used during pregnancy; use only if clearly needed.

Doxorubicin: May inhibit intracellular phosphorylation of stavudine; use with caution.

Hydroxyurea: Risk of hepatotoxicity or pancreatitis may be increased with concurrent use.

Ribavirin: May inhibit intracellular phosphorylation of stavudine; use with caution.

Zalcitabine: May increase risk of peripheral neuropathy; concurrent use not recommended.

Zidovudine: Inhibits intracellular phosphorylation of stavudine; concurrent use not recommended.

Dietary Considerations May be taken without regard to meals.

Dosage Forms

Capsule: 15 mg, 20 mg, 30 mg, 40 mg

Powder, for oral solution: 1 mg/mL (200 mL) [dye free; fruit flavor]

- ♦ **Stemetil® (Can)** *see* Prochlorperazine *on page 1061*
- ♦ **Sterapred®** *see* PredniSONE *on page 1050*
- ♦ **Sterapred® DS** *see* PredniSONE *on page 1050*
- ♦ **Stimate™** *see* Desmopressin *on page 363*
- ♦ **St. Joseph® Adult Aspirin [OTC]** *see* Aspirin *on page 129*
- ♦ **Streptase®** *see* Streptokinase *on page 1207*

Streptokinase (strep toe KYE nase)

Medication Safety Issues

High alert medication: The Institute for Safe Medication Practices (ISMP) includes this medication (I.V.) among its list of drugs which have a heightened risk of causing significant patient harm when used in error.

U.S. Brand Names Streptase®

Canadian Brand Names Streptase®

Synonyms SK

Pharmacologic Category Thrombolytic Agent

Generic Available No

Use Thrombolytic agent used in treatment of recent severe or massive deep vein thrombosis, pulmonary emboli, myocardial infarction, and occluded arteriovenous cannulas

Mechanism of Action Activates the conversion of plasminogen to plasmin by forming a complex, exposing plasminogen-activating site, and cleaving a peptide bond that converts plasminogen to plasmin; plasmin degrades fibrin, fibrinogen and other procoagulant proteins into soluble fragments; effective both outside and within the formed thrombus/embolus

Pharmacodynamics/Kinetics

Onset of action: Activation of plasminogen occurs almost immediately

Duration: Fibrinolytic effect: Several hours; Anticoagulant effect: 12-24 hours

Half-life elimination: 83 minutes

Excretion: By circulating antibodies and the reticuloendothelial system

Dosage I.V.:

Children: Safety and efficacy have not been not established. Limited studies have used 3500-4000 units/kg over 30 minutes followed by 1000-1500 units/kg/hour.

Clotted catheter: **Note:** Not recommended due to possibility of allergic reactions with repeated doses: 10,000-25,000 units diluted in NS to a final volume equivalent to catheter volume; instill into catheter and leave in place for 1 hour, then aspirate contents out of catheter and flush catheter with normal saline.

Adults: Antibodies to streptokinase remain for at least 3-6 months after initial dose: Administration requires the use of an infusion pump.

An intradermal skin test of 100 units has been suggested to predict allergic response to streptokinase. If a positive reaction is not seen after 15-20 minutes, a therapeutic dose may be administered.

(Continued)

Streptokinase *(Continued)*

Guidelines for acute myocardial infarction (AMI): 1.5 million units over 60 minutes

Administration:

Dilute two 750,000 unit vials of streptokinase with 5 mL dextrose 5% in water (D_5W) each, gently swirl to dissolve.

Add this dose of the 1.5 million units to 150 mL D_5W.

This should be infused over 60 minutes; an in-line filter ≥0.45 micron should be used.

Monitor for the first few hours for signs of anaphylaxis or allergic reaction. **Infusion should be slowed if blood pressure falls by 25 mm Hg or terminated if asthmatic symptoms appear.**

Following completion of streptokinase, initiate heparin, if directed, when aPTT returns to less than 2 times the upper limit of control; do not use a bolus, but initiate infusion adjusted to a target aPTT of 1.5-2 times the upper limit of control. If prolonged (>48 hours) heparin is required, infusion may be switched to subcutaneous therapy.

Guidelines for acute pulmonary embolism (APE): 3 million unit dose over 24 hours

Administration:

Dilute four 750,000 unit vials of streptokinase with 5 mL dextrose 5% in water (D_5W) each, gently swirl to dissolve.

Add this dose of 3 million units to 250 mL D_5W, an in-line filter ≥0.45 micron should be used.

Administer 250,000 units (23 mL) over 30 minutes followed by 100,000 units/hour (9 mL/hour) for 24 hours.

Monitor for the first few hours for signs of anaphylaxis or allergic reaction. **Infusion should be slowed if blood pressure is lowered by 25 mm Hg or if asthmatic symptoms appear.**

Begin heparin 1000 units/hour about 3-4 hours after completion of streptokinase infusion or when PTT is <100 seconds.

Monitor PT, PTT, and fibrinogen levels during therapy.

Thromboses: 250,000 units to start, then 100,000 units/hour for 24-72 hours depending on location.

Cannula occlusion: 250,000 units into cannula, clamp for 2 hours, then aspirate contents and flush with normal saline; **Not recommended; see Warnings/ Precautions**

Stability Streptokinase, a white lyophilized powder, may have a slight yellow color in solution due to the presence of albumin; intact vials should be stored at room temperature; reconstituted solutions should be refrigerated and are stable for 24 hours

Stability of parenteral admixture at room temperature (25°C): 8 hours; at refrigeration (4°C): 24 hours

Administration Avoid I.M. injections

Monitoring Parameters Blood pressure, PT, aPTT, platelet count, hematocrit, fibrinogen concentration, signs of bleeding

Reference Range

Partial thromboplastin time (aPTT) activated: 20.4-33.2 seconds

Prothrombin time (PT): 10.9-13.7 seconds (same as control)

Fibrinogen: 200-400 mg/dL

Anesthesia and Critical Care Concerns/Other Considerations Streptokinase can cause hypotension and anaphylaxis or allergic reaction. Heparin should be initiated several hours after completion of streptokinase therapy with close monitoring of the coagulation profile.

Antibodies to streptokinase (even if anistreplase was used) persist for up to 6 months after the initial dose. Therefore, an alternative thrombolytic approach (tissue plasminogen activator) should be used if thrombolytic therapy is needed. Furthermore, patients who have had a recent streptococcal infection (within 6 months) may also manifest hypersensitivity to streptokinase. a hypersensitivity response to urokinase.

Pregnancy Risk Factor C

Contraindications Hypersensitivity to anistreplase, streptokinase, or any component of the formulation; active internal bleeding; history of CVA; recent (within 2

months) intracranial or intraspinal surgery or trauma; intracranial neoplasm, arteriovenous malformation, or aneurysm; known bleeding diathesis; severe uncontrolled hypertension

Warnings/Precautions Concurrent heparin anticoagulation can contribute to bleeding; careful attention to all potential bleeding sites. I.M. injections and nonessential handling of the patient should be avoided. Venipunctures should be performed carefully and only when necessary. If arterial puncture is necessary, use an upper extremity vessel that can be manually compressed. If serious bleeding occurs then the infusion of streptokinase and heparin should be stopped.

For the following conditions the risk of bleeding is higher with use of thrombolytics and should be weighed against the benefits of therapy: recent (within 10 days) major surgery (eg, CABG, obstetrical delivery, organ biopsy, previous puncture of noncompressible vessels), cerebrovascular disease, recent (within 10 days) gastrointestinal or genitourinary bleeding, recent trauma (within 10 days) including CPR, hypertension (systolic BP >180 mm Hg and/or diastolic BP >110 mm Hg), high likelihood of left heart thrombus (eg, mitral stenosis with atrial fibrillation), acute pericarditis, subacute bacterial endocarditis, hemostatic defects including ones caused by severe renal or hepatic dysfunction, significant hepatic dysfunction, pregnancy, diabetic hemorrhagic retinopathy or other hemorrhagic ophthalmic conditions, septic thrombophlebitis or occluded AV cannula at seriously infected site, advanced age (eg, >75 years), patients receiving oral anticoagulants, any other condition in which bleeding constitutes a significant hazard or would be particularly difficult to manage because of location.

Coronary thrombolysis may result in reperfusion arrhythmias. Hypotension, occasionally severe, can occur (not from bleeding or anaphylaxis). Follow standard MI management. Rare anaphylactic reactions can occur. Cautious repeat administration in patients who have received anistreplase or streptokinase within 1 year (streptokinase antibody may decrease effectiveness or risk of allergic reactions). Safety and efficacy in pediatric patients have not been established.

Streptokinase is not indicated for restoration of patency of intravenous catheters. Serious adverse events relating to the use of streptokinase in the restoration of patency of occluded intravenous catheters have involved the use of high doses of streptokinase in small volumes (250,000 international units in 2 mL). Uses of lower doses of streptokinase in infusions over several hours, generally into partially occluded catheters, or local instillation into the catheter lumen and subsequent aspiration, have been described in the medical literature. Healthcare providers should consider the risk for potentially life-threatening reactions (hypersensitivity, apnea, bleeding) associated with the use of streptokinase in the management of occluded intravenous catheters.

Adverse Reactions As with all drugs which may affect hemostasis, bleeding is the major adverse effect associated with streptokinase. Hemorrhage may occur at virtually any site. Risk is dependent on multiple variables, including the dosage administered, concurrent use of multiple agents which alter hemostasis, and patient predisposition (including hypertension). Rapid lysis of coronary artery thrombi by thrombolytic agents may be associated with reperfusion-related atrial and/or ventricular arrhythmia.

>10%:
- Cardiovascular: Hypotension
- Local: Injection site bleeding

1% to 10%:
- Central nervous system: Fever (1% to 4%)
- Dermatologic: Bruising, rash, pruritus
- Gastrointestinal: Gastrointestinal hemorrhage, nausea, vomiting
- Genitourinary: Genitourinary hemorrhage
- Hematologic: Anemia
- Neuromuscular & skeletal: Muscle pain
- Ocular: Eye hemorrhage, periorbital edema
- Respiratory: Bronchospasm, epistaxis
- Miscellaneous: Diaphoresis

<1% (Limited to important or life-threatening): Acute tubular necrosis, allergic reactions, anaphylactic shock, anaphylactoid reactions, anaphylaxis, angioneurotic edema, ARDS, back pain (during infusion), cholesterol embolization, erysipelas-like rash, Guillain-Barré syndrome, hemarthrosis, intracranial hemorrhage, laryngeal edema, morbilliform, Parsonage-Turner syndrome, pericardial

(Continued)

Streptokinase *(Continued)*

hemorrhage, respiratory depression, retroperitoneal hemorrhage, splenic rupture, transaminases increased, urticaria

Additional cardiovascular events associated with use in MI: Asystole, AV block, cardiac arrest, cardiac tamponade, cardiogenic shock, electromechanical dissociation, heart failure, mitral regurgitation, myocardial rupture, pericardial effusion, pericarditis, pulmonary edema, recurrent ischemia/infarction, thromboembolism, ventricular tachycardia

Overdosage/Toxicology Symptoms of overdose include epistaxis, bleeding gums, hematoma, spontaneous ecchymoses, and oozing at the catheter site. If uncontrollable bleeding occurs, discontinue infusion. Whole blood or blood products may be used to reverse bleeding.

Drug Interactions

Aminocaproic acid (antifibrinolytic agent) may decrease effectiveness of thrombolytic agents.

Drugs which affect platelet function (eg, NSAIDs, dipyridamole, ticlopidine, clopidogrel, IIb/IIIa antagonists) may potentiate the risk of hemorrhage; use with caution.

Heparin and aspirin: Use with aspirin and heparin may increase bleeding over aspirin and heparin alone. However, aspirin and heparin were used concurrently in the majority of patients in some major clinical studies of streptokinase.

Warfarin or oral anticoagulants: Risk of bleeding may be increased during concurrent therapy.

Ethanol/Nutrition/Herb Interactions Herb/Nutraceutical: Avoid cat's claw, dong quai, evening primrose, feverfew, red clover, horse chestnut, garlic, green tea, ginseng, ginkgo (all have additional antiplatelet activity).

Dosage Forms [DSC] = Discontinued product

Injection, powder for reconstitution: 250,000 int. units; 750,000 int. units; 1,500,000 int. units [DSC]

- **Sublimaze®** *see* Fentanyl *on page 514*
- **Subutex®** *see* Buprenorphine *on page 198*

Succinylcholine (suks in il KOE leen)

Medication Safety Issues

High alert medication: The Institute for Safe Medication Practices (ISMP) includes this medication among its list of drugs which have a heightened risk of causing significant patient harm when used in error.

Related Information

Chronic Renal Failure *on page 1437*

Neuromuscular Blocking Agents *on page 1572*

U.S. Brand Names Quelicin®

Canadian Brand Names Quelicin®

Synonyms Succinylcholine Chloride; Suxamethonium Chloride

Pharmacologic Category Neuromuscular Blocker Agent, Depolarizing

Generic Available No

Use Adjunct to general anesthesia to facilitate both rapid sequence and routine endotracheal intubation and to relax skeletal muscles during surgery; to reduce the intensity of muscle contractions of pharmacologically- or electrically-induced convulsions; does not relieve pain or produce sedation

Mechanism of Action Acts similar to acetylcholine, produces depolarization of the motor endplate at the myoneural junction which causes sustained flaccid skeletal muscle paralysis produced by state of accommodation that developes in adjacent excitable muscle membranes

Pharmacodynamics/Kinetics

Onset of action: I.M.: 2-3 minutes; I.V.: Complete muscular relaxation: 30-60 seconds

Duration: I.M.: 10-30 minutes; I.V.: 4-6 minutes with single administration

Metabolism: Rapidly hydrolyzed by plasma pseudocholinesterase

Dosage I.M., I.V.: Dose to effect; doses will vary due to interpatient variability; use ideal body weight for obese patients

I.M.: 2.5-4 mg/kg, total dose should not exceed 150 mg

I.V.:

Children: Initial: 1-2 mg/kg; maintenance: 0.3-0.6 mg/kg every 5-10 minutes as needed; because of the risk of malignant hyperthermia, use of continuous infusions is not recommended in infants and children

Adults: 1-1.5 mg/kg, up to 150 mg total dose

Maintenance: 0.04-0.07 mg/kg every 5-10 minutes as needed

Continuous infusion: 10-100 mcg/kg/minute (or 0.5-10 mg/minute); dilute to concentration of 1-2 mg/mL in D_5W or NS

Note: Initial dose of succinylcholine must be increased when nondepolarizing agent pretreatment used because of the antagonism between succinylcholine and nondepolarizing neuromuscular blocking agents

Dosing adjustment in hepatic impairment: Dose should be decreased in patients with severe liver disease

Stability

Refrigerate at 2°C to 8°C (36°F to 46°F); however, remains stable for ≤3 months unrefrigerated; powder form does not require refrigeration

Stability of parenteral admixture at refrigeration temperature (4°C): 24 hours in D_5W or NS

I.V. form is **incompatible** when mixed with sodium bicarbonate, pentobarbital, thiopental

Administration May be administered by rapid I.V. injection without further dilution; I.M. injections should be made deeply, preferably high into deltoid muscle

Monitoring Parameters Cardiac monitor, blood pressure monitor, and ventilator required during administration; temperature, serum potassium and calcium, assisted ventilator status

Anesthesia and Critical Care Concerns/Other Considerations Classified as an ultra-short duration neuromuscular-blocking agent; some formulations may contain benzyl alcohol.

Critically-Ill Adult Patients: The 2002 ACCM/SCCM/ASHP clinical practice guidelines for sustained neuromuscular blockade in the adult critically-ill patient recommend:

Optimize sedatives and analgesics prior to initiation and monitor and adjust accordingly during course. Neuromuscular blockers do not relieve pain or produce sedation.

Protect patient's eyes from development of keratitis and corneal abrasion by administering ophthalmic ointment and taping eyelids closed or using eye patches. Reposition patient routinely to protect pressure points from breakdown. Address DVT prophylaxis.

Concurrent use of a neuromuscular blocker and corticosteroids appear to increase the risk of certain ICU myopathies; avoid or administer the corticosteroid at the lowest dose possible. Reassess need for neuromuscular blocker daily.

Using daily drug holidays (stopping neuromuscular-blocking agent until patient requires it again) may decrease the incidence of acute quadriplegic myopathy syndrome.

Tachyphylaxis can develop; switch to another neuromuscular blocker (taking into consideration the patient's organ function) if paralysis is still necessary.

Atracurium or cisatracurium is recommended for patients with significant hepatic or renal disease, due to organ-independent Hofmann elimination.

Monitor patients clinically and via "Train of Four" (TOF) testing with a goal of adjusting the degree of blockade to 1-2 twitches or based upon the patient's clinical condition.

Pregnancy Risk Factor C

Contraindications Hypersensitivity to succinylcholine or any component of the formulation; personal or familial history of malignant hyperthermia; myopathies associated with elevated serum creatine phosphokinase (CPK) values; narrow-angle glaucoma, penetrating eye injuries; disorders of plasma pseudocholinesterase

Warnings/Precautions [U.S. Boxed Warning]: Use with caution in pediatrics and adolescents secondary to undiagnosed skeletal muscle myopathy and potential for ventricular dysrhythmias and cardiac arrest resulting from hyperkalemia; use with caution in patients with pre-existing hyperkalemia, paraplegia, extensive or severe burns, extensive denervation of skeletal muscle because of disease or injury to the CNS or with degenerative or dystrophic neuromuscular disease; may increase vagal tone

(Continued)

Succinylcholine *(Continued)*

Adverse Reactions

>10%:

Ocular: Increased intraocular pressure

Miscellaneous: Postoperative stiffness

1% to 10%:

Cardiovascular: Bradycardia, hypotension, cardiac arrhythmia, tachycardia

Gastrointestinal: Intragastric pressure, salivation

<1% (Limited to important or life-threatening): Acute quadriplegic myopathy syndrome (prolonged use), apnea, bronchospasm, circulatory collapse, erythema, hyperkalemia, hypertension, itching, malignant hyperthermia, myalgia, myoglobinuria, myositis ossificans (prolonged use), rash

Overdosage/Toxicology

Symptoms of overdose include respiratory paralysis and cardiac arrest.

Bradyarrhythmias can often be treated with atropine 0.1 mg (infants). Do not treat with anticholinesterase drugs (eg, neostigmine, physostigmine) since this may worsen its toxicity by interfering with its metabolism.

Drug Interactions

Increased toxicity: Anticholinesterase drugs (neostigmine, physostigmine, or pyridostigmine) in combination with succinylcholine can cause cardiorespiratory collapse; cyclophosphamide, oral contraceptives, lidocaine, thiotepa, pancuronium, lithium, magnesium salts, aprotinin, chloroquine, metoclopramide, terbutaline, and procaine enhance and prolong the effects of succinylcholine

Prolonged neuromuscular blockade: Inhaled anesthetics; local anesthetics; calcium channel blockers; antiarrhythmics (eg, quinidine or procainamide); antibiotics (eg, aminoglycosides, tetracyclines, vancomycin, clindamycin); immunosuppressants (eg, cyclosporine)

Test Interactions Increased potassium (S)

Dosage Forms Injection, solution, as chloride: 20 mg/mL (5 mL, 10 mL); 50 mg/mL (10 mL); 100 mg/mL (10 mL)

♦ **Succinylcholine Chloride** *see* Succinylcholine *on page 1210*

Sucralfate (soo KRAL fate)

Medication Safety Issues

Sound-alike/look-alike issues:

Sucralfate may be confused with salsalate

Carafate® may be confused with Cafergot®

U.S. Brand Names Carafate®

Canadian Brand Names Apo-Sucralate®; Novo-Sucralate; Nu-Sucralate; PMS-Sucralate; Sulcrate®; Sulcrate® Suspension Plus

Synonyms Aluminum Sucrose Sulfate, Basic

Pharmacologic Category Gastrointestinal Agent, Miscellaneous

Generic Available Yes

Use Short-term management of duodenal ulcers; maintenance of duodenal ulcers

Unlabeled/Investigational Use Gastric ulcers; suspension may be used topically for treatment of stomatitis due to cancer chemotherapy and other causes of esophageal and gastric erosions; GERD, esophagitis; treatment of NSAID mucosal damage; prevention of stress ulcers; postsclerotherapy for esophageal variceal bleeding

Mechanism of Action Forms a complex by binding with positively charged proteins in exudates, forming a viscous paste-like, adhesive substance. This selectively forms a protective coating that protects the lining against peptic acid, pepsin, and bile salts.

Pharmacodynamics/Kinetics

Onset of action: Paste formation and ulcer adhesion: 1-2 hours

Duration: Up to 6 hours

Absorption: Oral: <5%

Distribution: Acts locally at ulcer sites; unbound in GI tract to aluminum and sucrose octasulfate

Metabolism: None

Excretion: Urine (small amounts as unchanged compounds)

Dosage Oral:

Children: Dose not established, doses of 40-80 mg/kg/day divided every 6 hours have been used

Stomatitis (unlabeled use): 2.5-5 mL (1 g/10 mL suspension), swish and spit or swish and swallow 4 times/day

Adults:

Stress ulcer prophylaxis: 1 g 4 times/day

Stress ulcer treatment: 1 g every 4 hours

Duodenal ulcer:

Treatment: 1 g 4 times/day on an empty stomach and at bedtime for 4-8 weeks, or alternatively 2 g twice daily; treatment is recommended for 4-8 weeks in adults, the elderly may require 12 weeks

Maintenance: Prophylaxis: 1 g twice daily

Stomatitis (unlabeled use): 1 g/10 mL suspension, swish and spit or swish and swallow 4 times/day

Dosage comment in renal impairment: Aluminum salt is minimally absorbed (<5%), however, may accumulate in renal failure

Stability Suspension: Shake well. Refrigeration is **not** necessary; do **not** freeze.

Administration Tablet may be broken or dissolved in water before ingestion. Administer with water on an empty stomach.

Pregnancy Risk Factor B

Contraindications Hypersensitivity to sucralfate or any component of the formulation

Warnings/Precautions Successful therapy with sucralfate should not be expected to alter the posthealing frequency of recurrence or the severity of duodenal ulceration; use with caution in patients with chronic renal failure who have an impaired excretion of absorbed aluminum. Because of the potential for sucralfate to alter the absorption of some drugs, separate administration (take other medication 2 hours before sucralfate) should be considered when alterations in bioavailability are believed to be critical

Adverse Reactions

1% to 10%: Gastrointestinal: Constipation

<1% (Limited to important or life-threatening): Bezoar formation, hypersensitivity (pruritus, urticaria, angioedema), rash

Overdosage/Toxicology Toxicity is minimal, may cause constipation

Drug Interactions Decreased effect: Digoxin, phenytoin (hydantoins), warfarin, ketoconazole, quinidine, ciprofloxacin, norfloxacin (quinolones), tetracycline, theophylline; because of the potential for sucralfate to alter the absorption of some drugs, separate administration (take other medications 2 hours before sucralfate) should be considered when alterations in bioavailability are believed to be critical

Note: When given with aluminum-containing antacids, may increase serum/body aluminum concentrations (see Warnings/Precautions)

Ethanol/Nutrition/Herb Interactions Food: Sucralfate may interfere with absorption of vitamin A, vitamin D, vitamin E, and vitamin K.

Dietary Considerations Administer with water on an empty stomach.

Dosage Forms [DSC] = Discontinued product

Suspension, oral: 1 g/10 mL (10 mL) [DSC]

Carafate®: 1 g/10 mL (420 mL)

Tablet (Carafate®): 1 g

References

Collard HR, Saint S, Matthay MA, "Prevention of Ventilator-Associated Pneumonia: An Evidence-Based Systematic Review," *Ann Intern Med*, 2003, 138(6):494-501.

Cook D, Guyatt G, Marshall J, et al, "A Comparison of Sucralfate and Ranitidine for the Prevention of Upper Gastrointestinal Bleeding in Patients Requiring Mechanical Ventilation. Canadian Critical Care Trials Group," *N Engl J Med*, 1998, 338(12):791-7.

♦ **Sudafed® [OTC]** *see* Pseudoephedrine *on page 1085*

♦ **Sudafed® 12 Hour [OTC]** *see* Pseudoephedrine *on page 1085*

♦ **Sudafed® 24 Hour [OTC]** *see* Pseudoephedrine *on page 1085*

♦ **Sudafed® Children's [OTC]** *see* Pseudoephedrine *on page 1085*

♦ **Sudafed® Decongestant (Can)** *see* Pseudoephedrine *on page 1085*

♦ **Sudafed PE™ [OTC]** *see* Phenylephrine *on page 1015*

♦ **Sudodrin [OTC]** *see* Pseudoephedrine *on page 1085*

♦ **SudoGest [OTC]** *see* Pseudoephedrine *on page 1085*

♦ **Sudo-Tab® [OTC]** *see* Pseudoephedrine *on page 1085*

♦ **Sufenta®** *see* Sufentanil *on page 1214*

Sufentanil (soo FEN ta nil)

Medication Safety Issues

Sound-alike/look-alike issues:

Sufentanil may be confused with alfentanil, fentanyl

Sufenta® may be confused with Alfenta®, Sudafed®, Survanta®

Related Information

Acute Postoperative Pain *on page 1388*
Anesthesia Considerations for Neurosurgery *on page 1401*
Chronic Pain Management *on page 1430*
Chronic Renal Failure *on page 1437*
Narcotic / Opioid Analgesics *on page 1568*
Opioids *on page 1535*
Substance Abuse and Anesthesia *on page 1496*

U.S. Brand Names Sufenta®

Canadian Brand Names Sufenta®; Sufentanil Citrate Injection, USP

Synonyms Sufentanil Citrate

Pharmacologic Category Analgesic, Narcotic; General Anesthetic

Restrictions C-II

Generic Available Yes

Use Analgesic supplement in maintenance of balanced general anesthesia

Mechanism of Action Binds to opioid receptors throughout the CNS. Once receptor binding occurs, effects are exerted by opening K+ channels and inhibiting Ca++ channels. These mechanisms increase pain threshold, alter pain perception, inhibit ascending pain pathways; short-acting narcotic

Pharmacodynamics/Kinetics

Onset of action: 1-3 minutes

Duration: Dose dependent

Metabolism: Primarily hepatic

Dosage

Children 2-12 years: 10-25 mcg/kg (10-15 mcg/kg most common dose) with 100% O_2, maintenance: up to 1-2 mcg/kg total dose

Adults: Dose should be based on body weight. **Note:** In obese patients (ie, >20% above ideal body weight), use lean body weight to determine dosage.

1-2 mcg/kg with N_2O/O_2 for endotracheal intubation; maintenance: 10-25 mcg as needed

2-8 mcg/kg with N_2O/O_2 more complicated major surgical procedures; maintenance: 10-50 mcg as needed

8-30 mcg/kg with 100% O_2 and muscle relaxant produces sleep; at doses ≥8 mcg/kg maintains a deep level of anesthesia; maintenance: 10-50 mcg as needed

Administration Parenteral: I.V.: Slow I.V. injection or by infusion

Anesthesia and Critical Care Concerns/Other Considerations Sufentanil is a short-acting narcotic, 5-10 times more potent than fentanyl; it is packaged in the same concentration as fentanyl (50 mcg/mL); keep in mind the differences in potency to prevent overdose with sufentanil. Sufentanil may be diluted to decrease concentration; this will decrease the potential for administering excessive doses.

Pregnancy Risk Factor C

Contraindications Hypersensitivity to sufentanil or any component of the formulation

Warnings/Precautions Sufentanil can cause severely compromised respiratory depression; use with caution in patients with head injuries, hepatic or renal impairment or with pulmonary disease; sufentanil shares the toxic potential of opiate agonists, precaution of opiate agonist therapy should be observed; rapid I.V. infusion may result in skeletal muscle and chest wall rigidity, impaired ventilation, respiratory distress/arrest; nondepolarizing skeletal muscle relaxant may be required

Adverse Reactions

>10%:

Cardiovascular: Bradycardia, hypotension

Central nervous system: Somnolence

Gastrointestinal: Nausea, vomiting

Respiratory: Respiratory depression

1% to 10%:
- Cardiovascular: Cardiac arrhythmia, orthostatic hypotension
- Central nervous system: CNS depression, confusion
- Gastrointestinal: Biliary spasm
- Ocular: Blurred vision

<1% (Limited to important or life-threatening): Bronchospasm, circulatory depression, convulsions, laryngospasm, mental depression, paradoxical CNS excitation or delirium, physical and psychological dependence with prolonged use, rash, urticaria

Overdosage/Toxicology Naloxone 2 mg I.V. (0.01 mg/kg for children) with repeat administration as necessary up to a total of 10 mg; supportive care includes establishment of respiratory change; naloxone may be used to treat respiratory depression; muscular rigidity may also respond to opiate antagonist therapy or to neuromuscular blocking agents

Drug Interactions Substrate of CYP3A4 (major)

CYP3A4 inhibitors: May increase the levels/effects of sufentanil. Example inhibitors include azole antifungals, clarithromycin, diclofenac, doxycycline, erythromycin, imatinib, isoniazid, nefazodone, nicardipine, propofol, protease inhibitors, quinidine, telithromycin, and verapamil.

Increased effect/toxicity with CNS depressants, beta-blockers

Dosage Forms Injection, solution [preservative free]: 50 mcg/mL (1 mL, 2 mL, 5 mL)

References

Bovill JG, Sebel PS, Blackburn CL, et al, "The Pharmacokinetics of Sufentanil in Surgical Patients," *Anesthesiology*, 1984, 61(5):502-6.

Bowdle TA, "Myoclonus Following Sufentanil Without EEG Seizure Activity," *Anesthesiology*, 1987, 67(4):593-5.

Guay J, Gaudreault P, Tang A, et al, "Pharmacokinetics of Sufentanil in Normal Children," *Can J Anaesth*, 1992, 39(1):14-20.

Gust R and Böhrer H, "Stiff-Man Syndrome Associated With Continuous Sufentanil Administration," *Anaesthesia*, 1995, 50(6):575.

Mokhlesi B, Leikin JB, Murray P, et al, "Adult Toxicology in Critical Care. Part 11: Specific Poisonings," *Chest*, 2003, 123(3):897-922.

Rosow CE, "Sufentanil Citrate: A New Opioid Analgesic for Use in Anaesthesia," *Pharmacotherapy*, 1984, 4(1):11-9.

Scholz J, Steinfath M, and Schulz M, "Clinical Pharmacokinetics of Alfentanil, Fentanyl, and Sufentanil. An Update," *Clin Pharmacokinet*, 1996, 31(4):275-92.

Seguin JH, Erenberg A, and Leff RD, "Safety and Efficacy of Sufentanil Therapy in the Ventilated Infant," *Neonatal Netw*, 1994, 13(4):37-40.

- **Sufentanil Citrate** *see* Sufentanil *on page 1214*
- **Sufentanil Citrate Injection, USP (Can)** *see* Sufentanil *on page 1214*
- **Sulbactam and Ampicillin** *see* Ampicillin and Sulbactam *on page 107*
- **Sulcrate® (Can)** *see* Sucralfate *on page 1212*
- **Sulcrate® Suspension Plus (Can)** *see* Sucralfate *on page 1212*

Sulfamethoxazole and Trimethoprim

(sul fa meth OKS a zole & trye METH oh prim)

Medication Safety Issues

Sound-alike/look-alike issues:
- Bactrim™ may be confused with bacitracin, Bactine®
- Co-trimoxazole may be confused with clotrimazole
- Septra® may be confused with Ceptaz®, Sectral®, Septa®

U.S. Brand Names Bactrim™; Bactrim™ DS; Septra®; Septra® DS

Canadian Brand Names Apo-Sulfatrim®; Novo-Trimel; Novo-Trimel D.S.; Nu-Cotrimox; Septra® Injection

Synonyms Co-Trimoxazole; SMZ-TMP; Sulfatrim; TMP-SMZ; Trimethoprim and Sulfamethoxazole

Pharmacologic Category Antibiotic, Miscellaneous; Antibiotic, Sulfonamide Derivative

Generic Available Yes

Use

Oral treatment of urinary tract infections due to *E. coli*, *Klebsiella* and *Enterobacter* sp, *M. morganii*, *P. mirabilis* and *P. vulgaris*; acute otitis media in children; acute exacerbations of chronic bronchitis in adults due to susceptible strains of *H. influenzae* or *S. pneumoniae*; treatment and prophylaxis of *Pneumocystis carinii* pneumonitis (PCP); traveler's diarrhea due to enterotoxigenic *E. coli*; treatment of enteritis caused by *Shigella flexneri* or *Shigella sonnei*

(Continued)

Sulfamethoxazole and Trimethoprim *(Continued)*

I.V. treatment or severe or complicated infections when oral therapy is not feasible, for documented PCP, empiric treatment of PCP in immune compromised patients; treatment of documented or suspected shigellosis, typhoid fever, *Nocardia asteroides* infection, or other infections caused by susceptible bacteria

Unlabeled/Investigational Use Cholera and *Salmonella*-type infections and nocardiosis; chronic prostatitis; as prophylaxis in neutropenic patients with *P. carinii* infections, in leukemics, and in patients following renal transplantation, to decrease incidence of PCP; treatment of *Cyclospora* infection, typhoid fever, *Nocardia asteroides* infection

Mechanism of Action Sulfamethoxazole interferes with bacterial folic acid synthesis and growth via inhibition of dihydrofolic acid formation from para-aminobenzoic acid; trimethoprim inhibits dihydrofolic acid reduction to tetrahydrofolate resulting in sequential inhibition of enzymes of the folic acid pathway

Pharmacodynamics/Kinetics

Absorption: Oral: Almost completely, 90% to 100%

Protein binding: SMX: 68%, TMP: 45%

Metabolism: SMX: N-acetylated and glucuronidated; TMP: Metabolized to oxide and hydroxylated metabolites

Half-life elimination: SMX: 9 hours, TMP: 6-17 hours; both are prolonged in renal failure

Time to peak, serum: Within 1-4 hours

Excretion: Both are excreted in urine as metabolites and unchanged drug

Effects of aging on the pharmacokinetics of both agents has been variable; increase in half-life and decreases in clearance have been associated with reduced creatinine clearance

Dosage Dosage recommendations are based on the trimethoprim component. Double-strength tablets are equivalent to sulfamethoxazole 800 mg and trimethoprim 160 mg.

Children >2 months:

General dosing guidelines:

Mild-to-moderate infections: Oral: 8-12 mg TMP/kg/day in divided doses every 12 hours

Serious infection:

Oral: 20 mg TMP/kg/day in divided doses every 6 hours

I.V.: 8-12 mg TMP/kg/day in divided doses every 6 hours

Acute otitis media: Oral: 8 mg TMP/kg/day in divided doses every 12 hours for 10 days

Urinary tract infection:

Treatment:

Oral: 6-12 mg TMP/kg/day in divided doses every 12 hours

I.V.: 8-10 mg TMP/kg/day in divided doses every 6, 8, or 12 hours for up to 4 days with serious infections

Prophylaxis: Oral: 2 mg TMP/kg/dose daily or 5 mg TMP/kg/dose twice weekly

Pneumocystis:

Treatment: Oral, I.V.: 15-20 mg TMP/kg/day in divided doses every 6-8 hours

Prophylaxis: Oral, 150 mg TMP/m^2/day in divided doses every 12 hours for 3 days/week; dose should not exceed trimethoprim 320 mg and sulfamethoxazole 1600 mg daily

Alternative prophylaxis dosing schedules include:

150 mg TMP/m^2/day as a single daily dose 3 times/week on consecutive days

or

150 mg TMP/m^2/day in divided doses every 12 hours administered 7 days/week

or

150 mg TMP/m^2/day in divided doses every 12 hours administered 3 times/week on alternate days

Shigellosis:

Oral: 8 mg TMP/kg/day in divided doses every 12 hours for 5 days

I.V.: 8-10 mg TMP/kg/day in divided doses every 6, 8, or 12 hours for up to 5 days

Cyclospora (unlabeled use): Oral, I.V.: 5 mg TMP/kg twice daily for 7-10 days

Adults:

Urinary tract infection:

Oral: One double-strength tablet every 12 hours

Duration of therapy: Uncomplicated: 3-5 days; Complicated: 7-10 days

Pyelonephritis: 14 days

Prostatitis: Acute: 2 weeks; Chronic: 2-3 months

I.V.: 8-10 mg TMP/kg/day in divided doses every 6, 8, or 12 hours for up to 14 days with severe infections

Chronic bronchitis: Oral: One double-strength tablet every 12 hours for 10-14 days

Meningitis (bacterial): I.V.: 10-20 mg TMP/kg/day in divided doses every 6-12 hours

Shigellosis:

Oral: One double strength tablet every 12 hours for 5 days

I.V.: 8-10 mg TMP/kg/day in divided doses every 6, 8, or 12 hours for up to 5 days

Travelers' diarrhea: Oral: One double strength tablet every 12 hours for 5 days

Sepsis: I.V.: 20 TMP/kg/day divided every 6 hours

Pneumocystis carinii:

Prophylaxis: Oral: 1 double strength tablet daily or 3 times/week

Treatment: Oral, I.V.: 15-20 mg TMP/kg/day in 3-4 divided doses

Cyclospora (unlabeled use): Oral, I.V.: 160 mg TMP twice daily for 7-10 days

Nocardia (unlabeled use): Oral, I.V.:

Cutaneous infections: 5 mg TMP/kg/day in 2 divided doses

Severe infections (pulmonary/cerebral): 10-15 mg TMP/kg/day in 2-3 divided doses. Treatment duration is controversial; an average of 7 months has been reported.

Note: Therapy for severe infection may be initiated I.V. and converted to oral therapy (frequently converted to approximate dosages of oral solid dosage forms: 2 DS tablets every 8-12 hours). Although not widely available, sulfonamide levels should be considered in patients with questionable absorption, at risk for dose-related toxicity, or those with poor therapeutic response.

Dosing adjustment in renal impairment: Oral, I.V.:

Cl_{cr} 15-30 mL/minute: Administer 50% of recommended dose

Cl_{cr} <15 mL/minute: Use is not recommended

Stability

Injection: Store at room temperature; do not refrigerate. Less soluble in more alkaline pH. Protect from light. Solution must be diluted prior to administration. Following dilution, store at room temperature; do not refrigerate. Manufacturer recommended dilutions and stability of parenteral admixture at room temperature (25°C):

5 mL/125 mL D_5W; stable for 6 hours

5 mL/100 mL D_5W; stable for 4 hours

5 mL/75 mL D_5W; stable for 2 hours

Studies have also confirmed limited stability in NS; detailed references should be consulted.

Suspension, tablet: Store at room temperature; protect from light

Administration I.V.: Infuse over 60-90 minutes, must dilute well before giving; may be given less diluted in a central line; not for I.M. injection

Oral: May be taken with food and water.

Pregnancy Risk Factor C/D (at term - expert analysis)

Contraindications Hypersensitivity to any sulfa drug, trimethoprim, or any component of the formulation; porphyria; megaloblastic anemia due to folate deficiency; infants <2 months of age; marked hepatic damage; severe renal disease; pregnancy (at term)

Warnings/Precautions Use with caution in patients with G6PD deficiency, impaired renal or hepatic function or potential folate deficiency (malnourished, chronic anticonvulsant therapy, or elderly); maintain adequate hydration to prevent crystalluria; adjust dosage in patients with renal impairment. Injection vehicle contains benzyl alcohol and sodium metabisulfite.

Chemical similarities are present among sulfonamides, sulfonylureas, carbonic anhydrase inhibitors, thiazides, and loop diuretics (except ethacrynic acid). Use in patients with sulfonamide allergy is specifically contraindicated in product labeling, however, a risk of cross-reaction exists in patients with allergy to any of these compounds; avoid use when previous reaction has been severe.

(Continued)

Sulfamethoxazole and Trimethoprim *(Continued)*

Fatalities associated with severe reactions including Stevens-Johnson syndrome, toxic epidermal necrolysis, hepatic necrosis, agranulocytosis, aplastic anemia and other blood dyscrasias; discontinue use at first sign of rash. Elderly patients appear at greater risk for more severe adverse reactions. May cause hypoglycemia, particularly in malnourished, or patients with renal or hepatic impairment. Use with caution in patients with porphyria or thyroid dysfunction. Slow acetylators may be more prone to adverse reactions. Caution in patients with allergies or asthma. May cause hyperkalemia (associated with high doses of trimethoprim). Incidence of adverse effects appears to be increased in patients with AIDS.

Adverse Reactions The most common adverse reactions include gastrointestinal upset (nausea, vomiting, anorexia) and dermatologic reactions (rash or urticaria). Rare, life-threatening reactions have been associated with co-trimoxazole, including severe dermatologic reactions and hepatotoxic reactions. Most other reactions listed are rare, however, frequency cannot be accurately estimated.

Cardiovascular: Allergic myocarditis

Central nervous system: Confusion, depression, hallucinations, seizure, aseptic meningitis, peripheral neuritis, fever, ataxia, kernicterus in neonates

Dermatologic: Rashes, pruritus, urticaria, photosensitivity; rare reactions include erythema multiforme, Stevens-Johnson syndrome, toxic epidermal necrolysis, exfoliative dermatitis, and Henoch-Schönlein purpura

Endocrine & metabolic: Hyperkalemia (generally at high dosages), hypoglycemia

Gastrointestinal: Nausea, vomiting, anorexia, stomatitis, diarrhea, pseudomembranous colitis, pancreatitis

Hematologic: Thrombocytopenia, megaloblastic anemia, granulocytopenia, eosinophilia, pancytopenia, aplastic anemia, methemoglobinemia, hemolysis (with G6PD deficiency), agranulocytosis

Hepatic: Hepatotoxicity (including hepatitis, cholestasis, and hepatic necrosis), hyperbilirubinemia, transaminases increased

Neuromuscular & skeletal: Arthralgia, myalgia, rhabdomyolysis

Renal: Interstitial nephritis, crystalluria, renal failure, nephrotoxicity (in association with cyclosporine), diuresis

Respiratory: Cough, dyspnea, pulmonary infiltrates

Miscellaneous: Serum sickness, angioedema, periarteritis nodosa (rare), systemic lupus erythematosus (rare)

Overdosage/Toxicology Symptoms of overdose include nausea, vomiting, GI distress, hematuria, and crystalluria. Bone marrow suppression may occur. Treatment is supportive. Adequate fluid intake is essential. Peritoneal dialysis is not effective and hemodialysis is only moderately effective in removing co-trimoxazole. Leucovorin 5-15 mg/day may accelerate hematologic recovery.

Drug Interactions

Sulfamethoxazole: **Substrate** of CYP2C9 (major), 3A4 (minor); **Inhibits** CYP2C9 (moderate)

Trimethoprim: **Substrate** (major) of CYP2C9, 3A4; **Inhibits** CYP2C8 (moderate) 2C9 (moderate)

ACE Inhibitors and angiotensin receptor antagonists: May increase the risk of hyperkalemia with sulfamethoxazole/trimethoprim.

Amantadine: Concurrent use with sulfamethoxazole/trimethoprim has been associated with toxic delirium (rare).

Cyclosporine: May result in an increased risk of nephrotoxicity when used with sulfamethoxazole/trimethoprim. Sulfonamides may decrease the serum concentrations of cyclosporine.

CYP2C9 inducers: May decrease the levels/effects of sulfamethoxazole and trimethoprim. Example inducers include carbamazepine, phenobarbital, phenytoin, rifampin, rifapentine, and secobarbital.

CYP2C8 Substrates: Trimethoprim may increase the levels/effects of CYP2C8 substrates. Example substrates include amiodarone, paclitaxel, pioglitazone, repaglinide, and rosiglitazone.

CYP2C9 Substrates: Sulfmethoxazole and trimethoprim may increase the levels/effects of CYP2C9 substrates. Example substrates include bosentan, dapsone, fluoxetine, glimepiride, glipizide, losartan, montelukast, nateglinide, paclitaxel, phenytoin, warfarin, and zafirlukast.

Dapsone: Trimethoprim may increase the serum concentration of dapsone.

Diuretics, potassium-sparing: May increase the risk of hyperkalemia with sulfamethoxazole/trimethoprim.

Leucovorin: Although occasionally recommended to limit or reverse hematologic toxicity of high-dose sulfamethoxazole/trimethoprim, concurrent use has been associated with a decreased effectiveness in treating *Pneumocystis carinii.*

Methotrexate: Sulfamethoxazole/trimethoprim may increase toxicity of methotrexate (due to displacement from binding sites and/or decreased renal secretion).

Phenytoin: Sulfamethoxazole/trimethoprim may increase phenytoin levels/ toxicity. Phenytoin may decrease sulfamethoxazole/trimethoprim levels.

Procainamide: Trimethoprim may decrease the excretion of procainamide.

Pyrimethamine: Concurrent therapy with pyrimethamine (in doses >25 mg/week) may be at increased risk of megaloblastic anemia.

Sulfonylureas: Sulfamethoxazole/trimethoprim may increase the hypoglycemic effect of sulfonylureas; monitor.

Warfarin: Sulfamethoxazole/trimethoprim may increase the hypoprothrombinemic effect of warfarin; monitor INR closely.

Ethanol/Nutrition/Herb Interactions Herb/Nutraceutical: Avoid dong quai, St John's wort (may also cause photosensitization).

Test Interactions Increased creatinine (Jaffé alkaline picrate reaction); increased serum methotrexate by dihydrofolate reductase method

Dietary Considerations Should be taken with 8 oz of water on empty stomach.

Dosage Forms Note: The 5:1 ratio (SMX:TMP) remains constant in all dosage forms.

Injection, solution: Sulfamethoxazole 80 mg and trimethoprim 16 mg per mL (5 mL, 10 mL, 30 mL) [contains propylene glycol ~400 mg/mL, alcohol, benzyl alcohol, and sodium metabisulfite]

Suspension, oral: Sulfamethoxazole 200 mg and trimethoprim 40 mg per 5 mL (480 mL) [contains alcohol]

Septra®: Sulfamethoxazole 200 mg and trimethoprim 40 mg per 5 mL (480 mL) [contains alcohol 0.26% and sodium benzoate; cherry and grape flavors]

Tablet: Sulfamethoxazole 400 mg and trimethoprim 80 mg

Bactrim™: Sulfamethoxazole 400 mg and trimethoprim 80 mg [contains sodium benzoate]

Septra®: Sulfamethoxazole 400 mg and trimethoprim 80 mg

Tablet, double strength: Sulfamethoxazole 800 mg and trimethoprim 160 mg

Bactrim™ DS: Sulfamethoxazole 800 mg and trimethoprim 160 mg [contains sodium benzoate]

Septra® DS: Sulfamethoxazole 800 mg and trimethoprim 160 mg

References

Gilbert DN, Moellering RC, Eliopoulos GM, et al, eds, *The Sanford Guide To Antimicrobial Therapy*, 2006, 36th ed, Hyde Park, VT: Antimicrobial Therapy, Inc, 2006, 6-7.

Tunkel AR, Hartman BJ, Kaplan SL, et al, "Practice Guidelines for the Management of Bacterial Meningitis," *Clin Infect Dis*, 2004, 39(9):1267-84.

♦ **Sulfamylon®** *see* Mafenide *on page 785*

♦ **Sulfatrim** *see* Sulfamethoxazole and Trimethoprim *on page 1215*

Sulindac (sul IN dak)

Medication Safety Issues

Sound-alike/look-alike issues:

Clinoril® may be confused with Cleocin®, Clozaril®, Oruvail®

Related Information

Chronic Pain Management *on page 1430*

U.S. Brand Names Clinoril®

Canadian Brand Names Apo-Sulin®; Novo-Sundac; Nu-Sundac

Pharmacologic Category Nonsteroidal Anti-inflammatory Drug (NSAID), Oral

Restrictions A medication guide should be dispensed with each prescription. A template for the required MedGuide can be found on the FDA website at: http://www.fda.gov/medwatch/SAFETY/2005/safety05.htm#NSAID

Generic Available Yes

Use Management of inflammatory disease, osteoarthritis, rheumatoid disorders, acute gouty arthritis, ankylosing spondylitis, bursitis/tendonitis of shoulder

Mechanism of Action Inhibits prostaglandin synthesis by decreasing the activity of the enzyme, cyclooxygenase, which results in decreased formation of prostaglandin precursors

Pharmacodynamics/Kinetics

Onset of action: Analgesic: ~1 hour

(Continued)

Sulindac *(Continued)*

Duration: 12-24 hours

Absorption: 90%

Metabolism: Hepatic; prodrug metabolized to sulfide metabolite (active) for therapeutic effects and to sulfone metabolites (inactive)

Half-life elimination: Parent drug: ~8 hours; Active metabolite: ~16 hours

Excretion: Urine (50%, primarily as inactive metabolites); feces (25%, primarily as metabolites)

Dosage Oral:

Children: Dose not established

Adults: **Note:** Maximum daily dose: 400 mg

Osteoarthritis, rheumatoid arthritis, ankylosing spondylitis: 150 mg twice/daily

Bursitis/tendonitis: 200 mg twice daily; usual treatment: 7-14 days

Acute gouty arthritis: 200 mg twice daily; usual treatment: 7 days

Dosing adjustment in renal impairment: Not recommended with advanced renal impairment; if required, decrease dose and monitor closely

Dosing adjustment in hepatic impairment: Dose reduction is necessary; discontinue if abnormal liver function tests occur

Administration Should be administered with food or milk.

Monitoring Parameters Liver enzymes, BUN, serum creatinine, CBC, blood pressure; signs and symptoms of GI bleeding

Anesthesia and Critical Care Concerns/Other Considerations The 2002 ACCM/SCCM guidelines for analgesia (critically-ill adult) suggest that NSAIDs may be used in combination with opioids in select patients for pain management. Concern about adverse events (increased risk of renal dysfunction, altered platelet function and gastrointestinal irritation) limits its use in patients who have other underlying risks for these events.

In short-term use, NSAIDs vary considerably in their effect on blood pressure. When NSAIDs are used in patients with hypertension, appropriate monitoring of blood pressure responses should be completed and the duration of therapy, when possible, kept short. The use of NSAIDs in the treatment of patients with congestive heart failure may be associated with an increased risk for fluid accumulation and edema; may precipitate renal failure in dehydrated patients.

Sulindac is associated with the highest incidence of upper GI bleeds among NSAIDs. It may be less likely to inhibit renal prostaglandin synthesis and adversely affect renal function than most other NSAIDs. Maximum therapeutic response may not be realized for up to 3 weeks.

Pregnancy Risk Factor C/D (3rd trimester)

Contraindications Hypersensitivity to sulindac, aspirin, other NSAIDs, or any component of the formulation; perioperative pain in the setting of coronary artery bypass surgery (CABG); pregnancy (3rd trimester)

Warnings/Precautions [U.S. Boxed Warning]: NSAIDs are associated with an increased risk of adverse cardiovascular events, including MI, stroke, and new onset or worsening of pre-existing hypertension. Risk may be increased with duration of use or pre-existing cardiovascular risk-factors or disease. Carefully evaluate individual cardiovascular risk profiles prior to prescribing. Use caution with fluid retention, CHF or hypertension.

Use of NSAIDs can compromise existing renal function. Renal toxicity can occur in patient with impaired renal function, dehydration, heart failure, liver dysfunction, those taking diuretics and ACEI and the elderly. Rehydrate patient before starting therapy. Monitor renal function closely. Sulindac is not recommended for patients with advanced renal disease. Use caution in patients with renal lithiasis; sulindac metabolites have been reported as components of renal stones. Use hydration in patients with a history of renal stones.

[U.S. Boxed Warning]: NSAIDs may increase risk of gastrointestinal irritation, ulceration, bleeding, and perforation. These events may occur at any time during therapy and without warning. Use caution with a history of GI disease (bleeding or ulcers), concurrent therapy with aspirin, anticoagulants and/or corticosteroids, smoking, use of alcohol, the elderly or debilitated patients.

Use the lowest effective dose for the shortest duration of time, consistent with individual patient goals, to reduce risk of cardiovascular or GI adverse events. Alternate therapies should be considered for patients at high risk.

NSAIDs may cause serious skin adverse events including exfoliative dermatitis, Stevens-Johnson syndrome (SJS) and toxic epidermal necrolysis (TEN). Anaphylactoid reactions may occur, even without prior exposure; patients with "aspirin triad" (bronchial asthma, aspirin intolerance, rhinitis) may be at increased risk. Do not use in patients who experience bronchospasm, asthma, rhinitis, or urticaria with NSAID or aspirin therapy.

Use with caution in patients with decreased hepatic function. Closely monitor patients with any abnormal LFT. Severe hepatic reactions (eg, fulminant hepatitis, liver failure) have occurred with NSAID use, rarely; discontinue if signs or symptoms of liver disease develop, or if systemic manifestations occur. May require dosage adjustment in hepatic dysfunction; sulfide and sulfone metabolites may accumulate.

Withhold for at least 4-6 half-lives prior to surgical or dental procedures.

Safety and efficacy in pediatric patients have not been established.

Adverse Reactions

1% to 10%:

Cardiovascular: Edema (1% to 3%)

Central nervous system: Dizziness (3% to 9%), headache (3% to 9%), nervousness (1% to 3%)

Dermatologic: Rash (3% to 9%), pruritus (1% to 3%)

Gastrointestinal: Gastrointestinal: GI pain (10%), constipation (3% to 9%), diarrhea (3% to 9%), dyspepsia (3% to 9%), nausea (3% to 9%), abdominal cramps (1% to 3%), anorexia (1% to 3%), flatulence (1% to 3%), vomiting (1% to 3%)

Otic: Tinnitus (1% to 3%)

<1% (Limited to important or life-threatening): Agranulocytosis, ageusia, alopecia, anaphylaxis, angioneurotic edema, aplastic anemia, arrhythmia, aseptic meningitis, bitter taste, blurred vision, bone marrow depression, bronchial spasm, cholestasis, colitis, CHF, crystalluria, depression, dry mucous membranes, dyspnea, dysuria, ecchymosis, epistaxis, erythema multiforme, exfoliative dermatitis, fever, gastritis, GI bleeding, GI perforation, glossitis, gynecomastia, hearing decreased, hematuria, hemolytic anemia, hepatitis, hepatic failure, hyperglycemia, hyperkalemia, hypersensitivity reaction, hypersensitivity vasculitis, hypertension, insomnia, intestinal stricture, interstitial nephritis, jaundice, leukopenia, metallic taste, necrotizing fascitis, nephrotic syndrome, neuritis, neutropenia, palpitation, pancreatitis, paresthesia, peptic ulcer, photosensitivity, proteinuria, psychosis, purpura, renal calculi, renal impairment, renal failure, retinal disturbances, seizures, somnolence, Stevens-Johnson syndrome, stomatitis, syncope, thrombocytopenia, toxic epidermal necrolysis, urine discoloration, vaginal bleeding, vertigo, weakness

Overdosage/Toxicology Symptoms of overdose include dizziness, vomiting, nausea, abdominal pain, hypotension, coma, stupor, metabolic acidosis, leukocytosis, and renal failure. Management of NSAID intoxication is supportive and symptomatic. Seizures tend to be short-lived and often do not require drug treatment.

Drug Interactions

ACE inhibitors: Antihypertensive effects may be decreased by concurrent therapy with NSAIDs; monitor blood pressure.

Aminoglycosides: NSAIDs may decrease the excretion of aminoglycosides.

Angiotensin II antagonists: Antihypertensive effects may be decreased by concurrent therapy with NSAIDs; monitor blood pressure.

Anticoagulants (warfarin, heparin, LMWHs): When used with NSAIDs can cause increased risk of bleeding.

Antiplatelet drugs (ticlopidine, clopidogrel, aspirin, abciximab, dipyridamole, eptifibatide, tirofiban): Concurrent use may cause an increased risk of bleeding.

Beta-blockers: NSAIDs may decrease the antihypertensive effect of beta-blockers. Monitor.

Bisphosphonates: NSAIDs may increase the risk of gastrointestinal ulceration.

Cholestyramine (and other bile acid sequestrants): May decrease the absorption of NSAIDs. Separate by at least 2 hours.

Corticosteroids: May increase the risk of GI ulceration; avoid concurrent use.

Cyclosporine: NSAIDs may increase serum creatinine, potassium, blood pressure, and cyclosporine levels; monitor cyclosporine levels and renal function carefully.

Dimethyl sulfoxide: May reduce plasma levels of sulindac's active metabolite. Combination may cause peripheral neuropathy; avoid concurrent use.

(Continued)

Sulindac *(Continued)*

Hydralazine's antihypertensive effect is decreased; avoid concurrent use.
Lithium: NSAIDs may increase lithium levels; avoid concurrent use if possible or monitor lithium levels and adjust dose. Sulindac may have the least effect. When NSAID is stopped, lithium will need adjustment again.
Loop diuretic: NSAIDs may decrease the efficacy (diuretic and antihypertensive effect) of loop diuretics.
Methotrexate: Severe bone marrow suppression, aplastic anemia, and GI toxicity have been reported with concomitant NSAID therapy. Avoid use during moderate or high-dose methotrexate (increased and prolonged methotrexate levels). NSAID use during low-dose treatment of rheumatoid arthritis has not been fully evaluated; extreme caution is warranted.
Pemetrexed: NSAIDs may decrease the excretion of pemetrexed. Patients with Cl_{cr} 45-79 mL/minute should avoid long-acting NSAIDs for 5 days before and 2 days after pemetrexed treatment.
Thiazides antihypertensive effects are decreased; avoid concurrent use.
Treprostinil: May enhance the risk of bleeding with concurrent use.
Vancomycin: NSAIDs may decrease the excretion of vancomycin.

Ethanol/Nutrition/Herb Interactions

Ethanol: Avoid ethanol (may enhance gastric mucosal irritation).
Food: Food may decrease the rate but not the extent of oral absorption. The therapeutic effect of sulindac may be decreased if taken with food.
Herb/Nutraceutical: Avoid alfalfa, anise, bilberry, bladderwrack, bromelain, cat's claw, celery, coleus, cordyceps, dong quai, evening primrose, feverfew, fenugreek, garlic, ginger, ginkgo biloba, red clover, horse chestnut, grapeseed, green tea, ginseng, guggul, horse chestnut seed, horseradish, licorice, prickly ash, red clover, reishi, SAMe, sweet clover, turmeric, white willow (all have additional antiplatelet activity).

Test Interactions Increased chloride (S), increased sodium (S), increased bleeding time

Dietary Considerations Drug may cause GI upset, bleeding, ulceration, perforation; take with food or milk to minimize GI upset.

Dosage Forms

Tablet: 150 mg, 200 mg
Clinoril®: 200 mg

Sumatriptan (soo ma TRIP tan)

Medication Safety Issues

Sound-alike/look-alike issues:
Sumatriptan may be confused with somatropin, zolmitriptan

U.S. Brand Names Imitrex®

Canadian Brand Names Apo-Sumatriptan®; CO Sumatriptan; Dom-Sumatriptan; Gen-Sumatriptan; Imitrex®; Imitrex® DF; Imitrex® Nasal Spray; Novo-Sumatriptan; PHL-Sumatriptan; PMS-Sumatriptan; ratio-Sumatriptan; Rhoxal-sumatriptan; Riva-Sumatriptan; Sandoz-Sumatriptan; Sumatryx

Synonyms Sumatriptan Succinate

Pharmacologic Category Serotonin 5-HT_{1D} Receptor Agonist

Generic Available No

Use

Oral, SubQ: Acute treatment of migraine with or without aura
SubQ: Acute treatment of cluster headache episodes

Mechanism of Action Selective agonist for serotonin (5-HT_{1D} receptor) in cranial arteries to cause vasoconstriction and reduces sterile inflammation associated with antidromic neuronal transmission correlating with relief of migraine

Pharmacodynamics/Kinetics

Onset of action: ~30 minutes
Distribution: V_d: 2.4 L/kg
Protein binding: 14% to 21%
Metabolism: Hepatic, primarily via MAO-A isoenzyme
Bioavailability: SubQ: 97% ± 16% of that following I.V. injection; Oral: 15%
Half-life elimination: Injection, tablet: 2.5 hours; Nasal spray: 2 hours
Time to peak, serum: 5-20 minutes
Excretion:
Injection: Urine (38% as indole acetic acid metabolite, 22% as unchanged drug)

Nasal spray: Urine (42% as indole acetic acid metabolite, 3% as unchanged drug)

Tablet: Urine (60% as indole acetic acid metabolite, 3% as unchanged drug); feces (40%)

Dosage Adults:

Oral: A single dose of 25 mg, 50 mg, or 100 mg (taken with fluids). If a satisfactory response has not been obtained at 2 hours, a second dose may be administered. Results from clinical trials show that initial doses of 50 mg and 100 mg are more effective than doses of 25 mg, and that 100 mg doses do not provide a greater effect than 50 mg and may have increased incidence of side effects. Although doses of up to 300 mg/day have been studied, the total daily dose should not exceed 200 mg. The safety of treating an average of >4 headaches in a 30-day period have not been established.

Intranasal: A single dose of 5 mg, 10 mg, or 20 mg administered in one nostril. A 10 mg dose may be achieved by administering a single 5 mg dose in each nostril. If headache returns, the dose may be repeated once after 2 hours, not to exceed a total daily dose of 40 mg. The safety of treating an average of >4 headaches in a 30-day period has not been established.

SubQ: Up to 6 mg; if side effects are dose-limiting, lower doses may be used. A second injection may be administered at least 1 hour after the initial dose, but not more than 2 injections in a 24-hour period.

Dosage adjustment in renal impairment: Dosage adjustment not necessary

Dosage adjustment in hepatic impairment: Bioavailability of oral sumatriptan is increased with liver disease. If treatment is needed, do not exceed single doses of 50 mg. The nasal spray has not been studied in patients with hepatic impairment, however, because the spray does not undergo first-pass metabolism, levels would not be expected to alter. Use of all dosage forms is contraindicated with severe hepatic impairment.

Stability Store at 2°C to 20°C (36°F to 86°F); protect from light

Administration

Oral: Should be taken with fluids as soon as symptoms appear

Injection solution: For SubQ administration; do not administer I.V.; may cause coronary vasospasm. An autoinjection device (STATdose System®) is available for use with the 4 mg and 6 mg cartridges.

Anesthesia and Critical Care Concerns/Other Considerations Sumatriptan should not be used in patients with a history of vasospastic disease, Prinzmetal's angina, or any critical vascular disease.

Pregnancy Risk Factor C

Contraindications Hypersensitivity to sumatriptan or any component of the formulation; patients with ischemic heart disease or signs or symptoms of ischemic heart disease (including Prinzmetal's angina, angina pectoris, myocardial infarction, silent myocardial ischemia); cerebrovascular syndromes (including strokes, transient ischemic attacks); peripheral vascular syndromes (including ischemic bowel disease); uncontrolled hypertension; use within 24 hours of ergotamine derivatives; use within 24 hours of another 5-HT_1 agonist; concurrent administration or within 2 weeks of discontinuing an MAO inhibitor, specifically MAO type A inhibitors; management of hemiplegic or basilar migraine; prophylactic treatment of migraine; severe hepatic impairment; not for I.V. administration

Warnings/Precautions Sumatriptan is indicated only in patients ≥18 years of age with a clear diagnosis of migraine or cluster headache.

Cardiac events (coronary artery vasospasm, transient ischemia, myocardial infarction, ventricular tachycardia/fibrillation, cardiac arrest and death), cerebral/subarachnoid hemorrhage and stroke have been reported with 5-HT_1 agonist administration.

Do not give to patients with risk factors for CAD until a cardiovascular evaluation has been performed; if evaluation is satisfactory, the healthcare provider should administer the first dose and cardiovascular status should be periodically evaluated.

Significant elevation in blood pressure, including hypertensive crisis, has also been reported on rare occasions in patients with and without a history of hypertension. Vasospasm-related reactions have been reported other than coronary artery vasospasm. Peripheral vascular ischemia and colonic ischemia with abdominal pain and bloody diarrhea have occurred.

Use with caution in patients with history of seizure disorder or in patients with a lowered seizure threshold. Safety and efficacy in pediatric patients have not been established.

(Continued)

Sumatriptan *(Continued)*

Adverse Reactions

Injection:

>10%:

Central nervous system: Dizziness (12%), warm/hot sensation (11%)
Local: Pain at injection site (59%)
Neuromuscular & skeletal: Paresthesia (14%)

1% to 10%:

Cardiovascular: Chest pain/tightness/heaviness/pressure (2% to 3%), hyper-/hypotension (1%)
Central nervous system: Burning (7%), feeling of heaviness (7%), flushing (7%), pressure sensation (7%), feeling of tightness (5%), drowsiness (3%), malaise/fatigue (1%), feeling strange (2%), headache (2%), tight feeling in head (2%), cold sensation (1%), anxiety (1%)
Gastrointestinal: Abdominal discomfort (1%), dysphagia (1%)
Neuromuscular & skeletal: Neck, throat, and jaw pain/tightness/pressure (2% to 5%), mouth/tongue discomfort (5%), weakness (5%), myalgia (2%); muscle cramps (1%), numbness (5%)
Ocular: Vision alterations (1%)
Respiratory: Throat discomfort (3%), nasal disorder/discomfort (2%)
Miscellaneous: Diaphoresis (2%)

Nasal spray:

>10%: Gastrointestinal: Bad taste (13% to 24%), nausea (11% to 13%), vomiting (11% to 13%)

1% to 10%:

Central nervous system: Dizziness (1% to 2%)
Respiratory: Nasal disorder/discomfort (2% to 4%), throat discomfort (1% to 2%)

Tablet:

1% to 10%:

Cardiovascular: Chest pain/tightness/heaviness/pressure (1% to 2%), hyper-/hypotension (1%), palpitation (1%), syncope (1%)
Central nervous system: Burning (1%), dizziness (>1%), drowsiness (>1%), malaise/fatigue (2% to 3%), headache (>1%), nonspecified pain (1% to 2%, placebo 1%), vertigo (<1% to 2%), migraine (>1%), sleepiness (>1%)
Gastrointestinal: Diarrhea (1%), nausea (>1%), vomiting (>1%), hyposalivation (>1%)
Genitourinary: Hematuria (1%)
Hematologic: Hemolytic anemia (1%)
Neuromuscular & skeletal: Neck, throat, and jaw pain/tightness/pressure (2% to 3%), paresthesia (3% to 5%), myalgia (1%), numbness (1%)
Otic: Ear hemorrhage (1%), hearing loss (1%), sensitivity to noise (1%), tinnitus (1%)
Respiratory: Allergic rhinitis (1%), dyspnea (1%), nasal inflammation (1%), nose/throat hemorrhage (1%), sinusitis (1%), upper respiratory inflammation (1%)
Miscellaneous: Hypersensitivity reactions (1%), nonspecified pressure/tightness/heaviness (1% to 3%, placebo 2%); warm/cold sensation (2% to 3%, placebo 2%)

Route unspecified: <1%: Postmarketing and uncontrolled studies (limited to important or life-threatening): Abdominal aortic aneurysm, abdominal discomfort, abnormal menstrual cycle, abnormal/elevated liver function tests, accommodation disorders, acute renal failure, agitation, anaphylactoid reaction, anaphylaxis, anemia, angioneurotic edema, arrhythmia, atrial fibrillation, bronchospasm, cerebral ischemia, cerebrovascular accident, convulsions, deafness, death, decreased appetite, dental pain, diarrhea, dyspeptic symptoms, dysphagia, dystonic reaction, ECG changes, fluid disturbances (including retention), flushing, gastrointestinal pain, hallucinations, heart block, hematuria, hemolytic anemia, hiccups, hypersensitivity reactions, intestinal obstruction, intracranial pressure increased, ischemic colitis, joint ache, muscle stiffness, nose/throat hemorrhage, numbness of tongue, optic neuropathy (ischemic), pancytopenia, paresthesia, phlebitis, photosensitivity, Prinzmetal's angina, pruritus, psychomotor disorders, pulmonary embolism, rash, Raynaud syndrome, sensation changes, shock, subarachnoid hemorrhage, swallowing disorders, syncope, thrombocytopenia, thrombophlebitis, thrombosis, transient myocardial ischemia, TSH increased, vasculitis, vision loss, xerostomia

Overdosage/Toxicology Single oral doses ≤400 mg, injectable doses ≤16 mg, and nasal doses of 40 mg have been reported without adverse effects. Treatment of overdose should be supportive and symptomatic. Monitor for at least 12 hours or until signs and symptoms subside. It is not known if hemodialysis or peritoneal dialysis is effective.

Drug Interactions Note: Use cautiously in patients receiving concomitant medications that can lower the seizure threshold.

Ergot-containing drugs: Prolong vasospastic reactions; do not use sumatriptan or ergot-containing drugs within 24 hours of each other.

MAO inhibitors (MAO type A inhibitors, nonspecific MAO inhibitors): Reduce sumatriptan clearance; concurrent use is contraindicated; wait at least 2 weeks after discontinuing MAO type A inhibitor to start sumatriptan.

Selegiline: Selegiline is a selective MAO type B inhibitor; while not specifically contraindicated, combination may best be avoided until further study.

SSRIs: Can lead to symptoms of hyper-reflexia, weakness, and incoordination; monitor.

Dosage Forms Note: Strength expressed as sumatriptan base

Injection, solution, as succinate: 8 mg/mL (0.5 mL) [disposable cartridge for use with STATdose System®]; 12 mg/mL (0.5 mL) [disposable cartridge for use with STATdose System® or vial]

Solution, intranasal spray: 5 mg (100 μL unit dose spray device); 20 mg (100 μL unit dose spray device)

Tablet, as succinate: 25 mg, 50 mg, 100 mg

- ♦ **Sumatriptan Succinate** *see* Sumatriptan *on page 1222*
- ♦ **Sumatryx (Can)** *see* Sumatriptan *on page 1222*
- ♦ **Summer's Eve® Medicated Douche [OTC]** *see* Povidone-Iodine *on page 1039*
- ♦ **Summer's Eve® SpecialCare™ Medicated Anti-Itch Cream [OTC]** *see* Hydrocortisone *on page 639*
- ♦ **Sun-Benz® (Can)** *see* Benzydamine *on page 167*
- ♦ **Supeudol® (Can)** *see* Oxycodone *on page 967*
- ♦ **Suprane®** *see* Desflurane *on page 357*
- ♦ **Sureprin 81™ [OTC]** *see* Aspirin *on page 129*
- ♦ **Surgicel®** *see* Cellulose (Oxidized Regenerated) *on page 258*
- ♦ **Surgicel® Fibrillar** *see* Cellulose (Oxidized Regenerated) *on page 258*
- ♦ **Surgicel® NuKnit** *see* Cellulose (Oxidized Regenerated) *on page 258*
- ♦ **Survanta®** *see* Beractant *on page 168*
- ♦ **Sustiva®** *see* Efavirenz *on page 441*
- ♦ **Suxamethonium Chloride** *see* Succinylcholine *on page 1210*
- ♦ **Symmetrel®** *see* Amantadine *on page 77*
- ♦ **Synacthen** *see* Cosyntropin *on page 333*
- ♦ **Syn-Diltiazem® (Can)** *see* Diltiazem *on page 394*
- ♦ **Synercid®** *see* Quinupristin and Dalfopristin *on page 1097*
- ♦ **Synthroid®** *see* Levothyroxine *on page 751*
- ♦ **Syntocinon® (Can)** *see* Oxytocin *on page 975*
- ♦ **Syrex** *see* Sodium Chloride *on page 1183*
- ♦ **T_3 Sodium (error-prone abbreviation)** *see* Liothyronine *on page 765*
- ♦ **T_4** *see* Levothyroxine *on page 751*
- ♦ **642® Tablet (Can)** *see* Propoxyphene *on page 1074*

Tacrolimus (ta KROE li mus)

Medication Safety Issues

Sound-alike/look-alike issues:

Prograf® may be confused with Gengraf®

U.S. Brand Names Prograf®; Protopic®

Canadian Brand Names Prograf®; Protopic®

Synonyms FK506

Pharmacologic Category Immunosuppressant Agent; Topical Skin Product

Restrictions An FDA-approved medication guide is available at http://www.fda.gov/cder/Offices/ODS/labeling.htm; distribute to each patient to whom the ointment is dispensed.

(Continued)

Tacrolimus *(Continued)*

Generic Available No

Use

Oral/injection: Potent immunosuppressive drug used in heart, kidney, or liver transplant recipients

Topical: Moderate-to-severe atopic dermatitis in patients not responsive to conventional therapy or when conventional therapy is not appropriate

Unlabeled/Investigational Use Potent immunosuppressive drug used in lung, small bowel transplant recipients; immunosuppressive drug for peripheral stem cell/bone marrow transplantation

Mechanism of Action Suppresses cellular immunity (inhibits T-lymphocyte activation), possibly by binding to an intracellular protein, FKBP-12

Pharmacodynamics/Kinetics

Absorption: Better in resected patients with a closed stoma; unlike cyclosporine, clamping of the T-tube in liver transplant patients does not alter trough concentrations or AUC

Oral: Incomplete and variable; food within 15 minutes of administration decreases absorption (27%)

Topical: Serum concentrations range from undetectable to 20 ng/mL (<5 ng/mL in majority of adult patients studied)

Protein binding: 99%

Metabolism: Extensively hepatic via CYP3A4 to eight possible metabolites (major metabolite, 31-demethyl tacrolimus, shows same activity as tacrolimus *in vitro*)

Bioavailability: Oral: Adults: 7% to 28%, Children: 10% to 52%; Topical: <0.5%; Absolute: Unknown

Half-life elimination: Variable, 21-61 hours in healthy volunteers

Time to peak: 0.5-4 hours

Excretion: Feces (~92%); feces/urine (<1% as unchanged drug)

Dosage

Oral:

Children: **Notes:** Patients without pre-existing renal or hepatic dysfunction have required (and tolerated) higher doses than adults to achieve similar blood concentrations. It is recommended that therapy be initiated at high end of the recommended adult I.V. and oral dosing ranges; dosage adjustments may be required. If switching from I.V. to oral, the oral dose should be started 8-12 hours after stopping the infusion. Adjunctive therapy with corticosteroids is recommended early post-transplant.

Liver transplant: Initial dose: 0.15-0.20 mg/kg/day in 2 divided doses, given every 12 hours; begin oral dose no sooner than 6 hours post-transplant

Adults: **Notes:** If switching from I.V. to oral, the oral dose should be started 8-12 hours after stopping the infusion. Adjunctive therapy with corticosteroids is recommended early post-transplant.

Heart transplant: Initial dose: 0.075 mg/kg/day in 2 divided doses, given every 12 hours; begin oral dose no sooner than 6 hours post-transplant

Kidney transplant: Initial dose: 0.2 mg/kg/day in 2 divided doses, given every 12 hours; initial dose may be given within 24 hours of transplant, but should be delayed until renal function has recovered; African-American patients may require larger doses to maintain trough concentration

Liver transplant: Initial dose: 0.1-0.15 mg/kg/day in 2 divided doses, given every 12 hours; begin oral dose no sooner than 6 hours post-transplant

I.V.: Children and Adults: **Note:** I.V. route should only be used in patients not able to take oral medications and continued only until oral medication can be tolerated; anaphylaxis has been reported. Begin no sooner than 6 hours post-transplant; adjunctive therapy with corticosteroids is recommended.

Heart transplant: Initial dose: 0.01 mg/kg/day as a continuous infusion

Kidney, liver transplant: Initial dose: 0.03-0.05 mg/kg/day as a continuous infusion

Prevention of graft-vs-host disease: 0.03 mg/kg/day as continuous infusion

Topical: Children ≥2 years and Adults: Atopic dermatitis (moderate to severe): Apply minimum amount of 0.03% or 0.1% ointment to affected area twice daily; rub in gently and completely. Discontinue use when symptoms have cleared. If no improvement within 6 weeks, patients should be re-examined to confirm diagnosis.

Dosing adjustment in renal impairment: Evidence suggests that lower doses should be used; patients should receive doses at the lowest value of the recommended I.V. and oral dosing ranges; further reductions in dose below these ranges may be required.

Tacrolimus therapy should usually be delayed up to 48 hours or longer in patients with postoperative oliguria.

Hemodialysis: Not removed by hemodialysis; supplemental dose is not necessary.

Peritoneal dialysis: Significant drug removal is unlikely based on physiochemical characteristics.

Dosing adjustment in hepatic impairment: Use of tacrolimus in liver transplant recipients experiencing post-transplant hepatic impairment may be associated with increased risk of developing renal insufficiency related to high whole blood levels of tacrolimus. The presence of moderate-to-severe hepatic dysfunction (serum bilirubin >2 mg/dL; Child-Pugh score ≥10) appears to affect the metabolism of tacrolimus. The half-life of the drug was prolonged and the clearance reduced after I.V. administration. The bioavailability of tacrolimus was also increased after oral administration. The higher plasma concentrations as determined by ELISA, in patients with severe hepatic dysfunction are probably due to the accumulation of metabolites of lower activity. These patients should be monitored closely and dosage adjustments should be considered. Some evidence indicates that lower doses could be used in these patients.

Stability

Injection: Prior to dilution, store at 5°C to 25°C (41°F to 77°F). Following dilution, stable for 24 hours in D_5W or NS in glass or polyolefin containers. Dilute with 5% dextrose injection or 0.9% sodium chloride injection to a final concentration between 0.004 mg/mL and 0.02 mg/mL.

Capsules and ointment: Store at room temperature of 15°C to 30°C (59°F to 86°F).

Administration

I.V.: Administer by I.V. continuous infusion only. Do not use PVC tubing when administering dilute solutions. Usually intended to be administered as a continuous infusion over 24 hours.

Oral: If dosed once daily (not common), administer in the morning. If dosed twice daily, doses should be 12 hours apart. If the morning and evening doses differ, the larger dose (differences are never >0.5-1 mg) should be given in the morning. If dosed 3 times/day, separate doses by 8 hours.

Topical: Do not use with occlusive dressings. Burning at the application site is most common in first few days; improves as atopic dermatitis improves. Limit application to involved areas. Continue as long as signs and symptoms persist; discontinue if resolution occurs; re-evaluate if symptoms persist >6 weeks.

Monitoring Parameters Renal function, hepatic function, serum electrolytes (especially potassium), glucose and blood pressure, measure 3 times/week for first few weeks, then gradually decrease frequency as patient stabilizes. Whole blood concentrations should be used for monitoring (trough for oral therapy). Signs/symptoms of anaphylactic reactions during infusion should also be monitored. Patients should be monitored during the first 30 minutes of the infusion, and frequently thereafter.

Reference Range

Heart: Typical whole blood trough concentrations:

One week to 3 months: 8-20 ng/mL

Months 3-18: 6-18 ng/mL

Kidney transplant: whole blood trough concentrations:

Months 1-3: 7-20 ng/mL

Months 4-12: 5-15 ng/mL

Liver transplant: whole blood trough concentrations: Months 1-12: 5-20 ng/mL

Anesthesia and Critical Care Concerns/Other Considerations

Additional dosing considerations:

Switch from I.V. to oral therapy: Threefold increase in dose

Pediatric patients: About 2 times higher dose compared to adults

Liver dysfunction: Decrease I.V. dose; decrease oral dose

Renal dysfunction: Does not affect kinetics; decrease dose to decrease levels if renal dysfunction is related to the drug

Tacrolimus is associated with more neurotoxicity, nephrotoxicity, and glucose intolerance but less hypertension, dyslipidemia, gingival hyperplasia, or hirsutism than cyclosporine.

Pregnancy Risk Factor C

(Continued)

Tacrolimus *(Continued)*

Contraindications Hypersensitivity to tacrolimus or any component of the formulation

Warnings/Precautions

Oral/injection: Insulin-dependent post-transplant diabetes mellitus (PTDM) has been reported (1% to 20%); risk increases in African-American and Hispanic kidney transplant patients. **[U.S. Boxed Warning]: Increased susceptibility to infection and the possible development of lymphoma may occur after administration of tacrolimus.** Nephrotoxicity and neurotoxicity have been reported, especially with higher doses; to avoid excess nephrotoxicity do not administer simultaneously with cyclosporine; monitoring of serum concentrations (trough for oral therapy) is essential to prevent organ rejection and reduce drug-related toxicity; tonic clonic seizures may have been triggered by tacrolimus. A period of 24 hours should elapse between discontinuation of cyclosporine and the initiation of tacrolimus. Use caution in renal or hepatic dysfunction, dosing adjustments may be required. Delay initiation if postoperative oliguria occurs. Use may be associated with the development of hypertension (common). Myocardial hypertrophy has been reported (rare). Each mL of injection contains polyoxyl 60 hydrogenated castor oil (HCO-60) (200 mg) and dehydrated alcohol USP 80% v/v. Anaphylaxis has been reported with the injection, use should be reserved for those patients not able to take oral medications.

Topical: [U.S. Boxed Warning]: Topical calcineurin inhibitors have been associated with rare cases of malignancy. Avoid use on malignant or skin conditions (eg cutaneous T-cell lymphoma). Topical calcineurin agents are considered second-line therapies in the treatment of atopic dermatitis/eczema, and should be limited to use in patients who have failed treatment with other therapies. **[U.S. Boxed Warning]: They should be used for short-term and intermittent treatment using the minimum amount necessary for the control of symptoms should be used.** Application should be limited to involved areas. Safety of intermittent use for >1 year has not been established.

Should not be used in immunocompromised patients. Do not apply to areas of active viral infection; infections at the treatment site should be cleared prior to therapy. Patients with atopic dermatitis are predisposed to skin infections, and tacrolimus therapy has been associated with risk of developing eczema herpeticum, varicella zoster, and herpes simplex. May be associated with development of lymphadenopathy; possible infectious causes should be investigated. Discontinue use in patients with unknown cause of lymphadenopathy or acute infectious mononucleosis. Not recommended for use in patients with skin disease which may increase systemic absorption (eg, Netherton's syndrome). Avoid artificial or natural sunlight exposure, even when Protopic® is not on the skin. Safety not established in patients with generalized erythroderma. **[U.S. Boxed Warning]: The use of Protopic® in children <2 years of age is not recommended,** particularly since the effect on immune system development is unknown.

Adverse Reactions

Oral, I.V.:

≥15%:

Cardiovascular: Chest pain, hypertension, pericardial effusion (heart transplant)

Central nervous system: Dizziness, headache, insomnia, tremor (headache and tremor are associated with high whole blood concentrations and may respond to decreased dosage)

Dermatologic: Pruritus, rash

Endocrine & metabolic: Diabetes mellitus, hyperglycemia, hyper-/hypokalemia, hyperlipemia, hypomagnesemia, hypophosphatemia

Gastrointestinal: Abdominal pain, constipation, diarrhea, dyspepsia, nausea, vomiting

Genitourinary: Urinary tract infection

Hematologic: Anemia, leukocytosis, leukopenia, thrombocytopenia

Hepatic: Ascites

Neuromuscular & skeletal: Arthralgia, back pain, paresthesia, tremor, weakness

Renal: Abnormal kidney function, BUN increased, creatinine increased, oliguria, urinary tract infection

Respiratory: Atelectasis, bronchitis, dyspnea, increased cough, pleural effusion

Miscellaneous: CMV infection, infection

<15%:

Cardiovascular: Abnormal ECG (QRS or ST segment abnormal), angina pectoris, cardiopulmonary failure, deep thrombophlebitis, heart rate decreased, hemorrhage, hemorrhagic stroke, hypervolemia, hypotension, generalized edema, peripheral vascular disorder, phlebitis, postural hypotension, tachycardia, thrombosis, vasodilation

Central nervous system: Abnormal dreams, abnormal thinking, agitation, amnesia, anxiety, chills, confusion, depression, dizziness, elevated mood, emotional lability, encephalopathy, hallucinations, nervousness, paralysis, psychosis, quadriparesis, seizure, somnolence

Dermatologic: Acne, alopecia, cellulitis, exfoliative dermatitis, fungal dermatitis, hirsutism, increased diaphoresis, photosensitivity reaction, skin discoloration, skin disorder, skin ulcer

Endocrine & metabolic: Acidosis, alkalosis, Cushing's syndrome, decreased bicarbonate, decreased serum iron, diabetes mellitus, hypercalcemia, hypercholesterolemia, hyperphosphatemia, hypoproteinemia, increased alkaline phosphatase

Gastrointestinal: Anorexia, appetite increased, cramps, duodenitis, dysphagia, enlarged abdomen, esophagitis (including ulcerative), flatulence, gastritis, gastroesophagitis, GI perforation/hemorrhage, ileus, oral moniliasis, pancreatic pseudocyst, rectal disorder, stomatitis, weight gain

Genitourinary: Bladder spasm, cystitis, dysuria, nocturia, oliguria, urge incontinence, urinary frequency, urinary incontinence, urinary retention, vaginitis

Hematologic: Bruising, coagulation disorder, decreased prothrombin, hypochromic anemia, polycythemia

Hepatic: Abnormal liver function tests, ALT/AST increased, bilirubinemia, cholangitis, cholestatic jaundice, GGT increased, hepatitis (including granulomatous), jaundice, liver damage, increase LDH

Neuromuscular & skeletal: Hypertonia, incoordination, joint disorder, leg cramps, myalgia, myasthenia, myoclonus, nerve compression, neuropathy, osteoporosis

Ocular: Abnormal vision, amblyopia

Otic: Ear pain, otitis media, tinnitus

Renal: Albuminuria, renal tubular necrosis, toxic nephropathy

Respiratory: Asthma, lung disorder, pharyngitis, pneumonia, pneumothorax, pulmonary edema, respiratory disorder, rhinitis, sinusitis, voice alteration

Miscellaneous: Abscess, abnormal healing, allergic reaction, crying, flu-like syndrome, generalized spasm, hernia, herpes simplex, peritonitis, sepsis, writing impaired

Topical:

>10%:

Central nervous system: Headache (5% to 20%), fever (1% to 21%)

Dermatologic: Skin burning (43% to 58%; tends to improve as lesions resolve), pruritus (41% to 46%), erythema (12% to 28%)

Respiratory: Increased cough (18% children)

Miscellaneous: Flu-like syndrome (23% to 28%), allergic reaction (4% to 12%)

Oral, I.V., topical: Postmarketing and/or case reports (limited to important or life-threatening): Acute renal failure, alopecia, anaphylaxis, anaphylactoid reaction, angioedema, ARDS, arrhythmia, atrial fibrillation, atrial flutter, bile duct stenosis, blindness, cardiac arrest, cerebral infarction, cerebrovascular accident, deafness, delirium, depression, DIC, hemiparesis, hemolytic-uremic syndrome, hemorrhagic cystitis, hepatic necrosis, hepatotoxicity, hyperglycemia, leukoencephalopathy, lymphoproliferative disorder (related to EBV), myocardial hypertrophy (associated with ventricular dysfunction; reversible upon discontinuation), MI, neutropenia, pancreatitis (hemorrhagic and necrotizing), pancytopenia, paresthesia, photosensitivity reaction (topical), quadriplegia, QT_c prolongation, respiratory failure, seizure, skin discoloration (topical), Stevens-Johnson syndrome, syncope, toxic epidermal necrolysis, thrombocytopenic purpura, torsade de pointes, TTP, veno-occlusive hepatic disease, venous thrombosis, ventricular fibrillation

Note: Calcineurin inhibitor-induced hemolytic uremic syndrome/thrombotic thrombocytopenic purpura/thrombotic microangiopathy (HUS/TTP/TMA) have been reported (with concurrent sirolimus).

Overdosage/Toxicology Symptoms are extensions of immunosuppressive activity and adverse effects. Symptomatic and supportive treatment is required. Hemodialysis is not effective.

(Continued)

Tacrolimus *(Continued)*

Drug Interactions Substrate of CYP3A4 (major); **Inhibits** CYP3A4 (weak)

Antacids: Separate administration by at least 2 hours

Anticonvulsants: Carbamazepine, phenobarbital, phenytoin: May decrease tacrolimus blood levels.

Calcium channel blockers: May increase tacrolimus serum concentrations; monitor.

Caspofungin: May decrease tacrolimus serum concentrations.

Cisapride (and metoclopramide): May increase serum concentration of tacrolimus

Cyclosporine: Concomitant use is associated with synergistic immunosuppression and increased nephrotoxicity; give first dose of tacrolimus no sooner than 24 hours after last cyclosporine dose. In the presence of elevated tacrolimus or cyclosporine concentration, dosing of the other usually should be delayed longer.

CYP3A4 inducers: CYP3A4 inducers may decrease the levels/effects of tacrolimus. Example inducers include aminoglutethimide, carbamazepine, nafcillin, nevirapine, phenobarbital, phenytoin, and rifamycins.

CYP3A4 inhibitors: May increase the levels/effects of tacrolimus. Example inhibitors include azole antifungals, clarithromycin, diclofenac, doxycycline, erythromycin, imatinib, isoniazid, nefazodone, nicardipine, propofol, protease inhibitors, quinidine, telithromycin, and verapamil.

Ganciclovir: Nephrotoxicity may be additive with tacrolimus; use caution.

Macrolides: May increase tacrolimus serum concentrations (limited documentation); monitor.

Potassium-sparing diuretics: Tacrolimus use may lead to hyperkalemia; avoid concomitant use

Rifabutin, rifampin: May decrease serum levels of tacrolimus.

Sirolimus: May decrease tacrolimus serum concentrations. Concurrent therapy may increase the risk of HUS/TTP/TMA.

St John's wort: May decrease tacrolimus serum concentrations; avoid concurrent use.

Sucralfate: Separate administration by at least 2 hours

Vaccines (live): Vaccine may be less effective; avoid vaccination during treatment if possible

Voriconazole: Tacrolimus serum concentrations may be increased; monitor serum concentrations and renal function. Decrease tacrolimus dosage by 66% when initiating voriconazole.

Ethanol/Nutrition/Herb Interactions

Ethanol: Localized flushing (redness, warm sensation) may occur at application site of topical tacrolimus following ethanol consumption.

Food: Decreases rate and extent of absorption. High-fat meals have most pronounced effect (35% decrease in AUC, 77% decrease in C_{max}). Grapefruit juice, CYP3A4 inhibitor, may increase serum level and/or toxicity of tacrolimus; avoid concurrent use.

Herb/Nutraceutical: St John's wort: May reduce tacrolimus serum concentrations (avoid concurrent use).

Dietary Considerations Capsule: Take on an empty stomach; be consistent with timing and composition of meals if GI intolerance occurs (per manufacturer).

Dosage Forms

Capsule (Prograf®): 0.5 mg, 1 mg, 5 mg

Injection, solution (Prograf®): 5 mg/mL (1 mL) [contains dehydrated alcohol 80% and polyoxyl 60 hydrogenated castor oil]

Ointment, topical (Protopic®): 0.03% (30 g, 60 g, 100 g); 0.1% (30 g, 60 g, 100 g)

References

Winkel E, DiSesa VJ, and Costanzo MR, "Advances in Heart Transplantation," *Dis Mon*, 1999, 45(3):62-87.

Tadalafil (tah DA la fil)

U.S. Brand Names Cialis®

Canadian Brand Names Cialis®

Synonyms GF196960

Pharmacologic Category Phosphodiesterase-5 Enzyme Inhibitor

Generic Available No

Use Treatment of erectile dysfunction

Mechanism of Action Does not directly cause penile erections, but affects the response to sexual stimulation. The physiologic mechanism of erection of the penis involves release of nitric oxide (NO) in the corpus cavernosum during sexual stimulation. NO then activates the enzyme guanylate cyclase, which results in increased levels of cyclic guanosine monophosphate (cGMP), producing smooth muscle relaxation and inflow of blood to the corpus cavernosum. Tadalafil enhances the effect of NO by inhibiting phosphodiesterase type 5 (PDE-5), which is responsible for degradation of cGMP in the corpus cavernosum; when sexual stimulation causes local release of NO, inhibition of PDE-5 by tadalafil causes increased levels of cGMP in the corpus cavernosum, resulting in smooth muscle relaxation and inflow of blood to the corpus cavernosum. At recommended doses, it has no effect in the absence of sexual stimulation.

Pharmacodynamics/Kinetics

Onset: Within 1 hour
Duration: Up to 36 hours
Distribution: V_d: 63 L
Protein binding: 94%
Metabolism: Hepatic, via CYP3A4 to metabolites (inactive)
Half-life elimination: 17.5 hours
Time to peak, plasma: 2 hours
Excretion: Feces (61%, as metabolites); urine (36%, as metabolites)

Dosage Oral: Adults: Erectile dysfunction: 10 mg prior to anticipated sexual activity (dosing range: 5-20 mg); to be given as one single dose and not given more than once daily. **Note:** Erectile function may be improved for up to 36 hours following a single dose; adjust dose.

Elderly: Dosage is based on renal function; refer to "Dosage adjustment in renal impairment"

Dosing adjustment with concomitant medications:

Alpha$_1$-blockers: If stabilized on either alpha blockers or tadalafil therapy, initiate new therapy with the other agent at the lowest possible dose.

CYP3A4 inhibitors: Dose reduction of tadalafil is recommended with strong CYP3A4 inhibitors. The dose of tadalafil should not exceed 10 mg, and tadalafil should not be taken more frequently than once every 72 hours. Examples of such inhibitors include amprenavir, atazanavir, clarithromycin, conivaptan, delavirdine, diclofenac, fosamprenavir, imatinib, indinavir, isoniazid, itraconazole, ketoconazole, miconazole, nefazodone, nelfinavir, nicardipine, propofol, quinidine, ritonavir, and telithromycin.

Dosage adjustment in renal impairment:

Cl_{cr} 31-50 mL/minute: Initial dose 5 mg once daily; maximum dose 10 mg not to be given more frequently than every 48 hours.

Cl_{cr} <30 mL/minute or hemodialysis: Maximum dose 5 mg.

Dosage adjustment in hepatic impairment:

Mild-to-moderate hepatic impairment (Child-Pugh class A or B): Dose should not exceed 10 mg once daily

Severe hepatic impairment: Use is not recommended

Stability Store at controlled room temperature of 15°C to 30°C (59°F to 86°F).

Administration May be administered with or without food, prior to anticipated sexual activity.

Monitoring Parameters Monitor for response and adverse effects.

Pregnancy Risk Factor B

Contraindications Hypersensitivity to tadalafil or any component of the formulation; concurrent use of organic nitrates (nitroglycerin) in any form

Warnings/Precautions There is a degree of cardiac risk associated with sexual activity; therefore, physicians may wish to consider the cardiovascular status of their patients prior to initiating any treatment for erectile dysfunction. Use caution in patients with left ventricular outflow obstruction (aortic stenosis or IHSS); may be more sensitive to hypotensive actions. Concurrent use with alpha-adrenergic antagonist therapy may cause symptomatic hypotension; patients should be hemodynamically stable prior to initiating tadalafil therapy at the lowest possible dose. Use caution in patients receiving strong CYP3A4 inhibitors, the elderly, or those with hepatic impairment or renal impairment; dosage adjustment/limitation is needed. Use caution in patients with peptic ulcer disease.

Agents for the treatment of erectile dysfunction should be used with caution in patients with anatomical deformation of the penis (angulation, cavernosal fibrosis, or Peyronie's disease), or in patients who have conditions which may predispose them to priapism (sickle cell anemia, multiple myeloma, leukemia). All patients

(Continued)

Tadalafil *(Continued)*

should be instructed to seek medical attention if erection persists >4 hours. The safety and efficacy of tadalafil with other treatments for erectile dysfunction have not been studied and are, therefore, not recommended as combination therapy.

Rare cases of nonarteritic ischemic optic neuropathy (NAION) have been reported; risk may be increased with history of vision loss. Other risk factors for NAION include heart disease, diabetes, hypertension, smoking, age >50 years, or history of certain eye problems.

Safety and efficacy have not been studied in patients with the following conditions, therefore, use in these patients is not recommended: Arrhythmias, hypotension, uncontrolled hypertension, unstable angina or angina during intercourse, cardiac failure (NYHA Class II or greater), myocardial infarction within the last 3 months, or stroke within the last 6 months. A minority of patients with retinitis pigmentosa have genetic disorders of retinal phosphodiesterases; use is not recommended. Safety and efficacy in children have not been established.

Adverse Reactions

>10%: Central nervous system: Headache (11% to 15%)

2% to 10%:

- Cardiovascular: Flushing (2% to 3%)
- Gastrointestinal: Dyspepsia (4% to 10%)
- Neuromuscular & skeletal: CPK increased (2%), back pain (3% to 6%), myalgia (1% to 4%), limb pain (1% to 3%)
- Respiratory: Nasal congestion (2% to 3%)

<2%, postmarketing, and/or case reports: Abdominal pain (upper), abnormal liver function tests, angina pectoris, arthralgia, blurred vision, chest pain, color perception change, color vision decreased, conjunctival hyperemia, conjunctivitis, diaphoresis, diarrhea, dizziness, dysphagia, dyspnea, epistaxis, esophagitis, exfoliative dermatitis, eye pain, eyelid swelling, facial edema, fatigue, gastritis, gastroesophageal reflux, hepatic enzymes increased, hyper-/hypotension, hypoesthesia, GGTP increased, insomnia, MI, nausea, nonarteritic ischemic optic neuropathy, pain, palpitation, paresthesia, pharyngitis, photophobia, postural hypotension, priapism (reported with drugs in this class), pruritus, rash, retinal artery occlusion, retinal vein occlusion, somnolence, Stevens-Johnson syndrome, stroke, sudden cardiac death, syncope, tachycardia, urticaria, vertigo, visual changes (color vision), visual field loss, vomiting, weakness, xerostomia

Overdosage/Toxicology Symptoms similar to those seen at lower doses (headache, back pain, myalgias). Treatment is symptomatic and supportive.

Drug Interactions Substrate of CYP3A4 (major)

Alpha$_1$-blockers: Phosphodiesterase-5 inhibitors may enhance the hypotensive effect of alpha$_1$-blockers.

Antifungal agents (imidazole): May decrease the metabolism, via CYP isoenzymes, of phosphodiesterase-5 inhibitors. Ketoconazole significantly increased tadalafil levels.

CYP3A4 inhibitors: May increase the levels/effects of tadalafil. Dose reduction of tadalafil is recommended with strong CYP3A4 inhibitors. The dose of tadalafil should not exceed 10 mg, and tadalafil should not be taken more frequently than once every 72 hours. Example inhibitors include azole antifungals, clarithromycin, diclofenac, doxycycline, erythromycin, grapefruit juice, imatinib, isoniazid, nefazodone, nicardipine, propofol, protease inhibitors, quinidine, telithromycin, and verapamil.

Macrolide antibiotics (clarithromycin, erythromycin, telithromycin, troleandomycin): May decrease the metabolism, via cyp isoenzymes, of phosphodiesterase-5 inhibitors.

Protease inhibitors (amprenavir, atazanavir, fosamprenavir, indinavir, lopinavir, nelfinavir, ritonavir, saquinavir): May decrease the metabolism, via cyp isoenzymes, of phosphodiesterase-5 inhibitors. Ritonavir increased tadalafil levels.

Vasodilators (organic nitrates): Concomitant use is contraindicated due to the potential for severe, life-threatening hypotension; separate doses by 48 hours.

Ethanol/Nutrition/Herb Interactions

Ethanol: Substantial consumption of ethanol may increase the risk of hypotension and orthostasis. Lower ethanol consumption has not been associated with significant changes in blood pressure or increase in orthostatic symptoms.

Food: Rate and extent of absorption are not affected by food. Grapefruit juice may increase serum levels/toxicity of tadalafil. Do not give more than a single 10 mg dose of tadalafil more frequently than every 72 hours in patients who regularly consume grapefruit juice.

Dietary Considerations May be taken with or without food.

Dosage Forms Tablet: 5 mg, 10 mg, 20 mg

- **Tagamet®** *see* Cimetidine *on page 281*
- **Tagamet® HB (Can)** *see* Cimetidine *on page 281*
- **Tagamet® HB 200 [OTC]** *see* Cimetidine *on page 281*
- **Tambocor™** *see* Flecainide *on page 527*
- **Tamiflu®** *see* Oseltamivir *on page 963*

Tamsulosin (tam SOO loe sin)

Medication Safety Issues

Sound-alike/look-alike issues:

Flomax® may be confused with Fosamax®, Volmax®

U.S. Brand Names Flomax®

Canadian Brand Names Flomax®; Flomax® CR

Synonyms Tamsulosin Hydrochloride

Pharmacologic Category Alpha$_1$ Blocker

Generic Available No

Use Treatment of signs and symptoms of benign prostatic hyperplasia (BPH)

Mechanism of Action Tamsulosin is an antagonist of alpha$_{1A}$ adrenoreceptors in the prostate. Smooth muscle tone in the prostate is mediated by alpha$_{1A}$ adrenoreceptors; blocking them leads to relaxation of smooth muscle in the bladder neck and prostate causing an improvement of urine flow and decreased symptoms of BPH. Approximately 75% of the alpha$_1$ receptors in the prostate are of the alpha$_{1A}$ subtype.

Pharmacodynamics/Kinetics

Absorption: >90%

Protein binding: 94% to 99%, primarily to alpha$_1$ acid glycoprotein (AAG)

Metabolism: Hepatic via CYP; metabolites undergo extensive conjugation to glucuronide or sulfate

Bioavailability: Fasting: 30% increase

Distribution: V_d: 16 L

Steady-state: By the fifth day of once-daily dosing

Half-life elimination: Healthy volunteers: 9-13 hours; Target population: 14-15 hours

Time to peak: Fasting: 4-5 hours; With food: 6-7 hours

Excretion: Urine (76%, <10% as unchanged drug); feces (21%)

Dosage Oral: Adults: 0.4 mg once daily ~30 minutes after the same meal each day; dose may be increased after 2-4 weeks to 0.8 mg once daily in patients who fail to respond. If therapy is interrupted for several days, restart with 0.4 mg once daily.

Dosage adjustment in renal impairment:

Cl_{cr} ≥10 mL/minute: No adjustment needed

Cl_{cr} <10 mL/minute: Not studied

Administration Capsules should be swallowed whole; do not crush, chew, or open.

Anesthesia and Critical Care Concerns/Other Considerations Tamsulosin may induce significant orthostatic hypotension with lightheadedness and possible loss of consciousness.

Pregnancy Risk Factor B

Contraindications Hypersensitivity to tamsulosin or any component of the formulation; concurrent use with phosphodiesterase-5 (PDE-5) inhibitors including sildenafil (>25 mg), tadalafil (if tamsulosin dose >0.4 mg/day), or vardenafil

Warnings/Precautions Not intended for use as an antihypertensive drug. May cause orthostasis, syncope or dizziness. Patients should avoid situations where injury may occur as a result of syncope. Rule out prostatic carcinoma before beginning therapy with tamsulosin. Intraoperative Floppy Iris Syndrome occurred most often in patients taking their alpha-1 blocker at the time of cataract surgery, but some cases occurred when the alpha-1 blocker blocker was stopped 2-14 days prior to surgery and as long as 5 weeks to 9 months prior to surgery. The benefit of stopping an alpha-1blocker prior to cataract surgery has not been established. Rarely, patients with a sulfa allergy have also developed an allergic reaction to tamsulosin; avoid use when previous reaction has been severe.

(Continued)

Tamsulosin *(Continued)*

Adverse Reactions

>10%:

Cardiovascular: Studies specific for orthostatic hypotension: Overall, at least one positive test was observed in 16% of patients receiving 0.4 mg and 19% of patients receiving the 0.8 mg dose. "First-dose" orthostatic hypotension following a 0.4 mg dose was reported as 7% at 4 hours postdose and 6% at 8 hours postdose.

Central nervous system: Headache (19% to 21%), dizziness (15% to 17%)

Genitourinary: Abnormal ejaculation (8% to 18%)

Respiratory: Rhinitis (13% to 18%)

1% to 10%:

Cardiovascular: Chest pain (~4%)

Central nervous system: Somnolence (3% to 4%), insomnia (1% to 2%), vertigo (0.6% to 1%)

Endocrine & metabolic: Libido decreased (1% to 2%)

Gastrointestinal: Diarrhea (4% to 6%), nausea (3% to 4%), stomach discomfort (2% to 3%), bitter taste (2% to 3%)

Neuromuscular & skeletal: Weakness (8% to 9%), back pain (7% to 8%)

Ocular: Amblyopia (0.2% to 2%)

Respiratory: Pharyngitis (5% to 6%), cough (3% to 5%), sinusitis (2% to 4%)

Miscellaneous: Infection (9% to 11%), tooth disorder (1% to 2%)

<1% (Limited to important or life-threatening): Allergic reactions (rash, angioedema, pruritus, urticaria) priapism; constipation, intraoperative floppy iris syndrome, orthostasis (symptomatic) (0.2% to 0.4%), palpitation, syncope (0.2% to 0.4%), transaminases increased, vomiting

Overdosage/Toxicology Symptoms of overdose include headache and hypotension. Treatment is supportive.

Drug Interactions Substrate (major) of CYP2D6, 3A4

Alpha-adrenergic blockers: Risk of hypotension may increase in combination with other alpha-adrenergic blocking agents.

Beta-blockers: Beta-blockers may increase risk of first-dose orthostatic hypotension of tamsulosin

Calcium channel blockers: Risk of hypotension may increase

Cimetidine: Cimetidine may decrease tamsulosin clearance.

CYP2D6 inhibitors: May increase the levels/effects of tamsulosin. Example inhibitors include chlorpromazine, delavirdine, fluoxetine, miconazole, paroxetine, pergolide, quinidine, quinine, ritonavir, and ropinirole.

CYP3A4 inducers: CYP3A4 inducers may decrease the levels/effects of tamsulosin. Example inducers include aminoglutethimide, carbamazepine, nafcillin, nevirapine, phenobarbital, phenytoin, and rifamycins.

CYP3A4 inhibitors: May increase the levels/effects of tamsulosin. Example inhibitors include azole antifungals, clarithromycin, diclofenac, doxycycline, erythromycin, imatinib, isoniazid, nefazodone, nicardipine, propofol, protease inhibitors, quinidine, telithromycin, and verapamil.

Sildenafil, tadalafil, vardenafil: Blood pressure-lowering effects are additive. Use of vardenafil is contraindicated by the manufacturer. Use sildenafil with extreme caution (dose ≤25 mg). Tadalafil may be used when tamsulosin dose is ≤0.4 mg/day.

Ethanol/Nutrition/Herb Interactions

Food: Fasting increases bioavailability by 30% and peak concentration 40% to 70%.

Herb/Nutraceutical: Avoid saw palmetto (due to limited experience with this combination).

Dietary Considerations Take once daily, 30 minutes after the same meal each day.

Dosage Forms Capsule, as hydrochloride: 0.4 mg

- **Tamsulosin Hydrochloride** *see* Tamsulosin *on page 1233*
- **Tantum® (Can)** *see* Benzydamine *on page 167*
- **Tapazole®** *see* Methimazole *on page 817*
- **Taro-Carbamazepine Chewable (Can)** *see* Carbamazepine *on page 225*
- **Taro-Ciprofloxacin (Can)** *see* Ciprofloxacin *on page 285*
- **Taro-Clindamycin (Can)** *see* Clindamycin *on page 304*
- **Taro-Simvastatin (Can)** *see* Simvastatin *on page 1174*
- **Taro-Sone® (Can)** *see* Betamethasone *on page 169*

- **Taro-Warfarin (Can)** *see* Warfarin *on page 1362*
- **Tazicef®** *see* Ceftazidime *on page 246*
- **Tazocin® (Can)** *see* Piperacillin and Tazobactam Sodium *on page 1029*
- **Taztia XT™** *see* Diltiazem *on page 394*
- **3TC® (Can)** *see* Lamivudine *on page 725*
- **Tears Again® Gel Drops™ [OTC]** *see* Carboxymethylcellulose *on page 230*
- **Tears Again® Night and Day™ [OTC]** *see* Carboxymethylcellulose *on page 230*
- **Tebamide™** *see* Trimethobenzamide *on page 1318*
- **Tegretol®** *see* Carbamazepine *on page 225*
- **Tegretol®-XR** *see* Carbamazepine *on page 225*

Telithromycin (tel ith roe MYE sin)

U.S. Brand Names Ketek®

Canadian Brand Names Ketek®

Synonyms HMR 3647

Pharmacologic Category Antibiotic, Ketolide

Generic Available No

Use Treatment of community-acquired pneumonia (mild-to-moderate) caused by susceptible strains of *Streptococcus pneumoniae* (including multidrug-resistant isolates), *Haemophilus influenzae, Chlamydia pneumoniae, Moraxella catarrhalis*, and *Mycoplasma pneumoniae*; treatment of bacterial exacerbation of chronic bronchitis caused by susceptible strains of *S. pneumoniae, H. influenzae* and *Moraxella catarrhalis*; treatment of acute bacterial sinusitis caused by *Streptococcus pneumoniae, Haemophilus influenzae, Moraxella catarrhalis*, and *Staphylococcus aureus*

Unlabeled/Investigational Use Approved in Canada for use in the treatment of tonsillitis/pharyngitis due to *S. pyogenes* (as an alternative to beta-lactam antibiotics when necessary/appropriate)

Mechanism of Action Inhibits bacterial protein synthesis by binding to two sites on the 50S ribosomal subunit. Telithromycin has also been demonstrated to alter secretion of IL-1alpha and TNF-alpha; the clinical significance of this immunomodulatory effect has not been evaluated.

Pharmacodynamics/Kinetics

Absorption: Rapid

Distribution: 2.9 L/kg

Protein binding: 60% to 70%

Metabolism: Hepatic, via CYP3A4 (50%) and non-CYP-mediated pathways

Bioavailability: 57% (significant first-pass metabolism)

Half-life elimination: 10 hours

Time to peak, plasma: 1 hour

Excretion: Urine (13% unchanged drug, remainder as metabolites); feces (7%)

Dosage Oral:

Children ≥13 years and Adults: Tonsillitis/pharyngitis (unlabeled U.S. indication): 800 mg once daily for 5 days

Adults:

Acute exacerbation of chronic bronchitis, acute bacterial sinusitis: 800 mg once daily for 5 days

Community-acquired pneumonia: 800 mg once daily for 7-10 days

Dosage adjustment in renal impairment:

U.S. product labeling: Cl_{cr} <30 mL/minute: 600 mg once daily; when renal impairment is accompanied by hepatic impairment, reduce dosage to 400 mg once daily

Canadian product labeling: Cl_{cr} <30 mL/minute: Reduce dose to 400 mg once daily

Hemodialysis: Administer following dialysis

Dosage adjustment in hepatic impairment: No adjustment recommended, unless concurrent severe renal impairment is present

Stability Store at room temperature between 15°C and 30°C.

Administration May be administered with or without food.

Monitoring Parameters Liver function tests, signs/symptoms of liver failure (eg, jaundice), visual acuity

Pregnancy Risk Factor C

(Continued)

Telithromycin *(Continued)*

Contraindications Hypersensitivity to telithromycin, macrolide antibiotics, or any component of the formulation; concurrent use of cisapride or pimozide

Warnings/Precautions May prolong QT_c interval, leading to a risk of ventricular arrhythmias; closely-related antibiotics have been associated with malignant ventricular arrhythmias and torsade de pointes. Avoid in patients with prolongation of QT_c interval due to congenital causes, history of long QT syndrome, uncorrected electrolyte disturbances (hypokalemia or hypomagnesemia), significant bradycardia (<50 bpm), or concurrent therapy with QT_c-prolonging drugs (eg, class Ia and class III antiarrhythmics). Avoid use in patients with a prior history of confirmed cardiogenic syncope or ventricular arrhythmias while receiving macrolide antibiotics or other QT_c-prolonging drugs. Limited case reports have documented the occurrence of jaundice and serious liver damage; use caution with hepatic impairment or previous history of jaundice, and discontinue with signs/symptoms of liver damage. Use caution in renal impairment. Use caution in patients with myasthenia gravis (use only if suitable alternatives are not available). Inform patients of potential for blurred vision, which may interfere with ability to operate machinery or drive; use caution until effects are known. Safety and efficacy not established in pediatric patients <13 years of age per Canadian approved labeling and <18 years of age per U.S. approved labeling. Pseudomembranous colitis has been reported.

Adverse Reactions

2% to 10%:

Central nervous system: Headache (2% to 6%), dizziness (3% to 4%)

Gastrointestinal: Diarrhea (10%), nausea (7% to 8%), vomiting (2% to 3%), loose stools (2%), dysgeusia (2%)

≥0.2% to <2%:

Central nervous system: Vertigo, fatigue, somnolence, insomnia

Dermatologic: Rash

Gastrointestinal: Abdominal distension, abdominal pain, anorexia, constipation, dyspepsia, flatulence, gastritis, gastroenteritis, GI upset, glossitis, stomatitis, watery stools, xerostomia

Genitourinary: Vaginal candidiasis

Hematologic: Platelets increased

Hepatic: Transaminases increased, hepatitis

Ocular: Blurred vision, accommodation delayed, diplopia

Miscellaneous: Candidiasis, diaphoresis increased, exacerbation of myasthenia gravis (rare)

<0.2%: Alkaline phosphatase increased, anxiety, bilirubin increased, bradycardia, eczema, eosinophilia, erythema multiforme, flushing, hypotension, paresthesia, pruritus, urticaria

Postmarketing and/or case reports: Anaphylaxis, angioedema, arrhythmia, edema (facial), hepatocellular injury, jaundice, liver failure, muscle cramps

Additional effects also reported with telithromycin: Abnormal dreams, anemia, appetite decreased, bundle branch block, cholestasis, coagulation disorder, esophagitis, hyperkalemia, hypersensitivity, hypokalemia, leukopenia, lymphopenia, nervousness, neutropenia, palpitation, pharyngolaryngeal pain, polyuria, pseudomembranous colitis, QT_c prolongation, reflux esophagitis, serum creatinine increased, thrombocytopenia, tooth discoloration, tremor, urine discoloration, vaginal irritation, vasculitis, weakness

Overdosage/Toxicology Treatment should be symptomatic and supportive. ECG and electrolytes should be monitored.

Drug Interactions **Substrate** of CYP1A2 (minor), 3A4 (major); **Inhibits** CYP2D6 (weak), 3A4 (strong)

Antiarrhythmics (class Ia and class III): Effect on QT_c prolongation may be additive; serious arrhythmias may occur; use caution.

Antipsychotic agents (mesoridazine and thioridazine): Risk of QT_c prolongation and malignant arrhythmias may be increased.

Benzodiazepines (those metabolized by CYP3A4, including alprazolam, midazolam, triazolam): Serum levels may be increased by telithromycin

Calcium channel blockers (felodipine, verapamil, and potentially others metabolized by CYP3A4): Serum levels may be increased by telithromycin; monitor.

Carbamazepine: Serum levels may be increased by telithromycin; monitor.

Cisapride: Serum levels may be increased by telithromycin; serious arrhythmias may occur; concurrent use is contraindicated.

Colchicine: Serum levels/effects may be increased by telithromycin. Avoid use, if possible.

CYP3A4 inhibitors: May increase the levels/effects of telithromycin. Example inhibitors include azole antifungals, clarithromycin, diclofenac, doxycycline, erythromycin, imatinib, isoniazid, nefazodone, nicardipine, propofol, protease inhibitors, quinidine, and verapamil.

CYP3A4 inducers: CYP3A4 inducers may decrease the levels/effects of telithromycin. Example inducers include aminoglutethimide, carbamazepine, nafcillin, nevirapine, phenobarbital, phenytoin, and rifamycins.

CYP3A4 substrates: Telithromycin may increase the levels/effects of CYP3A4 substrates. Example substrates include benzodiazepines, calcium channel blockers, mirtazapine, nateglinide, nefazodone, tacrolimus, and venlafaxine. Selected benzodiazepines (midazolam and triazolam), cisapride, ergot alkaloids, selected HMG-CoA reductase inhibitors (atorvastatin and lovastatin and simvastatin), and pimozide are generally contraindicated with strong CYP3A4 inhibitors.

Digoxin: Serum levels may be increased by telithromycin; monitor digoxin levels.

Ergot alkaloids: Concurrent use may lead to acute ergot toxicity (severe peripheral vasospasm and dysesthesia); concurrent use not recommended

HMG-CoA reductase inhibitors (atorvastatin, lovastatin, and simvastatin); Telithromycin may increase serum levels of "statins" metabolized by CYP3A4, increasing the risk of myopathy/rhabdomyolysis (does not include fluvastatin, pravastatin, and rosuvastatin). Switch to noninteracting drug or suspend treatment during course of telithromycin therapy.

Immunosuppressants (cyclosporine, sirolimus, tacrolimus): Serum levels may be increased by telithromycin; monitor serum levels.

Itraconazole, ketoconazole: May increase telithromycin levels; risk of telithromycin toxicity (eg, QT_c prolongation) may increase. No dosage adjustment recommended by manufacturer.

Neuromuscular-blocking agents: May be potentiated by telithromycin.

Pimozide: Serum levels may be increased by telithromycin; serious arrhythmias may occur; concurrent use contraindicated.

Quinolone antibiotics (sparfloxacin, gatifloxacin, or moxifloxacin): Concurrent use may increase the risk of malignant arrhythmias.

Rifampin: Rifampin may decrease the serum concentrations/effect of telithromycin; avoid concurrent use if possible.

Sildenafil, tadalafil, vardenafil: Serum levels may be increased by telithromycin. Do not exceed single sildenafil doses of 25 mg in 48 hours or single vardenafil dose of 2.5 mg in 24 hours. The dose of tadalafil should not exceed 10 mg, and tadalafil should not be taken more frequently than once every 72 hours.

Warfarin: Telithromycin may increase the effect of warfarin (limited data); monitor.

Dietary Considerations May be taken with or without food.

Dosage Forms

Tablet: 300 mg [not available in Canada], 400 mg

Ketek Pak™ [blister pack]: 400 mg (10s) [packaged as 10 tablets/card; 2 tablets/blister]

Telmisartan (tel mi SAR tan)

Related Information

Angiotensin Agents *on page 1544*

U.S. Brand Names Micardis®

Canadian Brand Names Micardis®

Pharmacologic Category Angiotensin II Receptor Blocker

Generic Available No

Use Treatment of hypertension; may be used alone or in combination with other antihypertensive agents

Mechanism of Action Angiotensin II acts as a vasoconstrictor. In addition to causing direct vasoconstriction, angiotensin II also stimulates the release of aldosterone. Once aldosterone is released, sodium as well as water are reabsorbed. The end result is an elevation in blood pressure. Telmisartan is a nonpeptide AT1 angiotensin II receptor antagonist. This binding prevents angiotensin II from binding to the receptor thereby blocking the vasoconstriction and the aldosterone secreting effects of angiotensin II.

Pharmacodynamics/Kinetics Orally active, not a prodrug

Onset of action: 1-2 hours

(Continued)

Telmisartan *(Continued)*

Peak effect: 0.5-1 hours
Duration: Up to 24 hours
Protein binding: >99.5%
Metabolism: Hepatic via conjugation to inactive metabolites; not metabolized via CYP
Bioavailability (dose dependent): 42% to 58%
Half-life elimination: Terminal: 24 hours
Excretion: Feces (97%)
Clearance: Total body: 800 mL/minute

Dosage Adults: Oral: Initial: 40 mg once daily; usual maintenance dose range: 20-80 mg/day. Patients with volume depletion should be initiated on the lower dosage with close supervision.

Dosage adjustment in hepatic impairment: Supervise patients closely.

Monitoring Parameters Supine blood pressure, electrolytes, serum creatinine, BUN, urinalysis, symptomatic hypotension, and tachycardia

Anesthesia and Critical Care Concerns/Other Considerations The angiotensin II receptor antagonists appear to have similar indications as the ACE inhibitors. In heart failure, the angiotensin II antagonists are especially useful in providing an alternative therapy in those patients who have intractable cough in response to ACE inhibitor therapy. Candesartan has been studied as an alternative therapy in chronic heart failure patients who cannot tolerate an ACE-I (CHARM-Alternative) and as an added therapy in heart failure patients who are maintained on an ACE-I (CHARM-Added). In both studies the combined endpoint of cardiovascular death or heart failure hospitalizations was significantly improved over the placebo treated group. Similar to ACE inhibitors, pre-existing volume depletion caused by diuretic therapy may potentiate hypotension in response to angiotensin II antagonists. Concomitant NSAID therapy may attenuate blood pressure control; use of NSAIDs should be avoided or limited, with monitoring of blood pressure control. In the setting of heart failure, NSAID use may be associated with an increased risk for fluid accumulation and edema.

Pregnancy Risk Factor C (1st trimester); D (2nd and 3rd trimesters)

Contraindications Hypersensitivity to telmisartan or any component of the formulation; hypersensitivity to other A-II receptor antagonists; bilateral renal artery stenosis; pregnancy (2nd and 3rd trimesters)

Warnings/Precautions **[U.S. Boxed Warning]: Based on human data, drugs that act on the angiotensin system can cause injury and death to the developing fetus when used in the second and third trimesters. Angiotensin receptor blockers should be discontinued as soon as possible once pregnancy is detected.** Avoid use or use a smaller dose in patients who are volume depleted; correct depletion first. Deterioration in renal function can occur with initiation. Use with caution in unilateral renal artery stenosis and pre-existing renal insufficiency; significant aortic/mitral stenosis. Use with caution in patients who have biliary obstructive disorders or hepatic dysfunction.

Adverse Reactions May be associated with worsening of renal function in patients dependent on renin-angiotensin-aldosterone system.

1% to 10%:
Cardiovascular: Hypertension (1%), chest pain (1%), peripheral edema (1%)
Central nervous system: Headache (1%), dizziness (1%), pain (1%), fatigue (1%)
Gastrointestinal: Diarrhea (3%), dyspepsia (1%), nausea (1%), abdominal pain (1%)
Genitourinary: Urinary tract infection (1%)
Neuromuscular & skeletal: Back pain (3%), myalgia (1%)
Respiratory: Upper respiratory infection (7%), sinusitis (3%), pharyngitis (1%), cough (2%)
Miscellaneous: Flu-like syndrome (1%)

<1% (Limited to important or life-threatening): Abnormal vision, allergic reaction, angina, angioedema, angioneurotic edema, atrial fibrillation, CHF, cramps, depression, dyspnea, edema, epistaxis, erectile dysfunction, erythema, facial edema, gout, hyperkalemia, hypersensitivity, hypotension, impotence, increased serum creatinine and BUN, insomnia, MI, migraine, muscle cramps, paresthesia, pruritus, rash, somnolence, syncope, tinnitus, urticaria, vertigo, weakness

Overdosage/Toxicology Symptoms of overdose may include hypotension, dizziness, and tachycardia. Vagal stimulation may result in bradycardia. Treatment is supportive.

Drug Interactions **Inhibits** CYP2C19 (weak)

Digoxin levels may be increased.

Lithium: Risk of toxicity may be increased by telmisartan; monitor lithium levels.

NSAIDs: May decrease angiotensin II antagonist efficacy; effect has been seen with losartan, but may occur with other medications in this class; monitor blood pressure

Potassium-sparing diuretics (amiloride, potassium, spironolactone, triamterene): Increased risk of hyperkalemia.

Potassium supplements may increase the risk of hyperkalemia.

Trimethoprim (high dose) may increase the risk of hyperkalemia.

Warfarin serum concentrations may be decreased (not associated with alteration in INR); monitor INR closely.

Ethanol/Nutrition/Herb Interactions Herb/Nutraceutical: Avoid dong quai if using for hypertension (has estrogenic activity). Avoid ephedra, yohimbe, ginseng (may worsen hypertension). Avoid garlic (may have increased antihypertensive effect).

Dietary Considerations May be taken without regard to food.

Dosage Forms Tablet: 20 mg, 40 mg, 80 mg

Temazepam (te MAZ e pam)

Medication Safety Issues

Sound-alike/look-alike issues:

Temazepam may be confused with flurazepam, lorazepam

Restoril® may be confused with Vistaril®, Zestril®

Related Information

Anesthesia Considerations for Neurosurgery *on page 1401*

Benzodiazepines *on page 1555*

U.S. Brand Names Restoril®

Canadian Brand Names Apo-Temazepam® ; CO Temazepam; Gen-Temazepam; Novo-Temazepam; Nu-Temazepam; PMS-Temazepam; ratio-Temazepam; Restoril®

Pharmacologic Category Hypnotic, Benzodiazepine

Restrictions C-IV

Generic Available Yes

Use Short-term treatment of insomnia

Unlabeled/Investigational Use Treatment of anxiety; adjunct in the treatment of depression; management of panic attacks

Mechanism of Action Binds to stereospecific benzodiazepine receptors on the postsynaptic GABA neuron at several sites within the central nervous system, including the limbic system, reticular formation. Enhancement of the inhibitory effect of GABA on neuronal excitability results by increased neuronal membrane permeability to chloride ions. This shift in chloride ions results in hyperpolarization (a less excitable state) and stabilization.

Pharmacodynamics/Kinetics

Distribution: V_d: 1.4 L/kg

Protein binding: 96%

Metabolism: Hepatic

Half-life elimination: 9.5-12.4 hours

Time to peak, serum: 2-3 hours

Excretion: Urine (80% to 90% as inactive metabolites)

Dosage Oral:

Adults: 15-30 mg at bedtime

Elderly or debilitated patients: 15 mg

Monitoring Parameters Respiratory and cardiovascular status

Reference Range Therapeutic: 26 ng/mL after 24 hours

Anesthesia and Critical Care Concerns/Other Considerations Chronic use of this agent may increase perioperative benzodiazepine dose needed to achieve desired effect. Abrupt discontinuation after sustained use (generally >10 days) may cause withdrawal symptoms. Benzodiazepines, as a class, may depress respiration; may exacerbate sleep-disordered breathing.

Pregnancy Risk Factor X

(Continued)

Temazepam *(Continued)*

Contraindications Hypersensitivity to temazepam or any component of the formulation (cross-sensitivity with other benzodiazepines may exist); narrow-angle glaucoma (not in product labeling, however, benzodiazepines are contraindicated); pregnancy

Warnings/Precautions Should be used only after evaluation of potential causes of sleep disturbance. Failure of sleep disturbance to resolve after 7-10 days may indicate psychiatric or medical illness. A worsening of insomnia or the emergence of new abnormalities of thought or behavior may represent unrecognized psychiatric or medical illness and requires immediate and careful evaluation.

Use with caution in elderly or debilitated patients, patients with hepatic disease (including alcoholics), or renal impairment. Use with caution in patients with respiratory disease, or impaired gag reflex. Avoid use inpatients with sleep apnea.

Causes CNS depression (dose-related) resulting in sedation, dizziness, confusion, or ataxia which may impair physical and mental capabilities. Patients must be cautioned about performing tasks which require mental alertness (eg, operating machinery or driving). Use with caution in patients receiving other CNS depressants or psychoactive agents. Effects with other sedative drugs or ethanol may be potentiated. Benzodiazepines have been associated with falls and traumatic injury and should be used with extreme caution in patients who are at risk of these events (especially the elderly).

Use caution in patients with depression, particularly if suicidal risk may be present. Use with caution in patients with a history of drug dependence. Benzodiazepines have been associated with dependence and acute withdrawal symptoms on discontinuation or reduction in dose (may occur after as little as 10 days). Acute withdrawal, including seizures, may be precipitated after administration of flumazenil to patients receiving long-term benzodiazepine therapy.

Benzodiazepines have been associated with anterograde amnesia. Paradoxical reactions, including hyperactive or aggressive behavior, have been reported with benzodiazepines, particularly in adolescent/pediatric or psychiatric patients. Does not have analgesic, antidepressant, or antipsychotic properties.

Adverse Reactions

1% to 10%:

Central nervous system: Confusion, dizziness, drowsiness, fatigue, anxiety, headache, lethargy, hangover, euphoria, vertigo
Dermatologic: Rash
Endocrine & metabolic: Decreased libido
Gastrointestinal: Diarrhea
Neuromuscular & skeletal: Dysarthria, weakness
Ocular: Blurred vision
Miscellaneous: Diaphoresis

<1% (Limited to important or life-threatening): Amnesia, ataxia, blood dyscrasias, drug dependence, paradoxical reactions, vomiting

Overdosage/Toxicology Symptoms of overdose include somnolence, confusion, coma, hypoactive reflexes, dyspnea, hypotension, slurred speech, and impaired coordination. Treatment for benzodiazepine overdose is supportive. Flumazenil has been shown to selectively block the binding of benzodiazepines to CNS receptors, resulting in a reversal of benzodiazepine-induced CNS depression but not always respiratory depression due to toxicity.

Drug Interactions Substrate (minor) of CYP2B6, 2C9, 2C19, 3A4

CNS depressants: Sedative effects and/or respiratory depression may be additive with CNS depressants; includes ethanol, barbiturates, narcotic analgesics, and other sedative agents; monitor for increased effect

Theophylline: May partially antagonize some of the effects of benzodiazepines; monitor for decreased response; may require higher doses for sedation

Ethanol/Nutrition/Herb Interactions

Ethanol: Avoid ethanol (may increase CNS depression).
Food: Serum levels may be increased by grapefruit juice.
Herb/Nutraceutical: St John's wort may decrease temazepam levels. Avoid valerian, St John's wort, kava kava, gotu kola (may increase CNS depression).

Dosage Forms

Capsule: 15 mg, 30 mg
Restoril®: 7.5 mg, 15 mg, 30 mg

♦ **Tempra® (Can)** *see* Acetaminophen *on page 26*

Tenecteplase (ten EK te plase)

Medication Safety Issues

Sound-alike/look-alike issues:

TNKase™ may be confused with t-PA

TNK (occasional abbreviation for TNKase™) is an error-prone abbreviation (mistaken as TPA)

High alert medication: The Institute for Safe Medication Practices (ISMP) includes this medication (I.V.) among its list of drugs which have a heightened risk of causing significant patient harm when used in error.

U.S. Brand Names TNKase™

Canadian Brand Names TNKase™

Pharmacologic Category Thrombolytic Agent

Generic Available No

Use Thrombolytic agent used in the management of acute myocardial infarction for the lysis of thrombi in the coronary vasculature to restore perfusion and reduce mortality.

Unlabeled/Investigational Use Acute MI — combination regimen of tenecteplase (unlabeled dose), abciximab, and heparin (unlabeled dose)

Mechanism of Action Initiates fibrinolysis by binding to fibrin and converting plasminogen to plasmin.

Pharmacodynamics/Kinetics

Distribution: V_d is weight related and approximates plasma volume

Metabolism: Primarily hepatic

Half-life elimination: 90-130 minutes

Excretion: Clearance: Plasma: 99-119 mL/minute

Dosage I.V.:

Adult: Recommended total dose should not exceed 50 mg and is based on patient's weight; administer as a bolus over 5 seconds

If patient's weight:

<60 kg, dose: 30 mg

≥60 to <70 kg, dose: 35 mg

≥70 to <80 kg, dose: 40 mg

≥80 to <90 kg, dose: 45 mg

≥90 kg, dose: 50 mg

All patients received 150-325 mg of aspirin as soon as possible and then daily. Intravenous heparin was initiated as soon as possible and aPTT was maintained between 50-70 seconds.

Elderly: Although dosage adjustments are not recommended, the elderly have a higher incidence of morbidity and mortality with the use of tenecteplase. The 30-day mortality in the ASSENT-2 trial was 2.5% for patients <65 years, 8.5% for patients 65-74 years, and 16.2% for patients ≥75 years. The intracranial hemorrhage rate was 0.4% for patients <65, 1.6 % for patients 65-74 years, and 1.7 % for patients ≥75 years. The risks and benefits of use should be weighted carefully in the elderly.

Combination regimen (unlabeled): Half-dose tenecteplase (15-25 mg based on weight) and abciximab 0.25 mg/kg bolus then 0.125 mcg/kg/minute (maximum 10 mcg/minute) for 12 hours with heparin dosing as follows: Concurrent bolus of 40 units/kg (maximum 3000 units), then 7 units/kg/hour (maximum 800 units/hour) as continuous infusion. Adjust to aPTT target of 50-70 seconds.

Dosage adjustment in renal impairment: No formal recommendations for renal impairment

Dosage adjustment in hepatic impairment: Severe hepatic failure is a relative contraindication. Recommendations were not made for mild to moderate hepatic impairment.

Stability Store at room temperature not to exceed 30°C (86°F) or under refrigeration 2°C to 8°C (36°F to 46°F). If reconstituted and not used immediately, store in refrigerator and use within 8 hours.

Administration Tenecteplase should be reconstituted using the supplied 10 mL syringe with TwinPak™ dual cannula device and 10 mL sterile water for injection. Do not shake when reconstituting. Slight foaming is normal and will dissipate if left standing for several minutes. The reconstituted solution is 5 mg/mL. Any unused

(Continued)

Tenecteplase *(Continued)*

solution should be discarded. Tenecteplase is **incompatible** with dextrose solutions. Dextrose-containing lines must be flushed with a saline solution before and after administration. Administer as a single I.V. bolus over 5 seconds. Avoid I.M. injections and nonessential handling of patient.

Monitoring Parameters CBC, aPTT, signs and symptoms of bleeding, ECG monitoring

Anesthesia and Critical Care Concerns/Other Considerations The 1999 ACC/AHA guidelines for the management of patients with acute myocardial infarction recommend prehospital thrombolysis in special circumstances (eg, transport time >90 minutes) (Class IIb recommendation). Efforts to quickly identify and safely treat appropriate candidates for therapy continue. Reducing treatment delays is very important to improve mortality. Tenecteplase has not shown to have a compelling advantage over alteplase. In ASSENT-2, 30-day mortality and rates of hemorrhage were similar between alteplase- and tenecteplase-treated patients.

Thrombolytic and GP IIb/IIIa Inhibitor: It has been demonstrated that full-dose thrombolytic and full-dose GP IIb/IIIa inhibitor result in patency, however, unacceptable bleeding (including cerebral bleeding) occurred.

Pregnancy Risk Factor C

Contraindications Hypersensitivity to tenecteplase or any component of the formulation; active internal bleeding; history of stroke; intracranial/intraspinal surgery or trauma within 2 months; intracranial neoplasm; arteriovenous malformation or aneurysm; bleeding diathesis; severe uncontrolled hypertension

Warnings/Precautions Stop antiplatelet agents and heparin if serious bleeding occurs. Avoid I.M. injections and nonessential handling of the patient for a few hours after administration. Monitor for bleeding complications. Venipunctures should be performed carefully and only when necessary. If arterial puncture is necessary, then use an upper extremity that can be easily compressed manually. For the following conditions, the risk of bleeding is higher with use of tenecteplase and should be weighed against the benefits: Recent major surgery, cerebrovascular disease, recent GI or GU bleed, recent trauma, uncontrolled hypertension (systolic BP ≥180 mm Hg and/or diastolic BP ≥110 mm Hg), suspected left heart thrombus, acute pericarditis, subacute bacterial endocarditis, hemostatic defects, severe hepatic dysfunction, pregnancy, hemorrhagic diabetic retinopathy or other hemorrhagic ophthalmic conditions, septic thrombophlebitis or occluded arteriovenous cannula at seriously infected site, advanced age (see Usual Dosing, Elderly), anticoagulants, recent administration of GP IIb/IIIa inhibitors. Coronary thrombolysis may result in reperfusion arrhythmias. Caution with readministration of tenecteplase. Safety and efficacy have not been established in pediatric patients. Cholesterol embolism has rarely been reported.

Adverse Reactions As with all drugs which may affect hemostasis, bleeding is the major adverse effect associated with tenecteplase. Hemorrhage may occur at virtually any site. Risk is dependent on multiple variables, including the dosage administered, concurrent use of multiple agents which alter hemostasis, and patient predisposition. Rapid lysis of coronary artery thrombi by thrombolytic agents may be associated with reperfusion-related arterial and/or ventricular arrhythmia.

>10%:

- Local: Hematoma (12% minor)
- Hematologic: Bleeding (22% minor: ASSENT-2 trial)

1% to 10%:

- Central nervous system: Stroke (2%)
- Gastrointestinal: GI hemorrhage (1% major, 2% minor), epistaxis (2% minor)
- Genitourinary: GU bleeding (4% minor)
- Hematologic: Bleeding (5% major; ASSENT-2 trial)
- Local: Bleeding at catheter puncture site (4% minor), hematoma (2% major)
- Respiratory: Pharyngeal (3% minor)

The incidence of stroke and bleeding increase with age above 65 years.

<1% (Limited to important or life-threatening): Anaphylaxis, angioedema, bleeding at catheter puncture site (<1% major), cholesterol embolism (clinical features may include livedo reticularis, "purple toe" syndrome, acute renal failure, gangrenous digits, hypertension, pancreatitis, MI, cerebral infarction,

spinal cord infarction, retinal artery occlusion, bowel infarction, rhabdomyolysis), GU bleeding (<1% major), intracranial hemorrhage (0.9%), laryngeal edema, rash, respiratory tract bleeding, retroperitoneal bleeding, urticaria

Additional cardiovascular events associated with use in MI: Arrhythmias, AV block, cardiac arrest, cardiac tamponade, cardiogenic shock, electromechanical dissociation, embolism, fever, heart failure, hypotension, mitral regurgitation, myocardial reinfarction, myocardial rupture, nausea, pericardial effusion, pericarditis, pulmonary edema, recurrent myocardial ischemia, thrombosis, vomiting

Overdosage/Toxicology Increased incidence of bleeding

Drug Interactions

Aminocaproic acid (antifibrinolytic agent) may decrease effectiveness.

Drugs which affect platelet function (eg, NSAIDs, dipyridamole, ticlopidine, clopidogrel, IIb/IIIa antagonists) may potentiate the risk of hemorrhage; use with caution.

Heparin and aspirin: Use with aspirin and heparin may increase bleeding. However, aspirin and heparin were used concomitantly with tenecteplase in the majority of patients in clinical studies.

Warfarin or oral anticoagulants: Risk of bleeding may be increased during concurrent therapy.

Dosage Forms Injection, powder for reconstitution, recombinant: 50 mg [packaged with diluent and syringe]

- **Tenolin (Can)** *see* Atenolol *on page 136*
- **Tenormin®** *see* Atenolol *on page 136*
- **Tensilon® (Can)** *see* Edrophonium *on page 439*
- **Tequin® [DSC]** *see* Gatifloxacin *on page 583*

Terazosin (ter AY zoe sin)

U.S. Brand Names Hytrin®

Canadian Brand Names Alti-Terazosin; Apo-Terazosin®; Hytrin®; Novo-Terazosin; Nu-Terazosin; PMS-Terazosin

Pharmacologic Category $Alpha_1$ Blocker

Generic Available Yes

Use Management of mild to moderate hypertension; alone or in combination with other agents such as diuretics or beta-blockers; benign prostate hyperplasia (BPH)

Mechanism of Action $Alpha_1$-specific blocking agent with minimal $alpha_2$ effects; this allows peripheral postsynaptic blockade, with the resultant decrease in arterial tone, while preserving the negative feedback loop which is mediated by the peripheral presynaptic $alpha_2$-receptors; terazosin relaxes the smooth muscle of the bladder neck, thus reducing bladder outlet obstruction

Pharmacodynamics/Kinetics

Onset of action: 1-2 hours

Absorption: Rapid

Protein binding: 90% to 95%

Metabolism: Extensively hepatic

Half-life elimination: 9.2-12 hours

Time to peak, serum: ~1 hour

Excretion: Feces (60%); urine (40%)

Dosage Oral: Adults:

Hypertension: Initial: 1 mg at bedtime; slowly increase dose to achieve desired blood pressure, up to 20 mg/day; usual dose range (JNC 7): 1-20 mg once daily

Dosage reduction may be needed when adding a diuretic or other antihypertensive agent; if drug is discontinued for greater than several days, consider beginning with initial dose and retitrate as needed; dosage may be given on a twice daily regimen if response is diminished at 24 hours and hypotensive is observed at 2-4 hours following a dose

Benign prostatic hyperplasia: Initial: 1 mg at bedtime, increasing as needed; most patients require 10 mg day; if no response after 4-6 weeks of 10 mg/day, may increase to 20 mg/day

Monitoring Parameters Standing and sitting/supine blood pressure, especially following the initial dose at 2-4 hours following the dose and thereafter at the trough point to ensure adequate control throughout the dosing interval; urinary symptoms

(Continued)

Terazosin *(Continued)*

Pregnancy Risk Factor C

Contraindications Hypersensitivity to quinazolines (doxazosin, prazosin, terazosin) or any component of the formulation; concurrent use with phosphodiesterase-5 (PDE-5) inhibitors including sildenafil (>25 mg), tadalafil, or vardenafil

Warnings/Precautions Can cause significant orthostatic hypotension and syncope, especially with first dose; anticipate a similar effect if therapy is interrupted for a few days, if dosage is rapidly increased, or if another antihypertensive drug (particularly vasodilators) or a PDE5 inhibitor is introduced. Patients should be cautioned about performing hazardous tasks when starting new therapy or adjusting dosage upward. Prostate cancer should be ruled out before starting for BPH. Use with caution in hepatic impairment. Intraoperative floppy iris syndrome has been observed in cataract surgery patients who were on or were previously treated with $alpha_1$ blockers. Causality has not been established and there appears to be no benefit in discontinuing alpha blocker therapy prior to surgery. Safety and efficacy in children have not been established.

Adverse Reactions Asthenia, postural hypotension, dizziness, somnolence, nasal congestion/rhinitis, and impotence were the only events noted in clinical trials to occur at a frequency significantly greater than placebo ($p < 0.05$).

>10%:
- Central nervous system: Dizziness, headache
- Neuromuscular & skeletal: Muscle weakness

1% to 10%:
- Cardiovascular: Edema, palpitation, chest pain, peripheral edema (3%), orthostatic hypotension (3% to 4%), tachycardia
- Central nervous system: Fatigue, nervousness, drowsiness
- Gastrointestinal: Dry mouth
- Genitourinary: Urinary incontinence
- Ocular: Blurred vision
- Respiratory: Dyspnea, nasal congestion

<1% (Limited to important or life-threatening): Allergic reactions, anaphylaxis, atrial fibrillation, priapism, sexual dysfunction, syncope (0.8%), thrombocytopenia

Overdosage/Toxicology Symptoms of overdose include hypotension, drowsiness, and shock. Treatment is supportive and symptomatic.

Drug Interactions
- ACE inhibitors: Hypotensive effect may be increased.
- Beta-blockers: Hypotensive effect may be increased.
- Calcium channel blockers: Hypotensive effect may be increased.
- NSAIDs may reduce antihypertensive efficacy.
- Sildenafil, tadalafil, vardenafil: Blood pressure-lowering effects are additive. Use of tadalafil or vardenafil is contraindicated by the manufacturer. Use sildenafil with extreme caution (dose ≤25 mg).

Ethanol/Nutrition/Herb Interactions Herb/Nutraceutical: Avoid dong quai if using for hypertension (has estrogenic activity). Avoid ephedra, yohimbe, ginseng (may worsen hypertension). Avoid saw palmetto. Avoid garlic (may have increased antihypertensive effect).

Dietary Considerations May be taken without regard to meals at the same time each day.

Dosage Forms Capsule: 1 mg, 2 mg, 5 mg, 10 mg

Terbutaline (ter BYOO ta leen)

Medication Safety Issues

Sound-alike/look-alike issues:
- Terbutaline may be confused with terbinafine, TOLBUTamide

U.S. Brand Names Brethine®

Canadian Brand Names Bricanyl®

Synonyms Brethaire [DSC]; Bricanyl [DSC]

Pharmacologic Category $Beta_2$-Adrenergic Agonist

Generic Available Yes

Use Bronchodilator in reversible airway obstruction and bronchial asthma

Unlabeled/Investigational Use Tocolytic agent (management of preterm labor)

Mechanism of Action Relaxes bronchial smooth muscle by action on $beta_2$-receptors with less effect on heart rate

Pharmacodynamics/Kinetics

Onset of action: Oral: 30-45 minutes; SubQ: 6-15 minutes

Protein binding: 25%

Metabolism: Hepatic to inactive sulfate conjugates

Bioavailability: SubQ doses are more bioavailable than oral

Half-life elimination: 11-16 hours

Excretion: Urine

Dosage

Children <12 years: Bronchoconstriction:

Oral: Initial: 0.05 mg/kg/dose 3 times/day, increased gradually as required; maximum: 0.15 mg/kg/dose 3-4 times/day or a total of 5 mg/24 hours

SubQ: 0.005-0.01 mg/kg/dose to a maximum of 0.3 mg/dose; may repeat in 15-20 minutes

Children ≥6 years and Adults: Bronchospasm (acute): Inhalation (Bricanyl® [CAN] MDI: 500 mcg/puff, *not labeled for use in the U.S.*): One puff as needed; may repeat with 1 inhalation (after 5 minutes); more than 6 inhalations should not be necessary in any 24 hour period. **Note:** If a previously effective dosage regimen fails to provide the usual relief, or the effects of a dose last for >3 hours, medical advice should be sought immediately; this is a sign of seriously worsening asthma that requires reassessment of therapy.

Children >12 years and Adults: Bronchoconstriction:

Oral:

12-15 years: 2.5 mg every 6 hours 3 times/day; not to exceed 7.5 mg in 24 hours

>15 years: 5 mg/dose every 6 hours 3 times/day; if side effects occur, reduce dose to 2.5 mg every 6 hours; not to exceed 15 mg in 24 hours

SubQ: 0.25 mg/dose; may repeat in 15-30 minutes (maximum: 0.5 mg/4-hour period)

Adults: Premature labor (tocolysis; unlabeled use):

Acute: I.V. 2.5-10 mcg/minute; increased gradually every 10-20 minutes; effective maximum dosages from 17.5-30 mcg/minute have been used with caution. Duration of infusion is at least 12 hours.

Maintenance: Oral: 2.5-10 mg every 4-6 hours for as long as necessary to prolong pregnancy depending on patient tolerance

Dosing adjustment/comments in renal impairment:

Cl_{cr} 10-50 mL/minute: Administer at 50% of normal dose

Cl_{cr} <10 mL/minute: Avoid use

Stability Store injection at room temperature; protect from heat, light, and from freezing; use only clear solutions. Store powder for inhalation (Bricanyl® Turbuhaler [CAN]) at room temperature between 15°C and 30°C (58°F and 86°F).

Administration

I.V.: Use infusion pump.

Oral: Administer around-the-clock to promote less variation in peak and trough serum levels

Monitoring Parameters Serum potassium, glucose; heart rate, blood pressure, respiratory rate; monitor for signs and symptoms of pulmonary edema (when used as a tocolytic); monitor FEV_1, peak flow, and/or other pulmonary function tests (when used as bronchodilator)

Anesthesia and Critical Care Concerns/Other Considerations $Beta_2$-selective agents lose much of their receptor selectivity when delivered parenterally or orally. Subcutaneous beta-agonist therapy has a deleterious therapeutic to toxicity ratio when compared with inhalation. There is no proven benefit of aerosolized over systemic therapy.

Pregnancy Risk Factor B

Contraindications Hypersensitivity to terbutaline or any component of the formulation; cardiac arrhythmias associated with tachycardia; tachycardia caused by digitalis intoxication

Warnings/Precautions When used for tocolysis, there is some risk of maternal pulmonary edema, which has been associated with the following risk factors, excessive hydration, multiple gestation, occult sepsis and underlying cardiac disease. To reduce risk, limit fluid intake to 2.5-3 L/day, limit sodium intake, maintain maternal pulse to <130 beats/minute.

Use caution in patients with cardiovascular disease (arrhythmia or hypertension or CHF), convulsive disorders, diabetes, glaucoma, hyperthyroidism, or hypokalemia. Beta agonists may cause elevation in blood pressure, heart rate, and result

(Continued)

Terbutaline *(Continued)*

in CNS stimulation/excitation. $Beta_2$ agonists may increase risk of arrhythmia, increase serum glucose, or decrease serum potassium.

When used as a bronchodilator, optimize anti-inflammatory treatment before initiating maintenance treatment with terbutaline. Do not use as a component of chronic therapy without an anti-inflammatory agent. Only the mildest form of asthma (Step 1 and/or exercise-induced) would not require concurrent use based upon asthma guidelines. Patient must be instructed to seek medical attention in cases where acute symptoms are not relieved or a previous level of response is diminished. The need to increase frequency of use may indicate deterioration of asthma, and treatment must not be delayed.

Do not exceed recommended dose; serious adverse events including fatalities, have been associated with excessive use of inhaled sympathomimetics. Rarely, paradoxical bronchospasm may occur with use of inhaled bronchodilating agents; this should be distinguished from inadequate response.

Adverse Reactions

>10%:

Central nervous system: Nervousness, restlessness
Endocrine & metabolic: Serum glucose increased, serum potassium decreased
Neuromuscular & skeletal: Trembling

1% to 10%:

Cardiovascular: Tachycardia, hypertension, pounding heartbeat
Central nervous system: Dizziness, lightheadedness, drowsiness, headache, insomnia
Gastrointestinal: Dry mouth, nausea, vomiting, bad taste in mouth
Neuromuscular & skeletal: Muscle cramps, weakness
Miscellaneous: Diaphoresis

<1% (Limited to important or life-threatening): Arrhythmia, chest pain, hypokalemia, paradoxical bronchospasm

Overdosage/Toxicology Symptoms of overdose include tachycardia, tremor, hypertension, angina, and seizures. Hypokalemia also may occur. Cardiac arrest and death may be associated with abuse of beta-agonist bronchodilators. Treatment includes immediate discontinuation and symptomatic and supportive therapies. Cautious use of beta-adrenergic blocking agents may be considered in severe cases.

Drug Interactions

Decreased effect with beta-blockers
Increased toxicity with MAO inhibitors, TCAs

Ethanol/Nutrition/Herb Interactions Herb/Nutraceutical: Avoid ephedra, yohimbe (may cause CNS stimulation).

Dosage Forms

Injection, solution, as sulfate: 1 mg/mL (1 mL)
Tablet, as sulfate: 2.5 mg, 5 mg

Additional dosage forms available in Canada: Powder for oral inhalation (Bricanyl® Turbuhaler): 500 mcg/actuation [50 or 200 metered doses]

References

National Asthma Education and Prevention Program, "Expert Panel Report: Guidelines for the Diagnosis and Management of Asthma - Update on Selected Topics 2002," Bethesda, MD: National Institutes of Health, National Heart, Lung, and Blood Institute; 2003. NIH publication 02-5074. Available at: http://www.nhlbi.nih.gov/guidelines/asthma/asthmafullrpt.pdf.

♦ **Terrell™** *see* Isoflurane *on page 702*

Tetanus Immune Globulin (Human)

(TET a nus i MYUN GLOB yoo lin HYU man)

U.S. Brand Names BayTet™

Canadian Brand Names BayTet™

Synonyms TIG

Pharmacologic Category Immune Globulin

Generic Available No

Use Passive immunization against tetanus; tetanus immune globulin is preferred over tetanus antitoxin for treatment of active tetanus; part of the management of an unclean, wound in a person whose history of previous receipt of tetanus toxoid is unknown or who has received less than three doses of tetanus toxoid; elderly may require TIG more often than younger patients with tetanus infection due to declining antibody titers with age

Mechanism of Action Passive immunity toward tetanus

Pharmacodynamics/Kinetics Absorption: Well absorbed

Dosage I.M.:

Prophylaxis of tetanus:

Children: 4 units/kg; some recommend administering 250 units to small children

Adults: 250 units

Treatment of tetanus:

Children: 500-3000 units; some should infiltrate locally around the wound

Adults: 3000-6000 units

Stability Refrigerate

Administration Do not administer I.V.; I.M. use only

Pregnancy Risk Factor C

Contraindications Hypersensitivity to tetanus immune globulin, thimerosal, or any component of the formulation

Warnings/Precautions Have epinephrine 1:1000 available for anaphylactic reactions. Use caution in patients with isolated immunoglobulin A deficiency or a history of systemic hypersensitivity to human immunoglobulins. As a product of human plasma, this product may potentially transmit disease; screening of donors, as well as testing and/or inactivation of certain viruses reduces this risk. Use caution in patients with thrombocytopenia or coagulation disorders (I.M. injections may be contraindicated). Not for intravenous administration.

Adverse Reactions

>10%: Local: Pain, tenderness, erythema at injection site

1% to 10%:

Central nervous system: Fever (mild)

Dermatologic: Urticaria, angioedema

Neuromuscular & skeletal: Muscle stiffness

Miscellaneous: Anaphylaxis reaction

<1% (Limited to important or life-threatening): Sensitization to repeated injections

Drug Interactions Never administer tetanus toxoid and TIG in same syringe (toxoid will be neutralized); toxoid may be given at a separate site; concomitant administration with Td may decrease its immune response, especially in individuals with low prevaccination antibody titers

Dosage Forms Injection, solution [preservative free]: 250 units/mL (1 mL) [prefilled syringe]

Tetanus Toxoid (Adsorbed) (TET a nus TOKS oyd, ad SORBED)

Medication Safety Issues

Sound-alike/look-alike issues:

Tetanus toxoid products may be confused with influenza virus vaccine and tuberculin products. Medication errors have occurred when tetanus toxoid products have been inadvertently administered instead of tuberculin skin tests (PPD) and influenza virus vaccine. These products are refrigerated and often stored in close proximity to each other.

Pharmacologic Category Toxoid

Generic Available No

Use Active immunization against tetanus when combination antigen preparations are not indicated. **Note:** Tetanus and diphtheria toxoids for adult use (Td) is the preferred immunizing agent for most adults and for children after their seventh birthday. Young children should receive trivalent DTaP (diphtheria/tetanus/acellular pertussis), as part of their childhood immunization program, unless pertussis is contraindicated, then TD is warranted.

Mechanism of Action Tetanus toxoid preparations contain the toxin produced by virulent tetanus bacilli (detoxified growth products of *Clostridium tetani*). The toxin has been modified by treatment with formaldehyde so that it has lost toxicity but still retains ability to act as antigen and produce active immunity; the aluminum salt, a mineral adjuvant, delays the rate of absorption and prolongs and enhances its properties; duration ~10 years.

Pharmacodynamics/Kinetics Duration: Primary immunization: ~10 years

Dosage Children ≥7 years and Adults: I.M.:

Primary immunization: 0.5 mL; repeat 0.5 mL at 4-8 weeks after first dose and at 6-12 months after second dose

Routine booster dose: Recommended every 10 years

(Continued)

Tetanus Toxoid (Adsorbed) *(Continued)*

Note: In most patients, Td is the recommended product for primary immunization, booster doses, and tetanus immunization in wound management

Stability Refrigerate, do not freeze

Administration Inject intramuscularly in the area of the vastus lateralis (midthigh laterally) or deltoid. Do not inject into gluteal area. Shake well prior to withdrawing dose; do not use if product does not form a suspension.

For patients at risk of hemorrhage following intramuscular injection, the ACIP recommends "it should be administered intramuscularly if, in the opinion of the physician familiar with the patients bleeding risk, the vaccine can be administered with reasonable safety by this route. If the patient receives antihemophilia or other similar therapy, intramuscular vaccination can be scheduled shortly after such therapy is administered. A fine needle (23 gauge or smaller) can be used for the vaccination and firm pressure applied to the site (without rubbing) for at least 2 minutes. The patient should be instructed concerning the risk of hematoma from the injection."

Pregnancy Risk Factor C

Contraindications Hypersensitivity to tetanus toxoid or any component of the formulation

Warnings/Precautions Not equivalent to tetanus toxoid fluid; the tetanus toxoid adsorbed is the preferred toxoid for immunization and Td, TD or DTaP are the preferred adsorbed forms; avoid injection into a blood vessel; allergic reactions may occur; epinephrine 1:1000 must be available; elderly may not mount adequate antibody titers following immunization. Patients who are immunocompromised may have reduced response; may be used in patients with HIV infection. May defer elective immunization during febrile illness or acute infection; defer elective immunization during outbreaks of poliomyelitis. In patients with a history of severe local reaction (Arthus-type) or temperature of >39.4°C (>103°F) following previous dose, do not give further routine or emergency doses of tetanus and diphtheria toxoids for 10 years. Use caution in patients on anticoagulants, with thrombocytopenia, or bleeding disorders (bleeding may occur following intramuscular injection). Contains thimerosal; vial stopper may contain natural latex rubber. This product is not indicated for use in children <7 years of age.

Adverse Reactions All serious adverse reactions must be reported to the U.S. Department of Health and Human Services (DHHS) Vaccine Adverse Event Reporting System (VAERS) 1-800-822-7967.

Frequency not defined.

Cardiovascular: Hypotension

Central nervous system: Brachial neuritis, fever, malaise, pain

Gastrointestinal: Nausea

Local: Edema, induration (with or without tenderness), rash, redness, urticaria, warmth

Neuromuscular: Arthralgia, Guillain-Barré syndrome

Miscellaneous: Anaphylactic reaction, Arthus-type hypersensitivity reaction

Drug Interactions

Corticosteroids: When used in greater than physiologic doses, corticosteroids lead to decreased effect of vaccine; consider deferring immunization for 1 month after steroid is discontinued.

Immunosuppressive agents: Decreased response to vaccine; consider deferring immunization for 1 month after immunosuppressive agent is discontinued.

Dosage Forms Injection, suspension: Tetanus 5 Lf units per 0.5 mL (0.5 mL) [contains trace amounts of thimerosal]; (5 mL) [contains thimerosal; vial stopper contains latex]

Tetracaine (TET ra kane)

Related Information

Local Anesthetics *on page 1532*

U.S. Brand Names Pontocaine®; Pontocaine® Niphanoid®

Canadian Brand Names Ametop™; Pontocaine®

Synonyms Amethocaine Hydrochloride; Tetracaine Hydrochloride

Pharmacologic Category Local Anesthetic

Generic Available Yes: Ophthalmic solution, solution for injection

Use Spinal anesthesia; local anesthesia in the eye for various diagnostic and examination purposes; topically applied to nose and throat for various diagnostic procedures

Mechanism of Action Ester local anesthetic blocks both the initiation and conduction of nerve impulses by decreasing the neuronal membrane's permeability to sodium ions, which results in inhibition of depolarization with resultant blockade of conduction

Pharmacodynamics/Kinetics

Onset of action: Anesthetic: Rhinolaryngology: 5-10 minutes

Duration: Rhinolaryngology: ~30 minutes

Metabolism: Hepatic; detoxified by plasma esterases to aminobenzoic acid

Excretion: Urine

Dosage Adults:

Ophthalmic: Short-term anesthesia of the eye: 0.5% solution: Instill 1-2 drops; prolonged use (especially for at-home self-medication) is not recommended

Injection: Spinal anesthesia: **Note:** Dosage varies with the anesthetic procedure, the degree of anesthesia required, and the individual patient response; it is administered by subarachnoid injection for spinal anesthesia.

Perineal anesthesia: 5 mg

Perineal and lower extremities: 10 mg

Anesthesia extending up to costal margin: 15 mg; doses up to 20 mg may be given, but are reserved for exceptional cases

Low spinal anesthesia (saddle block): 2-5 mg

Topical mucous membranes (rhinolaryngology): Used as a 0.25% or 0.5% solution by direct application or nebulization; total dose should not exceed 20 mg

Stability

Solution for injection: Store solution under refrigeration; protect from light.

Hyperbaric solution: May be made by mixing equal volumes of the 1% solution and $D_{10}W$.

Powder for injection: Following reconstitution, store solution under refrigeration; protect from light.

Hyperbaric solution: Dissolve 10 mg of Pontocaine® Niphanoid® in 1 mL $D_{10}W$; further dilute with equal volume of spinal fluid. Resulting solution is D_5W with tetracaine 5 mg/mL.

Hypobaric solution: Dissolve 1 mg of Pontocaine® Niphanoid® in 1 mL SWFI.

Ophthalmic and topical solutions: Store under refrigeration at 2°C to 8°C

Administration Before injection, withdraw syringe plunger to make sure injection is not into vein or artery

Anesthesia and Critical Care Concerns/Other Considerations Tetracaine is ~10 times more potent than procaine.

Pregnancy Risk Factor C

Contraindications Hypersensitivity to tetracaine, ester-type anesthetics, aminobenzoic acid, or any component of the formulation; injection should not be used when spinal anesthesia is contraindicated

Warnings/Precautions Use with caution in patients with cardiac disease, hyperthyroidism, abnormal or decreased levels of plasma esterases. Use of the lowest effective dose is recommended. Acutely ill, elderly, debilitated, obstetric patients, or patients with increased intra-abdominal pressure may require decreased doses. Products may contain sodium bisulfite which may cause allergic reactions in some individuals.

Ophthalmic: May delay wound healing. Prolonged use is not recommended. The anesthetized eye should be protected from irritation, foreign bodies, and rubbing to prevent inadvertent damage.

Adverse Reactions Frequency not defined.

Injection: Note: Adverse effects listed are those characteristics of local anesthetics.

Cardiovascular: Cardiac arrest, hypotension

Central nervous system: Chills, convulsions, dizziness, drowsiness, nervousness, unconsciousness

Gastrointestinal: Nausea, vomiting

Neuromuscular & skeletal: Tremors

Ocular: Blurred vision, pupil constriction

Otic: Tinnitus

Respiratory: Respiratory arrest

Miscellaneous: Allergic reaction

Ophthalmic: Ocular: Chemosis, lacrimation, photophobia, transient stinging

(Continued)

Tetracaine *(Continued)*

With chronic use: Corneal erosions, corneal healing retardation, corneal opacification (permanent), corneal scarring, keratitis (severe)

Overdosage/Toxicology Symptoms of overdose include seizures, respiratory depression, lacrimation, bradycardia, and hypotension. Treatment is supportive.

Dosage Forms [DSC] = Discontinued product

Injection, solution, as hydrochloride [preservative free] (Pontocaine®): 1% [10 mg/mL] (2 mL) [contains sodium bisulfite]

Injection, solution, as hydrochloride [premixed in dextrose 6%] (Pontocaine®): 0.3% [3 mg/mL] (5 mL) [DSC]

Injection, powder for reconstitution, as hydrochloride [preservative free] (Pontocaine® Niphanoid®): 20 mg

Solution, ophthalmic, as hydrochloride: 0.5% [5 mg/mL] (15 mL)

Solution, topical, as hydrochloride (Pontocaine®): 2% [20 mg/mL] (30 mL, 118 mL) [for rhinolaryngology]

References

Bartfield JM, Lee FS, Raccio-Robak N, et al, "Topical Tetracaine Attenuates the Pain of Infiltration of Buffered Lidocaine," *Acad Emerg Med*, 1996, 3(11):1001-5.

Bonadio WA, "Safe and Effective Method for Application of Tetracaine, Adrenaline, and Cocaine to Oral Lacerations," *Ann Emerg Med*, 1996, 28(4):396-8.

Duffin RM and Olson RJ, "Tetracaine Toxicity," *Ann Ophthalmol*, 1984, 16(9):836, 838.

Garfield JM, Andriole GL, Vetto JL, et al, "Prolonged Diabetes Insipidus Subsequent to an Episode of Chemical Meningitis," *Anesthesiology*, 1986, 64(2):253-4.

Grant SA and Hoffman RS, "Use of Tetracain, Epinephrine, and Cocaine as a Topical Anesthetic in the Emergency Department," *Ann Emerg Med*, 1992, 21(8):987-97.

Kintner JC, Grossniklaus HE, Lass JH, et al, "Infectious Crystalline Keratopathy Associated With Topical Anesthetic Abuse," *Cornea*, 1990, 9(1):77-80.

Skidmore RA, Patterson JD, and Tomsick RS, "Local Anesthetics," *Dermatol Surg*, 1996, 22(6):511-22.

van Kan JH, Egberts AC, Rijnvos WP, et al, "Tetracaine Versus Lidocaine-Prilocaine for Preventing Venipuncture-Induced Pain in Children," *Am J Health Syst Pharm*, 1997, 54(4):388-92.

♦ **Tetracaine Hydrochloride** *see* Tetracaine *on page 1248*

♦ **Tetracosactide** *see* Cosyntropin *on page 333*

♦ **Tetrahydrocannabinol** *see* Dronabinol *on page 430*

♦ **Teveten®** *see* Eprosartan *on page 469*

♦ **Tev-Tropin™** *see* Human Growth Hormone *on page 625*

♦ **Texacort®** *see* Hydrocortisone *on page 639*

Thalidomide (tha LI doe mide)

Medication Safety Issues

Sound-alike/look-alike issues:

Thalidomide may be confused with flutamide

U.S. Brand Names Thalomid®

Canadian Brand Names Thalomid®

Synonyms NSC-66847

Pharmacologic Category Angiogenesis Inhibitor; Immunosuppressant Agent; Tumor Necrosis Factor (TNF) Blocking Agent

Restrictions Thalidomide is approved for marketing only under a special distribution program. This program, called the "System for Thalidomide Education and Prescribing Safety" (STEPS® 1-888-423-5436), has been approved by the FDA. Prescribers and pharmacists must be registered with the program. No more than a 4-week supply should be dispensed. Blister packs should be dispensed intact (do not repackage capsules). Prescriptions must be filled within 7 days. Subsequent prescriptions may be filled only if fewer than 7 days of therapy remain on the previous prescription. A new prescription is required for further dispensing (a telephone prescription may not be accepted).

Generic Available No

Use Treatment of multiple myeloma (in combination with dexamethasone); treatment and maintenance of cutaneous manifestations of erythema nodosum leprosum (ENL)

Unlabeled/Investigational Use Treatment of Crohn's disease; graft-versus-host reactions after bone marrow transplantation; AIDS-related aphthous stomatitis; Behçet's syndrome; Waldenström's macroglobulinemia; Langerhans cell histiocytosis; may be effective in rheumatoid arthritis, discoid lupus erythematosus, and erythema multiforme

Mechanism of Action Has immunomodulatory and antiangiogenic characteristics. Immunologic effects may vary based on conditions; may suppress excessive tumor necrosis factor-alpha production in patients with ENL, yet may increase plasma tumor necrosis factor-alpha levels in HIV-positive patients. In multiple myeloma, thalidomide is associated with an increase in natural killer cells and increased levels of interleukin-2 and interferon gamma. Other proposed mechanisms of action include suppression of angiogenesis, prevention of free-radical-mediated DNA damage, increased cell mediated cytotoxic effects, and altered expression of cellular.

Pharmacodynamics/Kinetics

Distribution: V_d: 120 L

Protein binding: 55% to 66%

Metabolism: Nonenzymatic hydrolysis in plasma; forms multiple metabolites

Half-life elimination: 5-7 hours

Time to peak, plasma: 3-6 hours

Excretion: Urine (<1% as unchanged drug)

Dosage Oral:

Multiple myeloma: 200 mg once daily (with dexamethasone 40 mg daily on days 1-4, 9-12, and 17-20 of a 28-day treatment cycle)

Cutaneous ENL:

Initial: 100-300 mg/day taken once daily at bedtime with water (at least 1 hour after evening meal)

Patients weighing <50 kg: Initiate at lower end of the dosing range

Severe cutaneous reaction or patients previously requiring high dose may be initiated at 400 mg/day; doses may be divided, but taken 1 hour after meals

Maintenance: Dosing should continue until active reaction subsides (usually at least 2 weeks), then tapered in 50 mg decrements every 2-4 weeks

Patients who flare during tapering or with a history or requiring prolonged maintenance should be maintained on the minimum dosage necessary to control the reaction. Efforts to taper should be repeated every 3-6 months, in increments of 50 mg every 2-4 weeks.

Behçet's syndrome (unlabeled use): 100-400 mg/day

Graft-vs-host reactions (unlabeled use): 100-1600 mg/day; usual initial dose: 200 mg 4 times/day for use up to 700 days

AIDS-related aphthous stomatitis (unlabeled use): 200 mg twice daily for 5 days, then 200 mg/day for up to 8 weeks

Discoid lupus erythematosus (unlabeled use): 100-400 mg/day; maintenance dose: 25-50 mg

Stability Store at 15°C to 30°C (50°F to 86°F). Protect from light. Keep in original package.

Administration Oral: Administer with water, preferably at bedtime once daily, at least 1 hour after the evening meal. Avoid extensive handling of capsules; capsules should remain in blister pack until ingestion. If exposed to the powder content from broken capsules or body fluids from patients receiving thalidomide, the exposed area should be washed with soap and water.

Monitoring Parameters CBC with differential, platelets; signs of neuropathy monthly for the first 3 months, then periodically during treatment; consider monitoring of sensory nerve application potential amplitudes (at baseline and every 6 months) to detect asymptomatic neuropathy. In HIV-seropositive patients: viral load after 1 and 3 months, then every 3 months. Pregnancy testing (sensitivity of at least 50 mIU/mL) is required within 24 hours prior to initiation of therapy, weekly during the first 4 weeks, then every 4 weeks in women with regular menstrual cycles or every 2 weeks in women with irregular menstrual cycles.

Reference Range Therapeutic plasma thalidomide levels in graft-vs-host reactions are 5-8 mcg/mL, although it has been suggested that lower plasma levels (0.5-1.5 mcg/mL) may be therapeutic; peak serum thalidomide level after a 200 mg dose: 1.2 mcg/mL

Pregnancy Risk Factor X

Contraindications Hypersensitivity to thalidomide or any component of the formulation; neuropathy (peripheral); patient unable to comply with STEPS® program (including males); women of childbearing potential unless alternative therapies are inappropriate and adequate precautions are taken to avoid pregnancy; pregnancy

Warnings/Precautions Hazardous agent — use appropriate precautions for handling and disposal. **[U.S. Boxed Warning]: Thalidomide is a known teratogen; effective contraception must be used for at least 4 weeks before initiating therapy, during therapy, and for 4 weeks following discontinuation**

(Continued)

Thalidomide *(Continued)*

of thalidomide for women of childbearing potential. Use caution with drugs which may decrease the efficacy of hormonal contraceptives. May cause sedation; patients must be warned to use caution when performing tasks which require alertness. Use caution in patients with renal or hepatic impairment, neurological disorders, or constipation.

Thalidomide has been associated with the development of peripheral neuropathy, which may be irreversible; use caution with other medications which may cause peripheral neuropathy. Consider immediate discontinuation (if clinically appropriate) in patients who develop neuropathy. May cause seizures; use caution in patients with a history of seizures, concurrent therapy with drugs which alter seizure threshold, or conditions which predispose to seizures. May cause neutropenia; discontinue therapy if absolute neutrophil count decreases to <750/mm^3. Use caution in patients with HIV infection; has been associated with increased viral loads.

May cause orthostasis and/or bradycardia; use with caution in patients with cardiovascular disease or in patients who would not tolerate transient hypotensive episodes. Thrombotic events have been reported, generally in patients with other risk factors for thrombosis (neoplastic disease, inflammatory disease, or concurrent therapy with other drugs, including dexamethasone, which may cause thrombosis). **[U.S. Boxed Warning]: Use in multiple myeloma is associated with increased risk for deep vein thrombosis (DVT) and pulmonary embolism (PE), monitor for signs and symptoms of thromboembolism; patients at risk may benefit from prophylactic anticoagulation or aspirin.** Hypersensitivity, Stevens-Johnson syndrome (SJS) and toxic epidermal necrolysis (TEN) have been reported; withhold therapy and evaluate with skin rashes; permanently discontinued if rash is exfoliative, purpuric, bullous or if SJS or TEN is suspected. Safety and efficacy have not been established in children <12 years of age.

Adverse Reactions

>10%:

Cardiovascular: Edema (57%), thrombosis/embolism (23%; grade 3: 13%, grade 4: 9%), hypotension (16%)

Central nervous system: Fatigue (79%; grade 3: 3%, grade 4: 1%), somnolence (36% to 38%), dizziness (4% to 20%), sensory neuropathy (54%), confusion (28%), anxiety/agitation (9% to 26%), fever (19% to 23%), motor neuropathy (22%), headache (13% to 19%)

Dermatologic: Rash (21% to 31%), rash/desquamation (30%; grade 3: 4%), dry skin (21%), maculopapular rash (4% to 19%), acne (3% to 11%)

Endocrine & metabolic: Hypocalcemia (72%)

Gastrointestinal: Constipation (3% to 55%), anorexia (3% to 28%), nausea (4% to 24%), weight loss (23%), weight gain (22%), diarrhea (4% to 19%), oral moniliasis (4% to 11%)

Hematologic: Leukopenia (17% to 35%), neutropenia (31%), anemia (6% to 13%), lymphadenopathy (6% to 13%)

Hepatic: AST/SGOT increased (3% to 25%), bilirubin increased (14%)

Neuromuscular & skeletal: Muscle weakness (40%), tremor (4% to 26%), weakness (6% to 22%), myalgia (17%), paresthesia (6% to 16%), arthralgia (13%)

Renal: Hematuria (11%)

Respiratory: Dyspnea (42%)

Miscellaneous: Diaphoresis (13%)

1% to 10%:

Cardiovascular: Facial edema (4%), peripheral edema (3% to 8%)

Central nervous system: Insomnia (9%), nervousness (3% to 9%), malaise (8%), vertigo (8%), pain (3% to 8%)

Dermatologic: Dermatitis (fungal 4% to 9%), pruritus (3% to 8%), nail disorder (3% to 4%)

Endocrine & metabolic: Hyperlipemia (6% to 9%)

Gastrointestinal: Xerostomia (8% to 9%), flatulence (8%), tooth pain (4%)

Genitourinary: Impotence (3% to 8%)

Hepatic: LFTs abnormal (9%)

Neuromuscular & skeletal: Neuropathy (8%), back pain (4% to 6%), neck pain (4%), neck rigidity (4%)

Renal: Albuminuria (3% to 8%)

Respiratory: Pharyngitis (4% to 8%), rhinitis (4%), sinusitis (4% to 8%)

Miscellaneous: Infection (6% to 8%)

Postmarketing and/or case reports (limited to important or life-threatening): Acute renal failure, alkaline phosphatase increased, amenorrhea, aphthous stomatitis, arrhythmia, atrial fibrillation, bile duct obstruction, bradycardia, BUN increased, carpal tunnel, CML, creatinine clearance decreased, creatinine increased, deafness, depression, diplopia, dysesthesia, ECG abnormalities, electrolyte imbalances, enuresis, eosinophilia, epistaxis, erythema multiforme, erythema nodosum, erythroleukemia, exfoliative dermatitis, febrile neutropenia, foot drop, galactorrhea, granulocytopenia, gynecomastia, hepatomegaly, Hodgkin's disease, hypercalcemia, hyper-/hypokalemia, hypersensitivity, hypertension, hyper-/hypothyroidism, hyperuricemia, hypomagnesemia, hyponatremia, hypoproteinemia, intestinal obstruction, intestinal perforation, interstitial pneumonitis, LDH increased, lethargy, leukocytosis, lymphedema, lymphopenia, mental status changes, metrorrhagia, migraine, myxedema, nystagmus, oliguria, orthostatic hypotension, pancytopenia, paresthesia, petechiae, peripheral neuritis, photosensitivity, pleural effusion, prothrombin time changes, psychosis, pulmonary embolus, pulmonary hypertension, purpura, Raynaud's syndrome, seizure, SGPT increased, status epilepticus, Stevens-Johnson syndrome, stomach ulcer, stupor, suicide attempt, syncope, tachycardia, thrombocytopenia, toxic epidermal necrolysis, tumor lysis syndrome

Overdosage/Toxicology Doses of up to 14.4 g have been reported (in suicide attempts) without fatalities. Treatment is symptom-directed and supportive.

Drug Interactions

Abatacept: Thalidomide may be associated with increased risk of serious infection when used in combination with abatacept.

Anakinra: Thalidomide may be associated with increased risk of serious infection when used in combination with anakinra.

CNS depressants: Thalidomide may enhance the sedative activity of other drugs such as ethanol, barbiturates, reserpine, and chlorpromazine

Vaccine (dead organism): Thalidomide may decrease the effect of vaccines (dead organisms).

Vaccine (live organism): Thalidomide may increase the risk of vaccinal infection.

Ethanol/Nutrition/Herb Interactions

Ethanol: Avoid ethanol (may increase sedation).

Herb/Nutraceutical: Avoid cat's claw and echinacea (have immunostimulant properties; consider therapy modifications).

Dietary Considerations Should be taken at least 1 hour after the evening meal.

Dosage Forms

Capsule:

Thalomid®: 50 mg, 100 mg, 200 mg

- **Thalomid®** *see* Thalidomide *on page 1250*
- **THC** *see* Dronabinol *on page 430*
- **Theo-24®** *see* Theophylline *on page 1253*
- **TheoCap™** *see* Theophylline *on page 1253*
- **Theochron®** *see* Theophylline *on page 1253*
- **Theochron® SR (Can)** *see* Theophylline *on page 1253*
- **Theolair™ (Can)** *see* Theophylline *on page 1253*

Theophylline (thee OFF i lin)

Medication Safety Issues

Sound-alike/look-alike issues:

Theolair™ may be confused with Thiola®, Thyrolar®

Related Information

Anesthesia for Patients With Liver Disease *on page 1421*

U.S. Brand Names Elixophyllin®; Quibron®-T; Quibron®-T/SR; Theo-24®; TheoCap™; Theochron®; Uniphyl®

Canadian Brand Names Apo-Theo LA®; Novo-Theophyl SR; PMS-Theophylline; Pulmophylline; ratio-Theo-Bronc; Theochron® SR; Theolair™; Uniphyl® SRT

Synonyms Theophylline Anhydrous

Pharmacologic Category Theophylline Derivative

Generic Available Yes: Extended release capsule and tablet, infusion

Use Treatment of symptoms and reversible airway obstruction due to chronic asthma, chronic bronchitis, or COPD

Mechanism of Action Causes bronchodilatation, diuresis, CNS and cardiac stimulation, and gastric acid secretion by blocking phosphodiesterase which

(Continued)

Theophylline *(Continued)*

increases tissue concentrations of cyclic adenine monophosphate (cAMP) which in turn promotes catecholamine stimulation of lipolysis, glycogenolysis, and gluconeogenesis and induces release of epinephrine from adrenal medulla cells

Pharmacodynamics/Kinetics

Absorption: Oral: Dosage form dependent

Distribution: 0.45 L/kg based on ideal body weight

Metabolism: Children >1 year and Adults: Hepatic; involves CYP1A2, 2E1 and 3A4; forms active metabolites (caffeine and 3-methylxanthine)

Half-life elimination: Highly variable and dependent upon age, liver function, cardiac function, lung disease, and smoking history

Time to peak, serum:

Oral: Liquid: 1 hour; Tablet, enteric-coated: 5 hours; Tablet, uncoated: 2 hours

I.V.: Within 30 minutes

Excretion: Urine

Neonates: 50% unchanged

Children >3 months and Adults: 10% unchanged

Dosage Use ideal body weight for obese patients

I.V.: Initial: Maintenance infusion rates:

Children:

6 weeks to 6 months: 0.5 mg/kg/hour

6 months to 1 year: 0.6-0.7 mg/kg/hour

Children >1 year and Adults:

Acute bronchospasm: See table on next page.

Approximate I.V. maintenance dosages are based upon continuous infusions; bolus dosing (often used in children <6 months of age) may be determined by multiplying the hourly infusion rate by 24 hours and dividing by the desired number of doses/day. See the following:

Maintenance dose for acute symptoms: See table below.

Dosage should be adjusted according to serum level measurements during the first 12- to 24-hour period. See table on next page.

Oral theophylline: Initial dosage recommendation: Loading dose (to achieve a serum level of about 10 mcg/mL; loading doses should be given using a rapidly absorbed oral product **not** a sustained release product):

If no theophylline has been administered in the previous 24 hours: 4-6 mg/kg theophylline

Maintenance Dose for Acute Symptoms

Population Group	Oral Theophylline (mg/kg/day)	I.V. Aminophylline
Premature infant or newborn - 6 wk (for apnea/bradycardia)	4	5 mg/kg/day
6 wk - 6 mo	10	12 mg/kg/day or continuous I.V. infusion[1]
Infants 6 mo - 1 y	12-18	15 mg/kg/day or continuous I.V. infusion[1]
Children 1-9 y	20-24	1 mg/kg/h
Children 9-12 y, and adolescent daily smokers of cigarettes or marijuana, and otherwise healthy adult smokers <50 y	16	0.9 mg/kg/h
Adolescents 12-16 y (nonsmokers)	13	0.7 mg/kg/h
Otherwise healthy nonsmoking adults (including elderly patients)	10 (not to exceed 900 mg/day)	0.5 mg/kg/h
Cardiac decompensation, cor pulmonale, and/or liver dysfunction	5 (not to exceed 400 mg/day)	0.25 mg/kg/h

[1]For continuous I.V. infusion divide total daily dose by 24 = mg/kg/h.

Approximate I.V. Theophylline Dosage for Treatment of Acute Bronchospasm

Group	Dosage for Next 12 h[1]	Dosage After 12 h[1]
Infants 6 wk - 6 mo	0.5 mg/kg/h	
Children 6 mo - 1 y	0.6-0.7 mg/kg/h	
Children 1-9 y	0.95 mg/kg/h (1.2 mg/kg/h)	0.79 mg/kg/h (1 mg/kg/h)
Children 9-16 y and young adult smokers	0.79 mg/kg/h (1 mg/kg/h)	0.63 mg/kg/h (0.8 mg/kg/h)
Healthy, nonsmoking adults	0.55 mg/kg/h (0.7 mg/kg/h)	0.39 mg/kg/h (0.5 mg/kg/h)
Older patients and patients with cor pulmonale	0.47 mg/kg/h (0.6 mg/kg/h)	0.24 mg/kg/h (0.3 mg/kg/h)
Patients with congestive heart failure or liver failure	0.39 mg/kg/h (0.5 mg/kg/h)	0.08-0.16 mg/kg/h (0.1-0.2 mg/kg/h)

[1]Equivalent hydrous aminophylline dosage indicated in parentheses.

Dosage Adjustment After Serum Theophylline Measurement

Serum Theophylline		Guidelines
Within normal limits	10-20 mcg/mL	Maintain dosage if tolerated. Recheck serum theophylline concentration at 6- to 12-month intervals.[1]
Too high	20-25 mcg/mL	Decrease doses by about 10%. Recheck serum theophylline concentration after 3 days and then at 6- to 12-month intervals.[1]
	25-30 mcg/mL	Skip next dose and decrease subsequent doses by about 25%. Recheck serum theophylline.
	>30 mcg/mL	Skip next 2 doses and decrease subsequent doses by 50%. Recheck serum theophylline.
Too low	7.5-10 mcg/mL	Increase dose by about 25%.[2] Recheck serum theophylline concentration after 3 days and then at 6- to 12-month intervals.[1]
	5-7.5 mcg/mL	Increase dose by about 25% to the nearest dose increment[2] and recheck serum theophylline for guidance in further dosage adjustment (another increase will probably be needed, but this provides a safety check).

[1]Finer adjustments in dosage may be needed for some patients.

[2]Dividing the daily dose into 3 doses administered at 8-hour intervals may be indicated if symptoms occur repeatedly at the end of a dosing interval.

From Weinberger M and Hendeles L, "Practical Guide to Using Theophylline," *J Resp Dis*, 1981,2:12-27.

Oral Theophylline Dosage for Bronchial Asthma[1]

Age (y)	Initial 3 Days	Second 3 Days	Steady-State Maintenance
<1	0.2 x (age in weeks) + 5		0.3 x (age in weeks) + 8
1-9	16 up to a maximum of 400 mg/24 h	20	22
9-12	16 up to a maximum of 400 mg/24 h	16 up to a maximum of 600 mg/24 h	20 up to a maximum of 800 mg/24 h
12-16	16 up to a maximum of 400 mg/24 h	16 up to a maximum of 600 mg/24 h	18 up to a maximum of 900 mg/24 h
Adults	400 mg/24 h	600 mg/24 h	900 mg/24 h

[1]Dose in mg/kg/24 hours of theophylline.

Theophylline *(Continued)*

If theophylline has been administered in the previous 24 hours: administer 1/2 loading dose or 2-3 mg/kg theophylline can be given in emergencies when serum levels are not available

On the average, for every 1 mg/kg theophylline given, blood levels will rise 2 mcg/mL

Ideally, defer the loading dose if a serum theophylline concentration can be obtained rapidly. However, if this is not possible, exercise clinical judgment. If the patient is not experiencing theophylline toxicity, this is unlikely to result in dangerous adverse effects.

Oral theophylline dosage for bronchial asthma (by age): See table on previous page.

Increasing dose: The dosage may be increased in approximately 25% increments at 2- to 3-day intervals so long as the drug is tolerated or until the maximum dose is reached

Maintenance dose: In children and healthy adults, a slow-release product can be used; the total daily dose can be divided every 8-12 hours

Administration Oral: Long-acting preparations should be taken with a full glass of water, swallowed whole, or cut in half if scored. Do **not** crush. Extended release capsule forms may be opened and the contents sprinkled on soft foods; do **not** chew beads.

Pregnancy Risk Factor C

Contraindications Hypersensitivity to theophylline or any component of the formulation; premixed injection may contain corn-derived dextrose and its use is contraindicated in patients with allergy to corn-related products

Warnings/Precautions If a patient develops signs and symptoms of theophylline toxicity (eg, persistent, repetitive vomiting), a serum theophylline level should be measured and subsequent doses held. Due to potential saturation of theophylline clearance at serum levels in or (in some patients) less than the therapeutic range, dosage adjustment should be made in small increments (maximum: 25%). Due to wider interpatient variability, theophylline serum level measurements must be used to optimize therapy and prevent serious toxicity. Use with caution in patients with peptic ulcer, hyperthyroidism, seizure disorders, hypertension, and patients with cardiac arrhythmias (excluding bradyarrhythmias).

Adverse Reactions

Adverse reactions/theophylline serum level: (Adverse effects do not necessarily occur according to serum levels. Arrhythmia and seizure can occur without seeing the other adverse effects).

15-25 mcg/mL: GI upset, diarrhea, nausea/vomiting, abdominal pain, nervousness, headache, insomnia, agitation, dizziness, muscle cramp, tremor

25-35 mcg/mL: Tachycardia, occasional PVC

>35 mcg/mL: Ventricular tachycardia, frequent PVC, seizure

Uncommon at serum theophylline concentrations ≤20 mcg/mL:

1% to 10%:

Cardiovascular: Tachycardia

Central nervous system: Nervousness, restlessness

Gastrointestinal: Nausea, vomiting

<1% (Limited to important or life-threatening): Insomnia, irritability, seizure, tremor

Overdosage/Toxicology Symptoms of overdose include nausea, vomiting, insomnia, irritability, tachycardia, seizures, tonic-clonic seizures, insomnia, and circulatory failure. If seizures have not occurred, induce vomiting; ipecac syrup is preferred. Do not induce emesis in the presence of impaired consciousness. Repeated doses of charcoal have been shown to be effective in enhancing the total body clearance of theophylline. Do not repeat charcoal doses if an ileus is present. Charcoal hemoperfusion may be considered if serum theophylline levels exceed 40 mcg/mL, the patient is unable to tolerate repeat oral charcoal administrations, or if severe toxic symptoms are present. Clearance with hemoperfusion is better than clearance from hemodialysis. Administer a cathartic, especially if sustained release agents were used. Phenobarbital administered prophylactically may prevent seizures.

Drug Interactions Substrate of CYP1A2 (major), 2C9 (minor), 2D6 (minor), 2E1 (major), 3A4 (major); **Inhibits** CYP1A2 (weak)

CYP1A2 inducers: May decrease the levels/effects of theophylline. Example inducers include aminoglutethimide, carbamazepine, phenobarbital, and rifampin.

CYP1A2 inhibitors: May increase the levels/effects of theophylline. Example inhibitors include ciprofloxacin, fluvoxamine, ketoconazole, norfloxacin, ofloxacin, and rofecoxib.

CYP2E1 inhibitors: May increase the levels/effects of theophylline. Example inhibitors include disulfiram, isoniazid, and miconazole.

CYP3A4 inducers: CYP3A4 inducers may decrease the levels/effects of theophylline. Example inducers include aminoglutethimide, carbamazepine, nafcillin, nevirapine, phenobarbital, phenytoin, and rifamycins.

CYP3A4 inhibitors: May increase the levels/effects of theophylline. Example inhibitors include azole antifungals, clarithromycin, diclofenac, doxycycline, erythromycin, imatinib, isoniazid, nefazodone, nicardipine, propofol, protease inhibitors, quinidine, telithromycin, and verapamil.

Ethanol/Nutrition/Herb Interactions Food: Food does not appreciably affect the absorption of liquid, fast-release products, and most sustained release products; however, food may induce a sudden release (dose-dumping) of once-daily sustained release products resulting in an increase in serum drug levels and potential toxicity. Avoid excessive amounts of caffeine. Avoid extremes of dietary protein and carbohydrate intake. Changes in diet may affect the elimination of theophylline; charbroiled foods may increase elimination, reducing half-life by 50%.

Dietary Considerations Should be taken with water 1 hour before or 2 hours after meals. Premixed injection may contain corn-derived dextrose and its use is contraindicated in patients with allergy to corn-related products.

Dosage Forms

Capsule, extended release: 100 mg, 125 mg, 200 mg, 300 mg
- TheoCap™: 125 mg, 200 mg, 300 mg [12 hour]
- Theo-24®: 100 mg, 200 mg, 300 mg, 400 mg [24 hours]

Elixir:
- Elixophyllin®: 80 mg/15 mL (480 mL) [contains alcohol 20%; fruit flavor]

Infusion [premixed in D_5W]: 200 mg (50 mL, 100 mL); 400 mg (100 mL, 250 mL, 500 mL); 800 mg (250 mL, 500 mL, 1000 mL)

Tablet, controlled release:
- Uniphyl®: 400 mg, 600 mg [24 hours; contains cetostearyl alcohol]

Tablet, extended release: 100 mg, 200 mg, 300 mg, 450 mg
- Theochron®: 100 mg, 200 mg, 300 mg, 450 mg [12-24 hours]

Tablet, immediate release:
- Quibron®-T: 300 mg

Tablet, sustained release:
- Quibron®-T/SR: 300 mg [8-12 hours]

- ♦ **Theophylline Anhydrous** *see* Theophylline *on page 1253*
- ♦ **Theramycin Z®** *see* Erythromycin *on page 476*
- ♦ **Theratears®** *see* Carboxymethylcellulose *on page 230*
- ♦ **Thermazene®** *see* Silver Sulfadiazine *on page 1173*
- ♦ **Thiamazole** *see* Methimazole *on page 817*

Thiopental (thye oh PEN tal)

Related Information

Anesthesia Considerations for Neurosurgery *on page 1401*
Anesthesia for Patients With Liver Disease *on page 1421*
Chronic Renal Failure *on page 1437*
Intravenous Anesthetic Agents *on page 1531*

U.S. Brand Names Pentothal®

Canadian Brand Names Pentothal®

Synonyms Thiopental Sodium

Pharmacologic Category Anticonvulsant, Barbiturate; Barbiturate; General Anesthetic

Restrictions C-III

Generic Available No

Use Induction of anesthesia; adjunct for intubation in head injury patients; control of convulsive states; treatment of elevated intracranial pressure

Mechanism of Action Short-acting barbiturate with sedative, hypnotic, and anticonvulsant properties. Barbiturates depress the sensory cortex, decrease motor activity, alter cerebellar function, and produce drowsiness, sedation, and
(Continued)

Thiopental *(Continued)*

hypnosis. In high doses, barbiturates exhibit anticonvulsant activity; barbiturates produce dose-dependent respiratory depression.

Pharmacodynamics/Kinetics

Onset of action: Anesthetic: I.V.: 30-60 seconds

Duration: 5-30 minutes

Distribution: V_d: 1.4 L/kg

Protein binding: 72% to 86%

Metabolism: Hepatic, primarily to inactive metabolites but pentobarbital is also formed

Half-life elimination: 3-11.5 hours; decreased in children

Dosage I.V.:

Induction anesthesia:
- Infants: 5-8 mg/kg
- Children 1-12 years: 5-6 mg/kg
- Adults: 3-5 mg/kg

Maintenance anesthesia:
- Children: 1 mg/kg as needed
- Adults: 25-100 mg as needed

Increased intracranial pressure: Children and Adults: 1.5-5 mg/kg/dose; repeat as needed to control intracranial pressure

Seizures:
- Children: 2-3 mg/kg/dose; repeat as needed
- Adults: 75-250 mg/dose; repeat as needed

Dosing adjustment in renal impairment: Cl_{cr} <10 mL/minute: Administer at 75% of normal dose

Note: Accumulation may occur with chronic dosing due to lipid solubility; prolonged recovery may result from redistribution of thiopental from fat stores

Stability Reconstituted solutions remain stable for 3 days at room temperature and 7 days when refrigerated; solutions are alkaline and **incompatible** with drugs with acidic pH, such as succinylcholine, atropine sulfate, etc. I.V. form is **incompatible** when mixed with amikacin, benzquinamide, chlorpromazine, codeine, dimenhydrinate, diphenhydramine, glycopyrrolate, hydromorphone, insulin, levorphanol, meperidine, metaraminol, morphine, norepinephrine, penicillin G, prochlorperazine, succinylcholine, tetracycline

Administration Administer slowly over 20-30 seconds. Rapid I.V. injection may cause hypotension or decreased cardiac output; avoid extravasation, necrosis may occur. Check I.V. catheter placement prior to administration.

Monitoring Parameters Respiratory rate, heart rate, blood pressure

Reference Range Therapeutic: Hypnotic: 1-5 mcg/mL (SI: 4.1-20.7 µmol/L); Coma: 30-100 mcg/mL (SI: 124-413 µmol/L); Anesthesia: 7-130 mcg/mL (SI: 29-536 µmol/L); Toxic: >10 mcg/mL (SI: >41 µmol/L)

Anesthesia and Critical Care Concerns/Other Considerations Thiopental switches from linear to nonlinear pharmacokinetics following prolonged continuous infusions.

Pregnancy Risk Factor C

Contraindications Hypersensitivity to thiopental, barbiturates, or any component of the formulation; status asthmaticus; severe cardiovascular disease; porphyria (variegate or acute intermittent); should not be administered by intra-arterial injection

Warnings/Precautions Laryngospasm or bronchospasms may occur; use with extreme caution in patients with reactive airway diseases (asthma or COPD). Use with caution when the hypnotic may be prolonged or potentiated (excessive premedication, Addison's disease, hepatic or renal dysfunction, myxedema, increased blood urea, severe anemia, or myasthenia gravis). Potential for drug dependency exists, abrupt cessation may precipitate withdrawal, including status epilepticus in epileptic patients. Do not administer to patients in acute pain. Use caution in patients with unstable aneurysms, cardiovascular disease, renal impairment, or hepatic disease. Use caution in elderly, debilitated, or pediatric patients. May cause paradoxical responses, including agitation and hyperactivity, particularly in acute pain and pediatric patients. Effects with other sedative drugs or ethanol may be potentiated. May cause respiratory depression or hypotension. Use with caution in hemodynamically unstable patients (hypotension or shock) or patients with respiratory disease. Repeated dosing or continuous infusions may cause cumulative effects. Extravasation or intra-arterial injection causes necrosis due to pH of 10.6, ensure patient has intravenous access.

Adverse Reactions Frequency not defined.

Cardiovascular: Bradycardia, hypotension, syncope

Central nervous system: Drowsiness, lethargy, CNS excitation or depression, impaired judgment, "hangover" effect, confusion, somnolence, agitation, hyperkinesia, ataxia, nervousness, headache, insomnia, nightmares, hallucinations, anxiety, dizziness, shivering

Dermatologic: Rash, exfoliative dermatitis, Stevens-Johnson syndrome

Gastrointestinal: Nausea, vomiting, constipation

Hematologic: Agranulocytosis, thrombocytopenia, megaloblastic anemia, immune hemolytic anemia (rare)

Local: Pain at injection site, thrombophlebitis with I.V. use

Renal: Oliguria

Respiratory: Laryngospasm, respiratory depression, apnea (especially with rapid I.V. use), hypoventilation, sneezing, cough, bronchospasm

Miscellaneous: Gangrene with inadvertent intra-arterial injection, anaphylaxis, anaphylactic reactions

Overdosage/Toxicology Symptoms of overdose include respiratory depression, hypotension, shock. Hypotension should respond to I.V. fluids and placement of patient in Trendelenburg position; if necessary, pressors such as norepinephrine may be used; patient may require ventilatory support.

Drug Interactions

CNS depressants: Sedative effects and/or respiratory depression with barbiturates may be additive with other CNS depressants; monitor for increased effect; includes ethanol, sedatives, antidepressants, narcotic analgesics, and benzodiazepines

Felbamate may inhibit the metabolism of barbiturates and barbiturates may increase the metabolism of felbamate

Methoxyflurane: Barbiturates may enhance the nephrotoxic effects of methoxyflurane

Dietary Considerations Sodium content of 1 g (injection): 86.8 mg (3.8 mEq)

Dosage Forms Injection, powder for reconstitution, as sodium: 250 mg, 400 mg, 500 mg, 1 g

♦ **Thiopental Sodium** *see* Thiopental *on page 1257*

Thioridazine (thye oh RID a zeen)

Medication Safety Issues

Sound-alike/look-alike issues:

Thioridazine may be confused with thiothixene, Thorazine®

Mellaril® may be confused with Elavil®, Mebaral®

Canadian Brand Names Apo-Thioridazine®; Mellaril®

Synonyms Thioridazine Hydrochloride

Pharmacologic Category Antipsychotic Agent, Typical, Phenothiazine

Generic Available Yes

Use Management of schizophrenic patients who fail to respond adequately to treatment with other antipsychotic drugs, either because of insufficient effectiveness or the inability to achieve an effective dose due to intolerable adverse effects from those medications

Unlabeled/Investigational Use Psychosis

Mechanism of Action Thioridazine is a piperidine phenothiazine which blocks postsynaptic mesolimbic dopaminergic receptors in the brain; exhibits a strong alpha-adrenergic blocking effect and depresses the release of hypothalamic and hypophyseal hormones

Pharmacodynamics/Kinetics

Duration: 4-5 days

Half-life elimination: 21-25 hours

Time to peak, serum: ~1 hour

Dosage Oral:

Children >2-12 years: Range: 0.5-3 mg/kg/day in 2-3 divided doses; usual: 1 mg/kg/day; maximum: 3 mg/kg/day

Behavior problems: Initial: 10 mg 2-3 times/day, increase gradually

Severe psychoses: Initial: 25 mg 2-3 times/day, increase gradually

(Continued)

Thioridazine *(Continued)*

Children >12 years and Adults:

Schizophrenia/psychoses: Initial: 50-100 mg 3 times/day with gradual increments as needed and tolerated; maximum: 800 mg/day in 2-4 divided doses

Depressive disorders/dementia: Initial: 25 mg 3 times/day; maintenance dose: 20-200 mg/day

Elderly: Behavioral symptoms associated with dementia: Oral: Initial: 10-25 mg 1-2 times/day; increase at 4- to 7-day intervals by 10-25 mg/day; increase dose intervals (once daily, twice daily, etc) as necessary to control response or side effects. Maximum daily dose: 400 mg; gradual increases (titration) may prevent some side effects or decrease their severity.

Hemodialysis: Not dialyzable (0% to 5%)

Stability Protect from light

Administration Do not take antacid within 2 hours of taking drug.

Monitoring Parameters Baseline and periodic ECG; vital signs; serum potassium, lipid profile, fasting blood glucose and Hgb A_{1c}; BMI; mental status, abnormal involuntary movement scale (AIMS); periodic eye exam; do not initiate if QT_c >450 msec

Reference Range Toxic: >1 mg/mL; lethal: 2-8 mg/dL

Pregnancy Risk Factor C

Contraindications Hypersensitivity to thioridazine or any component of the formulation (cross-reactivity between phenothiazines may occur); severe CNS depression; circulatory collapse; severe hypotension; bone marrow suppression; blood dyscrasias; coma; in combination with other drugs that are known to prolong the QT_c interval; in patients with congenital long QT syndrome or a history of cardiac arrhythmias; concurrent use with medications that inhibit the metabolism of thioridazine (fluoxetine, paroxetine, fluvoxamine, propranolol, pindolol); patients known to have genetic defect leading to reduced levels of activity of CYP2D6

Warnings/Precautions [U.S. Boxed Warning]: Thioridazine has dose-related effects on ventricular repolarization leading to QT_c prolongation, a potentially life-threatening effect. Therefore, it should be reserved for patients with schizophrenia who have failed to respond to adequate levels of other antipsychotic drugs. May cause orthostatic hypotension - use with caution in patients at risk of this effect or those who would tolerate transient hypotensive episodes (cerebrovascular disease, cardiovascular disease, or other medications which may predispose).

Highly sedating, use with caution in disorders where CNS depression is a feature. Use with caution in Parkinson's disease. Caution in patients with hemodynamic instability; bone marrow suppression; predisposition to seizures; subcortical brain damage; severe cardiac, hepatic, renal, or respiratory disease. Esophageal dysmotility and aspiration have been associated with antipsychotic use - use with caution in patients at risk of pneumonia (ie, Alzheimer's disease). Caution in breast cancer or other prolactin-dependent tumors (may elevate prolactin levels). May alter temperature regulation or mask toxicity of other drugs due to antiemetic effects.

Phenothiazines may cause anticholinergic effects (confusion, agitation, constipation, xerostomia, blurred vision, urinary retention); therefore, they should be used with caution in patients with decreased gastrointestinal motility, urinary retention, BPH, xerostomia, or visual problems. Conditions which also may be exacerbated by cholinergic blockade include narrow-angle glaucoma (screening is recommended) and worsening of myasthenia gravis. Relative to other neuroleptics, thioridazine has a high potency of cholinergic blockade.

May cause extrapyramidal symptoms, including pseudoparkinsonism, acute dystonic reactions, akathisia, and tardive dyskinesia (risk of these reactions is low relative to other neuroleptics). May be associated with neuroleptic malignant syndrome (NMS). Doses exceeding recommended doses may cause pigmentary retinopathy.

Adverse Reactions Frequency not defined.

Cardiovascular: Hypotension, orthostatic hypotension, peripheral edema, ECG changes

Central nervous system: EPS (pseudoparkinsonism, akathisia, dystonias, tardive dyskinesia), dizziness, drowsiness, neuroleptic malignant syndrome (NMS), impairment of temperature regulation, lowering of seizure threshold

Dermatologic: Increased sensitivity to sun, rash, discoloration of skin (blue-gray)

Endocrine & metabolic: Changes in menstrual cycle, libido (changes in), breast pain, galactorrhea, amenorrhea
Gastrointestinal: Constipation, weight gain, nausea, vomiting, stomach pain, xerostomia, diarrhea
Genitourinary: Difficulty in urination, ejaculatory disturbances, urinary retention, priapism
Hematologic: Agranulocytosis, leukopenia
Hepatic: Cholestatic jaundice, hepatotoxicity
Neuromuscular & skeletal: Tremor, seizure
Ocular: Pigmentary retinopathy, blurred vision, cornea and lens changes
Respiratory: Nasal congestion

Overdosage/Toxicology Symptoms of overdose include deep sleep, coma, extrapyramidal symptoms, abnormal involuntary muscle movements, hypotension, and arrhythmias.

Immediate cardiac monitoring, including continuous electrocardiographic monitoring, to detect arrhythmias. Avoid use of medications that also prolong the QT_c interval, such as disopyramide, procainamide, and quinidine. Following initiation of essential overdose management, toxic symptom treatment and supportive treatment should be initiated. Hypotension usually responds to I.V. fluids or Trendelenburg positioning. If unresponsive to these measures, the use of a parenteral inotrope may be required (eg, norepinephrine 0.1-0.2 mcg/kg/minute titrated to response); do not use epinephrine or dopamine. Seizures commonly respond to diazepam (I.V. 5-10 mg bolus in adults every 15 minutes if needed up to a total of 30 mg; I.V. 0.25-0.4 mg/kg/dose up to a total of 10 mg in children) or to phenytoin. Avoid barbiturates (may potentiate respiratory depression). Neuroleptics often cause extrapyramidal symptoms (eg, dystonic reactions) requiring management with diphenhydramine 1-2 mg/kg (adults) up to a maximum of 50 mg I.M. or I.V. slow push followed by a maintenance dose for 48-72 hours. When these reactions are unresponsive to diphenhydramine, benztropine mesylate I.V. 1-2 mg (adults) may be effective. These agents are generally effective within 2-5 minutes.

Drug Interactions **Substrate** of CYP2C19 (minor), 2D6 (major); **Inhibits** CYP1A2 (weak), 2C9 (weak), 2D6 (moderate), 2E1 (weak)
Acetylcholinesterase inhibitors (central): May increase the risk of antipsychotic-related extrapyramidal symptoms; monitor.
Aluminum salts: May decrease the absorption of phenothiazines; monitor
Amphetamines: Efficacy may be diminished by antipsychotics; in addition, amphetamines may increase psychotic symptoms; avoid concurrent use
Anticholinergics: May inhibit the therapeutic response to phenothiazines and excess anticholinergic effects may occur; includes benztropine, trihexyphenidyl, biperiden, and drugs with significant anticholinergic activity (TCAs, antihistamines, disopyramide)
Antihypertensives: Concurrent use of phenothiazines with an antihypertensive may produce additive hypotensive effects (particularly orthostasis)
Beta-blockers: May increase the risk of arrhythmia; propranolol and pindolol are **contraindicated**
Bromocriptine: Phenothiazines inhibit the ability of bromocriptine to lower serum prolactin concentrations
Carvedilol: Serum concentrations may be increased, leading to hypotension and bradycardia; avoid concurrent use
CNS depressants: Sedative effects may be additive with phenothiazines; monitor for increased effect; includes barbiturates, benzodiazepines, narcotic analgesics, ethanol, and other sedative agents
CYP2D6 inhibitors: May increase the levels/effects of thioridazine. Example inhibitors include chlorpromazine, delavirdine, fluoxetine, miconazole, paroxetine, pergolide, quinidine, quinine, ritonavir, and ropinirole. **Thioridazine is contraindicated with inhibitors of this enzyme.**
CYP2D6 substrates: Thioridazine may increase the levels/effects of CYP2D6 substrates. Example substrates include amphetamines, selected beta-blockers, dextromethorphan, fluoxetine, lidocaine, mirtazapine, nefazodone, paroxetine, risperidone, ritonavir, tricyclic antidepressants, and venlafaxine.
CYP2D6 prodrug substrates: Thioridazine may decrease the levels/effects of CYP2D6 prodrug substrates. Example prodrug substrates include codeine, hydrocodone, oxycodone, and tramadol.
Epinephrine: Chlorpromazine (and possibly other low potency antipsychotics) may diminish the pressor effects of epinephrine
Guanethidine and guanadrel: Antihypertensive effects may be inhibited by phenothiazines

(Continued)

Thioridazine *(Continued)*

Levodopa: Phenothiazines may inhibit the antiparkinsonian effect of levodopa; avoid this combination

Lithium: Phenothiazines may produce neurotoxicity with lithium; this is a rare effect

Metoclopramide: May increase extrapyramidal symptoms (EPS) or risk.

Phenytoin: May reduce serum levels of phenothiazines; phenothiazines may increase phenytoin serum levels

Polypeptide antibiotics: Rare cases of respiratory paralysis have been reported with concurrent use of phenothiazines

Potassium-depleting agents: May increase the risk of serious arrhythmias with thioridazine; includes many diuretics, aminoglycosides, and amphotericin; monitor serum potassium closely

Propranolol: Serum concentrations of phenothiazines may be increased; propranolol also increases phenothiazine concentrations; may also occur with pindolol. **These agents are contraindicated with thioridazine.**

QT_c-prolonging agents: Effects on QT_c interval may be additive with phenothiazines, increasing the risk of malignant arrhythmias; includes type Ia antiarrhythmics, TCAs, and some quinolone antibiotics (sparfloxacin, moxifloxacin and gatifloxacin). **These agents are contraindicated with thioridazine.**

Sulfadoxine-pyrimethamine: May increase phenothiazine concentrations

Trazodone: Phenothiazines and trazodone may produce additive hypotensive effects

Tricyclic antidepressants: Concurrent use may produce increased toxicity or altered therapeutic response

Valproic acid: Serum levels may be increased by phenothiazines

Ethanol/Nutrition/Herb Interactions

Ethanol: Avoid ethanol (may increase CNS depression).

Herb/Nutraceutical: Avoid kava kava, valerian, St John's wort, gotu kola (may increase CNS depression). Avoid dong quai, St John's wort (may also cause photosensitization).

Test Interactions False-positives for phenylketonuria, urinary amylase, uroporphyrins, urobilinogen

Dosage Forms Tablet, as hydrochloride: 10 mg, 15 mg, 25 mg, 50 mg, 100 mg, 150 mg, 200 mg

◆ **Thioridazine Hydrochloride** *see* Thioridazine *on page 1259*

◆ **Thiosulfuric Acid Disodium Salt** *see* Sodium Thiosulfate *on page 1195*

◆ **Thrombate III®** *see* Antithrombin III *on page 115*

Tiagabine (tye AG a been)

Medication Safety Issues

Sound-alike/look-alike issues:

Tiagabine may be confused with tizanidine

Related Information

Perioperative Management of Patients on Antiseizure Medication *on page 1458*

U.S. Brand Names Gabitril®

Canadian Brand Names Gabitril®

Synonyms Tiagabine Hydrochloride

Pharmacologic Category Anticonvulsant, Miscellaneous

Generic Available No

Use Adjunctive therapy in adults and children ≥12 years of age in the treatment of partial seizures

Mechanism of Action The exact mechanism by which tiagabine exerts antiseizure activity is not definitively known; however, *in vitro* experiments demonstrate that it enhances the activity of gamma aminobutyric acid (GABA), the major neuroinhibitory transmitter in the nervous system; it is thought that binding to the GABA uptake carrier inhibits the uptake of GABA into presynaptic neurons, allowing an increased amount of GABA to be available to postsynaptic neurons; based on *in vitro* studies, tiagabine does not inhibit the uptake of dopamine, norepinephrine, serotonin, glutamate, or choline

Pharmacodynamics/Kinetics

Absorption: Rapid (45 minutes); prolonged with food

Protein binding: 96%, primarily to albumin and α_1-acid glycoprotein
Metabolism: Hepatic via CYP (primarily 3A4)
Bioavailability: Oral: Absolute: 90%
Half-life elimination: 2-5 hours when administered with enzyme inducers; 7-9 hours when administered without enzyme inducers
Time to peak, plasma: 45 minutes
Excretion: Feces (63%); urine (25%); 2% as unchanged drug; primarily as metabolites

Dosage Oral (administer with food):
Patients receiving enzyme-inducing AED regimens:
Children 12-18 years: 4 mg once daily for 1 week; may increase to 8 mg daily in 2 divided doses for 1 week; then may increase by 4-8 mg weekly to response or up to 32 mg daily in 2-4 divided doses
Adults: 4 mg once daily for 1 week; may increase by 4-8 mg weekly to response or up to 56 mg daily in 2-4 divided doses; usual maintenance: 32-56 mg/day
Patients **not** receiving enzyme-inducing AED regimens: The estimated plasma concentrations of tiagabine in patients not taking enzyme-inducing medications is twice that of patients receiving enzyme-inducing AEDs. Lower doses are required; slower titration may be necessary.

Monitoring Parameters A reduction in seizure frequency is indicative of therapeutic response to tiagabine in patients with partial seizures; complete blood counts, renal function tests, liver function tests, and routine blood chemistry should be monitored periodically during therapy

Reference Range Maximal plasma level after a 24 mg/dose: 552 ng/mL

Pregnancy Risk Factor C

Contraindications Hypersensitivity to tiagabine or any component of the formulation

Warnings/Precautions New-onset seizures and status epilepticus have been associated with tiagabine use when taken for unlabeled indications. Often these seizures have occurred shortly after the initiation of treatment or shortly after a dosage increase. Seizures have also occurred with very low doses or after several months of therapy. In most cases, patients were using concomitant medications (eg, antidepressants, antipsychotics, stimulants, narcotics). In these instances, the discontinuation of tiagabine, followed by an evaluation for an underlying seizure disorder, is suggested. Use for unapproved indications, however, has not been proven to be safe or effective and is not recommended. When tiagabine is used as an adjunct in partial seizures (an FDA-approved indication), it should not be abruptly discontinued because of the possibility of increasing seizure frequency, unless safety concerns require a more rapid withdrawal. Rarely, nonconvulsive status epilepticus has been reported following abrupt discontinuation or dosage reduction.

Use with caution in patients with hepatic impairment. Experience in patients not receiving enzyme-inducing drugs has been limited; caution should be used in treating any patient who is not receiving one of these medications (decreased dose and slower titration may be required). Weakness, sedation, and confusion may occur with tiagabine use. Patients must be cautioned about performing tasks which require mental alertness (eg, operating machinery or driving). Effects with other sedative drugs or ethanol may be potentiated. Animal studies suggest that tiagabine may bind to retina and uvea; however, no treatment-related ophthalmoscopic changes were seen long-term; periodic monitoring may be considered. May cause serious rash, including Stevens-Johnson syndrome. Safety and efficacy have not been established in children <12 years of age.

Adverse Reactions
>10%:
Central nervous system: Concentration decreased, dizziness, nervousness, somnolence
Gastrointestinal: Nausea
Neuromuscular & skeletal: Weakness, tremor
1% to 10%:
Cardiovascular: Chest pain, edema, hypertension, palpitation, peripheral edema, syncope, tachycardia, vasodilation
Central nervous system: Agitation, ataxia, chills, confusion, difficulty with memory, confusion, depersonalization, depression, euphoria, hallucination, hostility, insomnia, malaise, migraine, paranoid reaction, personality disorder, speech disorder
Dermatologic: Alopecia, bruising, dry skin, pruritus, rash

(Continued)

Tiagabine *(Continued)*

Gastrointestinal: Abdominal pain, diarrhea, gingivitis, increased appetite, mouth ulceration, stomatitis, vomiting, weight gain/loss

Neuromuscular & skeletal: Abnormal gait, arthralgia, dysarthria, hyper-/hypokinesia, hyper-/hypotonia, myasthenia, myalgia, myoclonus, neck pain, paresthesia, reflexes decreased, stupor, twitching, vertigo

Ocular: Abnormal vision, amblyopia, nystagmus

Otic: Ear pain, hearing impairment, otitis media, tinnitus

Respiratory: Bronchitis, cough, dyspnea, epistaxis, pneumonia

Miscellaneous: Allergic reaction, cyst, diaphoresis, flu-like syndrome, lymphadenopathy

<1% (Limited to important or life-threatening): Abortion, abscess, anemia, angina, apnea, asthma, blepharitis, blindness, cellulitis, cerebral ischemia, cholelithiasis, CNS neoplasm, coma, deafness, dehydration, dysphagia, dystonia, electrocardiogram abnormal, encephalopathy, hemorrhage, erythrocytes abnormal, leukopenia, fecal incontinence, herpes simplex/zoster, glossitis, goiter, hematuria, hemoptysis, hepatomegaly, hypercholesteremia, hyper-/hypoglycemia, hyperlipemia, hypokalemia, hyponatremia, hypotension, hypothyroidism, impotence, kidney failure, liver function tests abnormal, MI, neoplasm, peripheral vascular disorder, paralysis, photophobia, psychosis, petechia, photosensitivity, seizure (when used for unlabeled uses), sepsis, spasm, suicide attempt, thrombocytopenia, thrombophlebitis, urinary retention, urinary urgency, urticaria, visual field defect

Overdosage/Toxicology Somnolence, impaired consciousness, agitation, confusion, speech difficulty, hostility, depression, weakness, myoclonus, and seizures may occur. Treatment is supportive.

Drug Interactions Substrate of 3A4 (major)

CNS depressants: Sedative effects may be additive with other CNS depressants; monitor for increased effect; includes ethanol, sedatives, antidepressants, narcotic analgesics, other anticonvulsants, and benzodiazepines

CYP3A4 inducers: CYP3A4 inducers may decrease the levels/effects of tiagabine. Example inducers include aminoglutethimide, carbamazepine, nafcillin, nevirapine, phenobarbital, phenytoin, and rifamycins.

CYP3A4 inhibitors: May increase the levels/effects of tiagabine. Example inhibitors include azole antifungals, clarithromycin, diclofenac, doxycycline, erythromycin, imatinib, isoniazid, nefazodone, nicardipine, propofol, protease inhibitors, quinidine, telithromycin, and verapamil.

Valproate: Increased free tiagabine concentrations (*in vitro*) by 40%

Ethanol/Nutrition/Herb Interactions

Ethanol: Avoid ethanol (may increase CNS depression).

Food: Food reduces the rate but not the extent of absorption.

Herb/Nutraceutical: St John's wort may decrease tiagabine levels. Avoid valerian, St John's wort, kava kava, gotu kola (may increase CNS depression).

Dietary Considerations Take with food.

Dosage Forms Tablet, as hydrochloride: 2 mg, 4 mg, 6 mg, 8 mg, 10 mg, 12 mg, 16 mg

♦ **Tiagabine Hydrochloride** *see* Tiagabine *on page 1262*
♦ **Tiazac®** *see* Diltiazem *on page 394*
♦ **Tiazac® XC (Can)** *see* Diltiazem *on page 394*

Ticarcillin and Clavulanate Potassium

(tye kar SIL in & klav yoo LAN ate poe TASS ee um)

U.S. Brand Names Timentin®

Canadian Brand Names Timentin®

Synonyms Ticarcillin and Clavulanic Acid

Pharmacologic Category Antibiotic, Penicillin

Generic Available No

Use Treatment of infections of lower respiratory tract, urinary tract, skin and skin structures, bone and joint, and septicemia caused by susceptible organisms. Clavulanate expands activity of ticarcillin to include beta-lactamase producing strains of *S. aureus*, *H. influenzae*, *Bacteroides* species, and some other gram-negative bacilli

Mechanism of Action Inhibits bacterial cell wall synthesis by binding to one or more of the penicillin binding proteins (PBPs); which in turn inhibits the final transpeptidation step of peptidoglycan synthesis in bacterial cell walls, thus inhibiting cell wall biosynthesis. Bacteria eventually lyse due to ongoing activity of cell wall autolytic enzymes (autolysins and murein hydrolases) while cell wall assembly is arrested.

Pharmacodynamics/Kinetics

Ticarcillin: See Ticarcillin monograph.

Clavulanic acid:

Protein binding: 9% to 30%

Metabolism: Hepatic

Half-life elimination: 66-90 minutes

Excretion: Urine (45% as unchanged drug)

Clearance: Does not affect clearance of ticarcillin

Dosage

Usual dosage range:

Children and Adults <60 kg: I.V.: 75-300 mg of ticarcillin component/kg/day in divided doses every 4-6 hours

Children ≥60 kg and Adults: I.V.: 3.1 g (ticarcillin 3 g plus clavulanic acid 0.1 g) every 4-6 hours (maximum: 24 g/day)

Indication-specific dosing:

Children: I.V.:

Bite wounds (animal): 200 mg/kg/day in divided doses

Neutropenic fever: 75 mg/kg every 6 hours (maximum 3.1 g)

Pneumonia (nosocomial): 300 mg/kg/day in 4 divided doses (maximum: 18-24 g/day)

Children ≥60 kg and Adults: I.V.:

Amnionitis, cholangitis, diverticulitis, endometritis, epididymo-orchitis, mastoiditis, orbital cellulitis, peritonitis, pneumonia (aspiration): 3.1 g every 6 hours

Liver abscess, parafascial space infections, septic thrombophlebitis: 3.1 g every 4 hours

***Pseudomonas* infections:** 3.1 g every 4 hours

Urinary tract infections: 3.1 g every 6-8 hours

Dosing adjustment in renal impairment:

Cl_{cr} 30-60 mL/minute: Administer 2 g every 4 hours or 3.1 g every 8 hours

Cl_{cr} 10-30 mL/minute: Administer 2 g every 8 hours or 3.1 g every 12 hours

Cl_{cr} <10 mL/minute: Administer 2 g every 12 hours

Moderately dialyzable (20% to 50%)

Continuous arteriovenous or venovenous hemodiafiltration effects: Dose as for Cl_{cr} 10-50 mL/minute

Peritoneal dialysis: 3.1 g every 12 hours

Hemodialysis: 2 g every 12 hours; supplemented with 3.1 g after each dialysis

Dosing adjustment in hepatic dysfunction: Cl_{cr} <10 mL/minute: 2 g every 24 hours

Stability Reconstituted solution is stable for 6 hours at room temperature and 72 hours when refrigerated; for I.V. infusion in NS is stable for 24 hours at room temperature, 7 days when refrigerated or 30 days when frozen; after freezing, thawed solution is stable for 8 hours at room temperature; for I.V. infusion in D_5W solution is stable for 24 hours at room temperature, 3 days when refrigerated or 7 days when frozen; after freezing, thawed solution is stable for 8 hours at room temperature; darkening of drug indicates loss of potency of clavulanate potassium; **incompatible** with sodium bicarbonate, aminoglycosides

Administration Infuse over 30 minutes.

Some penicillins (eg, carbenicillin, ticarcillin and piperacillin) have been shown to inactivate aminoglycosides *in vitro*. This has been observed to a greater extent with tobramycin and gentamicin, while amikacin has shown greater stability against inactivation. Concurrent use of these agents may pose a risk of reduced antibacterial efficacy *in vivo*, particularly in the setting of profound renal impairment. However, definitive clinical evidence is lacking. If combination penicillin/aminoglycoside therapy is desired in a patient with renal dysfunction, separation of doses (if feasible), and routine monitoring of aminoglycoside levels, CBC, and clinical response should be considered.

Monitoring Parameters Observe for signs and symptoms of anaphylaxis during first dose.

Pregnancy Risk Factor B

Contraindications Hypersensitivity to ticarcillin, clavulanate, any penicillin, or any component of the formulation

(Continued)

Ticarcillin and Clavulanate Potassium *(Continued)*

Warnings/Precautions Not approved for use in children <12 years of age; use with caution and modify dosage in patients with renal impairment; use with caution in patients with a history of allergy to cephalosporins and in patients with CHF due to high sodium load

Adverse Reactions Frequency not defined.

Central nervous system: Confusion, convulsions, drowsiness, fever, Jarisch-Herxheimer reaction

Dermatologic: Rash, erythema multiforme, toxic epidermal necrolysis, Stevens-Johnson syndrome

Endocrine & metabolic: Electrolyte imbalance

Gastrointestinal: *Clostridium difficile* colitis

Hematologic: Bleeding, hemolytic anemia, leukopenia, neutropenia, positive Coombs' reaction, thrombocytopenia

Hepatic: Hepatotoxicity, jaundice

Local: Thrombophlebitis

Neuromuscular & skeletal: Myoclonus

Renal: Interstitial nephritis (acute)

Miscellaneous: Anaphylaxis, hypersensitivity reactions

Overdosage/Toxicology Symptoms of overdose include neuromuscular hypersensitivity and seizures. Hemodialysis may be helpful to aid in removal of the drug from blood; otherwise, treatment is supportive or symptom-directed.

Drug Interactions

Aminoglycosides: May be synergistic against selected organisms; physical inactivation of aminoglycosides in the presence of high concentrations of piperacillin and potential toxicity in patients with mild to moderate renal dysfunction

Heparin: Concomitant use with high-dose parenteral penicillins may result in increased risk of bleeding

Methotrexate: Penicillins may increase the exposure to methotrexate during concurrent therapy; monitor.

Neuromuscular blockers: May increase duration of blockade

Oral contraceptives: Anecdotal reports suggesting decreased contraceptive efficacy with penicillins have been refuted by more rigorous scientific and clinical data.

Probenecid: May increase levels of penicillins (ticarcillin)

Tetracyclines: May decrease effectiveness of penicillins (ticarcillin)

Warfarin: Effects of warfarin may be increased

Test Interactions Positive Coombs' test, false-positive urinary proteins

Some penicillin derivatives may accelerate the degradation of aminoglycosides *in vitro*, leading to a potential underestimation of aminoglycoside serum concentration.

Dietary Considerations Sodium content of 1 g: 4.51 mEq; potassium content of 1 g: 0.15 mEq

Dosage Forms

Infusion [premixed, frozen]: Ticarcillin 3 g and clavulanic acid 0.1 g (100 mL) [contains sodium 4.51 mEq and potassium 0.15 mEq per g]

Injection, powder for reconstitution: Ticarcillin 3 g and clavulanic acid 0.1 g (3.1 g, 31 g) [contains sodium 4.51 mEq and potassium 0.15 mEq per g]

- **Ticarcillin and Clavulanic Acid** *see* Ticarcillin and Clavulanate Potassium *on page 1264*
- **Ticlid®** *see* Ticlopidine *on page 1266*

Ticlopidine (tye KLOE pi deen)

U.S. Brand Names Ticlid®

Canadian Brand Names Alti-Ticlopidine; Apo-Ticlopidine®; Gen-Ticlopidine; Novo-Ticlopidine; Nu-Ticlopidine; Rhoxal-ticlopidine; Sandoz-Ticlopidine; Ticlid®

Synonyms Ticlopidine Hydrochloride

Pharmacologic Category Antiplatelet Agent

Generic Available Yes

Use Platelet aggregation inhibitor that reduces the risk of thrombotic stroke in patients who have had a stroke or stroke precursors. **Note:** Due to its association with life-threatening hematologic disorders, ticlopidine should be reserved for patients who are intolerant to aspirin, or who have failed aspirin therapy. Adjunctive therapy (with aspirin) following successful coronary stent implantation to reduce the incidence of subacute stent thrombosis.

Unlabeled/Investigational Use Protection of aortocoronary bypass grafts, diabetic microangiopathy, ischemic heart disease, prevention of postoperative DVT, reduction of graft loss following renal transplant

Mechanism of Action Ticlopidine is an inhibitor of platelet function with a mechanism which is different from other antiplatelet drugs. The drug significantly increases bleeding time. This effect may not be solely related to ticlopidine's effect on platelets. The prolongation of the bleeding time caused by ticlopidine is further increased by the addition of aspirin in *ex vivo* experiments. Although many metabolites of ticlopidine have been found, none have been shown to account for *in vivo* activity.

Pharmacodynamics/Kinetics

Onset of action: ~6 hours

Peak effect: 3-5 days; serum levels do not correlate with clinical antiplatelet activity

Metabolism: Extensively hepatic; has at least one active metabolite

Half-life elimination: 24 hours

Dosage Oral: Adults:

Stroke prevention: 250 mg twice daily with food

Coronary artery stenting (initiate after successful implantation): 250 mg twice daily with food (in combination with antiplatelet doses of aspirin) for up to 30 days

Administration Oral: Administer with food.

Monitoring Parameters Signs of bleeding; CBC with differential every 2 weeks starting the second week through the third month of treatment; more frequent monitoring is recommended for patients whose absolute neutrophil counts have been consistently declining or are 30% less than baseline values. The peak incidence of TTP occurs between 3-4 weeks, the peak incidence of neutropenia occurs at approximately 4-6 weeks, and the incidence of aplastic anemia peaks after 4-8 weeks of therapy. Few cases have been reported after 3 months of treatment. Liver function tests (alkaline phosphatase and transaminases) should be performed in the first 4 months of therapy if liver dysfunction is suspected.

Anesthesia and Critical Care Concerns/Other Considerations The adverse effect profile including neutropenia and thrombotic thrombocytopenia purpura (TTP), along with twice-daily dosing and GI upset, makes ticlopidine a less attractive option than clopidogrel. Neutropenia usually resolves within 1-3 weeks of discontinuation of therapy. TTP, although rare, is life-threatening and requires immediate plasma exchange.

Pregnancy Risk Factor B

Contraindications Hypersensitivity to ticlopidine or any component of the formulation; active pathological bleeding such as PUD or intracranial hemorrhage; severe liver dysfunction; hematopoietic disorders (neutropenia, thrombocytopenia, a past history of TTP)

Warnings/Precautions Use with caution in patients who may have an increased risk of bleeding (such as, ulcers). Consider discontinuing 10-14 days before elective surgery. Use caution in mixing with other antiplatelet drugs. Use with caution in patients with severe liver disease or severe renal impairment (experience is limited). **[U.S. Boxed Warning]: May cause life-threatening hematologic reactions, including neutropenia, agranulocytosis, thrombotic thrombocytopenia purpura (TTP), and aplastic anemia.** Routine monitoring is required (see Monitoring Parameters). Monitor for signs and symptoms of neutropenia including WBC count. Discontinue if the absolute neutrophil count falls to <1200/mm^3 or if the platelet count falls to <80,000/mm^3.

Adverse Reactions As with all drugs which may affect hemostasis, bleeding is associated with ticlopidine. Hemorrhage may occur at virtually any site. Risk is dependent on multiple variables, including the use of multiple agents which alter hemostasis and patient susceptibility.

>10%:

Endocrine & metabolic: Increased total cholesterol (increases of ~8% to 10% within 1 month of therapy)

Gastrointestinal: Diarrhea (13%)

1% to 10%: Central nervous system: Dizziness (1%)

Dermatologic: Rash (5%), purpura (2%), pruritus (1%)

(Continued)

Ticlopidine *(Continued)*

Gastrointestinal: Nausea (7%), dyspepsia (7%), gastrointestinal pain (4%), vomiting (2%), flatulence (2%), anorexia (1%)
Hematologic: Neutropenia (2%)
Hepatic: Abnormal liver function test (1%)
<1% (Limited to important or life-threatening): Agranulocytosis, anaphylaxis, angioedema, aplastic anemia, arthropathy, bone marrow suppression, bronchiolitis obliterans-organized pneumonia, chronic diarrhea, conjunctival bleeding, eosinophilia, erythema multiforme, erythema nodosum, exfoliative dermatitis, gastrointestinal bleeding, hematuria, hemolytic anemia, hepatic necrosis, hepatitis, hyponatremia, intracranial bleeding (rare), jaundice, maculopapular rash, menorrhagia, myositis, nephrotic syndrome, pancytopenia, peptic ulcer, peripheral neuropathy, pneumonitis (allergic), positive ANA, renal failure, sepsis, serum creatinine increased, serum sickness, Stevens-Johnson syndrome, systemic lupus erythematosus, thrombocytopenia (immune), thrombocytosis, thrombotic thrombocytopenic purpura, urticaria, vasculitis

Overdosage/Toxicology Symptoms of overdose include ataxia, seizures, vomiting, abdominal pain, and hematologic abnormalities. Specific treatments are lacking. Treatment is symptomatic and supportive.

Drug Interactions Substrate of CYP3A4 (major); **Inhibits** CYP1A2 (weak), 2C9 (weak), 2C19 (strong), 2D6 (moderate), 2E1 (weak), 3A4 (weak)
Antacids reduce absorption of ticlopidine (~18%).
Anticoagulants or other antiplatelet agents may increase the risk of bleeding; use with caution.
Carbamazepine blood levels may be increased by ticlopidine.
Cimetidine increases ticlopidine levels.
Cyclosporine blood levels may be reduced by ticlopidine.
CYP2C19 substrates: Ticlopidine may increase the levels/effects of CYP2C19 substrates. Example substrates include citalopram, diazepam, methsuximide, phenytoin, propranolol, and sertraline.
CYP2D6 substrates: Ticlopidine may increase the levels/effects of CYP2D6 substrates. Example substrates include amphetamines, selected beta-blockers, dextromethorphan, fluoxetine, lidocaine, mirtazapine, nefazodone, paroxetine, risperidone, ritonavir, thioridazine, tricyclic antidepressants, and venlafaxine.
CYP2D6 prodrug substrates: Ticlopidine may decrease the levels/effects of CYP2D6 prodrug substrates. Example prodrug substrates include codeine, hydrocodone, oxycodone, and tramadol.
CYP3A4 inducers: CYP3A4 inducers may decrease the levels/effects of ticlopidine. Example inducers include aminoglutethimide, carbamazepine, nafcillin, nevirapine, phenobarbital, phenytoin, and rifamycins.
Digoxin blood levels may be decreased by ticlopidine.
Phenytoin blood levels may be increased by ticlopidine (case reports).
Theophylline blood levels may be increased by ticlopidine.

Ethanol/Nutrition/Herb Interactions
Food: Ticlopidine bioavailability may be increased (20%) if taken with food. High-fat meals increase absorption, antacids decrease absorption.
Herb/Nutraceutical: Avoid cat's claw, dong quai, evening primrose, feverfew, garlic, ginkgo, ginger, red clover, horse chestnut, green tea, ginseng (all have additional antiplatelet activity).

Test Interactions Increased cholesterol (S), increased alkaline phosphatase, increased transaminases (S)

Dietary Considerations Should be taken with food to reduce stomach upset.

Dosage Forms Tablet, as hydrochloride: 250 mg

- **Ticlopidine Hydrochloride** *see* Ticlopidine *on page 1266*
- **TIG** *see* Tetanus Immune Globulin (Human) *on page 1246*
- **Tigan®** *see* Trimethobenzamide *on page 1318*
- **Tikosyn™** *see* Dofetilide *on page 409*
- **Tim-AK (Can)** *see* Timolol *on page 1268*
- **Timentin®** *see* Ticarcillin and Clavulanate Potassium *on page 1264*

Timolol (TYE moe lole)

Medication Safety Issues
Sound-alike/look-alike issues:
Timolol may be confused with atenolol, Tylenol®

Timoptic® may be confused with Talacen®, Viroptic®

Bottle cap color change:

Timoptic®: Both the 0.25% and 0.5% strengths are now packaged in bottles with yellow caps; previously, the color of the cap on the product corresponded to different strengths.

Related Information

Antiarrhythmic Drugs *on page 1548*
Beta-Blockers *on page 1557*
Preoperative Evaluation of the Cardiac Patient for Noncardiac Surgery *on page 1485*

U.S. Brand Names Betimol®; Blocadren®; Istalol™; Timoptic®; Timoptic® OcuDose®; Timoptic-XE®

Canadian Brand Names Alti-Timolol; Apo-Timol®; Apo-Timop®; Gen-Timolol; Nu-Timolol; Phoxal-timolol; PMS-Timolol; Sandoz-Timolol; Tim-AK; Timoptic®; Timoptic-XE®

Synonyms Timolol Hemihydrate; Timolol Maleate

Pharmacologic Category Beta-Adrenergic Blocker, Nonselective; Ophthalmic Agent, Antiglaucoma

Generic Available Yes: Excludes hemihydrate ophthalmic solutions

Use

Ophthalmic: Treatment of elevated intraocular pressure such as glaucoma or ocular hypertension

Oral: Treatment of hypertension and angina; to reduce mortality following myocardial infarction; prophylaxis of migraine

Mechanism of Action Blocks both $beta_1$- and $beta_2$-adrenergic receptors, reduces intraocular pressure by reducing aqueous humor production or possibly outflow; reduces blood pressure by blocking adrenergic receptors and decreasing sympathetic outflow, produces a negative chronotropic and inotropic activity through an unknown mechanism

Pharmacodynamics/Kinetics

Onset of action:
- Hypotensive: Oral: 15-45 minutes
  - Peak effect: 0.5-2.5 hours
- Intraocular pressure reduction: Ophthalmic: 30 minutes
  - Peak effect: 1-2 hours

Duration: ~4 hours; Ophthalmic: Intraocular: 24 hours

Protein binding: 60%

Metabolism: Extensively hepatic; extensive first-pass effect

Half-life elimination: 2-2.7 hours; prolonged with renal impairment

Excretion: Urine (15% to 20% as unchanged drug)

Dosage

Ophthalmic:

Children and Adults:
- Solution: Initial: Instill 1 drop (0.25% solution) into affected eye(s) twice daily; increase to 0.5% solution if response not adequate; decrease to 1 drop/day if controlled; do not exceed 1 drop twice daily of 0.5% solution
- Gel-forming solution (Timoptic-XE®): Instill 1 drop (either 0.25% or 0.5% solution) once daily

Adults: Solution (Istalol®): Instill 1 drop (0.5% solution) once daily in the morning

Oral: Adults:
- Hypertension: Initial: 10 mg twice daily, increase gradually every 7 days, usual dosage: 20-40 mg/day in 2 divided doses; maximum: 60 mg/day
- Prevention of myocardial infarction: 10 mg twice daily initiated within 1-4 weeks after infarction
- Migraine headache: Initial: 10 mg twice daily, increase to maximum of 30 mg/day

Stability Ophthalmic drops: Store at room temperature; protect from light and freezing

Timoptic Occudose®: Store in the protective foil wrap and use within 1 month after opening foil package

Administration Ophthalmic: Administer other topically-applied ophthalmic medications at least 10 minutes before Timoptic-XE®; wash hands before use; invert closed bottle and shake once before use; remove cap carefully so that tip does not touch anything; hold bottle between thumb and index finger; use index finger of other hand to pull down the lower eyelid to form a pocket for the eye drop and tilt head back; place the dispenser tip close to the eye and gently squeeze the

(Continued)

Timolol *(Continued)*

bottle to administer 1 drop; remove pressure after a single drop has been released; **do not allow the dispenser tip to touch the eye**; replace cap and store bottle in an upright position in a clean area; do **not** enlarge hole of dispenser; do **not** wash tip with water, soap, or any other cleaner. Some ophthalmic solutions contain benzalkonium chloride; wait at least 10 minutes after instilling solution before inserting soft contact lenses.

Monitoring Parameters Blood pressure, apical and radial pulses, fluid I & O, daily weight, respirations, mental status, and circulation in extremities before and during therapy; monitor for systemic effect of beta-blockade even when administering ophthalmic product

Anesthesia and Critical Care Concerns/Other Considerations It is important to recognize that timolol eye drops may have systemic effects, particularly when patients are also on oral beta-blocker therapy or therapy with other negative chronotropic agents.

Myocardial Infarction: Beta-blockers, in general without intrinsic sympathomimetic activity (ISA), have been shown to decrease morbidity and mortality when initiated in the acute treatment of myocardial infarction and continued long-term. In this setting, therapy should be avoided in patients with hypotension, cardiogenic shock, or heart block.

Surgery: Atenolol has also been shown to improve cardiovascular outcomes when used in the perioperative period in patients with underlying cardiovascular disease who are undergoing noncardiac surgery. Bisoprolol in high-risk patients undergoing vascular surgery reduced the perioperative incidence of death from cardiac causes and nonfatal myocardial infarction.

Withdrawal: Beta-blocker therapy should not be withdrawn abruptly, but gradually tapered to avoid acute tachycardia and hypertension.

Pregnancy Risk Factor C (manufacturer); D (2nd and 3rd trimesters - expert analysis)

Contraindications Hypersensitivity to timolol or any component of the formulation; sinus bradycardia; sinus node dysfunction; heart block greater than first degree (except in patients with a functioning artificial pacemaker); cardiogenic shock; uncompensated cardiac failure; bronchospastic disease; pregnancy (2nd and 3rd trimesters)

Warnings/Precautions Administer cautiously in compensated heart failure and monitor for a worsening of the condition. **[U.S. Boxed Warning]: Beta-blocker therapy should not be withdrawn abruptly (particularly in patients with CAD), but gradually tapered to avoid acute tachycardia, hypertension, and/or ischemia.** Use caution with concurrent use of beta-blockers and either verapamil or diltiazem; bradycardia or heart block can occur. Beta-blockers can aggravate symptoms in patients with PVD. Patients with bronchospastic disease should generally not receive beta-blockers; monitor closely if used in patients with potential risk of bronchospasm. Use cautiously in diabetics because it can mask prominent hypoglycemic symptoms. Can mask signs of thyrotoxicosis. Can cause fetal harm when administered in pregnancy. Use cautiously in severe renal impairment: marked hypotension can occur in patients maintained on hemodialysis. Use care with anesthetic agents which decrease myocardial function. Can worsen myasthenia gravis.

Ophthalmic: Systemic absorption and adverse effects may occur, including bradycardia and/or hypotension. Should not be used alone in angle-closure glaucoma (has no effect on pupillary constriction).

Adverse Reactions

Ophthalmic:

>10%: Ocular: Burning, stinging

1% to 10%:

Cardiovascular: Hypertension

Central nervous system: Headache

Ocular: Blurred vision, cataract, conjunctival injection, itching, visual acuity decreased

Miscellaneous: Infection

Systemic:

1% to 10%:

Cardiovascular: Bradycardia

Central nervous system: Fatigue, dizziness

Respiratory: Dyspnea

Frequency not defined (reported with any dosage form):

Cardiovascular: Angina pectoris, arrhythmia, bradycardia, cardiac failure, cardiac arrest, cerebral vascular accident, cerebral ischemia, edema, hypotension, heart block, palpitation, Raynaud's phenomenon

Central nervous system: Anxiety, confusion, depression, disorientation, dizziness, hallucinations, insomnia, memory loss, nervousness, nightmares, somnolence

Dermatologic: Alopecia, angioedema, pseudopemphigoid, psoriasiform rash, psoriasis exacerbation, rash, urticaria

Endocrine & metabolic: Hypoglycemia masked, libido decreased

Gastrointestinal: Anorexia, diarrhea, dyspepsia, nausea, xerostomia

Genitourinary: Impotence, retoperitoneal fibrosis

Hematologic: Claudication

Neuromuscular & skeletal: Myasthenia gravis exacerbation, paresthesia

Ocular: Blepharitis, conjunctivitis, corneal sensitivity decreased, cystoid macular edema, diplopia, dry eyes, foreign body sensation, keratitis, ocular discharge, ocular pain, ptosis, refractive changes, tearing, visual disturbances

Otic: Tinnitus

Respiratory: Bronchospasm, cough, dyspnea, nasal congestion, pulmonary edema, respiratory failure

Miscellaneous: Allergic reactions, cold hands/feet, Peyronie's disease, systemic lupus erythematosus

Overdosage/Toxicology Symptoms of intoxication include cardiac disturbances, CNS toxicity, bronchospasm, hypoglycemia and hyperkalemia. The most common cardiac symptoms include hypotension and bradycardia. Atrioventricular block, intraventricular conduction disturbances, cardiogenic shock, and asystole may occur with severe overdose, especially with membrane-depressant drugs (eg, propranolol). CNS effects including convulsions, coma, and respiratory arrest are commonly seen with propranolol and other membrane-depressant and lipid-soluble drugs. Treatment is symptom-directed and supportive. Timolol is not readily dialyzable.

Drug Interactions Substrate of CYP2D6 (major); **Inhibits** CYP2D6 (weak)

Albuterol (and other beta$_2$ agonists): Effects may be blunted by nonspecific beta-blockers.

Alpha-blockers (prazosin, terazosin): Concurrent use of beta-blockers may increase risk of orthostasis.

AV conduction-slowing agents (digoxin): Effects may be additive with beta-blockers.

Clonidine: Hypertensive crisis after or during withdrawal of either agent (not reported with timolol ophthalmic solution)

CYP2D6 inhibitors: May increase the levels/effects of timolol. Example inhibitors include chlorpromazine, delavirdine, fluoxetine, miconazole, paroxetine, pergolide, quinidine, quinine, ritonavir, and ropinirole.

Epinephrine (including local anesthetics with epinephrine): Timolol may cause hypertension.

Glucagon: Timolol may blunt hyperglycemic action.

Insulin and oral hypoglycemics: May mask symptoms of hypoglycemia.

NSAIDs (ibuprofen, indomethacin, naproxen, piroxicam) may reduce the antihypertensive effects of beta-blockers.

Salicylates may reduce the antihypertensive effects of beta-blockers.

Sulfonylureas: Beta-blockers may alter response to hypoglycemic agents.

Verapamil or diltiazem may have synergistic or additive pharmacological effects when taken concurrently with beta-blockers.

Dietary Considerations Oral product should be administered with food at the same time each day.

Dosage Forms Note: Unless otherwise specified, strength expressed as base.

Gel-forming solution, ophthalmic, as maleate: 0.25% (5 mL); 0.5% (2.5 mL, 5 mL)

Timoptic-XE®: 0.25% (5 mL); 0.5% (5 mL)

Solution, ophthalmic, as hemihydrate:

Betimol®: 0.25% (5 mL, 10 mL, 15 mL); 0.5% (5 mL, 10 mL, 15 mL) [contains benzalkonium chloride]

Solution, ophthalmic, as maleate: 0.25% (5 mL, 10 mL, 15 mL); 0.5% (5 mL, 10 mL, 15 mL) [contains benzalkonium chloride]

Istalol™: 0.5% (10 mL) [contains benzalkonium chloride and potassium sorbate]

Timoptic®: 0.25% (5 mL); 0.5% (5 mL, 10 mL) [contains benzalkonium chloride]

(Continued)

Timolol *(Continued)*

Solution, ophthalmic, as maleate [preservative free]:
Timoptic® OcuDose®: 0.25% (0.2 mL); 0.5% (0.2 mL) [single use]
Tablet, as maleate: 5 mg, 10 mg, 20 mg [strength expressed as salt]
Blocadren®: 20 mg [strength expressed as salt]

- ♦ **Timolol Hemihydrate** *see* Timolol *on page 1268*
- ♦ **Timolol Maleate** *see* Timolol *on page 1268*
- ♦ **Timoptic®** *see* Timolol *on page 1268*
- ♦ **Timoptic® OcuDose®** *see* Timolol *on page 1268*
- ♦ **Timoptic-XE®** *see* Timolol *on page 1268*

Tinzaparin (tin ZA pa rin)

U.S. Brand Names Innohep®

Canadian Brand Names Innohep®

Synonyms Tinzaparin Sodium

Pharmacologic Category Low Molecular Weight Heparin

Generic Available No

Use Treatment of acute symptomatic deep vein thrombosis, with or without pulmonary embolism, in conjunction with warfarin sodium

Mechanism of Action Standard heparin consists of components with molecular weights ranging from 4000-30,000 daltons with a mean of 16,000 daltons. Heparin acts as an anticoagulant by enhancing the inhibition rate of clotting proteases by antithrombin III, impairing normal hemostasis and inhibition of factor Xa. Low molecular weight heparins have a small effect on the activated partial thromboplastin time and strongly inhibit factor Xa. The primary inhibitory activity of tinzaparin is through antithrombin. Tinzaparin is derived from porcine heparin that undergoes controlled enzymatic depolymerization. The average molecular weight of tinzaparin ranges between 5500 and 7500 daltons which is distributed as (<10%) 2000 daltons (60% to 72%) 2000-8000 daltons, and (22% to 36%) >8000 daltons. The antifactor Xa activity is approximately 100 int. units/mg.

Pharmacodynamics/Kinetics

Onset of action: 2-3 hours
Distribution: 3-5 L
Half-life elimination: 3-4 hours
Metabolism: Partially metabolized by desulphation and depolymerization
Bioavailability: 87%
Time to peak: 4-5 hours
Excretion: Urine

Dosage SubQ:

Adults: 175 anti-Xa int. units/kg of body weight once daily. Warfarin sodium should be started when appropriate. Administer tinzaparin for at least 6 days and until patient is adequately anticoagulated with warfarin.

Note: To calculate the volume of solution to administer per dose: Volume to be administered (mL) = patient weight (kg) x 0.00875 mL/kg (may be rounded off to the nearest 0.05 mL)

Elderly: No significant differences in safety or response were seen when used in patients ≥65 years of age. However, increased sensitivity to tinzaparin in elderly patients may be possible due to a decline in renal function.

Dosage adjustment in renal impairment: Patients with severe renal impairment had a 24% decrease in clearance, use with caution.

Dosage adjustment in hepatic impairment: No specific dosage adjustment has been recommended.

Stability Store at 25°C (77°F); excursions permitted to 15°C to 30°C (59°F to 86°F)

Administration Patient should be lying down or sitting. Administer by deep SubQ injection, alternating between the left and right anterolateral and left and right posterolateral abdominal wall. Vary site daily. The entire needle should be introduced into the skin fold formed by the thumb and forefinger. Hold the skin fold until injection is complete. To minimize bruising, do not rub the injection site.

Monitoring Parameters CBC including platelet count and hematocrit or hemoglobin, and stool for occult blood; the monitoring of PT and/or aPTT is not necessary. Patients receiving both warfarin and tinzaparin should have their INR drawn just prior to the next scheduled dose of tinzaparin.

Pregnancy Risk Factor B

Contraindications Hypersensitivity to tinzaparin sodium, heparin, sulfites, benzyl alcohol, pork products, or any component of the formulation; active major bleeding; heparin-induced thrombocytopenia (current or history of)

Warnings/Precautions **[U.S. Boxed Warning]: Patients with recent or anticipated neuraxial anesthesia (epidural or spinal anesthesia) are at risk of spinal or epidural hematoma and subsequent paralysis.** Consider risk versus benefit prior to neuraxial anesthesia; risk is increased by concomitant agents which may alter hemostasis, as well as traumatic or repeated epidural or spinal puncture, and indwelling epidural catheters. Patient should be observed closely for signs and symptoms of neurological impairment. Not to be used interchangeably (unit for unit) with heparin or any other low molecular weight heparins.

Monitor patient closely for signs or symptoms of bleeding. Certain patients are at increased risk of bleeding. Risk factors include bacterial endocarditis; congenital or acquired bleeding disorders; active ulcerative or angiodysplastic GI diseases; severe uncontrolled hypertension; hemorrhagic stroke; use shortly after brain, spinal, or ophthalmologic surgery; patients treated concomitantly with platelet inhibitors; recent GI bleeding; thrombocytopenia or platelet defects; severe liver disease; hypertensive or diabetic retinopathy; or in patients undergoing invasive procedures. Monitor platelet count closely. Rare cases of thrombocytopenia have occurred. Manufacturer recommends discontinuation of therapy if platelets are <100,000/mm^3.

Safety and efficacy in pediatric patients has not been established. Use with caution in the elderly (delayed elimination may occur). Heparin can cause hyperkalemia by affecting aldosterone; similar reactions could occur with LMWHs. Monitor for hyperkalemia. For subcutaneous injection only, do not mix with other injections or infusions. Clinical experience is limited in patients with BMI >40 kg.

Adverse Reactions As with all anticoagulants, bleeding is the major adverse effect of tinzaparin. Hemorrhage may occur at virtually any site. Risk is dependent on multiple variables.

>10%:
- Hepatic: Increased ALT (13%)
- Local: Injection site hematoma (16%)

1% to 10%:
- Cardiovascular: Angina pectoris, chest pain (2%), hyper-/hypotension, tachycardia
- Central nervous system: Confusion, dizziness, fever (2%), headache (2%), insomnia, pain (2%)
- Dermatologic: Bullous eruption, pruritus, rash (1%), skin disorder
- Gastrointestinal: Constipation (1%), dyspepsia, flatulence, nausea (2%), nonspecified gastrointestinal disorder, vomiting (1%)
- Genitourinary: Dysuria, urinary retention, urinary tract infection (4%)
- Hematologic: Anemia, hematoma, hemorrhage (2%), thrombocytopenia (1%)
- Hepatic: Increased AST (9%)
- Local: Deep vein thrombosis
- Neuromuscular & skeletal: Back pain (2%)
- Renal: Hematuria (1%)
- Respiratory: Dyspnea (1%), epistaxis (2%), pneumonia, pulmonary embolism (2%), respiratory disorder
- Miscellaneous: Impaired healing, infection, unclassified reactions

<1% (Limited to important or life-threatening): Agranulocytosis, allergic purpura, allergic reaction, angioedema, arrhythmia, cholestatic hepatitis, epidermal necrolysis, gastrointestinal hemorrhage, granulocytopenia, hemarthrosis, hematoma, hemoptysis, intracranial hemorrhage, ischemic necrosis, major bleeding, MI, ocular hemorrhage, pancytopenia, priapism, purpura, rash, retroperitoneal/intra-abdominal bleeding, severe thrombocytopenia, skin necrosis, spinal epidural hematoma, Stevens-Johnson syndrome, urticaria, vaginal hemorrhage

Postmarketing and/or case reports: The following adverse effects have been reported in infants of women receiving tinzaparin during pregnancy (relationship has not been established): Cleft palate (one report), optic nerve hypoplasia (one report), trisomy 21 (one report), fetal death/miscarriage, fetal distress, neonatal hypotonia, cutis aplasia of the scalp

Overdosage/Toxicology Overdose may lead to bleeding; bleeding may occur at any site. In case of overdose, discontinue medication, apply pressure to bleeding site if possible, and replace volume and hemostatic blood elements as required. If

(Continued)

Tinzaparin *(Continued)*

these measures are ineffective, or if bleeding is severe, protamine sulfate may be administered at 1 mg per every 100 anti-Xa int. units of tinzaparin.

Drug Interactions

Drugs which affect platelet function (eg, aspirin, NSAIDs, dipyridamole, ticlopidine, clopidogrel, sulfinpyrazone, dextran) may potentiate the risk of hemorrhage.

Thrombolytic agents increase the risk of hemorrhage.

Warfarin: Risk of bleeding may be increased during concurrent therapy. Tinzaparin is commonly continued during the initiation of warfarin therapy to assure anticoagulation and to protect against possible transient hypercoagulability

Test Interactions Asymptomatic increases in AST (SGOT) (8.8%) and ALT (SGPT) (13%) have been reported. Elevations were >3 times the upper limit of normal and were reversible and rarely associated with increases in bilirubin.

Dosage Forms Injection, solution, as sodium: 20,000 anti-Xa int. units/mL (2 mL) [contains benzyl alcohol and sodium metabisulfite]

♦ **Tinzaparin Sodium** *see* Tinzaparin *on page 1272*

Tiotropium (ty oh TRO pee um)

Medication Safety Issues

Sound-alike/look-alike issues:

Spiriva® may be confused with Inspra™

Spiriva® capsules for inhalation are for administration via HandiHaler® device and are not for oral use

U.S. Brand Names Spiriva®

Canadian Brand Names Spiriva®

Synonyms Tiotropium Bromide Monohydrate

Pharmacologic Category Anticholinergic Agent

Use Maintenance treatment of bronchospasm associated with COPD (bronchitis and emphysema)

Mechanism of Action Blocks the action of acetylcholine at parasympathetic sites in bronchial smooth muscle causing bronchodilation

Pharmacodynamics/Kinetics

Absorption: Poorly absorbed from GI tract, systemic absorption may occur from lung

Distribution: V_d: 32 L/kg

Protein binding: 72%

Metabolism: Hepatic (minimal), via CYP2D6 and CYP3A4

Bioavailability: Following inhalation, 19.5%; oral solution: 2% to 3%

Half-life elimination: 5-6 days

Time to peak, plasma: 5 minutes (following inhalation)

Excretion: Urine (74% as unchanged drug)

Dosage Oral inhalation: Adults: Contents of 1 capsule (18 mcg) inhaled once daily using HandiHaler® device

Dosage adjustment in renal impairment: Plasma concentrations increase in renal impairment. Use caution; no specific dosage adjustment recommended.

Stability Store between 15°C and 25°C. Do not store capsules in HandiHaler® device. Capsules should be stored in the blister pack and only removed immediately before use. After first capsule in the strip is used, the 2 remaining capsules should be used over the next 2 days.

Administration Administer once daily at the same time each day. Remove capsule from foil blister immediately before use. Place capsule in the capsule-chamber in the base of the HandiHaler® Inhaler. Must only use the HandiHaler® Inhaler. Close mouthpiece until a click is heard, leaving dustcap open. Exhale fully. Do not exhale into inhaler. Tilt head slightly back and inhale (rapidly, steadily and deeply); the capsule vibration may be heard within the device. Hold breath as long as possible. If any powder remains in capsule, exhale and inhale again. Repeat until capsule is empty. Throw away empty capsule; do not leave in inhaler. Do not use a spacer with the HandiHaler® Inhaler. Always keep capsules and inhaler dry.

Delivery of dose: Instruct patient to place mouthpiece gently between teeth, closing lips around inhaler. Instruct patient to inhale deeply and hold breath held for 5-10 seconds. The amount of drug delivered is small, and the individual will not sense the medication as it is inhaled. Remove mouthpiece prior to exhalation. Patient should not breathe out through the mouthpiece.

Monitoring Parameters FEV_1, peak flow (or other pulmonary function studies)

Pregnancy Risk Factor C

Contraindications Hypersensitivity to tiotropium, its derivatives, or any component of the formulation (contains lactose); not for use as an acute ("rescue") bronchodilator

Warnings/Precautions Not indicated for the initial treatment of acute episodes of bronchospasm; use with caution in patients with myasthenia gravis, narrow-angle glaucoma, prostatic hyperplasia, or bladder neck obstruction; avoid inadvertent instillation of powder into the eyes. Immediate hypersensitivity reactions may occur. Use caution in renal impairment. Safety and efficacy have not been established in pediatric patients.

Adverse Reactions

>10%:

Gastrointestinal: Xerostomia (16%)

Respiratory: Upper respiratory tract infection (41% vs 37% with placebo), sinusitis (11% vs 9% with placebo), pharyngeal irritation (frequency not specified)

1% to 10%:

Cardiovascular: Angina, edema (dependent, 5%)

Central nervous system: Paresthesia, depression

Dermatologic: Rash (4%)

Endocrine & metabolic: Hypercholesterolemia, hyperglycemia

Gastrointestinal: Dyspepsia (6%), abdominal pain (5%), constipation (4%), vomiting (4%), reflux, ulcerative stomatitis

Genitourinary: Urinary tract infection (7%)

Neuromuscular & skeletal: Myalgia (4%), leg pain, skeletal pain

Ocular: Cataract

Respiratory: Pharyngitis (9%), rhinitis (6%), epistaxis (4%), dysphonia, laryngitis

Miscellaneous: Infection (4%), moniliasis (4%), allergic reaction, herpes zoster

<1% (Limited to important or life-threatening): Angioedema, blurred vision/pupil dilation (if powder comes in contact with eyes), hypersensitivity reactions, palpitation, paradoxical bronchospasm, pruritus, tachycardia, urinary retention, urticaria

Overdosage/Toxicology Conjunctivitis and xerostomia have been observed with doses up to 141 micrograms. Other symptoms of overdose include drying of respiratory secretions, cough, nausea, GI distress, blurred vision or impaired visual accommodation, headache, and nervousness. Acute overdose with tiotropium by inhalation is unlikely since it is so poorly absorbed. However, if poisoning occurs, it can be treated like any other anticholinergic toxicity. An anticholinergic overdose with severe life-threatening symptoms may be treated with physostigmine 1-2 mg SubQ or I.V. slowly.

Drug Interactions Substrate (minor) of CYP2D6, 3A4

Anticholinergic agents: Increased toxicity with anticholinergics or drugs with anticholinergic properties.

Dosage Forms Powder for oral inhalation [capsule]: 18 mcg/capsule [contains lactose; packaged in 6s or 30s with HandiHaler® device]

♦ **Tiotropium Bromide Monohydrate** *see* Tiotropium *on page 1274*

Tirofiban (tye roe FYE ban)

Medication Safety Issues

Sound-alike/look-alike issues:

Aggrastat® may be confused with Aggrenox®, argatroban

U.S. Brand Names Aggrastat®

Canadian Brand Names Aggrastat®

Synonyms MK383; Tirofiban Hydrochloride

Pharmacologic Category Antiplatelet Agent, Glycoprotein IIb/IIIa Inhibitor

Generic Available No

Use In combination with heparin, is indicated for the treatment of acute coronary syndrome, including patients who are to be managed medically and those undergoing PTCA or atherectomy. In this setting, it has been shown to decrease the rate of a combined endpoint of death, new myocardial infarction or refractory ischemia/repeat cardiac procedure.

(Continued)

Tirofiban *(Continued)*

Mechanism of Action A reversible antagonist of fibrinogen binding to the GP IIb/IIIa receptor, the major platelet surface receptor involved in platelet aggregation. When administered intravenously, it inhibits *ex vivo* platelet aggregation in a dose- and concentration-dependent manner. When given according to the recommended regimen, >90% inhibition is attained by the end of the 30-minute infusion. Platelet aggregation inhibition is reversible following cessation of the infusion.

Pharmacodynamics/Kinetics

Distribution: 35% unbound

Metabolism: Minimally hepatic

Half-life elimination: 2 hours

Excretion: Urine (65%) and feces (25%) primarily as unchanged drug

Clearance: Elderly: Reduced by 19% to 26%

Dosage Adults: I.V.: Initial rate of 0.4 mcg/kg/minute for 30 minutes and then continued at 0.1 mcg/kg/minute; dosing should be continued through angiography and for 12-24 hours after angioplasty or atherectomy. See table.

Tirofiban Dosing (Using 50 mcg/mL Concentration)

Patient Weight (kg)	Patients With Normal Renal Function		Patients With Renal Dysfunction	
	30-Min Loading Infusion Rate (mL/h)	Maintenance Infusion Rate (mL/h)	30-Min Loading Infusion Rate (mL/h)	Maintenance Infusion Rate (mL/h)
30-37	16	4	8	2
38-45	20	5	10	3
46-54	24	6	12	3
55-62	28	7	14	4
63-70	32	8	16	4
71-79	36	9	18	5
80-87	40	10	20	5
88-95	44	11	22	6
96-104	48	12	24	6
105-112	52	13	26	7
113-120	56	14	28	7
121-128	60	15	30	8
128-137	64	16	32	8
138-145	68	17	34	9
146-153	72	18	36	9

Dosing adjustment in severe renal impairment: Cl_{cr} <30 mL/minute: Reduce dose to 50% of normal rate.

Stability Store at 25°C (77°F); do not freeze. Protect from light during storage. Not compatible with diazepam.

Administration Intended for intravenous delivery using sterile equipment and technique. Do not add other drugs or remove solution directly from the bag with a syringe. Do not use plastic containers in series connections; such use can result in air embolism by drawing air from the first container if it is empty of solution. Discard unused solution 24 hours following the start of infusion. May be administered through the same catheter as heparin. Tirofiban injection must be diluted to a concentration of 50 mcg/mL (premixed solution does not require dilution). Infuse over 30 minutes.

Monitoring Parameters Platelet count. Hemoglobin and hematocrit should be monitored prior to treatment, within 6 hours following loading infusion, and at least daily thereafter during therapy. Platelet count may need to be monitored earlier in patients who received prior glycoprotein IIb/IIa antagonists. Persistent reductions of platelet counts <90,000/mm^3 may require interruption or discontinuation of infusion. Because tirofiban requires concurrent heparin therapy, aPTT levels should also be followed. Monitor vital signs and laboratory results prior to, during, and after therapy. Assess infusion insertion site during and after therapy (every 15 minutes or as institutional policy). Observe and teach patient bleeding precautions (avoid invasive procedures and activities that could result in injury). Monitor closely for signs of unusual or excessive bleeding (eg, CNS changes, blood in urine, stool, or vomitus, unusual bruising or bleeding). Breast-feeding is contraindicated.

Anesthesia and Critical Care Concerns/Other Considerations **Platelet Effects:** Tirofiban has a short duration of action and hemostasis is restored within about 4 hours after discontinuation in patients with normal renal function.

Pregnancy Risk Factor B

Contraindications Hypersensitivity to tirofiban or any component of the formulation; active internal bleeding or a history of bleeding diathesis within the previous 30 days; history of intracranial hemorrhage, intracranial neoplasm, arteriovenous malformation, or aneurysm; history of thrombocytopenia following prior exposure; history of CVA within 30 days or any history of hemorrhagic stroke; major surgical procedure or severe physical trauma within the previous month; history, symptoms, or findings suggestive of aortic dissection; severe hypertension (systolic BP >180 mm Hg and/or diastolic BP >110 mm Hg); concomitant use of another parenteral GP IIb/IIIa inhibitor; acute pericarditis

Warnings/Precautions Bleeding is the most common complication. Watch closely for bleeding, especially the arterial access site for the cardiac catheterization. Prior to pulling the sheath, heparin should be discontinued for 3-4 hours and ACT <180 seconds or aPTT <45 seconds. Use standard compression techniques after sheath removal. Watch the site closely afterwards for further bleeding. Use with extreme caution in patients with platelet counts <150,000/mm^3, patients with hemorrhagic retinopathy, and chronic dialysis patients. Use caution with administration of other drugs affecting hemostasis. Adjust the dose with severe renal dysfunction (Cl_{cr} <30 mL/minute). The use of tirofiban, aspirin and heparin together causes more bleeding than aspirin and heparin alone. Do not administer in the same I.V. line as diazepam.

Adverse Reactions Bleeding is the major drug-related adverse effect. Patients received background treatment with aspirin and heparin. Major bleeding was reported in 1.4% to 2.2%; minor bleeding in 10.5% to 12%; transfusion was required in 4% to 4.3%.

>1% (nonbleeding adverse events):
- Cardiovascular: Bradycardia (4%), coronary artery dissection (5%), edema (2%)
- Central nervous system: Dizziness (3%), fever (>1%), headache (>1%), vasovagal reaction (2%)
- Gastrointestinal: Nausea (>1%)
- Genitourinary: Pelvic pain (6%)
- Hematologic: Thrombocytopenia: <90,000/mm^3 (1.5%), <50,000/mm^3 (0.3%)
- Neuromuscular & skeletal: Leg pain (3%)
- Miscellaneous: Diaphoresis (2%)

<1% (Limited to important or life-threatening): Acutely decreased platelets in association with fever, anaphylaxis, GI bleeding (0.1% to 0.2%), GU bleeding (up to 0.1%), hemopericardium, intracranial bleeding (up to 0.1%), pulmonary alveolar hemorrhage, rash, retroperitoneal bleeding (up to 0.6%), severe (<10,000/mm^3) thrombocytopenia (rare), spinal-epidural hematoma

Overdosage/Toxicology The most frequent manifestation of overdose is bleeding. Treatment is cessation of therapy and assessment of transfusion. Tirofiban is dialyzable.

Drug Interactions

Cephalosporins which contain the MTT side chain may theoretically increase the risk of hemorrhage.

Drugs which affect platelet function (eg, aspirin, NSAIDs, dipyridamole, ticlopidine, clopidogrel) may potentiate the risk of hemorrhage.

Heparin and aspirin: Use with aspirin and heparin is associated with an increase in bleeding over aspirin and heparin alone. However, the concurrent use of aspirin and heparin has also improved the efficacy of tirofiban.

Levothyroxine and omeprazole increase tirofiban clearance; however, the clinical significance of this interaction remains to be demonstrated.

Thrombolytic agents theoretically may increase the risk of hemorrhage.

Warfarin and oral anticoagulants: Risk of bleeding may be increased during concurrent therapy.

Other IIb/IIIa antagonists: Concomitant use of other injectable glycoprotein IIb/IIIa antagonists is contraindicated (see Contraindications).

Dosage Forms

Infusion [premixed in sodium chloride]: 50 mcg/mL (100 mL, 250 mL)

Injection, solution: 250 mcg/mL (50 mL)

♦ **Tirofiban Hydrochloride** *see* Tirofiban *on page 1275*

♦ **Tisseel® VH** *see* Fibrin Sealant Kit *on page 523*

♦ **TMP-SMZ** *see* Sulfamethoxazole and Trimethoprim *on page 1215*

♦ **TNKase™** *see* Tenecteplase *on page 1241*

♦ **TOBI®** *see* Tobramycin *on page 1278*

Tobramycin (toe bra MYE sin)

Medication Safety Issues

Sound-alike/look-alike issues:

Tobramycin may be confused with Trobicin®

AKTob® may be confused with AK-Trol®

Nebcin® may be confused with Inapsine®, Naprosyn®, Nubain®

Tobrex® may be confused with TobraDex®

Related Information

Prevention of Wound Infection and Sepsis in Surgical Patients *on page 1588*

U.S. Brand Names AKTob®; TOBI®; Tobrex®

Canadian Brand Names Apo-Tobramycin®; PMS-Tobramycin; Sandoz-Tobramycin; TOBI®; Tobramycin Injection, USP; Tobrex®

Synonyms Tobramycin Sulfate

Pharmacologic Category Antibiotic, Aminoglycoside; Antibiotic, Ophthalmic

Generic Available Yes: Excludes ophthalmic ointment, solution for nebulization

Use Treatment of documented or suspected infections caused by susceptible gram-negative bacilli including *Pseudomonas aeruginosa*; topically used to treat superficial ophthalmic infections caused by susceptible bacteria. Tobramycin solution for inhalation is indicated for the management of cystic fibrosis patients (>6 years of age) with *Pseudomonas aeruginosa*

Mechanism of Action Interferes with bacterial protein synthesis by binding to 30S and 50S ribosomal subunits resulting in a defective bacterial cell membrane

Pharmacodynamics/Kinetics

Absorption: I.M.: Rapid and complete

Distribution: V_d: 0.2-0.3 L/kg; Pediatrics: 0.2-0.7 L/kg; to extracellular fluid including serum, abscesses, ascitic, pericardial, pleural, synovial, lymphatic, and peritoneal fluids; crosses placenta; poor penetration into CSF, eye, bone, prostate (see table)

Aminoglycoside Penetration Into Various Tissues

Site	Extent of Distribution
Eye	Poor
CNS	Poor (<25%)
Pleural	Excellent
Bronchial secretions	Poor
Sputum	Fair (10%-50%)
Pulmonary tissue	Excellent
Ascitic fluid	Variable (43%-132%)
Peritoneal fluid	Poor
Bile	Variable (25%-90%)
Bile with obstruction	Poor
Synovial fluid	Excellent
Bone	Poor
Prostate	Poor
Urine	Excellent
Renal tissue	Excellent

Protein binding: <30%

Half-life elimination:

Neonates: ≤1200 g: 11 hours; >1200 g: 2-9 hours

Adults: 2-3 hours; directly dependent upon glomerular filtration rate

Adults with impaired renal function: 5-70 hours

Time to peak, serum: I.M.: 30-60 minutes; I.V.: ~30 minutes

Excretion: Normal renal function: Urine (~90% to 95%) within 24 hours

Dosage Note: Dosage individualization is **critical** because of the low therapeutic index.

Use of ideal body weight (IBW) for determining the mg/kg/dose appears to be more accurate than dosing on the basis of total body weight (TBW). In morbid obesity, dosage requirement may best be estimated using a dosing weight of IBW + 0.4 (TBW - IBW).

Initial and periodic plasma drug levels (eg, peak and trough with conventional dosing) should be determined, particularly in critically-ill patients with serious infections or in disease states known to significantly alter aminoglycoside pharmacokinetics (eg, cystic fibrosis, burns, or major surgery).

Usual dosage range:

Infants and Children <5 years: I.M., I.V.: 2.5 mg/kg/dose every 8 hours

Children ≥5 years: I.M., I.V.: 2-2.5 mg/kg/dose every 8 hours

Note: Higher individual doses and/or more frequent intervals (eg, every 6 hours) may be required in selected clinical situations (cystic fibrosis) or serum levels document the need. Also see "Note" on monitoring and adjustment.

Children and Adults:

Inhalation: Children: 40-80 mg 2-3 times/day; Adults: 60-80 mg 3 times/day; Children ≥6 years and Adults: High-dose regimen: 300 mg every 12 hours (do not administer doses <6 hours apart); administer in repeated cycles of 28 days on drug followed by 28 days off drug

Intrathecal: 4-8 mg/day

Ophthalmic: Children ≥2 months:

Ointment: Instill ½" (1.25 cm) 2-3 times/day every 3-4 hours

Solution: Instill 1-2 drops every 2-4 hours, up to 2 drops every hour for severe infections

Topical: Apply 3-4 times/day to affected area

Adults: I.M., I.V.:

Conventional: 1-2.5 mg/kg/dose every 8-12 hours; to ensure adequate peak concentrations early in therapy, higher initial dosage may be considered in selected patients when extracellular water is increased (edema, septic shock, postsurgical, and/or trauma)

Once-daily: 4-7 mg/kg/dose once daily; some clinicians recommend this approach for all patients with normal renal function; this dose is at least as efficacious with similar, if not less, toxicity than conventional dosing.

Indication-specific dosing:

Children: I.M., I.V.:

Cystic fibrosis: 2.5-3.3 mg/kg every 6-8 hours; **Note:** Some patients may require larger or more frequent doses if serum levels document the need (eg, cystic fibrosis or febrile granulocytopenic patients). Also see "Note" on monitoring and adjustment.

Meningitis, neonatal:

0-7 days: <2000 g: 2.5 mg/kg every 18-24 hours; >2000 g: 2.5 mg/kg every 12 hours

8-28 days: <2000 g: 2.5 mg/kg every 8-12 hours; >2000 g: 2.5 mg/kg every 8 hours

Adults: I.M., I.V.:

Brucellosis: 240 mg (I.M.) daily or 5 mg/kg (I.V.) daily for 7 days; either regimen recommended in combination with doxycycline

Cholangitis: 4-6 mg/kg once daily with ampicillin

Diverticulitis, complicated: 1.5-2 mg/kg every 8 hours (with ampicillin and metronidazole)

Endocarditis prophylaxis (Dental, oral, upper respiratory procedures, GI/GU procedures): 1.5 mg/kg with ampicillin (50 mg/kg) 30 minutes prior to procedure

Endocarditis or synergy (for Gram-positive infections): 1 mg/kg every 8 hours (with ampicillin)

Meningitis *(Enterococcus or Pseudomonas aeruginosa)*: I.V.: Loading dose: 2 mg/kg, then 1.7 mg/kg/dose every 8 hours (administered with another bacteriocidal drug)

Pelvic inflammatory disease: Loading dose: 2 mg/kg, then 1.5 mg/kg every 8 hours **or** 4.5 mg/kg once daily

Plague *(Yersinia pestis)*: Treatment: 5 mg/kg/day, followed by postexposure prophylaxis with doxycycline

(Continued)

Tobramycin *(Continued)*

Pneumonia, hospital- or ventilator-associated: 7 mg/kg/day (with antipseudomonal beta-lactam or carbapenem)

Tularemia: 5 mg/kg/day divided every 8 hours for 1-2 weeks

Urinary tract infection: 1.5 mg/kg/dose every 8 hours

Dosing interval in renal impairment: I.M., I.V.:

Conventional dosing:

Cl_{cr} ≥60 mL/minute: Administer every 8 hours

Cl_{cr} 40-60 mL/minute: Administer every 12 hours

Cl_{cr} 20-40 mL/minute: Administer every 24 hours

Cl_{cr} 10-20 mL/minute: Administer every 48 hours

Cl_{cr} <10 mL/minute: Administer every 72 hours

High-dose therapy: Interval may be extended (eg, every 48 hours) in patients with moderate renal impairment (Cl_{cr} 30-59 mL/minute) and/or adjusted based on serum level determinations.

Hemodialysis: Dialyzable; 30% removal of aminoglycosides occurs during 4 hours of HD - administer dose after dialysis and follow levels

Continuous arteriovenous or venovenous hemofiltration: Dose as for Cl_{cr} of 10-40 mL/minute and follow levels

Administration in CAPD fluid:

Gram-negative infection: 4-8 mg/L (4-8 mcg/mL) of CAPD fluid

Gram-positive infection (ie, synergy): 3-4 mg/L (3-4 mcg/mL) of CAPD fluid

Administration IVPB/I.M.: Dose as for Cl_{cr} <10 mL/minute and follow levels

Dosing adjustment/comments in hepatic disease: Monitor plasma concentrations

Stability

Injection: Stable at room temperature both as the clear, colorless solution and as the dry powder. Reconstituted solutions remain stable for 24 hours at room temperature and 96 hours when refrigerated. Dilute in 50-100 mL NS, D_5W for I.V. infusion.

Separate administration of extended-spectrum penicillins (eg, carbenicillin, ticarcillin, piperacillin) from tobramycin in patients with severe renal impairment; tobramycin's efficacy may be reduced if given concurrently.

Ophthalmic solution: Store at 8°C to 27°C (46°F to 80°F).

Solution, for inhalation (TOBI®): Store under refrigeration at 2°C to 8°C (36°F to 46°F); may be stored in foil pouch at room temperature of 25°C (77°F) for up to 28 days. Avoid intense light. Solution may darken over time; however, do not use if cloudy or contains particles.

Administration

I.V.: Infuse over 30-60 minutes. Flush with saline before and after administration.

Inhalation (TOBI®): To be inhaled over ~15 minutes using a handheld nebulizer.

Ophthalmic: Contact lenses should not be worn during treatment of ophthalmic infections.

Ointment: Do not touch tip of tube to eye. Instill ointment into pocket between eyeball and lower lid; patient should look downward before closing eye.

Solution: Allow 5 minutes between application of "multiple-drop" therapy.

Suspension: Shake well before using; Tilt head back, instill suspension in conjunctival sac and close eye(s). Do not touch dropper to eye. Apply light finger pressure on lacrimal sac for 1 minute following instillation.

Some penicillins (eg, carbenicillin, ticarcillin and piperacillin) have been shown to inactivate aminoglycosides *in vitro*. This has been observed to a greater extent with tobramycin and gentamicin, while amikacin has shown greater stability against inactivation. Concurrent use of these agents may pose a risk of reduced antibacterial efficacy *in vivo*, particularly in the setting of profound renal impairment. However, definitive clinical evidence is lacking. If combination penicillin/aminoglycoside therapy is desired in a patient with renal dysfunction, separation of doses (if feasible), and routine monitoring of aminoglycoside levels, CBC, and clinical response should be considered.

Monitoring Parameters Urinalysis, urine output, BUN, serum creatinine, peak and trough plasma tobramycin levels; be alert to ototoxicity; hearing should be tested before and during treatment

Some penicillin derivatives may accelerate the degradation of aminoglycosides*in vitro*. This may be clinically-significant for certain penicillin (ticarcillin, piperacillin, carbenicillin) and aminoglycoside (gentamicin, tobramycin) combination therapy in patients with significant renal impairment. Close monitoring of aminoglycoside levels is warranted.

Reference Range

Timing of serum samples: Draw peak 30 minutes after 30-minute infusion has been completed or 1 hour following I.M. injection or beginning of infusion; draw trough immediately before next dose

Therapeutic levels:

Peak:

Serious infections: 6-8 mcg/mL (SI: 12-17 μmol/L)

Life-threatening infections: 8-10 mcg/mL (SI: 17-21 μmol/L)

Urinary tract infections: 4-6 mcg/mL (SI: 7-12 μmol/L)

Synergy against gram-positive organisms: 3-5 mcg/mL

Trough:

Serious infections: 0.5-1 mcg/mL

Life-threatening infections: 1-2 mcg/mL

The American Thoracic Society (ATS) recommends trough levels of <1 mcg/mL for patients with hospital-acquired pneumonia.

Monitor serum creatinine and urine output; obtain drug levels after the third dose unless otherwise directed

Inhalation: Serum levels are ~1 mcg/mL one hour following a 300 mg dose in patients with normal renal function.

Pregnancy Risk Factor D (injection, inhalation); B (ophthalmic)

Contraindications Hypersensitivity to tobramycin, other aminoglycosides, or any component of the formulation; pregnancy (injection/inhalation)

Warnings/Precautions [U.S. Boxed Warning]: Aminoglycosides may cause neurotoxicity and/or nephrotoxicity; usual risk factors include prexisiting renal impairment, concomitant neuro-/nephrotoxic medications, advanced age and dehydration. Ototoxicity may be directly proportional to the amount of drug given and the duration of treatment; tinnitus or vertigo are indications of vestibular injury and impending hearing loss; renal damage is usually reversible

Not intended for long-term therapy due to toxic hazards associated with extended administration; use caution in pre-existing renal insufficiency, vestibular or cochlear impairment, myasthenia gravis, hypocalcemia, conditions which depress neuromuscular transmission. Dosage modification required in patients with impaired renal function

Adverse Reactions

Injection: Frequency not defined:

Central nervous system: Confusion, disorientation, dizziness, fever, headache, lethargy, vertigo

Dermatologic: Exfoliative dermatitis, itching, rash, urticaria

Endocrine & metabolic: Serum calcium, magnesium, potassium, and/or sodium decreased

Gastrointestinal: Diarrhea, nausea, vomiting

Hematologic: Anemia, eosinophilia, granulocytopenia, leukocytosis, leukopenia, thrombocytopenia

Hepatic: ALT, AST, bilirubin, and/or LDH increased

Local: Pain at the injection site

Otic: Hearing loss, tinnitus, ototoxicity (auditory), ototoxicity (vestibular), roaring in the ears

Renal: BUN increased, cylindruria, serum creatinine increased, oliguria, proteinuria

Inhalation:

>10%:

Gastrointestinal: Sputum discoloration (21%)

Respiratory: Voice alteration (13%)

1% to 10%:

Central nervous system: Malaise (6%)

Otic: Tinnitus (3%)

Postmarketing and/or case reports: Hearing loss

Ophthalmic: <1% (Limited to important or life-threatening): Ocular: Conjunctival erythema, lid itching, lid swelling

Overdosage/Toxicology Symptoms of overdose include ototoxicity, nephrotoxicity, and neuromuscular toxicity. Treatment of choice following a single acute overdose appears to be maintenance of urine output of at least 3 mL/kg/hour during the acute treatment phase. Dialysis is of questionable value in enhancing aminoglycoside elimination. If required, hemodialysis is preferred over peritoneal

(Continued)

Tobramycin *(Continued)*

dialysis in patients with normal renal function. Chelation with penicillins is investigational.

Drug Interactions

Increased effect: Extended spectrum penicillins (synergistic)

Increased toxicity:

Aminoglycosides may potentiate the effects of neuromuscular-blocking agents

Amphotericin B, cephalosporins, loop diuretics, and vancomycin may increase risk of nephrotoxicity

Decreased effect: Tobramycin's efficacy reduced when given concurrently with carbenicillin, ticarcillin, or piperacillin to patients with severe renal impairment (inactivation). Separate administration.

Test Interactions Some penicillin derivatives may accelerate the degradation of aminoglycosides *in vitro*, leading to a potential underestimation of aminoglycoside serum concentration.

Dietary Considerations May require supplementation of calcium, magnesium, potassium.

Dosage Forms

Infusion [premixed in NS]: 60 mg (50 mL); 80 mg (100 mL)

Injection, powder for reconstitution: 1.2 g

Injection, solution: 10 mg/mL (2 mL, 8 mL); 40 mg/mL (2 mL, 30 mL, 50 mL) [may contain sodium metabisulfite]

Ointment, ophthalmic (Tobrex®): 0.3% (3.5 g)

Solution for nebulization [preservative free] (TOBI®): 60 mg/mL (5 mL)

Solution, ophthalmic (AKTob®, Tobrex®): 0.3% (5 mL) [contains benzalkonium chloride]

References

American Thoracic Society and Infectious Diseases Society of America, "Guidelines for the Management of Adults With Hospital-Acquired, Ventilator-Associated, and Healthcare-Associated Pneumonia," *Am J Respir Crit Care Med*, 2005, 171(4):388-416.

Kahler DA, Schowengerdt KO, Fricker FJ, et al, "Toxic Serum Trough Concentrations After Administration of Nebulized Tobramycin," *Pharmacotherapy*, 2003, 23(4):543-5.

Ramsey BW, Burns J, Smith A, et al, "Safety and Efficacy of Tobramycin for Inhalation in Patients With Cystic Fibrosis: The Results of Two Phase III Placebo Controlled Clinical Trials," *Pediatr Pulmonol*, 1997, (Suppl 14):137-8, S10.3.

Ramsey BW, Dorkin HL, Eisenberg JD, et al, "Efficacy of Aerosolized Tobramycin in Patients With Cystic Fibrosis," *N Engl J Med*, 1993, 328(24):1740-6.

Shaw PK, Braun TL, Liebergen A, et al, "Aerosolized Tobramycin Pharmacokinetics in Cystic Fibrosis Patients," *J Pediatr Pharm Pract*, 1997, 2(1):23-6.

Tunkel AR, Hartman BJ, Kaplan SL, et al, "Practice Guidelines for the Management of Bacterial Meningitis," *Clin Infect Dis*, 2004, 39(9):1267-84.

♦ **Tobramycin Injection, USP (Can)** *see* Tobramycin *on page 1278*
♦ **Tobramycin Sulfate** *see* Tobramycin *on page 1278*
♦ **Tobrex®** *see* Tobramycin *on page 1278*
♦ **Tofranil®** *see* Imipramine *on page 663*
♦ **Tofranil-PM®** *see* Imipramine *on page 663*
♦ **Tolectin®** *see* Tolmetin *on page 1282*

Tolmetin (TOLE met in)

Related Information

Chronic Pain Management *on page 1430*

U.S. Brand Names Tolectin®

Synonyms Tolmetin Sodium

Pharmacologic Category Nonsteroidal Anti-inflammatory Drug (NSAID), Oral

Restrictions A medication guide should be dispensed with each prescription. A template for the required MedGuide can be found on the FDA website at: http://www.fda.gov/medwatch/SAFETY/2005/safety05.htm#NSAID

Generic Available Yes

Use Treatment of rheumatoid arthritis and osteoarthritis, juvenile rheumatoid arthritis

Mechanism of Action Inhibits prostaglandin synthesis by decreasing the activity of the enzyme, cyclooxygenase, which results in decreased formation of prostaglandin precursors

Pharmacodynamics/Kinetics

Onset of action: Analgesic: 1-2 hours; Anti-inflammatory: Days to weeks

Absorption: Well absorbed

Bioavailability: Reduced 16% with food or milk
Half-life elimination: Biphasic: Rapid: 1-2 hours; Slow: 5 hours
Time to peak, serum: 30-60 minutes
Excretion: Urine (as inactive metabolites or conjugates) within 24 hours

Dosage Oral:
Children ≥2 years:
Anti-inflammatory: Initial: 20 mg/kg/day in 3 divided doses, then 15-30 mg/kg/day in 3 divided doses
Analgesic: 5-7 mg/kg/dose every 6-8 hours
Adults: 400 mg 3 times/day; usual dose: 600 mg to 1.8 g/day; maximum: 2 g/day

Monitoring Parameters Occult blood loss, CBC, liver enzymes, BUN, serum creatinine, periodic liver function test

Anesthesia and Critical Care Concerns/Other Considerations The 2002 ACCM/SCCM guidelines for analgesia (critically-ill adult) suggest that NSAIDs may be used in combination with opioids in select patients for pain management. Concern about adverse events (increased risk of renal dysfunction, altered platelet function and gastrointestinal irritation) limits its use in patients who have other underlying risks for these events.

In short-term use, NSAIDs vary considerably in their effect on blood pressure. When NSAIDs are used in patients with hypertension, appropriate monitoring of blood pressure responses should be completed and the duration of therapy, when possible, kept short. The use of NSAIDs in the treatment of patients with congestive heart failure may be associated with an increased risk for fluid accumulation and edema; may precipitate renal failure in dehydrated patients.

Pregnancy Risk Factor C/D (3rd trimester)

Contraindications Hypersensitivity to tolmetin, aspirin, other NSAIDs, or any component of the formulation; perioperative pain in the setting of coronary artery bypass surgery (CABG); pregnancy (3rd trimester or near term)

Warnings/Precautions **[U.S. Boxed Warning]: NSAIDs are associated with an increased risk of adverse cardiovascular events, including MI, stroke, and new onset or worsening of pre-existing hypertension.** Risk may be increased with duration of use or pre-existing cardiovascular risk-factors or disease. Carefully evaluate individual cardiovascular risk profiles prior to prescribing. Use caution with fluid retention, CHF or hypertension.

Use of NSAIDs can compromise existing renal function. Renal toxicity can occur in patient with impaired renal function, dehydration, heart failure, liver dysfunction, those taking diuretics and ACEI and the elderly. Rehydrate patient before starting therapy. Monitor renal function closely. Use caution in patients with advanced renal disease.

[U.S. Boxed Warning]: NSAIDs may increase risk of gastrointestinal irritation, ulceration, bleeding, and perforation. These events may occur at any time during therapy and without warning. Use caution with a history of GI disease (bleeding or ulcers), concurrent therapy with aspirin, anticoagulants and/or corticosteroids, smoking, use of alcohol, the elderly or debilitated patients.

Use the lowest effective dose for the shortest duration of time, consistent with individual patient goals, to reduce risk of cardiovascular or GI adverse events. Alternate therapies should be considered for patients at high risk.

NSAIDs may cause serious skin adverse events including exfoliative dermatitis, Stevens-Johnson syndrome (SJS) and toxic epidermal necrolysis (TEN). Anaphylactoid reactions may occur, even without prior exposure; patients with "aspirin triad" (bronchial asthma, aspirin intolerance, rhinitis) may be at increased risk. Do not use in patients who experience bronchospasm, asthma, rhinitis, or urticaria with NSAID or aspirin therapy.

Use with caution in patients with decreased hepatic function. Closely monitor patients with any abnormal LFT. Severe hepatic reactions (eg, fulminant hepatitis, liver failure) have occurred with NSAID use, rarely; discontinue if signs or symptoms of liver disease develop, or if systemic manifestations occur.

The elderly are at increased risk for adverse effects (especially peptic ulceration, CNS effects, renal toxicity) from NSAIDs even at low doses.

Withhold for at least 4-6 half-lives prior to surgical or dental procedures. Safety and efficacy have not been established in children <2 years of age.

Adverse Reactions
1% to 10%:
Cardiovascular: Chest pain, hypertension, edema

(Continued)

Tolmetin *(Continued)*

Central nervous system: Headache, dizziness, drowsiness, depression
Dermatologic: Skin irritation
Endocrine & metabolic: Weight gain/loss
Gastrointestinal: Heartburn, abdominal pain, diarrhea, flatulence, vomiting, constipation, gastritis, peptic ulcer, nausea
Genitourinary: Urinary tract infection
Hematologic: Elevated BUN, transient decreases in hemoglobin/hematocrit
Ocular: Visual disturbances
Otic: Tinnitus

<1% (Limited to important or life-threatening): Abnormal LFTs, agranulocytosis, bronchospasm, CHF, dyspnea, erythema multiforme, GI bleeding, granulocytopenia, hematuria, hemolytic anemia, hepatitis, proteinuria, renal failure, thrombocytopenia, toxic epidermal necrolysis

Overdosage/Toxicology Symptoms of overdose include lethargy, mental confusion, dizziness, leukocytosis, and renal failure. Management of NSAID intoxication is supportive and symptomatic. Since many NSAIDs undergo enterohepatic cycling, multiple doses of charcoal may be needed to reduce the potential for delayed toxicities.

Drug Interactions

ACE inhibitors: Antihypertensive effects may be decreased by concurrent therapy with NSAIDs; monitor blood pressure.

Angiotensin II antagonists: Antihypertensive effects may be decreased by concurrent therapy with NSAIDs; monitor blood pressure.

Anticoagulants (warfarin, heparin, LMWHs) in combination with NSAIDs can cause increased risk of bleeding.

Antiplatelet drugs (ticlopidine, clopidogrel, aspirin, abciximab, dipyridamole, eptifibatide, tirofiban) can cause an increased risk of bleeding.

Beta-blockers: NSAIDs may decrease the antihypertensive effect of beta-blockers. Monitor.

Cholestyramine (and other bile acid sequestrants): May decrease the absorption of NSAIDs. Separate by at least 2 hours.

Corticosteroids may increase the risk of GI ulceration; avoid concurrent use.

Cyclosporine: NSAIDs may increase serum creatinine, potassium, blood pressure, and cyclosporine levels; monitor cyclosporine levels and renal function carefully.

Hydralazine's antihypertensive effect is decreased; avoid concurrent use.

Lithium levels can be increased; avoid concurrent use if possible or monitor lithium levels and adjust dose. Sulindac may have the least effect. When NSAID is stopped, lithium will need adjustment again.

Loop diuretics efficacy (diuretic and antihypertensive effect) may be reduced.

Methotrexate: Severe bone marrow suppression, aplastic anemia, and GI toxicity have been reported with concomitant NSAID therapy. Avoid use during moderate or high-dose methotrexate (increased and prolonged methotrexate levels). NSAID use during low-dose treatment of rheumatoid arthritis has not been fully evaluated; extreme caution is warranted.

Thiazides antihypertensive effects are decreased; avoid concurrent use.

Warfarin's INRs may be increased by piroxicam. Other NSAIDs may have the same effect depending on dose and duration. Monitor INR closely. Use the lowest dose of NSAIDs possible and for the briefest duration.

Ethanol/Nutrition/Herb Interactions

Ethanol: Avoid ethanol (may enhance gastric mucosal irritation).

Food: Tolmetin peak serum concentrations may be decreased if taken with food or milk.

Herb/Nutraceutical: Avoid alfalfa, anise, bilberry, bladderwrack, bromelain, cat's claw, celery, coleus, cordyceps, dong quai, evening primrose, feverfew, fenugreek, garlic, ginger, ginkgo biloboa, red clover, horse chestnut, grapeseed, green tea, ginseng, guggul, horse chestnut seed, horseradish, licorice, prickly ash, red clover, reishi, SAMe, sweet clover, turmeric, white willow (all have additional antiplatelet activity).

Dietary Considerations Should be taken with food, milk, or antacids to decrease GI adverse effects. Sodium content of 200 mg: 0.8 mEq.

Dosage Forms

Capsule: 400 mg
Tablet: 200 mg, 600 mg
Tolectin®: 600 mg [contains sodium 54 mg (2.35 mEq)]

♦ **Tolmetin Sodium** *see* Tolmetin *on page 1282*

Tolterodine (tole TER oh deen)

Medication Safety Issues

Sound-alike/look-alike issues:

Detrol® may be confused with Ditropan®

U.S. Brand Names Detrol®; Detrol® LA

Canadian Brand Names Detrol®; Detrol® LA; Unidet®

Synonyms Tolterodine Tartrate

Pharmacologic Category Anticholinergic Agent

Generic Available No

Use Treatment of patients with an overactive bladder with symptoms of urinary frequency, urgency, or urge incontinence

Mechanism of Action Tolterodine is a competitive antagonist of muscarinic receptors. In animal models, tolterodine demonstrates selectivity for urinary bladder receptors over salivary receptors. Urinary bladder contraction is mediated by muscarinic receptors. Tolterodine increases residual urine volume and decreases detrusor muscle pressure.

Pharmacodynamics/Kinetics

Absorption: Immediate release tablet: Rapid; ≥77%

Distribution: I.V.: V_d: 113 ± 27 L

Protein binding: >96% (primarily to $alpha_1$-acid glycoprotein)

Metabolism: Extensively hepatic, primarily via CYP2D6 (some metabolites share activity) and 3A4 usually (minor pathway). In patients with a genetic deficiency of CYP2D6, metabolism via 3A4 predominates. Forms three active metabolites.

Bioavailability: Immediate release tablet: Increased 53% with food

Half-life elimination:

Immediate release tablet: Extensive metabolizers: ~2 hours; Poor metabolizers: ~10 hours

Extended release capsule: Extensive metabolizers: ~7 hours; Poor metabolizers: ~18 hours

Time to peak: Immediate release tablet: 1-2 hours; Extended release tablet: 2-6 hours

Excretion: Urine (77%); feces (17%); excreted primarily as metabolites (<1% unchanged drug) of which the active 5-hydroxymethyl metabolite accounts for 5% to 14% (<1% in poor metabolizers)

Dosage

Oral: Adults: Treatment of overactive bladder:

Immediate release tablet: 2 mg twice daily; the dose may be lowered to 1 mg twice daily based on individual response and tolerability

Dosing adjustment in patients concurrently taking CYP3A4 inhibitors: 1 mg twice daily

Extended release capsule: 4 mg once a day; dose may be lowered to 2 mg daily based on individual response and tolerability

Dosing adjustment in patients concurrently taking CYP3A4 inhibitors: 2 mg daily

Elderly: Safety and efficacy in patients >64 years was found to be similar to that in younger patients; no dosage adjustment is needed based on age

Dosing adjustment in renal impairment: Use with caution (studies conducted in patients with Cl_{cr} 10-30 mL/minute):

Immediate release tablet: 1 mg twice daily

Extended release capsule: 2 mg daily

Dosing adjustment in hepatic impairment:

Immediate release tablet: 1 mg twice daily

Extended release capsule: 2 mg daily

Stability Store at 15°C to 30°C (59°F to 86°F); protect from light

Administration Extended release capsule: Swallow whole; do not crush, chew, or open

Pregnancy Risk Factor C

Contraindications Hypersensitivity to tolterodine or any component of the formulation; urinary retention; gastric retention; uncontrolled narrow-angle glaucoma; myasthenia gravis

Warnings/Precautions Use with caution in patients with bladder flow obstruction, may increase the risk of urinary retention. Use with caution in patients with

(Continued)

Tolterodine *(Continued)*

gastrointestinal obstructive disorders (ie, pyloric stenosis), may increase the risk of gastric retention. Use with caution in patients with controlled (treated) narrow-angle glaucoma; metabolized in the liver and excreted in the urine and feces, dosage adjustment is required for patients with renal or hepatic impairment. Tolterodine has been associated with QT_c prolongation at high (supratherapeutic) doses. The manufacturer recommends caution in patients with congenital prolonged QT or in patients receiving concurrent therapy with QT_c-prolonging drugs (class Ia or III antiarrhythmics). However, the extent of QT_c prolongation even at supratherapeutic dosages was less than 15 msec. Individuals who are poor metabolizers via CYP2D6 or in the presence of inhibitors of CYP2D6 and CYP3A4 may be more likely to exhibit prolongation. Dosage adjustment is recommended in patients receiving CYP3A4 inhibitors (a lower dose of tolterodine is recommended). Safety and efficacy in pediatric patients have not been established.

Adverse Reactions As reported with immediate release tablet, unless otherwise specified

>10%: Gastrointestinal: Dry mouth (35%; extended release capsules 23%)

1% to 10%:

Cardiovascular: Chest pain (2%)

Central nervous system: Headache (7%; extended release capsules 6%), somnolence (3%; extended release capsules 3%), fatigue (4%; extended release capsules 2%), dizziness (5%; extended release capsules 2%), anxiety (extended release capsules 1%)

Dermatologic: Dry skin (1%)

Gastrointestinal: Abdominal pain (5%; extended release capsules 4%), constipation (7%; extended release capsules 6%), dyspepsia (4%; extended release capsules 3%), diarrhea (4%), weight gain (1%)

Genitourinary: Dysuria (2%; extended release capsules 1%)

Neuromuscular & skeletal: Arthralgia (2%)

Ocular: Abnormal vision (2%; extended release capsules 1%), dry eyes (3%; extended release capsules 3%)

Respiratory: Bronchitis (2%), sinusitis (extended release capsules 2%)

Miscellaneous: Flu-like syndrome (3%), infection (1%)

<1% (Limited to important or life-threatening): Anaphylactoid reactions, angioedema, hallucinations, palpitation, peripheral edema, QT_c prolongation, tachycardia

Overdosage/Toxicology Overdosage with tolterodine can potentially result in severe central anticholinergic effects and should be treated accordingly. ECG monitoring is recommended in the event of overdosage. QT_c prolongation has been observed at supratherapeutic doses; particularly in CYP2D6 poor metabolizers.

Drug Interactions **Substrate** of CYP2C9 (minor), 2C19 (minor), 2D6 (major), 3A4 (major)

Acetylcholinesterase inhibitors (central): May reduce the therapeutic efficacy of tolterodine.

Anticholinergic agents: Concomitant use with tolterodine may increase the risk of anticholinergic side effects.

Antifungal agents (eg, ketoconazole, fluconazole): May increase the levels/effects of tolterodine; monitor.

CYP2D6 inhibitors: May increase the levels/effects of tolterodine, which may include QT_c prolongation. Example inhibitors include chlorpromazine, delavirdine, fluoxetine, miconazole, paroxetine, pergolide, quinidine, quinine, ritonavir, and ropinirole.

CYP3A4 inducers: CYP3A4 inducers may decrease the levels/effects of tolterodine. Example inducers include aminoglutethimide, carbamazepine, nafcillin, nevirapine, phenobarbital, phenytoin, and rifamycins.

CYP3A4 inhibitors: May increase the levels/effects of tolterodine, which may include QT_c prolongation. Example inhibitors include azole antifungals, clarithromycin, diclofenac, doxycycline, erythromycin, imatinib, isoniazid, nefazodone, nicardipine, propofol, protease inhibitors, quinidine, telithromycin, and verapamil.

Pramlintide: Concomitant use with tolterodine may increase the risk of anticholinergic gastrointestinal adverse effects (eg, reduced gut motility).

Ethanol/Nutrition/Herb Interactions

Food: Increases bioavailability (~53% increase) of tolterodine tablets, but does not affect the pharmacokinetics of tolterodine extended release capsules; adjustment of dose is not needed. As a CYP3A4 inhibitor, grapefruit juice may increase the serum level and/or toxicity of tolterodine, but unlikely secondary to high oral bioavailability.

Herb/Nutraceutical: St John's wort (*Hypericum*) appears to induce CYP3A enzymes.

Dosage Forms

Capsule, extended release, as tartrate (Detrol® LA): 2 mg, 4 mg

Tablet, as tartrate (Detrol®): 1 mg, 2 mg

- **Tolterodine Tartrate** *see* Tolterodine *on page 1285*
- **Topamax®** *see* Topiramate *on page 1287*
- **Topicaine® [OTC]** *see* Lidocaine *on page 755*
- **Topilene® (Can)** *see* Betamethasone *on page 169*

Topiramate (toe PYRE a mate)

Medication Safety Issues

Sound-alike/look-alike issues:

Topamax® may be confused with Tegretol®, Tegretol®-XR, Toprol-XL®

Related Information

Chronic Pain Management *on page 1430*

Perioperative Management of Patients on Antiseizure Medication *on page 1458*

U.S. Brand Names Topamax®

Canadian Brand Names Dom-Topiramate; Gen-Topiramate; Novo-Topiramate; PHL-Topiramate; PMS-Topiramate; ratio-Topiramate; Rhoxal-topiramate; Sandoz-Topiramate; Topamax®

Pharmacologic Category Anticonvulsant, Miscellaneous

Generic Available No

Use Monotherapy or adjunctive therapy for partial onset seizures and primary generalized tonic-clonic seizures; adjunctive treatment of seizures associated with Lennox-Gastaut syndrome; prophylaxis of migraine headache

Unlabeled/Investigational Use Infantile spasms, neuropathic pain, cluster headache

Mechanism of Action Anticonvulsant activity may be due to a combination of potential mechanisms: Blocks neuronal voltage-dependent sodium channels, enhances GABA(A) activity, antagonizes AMPA/kainate glutamate receptors, and weakly inhibits carbonic anhydrase.

Pharmacodynamics/Kinetics

Absorption: Good, rapid; unaffected by food

Protein binding: 15% to 41% (inversely related to plasma concentrations)

Metabolism: Hepatic via P450 enzymes

Bioavailability: 80%

Half-life elimination: Mean: Adults: Normal renal function: 21 hours; shorter in pediatric patients; clearance is 50% higher in pediatric patients

Time to peak, serum: ~2-4 hours

Excretion: Urine (~70% to 80% as unchanged drug)

Dialyzable: ~30%

Dosage Oral: **Note:** Do not abruptly discontinue therapy; taper dosage gradually to prevent rebound seizure.

Monotherapy: Children ≥10 years and Adults: Partial onset seizure and primary generalized tonic-clonic seizure: Initial: 25 mg twice daily; may increase weekly by 50 mg/day up to 100 mg twice daily (week 4 dose); thereafter, may further increase weekly by 100 mg/day up to the recommended maximum of 200 mg twice daily.

Adjunctive therapy:

Children 2-16 years:

Partial onset seizure or seizure associated with Lennox-Gastaut syndrome: Initial dose titration should begin at 25 mg (or less, based on a range of 1-3 mg/kg/day) nightly for the first week; dosage may be increased in increments of 1-3 mg/kg/day (administered in 2 divided doses) at 1- or 2-week intervals to a total daily dose of 5-9 mg/kg/day

(Continued)

Topiramate *(Continued)*

Primary generalized tonic-clonic seizure: Use initial dose listed above, but use slower initial titration rate; titrate to recommended maintenance dose by the end of 8 weeks

Adolescents ≥17 years and Adults:

Partial onset seizures: Initial: 25-50 mg/day (given in 2 divided doses) for 1 week; increase at weekly intervals by 25-50 mg/day until response; usual maintenance dose: 100-200 mg twice daily. Doses >1600 mg/day have not been studied.

Primary generalized tonic-clonic seizures: Use initial dose as listed above for partial onset seizures, but use slower initial titration rate; titrate upwards to recommended dose by the end of 8 weeks; usual maintenance dose: 200 mg twice daily. Doses >1600 mg/day have not been studied.

Adults:

Migraine prophylaxis: Initial: 25 mg/day (in the evening), titrated at weekly intervals in 25 mg increments, up to the recommended total daily dose of 100 mg/day given in 2 divided doses

Cluster headache (unlabeled use): Initial: 25 mg/day, titrated at weekly intervals in 25 mg increments, up to 200 mg/day

Neuropathic pain (unlabeled use): Initial: 25 mg/day, titrated at weekly intervals in 25-50 mg increments to target dose of 400 mg daily in 2 divided doses. Reported dosage range studied: 25-800 mg/day

Dosing adjustment in renal impairment: Cl_{cr} <70 mL/minute: Administer 50% dose and titrate more slowly

Hemodialysis: Supplemental dose may be needed during hemodialysis

Dosing adjustment in hepatic impairment: Clearance may be reduced

Stability Store at room temperature of 15°C to 30°C (59°F to 86°F); protect from moisture

Administration Oral: May be administered without regard to meals

Capsule sprinkles: May be swallowed whole or opened to sprinkle the contents on soft food (drug/food mixture should not be chewed).

Tablet: Because of bitter taste, tablets should not be broken.

Monitoring Parameters Seizure frequency, hydration status; electrolytes (recommended monitoring includes serum bicarbonate at baseline and periodically during treatment); monitor for symptoms of acute acidosis and complications of long-term acidosis (nephrolithiasis, osteomalacia, and reduced growth rates in children); ammonia level in patients with unexplained lethargy, vomiting, or mental status changes; symptoms of secondary angle closure glaucoma

Pregnancy Risk Factor C

Contraindications Hypersensitivity to topiramate or any component of the formulation

Warnings/Precautions

Key Adverse Reactions:

- Metabolic acidosis (hyperchloremic, nonanion gap): Topiramate may decrease serum bicarbonate concentrations, due to inhibition of carbonic anhydrase and increased renal bicarbonate loss. Decreases in serum bicarbonate are relatively common (7% to 67%) but usually mild to moderate (average decrease of 4 mEq/L at dose of 400 mg/day in adults and 6 mg/kg/day in children). Treatment-emergent metabolic acidosis is less common; however, risk may be increased in patients with a predisposing condition (renal, respiratory and/or hepatic impairment), ketogenic diet, or concurrent treatment with other drugs which may cause acidosis. Metabolic acidosis may occur at dosages as low as 50 mg/day. Serum bicarbonate should be monitored, as well as potential complications of chronic acidosis (nephrolithiasis, osteomalacia, and reduced growth rates in children). Dose reduction or discontinuation (by tapering dose) should be considered in patients with persistent or severe metabolic acidosis. If treatment is continued, alkali supplementation should be considered.
- Kidney stones: The risk of kidney stones is about 2-4 times that of the untreated population, the risk of this event may be reduced by increasing fluid intake.
- Hyperthermia: May be associated (rarely) with severe oligohydrosis and hyperthermia, most frequently in children; use caution and monitor closely during strenuous exercise, during exposure to high environmental temperature, or in patients receiving drugs with anticholinergic activity.

- CNS Effects: Cognitive dysfunction, psychiatric disturbances (mood disorders), and sedation (somnolence or fatigue) may occur with topiramate use; incidence may be related to rapid titration and higher doses. Topiramate may also cause paresthesia and ataxia.
- Withdrawal: Avoid abrupt withdrawal of topiramate therapy, it should be withdrawn/tapered slowly to minimize the potential of increased seizure frequency.

Concurrent Disease:

- Organ dysfunction: Use cautiously in patients with hepatic or renal impairment; dosage adjustment may be required
- Glaucoma: Has been associated with secondary angle-closure glaucoma in adults and children, typically within 1 month of initiation. Discontinue in patients with acute onset of decreased visual acuity or ocular pain.

Concurrent Drug Therapy:

- Valproate: Hyperammonemia with or without encephalopathy may occur and has been documented in patients who have tolerated each drug alone. Risk may be increased in patients with inborn errors of metabolism or decreased hepatic mitochondrial activity. Monitor for lethargy, vomiting, or unexplained changes in mental status.

Special populations:

- Safety and efficacy have not been established in children <2 years of age for adjunctive treatment and <10 years of age for monotherapy.
- Pregnancy: No adequate and well-controlled studies have been conducted; use only if benefit clearly outweighs risk

Adverse Reactions Adverse events are reported for placebo-controlled trials of adjunctive therapy in adult and pediatric patients. Unless otherwise noted, the percentages refer to incidence in epilepsy trials. Note: A wide range of dosages were studied; incidence of adverse events was frequently lower in the pediatric population studied.

>10%:

Central nervous system: Dizziness (4% to 32%), ataxia (6% to 16%), somnolence (15% to 29%), psychomotor slowing (3% to 21%), nervousness (9% to 19%), memory difficulties (2% to 14%), speech problems (2% to 13%), fatigue (9% to 30%), difficulty concentrating (5% to 14%), depression (9% to 13%), confusion (4% to 14%)

Endocrine & metabolic: Serum bicarbonate decreased (dose-related: 7% to 67%; marked reductions [to <17 mEq/L] 1% to 11%)

Gastrointestinal: Nausea (6% to 12%; migraine trial: 14%), weight loss (8% to 13%), anorexia (4% to 24%)

Neuromuscular & skeletal: Paresthesia (1% to 19%; migraine trial: 35% to 51%)

Ocular: Nystagmus (10% to 11%), abnormal vision (<1% to 13%)

Respiratory: Upper respiratory infection (migraine trial: 12% to 13%)

Miscellaneous: Injury (6% to 14%)

1% to 10%:

Cardiovascular: Chest pain (2% to 4%), edema (1% to 2%), bradycardia (1%), pallor (up to 1%), hypertension (1% to 2%)

Central nervous system: Abnormal coordination (4%), hypoesthesia (1% to 2%; migraine trial: 8%), convulsions (1%), depersonalization (1% to 2%), apathy (1% to 3%), cognitive problems (3%), emotional lability (3%), agitation (3%), aggressive reactions (2% to 9%), tremor (3% to 9%), stupor (1% to 2%), mood problems (4% to 9%), anxiety (2% to 10%), insomnia (4% to 8%), appetite increased (1%), neurosis (1%), vertigo (1% to 2%)

Dermatologic: Pruritus (migraine trial: 2% to 4%), skin disorder (1% to 3%), alopecia (2%), dermatitis (up to 2%), hypertrichosis (up to 2%), rash erythematous (up to 2%), eczema (up to 1%), seborrhea (up to 1%), skin discoloration (up to 1%)

Endocrine & metabolic: Hot flashes (1% to 2%); metabolic acidosis (hyperchloremia, nonanion gap), dehydration, breast pain (up to 4%), menstrual irregularities (1% to 2%), hypoglycemia (1%), libido decreased (<1% to 2%)

Gastrointestinal: Dyspepsia (2% to 7%), abdominal pain (5% to 7%), constipation (3% to 5%), xerostomia (2% to 4%), fecal incontinence (1%), gingivitis (1%), diarrhea (2%; migraine trial: 11%), vomiting (1% to 3%), gastroenteritis (1% to 3%), GI disorder (1%), (2% to 4%; migraine trial: 12% to 15%), dysphagia (1%), flatulence (1%), GERD (1%), glossitis (1%), gum hyperplasia (1%), weight increase (1%)

(Continued)

Topiramate *(Continued)*

Genitourinary: Impotence, dysuria/incontinence (<1% to 4%), prostatic disorder (2%), UTI (2% to 3%), premature ejaculation (migraine trial: 3%), cystitis (2%)
Hematologic: Leukopenia (1% to 2%), purpura (8%), hematoma (1%), prothrombin time increased (1%), thrombocytopenia (1%)
Neuromuscular & skeletal: Myalgia (2%), weakness (3% to 6%), back pain (1% to 5%), leg pain (2% to 4%), rigors (1%), hypertonia, arthralgia (1% to 7%), gait abnormal (2% to 8%), involuntary muscle contractions (2%; migraine trial: 4%), skeletal pain (1%), hyperkinesia (up to 5%), hyporeflexia (up to 2%)
Ocular: Conjunctivitis (1%), diplopia (2% to 10%), myopia (up to 1%)
Otic: Hearing decreased (1% to 2%), tinnitus (1% to 2%), otitis media (migraine trial: 1% to 2%)
Renal: Nephrolithiasis, renal calculus (migraine trial: 2%), hematuria (<1% to 2%)
Respiratory: Pharyngitis (3% to 6%), sinusitis (4% to 6%; migraine trial: 8% to 10%), epistaxis (1% to 4%) , rhinitis (4% to 7%), dyspnea (1% to 2%), pneumonia (5%), coughing (migraine trial: 2% to 3%), bronchitis (migraine trial: 3%)
Miscellaneous: Flu-like symptoms (3% to 7%), allergy (2% to 3%), body odor (up to 1%), fever (migraine trial: 1% to 2%), viral infection (migraine trial: 3% to 4%), infection (<1% to 2%), diaphoresis (≤1%), thirst (2%)

<1% (Limited to important or life-threatening): Accommodation abnormality, allergic reactions, alopecia, anemia, angina, apraxia, AV block, bone marrow depression, deep vein thrombosis, dehydration, delirium, diabetes mellitus, dyskinesia, electrolyte imbalance, encephalopathy (with valproate therapy), eosinophilia, erythema multiforme, euphoria, eye pain, granulocytopenia, hepatic failure, hepatitis, hyperammonemia (with valproate therapy), hyperthermia (severe), hypotension, liver enzymes increased, lymphadenopathy, lymphopenia, manic reaction, migraine aggravated, neuropathy, oligohydrosis, pancreatitis, pancytopenia, paranoid reaction, pemphigus, photosensitivity, psychosis, pulmonary embolism, rash. renal tubular acidosis, Stevens-Johnson syndrome, suicidal behavior, syncope, syndrome of acute myopia/secondary angle-closure glaucoma, tongue edema, toxic epidermal necrolysis, tremor, vertigo

Overdosage/Toxicology Signs and symptoms of overdose include convulsions, drowsiness, speech disturbance, blurred vision, diplopia, impaired mentation, lethargy, and metabolic acidosis. Activated charcoal has not been shown to adsorb topiramate and is, therefore, not recommended; gastric contents should be emptied via lavage or emesis. Hemodialysis can remove approximately ~30% of the drug; however, most cases do not require removal and instead are best treated with supportive measures.

Drug Interactions Inhibits CYP2C19 (weak); **Induces** CYP3A4 (weak)
Acetazolamide: Coadministration may increase the chance of nephrolithiasis and/or hyperthermia.
Anticholinergic drugs: Concurrent administration may increase the risk of oligohydrosis and/or hyperthermia; includes drugs with high anticholinergic activity such as antihistamines, cyclic antidepressants, and antipsychotics; use caution
Carbamazepine: May reduce topiramate levels 40%
CNS depressants: Sedative effects may be additive with topiramate; monitor for increased effect; includes barbiturates, benzodiazepines, narcotic analgesics, ethanol, and other sedative agents.
Digoxin: Blood levels of digoxin are decreased when coadministered with topiramate.
Estrogens: Blood levels of estrogens are decreased when coadministered with topiramate, this may lead to a loss of efficacy.
Oral contraceptives: See interaction with Estrogens; use of alternative nonhormonal contraception is recommended.
Phenytoin: May decrease topiramate levels by as much as 48%; topiramate may increase phenytoin concentration by 25%
Valproic acid: Hyperammonemia with or without encephalopathy has been reported in patients who tolerated either drug alone. These drugs may modestly decrease the serum concentrations of the other drug.

Ethanol/Nutrition/Herb Interactions
Ethanol: Avoid ethanol (may increase CNS depression).
Food: Ketogenic diet may increase the possibility of acidosis.

Herb/Nutraceutical: Avoid evening primrose (seizure threshold decreased).

Dosage Forms

Capsule, sprinkle: 15 mg, 25 mg

Tablet: 25 mg, 50 mg, 100 mg, 200 mg

- ♦ **Topisone® (Can)** *see* Betamethasone *on page 169*
- ♦ **Toprol-XL®** *see* Metoprolol *on page 839*
- ♦ **Toradol®** *see* Ketorolac *on page 717*
- ♦ **Toradol® IM (Can)** *see* Ketorolac *on page 717*

Torsemide (TORE se mide)

Medication Safety Issues

Sound-alike/look-alike issues:

Torsemide may be confused with furosemide

Demadex® may be confused with Denorex®

Related Information

Diuretics, Loop *on page 1565*

Heart Failure (Systolic) *on page 1607*

U.S. Brand Names Demadex®

Pharmacologic Category Diuretic, Loop

Generic Available Yes: Tablet

Use Management of edema associated with congestive heart failure and hepatic or renal disease; used alone or in combination with antihypertensives in treatment of hypertension; I.V. form is indicated when rapid onset is desired

Mechanism of Action Inhibits reabsorption of sodium and chloride in the ascending loop of Henle and distal renal tubule, interfering with the chloride-binding cotransport system, thus causing increased excretion of water, sodium, chloride, magnesium, and calcium; does not alter GFR, renal plasma flow, or acid-base balance

Pharmacodynamics/Kinetics

Onset of action: Diuresis: 30-60 minutes

Peak effect: 1-4 hours

Duration: ~6 hours

Absorption: Oral: Rapid

Protein binding, plasma: ~97% to 99%

Metabolism: Hepatic (80%) via CYP

Bioavailability: 80% to 90%

Half-life elimination: 2-4; Cirrhosis: 7-8 hours

Excretion: Urine (20% as unchanged drug)

Dosage Adults: Oral, I.V.:

Congestive heart failure: 10-20 mg once daily; may increase gradually for chronic treatment by doubling dose until the diuretic response is apparent (for acute treatment, I.V. dose may be repeated every 2 hours with double the dose as needed). **Note:** ACC/AHA 2005 guidelines for chronic heart failure recommend a maximum daily oral dose of 200 mg; maximum single I.V. dose of 100-200 mg

Continuous I.V. infusion: 20 mg I.V. load then 5-20 mg/hour

Chronic renal failure: 20 mg once daily; increase as described above

Hepatic cirrhosis: 5-10 mg once daily with an aldosterone antagonist or a potassium-sparing diuretic; increase as described above

Hypertension: 2.5-5 mg once daily; increase to 10 mg after 4-6 weeks if an adequate hypotensive response is not apparent; if still not effective, an additional antihypertensive agent may be added

Stability If torsemide is to be administered via continuous infusion, stability has been demonstrated through 24 hours at room temperature in plastic containers for the following fluids and concentrations:

200 mg torsemide (10 mg/mL) added to 250 mL D_5W, 250 mL NS or 500 mL 0.45% sodium chloride

50 mg torsemide (10 mg/mL) added to 500 mL D_5W, 250 mL NS or 500 mL 0.45% sodium chloride

Administration I.V. injections should be administered over ≥2 minutes; the oral form may be administered regardless of meal times; patients may be switched from the I.V. form to the oral and vice-versa with no change in dose; no dosage adjustment is needed in the elderly or patients with hepatic impairment

To administer as a continuous infusion: 50 mg or 200 mg torsemide should be diluted in 250 mL or 500 mL of compatible solution in plastic containers

(Continued)

Torsemide *(Continued)*

Monitoring Parameters Renal function, electrolytes, and fluid status (weight and I & O), blood pressure

Anesthesia and Critical Care Concerns/Other Considerations If given the morning of surgery, it may render the patient volume depleted and blood pressure may be labile during general anesthesia. Torsemide may induce potent diuretic effects and, as with other potent diuretics, electrolytes and volume status needs to be closely monitored.

Equivalent dosing: Torsemide 10-20 mg is approximately equivalent to furosemide 40 mg or bumetanide 1 mg.

Pregnancy Risk Factor B

Contraindications Hypersensitivity to torsemide, any component of the formulation, or any sulfonylureas; anuria

Warnings/Precautions Adjust dose to avoid dehydration. In cirrhosis, avoid electrolyte and acid/base imbalances that might lead to hepatic encephalopathy. Ototoxicity is associated with rapid I.V. administration of other loop diuretics and has been seen with oral torsemide. Do not administer intravenously in less than 2 minutes; single doses should not exceed 200 mg. Hypersensitivity reactions can rarely occur. Monitor fluid status and renal function in an attempt to prevent oliguria, azotemia, and reversible increases in BUN and creatinine. Close medical supervision of aggressive diuresis is required. Monitor closely for electrolyte imbalances particularly hypokalemia and correct when necessary. Coadministration with antihypertensives may increase the risk of hypotension.

Chemical similarities are present among sulfonamides, sulfonylureas, carbonic anhydrase inhibitors, thiazides, and loop diuretics (except ethacrynic acid). Use in patients with sulfonylurea allergy is specifically contraindicated in product labeling, however, a risk of cross-reaction exists in patients with allergy to any of these compounds; avoid use when previous reaction has been severe.

Adverse Reactions

1% to 10%:

- Cardiovascular: Edema (1.1%), ECG abnormality (2%), chest pain (1.2%)
- Central nervous system: Headache (7.3%), dizziness (3.2%), insomnia (1.2%), nervousness (1%)
- Endocrine & metabolic: Hyperglycemia, hyperuricemia, hypokalemia
- Gastrointestinal: Diarrhea (2%), constipation (1.8%), nausea (1.8%), dyspepsia (1.6%), sore throat (1.6%)
- Genitourinary: Excessive urination (6.7%)
- Neuromuscular & skeletal: Weakness (2%), arthralgia (1.8%), myalgia (1.6%)
- Respiratory: Rhinitis (2.8%), cough increase (2%)

<1% (Limited to important or life-threatening): Angioedema, atrial fibrillation, GI hemorrhage, hypernatremia hypotension, hypovolemia, rash, rectal bleeding, shunt thrombosis, syncope, ventricular tachycardia

Overdosage/Toxicology Symptoms include electrolyte depletion, volume depletion, hypotension, dehydration, and circulatory collapse. Electrolyte depletion may manifest as weakness, dizziness, mental confusion, anorexia, lethargy, vomiting, and cramps. Treatment is supportive.

Drug Interactions **Substrate** of CYP2C8 (minor), 2C9 (major); **Inhibits** CYP2C19 (weak)

ACE inhibitors: Hypotensive effects and/or renal effects are potentiated by hypovolemia.

Aminoglycosides: Ototoxicity may be increased.

Anticoagulant activity is enhanced.

Antidiabetic agents: Glucose tolerance may be decreased.

Antihypertensive agents: Effects may be enhanced.

Beta-blockers: Plasma concentrations of beta-blockers may be increased with torsemide.

Chloral hydrate: Transient diaphoresis, hot flashes, hypertension may occur.

Cisplatin: Ototoxicity may be increased.

CYP2C9 inducers: May decrease the levels/effects of torsemide. Example inducers include carbamazepine, phenobarbital, phenytoin, rifampin, rifapentine, and secobarbital.

Digitalis: Arrhythmias may occur with diuretic-induced electrolyte disturbances.

Lithium: Plasma concentrations of lithium may be increased; monitor lithium levels.

NSAIDs: Torsemide efficacy may be decreased.

Probenecid: Torsemide action may be reduced.
Salicylates: Diuretic action may be impaired in patients with cirrhosis and ascites.
Thiazides: Synergistic effects may result.

Ethanol/Nutrition/Herb Interactions Herb/Nutraceutical: Avoid dong quai if using for hypertension (has estrogenic activity). Avoid ephedra, yohimbe, ginseng (may worsen hypertension). Avoid garlic (may have increased antihypertensive effect).

Dosage Forms
Injection, solution: 10 mg/mL (2 mL, 5 mL)
Tablet: 5 mg, 10 mg, 20 mg, 100 mg

Total Parenteral Nutrition (TOE tal par EN ter al noo TRISH un)

Related Information
Fat Emulsion *on page 508*

Synonyms Hyperal; Hyperalimentation; Parenteral Nutrition; PN; TPN

Pharmacologic Category Caloric Agent; Intravenous Nutritional Therapy

Use Infusion of nutrient solutions into the bloodstream to support nutritional needs during a time when patient is unable to absorb nutrients via the gastrointestinal tract, cannot take adequate nutrition orally or enterally, or have had (or are expected to have) inadequate oral intake for 7-14 days

Dosage PN is a highly-individualized therapy. The following general guidelines may be used in the estimation of needs. Electrolytes, vitamins, and trace minerals should be added to TPN mixtures based on patients individualized needs.

Neonates: I.V.: **Note:** When indicated for premature neonates, start on day 1 of life if possible.

Total calories:
Term: 85-105 kcal/kg/day
Preterm (stable): 90-120 kcal/kg/day

Fluid:
<1.5 kg: 130-150 mL/kg/day
1.5-2 kg: 110-130 mL/kg/day
2-10 kg: 100 mL/kg/day

Carbohydrate (dextrose): 40% to 50 % of caloric intake; advance as tolerated
Term: Initial: 6-8 mg/kg/minute; goal: 10-14 mg/kg/minute
Premature: Initial: 6 mg/kg/minute; goal: 10-13 mg/kg/minute

Protein (amino acids):
Term: Initial: 2.5 g/kg/day; goal: 3 g/kg/day
Extremely (<1000 g) and very (<1500 g) low-birth-weight (stable): Initial: 1-1.5 g/kg/day; goal: 3.5-3.85 g/kg/day to promote utero growth rates.
Sepsis, hypoxia: Initial: 1 g/kg/day; goal: 3-3.85 g/kg/day

Fat:
Term: Initial: 0.5-1 g/kg/day (maximum: 3 g/kg/day); administer over 24 hours
Preterm: Initial: 0.25-0.5 g/kg/day (maximum: 3 g/kg/day or 1 g/kg/day if on phototherapy); administer over 24 hours
Note: Monitor triglycerides while receiving intralipids. If triglycerides >200 mg/dL, stop infusion and restart at 0.5-1g/kg/day

Heparin: 1 unit/mL of parenteral nutrition fluids should be added to enhance clearance of lipid emulsions

Children: I.V.: **Note:** Give within 5-7 days if unable to meet needs orally or with enteral nutrition:

Total calories:
<6 months: 85-105 kcal/kg/day
6-12 months: 80-100 kcal/kg/day
1-7 years: 75-90 kcal/kg/day
7-12 years: 50-75 kcal/kg/day
12-18 years: 30-50 kcal/kg/day

Fluid:
2-10 kg: 100 mL/kg
>10-20 kg: 1000 mL for 10 kg plus 50 mL/kg for each kg >10
>20 kg: 1500 mL for 10 kg plus 20 mL/kg for each kg >20

Carbohydrate (dextrose): 40% to 50% of caloric intake
<1 year: Initial: 6-8 mg/kg/minute; goal: 10-14 mg/kg/minute
1-10 years: Initial: 10% to 12.5%; daily increase: 5% increments (maximum: 15 mg/kg/minute)

(Continued)

Total Parenteral Nutrition *(Continued)*

>10 years: Initial: 10% to 15%; daily increase: 5% increments (maximum: 8.5 mg/kg/minute)

Protein (amino acids):

1-12 months: Initial: 2-3 g/kg/day; daily increase: 1 g/kg/day (maximum: 3 g/kg/day)

1-10 years: Initial: 1-2 g/kg/day; daily increase: 1 g/kg/day (maximum: 2-2.5 g/kg/day)

>10 years: Initial: 0.8-1.5 g/kg/day; daily increase: 1 g/kg/day (maximum: 1.5-2 g/kg/day)

Fat: Initial: 1 g/kg/day; daily increase: 1 g/kg/day (maximum: 3 g/kg/day); **Note:** Monitor triglycerides while receiving intralipids.

Adults: I.V.:

Total calories: Calculate using Harris-Benedict equation or based on stress level as indicated below:

Harris-Benedict Equation (BEE):

Females: 655.1 + [(9.56 x W) + (1.85 x H) - (4.68 x A)]

Males: 66.47 + [(13.75 x W) + (5 x H) - (6.76 x A)]

Then multiply BEE x (activity factor) x (stress factor)

W = weight in kg; H = height in cm; A = age in years

Activity factor = 1.2 sedentary, 1.3 normal activity, 1.4 active, 1.5 very active

Stress factor = 1.5 for trauma, stressed, or surgical patients and underweight (to promote weight gain); 2.0 for severe burn patients

Stress level:

Normal/mild stress level: 20-25 kcal/kg/day

Moderate stress level: 25-30 kcal/kg/day

Severe stress level: 30-40 kcal/kg/day

Pregnant women in second or third trimester: Add an additional 300 kcal/day

Fluid: mL/day = 30-40 mL/kg

Carbohydrate (dextrose):

5 g/kg/day or 3.5 mg/kg/minute (maximum rate: 4-7 mg/kg/minute)

Minimum recommended amount: 400 calories/day or 100 g/day

Protein (amino acids):

Maintenance: 0.8-1 g/kg/day

Normal/mild stress level: 1-1.2 g/kg/day

Moderate stress level: 1.2-1.5 g/kg/day

Severe stress level: 1.5-2 g/kg/day

Burn patients (severe): Increase protein until significant wound healing achieved

Solid organ transplant: Perioperative: 1.5-2 g/kg/day

Renal failure:

Acute (severely malnourished or hypercatabolic): 1.5-1.8 g/kg/day

Chronic, with dialysis: 1.2-1.3 g/kg/day

Chronic, without dialysis: 0.6-0.8 g/kg/day

Continuous hemofiltration: ≥1 g/kg/day

Hepatic failure:

Acute management when other treatments have failed:

With encephalopathy: 0.6-1 g/kg/day

Without encephalopathy: 1-1.5 g/kg/day

Chronic encephalopathy: Use branch chain amino acid enriched diets only if unresponsive to pharmacotherapy

Pregnant women in second or third trimester: Add an additional 10-14 g/day

Fat:

Initial: 20% to 40 % of total calories (maximum: 60% of total calories or 2.5 g/kg/day); **Note:** Monitor triglycerides while receiving intralipids.

Safe for use in pregnancy

I.V. lipids are safe in adults with pancreatitis if triglyceride levels <400 mg/dL

Stability USP Chapter 797 Guidelines consider TPN a medium-risk preparation and state that (in the absence of passing a sterility test) storage period should not exceed 30 hours at room temperature, 7 days at cold temperature, and 45 days in a solid frozen state at -20°C or colder. For patients on home TPN, multiple vitamins should be added prior to TPN administration, due to limited stability of multiple vitamins.

Administration For I.V. administration only, usually via a central venous catheter; can be administered by continuous infusion over 24 hours or cyclic infusion over 12-14 hours. Cyclic infusion is used with a tapering-up period at the beginning and a tapering-down period at the end to avoid hyper-/hypoglycemia. For infants <2 years, taper over 1-2 hours. Change tubing after each infusion. Hang fat emulsion higher than other fluids (has low specific gravity and could run up into other lines). Infuse via pump using either peripheral or central venous line. Do not use in-line filter.

Monitoring Parameters

Electrolytes: Sodium, potassium, chloride, and bicarbonate should be monitored frequently upon initiation and until stable; phosphate should be monitored closely in patients with pulmonary disease.

Efficacy: Nutrition and outcome parameters should be measured serially.

Glucose: In diabetics or patients with glucose intolerance risk factors, monitor closely. Monitor frequently upon initiation of therapy and with any changes in insulin dose or renal function.

Line site: Monitor for signs and symptoms of infection.

Liver function tests: Monitor periodically.

Triglycerides: Before initiation of lipid therapy and at least weekly during therapy.

Refeeding syndrome: Patients at risk should have phosphorus, magnesium, potassium, and glucose levels monitored closely at initiation.

Bone densitometry: Perform upon initiation of long-term therapy.

Vitamin A status: Should be carefully monitored in patients with chronic renal failure.

Neonates: Sodium, calcium and phosphate should be monitored closely. Frequent (some advise daily) platelet counts should be performed in neonatal patients receiving parenteral lipids.

Contraindications Varies by composition:

Lipid-containing formulations are contraindicated in patients with hypersensitivity to fat emulsion or any component of the formulation; severe egg or legume (soybean) allergies; pathologic hyperlipidemia, lipoid nephrosis, pancreatitis with hyperlipemia

Dextrose is contraindicated in patients with hypersensitivity to corn or corn products; hypertonic solutions in patients with intracranial or intraspinal hemorrhage; glucose-galactose malabsorption syndrome

Amino acids are contraindicated in patients with hypersensitivity to one or more amino acids; severe liver disease or hepatic coma

Warnings/Precautions Monitor fluid and electrolyte status carefully. Use with caution in patients at risk for refeeding syndrome. Refeeding syndrome is a medical emergency; it can consist of electrolyte disturbances (eg, potassium, phosphorus), respiratory distress, and cardiac arrhythmias, resulting in cardiopulmonary arrest. It is usually seen in patients with long-standing or severe malnutrition; initiate cautiously; approach goals slowly. Do not overfeed patients; caloric replacement should match as closely as possible to intake. Use caution in patients with diabetes or insulin resistance. Use caution in patients who may be sensitive to volume overload (eg, CHF, renal failure, hepatic failure). Use caution and limit protein in patients with hepatic disease. If TPN is discontinued abruptly, infuse 10% dextrose at same rate and monitor blood glucose for hypoglycemia.

Adverse Reactions Frequency not defined (unless noted).

Endocrine & metabolic: Fluid overload, hypercapnia, hyperglycemia, hyper-/hypokalemia, hyper-/hypophosphatemia, metabolic bone disease, nonanion gap metabolic acidosis, refeeding syndrome

Hepatic: Cholestasis, cirrhosis (<1%), gallstones, liver function tests increased, pancreatitis, steatosis, triglycerides increased

Renal: Azotemia, BUN increased

Miscellaneous: Bacteremia, catheter-induced infection, exit-site infections

Dosage Forms TPN is usually compounded from optimal combinations of macronutrients (water, protein, dextrose, and lipids) and micronutrients (electrolytes, trace elements, and vitamins) to meet the specific nutritional requirements of a patient. Individual hospitals may have designated standard TPN formulas. There are a few commercially-available amino acids with electrolytes solutions; however, these products may not meet an individual's specific nutrition requirements.

References

ASPEN Board of Directors and the Clinical Guidelines Task Force, "Guidelines for the Use of Parenteral and Enteral Nutrition in Adult and Pediatric Patients," *JPEN J Parenter Enteral Nutr*, 2002, 26(1 Suppl):1-138.

(Continued)

Total Parenteral Nutrition *(Continued)*

Dersch D and Schoen J, "Weight-Based Ordering: An Evaluation of Increased Guideline Use in Hospital Total Parenteral Nutrition Dosing," *Nutr Clin Pract*, 2002, 17(5):296-303.

Fulford A, Scolapio JS, and Aranda-Michel J, "Parenteral Nutrition-Associated Hepatotoxicity," *Nutr Clin Pract*, 2004, 19(3):274-83.

Howard L, "Enteral and Parenteral Nutrition Therapy," *Harrison's Principles of Internal Medicine*, 14th ed, Chapter 78, Fauci AS, Braunwald E, Isselbacher KJ, et al, eds, New York, NY: McGraw-Hill, 1998, 472-80.

Ireton-Jones C, DeLegge MH, Epperson LA, et al, "Management of the Home Parenteral Nutrition Patient," *Nutr Clin Pract*, 2003, 18(4):310-17.

Mayhew SL and Gonzalez ER, "Neonatal Nutrition: A Focus on Parenteral Nutrition and Early Enteral Nutrition," *Nutr Clin Pract*, 2003, 18(5):406-13.

Mattox T, "Parenteral Nutrition," *Pharmacotherapy: A Pathophysiologic Approach*, 4th ed, Chapter 128, Dipiro JT, Talbert RL, Yee GC, et al, eds, Stamford, CT: Appleton & Lange, 1999, 2247-65.

Mirtallo J, Canada T, Johnson D, et al, "Safe Practices for Parenteral Nutrition. Task Force for the Revision of Safe Practices for Parenteral Nutrition," *JPEN J Parenter Enteral Nutr*, 2004, 28(6):S39-70.

U.S. Pharmacopeial Convention, Inc, U.S. Pharmacopeia 27, Chapter <797> Pharmaceutical Compounding — Sterile Preparations. Rockville, MD: U.S. Pharmacopeial Convention, Inc, 2003, 2350-70.

♦ **tPA** *see* Alteplase *on page 72*

♦ **TPN** *see* Total Parenteral Nutrition *on page 1293*

Trace Metals (trase MET als)

U.S. Brand Names Iodopen®; Molypen®; M.T.E.-4®; M.T.E.-5®; M.T.E.-6®; M.T.E.-7®; Multitrace™-4; Multitrace™-4 Neonatal; Multitrace™-4 Pediatric; Multitrace™-5; Neotrace-4®; Pedtrace-4®; P.T.E.-4®; P.T.E.-5®; Selepen®

Synonyms Chromium; Copper; Iodine; Manganese; Molybdenum; Neonatal Trace Metals; Selenium; Zinc

Pharmacologic Category Trace Element, Parenteral

Generic Available Yes

Use Prevention and correction of trace metal deficiencies

Dosage Recommended daily parenteral dosage: See table.

Recommended Daily Parenteral Dosage

	Infants	Children	Adults
Chromium[1]	0.2 mcg/kg	0.2 mcg/kg (max: 5 mcg)	10-15 mcg
Copper[2]	20 mcg/kg	20 mcg/kg (max: 300 mcg)	0.5-1.5 mg
Manganese[2,3]	1 mcg/kg	1 mcg/kg (max: 50 mcg)	150-800 mcg
Molybdenum[1,4]	0.25 mcg/kg	0.25 mcg/kg (max: 5 mcg)	20-120 mcg
Selenium[1,4]	2 mcg/kg	2 mcg/kg (max: 30 mcg)	20-40 mcg
Zinc		50 mcg/kg (max: 5 mg)	2.5-4 mg
preterm	400 mcg/kg		
term <3 mo	250 mcg/kg		
term >3 mo	100 mcg/kg		

[1]Omit in patients with renal dysfunction.

[2]Omit in patients with obstructive jaundice.

[3]Current available commercial products are not in appropriate ratios to maintain this recommendation — doses of up to 10 mcg/kg have been used.

[4]Indicated for use in long-term parenteral nutrition patients.

Administration Must be diluted prior to use and infused as component of parenteral nutrition or parenteral solutions

Pregnancy Risk Factor C

Ethanol/Nutrition/Herb Interactions Food: Decreased absorption of oral zinc when administered with bran products, protein, and phytates.

Dosage Forms

Injection, solution [combination products]:

M.T.E.-4®: Chromium 4 mcg, copper 0.4 mg, manganese 0.1 mg, and zinc 1 mg per mL (3 mL, 10 mL, 30 mL) [30 mL contains benzyl alcohol]

M.T.E.-4® Concentrate: Chromium 10 mcg, copper 1 mg, manganese 0.5 mg, and zinc 5 mg per mL (1 mL, 10 mL) [10 mL contains benzyl alcohol]
M.T.E.-5® [preservative free]: Chromium 4 mcg, copper 0.4 mg, manganese 0.1 mg, selenium 20 mcg, and zinc 1 mg per mL (10 mL)
M.T.E.-5® Concentrate: Chromium 10 mcg, copper 1 mg, manganese 0.5 mg, selenium 60 mcg, and zinc 5 mg per mL (1 mL, 10 mL) [10 mL contains benzyl alcohol]
M.T.E.-6® [preservative free]: Chromium 4 mcg, copper 0.4 mg, iodide 25 mcg, manganese 0.1 mg, selenium 20 mcg, and zinc 1 mg per mL (10 mL)
M.T.E.-6® Concentrate: Chromium 10 mcg, copper 1 mg, iodide 75 mcg, manganese 0.5 mg, selenium 60 mcg, and zinc 5 mg per mL (10 mL) [contains benzyl alcohol]
M.T.E.-7® [preservative free]: Chromium 4 mcg, copper 0.4 mg, iodide 25 mcg, manganese 0.1 mg, molybdenum 25 mcg, selenium 20 mcg, and zinc 1 mg per mL (10 mL)
Multitrace™-4: Chromium 4 mcg, copper 0.4 mg, manganese 0.1 mg, and zinc 1 mg per mL (10 mL) [contains benzyl alcohol]
Multitrace™-4 Neonatal: Chromium 0.85 mcg, copper 0.1 mg, manganese 0.025 mg, and zinc 1.5 mg per mL (2 mL)
Multitrace™-4 Pediatric: Chromium 1 mcg, copper 0.1 mg, manganese 0.025 mg, and zinc 1 mg per mL (3 mL)
Multitrace™-4 Concentrate: Chromium 10 mcg, copper 1 mg, manganese 0.5 mg, and zinc 5 mg per mL (1 mL, 10 mL) [10 mL contains benzyl alcohol]
Multitrace™-5: Chromium 4 mcg, copper 0.4 mg, manganese 0.1 mg, selenium 20 mcg, and zinc 1 mg per mL (10 mL) [contains benzyl alcohol]
Multitrace™-5 Concentrate: Chromium 10 mcg, copper 1 mg, manganese 0.5 mg, selenium 60 mcg, and zinc 5 mg per mL (1 mL, 10 mL) [10 mL contains benzyl alcohol]
Neotrace-4® [preservative free]: Chromium 0.85 mcg, copper 0.1 mg, manganese 0.025 mg, and zinc 1.5 mg per mL (2 mL)
Pedtrace-4® [preservative free]: Chromium 0.85 mcg, copper 0.1 mg, manganese 0.025 mg, and zinc 0.5 mg per mL (3 mL, 10 mL)
P.T.E.-4® [preservative free]: Chromium 1 mcg, copper 0.1 mg, manganese 0.025 mg, and zinc 1 mg per mL (3 mL)
P.T.E.-5® [preservative free]: Chromium 1 mcg, copper 0.1 mg, manganese 0.025 mg, selenium 15 mcg, and zinc 1 mg per mL (3 mL)
Trace elements pediatric: Chromium 1 mcg, copper 0.1 mg, manganese 0.03 mg, and zinc 0.5 mg per mL (10 mL) [contains benzyl alcohol]

Injection, solution [elemental equivalence]:
Chromium, as chromic chloride (hexahydrate) [preservative free]: 0.0205 mg/mL [0.004 mg/mL] (10 mL)
Copper, as cupric chloride: 1.07 mg/mL [0.4 mg/mL] (10 mL)
Iodine, as iodine sodium (Iodopen®): 0.118 mg/mL [0.1 mg/mL] (10 mL)
Manganese:
As chloride: 0.36 mg/mL [0.1 mg/mL] (10 mL)
As sulfate [preservative free]: 0.31 mg/mL [0.1 mg/mL] (10 mL)
Molybdenum, as ammonium molybdate (tetrahydrate) (Molypen®): 46 mcg/mL [25 mcg/mL] (10 mL)
Selenium, as selenious acid: 0.0654 mg/mL [0.04 mg/mL] (10 mL)
Selepen®: 0.0654 mg/mL [0.04 mg/mL] (10 mL, 30 mL) [30 mL contains benzyl alcohol]
Zinc:
As chloride: 2.09 mg/mL [1 mg/mL] (10 mL, 50 mL)
As sulfate, anhydrous [preservative free]: 2.46 mg/mL [1 mg/mL] (10 mL)
As sulfate, anhydrous, concentrate [preservative free]: 12.32 mg/mL [5 mg/mL] (5 mL)

♦ **Tracleer®** *see* Bosentan *on page 182*
♦ **Tracrium®** *see* Atracurium *on page 141*

Tramadol (TRA ma dole)

Medication Safety Issues

Sound-alike/look-alike issues:
Tramadol may be confused with Toradol®, Trandate®, Voltaren®
Ultram® may be confused with Ultane®, Voltaren®

(Continued)

Tramadol *(Continued)*

Related Information

Acute Postoperative Pain *on page 1388*
Angiotensin Agents *on page 1544*
Chronic Pain Management *on page 1430*

U.S. Brand Names Ultram®; Ultram® ER

Canadian Brand Names Ultram®

Synonyms Tramadol Hydrochloride

Pharmacologic Category Analgesic, Non-narcotic

Generic Available Yes: Excludes extended release tablet

Use Relief of moderate to moderately-severe pain

Mechanism of Action Binds to μ-opiate receptors in the CNS causing inhibition of ascending pain pathways, altering the perception of and response to pain; also inhibits the reuptake of norepinephrine and serotonin, which also modifies the ascending pain pathway

Pharmacodynamics/Kinetics

Onset of action: ~1 hour
Duration of action: 9 hours
Absorption: Rapid and complete
Distribution: V_d: 2.5-3 L/kg
Protein binding, plasma: 20%
Metabolism: Extensively hepatic via demethylation, glucuronidation, and sulfation; has pharmacologically active metabolite formed by CYP2D6 (M1; O-desmethyl tramadol)
Bioavailability: Immediate release: 75%; Extended release: 85% to 90% as compared to immediate release.
Half-life elimination: Tramadol: ~6-8 hours; Active metabolite: 7-9 hours; prolonged in elderly, hepatic or renal impairment
Time to peak: Immediate release: 2 hours; Extended release: 12 hours
Excretion: Urine (30% as unchanged drug; 60% as metabolites)

Dosage Moderate-to-severe chronic pain: Oral:

Adults:

Immediate release formulation: 50-100 mg every 4-6 hours (not to exceed 400 mg/day)

For patients not requiring rapid onset of effect, tolerability may be improved by starting dose at 25 mg/day and titrating dose by 25 mg every 3 days, until reaching 25 mg 4 times/day. Dose may then be increased by 50 mg every 3 days as tolerated, to reach dose of 50 mg 4 times/day.

Extended release formulation: 100 mg once daily; titrate every 5 days (maximum: 300 mg/day)

Elderly: >75 years:

Immediate release: 50 mg every 6 hours (not to exceed 300 mg/day); see dosing adjustments for renal and hepatic impairment.

Extended release formulation: Use with great caution. See adult dosing.

Dosing adjustment in renal impairment:

Immediate release: Cl_{cr} <30 mL/minute: Administer 50-100 mg dose every 12 hours (maximum: 200 mg/day)

Extended release: Should not be used in patients with Cl_{cr} < 30 mL/minute

Dosing adjustment in hepatic impairment:

Immediate release: Cirrhosis: Recommended dose: 50 mg every 12 hours

Extended release: Should not be used in patients with severe (Child-Pugh Class C) hepatic dysfunction

Stability Store at 15°C to 30°C (59°F to 86°F).

Administration Do not crush or chew extended release tablet.

Monitoring Parameters Pain relief, respiratory rate, blood pressure, and pulse; signs of tolerance or abuse

Reference Range 100-300 ng/mL; however, serum level monitoring is not required

Anesthesia and Critical Care Concerns/Other Considerations Tramadol 50 mg is comparable to codeine 60 mg; tramadol 100 mg is comparable to aspirin 650 mg/codeine 60 mg. Tramadol is 5-10 times less potent than morphine and reported to cause less respiratory depression.

Pregnancy Risk Factor C

Contraindications Hypersensitivity to tramadol, opioids, or any component of the formulation; opioid-dependent patients; acute intoxication with alcohol, hypnotics, centrally-acting analgesics, opioids, or psychotropic drugs

Ultram® ER (extended release formulation): Additional contraindications: Severe (Cl_{cr} <30 mL/minute) renal dysfunction, severe (Child-Pugh Class C) hepatic dysfunction

Warnings/Precautions Should be used only with extreme caution in patients receiving MAO inhibitors. May cause CNS depression and/or respiratory depression, particularly when combined with other CNS depressants. Use with caution and reduce dosage when administered to patients receiving other CNS depressants. An increased risk of seizures may occur in patients receiving serotonin reuptake inhibitors (SSRIs or anorectics), tricyclic antidepressants, other cyclic compounds (including cyclobenzaprine, promethazine), neuroleptics, MAO inhibitors, or drugs which may lower seizure threshold. Patients with a history of seizures, or with a risk of seizures (head trauma, metabolic disorders, CNS infection, or malignancy, or during ethanol/drug withdrawal) are also at increased risk.

Elderly patients and patients with chronic respiratory disorders may be at greater risk of adverse events. Use with caution in patients with increased intracranial pressure or head injury. Avoid use in patients who are suicidal or addiction prone. Use caution in heavy alcohol users. Use caution in treatment of acute abdominal conditions; may mask pain. Use tramadol with caution and reduce dosage in patients with liver disease or renal dysfunction. Not recommended during pregnancy or in nursing mothers. Tolerance or drug dependence may result from extended use (withdrawal symptoms have been reported); abrupt discontinuation should be avoided. Tapering of dose at the time of discontinuation limits the risk of withdrawal symptoms. Safety and efficacy in pediatric patients <18 years of age have not been established; use in this population is not recommended.

Adverse Reactions

>10%:

Cardiovascular: Flushing (8% to 16%)

Central nervous system: Dizziness (16% to 33%), headache (8% to 32%), insomnia (7% to 11%), somnolence (7% to 25%)

Dermatologic: Pruritus (6% to 12%)

Gastrointestinal: Constipation (12% to 46%), nausea (15% to 40%)

Neuromuscular & skeletal: Weakness (4% to 12%)

1% to 10%:

Cardiovascular: Chest pain (1% to <5%), postural hypotension (2% to 5%), vasodilation (1% to <5%)

Central nervous system: Agitation, anxiety (1% to <5%), confusion (1% to <5%), coordination impaired (1% to <5%), depression (1% to <5%), emotional lability, euphoria, hallucinations, hypoesthesia, lethargy, malaise, nervousness (1% to <5%), pain, pyrexia, restlessness

Dermatologic: Dermatitis, rash

Endocrine & metabolic: Hot flashes (2% to 9%), menopausal symptoms (1% to <5%)

Gastrointestinal: Abdominal pain, anorexia (<6%), diarrhea (5% to 10%), dry mouth (5% to 10%), dyspepsia, flatulence, vomiting (5% to 9%), weight loss

Genitourinary: Urinary frequency (1% to <5%), urinary retention (1% to <5%), urinary tract infection (1% to <5%)

Neuromuscular & skeletal: Arthralgia (1% to <5%), hypertonia (1% to <5%), rigors (<4%), paresthesia (1% to <5%), spasticity (1% to <5%), tremor (1% to <5%), creatinine phosphokinase increased

Ocular: Blurred vision (1% to <5%), miosis (1% to <5%)

Respiratory: Bronchitis (1% to <5%), cough (1% to <5%), dyspnea (1% to <5%), pharyngitis (1% to <5%), rhinorrhea (1% to <5%), sinusitis (1% to <5%)

Miscellaneous: Diaphoresis (2% to 6%), flu-like syndrome (<2%)

<1% (Limited to important or life-threatening): Allergic reaction, amnesia, anaphylactoid reactions, anaphylaxis, angioedema, bronchospasm, cataracts, cholecystitis, cholelithiasis, cognitive dysfunction, concentration difficulty, creatinine increased, deafness, gastrointestinal bleeding, hepatitis, hyper-/hypotension, liver failure, MI, migraine, myocardial ischemia, night sweats, pancreatitis, peripheral ischemia, pulmonary edema, pulmonary embolism, seizure, serotonin syndrome, Stevens-Johnson syndrome, suicidal tendency, syncope, toxic epidermal necrolysis, vertigo

A withdrawal syndrome may occur with abrupt discontinuation; includes anxiety, diarrhea, hallucinations (rare), nausea, pain, piloerection, rigors, sweating, and

(Continued)

Tramadol *(Continued)*

tremor. Uncommon discontinuation symptoms may include severe anxiety, panic attacks, or paresthesia.

Overdosage/Toxicology Symptoms of overdose include CNS and respiratory depression, lethargy, coma, miosis, seizure, cardiac arrest, and death. Treatment may be symptom-directed and supportive. Naloxone may reverse some overdose symptoms, but may increase the risk of seizures. Hemodialysis is not helpful in removal of tramadol.

Drug Interactions Substrate of CYP2B6 (minor), 2D6 (major), 3A4 (minor)

Carbamazepine: Tramadol metabolism is increased by carbamazepine. Avoid concurrent use; increases risk of seizures.

Cyclobenzaprine: May enhance the neuroexcitatory and/or seizure-potentiating effect of tramadol.

CYP2D6 inhibitors: May decrease the effects of tramadol. Example inhibitors include chlorpromazine, delavirdine, fluoxetine, miconazole, paroxetine, pergolide, quinidine, quinine, ritonavir, and ropinirole.

Ethanol: Tramadol may enhance the CNS depressant effect of ethanol.

MAO inhibitors: May increase the neuroexcitatory effects or risk of seizures. Examples of inhibitors include isocarboxazid, linezolid, phenelzine, selegiline, and tranylcypromine.

Naloxone: May increase the risk of seizures (if administered in tramadol overdose).

Quinidine: May increase the tramadol serum concentrations and decrease serum concentrations of M1

SSRIs: May increase the neuroexcitatory effects or risk of seizures with tramadol. Examples of SSRIs include citalopram, escitalopram, fluoxetine, fluvoxamine, paroxetine, sertraline.

Serotonin modulators: May enhance the adverse/toxic effects of tramadol. The development of serotonin syndrome may occur.

Sibutramine: May enhance the serotonergic effects of tramadol. Avoid concurrent use.

Tricyclic antidepressants: May increase the risk of seizures.

Ethanol/Nutrition/Herb Interactions

Ethanol: Avoid ethanol (may increase CNS depression).

Food:

Immediate release: Does not affect the rate or extent of absorption.

Extended release: Reduced C_{max} and AUC and T_{max} occurred 3 hours earlier when taken with a high-fat meal.

Herb/Nutraceutical: Avoid valerian, St John's wort, kava kava, gotu kola (may increase CNS depression).

Dietary Considerations May be taken with or without food. Extended release formulation: Be consistent; always give with food or always give on an empty stomach.

Dosage Forms

Tablet, as hydrochloride: 50 mg

Ultram®: 50 mg

Tablet, extended release, as hydrochloride:

Ultram® ER: 100 mg, 200 mg, 300 mg

- **Tramadol Hydrochloride** *see* Tramadol *on page 1297*
- **Trandate®** *see* Labetalol *on page 721*

Trandolapril (tran DOE la pril)

Related Information

Angiotensin Agents *on page 1544*

U.S. Brand Names Mavik®

Canadian Brand Names Mavik™

Pharmacologic Category Angiotensin-Converting Enzyme (ACE) Inhibitor

Generic Available No

Use Management of hypertension alone or in combination with other antihypertensive agents; treatment of left ventricular dysfunction after myocardial infarction

Unlabeled/Investigational Use As a class, ACE inhibitors are recommended in the treatment of systolic congestive heart failure

Mechanism of Action Trandolapril is an ACE inhibitor which prevents the formation of angiotensin II from angiotensin I. Trandolapril must undergo enzymatic hydrolysis, mainly in liver, to its biologically active metabolite, trandolaprilat. A CNS mechanism may also be involved in the hypotensive effect as angiotensin II increases adrenergic outflow from the CNS. Vasoactive kallikrein's may be decreased in conversion to active hormones by ACE inhibitors, thus, reducing blood pressure.

Pharmacodynamics/Kinetics

Onset of action: 1-2 hours

Peak effect: Reduction in blood pressure: 6 hours

Duration: Prolonged; 72 hours after single dose

Absorption: Rapid

Distribution: Trandolaprilat (active metabolite) is very lipophilic in comparison to other ACE inhibitors

Protein binding: 80%

Metabolism: Hepatically hydrolyzed to active metabolite, trandolaprilat

Half-life elimination:

Trandolapril: 6 hours; Trandolaprilat: Effective: 10 hours, Terminal: 24 hours

Time to peak: Parent: 1 hour; Active metabolite trandolaprilat: 4-10 hours

Excretion: Urine (as metabolites)

Clearance: Reduce dose in renal failure; creatinine clearances ≤30 mL/minute result in accumulation of active metabolite

Dosage Adults: Oral:

Hypertension: Initial dose in patients not receiving a diuretic: 1 mg/day (2 mg/day in black patients). Adjust dosage according to the blood pressure response. Make dosage adjustments at intervals of ≥1 week. Most patients have required dosages of 2-4 mg/day. There is a little experience with doses >8 mg/day. Patients inadequately treated with once daily dosing at 4 mg may be treated with twice daily dosing. If blood pressure is not adequately controlled with trandolapril monotherapy, a diuretic may be added.

Usual dose range (JNC 7): 1-4 mg once daily

Heart failure postmyocardial infarction or left ventricular dysfunction postmyocardial infarction: Initial: 1 mg/day; titrate patients (as tolerated) towards the target dose of 4 mg/day. If a 4 mg dose is not tolerated, patients can continue therapy with the greatest tolerated dose.

Dosing adjustment in renal impairment: Cl_{cr} ≤30 mL/minute: Recommended starting dose: 0.5 mg/day.

Dosing adjustment in hepatic impairment: Cirrhosis: Recommended starting dose: 0.5 mg/day.

Monitoring Parameters Serum potassium, renal function, serum creatinine, BUN, CBC; observe for hypotensive effects within 1-3 hours of first dose or new higher dose

Pregnancy Risk Factor C (1st trimester)/D (2nd and 3rd trimesters)

Contraindications Hypersensitivity to trandolapril or any component of the formulation; history of angioedema-related to previous treatment with an ACE inhibitor; bilateral renal artery stenosis; pregnancy (2nd and 3rd trimesters)

Warnings/Precautions Anaphylactic reactions can occur. Angioedema can occur at any time during treatment (especially following first dose). It may involve head and neck (potentially affecting the airway) or the intestine (presenting with abdominal pain). Prolonged monitoring may be required especially if tongue, glottis, or larynx are involved as they are associated with airway obstruction. Those with a history of airway surgery in this situation have a higher risk. Careful blood pressure monitoring with first dose (hypotension can occur especially in volume-depleted patients). **[U.S. Boxed Warning]: Based on human data, ACEIs can cause injury and death to the developing fetus when used in the second and third trimesters. ACEIs should be discontinued as soon as possible once pregnancy is detected.** Dosage adjustment needed in severe renal dysfunction (Cl_{cr} <30 mL/minute) or in hepatic cirrhosis. Use with caution in hypovolemia; collagen vascular diseases; valvular stenosis (particularly aortic stenosis); hyperkalemia; or before, during, or immediately after anesthesia. Avoid rapid dosage escalation, which may lead to renal insufficiency. Rare toxicities associated with ACE inhibitors include cholestatic jaundice (which may progress to hepatic necrosis) and neutropenia/agranulocytosis with myeloid hyperplasia. If patient has renal impairment then a baseline WBC with differential and serum creatinine should be evaluated and monitored closely during the first 3 months of therapy. Use with caution in unilateral renal artery stenosis and pre-existing renal insufficiency.

Adverse Reactions Note: Frequency ranges include data from hypertension and heart failure trials. Higher rates of adverse reactions have generally been noted in

(Continued)

Trandolapril *(Continued)*

patients with CHF. However, the frequency of adverse effects associated with placebo is also increased in this population.

>1%:

Cardiovascular: Hypotension (<1% to 11%), bradycardia (<1% to 4.7%), intermittent claudication (3.8%), stroke (3.3%), syncope (5.9%)

Central nervous system: Dizziness (1.3% to 23%), asthenia (3.3%)

Endocrine & metabolic: Elevated uric acid (15%), hyperkalemia (5.3%), hypocalcemia (4.7%)

Gastrointestinal: Dyspepsia (6.4%), gastritis (4.2%)

Neuromuscular & skeletal: Myalgia (4.7%)

Renal: Elevated BUN (9%), elevated serum creatinine (1.1% to 4.7%)

Respiratory: Cough (1.9% to 35%)

<1% (Limited to important or life-threatening): Angina, angioedema, anxiety, AV block (first-degree), dyspnea, gout, impotence, increased ALT, increased serum creatinine, insomnia, laryngeal edema, muscle pain, neutropenia, pancreatitis, paresthesia, pruritus, rash, symptomatic hypotension, thrombocytopenia, vertigo. Worsening of renal function may occur in patients with bilateral renal artery stenosis or in hypovolemic patients. In addition, a syndrome which may include fever, myalgia, arthralgia, interstitial nephritis, vasculitis, rash, eosinophilia and positive ANA, and elevated ESR has been reported with ACE inhibitors.

Overdosage/Toxicology Mild hypotension has been the primary toxic effect seen with acute overdose. Bradycardia may also occur. Hyperkalemia occurs even with therapeutic doses, especially in patients with renal insufficiency and those taking NSAIDs. Treatment is symptom-directed and supportive.

Drug Interactions

Alpha$_1$ blockers: Hypotensive effect increased.

Aspirin: The effects of ACE inhibitors may be blunted by aspirin administration, particularly at higher dosages and/or increase adverse renal effects.

Diuretics: Hypovolemia due to diuretics may precipitate acute hypotensive events or acute renal failure.

Insulin: Risk of hypoglycemia may be increased.

Lithium: Risk of lithium toxicity may be increased; monitor lithium levels, especially the first 4 weeks of therapy.

Mercaptopurine: Risk of neutropenia may be increased.

NSAIDs: May attenuate hypertensive efficacy; effect has been seen with captopril and may occur with other ACE inhibitors; monitor blood pressure. May increase adverse renal effects.

Potassium-sparing diuretics (amiloride, potassium, spironolactone, triamterene): Increased risk of hyperkalemia.

Potassium supplements may increase the risk of hyperkalemia.

Trimethoprim (high dose) may increase the risk of hyperkalemia.

Ethanol/Nutrition/Herb Interactions Herb/Nutraceutical: Avoid dong quai if using for hypertension (has estrogenic activity). Avoid ephedra, yohimbe, ginseng (may worsen hypertension). Avoid garlic (may have increased antihypertensive effect).

Dosage Forms Tablet: 1 mg, 2 mg, 4 mg

- **Transamine Sulphate** *see* Tranylcypromine *on page 1302*
- **Transderm-Nitro® (Can)** *see* Nitroglycerin *on page 928*
- **Transderm Scōp®** *see* Scopolamine *on page 1152*
- **Transderm-V® (Can)** *see* Scopolamine *on page 1152*
- **Tranxene® SD™** *see* Clorazepate *on page 321*
- **Tranxene® SD™-Half Strength** *see* Clorazepate *on page 321*
- **Tranxene® T-Tab®** *see* Clorazepate *on page 321*

Tranylcypromine (tran il SIP roe meen)

Related Information

Antidepressant Agents *on page 1551*

U.S. Brand Names Parnate®

Canadian Brand Names Parnate®

Synonyms Transamine Sulphate; Tranylcypromine Sulfate

Pharmacologic Category Antidepressant, Monoamine Oxidase Inhibitor

Restrictions A medication guide concerning the use of antidepressants in children and teenagers can be found on the FDA website at http://www.fda.gov/cder/Offices/ODS/labeling.htm. It should be dispensed to parents or guardians of children and teenagers receiving this medication.

Generic Available No

Use Treatment of major depressive episode without melancholia

Unlabeled/Investigational Use Post-traumatic stress disorder

Mechanism of Action Tranylcypromine is a nonhydrazine monoamine oxidase inhibitor. It increases endogenous concentrations of epinephrine, norepinephrine, dopamine, and serotonin through inhibition of the enzyme (monoamine oxidase) responsible for the breakdown of these neurotransmitters.

Pharmacodynamics/Kinetics

Onset of action: Therapeutic: 2 days to 3 weeks continued dosing

Half-life elimination: 90-190 minutes

Time to peak, serum: ~2 hours

Excretion: Urine

Dosage Adults: Oral: 10 mg twice daily, increase by 10 mg increments at 1- to 3-week intervals; maximum: 60 mg/day; usual effective dose: 30 mg/day

Monitoring Parameters Blood pressure, mental status

Pregnancy Risk Factor C

Contraindications Hypersensitivity to tranylcypromine, other MAO inhibitors, dibenzazepine derivatives, or any component of the formulation; antiparkinson drugs, cardiovascular disease; cerebrovascular defect; headache history; hepatic disease; hypertension; pheochromocytoma; renal disease; concurrent use of antihistamines, antihypertensives, bupropion, buspirone, CNS depressants, dexfenfluramine, dextromethorphan, diuretics, ethanol, meperidine, SSRIs, and sympathomimetics; general anesthesia (discontinue 10 days prior to elective surgery); local vasoconstrictors; spinal anesthesia (hypotension may be exaggerated); foods which are high in tyramine, tryptophan, or dopamine, chocolate, or caffeine

Warnings/Precautions **Risk of suicide: [U.S. Boxed Warning]: Antidepressants increase the risk of suicidal thinking and behavior in children and adolescents with major depressive disorder (MDD) and other depressive disorders;** consider risk prior to prescribing. Closely monitor for clinical worsening, suicidality, or unusual changes in behavior such as anxiety, agitation, panic attacks, insomnia, irritability, hostility, impulsivity, akathisia, hypomania, and mania. The child's family or caregiver should be instructed to closely observe the patient and communicate condition with healthcare provider. Such observation would generally include at least weekly face-to-face contact with patients or their family members or caregivers during the first 4 weeks of treatment, then every other week visits for the next 4 weeks, then at 12 weeks, and as clinically indicated beyond 12 weeks. Additional contact by telephone may be appropriate between face-to-face visits. A medication guide should be dispensed with each prescription. **Tranylcypromine is not FDA approved for treatment of children and adolescents.**

Adults treated with antidepressants should be observed similarly for clinical worsening and suicidality, especially during the initial few months of a course of drug therapy, or at times of dose changes, either increases or decreases. The possibility of a suicide attempt is inherent in major depression and may persist until remission occurs. Worsening depression and severe abrupt suicidality that are not part of the presenting symptoms may require discontinuation or modification of drug therapy. Use caution in high-risk patients during initiation of therapy. Prescriptions should be written for the smallest quantity consistent with good patient care.

Disease state precautions: Use with caution in patients who are hyperactive, hyperexcitable, or who have glaucoma, hyperthyroidism, diabetes or hypotension. May cause orthostatic hypotension (especially at dosages >30 mg/day); use with caution in patients who would not tolerate transient hypotensive episodes. Use with caution in patients at risk of seizures, or in patients receiving other drugs which may lower seizure threshold. Discontinue at least 48 hours prior to myelography. May increase the risks associated with electroconvulsive therapy.
(Continued)

Tranylcypromine *(Continued)*

Consider discontinuing, when possible, prior to elective surgery. Use with caution in patients with renal impairment. May worsen psychosis in some patients or precipitate a shift to mania or hypomania in patients with bipolar disorder. Monotherapy in patients with bipolar disorder should be avoided. Patients presenting with depressive symptoms should be screened for bipolar disorder. **Tranylcypromine is not FDA approved for the treatment of bipolar depression.**

Drug interactions: Hypertensive crisis may occur with tyramine, tryptophan, or dopamine-containing foods. Should not be used in combination with other antidepressants. Do not use within 5 weeks of fluoxetine discontinuation or 2 weeks of other antidepressant discontinuation. Hypotensive effects of antihypertensives (beta-blockers, thiazides) may be exaggerated. Orthostasis may be additive when used with other agents also known to cause it (eg, phenothiazines). Use with caution in patients receiving disulfiram.

Elderly patients: The MAO inhibitors are effective and generally well tolerated by older patients. It is the potential interactions with tyramine or tryptophan-containing foods and other drugs, and their effects on blood pressure that have limited their use.

Adverse Reactions Frequency not defined.

Cardiovascular: Edema, orthostatic hypotension, palpitations, tachycardia

Central nervous system: Agitation, akinesia, anxiety, ataxia, chills, confusion, disorientation, dizziness, drowsiness, fatigue, headache, hyper-reflexia, insomnia, mania, memory loss, restlessness, sleep disturbances, twitching

Dermatologic: Alopecia, cystic acne (flare), pruritus, rash, urticaria, scleroderma (localized)

Endocrine & metabolic: Hypernatremia, hypermetabolic syndrome; sexual dysfunction (anorgasmia, ejaculatory disturbances, impotence); SIADH

Gastrointestinal: Abdominal pain, anorexia, constipation, diarrhea, nausea, vomiting, weight gain, xerostomia

Genitourinary: Incontinence, urinary retention

Hematologic: Agranulocytosis, anemia, leukopenia, thrombocytopenia

Hepatic: Hepatitis

Neuromuscular & skeletal: Akinesis, muscle spasm, myoclonus, numbness, paresthesia, tremor, weakness

Ocular: Blurred vision, glaucoma

Otic: Tinnitus

Miscellaneous: Diaphoresis

Overdosage/Toxicology Symptoms of overdose include headache, tachycardia or bradycardia, neck stiffness, nausea, vomiting, chest pain, sweating, photophobia, palpitations, muscle twitching, seizures, insomnia, orthostatic hypotension, hypertension, hypertensive crisis, hyperpyrexia, and coma. Treatment is symptom-directed and supportive. The manufacturer suggests phentolamine (5 mg given slowly I.V.) for treatment of hypertensive crisis. Other useful agents may be labetalol or nitroprusside.

Drug Interactions Inhibits CYP1A2 (moderate), 2A6 (strong), 2C8 (weak), 2C9 (weak), 2C19 (moderate), 2D6 (moderate), 2E1 (weak), 3A4 (weak)

Acetylcholinesterase inhibitors: May diminish the anticholinergic side effects of tranylcypromine.

Alpha-/beta-agonists: MAO inhibitors may enhance the vasopressor effect. Alpha-/beta-agonists (indirect-acting): MAO inhibitors may enhance the vasopressor effect.

Alpha$_1$-agonist: MAO inhibitors may enhance the hypertensive effects.

Altretamine: May enhance the orthostatic effect of MAO inhibitors.

Amphetamines: MAO inhibitors in combination with amphetamines may result in severe hypertensive reaction; these combinations are best avoided.

Anesthetics, general: Discontinue tranylcypromine 10 days prior to elective surgery.

Anorexiants: Concurrent use of anorexiants may result in serotonin syndrome; contraindicated with dexfenfluramine; avoid use with fenfluramine or sibutramine.

Anticholinergics: May enhance the adverse/toxic anticholinergic effects of tranylcypromine.

Atomoxetine: MAO Inhibitors may enhance the neurotoxic (central) effect of atomoxetine. Avoid combination. Atomoxetine should not be used within 14 days of an MAO inhibitor.

Bupropion: May cause hypertensive crisis; at least 14 days should elapse before initiating bupropion; concurrent use with an MAO inhibitor is contraindicated.

Buspirone: May cause increased blood pressure; concurrent use with an MAO inhibitor should be avoided.

COMT Inhibitors: May enhance the adverse/toxic effect of MAO inhibitors. Avoid concurrent use.

Cyclobenzaprine: May enhance the serotonergic effect of MAO Inhibitors. This could result in serotonin syndrome. Avoid combination.

CYP1A2 substrates: Tranylcypromine may increase the levels/effects of CYP1A2 substrates. Example substrates include aminophylline, fluvoxamine, mexiletine, mirtazapine, ropinirole, theophylline, and trifluoperazine.

CYP2A6 substrates: Tranylcypromine may increase the levels/effects of CYP2A6 substrates. Example substrates include dexmedetomidine and ifosfamide.

CYP2C19 substrates: Tranylcypromine may increase the levels/effects of CYP2C19 substrates. Example substrates include citalopram, diazepam, methsuximide, phenytoin, and trimipramine.

CYP2D6 substrates: Tranylcypromine may increase the levels/effects of CYP2D6 substrates. Example substrates include amphetamines, selected beta-blockers, dextromethorphan, fluoxetine, lidocaine, mirtazapine, nefazodone, paroxetine, risperidone, thioridazine, tricyclic antidepressants, and venlafaxine.

CYP2D6 prodrug substrates: Tranylcypromine may decrease the levels/effects of CYP2D6 prodrug substrates. Example prodrug substrates include codeine, hydrocodone, oxycodone, and tramadol.

Dexmethylphenidate: MAO inhibitors may enhance the hypertensive effect of dexmethylphenidate; avoid concurrent use.

Dextromethorphan: Concurrent use of MAO inhibitors may result in serotonin syndrome; concurrent use is contraindicated.

Disulfiram: MAO inhibitors may produce delirium in patients receiving disulfiram; monitor.

Ethanol: Tranylcypromine may enhance CNS depressant effect of ethanol.

False neurotransmitters: MAO inhibitors inhibit the antihypertensive response to guanadrel or methyldopa; monitor therapy.

Levodopa: MAO inhibitors in combination with levodopa may result in hypertensive reactions; monitor.

Lithium: MAO inhibitors in combination with lithium have resulted in CNS toxicity (malignant hyperpyrexia, tardive dyskinesias); monitor therapy.

Meperidine: May cause serotonin syndrome when combined with an MAO inhibitor; concurrent use is contraindicated; should not be used within 14 days of an MAO inhibitor.

Methylphenidate: MAO inhibitors may enhance the hypertensive effect of methylphenidate. Avoid combination.

Mirtazapine: MAO inhibitors may enhance the neurotoxic (central) effect of mirtazapine. Avoid combination.

Pramlintide: Pramlintide may enhance the anticholinergic effect of tranylcypromine. Additive effects on reduced GI motility may occur.

Rauwolfia alkaloids: MAO inhibitors may enhance the adverse/toxic effect of rauwolfia alkaloids. If a rauwolfia alkaloid is added to existing MAOI therapy, a burst of catecholamine stimulation (eg, excitation, hypertension) may occur.

Serotonin/norepinephrine reuptake inhibitors (SNRIs): MAO inhibitors may enhance the serotonergic effect of SNRI antidepressants. This may cause serotonin syndrome.

Selective serotonin reuptake inhibitors (SSRIs): MAO Inhibitors may enhance the serotonergic effect of SSRIs. This may cause serotonin syndrome. Avoid concurrent use. Do not use within 5 weeks of fluoxetine discontinuation or 2 weeks of other antidepressant discontinuation.

Serotonin 5-HT_{1D} receptor agonists: May increase the risk of serotonin syndrome. The manufacturers of rizatriptan, sumatriptan, and zolmitriptan state that concurrent use (or use within 2 weeks of MAO therapy) is contraindicated.

Serotonin modulators: May enhance the adverse/toxic effect of other serotonin modulators, such as tranylcypromine. The development of serotonin syndrome may occur.

Sibutramine: May enhance the serotonergic effect of tranylcypromine. This may cause serotonin syndrome. Avoid concurrent use.

(Continued)

Tranylcypromine *(Continued)*

Thioridazine: Tranylcypromine may decrease the metabolism of thioridazine. Avoid concurrent use.

Tramadol: May enhance the neuroexcitatory and/or seizure-potentiating effect of MAO Inhibitors.

Tricyclic antidepressants: MAO inhibitors may enhance the serotonergic effect of tricyclic antidepressants. This may cause serotonin syndrome. Avoid concurrent use.

Ethanol/Nutrition/Herb Interactions

Ethanol: Avoid ethanol (many contain tyramine).

Food: Clinically-severe elevated blood pressure may occur if tranylcypromine is taken with tyramine-containing food. Avoid foods containing tryptophan or dopamine, chocolate or caffeine.

Herb/Nutraceutical: Avoid valerian, St John's wort, SAMe, ginseng. Avoid ginkgo (may lead to MAO inhibitor toxicity). Avoid ephedra, yohimbe (can cause hypertension).

Dietary Considerations Avoid food which contains high amounts of tyramine. Avoid foods containing tryptophan or dopamine, including chocolate and caffeine.

Dosage Forms Tablet: 10 mg

♦ **Tranylcypromine Sulfate** *see* Tranylcypromine *on page 1302*

♦ **Trasylol®** *see* Aprotinin *on page 123*

Trazodone (TRAZ oh done)

Medication Safety Issues

Sound-alike/look-alike issues:

Desyrel® may be confused with Demerol®, Delsym®, Zestril®

Related Information

Antidepressant Agents *on page 1551*

Chronic Pain Management *on page 1430*

U.S. Brand Names Desyrel®

Canadian Brand Names Alti-Trazodone; Apo-Trazodone®; Apo-Trazodone D®; Desyrel®; Gen-Trazodone; Novo-Trazodone; Nu-Trazodone; PMS-Trazodone; ratio-Trazodone; Trazorel®

Synonyms Trazodone Hydrochloride

Pharmacologic Category Antidepressant, Serotonin Reuptake Inhibitor/Antagonist

Restrictions A medication guide concerning the use of antidepressants in children and teenagers can be found on the FDA website at http://www.fda.gov/cder/Offices/ODS/labeling.htm. It should be dispensed to parents or guardians of children and teenagers receiving this medication.

Generic Available Yes

Use Treatment of depression

Unlabeled/Investigational Use Potential augmenting agent for antidepressants, hypnotic

Mechanism of Action Inhibits reuptake of serotonin, causes adrenoreceptor subsensitivity, and induces significant changes in 5-HT presynaptic receptor adrenoreceptors. Trazodone also significantly blocks histamine (H_1) and alpha$_1$-adrenergic receptors.

Pharmacodynamics/Kinetics

Onset of action: Therapeutic (antidepressant): 1-3 weeks; sleep aid: 1-3 hours

Protein binding: 85% to 95%

Metabolism: Hepatic via CYP3A4 to an active metabolite (mCPP)

Half-life elimination: 7-8 hours, two compartment kinetics

Time to peak, serum: 30-100 minutes; delayed with food (up to 2.5 hours)

Excretion: Primarily urine; secondarily feces

Dosage Oral: Therapeutic effects may take up to 6 weeks to occur; therapy is normally maintained for 6-12 months after optimum response is reached to prevent recurrence of depression

Children 6-12 years: Depression (unlabeled use): Initial: 1.5-2 mg/kg/day in divided doses; increase gradually every 3-4 days as needed; maximum: 6 mg/kg/day in 3 divided doses

Adolescents: Depression (unlabeled use): Initial: 25-50 mg/day; increase to 100-150 mg/day in divided doses

Adults:

Depression: Initial: 150 mg/day in 3 divided doses (may increase by 50 mg/day every 3-7 days); maximum: 600 mg/day

Sedation/hypnotic (unlabeled use): 25-50 mg at bedtime (often in combination with daytime SSRIs); may increase up to 200 mg at bedtime

Elderly: 25-50 mg at bedtime with 25-50 mg/day dose increase every 3 days for inpatients and weekly for outpatients, if tolerated; usual dose: 75-150 mg/day

Administration Dosing after meals may decrease lightheadedness and postural hypotension

Reference Range

Plasma levels do not always correlate with clinical effectiveness

Therapeutic: 0.5-2.5 mcg/mL

Potentially toxic: >2.5 mcg/mL

Toxic: >4 mcg/mL

Pregnancy Risk Factor C

Contraindications Hypersensitivity to trazodone or any component of the formulation

Warnings/Precautions [U.S. Boxed Warning]: Antidepressants increase the risk of suicidal thinking and behavior in children and adolescents with major depressive disorder (MDD) and other depressive disorders; consider risk prior to prescribing. Closely monitor for clinical worsening, suicidality, or unusual changes in behavior; the child's family or caregiver should be instructed to closely observe the patient and communicate condition with healthcare provider. Such observation would generally include at least weekly face-to-face contact with patients or their family members or caregivers during the first 4 weeks of treatment, then every other week visits for the next 4 weeks, then at 12 weeks, and as clinically indicated beyond 12 weeks. Additional contact by telephone may be appropriate between face-to-face visits. Adults treated with antidepressants should be observed similarly for clinical worsening and suicidality, especially during the initial few months of a course of drug therapy, or at times of dose changes, either increases or decreases. A medication guide should be dispensed with each prescription. **Trazodone is not FDA approved for use in children.**

The possibility of a suicide attempt is inherent in major depression and may persist until remission occurs. Monitor for worsening of depression or suicidality, especially during initiation of therapy or with dose increases or decreases. Worsening depression and severe abrupt suicidality that are not part of the presenting symptoms may require discontinuation or modification of drug therapy. Use caution in high-risk patients during initiation of therapy. Prescriptions should be written for the smallest quantity consistent with good patient care. The patient's family or caregiver should be alerted to monitor patients for the emergence of suicidality and associated behaviors such as anxiety, agitation, panic attacks, insomnia, irritability, hostility, impulsivity, akathisia, hypomania, and mania; patients should be instructed to notify their healthcare provider if any of these symptoms or worsening depression occur.

May worsen psychosis in some patients or precipitate a shift to mania or hypomania in patients with bipolar disorder. Monotherapy in patients with bipolar disorder should be avoided. Patients presenting with depressive symptoms should be screened for bipolar disorder. **Trazodone is not FDA approved for the treatment of bipolar depression.**

Priapism, including cases resulting in permanent dysfunction, has occurred with the use of trazodone. Not recommended for use in a patient during the acute recovery phase of MI. Trazodone should be initiated with caution in patients who are receiving concurrent or recent therapy with a MAO inhibitor. May cause sedation, resulting in impaired performance of tasks requiring alertness (eg, operating machinery or driving). Sedative effects may be additive with other CNS depressants and ethanol. The degree of sedation is very high relative to other antidepressants. May increase the risks associated with electroconvulsive therapy. Consider discontinuing, when possible, prior to elective surgery. Therapy should not be abruptly discontinued in patients receiving high doses for prolonged periods.

Use with caution in patients at risk of hypotension or in patients where transient hypotensive episodes would be poorly tolerated (cardiovascular disease or cerebrovascular disease). The risk of postural hypotension is high relative to other antidepressants.

(Continued)

Trazodone *(Continued)*

Use caution in patients with a previous seizure disorder or condition predisposing to seizures such as brain damage, alcoholism, or concurrent therapy with other drugs which lower the seizure threshold. Use with caution in patients with hepatic or renal dysfunction and in elderly patients. Use with caution in patients with a history of cardiovascular disease (including previous MI, stroke, tachycardia, or conduction abnormalities). However, the risk of conduction abnormalities with this agent is low relative to other antidepressants.

Adverse Reactions

>10%:

Central nervous system: Dizziness, headache, sedation
Gastrointestinal: Nausea, xerostomia
Ocular: Blurred vision

1% to 10%:

Cardiovascular: Syncope, hyper-/hypotension, edema
Central nervous system: Confusion, decreased concentration, fatigue, incoordination
Gastrointestinal: Diarrhea, constipation, weight gain/loss
Neuromuscular & skeletal: Tremor, myalgia
Respiratory: Nasal congestion

<1% (Limited to important or life-threatening): Agitation, allergic reactions, alopecia, anxiety, bradycardia, extrapyramidal symptoms, hepatitis, priapism, rash, seizure, speech impairment, tachycardia, urinary retention

Overdosage/Toxicology Symptoms of overdose include drowsiness, vomiting, hypotension, tachycardia, incontinence, coma, and priapism. Treatment is symptom-directed and supportive.

Drug Interactions Substrate of CYP2D6 (minor), 3A4 (major); **Inhibits** CYP2D6 (moderate), 3A4 (weak)

Antipsychotics: Trazodone, in combination with other psychotropics (low potency antipsychotics), may result in additional hypotension (isolated case reports); monitor.

Azole antifungals: Serum concentrations of trazodone may be increased by azole antifungals, via inhibition of CYP3A4. Ketoconazole has been specifically studied. Consider a lower dose of trazodone.

Buspirone: Serotonergic effects may be additive (limited documentation); monitor.

Carbamazepine: Serum concentrations of trazodone may be decreased by carbamazepine, due to induction of CYP3A4. Other CYP inducers are likely to share this effect.

CNS depressants: Sedative effects may be additive with CNS depressants. Includes ethanol, barbiturates, benzodiazepines, narcotic analgesics, and other sedative agents; monitor for increased effect

CYP2D6 substrates: Trazodone may increase the levels/effects of CYP2D6 substrates. Example substrates include amphetamines, selected beta-blockers, dextromethorphan, fluoxetine, lidocaine, mirtazapine, nefazodone, paroxetine, risperidone, ritonavir, thioridazine, tricyclic antidepressants, and venlafaxine.

CYP2D6 prodrug substrates: Trazodone may decrease the levels/effects of CYP2D6 prodrug substrates. Example prodrug substrates include codeine, hydrocodone, oxycodone, and tramadol.

CYP3A4 inducers: CYP3A4 inducers may decrease the levels/effects of trazodone. Example inducers include aminoglutethimide, carbamazepine, nafcillin, nevirapine, phenobarbital, phenytoin, and rifamycins.

CYP3A4 inhibitors: May increase the levels/effects of trazodone. Example inhibitors include azole antifungals, clarithromycin, diclofenac, doxycycline, erythromycin, imatinib, isoniazid, nefazodone, nicardipine, propofol, protease inhibitors, quinidine, telithromycin, and verapamil.

Linezolid: Due to MAO inhibition (see note on MAO inhibitors), this combination should be avoided

MAO inhibitors: Concurrent use may lead to serotonin syndrome; avoid concurrent use or use within 14 days

Meperidine: Combined use, theoretically, may increase the risk of serotonin syndrome

Protease inhibitors: Serum concentrations of trazodone may be increased by protease inhibitors, via inhibition of CYP3A4. Consider a lower dose of trazodone.

Serotonin agonists: Theoretically, may increase the risk of serotonin syndrome; includes sumatriptan, naratriptan, rizatriptan, and zolmitriptan

SSRIs: Combined use of trazodone with an SSRI may, theoretically, increase the risk of serotonin syndrome; in addition, some SSRIs may inhibit the metabolism of trazodone resulting in elevated plasma levels and increased sedation; includes fluoxetine and fluvoxamine (see CYP inhibition); low doses of trazodone appear to represent little risk

Venlafaxine: Combined use with trazodone may increase the risk of serotonin syndrome

Ethanol/Nutrition/Herb Interactions

Ethanol: Avoid ethanol (may increase CNS depression).

Food: Time to peak serum levels may be increased if trazodone is taken with food.

Herb/Nutraceutical: Avoid valerian, St John's wort, SAMe, kava kava (may increase risk of serotonin syndrome and/or excessive sedation).

Dosage Forms Tablet, as hydrochloride: 50 mg, 100 mg, 150 mg, 300 mg

- **Trazodone Hydrochloride** *see* Trazodone *on page 1306*
- **Trazorel® (Can)** *see* Trazodone *on page 1306*

Treprostinil (tre PROST in il)

Related Information

Heart Failure (Systolic) *on page 1607*

U.S. Brand Names Remodulin®

Canadian Brand Names Remodulin®

Synonyms Treprostinil Sodium

Pharmacologic Category Vasodilator

Generic Available No

Use Treatment of pulmonary arterial hypertension (PAH) in patients with NYHA Class II-IV symptoms to decrease exercise-associated symptoms; to diminish clinical deterioration when transitioning from epoprostenol (I.V.)

Mechanism of Action Treprostinil is a direct dilator of both pulmonary and systemic arterial vascular beds; also inhibits platelet aggregation.

Pharmacodynamics/Kinetics

Absorption: SubQ: Rapidly and completely

Distribution: 14 L/70 kg lean body weight

Protein binding: 91%

Metabolism: Hepatic (enzymes unknown); forms metabolites

Bioavailability: 100%

Half-life elimination: Terminal: 2-4 hours

Excretion: Urine (79%; 4% as unchanged drug, 64% as metabolites); feces (13%)

Dosage SubQ or I.V. infusion:

Adults: PAH:

Initial: New to prostacyclin therapy: 1.25 ng/kg/minute continuous; if dose cannot be tolerated, reduce to 0.625 ng/kg/minute. Increase at rate not >1.25 ng/kg/minute per week for first 4 weeks, and not >2.5 ng/kg/minute per week

Transitioning From Epoprostenol to Treprostinil

Step	Epoprostenol Dose	Treprostinil Dose
1	Maintain current dose	Initiate at 10% initial epoprostenol dose
2	Decrease to 80% initial dose	Increase to 30% initial epoprostenol dose
3	Decrease to 60% initial dose	Increase to 50% initial epoprostenol dose
4	Decrease to 40% initial dose	Increase to 70% initial epoprostenol dose
5	Decrease to 20% initial dose	Increase to 90% initial epoprostenol dose
6	Decrease to 5% initial dose	Increase to 110% initial epoprostenol dose
7	Discontinue epoprostenol	Maintain current dose plus additional 5% to 10% as needed

(Continued)

Treprostinil *(Continued)*

for remainder of therapy. Limited experience with doses >40 ng/kg/minute. **Note:** Dose must be carefully and individually titrated (symptom improvement with minimal adverse effects). Avoid abrupt withdrawal.

Transitioning from epoprostenol (see table on previous page): I.V. Infusion: **Note:** Transition should occur in a hospital setting to follow response (eg, walking distance, sign/symptoms of disease progression). May take 24-48 hours to transition.

Elderly: Limited experience in patients >65 years; refer to adult dosing; use caution

Dosage adjustment in renal impairment: No specific dosage adjustment recommended; use with caution.

Dosage adjustment in hepatic impairment:

Mild to moderate: Initial: 0.625 ng/kg/minute; increase with caution.

Severe: No data available.

Stability Store at 15°C to 30°C (59°F to 86°F). Product does not need dilution prior to SubQ use. For I.V. infusion, dilute in SWFI or NS to a final volume of either 50 mL or 100 mL (dependent on system reservoir and calculated dose). Stability for up to 48 hours has been shown for concentrations as low as 4000 ng/mL. Contents of a single-reservoir syringe of treprostinil can be administered up to 72 hours at 37°C; diluted solutions can be used up to 48 hours at 37°C. Contents of a vial should not be used past 30 days after the initial needle access into the vial.

Administration

I.V. infusion: Solution must be diluted in SWFI or NS prior to use and administered by continuous infusion using a central indwelling catheter and infusion pump. A backup infusion pump and infusion set should be immediately available in order to avoid therapy interruption. I.V. use is recommended when SubQ infusion is not tolerated. Infusion site reactions may be helped by moving the infusion site every 3 days, local application of topical hot and cold packs, topical or oral analgesics. Injection site pain and erythema may improve after several months of therapy.

SubQ infusion: Administer via continuous SubQ infusion using an appropriately-designed infusion pump. Patients must be assessed regarding their ability to manage such a delivery system.

Monitoring Parameters Dyspnea, fatigue, activity tolerance, symptoms of excessive dose (eg, headache, nausea, vomiting)

Pregnancy Risk Factor B

Contraindications Hypersensitivity to treprostinil or any component of formulation

Warnings/Precautions Use caution in hepatic insufficiency, dose modification may be warranted; use caution in renal impairment; abrupt withdrawal/large dosage reductions may worsen symptoms of PAH. Safety and efficacy have not been established in patients ≤16 years of age.

Adverse Reactions

>10%:

Cardiovascular: Vasodilation (11%)

Central nervous system: Headache (27%)

Dermatologic: Rash (14%)

Gastrointestinal: Diarrhea (25%), nausea (22%)

Local: Infusion site pain (SubQ 85%, may improve after several months of therapy); infusion site reaction (SubQ 83%)

Miscellaneous: Jaw pain (13%)

1% to 10%:

Cardiovascular: Edema (9%), hypotension (4%)

Central nervous system: Dizziness (9%)

Dermatologic: Pruritus (8%)

Postmarketing and/or case reports: Arm swelling, hematoma, I.V. line infections, pain, paresthesia, sepsis

Overdosage/Toxicology Symptoms of overdose may include flushing, headache, hypotension, nausea, vomiting, diarrhea and seizure-like activity. Dosage reduction will likely coincide with symptom resolution. Treatment is symptom-directed and supportive.

Drug Interactions

Anticoagulants: Treprostinil inhibits platelet aggregation. Concomitant use with anticoagulants may increase the risk of bleeding.

Antiplatelet agents: Treprostinil inhibits platelet aggregation. Concomitant use with antiplatelet agents may increase the risk of bleeding.

NSAIDs: Treprostinil inhibits platelet aggregation. Concomitant use with NSAIDs may increase the risk of bleeding.

Salicylates: Treprostinil inhibits platelet aggregation. Concomitant use with salicylates may increase the risk of bleeding.

Dietary Considerations Sodium chloride content of solution for injection:

1 mg/mL, 2.5 mg/mL, and 5 mg/mL each contain sodium chloride 5.3 mg/mL

10 mg/mL contains sodium chloride 4 mg/mL

Dosage Forms Injection, solution: 1 mg/mL (20 mL) [contains sodium chloride 5.3 mg/mL]; 2.5 mg/mL (20 mL) [contains sodium chloride 5.3 mg/mL]; 5 mg/mL (20 mL) [contains sodium chloride 5.3 mg/mL]; 10 mg/mL (20 mL) [contains sodium chloride 4 mg/mL]

References

Badesch DB, Abman SH, Ahearn GS, et al, "Medical Therapy for Pulmonary Arterial Hypertension: ACCP Evidence-Based Clinical Practice Guidelines," *Chest*, 2004, 126(1 Suppl):35-62.

Gildea TR, Arroliga AC, and Minai OA, "Treatments and Strategies to Optimize the Comprehensive Management of Patients With Pulmonary Arterial Hypertension," *Cleve Clin J Med*, 2003, 70(Suppl 1):18-27.

Gomberg-Maitland M, Tapson VF, Benza RL, et al, "Transition from Intravenous Epoprostenol to Intravenous Treprostinil in Pulmonary Hypertension," *Am J Respir Crit Care Med*, 2005, 172(12):1586-9.

Humbert M, Sitbon O, and Simmoneau G, "Treatment of Pulmonary Arterial hypertension," *N Engl J Med*, 2004, 351(14):1425-36.

McLaughlin VV, Gaine SP, Barst RJ, et al, "Efficacy and Safety of Treprostinil: An Epoprostenol Analog for Primary Pulmonary Hypertension," *J Cardiovasc Pharmacol*, 2003, 41(2):293-9.

♦ **Treprostinil Sodium** *see* Treprostinil *on page 1309*

♦ **Trexall**™ *see* Methotrexate *on page 821*

♦ **Triaderm (Can)** *see* Triamcinolone *on page 1311*

Triamcinolone (trye am SIN oh lone)

Medication Safety Issues

Sound-alike/look-alike issues:

Kenalog® may be confused with Ketalar®

Nasacort® may be confused with NasalCrom®

TAC (occasional abbreviation for triamcinolone) is an error-prone abbreviation (mistaken as tetracaine-adrenaline-cocaine)

Related Information

Asthma *on page 1594*

Corticosteroids *on page 1561*

Stress Replacement of Corticosteroids *on page 1494*

U.S. Brand Names Aristocort®; Aristocort® A; Aristospan®; Azmacort®; Kenalog®; Kenalog-10®; Kenalog-40®; Nasacort® AQ; Triderm®; Tri-Nasal®

Canadian Brand Names Aristospan®; Kenalog®; Kenalog® in Orabase; Nasacort® AQ; Oracort; Triaderm; Trinasal®

Synonyms Triamcinolone Acetonide, Aerosol; Triamcinolone Acetonide, Parenteral; Triamcinolone Diacetate, Oral; Triamcinolone Diacetate, Parenteral; Triamcinolone Hexacetonide; Triamcinolone, Oral

Pharmacologic Category Corticosteroid, Adrenal; Corticosteroid, Inhalant (Oral); Corticosteroid, Nasal; Corticosteroid, Systemic; Corticosteroid, Topical

Generic Available Yes: Cream, lotion, ointment, paste

Use

Nasal inhalation: Management of seasonal and perennial allergic rhinitis in patients ≥6 years of age

Oral inhalation: Control of bronchial asthma and related bronchospastic conditions

Oral topical: Adjunctive treatment and temporary relief of symptoms associated with oral inflammatory lesions and ulcerative lesions resulting from trauma

Systemic: Adrenocortical insufficiency, rheumatic disorders, allergic states, respiratory diseases, systemic lupus erythematosus (SLE), and other diseases requiring anti-inflammatory or immunosuppressive effects

Topical: Inflammatory dermatoses responsive to steroids

Mechanism of Action Decreases inflammation by suppression of migration of polymorphonuclear leukocytes and reversal of increased capillary permeability; suppresses the immune system by reducing activity and volume of the lymphatic system; suppresses adrenal function at high doses

(Continued)

Triamcinolone *(Continued)*

Pharmacodynamics/Kinetics

Duration: Oral: 8-12 hours
Absorption: Topical: Systemic
Time to peak: I.M.: 8-10 hours
Half-life elimination: Biologic: 18-36 hours

Dosage The lowest possible dose should be used to control the condition; when dose reduction is possible, the dose should be reduced gradually. Parenteral dose is usually 1/3 to 1/2 the oral dose given every 12 hours. In life-threatening situations, parenteral doses larger than the oral dose may be needed.

Injection:

Acetonide:
- Intra-articular, intrabursal, tendon sheaths: Adults: Initial: Smaller joints: 2.5-5 mg, larger joints: 5-15 mg
- Intradermal: Adults: Initial: 1 mg
- I.M.: Range: 2.5-60 mg/day
  - Children 6-12 years: Initial: 40 mg
  - Children >12 years and Adults: Initial: 60 mg

Hexacetonide: Adults:
- Intralesional, sublesional: Up to 0.5 mg/square inch of affected skin
- Intra-articular: Range: 2-20 mg

Triamcinolone Dosing

	Acetonide	Hexacetonide
Intrasynovial	5-40 mg	
Intralesional	1-30 mg (usually 1 mg per injection site); 10 mg/mL suspension usually used	Up to 0.5 mg/sq inch affected area
Sublesional	1-30 mg	
Systemic I.M.	2.5-60 mg/dose (usual adult dose: 60 mg; may repeat with 20-100 mg dose when symptoms recur)	
Intra-articular	2.5-40 mg	2-20 mg average
large joints	5-15 mg	10-20 mg
small joints	2.5-5 mg	2-6 mg
Tendon sheaths	2.5-10 mg	
Intradermal	1 mg/site	

Intranasal: Perennial allergic rhinitis, seasonal allergic rhinitis:

Nasal spray:
- Children 6-11 years: 110 mcg/day as 1 spray in each nostril once daily.
- Children ≥12 years and Adults: 220 mcg/day as 2 sprays in each nostril once daily

Nasal inhaler:
- Children 6-11 years: Initial: 220 mcg/day as 2 sprays in each nostril once daily
- Children ≥12 years and Adults: Initial: 220 mcg/day as 2 sprays in each nostril once daily; may increase dose to 440 mcg/day (given once daily or divided and given 2 or 4 times/day)

Oral: Adults:
- Acute rheumatic carditis: Initial: 20-60 mg/day; reduce dose during maintenance therapy
- Acute seasonal or perennial allergic rhinitis: 8-12 mg/day
- Adrenocortical insufficiency: Range 4-12 mg/day
- Bronchial asthma: 8-16 mg/day
- Dermatological disorders, contact/atopic dermatitis: Initial: 8-16 mg/day

Ophthalmic disorders: 12-40 mg/day

Rheumatic disorders: Range: 8-16 mg/day

SLE: Initial: 20-32 mg/day, some patients may need initial doses ≥48 mg; reduce dose during maintenance therapy

Oral inhalation: Asthma:

Children 6-12 years: 100-200 mcg 3-4 times/day **or** 200-400 mcg twice daily; maximum dose: 1200 mcg/day

Children >12 years and Adults: 200 mcg 3-4 times/day **or** 400 mcg twice daily; maximum dose: 1600 mcg/day

Oral topical: Oral inflammatory lesions/ulcers: Press a small dab (about 1/4 inch) to the lesion until a thin film develops. A larger quantity may be required for coverage of some lesions. For optimal results use only enough to coat the lesion with a thin film; do not rub in.

Topical:

Cream, Ointment: Apply thin film to affected areas 2-4 times/day

Spray: Apply to affected area 3-4 times/day

Stability Store at room temperature; avoid freezing

Injection, suspension: Shake well prior to use

Hexacetonide suspension: Avoid diluents containing parabens or preservatives (may cause flocculation). Diluted suspension stable ~1 week. Suspension for intralesional use, may be diluted with D_5NS, $D_{10}NS$ or SWFI to a 1:1, 1:2, or 1:4 concentration. Solutions for intra-articular use, may be diluted with lidocaine 1% or 2%.

Topical spray: Avoid excessive heat

Administration

Injection: Avoid injecting into a previously infected joint; do not inject into unstable joints

I.M.: Inject deep in large muscle mass, avoid deltoid.

SubQ: Avoid subcutaneous administration.

Nasal spray, inhalation: Shake well prior to use. Gently blow nose to clear nostrils.

Oral inhalation: Shake well prior to use. Rinse mouth and throat after using inhaler to prevent candidiasis. Use spacer device provided with Azmacort®.

Oral topical: Apply small dab to lesion until a thin film develops; do not rub in. Apply at bedtime or after meals if applications are needed throughout the day.

Tablet: Once-daily doses should be given in the morning.

Topical: Apply a thin film sparingly and avoid topical application on the face. Do not use on open skin or wounds. Do not occlude area unless directed.

Anesthesia and Critical Care Concerns/Other Considerations Triamcinolone is a long-acting corticosteroid with minimal sodium-retaining potential.

Neuromuscular Effects: ICU-acquired paresis was recently studied in 5 ICUs (3 medical and 2 surgical ICUs) at 4 French hospitals. All ICU patients without pre-existing neuromuscular disease admitted from March 1999 through June 2000 were evaluated (De Jonghe B, 2002). Each patient had to be mechanically ventilated for ≥7 days and was screened daily for awakening. The first day the patient was considered awake was Study Day 1. Patients with severe muscle weakness on Study Day 7 were considered to have ICU-acquired paresis. Among the 95 patients who were evaluable, about 25% developed ICU-acquired paresis. Independent predictors included female gender, the number of days with ≥2 organ dysfunction, and administration of corticosteroids. Further studies may be required to verify and characterize the association between the development of ICU-acquired paresis and use of corticosteroids. Concurrent use of a corticosteroid and muscle relaxant appear to increase the risk of certain ICU myopathies; avoid or administer the corticosteroid at the lowest dose possible.

Adrenal Insufficiency: Patients will often have steroid-induced adverse effects on glucose tolerance and lipid profiles. When discontinuing steroid therapy in patients on long-term steroid supplementation, it is important that the steroid therapy be discontinued gradually. Abrupt withdrawal may result in adrenal insufficiency with hypotension and hyperkalemia. Patients on long-term steroid supplementation will require higher corticosteroid doses when subject to stress (ie, trauma, surgery, severe infection). Guidelines for glucocorticoid replacement during various surgical procedures have been published (Salem M, 1994, Coursin DB, 2002).

Septic Shock: A recent randomized, double-blind, placebo controlled trial assessed whether low dose corticosteroid administration could improve 28-day

(Continued)

Triamcinolone *(Continued)*

survival in patients with septic shock and relative adrenal insufficiency. Relative adrenal insufficiency was defined as an inappropriate response to corticotropin administration (increase of serum cortisol of ≤9 mcg/dL from baseline). Cortisol levels were drawn immediately before corticotropin administration and 30 to 60 minutes afterwards. Three hundred adult septic shock patients requiring mechanical ventilation and vasopressor support were randomized to either hydrocortisone (50 mg IVP every 6 hours) and fludrocortisone (50 mcg tablet daily via nasogastric tube) or matching placebos for 7 days. In patients who did not appropriately respond to corticotropin (nonresponders), there were significantly fewer deaths in the active treatment group. Vasopressor therapy was withdrawn more frequently in this subset of the active treatment group. Adverse events were similar in both groups. Patients who lack adrenal reserve and thus have relative adrenal insufficiency during the stress of septic shock may benefit from physiologic steroid replacement. However, there was a trend for increased mortality in patients who responded to the corticotropin test (increase serum cortisol >9 mcg/dL from baseline). These patients may not benefit from physiologic steroid replacement. Further study is required to better characterize the patient populations who may benefit.

Pregnancy Risk Factor C

Contraindications Hypersensitivity to triamcinolone or any component of the formulation; systemic fungal infections; serious infections (except septic shock or tuberculous meningitis); primary treatment of status asthmaticus; fungal, viral, or bacterial infections of the mouth or throat (oral topical formulation)

Warnings/Precautions May cause suppression of hypothalamic-pituitary-adrenal (HPA) axis, particularly in younger children or in patients receiving high doses for prolonged periods. Particular care is required when patients are transferred from systemic corticosteroids to inhaled products due to possible adrenal insufficiency or withdrawal from steroids, including an increase in allergic symptoms. Patients receiving 20 mg per day of prednisone (or equivalent) may be most susceptible. Fatalities have occurred due to adrenal insufficiency in asthmatic patients during and after transfer from systemic corticosteroids to aerosol steroids; aerosol steroids do **not** provide the systemic steroid needed to treat patients having trauma, surgery, or infections. Withdrawal and discontinuation of the corticosteroid should be done slowly and carefully

Use with caution in patients with hypothyroidism, cirrhosis, nonspecific ulcerative colitis and patients at increased risk for peptic ulcer disease. Corticosteroids should be used with caution in patients with diabetes, hypertension, osteoporosis, glaucoma, cataracts, or tuberculosis. Use caution in hepatic impairment. Do not use occlusive dressings on weeping or exudative lesions and general caution with occlusive dressings should be observed; discontinue if skin irritation or contact dermatitis should occur; do not use in patients with decreased skin circulation; avoid the use of high potency steroids on the face.

Because of the risk of adverse effects, systemic corticosteroids should be used cautiously in the elderly, in the smallest possible dose, and for the shortest possible time. Azmacort® (metered dose inhaler) comes with its own spacer device attached and may be easier to use in older patients.

Controlled clinical studies have shown that orally-inhaled and intranasal corticosteroids may cause a reduction in growth velocity in pediatric patients. (In studies of orally-inhaled corticosteroids, the mean reduction in growth velocity was approximately 1 centimeter per year [range 0.3-1.8 cm per year] and appears to be related to dose and duration of exposure.) The growth of pediatric patients receiving inhaled corticosteroids, should be monitored routinely (eg, via stadiometry). To minimize the systemic effects of orally-inhaled and intranasal corticosteroids, each patient should be titrated to the lowest effective dose.

May suppress the immune system, patients may be more susceptible to infection. Use with caution in patients with systemic infections or ocular herpes simplex. Avoid exposure to chickenpox and measles. Injection suspension contains benzyl alcohol; benzyl alcohol has been associated with the "gasping syndrome" in neonates and low-birth-weight infants.

Oral topical: Discontinue if local irritation or sensitization should develop. If significant regeneration or repair of oral tissues has not occurred in seven days, re-evaluation of the etiology of the oral lesion is advised.

Adverse Reactions

Systemic: Frequency not defined:

Cardiovascular: Angioedema, bradycardia, CHF, hypertension, myocardial rupture (following recent MI), thrombophlebitis, vasculitis

Central nervous system: Convulsions, depression, emotional instability, fever, headache, intracranial pressure increased, neuropathy, paresthesia, personality changes, vertigo

Dermatologic: Acne, allergic dermatitis, bruising, cutaneous atrophy, dry/scaly skin, ecchymoses, facial erythema, petechiae, photosensitivity, rash, striae, thin/fragile skin, wound healing impaired

Endocrine & metabolic: Adrenocortical/pituitary unresponsiveness (particularly during stress), carbohydrate tolerance decreased, cushingoid state, diabetes mellitus (manifestations of latent disease), fluid retention, growth suppression (children), hirsutism, hypokalemic alkalosis, menstrual irregularities, negative nitrogen balance, potassium loss, sodium retention

Gastrointestinal: Abdominal distention, bowel perforation, diarrhea, dyspepsia, nausea, oral *Monilia* (oral inhaler), pancreatitis, peptic ulcer, ulcerative esophagitis, weight gain

Hepatic: Hepatomegaly

Local: Skin atrophy (at the injection site)

Neuromuscular & skeletal: Calcinosis (following intra-articular or intralesional injection), Charcot-like arthropathy, femoral/humeral head aseptic necrosis, muscle mass decreased, muscle weakness, osteoporosis, pathologic fracture of long bones, steroid myopathy, tendon rupture, vertebral compression fractures

Ocular: Blindness (periocular injections), cataracts, intraocular pressure increased, exophthalmos, glaucoma, subcapsular cataract

Respiratory: Cough increased (nasal spray), epistaxis (nasal inhaler/spray), pharyngitis (nasal spray/oral inhaler), sinusitis (oral inhaler), voice alteration (oral inhaler)

Miscellaneous: Abnormal fat deposition (moon face), anaphylactoid reaction, anaphylaxis, diaphoresis increased, suppression to skin tests

Topical: Frequency not defined:

Dermatologic: Itching, allergic contact dermatitis, dryness, folliculitis, skin infection (secondary), itching, hypertrichosis, acneiform eruptions, hypopigmentation, skin maceration, skin atrophy, striae, miliaria, perioral dermatitis, atrophy of oral mucosa

Local: Burning, irritation

Overdosage/Toxicology When consumed in high doses for prolonged periods, systemic hypercorticism and adrenal suppression may occur. In those cases, discontinuation of the corticosteroid should be done judiciously.

Drug Interactions

Decreased effect: Barbiturates, phenytoin, rifampin increase metabolism of triamcinolone; vaccine and toxoid effects may be reduced

Increased effect: Salmeterol: The addition of salmeterol has been demonstrated to improve response to inhaled corticosteroids (as compared to increasing steroid dosage).

Increased toxicity: Salicylates may increase risk of GI ulceration

Ethanol/Nutrition/Herb Interactions

Ethanol: Avoid ethanol (may enhance gastric mucosal irritation).

Food: Triamcinolone interferes with calcium absorption.

Herb/Nutraceutical: Avoid cat's claw, echinacea (have immunostimulant properties).

Dietary Considerations May be taken with food to decrease GI distress.

Dosage Forms

Aerosol for oral inhalation, as acetonide (Azmacort®): 100 mcg per actuation (20 g) [240 actuations]

Aerosol, topical, as acetonide (Kenalog®): 0.2 mg/2-second spray (63 g)

Cream, as acetonide: 0.025% (15 g, 80 g, 454 g); 0.1% (15 g, 80 g, 454 g, 2270 g); 0.5% (15 g)

Aristocort® A: 0.025% (15 g, 60 g); 0.1% (15 g, 60 g); 0.5% (15 g) [contains benzyl alcohol]

Triderm®: 0.1% (30 g, 85 g)

Injection, suspension, as acetonide:

Kenalog-10®: 10 mg/mL (5 mL) [contains benzyl alcohol; not for I.V. or I.M. use]

(Continued)

Triamcinolone *(Continued)*

Kenalog-40®: 40 mg/mL (1 mL, 5 mL, 10 mL) [contains benzyl alcohol; not for I.V. or intradermal use]

Injection, suspension, as hexacetonide (Aristospan®): 5 mg/mL (5 mL); 20 mg/mL (1 mL, 5 mL) [contains benzyl alcohol; not for I.V. use]

Lotion, as acetonide: 0.025% (60 mL); 0.1% (60 mL)

Ointment, topical, as acetonide: 0.025% (15 g, 80 g, 454 g); 0.1% (15 g, 80 g, 454 g); 0.5% (15 g)

Aristocort® A: 0.1% (15 g, 60 g)

Paste, oral, topical, as acetonide: 0.1% (5 g)

Solution, intranasal, as acetonide [spray] (Tri-Nasal®): 50 mcg/inhalation (15 mL) [120 doses]

Suspension, intranasal, as acetonide [spray] (Nasacort® AQ): 55 mcg/inhalation (16.5 g) [120 doses]

Tablet (Aristocort®): 4 mg [contains lactose and sodium benzoate]

References

Abraham E and Evans T, "Corticosteroids and Septic Shock (editorial)," *JAMA*, 2002, 288(7):886-7.

American Academy of Pediatrics Committee on Drugs: "Transfer of Drugs and Other Chemicals into Human Milk," *Pediatrics*, 2001, 108(3):776-89.

Annane D, Sebille V, Charpentier C, et al, "Effect of Treatment With Low Doses of Hydrocortisone and Fludrocortisone on Mortality in Patients With Septic Shock," *JAMA*, 2002, 288(7):862-71.

Cooper MS and Stewart PM, "Corticosteroid Insufficiency in Acutely Ill Patients," *N Engl J Med*, 2003, 348(8):727-34.

Coursin DB and Wood KE, "Corticosteroid Supplementation for Adrenal Insufficiency," *JAMA*, 2002, 287(2):236-40.

De Jonghe B, Sharshar T, Lefaucheur JP, et al, "Paresis Acquired in the Intensive Care Unit. A Prospective Multicenter Study," *JAMA*, 2002, 288(22):2859-67.

Hotchkiss RS and Karl IE, "The Pathophysiology and Treatment of Sepsis," *N Engl J Med*, 2003, 348(2):138-50.

Salem M, Tainsh RE, Jr, Bromberg J, et al, "Perioperative Glucocorticoid Coverage: A Reassessment 42 Years After Emergence of a Problem," *Ann Surg*, 1994, 219(4):416-25.

♦ **Triamcinolone Acetonide, Aerosol** *see* Triamcinolone *on page 1311*
♦ **Triamcinolone Acetonide, Parenteral** *see* Triamcinolone *on page 1311*
♦ **Triamcinolone Diacetate, Oral** *see* Triamcinolone *on page 1311*
♦ **Triamcinolone Diacetate, Parenteral** *see* Triamcinolone *on page 1311*
♦ **Triamcinolone Hexacetonide** *see* Triamcinolone *on page 1311*
♦ **Triamcinolone, Oral** *see* Triamcinolone *on page 1311*
♦ **Triaminic® Thin Strips™ Cough and Runny Nose [OTC]** *see* DiphenhydrAMINE *on page 399*
♦ **Triatec-8 (Can)** *see* Acetaminophen and Codeine *on page 29*
♦ **Triatec-8 Strong (Can)** *see* Acetaminophen and Codeine *on page 29*
♦ **Triatec-30 (Can)** *see* Acetaminophen and Codeine *on page 29*

Triazolam (trye AY zoe lam)

Medication Safety Issues

Sound-alike/look-alike issues:

Triazolam may be confused with alprazolam

Halcion® may be confused with halcinonide, Haldol®

Related Information

Benzodiazepines *on page 1555*

U.S. Brand Names Halcion®

Canadian Brand Names Apo-Triazo®; Gen-Triazolam; Halcion®

Pharmacologic Category Hypnotic, Benzodiazepine

Restrictions C-IV

Generic Available Yes

Use Short-term treatment of insomnia

Mechanism of Action Binds to stereospecific benzodiazepine receptors on the postsynaptic GABA neuron at several sites within the central nervous system, including the limbic system, reticular formation. Enhancement of the inhibitory effect of GABA on neuronal excitability results by increased neuronal membrane permeability to chloride ions. This shift in chloride ions results in hyperpolarization (a less excitable state) and stabilization.

Pharmacodynamics/Kinetics

Onset of action: Hypnotic: 15-30 minutes

Duration: 6-7 hours

Distribution: V_d: 0.8-1.8 L/kg

Protein binding: 89%
Metabolism: Extensively hepatic
Half-life elimination: 1.7-5 hours
Excretion: Urine as unchanged drug and metabolites

Dosage Oral (onset of action is rapid, patient should be in bed when taking medication):
Children <18 years: Dosage not established
Adults:
Hypnotic: 0.125-0.25 mg at bedtime (maximum dose: 0.5 mg/day)
Preprocedure sedation (dental): 0.25 mg taken the evening before oral surgery; or 0.25 mg 1 hour before procedure
Elderly: Insomnia (short-term use): 0.0625-0.125 mg at bedtime; maximum dose: 0.25 mg/day (see Geriatric Considerations)
Dosing adjustment/comments in hepatic impairment: Reduce dose or avoid use in cirrhosis

Administration May take with food. Tablet may be crushed or swallowed whole. Onset of action is rapid, patient should be in bed when taking medication.

Monitoring Parameters Respiratory and cardiovascular status

Anesthesia and Critical Care Concerns/Other Considerations Chronic use of this agent may increase the perioperative benzodiazepine dose needed to achieve desired effect. Abrupt discontinuation after sustained use (generally >10 days) may cause withdrawal symptoms.

Pregnancy Risk Factor X

Contraindications Hypersensitivity to triazolam or any component of the formulation (cross-sensitivity with other benzodiazepines may exist); concurrent therapy with atazanavir, ketoconazole, itraconazole, nefazodone, and ritonavir; pregnancy

Warnings/Precautions Should be used only after evaluation of potential causes of sleep disturbance. Failure of sleep disturbance to resolve after 7-10 days may indicate psychiatric or medical illness. A worsening of insomnia or the emergence of new abnormalities of thought or behavior may represent unrecognized psychiatric or medical illness and requires immediate and careful evaluation. Prescription should be written for a maximum of 7-10 days and should not be prescribed in quantities exceeding a 1-month supply. Abrupt discontinuation after sustained use (generally >10 days) may cause withdrawal symptoms.

An increase in daytime anxiety may occur after as few as 10 days of continuous use, which may be related to withdrawal reaction in some patients. Anterograde amnesia may occur at a higher rate with triazolam than with other benzodiazepines. Use with caution in elderly or debilitated patients, patients with hepatic disease (including alcoholics), or renal impairment. Use with caution in patients with respiratory disease or impaired gag reflex. Avoid use in patients with sleep apnea.

Causes CNS depression (dose-related) resulting in sedation, dizziness, confusion, or ataxia which may impair physical and mental capabilities. Patients must be cautioned about performing tasks which require mental alertness (eg, operating machinery or driving). Use with caution in patients receiving other CNS depressants or psychoactive agents. Effects with other sedative drugs or ethanol may be potentiated. Benzodiazepines have been associated with falls and traumatic injury and should be used with extreme caution in patients who are at risk of these events (especially the elderly).

Use caution with potent CYP3A4 inhibitors, as they may significantly decreased the clearance of triazolam. Use caution in patients with depression, particularly if suicidal risk may be present. Use with caution in patients with a history of drug dependence. Benzodiazepines have been associated with dependence and acute withdrawal symptoms on discontinuation or reduction in dose. Acute withdrawal, including seizures, may be precipitated after administration of flumazenil to patients receiving long-term benzodiazepine therapy.

Paradoxical reactions, including hyperactive or aggressive behavior have been reported with benzodiazepines, particularly in adolescent/pediatric or psychiatric patients. Does not have analgesic, antidepressant, or antipsychotic properties.

Adverse Reactions
>10%: Central nervous system: Drowsiness, anteriograde amnesia
1% to 10%:
Central nervous system: Headache, dizziness, nervousness, lightheadedness, ataxia

(Continued)

Triazolam *(Continued)*

Gastrointestinal: Nausea, vomiting

<1% (Limited to important or life-threatening): Confusion, depression, euphoria, memory impairment

Overdosage/Toxicology Symptoms of overdose include somnolence, confusion, coma, diminished reflexes, dyspnea, and hypotension. Treatment for benzodiazepine overdose is supportive. Flumazenil has been shown to selectively block the binding of benzodiazepines to CNS receptors, resulting in reversal of benzodiazepine-induced CNS depression but not always respiratory depression.

Drug Interactions **Substrate** of CYP3A4 (major); **Inhibits** CYP2C8 (weak), 2C9 (weak)

CNS depressants: Sedative effects and/or respiratory depression may be additive with CNS depressants; includes ethanol, barbiturates, narcotic analgesics, and other sedative agents; monitor for increased effect

CYP3A4 inducers: CYP3A4 inducers may decrease the levels/effects of triazolam. Example inducers include aminoglutethimide, carbamazepine, nafcillin, nevirapine, phenobarbital, phenytoin, and rifamycins.

CYP3A4 inhibitors: May increase the levels/effects of triazolam. Example inhibitors include azole antifungals, clarithromycin, diclofenac, doxycycline, erythromycin, imatinib, isoniazid, nefazodone, nicardipine, propofol, protease inhibitors, quinidine, telithromycin, and verapamil.

Isoniazid: Isoniazid may increase triazolam levels.

Levodopa: Therapeutic effects may be diminished in some patients following the addition of a benzodiazepine; limited/inconsistent data

Oral contraceptives: May decrease the clearance and increase the half-life of triazolam; monitor for increased triazolam effect

Ranitidine: Ranitidine may increase triazolam levels.

Theophylline: May partially antagonize some of the effects of benzodiazepines; monitor for decreased response; may require higher doses for sedation

Ethanol/Nutrition/Herb Interactions

Ethanol: Avoid ethanol (may increase CNS depression).

Food: Food may decrease the rate of absorption. Triazolam serum concentration may be increased by grapefruit juice; avoid concurrent use.

Herb/Nutraceutical: St John's wort may decrease levels. Avoid valerian, St John's wort, kava kava, gotu kola (may increase CNS depression).

Dosage Forms Tablet: 0.125 mg, 0.25 mg [contains sodium benzoate]

- **Tribavirin** *see* Ribavirin *on page 1116*
- **Trichloroacetaldehyde Monohydrate** *see* Chloral Hydrate *on page 261*
- **Tricosal** *see* Choline Magnesium Trisalicylate *on page 276*
- **Triderm®** *see* Triamcinolone *on page 1311*
- **Trikacide (Can)** *see* Metronidazole *on page 842*
- **Trilisate® [DSC]** *see* Choline Magnesium Trisalicylate *on page 276*
- **Trimazide [DSC]** *see* Trimethobenzamide *on page 1318*

Trimethobenzamide (trye meth oh BEN za mide)

Medication Safety Issues

Sound-alike/look-alike issues:

Tigan® may be confused with Tiazac®, Ticar®

Related Information

Postoperative Nausea and Vomiting *on page 1477*

U.S. Brand Names Tebamide™; Tigan®; Trimazide [DSC]

Canadian Brand Names Tigan®

Synonyms Trimethobenzamide Hydrochloride

Pharmacologic Category Anticholinergic Agent; Antiemetic

Generic Available Yes

Use Treatment of nausea and vomiting

Mechanism of Action Acts centrally to inhibit the medullary chemoreceptor trigger zone

Pharmacodynamics/Kinetics

Onset of action: Antiemetic: Oral: 10-40 minutes; I.M.: 15-35 minutes

Duration: 3-4 hours

Absorption: Rectal: ~60%

Bioavailability: Oral: 60% to 100%

Half-life elimination: 7-9 hours
Time to peak: Oral: 45 minutes; I.M.: 30 minutes
Excretion: Urine (30% to 50%)

Dosage Rectal use is contraindicated in neonates and premature infants

Children:
- <14 kg: Rectal: 100 mg 3-4 times/day
- 14-40 kg: Rectal: 100-200 mg 3-4 times/day
- >40 kg:
  - Oral: 300 mg 3-4 times/day
  - Rectal: 200 mg 3-4 times/day

Adults:
- Oral: 300 mg 3-4 times/day
- I.M., rectal: 200 mg 3-4 times/day
  - Postoperative nausea and vomiting (PONV): I.M.: 200 mg, followed 1 hour later by a second 200 mg dose

Stability Store capsules, injection solution, and suppositories at room temperature.

Administration Administer I.M. only; not for I.V. administration. Inject deep into upper outer quadrant of gluteal muscle.

Pregnancy Risk Factor C

Contraindications Hypersensitivity to trimethobenzamide, benzocaine (or similar local anesthetics), or any component of the formulation; injection contraindicated in children; suppositories contraindicated in premature infants or neonates

Warnings/Precautions May mask emesis due to Reye's syndrome or mimic CNS effects of Reye's syndrome in patients with emesis of other etiologies; use in patients with acute vomiting should be avoided. May cause drowsiness; patient should avoid tasks requiring alertness (eg, driving, operating machinery). May cause extrapyramidal symptoms (EPS) which may be confused with CNS symptoms of primary disease responsible for emesis. Risk of adverse effects (eg, EPS, seizure) may be increased in patients with acute febrile illness, dehydration, or electrolyte imbalance; use caution.

Adverse Reactions Frequency not defined.

Cardiovascular: Hypotension
Central nervous system: Coma, depression, disorientation, dizziness, drowsiness, EPS, headache, opisthotonos, Parkinson-like syndrome, seizure
Gastrointestinal: Diarrhea
Hematologic: Blood dyscrasias
Hepatic: Jaundice
Neuromuscular & skeletal: Muscle cramps
Ocular: Blurred vision
Miscellaneous: Hypersensitivity reactions

Overdosage/Toxicology Symptoms of overdose include hypotension, seizures, CNS depression, cardiac arrhythmias, disorientation, and confusion. Treatment is symptom-directed and supportive.

Ethanol/Nutrition/Herb Interactions Ethanol: Concomitant use should be avoided (sedative effects may be additive).

Dosage Forms

Capsule, as hydrochloride (Tigan®): 300 mg
Injection, solution, as hydrochloride: 100 mg/mL (2 mL)
  Tigan®: 100 mg/mL (2 mL [preservative free], 20 mL)
Suppository, rectal, as hydrochloride: 100 mg, 200 mg
  Tebamide™: 100 mg, 200 mg [contains benzocaine]
  Tigan®, Trimazide [DSC]: 200 mg [contains benzocaine]

- ♦ **Trimethobenzamide Hydrochloride** *see* Trimethobenzamide *on page 1318*
- ♦ **Trimethoprim and Sulfamethoxazole** *see* Sulfamethoxazole and Trimethoprim *on page 1215*
- ♦ **Tri-Nasal®** *see* Triamcinolone *on page 1311*
- ♦ **Trinipatch® 0.2 (Can)** *see* Nitroglycerin *on page 928*
- ♦ **Trinipatch® 0.4 (Can)** *see* Nitroglycerin *on page 928*
- ♦ **Trinipatch® 0.6 (Can)** *see* Nitroglycerin *on page 928*
- ♦ **Triostat®** *see* Liothyronine *on page 765*
- ♦ **Trombovar® (Can)** *see* Sodium Tetradecyl *on page 1194*
- ♦ **Tronolane® Suppository [OTC]** *see* Phenylephrine *on page 1015*
- ♦ **Tropicacyl®** *see* Tropicamide *on page 1320*

Tropicamide (troe PIK a mide)

Related Information

Cycloplegic Mydriatics *on page 1564*

U.S. Brand Names Mydral™; Mydriacyl®; Tropicacyl®

Canadian Brand Names Diotrope®; Mydriacyl®

Synonyms Bistropamide

Pharmacologic Category Ophthalmic Agent, Mydriatic

Generic Available Yes

Use Short-acting mydriatic used in diagnostic procedures; as well as preoperatively and postoperatively; treatment of some cases of acute iritis, iridocyclitis, and keratitis

Mechanism of Action Prevents the sphincter muscle of the iris and the muscle of the ciliary body from responding to cholinergic stimulation

Pharmacodynamics/Kinetics

Onset of action: Mydriasis: ~20-40 minutes; Cycloplegia: ~30 minutes

Duration: Mydriasis: ~6-7 hours; Cycloplegia: <6 hours

Dosage Ophthalmic: Children and Adults (individuals with heavily pigmented eyes may require larger doses):

Cycloplegia: Instill 1-2 drops (1%); may repeat in 5 minutes

Exam must be performed within 30 minutes after the repeat dose; if the patient is not examined within 20-30 minutes, instill an additional drop

Mydriasis: Instill 1-2 drops (0.5%) 15-20 minutes before exam; may repeat every 30 minutes as needed

Stability Store in tightly closed containers

Monitoring Parameters Ophthalmic exam

Pregnancy Risk Factor C

Contraindications Hypersensitivity to tropicamide or any component of the formulation; glaucoma

Warnings/Precautions Use with caution in infants and children since tropicamide may cause potentially dangerous CNS disturbances; tropicamide may cause an increase in intraocular pressure

Adverse Reactions Frequency not defined.

Cardiovascular: Edema, tachycardia, vascular congestion

Central nervous system: Headache, parasympathetic stimulations, somnolence

Dermatologic: Eczematoid dermatitis

Gastrointestinal: Dryness of the mouth

Local: Transient stinging

Ocular: Blurred vision, follicular conjunctivitis, increased intraocular pressure, photophobia with or without corneal staining

Overdosage/Toxicology

Symptoms of overdose include blurred vision, urinary retention, tachycardia, cardiorespiratory collapse

Antidote is physostigmine, pilocarpine; anticholinergic toxicity is caused by strong binding of the drug to cholinergic receptors. For anticholinergic overdose with severe life-threatening symptoms, physostigmine 1-2 mg (0.5 mg or 0.02 mg/kg for children) SubQ or I.V., slowly may be given to reverse systemic effects.

Dosage Forms

Solution, ophthalmic: 0.5% (15 mL); 1% (2 mL, 15 mL) [contains benzalkonium chloride]

Mydriacyl®: 1% (3 mL, 15 mL) [contains benzalkonium chloride]

Mydral™, Tropicacyl®: 0.5% (15 mL); 1% (15 mL) [contains benzalkonium chloride]

Trovafloxacin (TROE va floks a sin)

Medication Safety Issues

Sound-alike/look-alike issues:

Trovan® may be confused with Tenormin®

U.S. Brand Names Trovan® [DSC]

Synonyms Alatrofloxacin Mesylate; CP-99,219-27

Pharmacologic Category Antibiotic, Quinolone

Generic Available No

Use Should be used only in life- or limb-threatening infections

Treatment of nosocomial pneumonia, community-acquired pneumonia, complicated intra-abdominal infections, gynecologic/pelvic infections, complicated skin and skin structure infections

Mechanism of Action Inhibits DNA-gyrase in susceptible organisms; inhibits relaxation of supercoiled DNA and promotes breakage of double-stranded DNA

Pharmacodynamics/Kinetics

Distribution: Concentration in most tissues greater than plasma or serum

Protein binding: 76%

Metabolism: Hepatic conjugation; glucuronidation 13%, acetylation 9%

Bioavailability: 88%

Half-life elimination: 9-12 hours

Time to peak, serum: Oral: Within 2 hours

Excretion: Feces (43% as unchanged drug); urine (6% as unchanged drug)

Dosage Adults:

Nosocomial pneumonia: I.V.: 300 mg single dose followed by 200 mg/day orally for a total duration of 10-14 days

Community-acquired pneumonia: Oral, I.V.: 200 mg/day for 7-14 days

Complicated intra-abdominal infections, including postsurgical infections/gynecologic and pelvic infections: I.V.: 300 mg as a single dose followed by 200 mg/day orally for a total duration of 7-14 days

Skin and skin structure infections, complicated, including diabetic foot infections: Oral, I.V.: 200 mg/day for 10-14 days

Dosage adjustment in renal impairment: No adjustment is necessary

Dosage adjustment for hemodialysis: None required; trovafloxacin not sufficiently removed by hemodialysis

Dosage adjustment in hepatic impairment:

Mild to moderate cirrhosis:

Initial dose for normal hepatic function: 300 mg I.V.; 200 mg I.V. or oral; 100 mg oral

Reduced dose: 200 mg I.V.; 100 mg I.V. or oral; 100 mg oral

Severe cirrhosis: No data available

Stability Store undiluted vials of solution at 15°C to 30°C (50°F to 86°F). Diluted solutions are stable for up to 7 days when refrigerated and up to 3 days at room temperature. Trovan® I.V. should not be diluted with 0.9% sodium chloride injection, USP (normal saline), alone or in combination with other diluents. A precipitate may form under these conditions. In addition, Trovan® I.V. should not be diluted with lactated Ringer's, USP.

Dilute to a concentration of 0.5-2 mg/mL in dextrose 5% in water, 0.45% sodium chloride, dextrose 5% in water and 0.45% sodium chloride, dextrose 5% in water and 0.2% sodium chloride, or lactated Ringer's in dextrose 5% in water.

Administration

Oral: Administer without regard to meals.

I.V.: Not for I.M. or SubQ; administer IVPB over 60 minutes

Monitoring Parameters Periodic assessment of liver function tests should be considered

Anesthesia and Critical Care Concerns/Other Considerations Trovafloxacin should only be used in severe life or limb threatening infections. If treatment is >14 days, monitor LFTs. *In vitro* trovafloxacin was more active than sparfloxacin, ofloxacin, ciprofloxacin, ceftriaxone, erythromycin, and vancomycin against *S. pneumoniae*. It was also more active against penicillin-resistant strains than ceftriaxone, erythromycin, or vancomycin. It has good activity against resistant organisms, and penetration of the cerebral spinal fluid giving potential in the treatment of central nervous system infections.

Pregnancy Risk Factor C

Contraindications History of hypersensitivity to trovafloxacin, alatrofloxacin, quinolone antimicrobial agents, or any component of the formulation

Warnings/Precautions For use only in serious life- or limb-threatening infections. Initiation of therapy must occur in an inpatient healthcare facility. May alter GI flora resulting in pseudomembranous colitis due to *Clostridium difficile*; use with caution in patients with seizure disorders or severe cerebral atherosclerosis; photosensitivity; CNS stimulation may occur which may lead to tremor, restlessness, confusion, hallucinations, paranoia, depression, nightmares, insomnia, or lightheadedness. Hepatic reactions have resulted in death. Risk of hepatotoxicity is increased if therapy exceeds 14 days. Tendon inflammation and/or rupture have been reported with other quinolone antibiotics. Risk may be increased with

(Continued)

Trovafloxacin *(Continued)*

concurrent corticosteroids, particularly in the elderly. Discontinue at first sign of tendon inflammation or pain.

Severe hypersensitivity reactions, including anaphylaxis, have occurred with quinolone therapy. If an allergic reaction occurs (itching, urticaria, dyspnea, facial edema, loss of consciousness, tingling, cardiovascular collapse), discontinue drug immediately. Prolonged use may result in superinfection; pseudomembranous colitis may occur and should be considered in all patients who present with diarrhea. Quinolones may exacerbate myasthenia gravis, use with caution (rare, potentially life-threatening weakness of respiratory muscles may occur).

Adverse Reactions Note: Fatalities have occurred in patients developing hepatic necrosis.

1% to 10% (range reported in clinical trials):
- Central nervous system: Dizziness (2% to 11%), lightheadedness (<1% to 4%), headache (1% to 5%)
- Dermatologic: Rash (<1% to 2%), pruritus (<1% to 2%)
- Gastrointestinal: Nausea (4% to 8%), abdominal pain (<1% to 1%), vomiting, diarrhea
- Genitourinary: Vaginitis (<1% to 1%)
- Hepatic: Increased LFTs
- Local: Injection site reaction, pain, or inflammation

<1% (Limited to important or life-threatening): Allergic/anaphylactoid reaction, anaphylaxis, bronchospasm, convulsions, dyskinesia, hepatic necrosis, interstitial nephritis, pancreatitis, phototoxicity, pseudomembranous colitis, Stevens-Johnson syndrome, tendonitis; quinolones have been associated with tendon rupture,

Overdosage/Toxicology Empty the stomach by vomiting or gastric lavage. Observe carefully and give symptomatic and supportive treatment; maintain adequate hydration.

Drug Interactions

Corticosteroids: Concurrent use may increase the risk of tendon rupture, particularly in elderly patients (overall incidence rare).

Glyburide: Quinolones may increase the effect of glyburide; monitor.

Metal cations (aluminum, calcium, iron, magnesium, and zinc) bind quinolones in the gastrointestinal tract and inhibit absorption. Concurrent administration of most antacids, oral electrolyte supplements, quinapril, sucralfate, some didanosine formulations (chewable/buffered tablets and pediatric powder for oral suspension), and other highly-buffered oral drugs, should be avoided. Trovafloxacin should be administered 2 hours before or 2 hours after these agents.

Probenecid: May decrease renal secretion of trovafloxacin.

Warfarin: The hypoprothrombinemic effect of warfarin may be enhanced by some quinolone antibiotics; monitor INR.

Ethanol/Nutrition/Herb Interactions

Food: Dairy products such as milk or yogurt may reduce absorption of oral trovafloxacin; avoid concurrent use. Enteral feedings may also limit absorption.

Herb/Nutraceutical: Avoid dong quai, St John's wort (may also cause photosensitization).

Dosage Forms

Injection, solution, as mesylate [alatrofloxacin]: 5 mg/mL (40 mL, 60 mL)

Tablet, as mesylate [trovafloxacin]: 100 mg, 200 mg

- **Trovan® [DSC]** *see* Trovafloxacin *on page 1320*
- **T-Stat® [DSC]** *see* Erythromycin *on page 476*
- **Tucks® Anti-Itch [OTC]** *see* Hydrocortisone *on page 639*
- **Twilite® [OTC]** *see* DiphenhydrAMINE *on page 399*
- **Twinject™** *see* Epinephrine *on page 457*
- **Twinrix®** *see* Hepatitis A Inactivated and Hepatitis B (Recombinant) Vaccine *on page 615*
- **Tycolene [OTC]** *see* Acetaminophen *on page 26*
- **Tycolene Maximum Strength [OTC]** *see* Acetaminophen *on page 26*
- **Tylenol® [OTC]** *see* Acetaminophen *on page 26*
- **Tylenol® 8 Hour [OTC]** *see* Acetaminophen *on page 26*
- **Tylenol® Arthritis Pain [OTC]** *see* Acetaminophen *on page 26*
- **Tylenol® Children's [OTC]** *see* Acetaminophen *on page 26*

- **Tylenol® Children's with Flavor Creator [OTC]** *see* Acetaminophen *on page 26*
- **Tylenol Elixir with Codeine (Can)** *see* Acetaminophen and Codeine *on page 29*
- **Tylenol® Extra Strength [OTC]** *see* Acetaminophen *on page 26*
- **Tylenol® Infants [OTC]** *see* Acetaminophen *on page 26*
- **Tylenol® Junior [OTC]** *see* Acetaminophen *on page 26*
- **Tylenol No. 1 (Can)** *see* Acetaminophen and Codeine *on page 29*
- **Tylenol No. 1 Forte (Can)** *see* Acetaminophen and Codeine *on page 29*
- **Tylenol No. 2 with Codeine (Can)** *see* Acetaminophen and Codeine *on page 29*
- **Tylenol No. 3 with Codeine (Can)** *see* Acetaminophen and Codeine *on page 29*
- **Tylenol No. 4 with Codeine (Can)** *see* Acetaminophen and Codeine *on page 29*
- **Tylenol® With Codeine** *see* Acetaminophen and Codeine *on page 29*
- **Tylox®** *see* Oxycodone and Acetaminophen *on page 969*
- **Tysabri®** *see* Natalizumab *on page 904*
- **UK** *see* Urokinase *on page 1323*
- **UK92480** *see* Sildenafil *on page 1169*
- **UK109496** *see* Voriconazole *on page 1358*
- **Ulcerease® [OTC]** *see* Phenol *on page 1012*
- **Ulcidine (Can)** *see* Famotidine *on page 506*
- **Ultane®** *see* Sevoflurane *on page 1166*
- **Ultiva®** *see* Remifentanil *on page 1109*
- **Ultram®** *see* Tramadol *on page 1297*
- **Ultram® ER** *see* Tramadol *on page 1297*
- **Ultraprin [OTC]** *see* Ibuprofen *on page 651*
- **Unasyn®** *see* Ampicillin and Sulbactam *on page 107*
- **Unidet® (Can)** *see* Tolterodine *on page 1285*
- **Unipen® (Can)** *see* Nafcillin *on page 890*
- **Uniphyl®** *see* Theophylline *on page 1253*
- **Uniphyl® SRT (Can)** *see* Theophylline *on page 1253*
- **Unisom® Maximum Strength SleepGels® [OTC]** *see* DiphenhydrAMINE *on page 399*
- **Unithroid®** *see* Levothyroxine *on page 751*
- **Univasc®** *see* Moexipril *on page 862*

Urokinase (yoor oh KIN ase)

U.S. Brand Names Abbokinase® [DSC]

Synonyms UK

Pharmacologic Category Thrombolytic Agent

Generic Available No

Use Thrombolytic agent for the lysis of acute massive pulmonary emboli or pulmonary emboli with unstable hemodynamics

Unlabeled/Investigational Use Thrombolytic agent used in treatment of recent severe or massive deep vein thrombosis, myocardial infarction, and occluded I.V. or dialysis cannulas

Mechanism of Action Promotes thrombolysis by directly activating plasminogen to plasmin, which degrades fibrin, fibrinogen, and other procoagulant plasma proteins

Pharmacodynamics/Kinetics

Onset of action: I.V.: Fibrinolysis occurs rapidly

Duration: ≥4 hours

Distribution: 11.5 L

Half-life elimination: 6.4-18.8 minutes

Excretion: Urine and feces (small amounts)

Dosage

Children and Adults: Deep vein thrombosis (unlabeled use): I.V.: Loading: 4400 units/kg over 10 minutes, then 4400 units/kg/hour for 12 hours

(Continued)

Urokinase *(Continued)*

Adults:

Acute pulmonary embolism: I.V.: Loading: 4400 int. units/kg over 10 minutes; maintenance: 4400 int. units/kg/hour for 12 hours. Following infusion, anticoagulation treatment is recommended to prevent recurrent thrombosis. Do not start anticoagulation until aPTT has decreased to less than twice the normal control value. If heparin is used, do not administer loading dose. Treatment should be followed with oral anticoagulants.

Myocardial infarction (unlabeled use): Intracoronary: 750,000 units over 2 hours (6000 units/minute over up to 2 hours)

Occluded I.V. catheters (unlabeled use):

5000 units in each lumen over 1-2 minutes, leave in lumen for 1-4 hours, then aspirate; may repeat with 10,000 units in each lumen if 5000 units fails to clear the catheter; **do not infuse into the patient**; volume to instill into catheter is equal to the volume of the catheter

I.V. infusion: 200 units/kg/hour in each lumen for 12-48 hours at a rate of at least 20 mL/hour

Dialysis patients: 5000 units is administered in each lumen over 1-2 minutes; leave urokinase in lumen for 1-2 days, then aspirate

Stability Prior to reconstitution, store in refrigerator at 2°C to 8°C (36°F to 46°F). Reconstitute vial with 5 mL sterile water for injection (preservative free) by gently rolling and tilting; do not shake; contains no preservatives, should not be reconstituted until immediately before using, discard unused portion; solution will look pale and straw colored; may filter through ≤0.45 micron filter

Prior to infusion, solution should be further diluted in D_5W or NS.

Administration Solution may be filtered using a 0.22 or 0.45 micron filter during I.V. therapy. Administer using a pump which can deliver a total volume of 195 mL. The loading dose should be administered at 90 mL/hour over 10 minutes. The maintenance dose should be administered at 15 mL/hour over 12 hours. I.V. tubing should be flushed with NS or D_5W to ensure total dose is administered.

Monitoring Parameters Blood pressure, pulse; CBC, platelet count, aPTT, urinalysis

Anesthesia and Critical Care Concerns/Other Considerations When using thrombolytic therapy in an institution, it is important that the protocol for that institution be followed closely, particularly in terms of dosage, adjunctive heparin therapy, and standard myocardial infarction therapy (eg, aspirin, beta-blocker, ACE inhibitor). Preceding recent thrombolytic therapy must be taken into account when invasive procedures (particularly intravascular procedures) are undertaken. Close clinical monitoring is required to ensure efficacy of therapy. Failure of therapy may require emergent cardiac catheterization and interventional therapy. Reperfusion after successful thrombolysis may be associated with rapid resolution of ECG changes and restoration of cardiac function. However, reperfusion arrhythmias may also manifest.

Pregnancy Risk Factor B

Contraindications Hypersensitivity to urokinase or any component of the formulation; active internal bleeding; history of CVA; recent (within 2 months) intracranial or intraspinal surgery or trauma; intracranial neoplasm, arteriovenous malformation, or aneurysm; known bleeding diathesis; severe uncontrolled hypertension

Warnings/Precautions Concurrent heparin anticoagulation can contribute to bleeding; careful attention to all potential bleeding sites. I.M. injections and nonessential handling of the patient should be avoided. Venipunctures should be performed carefully and only when necessary. If arterial puncture is necessary, use an upper extremity vessel that can be manually compressed. If serious bleeding occurs, then the infusion of urokinase and heparin should be stopped.

For the following conditions the risk of bleeding is higher with use of thrombolytics and should be weighed against the benefits of therapy: recent (within 10 days) major surgery (eg, CABG, obstetrical delivery, organ biopsy, previous puncture of noncompressible vessels), cerebrovascular disease, recent (within 10 days) gastrointestinal or genitourinary bleeding, recent trauma (within 10 days) including CPR, hypertension (systolic BP >180 mm Hg and/or diastolic BP >110 mm Hg), high likelihood of left heart thrombus (eg, mitral stenosis with atrial fibrillation), acute pericarditis, subacute bacterial endocarditis, hemostatic defects including ones caused by severe renal or hepatic dysfunction, significant hepatic dysfunction, pregnancy, diabetic hemorrhagic retinopathy or other hemorrhagic ophthalmic conditions, septic thrombophlebitis or occluded AV cannula at seriously infected site, advanced age (eg, >75 years), patients receiving oral anticoagulants, any other condition in which bleeding constitutes a significant hazard or would be particularly difficult to manage because of location.

Coronary thrombolysis may result in reperfusion arrhythmias. Follow standard MI management. Rare anaphylactoid reactions can occur. Formulated in human albumin; products made from human sources have a theoretical risk of transmitting infectious agents. Safety and efficacy in pediatric patients have not been established.

Adverse Reactions As with all drugs which may affect hemostasis, bleeding is the major adverse effect associated with urokinase. Hemorrhage may occur at virtually any site. Risk is dependent on multiple variables, including the dosage administered, concurrent use of multiple agents which alter hemostasis, and patient predisposition.

>10%: Local: Injection site: Bleeding (5% decrease in hematocrit reported in 37% patients; most bleeding occurring at external incisions or injection sites, but also reported in other areas)

<1% (Limited to important or life-threatening): Allergic reaction (includes bronchospasm, orolingual edema, urticaria, skin rash, pruritus); cardiac arrest, cerebral vascular accident, chest pain, cholesterol embolism, diaphoresis, hemiplegia, intracranial hemorrhage, retroperitoneal hemorrhage, MI, pulmonary edema, recurrent pulmonary embolism, reperfusion ventricular arrhythmia, stroke, substernal pain, thrombocytopenia, vascular embolization (cerebral and distal); infusion reactions (most occurring within 1 hour) including acidosis, back pain, chills, cyanosis, dyspnea, fever, hyper-/hypotension, hypoxia, nausea, rigors, tachycardia, vomiting

Overdosage/Toxicology Symptoms of overdose include epistaxis, bleeding gums, hematoma, spontaneous ecchymoses, and oozing at the catheter site. In the event of overdose, stop the infusion and reverse bleeding with blood products that contain clotting factors.

Drug Interactions

Aminocaproic acid (antifibrinolytic agent) may decrease effectiveness.

Drugs which affect platelet function (eg, aspirin, NSAIDs, dipyridamole, ticlopidine, clopidogrel, IIb/IIIa antagonists) may potentiate the risk of hemorrhage; use with caution.

Heparin: Concurrent use may increase risk of bleeding; use caution.

Warfarin or oral anticoagulants: Risk of bleeding may be increased during concurrent therapy.

Dosage Forms [DSC] = Discontinued product

Injection, powder for reconstitution: 250,000 int. units [contains human albumin 250 mg and mannitol 25 mg] [DSC]

♦ **Urolene Blue®** *see* Methylene Blue *on page 828*
♦ **Uroxatral®** *see* Alfuzosin *on page 58*
♦ **Utradol™ (Can)** *see* Etodolac *on page 496*
♦ **Vagi-Gard® [OTC]** *see* Povidone-Iodine *on page 1039*
♦ **Valcyte™** *see* Valganciclovir *on page 1327*

Valdecoxib (val de KOKS ib)

U.S. Brand Names Bextra® *[Withdrawn from Market]*

Pharmacologic Category Nonsteroidal Anti-inflammatory Drug (NSAID), COX-2 Selective

Generic Available No

Use Relief of signs and symptoms of osteoarthritis and adult rheumatoid arthritis; treatment of primary dysmenorrhea

Mechanism of Action Inhibits prostaglandin synthesis by decreasing the activity of the enzyme, cyclooxygenase-2 (COX-2), which results in decreased formation of prostaglandin precursors. Does not affect platelet function.

Pharmacodynamics/Kinetics

Onset of action: Dysmenorrhea: 60 minutes

Distribution: V_d: 86 L

Protein binding: 98%

Metabolism: Extensively hepatic via CYP3A4 and 2C9; glucuronidation; forms metabolite (active)

Bioavailability: 83%

(Continued)

Valdecoxib *(Continued)*

Half-life elimination: 8-11 hours
Time to peak: 2.25-3 hours
Excretion: Primarily urine (as metabolites)

Dosage Oral: Adults:

Osteoarthritis and rheumatoid arthritis: 10 mg once daily; **Note:** No additional benefits seen with 20 mg/day

Primary dysmenorrhea: 20 mg twice daily as needed

Dosage adjustment in renal impairment: Not recommended for use in advanced disease

Dosage adjustment in hepatic impairment: Not recommended for use in advanced liver dysfunction (Child-Pugh Class C)

Stability Store at 15°C to 30°C (59°F to 86°F).

Administration Avoid dehydration. Encourage patient to drink plenty of fluids.

Monitoring Parameters If used in patients with advanced renal disease, monitor serum creatinine closely; signs and symptoms of GI bleeding

Anesthesia and Critical Care Concerns/Other Considerations Valdecoxib does not inhibit platelets or prolong bleeding time.

Pregnancy Risk Factor C/D (3rd trimester)

Contraindications Hypersensitivity to valdecoxib, sulfonamides, or any component of the formulation; patients who have experienced asthma, urticaria, or allergic-type reactions to aspirin or NSAIDs; acute pain following CABG; pregnancy (3rd trimester)

Warnings/Precautions Gastrointestinal irritation, ulceration, bleeding, and perforation may occur with NSAIDs (it is unclear whether valdecoxib is associated with rates of these events which are similar to nonselective NSAIDs). Use with caution in patients with a history of GI disease (bleeding or ulcers) or risk factor for GI bleeding, use lowest dose for shortest time possible. Anaphylactic/anaphylactoid reactions may occur, even with no prior exposure to valdecoxib. Serious dermatologic reactions (including life-threatening Stevens-Johnson syndrome and erythema multiforme) have been reported; discontinue immediately in any patients who develop rash or any signs of hypersensitivity. Risk may be greatest in the first 2 weeks of therapy and in patients with prior sulfonamide allergy. Use with caution in patients with decreased renal function, hepatic disease, CHF, hypertension, fluid retention, dehydration, or asthma. Carefully evaluate individual cardiovascular risk profiles prior to prescribing COX-2 inhibitors. COX-2 inhibitors may not be appropriate in patients with cardiovascular disease or in patients with significant risk factors for cardiovascular disease. Use caution in patients with known or suspected deficiency of cytochrome P450 isoenzyme 2C9. Use in patients with severe hepatic impairment (Child-Pugh Class C) is not recommended. Use in patients following CABG has been associated with an increase in thromboembolic events, including MI, stroke, DVT, and PE. Safety and efficacy have not been established for patients <18 years of age.

Adverse Reactions

2% to 10%:

Cardiovascular: Peripheral edema (2% to 3%), hypertension (2%)
Central nervous system: Headache (5% to 9%), dizziness (3%)
Dermatologic: Rash (1% to 2%)
Gastrointestinal: Dyspepsia (8% to 9%), abdominal pain (7% to 8%), nausea (6% to 7%), diarrhea (5% to 6%), flatulence (3% to 4%), abdominal fullness (2%)
Neuromuscular & skeletal: Back pain (2% to 3%), myalgia (2%)
Otic: Earache, tinnitus
Respiratory: Upper respiratory tract infection (6% to 7%), sinusitis (2% to 3%)
Miscellaneous: Influenza-like symptoms (2%)

<2% (Limited to important or life threatening): Allergy, anaphylaxis, aneurysm, angina, angioedema, aortic stenosis, arrhythmia, atrial fibrillation, bradycardia, breast neoplasm, cardiomyopathy, carotid stenosis, colitis, CHF, convulsion, coronary thrombosis, depression exacerbation, diabetes mellitus, diverticulosis, duodenal ulcer, emphysema, erythema multiforme, esophageal perforation, exfoliative dermatitis, facial edema, gastric ulcer, gastroesophageal reflux, gastrointestinal bleeding, gout, heart block, hepatitis, hiatal hernia, hyperlipemia, hyperparathyroidism, hypertension exacerbation, hypertensive encephalopathy, hypotension, impotence, intermittent claudication, liver function tests increased, lymphadenopathy, lymphangitis, lymphopenia, migraine, mitral insufficiency, MI, myocardial ischemia, neuropathy, osteoporosis, ovarian cyst

(malignant), pancreatitis, pericarditis, periorbital swelling, photosensitivity, pneumonia, rash (erythematous, maculopapular, psoriaform), Stevens-Johnson syndrome, syncope, tachycardia, thrombocytopenia, thrombophlebitis, toxic epidermal necrolysis, unstable angina, urinary tract infection, vaginal hemorrhage, ventricular fibrillation, vertigo

Overdosage/Toxicology Symptoms of overdose may include epigastric pain, drowsiness, lethargy, nausea, and vomiting; gastrointestinal bleeding may occur. Rare manifestations include hypertension, respiratory depression, coma, and acute renal failure. Treatment is symptomatic and supportive. Forced diuresis, hemodialysis, hemoperfusion, and/or urinary alkalinization may not be useful.

Drug Interactions Substrate (minor) of CYP2C9, 3A4; **Inhibits** CYP2C8 (weak), 2C9 (weak), 2C19 (weak)

ACE inhibitors: Antihypertensive effects may be decreased by concurrent therapy with NSAIDs; monitor blood pressure.

Angiotensin II antagonists: Antihypertensive effects may be decreased by concurrent therapy with NSAIDs; monitor blood pressure.

Anticoagulants (warfarin, heparin, LMWHs): In combination with NSAIDs, can cause increased risk of bleeding.

Antiplatelet drugs (ticlopidine, clopidogrel, aspirin, abciximab, dipyridamole, eptifibatide, tirofiban): Can cause an increased risk of bleeding.

Azole antifungals: May increase valdecoxib concentrations.

Corticosteroids: May increase the risk of GI ulceration; avoid concurrent use

Cyclosporine: NSAIDs may increase serum creatinine, potassium, blood pressure, and cyclosporine levels; monitor cyclosporine levels and renal function carefully.

Hydralazine: Antihypertensive effect is decreased; avoid concurrent use

Lithium levels can be increased; avoid concurrent use if possible or monitor lithium levels and adjust dose. When NSAID is stopped, lithium will need adjustment again.

Loop diuretics: Diuretic and antihypertensive efficacy is reduced. May be anticipated with any NSAID.

Methotrexate: Severe bone marrow suppression, aplastic anemia, and GI toxicity have been reported with concomitant NSAID therapy. Selective COX-2 inhibitors appear to have a lower risk of this toxicity, however, caution is warranted.

Thiazides: Diuretic efficacy is reduced.

Warfarin: Valdecoxib (40 mg twice daily) may increase plasma warfarin exposure (12% R-warfarin, 15% S-warfarin). May increase the anticoagulant effects of warfarin. Monitor INR closely.

Ethanol/Nutrition/Herb Interactions

Ethanol: Avoid ethanol (may enhance gastric mucosal irritation).

Food: Time to peak level is delayed by 1-2 hours when taken with high-fat meal, but other parameters are unaffected.

Herb/Nutraceutical: Avoid cat's claw, dong quai, evening primrose, feverfew, garlic, ginger, ginkgo, red clover, horse chestnut, green tea, ginseng (may cause increased risk of bleeding).

Dietary Considerations May be taken with or without food.

Dosage Forms Tablet: 10 mg, 20 mg

Valganciclovir (val gan SYE kloh veer)

Medication Safety Issues

Sound-alike/look-alike issues:

Valcyte™ may be confused with Valium®, Valtrex®

Valganciclovir may be confused with valacyclovir

U.S. Brand Names Valcyte™

Canadian Brand Names Valcyte™

Synonyms Valganciclovir Hydrochloride

Pharmacologic Category Antiviral Agent

Generic Available No

Use Treatment of cytomegalovirus (CMV) retinitis in patients with acquired immunodeficiency syndrome (AIDS); prevention of CMV disease in high-risk patients (donor CMV positive/recipient CMV negative) undergoing kidney, heart, or kidney/pancreas transplantation

Mechanism of Action Valganciclovir is rapidly converted to ganciclovir in the body. The bioavailability of ganciclovir from valganciclovir is increased 10-fold compared to the oral ganciclovir. A dose of 900 mg achieved systemic exposure

(Continued)

Valganciclovir *(Continued)*

of ganciclovir comparable to that achieved with the recommended doses of intravenous ganciclovir of 5 mg/kg. Ganciclovir is phosphorylated to a substrate which competitively inhibits the binding of deoxyguanosine triphosphate to DNA polymerase resulting in inhibition of viral DNA synthesis.

Pharmacodynamics/Kinetics

Absorption: Well absorbed; high-fat meal increases AUC by 30%

Distribution: Ganciclovir: V_d: 15.26 L/1.73 m^2; widely to all tissues including CSF and ocular tissue

Protein binding: 1% to 2%

Metabolism: Converted to ganciclovir by intestinal mucosal cells and hepatocytes

Bioavailability: With food: 60%

Half-life elimination: Ganciclovir: 4.08 hours; prolonged with renal impairment; Severe renal impairment: Up to 68 hours

Excretion: Urine (primarily as ganciclovir)

Dosage Oral: Adults:

CMV retinitis:

Induction: 900 mg twice daily for 21 days (with food)

Maintenance: Following induction treatment, or for patients with inactive CMV retinitis who require maintenance therapy: Recommended dose: 900 mg once daily (with food)

Prevention of CMV disease following transplantation: 900 mg once daily (with food) beginning within 10 days of transplantation; continue therapy until 100 days post-transplantation

Dosage adjustment in renal impairment:

Induction dose:

Cl_{cr} 40-59 mL/minute: 450 mg twice daily

Cl_{cr} 25-39 mL/minute: 450 mg once daily

Cl_{cr} 10-24 mL/minute: 450 mg every 2 days

Maintenance dose:

Cl_{cr} 40-59 mL/minute: 450 mg once daily

Cl_{cr} 25-39 mL/minute: 450 mg every 2 days

Cl_{cr} 10-24 mL/minute: 450 mg twice weekly

Note: Valganciclovir is not recommended in patients receiving hemodialysis. For patients on hemodialysis (Cl_{cr} <10 mL/minute), it is recommended that ganciclovir be used (dose adjusted as specified for ganciclovir).

Stability Store at 25°C (77°F), excursions permitted to 15°C to 30°C (59°F to 86°F).

Administration Avoid direct contact with broken or crushed tablets. Consideration should be given to handling and disposal according to guidelines issued for antineoplastic drugs. However, there is no consensus on the need for these precautions.

Monitoring Parameters Retinal exam (at least every 4-6 weeks), CBC, platelet counts, serum creatinine

Pregnancy Risk Factor C

Contraindications Hypersensitivity to valganciclovir, ganciclovir, acyclovir, or any component of the formulation; absolute neutrophil count <500/mm^3; platelet count <25,000/mm^3; hemoglobin <8 g/dL

Warnings/Precautions **[U.S. Boxed Warning]: May cause dose or therapy limiting granulocytopenia, anemia, and/or thrombocytopenia;** use with caution in patients with pre-existing bone marrow suppression, cytopenias, or in those receiving myelosuppressive drugs/irradiation. Use with caution in patients with impaired renal function (dosage adjustment required). **[U.S. Boxed Warning]: Ganciclovir may adversely affect spermatogenesis and fertility;** due to its mutagenic potential, contraceptive precautions for female and male patients need to be followed during and for at least 90 days after therapy with the drug. Due to differences in bioavailability, valganciclovir tablets cannot be substituted for ganciclovir capsules on a one-to-one basis. Not indicated for use in liver transplant patients (higher incidence of tissue-invasive CMV relative to oral ganciclovir was observed in trials). Safety and efficacy have not been established in pediatric patients.

Adverse Reactions

>10%:

Central nervous system: Fever (31%), headache (9% to 22%), insomnia (16%)

Gastrointestinal: Diarrhea (16% to 41%), nausea (8% to 30%), vomiting (21%), abdominal pain (15%)

Hematologic: Granulocytopenia (11% to 27%), anemia (8% to 26%)
Ocular: Retinal detachment (15%)

1% to 10%:

Central nervous system: Peripheral neuropathy (9%), paresthesia (8%), seizure (<5%), psychosis, hallucinations (<5%), confusion (<5%), agitation (<5%)
Hematologic: Thrombocytopenia (8%), pancytopenia (<5%), bone marrow depression (<5%), aplastic anemia (<5%), bleeding (potentially life-threatening due to thrombocytopenia <5%)
Renal: Decreased renal function (<5%)
Miscellaneous: Local and systemic infection, including sepsis (<5%); allergic reaction (<5%)

<1% (Limited to important or life-threatening): Valganciclovir is expected to share the toxicities which may occur at a low incidence or due to idiosyncratic reactions which have been associated with ganciclovir

Overdosage/Toxicology Symptoms of overdose with ganciclovir include neutropenia, vomiting, hypersalivation, bloody diarrhea, cytopenia, and testicular atrophy. Treatment is supportive. Hemodialysis removes 50% of the drug. Hydration may be of some benefit.

Drug Interactions Note: Drug interaction studies have not been conducted with valganciclovir. The following interactions have been described for ganciclovir.

Decreased effect: Didanosine: A decrease in steady-state ganciclovir AUC may occur

Increased toxicity:

Didanosine levels are increased with concurrent ganciclovir
Immunosuppressive agents may increase cytotoxicity of ganciclovir
Imipenem/cilastatin may increase seizure potential
Probenecid: The renal clearance of ganciclovir is decreased in the presence of probenecid
Other nephrotoxic drugs (eg, amphotericin and cyclosporine) may have additive nephrotoxicity with ganciclovir
Zidovudine: Oral ganciclovir increased the AUC of zidovudine, although zidovudine decreases steady state levels of ganciclovir. Since both drugs have the potential to cause neutropenia and anemia, some patients may not tolerate concomitant therapy with these drugs at full dosage.

Ethanol/Nutrition/Herb Interactions Food: Coadministration with a high-fat meal increased AUC by 30%.

Dietary Considerations Should be taken with meals.

Dosage Forms Tablet, as hydrochloride: 450 mg [valganciclovir hydrochloride 496.3 mg equivalent to valganciclovir 450 mg]

♦ **Valganciclovir Hydrochloride** *see* Valganciclovir *on page 1327*
♦ **Valisone® Scalp Lotion (Can)** *see* Betamethasone *on page 169*
♦ **Valium®** *see* Diazepam *on page 374*
♦ **Valorin [OTC]** *see* Acetaminophen *on page 26*
♦ **Valorin Extra [OTC]** *see* Acetaminophen *on page 26*
♦ **Valproate Semisodium** *see* Valproic Acid and Derivatives *on page 1329*
♦ **Valproate Sodium** *see* Valproic Acid and Derivatives *on page 1329*
♦ **Valproic Acid** *see* Valproic Acid and Derivatives *on page 1329*

Valproic Acid and Derivatives

(val PROE ik AS id & dah RIV ah tives)

Medication Safety Issues

Sound-alike/look-alike issues:

Depakene® may be confused with Depakote®
Depakote® may be confused with Depakene®, Depakote® ER, Senokot®

Related Information

Chronic Pain Management *on page 1430*
Chronic Renal Failure *on page 1437*
Epilepsy *on page 1604*
Perioperative Management of Patients on Antiseizure Medication *on page 1458*

U.S. Brand Names Depacon®; Depakene®; Depakote® Delayed Release; Depakote® ER; Depakote® Sprinkle®

(Continued)

Valproic Acid and Derivatives *(Continued)*

Canadian Brand Names Alti-Divalproex; Apo-Divalproex®; Depakene®; Epival® I.V.; Gen-Divalproex; Novo-Divalproex; Nu-Divalproex; PMS-Valproic Acid; PMS-Valproic Acid E.C.; Rhoxal-valproic; Sandoz-Valproic

Synonyms Dipropylacetic Acid; Divalproex Sodium; DPA; 2-Propylpentanoic Acid; 2-Propylvaleric Acid; Valproate Semisodium; Valproate Sodium; Valproic Acid

Pharmacologic Category Anticonvulsant, Miscellaneous

Generic Available Yes: Capsule (excluding sprinkle), injection, syrup

Use Monotherapy and adjunctive therapy in the treatment of patients with complex partial seizures; monotherapy and adjunctive therapy of simple and complex absence seizures; adjunctive therapy patients with multiple seizure types that include absence seizures; treatment of acute or mixed manic episodes associated with bipolar disorder; migraine prophylaxis

Mania associated with bipolar disorder (Depakote®)

Migraine prophylaxis (Depakote®, Depakote® ER)

Unlabeled/Investigational Use Behavior disorders (eg, agitation, aggression) in patients with dementia (based on the results of several randomized, controlled trials, there is little evidence to support this use); status epilepticus

Mechanism of Action Causes increased availability of gamma-aminobutyric acid (GABA), an inhibitory neurotransmitter, to brain neurons or may enhance the action of GABA or mimic its action at postsynaptic receptor sites

Pharmacodynamics/Kinetics

Distribution: Total valproate: 11 L/1.73 m^2; free valproate 92 L/1.73 m^2

Protein binding (dose dependent): 80% to 90%

Metabolism: Extensively hepatic via glucuronide conjugation and mitochondrial beta-oxidation. The relationship between dose and total valproate concentration is nonlinear; concentration does not increase proportionally with the dose, but increases to a lesser extent due to saturable plasma protein binding. The kinetics of unbound drug are linear.

Bioavailability: Extended release: 90% of I.V. dose and 81% to 90% of delayed release dose

Half-life elimination: (increased in neonates and with liver disease): Children: 4-14 hours; Adults: 9-16 hours

Time to peak, serum: 1-4 hours; Divalproex (enteric coated): 3-5 hours

Excretion: Urine (30% to 50% as glucuronide conjugate, 3% as unchanged drug)

Dosage

Seizures:

Children ≥10 years and Adults:

Oral: Initial: 10-15 mg/kg/day in 1-3 divided doses; increase by 5-10 mg/kg/day at weekly intervals until therapeutic levels are achieved; maintenance: 30-60 mg/kg/day. Adult usual dose: 1000-2500 mg/day. **Note:** Regular release and delayed release formulations are usually given in 2-4 divided doses/day, extended release formulation (Depakote® ER) is usually given once daily. Conversion to Depakote® ER from a stable dose of Depakote® may require an increase in the total daily dose between 8% and 20% to maintain similar serum concentrations.

Children receiving more than one anticonvulsant (ie, polytherapy) may require doses up to 100 mg/kg/day in 3-4 divided doses

I.V.: Administer as a 60-minute infusion (≤20 mg/minute) with the same frequency as oral products; switch patient to oral products as soon as possible. Alternatively, rapid infusions have been given: ≤15 mg/kg over 5-10 minutes (1.5-3 mg/kg/minute).

Rectal (unlabeled): Dilute syrup 1:1 with water for use as a retention enema; loading dose: 17-20 mg/kg one time; maintenance: 10-15 mg/kg/dose every 8 hours

Status epilepticus (unlabeled use): Adults:

Loading dose: I.V.: 15-25 mg/kg administered at 3 mg/kg/minute.

Maintenance dose: I.V. infusion: 1-4 mg/kg/hour; titrate dose as needed based upon patient response and evaluation of drug-drug interactions

Mania: Adults: Oral: 750-1500 mg/day in divided doses; dose should be adjusted as rapidly as possible to desired clinical effect; a loading dose of 20 mg/kg may be used; maximum recommended dosage: 60 mg/kg/day

Extended release tablets: Initial: 25 mg/kg/day given once daily; dose should be adjusted as rapidly as possible to desired clinical effect; maximum recommended dose: 60 mg/kg/day.

Migraine prophylaxis: Adults: Oral:

Extended release tablets: 500 mg once daily for 7 days, then increase to 1000 mg once daily; adjust dose based on patient response; usual dosage range 500-1000 mg/day

Delayed release tablets: 250 mg twice daily; adjust dose based on patient response, up to 1000 mg/day

Elderly: Elimination is decreased in the elderly. Studies of elderly patients with dementia show a high incidence of somnolence. In some patients, this was associated with weight loss. Starting doses should be lower and increases should be slow, with careful monitoring of nutritional intake and dehydration. Safety and efficacy for use in patients >65 years have not been studied for migraine prophylaxis.

Dosing adjustment in renal impairment: A 27% reduction in clearance of unbound valproate is seen in patients with Cl_{cr} <10 mL/minute. Hemodialysis reduces valproate concentrations by 20%, therefore no dose adjustment is needed in patients with renal failure. Protein binding is reduced, monitoring only total valproate concentrations may be misleading.

Dosing adjustment/comments in hepatic impairment: Reduce dose. Clearance is decreased with liver impairment. Hepatic disease is also associated with decreased albumin concentrations and 2- to 2.6-fold increase in the unbound fraction. Free concentrations of valproate may be elevated while total concentrations appear normal.

Stability Injection should be diluted in 50 mL of a compatible diluent; is physically compatible and chemically stable in D_5W, NS, and LR for at least 24 hours when stored in glass or PVC; store vials at room temperature 15°C to 30°C (59°F to 86°F)

Administration

Depakote® ER: Swallow whole, do not crush or chew. Patients who need dose adjustments smaller than 500 mg/day for migraine prophylaxis should be changed to Depakote® delayed release tablets. Sprinkle capsules may be swallowed whole or open cap and sprinkle on small amount (1 teaspoonful) of soft food and use immediately (do not store or chew).

Depacon®: Following dilution to final concentration, administer over 60 minutes at a rate of ≤20 mg/minute. Alternatively, single doses up to 15 mg/kg have been administered as a rapid infusion over 5-10 minutes (1.5-3 mg/kg/minute).

Monitoring Parameters Liver enzymes, CBC with platelets, PT/PTT, serum ammonia (with symptoms of lethargy, mental status change)

Reference Range

Therapeutic:

Epilepsy: 50-100 mcg/mL (SI: 350-690 μmol/L)

Mania: 50-125 mcg/mL (SI: 350-860 μmol/L)

Toxic: Some laboratories may report >200 mcg/mL (SI: >1390 μmol/L) as a toxic threshold, although clinical toxicity can occur at lower concentrations.

Seizure control: May improve at levels >100 mcg/mL (SI: 690 μmol/L), but toxicity may occur at levels of 100-150 mcg/mL (SI: 690-1040 μmol/L)

Mania: Clinical response seen with trough levels between 50-125 mcg/mL; risk of toxicity increases at levels >125 mcg/mL

Anesthesia and Critical Care Concerns/Other Considerations Extended release tablets have 10% to 20% less fluctuation in serum concentration than delayed release tablets. Extended release tablets are not bioequivalent to delayed release tablets.

Symptoms of overdose include coma, somnolence, motor restlessness, visual hallucinations, and heart block. Naloxone has been used to reverse toxic CNS depressant effects but may block anticonvulsant effects.

Pregnancy Risk Factor D

Contraindications Hypersensitivity to valproic acid, derivatives, or any component of the formulation; hepatic dysfunction; urea cycle disorders

Warnings/Precautions

[US Boxed Warning]: Hepatic failure resulting in fatalities has occurred in patients; children <2 years of age are at considerable risk. Other risk factors include organic brain disease, mental retardation with severe seizure disorders, congenital metabolic disorders, and patients on multiple anticonvulsants. Hepatotoxicity has been reported after 3 days to 6 months of therapy. Monitor patients closely for appearance of malaise, weakness, facial edema, anorexia, jaundice, and vomiting.

(Continued)

Valproic Acid and Derivatives *(Continued)*

[US Boxed Warning]: May cause teratogenic effects such as neural tube defects (eg, spina bifida). Use in women of childbearing potential requires that benefits of use in mother be weighed against the potential risk to fetus, especially when used for conditions not associated with permanent injury or risk of death (eg, migraine).

May cause severe thrombocytopenia, inhibition of platelet aggregation and bleeding; tremors may indicate overdosage; use with caution in patients receiving other anticonvulsants. Cases of life-threatening pancreatitis, occurring at the start of therapy or following years of use, have been reported in adults and children. Some cases have been hemorrhagic with rapid progression of initial symptoms to death. Hypersensitivity reactions affecting multiple organs have been reported in association with valproic acid use; may include dermatologic and/or hematologic changes (eosinophilia, neutropenia, thrombocytopenia) or symptoms of organ dysfunction.

Hyperammonemia and/or encephalopathy, sometimes fatal, have been reported following the initiation of valproate therapy and may be present with normal transaminase levels. Ammonia levels should be measured in patients who develop unexplained lethargy and vomiting, or changes in mental status. Discontinue therapy if ammonia levels are increased and evaluate for possible urea cycle disorder (UCD). Although rare genetic disorders, UCD evaluation should be considered for the following patients, prior to the start of therapy: History of unexplained encephalopathy or coma; encephalopathy associated with protein load; pregnancy or postpartum encephalopathy; unexplained mental retardation; history of elevated plasma ammonia or glutamine; history of cyclical vomiting and lethargy; episodic extreme irritability, ataxia; low BUN or protein avoidance; family history of UCD or unexplained infant deaths (particularly male); signs or symptoms of UCD (hyperammonemia, encephalopathy, respiratory alkalosis).

In vitro studies have suggested valproate stimulates the replication of HIV and CMV viruses under experimental conditions. The clinical consequence of this is unknown, but should be considered when monitoring affected patients.

Anticonvulsants should not be discontinued abruptly because of the possibility of increasing seizure frequency; valproate should be withdrawn gradually to minimize the potential of increased seizure frequency, unless safety concerns require a more rapid withdrawal. Concomitant use with clonazepam may induce absence status.

CNS depression may occur with valproate use. Patients must be cautioned about performing tasks which require mental alertness (operating machinery or driving). Effects with other sedative drugs or ethanol may be potentiated.

Adverse Reactions

Adverse reactions reported when used as monotherapy for complex partial seizure:

>10%:

- Central nervous system: Headache (up to 31%), somnolence (7% to 30%), dizziness (12% to 25%), insomnia (1% to 15%), nervousness (1% to 11%), pain (up to 11%)
- Dermatologic: Alopecia (6% to 24%)
- Gastrointestinal: Nausea (15% to 48%), vomiting (7% to 27%), diarrhea (7% to 23%), abdominal pain (7% to 23%), dyspepsia (7% to 23%), anorexia (11% to 12%)
- Hematologic: Thrombocytopenia (1% to 24%)
- Neuromuscular & skeletal: Tremor (1% to 57%), weakness (6% to 27%)
- Ocular: Diplopia (up to 16%), amblyopia/blurred vision (8% to 12%)
- Miscellaneous: Infection (1% to 20%), flu-like symptoms (1% to 12%)

1% to 10%:

- Cardiovascular: Arrhythmia, chest pain, edema, hyper-/hypotension, palpitation, peripheral edema (1% to 8%), postural hypotension, tachycardia, vasodilatation
- Central nervous system: Abnormal dreams, agitation, amnesia (5% to 7%), anxiety, catatonic reaction, chills, confusion, depression, emotional lability, hallucinations, hypokinesia, malaise, personality disorder, psychosis, reflexes increased, sleep disorder, speech disorder, tardive dyskinesia, thinking abnormal (up to 6%), vertigo

Dermatologic: Bruising, discoid lupus erythematosus, dry skin, erythema nodosum, furunculosis, macropapular rash, petechia, pruritus, rash, seborrhea, vesiculobullous rash

Endocrine & metabolic: Amenorrhea, dysmenorrhea, hypoproteinemia, metrorrhagia

Gastrointestinal: Dysphagia, eructation, fecal incontinence, flatulence, gastroenteritis, glossitis, gum hemorrhage, hematemesis, appetite increased, mouth ulceration, pancreatitis, periodontal abscess, taste perversion, weight gain (1% to 9%), stomatitis, constipation, dry mouth, tooth disorder, weight loss (up to 6%)

Genitourinary: Cystitis, urinary frequency, urinary incontinence, UTI, vaginitis

Hematologic: Anemia, bleeding time increased, leukopenia

Hepatic: AST/ALT increased

Neuromuscular & skeletal: Abnormal gait, arthralgia, arthrosis, ataxia (up to 8%), back pain (1% to 8%), hypertonia, leg cramps, myalgia, myasthenia, neck rigidity, paresthesia, twitching

Ocular: Abnormal vision, conjunctivitis, dry eye, eye pain, nystagmus (7% to 8%), photophobia

Otic: Deafness, otitis media, tinnitus (1% to 7%)

Respiratory: Bronchitis, epistaxis, hiccup, increased cough, pneumonia, rhinitis, sinusitis

Additional adverse effects: Frequency not defined:

Cardiovascular: Bradycardia

Central nervous system: Aggression, behavioral deterioration, cerebral atrophy (reversible), dementia, encephalopathy (rare), hostility, hyperactivity, hypoesthesia, parkinsonism

Dermatologic: Cutaneous vasculitis, erythema multiforme, photosensitivity, Stevens-Johnson syndrome, toxic epidermal necrolysis (rare)

Endocrine & metabolic: Breast enlargement, galactorrhea, hyperammonemia, hyponatremia, inappropriate ADH secretion, parotid gland swelling, polycystic ovary disease (rare), abnormal thyroid function tests

Genitourinary: Enuresis

Hematologic: Anemia, aplastic anemia, bone marrow suppression, eosinophilia, hematoma formation, hemorrhage, hypofibrinogenemia, intermittent porphyria, lymphocytosis, macrocytosis, pancytopenia

Hepatic: Bilirubin increased, hyperammonemic encephalopathy (in patients with UCD)

Neuromuscular & skeletal: Asterixis, bone pain, dysarthria

Ocular: Seeing "spots before the eyes"

Renal: Fanconi-like syndrome (rare, in children)

Miscellaneous: Anaphylaxis, carnitine decreased, hyperglycinemia, lupus

Postmarketing and/or case reports: Life-threatening pancreatitis (2 cases out of 2416 patients), occurring at the start of therapy or following years of use, has been reported in adults and children. Some cases have been hemorrhagic with rapid progression of initial symptoms to death. Cases have also been reported upon rechallenge. Severe hypersensitivity reactions with organ dysfunction have been reported; symptoms include fever and rash along with organ dysfunction, eosinophilia, and hematologic depression (thrombocytopenia, neutropenia).

Overdosage/Toxicology Symptoms of overdose include coma, deep sleep, motor restlessness, and visual hallucinations. Supportive treatment is necessary. Naloxone has been used to reverse CNS depressant effects, but may block the action of other anticonvulsants.

Drug Interactions For valproic acid: **Substrate** (minor) of CYP2A6, 2B6, 2C9, 2C19, 2E1; **Inhibits** CYP2C9 (weak), 2C19 (weak), 2D6 (weak), 3A4 (weak); **Induces** CYP2A6 (weak)

Carbamazepine: Valproic acid may increase, decrease, or have no effect on carbamazepine levels; valproic acid may increase serum concentrations of carbamazepine - epoxide (active metabolite); valproic acid may induce the metabolism of carbamazepine; monitor.

Carbapenem antibiotics (ertapenem, imipenem, meropenem): May decrease valproic acid concentrations to subtherapeutic levels; monitor.

Felbamate: May increase the levels/effects of valproic acid; monitor.

Isoniazid: May decrease valproic acid metabolism (limited documentation).

Lamotrigine: Valproic acid inhibits the metabolism of lamotrigine; combination therapy has been proposed to increase the risk of toxic epidermal necrolysis; monitor.

(Continued)

Valproic Acid and Derivatives *(Continued)*

Macrolide antibiotics: May decrease valproic acid metabolism (limited documentation); includes clarithromycin, erythromycin, troleandomycin; monitor.

Primidone, phenobarbital: Valproic acid appears to inhibit the metabolism of phenobarbital; monitor for increased effect.

Salicylates: May displace valproic acid from plasma proteins, leading to acute toxicity.

Topiramate: Hyperammonemia with or without encephalopathy has been reported in patients who tolerated either drug alone. These drugs may modestly decrease the serum concentrations of the other drug.

Tricyclic antidepressants: Valproate may increase serum concentrations and/or toxicity of tricyclic antidepressants.

Zidovudine: Valproic acid may increase the levels/effects of zidovudine; monitor.

Ethanol/Nutrition/Herb Interactions

Ethanol: Avoid ethanol (may increase CNS depression).

Food: Food may delay but does not affect the extent of absorption. Valproic acid serum concentrations may be decreased if taken with food. Milk has no effect on absorption.

Herb/Nutraceutical: Avoid evening primrose (seizure threshold decreased)

Test Interactions False-positive result for urine ketones; accuracy of thyroid function tests

Dietary Considerations Valproic acid may cause GI upset; take with large amount of water or food to decrease GI upset. May need to split doses to avoid GI upset.

Coated particles of divalproex sodium may be mixed with semisolid food (eg, applesauce or pudding) in patients having difficulty swallowing; particles should be swallowed and not chewed

Valproate sodium oral solution will generate valproic acid in carbonated beverages and may cause mouth and throat irritation; do not mix valproate sodium oral solution with carbonated beverages; sodium content of valproate sodium syrup (5 mL): 23 mg (1 mEq)

Dosage Forms Note: Strength expressed as valproic acid

Capsule, as valproic acid (Depakene®): 250 mg

Capsule, sprinkles, as divalproex sodium (Depakote® Sprinkle®): 125 mg

Injection, solution, as valproate sodium (Depacon®): 100 mg/mL (5 mL) [contains edetate disodium]

Syrup, as valproic acid: 250 mg/5 mL (480 mL)

Depakene®: 250 mg/5 mL (480 mL)

Tablet, delayed release, as divalproex sodium (Depakote®): 125 mg, 250 mg, 500 mg

Tablet, extended release, as divalproex sodium (Depakote® ER): 250 mg, 500 mg

References

Chez MG, Hammer MS, Loeffel M, et al, "Clinical Experience of Three Pediatric and One Adult Case of Spike-and-Wave Status Epilepticus Treated With Injectable Valproic Acid," *J Child Neurol*, 1999, 14(4):239-42.

Hovinga CA, Chicella MF, Rose DF, et al, "Use of Intravenous Valproate in Three Pediatric Patients With Nonconvulsive or Convulsive Status Epilepticus," *Ann Pharmacother*, 1999, 33(5):579-84.

Manno EM, "New Management Strategies in the Treatment of Status Epilepticus," *Mayo Clin Proc*, 2003, 78(4):508-18.

Venkataraman V and Wheless JW, "Safety of Rapid Intravenous Infusion of Valproate Loading Doses in Epilepsy Patients," *Epilepsy Res*, 1999, 35(2):147-53.

Valsartan (val SAR tan)

Medication Safety Issues

Sound-alike/look-alike issues:

Valsartan may be confused with losartan, Valstar™

Diovan® may be confused with Darvon®, Dioval®, Zyban®

Related Information

Angiotensin Agents *on page 1544*

U.S. Brand Names Diovan®

Canadian Brand Names Diovan®

Pharmacologic Category Angiotensin II Receptor Blocker

Generic Available No

Use Alone or in combination with other antihypertensive agents in the treatment of essential hypertension; treatment of heart failure (NYHA Class II-IV); reduction of cardiovascular mortality in patients with left ventricular dysfunction postmyocardial infarction

Mechanism of Action Valsartan produces direct antagonism of the angiotensin II (AT2) receptors, unlike the ACE inhibitors. It displaces angiotensin II from the AT1 receptor and produces its blood pressure lowering effects by antagonizing AT1-induced vasoconstriction, aldosterone release, catecholamine release, arginine vasopressin release, water intake, and hypertrophic responses. This action results in more efficient blockade of the cardiovascular effects of angiotensin II and fewer side effects than the ACE inhibitors.

Pharmacodynamics/Kinetics

Onset of antihypertensive effect: 2 weeks (maximal: 4 weeks)

Distribution: V_d: 17 L (adults)

Protein binding: 95%, primarily albumin

Metabolism: To inactive metabolite

Bioavailability: 25% (range 10% to 35%)

Half-life elimination: 6 hours

Time to peak, serum: 2-4 hours

Excretion: Feces (83%) and urine (13%) as unchanged drug

Dosage Adults: Oral:

Hypertension: Initial: 80 mg or 160 mg once daily (in patients who are not volume depleted); dose may be increased to achieve desired effect; maximum recommended dose: 320 mg/day

Heart failure: Initial: 40 mg twice daily; titrate dose to 80-160 mg twice daily, as tolerated; maximum daily dose: 320 mg

Left ventricular dysfunction after MI: Initial: 20 mg twice daily; titrate dose to target of 160 mg twice daily as tolerated; may initiate ≥12 hours following MI

Dosing adjustment in renal impairment: No dosage adjustment necessary if Cl_{cr} >10 mL/minute.

Dosing adjustment in hepatic impairment (mild - moderate): ≤80 mg/day

Dialysis: Not significantly removed

Stability Store at controlled room temperature of 15°C to 30°C (59°F to 86°F); protect from moisture

Administration Administer with or without food.

Monitoring Parameters Baseline and periodic electrolyte panels, renal function, BP; in CHF, serum potassium during dose escalation and periodically thereafter

Anesthesia and Critical Care Concerns/Other Considerations The angiotensin II receptor antagonists appear to have similar indications as the ACE inhibitors. In heart failure, the angiotensin II antagonists are especially useful in providing an alternative therapy in those patients who have intractable cough in response to ACE inhibitor therapy. Candesartan has been studied as an alternative therapy in chronic heart failure patients who cannot tolerate an ACE-I (CHARM-Alternative) and as an added therapy in heart failure patients who are maintained on an ACE-I (CHARM-Added). In both studies the combined endpoint of cardiovascular death or heart failure hospitalizations was significantly improved over the placebo treated group. Similar to ACE inhibitors, pre-existing volume depletion caused by diuretic therapy may potentiate hypotension in response to angiotensin II antagonists. Concomitant NSAID therapy may attenuate blood pressure control; use of NSAIDs should be avoided or limited, with monitoring of blood pressure control. In the setting of heart failure, NSAID use may be associated with an increased risk for fluid accumulation and edema.

Pregnancy Risk Factor C/D (2nd and 3rd trimesters)

Contraindications Hypersensitivity to valsartan or any component of the formulation; hypersensitivity to other A-II receptor antagonists; bilateral renal artery stenosis; pregnancy (2nd and 3rd trimesters)

Warnings/Precautions [U.S. Boxed Warning]: Based on human data, drugs that act on the angiotensin system can cause injury and death to the developing fetus when used in the second and third trimesters. Angiotensin receptor blockers should be discontinued as soon as possible once pregnancy is detected. During the initiation of therapy, hypotension may occur, particularly in patients with heart failure or post-MI patients. Avoid use or use a smaller dose in patients who are volume depleted; correct depletion first.

Deterioration in renal function can occur with initiation. Use with caution in unilateral renal artery stenosis and pre-existing renal insufficiency; significant aortic/mitral stenosis. Use caution in patients with severe renal impairment or significant hepatic dysfunction. Monitor renal function closely in patients with severe heart

(Continued)

Valsartan *(Continued)*

failure; changes in renal function should be anticipated and dosage adjustments of valsartan or concomitant medications may be needed.

Adverse Reactions

>10%: Central nervous system: Dizziness (2% to 17%)

1% to 10%:

Cardiovascular: Hypotension (6% to 7%), postural hypotension (2%)

Central nervous system: Fatigue (2% to 3%)

Endocrine & metabolic: Serum potassium increased (4% to 10%), hyperkalemia (<1% to 2%)

Gastrointestinal: Diarrhea (5%), abdominal pain (2%)

Hematologic: Neutropenia (2%)

Neuromuscular & skeletal: Arthralgia (3%), back pain (3%)

Renal: Creatinine increased >50% (4%)

Respiratory: Cough (3%)

Miscellaneous: Viral infection (3%)

All indications:

<1% (Limited to important or life-threatening): Allergic reactions, anemia, angioedema, anorexia, anxiety, asthenia, back pain, chest pain, constipation, dyspepsia, dyspnea, flatulence, hematocrit/hemoglobin decreased, hepatitis, impaired renal function, impotence, insomnia, muscle cramps, myalgia, palpitation, paresthesia, pruritus, rhabdomyolysis (rare), rash, renal dysfunction, somnolence, syncope, transaminases increased, vertigo, vomiting, xerostomia

Overdosage/Toxicology Only mild toxicity (hypotension, bradycardia, hyperkalemia) has been reported with large overdoses (up to 5 g of captopril and 300 mg of enalapril). No fatalities have been reported. Treatment is symptomatic. Not removed by hemodialysis.

Drug Interactions Inhibits CYP2C9 (weak)

Lithium: Risk of toxicity may be increased by valsartan; monitor lithium levels.

NSAIDs: May decrease angiotensin II antagonist efficacy; effect has been seen with losartan, but may occur with other medications in this class; monitor blood pressure

Potassium-sparing diuretics (amiloride, potassium, spironolactone, triamterene): Increased risk of hyperkalemia.

Potassium supplements may increase the risk of hyperkalemia.

Trimethoprim (high dose) may increase the risk of hyperkalemia.

Ethanol/Nutrition/Herb Interactions

Food: Decreases rate and extent of absorption by 50% and 40%, respectively.

Herb/Nutraceutical: Avoid dong quai if using for hypertension (has estrogenic activity). Avoid ephedra, yohimbe, ginseng (may worsen hypertension). Avoid garlic (may have increased antihypertensive effect).

Dietary Considerations Avoid salt substitutes which contain potassium. May be taken with or without food.

Dosage Forms Tablet: 40 mg, 80 mg, 160 mg, 320 mg

- **Vanceril® AEM (Can)** *see* Beclomethasone *on page 161*
- **Vancocin®** *see* Vancomycin *on page 1336*

Vancomycin (van koe MYE sin)

Medication Safety Issues

Sound-alike/look-alike issues:

I.V. vancomycin may be confused with Invanz®

Vancomycin may be confused with vecuronium

Related Information

Anesthesia for Patients With Liver Disease *on page 1421*

Prevention of Bacterial Endocarditis *on page 1583*

Prevention of Wound Infection and Sepsis in Surgical Patients *on page 1588*

U.S. Brand Names Vancocin®

Canadian Brand Names Vancocin®

Synonyms Vancomycin Hydrochloride

Pharmacologic Category Antibiotic, Miscellaneous

Generic Available Yes: Injection

Use Treatment of patients with infections caused by staphylococcal species and streptococcal species; used orally for staphylococcal enterocolitis or for antibiotic-associated pseudomembranous colitis produced by *C. difficile*

Mechanism of Action Inhibits bacterial cell wall synthesis by blocking glycopeptide polymerization through binding tightly to D-alanyl-D-alanine portion of cell wall precursor

Pharmacodynamics/Kinetics

Absorption: Oral: Poor; I.M.: Erratic; Intraperitoneal: ~38%

Distribution: Widely in body tissues and fluids. except for CSF

Relative diffusion from blood into CSF: Good only with inflammation (exceeds usual MICs)

CSF:blood level ratio: Normal meninges: Nil; Inflamed meninges: 20% to 30%

Protein binding: 10% to 50%

Half-life elimination: Biphasic: Terminal:

Newborns: 6-10 hours

Infants and Children 3 months to 4 years: 4 hours

Children >3 years: 2.2-3 hours

Adults: 5-11 hours; significantly prolonged with renal impairment

End-stage renal disease: 200-250 hours

Time to peak, serum: I.V.: 45-65 minutes

Excretion: I.V.: Urine (80% to 90% as unchanged drug); Oral: Primarily feces

Dosage Initial dosage recommendation:

Neonates: I.V.:

Postnatal age ≤7 days:

<1200 g: 15 mg/kg/dose every 24 hours

1200-2000 g: 10 mg/kg/dose every 12 hours

>2000 g: 15 mg/kg/dose every 12 hours

Postnatal age >7 days:

<1200 g: 15 mg/kg/dose every 24 hours

≥1200 g: 10 mg/kg/dose every 8 hours

Infants >1 month and Children: I.V.:

40 mg/kg/day in divided doses every 6 hours

Prophylaxis for bacterial endocarditis:

Dental, oral, or upper respiratory tract surgery: 20 mg/kg 1 hour prior to the procedure

GI/GU procedure: 20 mg/kg plus gentamicin 2 mg/kg 1 hour prior to surgery

Infants >1 month and Children with staphylococcal central nervous system infection: I.V.: 60 mg/kg/day in divided doses every 6 hours

Adults: I.V.:

With normal renal function: 1 g **or** 10-15 mg/kg/dose every 12 hours

Hospital"acquired pneumonia (HAP): 15 mg/kg/dose every 12 hours (American Thoracic Society/ATS guidelines)

Meningitis *(Pneumococcus* or *Staphylococcus)*: 30-45 mg/kg/day in divided doses every 8-12 hours **or** 500-750 mg every 6 hours (with third-generation cephalosporin for PCN-resistant *Streptococcus pneumoniae*); maximum dose: 2-3 g/day

Prophylaxis for bacterial endocarditis:

Dental, oral, or upper respiratory tract surgery: 1 g 1 hour before surgery

GI/GU procedure: 1 g plus 1.5 mg/kg gentamicin 1 hour prior to surgery

Antibiotic lock technique (for catheter infections): 2 mg/mL in SWI/NS or D_5W; instill 3-5 mL into catheter port as a flush solution instead of heparin lock (**Note:** Do not mix with any other solutions)

Intrathecal: Vancomycin is available as a powder for injection and may be diluted to 1-5 mg/mL concentration in preservative-free 0.9% sodium chloride for administration into the CSF

Neonates: 5-10 mg/day

Children: 5-20 mg/day

Adults: Up to 20 mg/day

Oral: Pseudomembranous colitis produced by *C. difficile*:

Neonates: 10 mg/kg/day in divided doses

Children: 40 mg/kg/day in divided doses, added to fluids

Adults: 125 mg 4 times/day for 10 days

Dosing interval in renal impairment (vancomycin levels should be monitored in patients with any renal impairment):

Cl_{cr} >60 mL/minute: Start with 1 g or 10-15 mg/kg/dose every 12 hours

Cl_{cr} 40-60 mL/minute: Start with 1 g or 10-15 mg/kg/dose every 24 hours

(Continued)

Vancomycin *(Continued)*

Cl_{cr} <40 mL/minute: Will need longer intervals; determine by serum concentration monitoring

Hemodialysis: Not dialyzable (0% to 5%); generally not removed; exception minimal-moderate removal by some of the newer high-flux filters; dose may need to be administered more frequently; monitor serum concentrations

Continuous ambulatory peritoneal dialysis (CAPD): Not significantly removed; administration via CAPD fluid: 15-30 mg/L (15-30 mcg/mL) of CAPD fluid

Continuous arteriovenous hemofiltration: Dose as for Cl_{cr} 10-40 mL/minute

Stability Reconstituted 500 mg and 1 g vials are stable for at either room temperature or under refrigeration for 14 days. **Note:** Vials contain no bacteriostatic agent. Solutions diluted for administration in either D_5W or NS are stable under refrigeration for 14 days or at room temperature for 7 days. Reconstitute vials with 20 mL of SWFI for each 1 g of vancomycin (10 mL/500 mg vial; 20 mL/1 g vial; 100 mL/5 g vial; 200 mL/10 g vial). The reconstituted solution must be further diluted with at least 100 mL of a compatible diluent per 500 mg of vancomycin prior to parenteral administration.

Intrathecal: Vancomycin is available as a powder for injection and may be diluted to 1-5 mg/mL concentration in preservative free 0.9% sodium chloride for administration into the CSF.

Administration Administer vancomycin by I.V. intermittent infusion over at least 60 minutes at a final concentration not to exceed 5 mg/mL. If a maculopapular rash appears on the face, neck, trunk, and/or upper extremities (Red man syndrome), slow the infusion rate to over 1½ to 2 hours and increase the dilution volume. Hypotension, shock, and cardiac arrest (rare) have also been reported with too rapid of infusion. Reactions are often treated with antihistamines and steroids.

Extravasation treatment: Monitor I.V. site closely; extravasation will cause serious injury with possible necrosis and tissue sloughing. Rotate infusion site frequently.

Monitoring Parameters Periodic renal function tests, urinalysis, serum vancomycin concentrations, WBC, audiogram

Reference Range

Timing of serum samples: Draw peak 1 hour after 1-hour infusion has completed; draw trough just before next dose

Therapeutic levels: Peak: 25-40 mcg/mL; Trough: 5-12 mcg/mL

Toxic: >80 mcg/mL (SI: >54 μmol/L)

The ATS guidelines recommend trough levels of 15-20 mcg/mL for hospital-acquired pneumonia. The Infectious Disease Society of America (ISDA) meningitis guidelines recommend trough levels of 15-20 mcg/mL.

Anesthesia and Critical Care Concerns/Other Considerations The "red man syndrome" (characterized by skin rash and hypotension) is not an allergic reaction, but rather is associated with infusion administered too rapidly. To alleviate or prevent the reaction, infuse vancomycin at a rate of ≥30 minutes for each 500 mg of drug being administered (eg, 1 g over ≥60 minutes; 1.5 g over ≥90 minutes). CVVHD clears vancomycin from the circulation while conventional hemodialysis does not.

Limitations which may contribute to clinical failure include poor lung penetration, slow bactericidal activity against *S. aureus*, limited CNS penetration, high-level resistance to enterococci and *S. aureus*, and limited activity against bacteria that coat prosthetic devices.

Pregnancy Risk Factor C

Contraindications Hypersensitivity to vancomycin or any component of the formulation; avoid in patients with previous severe hearing loss

Warnings/Precautions Use with caution in patients with renal impairment or those receiving other nephrotoxic or ototoxic drugs; dosage modification required in patients with impaired renal function (especially elderly)

Adverse Reactions

Oral:

>10%: Gastrointestinal: Bitter taste, nausea, vomiting, stomatitis

1% to 10%:

Central nervous system: Chills, drug fever

Hematologic: Eosinophilia

<1% (Limited to important or life-threatening): Interstitial nephritis, ototoxicity, renal failure, skin rash, thrombocytopenia, vasculitis

Parenteral:

>10%:

Cardiovascular: Hypotension accompanied by flushing

Dermatologic: Erythematous rash on face and upper body (red neck or red man syndrome)

1% to 10%:

Central nervous system: Chills, drug fever

Hematologic: Eosinophilia

<1% (Limited to important or life-threatening): Ototoxicity, renal failure, thrombocytopenia, vasculitis

Overdosage/Toxicology Symptoms of overdose include ototoxicity and nephrotoxicity. There is no specific therapy for overdose with vancomycin. Care is symptomatic and supportive. Peritoneal filtration and hemofiltration (not dialysis) have been shown to reduce the serum concentration of vancomycin. High flux dialysis may remove up to 25% of the drug.

Drug Interactions Increased toxicity: Anesthetic agents; other ototoxic or nephrotoxic agents

Dietary Considerations May be taken with food.

Dosage Forms

Capsule (Vancocin®): 125 mg, 250 mg

Infusion [premixed in iso-osmotic dextrose] (Vancocin®): 500 mg (100 mL); 1 g (200 mL)

Injection, powder for reconstitution: 500 mg, 1 g, 5 g, 10 g

References

American Thoracic Society and Infectious Diseases Society of America, "Guidelines for the Management of Adults With Hospital-Acquired, Ventilator-Associated, and Healthcare-Associated Pneumonia," *Am J Respir Crit Care Med*, 2005, 171(4):388-416.

Gilbert DN, Moellering RC, Eliopoulos GM, et al, eds, *The Sanford Guide To Antimicrobial Therapy*, 2006, 36th ed, Hyde Park, VT: Antimicrobial Therapy, Inc, 2006, 6-7.

Joy MS, Matzke GR, Frye RF, et al, "Determinants of Vancomycin Clearance by Continuous Veno-Venous Hemofiltration and Continuous Veno-Venous Hemodialysis," *Am J Kidney Dis*, 1998, 31(6):1019-27.

Murray BE, "Vancomycin-Resistant Enterococcal Infections," *N Engl J Med*, 2000, 342(10):710-21.

Tunkel AR, Hartman BJ, Kaplan SL, et al, "Practice Guidelines for the Management of Bacterial Meningitis," *Clin Infect Dis*, 2004, 39(9):1267-84.

♦ **Vancomycin Hydrochloride** *see* Vancomycin *on page 1336*

♦ **Vandazole™** *see* Metronidazole *on page 842*

♦ **Vaprisol®** *see* Conivaptan *on page 331*

♦ **VAQTA®** *see* Hepatitis A Vaccine *on page 616*

Vardenafil (var DEN a fil)

Medication Safety Issues

Sound-alike/look-alike issues:

Levitra® may be confused with Lexiva®

U.S. Brand Names Levitra®

Canadian Brand Names Levitra®

Synonyms Vardenafil Hydrochloride

Pharmacologic Category Phosphodiesterase-5 Enzyme Inhibitor

Generic Available No

Use Treatment of erectile dysfunction

Mechanism of Action Does not directly cause penile erections, but affects the response to sexual stimulation. The physiologic mechanism of erection of the penis involves release of nitric oxide (NO) in the corpus cavernosum during sexual stimulation. NO then activates the enzyme guanylate cyclase, which results in increased levels of cyclic guanosine monophosphate (cGMP), producing smooth muscle relaxation and inflow of blood to the corpus cavernosum. Vardenafil enhances the effect of NO by inhibiting phosphodiesterase type 5 (PDE-5), which is responsible for degradation of cGMP in the corpus cavernosum; when sexual stimulation causes local release of NO, inhibition of PDE-5 by vardenafil causes increased levels of cGMP in the corpus cavernosum, resulting in smooth muscle relaxation and inflow of blood to the corpus cavernosum; at recommended doses, it has no effect in the absence of sexual stimulation.

Pharmacodynamics/Kinetics

Absorption: Rapid

Distribution: V_d: 208 L; <0.01% found in semen 1.5 hours after dose

(Continued)

Vardenafil *(Continued)*

Metabolism: Hepatic via CYP3A4 (major), CYP2C and 3A5 (minor); forms metabolite (active)
Bioavailability: 15%; Elderly (≥65 years): 52%; Hepatic impairment (Child-Pugh class B): 160%
Half-life elimination: Terminal: Vardenafil and metabolite: 4-5 hours
Time to peak, plasma: 0.5-2 hours
Excretion: Feces (91% to 95% as metabolites); urine (2% to 6%)
Clearance: 56 L/hour

Dosage Oral: Adults: Erectile dysfunction: 10 mg 60 minutes prior to sexual activity; dosing range: 5-20 mg; to be given as one single dose and not given more than once daily

Dosing adjustment with concomitant medications:

Alpha blocker (dose should be stable at time of vardenafil initiation): Initial vardenafil dose: 5 mg/24 hours; if an alpha blocker is added to vardenafil therapy, it should be initiated at the smallest possible dose, and titrated carefully.

Erythromycin: Maximum vardenafil dose: 5 mg/24 hours
Indinavir: Maximum vardenafil dose: 2.5 mg/24 hours
Itraconazole:
200 mg/day: Maximum vardenafil dose: 5 mg/24 hours
400 mg/day: Maximum vardenafil dose: 2.5 mg/24 hours
Ketoconazole:
200 mg/day: Maximum vardenafil dose: 5 mg/24 hours
400 mg/day: Maximum vardenafil dose: 2.5 mg/24 hours
Ritonavir: Maximum vardenafil dose: 2.5 mg/72 hours

Elderly ≥65 years: Initial: 5 mg 60 minutes prior to sexual activity; to be given as one single dose and not given more than once daily

Dosage adjustment in renal impairment: Dose adjustment not needed for mild, moderate, or severe impairment; use has not been studied in patients on renal dialysis

Dosage adjustment in hepatic impairment: Child-Pugh class B: Initial: 5 mg 60 minutes prior to sexual activity (maximum dose: 10 mg); to be given as one single dose and not given more than once daily

Stability Store at controlled room temperature of 15°C to 30°C (59°F to 86°F).

Administration May be administered with or without food, 60 minutes prior to sexual activity.

Monitoring Parameters Monitor for response and adverse reactions.

Anesthesia and Critical Care Concerns/Other Considerations

Cardiovascular effects of PDE-5 inhibitors may be potentially hazardous in patients with:

- active coronary ischemia (not on nitrates)
- heart failure and with low blood pressure and low volume status
- complicated, multidrug antihypertensive regimens
- potential for drug-drug interactions that may prolong PDE-5 inhibitor half-life (eg, drugs that inhibit CYP3A4)

Vardenafil is selective for PDE-5 and has limited effect on PDE3, which controls cardiac contractility.

Pregnancy Risk Factor B

Contraindications Hypersensitivity to vardenafil or any component of the formulation; concurrent use of organic nitrates (nitroglycerin; scheduled dosing or as needed)

Warnings/Precautions There is a degree of cardiac risk associated with sexual activity; therefore, physicians may wish to consider the patient's cardiovascular status prior to initiating any treatment for erectile dysfunction. Use caution in patients with anatomical deformation of the penis (angulation, cavernosal fibrosis, or Peyronie's disease) and in patients who have conditions which may predispose them to priapism (sickle cell anemia, multiple myeloma, leukemia). Patients should be instructed to seek medical attention if erection persists >4 hours.

Not recommended for use in patients with congenital QT prolongation or those taking Class Ia or III antiarrhythmics. Concomitant use with alpha blockers may cause hypotension; safety of this combination may be affected by other antihypertensives and intravascular volume depletion. Patients should be hemodynamically stable prior to initiating therapy. Use caution with alpha blockers, effective CYP3A4 inhibitors, the elderly, or those with hepatic impairment (Child-Pugh class B); dosage adjustment is needed.

Rare cases of nonarteritic ischemic optic neuropathy (NAION) have been reported; risk may be increased with history of vision loss. Other risk factors for NAION include heart disease, diabetes, hypertension, smoking, age >50 years, or history of certain eye problems.

Safety and efficacy have not been studied in patients with the following conditions, therefore, use in these patients is not recommended at this time: Hypotension, uncontrolled hypertension, unstable angina, severe cardiac failure; a life-threatening arrhythmia, myocardial infarction, or stroke within the last 6 months; severe hepatic impairment (Child-Pugh class C); end-stage renal disease requiring dialysis; retinitis pigmentosa or other degenerative retinal disorders. The safety and efficacy of vardenafil with other treatments for erectile dysfunction have not been studied and are not recommended as combination therapy.

Adverse Reactions

>10%:

- Cardiovascular: Flushing (11%)
- Central nervous system: Headache (15%)

2% to 10%:

- Central nervous system: Dizziness (2%)
- Gastrointestinal: Dyspepsia (4%), nausea (2%)
- Neuromuscular & skeletal: CPK increased (2%)
- Respiratory: Rhinitis (9%), sinusitis (3%)
- Miscellaneous: Flu-like syndrome (3%)

<2% (Limited to important or life-threatening): Abnormal ejaculation, anaphylactic reaction, angina, arthralgia, dyspnea, hyper-/hypotension, insomnia, liver function tests abnormal, MI, myalgia, nonarteritic ischemic optic neuropathy (NAION), pain, photophobia, photosensitivity, postural hypotension, priapism, pruritus, rash, somnolence, syncope, tachycardia, tinnitus, vertigo, vision changes (including blurred vision, color changes, dimming)

Overdosage/Toxicology Doses of up to 120 mg caused back pain, myalgia, and/or abnormal vision in healthy volunteers. Treatment should be symptomatic and supportive.

Drug Interactions Substrate of CYP2C (minor), 3A5 (minor), 3A4 (major)

Alpha-blockers: May lead to significant hypotension in some patients; initiate vardenafil at lowest possible dose if patient is stabilized on alpha blocker. Initiate alpha-blocker at lowest possible dose and titrate cautiously in patients on a stable dose of vardenafil.

CYP3A4 inhibitors: May increase the levels/effects of vardenafil. Example inhibitors include azole antifungals, clarithromycin, diclofenac, doxycycline, erythromycin, imatinib, isoniazid, nefazodone, nicardipine, propofol, protease inhibitors, quinidine, telithromycin, and verapamil.

Erythromycin: Serum concentrations of vardenafil are increased fourfold when given with erythromycin. Dose of vardenafil should not exceed 5 mg/24 hours.

Indinavir: Serum concentrations of vardenafil are increased 16-fold; half-life is also increased. Dose of vardenafil should not exceed 2.5 mg/24 hours. Serum concentrations of indinavir may be decreased by vardenafil.

Itraconazole: Serum concentrations of vardenafil are increased. Dose of vardenafil should not exceed 5 mg/24 hours when used with itraconazole 200 mg/day or 2.5 mg/24 hours when used with itraconazole 400 mg/day

Ketoconazole: Serum concentrations of vardenafil are increased 10-fold when given with ketoconazole 200 mg/day. Dose of vardenafil should not exceed 5 mg/24 hours when used with ketoconazole 200 mg/day or 2.5 mg/24 hours when used with ketoconazole 400 mg/day

Nitroglycerin (or other nitrates): Concomitant use is contraindicated due to the potential for severe, potentially fatal, hypotensive responses.

Ritonavir: Serum concentrations of vardenafil are increased 49-fold; half-life of vardenafil is prolonged to 26 hours. Dose of vardenafil should not exceed 2.5 mg/72 hours. Serum concentrations of ritonavir may be decreased by vardenafil.

Ethanol/Nutrition/Herb Interactions

Food: High-fat meals decrease maximum serum concentration 18% to 50%. Serum concentrations/toxicity may be increased with grapefruit juice; avoid concurrent use.

Dietary Considerations May take with or without food

Dosage Forms Tablet: 2.5 mg, 5 mg, 10 mg, 20 mg

- **Vardenafil Hydrochloride** *see* Vardenafil *on page 1339*

Vasopressin (vay soe PRES in)

Medication Safety Issues

Sound-alike/look-alike issues:

Pitressin® may be confused with Pitocin®

U.S. Brand Names Pitressin®

Canadian Brand Names Pressyn®; Pressyn® AR

Synonyms ADH; Antidiuretic Hormone; 8-Arginine Vasopressin

Pharmacologic Category Antidiuretic Hormone Analog; Hormone, Posterior Pituitary

Generic Available No

Use Treatment of diabetes insipidus; prevention and treatment of postoperative abdominal distention; differential diagnosis of diabetes insipidus

Unlabeled/Investigational Use Adjunct in the treatment of GI hemorrhage and esophageal varices; pulseless arrest (ventricular tachycardia [VT]/ventricular fibrillation [VF], asystole/pulseless electrical activity [PEA]); vasodilatory shock (septic shock)

Mechanism of Action Increases cyclic adenosine monophosphate (cAMP) which increases water permeability at the renal tubule resulting in decreased urine volume and increased osmolality; causes peristalsis by directly stimulating the smooth muscle in the GI tract; direct vasoconstrictor without inotropic or chronotropic effects

Pharmacodynamics/Kinetics

Onset of action: Nasal: 1 hour

Duration: Nasal: 3-8 hours; I.M., SubQ: 2-8 hours

Metabolism: Nasal/Parenteral: Hepatic, renal

Half-life elimination: Nasal: 15 minutes; Parenteral: 10-20 minutes

Excretion: Nasal: Urine; SubQ: Urine (5% as unchanged drug) after 4 hours

Dosage

Diabetes insipidus (highly variable dosage; titrated based on serum and urine sodium and osmolality in addition to fluid balance and urine output):

I.M., SubQ:

Children: 2.5-10 units 2-4 times/day as needed

Adults: 5-10 units 2-4 times/day as needed (dosage range 5-60 units/day)

Continuous I.V. infusion: Children and Adults: 0.5 milliunit/kg/hour (0.0005 unit/kg/hour); double dosage as needed every 30 minutes to a maximum of 0.01 unit/kg/hour

Intranasal: Administer on cotton pledget, as nasal spray, or by dropper

Abdominal distention: Adults: I.M.: 5 units stat, 10 units every 3-4 hours

GI hemorrhage (unlabeled use): I.V. infusion: Dilute in NS or D_5W to 0.1-1 unit/mL

Children: Initial: 0.002-0.005 units/kg/minute; titrate dose as needed; maximum: 0.01 unit/kg/minute; continue at same dosage (if bleeding stops) for 12 hours, then taper off over 24-48 hours

Adults: Initial: 0.2-0.4 unit/minute, then titrate dose as needed, if bleeding stops; continue at same dose for 12 hours, taper off over 24-48 hours

Pulseless arrest (unlabeled use) [ACLS protocol]: Adults: I.V; I.O.: 40 units; may give one dose to replace first or second dose of epinephrine. I.V./I.O. drug administration is preferred, but if no access, may give endotracheally at 2 to 2 ½ times the I.V. dose. Mix with 5-10 mL of water or normal saline, and administer down the endotracheal tube.

Vasodilatory shock/septic shock (unlabeled use): Adults: I.V.: 0.01-0.04 units/minute for the treatment of septic shock. Doses >0.04 units/minute may have more cardiovascular side effects. Most case reports have used 0.04 units/minute continuous infusion as a fixed dose.

Dosing adjustment in hepatic impairment: Some patients respond to much lower doses with cirrhosis

Stability Store injection at room temperature; protect from heat and from freezing; use only clear solutions

Administration

I.V.: Use extreme caution to avoid extravasation because of risk of necrosis and gangrene. In treatment of varices, infusions are often supplemented with nitroglycerin infusions to minimize cardiac effects.

GI hemorrhage: Administration requires the use of an infusion pump and should be administered in a peripheral line.

Vasodilatory shock: Administration through a central catheter is recommended.

Infusion rates: 100 units in 500 mL D_5W rate

0.1 unit/minute: 30 mL/hour
0.2 unit/minute: 60 mL/hour
0.3 unit/minute: 90 mL/hour
0.4 unit/minute: 120 mL/hour
0.5 unit/minute: 150 mL/hour
0.6 unit/minute: 180 mL/hour

Intranasal (topical administration on nasal mucosa): Administer injectable vasopressin on cotton plugs, as nasal spray, or by dropper. Should not be inhaled.

Endotreacheal: If no I.V. /I.O. access may give endotracheally at 2 to 2½ times the I.V. dose. Mix with 5-10 mL of water or normal saline, and administer down the endotracheal tube.

Monitoring Parameters Serum and urine sodium, urine specific gravity, urine and serum osmolality; urine output, fluid input and output, blood pressure, heart rate

Reference Range Plasma: 0-2 pg/mL (SI: 0-2 ng/L) if osmolality <285 mOsm/L; 2-12 pg/mL (SI: 2-12 ng/L) if osmolality >290 mOsm/L

Anesthesia and Critical Care Concerns/Other Considerations

Shock: Low-dose vasopressin may be effective for the management of vasodilator shock. Vasopressin binds to different receptors than the catecholamine pressors. Vasoconstrictor effects are through the V_1 vascular receptors. In clinical studies and case reports, vasopressin increased blood pressure, systemic vascular resistance, and urine output. Vasopressin may decrease heart rate and cardiac output, especially at higher doses. Vasopressin has been used in doses of 0.01-0.1 units/minute. Doses >0.04 units/minute may have more cardiovascular effects (decreased cardiac output, asystole, cardiac ischemia). Use caution in patients with underlying cardiac dysfunction. Vasoconstriction appears to remain effective in severe acidosis. When possible, low-dose vasopressin should be infused via central catheter for the management of vasodilatory shock; peripheral administration has been associated with skin necrosis. The 2004 Surviving Sepsis Campaign Guidelines (Dellinger, 2004) suggest vasopressin use may be considered in patients with refractory shock despite adequate fluid resuscitation and high-dose conventional vasopressors. Pending the outcome of ongoing trials, it is not recommended as a replacement for norepinephrine or dopamine as a first-line agent.

Pulseless Arrest: A multicenter, double-blind, randomized, controlled trial evaluated the efficacy of vasopressin or epinephrine when administered to adult patients who suffered an out-of-hospital cardiac arrest (Wenzel V, 2004). For inclusions, patients presented with ventricular fibrillation, pulseless electrical activity, or asystole. They were excluded if they were successfully defibrillated without the administration of a vasopressor, had a terminal illness or had a DNR order, a lack of intravenous access, hemorrhagic shock, pregnancy, cardiac arrest due to trauma or were <18 years of age. Eligible patients were randomized to intravenous vasopressin (40 units) or epinephrine (1 mg). Each patient received an injection of the study drug, if spontaneous circulation was not restored in 3 minutes they received a second dose (same amount) of the same study drug. If there was no response, the managing physician had the option of giving epinephrine. Patients with ventricular fibrillation were randomized if the first three attempts at defibrillation failed; all others were randomized immediately. The primary endpoint was survival to hospital admission; the secondary endpoint was survival to hospital discharge. Five hundred and eighty-nine patients were randomized to vasopressin and 597 patients were randomized to epinephrine. There was no significant difference in the rate of hospital admission between the vasopressin group and the epinephrine group if they had ventricular fibrillation (46.2% vs 43% respectively, p: 0.48) or pulseless electrical activity (33.7% vs 30.5% respectively, p: 0.65). Patients with asystole responded significantly better to vasopressin; having higher rates of hospital admission (29% vs 20.3% in the epinephrine group, p: 0.02) and hospital discharge (4.7% vs 1.5% in the epinephrine group, p: 0.04). Patients who failed vasopressin therapy and received additional epinephrine had significant improvement in survival to hospital admission (25.7% vs 16.4% in the epinephrine group, p: 0.002) and discharge (6.2% vs 1.7%, p: 0.002). Similar patients who were randomized to epinephrine and failed to respond did not improve with additional epinephrine. Cerebral performance among all patients who survived to discharge was similar in both groups. In this trial, vasopressin was superior to epinephrine in patients with asystole. Vasopressin followed by epinephrine may be more effective than epinephrine alone in refractory out-of-hospital cardiac arrest.

(Continued)

Vasopressin *(Continued)*

A small in-hospital cardiac arrest study evaluated the efficacy of vasopressin or epinephrine in 200 patients. These investigators did not find any differences between the two treatment groups with regard to survival, discharge, or cerebral performance (Stiell, 2001).

Pregnancy Risk Factor C

Contraindications Hypersensitivity to vasopressin or any component of the formulation

Warnings/Precautions Use with caution in patients with seizure disorders, migraine, asthma, vascular disease, renal disease, cardiac disease; chronic nephritis with nitrogen retention. Goiter with cardiac complications, arteriosclerosis; I.V. infiltration may lead to severe vasoconstriction and localized tissue necrosis; also, gangrene of extremities, tongue, and ischemic colitis. Elderly patients should be cautioned not to increase their fluid intake beyond that sufficient to satisfy their thirst in order to avoid water intoxication and hyponatremia; under experimental conditions, the elderly have shown to have a decreased responsiveness to vasopressin with respect to its effects on water homeostasis

Adverse Reactions Frequency not defined.

Cardiovascular: Arrhythmia, asystole (>0.4 units/minute), blood pressure increased, cardiac output decreased (>0.4 units/minute), chest pain, MI, vasoconstriction (with higher doses), venous thrombosis

Central nervous system: Pounding in the head, fever, vertigo

Dermatologic: Ischemic skin lesions, circumoral pallor, urticaria

Gastrointestinal: Abdominal cramps, flatulence, mesenteric ischemia, nausea, vomiting

Genitourinary: Uterine contraction

Neuromuscular & skeletal: Tremor

Respiratory: Bronchial constriction

Miscellaneous: Diaphoresis

Overdosage/Toxicology Symptoms of overdose include drowsiness, weight gain, confusion, listlessness, and water intoxication. Water intoxication requires withdrawal of the drug. Severe intoxication may require osmotic diuresis and loop diuretics.

Drug Interactions

Decreased effect: Lithium, epinephrine, demeclocycline, heparin, and ethanol block antidiuretic activity to varying degrees

Increased effect: Chlorpropamide, phenformin, urea and fludrocortisone potentiate antidiuretic response

Ethanol/Nutrition/Herb Interactions Ethanol: Avoid ethanol (due to effects on ADH).

Dosage Forms

Injection, solution: 20 units/mL (0.5 mL, 1 mL, 10 mL)

Pitressin®: 20 units/mL (1 mL)

References

"2005 American Heart Association Guidelines for Cardiopulmonary Resuscitation and Emergency Cardiovascular Care," *Circulation*, 2005, 112(24 Suppl): 1-211.

Aung K and Htay T, "Vasopressin for Cardiac Arrest: A Systematic Review and Meta-Analysis," *Arch Intern Med*, 2005, 165(1):17-24.

Dellinger RP, Carlet JM, Masur H, et al, "Surviving Sepsis Campaign Guidelines for Management of Severe Sepsis and Septic Shock," *Crit Care Med*, 2004, 32(3):858-73.

Dunser MW, Mayr AJ, Ulmer H, et al, "The Effects of Vasopressin on Systemic Hemodynamics in Catecholamine-Resistant Septic and Postcardiotomy Shock: A Retrospective Analysis," *Anest Analg*, 2001, 93(1):7-13.

Gazmuri RJ and Shakeri SA, "Low-Dose Vasopressin for Reversing Vasodilation During Septic Shock," *Crit Care Med*, 2001, 29(3):673-5.

Holmes CL, Walley KR, Chittock DR, et al, "The Effects of Vasopressin on Hemodynamics and Renal Function in Severe Septic Shock: A Case Series," *Inten Care Med*, 2001, 27(8):1416-21.

Kahn JM, Kress JP, and Hall JB, "Skin Necrosis After Extravasation of Low-Dose Vasopressin Administered for Septic Shock," *Crit Care Med*, 2002, 30(8):1899-901.

Landry DW, Levin HR, Gallant EM, et al, "Vasopressin Deficiency Contributes to the Vasodilation of Septic Shock," *Circulation*, 1997, 95(5):1122-5.

Malay MB, Ashton RC, Landry DW, et al, "Low-Dose Vasopressin in the Treatment of Vasodilatory Septic Shock," *J Trauma*, 1999, 47(4):699-705.

Reid IA, "Role of Vasopressin Deficiency in the Vasodilation of Septic Shock," *Circulation*, 1997, 95(5):1108-10.

Rozenfeld V and Cheng JW, "The Role of Vasopressin in the Treatment of Vasodilation in Shock States," *Ann Pharmacother*, 2000, 34(2):250-4.

Stiell IG, Hebert PC, Wells GA, et al, "Vasopressin Versus Epinephrine for in Hospital Cardiac Arrest: A Randomised Controlled Trial," *Lancet*, 2001, 358(9276):105-9.

Tsuneyoshi I, Yamada H, Kakihana Y, et al, "Hemodynamic and Metabolic Effects of Low-Dose Vasopressin Infusions in Vasodilatory Septic Shock," *Crit Care Med*, 2001, 29(3):487-93.

Tuggle DW, Bennett KG, Scott J, et al, "Intravenous Vasopressin and Gastrointestinal Hemorrhage in Children," *J Pediatr Surg*, 1988, 23(7):627-9.

Wenzel V, Krismer AC, Arntz HR, et al, "A Comparison of Vasopressin and Epinephrine for Out-of-Hospital Cardiopulmonary Resuscitation," *N Engl J Med*, 2004, 350(2):105-13.

♦ **Vasotec®** *see* Enalapril *on page 446*

Vecuronium (ve KYOO roe ni um)

Medication Safety Issues

Sound-alike/look-alike issues:

Vecuronium may be confused with vancomycin

Norcuron® may be confused with Narcan®

High alert medication: The Institute for Safe Medication Practices (ISMP) includes this medication among its list of drugs which have a heightened risk of causing significant patient harm when used in error.

Related Information

Chronic Renal Failure *on page 1437*

Neuromuscular Blocking Agents *on page 1572*

U.S. Brand Names Norcuron® [DSC]

Canadian Brand Names Norcuron®

Synonyms ORG NC 45

Pharmacologic Category Neuromuscular Blocker Agent, Nondepolarizing

Generic Available Yes

Use Adjunct to general anesthesia to facilitate endotracheal intubation and to relax skeletal muscles during surgery; to facilitate mechanical ventilation in ICU patients; does not relieve pain or produce sedation

Mechanism of Action Blocks acetylcholine from binding to receptors on motor endplate inhibiting depolarization

Pharmacodynamics/Kinetics

Onset of action:

Good intubation conditions: Within 2.5-3 minutes

Maximum neuromuscular blockade: Within 3-5 minutes

Duration: 20-40 minutes

Metabolism: Active metabolite: 3-desacetyl vecuronium (1/2 the activity of parent drug)

Half-life elimination: 51-80 minutes

Excretion: Primarily feces (40% to 75%); urine (30% as unchanged drug and metabolites)

Dosage Administer I.V.; dose to effect; doses will vary due to interpatient variability; use ideal body weight for obese patients

Surgery:

Neonates: 0.1 mg/kg/dose; maintenance: 0.03-0.15 mg/kg every 1-2 hours as needed

Infants >7 weeks to 1 year: Initial: 0.08-0.1 mg/kg/dose; maintenance: 0.05-0.1 mg/kg every 60 minutes as needed

Children >1 year and Adults: Initial: 0.08-0.1 mg/kg or 0.04-0.06 mg/kg after initial dose of succinylcholine for intubation; maintenance: 0.01-0.015 mg/kg 25-40 minutes after initial dose, then 0.01-0.015 mg/kg every 12-15 minutes (higher doses will allow less frequent maintenance doses); may be administered as a continuous infusion at 0.8-2 mcg/kg/minute

Pretreatment/priming: Adults: 10% of intubating dose given 3-5 minutes before initial dose

ICU: Adults: 0.05-0.1 mg/kg bolus followed by 0.8-1.7 mcg/kg/minute once initial recovery from bolus observed or 0.1-0.2 mg/kg/dose every 1 hour

Note: Children (1-10 years) may require slightly higher initial doses and slightly more frequent supplementation; infants >7 weeks to 1 year may be more sensitive to vecuronium and have a longer recovery time

Dosing adjustment in renal impairment: Prolongation of blockade

Dosing adjustment in hepatic impairment: Dose reductions are necessary in patients with cirrhosis or cholestasis

Stability Store intact vials of powder for injection at room temperature 15°C to 30°C (59°F to 86°F). Vials reconstituted with bacteriostatic water for injection (BWFI) may be stored for 5 days under refrigeration or at room temperature. Vials reconstituted with other compatible diluents (nonbacteriostatic) should be stored

(Continued)

Vecuronium *(Continued)*

under refrigeration and used within 24 hours. Reconstitute with compatible solution for injection to final concentration of 1 mg/mL. Stable in D_5W, D_5NS, LR, NS, SWI, BWFI.

Administration Concentration of 1 mg/mL may be administered by rapid I.V. injection. May further dilute reconstituted vial to 0.1-0.2 mg/mL in a compatible solution for I.V. infusion. Concentration of 1 mg/mL may be used for I.V. infusion in fluid-restricted patients.

Monitoring Parameters Blood pressure, heart rate

Anesthesia and Critical Care Concerns/Other Considerations Classified as an intermediate duration neuromuscular-blocking agent; produces minimal, if any, histamine release.

Critically-Ill Adult Patients:

The 2004 Surviving Sepsis Campaign guidelines recommend avoiding use of neuromuscular blockers if at all possible in the septic patient due to the risk of prolonged neuromuscular blockade following discontinuation. If one is required, monitor carefully and observe the following recommendations.

The 2002 ACCM/SCCM/ASHP clinical practice guidelines for sustained neuromuscular blockade in the adult critically-ill patient recommend:

Optimize sedatives and analgesics prior to initiation and monitor and adjust accordingly during course. Neuromuscular blockers do not relieve pain or produce sedation.

Protect patient's eyes from development of keratitis and corneal abrasion by administering ophthalmic ointment and taping eyelids closed or using eye patches. Reposition patient routinely to protect pressure points from breakdown. Address DVT prophylaxis.

Concurrent use of a neuromuscular blocker and corticosteroids appear to increase the risk of certain ICU myopathies; avoid or administer the corticosteroid at the lowest dose possible. Reassess need for neuromuscular blocker daily.

Using daily drug holidays (stopping neuromuscular-blocking agent until patient requires it again) may decrease the incidence of acute quadriplegic myopathy syndrome.

Tachyphylaxis can develop; switch to another neuromuscular blocker (taking into consideration the patient's organ function) if paralysis is still necessary.

Atracurium or cisatracurium is recommended for patients with significant hepatic or renal disease, due to organ-independent Hofmann elimination.

Monitor patients clinically and via "Train of Four" (TOF) testing with a goal of adjusting the degree of blockade to 1-2 twitches or based upon the patient's clinical condition.

Pregnancy Risk Factor C

Contraindications Hypersensitivity to vecuronium or any component of the formulation

Warnings/Precautions Ventilation must be supported during neuromuscular blockade; certain clinical conditions may result in potentiation or antagonism of neuromuscular blockade:

Potentiation: Electrolyte abnormalities, severe hyponatremia, severe hypocalcemia, severe hypokalemia, hypermagnesemia, neuromuscular diseases, acidosis, acute intermittent porphyria, renal failure, hepatic failure

Antagonism: Alkalosis, hypercalcemia, demyelinating lesions, peripheral neuropathies, diabetes mellitus

Increased sensitivity in patients with myasthenia gravis, Eaton-Lambert syndrome; resistance in burn patients (>30% of body) for period of 5-70 days postinjury; resistance in patients with muscle trauma, denervation, immobilization, infection; use with caution in patients with hepatic or renal impairment; does not counteract bradycardia produced by anesthetics/vagal stimulation. Cross-sensitivity with other neuromuscular-blocking agents may occur; use extreme caution in patients with previous anaphylactic reactions.

Adverse Reactions <1% (Limited to important or life-threatening): Bradycardia, circulatory collapse, edema, flushing, hypersensitivity reaction, hypotension, itching, rash, tachycardia, acute quadriplegic myopathy syndrome (prolonged use), myositis ossificans (prolonged use)

Overdosage/Toxicology

Symptoms of overdose include prolonged skeletal muscle weakness and apnea cardiovascular collapse.

Use neostigmine, edrophonium, or pyridostigmine with atropine to antagonize skeletal muscle relaxation; support of ventilation and the cardiovascular system through mechanical means, fluids, and pressors may be necessary.

Drug Interactions Increased toxicity/effect with aminoglycosides, ketamine, magnesium sulfate, verapamil, quinidine, clindamycin, furosemide

Dosage Forms Injection, powder for reconstitution, as bromide: 10 mg, 20 mg [may be supplied with diluent containing benzyl alcohol]

References

Dellinger RP, Carlet JM, Masur H, et al, "Surviving Sepsis Campaign Guidelines for Management of Severe Sepsis and Septic Shock," *Crit Care Med*, 2004, 32(3):858-73.

Murray MJ, Cowen J, DeBlock H, et al, "Clinical Practice Guidelines for Sustained Neuromuscular Blockade in the Adult Critically Ill Patient. Task Force of the American College of Critical Care Medicine (ACCM) of the Society of Critical Care Medicine (SCCM), American Society of Health-System Pharmacists, American College of Chest Physicians," *Crit Care Med*, 2002, 30(1):142-56; viewable at http://www.sccm.org/pdf/NeuromuscularBlockade.pdf.

Venlafaxine (VEN la faks een)

Related Information

Antidepressant Agents *on page 1551*
Chronic Pain Management *on page 1430*

U.S. Brand Names Effexor®; Effexor® XR

Canadian Brand Names Effexor® XR

Pharmacologic Category Antidepressant, Serotonin/Norepinephrine Reuptake Inhibitor

Restrictions A medication guide concerning the use of antidepressants in children and teenagers can be found on the FDA website at http://www.fda.gov/cder/Offices/ODS/labeling.htm. It should be dispensed to parents or guardians of children and teenagers receiving this medication.

Generic Available No

Use Treatment of major depressive disorder; generalized anxiety disorder (GAD), social anxiety disorder (social phobia); panic disorder

Unlabeled/Investigational Use Obsessive-compulsive disorder (OCD); hot flashes; neuropathic pain; attention-deficit/hyperactivity disorder (ADHD)

Mechanism of Action Venlafaxine and its active metabolite o-desmethylvenlafaxine (ODV) are potent inhibitors of neuronal serotonin and norepinephrine reuptake and weak inhibitors of dopamine reuptake. Venlafaxine and ODV have no significant activity for muscarinic cholinergic, H_1-histaminergic, or alpha$_2$-adrenergic receptors. Venlafaxine and ODV do not possess MAO-inhibitory activity.

Pharmacodynamics/Kinetics

Absorption: Oral: 92% to 100%; food has no significant effect on the absorption of venlafaxine or formation of the active metabolite O-desmethylvenlafaxine (ODV)

Distribution: At steady state: Venlafaxine 7.5 ± 3.7 L/kg, ODV 5.7 ± 1.8 L/Kg

Protein binding: Bound to human plasma protein: Venlafaxine 27%, ODV 30%

Metabolism: Hepatic via CYP2D6 to active metabolite, O-desmethylvenlafaxine (ODV); other metabolites include N-desmethylvenlafaxine and N,O-didesmethylvenlafaxine

Bioavailability: Absolute: ~45%

Half-life elimination: Venlafaxine: 3-7 hours; ODV: 9-13 hours; Steady-state, plasma: Venlafaxine/ODV: Within 3 days of multiple-dose therapy; prolonged with cirrhosis (Adults: Venlafaxine: ~30%, ODV: ~60%) and with dialysis (Adults: Venlafaxine: ~180%, ODV: ~142%)

Time to peak:

- Immediate release: Venlafaxine: 2 hours, ODV: 3 hours
- Extended release: Venlafaxine: 5.5 hours, ODV: 9 hours

Excretion: Urine (~87%, 5% as unchanged drug, 29% as unconjugated ODV, 26% as conjugated ODV, 27% as minor inactive metabolites) within 48 hours

Clearance at steady state: Venlafaxine: 1.3 ± 0.6 L/hour/kg, ODV: 0.4 ± 0.2 L/hour/kg

Clearance decreased with:

- Cirrhosis: Adults: Venlafaxine: ~50%, ODV: ~30%
- Severe cirrhosis: Adults: Venlafaxine: ~90%
- Renal impairment (Cl_{cr} 10-70 mL/minute): Adults: Venlafaxine: ~24%
- Dialysis: Adults: Venlafaxine: ~57%, ODV: ~56%; due to large volume of distribution, a significant amount of drug is not likely to be removed.

(Continued)

Venlafaxine *(Continued)*

Dosage Oral:

Children and Adolescents:

ADHD (unlabeled use): Initial: 12.5 mg/day

Children <40 kg: Increase by 12.5 mg/week to maximum of 50 mg/day in 2 divided doses

Children ≥40 kg: Increase by 25 mg/week to maximum of 75 mg/day in 3 divided doses.

Mean dose: 60 mg or 1.4 mg/kg administered in 2-3 divided doses

Adults:

Depression:

Immediate-release tablets: 75 mg/day, administered in 2 or 3 divided doses, taken with food; dose may be increased in 75 mg/day increments at intervals of at least 4 days, up to 225-375 mg/day

Extended-release capsules: 75 mg once daily taken with food; for some new patients, it may be desirable to start at 37.5 mg/day for 4-7 days before increasing to 75 mg once daily; dose may be increased by up to 75 mg/day increments every 4 days as tolerated, up to a maximum of 225 mg/day

GAD, social anxiety disorder: Extended-release capsules: 75 mg once daily taken with food; for some new patients, it may be desirable to start at 37.5 mg/day for 4-7 days before increasing to 75 mg once daily; dose may be increased by up to 75 mg/day increments every 4 days as tolerated, up to a maximum of 225 mg/day

Panic disorder: Extended-release capsules: 37.5 mg once daily for 1 week; may increase to 75 mg daily, with subsequent weekly increases of 75 mg/day up to a maximum of 225 mg/day.

Obsessive-compulsive disorder (unlabeled use): Titrate to usual dosage range of 150-300 mg/day; however, doses up to 375 mg daily have been used; response may be seen in 4 weeks

Neuropathic pain (unlabeled use): Dosages evaluated varied considerably based on etiology of chronic pain, but efficacy has been shown for many conditions in the range of 75-225 mg/day; onset of relief may occur in 1-2 weeks, or take up to 6 weeks for full benefit.

Hot flashes (unlabeled use): Doses of 37.5-75 mg/day have demonstrated significant improvement of vasomotor symptoms after 4-8 weeks of treatment; in one study, doses >75 mg/day offered no additional benefit; however, higher doses (225 mg/day) may be beneficial in patients with perimenopausal depression.

Attention-deficit disorder (unlabeled use): Initial: Doses vary between 18.75 to 75 mg/day; may increase after 4 weeks to 150 mg/day; if tolerated, doses up to 225 mg/day have been used

Note: When discontinuing this medication after more than 1 week of treatment, it is generally recommended that the dose be tapered. If venlafaxine is used for 6 weeks or longer, the dose should be tapered over 2 weeks when discontinuing its use.

Dosing adjustment in renal impairment: Cl_{cr} 10-70 mL/minute: Decrease dose by 25%; decrease total daily dose by 50% if dialysis patients; dialysis patients should receive dosing after completion of dialysis

Dosing adjustment in moderate hepatic impairment: Reduce total daily dosage by 50%

Administration Administer with food.

Extended release capsule: Swallow capsule whole; do not crush or chew. Alternatively, contents may be sprinkled on a spoonful of applesauce and swallowed immediately without chewing; followed with a glass of water to ensure complete swallowing of the pellets.

Monitoring Parameters Blood pressure should be regularly monitored, especially in patients with a high baseline blood pressure; may cause mean increase in heart rate of 4-9 beats/minute; cholesterol; mental status for depression, suicidal ideation (especially at the beginning of therapy or when doses are increased or decreased), anxiety, social functioning, mania, panic attacks; height and weight should be monitored in children

Reference Range Peak serum level of 163 ng/mL (325 ng/mL of ODV metabolite) obtained after a 150 mg oral dose

Pregnancy Risk Factor C

Contraindications Hypersensitivity to venlafaxine or any component of the formulation; use of MAO inhibitors within 14 days; should not initiate MAO inhibitor within 7 days of discontinuing venlafaxine

Warnings/Precautions

Major psychiatric warnings:

- **[U.S. Boxed Warning]: Antidepressants increase the risk of suicidal thinking and behavior in children and adolescents with major depressive disorder (MDD) and other depressive disorders;** consider risk prior to prescribing. Closely monitor for clinical worsening, suicidality, or unusual changes in behavior; the child's family or caregiver should be instructed to closely observe the patient and communicate condition with healthcare provider. A medication guide concerning the use of antidepressants in children and teenagers should be dispensed with each prescription. **Venlafaxine is not FDA approved for use in children.**
- The possibility of a suicide attempt is inherent in major depression and may persist until remission occurs. Patients treated with antidepressants should be observed for clinical worsening and suicidality, especially during the initial few months of a course of drug therapy, or at times of dose changes, either increases or decreases. Worsening depression and severe abrupt suicidality that are not part of the presenting symptoms may require discontinuation or modification of drug therapy. Use caution in high-risk patients during initiation of therapy.
- Prescriptions should be written for the smallest quantity consistent with good patient care. The patient's family or caregiver should be alerted to monitor patients for the emergence of suicidality and associated behaviors such as anxiety, agitation, panic attacks, insomnia, irritability, hostility, impulsivity, akathisia, hypomania, and mania; patients should be instructed to notify their healthcare provider if any of these symptoms or worsening depression or psychosis occur.
- May worsen psychosis in some patients or precipitate a shift to mania or hypomania in patients with bipolar disorder. Monotherapy in patients with bipolar disorder should be avoided. Patients presenting with depressive symptoms should be screened for bipolar disorder. **Venlafaxine is not FDA approved for the treatment of bipolar depression.**

Key adverse effects:

- CNS depression: Has a low potential to impair cognitive or motor performance; caution operating hazardous machinery or driving.
- SIADH and hyponatremia: Has been associated with the development of SIADH; hyponatremia has been reported rarely, predominately in the elderly
- Weight loss and anorectic effects: Have been observed in both pediatric and adult patients; weight loss was not limited to those experiencing reduced appetite
- Reduced growth rate (pediatric): Small differences in height have been observed in pediatric patients receiving venlafaxine, particularly those <12 years of age, compared to placebo

Concurrent disease:

- Anxiety/Insomnia: May cause increase in anxiety, nervousness, and insomnia.
- Hepatic impairment: Use caution; clearance is decreased and plasma concentrations are increased; a lower dosage may be needed.
- Hypercholesterolemia: May cause increases to serum cholesterol.
- Hypertension/Tachycardia: May cause sustained increase in blood pressure or tachycardia. Control pre-existing hypertension perior to initiation of venlafaxine. Use caution in patients with recent history of MI, unstable heart disease, or hyperthyroidism. Effect is dose related and increases are generally modest (12-15 mmHg diastolic).
- Narrow-angle glaucoma: May cause mydriasis; use caution in patients with increased intraocular pressure or at risk of acute narrow-angle glaucoma.
- Platelet aggregation: May impair platelet aggregation, resulting in bleeding.
- Renal impairment: Use caution; clearance is decreased and plasma concentrations are increased; a lower dosage may be needed.
- Seizure disorders: Use caution with a previous seizure disorder or condition predisposing to seizures such as brain damage or alcoholism.
- Sexual dysfunction: May cause or exacerbate sexual dysfunction.
- Weight loss: May cause weight loss; use caution in patients where weight loss is undesirable.

(Continued)

Venlafaxine *(Continued)*

Concurrent drug therapy:

- Agents which lower seizure threshold: Concurrent therapy with other drugs which lower the seizure threshold.
- Anticoagulants/Antiplatelets: Use caution with concomitant use of NSAIDs, ASA, or other drugs that affect coagulation; the risk of bleeding is potentiated.
- CNS depressants: Use caution with concomitant therapy.
- MAO inhibitors: Potential for severe reaction when used with MAO inhibitors; autonomic instability, coma, death, delirium, diaphoresis, hyperthermia, mental status changes/agitation, muscular rigidity, myoclonus, neuroleptic malignant syndrome features, and seizures may occur.
- Agents causing weight loss or anorectic effects should be avoided.

Special notes:

- Electroconvulsive therapy: May increase the risks associated with electroconvulsive therapy; consider discontinuing, when possible, prior to ECT treatment.
- Withdrawal syndrome: May cause dysphoric mood, irritability, agitation, dizziness, sensory disturbances, anxiety, confusion, headache, lethargy, emotional lability, insomnia, hypomania, tinnitus, and seizures. Upon discontinuation of venlafaxine therapy, gradually taper dose. If intolerable symptoms occur following a decrease in dosage or upon discontinuation of therapy, then resuming the previous dose with a more gradual taper should be considered.

Adverse Reactions

>10%:

Central nervous system: Headache (25% to 34%), insomnia (15% to 23%), somnolence (12% to 23%), dizziness (11% to 20%), nervousness (6% to 13%)

Gastrointestinal: Nausea (21% to 37%), xerostomia (12% to 22%), anorexia (8% to 20%), constipation (8% to 15%)

Genitourinary: Abnormal ejaculation/orgasm (2% to 16%)

Neuromuscular & skeletal: Weakness (8% to 17%)

Miscellaneous: Diaphoresis (10% to 14%)

1% to 10%:

Cardiovascular: Hypertension (dose related; 3% in patients receiving <100 mg/day, up to 13% in patients receiving >300 mg/day); vasodilation (3% to 4%); palpitation (3%), tachycardia (2%), chest pain (2%), postural hypotension (1%), edema

Central nervous system: Abnormal dreams (3% to 7%), anxiety (5% to 6%), yawning (3% to 5%), agitation (2% to 4%), chills (3%), confusion (2%), abnormal thinking (2%), depersonalization (1%), depression (1% to 3%), fever, migraine, amnesia, hypoethesia, trismus, vertigo

Dermatologic: Rash (3%), pruritus (1%), bruising

Endocrine & metabolic: Libido decreased (3% to 9%)

Gastrointestinal: Diarrhea (6% to 8%), vomiting (3% to 6%), dyspepsia (5%), abdominal pain (4%), flatulence (3% to 4%), taste perversion (2%), weight loss (1% to 4%), appetite increased, weight gain

Genitourinary: Impotence (4% to 10%), urinary frequency (3%), impaired urination (2%), urinary retention (1%), prostatic disorder

Neuromuscular & skeletal: Tremor (4% to 5%), hypertonia (3%), paresthesia (2% to 3%), twitching (1% to 2%), neck pain, arthralgia

Ocular: Abnormal or blurred vision (4% to 6%), mydriasis (2%)

Otic: Tinnitus (2%)

Respiratory: Pharyngitis (7%), sinusitis (2%), cough increased, dyspnea

Miscellaneous: Infection (6%), flu-like syndrome (6%), trauma (2%)

<1% (Limited to important or life-threatening): Agranulocytosis, anaphylaxis, aplastic anemia, aneurysm, angina pectoris, anuria; arrhythmia (including atrial and ventricular tachycardia, fibrillation and torsade de pointes); arteritis, asthma, ataxia, atelectasis, atrioventricular block, bacteremia, basophilia, bigeminy, biliary pain, bilirubinemia, bleeding time increased, bradycardia, bradykinesia, BUN increased, bundle branch block, carcinoma, cardiovascular disorder (mitral valve and circulatory disturbance), cataract, catatonia, cellulitis, cerebral ischemia, cholelithiasis, congestive heart failure, coronary artery disease, creatinine increased, crystalluria, cyanosis, deafness, DVT, dehydration, delusions, dementia, diabetes mellitus, dystonia, EKG abnormalities (including QT prolongation), electrolyte abnormalities, embolus, eosinophilia,

exfoliative dermatitis, erythema multiforme, extrapyramidal symptoms, extrasystoles, facial paralysis, fasciitis, gastrointestinal ulcer, glaucoma, Guillain-Barré syndrome, heart arrest, hematemesis, hematoma; hemorrhage (eye, GI, mucocutaneous, rectal); hepatitis, homicidal ideation, hostility, hyperacusis, hypercalcinuria, hyperchlorhydria, hyper-/hypocholesteremia, hyper-/hypoglycemia, hyperlipemia, hyper-/hypothyroidism, hyperuricemia, hypokalemia, hyponatremia, hypophosphatemia, hypoproteinemia, hypotension, intestinal obstruction, jaundice, kidney function abnormal, larynx edema, leukocytosis, leukoderma, leukopenia, liver enzymes increased, loss of consciousness, lymphadenopathy, lymphocytosis, maculopapular rash, menstrual abnormalities, miliaria, moniliasis, multiple myeloma, myasthenia, myocardial infarct, myoclonus, myopathy, neck rigidity, neuroleptic malignant-like syndrome, neuropathy, neutropenia, osteoporosis, pancytopenia, pleurisy, pneumonia, pyelonephritis, pyuria, rhabdomyolysis, rheumatoid arthritis, seizure, serotonin syndrome, SIADH, skin atrophy, Stevens-Johnson syndrome, suicidal ideation (reported at a frequency up to 2% in children/adolescents with major depressive disorder), suicide attempt, syncope, tendon rupture, thrombocythemia, thrombocytopenia, thrombophlebitis, toxic epidermal necrolysis, withdrawal syndrome

Overdosage/Toxicology Symptoms of overdose include somnolence and occasionally tachycardia. Predominantly occurs in combination with ethanol and/or other drug use. Most overdoses resolve with only supportive treatment, though ECG monitoring would be prudent considering the risk of arrythmia. Use of activated charcoal, inductions of emesis, or gastric lavage should be considered for acute ingestion. Forced diuresis, dialysis, and hemoperfusion not effective due to large volume of distribution.

Drug Interactions **Substrate** of CYP2C9 (minor), 2C19 (minor), 2D6 (major), 3A4 (major); **Inhibits** CYP2B6 (weak), 2D6 (weak), 3A4 (weak)

Buspirone: Concurrent use may result in serotonin syndrome; these combinations are best avoided

Clozapine: Addition of venlafaxine has been associated with case reports of increased clozapine serum concentrations and seizures.

CYP2D6 inhibitors: May increase the levels/effects of venlafaxine. Example inhibitors include chlorpromazine, delavirdine, fluoxetine, miconazole, paroxetine, pergolide, quinidine, quinine, ritonavir, and ropinirole.

CYP3A4 inducers: CYP3A4 inducers may decrease the levels/effects of venlafaxine. Example inducers include aminoglutethimide, carbamazepine, nafcillin, nevirapine, phenobarbital, phenytoin, and rifamycins.

CYP3A4 inhibitors: May increase the levels/effects of venlafaxine. Example inhibitors include azole antifungals, clarithromycin, diclofenac, doxycycline, erythromycin, imatinib, isoniazid, nefazodone, nicardipine, propofol, protease inhibitors, quinidine, telithromycin, and verapamil.

Haloperidol: Serum levels may be increased during concurrent administration; AUC may be increased by as much as 70%

Indinavir: Serum levels may be reduced by venlafaxine (AUC reduced by 28%); clinical significance unknown

Lithium: Concurrent use may increase risk of serotonin syndrome.

MAO inhibitors: Serotonin syndrome may result when venlafaxine is used in combination or within 2 weeks of an MAO inhibitor; these combinations should be avoided

Meperidine: Concurrent use may increase risk of serotonin syndrome

Mirtazapine: Concurrent use may increase risk of serotonin syndrome

Nefazodone: Concurrent use may increase risk of serotonin syndrome; in addition, nefazodone may inhibit the metabolism of venlafaxine

Selegiline: Concurrent use may predispose to serotonin syndrome; avoid concurrent use.

Serotonin agonists: Theoretically, may increase the risk of serotonin syndrome; includes sumatriptan, naratriptan, rizatriptan, and zolmitriptan

Sibutramine: Concurrent use may increase risk of serotonin syndrome; avoid concomitant use.

SSRIs: Concurrent use may increase risk of serotonin syndrome.

Tramadol: Concurrent use may increase risk of serotonin syndrome.

Trazodone: Concurrent use may increase risk of serotonin syndrome.

Tricyclic antidepressants: Concurrent use may increase risk of serotonin syndrome

Warfarin: Case reports of increased INR when venlafaxine was added to therapy.

(Continued)

Venlafaxine *(Continued)*

Ethanol/Nutrition/Herb Interactions

Ethanol: Avoid ethanol (may increase CNS effects).

Herb/Nutraceutical: Avoid valerian, St John's wort, SAMe, kava kava, tryptophan (may increase risk of serotonin syndrome and/or excessive sedation).

Dietary Considerations Should be taken with food.

Dosage Forms

Capsule, extended release (Effexor® XR): 37.5 mg, 75 mg, 150 mg
Tablet (Effexor®): 25 mg, 37.5 mg, 50 mg, 75 mg, 100 mg

- ♦ **Ventavis™** *see* Iloprost *on page 658*
- ♦ **Ventolin® (Can)** *see* Albuterol *on page 50*
- ♦ **Ventolin® Diskus (Can)** *see* Albuterol *on page 50*
- ♦ **Ventolin® HFA** *see* Albuterol *on page 50*
- ♦ **Ventrodisk (Can)** *see* Albuterol *on page 50*

Verapamil (ver AP a mil)

Medication Safety Issues

Sound-alike/look-alike issues:

Verapamil may be confused with Verelan®
Calan® may be confused with Colace®
Covera-HS® may be confused with Provera®
Isoptin® may be confused with Isopto® Tears
Verelan® may be confused with verapamil, Virilon®, Voltaren®

Related Information

Anesthesia for Patients With Liver Disease *on page 1421*
Antiarrhythmic Drugs *on page 1548*
Calcium Channel Blockers *on page 1559*
Hypertension *on page 1620*

U.S. Brand Names Calan®; Calan® SR; Covera-HS®; Isoptin® SR; Verelan®; Verelan® PM

Canadian Brand Names Alti-Verapamil; Apo-Verap®; Calan®; Chronovera®; Covera®; Covera-HS®; Gen-Verapamil; Gen-Verapamil SR; Isoptin® SR; Novo-Veramil SR; Nu-Verap; Riva-Verapamil SR; Verapamil Hydrochloride Injection, USP

Synonyms Iproveratril Hydrochloride; Verapamil Hydrochloride

Pharmacologic Category Antiarrhythmic Agent, Class IV; Calcium Channel Blocker

Generic Available Yes: Excludes controlled onset products

Use Orally for treatment of angina pectoris (vasospastic, chronic stable, unstable) and hypertension; I.V. for supraventricular tachyarrhythmias (PSVT, atrial fibrillation, atrial flutter)

Unlabeled/Investigational Use Migraine; hypertrophic cardiomyopathy; bipolar disorder (manic manifestations)

Mechanism of Action Inhibits calcium ion from entering the "slow channels" or select voltage-sensitive areas of vascular smooth muscle and myocardium during depolarization; produces a relaxation of coronary vascular smooth muscle and coronary vasodilation; increases myocardial oxygen delivery in patients with vasospastic angina; slows automaticity and conduction of AV node.

Pharmacodynamics/Kinetics

Onset of action: Peak effect: Oral: Immediate release: 1-2 hours; I.V.: 1-5 minutes
Duration: Oral: Immediate release tablets: 6-8 hours; I.V.: 10-20 minutes
Protein binding: 90%
Metabolism: Hepatic via multiple CYP isoenzymes; extensive first-pass effect
Bioavailability: Oral: 20% to 35%
Half-life elimination: Infants: 4.4-6.9 hours; Adults: Single dose: 2-8 hours, Multiple doses: 4.5-12 hours; prolonged with hepatic cirrhosis
Excretion: Urine (70%, 3% to 4% as unchanged drug); feces (16%)

Dosage

Children: SVT:

I.V.:

<1 year: 0.1-0.2 mg/kg over 2 minutes; repeat every 30 minutes as needed

1-15 years: 0.1-0.3 mg/kg over 2 minutes; maximum: 5 mg/dose, may repeat dose in 15 minutes if adequate response not achieved; maximum for second dose: 10 mg/dose

Oral (dose not well established):

1-5 years: 4-8 mg/kg/day in 3 divided doses **or** 40-80 mg every 8 hours

>5 years: 80 mg every 6-8 hours

Adults:

SVT: I.V.: 2.5-5 mg (over 2 minutes); second dose of 5-10 mg (~0.15 mg/kg) may be given 15-30 minutes after the initial dose if patient tolerates, but does not respond to initial dose; maximum total dose: 20 mg

Angina: Oral: Initial dose: 80-120 mg 3 times/day (elderly or small stature: 40 mg 3 times/day); range: 240-480 mg/day in 3-4 divided doses

Hypertension: Oral:

Immediate release: 80 mg 3 times/day; usual dose range (JNC 7): 80-320 mg/day in 2 divided doses

Sustained release: 240 mg/day; usual dose range (JNC 7): 120-360 mg/day in 1-2 divided doses; 120 mg/day in the elderly or small patients (no evidence of additional benefit in doses >360 mg/day).

Extended release:

Covera-HS®: Usual dose range (JNC 7): 120-360 mg once daily (once-daily dosing is recommended at bedtime)

Verelan® PM: Usual dose range: 200-400 mg once daily at bedtime

Dosing adjustment in renal impairment: Cl_{cr} <10 mL/minute: Administer at 50% to 75% of normal dose.

Dialysis: Not dialyzable (0% to 5%) via hemo- or peritoneal dialysis; supplemental dose is not necessary.

Dosing adjustment/comments in hepatic disease: Reduce dose in cirrhosis, reduce dose to 20% to 50% of normal and monitor ECG.

Stability Store injection at room temperature; protect from heat and from freezing; use only clear solutions; **compatible** in solutions of pH of 3-6, but may precipitate in solutions having a pH ≥6

Administration

Oral: Do not crush or chew sustained or extended release products.

Calan® SR, Isoptin® SR: Administer with food.

Verelan®, Verelan® PM: Capsules may be opened and the contents sprinkled on 1 tablespoonful of applesauce, then swallowed without chewing.

I.V.: Rate of infusion: Over 2 minutes.

Monitoring Parameters Monitor blood pressure closely

Reference Range Therapeutic: 50-200 ng/mL (SI: 100-410 nmol/L) for parent; under normal conditions norverapamil concentration is the same as parent drug. Toxic: >90 mcg/mL

Anesthesia and Critical Care Concerns/Other Considerations I.V. administration, hypertrophic cardiomyopathy, sick sinus syndrome, moderate to severe congestive heart failure, concomitant therapy with beta-blockers or digoxin can all increase incidence of adverse effects. Verapamil should be avoided in patients with left ventricular dysfunction, pulmonary congestion, or heart failure. Verapamil may be administered intravenously in the acute setting to attain ventricular rate control in patients with atrial fibrillation or flutter. Patients that respond, defined in general as at least a 20% decrease in ventricular response rate or attaining a rate <100 beats/minute, can be continued on oral therapy to maintain control. It is important to consider the potential drug interaction with digoxin, as these agents are both used in this setting.

Pregnancy Risk Factor C

Contraindications Hypersensitivity to verapamil or any component of the formulation; severe left ventricular dysfunction; hypotension (systolic pressure <90 mm Hg) or cardiogenic shock; sick sinus syndrome (except in patients with a functioning artificial pacemaker); second- or third-degree AV block (except in patients with a functioning artificial pacemaker); atrial flutter or fibrillation and an accessory bypass tract (WPW, Lown-Ganong-Levine syndrome)

Warnings/Precautions Avoid use in heart failure; can exacerbate condition. Can cause hypotension. Rare increases in liver function tests can be observed. Can cause first-degree AV block or sinus bradycardia. Other conduction abnormalities are rare. Use caution when using verapamil together with a beta-blocker. Avoid use of I.V. verapamil with an I.V. beta-blocker; can result in asystole. Use caution in patients with hypertrophic cardiomyopathy (IHSS). Use with caution in patients with attenuated neuromuscular transmission (Duchenne's muscular dystrophy, myasthenia gravis). Adjust the dose in severe renal dysfunction and hepatic

(Continued)

Verapamil *(Continued)*

dysfunction. Verapamil significantly increases digoxin serum concentrations (adjust digoxin's dose). May prolong recovery from nondepolarizing neuromuscular-blocking agents.

Adverse Reactions

>10%: Gastrointestinal: Gingival hyperplasia (up to 19%), constipation (12% up to 42% in clinical trials)

1% to 10%:

Cardiovascular: Bradycardia (1.2 to 1.4%), first-, second-, or third-degree AV block (1.2%), CHF (1.8%), hypotension (2.5% to 3%), peripheral edema (1.9%), symptomatic hypotension (1.5% I.V.), severe tachycardia (1%)

Central nervous system: Dizziness (1.2% to 3.3%), fatigue (1.7%), headache (1.2% to 2.2%)

Dermatologic: Rash (1.2%)

Gastrointestinal: Nausea (0.9% to 2.7%)

Respiratory: Dyspnea (1.4%)

<1% (Limited to important or life-threatening): Alopecia, angina, arthralgia, asystole, atrioventricular dissociation, bronchial/laryngeal spasm, cerebrovascular accident, chest pain, claudication, confusion, diarrhea, dry mouth, ecchymosis, electrical mechanical dissociation (EMD), emotional depression, eosinophilia, equilibrium disorders, erythema multiforme, exanthema, exfoliative dermatitis, galactorrhea/hyperprolactinemia, GI obstruction, gingival hyperplasia, gynecomastia, hair color change, impotence, muscle cramps, MI, myoclonus, paresthesia, Parkinsonian syndrome, psychotic symptoms, purpura (vasculitis), rash, respiratory failure, rotary nystagmus, shakiness, shock, somnolence, Stevens-Johnson syndrome, syncope, urticaria, ventricular fibrillation, vertigo

Overdosage/Toxicology Primary cardiac symptoms of calcium blocker overdose include hypotension and bradycardia (second- or third-degree atrioventricular block, or sinus arrest with junctional rhythm). Intraventricular conduction is usually not affected so QRS duration is normal (verapamil does prolong the PR interval).

Noncardiac symptoms include confusion, stupor, nausea, vomiting, metabolic acidosis and hyperglycemia. Following initial gastric decontamination, if possible, repeated calcium administration may promptly reverse depressed cardiac contractility (but not sinus node depression or peripheral vasodilation). Large doses of calcium chloride (up to 1 g/hour for 24 hours) have been used in refractory cases. Glucagon, epinephrine, and amrinone may treat refractory hypotension. Glucagon and epinephrine also increase heart rate (outside the U.S., 4-aminopyridine may be available as an antidote). Dialysis and hemoperfusion are not effective in enhancing elimination although repeat-dose activated charcoal may serve as an adjunct with sustained-release preparations.

Drug Interactions **Substrate** of CYP1A2 (minor), 2B6 (minor), 2C9 (minor), 2C18 (minor), 2E1 (minor), 3A4 (major); **Inhibits** CYP1A2 (weak), 2C9 (weak), 2D6 (weak), 3A4 (moderate)

Alfentanil's plasma concentration is increased. Fentanyl and sufentanil may be affected similarly.

Amiodarone use may lead to bradycardia and decreased cardiac output. Monitor closely if using together.

Aspirin and concurrent verapamil use may increase bleeding times; monitor closely, especially if on other antiplatelet agents or anticoagulants.

Azole antifungals may inhibit the calcium channel blocker's metabolism; avoid this combination. Try an antifungal like terbinafine (if appropriate) or monitor closely for altered effect of the calcium channel blocker.

Barbiturates reduce the plasma concentration of verapamil. May require much higher dose of verapamil.

Beta-blockers may have increased pharmacodynamic interactions with verapamil (see Warnings/Precautions).

Buspirone's serum concentration may increase. May require dosage adjustment.

Calcium may reduce the calcium channel blocker's effects, particularly hypotension.

Carbamazepine's serum concentration is increased and toxicity may result; avoid this combination.

Cimetidine reduced verapamil's metabolism; consider an alternative H_2 antagonist.

Colchicine: Verapamil may increase colchicine toxicity (especially nephrotoxicity).

Cyclosporine's serum concentrations are increased by verapamil; avoid this combination. Use another calcium channel blocker or monitor cyclosporine trough levels and renal function closely.

CYP3A4 inducers: CYP3A4 inducers may decrease the levels/effects of verapamil. Example inducers include aminoglutethimide, carbamazepine, nafcillin, nevirapine, phenobarbital, phenytoin, and rifamycins.

CYP3A4 inhibitors: May increase the levels/effects of verapamil. Example inhibitors include azole antifungals, clarithromycin, diclofenac, doxycycline, erythromycin, imatinib, isoniazid, nefazodone, nicardipine, propofol, protease inhibitors, telithromycin, and quinidine.

CYP3A4 substrates: Verapamil may increase the levels/effects of CYP3A4 substrates. Example substrates include benzodiazepines, calcium channel blockers, cyclosporine, mirtazapine, nateglinide, nefazodone, sildenafil (and other PDE-5 inhibitors), tacrolimus, and venlafaxine. Selected benzodiazepines (midazolam and triazolam), cisapride, ergot alkaloids, selected HMG-CoA reductase inhibitors (lovastatin and simvastatin), and pimozide are generally contraindicated with strong CYP3A4 inhibitors.

Digoxin's serum concentration is increased; reduce digoxin's dose when adding verapamil.

Doxorubicin's clearance was reduced; monitor for altered doxorubicin's effect.

Erythromycin may increase verapamil's effects; monitor altered verapamil effect.

Ethanol's effects may be increased by verapamil; reduce ethanol consumption.

Flecainide may have additive negative effects on conduction and inotropy.

Grapefruit juice: Verapamil serum concentrations may be increased by grapefruit juice. Avoid concurrent use.

HMG-CoA reductase inhibitors (atorvastatin, cerivastatin, lovastatin, simvastatin): Serum concentration will likely be increased; consider pravastatin/fluvastatin or a dihydropyridine calcium channel blocker. If concurrent use with lovastatin is unavoidable, dose of lovastatin should not exceed 40 mg/day.

Lithium neurotoxicity may result when verapamil is added; monitor lithium levels.

Midazolam's plasma concentration is increased by verapamil; monitor for prolonged CNS depression.

Nafcillin decreases plasma concentration of verapamil; avoid this combination.

Nondepolarizing muscle relaxant: Neuromuscular blockade may be prolonged. Monitor closely.

Prazosin's serum concentration increases; monitor blood pressure.

Quinidine's serum concentration is increased; adjust quinidine's dose as necessary.

Rifampin increases the metabolism of calcium channel blockers; adjust the dose of the calcium channel blocker to maintain efficacy.

Risperidone: Verapamil may increase the levels and effects of risperidone.

Sildenafil, tadalafil, vardenafil: Blood pressure-lowering effects may be additive; use caution.

Tacrolimus's serum concentrations are increased by verapamil; avoid the combination. Use another calcium channel blocker or monitor tacrolimus trough levels and renal function closely.

Theophylline's serum concentration may be increased by verapamil. Those at increased risk include children and cigarette smokers.

Ethanol/Nutrition/Herb Interactions

Ethanol: Avoid or limit ethanol (may increase ethanol levels).

Food: Grapefruit juice may increase the serum concentration of verapamil; avoid concurrent use.

Herb/Nutraceutical: St John's wort may decrease levels. Avoid dong quai if using for hypertension (has estrogenic activity). Avoid ephedra, yohimbe, ginseng (may worsen arrhythmia or hypertension). Avoid garlic (may have increased antihypertensive effect).

Dietary Considerations Calan® SR and Isoptin® SR products may be taken with food or milk, other formulations may be administered without regard to meals; sprinkling contents of Verelan® or Verelan® PM capsule onto applesauce does not affect oral absorption.

Dosage Forms

Caplet, sustained release: 120 mg, 180 mg, 240 mg
  Calan® SR: 120 mg, 180 mg, 240 mg

Capsule, extended release, controlled onset, as hydrochloride:
  Verelan® PM: 100 mg, 200 mg, 300 mg

Capsule, sustained release, as hydrochloride: 120 mg, 180 mg, 240 mg, 360 mg
  Verelan®: 120 mg, 180 mg, 240 mg, 360 mg

(Continued)

Verapamil *(Continued)*

Injection, solution, as hydrochloride: 2.5 mg/mL (2 mL, 4 mL)
Tablet, as hydrochloride: 80 mg, 120 mg
Calan®: 40 mg, 80 mg, 120 mg
Tablet, extended release: 120 mg, 180 mg, 240 mg
Tablet, extended release, controlled onset, as hydrochloride:
Covera-HS®: 180 mg, 240 mg
Tablet, sustained release, as hydrochloride: 120 mg, 180 mg, 240 mg
Isoptin® SR: 120 mg, 180 mg, 240 mg

- ♦ **Verapamil Hydrochloride** *see* Verapamil *on page 1352*
- ♦ **Verapamil Hydrochloride Injection, USP (Can)** *see* Verapamil *on page 1352*
- ♦ **Verelan®** *see* Verapamil *on page 1352*
- ♦ **Verelan® PM** *see* Verapamil *on page 1352*
- ♦ **Versed** *see* Midazolam *on page 847*
- ♦ **Versiclear™** *see* Sodium Thiosulfate *on page 1195*
- ♦ **VESIcare®** *see* Solifenacin *on page 1196*
- ♦ **VFEND®** *see* Voriconazole *on page 1358*
- ♦ **Viagra®** *see* Sildenafil *on page 1169*
- ♦ **Vibramycin®** *see* Doxycycline *on page 426*
- ♦ **Vibra-Tabs®** *see* Doxycycline *on page 426*
- ♦ **Vicks Sinex® 12 Hour [OTC]** *see* Oxymetazoline *on page 973*
- ♦ **Vicks Sinex® 12 Hour Ultrafine Mist [OTC]** *see* Oxymetazoline *on page 973*
- ♦ **Vicks® Sinex® Nasal Spray [OTC]** *see* Phenylephrine *on page 1015*
- ♦ **Vicks® Sinex® UltraFine Mist [OTC]** *see* Phenylephrine *on page 1015*
- ♦ **Vicodin®** *see* Hydrocodone and Acetaminophen *on page 636*
- ♦ **Vicodin® ES** *see* Hydrocodone and Acetaminophen *on page 636*
- ♦ **Vicodin® HP** *see* Hydrocodone and Acetaminophen *on page 636*
- ♦ **Videx®** *see* Didanosine *on page 382*
- ♦ **Videx® EC** *see* Didanosine *on page 382*
- ♦ **Vigamox™** *see* Moxifloxacin *on page 873*

VinBLAStine (vin BLAS teen)

Medication Safety Issues

Sound-alike/look-alike issues:
VinBLAStine may be confused with vinCRIStine, vinorelbine

Note: Must be dispensed in overwrap which bears the statement **"Do not remove covering until the moment of injection. Fatal if given intrathecally. For I.V. use only."** Syringes should be labeled: **"Fatal if given intrathecally. For I.V. use only."**

Synonyms NSC-49842; Vinblastine Sulfate; VLB

Pharmacologic Category Antineoplastic Agent, Natural Source (Plant) Derivative; Antineoplastic Agent, Vinca Alkaloid

Generic Available Yes

Use Treatment of Hodgkin's and non-Hodgkin's lymphoma, testicular, lung, head and neck, breast, and renal carcinomas, Mycosis fungoides, Kaposi's sarcoma, histiocytosis, choriocarcinoma, and idiopathic thrombocytopenic purpura

Mechanism of Action Vinblastine binds to tubulin and inhibits microtubule formation, therefore, arresting the cell at metaphase by disrupting the formation of the mitotic spindle; it is specific for the M and S phases. Vinblastine may also interfere with nucleic acid and protein synthesis by blocking glutamic acid utilization.

Pharmacodynamics/Kinetics

Distribution: V_d: 27.3 L/kg; binds extensively to tissues; does not penetrate CNS or other fatty tissues; distributes to liver
Protein binding: 99%
Metabolism: Hepatic to active metabolite
Half-life elimination: Biphasic: Initial: 0.164 hours; Terminal: 25 hours
Excretion: Feces (95%); urine (<1% as unchanged drug)

Dosage Refer to individual protocols.

Children and Adults: I.V.: 4-20 mg/m^2 (0.1-0.5 mg/kg) every 7-10 days **or** 5-day continuous infusion of 1.5-2 mg/m^2/day **or** 0.1-0.5 mg/kg/week

Dosing adjustment in hepatic impairment:

Serum bilirubin 1.5-3.0 mg/dL or AST 60-180 units: Administer 50% of normal dose

Serum bilirubin 3.0-5.0 mg/dL: Administer 25% of dose

Serum bilirubin >5.0 mg/dL or AST >180 units: Omit dose

Stability Store intact vials under refrigeration (2°C to 8°C) and protect from light. Reconstitute to a concentration of 1 mg/mL with bacteriostatic water, bacteriostatic NS, SWFI, NS, or D_5W; for infusion, may be diluted with 50-1000 mL Ns or D_5W. Solutions reconstituted in bacteriostatic water or bacteriostatic NS are stable for 21 days at room temperature or under refrigeration.

Note: Must be dispensed in overwrap which bears the statement "Do not remove covering until the moment of injection. Fatal if given intrathecally. For I.V. use only." Syringes should be labeled: "Fatal if given intrathecally. For I.V. use only."

Administration FATAL IF GIVEN INTRATHECALLY. For I.V. administration only, usually as a slow (2-3 minutes) push, or a bolus (5- to 15-minute) infusion. It is occasionally given as a 24-hour continuous infusion.

Extravasation management: Mix 250 units hyaluronidase with 6 mL of NS. Inject the hyaluronidase solution subcutaneously through 6 clockwise injections into the infiltrated area using a 25-gauge needle; change the needle with each new injection. Apply heat immediately for 1 hour. Repeat 4 times/day for 3-5 days. Elevate extremity. Application of cold or hydrocortisone is contraindicated.

Monitoring Parameters CBC with differential and platelet count, serum uric acid, hepatic function tests

Pregnancy Risk Factor D

Contraindications For I.V. use only; **I.T. use may result in death**; hypersensitivity to vinblastine or any component of the formulation; pregnancy

Warnings/Precautions Hazardous agent - use appropriate precautions for handling and disposal. **[U.S. Boxed Warning]: Vinblastine is a moderate vesicant; avoid extravasation.** Dosage modification required in patients with impaired liver function and neurotoxicity. Using small amounts of drug daily for long periods may cause neurotoxicity and is therefore not advised. **[U.S. Boxed Warning]: For I.V. use only. Intrathecal administration may result in death.** Monitor closely for shortness of breath or bronchospasm in patients receiving mitomycin C. **[U.S. Boxed Warning]: Should be administered under the supervision of an experienced cancer chemotherapy physician.**

Adverse Reactions

>10%:

- Dermatologic: Alopecia
- Endocrine & metabolic: SIADH
- Gastrointestinal: Diarrhea (less common), stomatitis, anorexia, metallic taste
- Hematologic: May cause severe bone marrow suppression and is the dose-limiting toxicity of VLB (unlike vincristine); severe granulocytopenia and thrombocytopenia may occur following the administration of VLB and nadir 5-10 days after treatment
- Myelosuppression (primarily leukopenia, may be dose limiting)
  - Onset: 4-7 days
  - Nadir: 5-10 days
  - Recovery: 4-21 days

1% to 10%:

- Cardiovascular: Hypertension, Raynaud's phenomenon
- Central nervous system: Depression, malaise, headache, seizure
- Dermatologic: Rash, photosensitivity, dermatitis
- Endocrine & metabolic: Hyperuricemia
- Gastrointestinal: Constipation, abdominal pain, nausea (mild), vomiting (mild), paralytic ileus, stomatitis
- Genitourinary: Urinary retention
- Neuromuscular & skeletal: Jaw pain, myalgia, paresthesia
- Respiratory: Bronchospasm

<1% (Limited to important or life-threatening): Hemorrhagic colitis, neurotoxicity (rare; symptoms may include peripheral neuropathy, loss of deep tendon reflexes, headache, weakness, urinary retention, GI symptoms, tachycardia, orthostatic hypotension, convulsions), rectal bleeding

Overdosage/Toxicology Symptoms of overdose include bone marrow suppression, mental depression, paresthesia, loss of deep tendon reflexes, and neurotoxicity. There are no antidotes for vinblastine. Treatment is supportive and

(Continued)

VinBLAStine *(Continued)*

symptomatic, including fluid restriction or hypertonic saline (3% sodium chloride) for drug-induced secretion of inappropriate antidiuretic hormone (SIADH).

Drug Interactions Substrate of CYP2D6 (minor), 3A4 (major); **Inhibits** CYP2D6 (weak), 3A4 (weak)

CYP3A4 inducers: CYP3A4 inducers may decrease the levels/effects of vinblastine. Example inducers include aminoglutethimide, carbamazepine, nafcillin, nevirapine, phenobarbital, phenytoin, and rifamycins.

CYP3A4 inhibitors: May increase the levels/effects of vinblastine. Example inhibitors include azole antifungals, clarithromycin, diclofenac, doxycycline, erythromycin, imatinib, isoniazid, nefazodone, nicardipine, propofol, protease inhibitors, quinidine, telithromycin, and verapamil.

Mitomycin-C: Previous or simultaneous use with mitomycin-C has resulted in acute shortness of breath and severe bronchospasm within minutes or several hours after vinca alkaloid injection and may occur up to 2 weeks after the dose of mitomycin. Mitomycin-C, in combination with administration of VLB, may cause acute shortness of breath and severe bronchospasm, onset may be within minutes or several hours after VLB injection

Phenytoin may reduce vinblastine serum concentrations.

Ethanol/Nutrition/Herb Interactions Herb/Nutraceutical: St John's wort may decrease vinblastine levels. Avoid black cohosh, dong quai in estrogen-dependent tumors.

Dosage Forms

Injection, powder for reconstitution, as sulfate: 10 mg

Injection, solution, as sulfate: 1 mg/mL (10 mL) [contains benzyl alcohol]

- **Vinblastine Sulfate** *see* VinBLAStine *on page 1356*
- **Vioxx® [DSC]** *see* Rofecoxib *on page 1138*
- **Viracept®** *see* Nelfinavir *on page 906*
- **Viramune®** *see* Nevirapine *on page 915*
- **Virazole®** *see* Ribavirin *on page 1116*
- **Visicol®** *see* Sodium Phosphates *on page 1189*
- **Visine® L.R. [OTC]** *see* Oxymetazoline *on page 973*
- **Vitamin B_6** *see* Pyridoxine *on page 1090*
- **Vitamin K_1** *see* Phytonadione *on page 1027*
- **Vitrase®** *see* Hyaluronidase *on page 631*
- **Vitrasert®** *see* Ganciclovir *on page 581*
- **Vivarin® [OTC]** *see* Caffeine *on page 211*
- **Vivitrol™** *see* Naltrexone *on page 897*
- **VLB** *see* VinBLAStine *on page 1356*
- **Voltaren®** *see* Diclofenac *on page 378*
- **Voltaren Ophtha® (Can)** *see* Diclofenac *on page 378*
- **Voltaren Ophthalmic®** *see* Diclofenac *on page 378*
- **Voltaren Rapide® (Can)** *see* Diclofenac *on page 378*
- **Voltaren®-XR** *see* Diclofenac *on page 378*
- **Voluven® (Can)** *see* Hetastarch *on page 623*

Voriconazole (vor i KOE na zole)

Related Information

Antifungal Agents *on page 1554*

U.S. Brand Names VFEND®

Canadian Brand Names VFEND®

Synonyms UK109496

Pharmacologic Category Antifungal Agent, Oral; Antifungal Agent, Parenteral

Generic Available No

Use Treatment of invasive aspergillosis; treatment of esophageal candidiasis; treatment of candidemia (in non-neutropenic patients); treatment of *Candida* deep tissue infections; treatment of serious fungal infections caused by *Scedosporium apiospermum* and *Fusarium* spp (including *Fusarium solani*) in patients intolerant of, or refractory to, other therapy

Mechanism of Action Interferes with fungal cytochrome P450 activity, decreasing ergosterol synthesis (principal sterol in fungal cell membrane) and inhibiting fungal cell membrane formation.

Pharmacodynamics/Kinetics

Absorption: Well absorbed after oral administration
Distribution: V_d: 4.6 L/kg
Protein binding: 58%
Metabolism: Hepatic, via CYP2C19 (major pathway) and CYP2C9 and CYP3A4 (less significant); saturable (may demonstrate nonlinearity)
Bioavailability: 96%
Half-life elimination: Variable, dose-dependent
Time to peak: 1-2 hours
Excretion: Urine (as inactive metabolites)

Dosage

Usual dosage ranges:

Children <12 years: Dosage not established
Children ≥12 years and Adults:
Oral: 100-300 mg every 12 hours
I.V.: 6 mg/kg every 12 hours for 2 doses; followed by maintenance dose of 4 mg/kg every 12 hours

Indication-specific dosing: Children ≥12 years and Adults:

Aspergillosis (invasive) and other serious fungal infections: I.V.: Initial: Loading dose: 6 mg/kg every 12 hours for 2 doses; followed by maintenance dose of 4 mg/kg every 12 hours

Candidemia and other deep tissue *Candida* infections: I.V.: Initial: Loading dose 6 mg/kg every 12 hours for 2 doses; followed by maintenance dose of 3-4 mg/kg every 12 hours

Note: Conversion to oral dosing:
Patients <40 kg: 100 mg every 12 hours; increase to 150 mg every 12 hours in patients who fail to respond adequately
Patients ≥40 kg: 200 mg every 12 hours; increase to 300 mg every 12 hours in patients who fail to respond adequately

Endophthalmitis, fungal: I.V.: 6 mg/kg every 12 hours for 2 doses, then 200 mg orally twice daily

Esophageal candidiasis: Oral:
Patients <40 kg: 100 mg every 12 hours
Patients ≥40 kg: 200 mg every 12 hours
Note: Treatment should continue for a minimum of 14 days, and for at least 7 days following resolution of symptoms.

Dosage adjustment in patients unable to tolerate treatment:

I.V.: Dose may be reduced to 3 mg/kg every 12 hours
Oral: Dose may be reduced in 50 mg increments to a minimum dosage of 200 mg every 12 hours in patients weighing ≥40 kg (100 mg every 12 hours in patients <40 kg)

Dosage adjustment in patients receiving concomitant phenytoin:

I.V.: Increase maintenance dosage to 5 mg/kg every 12 hours
Oral: Increase dose from 200 mg to 400 mg every 12 hours in patients ≥40 kg (100 mg to 200 mg every 12 hours in patients <40 kg)

Dosage adjustment in patients receiving concomitant cyclosporine: Reduce cyclosporine dose by ½ and monitor closely.

Dosage adjustment in renal impairment: In patients with Cl_{cr} <50 mL/minute, accumulation of the intravenous vehicle (SBECD) occurs. After initial loading dose, oral voriconazole should be administered to these patients, unless an assessment of the benefit:risk to the patient justifies the use of I.V. voriconazole. Monitor serum creatinine and change to oral voriconazole therapy when possible.
Hemodialysis: Oral dosage adjustment not required.

Dosage adjustment in hepatic impairment:

Mild-to-moderate hepatic dysfunction (Child-Pugh Class A and B): Following standard loading dose, reduce maintenance dosage by 50%
Severe hepatic impairment: Should only be used if benefit outweighs risk; monitor closely for toxicity

Stability

Powder for injection: Store at 15°C to 30°C (59°F to 86°F). Reconstitute 200 mg vial with 19 mL of sterile water for injection (use of automated syringe is not recommended). Resultant solution (20 mL) has a concentration of 10 mg/mL. Prior to infusion, must dilute to 0.5-5 mg/mL with NS, LR, D_5WLR, D_5½NS, D_5W, D_5W with KCl 20 mEq, ½NS, or D_5WNS. Do not dilute with 4.2% sodium

(Continued)

Voriconazole *(Continued)*

bicarbonate infusion. Reconstituted solutions are stable for up to 24 hours under refrigeration at 2°C to 8°C (36°F to 46°F).

Powder for oral suspension: Store at 2°C to 8°C (36°F to 46°F). Add 46 mL of water to the bottle to make 40 mg/mL suspension. Reconstituted oral suspension may be stored at 15°C to 30°C (59°F to 86°F). Discard after 14 days.

Tablets: Store at 15°C to 30°C (59°F to 86°F).

Administration

Oral: Administer 1 hour before or 1 hour after a meal.

I.V.: Infuse over 1-2 hours (rate not to exceed 3 mg/kg/hour). Do not infuse concomitantly into same line or cannula with other drug infusions, including TPN.

Monitoring Parameters Hepatic function at initiation and during course of treatment; visual function if treatment course continues >28 days; renal function

Anesthesia and Critical Care Concerns/Other Considerations Based on high oral bioavailability, switching between I.V. and oral administration is appropriate when clinically indicated. Infusions of blood products and any electrolyte supplementation must not occur simultaneously with intravenous voriconazole. Voriconazole I.V. must not be infused into the same line or cannula concomitantly with other drug infusions.

Pregnancy Risk Factor D

Contraindications Hypersensitivity to voriconazole or any component of the formulation (cross-reaction with other azole antifungal agents may occur but has not been established, use caution); coadministration of CYP3A4 substrates which may lead to QT_c prolongation (cisapride, pimozide, or quinidine); coadministration with barbiturates (long acting), carbamazepine, efavirenz, ergot alkaloids, rifampin, rifabutin, ritonavir (≥800 mg/day), and sirolimus; pregnancy (unless risk:benefit justifies use)

Warnings/Precautions Visual changes are commonly associated with treatment, including blurred vision, changes in visual acuity, color changes, and photophobia. Patients should be warned to avoid tasks which depend on vision, including operating machinery or driving. Changes are reversible on discontinuation following brief exposure/treatment regimens (≤28 days); reversibility following long-term administration has not been evaluated.

Serious hepatic reactions (including hepatitis, cholestasis, and fulminant hepatic failure) have occurred during treatment, primarily in patients with serious concomitant medical conditions, including hematological malignancy. However, hepatotoxicity has occurred in patients with no identifiable risk factors. Use caution in patients with pre-existing hepatic impairment (dose adjustment required).

Voriconazole tablets contain lactose; avoid administration in hereditary galactose intolerance, Lapp lactase deficiency, or glucose-galactose malabsorption. Suspension contains sucrose; use caution with fructose intolerance, sucrose-isomaltase deficiency, or glucose-galactose malabsorption. Avoid/limit use of intravenous formulation in patients with renal impairment; intravenous formulation contains excipient sulfobutyl ether beta-cyclodextrin (SBECD), which may accumulate in renal insufficiency. Infusion-related reactions may occur with intravenous dosing. Consider discontinuation of infusion if reaction is severe.

Use caution in patients with an increased risk of arrhythmia (concurrent QT_c-prolonging drugs, hypokalemia, cardiomyopathy, or prior cardiotoxic therapy). Correct electrolyte abnormalities (eg, hypokalemia, hypomagnesemia, hypocalcemia) before initiating therapy. Use caution in patients receiving concurrent non-nucleoside reverse transcriptase inhibitors (efavirenz is contraindicated).

Avoid use in pregnancy, unless an evaluation of the potential benefit justifies possible risk to the fetus. Safety and efficacy have not been established in children <12 years of age.

Adverse Reactions

>10%: Ocular: Visual changes (photophobia, color changes, increased or decreased visual acuity, or blurred vision occur in ~21%)

1% to 10%:

Cardiovascular: Tachycardia (2% to 3%), hyper-/hypotension (2%), vasodilation (2%), peripheral edema (1%)

Central nervous system: Fever (6%), chills (4%), headache (3%), hallucinations (3%), dizziness (1%)

Dermatologic: Rash (6%), pruritus (1%)

Endocrine & metabolic: Hypokalemia (2%), hypomagnesemia (1%)

Gastrointestinal: Nausea (5% to 6%), vomiting (4% to 5%), abdominal pain (2%), diarrhea (1%), xerostomia (1%)

Hematologic: Thrombocytopenia (1%)

Hepatic: Alkaline phosphatase increased (4%), transaminases increased (2% to 3%), AST increased (2%), ALT increased (2%), cholestatic jaundice (1%)

Ocular: Chromatopsia (1%), photophobia (2% to 3%)

<1% (Limited to important or life-threatening): Acute tubular necrosis, adrenal cortical insufficiency, agranulocytosis, allergic reaction, anaphylactoid reaction; anemia (aplastic, macrocytic, megaloblastic, or microcytic); angioedema, ataxia, atrial arrhythmia, atrial fibrillation, AV block, bone marrow depression, bone necrosis, bradycardia, brain edema, bundle branch block, cardiac arrest, cerebral hemorrhage, cholecystitis, cholelithiasis, coma, CHF, convulsion, delirium, dementia, depression, DIC, discoid lupus erythematosus, duodenal ulcer perforation, encephalopathy, erythema multiforme, exfoliative dermatitis, extrapyramidal symptoms, fixed drug eruption, gastrointestinal hemorrhage, grand mal seizure, Guillain-Barré syndrome, hematemesis, hemolytic anemia, hepatic coma, hepatic failure, hepatitis, intestinal perforation, intracranial hypertension, kidney dysfunction, lung edema, myasthenia, MI, neuropathy, night blindness, optic atrophy, optic neuritis, pancreatitis, pancytopenia, papilledema, paresthesia, photosensitivity, psychosis, pulmonary embolus, QT-interval prolongation, renal failure (acute), respiratory distress syndrome, sepsis, Stevens-Johnson syndrome, suicidal ideation, supraventricular tachycardia, syncope, thrombotic thrombocytopenic purpura, toxic epidermal necrolysis, ventricular arrhythmia, ventricular fibrillation, ventricular tachycardia, torsade de pointes, vertigo

Overdosage/Toxicology Visual changes may occur; one patient had photophobia for 10 minutes. Treatment is symptom-directed and supportive. Following intravenous overdose, toxicity from the vehicle, SBECD, may also occur. Both voriconazole and the intravenous vehicle may be eliminated via hemodialysis.

Drug Interactions Substrate of CYP2C9 (major), 2C19 (major), 3A4 (minor); **Inhibits** CYP2C9 (weak), 2C19 (weak), 3A4 (moderate)

Barbiturates (phenobarbital, secobarbital): May decrease the serum levels/effects of voriconazole; concurrent use is contraindicated.

Benzodiazepines (metabolized by oxidation): Alprazolam, diazepam, temazepam, triazolam, and midazolam serum concentrations/toxicity may be increased. Manufacturer suggests adjustment of benzodiazepine dose be considered.

Buspirone: Serum concentrations may be increased; monitor for sedation.

Busulfan: Serum concentrations may be increased; avoid concurrent use.

Calcium channel blockers: Serum levels may be increased (applies to those agents metabolized by CYP3A4, including felodipine, nifedipine, and verapamil).

Carbamazepine: May decrease the serum levels/effects of voriconazole; concurrent use is contraindicated.

Cisapride: Serum concentrations may be increased which may lead to malignant arrhythmias; concurrent use is contraindicated.

CYP2C9 inducers: May decrease the levels/effects of voriconazole. Example inducers include carbamazepine, phenobarbital, phenytoin, rifampin, rifapentine, and secobarbital.

CYP2C19 inducers: May decrease the levels/effects of voriconazole. Example inducers include aminoglutethimide, carbamazepine, phenytoin, and rifampin.

CYP3A4 substrates: Voriconazole may increase the levels/effects of CYP3A4 substrates. Example substrates include benzodiazepines, calcium channel blockers, cyclosporine, mirtazapine, nateglinide, nefazodone, sildenafil (and other PDE-5 inhibitors), tacrolimus, and venlafaxine. Selected benzodiazepines (midazolam and triazolam), cisapride, ergot alkaloids, selected HMG-CoA reductase inhibitors (lovastatin and simvastatin), and pimozide are generally contraindicated with strong CYP3A4 inhibitors.

Cyclosporine: Voriconazole increases the serum levels/effects of cyclosporine. Decrease cyclosporine dose and monitor. Readjust dose when voriconazole is discontinued.

Efavirenz: Serum levels/effects of voriconazole may be reduced, and efavirenz levels increased during therapy; concurrent use is contraindicated.

Ergot alkaloids: Serum levels may be increased by voriconazole, leading to ergot toxicity; concurrent use is contraindicated.

HMG-CoA reductase inhibitors (except pravastatin and fluvastatin): Serum levels/effects may be increased. The risk of myopathy/rhabdomyolysis may be increased. Switch to pravastatin/fluvastatin or monitor for development of myopathy. Manufacturer suggests that dosage adjustment of HMG-CoA reductase inhibitor may be necessary with concurrent use.

(Continued)

Voriconazole *(Continued)*

Methadone: Serum levels and duration/effects may be increased significantly; monitor and reduce methadone dose if necessary.

Omeprazole: Voriconazole may increase omeprazole serum levels. In patients taking ≥40 mg of omeprazole per day, dose should be reduced by half.

Oral (hormonal) contraceptives: May increase the levels/effects of voriconazole. Conversely, voriconazole may increase the levels/effects of ethinyl estradiol and norethindrone; monitor for adverse effects.

Phenytoin: Serum levels/effects of voriconazole may be decreased; adjust dose of voriconazole. Phenytoin levels may be increased; monitor phenytoin levels and adjust dose as needed.

Pimozide: Serum levels/toxicity may be increased; concurrent use is contraindicated.

QT_c-prolonging agents: Risk of arrhythmia (torsade de pointes) may be increased.

Quinidine: Serum levels may be increased; concurrent use is contraindicated.

Rifabutin: Rifabutin serum levels are increased by voriconazole; concurrent use is contraindicated.

Rifampin: Rifampin decreases voriconazole's serum concentration to levels which are no longer effective; concurrent use is contraindicated.

Ritonavir: Serum levels/effects of voriconazole are reduced; concurrent use of ritonavir ≥800 mg/day is contraindicated. Use caution with smaller doses (<800 mg/day) of ritonavir.

Sirolimus: Serum levels may be increased by voriconazole; concurrent use in contraindicated.

Sulfonylureas: Serum levels may be increased by voriconazole, potentially leading to hypoglycemia; monitor.

Tacrolimus: Serum levels may be increased by voriconazole. Reduce tacrolimus dose to $^1/_3$ of original dose and monitor. Readjust dose when voriconazole is discontinued.

Trimetrexate: Serum concentrations may be increased; monitor.

Warfarin: Anticoagulant effects may be increased; monitor INR.

Vinca alkaloids: Serum concentrations may be increased; consider reduced dosage of vinca alkaloid.

Ethanol/Nutrition/Herb Interactions

Food: May decrease voriconazole absorption. Voriconazole should be taken 1 hour before or 1 hour after a meal.

Herb/Nutraceutical: St John's wort may decrease voriconazole levels.

Dietary Considerations Oral: Should be taken 1 hour before or 1 hour after a meal. Voriconazole tablets contain lactose; avoid administration in hereditary galactose intolerance, Lapp lactase deficiency, or glucose-galactose malabsorption. Suspension contains sucrose; use caution with fructose intolerance, sucrose-isomaltase deficiency, or glucose-galactose malabsorption.

Dosage Forms

Injection, powder for reconstitution: 200 mg [contains SBECD 3200 mg]

Powder for oral suspension: 200 mg/5 mL (70 mL) [contains sodium benzoate and sucrose; orange flavor]

Tablet: 50 mg, 200 mg [contains lactose]

- **VoSpire ER®** *see* Albuterol *on page 50*
- **Vusion™** *see* Miconazole and Zinc Oxide *on page 847*

Warfarin (WAR far in)

Medication Safety Issues Sound-alike/look-alike issues:

Coumadin® may be confused with Avandia®, Cardura®, Compazine®, Kemadrin®

High alert medication: The Institute for Safe Medication Practices (ISMP) includes this medication among its list of drugs which have a heightened risk of causing significant patient harm when used in error.

U.S. Brand Names Coumadin®; Jantoven™

Canadian Brand Names Apo-Warfarin®; Coumadin®; Gen-Warfarin; Novo-Warfarin; Taro-Warfarin

Synonyms Warfarin Sodium

Pharmacologic Category Anticoagulant, Coumarin Derivative

Generic Available Yes: Tablet

Use Prophylaxis and treatment of venous thrombosis, pulmonary embolism and thromboembolic disorders; atrial fibrillation with risk of embolism and as an adjunct in the prophylaxis of systemic embolism after myocardial infarction

Unlabeled/Investigational Use Prevention of recurrent transient ischemic attacks and to reduce risk of recurrent myocardial infarction

Mechanism of Action Interferes with hepatic synthesis of vitamin K-dependent coagulation factors (II, VII, IX, X)

Pharmacodynamics/Kinetics

Onset of action: Anticoagulation: Oral: 36-72 hours

Peak effect: Full therapeutic effect: 5-7 days; INR may increase in 36-72 hours

Duration: 2-5 days

Absorption: Oral: Rapid

Metabolism: Hepatic

Half-life elimination: 20-60 hours; Mean: 40 hours; highly variable among individuals

Dosage

Oral:

Infants and Children: 0.05-0.34 mg/kg/day; infants <12 months of age may require doses at or near the high end of this range; consistent anticoagulation may be difficult to maintain in children <5 years of age

Adults: Initial dosing must be individualized. Consider the patient (hepatic function, cardiac function, age, nutritional status, concurrent therapy, risk of bleeding) in addition to prior dose response (if available) and the clinical situation. Start 5-10 mg daily for 2 days. Adjust dose according to INR results; usual maintenance dose ranges from 2-10 mg daily (individual patients may require loading and maintenance doses outside these general guidelines).

Note: Lower starting doses may be required for patients with hepatic impairment, poor nutrition, CHF, elderly, high risk of bleeding, or patients that are debilitated. Higher initial doses may be reasonable in selected patients (ie, receiving enzyme-inducing agents and with low risk of bleeding).

I.V. (administer as a slow bolus injection): 2-5 mg/day

Dosing adjustment/comments in hepatic disease: Monitor effect at usual doses; the response to oral anticoagulants may be markedly enhanced in obstructive jaundice (due to reduced vitamin K absorption) and also in hepatitis and cirrhosis (due to decreased production of vitamin K-dependent clotting factors); prothrombin index should be closely monitored

Stability Protect from light; injection is stable for 4 hours at room temperature after reconstitution with 2.7 mL of sterile water (yields 2 mg/mL solution)

Administration

Oral: Do not take with food. Take at the same time each day.

I.V.: Administer as a slow bolus injection over 1-2 minutes; avoid all I.M. injections

Monitoring Parameters Prothrombin time, hematocrit, INR

INR Ranges Based Upon Indication

Indication	Targeted INR	Targeted INR Range
Acute myocardial infarction (high-risk)	2.5	2.0-3.0 [1,2,3]
Atrial fibrillation	2.5	2.0-3.0
St Jude Medical bileaflet mechanical aortic valve	2.5	2.0-3.0
Bileaflet or tilting disk mechanical aortic valve	3	2.5-3.5
Caged ball or caged disk mechanical valve	3	2.5-3.5[1]
Mechanical prosthetic valve with systemic embolism despite adequate anticoagulation	3	2.5-3.5[1]
Carbomedics bileaflet/Medtronic Hall tilting disk mechanical aortic valve (NSR, NI LA size)	2.5	2.0-3.0
Mechanical valve and risk factors (atrial fibrillation, MI, left atrial enlargement, low EF, endocardial damage)	3	2.5-3.5[1]
Bioprosthetic mitral valve	2.5	2.0-3.0[2]
Bioprosthetic aortic valve	2.5	2.0-3.0[2] (or aspirin 81 mg/day)
Bioprosthetic mitral or aortic valve with atrial fibrillation	2.5	2.0-3.0
Rheumatic mitral valve disease and NSR (left atrial diameter >5.5 cm)	2.5	2.0-3.0
Venous thromboembolism	2.5	2.0-3.0
Lupus inhibitor (no other risk factors)	2.5	2.0-3.0
Lupus inhibitor and recurrent thromboembolism	3	2.5-3.5

[1]Combine with aspirin 81 mg/day

[2]Maintain anticoagulation for 3 months

[3]High-risk includes a large anterior MI, significant heart failure, intracardiac thrombus, thromboembolism

(Continued)

Warfarin *(Continued)*

Reference Range

INR = patient prothrombin time/mean normal prothrombin time

ISI = international sensitivity index

INR should be increased by 2-3½ times depending upon indication.

INR ranges based upon indication: See table on previous page.

Warfarin levels are not used for monitoring degree of anticoagulation. They may be useful if a patient with unexplained coagulopathy is using the drug surreptitiously or if it is unclear whether clinical resistance is due to true drug resistance or lack of drug intake.

Normal prothrombin time (PT): 10.9-12.9 seconds. Healthy premature newborns have prolonged coagulation test screening results (eg, PT, aPTT, TT) which return to normal adult values at approximately 6 months of age. Healthy prematures, however, do not develop spontaneous hemorrhage or thrombotic complications because of a balance between procoagulants and inhibitors

Anesthesia and Critical Care Concerns/Other Considerations

Tube-feeding formulas are often a rich source of vitamin K.

Management of oral anticoagulation prior to surgery: Patients with low risk of thromboembolism: Stop warfarin therapy approximately 4 days before surgery, allow the INR to return to a near normal level, briefly administer postoperative prophylaxis (if the intervention itself creates a higher risk of thrombosis) using low-dose heparin or LMWH, and simultaneously begin warfarin therapy after surgery.

Patients with intermediate risk of thromboembolism: Stop warfarin therapy approximately 4 days before surgery, allow the INR to fall. Initiate low-dose heparin or prophylactic dose of LMWH beginning 2 days before surgery. Then commence full-dose heparin or LMWH, and warfarin therapy after surgery.

Patients with high risk of thromboembolism (eg, a recent [<3 months] history of venous thromboembolism, a mechanical cardiac valve in the mitral position; or an old model of cardiac valve [ball/cage]): Stop warfarin therapy approximately 4 days before surgery, allow the INR to return to a normal level, begin therapy with full-dose heparin or full-dose LMWH as the INR falls (approximately 2 days before surgery). Heparin can be administered as a SubQ injection on an outpatient basis, can then be given as a continuous I.V. infusion after hospital admission in preparation for surgery, and can be discontinued 5 hours before surgery with the expectation that the anticoagulant effect will have worn off at the time of surgery. It is also possible to continue the administration of SubQ heparin or LMWH and to stop therapy 12-24 hours before surgery with the expectation that the anticoagulant effect will be very low or will have worn off by the time of surgery.

Patients with low risk of bleeding: Continue warfarin therapy at a lower dose and operate at an INR of 1.3-1.5, an intensity that has been shown to be safe in randomized trials of gynecologic and orthopedic surgical patients. The dose of warfarin can be lowered 4-5 days before surgery. Warfarin therapy then can be restarted after surgery and supplemented with low-dose heparin or LMWH if necessary.

Heparin-induced Thrombocytopenia (HIT) or Heparin-induced Thrombotic Thrombocytopenia Syndrome (HITTS): When a patient develops HIT/HITTS, do not start warfarin. Rather, a direct thrombin inhibitor should be initiated and continued until platelets return. Warfarin anticoagulation should be postponed in the patient with HIT until substantial recovery of the platelet count has occurred.

Pregnancy Risk Factor X

Contraindications Hypersensitivity to warfarin or any component of the formulation; hemorrhagic tendencies; hemophilia; thrombocytopenia purpura; leukemia; recent or potential surgery of the eye or CNS; major regional lumbar block anesthesia or surgery resulting in large, open surfaces; patients bleeding from the GI, respiratory, or GU tract; threatened abortion; aneurysm; ascorbic acid deficiency; history of bleeding diathesis; prostatectomy; continuous tube drainage of the small intestine; polyarthritis; diverticulitis; emaciation; malnutrition; cerebrovascular hemorrhage; eclampsia/pre-eclampsia; blood dyscrasias; severe uncontrolled or malignant hypertension; severe hepatic disease; pericarditis or pericardial effusion; subacute bacterial endocarditis; visceral carcinoma; following spinal puncture and other diagnostic or therapeutic procedures with potential for significant bleeding; history of warfarin-induced necrosis; an unreliable, noncompliant patient; alcoholism; patient who has a history of falls or is a significant fall risk; pregnancy

Warnings/Precautions Use care in the selection of patients appropriate for this treatment. Ensure patient cooperation especially from the alcoholic, illicit drug user, demented, or psychotic patient. Use with caution in trauma, acute infection (antibiotics and fever may alter affects), renal insufficiency, prolonged dietary insufficiencies (vitamin K deficiency), moderate-severe hypertension, polycythemia vera, vasculitis, open wound, active TB, history of PUD, anaphylactic disorders, indwelling catheters, severe diabetes, thyroid disease, severe renal disease, and menstruating and postpartum women. Use with caution in protein C deficiency.

Hemorrhage is the most serious risk of therapy. Patient must be instructed to report bleeding, accidents, or falls. Patient must also report any new or discontinued medications, herbal or alternative products used, significant changes in smoking or dietary habits. Necrosis or gangrene of the skin and other tissues can occur (rarely) due to early hypercoagulability. "Purple toes syndrome," due to cholesterol microembolization, may rarely occur (often after several weeks of therapy). Women may be at risk of developing ovarian hemorrhage at the time of ovulation. The elderly may be more sensitive to anticoagulant therapy.

Adverse Reactions As with all anticoagulants, bleeding is the major adverse effect of warfarin. Hemorrhage may occur at virtually any site. Risk is dependent on multiple variables, including the intensity of anticoagulation and patient susceptibility.

Additional adverse effects are often related to idiosyncratic reactions, and the frequency cannot be accurately estimated.

Cardiovascular: Vasculitis, edema, hemorrhagic shock

Central nervous system: Fever, lethargy, malaise, asthenia, pain, headache, dizziness, stroke

Dermatologic: Rash, dermatitis, bullous eruptions, urticaria, pruritus, alopecia

Gastrointestinal: Anorexia, nausea, vomiting, stomach cramps, abdominal pain, diarrhea, flatulence, gastrointestinal bleeding, taste disturbance, mouth ulcers

Genitourinary: Priapism, hematuria

Hematologic: Hemorrhage, leukopenia, unrecognized bleeding sites (eg, colon cancer) may be uncovered by anticoagulation, retroperitoneal hematoma, agranulocytosis

Hepatic: Hepatic injury, jaundice, transaminases increased

Neuromuscular & skeletal: Paresthesia, osteoporosis

Respiratory: Hemoptysis, epistaxis, pulmonary hemorrhage, tracheobronchial calcification

Miscellaneous: Hypersensitivity/allergic reactions

Skin necrosis/gangrene, due to paradoxical local thrombosis, is a known but rare risk of warfarin therapy. Its onset is usually within the first few days of therapy and is frequently localized to the limbs, breast or penis. The risk of this effect is increased in patients with protein C or S deficiency.

"Purple toes syndrome," caused by cholesterol microembolization, also occurs rarely. Typically, this occurs after several weeks of therapy, and may present as a dark, purplish, mottled discoloration of the plantar and lateral surfaces. Other manifestations of cholesterol microembolization may include rash; livedo reticularis; gangrene; abrupt and intense pain in lower extremities; abdominal, flank, or back pain; hematuria, renal insufficiency; hypertension; cerebral ischemia; spinal cord infarction; or other symptom of vascular compromise.

Overdosage/Toxicology Symptoms of overdose include internal or external hemorrhage and hematuria. Avoid emesis and lavage to avoid possible trauma and incidental bleeding. When an overdose occurs, the drug should be immediately discontinued and vitamin K_1 (phytonadione) may be administered, up to 25 mg I.V. for adults. When hemorrhage occurs, fresh frozen plasma transfusions can help control bleeding by replacing clotting factors. In urgent bleeding, prothrombin complex concentrates may be needed.

Management of elevated INR: See table on page 1368.

Drug Interactions **Substrate** of CYP1A2 (minor), 2C9 (major), 2C19 (minor), 3A4 (minor); **Inhibits** CYP2C9 (moderate), 2C19 (weak)

Acetaminophen: May enhance the anticoagulant effect of warfarin. Most likely to occur with daily acetaminophen doses >1.3 g for >1 week.

Allopurinol: May enhance the anticoagulant effect of warfarin. Reductions in warfarin will likely be required.

Aminoglutethimide: May increase the metabolism, via CYP isoenzymes, of warfarin. Monitor therapy for decreased warfarin effect.

Amiodarone: May enhance the anticoagulant effect of warfarin. An empiric warfarin dosage reduction of 30% to 50% at the initiation of warfarin may be considered.

Androgens: May enhance the anticoagulant effect of warfarin. Significant reductions in warfarin dosage may be needed during concomitant therapy.

Antifungal agents (imidazole): May decrease the metabolism, via CYP isoenzymes, of warfarin. Monitor for increased therapeutic/toxic effects of warfarin.

(Continued)

Warfarin *(Continued)*

Antithyroid agents: May diminish the anticoagulant effects of warfarin. Monitor for decreased therapeutic effects.

Aprepitant: May decrease the serum concentration of warfarin. Monitor closely for 2 weeks following each course of aprecitant.

Azathioprine: May decrease the anticoagulant effect of warfarin. An adjustment in warfarin dose may be needed.

Barbiturates: May increase the metabolism, via CYP isoenzymes, of warfarin. Monitor for decreased therapeutic effect of warfarin. Anticoagulation dosage increase of 30% to 60% may be needed based upon monitored PT.

Bile acid sequestrants: May decrease absorption of warfarin. Separating the administration of doses by >2 hours may reduce the risk of interaction.

Bosentan: May increase metabolism, via CYP isoenzymes, of warfarin. Monitor for decreased effects.

Capecitabine: May decrease metabolism of warfarin. Monitor for evidence of excess anticoagulation.

Carbamazepine: May increase the metabolism, via CYP isoenzymes, of warfarin. Monitor for decreased therapeutic effect of warfarin.

Cephalosporins: May enhance the anticoagulant effect of warfarin. Monitor for increased evidence of bleeding especially in cephalosporins that have NMTT side chain.

Cimetidine: May enhance the anticoagulant effect of warfarin. Monitor for increased therapeutic effects of warfarin.

Contraceptives, hormonal (estrogens and progestins): May diminish the anticoagulant effect of warfarin. Monitor for changes in coagulation status.

COX-2 inhibitor: May enhance the anticoagulant effect of warfarin. Monitor for increased signs and symptoms of bleeding.

CYP2C9 inducers (strong): May increase the metabolism of warfarin. Examples of inducers include: Carbamazepine, fosphenytoin, phenobarbital, phenytoin, primidone, rifampin, rifapentine, secobarbital. Monitor for decreased effect of warfarin.

CYP2C9 Inhibitors may increase the levels/effects of warfarin. Example inhibitors include delavirdine, fluconazole, gemfibrozil, ketoconazole, nicardipine, NSAIDs, sulfonamides and tolbutamide.

Dicloxacillin: May increase the metabolism, via CYP isoenzymes, of warfarin. Monitor for decreased therapeutic effect of warfarin.

Disulfiram: May increase the serum concentration of warfarin. Monitor for increased therapeutic effects of warfarin.

Drotrecogin Alfa: Warfarin may enhance the adverse/toxic effect of drotrecogin alfa. Monitor for increased risk of bleeding during concomitant therapy. If possible, avoid use of drotrecogin within 7 days of warfarin therapy, or if INR ≥3.

Etoposide: May enhance the anticoagulant effect of warfarin. Monitor for increased effects of warfarin.

Fibric acid derivatives: May enhance the anticoagulant effect of warfarin. Monitor for toxic effects of warfarin; may warrant a 25% to 33% reduction in the warfarin dosage.

Fluconazole: May decrease the metabolism, via CYP isoenzymes, of warfarin. Monitor for increased therapeutic/toxic effects warfarin.

Fluorouracil: May enhance the anticoagulant effect of warfarin. Monitor for increased effects of warfarin.

Glucagon: May enhance the anticoagulant effect of warfarin. Monitor for toxic effects of warfarin, especially if glucagon is administered in high doses.

Glutethimide: May increase the metabolism, via CYP isoenzymes, of warfarin. Consider alternative sedative-hypnotic. Monitor for decreased therapeutic effects of warfarin.

Griseofulvin: May increase the metabolism, via CYP isoenzymes, of warfarin. Monitor for decreased therapeutic effects of warfarin.

HMG-CoA reductase inhibitors: May enhance the anticoagulant effect of warfarin. Monitor for increased effects of warfarin.

Ifosfamide: May enhance the anticoagulant effect of warfarin. Monitor for increased effects of warfarin.

Leflunomide: May enhance the anticoagulant effect of warfarin. Monitor for increased effects of warfarin.

Macrolide antibiotics: May decrease the metabolism, via CYP isoenzymes, of warfarin. Monitor for increased therapeutic effects of warfarin. CYP inhibitors (eg, clarithromycin, erythromycin, and troleandomycin) appear to pose the greatest risk. Azithromycin and telithromycin have also been implicated in a few cases.

Mercaptopurine: May diminish the anticoagulant effect of warfarin. Monitor for decreased therapeutic effects of warfarin.

Metronidazole: May decrease the metabolism, via CYP isoenzymes, of warfarin. If concomitant therapy is necessary, consider an empiric reduction in warfarin dosage of approximately one-third. Monitor for increased therapeutic/toxic effects of warfarin.

Nafcillin: May increase the metabolism of warfarin. Consider choosing an alternative antibiotic if available. Monitor for decreased therapeutic effect of warfarin if nafcillin is initiated. The effects on warfarin dosing may persist long after the nafcillin is discontinued. Close monitoring is required even after nafcillin is discontinued.

NSAID (nonselective): May enhance the anticoagulant effect of warfarin. Monitor for increased signs and symptoms of bleeding.

Orlistat: May enhance the anticoagulant effect of warfarin. Monitor for changes in effects of warfarin.

Phenytoin: May enhance the anticoagulant effect of warfarin. Warfarin may increase the serum concentration of phenytoin. Monitor for increased effects of warfarin and for increased serum concentrations/toxic effects of phenytoin.

Phytonadione: May antagonize the effects of warfarin. Monitor for decreased therapeutic effect of warfarin.

Propafenone: May increase the serum concentration of warfarin. Monitor for increased prothrombin times (PT)/therapeutic effects of warfarin.

Propoxyphene: May decrease the metabolism, via CYP isoenzymes, of warfarin. Monitor for increased prothrombin time/toxic effects of warfarin.

Proton pump inhibitors (omeprazole): May increase the serum concentration of warfarin. Monitor for increased effects of warfarin.

Quinidine: May enhance the anticoagulant effect of warfarin. Monitor for increased prothrombin times (PT)/therapeutic effects of warfarin.

Quinolone antibiotics: May enhance the anticoagulant effect of warfarin. Monitor for increased prothrombin time/toxic effects of warfarin.

Rifamycin derivatives: May increase the metabolism, via CYP isoenzymes, of warfarin. Monitor for decreased prothrombin times (PT)/therapeutic effects of warfarin.

Ropinirole: May enhance the anticoagulant effect of warfarin. Monitor for increased INR/effects of warfarin.

Salicylates: May enhance the anticoagulant effect of warfarin. Monitor for increased signs and symptoms of bleeding if used concomitantly.

Selective serotonin reuptake inhibitors (SSRIs): May enhance the anticoagulant effect of warfarin. Monitor for increased therapeutic/toxic effects of warfarin.

Sulfasalazine: May diminish the anticoagulant effect of warfarin. Monitor for decreased INR/effects of warfarin

Sulfinpyrazone: May decrease the metabolism, via CYP isoenzymes, of warfarin and may decrease the protein binding of warfarin. Monitor for increased prothrombin time (PT)/toxic effects of warfarin.

Sulfonamide derivatives: May enhance the anticoagulant effect of warfarin. Monitor for increased prothrombin time (PT)/toxic effects of warfarin.

Tetracycline derivatives: May enhance the anticoagulant effect of warfarin. Monitor for toxic effects of warfarin.

Thyroid products: May enhance the anticoagulant effect of warfarin. Monitor for increased hypoprothrombinemic effects of warfarin.

Tigecycline: May increase the serum concentration of warfarin. Monitor for increased effects of warfarin.

Treprostinil: May enhance the adverse/toxic effect of warfarin. Monitor for increased risk of bleeding when used concomitantly.

Tricyclic antidepressants: May enhance the anticoagulant effect of warfarin. Monitor for increased prothrombin times (PT)/toxic effects of warfarin.

Vitamin A: May enhance the anticoagulant effect of warfarin. Monitor for increased prothrombin time (PT)/effects of warfarin.

Vitamin E: May enhance the anticoagulant effect of warfarin. Monitor for increased prothrombin time (PT)/effects of warfarin. Likely only of significant concern with higher doses of vitamin E (eg, 1200 int. units/day).

Voriconazole: May increase the serum concentration of warfarin. Monitor for increased effects (eg, INR, bleeding) of warfarin.

Zafirlukast: May decrease the metabolism, via CYP isoenzymes, of warfarin. Monitor for increased prothrombin time (PT)/effects of warfarin.

Zileuton: May increase the serum concentration of warfarin. Monitor for increased effects of warfarin.

Ethanol/Nutrition/Herb Interactions

Ethanol: Avoid ethanol. Acute ethanol ingestion (binge drinking) decreases the metabolism of warfarin and increases PT/INR. Chronic daily ethanol use increases the metabolism of warfarin and decreases PT/INR.

Food: The anticoagulant effects of warfarin may be decreased if taken with foods rich in vitamin K. Vitamin E may increase warfarin effect. Cranberry juice may increase warfarin effect.

(Continued)

Warfarin *(Continued)*

Herb/Nutraceutical: Cranberry, fenugreek, ginkgo biloba, glucosamine, may enhance bleeding or increase warfarin's effect. Ginseng (American), coenzyme Q_{10}, and St John's wort may decrease warfarin levels and effects. Avoid alfalfa, anise, bilberry, bladderwrack, bromelain, cat's claw, celery, coleus, cordyceps, dong quai, evening primrose oil, fenugreek, feverfew, garlic, ginger, ginkgo biloba, ginseng (American), ginseng (Panax), ginseng (Siberian), grape seed, green tea, guggul, horse chestnut seed, horseradish, licorice, prickly ash, red clover, reishi, same (s-adenosylmethionine), sweet clover, turmeric,and white willow (all have additional antiplatelet activity).

Management of Elevated INR

INR	Symptom	Action
Above therapeutic range to <5	No significant bleeding	Lower or hold the next dose and monitor frequently; when INR approaches desired range, may resume dosing with a lower dose if INR was significantly above therapeutic range.
≥5 and <9	No significant bleeding	Omit the next 1or 2 doses; monitor INR and resume with a lower dose when the INR approaches the desired range. Alternatively, if there are other risk factors for bleeding, omit the next dose and give vitamin K_1 orally ≤5 mg; resume with a lower dose when the INR approaches the desired range. If rapid reversal is required for surgery, then given vitamin K_1 orally 2-4 mg and hold warfarin. Expect a response within 24 hours; another 1-2 mg may be given orally if needed.
≥9	No significant bleeding	Hold warfarin, give vitamin K_1 orally 5-10 mg, expect the INR to be reduced within 24-48 hours; monitor INR and administer additional vitamin K if necessary. Resume warfarin at lower doses when INR is in the desired range.
Any INR elevation	Serious bleeding	Hold warfarin, give vitamin K_1 (10 mg by slow I.V. infusion), and supplement with fresh plasma transfusion or prothrombin complex concentrate (Factor X complex); recombinant factor VIIa is an alternative to prothrombin complex concentrate. Vitamin K_1 injection can be repeated every 12 hours.
Any INR elevation	Life-threatening bleeding	Hold warfarin, give prothrombin complex concentrate, supplemented with vitamin K_1 (10 mg by slow I.V. infusion); repeat if necessary. Recombinant factor VIIa is an alternative to prothrombin complex concentrate.

Note: Use of high doses of vitamin K_1 (10-15 mg) may cause resistance to warfarin for up to a week. Heparin or low molecular weight heparin can be given until the patient becomes respon sive to warfarin.

Reference: Ansell J, Hirsh J, Poller L et al. "The Pharmacology and Management of the Vitamin K Antagonists," *Chest*, 2004, 126 (3 Suppl):204-33.

Dietary Considerations Foods high in vitamin K (eg, beef liver, pork liver, green tea and leafy green vegetables) inhibit anticoagulant effect. Do not change dietary habits once stabilized on warfarin therapy; a balanced diet with a consistent intake of vitamin K is essential; avoid large amounts of alfalfa, asparagus, broccoli, Brussels sprouts, cabbage, cauliflower, green teas, kale, lettuce, spinach, turnip greens, watercress decrease efficacy of warfarin. It is recommended that the diet contain a CONSISTENT vitamin K content of 70-140 mcg/day. Check with healthcare provider before changing diet.

Dosage Forms

Injection, powder for reconstitution, as sodium (Coumadin®): 5 mg

Tablet, as sodium (Coumadin®, Jantoven™): 1 mg, 2 mg, 2.5 mg, 3 mg, 4 mg, 5 mg, 6 mg, 7.5 mg, 10 mg

References

Hirsh J, Guyatt G, Albers GW, et al, "The Seventh ACCP Conference on Antithrombotic and Thrombolytic Therapy: Evidence-Based Guidelines," *Chest*, 2004, 126(3 Suppl):163S-608S.

♦ **Warfarin Sodium** *see* Warfarin *on page 1362*

♦ **4-Way® 12 Hour [OTC]** *see* Oxymetazoline *on page 973*

♦ **4-Way® Saline Moisturizing Mist [OTC]** *see* Sodium Chloride *on page 1183*

- **Wellbutrin®** *see* BuPROPion *on page 201*
- **Wellbutrin XL™** *see* BuPROPion *on page 201*
- **Wellbutrin SR®** *see* BuPROPion *on page 201*
- **Westcort®** *see* Hydrocortisone *on page 639*
- **Winpred™ (Can)** *see* PredniSONE *on page 1050*
- **Wound Wash Saline™ [OTC]** *see* Sodium Chloride *on page 1183*
- **Xanax®** *see* Alprazolam *on page 65*
- **Xanax TS™ (Can)** *see* Alprazolam *on page 65*
- **Xanax XR®** *see* Alprazolam *on page 65*
- **Xatral (Can)** *see* Alfuzosin *on page 58*
- **Xigris®** *see* Drotrecogin Alfa *on page 434*
- **Xolair®** *see* Omalizumab *on page 955*
- **Xopenex®** *see* Levalbuterol *on page 739*
- **Xopenex HFA™** *see* Levalbuterol *on page 739*
- **Xylocaine®** *see* Lidocaine *on page 755*
- **Xylocaine® MPF** *see* Lidocaine *on page 755*
- **Xylocaine® Viscous** *see* Lidocaine *on page 755*
- **Xylocard® (Can)** *see* Lidocaine *on page 755*
- **Xyrem®** *see* Sodium Oxybate *on page 1187*
- **YM087** *see* Conivaptan *on page 331*

Zanamivir (za NA mi veer)

U.S. Brand Names Relenza®

Canadian Brand Names Relenza®

Pharmacologic Category Antiviral Agent; Neuraminidase Inhibitor

Generic Available No

Use Treatment of uncomplicated acute illness due to influenza virus A and B; treatment should only be initiated in patients who have been symptomatic for no more than 2 days. Prophylaxis against influenza virus A and B

Mechanism of Action Zanamivir inhibits influenza virus neuraminidase enzymes, potentially altering virus particle aggregation and release.

Pharmacodynamics/Kinetics

Absorption: Inhalation: 4% to 17%

Protein binding, plasma: <10%

Metabolism: None

Half-life elimination, serum: 2.5-5.1 hours

Excretion: Urine (as unchanged drug); feces (unabsorbed drug)

Dosage Oral inhalation:

Children ≥5 years and Adults: Prophylaxis (household setting): Two inhalations (10 mg) once daily for 10 days. Begin within 1 ½ days following onset of signs or symptoms of index case.

Children ≥7 years and Adults: Treatment: Two inhalations (10 mg total) twice daily for 5 days. Doses on first day should be separated by at least 2 hours; on subsequent days, doses should be spaced by ~12 hours. Begin within 2 days of signs or symptoms.

Adolescents and Adults: Prophylaxis (community outbreak): Two inhalations (10 mg) once daily for 28 days. Begin within 5 days of outbreak.

Stability Store at room temperature (25°C) 77°F; do not puncture blister until taking a dose using the Diskhaler®

Administration Inhalation: Must be used with Diskhaler® delivery device. Patients who are scheduled to use an inhaled bronchodilator should use their bronchodilator prior to zanamivir. With the exception of the initial dose when used for treatment, administer at the same time each day.

Anesthesia and Critical Care Concerns/Other Considerations Patients with asthma or COPD should be informed of the risk of bronchospasm and should have a fast-acting bronchodilator available when treated with zanamivir. Majority of patients included in clinical trials were infected with influenza A, however, a number of patients with influenza B infections were also enrolled. Patients with lower temperature or less severe symptoms appeared to derive less benefit from therapy. No consistent treatment benefit was demonstrated in patients with chronic underlying medical conditions.

(Continued)

Zanamivir *(Continued)*

Pregnancy Risk Factor C

Contraindications Hypersensitivity to zanamivir or any component of the formulation

Warnings/Precautions Patients must be instructed in the use of the delivery system. No data are available to support the use of this drug in patients who begin use for treatment after 48 hours of symptoms. Effectiveness has not been established in patients with significant underlying medical conditions or for prophylaxis of influenza in nursing home patients. Not recommended for use in patients with underlying respiratory disease, such as asthma or COPD, due to lack of efficacy and risk of serious adverse effects. Bronchospasm, decreased lung function, and other serious adverse reactions, including those with fatal outcomes, have been reported in patients with and without airway disease; discontinue with bronchospasm or signs of decreased lung function. For a patient with an underlying airway disease where a medical decision has been made to use zanamivir, a fast-acting bronchodilator should be made available, and used prior to each dose. Not a substitute for the flu vaccine. Consider primary or concomitant bacterial infections. Powder for oral inhalation contains lactose. Safety and efficacy of repeated courses or use with severe renal impairment have not been established; efficacy in children <5 years of age have not been established.

Adverse Reactions Most adverse reactions occurred at a frequency which was less than or equal to the control (lactose vehicle).

>10%:

Central nervous system: Headache (prophylaxis 13% to 24%; treatment 2%)
Gastrointestinal: Throat/tonsil discomfort/pain (prophylaxis 8% to 19%)
Respiratory: Cough (prophylaxis 7% to 17%; treatment ≤2%), nasal signs and symptoms (prophylaxis 12%; treatment 2%)
Miscellaneous: Viral infection (prophylaxis 3% to 13%)

1% to 10%:

Central nervous system: Fever/chills (prophylaxis 5% to 9%; treatment <1.5%), fatigue (prophylaxis 5% to 8%; treatment <1.5%), malaise (prophylaxis 5% to 8%; treatment <1.5%), dizziness (treatment 1% to 2%)
Dermatologic: Urticaria (treatment <1.5%)
Gastrointestinal: Anorexia/appetite decreased (prophylaxis 2% to 4%), nausea (prophylaxis 1% to 2%; treatment ≤3%), diarrhea (prophylaxis 2%; treatment 2% to 3%), vomiting (prophylaxis 1% to 2%; treatment 1% to 2%) abdominal pain (treatment <1.5%)
Neuromuscular & skeletal: Muscle pain (prophylaxis 3% to 8%), musculoskeletal pain (prophylaxis 6%), arthralgia/articular rheumatism (prophylaxis 2%), arthralgia (treatment <1.5%), myalgia (treatment <1.5%)
Respiratory: Infection (ear/nose/throat; prophylaxis 2%; treatment 2% to 5%), sinusitis (treatment 3%), bronchitis (treatment 2%), nasal inflammation (prophylaxis 1%)

<1% (Limited to important or life-threatening): Allergic or allergic-like reaction (including oropharyngeal edema), arrhythmia, asthma, bronchospasm, dyspnea, facial edema, hemorrhage (ear/nose/throat), rash (including serious cutaneous reactions), seizure, syncope

Overdosage/Toxicology Information is limited, and symptoms appear similar to reported adverse events from clinical studies. Treatment should be symptom-directed and supportive

Drug Interactions Influenza virus vaccine: Zanamivir may diminish the therapeutic effect of live, attentuated influenza virus vaccine (FluMist™). The manufacturer of FluMist™ recommends that the administration of anti-influenza virus medications be avoided during the period beginning 48 hours prior to vaccine administration and ending 2 weeks after vaccine.

Dosage Forms Powder for oral inhalation: 5 mg/blister (20s) [4 blisters per Rotadisk® foil pack, 5 Rotadisk® per package; packaged with Diskhaler® inhalation device; contains lactose]

- **Zantac®** *see* Ranitidine *on page 1105*
- **Zantac® EFFERdose®** *see* Ranitidine *on page 1105*
- **Zaroxolyn®** *see* Metolazone *on page 837*
- **ZDV** *see* Zidovudine *on page 1371*
- **Zebeta®** *see* Bisoprolol *on page 176*
- **Zeldox** *see* Ziprasidone *on page 1374*
- **Zemuron®** *see* Rocuronium *on page 1135*

- **Zenapax®** *see* Daclizumab *on page 346*
- **Zeneca 182,780** *see* Fulvestrant *on page 571*
- **Zerit®** *see* Stavudine *on page 1205*
- **Zestril®** *see* Lisinopril *on page 767*
- **Ziagen®** *see* Abacavir *on page 22*

Zidovudine (zye DOE vyoo deen)

Medication Safety Issues

Sound-alike/look-alike issues:

Azidothymidine may be confused with azathioprine, aztreonam

Retrovir® may be confused with ritonavir

AZT is an error-prone abbreviation (mistaken as azathioprine, aztreonam)

U.S. Brand Names Retrovir®

Canadian Brand Names AZT™; Retrovir®

Synonyms Azidothymidine; AZT (error-prone abbreviation); Compound S; ZDV

Pharmacologic Category Antiretroviral Agent, Reverse Transcriptase Inhibitor (Nucleoside)

Generic Available Yes: Tablet

Use Management of patients with HIV infections in combination with at least two other antiretroviral agents; for prevention of maternal/fetal HIV transmission as monotherapy

Unlabeled/Investigational Use Postexposure prophylaxis for HIV exposure as part of a multidrug regimen

Mechanism of Action Zidovudine is a thymidine analog which interferes with the HIV viral RNA dependent DNA polymerase resulting in inhibition of viral replication; nucleoside reverse transcriptase inhibitor

Pharmacodynamics/Kinetics

Distribution: Significant penetration into the CSF; crosses placenta

V_d: 1-2.2 L/kg

Relative diffusion from blood into CSF: Adequate with or without inflammation (exceeds usual MICs)

CSF:blood level ratio: Normal meninges: ~60%

Protein binding: 25% to 38%

Metabolism: Hepatic via glucuronidation to inactive metabolites; extensive first-pass effect

Bioavailability: 54% to 74%

Half-life elimination: Terminal: 0.5-3 hours

Time to peak, serum: 30-90 minutes

Excretion:

Oral: Urine (72% to 74% as metabolites, 14% to 18% as unchanged drug)

I.V.: Urine (45% to 60% as metabolites, 18% to 29% as unchanged drug)

Dosage

Prevention of maternal-fetal HIV transmission:

Neonatal: **Note:** Dosing should begin 8-12 hours after birth and continue for the first 6 weeks of life.

Oral:

Full-term infants: 2 mg/kg/dose every 6 hours

Infants ≥30 weeks and <35 weeks gestation at birth: 2 mg/kg/dose every 12 hours; at 2 weeks of age, advance to 2 mg/kg/dose every 8 hours

Infants <30 weeks gestation at birth: 2 mg/kg/dose every 12 hours; at 4 weeks of age, advance to 2 mg/kg/dose every 8 hours

I.V.: Infants unable to receive oral dosing:

Full term: 1.5 mg/kg/dose every 6 hours

Infants ≥30 weeks and <35 weeks gestation at birth: 1.5 mg/kg/dose every 12 hours; at 2 weeks of age, advance to 1.5 mg/kg/dose every 8 hours

Infants <30 weeks gestation at birth: 1.5 mg/kg/dose every 12 hours; at 4 weeks of age, advance to 1.5 mg/kg/dose every 8 hours

Maternal: Oral (per AIDSinfo guidelines): 100 mg 5 times/day **or** 200 mg 3 times/day **or** 300 mg twice daily. Begin at 14-34 weeks gestation and continue until start of labor.

During labor and delivery, administer zidovudine I.V. at 2 mg/kg over 1 hour followed by a continuous I.V. infusion of 1 mg/kg/hour until the umbilical cord is clamped

Treatment of HIV infection:

Children 6 weeks to 12 years:

Oral: 160 mg/m²/dose every 8 hours (maximum: 200 mg every 8 hours);

(Continued)

Zidovudine *(Continued)*

some Working Group members use a dose of 180 mg/m² to 240 mg/m² every 12 hours when using in drug combinations with other antiretroviral compounds, but data on this dosing in children is limited

I.V. continuous infusion: 20 mg/m²/hour

I.V. intermittent infusion: 120 mg/m²/dose every 6 hours

Adults:

Oral: 300 mg twice daily or 200 mg 3 times/day

I.V.: 1-2 mg/kg/dose (infused over 1 hour) administered every 4 hours around-the-clock (6 doses/day)

Prevention of HIV following needlesticks (unlabeled use): Oral: Adults: 200 mg 3 times/day plus lamivudine 150 mg twice daily; a protease inhibitor (eg, indinavir) may be added for high risk exposures; begin therapy within 2 hours of exposure if possible

Patients should receive I.V. therapy only until oral therapy can be administered

Dosing adjustment for hematologic toxicity: Consider dose interruption for significant anemia (hemoglobin <7.5 g/dL or >25% reduction from baseline) and/or neutropenia (granulocyte count <750 cells/mm³ or >50% reduction from baseline) until evidence of recovery. Anemia associated with chronic zidovudine may warrant dose reduction.

Dosing adjustment in renal impairment: Cl_{cr} <15 mL/minute: May require minor dose adjustment

Hemodialysis/peritoneal dialysis: 100 mg every 6-8 hours

Continuous arteriovenous or venovenous hemodiafiltration effects: Administer 100 mg every 8 hours

Dosing adjustment in hepatic impairment: Reduce dose by 50% or double dosing interval in patients with cirrhosis

Stability Solution for injection should be diluted with D_5W to a concentration of ≤4 mg/mL; the solution is physically and chemically stable for 24 hours at room temperature and 48 hours if refrigerated; attempt to administer diluted solution within 8 hours, if stored at room temperature or 24 hours if refrigerated to minimize potential for microbially contaminated solutions; store undiluted vials at room temperature and protect from light

Administration

Oral: Administer around-the-clock to promote less variation in peak and trough serum levels; may be administered without regard to food

I.M.: Do not administer I.M.

I.V.: Avoid rapid infusion or bolus injection

Neonates: Infuse over 30 minutes

Adults: Infuse over 1 hour

Monitoring Parameters Monitor CBC and platelet count at least every 2 weeks, liver function tests, MCV, serum creatinine kinase, viral load, and CD4 count; observe for appearance of opportunistic infections

Anesthesia and Critical Care Concerns/Other Considerations Does not reduce risk of transmitting HIV infections. Potential compliance problems, frequency of administration and adverse effects should be discussed with patients before initiating therapy to help prevent the emergence of resistance.

Pregnancy Risk Factor C

Contraindications Life-threatening hypersensitivity to zidovudine or any component of the formulation

Warnings/Precautions [U.S. Boxed Warning]: Often associated with hematologic toxicity including granulocytopenia, severe anemia requiring transfusions, or (rarely) pancytopenia. Use with caution in patients with bone marrow compromise (granulocytes <1000 cells/mm³ or hemoglobin <9.5 mg/dL); dosage adjustment may be required in patients who develop anemia or neutropenia. **[U.S. Boxed Warning]: Lactic acidosis and severe hepatomegaly with steatosis have been reported, including fatal cases;** use with caution in patients with risk factors for liver disease (risk may be increased in obese patients or prolonged exposure) and suspend treatment with zidovudine in any patient who develops clinical or laboratory findings suggestive of lactic acidosis (transaminase elevation may/may not accompany hepatomegaly and steatosis). Use caution in combination with interferon alfa with or without ribavirin in HIV/HBV coinfected patients; monitor closely for hepatic decompensation, anemia, or neutropenia. Prolonged use has been associated with symptomatic myopathy and myositis. Immune reconstitution syndrome may develop resulting in the occurrence of an inflammatory response to an indolent or residual opportunistic infection; further evaluation and treatment may be required. Reduce dose in patients with severe renal impairment.

Adverse Reactions As reported in adult patients with asymptomatic HIV infection. Frequency and severity may increase with advanced disease.

>10%:
- Central nervous system: Headache (63%), malaise (53%)
- Gastrointestinal: Nausea (51%), anorexia (20%), vomiting (17%)

1% to 10%:
- Gastrointestinal: Constipation (6%)
- Hematologic: Granulocytopenia (2%), anemia (1%)
- Hepatic: Transaminases increased (1% to 3%)
- Neuromuscular & skeletal: Weakness (9%)

Frequency not defined:
- Cardiovascular: Cardiomyopathy, chest pain, syncope, vasculitis
- Central nervous system: Anxiety, chills, confusion, depression, dizziness, fatigue, insomnia, loss of mental acuity, mania, seizures, somnolence, vertigo
- Dermatologic: Pruritus, rash, skin/nail pigmentation changes, Stevens-Johnson syndrome, toxic epidermal necrolysis, urticaria
- Endocrine & metabolic: Body fat redistribution, gynecomastia
- Gastrointestinal: Abdominal cramps, abdominal pain, dyspepsia, dysphagia, flatulence, mouth ulcer, oral mucosa pigmentation, pancreatitis, taste perversion
- Genitourinary: Urinary frequency, urinary hesitancy
- Hematologic: Aplastic anemia, hemolytic anemia, leukopenia, lymphadenopathy, pancytopenia with marrow hypoplasia, pure red cell aplasia
- Hepatic: Hepatitis, hepatomegaly with steatosis, hyperbilirubinemia, jaundice, lactic acidosis
- Neuromuscular & skeletal: Arthralgia, back pain, CPK increased, LDH increased, musculoskeletal pain, myalgia, neuropathy, muscle spasm, myopathy, myositis, paresthesia, rhabdomyolysis, tremor
- Ocular: Amblyopia, macular edema, photophobia
- Otic: Hearing loss
- Respiratory: Cough, dyspnea, rhinitis, sinusitis
- Miscellaneous: Allergic reactions, anaphylaxis, angioedema, diaphoresis, flu-like syndrome

Overdosage/Toxicology Acute overdoses up to 50 g have been reported. Symptoms of overdose include nausea, vomiting, ataxia, and granulocytopenia. Treatment is symptom-directed and supportive. Dialysis does not appear to significantly remove zidovudine, but does improve clearance of the primary metabolite.

Drug Interactions **Substrate** (minor) of CYP2A6, 2C9, 2C19, 3A4

- Bone marrow suppressants/cytotoxic agents: Concomitant use may increase risk of hematologic toxicity. (May be seen with adriamycin, dapsone, flucytosine, vincristine, vinblastine.)
- Fluconazole: Fluconazole may decrease clearance and metabolism of zidovudine
- Ganciclovir, valganciclovir: Concomitant use may increase risk of hematologic toxicities; monitor hemoglobin, hematocrit, and white blood cell count with differential frequently; dose reduction or interruption of either agent may be needed
- Interferon-alfa: Concomitant use may increase risk of hematologic toxicities; monitor hemoglobin, hematocrit, and white blood cell count with differential frequently; dose reduction or interruption of either agent may be needed.
- Methadone: May increase serum levels/effects of zidovudine; monitor.
- Probenecid: Probenecid may increase zidovudine levels. Myalgia, malaise, and/or fever and maculopapular rash have been reported with concomitant use.
- Ribavirin: Concomitant use of ribavirin and nucleoside analogues may increase the risk of developing lactic acidosis (includes adefovir, didanosine, lamivudine, stavudine, zalcitabine, zidovudine). May decrease the antiviral activity of zidovudine (based on *in vitro* data); avoid concurrent use.
- Rifampin: May decrease levels of zidovudine; monitor.
- Stavudine: Zidovudine may decrease the antiviral activity of stavudine (based on *in vitro* data). Avoid concurrent use.
- Trimetrexate: Zidovudine may increase the myelosuppressive effects of trimetrexate; avoid concomitant use.
- Valproic acid: Valproic acid may increase plasma levels of zidovudine; monitor for possible increase in side effects (AUC increased by 80%)

Dietary Considerations May be taken without regard to food.

(Continued)

Zidovudine *(Continued)*

Dosage Forms

Capsule (Retrovir®): 100 mg

Injection, solution [preservative free] (Retrovir®): 10 mg/mL (20 mL)

Syrup (Retrovir®): 50 mg/5 mL (240 mL) [contains sodium benzoate; strawberry flavor]

Tablet (Retrovir®): 300 mg

- **Zilactin® (Can)** *see* Lidocaine *on page 755*
- **Zilactin-L® [OTC]** *see* Lidocaine *on page 755*
- **Zinacef®** *see* Cefuroxime *on page 253*
- **Zinc** *see* Trace Metals *on page 1296*
- **Zinc Oxide and Miconazole Nitrate** *see* Miconazole and Zinc Oxide *on page 847*

Ziprasidone (zi PRAY si done)

U.S. Brand Names Geodon®

Synonyms Zeldox; Ziprasidone Hydrochloride; Ziprasidone Mesylate

Pharmacologic Category Antipsychotic Agent, Atypical

Generic Available No

Use Treatment of schizophrenia; treatment of acute manic or mixed episodes associated with bipolar disorder with or without psychosis; acute agitation in patients with schizophrenia

Unlabeled/Investigational Use Tourette's syndrome

Mechanism of Action Ziprasidone is a benzylisothiazolylpiperazine antipsychotic. The exact mechanism of action is unknown. However, *in vitro* radioligand studies show that ziprasidone has high affinity for D_2, D_3, 5-HT_{2A}, 5-HT_{1A}, 5-HT_{2C}, 5-HT_{1D}, and $alpha_1$ adrenergic; moderate affinity for histamine H_1 receptors; and no appreciable affinity for $alpha_2$ adrenergic receptors, beta adrenergic, 5-HT_3, 5-HT_4, cholinergic, mu, sigma, or benzodiazepine receptors. Ziprasidone functions as an antagonist at the D_2, 5-HT_{2A}, and 5-HT_{1D} receptors and as an agonist at the 5-HT_{1A} receptor. Ziprasidone moderately inhibits the reuptake of serotonin and norepinephrine.

Pharmacodynamics/Kinetics

Absorption: Well absorbed

Distribution: V_d: 1.5 L/kg

Protein binding: 99%, primarily to albumin and $alpha_1$-acid glycoprotein

Metabolism: Extensively hepatic, primarily via aldehyde oxidase; less than ⅓ of total metabolism via CYP3A4 and CYP1A2 (minor)

Bioavailability: Oral (with food): 60% (up to twofold increase with food); I.M.: 100%

Half-life elimination: Oral: 7 hours; I.M.: 2-5 hours

Time to peak: Oral: 6-8 hours; I.M.: ≤60 minutes

Excretion: Feces (66%) and urine (20%) as metabolites; little as unchanged drug (1% urine, 4% feces)

Clearance: 7.5 mL/minute/kg

Dosage

Children and Adolescents: Tourette's syndrome (unlabeled use): Oral: 5-40 mg/day

Adults:

Bipolar mania: Oral: Initial: 40 mg twice daily (with food)

Adjustment: May increase to 60 or 80 mg twice daily on second day of treatment; average dose 40-80 mg twice daily

Schizophrenia: Oral: Initial: 20 mg twice daily (with food)

Adjustment: Increases (if indicated) should be made no more frequently than every 2 days; ordinarily patients should be observed for improvement over several weeks before adjusting the dose

Maintenance: Range 20-100 mg twice daily; however, dosages >80 mg twice daily are generally not recommended

Acute agitation (schizophrenia): I.M.: 10 mg every 2 hours **or** 20 mg every 4 hours; maximum: 40 mg/day; oral therapy should replace I.M. administration as soon as possible

Elderly: No dosage adjustment is recommended; consider initiating at a low end of the dosage range, with slower titration

Dosage adjustment in renal impairment:

Oral: No dosage adjustment is recommended

I.M.: Cyclodextrin, an excipient in the I.M. formulation, is cleared by renal filtration; use with caution.

Ziprasidone is not removed by hemodialysis.

Dosage adjustment in hepatic impairment: No dosage adjustment is recommended

Stability

Capsule: Store at controlled room temperature of 15°C to 30°C (59°F to 86°F).

Vials for injection: Store at controlled room temperature of 15°C to 30°C (59°F to 86°F); protect from light. Each vial should be reconstituted with 1.2 mL SWI; shake vigorously; will form a pale, pink solution containing 20 mg/mL ziprasidone. Following reconstitution, injection may be stored at room temperature up to 24 hours, or up to 7 days if refrigerated; protect from light.

Administration

Oral: Administer with food.

Injection: For I.M. administration only.

Monitoring Parameters Vital signs; serum potassium and magnesium; fasting lipid profile and fasting blood glucose/Hgb A_{1c} (prior to treatment, at 3 months, then annually); BMI, personal/family history of obesity, waist circumference; blood pressure; mental status, abnormal involuntary movement scale (AIMS), extrapyramidal symptoms. Weight should be assessed prior to treatment, at 4 weeks, 8 weeks, 12 weeks, and then at quarterly intervals. Consider titrating to a different antipsychotic agent for a weight gain ≥5% of the initial weight. The value of routine ECG screening or monitoring has not been established.

Pregnancy Risk Factor C

Contraindications Hypersensitivity to ziprasidone or any component of the formulation; history (or current) prolonged QT; congenital long QT syndrome; recent myocardial infarction; history of arrhythmias; uncompensated heart failure; concurrent use of other QT_c-prolonging agents including amiodarone, arsenic trioxide, bretylium, chlorpromazine, cisapride, class Ia antiarrhythmics (quinidine, procainamide), dofetilide, dolasetron, droperidol, halofantrine, ibutilide, levomethadyl, mefloquine, mesoridazine, pentamidine, pimozide, probucol, some quinolone antibiotics (moxifloxacin, sparfloxacin, gatifloxacin), sotalol, tacrolimus, and thioridazine

Warnings/Precautions [U.S. Boxed Warning]: Patients with dementia-related behavioral disorders treated with atypical antipsychotics are at an increased risk of death compared to placebo. Ziprasidone is not approved for this indication.

May result in QT_c prolongation (dose-related), which has been associated with the development of malignant ventricular arrhythmias (torsade de pointes) and sudden death. Observed prolongation was greater than with other atypical antipsychotic agents (risperidone, olanzapine, quetiapine), but less than with thioridazine. Avoid hypokalemia, hypomagnesemia. Use caution in patients with bradycardia. Discontinue in patients found to have persistent QT_c intervals >500 msec. Patients with symptoms of dizziness, palpitations, or syncope should receive further cardiac evaluation.

May cause extrapyramidal symptoms, including pseudoparkinsonism, acute dystonic reactions, akathisia, and tardive dyskinesia. Disturbances of temperature regulation have been reported with antipsychotics (not reported in premarketing trials of ziprasidone). Antipsychotic use may also be associated with neuroleptic malignant syndrome (NMS). Use with caution in patients at risk of seizures, including those with a history of seizures, head trauma, brain damage, alcoholism, or concurrent therapy with medications which may lower seizure threshold. Elderly patients may be at increased risk of seizures due to an increased prevalence of predisposing factors.

May cause orthostatic hypotension; use with caution in patients at risk of this effect or in those who would tolerate transient hypotensive episodes (cerebrovascular disease, cardiovascular disease, hypovolemia, or other medications which may predispose).

Atypical antipsychotics have been associated with development of hyperglycemia; in some cases, may be extreme and associated with ketoacidosis, hyperosmolar coma, or death. There is limited documentation with ziprasidone and specific risk associated with this agent is not known. Use caution in patients with diabetes or other disorders of glucose regulation; monitor for worsening of glucose control.

(Continued)

Ziprasidone *(Continued)*

Cognitive and/or motor impairment (sedation) is common with ziprasidone, resulting in impaired performance of tasks requiring alertness (eg, operating machinery or driving). Use with caution in disorders where CNS depression is a feature. Use with caution in Parkinson's disease. Esophageal dysmotility and aspiration have been associated with antipsychotic use; use with caution in patients at risk of aspiration pneumonia (ie, Alzheimer's disease). Caution in breast cancer or other prolactin-dependent tumors (may elevate prolactin levels). Use caution in patients with renal or hepatic impairment. Ziprasidone has been associated with a fairly high incidence of rash (5%); discontinue if alternative etiology is not identified. Safety and efficacy have not been established in pediatric patients.

The possibility of a suicide attempt is inherent in psychotic illness or bipolar disorder; use caution in high-risk patients during initiation of therapy. Prescriptions should be written for the smallest quantity consistent with good patient care.

Adverse Reactions Note: Although minor QT_c prolongation (mean 10 msec at 160 mg/day) may occur more frequently (incidence not specified), clinically-relevant prolongation (>500 msec) was rare (0.06%) and less than placebo (0.23%).

>10%:

- Central nervous system: Extrapyramidal symptoms (2% to 31%), somnolence (8% to 31%), headache (3% to 18%), dizziness (3% to 16%)
- Gastrointestinal: Nausea (4% to 12%)

1% to 10%:

- Cardiovascular: Chest pain (5%), postural hypotension (5%), hypertension (2% to 3%), bradycardia (2%), tachycardia (2%), vasodilation (1%), facial edema, orthostatic hypotension
- Central nervous system: Akathisia (2% to 10%), anxiety (2% to 5%) insomnia (3%), agitation (2%), speech disorder (2%), personality disorder (2%), psychosis (1%), akinesia, amnesia, ataxia, chills, confusion, coordination abnormal, delirium, dystonia, fever, hostility, hypothermia, oculogyric crisis, vertigo
- Dermatologic: Rash (4%), fungal dermatitis (2%)
- Endocrine & metabolic: Dysmenorrhea (2%)
- Gastrointestinal: Weight gain (10%), constipation (2% to 9%), dyspepsia (1% to 8%), diarrhea (3% to 5%), vomiting (3% to 5%), salivation increased (4%), xerostomia (1% to 5%), tongue edema (3%), abdominal pain (2%), anorexia (2%), dysphagia (2%), rectal hemorrhage (2%), tooth disorder (1%), buccoglossal syndrome
- Genitourinary: Priapism (1%)
- Local: Injection site pain (7% to 9%)
- Neuromuscular & skeletal: Weakness (2% to 6%), hypoesthesia (2%), myalgia (2%), paresthesia (2%), back pain (1%), cogwheel rigidity (1%), hypertonia (1%), abnormal gait, choreoathetosis, dysarthria, dyskinesia, hyper-/hypokinesia, hypotonia, neuropathy, tremor, twitching
- Ocular: Vision abnormal (3% to 6%), diplopia
- Respiratory: Infection (8%), rhinitis (1% to 4%), cough (3%), pharyngitis (3%), dyspnea (2%)
- Miscellaneous: Diaphoresis (2%), furunculosis (2%), flu-like syndrome (1%), photosensitivity reaction, withdrawal syndrome

<1% (Limited to important or life-threatening): Akinesia, allergic reaction, angina, atrial fibrillation, ataxia, AV block (first degree), bundle branch block, cerebral infarction, cholestatic jaundice, choreoathetosis, delirium, dysarthria, dysphagia, eosinophilia, exfoliative dermatitis, galactorrhea, gout, gynecomastia, hemorrhage, hepatitis, jaundice, myocarditis, neuroleptic malignant syndrome, neuropathy, opisthotonos, photophobia, pneumonia, pulmonary embolism, QT_c prolongation >500 msec (0.06%), seizure (0.4%), sexual dysfunction (male and female), stroke, syncope (0.6%), tenosynovitis, thrombocytopenia, thyroiditis, torsade de pointes, torticollis, urinary retention

Overdosage/Toxicology Reported symptoms include somnolence, slurring of speech, tremor, and anxiety. Acute extrapyramidal symptoms may also occur. Cardiac monitoring should be initiated immediately. Treatment is symptom-directed and supportive. Not removed by dialysis.

Drug Interactions Substrate (minor) of CYP1A2, 3A4; **Inhibits** CYP2D6 (weak), 3A4 (weak)

Acetylcholinesterase inhibitors (central): May increase the risk of antipsychotic-related extrapyramidal symptoms; monitor.

Amphetamines: Efficacy may be diminished by antipsychotics; in addition, amphetamines may increase psychotic symptoms; avoid concurrent use

Antihypertensives: Concurrent use of ziprasidone with an antihypertensive may produce additive hypotensive effects (particularly orthostasis)

Carbamazepine: May decrease serum concentrations of ziprasidone (AUC is decreased by 35%); other enzyme-inducing agents may share this potential

CNS depressants: Sedative effects may be additive with ziprasidone; monitor for increased effect; includes barbiturates, benzodiazepines, narcotic analgesics, ethanol, and other sedative agents

Ketoconazole: May increase serum concentrations of ziprasidone (AUC is increased by 35% to 40%); other CYP3A4 inhibitors may share this potential. QT_c prolongation was not demonstrated.

Levodopa: Ziprasidone may inhibit the antiparkinsonian effect of levodopa; avoid this combination

Metoclopramide: May increase extrapyramidal symptoms (EPS) or risk.

Potassium- or magnesium-depleting agents: May increase the risk of serious arrhythmias with ziprasidone; includes many diuretics, aminoglycosides, cyclosporine, and amphotericin; monitor serum potassium and magnesium levels closely

QT_c-prolonging agents: May result in additive effects on cardiac conduction, potentially resulting in malignant or lethal arrhythmias; concurrent use is contraindicated. Includes amiodarone, arsenic trioxide, bretylium, chlorpromazine, cisapride; class Ia antiarrhythmics (quinidine, procainamide); dofetilide, dolasetron, droperidol, halofantrine, ibutilide, levomethadyl, mefloquine, mesoridazine, pentamidine, pimozide, probucol; some quinolone antibiotics (moxifloxacin, sparfloxacin, gatifloxacin); sotalol, tacrolimus, and thioridazine.

Ethanol/Nutrition/Herb Interactions

Ethanol: Avoid ethanol (may increase CNS depression).

Food: Administration with food increases serum levels twofold. Grapefruit juice may increase serum concentration of ziprasidone.

Herb/Nutraceutical: St John's wort may decrease serum levels of ziprasidone, due to a potential effect on CYP3A4. This has not been specifically studied. Avoid kava kava, chamomile (may increase CNS depression).

Dosage Forms

Capsule, as hydrochloride: 20 mg, 40 mg, 60 mg, 80 mg

Injection, powder for reconstitution, as mesylate: 20 mg

- ♦ **Ziprasidone Hydrochloride** *see* Ziprasidone *on page 1374*
- ♦ **Ziprasidone Mesylate** *see* Ziprasidone *on page 1374*
- ♦ **Zithromax®** *see* Azithromycin *on page 149*
- ♦ **Zithromax® TRI-PAK™** *see* Azithromycin *on page 149*
- ♦ **Zithromax® Z-PAK®** *see* Azithromycin *on page 149*
- ♦ **ZM-182,780** *see* Fulvestrant *on page 571*
- ♦ **Zmax™** *see* Azithromycin *on page 149*
- ♦ **Zocor®** *see* Simvastatin *on page 1174*
- ♦ **Zofran®** *see* Ondansetron *on page 959*
- ♦ **Zofran® ODT** *see* Ondansetron *on page 959*
- ♦ **Zoledronate** *see* Zoledronic Acid *on page 1377*

Zoledronic Acid (ZOE le dron ik AS id)

U.S. Brand Names Zometa®

Canadian Brand Names Aclasta®; Zometa®

Synonyms CGP-42446; NSC-721517; Zoledronate

Pharmacologic Category Antidote; Bisphosphonate Derivative

Generic Available No

Use Treatment of hypercalcemia of malignancy, multiple myeloma, bone metastases of solid tumors

Unlabeled/Investigational Use Treatment of metabolic bone diseases

Mechanism of Action A bisphosphonate which inhibits bone resorption via actions on osteoclasts or on osteoclast precursors; inhibits osteoclastic activity and skeletal calcium release induced by tumors. Decreases serum calcium and phosphorus, and increases their elimination.

(Continued)

Zoledronic Acid *(Continued)*

Pharmacodynamics/Kinetics

Onset of action: Maximum effect may not been seen for 7 days

Distribution: Binds to bone

Protein binding: ~22%

Half-life elimination: Triphasic; Terminal: 146 hours

Excretion: Urine (39% ± 16% as unchanged drug) within 24 hours; feces (<3%)

Dosage I.V.: Adults:

Hypercalcemia of malignancy (albumin-corrected serum calcium ≥12 mg/dL): 4 mg (maximum) given as a single dose. Wait at least 7 days before considering retreatment. Dosage adjustment may be needed in patients with decreased renal function following treatment.

Multiple myeloma or metastatic bone lesions from solid tumors: 4 mg every 3-4 weeks

Note: Patients should receive a daily calcium supplement and multivitamin containing vitamin D

Paget's disease (Aclasta®, not available in U.S.): 5 mg infused over at least 15 minutes. **Note:** Data concerning retreatment is not available.

Dosage adjustment in renal impairment (at treatment initiation):

Zometa®: Multiple myeloma and bone metastases:

- Cl_{cr} >60 mL/minute: 4 mg
- Cl_{cr} 50-60 mL/minute: 3.5 mg
- Cl_{cr} 40-49 mL/minute: 3.3 mg
- Cl_{cr} 30-39 mL/minute: 3 mg
- Cl_{cr} <30 mL/minute: Not recommended

Zometa®: Hypercalcemia of malignancy:

- Mild-to-moderate impairment: No adjustment necessary
- Severe impairment (serum creatinine >4.5 mg/dL): Evaluate risk versus benefit

Aclasta® [not available in U.S.]: Cl_{cr} >30 mL/minute: No adjustment recommended

Dosage adjustment for renal toxicity (during treatment):

Hypercalcemia of malignancy: Evidence of renal deterioration: Evaluate risk versus benefit.

Multiple myeloma and bone metastases: Evidence of renal deterioration: Withhold dose until renal function returns to within 10% of baseline: renal deterioration defined as follows:

- Normal baseline creatinine: Increase of 0.5 mg/dL
- Abnormal baseline creatinine: Increase of 1 mg/dL

Reinitiate dose at the same dose administered prior to treatment interruption.

Dosage adjustment in hepatic impairment: Specific guidelines are not available.

Stability Store vials at 15°C to 30°C (59°F to 86°F). Dilute solution for injection in 100 mL NS or D_5W prior to administration. Solutions for infusion may be stored for 24 hours at 15°C to 30°C (59°F to 86°F). Infusion of solution must be completed within 24 hours.

Administration Infuse over 15-30 minutes; do not infuse over <15 minutes. Infuse in a line separate from other medications. Patients should be appropriately hydrated prior to treatment.

Monitoring Parameters Prior to initiation of therapy, dental exam and preventative dentistry for patients at risk for osteonecrosis; serum creatinine prior to each dose; serum electrolytes, phosphate, magnesium, and hemoglobin/hematocrit should be evaluated regularly. Monitor serum calcium to assess response and avoid overtreatment.

Pregnancy Risk Factor D

Contraindications Hypersensitivity to zoledronic acid, other bisphosphonates, or any component of the formulation; pregnancy

Warnings/Precautions Bisphosphonate therapy has been associated with osteonecrosis, primarily of the jaw; this has been observed mostly in cancer patients, but also in patients with postmenopausal osteoporosis and other diagnoses. Risk factors include a diagnosis of cancer, with concomitant chemotherapy, radiotherapy or corticosteroids; anemia, coagulopathy, infection or pre-existing dental disease. Symptoms included nonhealing extraction socket or an exposed jawbone. There are no data addressing whether discontinuation of therapy reduces the risk of developing osteonecrosis. However, as a precautionary measure, dental exams and preventative dentistry should be performed prior to placing patients with risk factors on chronic bisphosphonate therapy. Invasive dental procedures should be avoided during treatment.

Use caution in renal dysfunction; dosage adjustment required. In cancer patients, renal toxicity has been reported with doses >4 mg or infusions administered over 15 minutes. Risk factors for renal deterioration include pre-existing renal insufficiency and repeated doses of zoledronic acid and other bisphosphonates. Dehydration and the use of other nephrotoxic drugs which may contribute to renal deterioration should be identified and managed. Use is not recommended in patients with severe renal impairment (serum creatinine >3 mg/dL) and bone metastases (limited data); use in patients with hypercalcemia of malignancy and severe renal impairment should only be done if the benefits outweigh the risks. Renal function should be assessed prior to treatment; if decreased after treatment, additional treatments should be withheld until renal function returns to within 10% of baseline. Adequate hydration is required during treatment (urine output ~2 L/day); avoid overhydration, especially in patients with heart failure; diuretics should not be used before correcting hypovolemia. Renal deterioration, resulting in renal failure and dialysis has occurred in patients treated with zoledronic acid after single and multiple infusions at recommended doses of 4 mg over 15 minutes. **Note:** When used in the treatment of Paget's disease (Aclasta® — not available in the U.S.), significant renal deterioration has not been observed with the usual 5 mg unit-dose.

Infrequent reports of severe (and occasionally debilitating) bone, joint, and/or muscle pain during bisphosphonate treatment; onset of pain ranged from a single day to several months, with relief in most cases upon discontinuation of the drug. Some patients experienced recurrence when rechallenged with same drug or another bisphosphonate.

Use caution in patients with aspirin-sensitive asthma (may cause bronchoconstriction), hepatic dysfunction, and the elderly. Women of childbearing age should be advised against becoming pregnant. Safety and efficacy in pediatric patients have not been established.

Adverse Reactions

>10%:

- Cardiovascular: Leg edema (5% to 21%), hypotension (11%)
- Central nervous system: Fatigue (39%), fever (32% to 44%), headache (5% to 19%), dizziness (18%), insomnia (15% to 16%), anxiety (11% to 14%), depression (14%), agitation (13%), confusion (7% to 13%), hypoesthesia (12%)
- Dermatologic: Alopecia (12%), dermatitis (11%)
- Endocrine & metabolic: Dehydration (5% to 14%), hypophosphatemia (12% to 13%), hypokalemia (12%), hypomagnesemia (11%)
- Gastrointestinal: Nausea (29% to 46%), constipation (27% to 31%), vomiting (14% to 32%), diarrhea (17% to 24%), anorexia (9% to 22%), abdominal pain (14% to 16%), weight loss (16%), appetite decreased (13%)
- Genitourinary: Urinary tract infection (12% to 14%)
- Hematologic: Anemia (22% to 33%), neutropenia (12%)
- Neuromuscular & skeletal: Bone pain (55%), weakness (5% to 24%), myalgia (23%), arthralgia (5% to 21%), back pain (15%), paresthesia (15%), limb pain (14%), skeletal pain (12%), rigors (11%)
- Renal: Renal deterioration (8% to 17%; up to 40% in patients with abnormal baseline creatinine)
- Respiratory: Dyspnea (22% to 27%), cough (12% to 22%)
- Miscellaneous: Cancer progression (16%), moniliasis (12%)

1% to 10%:

- Cardiovascular: Chest pain (5% to 10%)
- Central nervous system: Somnolence (5% to 10%)
- Endocrine & metabolic: Hypocalcemia (1% to 10%), hypermagnesemia (2%)
- Gastrointestinal: Dysphagia (5% to 10%), dyspepsia (10%), mucositis (5% to 10%), stomatitis (8%), sore throat (8%)
- Hematologic: Thrombocytopenia (5% to 10%), pancytopenia (5% to 10%), granulocytopenia (5% to 10%)
- Renal: Serum creatinine increased (grades 3/4: 2%)
- Respiratory: Pleural effusion, upper respiratory tract infection (10%)
- Miscellaneous: Metastases (5% to 10%), nonspecifc infection (5% to 10%)

<1% (Limited to important or life-threatening): Angioneurotic edema, blurred vision, bradycardia, conjunctivitis, diaphoresis, episcleritis, flu-like syndrome, hematuria, hyperesthesia, hyperkalemia, hypernatremia, hypersensitivity, hypertension, injection-site reaction, joint and/or muscle pain, muscle cramps,

(Continued)

Zoledronic Acid *(Continued)*

osteonecrosis (primarily of the jaws), proteinuria, pruritus, rash, renal failure, renal impairment, taste perversion, tremor, uveitis, weight gain, xerostomia

Overdosage/Toxicology Clinically-significant hypocalcemia, hypophosphatemia, and hypomagnesemia may occur. Doses >4 mg and infusion times <15 minutes are associated with a risk of renal toxicity. Treatment is symptom-directed and supportive.

Drug Interactions

Aminoglycosides: May lower serum calcium levels with prolonged administration. Concomitant use may have an additive hypocalcemic effect.

Antacids: May decrease the absorption of bisphosphonate derivatives; should be administered at a different time of the day. Antacids containing aluminum, calcium, or magnesium are of specific concern.

Calcium salts: May decrease the absorption of bisphosphonate derivatives. Separate oral dosing in order to minimize risk of interaction.

Iron salts: May decrease the absorption of bisphosphonate derivatives. Only oral iron salts and oral bisphosphonates are of concern.

Magnesium salts: May decrease the absorption of bisphosphonate derivatives. Only oral magnesium salts and oral bisphosphonates are of concern.

Nonsteroidal anti-inflammatory drugs (NSAIDs): May enhance the gastrointestinal adverse/toxic effects (increased incidence of GI ulcers) of bisphosphonate derivatives.

Phosphate supplements: Bisphosphonate derivatives may enhance the hypocalcemic effect of phosphate supplements.

Test Interactions Bisphosphonates may interfere with diagnostic imaging agents such as technetium-99m-diphosphonate in bone scans.

Dietary Considerations Multiple myeloma or metastatic bone lesions from solid tumors: Take daily calcium supplement (500 mg) and daily multivitamin (with 400 int. units vitamin D).

Dosage Forms [CAN] = Canadian brand name

Infusion, solution [premixed]:

Aclasta® [CAN]: 5 mg (100 mL) [not available in U.S.]

Injection, solution:

Zometa®: 4 mg/5 mL (5 mL) [as monohydrate 4.264 mg]

Zolmitriptan (zohl mi TRIP tan)

Medication Safety Issues

Sound-alike/look-alike issues:

Zolmitriptan may be confused with sumatriptan

U.S. Brand Names Zomig®; Zomig-ZMT™

Canadian Brand Names Zomig®; Zomig® Nasal Spray; Zomig® Rapimelt

Synonyms 311C90

Pharmacologic Category Serotonin 5-HT_{1D} Receptor Agonist

Generic Available No

Use Acute treatment of migraine with or without aura

Mechanism of Action Selective agonist for serotonin (5-HT_{1B} and 5-HT_{1D} receptors) in cranial arteries to cause vasoconstriction and reduce sterile inflammation associated with antidromic neuronal transmission correlating with relief of migraine

Pharmacodynamics/Kinetics

Onset of action: 0.5-1 hour

Absorption: Well absorbed

Distribution: V_d: 7 L/kg

Protein binding: 25%

Metabolism: Converted to an active N-desmethyl metabolite (2-6 times more potent than zolmitriptan)

Half-life elimination: 2.8-3.7 hours

Bioavailability: 40%

Time to peak, serum: Tablet: 1.5 hours; Orally-disintegrating tablet and nasal spray: 3 hours

Excretion: Urine (~60% to 65% total dose); feces (30% to 40%)

Dosage Oral:

Children: Safety and efficacy have not been established

Adults: Migraine:

Tablet: Initial: ≤2.5 mg at the onset of migraine headache; may break 2.5 mg tablet in half

Orally-disintegrating tablet: Initial: 2.5 mg at the onset of migraine headache

Nasal spray: Initial: 1 spray (5 mg) at the onset of migraine headache

Note: Use the lowest possible dose to minimize adverse events. If the headache returns, the dose may be repeated after 2 hours; do not exceed 10 mg within a 24-hour period. Controlled trials have not established the effectiveness of a second dose if the initial one was ineffective

Elderly: No dosage adjustment needed but elderly patients are more likely to have underlying cardiovascular disease and should have careful evaluation of cardiovascular system before prescribing.

Dosage adjustment in renal impairment: No dosage adjustment recommended. There is a 25% reduction in zolmitriptan's clearance in patients with severe renal impairment (Cl_{cr} 5-25 mL/minute)

Dosage adjustment in hepatic impairment: Administer with caution in patients with liver disease, generally using doses <2.5 mg. Patients with moderate-to-severe hepatic impairment may have decreased clearance of zolmitriptan, and significant elevation in blood pressure was observed in some patients.

Stability Store at 20°C to 25°C (68°F to 77°F); protect from light and moisture

Administration Administer as soon as migraine headache starts.

Tablet: May be broken

Orally-disintegrating tablet: Must be taken whole; do not break, crush or chew; place on tongue and allow to dissolve; administration with liquid is not required

Nasal spray: Blow nose gently prior to use. After removing protective cap, instill device into nostril. Block opposite nostril; breathe in gently through nose while pressing plunger of spray device. One dose (5 mg) is equal to 1 spray in 1 nostril.

Anesthesia and Critical Care Concerns/Other Considerations Zolmitriptan should not be used in patients with a history of vasospastic disease, Prinzmetal's angina, or any critical vascular disease.

Pregnancy Risk Factor C

Contraindications Hypersensitivity to zolmitriptan or any component of the formulation; ischemic heart disease or Prinzmetal's angina; signs or symptoms of ischemic heart disease; uncontrolled hypertension; symptomatic Wolff-Parkinson-White syndrome or arrhythmias associated with other cardiac accessory conduction pathway disorders; use with ergotamine derivatives (within 24 hours of); use within 24 hours of another $5-HT_1$ agonist; concurrent administration or within 2 weeks of discontinuing an MAO inhibitor; management of hemiplegic or basilar migraine

Warnings/Precautions Zolmitriptan is indicated only in patient populations with a clear diagnosis of migraine. Not for prophylactic treatment of migraine headaches. Cardiac events (coronary artery vasospasm, transient ischemia, myocardial infarction, ventricular tachycardia/fibrillation, cardiac arrest, and death) have been reported with $5-HT_1$ agonist administration. Should not be given to patients who have risk factors for CAD (eg, hypertension, hypercholesterolemia, smoker, obesity, diabetes, strong family history of CAD, menopause, male >40 years of age) without adequate cardiac evaluation. Patients with suspected CAD should have cardiovascular evaluation to rule out CAD before considering zolmitriptan's use; if cardiovascular evaluation negative, first dose would be safest if given in the healthcare provider's office. Periodic evaluation of those without cardiovascular disease, but with continued risk factors should be done. Significant elevation in blood pressure, including hypertensive crisis, has also been reported on rare occasions in patients with and without a history of hypertension. Vasospasm-related reactions have been reported other than coronary artery vasospasm. Peripheral vascular ischemia and colonic ischemia with abdominal pain and bloody diarrhea have occurred. Use with caution in patients with hepatic impairment. Zomig-ZMT™ tablets contain phenylalanine. Safety and efficacy not established in patients <18 years of age.

Adverse Reactions Percentages noted from oral preparations.

1% to 10%:

Cardiovascular: Chest pain (2% to 4%), palpitation (up to 2%)

Central nervous system: Dizziness (6% to 10%), somnolence (5% to 8%), pain (2% to 3%), vertigo (≤2%)

Gastrointestinal: Nausea (4% to 9%), xerostomia (3% to 5%), dyspepsia (1% to 3%), dysphagia (≤2%)

(Continued)

Zolmitriptan *(Continued)*

Neuromuscular & skeletal: Paresthesia (5% to 9%), weakness (3% to 9%), warm/cold sensation (5% to 7%), hypoesthesia (1% to 2%), myalgia (1% to 2%), myasthenia (up to 2%)

Miscellaneous: Neck/throat/jaw pain (4% to 10%), diaphoresis (up to 3%), allergic reaction (up to 1%)

<1% (Limited to important or life-threatening): Anaphylactoid reaction, anaphylaxis, angina, apnea, arrhythmia, ataxia, bronchospasm, cerebral ischemia, coronary artery vasospasm, cyanosis, eosinophilia, esophagitis, gastrointestinal infarction/necrosis, hallucinations, headache, hematemesis, hypertension, hypertensive crisis, ischemic colitis, melena, miscarriage, MI, myocardial ischemia, pancreatitis, photosensitivity, QT prolongation, rash, splenic infarction, syncope, tetany, thrombocytopenia, tinnitus, ulcer, urticaria

Events related to other serotonin 5-HT_{1D} receptor agonists: Cardiac arrest, cerebral hemorrhage, peripheral vascular ischemia, stroke, subarachnoid hemorrhage, ventricular fibrillation

Overdosage/Toxicology Treatment is symptom-directed and supportive. It is not known if hemodialysis or peritoneal dialysis is effective.

Drug Interactions Substrate of CYP1A2 (minor)

Cimetidine: Zolmitriptan serum levels increased; avoid concurrent use

Ergot-containing drugs (dihydroergotamine, methysergide): Concurrent use may lead to vasospastic reactions; separate use by at least 24 hours.

MAO inhibitors: Increases systemic exposure to zolmitriptan. Avoid concurrent use and use within 2 weeks of discontinuing a MAO inhibitor. Selegiline (selective MAO type B inhibitor) does not affect zolmitriptan levels.

Oral contraceptives: Zolmitriptan serum levels increased with concurrent use.

Propranolol: Increased zolmitriptan toxicity

Selective serotonin reuptake inhibitors (SSRIs): Concurrent use may lead to serotonin syndrome.

Sibutramine: Concurrent use may lead to serotonin syndrome.

Ethanol/Nutrition/Herb Interactions Ethanol: Limit use (may have additive CNS toxicity).

Dosage Forms

Solution, nasal spray [single dose] (Zomig®): 5 mg/0.1 mL (0.1 mL)

Tablet (Zomig®): 2.5 mg, 5 mg

Tablet, orally disintegrating (Zomig-ZMT™): 2.5 mg [contains phenylalanine 2.81 mg/tablet; orange flavor]; 5 mg [contains phenylalanine 5.62 mg/tablet; orange flavor]

♦ **Zoloft**® *see* Sertraline *on page 1161*

Zolpidem (zole PI dem)

Medication Safety Issues

Sound-alike/look-alike issues:

Ambien® may be confused with Ambi 10®

U.S. Brand Names Ambien®; Ambien CR™

Synonyms Zolpidem Tartrate

Pharmacologic Category Hypnotic, Nonbenzodiazepine

Restrictions C-IV; not available in Canada

Generic Available No

Use Short-term treatment of insomnia (sleep onset and/or sleep maintenance)

Mechanism of Action Structurally dissimilar to benzodiazepines. Selective hypnotic effects (with minor anxiolytic, myorelaxant and anticovulsant properties) mediated through selective affinity for the alpha-1 subunit of the omega-1 (benzodiazepine) receptor located on the $GABA_A$ receptor complex. Agonism at this site enhances GABA-ergic chloride conductance hyperpolarizing neuronal membranes thereby reducing the responsiveness to excitatory signals.

Pharmacodynamics/Kinetics

Onset of action: 30 minutes

Duration: 6-8 hours

Absorption: Rapid

Distribution: Very low amounts enter breast milk

Protein binding: 92%

Metabolism: Hepatic, primarily via CYP3A4 (~60%), to inactive metabolites

Half-life elimination: 2.5-2.8 hours (range 1.4-4.5 hours); Cirrhosis: Up to 9.9 hours

Time to peak, plasma: 2 hours; 4 hours with food

Excretion: As metabolites in urine, bile, feces

Dosage Oral:

Adults:

Ambien®: 10 mg immediately before bedtime; maximum dose: 10 mg

Ambien CR™: 12.5 mg immediately before bedtime

Elderly:

Ambien®: 5 mg immediately before bedtime

Ambien CR™: 6.25 mg immediately before bedtime

Dosing adjustment in renal impairment: Dose adjustment not required; monitor closely

Hemodialysis: Not dialyzable

Dosing adjustment in hepatic impairment:

Ambien®: 5 mg

Ambien CR™: 6.25 mg

Administration Ingest immediately before bedtime due to rapid onset of action. Ambien CR™ tablets should not be divided, crushed, or chewed.

Monitoring Parameters Daytime alertness; respiratory and cardiac status; behavior profile

Reference Range 80-150 ng/mL

Anesthesia and Critical Care Concerns/Other Considerations Causes less disturbances in sleep stages as compared to benzodiazepines; time spent in sleep stages 3 and 4 are maintained. Zolpidem decreases sleep latency; should not be prescribed in quantities exceeding a 1-month supply.

Pregnancy Risk Factor C

Contraindications Hypersensitivity to zolpidem or any component of the formulation

Warnings/Precautions Should be used only after evaluation of potential causes of sleep disturbance. Failure of sleep disturbance to resolve after 7-10 days may indicate psychiatric or medical illness. Use with caution in patients with depression. Abnormal thinking and behavioral changes have been associated with sedative-hypnotics. Sedative/hypnotics may produce withdrawal symptoms following abrupt discontinuation. Causes CNS depression, which may impair physical and mental capabilities. Effects with other sedative drugs or ethanol may be potentiated. Use caution in the elderly; dose adjustment recommended. Closely monitor elderly or debilitated patients for impaired cognitive or motor performance. Avoid use in patients with sleep apnea or a history of sedative-hypnotic abuse. Use caution with hepatic impairment; dose adjustment required. Prescriptions should be written for the smallest effective dose (especially in the elderly) and for the smallest quantity consistent with good patient care (especially with depression). Safety and efficacy have not been established in pediatric patients.

Adverse Reactions Actual frequency may be dosage form, dose and/or age dependent

>10%: Central nervous system: Dizziness, headache, somnolence

1% to 10%:

Cardiovascular: Blood pressure increased, chest discomfort, palpitation

Central nervous system: Anxiety, apathy, amnesia, ataxia, attention disturbance, body temperature increased, confusion, depersonalization, depression, disinhibition, disorientation, drowsiness, drugged feeling, euphoria, fatigue, fever, hallucinations, hypoesthesia, insomnia, memory disorder, lethargy, lightheadedness, mood swings, stress

Dermatologic: Rash, urticaria, wrinkling

Endocrine & metabolic: Menorrhagia

Gastrointestinal: Abdominal discomfort, abdominal pain, abdominal tenderness, appetite disorder, constipation, diarrhea, dyspepsia, flatulence, gastroenteritis, gastroesophageal reflux, hiccup, nausea, vomiting, xerostomia

Genitourinary: Urinary tract infection

Neuromuscular & skeletal: Arthralgia, back pain, balance disorder, myalgia, neck pain, paresthesia, psychomotor retardation, tremor, weakness

Ocular: Asthenopia, blurred vision, depth perception altered, diplopia, red eye, visual disturbance

Otic: Labyrinthitis, tinnitus, vertigo

Renal: Dysuria

Respiratory: Pharyngitis, sinusitis, throat irritation, upper respiratory tract infection

(Continued)

Zolpidem *(Continued)*

Miscellaneous: Allergy, binge eating, flu-like symptoms

<1% (Limited to important or life-threatening): Abnormal dreams, agitation, anorexia, arthritis, bronchitis, chest pain, cognition decreased, concentrating difficulty, constipation, cough, cystitis, diaphoresis increased, dysarthria, dysphagia, edema, emotional lability, eye irritation, falling, hepatic function abnormalities, hyperglycemia, hypoesthesia, illusion, leg cramps, menstrual disorder, nervousness, pallor, postural hypotension, pruritus, scleritis, somnambulism (sleepwalking), speech disorder, stupor, syncope, tachycardia, taste perversion, thirst, urinary incontinence, vaginitis

Overdosage/Toxicology Symptoms of overdose include coma and hypotension. Treatment for overdose is supportive. Rarely is mechanical ventilation required. Flumazenil has been shown to selectively block binding to CNS receptors, resulting in a reversal of CNS depression, but not always respiratory depression. Hemodialysis is not likely to be of benefit.

Drug Interactions Substrate of CYP1A2 (minor), 2C9 (minor), 2C19 (minor), 2D6 (minor), 3A4 (major)

Antipsychotics: Sedative effects may be additive with antipsychotics, including phenothiazines; monitor for increased effect

CNS depressants: Sedative effects may be additive with other CNS depressants; monitor for increased effect; includes barbiturates, benzodiazepines, narcotic analgesics, ethanol, and other sedative agents

CYP3A4 inducers: CYP3A4 inducers may decrease the levels/effects of zolpidem. Example inducers include aminoglutethimide, carbamazepine, nafcillin, nevirapine, phenobarbital, phenytoin, and rifamycins.

CYP3A4 inhibitors: May increase the levels/effects of zolpidem. Example inhibitors include azole antifungals, clarithromycin, diclofenac, doxycycline, erythromycin, imatinib, isoniazid, nefazodone, nicardipine, propofol, protease inhibitors, quinidine, telithromycin, troleandomycin, and verapamil.

Rifamycin derivatives: May decrease levels/effects of zolpidem.

Ethanol/Nutrition/Herb Interactions

Ethanol: Avoid ethanol (may increase CNS depression).

Food: Maximum plasma concentration and bioavailability are decreased with food; time to peak plasma concentration is increased; half-life remains unchanged.

Herb/Nutraceutical: St John's wort may decrease zolpidem levels. Avoid valerian, St John's wort, kava kava, gotu kola (may increase CNS depression).

Dietary Considerations For faster sleep onset, do not administer with (or immediately after) a meal.

Dosage Forms [DSC] = Discontinued product

Tablet, as tartrate:

Ambien®: 5 mg, 10 mg

Ambien® PAK™ [dose pack]: 5 mg (30s); 10 mg (30s) [DSC]

Tablet, extended release, as tartrate (Ambien CR™): 6.25 mg, 12.5 mg

- **Zolpidem Tartrate** *see* Zolpidem *on page 1382*
- **Zometa®** *see* Zoledronic Acid *on page 1377*
- **Zomig®** *see* Zolmitriptan *on page 1380*
- **Zomig® Nasal Spray (Can)** *see* Zolmitriptan *on page 1380*
- **Zomig® Rapimelt (Can)** *see* Zolmitriptan *on page 1380*
- **Zomig-ZMT™** *see* Zolmitriptan *on page 1380*
- **Zomorph® (Can)** *see* Morphine Sulfate *on page 867*
- **Zonalon®** *see* Doxepin *on page 422*
- **Zonegran®** *see* Zonisamide *on page 1384*

Zonisamide (zoe NIS a mide)

Related Information

Perioperative Management of Patients on Antiseizure Medication *on page 1458*

U.S. Brand Names Zonegran®

Canadian Brand Names Zonegran®

Pharmacologic Category Anticonvulsant, Miscellaneous

Generic Available Yes

Use Adjunct treatment of partial seizures in children >16 years of age and adults with epilepsy

Unlabeled/Investigational Use Bipolar disorder

Mechanism of Action The exact mechanism of action is not known. May stabilize neuronal membranes and suppress neuronal hypersynchronization through action at sodium and calcium channels. Does not affect GABA activity.

Pharmacodynamics/Kinetics

Distribution: V_d: 1.45 L/kg

Protein binding: 40%

Metabolism: Hepatic via CYP3A4; forms N-acetyl zonisamide and 2-sulfamoylacetyl phenol (SMAP)

Half-life elimination: 63 hours

Time to peak: 2-6 hours

Excretion: Urine (62%, 35% as unchanged drug, 65% as metabolites); feces (3%)

Dosage Oral:

Children >16 years and Adults:

Adjunctive treatment of partial seizures: Initial: 100 mg/day; dose may be increased to 200 mg/day after 2 weeks. Further dosage increases to 300 mg/day and 400 mg/day can then be made with a minimum of 2 weeks between adjustments, in order to reach steady state at each dosage level. Doses of up to 600 mg/day have been studied, however, there is no evidence of increased response with doses above 400 mg/day.

Mania (unlabeled use): Initial: 100-200 mg/day; maximum: 600 mg/day (Kanba, 1994)

Elderly: Data from clinical trials is insufficient for patients >65 years; begin dosing at the low end of the dosing range.

Dosage adjustment in renal/hepatic impairment: Slower titration and frequent monitoring are indicated in patients with renal or hepatic disease. There is insufficient experience regarding dosing/toxicity in patients with estimated GFR <50 mL/minute. Marked renal impairment (Cl_{cr} <20 mL/minute) was associated with a 35% increase in AUC.

Stability Store at controlled room temperature 25°C (77°F). Protect from moisture and light.

Administration Capsules should be swallowed whole. Dose may be administered once or twice daily. Doses of 300 mg/day and higher are associated with increased side effects. Steady-state levels are reached in 14 days.

Monitoring Parameters Monitor BUN and serum creatinine

Pregnancy Risk Factor C

Contraindications Hypersensitivity to zonisamide, sulfonamides, or any component of the formulation

Warnings/Precautions Rare, but potentially fatal sulfonamide reactions have occurred following the use of zonisamide. These reactions include Stevens-Johnson syndrome and toxic epidermal necrolysis, usually appearing within 2-16 weeks of drug initiation. Discontinue zonisamide if rash develops. Chemical similarities are present among sulfonamides, sulfonylureas, carbonic anhydrase inhibitors, thiazides, and loop diuretics (except ethacrynic acid). Use in patients with sulfonamide allergy is specifically contraindicated in product labeling, however, a risk of cross-reaction exists in patients with allergy to any of these compounds; avoid use when previous reaction has been severe.

Decreased sweating (oligohydrosis) and hyperthermia requiring hospitalization have been reported in children. Discontinue zonisamide in patients who develop acute renal failure or a significant sustained increase in creatinine/BUN concentration. Kidney stones have been reported. Use cautiously in patients with renal or hepatic dysfunction. Significant CNS effects include psychiatric symptoms, psychomotor slowing, and fatigue or somnolence. Fatigue and somnolence occur within the first month of treatment, most commonly at doses of 300-500 mg/day. Abrupt withdrawal may precipitate seizures; discontinue or reduce doses gradually. Safety and efficacy in children <16 years of age has not been established.

Adverse Reactions Adjunctive Therapy: Frequencies noted in patients receiving other anticonvulsants:

>10%:

Central nervous system: Somnolence (17%), dizziness (13%)

Gastrointestinal: Anorexia (13%)

1% to 10%:

Central nervous system: Headache (10%), agitation/irritability (9%), fatigue (8%), tiredness (7%), ataxia (6%), confusion (6%), decreased concentration

(Continued)

Zonisamide *(Continued)*

(6%), memory impairment (6%), depression (6%), insomnia (6%), speech disorders (5%), mental slowing (4%), anxiety (3%), nervousness (2%), schizophrenic/schizophreniform behavior (2%), difficulty in verbal expression (2%), status epilepticus (1%), tremor (1%), convulsion (1%), hyperesthesia (1%), incoordination (1%)

Dermatologic: Rash (3%), bruising (2%), pruritus (1%)

Gastrointestinal: Nausea (9%), abdominal pain (6%), diarrhea (5%), dyspepsia (3%), weight loss (3%), constipation (2%), dry mouth (2%), taste perversion (2%), vomiting (1%)

Neuromuscular & skeletal: Paresthesia (4%), weakness (1%), abnormal gait (1%)

Ocular: Diplopia (6%), nystagmus (4%), amblyopia (1%)

Otic: Tinnitus (1%)

Respiratory: Rhinitis (2%), pharyngitis (1%), increased cough (1%)

Miscellaneous: Flu-like syndrome (4%) accidental injury (1%)

<1% (Limited to important or life threatening symptoms): Agranulocytosis, allergic reaction, alopecia, aplastic anemia, apnea, atrial fibrillation, bladder calculus, cholangitis, cholecystitis, cholestatic jaundice, colitis, deafness, duodenitis, dysarthria, dyskinesia, dyspnea, dystonia, encephalopathy, esophagitis, facial paralysis, gingival hyperplasia, glaucoma, gum hemorrhage, gynecomastia, heart failure, hematemesis, hemoptysis, hirsutism, hyperthermia, impotence, leukopenia, lupus erythematosus, menorrhagia, movement disorder, myoclonus, nephrolithiasis, neuropathy, oculogyric crisis, oligohydrosis, paresthesia, peripheral neuritis, pulmonary embolus, rash, rectal hemorrhage, Stevens-Johnson syndrome, stroke, syncope, thrombocytopenia, toxic epidermal necrolysis, urinary retention, urticaria

Overdosage/Toxicology No specific antidotes are available; experience with doses >800 mg/day is limited. Emesis or gastric lavage, with airway protection, should be done following a recent overdose. General supportive care and close observation are indicated. Renal dialysis may not be effective due to low protein binding (40%).

Drug Interactions Substrate of CYP2C19 (minor), 3A4 (major)

CNS depressants: Sedative effects may be additive with other CNS depressants; monitor for increased effect; includes barbiturates, benzodiazepines, narcotic analgesics, ethanol, and other sedative agents.

CYP3A4 inducers: CYP3A4 inducers may decrease the levels/effects of zonisamide. Example inducers include aminoglutethimide, carbamazepine, nafcillin, nevirapine, phenobarbital, phenytoin, and rifamycins.

CYP3A4 inhibitors: May increase the levels/effects of zonisamide. Example inhibitors include azole antifungals, clarithromycin, diclofenac, doxycycline, erythromycin, imatinib, isoniazid, nefazodone, nicardipine, propofol, protease inhibitors, quinidine, telithromycin, and verapamil.

Ethanol/Nutrition/Herb Interactions

Ethanol: Avoid ethanol (may increase CNS depression).

Food: Food delays time to maximum concentration, but does not affect bioavailability.

Dietary Considerations May be taken with or without food.

Dosage Forms [DSC] = Discontinued product

Capsule: 25 mg, 50 mg, 100 mg

Zonegran®: 25 mg, 50 mg [DSC], 100 mg

- **Zorbtive™** *see* Human Growth Hormone *on page 625*
- **ZORprin®** *see* Aspirin *on page 129*
- **Zosyn®** *see* Piperacillin and Tazobactam Sodium *on page 1029*
- **Zovirax®** *see* Acyclovir *on page 39*
- **Zyban®** *see* BuPROPion *on page 201*
- **Zydone®** *see* Hydrocodone and Acetaminophen *on page 636*
- **Zyloprim®** *see* Allopurinol *on page 59*
- **Zymar™** *see* Gatifloxacin *on page 583*
- **Zyvox™** *see* Linezolid *on page 762*
- **Zyvoxam® (Can)** *see* Linezolid *on page 762*

SPECIAL TOPICS / ISSUES

TABLE OF CONTENTS

ACUTE POSTOPERATIVE PAIN

Pain in a surgical patient can be due to preexisting disease, the surgical procedure (surgical incision, related drains and tubes, body positioning, immobility, excessive stretching or trauma to a peripheral nerve, postoperative ileus), or a combination of preexisting disease and procedure-related causes. Pain can occur at rest and/or with movement or physical activity. Effective postoperative pain management should provide subjective pain relief, minimize the risk for adverse effects, and allow the patient to return to normal daily activities as soon as possible. In addition, postoperative pain management should minimize the detrimental effects from unrelieved pain which include: thromboembolic and pulmonary complications; impairment of immune function; unnecessary fear, anxiety, and/or suffering; and development of chronic pain.

Preparation should begin before the surgical procedure by performing a pain history and physical exam; treating pre-existing pain and anxiety; and educating the patient about his or her role in reporting pain, reporting analgesic adverse effects, and properly using analgesic modalities (eg, patient controlled analgesia) and nonpharmacological techniques. Then, the pain management plan can be made. The inclusion of pre- and intraoperative analgesics has been shown to provide better pain relief and reduce the need for potent opioid analgesics following surgery.

It is now recommended to utilize a combination of analgesic agents and techniques that work by different mechanisms to provide postoperative analgesia (balanced or multimodal analgesia). Combining analgesics and analgesic techniques provides additive or synergistic analgesia with lower doses compared to monotherapy, potentially minimizing adverse effects. Examples of balanced or multimodal analgesia include a nonsteroidal anti-inflammatory drug (NSAID) or acetaminophen combined with an opioid following outpatient surgery, epidural analgesia with an opioid and a local anesthetic following major abdominal or thoracic surgery, and a peripheral nerve block (using a local anesthetic) with an opioid following shoulder surgery. In some cases, therapy for postoperative pain management actually begins before surgery (eg, preemptive analgesia, peripheral nerve block).

Analgesic drugs can be divided into opioid and nonopioid drugs. Nonopioid analgesics are used alone to manage mild and moderate pain and in combination with opioids for more severe pain. Examples of nonopioid analgesics commonly used to manage postoperative pain include acetaminophen, NSAIDs, and local anesthetics. Anticonvulsants have analgesic properties and are routinely used to manage chronic neuropathic pain. Traditionally, it was thought that postoperative pain was nociceptive in nature, but a recent review by Dahl, et al, suggested that postoperative pain may be accompanied by a short-term type of neuropathic pain. Using that premise, Turan et al, compared the analgesic effect of gabapentin, rofecoxib, gabapentin and rofecoxib, and placebo for short-term perioperative pain management. When compared to placebo, gabapentin was as effective as rofecoxib in reducing postoperative morphine consumption and pain scores following abdominal hysterectomy. Opioids, however, remain the mainstay of analgesic therapy for moderate and severe pain. This chapter will review the commonly used drugs in the management of acute postoperative pain.

ACETAMINOPHEN

Acetaminophen, alone or in combination with an opioid or NSAID, is frequently used for treatment of mild to moderate postoperative pain. Acetaminophen most likely provides analgesia by interrupting prostaglandin synthesis in the central nervous system, with no peripheral anti-inflammatory effects. Acetaminophen is generally well tolerated when administered in a daily maximum dose of 4 grams for short-term pain management in adults with normal liver function.

NONSTEROIDAL ANTI-INFLAMMATORY DRUGS (NSAIDs)

NSAIDs are commonly used for postoperative pain management. These agents are frequently the first-line therapy for mild to moderate postoperative pain. The use of NSAIDs for the management of postoperative pain has seen an exponential increase in the past decade, with the entrance of ketorolac (the only parenteral NSAID with an indication for pain) onto the market, and the increase in ambulatory surgical procedures. NSAIDs inhibit the production of prostaglandins by inhibiting cyclooxygenase. These agents have both a peripheral and central effect, with their central effect providing a significant portion of the analgesia and their peripheral effect suppressing postinjury inflammation and subsequent pain. NSAIDs are known to have a morphine-sparing effect and are most beneficial when used in combination with opioids for postoperative pain management.

Adverse Effects

Traditionally, the most common perioperative limitation of nonselective NSAIDs (eg, ketorolac, ibuprofen, naproxen) was their ability to impair platelet aggregation, which can increase bleeding. An additional concern in the perioperative setting is the effects of inhibiting renal prostaglandins, which are involved in maintaining renal function for at least the first postoperative day. Short-term use of NSAIDs (celecoxib or a nonselective agent) in healthy adults who are not expected to become hypovolemic during surgery would not be anticipated to cause clinically significant renal dysfunction. However, it is possible that patients with pre-existing impaired renal blood flow (eg, elderly patients, patients with heart failure) could be at risk for postoperative renal failure from NSAIDs. Recently, the FDA has strengthened its warnings of increased risk for serious cardiovascular thrombotic events and/or gastrointestinal adverse events with the use of NSAIDs (celecoxib or a nonselective agent). This risk may increase with the duration of use, in patients already at risk for cardiovascular disease, and in elderly or debilitated patients. Careful patient screening for cardiovascular disease, renal dysfunction, gastritis, gastric ulcers, or bleeding disorders and short-term use of the lowest effective dose should minimize the risk of these major complications from NSAID therapy. NSAIDs (celecoxib and nonselective agents) are contraindicated in the treatment of perioperative pain associated with CABG surgery.

Overall, the risk of adverse effects from NSAID use in postoperative pain management is small and the benefit (good analgesia) is substantial. When considering dosing, analgesia is provided at lower doses (eg, 200 or 400 mg ibuprofen), whereas higher doses (eg, 600 or 800 mg ibuprofen) are necessary to suppress inflammation. If inflammation and swelling are not present, lower analgesic doses of NSAIDs should be used to minimize the occurrence of adverse effects. Similarly, to minimize the risk of serious adverse effects from ketorolac, adult patients who are >65 years old, <50 kg, or renally impaired should receive 15 mg of I.V. ketorolac rather than 30 mg.

TRAMADOL

Tramadol provides analgesia primarily by inhibiting reuptake of norepinephine and serotonin and secondarily by binding to mu-opioid receptors. Similar to oral opioid-acetaminophen combinations products, tramadol is effective for treating moderate pain associated with surgery. Adverse effects that can occur with tramadol include nausea, vomiting, dizziness, tiredness, sweating, and dry mouth. Tramadol should be used with caution in patients with a history of seizure disorder, at risk for seizures, or taking concurrent medications that reduce the seizure threshold. Tramadol has less of an effect on respiratory or cardiovascular parameters than opioids, but caution is recommended when tramadol is combined with other CNS depressant drugs. Although tramadol has a low risk for abuse, physical dependence on and abuse of tramadol have been reported (primarily in patients with a previous history of abuse).

ACUTE POSTOPERATIVE PAIN *(Continued)*

Table 1. Nonopioid Analgesic Agents

Drug	Usual Dose for Adults >50 kg Body Weight	Usual Dose for Adults <50 kg Body Weight
Acetaminophen (Tylenol®)	650 mg q4h or 1000 mg q6h	10-15 mg/kg q4h maximum of 4 g/day
Ibuprofen (Motrin®, others)	400-600 mg q6h	10 mg/kg q6-8h
Ketorolac tromethamine tablets[1] (Toradol®)	10 mg q4-6h to a maximum of 40 mg/d	
Naproxen (Naprosyn®)	250-275 mg q6-8h	5 mg/kg q8h
Naproxen sodium (Anaprox®)	275 mg q6-8h	
Ketorolac tromethamine injection (Toradol®)	60 mg I.M. or 30 mg I.V. initially, then 30 mg q6h, not to exceed 5 days	30 mg I.M. or 15 mg I.V. initially, then 15 mg q6h, not to exceed 5 days
Tramadol	50-100 mg q4-6h[2]	–

[1]For short-term use only.

[2]Not to exceed 400 mg/day in adults or 300 mg/day in patients ≥75 years of age.

Note: Only the above NSAIDs have FDA approval for use as simple analgesics, but clinical experience has been gained with other drugs as well. Doses are for patients with normal renal and hepatic function. Carefully screen patient for cardiovascular disease, renal dysfunction, gastritis, gastric ulcers, or bleeding disorders before initiating therapy.

OPIOIDS

Opioids are the mainstay of treatment for moderate to severe postoperative pain management. They are commonly used as the initial analgesic agent in the immediate postoperative period and are continued postoperatively, for days to weeks, for moderate or severe pain. Opioids are administered by the oral, parenteral, or neuraxial route, with the severity of pain and type of surgical procedure dictating the method in which they are administered. Oral opioids, either alone or in combination with acetaminophen, are frequently administered for moderate pain. Parenteral and neuraxial opioids are usually administered for severe pain.

Opioids exert their effects by binding to central opioid receptors, thereby decreasing the rate of release of neurotransmitters (such as substance P and acetylcholine) to reduce the perception of pain. The choice of opioid is based upon potency, safety, and patient characteristics. Propoxyphene is the least potent agent, with comparable efficacy to a nonopioid analgesic such as acetaminophen. Hydrocodone and codeine are less potent opioids that are administered in combination with a nonopioid (most commonly acetaminophen). These combination products are indicated for mild to moderate pain. For severe pain, higher doses would be needed and result in an acetaminophen overdose. Morphine, hydromorphone, and fentanyl are potent opioids that, when used alone, will treat moderate and severe pain. Oxycodone can be used for moderate or severe pain, depending upon the product formulation. When combined with acetaminophen or aspirin, the dose is limited by the amount of nonopioid in the product. Therefore, the dose of oxycodone needed to treat severe pain could not be provided with the combination product. Meperidine undergoes extensive first-pass metabolism, limiting its usefulness as an oral analgesic. High levels of its metabolite, normeperidine, can result in central nervous system excitation ranging from agitation to seizures. Meperidine also inhibits serotonin reuptake, raising concerns about the development of the serotonin syndrome if a second serotonergic agent (eg, paroxetine, fluoxetine, or any selective serotonin reuptake inhibitor) is concurrently administered. So, for safety reasons, many hospitals limit the use or dose of meperidine for analgesia. For patients with renal and/or hepatic insufficiency, the doses of most opioids should be reduced. Table 2 represents the most frequently prescribed oral opioids for acute postoperative pain management.

Table 2. Oral Opioids for Acute Postoperative Pain

Drug	Equianalgesic Dose	Effective Adult Dosing[1]	Indication
Hydromorphone	7.5 mg	2-4 mg q4-6h	Severe pain
Codeine[2]	200 mg	15-60 mg q4-6h	Moderate pain
Hydrocodone[3]	30 mg	5-10 mg q4-6h	Moderate pain
Oxycodone[2]	20 mg	5-10 mg q4-6h	Moderate pain
Oxycodone[4]		10-15 mg (IR) q4-6h 20-30 mg (CR) q12h	Moderate-severe pain

[1]For patients with normal renal and hepatic function.
[2]When combined with acetaminophen or aspirin.
[3]When combined with acetaminophen or ibuprofen.
[4]Alone, immediate release (IR) or controlled release (CR).

Parenteral opioids remain an important component of any analgesic regimen for managing severe postoperative pain in the inpatient and ambulatory setting. Fentanyl, hydromorphone, and morphine are the most commonly used agents. Onset and duration of action from a single dose is determined by lipid solubility. Fentanyl, the most lipid soluble, has the fastest onset (1-2 minutes) and shortest duration (~1 hour) of action. Morphine, the least lipid soluble, has the slowest onset (5-6 minutes) and a longer duration of action (~2 hours). Hydromorphone has intermediate lipid solubility, with an onset of action 2-3 minutes and a duration of action of ~2 hours. These agents should be administered I.V., avoiding the pain on injection, variability of absorption, and longer time to peak effect with I.M. injection.

Patient-controlled analgesia (PCA), the self-administered intermittent I.V. administration of an opioid, is the preferred method for administering I.V. opioids for managing moderate to severe postoperative pain. The key to using PCA appropriately is patient selection and education. The patient must be willing to assume control of their analgesia, understand the concept of PCA, be able to press the button, and not be obtunded or sedated by their illness or medication.

An individually titrated loading dose is often necessary to provide initial analgesia. This loading dose can often be used to evaluate the patient's individual response and predict future opioid requirements. When choosing the PCA dose, patients with a history of previous opioid use would be anticipated to have increased opioid requirements, whereas elderly or very sick patients generally require less opioid to maintain good analgesia. Continuous infusion of the opioid is not routine, but may be useful for patients who were on prior opioids, patients with high opioid requirements, or patients whose pain is constant and intense or wake up with severe pain at night. For an opioid-naïve patient, the continuous infusion of opioid should not supply more than 30% to 50% of the patient's total daily opioid requirement. On the other hand, the continuous infusion should supply most (60% to 80%) of the total daily opioid requirement in an opioid-tolerant patient. Table 3 represents the usual PCA doses of common opioids for the treatment of moderate or severe acute postoperative pain.

ACUTE POSTOPERATIVE PAIN *(Continued)*

Table 3. Usual Adult PCA Opioid Dosing[1]

Drug	Equianalgesic Dose	Loading Dose[2]	PCA Dose	Lockout Interval
Fentanyl	20 mcg	25-100 mcg	20-40 mcg	4-8 min
Hydromorphone (Dilaudid®)	0.2 mg	0.2-1 mg	0.2-0.4 mg	5-10 min
Morphine	1 mg	2-10 mg	1-2 mg	5-10 min

[1]In patients with normal renal and hepatic function.

[2]Titrate in increments to desired level of analgesia or occurrence of excessive adverse effects.

If the patient is complaining about inadequate analgesia, assess the patient for number of PCA doses successfully received per hour, level of sedation, and respiratory status. If the patient has received 2-4 demands per hour and is not bradypneic or oversedated, a bolus dose should be administered and the demand dose increased by 50% to 100%. Consider adding a nonopioid adjunct (eg, acetaminophen, NSAID). It is important to assess if the patient's opioid requirements are increasing when they should be decreasing. An abrupt increase in pain several days following surgery should be evaluated because it could be a sign of a surgical complication.

Neuraxial opioid administration is another route that is used for management of moderate or severe acute postoperative pain. Neuraxial administration of opioids works by binding to opioid receptors on the spinal cord. This type of opioid administration can be used to provide analgesia for major abdominal, thoracic, and pelvic procedures, as well as total knee replacements. In these types of surgeries, epidural analgesia often provides better postoperative analgesia than parenteral opioids. Epidural administration of opioids is much more common than intrathecal administration for postoperative pain management. Table 4 represents neuraxial analgesic doses of opioid agonists for the treatment of moderate or severe acute postoperative pain.

Table 4. Usual Neuraxial Opioid Dosing in Adults

Agent	Epidural Bolus Dose	Epidural Continuous Infusion	Intrathecal Bolus Dose
Fentanyl	25-100 mcg	25-100 mcg/h	5-25 mcg
Hydromorphone	1 mg	0.1-0.2 mg/h	–
Morphine	5 mg	0.1-1 mg/h	0.1-0.3 mg
Morphine extended-release liposome injection[1]	10-15 mg	–	–
Sufentanil	10-50 mcg	5-30 mcg/h	0.02-0.05 mcg/kg

[1]Indicated for lumbar epidural injection for the treatment of pain for up to 48 hours following major surgery or elective cesarean section.

[2]10 mg for elective cesarean section; 15 mg for major orthopedic surgery of the lower extremity

Adverse Effects

Adverse effects of oral, parenteral, and neuraxial opioid therapy for treatment of acute postoperative pain include sedation, dizziness, nausea, vomiting, pruritus, urinary retention, and respiratory depression. Risk factors for respiratory depression include large doses administered to an opioid-naïve patient, respiratory dysfunction or compromise (eg, asthma, obstructive sleep apnea), obesity, low body weight, and concurrent medications that potentiate the respiratory depressant effect of the opioid. The potential for excessive sedation and respiratory depression to occur is greater when parenteral or neuraxial opioids are administered. Monitoring the patient's sedation level is the most effective way to prevent significant opioid-induced respiratory depression.

LOCAL ANESTHETICS

Local anesthetics provide good postoperative analgesia. These agents can be administered by the neuraxial route, as a peripheral nerve block (PNB), or directly into and around the wound via infiltration. Neuraxial administration is commonly used for acute postoperative pain management for the inpatient who has undergone major surgery, whereas PNB and wound infiltration are commonly used for the ambulatory surgery patient.

Peripheral nerve blocks of upper and lower extremities (eg, interscalene block, femoral nerve block) are often performed to provide intraoperative anesthesia and/or postoperative analgesia. A local anesthetic is injected near or around a nerve or nerve plexus to stop the pain impulses that originate from the surgical site. In addition to sensory fibers, motor and sympathetic fibers are also affected by injection of the local anesthetic solution. Patients undergoing more extensive, and therefore more painful, shoulder, elbow, knee, foot, or ankle surgeries are potential candidates for PNBs. These nerve blocks can be provided by a single injection, with or without a continuous infusion of a local anesthetic to provide postoperative analgesia. Local anesthetic wound infiltration (single injection with or without a postoperative continuous infusion) before, during, and after surgical procedures has been shown to decrease postoperative pain. Local anesthetics administered epidurally or intrathecally are frequently combined with opioids to provide "balanced analgesia." The most common local anesthetic agents used for intra- and postoperative analgesia are lidocaine, mepivacaine, bupivacaine, and ropivacaine. (Table 5)

Table 5. Common Local Anesthetic Agents and Doses for Intra- and Postoperative Analgesia

Agent	Local Infiltration	Peripheral Nerve Block[1]	Continuous Peripheral Nerve Block	Continuous Epidural Analgesia
Lidocaine	0.5%-1%, 1-50 mL	1%-1.5%, 20 mL	–	–
Bupivacaine	0.25%, 1-50 mL	0.25%-0.5%, 30 mL	0.1%-0.2% at 5-10 mL/h[2]	0.05%-0.125% at 4-10 mL/h[3]
Ropivacaine	0.5%, 1-40 mL	0.5%-0.75%, 15-40 mL	0.17%-0.2% at 5-10 mL/h[2]	0.1%-0.2% at 4-10 mL/h
Mepivacaine	0.5%-1%, 1-50 mL	1.5%-2%, 30 mL	–	–

[1]For a 70 kg patient – doses vary with the type of block and should not exceed the maximum recommended single dose.

[2]For 24-72 hours; some studies have added clonidine 1 mcg/mL.

[3]When administered in combination with fentanyl, sufentanil, hydromorphone, or morphine.

Adverse Effects

The adverse effects most commonly seen with analgesic doses of local anesthetics include hypotension (secondary to sympathetic blockade) and dose-related motor blockade. The potential for CNS and cardiovascular toxicity exists if a large amount of the local anesthetic agent is inadvertently administered systemically (eg, inadvertent intravascular injection, migration of the catheter into a blood vessel). Symptoms of high plasma levels of local anesthetic include unusual drowsiness, dizziness, blurred vision, slurred speech, poor balance, tingling around the lips or mouth, and seizure. Complications of the peripheral nerve catheter include inflammation and/or pain at the catheter entry site, blood in the catheter, the catheter can become dislodged, Horner syndrome, and with upper extremity catheters, hoarseness and dyspnea can occur.

SUMMARY

The goal of acute postoperative pain management is to provide good analgesia with minimal adverse effects. Oftentimes, this is best accomplished with the use of a combination of analgesic agents and techniques that provide analgesia by different mechanisms.

ACUTE POSTOPERATIVE PAIN *(Continued)*

REFERENCES AND RECOMMENDED READING

American Society of Anesthesiologists Task Force on Acute Pain Management, "Practice Guidelines for Acute Pain Management in the Perioperative Setting," *Anesthesiology*, 2004, 100(6):1573-81.

Block BM, Liu SS, Rowlingson AJ, et al, "Efficacy of Postoperative Epidural Analgesia: A Meta-Analysis," *JAMA*, 2003, 290(18):2455-63.

Boezaart AP, et al, Regional Anesthesia Study Center of Iowa, Department of Anesthesia, University of Iowa. http://www.anesth.uiowa.edu/rasci/index.html

Boezaart AP, "Perineural Infusion of Local Anesthetics," *Anesthesiology*, 2006, 104(4):872-80.

Capdevila X, Pirat P, Bringuier S, et al, "Continuous Peripheral Nerve Blocks in Hospital Wards After Orthopedic Surgery: A Multicenter Prospective Analysis of the Quality of Postoperative Analgesia and Complications in 1,416 patients," *Anesthesiology*, 2005, 103(5):1035-45.

Chelly J, Fanelli G, and Casati A, *Continuous Peripheral Nerve Blocks – An Illustrated Guide*, Mosby, 2001 (e-book) **(http://www.harcourt-international.com/e-books/viewbook.cfm?ID=252)**.

Gilron I, Milne B, and Hong M, "Cyclooxygenase-2 Inhibitors in Postoperative Pain Management: Current Evidence and Future Directions," *Anesthesiology*, 2003, 99(5):1198-208.

Grass JA, "Patient-Controlled Analgesia," *Anesth Analg*, 2005, 101(5 Suppl):S44-61.

Lee A, Cooper MG, Craig JC, et al, "The Effects of Nonsteroidal Anti-Inflammatory Drugs (NSAIDs) on Postoperative Renal Function: A Meta-Analysis," *Anaesth Intensive Care*, 1999, 27(6):574-80.

Macintyre PE, "Intravenous Patient-Controlled Analgesia: One Size Does Not Fit All," *Anesthesiol Clin North America*, 2005, 23(1):109-23.

Reuben SS, Connelly NR, and Maciolek H, "Postoperative Analgesia With Controlled-Release Oxycodone for Outpatient Anterior Cruciate Ligament Surgery," *Anesth Analg*, 1999, 88(6):1286-91.

Scott LJ and Perry CM, "Tramadol: A Review of its Use in Perioperative Pain," *Drugs*, 2000, 60(1):139-76.

Strassels SA, McNicol E, and Suleman R, "Postoperative Pain Management: A Practical Review, Part 1," *Am J Health Syst Pharm*, 2005, 62(18):1904-16.

Strassels SA, McNicol E, and Suleman R, "Postoperative Pain Management: A Practical Review, Part 2," *Am J Health Syst Pharm*, 2005, 62(19):2019-25.

Sunshine A, Olson NZ, Colon A, et al, "Analgesic Efficacy of Controlled-Release Oxycodone in Postoperative Pain," *J Clin Pharmacol*, 1996, 36(7):595-603.

Turan A, White PF, Karamanlioglu B, et al, "Gabapentin: An Alternative to the Cyclooxygenase-2 Inhibitors for Perioperative Pain Management," *Anesth Analg*, 2006, 102(1):175-81.

ALLERGIC REACTIONS

An allergic drug reaction can be considered an adverse effect involving immunologic mechanisms. True allergic reactions are much less common than nonallergic responses such as side effects and drug-drug interactions. As a result, it is important to carefully evaluate patients who present with allergies to drugs. Patients frequently state an allergy to a drug when the reaction was a predictable side effect (eg, nausea/vomiting with codeine). If a patient presents a history of one or more of the following signs or symptoms after drug administration, an allergic reaction should be assumed until proven otherwise: Skin manifestations (pruritus with hives or flushing), facial or oral swelling, shortness of breath, choking, wheezing, and vascular collapse. In these situations, an alternate agent should be selected.

CLASSIFICATION OF ALLERGIC REACTIONS

Allergic reactions can be classified into one of four immunopathologic categories (types I through IV) using the Coombs and Gell Classification System. The following table summarizes the key characteristics of each type of reaction.

Type	Characteristics	Usual Onset	Examples
I - Anaphylactic (IgE mediated)	Requires the presence of IgE specific for drug antigen or other allergen; allergen binds to IgE on basophils and mast cells resulting in release of inflammatory mediators (eg, histamine, serotonin, proteases, bradykinin generating factor, eosinophil chemotactic factors, neutrophil chemotactic factor, leukotrienes, prostaglandins, thromboxanes)	Within 30 minutes	Immediate penicillin reaction Immediate latex reaction Blood products Vaccines Dextran Polypeptide hormones
II - Cytotoxic	Destruction of host cells; cell-associated antigen initiates cytolysis by antigen-specific antibody (IgG or IgM); most often involves blood elements (eg, erythrocytes, leukocytes, platelets)	Usually 5-12 hours	Penicillin, quinidine, phenylbutazone, thiouracils, sulfonamides, methyldopa
III - Immune complex	Antigen-antibody complexes form and deposit on blood vessel walls and activate complement. Result is a serum-sickness-like syndrome.	3-8 hours	Serum sickness; may be caused by penicillins, sulfonamides, I.V. contrast media, hydantoins
IV - Cell mediated (delayed)	Antigens cause activation of lymphocytes (T cells), which release inflammatory mediators	24-48 hours	Graft rejection Latex contact dermatitis Tuberculin reaction

Modified from DiPiro JT and Stafford CT, "Allergic and Pseudoallergic Drug Reactions," *Pharmacotherapy: A Pathophysiologic Approach*, 3rd ed, Stamford CT: Appleton and Lange, 1997, 1675-88.

ANESTHESIA-RELATED AGENTS ASSOCIATED WITH ALLERGY

Certain agents are most often responsible for allergic reactions in surgical patients. These include neuromuscular blocking agents, latex, colloids, hypnotics, antibiotics, benzodiazepines, opioids, local anesthetics, I.V. contrast media, and blood products. The antibiotics most commonly associated with allergic reactions are the sulfonamides, penicillins, and cephalosporins. Propofol contains soybean oil and egg yolk components; in patients with allergies to these items, propofol should be avoided. The ester-type local anesthetics can produce allergic reactions secondary to the metabolite para-aminobenzoic acid. The methylparaben preservative in amide-type local anesthetics may also produce an allergic reaction in

ALLERGIC REACTIONS *(Continued)*

patients sensitive to para-aminobenzoic acid. Sulfites, which are used as preservatives in various drug products, can produce pulmonary complications in patients, occurring more frequently in asthmatics. Cross allergenicity exists between shellfish/seafood and protamine and I.V. contrast media; care should be taken when using these agents in patients with these types of allergies. Special consideration should be given to a patient who presents a personal or family history of allergy to halothane or succinylcholine as this may actually represent an occurrence of malignant hyperthermia.

ANAPHYLAXIS

Anaphylaxis is the most severe form of allergic reaction. It can present as an acute, life-threatening reaction with multiple organ system involvement or it can be more localized in appearance. It has been estimated that 1 in every 2700 hospitalized patients experience drug-induced anaphylaxis. When antibodies are not involved in the process, the reaction is termed anaphylactoid. It is not possible through clinical observation to distinguish between anaphylactic and anaphylactoid reactions. Life-threatening reactions are more likely to occur in patients with a history of allergy, atopy, or asthma. Although these patients are frequently pretreated with corticosteroids, there is no evidence to suggest this practice is effective for preventing true anaphylactic reactions. In a survey examining the incidence of intraoperative anaphylaxis, 70.2% were due to neuromuscular blocking agents, 12.5% due to latex, 4.6% due to colloids, 3.6% due to hypnotics, 2.6% due to antibiotics, 2% due to benzodiazepines, 1.7% due to opioids, 0.7% due to local anesthetics, and 2.8% due to other agents.

Pathophysiology

Anaphylaxis is initiated by an antigen binding to IgE antibodies; however, prior exposure to the antigen or a substance with a similar structure is first required to sensitize the patient to the antigen. The binding of the antigen to the IgE antibodies on the surface of basophils and mast cells causes release of histamine and the chemotactic factors of anaphylaxis. Other chemical mediators (leukotrienes, prostaglandins, kinins) are also released in response to cellular activation. The liberated mediators produce bronchospasm, upper airway edema, vasodilation, increased capillary permeability, and urticaria. The effects of multiple mediators on the heart and peripheral vasculature cause the cardiovascular collapse seen during anaphylaxis. Antigenic challenge in a sensitized individual usually produces immediate clinical manifestations of anaphylaxis; however, the onset may be delayed by up to 30 minutes. The reaction can vary in severity, from minor clinical changes to acute cardiopulmonary collapse.

Signs / Symptoms of Anaphylactic Reaction

The following table lists the signs and symptoms that may indicate an anaphylactic reaction during anesthesia.

Systems	Symptoms	Signs
Cutaneous	Itching, burning	Urticaria (hives), flushing, periorbital edema, perioral edema
Respiratory	Dyspnea, chest tightness	Coughing, wheezing, sneezing, laryngeal edema, decreased pulmonary compliance, pulmonary edema, acute respiratory distress, bronchospasm
Cardiovascular	Dizziness, malaise, retrosternal oppression	Disorientation, diaphoresis, loss of consciousness, hypotension, tachycardia, dysrhythmias, decreased systemic vascular resistance, pulmonary hypertension, cardiovascular collapse

Modified from Levy JH, *Anaphylactic Reactions in Anesthesia and Intensive Care*, Stoneham, Butterworth-Heinemann, 1992.

Treatment of Anaphylactic Reaction

Treatment of a severe, life-threatening anaphylactic reaction must be immediate. Initial therapy should consist of: 1) stop administration of precipitating drug; 2) maintain airway with 100% oxygen; 3) discontinue all anesthetic agents; 4) intravascular volume expansion with crystalloid solution; and 5) epinephrine administration. Secondary therapy consists of administration of antihistamines (eg, diphenhydramine), catecholamine infusions (eg, norepinephrine, epinephrine), inhaled bronchodilators (eg, albuterol) for bronchospasm, corticosteroids (eg, hydrocortisone, methylprednisolone, dexamethasone), and sodium bicarbonate. Patients should be admitted to an ICU for 24 hours following an anaphylactic reaction because of the possibility of recurrent "late-phase" reactions.

REFERENCES AND RECOMMENDED READING

DiPiro JT and Stafford CT, "Allergic and Pseudoallergic Drug Reactions," *Pharmacotherapy: A Pathophysiologic Approach*, 3rd ed, Stamford, CT: Appleton and Lange, 1997, 1675-88.

Levy JH, "Allergy and Anesthesia," Paper presented at the ASA 1996 Annual Refresher Course Lectures, New Orleans, LA, 1996 Oct 20.

LATEX ALLERGY

The incidence of latex allergy is increasing. This increase has been suggested to be due in part to the implementation of universal precautions by the CDC in 1987 secondary to the AIDS epidemic. **Because of the increased incidence of latex allergy, all patients should be asked about allergic responses to latex products.** For example, patients should be questioned about the presence of swelling or itching of the hands or other areas after contact with rubber gloves, condoms, diaphragms, toys, or other rubber products and about itching or swelling of the lips or mouth after dental exams, blowing up balloons, or after eating bananas, chestnuts, and avocados.

It is important today for healthcare institutions to have a comprehensive plan (including a perioperative component) in place for dealing with the latex allergic patient.

Hypersensitivity Reactions Caused by Latex

Latex-containing products can produce type I and type IV hypersensitivity reactions.

The type I hypersensitivity reaction is the true "allergic" reaction seen with latex products. Proteins found in the latex promote the production of an antibody of the IgE class which attaches to basophils and mast cells. When the antigen (protein) is encountered again, histamine and other physiologically active mediators are released from mast cells and basophils. The clinical manifestations can include single or multiple system involvement, be mild or severe, range from itching to edema, and from mild hypotension to shock. It has been estimated that 10% of the true anaphylactic reactions during anesthesia are due to latex allergy. These reactions are usually seen 5-30 minutes after induction of anesthesia and start of surgery.

In the type IV reaction, a contact dermatitis is seen. The preservatives, stabilizers, accelerators, and antioxidants used in the latex manufacturing process serve as the antigens for T-cell lymphocytes. The dermatitis produced can be uncomfortable but is not life-threatening.

Routes of Exposure to Latex Proteins

It is important to consider the route of exposure of the latex protein in allergic patients as this can be a determinant of the type of reaction produced. The following table summarizes major routes of exposure.

Type of Exposure	Reaction
Direct skin contact	Localized or generalized urticaria
Mucous membrane	Rhinitis, conjunctivitis, stomatitis, angioedema; severe anaphylactic reactions and death reported
Inhalation of airborne starch-protein particles	Wheezing, bronchospasm, reduced lung compliance, episodes of desaturation and/or severe hypoxemia
Intravascular absorption of water soluble latex particles from surgical gloves	Sudden tachycardia, severe hypotension, cardiorespiratory collapse

ANESTHESIA CONSIDERATIONS FOR NEUROSURGERY

Various factors must be taken into account for the patient undergoing neurosurgery. These include the surgical procedure being performed; the type of anesthesia to be used; the need for special anesthetic techniques (eg, controlled hypotension); and the effects of the anesthetic agents on brain physiology (cerebral blood flow, cerebral metabolic oxygen requirements, and cerebral vasodilation). This section will review key aspects of the anesthetic management of neurosurgical patients.

PHYSIOLOGY

Cerebral Blood Flow

Cerebral blood flow (CBF) is equal to cerebral perfusion pressure divided by the cerebral vascular resistance. Cerebral perfusion pressure is defined as the difference between mean arterial pressure (MABP) and the greater of intracranial pressure (ICP) or central venous pressure. Autoregulation maintains CBF at a constant level (50 mL/100 g brain/minute) between the MABP of 50 and 150 mm Hg (see Figure A). Various conditions and/or medications can attenuate or abolish autoregulation, making blood flow dependent on MABP; these include the volatile inhalation agents, hypoxia, hypercarbia, and cerebral ischemia. Hypoxia causes cerebral vasodilation and an increase in CBF (see Figure B) while hypocarbia causes a linear decrease in CBF between $PaCO_2$ of 20 and 80 mm Hg (see Figure C).

Cerebral Metabolic Rate

Cerebral metabolic rate ($CMRO_2$) and CBF are directly related; as $CMRO_2$ increases, so does CBF to ensure sufficient substrate is available for metabolic demand (see Figure D). Conditions and/or medications that influence $CMRO_2$ include seizures (↑ $CMRO_2$), temperature (hypothermia ↓ $CMRO_2$), and various anesthetics (eg, volatile inhalation agents ↓ $CMRO_2$).

The Brain's Protective Mechanisms

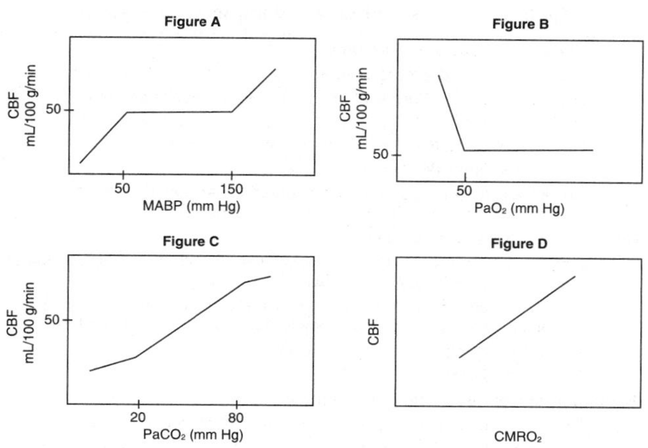

ANESTHESIA CONSIDERATIONS FOR NEUROSURGERY *(Continued)*

Intracranial Pressure

Normal ICP values are between 5 and 15 mm Hg and reflect the relationship between the volume of the cranial vault and intracranial contents. Since the cranial vault is rigid, the capacity of the intracranial contents to adjust to an increasing volume (compliance) will ultimately be exceeded, resulting in a marked increase in ICP with a small increase in volume. Signs and symptoms of increased ICP are found in Table 1. It must be kept in mind that a patient with an increased intracranial volume as a result of a tumor, for example, may be especially sensitive to volume increases secondary to cerebral vasodilation caused by factors such as CO_2 retention or volatile inhalational anesthetic agents. Elevated ICP can be treated by reducing cerebral blood volume, reducing brain tissue volume, or reducing cerebrospinal fluid (CSF) volume (Table 2).

Table 1. Signs and Symptoms of Increased Intracranial Pressure

- Headache
- Nausea/vomiting
- Decreased level of consciousness
- Hypertension
- Bradycardia
- Irregular breathing
- Oculomotor (third cranial) nerve palsy
- Pupillary dilation
- Abducens (sixth cranial) nerve palsy
- Hemiparesis or hemiplegia
- Coma
- Respiratory arrest

Table 2. Treatment of Elevated Intracranial Pressure

Reduction of Cerebral Blood Volume

- Avoid hypoxia and hypercarbia, as they cause cerebral vasodilation
- Hyperventilate to a $PaCO_2$ of 25-30 mm Hg (produces cerebral vasoconstriction)
- Promote venous drainage (eg, elevate head 30 degrees)
- Treat severe hypertension
- Administer medications to produce cerebral vasoconstriction (eg, barbiturates, propofol, etomidate, benzodiazepines)

Reduction of Brain Tissue Volume

- Increase serum osmolality to 305-320 mOsm/L with the administration of mannitol (0.2-1 g/kg I.V.), urea, hypertonic saline
- Administer furosemide (0.5-1 mg/kg I.V.); optimal results seen when combined with mannitol ($\downarrow$ furosemide dose to 0.15-0.3 mg/kg I.V.)
- Administer steroids (effective for tumors)
- Resection of brain

Reduction of Cerebrospinal Fluid Volume

- Drain CSF through lumbar subarachnoid or ventriculostomy catheter
- Decrease CSF production (furosemide, acetazolamide) and/or increase CSF reabsorption

Cerebrospinal Fluid

The CSF volume in an adult is approximately 150 mL. It is formed in the choroid plexus of the cerebral ventricles (0.35 mL/minute) by the transport of sodium, chloride, and bicarbonate with osmotic movement of water. CSF is absorbed into the venous system of the brain through arachnoid membrane villi. Furosemide and acetazolamide can reduce CSF formation by inhibiting the combined transport of sodium and chloride and by reducing bicarbonate transport, respectively.

EFFECTS OF MEDICATIONS ON BRAIN PHYSIOLOGY

Table 3 lists the effects of select anesthetic agents on cerebral blood flow, cerebral metabolic oxygen requirements, and cerebral vasodilation. In general, inhalational anesthetics decrease cerebral metabolism and increase CBF whereas intravenous agents decrease both cerebral metabolism and blood flow. Of note, ketamine increases oxygen demand and as a result is not commonly used in neuroanesthesia. Isoflurane continues to be an excellent choice for a volatile inhalation agent. Its mild direct vasodilating action is partly offset by its ability to reduce cerebral metabolic rate and subsequently CBF, thereby limiting the net increase in CBF. The newer volatile inhalation agents desflurane and sevoflurane generally appear to act similarly. The nondepolarizing neuromuscular blocking (NMB) agents have no direct effects on CBF and $CMRO_2$ as they do not cross the blood brain barrier; they may have an indirect effect secondary to their effects on heart rate (eg, pancuronium) and blood pressure (eg, tubocurarine) if autoregulation has been abolished. Succinylcholine does increase CBF and $CMRO_2$, but this has minimal clinical impact if administered after a defasciculating dose of a nondepolarizing NMB agent or induction of adequate anesthesia. The vasopressors epinephrine, phenylephrine, and norepinephrine also have no direct cerebral effects but may indirectly increase CBF by increasing cerebral perfusion pressure. The vasodilators nitroglycerin, sodium nitroprusside, and hydralazine can increase CBF and ICP via direct cerebral vasodilation if arterial blood pressure is maintained. Beta-blockers (esmolol, labetalol) do not alter cerebral metabolism or vascular tone.

Table 3. Effects of Anesthetic Agents on Brain Physiology

Medication	Cerebral Blood Flow	Cerebral Metabolic Rate	Direct Cerebral Vasodilation
Inhalation Anesthetic Agents			
Desflurane	↑	↓↓	Yes
Enflurane	↑↑	↓	Yes
Halothane	↑↑↑	↓	Yes
Isoflurane	↑	↓↓	Yes
Nitrous oxide	↑↑/0	↑/0	–
Nitrous oxide with volatile inhalation agent	↑	↑/0	–
Nitrous oxide with intravenous anesthetic agent	0	0	–
Sevoflurane	↑	↓↓	Yes
Intravenous Anesthetic Agents			
Barbiturates	↓↓↓	↓↓↓	No
Etomidate	↓↓↓	↓↓↓	No
Fentanyl	↓/0	↓/0	No
Ketamine	↑↑	↑	Yes
Midazolam	↓↓	↓↓	No
Propofol	↓↓	↓↓	No

ANESTHESIA CONSIDERATIONS FOR NEUROSURGERY
(Continued)

ELECTROPHYSIOLOGIC MONITORING

Electroencephalogram

The electroencephalogram (EEG) is used to monitor cerebral electrical activity and may allow early detection of ischemia before CBF is not sufficient to maintain tissue viability. It can also be used for localization of epileptic foci. As a general rule, anesthetic effects on the EEG are global in nature in contrast to the focal changes seen with ischemia (see Table 4).

Table 4. EEG Rhythms

Wave Forms	Frequency	Activity
Delta	0-0.4 Hz	Deep sleep Deep anesthesia Ischemia
Theta	4-8 Hz	Light sleep Light anesthesia
Alpha	8-13 Hz	Resting and alert
Beta	13-30 Hz	Mental concentration Light sedation

Evoked Potentials

Evoked potentials monitor the functional integrity of ascending sensory pathways and descending motor pathways. Sensory evoked potentials are recorded from the cerebral cortex following peripheral (sensory nerve) stimulation. Motor evoked potentials are recorded from peripheral muscle activity initiated by stimulation of the motor cortex. Evoked potentials are classified by the nerve tract being evaluated (somatosensory, auditory, visual, motor) (see Table 5). The type of evoked potential monitored depends on the area of CNS at risk for intraoperative injury. Evoked potentials are measured in terms of latency (how long it takes the stimulus to reach the recording device) and amplitude (the peak to trough height of the recorded waveform). Because anesthetic agents affect the latency and/or amplitude measurements (Table 6) it is important to obtain a baseline measurement after establishment of anesthesia. Thereafter, the anesthetic regimen should not be altered so that any subsequent decrease in amplitude or increase in latency reflects neuronal ischemia, not a change in depth of anesthesia. Maintaining an adequate depth of anesthesia when monitoring MEPs is difficult, especially since muscle relaxants must be used sparingly to preserve the motor response. Other factors that can alter evoked potentials include hypotension, hypoxia, and hypothermia.

The reader is referred to any major anesthesia text for a further discussion of electrophysiologic monitoring.

Table 5. Evoked Potentials and the Neuronal Tracts They Monitor

Evoked Potential	CNS Tract	Surgical Procedures
SSEP (somatosensory evoked potential)	Sensory neural axis from peripheral nerves to brainstem and cortex	Spinal cord surgery (tumor, scoliosis), carotid endarterectomy, aortic surgery, cerebral aneurysm
BAER (brainstem auditory evoked response)	Brain stem	Acoustic neuroma, posterior fossa lesions, surgery involving cranial nerve VIII or auditory canal
VER (visual evoked response)	Retina, optic chiasm, optic radiation, occipital cortex	Orbit tumors, sphenoid wing meningiomas, supracellular/pituitary tumors, surgery around optic nerve or occipital cortex
MEP (motor evoked potential)	Motor cortex and descending motor tracts	Spinal cord surgery (tumor, scoliosis)

Table 6. Drug Effects on Evoked Potentials

	Amplitude	Latency
I.V. Drugs		
Barbiturates	↓	↑
Benzodiazepines	↓	↑
Droperidol	↓	↑
Etomidate	↑,→	↑,→
Ketamine	↑	→
Narcotics	↓	↑,→
Propofol	↓	↑
Anesthetic Gases		
Inhalational agents (0.5 MAC)	→	→
Inhalational agents (>1 MAC)	↓	↑
Nitrous oxide	↓	→

NEUROSURGICAL PROCEDURES

The following information should be considered when anesthetizing patients undergoing neurosurgical procedures.

Intracranial Tumors

- Assess fluid and electrolyte status. Hypovolemia, which is not uncommon in patients who have been at bedrest and/or treated with mannitol, can predispose the patient to hypotension during induction of anesthesia.
- Care should be taken in premedicating patients as they may be especially sensitive to central nervous system (CNS) depressant drugs; sedatives/analgesics are often not administered until the patient is in the operating room.
- Monitoring should include measurement of arterial blood gases, intra-arterial blood pressure, central venous pressure, and urinary output in addition to the standard monitoring.
- Goals of anesthesia management: Avoid hypertension, hypotension, hypoxia, hypercarbia, and coughing; ICP should not be increased nor CBF compromised.
  - Thiopental, propofol, etomidate, or midazolam are all suitable induction agents.
  - An opioid can be administered to blunt the response to induction.
  - A nondepolarizing NMB agent with minimal cardiovascular effects (eg, vecuronium) should be used if airway management is not considered problematic.
  - A deep level of anesthesia should be established before laryngoscopy/intubation to minimize increases in ICP due to sympathetic stimulation.
  - Hyperventilation to a $PaCO_2$ of 25-30 mm Hg produces cerebral vasoconstriction and decreases intracranial pressure without producing cerebral ischemia.
  - $PaCO_2$ should be normalized near the end of surgery.
  - Long-acting agents should be avoided for the last 1-2 hours of surgery to prevent prolonged wakeup and allow a neurologic examination at the end of surgery.
  - Consider administering lidocaine I.V. 90 seconds before suctioning/extubation to minimize coughing, straining, and hypertension.
  - Before extubation, the patient's ability to protect his/her airway and the adequacy of respiration should be assessed.
  - Hypertension should be treated to minimize bleeding, prevent brain edema, and hematoma; esmolol, sodium nitroprusside, nitroglycerin, nicardipine, and labetalol are suitable options.
  - A neurologic exam should be performed after the patient is extubated.

ANESTHESIA CONSIDERATIONS FOR NEUROSURGERY *(Continued)*

Pituitary Tumors

- ICP may be less of a concern if the tumor is small.
- Endocrine function should be assessed preoperatively.
- Supplemental, short-acting corticosteroid therapy may need to be administered perioperatively.
- With the transcranial approach, ICP may be a concern; measures to control ICP intraoperatively should be instituted.
- Hypertension, tachycardia, arrhythmias, and myocardial ischemia may be seen when phenylephrine and cocaine are used to prepare the nares for the transphenoidal approach.
- At the end of transphenoidal surgery, nasal breathing will not be possible due to nasal packing; make sure the patient is fully conscious before extubation.
- Diabetes insipidus frequently occurs after surgery (within first 12 hours) requiring treatment with I.V. fluids or vasopressin.

Intracranial Aneurysms

- Complications of subarachnoid hemorrhage include increased ICP, aneurysm rebleed, vasospasm, and hydrocephalus.
- Thiopental, propofol, opioids, and volatile inhalation agents (eg, isoflurane) can be used to induce/maintain anesthesia.
- Lidocaine, esmolol, or labetalol can be used during induction to reduce the risk of hypertension and rupture of the aneurysm.
- Following induction, $PaCO_2$ should be maintained between 25 and 35 mm Hg.
- In addition to hyperventilation, osmotic diuresis and CSF drainage may be used to provide a "slack" brain.
- Controlled hypotension may be considered during dissection of the aneurysm.
- Normotension or a slight increase in blood pressure may be employed with temporary "trapping" of the aneurysm.
- EEG or evoked potentials may be used to monitor the safety of temporary occlusion of arteries.
- Mild hypothermia (32°C to 34°C) can improve the brain's ability to tolerate ischemia.
- Treat hyperglycemia because ischemic damage is worse when it occurs with elevated blood glucose levels (>150-180 mg/dL).
- Minimize coughing, straining, hypertension at extubation.
- A neurologic exam should be performed in the operating room.

REFERENCES AND RECOMMENDED READING

Albin MS, ed, *Textbook of Neuroanesthesia With Neurosurgical and Neuroscience Perspectives*, New York, NY: McGraw-Hill, 1997.

Barash PG, Cullen BF, and Stoelting RK, "Neurophysiology and Neuroanesthesia," *Handbook of Clinical Anesthesia*, 2nd ed, Philadelphia, PA: JB Lippincott, 1993, 256-76.

Bendo AA, Kass IS, Hartung J, et al. "Anesthesia for Neurosurgery," Barash PG, Cullen BF, Stoelting RK, eds, *Clinical Anesthesia*, 3rd ed, Philadelphia, PA: Lippincott-Raven, 1997, 699-745.

Cottrell JE and Smith DS, *Anesthesia and Neurosurgery*, 3rd ed, St Louis, MO: Mosby Co, 1994.

Goto T and Kliewer D, "Anesthesia for Neurosurgery," Davison JK, Eckhardt III WF, Perese DA, eds, *Clinical Anesthesia Procedures of the Massachusetts General Hospital*, 4th ed, Boston, MA: Little, Brown and Company, 1993, 368-89.

Shapiro HM and Drummond JC, "Neurosurgical Anesthesia," Miller RD, ed, *Anesthesia*, 4th ed, New York, NY: Churchill Livingstone, 1994, 1897-946.

ANESTHESIA FOR GERIATRIC PATIENTS

"No skill or art is needed to grow old, but the trick is to endure it." – Goethe

In 1980, people 65 years of age and older made up 12% of the population in the United States but consumed 30% of the healthcare expenditures. By 2040, the elderly will make up about 25% of the population and account for 50% of health-care costs. Because at least half will require surgery, understanding physiologic and pathologic changes in the geriatric population is important to reduce perioperative morbidity and mortality.

In 1961, the perioperative mortality rate in geriatric patients approached 20%. Because of increased understanding of the physiology of aging and improved perianesthetic monitoring, the mortality rate decreased to <5% by 1980, although the mortality associated with emergency surgery is 3-10 times greater than when the same surgery is performed on an elective basis. Improvements in preoperative evaluation, intraoperative management, and postoperative treatment have further reduced morbidity and mortality in geriatric patients.

As a general rule, older people have more pre-existing diseases than younger people do. In addition, geriatric patients have significant alterations in anatomy, physiology, pharmacokinetics, pharmacodynamics, recovery ability, and psychological coping mechanisms. The purpose of this chapter is to identify those major changes which necessitate a modification in perioperative practice. A brief review of major organ systems highlights the natural aging process and the common disease processes that compromise the elderly person.

Figure 1: Changes in physiologic function with age in humans expressed as percentage of mean value at age 30 years.

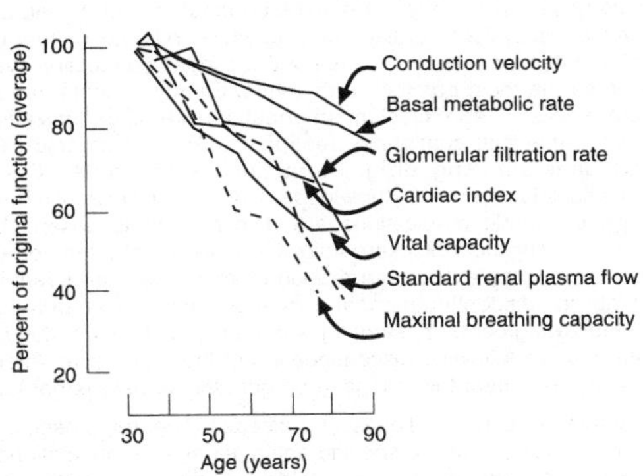

With permission from Miller RD, "Anesthesia for the Elderly," *Anesthesia*, 2nd ed, Miller RD, ed, New York, NY: Churchill Livingstone, 1986, 1802.

CARDIOVASCULAR SYSTEM

Hypertension and atherosclerotic cardiovascular disease occur in more than half of the elderly. Loss of elasticity in arterial walls increases vascular resistance

ANESTHESIA FOR GERIATRIC PATIENTS *(Continued)*

leading to an increase in systolic blood pressure which, in time, produces left ventricular hypertrophy. With aging, the vascular muscular layer is replaced with fibrous tissue and plaque, which cannot stretch, exaggerating the blood pressure rise during systole and fall during diastole. This widened pulse pressure is a marker of compromised compliance in the vessel wall and is associated with increased risk of coronary events.

A decrease in adrenergic activity leads to a slower resting heart rate, a lower maximal heart rate, and a depressed baroreceptor reflex. These physiologic changes associated with aging impair a person's ability to respond to hypovolemia, hypotension, or hypoxemia by attenuating increases in heart rate and cardiac output. A slow circulation time, frequently found in geriatric patients, prolongs onset of action for I.V. drugs (eg, thiopental, propofol, fentanyl), while speeding the induction of anesthesia using inhalational agents (eg, sevoflurane, isoflurane).

Normal Physiologic Changes	Pathophysiologic Changes
Decreased elasticity	Atherosclerosis
Increased afterload	Coronary artery disease
Increased left ventricular hypertrophy	Hypertension
Increased systolic blood pressure	Congestive heart failure
Decreased diastolic blood pressure	Arrhythmias
Decreased adrenergic activity	
Decreased resting heart rate	
Decreased maximum heart rate	
Decreased baroreceptor reflex	
Slowed circulation time	

The development of atherosclerosis is a pathologic process which produces critical coronary stenosis. The development of congestive heart failure and myocardial ischemia compromises cardiac function, which influences other organ systems. Onset of arrhythmias reflects disease of the cardiac conduction system, with atrial fibrillation as the most common arrhythmia. Elderly patients frequently take nitrates, beta-blockers, and calcium channel blockers. Optimization of cardiac function preoperatively, continuing treatment with most chronic cardiac medications, and understanding drug interactions with anesthetics and perioperative medications is important. Knowledge of not only drug action but also physiologic reaction if chronic medications are discontinued is essential. For example, a person receiving beta-blockers following myocardial infarction or for treatment of hypertension may experience rebound hypertension and ventricular arrhythmias with abrupt discontinuation of this medication. The duration of antiplatelet therapy following coronary stenting is not completely understood, with reports of acute thrombosis following discontinuation of the drugs even after one year of administration. The effect this will have on geriatric surgery is not known.

Hypertension is another common cardiovascular disease. Therapy crosses many drug categories. Knowledge about the specific antihypertensive medications and their interactions with anesthetic drugs (eg, clonidine decreases anesthetic drug requirements) is important. Discontinuation of antihypertensive medication can produce preoperative hypertension, with enhanced hemodynamic instability. The decision to continue diuretic therapy preoperatively depends on the patient. Patients prone to congestive heart failure should be maintained on their diuretic therapy, whereas a chronic hypertensive patient receiving a bowel prep for GI surgery does not need additional loss of intravascular volume prior to surgery. Serum potassium may be low in patients taking a thiazide diuretic. This is especially important for people taking digitalis. Although anesthesiologists, cardiologists, and intensivists have over the years expressed concern that maintenance of chronic drug therapy (ie, beta-blockers, calcium channel blockers, ACE inhibitors) may produce complications when combined with anesthetic drugs, current thinking is that maintaining the patient in his optimal state of preoperative hemodynamic control provides the best situation for perianesthetic management. Recently, anesthesiologists echo cardiologists in suggesting that initiation of perioperative beta-blocker therapy for geriatric patients with cardiovascular disease decreases operative morbidity and mortality. Aging also leads to abnormal response to endothelium-dependent vasodilators (ie, acetylcholine) and decreased production of endothelial-derived vasodilator substances (ie, nitric oxide). A poorly controlled hypertensive patient may have a reduced blood volume and will experience tremendous swings in blood pressure during anesthesia and surgery.

RESPIRATORY SYSTEM

A carefully performed history and physical examination can identify patients whose normal pulmonary aging changes have become a pathophysiologic risk. History of recurrent pulmonary infections, smoking, asthma, COPD, and emphysema place patients at high risk for pulmonary complications. Preoperative optimization of pulmonary function (treat infection, stop smoking, bronchodilators) and instruction in the use and importance of incentive spirometry can improve the perioperative pulmonary course. Pulmonary function tests add little to the preoperative evaluation, except for lung resection surgery.

Smoking is a serious problem for the general population. It is more serious in the geriatric population because they have more years of tobacco exposure and more pulmonary damage. Cessation of smoking the day before surgery does two things: a) decreases the level of carbon monoxide in the blood and therefore enhances oxygen carrying capacity, and b) increases bronchial reactivity to stimuli due to the acute withdrawal of nicotine. To improve pulmonary function, the patient must stop smoking at least 6 weeks before surgery. Anatomic and physiologic damage are not reversed, however, the rate of continuing organ dysfunction is reduced to reflect the normal aging process. Supplemental oxygen may be needed in the immediate postoperative period.

Normal Physiologic Changes	Pathophysiologic Changes
Decreased pulmonary elasticity	Emphysema
Decreased alveolar surface, FEV	Chronic bronchitis
Increased V_d, RV, FRC	Pneumonia
Increased closing capacity	Lung cancer
V/Q mismatching	Tuberculosis
Decreased arterial oxygenation	
Increased chest wall rigidity	
Decreased cough	
Blunted response to hypercapnia/ hypoxia	
Progressive kyphosis/scoliosis	
Decreased total lung capacity	

Reduction in elastic recoil of the lung and chest wall, in addition to a decrease in pulmonary blood flow, leads to changes in ventilation:perfusion ratio. Dead space (V_d) increases and small airway collapse occurs during tidal volume ventilation, resulting in decreased gas exchange. This leads to an increase in the alveolar/arterial oxygen gradient and a decrease in arterial oxygen tension. Residual volume (RV) and functional residual capacity (FRC) increase as lung elasticity decreases with a concomitant decrease in forced expiratory volume (FEV). A "rule of thumb" for the normal deterioration of pulmonary function to predict expected change in arterial oxygenation while breathing room air is:

PaO_2 (expected) = 100 - age/4 **or** PaO_2 decreases 0.35 mm Hg per year

ANESTHESIA FOR GERIATRIC PATIENTS *(Continued)*

CENTRAL NERVOUS SYSTEM

With aging, there is a progressive decrease in cerebral cortical mass and an increase in brain sensitivity to anesthetic agents. The MAC of inhalational anesthetics decreases 40% to 60% by 80 years of age. This occurs not only with inhalational anesthetic gases, but also with intravenous, intrathecal, and epidural drugs. For example, the induction dose of sodium thiopental decreases from 5 mg/kg to 2 mg/kg in the 70 year old patient.

Figure 2: Refers to inhalation, intravenous, and spinal/epidural anesthetic doses

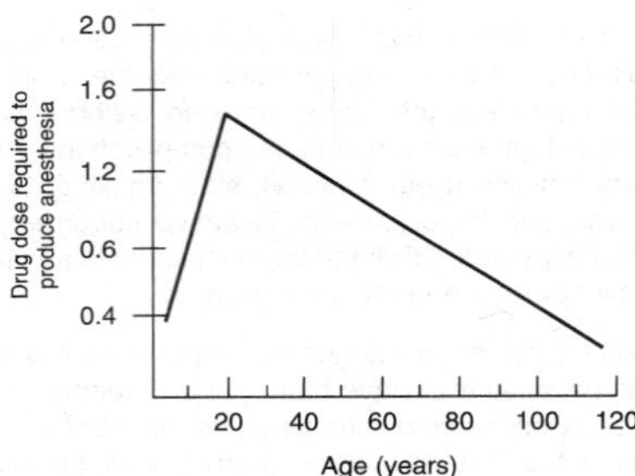

Therefore, it is easy to overdose elderly patients who do not have reserve capacity to overcome the profound side effects of "normal" anesthetic doses. The duration of anesthetics is also prolonged, slowing recovery and increasing postoperative confusion, often for days.

Normal Physiologic Changes	Pathophysiologic Changes
Decreased cerebral cortex	Stroke
Decreased cerebral blood flow (CBF)	Dementia
Decreased cerebral metabolic rate (CMR O_2)	Alzheimer's disease
Prolonged CNS recovery	Memory impairment
Postop confusion	

The blood pressure of patients with cerebrovascular disease should be maintained in the the patient's normal range during and after surgery. Head position should be maintained in the neutral position to prevent occlusion of the carotid or vertebral circulation. Patients with Parkinsonism should continue taking levodopa up to the time of surgery. Drugs with antidopaminergic effects are to be avoided (ie, phenothiazines, butyrophenones). Surgery for patients with recent stroke should be delayed at least 6 weeks to allow for restabilization of the blood-brain barrier and resumption of cerebral autoregulation.

ENDOCRINE SYSTEM

Normal Physiologic Changes	Pathophysiologic Changes
Decreased insulin secretion	Obesity
Increased insulin resistance	Type 2 diabetes mellitus
Decreased thyroid function	Poor wound healing
	Decreased leukocyte function

Adult onset diabetes is a common geriatric disease. It affects approximately 35 million people in the United States and is predicted to increase 200% over the next several decades. The severity of the disease and success of glucose management predict end-organ damage. Historically, tight glucose control, the medical management goal for diabetes, could be relaxed in the perioperative period. However, recently there is evidence that tight glucose control in the perioperative and ICU periods improves outcome. These studies show a striking increase in cardiovascular risk with a mild increase in blood glucose concentration. Whether tight glucose control to <110 mg/dL is also important for outpatient surgical patients is not known. It is well known that hyperglycemia decreases wound healing and increases infection; hyperglycemia will also increase the amount of cerebral injury should ischemia occur. However, hypoglycemia can cause cerebral and myocardial ischemia.

For the insulin-controlled diabetic, there is no ideal management protocol. Therapy ranges from withholding all insulin preoperatively vs administering a fraction of the usual dose vs initiation of a continuous dextrose/insulin infusion. Surgery is stressful and blood glucose increases. Without insulin an osmotic glucose diuresis can occur, producing dehydration. Some clinicians feel that the administration of exogenous insulin improves patient outcome by providing the body with a source of energy during this time of stress. The critical aspect of any management regimen is the frequent evaluation of blood glucose levels and appropriate treatment of hyper- or hypoglycemia.

UROLOGIC SYSTEM

Aging decreases renal function as reflected by a reduction in glomerular filtration rate and creatinine clearance. An increase in serum creatinine may not be evident on laboratory tests because total body muscle mass and creatinine production decrease with aging. However, BUN increases on an average of 0.2 mg/dL/year. Decreased ability to concentrate/dilute urine puts the geriatric patient at risk for dehydration/fluid overload. The patient's capacity to metabolize and excrete drugs is also affected.

Normal Physiologic Changes	Pathophysiologic Changes
Decreased renal blood flow	Diabetic nephropathy
Decreased kidney mass	Hypertensive nephropathy
Decreased tubular function	Prostatic enlargement

Elderly males with benign prostatic hypertrophy may experience bladder distention with loss of detrusor muscle tone leading to urinary retention. This can occur with general anesthesia, but is more common with spinal/epidural anesthesia. Neuraxial anesthesia decreases detrusor tone while increasing sphincter tone. Because neuraxial anesthesia produces a sympathectomy and a decrease in blood pressure, fluid administration to maintain normal blood pressure frequently complicates the situation by overdistending the urinary bladder.

Renal blood flow decreases with aging, with a 50% reduction by age 75. This places the geriatric patient at greater risk for perioperative renal damage/failure. Hypotension during anesthesia can further decrease renal perfusion, which can lead to additional renal damage. Maintenance of 0.5 mL/kg/hour urine output is recommended. A decrease in renal blood flow reduces clearance of many drugs, which can prolong drug action and may necessitate a reduction in drug dosage and/or frequency of administration.

GASTROINTESTINAL SYSTEM

Hepatic blood flow decreases with age, as does hepatic protein synthesis and drug metabolism. Gastric emptying also slows, decreasing absorption of orally administered drugs. Many drugs are highly protein bound, therefore a decrease in albumin significantly increases the amount of free drug. Because many drugs are metabolized by the liver, clearance can be decreased. See Pharmacokinetic/ Pharmacodynamic section.

ANESTHESIA FOR GERIATRIC PATIENTS *(Continued)*

MUSCULOSKELETAL SYSTEM

Normal Physiologic Changes	Pathophysiologic Changes
Decreased muscle mass	Weakness
Decreased joint mobility	Arthritis
Decreased dentition	Airway management problems
Increase osteoporosis	Bone fractures

Changes in the musculoskeletal system pose significant problems in positioning elderly patients. Alterations in skin elasticity and perfusion put patients at risk for ischemic ulcers at pressure points. Restricted joint mobility compounds this problem.

Many geriatric patients are edentulous, which facilitates intubation; however, many others have poor dentition or only a few teeth left, which are critical in supporting their dental bridges. Poor dentition increases the risk of dental trauma. Loss of mandibular bone contour can complicate adequate mask fit, making positive pressure ventilation difficult. Cervical arthritis and temporomandibular problems are not uncommon, as are gastroesophageal reflux and hiatal hernia, which put the patient at risk for inadequate ventilation or aspiration.

Osteoporosis reduces bone density and produces skeletal fragility, especially in postmenopausal women (40% in white females). Hormone replacement therapy in addition to calcium, vitamin D, and exercise, lowers the likelihood of osteoporotic fractures by at least 25%. Estrogen blocks bone resorption by inhibiting cytokine signals necessary for recruitment of bone-resorbing osteoclasts, but has been associated with increased cardiovascular adverse events. Drug therapy (ie, alendronate) also interferes with bone resorption.

The initial dose of muscle relaxant drugs is unchanged, but elderly patients require a decrease in frequency of redosing (due to prolonged elimination). The exceptions to this general rule are drugs that are metabolized in the blood by Hoffman elimination or nonspecific esterases (atracurium, mivacurium, and cisatracurium).

HYPOTHERMIA

Geriatric patients experience more intraoperative hypothermia than younger patients do. The consequences of this include prolonged awakening, slower drug elimination, increased shivering, enhanced coagulation, and increased postoperative metabolic demand associated with increased catabolism. Oxygen demand is increased, and if pulmonary and cardiovascular systems are unable to handle this increased workload, the potential for myocardial ischemia increases. Myocardial oxygen consumption can increase up to 500% with postoperative shivering. Maintenance of intraoperative temperature has been associated with significantly improved wound healing and outcome.

PHARMACOKINETICS / PHARMACODYNAMICS

Gastrointestinal absorption of orally administered drugs is affected by aging. There are changes in gastric acidity, intestinal motility, and intestinal perfusion.

Figure 3: Example of increased half-life of diazepam

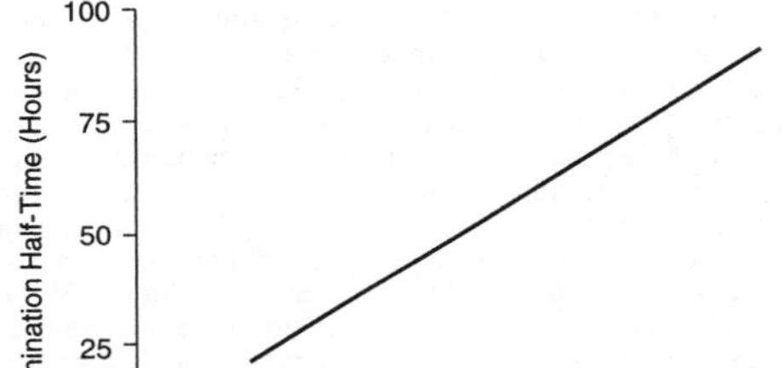

Once a drug is absorbed, its pharmacologic action is altered by decreased total body water and increased body fat concentration. Redistribution of drugs from the vessel-rich group is slowed, especially for highly lipid soluble drugs. Decreased hepatic perfusion and drug metabolism by liver microsomal enzymes combined with a reduced renal excretion of drug and/or metabolites can lead to an increased and prolonged drug effect. A decreased number of receptors leads to receptor saturation at substantially lower serum concentration. A decrease in both the amount of plasma protein and the quality of drug-protein binding leads to an increase in free fraction of the drug.

Drug Dosing Adjustments in the Elderly

Drug	Action	Mechanism
Inhalational anesthetics	Decrease dose 40%	↑ sensitivity
I.V. induction drugs[1]	Decrease dose 50%	↑ sensitivity, ↓ clearance/half-life
Antibiotics		
Initial dose	No change	
Repeat doses	Decrease frequency	↓ clearance, ↑ half-life
Muscle relaxants[2]		
Initial bolus	No change	
Repeat bolus	Decrease frequency	↓ clearance, ↑ half-life
Infusion	Decrease dose	↓ clearance, ↑ half-life
Narcotics[3]		
Initial bolus	Decrease dose 50%	↑ sensitivity
Infusion	Decrease dose 30%	↓ clearance, ↑ half-life

[1]Sodium thiopental, propofol, midazolam, etomidate, methohexital.

[2]This does not include muscle relaxants that are metabolized by Hoffman elimination.

[3]This does not include remifentanil.

ANESTHESIA FOR GERIATRIC PATIENTS *(Continued)*

TYPE OF ANESTHESIA: GENERAL vs REGIONAL

The debate between regional vs general anesthesia continues to be a topic for discussion, for no single anesthetic technique has been shown to be better for either the young or the geriatric patient. The type of anesthesia depends on the patient, concurrent medical diseases, underlying physiology, type of surgery, and the patient's expectations/wishes. There are several surgeries where the above statement is debated: transurethral resection of the prostate (TURP), cataract extraction, and knee surgery. Traditionally, TURP surgery is performed with regional anesthesia so that mental status changes associated with TURP syndrome can be elicited early. Cataract surgery is minimally invasive, with local ophthalmic analgesia providing adequate anesthesia for the procedure and thereby avoiding the physiologic transgressions associated with general anesthesia. Patients with hip and knee surgery performed with regional anesthesia experience an initial 50% reduction in the incidence of deep vein thrombosis and pulmonary embolus; however, the 3- to 6-month outcomes were similar. These studies were performed before the intra-/postoperative use of lower extremity compression sleeves and low molecular weight heparin. A modern day comparison has not been made.

Postoperative mental changes attributed to general anesthesia are not uncommon in the elderly; however, the use of heavy sedation during regional or local anesthesia can also produce a similar prolonged alteration of mental status. The incidence of postoperative cognitive decline (POCD) increases with advanced age. Recent studies suggest that long tern postoperative morbidity and mortality is associated with (1) extent of comorbidities, (2) duration of intraoperative hypotension, and (3) duration of deep general anesthesia. Drug metabolism and elimination are slowed, producing prolonged sedative effects. It has been proposed that outpatient surgery may disrupt daily habits less and the elderly may actually return to normal faster when in a familiar environment.

EDUCATION FOR GERIATRIC ANESTHESIA

The Anesthesiology Residency Review Committee has mandated that each program provide didactic instruction and clinical experience in managing the geriatric surgical population. The Society for the Advancement of Geriatric Anesthesia (SAGA) was established in 2000 to improve the care of the older person having surgery. There is a joint project between the ASA committee on Geriatric Anesthesia, SAGA, and the American Geriatrics Society (AGS) to develop a curriculum for geriatric anesthesia education. These educational materials can be accessed via the internet.

SUMMARY

The aging process is a progressive alteration of normal physiology over time. This deterioration can significantly alter the patient's response to anesthetics and perioperative medications. Frequently, coexistent with this progressive depression of organ function are superimposed disease processes, which further impair organ function. Geriatric patients present a significant challenge to the physician.

REFERENCES AND RECOMMENDED READING

Apfelbaum JL, Kallar SK, and Wetchler BV, "Adult and Geriatric Patients," *Anesthesia for Ambulatory Surgery*, 2nd ed, Chapter 5, Wetchler BV, ed, JB Lippincott Co, 1995, 272-307.

Bode RH Jr, Lewis KP, Zarich SW, et al, "Cardiac Outcome After Peripheral Vascular Surgery. Comparison of General and Regional Anesthesia," *Anesthesiology*, 1996, 84(1):3-13.

Campbell DN, Lim M, Muir MK, et al, "A Prospective Randomised Study of Local Versus General Anesthesia for Cataract Surgery," *Anaesthesia*, 1993, 48(5):422-8.

Dodds C and Allison J, "Postoperative Cognitive Deficit in the Elderly Surgical Patient," *Br J Anesth*, 1998, 81(3):449-62.

Gottlieb SS, McCarter RJ, and Vogel RA, "Effect of Beta-Blockade on Mortality Among High-Risk and Low-Risk Patients After Myocardial Infarction," *N Engl J Med*, 1998, 339(8):489-97.

Gu W, Pagel PS, Warltier DC, et al, "Modifying Cardiovascular Risk in Diabetes Mellitus," *Anesthesiology*, 2003, 98(3):774-9.

Kurz A, Sessler DI, and Lenhardt R, "Perioperative Normothermia to Reduce the Incidence of Surgical-Wound Infection and Shorten Hospitalization," *N Engl J Med*, 1996, 334(19):1209-15.

Monk TG, Saini V, Weldon BC, et al, "Anesthetic Management and One-Year Mortality After Noncardiac Surgery," *Anesth Analg*, 2005, 100(1):4-10.

Modig J, Borg T, Karlstrom G, et al, "Thromboembolism After Total Hip Replacement: Role of Epidural and General Anesthesia," *Anesth Analg*, 1983, 62(2):174-80.

Priebe HJ, "The Aged Cardiovascular Risk Patient," *Br J Anaesth*, 2000, 85(5):763-78.

Tuman KJ, McCarthy RJ, March RJ, et al, "Effects of Epidural Anesthesia and Analgesia on Coagulation and Outcome After Major Vascular Surgery," *Anesth Analg*, 1991, 73(6):696-704.

Wallace A, Layug B, Tateo I, et al, "Prophylactic Atenolol Reduces Postoperative Myocardial Ischemia. McSPI Research Group," *Anesthesiology*, 1998, 88(1):7-17

ANESTHESIA FOR OBSTETRIC PATIENTS IN NONOBSTETRIC SURGERY

Every year 0.75% to 2% of pregnant women undergo a nonobstetric surgical procedure. The major indications for these approximately 75,000 anesthetics are trauma, ovarian cysts, appendicitis, breast tumors, and cervical incompetence. More serious procedures such as cardiopulmonary bypass and cerebral aneurysm clipping are not uncommon. Preoperative, intraoperative, and postoperative care of the pregnant patient is unique because the physician must be concerned about two patients (the mother and the fetus), each with its own special needs.

The physician must take into account the normal physiologic changes of pregnancy, and the possibility of pregnancy-related disease (eg, preeclampsia, HELLP, gestational hypertension, gestational diabetes). Two additional major concerns that must continually be attended to during nonobstetric surgery are the maintenance of uterine perfusion and the prevention of premature labor. In order to understand the importance of these factors, a brief review of the physiologic changes of pregnancy is required.

PHYSIOLOGY OF PREGNANCY

Cardiovascular

Intravascular volume and cardiac output begin to increase during the first trimester and become 30% to 40% above the nonpregnant state by 28 weeks gestational age. Despite this increase in intravascular volume, the mother and fetus are at risk for hypotension which is caused by the gravid uterus compressing the aorta and/or inferior vena cava. This significantly reduces venous return and is called the supine hypotension syndrome. It occurs starting at 20 weeks gestation. The reduction in venous return may or may not be evident as maternal hypotension and puts the fetus at substantial risk of inadequate uteroplacental perfusion even in the asymptomatic mother. The most effective therapy is uterine displacement (ie, lateral position or displace the uterus to the left manually or with a wedge under the right hip). Correct positioning of the pregnant woman is critically important in maintaining adequate uterine blood flow.

Pregnant women are anemic despite a 35% increase in red blood cell mass. This happens because plasma volume, and therefore total blood volume, increases by 50% to 55%, producing a condition called physiologic anemia of pregnancy. Leukocytosis is also present in pregnant women, making the diagnosis of infection more difficult.

Respiratory

During pregnancy, the female experiences a 20% decrease in functional residual capacity concurrent with a 60% increase in oxygen consumption. This places the pregnant female and her infant at risk for hypoxia. Minute ventilation normally increases 50%, with most of this due to an increase in tidal volume. Closing volume (the lung volume at which airways collapse) moves from functional residual capacity into tidal volume ventilation in 30% of parturients, futher increasing the risk of hypoxia. Mild hyperventilation reduces $PaCO_2$ by 10 mm Hg with a compensatory decrease in bicarbonate, maintaining a normal pH; therefore, mechanical ventilation with a $PaCO_2$ of 40 mm Hg will produce respiratory acidosis. Positive pressure ventilation can decrease uterine blood flow 25% by reducing venous return. Therefore adequacy of uterine perfusion needs to be evaluated in pregnant women who are mechanically ventilated by monitoring fetal heart tones (eg, looking for loss of beat-to-beat variability, decelerations, fetal bradycardia).

Capillary engorgement increases the possibility of bleeding with the use of oral and nasal airways. The probability of a difficult intubation increases 8-fold during pregnancy; therefore, a smaller size endotracheal tube (6 or 6.5) should be used. Nasal intubations and nasogastric tubes should be avoided if possible.

Gastrointestinal

Pregnant women are at risk for aspiration after the first trimester because of increased gastric volume. Gastric emptying is similar in pregnant and nonpregnant patients. It is delayed only during labor, largely because of administration of narcotics. Pregnant patients are at risk for aspiration because of elevation of the stomach and rotation on its axis to the right by the gravid uterus. This leads to incompetence of the lower esophageal sphincter. Up to 80% of pregnant patients experience heartburn.

Use of an oral nonparticulate antacid (ie, sodium citrate, 30 mL) is recommended immediately prior to induction of general anesthesia. Histamine-2 receptor blocker (ie, cimetidine 300 mg I.V., ranitidine 50 mg I.V.) should be given 60-90 minutes prior to induction of general anesthesia to decrease acid production. Metoclopramide (10 mg I.V.) is given to enhance gastric emptying. Intubation should be performed by rapid sequence with cricoid pressure to prevent regurgitation and aspiration.

Renal

Because pregnant females experience an increase in glomerular filtration rate (GFR), their blood urea nitrogen (BUN) and creatinine (Cr) levels are decreased. Therefore, a pregnant woman with high-normal values may have renal insufficiency.

Coagulation

Pregnant women are hypercoagulable with an increase in factors V, VII, VIII, IX, X, XII, and fibrinogen and a decrease in factor XI, XIII, and antithrombin III. Platelet turnover is also increased. They are at risk for deep vein thrombosis (DVT) and pulmonary embolism which accounts for 25% of maternal deaths in the United States annually.

Neurology

Pregnant women have an increased sensitivity to anesthetic agents and other sedative/hypnotic/analgesic drugs because of increased levels of endorphins. Minimum alveolar concentration (MAC) for inhalational anesthetics is decreased 40% and the dose of spinal/epidural drugs also needs to be decreased by a similar amount because of engorgement of epidural veins. It is also thought that the elevated level of circulating progesterone increases neuronal sensitivity (both central and peripheral) to anesthetic/analgesic drugs.

TERATOGENICITY

The incidence of both major and minor anatomic birth defects ranges as high as 7% to 10%. Drug exposure accounts for 2% to 3% and genetic abnormalities for 25% of birth defects, while the etiology for the rest remains unknown. The fetus is most vulnerable to teratogenic drug effects from day 15 to 90 of gestation, when organogenesis is occurring. Unfortunately, many women do not know that they are pregnant during this period.

Drugs are routinely tested in animal teratologic studies; however, there are many examples where extensive animal testing does not correlate with human results. For example, thalidomide was tested in both rats and mice and was not found to be teratogenic; however, the teratogenic effects in the human fetus are profound, especially since no signs of toxicity are present in the mother. Conversely, drugs that are teratogenic in certain animal models, such as steroid therapy, have not exhibited any significant effect on the human fetus. A general statement is that most drugs, at some dose, can be teratogenic in some animal model but few drugs have a proven, clinically significant, teratogenic potential. See FDA Pregnancy Categories *on page 17*.

ANESTHESIA FOR OBSTETRIC PATIENTS IN NONOBSTETRIC SURGERY *(Continued)*

Possible Teratogens

Alcohol: This teratogen produces fetal alcohol syndrome with an incidence of 2/1000 live births, which is probably an underestimate of the real number. There is a twofold increase in spontaneous abortion, which increases to 5% with heavy alcohol consumption. Gestational alcohol consumption is a leading cause of mental retardation, which exceeds that found with Down syndrome and cerebral palsy. Hyperactivity, speech, language, and hearing difficulties, microcephaly, and abnormal brain development are also common.

Anesthetics: Although there is great concern that anesthetic agents may injure the developing fetus, there is little solid evidence for this. Nitrous oxide inhibits methionine synthetase activity which is involved in thymidine production and subsequent DNA synthesis and cell division. However, recent human studies have shown no effect on fetal outcome. Despite these negative studies, it is still wise to postpone surgery or unnecessary drug therapy until after delivery if possible.

Anticonvulsants: The risk of birth defects increases to 7% in women taking antiepileptic drugs during pregnancy (vs 2% to 3% in controls). The incidence increases in mothers taking higher doses and/or multiple antiseizure drugs. The epoxide metabolites of these drugs appear to produce the fetal abnormalities. Discontinuation of antiseizure drugs may also be dangerous if the fetus is exposed to hypoxia due to maternal seizures.

Benzodiazepines: Retrospective studies from the 1970s showed an increased incidence of cleft lip and palate in infants of mothers who were using benzodiazepines during pregnancy. However, recent epidemiologic studies have been unable to demonstrate this association.

Caffeine: There is no convincing data that caffeine is teratogenic in humans.

Cocaine: Cocaine and heroin exposure of both the mother and the father is associated with fetal microcephaly and other neurologic abnormalities.

Hyperglycemia: Diabetic mothers have a 4% to 12% incidence of major congenital anomalies, which can be significantly reduced to 1.2% when blood glucose levels are tightly controlled during pregnancy.

Marijuana: The placenta acts as a barrier to fetal marijuana exposure. Several studies have demonstrated maternal blood levels of marijuana with nondetectable drug concentration in the cord blood. Cannabinoids are also nonteratogenic in animals.

Retinoids (tretinoin, isotretinoin, etretinate): These drugs are used to treat acne, gram-negative folliculitis, hidradenitis suppurativa, and psoriasis. Teratogenic effects include CNS, cardiac, thymus, craniofacial abnormalities, and spontaneous abortion. Birth control must be practiced when using this class of drugs.

Tobacco: Cigarette smoking during pregnancy is associated with growth retardation. Reports of anencephaly, congenital heart defects, and orofacial clefts have not been confirmed.

Warfarin: Because of its small molecular weight, warfarin easily crosses the placenta. Administration between the 6th and 9th weeks of pregnancy can produce the warfarin embryopathy syndrome which consists of nasal hypoplasia, stippling of uncalcified epiphysis, shortened fingers with nail hypoplasia, low birth weight, and mental retardation in 13% of exposed fetuses.

The two most important factors affecting fetal development are decreased uterine perfusion and hypoxia.

GESTATIONAL PHARMACOKINETICS AND PHARMACODYNAMICS

Drugs cross the placenta by simple diffusion. Lipid soluble drugs with low molecular weight (ie, fentanyl, thiopental, isoflurane) cross easily while highly polar water soluble drugs (ie, neuromuscular blocking agents) do not readily cross the placenta. Because fetal pH is lower than maternal pH, the ionized fraction of weak bases (ie, narcotics, local anesthetics) is higher in the fetus than in the mother. This is called "ion trapping." Ion trapping increases total fetal drug level, which will prolong clearance of the drug from the fetus. Ion trapping has been connected with lidocaine (a weak base) and fetal acidosis, leading to "floppy baby syndrome."

PRINCIPLES OF SURGICAL MANAGEMENT

1. **The most important thing is to notify your hospital obstetrician about the case before starting it.**
2. Postpone surgery until the second trimester or delay until after delivery, if possible.
3. Use a nonparticulate antacid preoperatively.
4. Maintain maternal oxygenation and blood pressure.
5. Document fetal heart tones before and after surgery.
6. Monitor for uterine contraction and fetal heart rate intraoperatively whenever possible.
7. Use left uterine displacement during the entire perioperative period.
8. Consider the use of prophylactic tocolytic agents (note that inhalational anesthetic gases are tocolytics)
9. Nonsteroidal anti-inflammatory drugs should not be used after 32 weeks gestational age because of the concern that the ductus may close.
10. Based on gestational age, the obstetrician may give betamethasone prior to surgery to promote fetal lung maturity in case of premature delivery.

The reason to monitor fetal heart tones and uterine contractions is to provide the physician with the opportunity to prevent fetal hypoxia and/or early delivery. Monitoring fetal heart rate will allow the physician to optimize the fetal environment by augmenting oxygen delivery if fetal bradycardia or loss of heart rate variability occurs. Because most anesthetic drugs depress fetal beat-to-beat variability, this monitor of fetal well-being cannot be relied upon until the drug is cleared from the fetus.

Taking care of the pregnant patient for nonobstetric surgery requires recognition of the physiologic changes that accompany pregnancy and the need to treat two patients – the mother and the baby.

Physiologic Changes of Pregnancy

Cardiovascular	Increased cardiac output 50% Increased red blood cell mass 35% Increased plasma volume 55% Physiologic anemia of pregnancy
Pulmonary	Decreased functional reserve capacity (FRC) 20% Increased oxygen consumption (VO_2) 60% Increased minute ventilation (MV) 50% Increased respiratory rate (RR) 10% Increased tidal volume (V_T) 40% Decreased $PaCO_2$ by 10 mm Hg
Gastrointestinal	Increased gastric volume Decreased gastric pH Incompetent lower esophageal sphincter
Renal	Increased glomerular filtration rate (GFR) Decreased blood urea nitrogen (BUN) Decreased creatinine (Cr)
Coagulation	Increased factors V, VII, VIII, X, XII Increased fibrinogen Decreased factor XI, XIII, and antithrombin III Increased platelet turnover
Neurology	Decreased anesthesia/analgesia drug requirements (35% to 40%) Increased circulating endorphins

ANESTHESIA FOR OBSTETRIC PATIENTS IN NONOBSTETRIC SURGERY *(Continued)*

REFERENCES AND RECOMMENDED READING

Brodsky JB, Cohen EN, Brown BW Jr, et al, "Surgery During Pregnancy and Fetal Outcome," *Am J Obstet Gynecol*, 1980, 138(8):1165-7.

Chestnut DH, *Obstetric Anesthesia: Principles and Practice*, 2nd ed, Chapter 16, Cohen SE, "Nonobstetric Surgery During Pregnancy," Mosby: Philadelphia, 1999, 279-302.

Cohen EN, Bellville JW, and Brown BS, "Anesthesia, Pregnancy and Miscarriage: A Study of Operating Room Nurses and Anesthetists," *Anesthesiology*, 1971, 35(4):343-7.

Dewan DM and Hoad DD, *Practical Obstetric Anesthesia*, Chapter 20, "Anesthesia for Non-Birth Related Surgery During Pregnancy," WB Saunders Company, Philadelphia: Pennsylvania, 1997, 309-20.

Duncan PG, Pope WD, Cohen MM, et al, "Fetal Risk of Anesthesia and Surgery During Pregnancy," *Anesthesiology*, 1986, 64(6):790-4.

Kaneko M, Saito Y, Kirihara Y, et al, "Pregnancy Enhances the Antinociceptive Effects of Extradural Lignocaine in the Rat," *Br J Anaesth*, 1994, 72(6):657-61.

Liu PL, Warren TM, Ostheimer GW, et al, "Foetal Monitoring in Parturients Undergoing Surgery Unrelated to Pregnancy," *Can Anaesth Soc J*, 1985, 32(5):525-32.

Mazze RI and Kallen B, "Reproductive Outcome After Anesthesia and Operation During Pregnancy: A Register Study of 5405 Cases," *Am J Obstet Gynecol*, 1989, 161(5):1178-85.

Medina VM, Dawson-Basoa ME, and Gintzler AR, "17 Beta-Estradiol and Progesterone Positively Modulate Spinal Cord Dynorphin: Relevance to the Analgesia of Pregnancy," *Neuroendocrinology*, 1993, 58(3):310-5.

Niebyl JR, ed, *Drug Use in Pregnancy*, Philadelphia, PA; Lea & Febiger, 1988.

Palahniuk FJ, Schnider SM, and Eger EI, "Pregnancy Decreases the Requirement for Inhaled Anesthetic Agents," *Anesthesiology*, 1974, 41:82-3.

Pedersen H and Finster M, "Anesthetic Risk in the Pregnant Surgical Patient," *Anesthesiology*, 1979, 51(5):439-51.

Rosenberg L, Mitchell AA, Parsells JL, et al, "Lack of Relation of Oral Clefts to Diazepam Use During Pregnancy," *N Engl J Med*, 1983, 309(21):1282-5.

Schnider SM and Webster GM, "Maternal and Fetal Hazards of Surgery During Pregnancy," *Am J Obstet Gynecol*, 1965, 92:891.

Selye H, "Anesthetic Effect of Steroid Hormones," *Proc Soc Exp Biol Med*, 1941, 46:116-21.

ANESTHESIA FOR PATIENTS WITH LIVER DISEASE

Patients with liver disease pose a significant problem to the perioperative physician. Although the prevalence of clinically significant unsuspected liver disease is 1%, abnormal liver function tests may occur in 33% of screened patients.

The liver is the largest gland in the body, receiving 25% of the cardiac output. While the hepatic artery supplies 25% of the blood flow (and 45% to 50% of the hepatic oxygen supply), the portal vein provides 75% of the blood flow (but only 50% of the oxygen delivery). This unique blood flow circuitry puts the liver at risk for ischemia since half of its oxygen supply is provided by venous blood. Oxygen delivery to this essential organ can be decreased by either an increase in oxygen extraction (reducing portal vein oxygen concentration) or a decrease in arterial blood pressure resulting in a decrease in hepatic artery blood flow.

FUNCTIONS OF THE LIVER

- Glucose homeostasis
  - Glycogen storage
  - Gluconeogenesis
- Fat metabolism (beta oxidation)
- Protein synthesis
  - Albumin, gamma globulin, alpha$_1$-glycoprotein
  - Drug binding
  - Coagulation factors
  - Hydrolysis of ester linkage
- Drug and hormone metabolism
- Bilirubin formation and excretion
- Phagocytize bacteria

PATHOPHYSIOLOGY OF LIVER INJURY

To simplify this presentation, liver disease is divided into two categories: 1) cholestatic disease and 2) parenchymal disease, including acute and chronic hepatitis and cirrhosis.

1. With cholestasis (obstructive jaundice), the liver is unable to secrete bile because of either hepatocellular dysfunction or extrahepatic obstruction. Bilirubin accumulation affects cellular respiration; heme biosynthesis; metabolism of lipids, amino acids, and proteins; and alteration of drug/albumin binding. Coagulation defects occur because of deficient production of vitamin K-dependent factors by the dysfunctional hepatocytes.

   Drugs/conditions that cause cholestasis:
   - Primary biliary cirrhosis
   - Estrogens
   - Methyltestosterone
   - Bile duct gallstones
   - Bile duct stricture
   - Pancreatic cancer obstructing bile duct

2. Hepatic parenchymal disease (ie, hepatitis, cirrhosis) is associated with a hyperdynamic cardiovascular state. Cardiac output increases due to arteriovenous fistulae which decrease systemic vascular resistance and lead to an increased intravascular volume. Blood pressure and heart rate remain normal but portal vein blood flow to the liver is decreased. Hypoxemia occurs because of intrapulmonary shunting (hepatopulmonary syndrome) and ascites can limit diaphragm excursion. The oxygen dissociation curve is shifted to the right and hypoxic pulmonary vasoconstriction is blunted. The patient is anemic due to increased plasma volume, GI bleeding, hemolysis, and malnutrition. Thrombocytopenia occurs from bone marrow depression and hypersplenism. The depressed synthetic function of the liver is manifested by decreased albumin production and prolonged PT and PTT due to

ANESTHESIA FOR PATIENTS WITH LIVER DISEASE *(Continued)*

decreased production of factors II, VII, IX, and X. The encephalopathy that appears with acute liver failure is probably due to cerebral edema, while chronic encephalopathy may be caused by decreased elimination of nitrogenous compounds (ie, ammonia). GI bleeding, infection, and excessive use of diuretics increases blood urea nitrogen (BUN). Ascites and peripheral edema are produced by hypoabluminemia and renal reabsorption of urinary sodium. As hepatic dysfunction progresses, hepatorenal syndrome may develop in patients with portal hypertension and ascites. This renal failure is produced by multiple reasons and can be cured by liver transplant.

SOME CAUSES OF HEPATIC INJURY

Viral	Infection
Drugs	NSAIDs
	ACE inhibitors
	Sulfonamides
Other	Reye's syndrome
	Wilson's disease
	Acute fatty liver of pregnancy
	Hemochromatosis
	Cystic fibrosis
	Alpha$_1$-antitrypsin deficiency
	Total parenteral nutrition

LIVER FUNCTION TESTS AND DIFFERENTIAL DIAGNOSIS

Diagnostic Factors	Cholestatic Intrahepatic	Cholestatic Extrahepatic	Parenchymal Hepatocellular
Symptom	Deep jaundice, dark urine, light stools, pruritus	Deep jaundice, dark urine, light stools, pruritus, biliary cholic, cholangitis	Nausea, vomit, fever, anorexia
Physical findings	Tender hepatomegaly	Hepatomegaly, palpable gallbladder	Tender hepatomegaly, ± splenomegaly
Bilirubin, total	>30 mg/dL	<30 mg/dL	↑ conjugated
Transaminases	2-5 fold ↑	>2-3 fold ↑	>5 fold ↑
Alkaline phosphatase	>3-5 fold ↑	<3-5 fold ↑	2-3 fold ↑
Prothrombin time	Prolonged	Prolonged	Prolonged
PT correct with vitamin K	Variable	Yes	No
Causes	Stones, sepsis	Hemolysis, hematoma reabsorption, bili overload from whole blood transfusion	Viral, drugs, sepsis, hypoxemia, cirrhosis

THE EFFECTS OF ANESTHESIA AND SURGERY ON LIVER FUNCTION

Liver injury can occur during surgery either from decreased hepatic oxygen delivery or direct drug toxicity. The most injurious conditions in the perioperative period are hypotension, hypoxemia, and hypovolemia, all which decrease hepatic oxygen delivery. Surgical stress carries a high mortality in patients with severe liver disease, with the greatest insult to the liver occurring with upper abdominal surgery.

Management of the patient with hepatic parenchymal injury requires maintenance of arterial blood pressure and cardiac output to assure adequate hepatic oxygen delivery. When blood flow decreases, the body extracts more oxygen to maintain adequate tissue oxygenation. In the normal person, when portal blood flow decreases, hepatic arterial blood flow increases, thereby ensuring adequate oxygen delivery. In the patient with severe hepatic dysfunction, this vascular autoregulation does not occur, leading to reduced hepatic oxygenation.

CLASSIFICATION OF SURGICAL RISK

	Minimal	**Mild**	**Severe**
Bilirubin (mg/dL)	<2	2-3	>3
Albumin (g/dL)	>3.5	3-3.5	<3
Prothrombin time (sec prolonged)	1-4	4-6	>6
Encephalopathy	None	Moderate	Severe
Nutrition	Excellent	Good	Poor
Ascites	None	Moderate	Marked

Anesthetic concerns with regional anesthesia include coagulopathy and hypotension. "Halothane hepatitis" is a concern with repeat halothane exposure, with several case reports implicating other inhalational anesthetics. Halothane hepatitis is an immune-mediated response which requires previous exposure and antibody formation against an oxidative trifluoroacetyl halide metabolite of halothane. Genetic susceptibility is probable and it can be fatal.

PHARMACOKINETICS

There are significant changes in the pharmacokinetic profiles of many drugs in the patient with liver disease because the liver is important in metabolism and elimination of drugs. Multiple hepatic enzymes are responsible for drug metabolism, with the cytochrome P450 family of enzymes important in mixed function oxidative reactions.

Albumin is produced solely by the liver, therefore, a decrease in albumin concentration can indicate significant liver disease or malnutrition. Prothrombin time is considered a more sensitive indicator of liver disease than albumin because severe liver disease can affect hepatic synthetic function sufficiently to prolong prothrombin time within 24 hours.

Hepatic drug metabolism and elimination can be classified based on alterations in hepatic blood flow, volume of distribution, and protein binding.

Hepatic blood flow patterns change with hepatic injury. As the liver architecture changes with the development of cirrhosis, portal venous blood is shunted from the liver by collateral channels into the systemic circulation. This blood, along with orally administered drugs absorbed from the GI tract, avoids the hepatic first-pass effect preventing the initial drug metabolism and increasing the amount of drug presented to the central circulation. Blood that passes through the liver has decreased exposure to hepatocyte enzymes because of increased fibrosis and a decrease in number and size of loose endothelial junctions, which limits blood exposure to hepatocytes for drug metabolism. If clearance is high, then changes in hepatic blood flow will significantly alter drug elimination (flow limited drugs). Conversely, clearance is not affected by a decrease in hepatic blood flow for enzyme-limited drugs. The clearance of enzyme-limited drugs may either be protein-binding sensitive (>85% bound) or protein-binding insensitive (<50% bound).

ANESTHESIA FOR PATIENTS WITH LIVER DISEASE *(Continued)*

Volume of distribution (V_d) is altered by the development of ascites (which increases the body's total fluid component) and altered hepatic production of plasma proteins. As the volume of distribution increases, drug concentration at steady state decreases. For example, V_d of propranolol and verapamil is doubled in patients with ascites. This condition may lead to an increase in drug half-life and a decrease in drug clearance.

Protein binding is altered with cirrhosis because of a decrease in serum albumin and an accumulation of substances that displace drugs from albumin-binding sites. In this circumstance, the availability of unbound drug increases, leading to greater drug effect. For example, phenytoin is 90% albumin bound. With hypoalbuminemia, the free fraction increases 20% to 30%, which can double or triple unbound active phenytoin, producing drug toxicity; however, this effect may be countered if there is an increase in volume of distribution (V_d) due to ascites. An increase in free unbound drug may also increase clearance, because more drug is available to be metabolized, which can shorten its half-life. The effect of altered protein binding on drug pharmacokinetics is difficult to predict. A simple rule of thumb is that a change in protein binding has a greater effect on drugs that are normally highly protein bound (>60%) compared to poorly bound drugs.

Drug Characteristics in Normal Subjects and Liver Failure Patients

Drug	Protein Binding (%)	Volume of Distribution (V_d) (L/kg)	Half-life (h)	Clearance (Cl) (mL/min)	Effect of Liver Disease on Drug Disposition	Adjustment of Dose
Antibiotics / Antiviral / Antifungal						
Ampicillin	30	0.28	1.0	340	Half-life ↑; V_d ↑; Cl →	None
Cefazolin	84	0.15	1.8	68	Half-life ↓; f_p ↑	None
Cefotetan	83	0.15	3.7	39.5	Negligible unless renal function decreased	None
Cefoxitin	73	0.12	1.0	98	Negligible unless renal function decreased	None
Clindamycin	79	0.58	2.0	160	Half-life slight ↑; V_d →; Cl ↓ 23%; f_p →	Decrease dose in severe cases
Erythromycin	80	0.77	1.6	600	Half-life ↑	Decrease dose in moderate or severe disease
Gentamicin	<5	0.25	2.0	100	Negligible unless renal function decreased	None
Nafcillin	90	0.4	1.0	580	Half-life ↑ but little change; V_d ↓; Cl ↓ 50% to 60%; f_p ?→	Decrease dose in moderate or severe disease
Vancomycin	55	0.4	5.0	80	Half-life ↑; V_d →; Cl ↓	Decrease dose
Analgesic						
Alfentanil	90	0.28	1.5	200	Half-life ↑; V_d →; Cl ↓; f_p ↑ (dose-dependent)	Decrease dose
Fentanyl	80	3.5	4.0	750	Half-life →; V_d →; Cl →	None
Meperidine	65	4.5	4.5	900	Half-life ↑; V_d →; Cl ↓ 50%; f_p →	Decrease oral dose by 50% in cirrhosis or acute viral hepatitis
Methadone	80	4.0	28	150	Half-life ↑ with severe liver disease; Cl →	None or decrease
Morphine	35	3.7	2.0	1200	Half-life →; V_d →; Cl →; f_p →, by some reports f_p ↑	None, but avoid in severe liver disease

ANESTHESIA FOR PATIENTS WITH LIVER DISEASE
(Continued)

Drug Characteristics in Normal Subjects and Liver Failure Patients *(continued)*

Drug	Protein Binding (%)	Volume of Distribution (V_d) (L/kg)	Half-life (h)	Clearance (Cl) (mL/min)	Effect of Liver Disease on Drug Disposition	Adjustment of Dose
Antiepileptic						
Phenytoin	92	0.65	15.0 nonlinear	40	AVH half-life →; Cl →; f_p ↑. Cirrhosis f_p ↑	Decrease dose in moderate to severe liver disease
Phenobarbital	50	0.8	100	8	Half-life ↑; presumed Cl ↓	Decrease with severe liver disease
Antipyretic / Anti-inflammatory						
Dexamethasone	68	0.75	3.25	260	f_p →; V_d →; half-life ↑; Cl ↓	Decrease dose
Ibuprofen	>99	0.15 V area F	2.0	52	Half-life slightly ↑ in severe LD; V_d ?; Cl ?	Decrease in severe liver disease if high doses
Cardiovascular						
Atenolol	<5	0.55	6.5	55-130	Half-life →; V_d →; Cl →	None
Digoxin	30	6.0	35	150	Appears negligible	None
Esmolol	55	1.2	0.15	310/kg	Negligible	None
Labetalol	50	11.5	3.0	1600	Half-life →; V_d ↓; Cl → or ↓; f_p ?, assume ↑	Decrease oral dose; decrease I.V. dose to much smaller extent
Lidocaine	65 nonlinear	1.1	2.0	1000	Half-life ↑; V_d ↑ or →; Cl ↓ ~50%; f_p ? Low therapeutic ratio; decrease in Cl depends on severity of disease	Decrease dose by 50% in severe liver disease
Metoprolol	10	3.2	4.0	800	Half-life ↑; V_d ↑ slightly; Cl ↓ 23%; f_p ?	Decrease dose slightly
Propranolol	95	4.0	4.0	850	Half-life ↑; V_d ↑; Cl ↓ ~60%; f_p ↑. Tremendous decrease in Cl_{int}. Flow/enzyme-limited in cirrhosis	Decrease dose depending on extent of damage
Verapamil	92	6.7	3.5	1570	Half-life ↑; V_d ↑; Cl ↓ 60%; f_p →. Cl_{int} decreases even more than 60%.	Decrease dose by 50% in severe liver disease

Drug Characteristics in Normal Subjects and Liver Failure Patients *(continued)*

Drug	Protein Binding (%)	Volume of Distribution (V_d) (L/kg)	Half-life (h)	Clearance (Cl) (mL/min)	Effect of Liver Disease on Drug Disposition	Adjustment of Dose
Diuretic						
Furosemide	95	0.15	1.0	170	Half-life ↑ or →; V_d ↑ or →; Cl →; f_p ↑; the change in f_p compensates for decrease in Cl_{int} of liver	None or slight decrease in severe cases
Sedative / Hypnotic						
Diazepam	99	1.2	45	28	Half-life ↑; V_d ↑; Cl ↓ 50%; f_p ↑. AVH and cirrhosis increase half-life. Large therapeutic index — safe	Single dose, no change; chronic, decrease dose
Flumazenil	40	0.85	0.8	1201	Half-life, Cl, V_d	? Decrease dose
Lorazepam	90	1.3	12.0	53	Half-life ↑; V_d ↑; Cl→; f_p ↑. Neither AVH nor cirrhosis affects drug dosing	None
Methohexital	—	61	2.0	829	No data; assume Cl ↓, half-life↑	Probably decrease dose
Thiopental	85	2.3	9.0	275	Half-life →; V_d →; Cl →; f_p ↑	Uncertain; may need to decrease dose
Midazolam	—	1.3	1.6	624	Half-life ↑; V_d slightly ↑; Cl ↓	Decrease dose

ANESTHESIA FOR PATIENTS WITH LIVER DISEASE
(Continued)

Drug Characteristics in Normal Subjects and Liver Failure Patients *(continued)*

Drug	Protein Binding (%)	Volume of Distribution (V_d) (L/kg)	Half-life (h)	Clearance (Cl) (mL/min)	Effect of Liver Disease on Drug Disposition	Adjustment of Dose
Others						
Atracurium	—	0.16	0.33	385	Half-life →; V_d ↑; Cl →; long half-life of metabolite	Decrease dose if long-term use
Cimetidine	20	1.1	2.3	550	Half-life →; V_d ↑ or ↓ or →; Cl → or ↓; f_p changes assumed unimportant. Drug associated with increased incidence of mental confusion in cirrhotics.	Decrease dose to severe liver disease
Ranitidine	15	1.5	2.3	600	Half-life →; V_d →; Cl →	None
Theophylline	52	0.5	8.0	45	Half-life ↑; V_d → cirrhosis, ↑ hepatitis and cholestasis; Cl ↓ 55%; f_p ↑. Low therapeutic index caution.	Decrease dose by 50%

AVH = acute viral hepatitis; LD = liver disease; fp = fraction of unbound drug; Cl_{int} = intrinsic clearance.

REFERENCES AND RECOMMENDED READING

Barash PG, Cullen BF, and Stoelting RK, "Anesthesia and the Liver," *Handbook of Clinical Anesthesia*, Philadelphia, PA: JB Lippincott, 1991, 314-24.

Jalan R and Hayes PC, "Hepatic Encephalopathy and Ascites," *Lancet*, 1997, 350(9087):1309-15.

Gelman S, Dillard E, and Bradley EL Jr, "Hepatic Circulation During Surgical Stress and Anesthesia With Halothane, Isoflurane, or Fentanyl," *Anesth Anal*, 1987, 66(10):936-43.

Gelman S and Ernst E, "Role of pH, PCO_2, and O_2 Content of Portal Blood in Hepatic Autoregulation," *Am J Physiol*, 1977, 233(4):E255.

Gelman S, "General Anesthesia and Hepatic Circulation," *Can J Physiol Pharmacol*, 1987, 65(8):1762-79.

Kamath PS, "Clinical Approach to the Patient With Abnormal Liver Test Results," *Mayo Clin Proc*, 1996, 71(11):1089-94.

Krowka MJ, Porayko MK, Plevak DJ, et al, "Hepatopulmonary Syndrome With Progressive Hypoxemia as an Indication for Liver Transplantation: Case Reports and Literature Review," *Mayo Clin Proc*, 1997, 72(1):44-53.

Kubisty CA, Arns RA, Wedlund PJ, et al, "Adjustment of Medication in Liver Failure," *The Pharmacologic Approach to the Critically Ill Patient*, Chernow B, ed, 3rd ed, Baltimore, MD: Williams & Wilkins, 1994, 95-113.

Merritt WT and Gelman S, "Anesthesia for Liver Surgery," *Principles and Practice of Anesthesiology*, Rogers MC, Tinker JH, and Covino BG, eds, Longnecker, DE: Mosby, 1992, 1991-2034.

Neal E, Meffin P, Gregory P, et al, "Enhanced Bioavailability and Decreased Clearance of Analgesics in Patients With Cirrhosis," *Gastroenterology*, 1979, 77(1):96-102.

Powell-Jackson P, Greenway B, and Williams R, "Adverse Effects of Exploratory Laparotomy in Patients With Suspected Liver Disease," *Br J Surg*, 1982, 69(8):449-51.

CHRONIC PAIN MANAGEMENT

Chronic pain is a common problem that is considered one of the least effectively treated disease states in society today. Chronic pain is defined as pain that persists beyond the usual course of an acute disease or after a reasonable time for healing to occur (eg, at least 3-6 months). Unlike acute pain, the origin of chronic pain cannot always be delineated. Chronic pain can be neuropathic, nociceptive, or mixed nociceptive and neuropathic in nature. Chronic pain is a condition that can cause patients to have functional loss, psychological problems, and may interfere not only with their livelihood, but also with some normal activities of daily living.

Chronic pain is most successfully treated by a multidisciplinary, multimodality method. The involvement of the anesthesiologist, as the pain specialist, in the management of chronic pain is becoming increasingly evident, therefore, it is important for the anesthesiologist to have a solid background in physiology and pharmacology. Specifically, knowledge of the type, dosage, and side effects of the pharmacologic agents recommended for the treatment of chronic pain is necessary.

When treating chronic pain, many analgesic medications are used. These agents include nonsteroidal anti-inflammatory drugs (NSAIDs), antidepressants, anticonvulsants, corticosteroids, local anesthetics, and others. All of the agents, except the NSAIDs, are considered to be adjuvant agents and are frequently grouped together under that term. These agents are preferable over opioids when chronic pain is not of malignant origin. The initial choice of agent depends upon the severity and the pathophysiology and etiology of the pain (nociceptive, neuropathic, psychogenic). When treating neuropathic pain, it usually takes weeks before beneficial effects from these agents are seen.

Opioids are used in the treatment of chronic pain when the pain is malignant or when other conservative or procedure-type approaches have failed and the pain is causing the patients' quality of life to be poor. Using equianalgesic conversions as a guide, followed by careful titration and monitoring, opioids can effectively manage many types of chronic pain without intolerable adverse effects.

This section reviews the agents, doses, and dosing regimens of the adjuvant agents and the common opioids used for the treatment of chronic pain.

NONSTEROIDAL ANTI-INFLAMMATORY AGENTS

The nonsteroidal anti-inflammatory drugs (NSAIDs) are considered first-line agents for mild to moderate pain. NSAIDs have anti-inflammatory, analgesic, and antipyretic properties. Their analgesic effects are produced by central and peripheral mechanisms. NSAIDs work by inhibiting cyclooxygenase activity peripherally and preventing the formation of prostaglandins. When administered with an opioid for treating moderate to severe pain, NSAIDs are opioid-sparing. NSAIDs, however, are not effective for managing neuropathic pain. Individual patient characteristics may favor the selection of one NSAID over another. Careful patient screening for age, cardiovascular disease, renal dysfunction, gastritis, gastric ulcers, or bleeding disorders due to platelet dysfunction and use of the lowest effective dose for the least amount of time is important for minimizing the risk of serious cardiovascular thrombotic events and/or gastrointestinal adverse events. NSAIDs are contraindicated in patients who have experienced asthma, urticaria, or allergic-type reactions after taking aspirin or other NSAIDs.

Refer to the table Nonsteroidal Anti-Inflammatory Agents *on page 1575* in Comparative Drug Charts section.

ANTIDEPRESSANTS

Antidepressant agents have been used to treat chronic pain for many years. These agents have an analgesic effect that occurs at a dose lower than the dose needed for their antidepressant effect. It is theorized that antidepressants may work in the treatment of pain by altering a biochemical mechanism (through inhibition of norepinephrine and/or serotonin reuptake) that may be related to both depression and pain or by enhancing or modulating endogenous opioid analgesia.

Several antidepressants are used for chronic pain management. These agents are considered first- or second-line therapy for neuropathic pain. Although tricyclic antidepressants (TCAs) effectively treat neuropathic pain, their adverse effect profile is problematic. Anticholinergic effects (dry mouth, constipation, blurred vision, sedation, dizziness, urinary retention) can occur, particularly when the tertiary amine amitriptyline is used. Secondary amines such as nortriptyline and desipramine cause less sedation and anticholinergic effects than amitriptyline, making them a better choice for older or debilitated patients. Cardiovascular effects of TCAs include orthostatic hypotension, conduction defects, and arrhythmias due to their quinidine-like effect. Cardiovascular effects may be most concerning when amitriptyline is used. Selective serotonin reuptake inhibitors (SSRIs) are better tolerated than TCAs but have not consistently been shown to effectively manage neuropathic pain symptoms in nondepressed patients.

Duloxetine, an antidepressant that acts by highly specific inhibition of serotonin and norepinephrine reuptake, has been shown to effectively manage painful diabetic neuropathy. Somnolence and constipation are its most common adverse effects.

Venlafaxine, a bicyclic antidepressant, inhibits the reuptake of serotonin at low doses and norepinephrine at moderate doses. Adverse effects are similar to that of SSRIs. Venlafaxine may be considered for neuropathic pain that does not respond to TCAs, duloxetine, or anticonvulsants. All of the antidepressants require anywhere from one (eg, duloxetine) to three weeks (eg, TCAs) for an adequate trial for managing neuropathic pain.

Antidepressants

Drug	Starting Dose (mg/day)	Dose Range (mg/day)	Adverse Effects
Amitriptyline (TCA)	10-25	75-150	Dry mouth, constipation, blurred vision, sedation, weight gain, sexual dysfunction, orthostatic hypotension, cardiac conduction abnormalities[1]
Citalopram (SSRI)	10	20-60	Nausea, insomnia, anxiety, tremor
Desipramine (TCA)	25-50	75-200	Dry mouth, constipation, blurred vision, sedation, weight gain, sexual dysfunction, orthostatic hypotension, cardiac conduction abnormalities[1]
Duloxetine (SNRI)	60	60-120	Somnolence, constipation, nausea, dry mouth, dizziness, sweating, anorexia
Fluoxetine (SSRI)	10	10-20	Insomnia, anxiety, restlessness, nervousness, gastrointestinal symptoms, sexual dysfunction
Nortriptyline (TCA)	10-25	75-150	Dry mouth, constipation, blurred vision, sedation, weight gain, sexual dysfunction, orthostatic hypotension, cardiac conduction abnormalities[1]

(Continued)

CHRONIC PAIN MANAGEMENT *(Continued)*

Antidepressants *(continued)*

Drug	Starting Dose (mg/day)	Dose Range (mg/day)	Adverse Effects
Venlafaxine (SNRI)	37.5	150-375	Nausea, dizziness, insomnia, sedation, dry mouth, sweating, impotence

[1]Amitriptyline, a tertiary amine, is more likely to cause these adverse effects than desipramine or nortriptyline (secondary amines).

Key: TCA = tricyclic antidepressant; SSRI = selective serotonin reuptake inhibitor; SNRI = serotonin and norepinephrine reuptake inhibitor

ANTICONVULSANTS

Anticonvulsant agents are another class of drugs that have been used as adjuvants for chronic pain management. These agents may be used as first-line therapy for neuropathic pain, exerting their analgesic effects by blocking sodium or calcium channels to prevent sensory nerve firing. Newer agents (gabapentin, pregabalin) are less toxic than the older agents (carbamazepine, phenytoin, and valproic acid) and are preferred. When anticonvulsants are used as analgesic agents, their efficacy does not correlate with therapeutic serum concentrations. Lamotrigine also has antidepressant properties. Strict dose titration of lamotrigine is necessary to minimize the risk of serious adverse effects such as Stevens-Johnson Syndrome and toxic epidermal necrosis. Discontinue lamotrigine with the first sign of a rash. Although not a first-line agent, clonazepam has been effectively used for trigeminal neuralgia, post-traumatic neuralgia, paroxysmal postlaminectomy pain, and lancinating phantom limb pain. Like other benzodiazepines, drowsiness is common and withdrawal symptoms may occur following abrupt discontinuation.

Anticonvulsants

Drug	Starting Dose (mg/day)	Dose Range (mg/day)
Carbamazepine	200	1000-1600
Clonazepam	0.5	5-20
Gabapentin	900	1800-3600
Lamotrigine	50	200-600
Phenytoin	100	300-500
Pregabalin	150	150-300
Tiagabine	4	12-60
Topiramide	25	100-400

OTHER ADJUVANTS

The systemic delivery of sodium channel blockers such as lidocaine and mexiletine has been shown to have analgesic efficacy in a variety of neuropathic pain conditions and lowers intraoperative anesthetic requirements. Mexiletine, an oral local anesthetic, produces analgesia by suppressing abnormal electrical activity or hypersensitivity in damaged neurons. It has been used as a third-line agent for neuropathic pain, although its efficacy is not well-established and adverse effects are problematic. Dizziness, paresthesias, or tremor may occur at lower concentrations, whereas seizures and cardiac conduction abnormalities can occur at higher plasma concentrations. In patients with cancer, corticosteroids can be added to elevate mood, stimulate appetite, reduce nausea and vomiting, and reduce inflammation. Because of their potent anti-inflammatory effects, corticosteroids can be effective for pain caused by soft tissue infiltration, visceral distension, or increased intracranial pressure. Oral muscle relaxants (eg, cyclobenzaprine, carisoprodol, methocarbamol) exert their effects by depressing spinal polysynaptic pathways and producing sedation. These agents are most helpful in acute musculoskeletal conditions such as neck and back pain. Efficacy from long-term administration has not been demonstrated and abrupt discontinuation following prolonged administration can cause withdrawal symptoms. Tizanidine's exact mechanism of action is unknown, but it has been shown to have antinociceptive, anti-inflammatory, and $alpha_2$ agonist properties. Tizanidine requires gradual dose titration over 2-4 weeks and is best used to treat chronic muscle spasticity, such as that seen with multiple sclerosis. Baclofen, an agonist at the GABA-B receptor, acts at the spinal end of the upper motor neurons to cause muscle relaxation. It has been used to treat trigeminal neuralgia and other neuropathic pain, as well as muscle spasms from conditions such as multiple sclerosis or spinal cord lesions. Adverse effects can be minimized by gradual dose titration over several days to weeks. Baclofen should be tapered and not abruptly discontinued because of the risk for serious withdrawal symptoms such as delirium and seizures. Clonidine, a centrally-acting $alpha_2$ agonist, provides analgesia by blocking transmission of noxious sensory information in the dorsal horn of the spinal cord. When administered transdermally, clonidine may also have a peripheral site of action. Limited data supports the efficacy of transdermal clonidine in certain patients with painful diabetic neuropathy. Tramadol provides analgesia by inhibiting reuptake of norepinephrine and serotonin within (central nervous system) pain pathways and is a weak mu-opioid receptor agonist. It has been effectively used for short-term (eg, flare-ups from osteoarthritis) and long-term (eg, low back, osteoarthritis, or cancer pain) treatment of chronic pain.

Other Adjuvants

Drug	Starting Dose (mg/day)	Dose Range (mg/day)	Adverse Effects
Baclofen	15	40-80	Nausea, constipation, weakness, confusion, dizziness, drowsiness
Clonidine (transdermal)	0.1	0.1	Drowsiness, dry mouth, fatigue, headache, local skin reaction, hypotension
Dexamethasone	1	4	Edema, hyperglycemia, immunosuppression, euphoria, depression, cognitive impairment
Mexiletine	150	600-1200	Nausea, heartburn, lightheadedness, dizziness, tremor, ataxia, confusion, palpitations
Prednisone	5	20	Edema, hyperglycemia, immunosuppression, euphoria, depression, cognitive impairment
Tizanidine	4	6-36	Drowsiness, insomnia, dizziness, fatigue, dry mouth, hypotension, elevated liver function tests
Tramadol	25 (100 mg extended release formulation)	150-300	Nausea, dizziness, vomiting, drowsiness

CHRONIC PAIN MANAGEMENT *(Continued)*

TOPICAL AGENTS

When the pain is localized, topical agents can be effective for chronic conditions such as arthritic and neuropathic pain. Capsaicin initially releases substance P, which results in an initial burning sensation and heat hyperalgesia during the first few days of its use. After several weeks of continued application, substance P becomes depleted from the nerve terminals, C-fibers are desensitized (superficial fibers may be killed), and analgesia occurs. Studies evaluating its efficacy have not been overwhelmingly favorable, but some patients with postherpetic neuralgia and diabetic neuropathy have reported modest pain relief from capsaicin. When administered topically, lidocaine acts directly at the local site through inhibition of sodium channels in nerve endings to reduce neuropathic pain transmission.

Topical Agents

Drug	Starting Dose	Dose Range	Adverse Effects
Capsaicin	0.025% applied 3-4 times a day[1]	0.025% to 0.075% applied 3-4 times a day[1]	Burning, stinging, redness of the skin
Lidocaine	5% patch	Up to three 5% patches at one time for ≤12 hours within a 24 hour period	Localized skin reaction, burning or abnormal sensation, skin discoloration, pruritus

[1]A minimum of 4 weeks is required to determine effectiveness

OPIOIDS

Opioids are routinely used in the treatment of cancer pain. However, opioids can also be effective as a component of chronic noncancer pain management when other agents are not sufficient and even when the pain is neuropathic in nature. In fact, combining morphine with gabapentin allows lower doses to be used with improved analgesia from that provided by either agent alone in patients with diabetic neuropathy or postherpetic neuralgia pain (Gilron, 2005). The primary care physician or pain specialist will decide whether an opioid could be successful for the chronic pain patient on a patient-specific basis.

Many opioid agents, formulations, and routes of administration are available for chronic pain management. Morphine, oxycodone, and hydromorphone are commonly used and available in short-acting formulations. Long-acting agents include oxycodone, morphine, transdermal fentanyl, and methadone. Opioid therapy is usually initiated using short-acting formulations to provide immediate pain relief and allow titration to a minimal effective dose, then switched to a long-acting agent to provide a longer duration of effective analgesia, minimize adverse effects, and improve compliance. For patients who are unable to take oral tablets, morphine can be administered as an oral liquid, rectally, or intravenously, whereas fentanyl can be administered transdermally or transmucosally. I.M. or SubQ administration may cause pain on injection and delayed absorption, especially with impaired tissue perfusion. These routes should only be used when absolutely necessary. Many opioids undergo a significant first-pass effect. All are metabolized by the liver (several to an active metabolite) and excreted in the urine. Meperidine is metabolized to normeperidine, a renally-eliminated metabolite that can cause anxiety, tremors, myoclonus, and seizures when the dose of meperidine is high and/or repeated doses are administered. Meperidine also has serotonergic activity which, when combined with other serotonin reuptake inhibitors (eg, MAOI, SSRI), can produce a serious serotonin toxicity reaction. Oral merperidine undergoes extensive first-pass metabolism, with significant amounts of normeperidine formed. For these reasons, meperidine has no place in chronic pain management. Pentazocine, an oral agonist at the kappa-opioid receptor and antagonist at the mu-receptor, offers no advantages over agonists such as morphine. In fact, pentazocine can cause undesirable psychotomimetic effects. Butorphanol is a mixed agonist-antagonist that is administered as a nasal spray for the treatment of migraines.

Opioids

Drug	Approximate Equianalgesic Parenteral Dose	Approximate Equianalgesic Oral Dose	Usual Oral Starting Dose for Opioid-Naïve Adults
Morphine[1]	10 mg	30 mg	30 mg q3-4 hours
Hydromorphone[1] (Dilaudid®)	1.5 mg	7.5 mg	6 mg q3-4 hours
Levorphanol (Levo-Dromoran®)	2 mg	4 mg	4 mg q6-8 hours
Methadone[2] (Dolophine®, others)	10 mg	3-5 mg	10 mg q6-8 hours
Oxycodone Roxicodone®, others)	Not available	20 mg	10 mg q3-4 hours

Combination Opioid Preparations[3]

Drug	Approximate Equianalgesic Oral Dose	Usual Oral Starting Dose for Opioid-Naïve Adults
Codeine (Tylenol® with codeine, others)	200 mg	60 mg q3-4 hours
Hydrocodone (Lorcet®, Lortab®, Norco®, Vicodin®, Vicoprofen®, others)	30 mg	10 mg q3-4 hours
Oxycodone (Percocet®, Percodan®, Tylox®, others)	20 mg	10 mg q3-4 hours

Note: Tables vary in the suggested doses that are equianalgesic to morphine. Furthermore, when a patient has been taking a very large dose of an opioid for a long time, equianalgesic dosing may be quite different. Therefore, clinical response is the criterion that must be applied for each patient; titration to clinical response is necessary. Because there is not complete cross tolerance among these drugs, it is usually necessary to use a lower than equianalgesic dose when changing drugs and to retitrate to response.

Caution: Recommended doses do not apply to patients with renal or hepatic insufficiency or other conditions affecting drug metabolism and pharmacokinetics.

[1]**Caution:** For morphine and hydromorphone, rectal administration is an alternate route for patients unable to take oral medications. Equianalgesic doses for rectal administration may differ from oral and parenteral doses because of pharmacokinetic differences. **Note:** A short-acting opioid should be used for initial therapy of moderate to severe pain, and then switched to a long-acting preparation once the optimal dose has been reached.

[2]Although many equianalgesic tables list 20 mg as the methadone equianalgesic oral dose, recent data suggest methadone is significantly more potent with repetitive dosing (due to its active metabolite). Ratios between oral morphine and oral methadone can range from 4:1 to 14:1.

[3]The maximum dose of these combination products is limited by the acetaminophen, aspirin, or ibuprofen in each tablet. For that reason, these combination products should not be used for severe pain.

REFERENCES AND RECOMMENDED READING

Ables AZ and Baughman OL, "Antidepressants: Update on New Agents and Indications," *Am Fam Physician*, 2003, 67(3):547-54.

Argoff CE, Backonja MM, Belgrade MJ, et al, "Consensus Guidelines: Treatment Planning and Options. Diabetic Peripheral Neuropathic Pain," *Mayo Clin Proc*, 2006, 81(4 Suppl):S12-25.

Backonja MM, "Use of Anticonvulsants for Treatment of Neuropathic Pain," *Neurology*, 2002, 59(5 Suppl 2):S14-7.

Beebe FA, Barkin RL, Barkin S, et al, "A Clinical and Pharmacologic Review of Skeletal Muscle Relaxants for Musculoskeletal Conditions," *Am J Ther*, 2005, 12(2):151-71.

Bonezzi C and Demartini L, "Treatment Options in Postherpetic Neuralgia," *Acta Neurol Scand Suppl*, 1999, 173:25-35.

Eisenberg E, McNicol ED, and Carr DB, "Efficacy and Safety of Opioid Agonists in the Treatment of Neuropathic Pain of Nonmalignant Origin," *JAMA*, 2005, 293(24):3043-52.

Galer BS, "Neuropathic Pain of Peripheral Origin: Advances in Pharmacologic Treatment," *Neurology*, 1995, 45(12 Suppl 9):S17-25.

Gardner-Nix J, "Principles of Opioid Use in Chronic Noncancer Pain," *CMAJ*, 2003, 169(1):38-43.

Gilron I, Bailey JM, Tu D, et al, "Morphine, Gabapentin, or Their Combination for Neuropathic Pain," *N Engl J Med*, 2005, 352(13):1324-34.

CHRONIC PAIN MANAGEMENT *(Continued)*

Guay DR, "Adjunctive Agents in the Management of Chronic Pain," *Pharmacotherapy*, 2001, 21(9):1070-81.

Jackson KC and St. Onge EL, "Antidepressant Pharmacotherapy: Considerations for the Pain Clinician," *Pain Practice*, 2003, 3(2):135-43.

"Principles of Analgesic Use in the Treatment of Acute Pain and Cancer Pain," 5th ed, Glenview, IL: American Pain Society, 2003.

CHRONIC RENAL FAILURE

In chronic renal failure, there is a progressive loss of nephron function. Depending upon the extent of loss, signs, symptoms, and biochemical abnormalities may or may not be present. Signs of renal failure (eg, nocturia) begin to appear when the number of functioning nephrons decreases to 10% to 40%. This stage of renal failure is referred to as renal insufficiency. Patients at this stage have little or no renal reserve; the ability to metabolize and excrete certain drugs is impaired as is the ability to eliminate large quantities of protein catabolic products. Serum creatinine (Cr) and blood urea nitrogen (BUN) are increased. The loss of approximately 95% of functioning nephrons results in the uremic syndrome. Acid-base, hematologic, and electrolyte abnormalities (hyperkalemia, hyponatremia, hypercalcemia, hypocalcemia, hypermagnesemia, hyperphosphatemia) are routinely seen as is fluid overload, which can result in CHF, hypertension, and left ventricular hypertrophy. Hyperkalemia is an important consideration because of its ability to precipitate fatal cardiac arrhythmias. Gastrointestinal disorders (eg, nausea, vomiting, anorexia, GI bleeding), chronic anemia, and an altered immune system are also present.

EFFECT ON DRUG DISPOSITION

Bioavailability

Several factors affect drug absorption in renal failure patients. Absorption of drugs can be decreased in uremic patients who have nausea, vomiting, diarrhea, gastritis, and pancreatitis. Uremia can result in an increase in gastric pH, thereby reducing the bioavailability of drugs requiring an acidic medium for absorption. An increase in gastric pH can also occur secondary to antacid use, which is often needed by renal failure patients. Antacids bind to other drugs, reducing their absorption. Gastric emptying time, gastric mobility, and intestinal motility can be decreased in the uremic patient, which can influence drug absorption.

Protein Binding

A drug's effect is produced by its free or unbound fraction. In renal failure patients, protein binding is reduced, which increases the amount of unbound drug. For example, this is seen with acidic drugs normally bound to albumin; since albumin is frequently decreased in renal failure, a greater free fraction of drug is seen. This effect is most important for drugs with high protein binding (>80%), such as phenytoin and valproic acid. The increase in free fraction can increase clearance of phenytoin since it is a low extraction ratio drug. Increased free drug can also result from the displacement of acidic drugs from albumin binding sites by acidic by-products seen in uremia and as a result of conformational changes in albumin which reduce the number/affinity of binding sites for drugs. Decreased tissue protein binding of digoxin decreases its volume of distribution, necessitating smaller loading digoxin loading doses in renal failure.

Metabolism

Renal failure significantly impacts on drug metabolism in a number of organs. The kidney houses the renal cytochrome P450 system which contributes to the metabolism of a number of drugs. Renal failure has been demonstrated to potentially increase, decrease, or have no effect on drug metabolism. Renal failure can also impact on drugs, which are metabolized by the liver to active metabolites. If these metabolites are renally eliminated, they accumulate in renal failure leading to increased activity and/or adverse effects. Meperidine (normeperidine), morphine (morphine-6-glucuronide), procainamide (N-acetylprocainamide), and allopurinol (oxypurinol) are four examples of such drugs. Dosages of these drugs should be carefully titrated in renal failure patients, and potential toxic effects should be monitored.

Elimination

The degree of renal impairment and the percentage of drug normally excreted unchanged in the urine will determine the impact of renal failure on elimination.

CHRONIC RENAL FAILURE *(Continued)*

Drugs are eliminated by the kidney via either filtration or active secretion. Molecular size and protein binding will determine a drug's filterability; low protein bound and small drugs are filtered more easily. Renal secretion is dependent on the anionic and cationic pathways. Depending on the cause of the renal disease, alterations in secretion and filtration can occur independently of each other. Estimates of GFR such as creatinine clearance are generally used to estimate renal function. But estimates of GFR may not predict alterations in clearance due to tubular dysfunction and altered secretion. Therefore close monitoring for efficacy and toxicity of renally eliminated drugs is necessary even when appropriate dosage alterations based on estimates of creatinine clearance have been performed.

Renal Dosing

Individualized drug dosage regimens for patients with renal failure generally utilize a correlation between creatinine clearance and drug clearance. Creatinine clearance is best estimated from a stable serum creatinine in patients with normal muscle mass and weight. A number of equations to estimate creatinine clearance are available. Multiple methods of renal dosage modification may be available, and they generally include increasing the interval or decreasing the dose. Both of these methods maintain the same steady state serum concentrations. Increasing the interval maintains similar peaks and troughs as usual dosing. Decreasing the dose results in lower peaks and higher troughs. This method is useful for antibiotics such as cephalosporins where the lack of postantibiotic effect necessitates maintenance of serum concentrations above the MIC.

Drug Dosing in Renal Replacement Therapy

Drug removal by hemodialysis is impacted by numerous drug-related factors. Molecular weight less than 500 daltons is generally associated with drug removal by traditional hemodialysis methods. However, high-flux filters can remove drugs of 5,000 daltons or greater. Water soluble drugs are more likely to be removed than drugs of poor solubility in aqueous media. Protein binding is an additional significant factor, since only free drug is available to diffuse across the semi-permeable membrane. Volume of distribution also correlates well, as drugs with smaller volumes of distribution are more likely to come in contact with the semi-permeable membrane and are more significantly dialyzed than drugs with large volumes of distribution that are largely distributed to tissue.

Characteristics of the dialysis procedure also impact on the amount of drug removed. A variety of dialysis filters of various compositions are available. Significant differences in drug clearances with different dialysis membranes and filters have been described. In addition blood and dialysate flow rates vary along with the length of the dialysis session. Therefore, drug clearances can vary significantly based on the specific dialysis prescription.

The need for supplemental dosing after dialysis is based on the relative amount of drug removed by a typical dialysis session. When >25% to 30% of a dose is removed by a typical 4-hour dialysis session, it is generally recommended that a supplemental dose be administered. Use of high-flux membranes may necessitate more aggressive supplementation, especially for some drugs that are not removed by typical procedures (eg, vancomycin). Given the multitude of factors impacting the potential amount of drug removed, close monitoring for efficacy and toxicity is necessary.

PREOPERATIVE EVALUATION OF THE CHRONIC RENAL FAILURE PATIENT

Assessment of renal function should be part of the comprehensive preoperative evaluation of the chronic renal failure patient. Tests are used in an attempt to quantify renal function and include BUN, serum creatinine, measured creatinine clearance, and estimated creatinine clearance. The following table lists the advantages and disadvantages for each test as well as their normal values.

Test	Normal Values	Advantages / Disadvantages
BUN	8-20 mg/dL	- Rapid, inexact estimate of creatinine clearance - BUN is increased by high protein intake, blood in GI tract, accelerated catabolism - Hepatic dysfunction decreases BUN concentration - Reabsorption of urea is greater when urinary flow is low
S_{cr}	0.5-1.2 mg/dL	- Rapid, inexact estimate of creatinine clearance - Creatinine is produced at a lower rate in elderly and in females; levels may fail to accurately reflect degree of nephron loss - Patients with muscle wasting from chronic disease may have low serum creatinine levels - Heavily muscled patients or acutely catabolic patients may have higher than normal serum creatinine levels secondary to more rapid muscle breakdown
Cl_{cr} (measured)	120 mL/minute	- Best overall indicator of GFR - Must accurately record urinary volume - Hydration can influence GFR determination
Cl_{cr} (estimated)	120 mL/minute	- Superior to BUN or serum creatinine for quantification of renal reserve - Same disadvantages as serum creatinine

Urinalysis assesses urinary pH as well as the presence of hematuria, pyuria, cellular casts, and proteinuria. The patient's cardiovascular status, hemoglobin concentration, and adequacy of dialysis therapy should also be assessed.

INTRAOPERATIVE MANAGEMENT OF THE CHRONIC RENAL FAILURE PATIENT

Monitoring

Intraoperative monitoring should include blood pressure, heart rate, EKG, oxygen saturation (via pulse oximeter), carbon dioxide (via capnometry), and degree of neuromuscular blockade (via a peripheral nerve stimulator). Invasive cardiovascular monitoring should be performed as needed.

Fluid Management

Fluid management must take into consideration the chronic renal failure patient's inability to excrete excess sodium and water. In those patients not requiring hemodialysis, a urine output >0.5 mL/kg/hour can usually be maintained by administration of a balanced salt solution at a rate of 3-5 mL/kg/hour. If necessary, the patient can be dialyzed postoperatively if intravascular volume is increased to an unsatisfactory level intraoperatively.

Selection of Anesthetic Agents

A knowledge of drug action in renal failure is important in determining an appropriate drug regimen (drug and dose). The reader is referred to the drugs' individual monographs to determine dosing in renal failure. Several examples follow.

I.V. anesthetic agents. Thiopental is highly bound to plasma proteins. Since protein binding is reduced in renal failure, a larger fraction of unbound thiopental is available. Further, a greater proportion of thiopental is found in the nonionized,

CHRONIC RENAL FAILURE *(Continued)*

unbound form secondary to the acidic pH seen in renal failure. Finally, uremia alters the blood-brain barrier, which results in an increased sensitivity to thiopental. Because of these factors, a lower induction dose of thiopental is needed for uremic patients.

Induction doses of ketamine and benzodiazepines require less reduction since they are less protein-bound than thiopental. Normal benzodiazepine doses, however, may show an exaggerated response in debilitated renal failure patients. Ketamine, because of its ability to increase blood pressure and cardiac output, may worsen the hypertension seen with renal failure.

Morphine's elimination half-life and clearance are not changed in renal failure. As already alluded to, its glucuronide metabolite accumulates in renal failure and can cause prolonged respiratory depression The synthetic opioids, fentanyl, sufentanil, and alfentanil are hepatically metabolized with their metabolites renally excreted. The rapid tissue redistribution seen with these agents after small doses should result in a short duration of action in both normal and renal failure patients. Sufentanil does, however, have an active metabolite which can accumulate in chronic renal failure patients. Remifentanil, because of its metabolism by nonspecific esterases in blood and tissue, is not affected by renal failure. Dosing remains the same as in normal patients.

Inhalational agents. The major route of elimination of these agents is via the lungs, not the kidneys. Metabolism of some of these agents can result in renally excreted metabolites. Enflurane and sevoflurane are metabolized to inorganic fluoride, which can accumulate in renal failure patients. Sevoflurane is currently not recommended for use in patients with a serum creatinine >1.5 mg/dL. An advantage of the volatile inhalation agents is that they produce neuromuscular blockade, which can reduce the dose of neuromuscular blocking agent required.

Neuromuscular-blocking agents. The depolarizing neuromuscular blocking agent succinylcholine causes a transient increase in serum potassium of approximately 0.5-1 mEq/L. This may become a problem in uremic patients who have an elevated serum potassium; the increase may be enough to produce cardiac arrhythmias. Plasma cholinesterase levels are sufficient in renal failure patients so that no clinically significant prolongation of succinylcholine's effect should be expected.

The elimination of nondepolarizing neuromuscular blocking agents is dependent to varying degrees on renal excretion. The following table lists the elimination profiles of the commercially available nondepolarizing agents. The elimination half-lives of agents primarily eliminated renally are increased in patients with renal failure. Atracurium and cisatracurium, because of their primarily nonrenal elimination, are ideal agents to use in renal failure patients. Both pancuronium and vecuronium have active metabolites that can accumulate in renal failure. One of atracurium's metabolites, laudanosine, can also accumulate in renal failure. Laudanosine has no neuromuscular blocking activity but has been shown to cause CNS excitation in animals; this effect has not been demonstrated in humans.

Agent	Renal	Hepatic	Biliary	Plasma
Atracurium	<5%	—	—	Hofmann elimination Ester hydrolysis
Cisatracurium	R/H <20%	R/H <20%	—	Hofmann elimination
Doxacurium	80% to 100%	—	Yes	—
Gallamine	95% to 100%	—	<1%	—
Mivacurium	<10%	—	Minor	Plasma cholinesterase
Pancuronium	60% to 80%	15% to 40%	5% to 10%	—
Rocuronium	30%	—	50%	—
Vecuronium	30%	20% to 30%	40% to 75%	—

R/H = renal/hepatic metabolism.

Renal failure increases the duration of action of the anticholinesterase agents (neostigmine, pyridostigmine, edrophonium) commonly used to reverse the residual effects of neuromuscular blockade by 100% or more (secondary to their elimination primarily by the kidneys). This makes the possibility of recurarization unlikely. Other factors which influence reversal of neuromuscular blockade in the renal failure patient include acid-base status, electrolyte levels, concomitant use of potentiating drugs (eg, aminoglycosides), and temperature.

POSTOPERATIVE MANAGEMENT OF THE CHRONIC RENAL FAILURE PATIENT

Hypertension is frequently seen in the postoperative period. Vasodilators (eg, esmolol, fenoldopam, labetalol, nicardipine) may be useful as initial therapy. Nitroprusside can be used transiently, but large doses or prolonged use could be associated with thiocyanate toxicity in renal failure. If hypervolemia is the cause, dialysis can be used to remove excess fluid if it is an option. Supplemental oxygen should be considered if anemia is present, continuous monitoring of the EKG is warranted if arrhythmias are a concern in a hyperkalemic patient, and caution should be used when administering opioids for pain secondary to the potential for CNS depression and hypoventilation.

REFERENCES AND RECOMMENDED READING

Quan DJ and Aweeka FT, "Dosing of Drugs in Renal Failure," *Applied Therapeutics: The Clinical Use of Drugs*, Young LY and Koda-Kimble MA, eds, 8th ed, Vancouver, WA: Applied Therapeutics Inc, 2004, 32(1)-(26).

Matzke GR and Frye RF, "Drug Therapy Individualization for Patients With Renal Insufficiency," *Pharmacotherapy: A Pathophysiologic Approach*, DiPiro JT, Talbert RL, Yess GC, et al, eds, 5th ed, Stamford, CT: Appleton and Lange, 2002, 939-52.

Monk TG and Weldon BC, "The Renal System and Anesthesia for Urologic Surgery," *Clinical Anesthesia*, Barash PG, Cullen BF, Stoelting RK, eds, 3rd ed, Philadelphia, PA: Lippincott Williams & Wilkins, 1996, 945-73.

Stoelting RK and Dierdorf SF, "Renal Disease," *Anesthesia and Co-Existing Disease*, 3rd ed, New York, NY: Churchill Livingstone, 1993, 289-312.

MODERATE SEDATION

The goal of conscious sedation is to produce a state where: 1) patients are able to tolerate unpleasant procedures; 2) adequate cardiorespiratory function is maintained; and 3) patients are able to respond purposefully to verbal commands and/or tactile stimulation. It is important to remember that sedation occurs over a continuum that can unintentionally progress to deep sedation or even general anesthesia. The American Society of Anesthesiologists (ASA) Task Force on Sedation and Analgesia by Non-Anesthesiologists has recommended that the term "conscious sedation" be replaced with "sedation and analgesia" as this more accurately describes the therapeutic goal desired. The ASA Practice Guidelines for Sedation and Analgesia by Non-Anesthesiologists state that sedation/analgesia should "provide benefits of sedation/analgesia while minimizing the associated risks. In children and uncooperative adults, sedation/analgesia may expedite the conduct of procedures that are not particularly uncomfortable but require that the patient not move." Similar to that used by the ASA Task Force, the Joint Commission on Accreditation of Healthcare Organizations' standards and intents for sedation and anesthesia care uses the terminology "moderate sedation/analgesia" instead of conscious sedation. The JCAHO definition of "moderate sedation/analgesia" states that the patient should be able to respond purposefully to verbal commands, either alone or accompanied by tactile stimulation. It further states that no interventions are required to maintain a patent airway, that spontaneous ventilation is adequate, and that cardiovascular function is usually maintained.

Nonanesthesiologist clinicians who wish to order/administer medications for sedation/analgesia must be trained, demonstrate competency, and receive medical staff privileges to do so. Often times, CPR training is required. Personnel who assist the licensed independent practitioners must be trained to appropriately document and monitor patient status.

PATIENT EVALUATION

A presedation assessment, including a relevant patient history and pertinent physical exam, should be performed. The presedation assessment should include:

- Chief complaint/present illness
- Relevant medical/surgical history
- Relevant family history
- Medication history
- Pregnancy status, if appropriate
- Baseline mental status
- Airway assessment
- ASA classification
- Allergies
- Patient's weight and vital signs (HR and rhythm, blood pressure, respiratory rate, temperature, oxygen saturation)
- Previous adverse effects/complications from sedation/analgesia, regional anesthesia, or general anesthesia
- Time/nature of last oral intake (eg, clear liquids >2-3 hours, solids >6-8 hours)
- History of alcohol, tobacco, illicit drug use
- Review of systems (eg, any abnormalities of major organ function)
- Cardiopulmonary physical examination

A thorough medication history is important to prevent potential drug interactions. For example, meperidine is contraindicated in a patient taking a monoamine oxidase inhibitor (MAOI). Opioids and CNS depressants can increase the potential for apnea and oversedation when administered with a benzodiazepine. Other drugs also have the potential to interact with medications used for sedation and analgesia. For example, the clearance of diazepam, but not midazolam, is decreased and its half-life increased with cimetidine. Ritonavir can inhibit the metabolism of midazolam, potentially causing extreme sedation and respiratory depression.

SEDATION AND ANALGESIA PLAN

A sedation and analgesia plan must be developed and communicated to the patient, family, and other healthcare providers involved with the procedure as well as be documented in the patient's medical record. The plan should be re-evaluated immediately prior to beginning sedation and analgesia. Pre-procedure fasting should occur prior to sedative administration.

PATIENT COUNSELING

Patients should be informed of the risks, benefits, and limitations of sedation/analgesia and of potential alternatives. An informed consent form needs to be signed by the patient (or guardian) before proceeding with sedation and analgesia.

MONITORING

Monitoring of the patient during moderate sedation is necessary to assure adequacy of oxygenation, circulation, and level of consciousness during the procedure. The following data should be recorded starting before the procedure and continued during the procedure and recovery period:

- Drugs administered (drug, route, site, time, dose)
- Oxygen saturation (via pulse oximetry)
- Type and amount of I.V. fluid
- Level of consciousness
- Pulmonary ventilation (through observation of spontaneous respiratory activity or auscultation of breath sounds)
- Blood pressure, temperature (pre- and postprocedure), heart rate, and respiratory rate
- ECG for patients with significant cardiovascular disease, ASA class III or IV patients
- Unexpected events
- Status of patient upon completion of the procedure and the start of the recovery period

Minimally, the patient's hemodynamic variables (heart rate, blood pressure), ventilatory status (respiratory rate), and oxygenation status (pulse oximetry) should be documented before the beginning of the procedure, after administration of sedative/analgesic agents, at completion of the procedure, during initial recovery, and at discharge. However, these variables are normally recorded at regular intervals (eg, every 5 minutes) during the procedure. The frequency of vital signs monitoring may need to be individualized on a case-to-case basis. Patients who are chronically or acutely ill or debilitated, or those who deteriorate during the diagnostic or therapeutic procedure may require more frequent measurements of vital signs. The conduct of the procedure may practically preclude monitoring/recording of a given vital sign at a routine interval. Sicker patients (ASA class III or IV) should have ECG monitoring.

Signs and symptoms of toxicity associated with sedation/analgesia include deep sedation, somnolence, confusion, respiratory depression, apnea, respiratory arrest, hypotension, cardiac arrest, nausea and vomiting, diminished reflexes, impaired coordination, and severe changes in vital signs.

It is critical that an appropriately trained individual other than the person performing the procedure be present to continuously monitor the patient throughout the procedure and recovery.

MODERATE SEDATION *(Continued)*

EQUIPMENT REQUIREMENTS

The following equipment and supplies should be present or readily available (within or adjacent to the procedure room).

- Oxygen source and administration equipment of various types and sizes; supplemental oxygen should be administered when clinically indicated (eg, hypoxemia)
- Suction
- Emergency airway equipment (variety of laryngoscope blades and handles, oral and nasal airways, and various sizes of endotracheal tubes with stylets)
- Means of positive-pressure ventilation (eg, ambu or other resuscitation bag)
- Emergency resuscitation drugs (eg, drugs recommended in the current ACLS guidelines)
- Pharmacologic antagonists (eg, naloxone for opioids, flumazenil for benzodiazepines)
- Intravenous equipment; for patients receiving drugs intravenously, I.V. access should be maintained throughout the whole procedure and until the patient is not at risk for serious adverse events from the drugs administered (eg, cardiorespiratory depression).
- Pulse oximetry
- Noninvasive blood pressure equipment
- ECG
- Telephone
- Device for measuring temperature

AGENT SELECTION / DOSE TITRATION

Sedatives (eg, midazolam, diazepam, chloral hydrate) are routinely used to decrease anxiety and promote somnolence. Analgesics (eg, morphine, fentanyl) are routinely used to relieve pain. Combinations of opioids and sedatives may increase the incidence of adverse effects. Propofol should be administered by a person trained in the administration of general anesthesia who is not involved in performing the procedure. Propofol must be titrated because a patient can go from breathing normally to a respiratory arrest very rapidly and without warning.

When given intravenously, sedative/analgesic drugs should be administered in small, incremental doses until the desired effect is achieved (titrate to effect). Please refer to the individual drug monographs for appropriate dosing guidelines. Care must be taken to allow a sufficient time between doses to allow the effect of each dose to be seen. Dosage reductions are often required in the chronically ill or elderly as well as with the concomitant administration of an opioid and sedative agent (eg, benzodiazepine). Additional time should be allowed between doses when drugs are administered by nonintravenous routes (eg, oral, rectal, I.M.) secondary to the time required for drug absorption.

RECOVERY

Patients may continue to be at risk for complications after the procedure and must be monitored (level of consciousness, vital signs, respiratory function) throughout the recovery period until meeting discharge criteria. If a reversal agent has been administered, an appropriate time (up to 2 hours) should have elapsed to ensure that resedation does not occur secondary to the reversal agent's short duration of action when compared to the sedation/analgesia agent's duration of action. Patients must be discharged with an accompanying responsible adult. The patient and accompanying adult should be advised (both verbally and in writing) regarding any limitations on the patient's activity (eg, do not operate machinery or drive an automobile for 24 hours), diet, and medication use. In addition, the patient should be given a 24-hour emergency contact telephone number in case problems arise.

QUALITY ASSURANCE

Any unusual occurrences or adverse drug reactions should be reported via the quality assurance program in place for sedation/analgesia. These could include:

- Assisted ventilation required, respiratory rate <8 or periods of apnea at any time during the procedure
- Oxygen saturation decrease ≥10% from preprocedure for ≥5 minutes
- Arrhythmia or hemodynamic instability
- Use of reversal agent
- Procedure stopped or interrupted due to excessive sedation or adverse drug reaction
- Delayed recovery from sedation
- Unanticipated hospital admission or transfer to a higher level of care
- Other clinically significant changes from preprocedure baseline not noted above

REFERENCES AND RECOMMENDED READING

Cravero JP and Blike GT, "Review of Pediatric Sedation," *Anesth Analg*, 2004, 99(5):1355-64.

Holland CA, "Conscious Sedation Policy Development and Review," *AANA J*, 1995, 63(3):196-7.

Holzman RS, Cullen DJ, Eichhorn JH, et al, "Guidelines for Sedation by Nonanesthesiologists During Diagnostic and Therapeutic Procedures. The Risk Management Committee of the Department of Anesthesia of Harvard Medical School," *J Clin Anesth*, 1994, 6(4):265-76.

Malviya S and Voepel-Lewis T, "Sedation of Children Outside the Operating Room," *Progress in Anesthesiology*, 1995, 9:399-411.

"Practice Guidelines for Sedation and Analgesia by Non-Anesthesiologists. An Updated Report by the American Society of Anesthesiologists Task Force on Sedation and Analgesia by Nonanesthesiologists," *Anesthesiology*, 2002, 96(4):1004-17.

Revisions to Anesthesia Care Standards, *Comprehensive Accreditation Manual for Hospitals*: Standards and Intents for Sedation and Anesthesia Care, January 1, 2001. Available at: http://www.jcrinc.com/generic.asp?durki=405.

Smetzer JL and Cohen MR, "Propofol Sedation: Who Should Administer?," *Jt Comm J Qual Patient Saf*, 2006, 32(5):293-5.

MODERATE SEDATION *(Continued)*

Most Commonly Used Agents for Moderate Sedation in Adults

Medication	Onset of Action	Duration of Action	Adult Dose	Reversal Agent	Comments
Diazepam	P.O.15-30 min I.V.: 3-10 min	P.O./I.V.: 6-8 h	P.O.: 10 mg I.V.: 2-5 mg Repeat dosage q10min prn; Max: 0.1-0.2 mg/kg (10 mg)	Flumazenil	
Fentanyl	I.V.: 1-2 min	I.V.: 30-60 min	I.V.: 25-50 mcg Repeat dosage q3-5min prn; Max: 500 mcg/4 h	Naloxone	
Flumazenil	I.V.: 1-2 min	I.V.: 1-2 h	I.V.: 0.2 mg Repeat dosage q1min prn; Max: 1 mg		Reversal agent for BZD
Lorazepam	I.V.: 5-10 min P.O.: 20-30 min	I.V.: 4-6 h P.O.: 6-8 h	Slow I.V.: 0.5-2 mg P.O.: 2 mg Repeat dosage q20min prn; Max: 4 mg	Flumazenil	Hypotension and bradycardia with fast injection
Methohexital	Immediate	I.V.: 10-20 min	50-120 mg Repeat 20-40 mg q4-7min prn	None	Use with caution if CV instability, severe liver disease, or asthma
Midazolam	I.V.: 1-5 min	I.V.: 30-120 min	**<60 y:** Slow I.V.: 1-2 mg Repeat dosage q2min prn; Max: 0.1 mg/kg (10 mg)/h **>60 y or debilitated:** I.V.: 0.5 mg Repeat dosage q3min prn; Max: 0.05 mg/kg (5 mg)/h	Flumazenil	Hypotension and bradycardia with fast injection
Morphine	I.V.: 5-10 min	I.V.: 2-4 h	I.V.: 1-2 mg Repeat dosage q3-5min prn; Max: 20 mg	Naloxone	Hypotension due to histamine release
Naloxone	I.V.: 1-2 min	I.V.: 30-60 min	I.V.: 40 mcg Repeat dosage q2-3min prn; Max: 2 mg		Reversal agent for opioids
Propofol	Immediate	I.V.: 3-10 min	5-10 mcg/kg/min infusion Titrate q5min prn; Max: 75 mcg/kg/min	None	Do not bolus (severe hypotension, bradycardia)

CONTINUOUS RENAL REPLACEMENT THERAPY

Continuous renal replacement therapy (CRRT) has evolved over the last 25 years as a means of providing safe and effective renal replacement therapy to critically ill patients with fluid overload and/or renal failure who may not tolerate the hemodynamic disturbances that accompany traditional intermittent hemodialysis. CRRT provides additional benefits by decreasing fluid and electrolyte shifts, improving dialysis adequacy, and providing the potential for unlimited fluid administration to accommodate optimal nutrition. More recently, CRRT has also been investigated for removal of inflammatory substances or mediators in conditions such as acute respiratory distress syndrome or sepsis. Although CRRT has been found to remove these substances, its clinical impact has not yet been defined.

CRRT procedures utilize diffusion, filtration (convection), or combined diffusion/filtration techniques which assist in the management of fluid volume, electrolytes, and acid base status. Vascular access for these procedures can be either arterial or venous. Whereas arterial access utilizes the patient's own blood pressure for the maintenance of filtration pressure, venous access systems incorporating a blood pump are utilized more frequently as they result in higher solute clearance. Procedures offering only fluid volume control include slow continuous ultrafiltration (SCUF), and continuous arterio-and venovenous hemofiltration (CAVH and CVVH). Procedures which provide both solute and fluid volume control include continuous arterio- and venovenous hemodialysis (CAVHD and CVVHD), and continuous arterio- and venovenous hemodiafiltration (CAVHDF and CVVHDF). The method selected is determined by the patient's clinical needs.

Continuous Renal Replacement Therapies

Therapy	Abbreviation	Definition	Volume Control	Solute Control
Ultrafiltration	SCUF	Plasma water removal	Effective	Ineffective
Hemofiltration	CAVH CVVH	Convective process using semi-permeable membrane	Effective	Ineffective
Hemodialysis	CAVHD CVVHD	Diffusion using dialysate and semipermeable membrane	Effective	Effective
Hemodiafiltration	CAVHDF CVVHDF	Diffusion and convection	Effective	Effective

ANTICOAGULATION IN CRRT

All hemodialysis procedures are prone to clotting of the blood lines and/or hemofilter due to platelet activation. Clotting is more likely to occur in an arteriovenous procedure since the blood flow rates are lower than in a venovenous one.

Numerous anticoagulation schemes are employed which provide safe and effective CRRT with filter survival times often >48 hours.

Anticoagulants Used In CRRT

Drug	Dose	Monitoring Goal
Heparin	500-1000 units bolus, then 5-10 units/kg/h	aPTT 35-45 seconds
Dalteparin	20 units/kg bolus, then 10 units/kg/h	
Prostacyclin (PGI_2, epoprostenol)	2-10 ng/kg/min	
Hirudin	0.01 mg/kg bolus, then 0.005 mg/kg/h	
Argatroban	0.9 mcg/kg/min	aPTT 2-2.5 x normal

Unfractionated heparin is the most commonly used anticoagulant in CRRT procedures due to its lack of renal elimination and poor dialyzability. Critically ill patients are often at risk of bleeding due to concomitant organ failure and

CONTINUOUS RENAL REPLACEMENT THERAPY
(Continued)

coagulopathies. Even with low dose regimens and monitoring, bleeding rates have been reported to be as high as 50%. Heparin-induced thrombocytopenia (HIT) is another potential complication of this therapy.

Low molecular weight heparins have been useful anticoagulants in chronic hemodialysis, and have been investigated in CRRT. Dalteparin provides comparable filter patency and bleeding rates to heparin, but has significant renal elimination, may accumulate in renal failure, and is not removed by filtration. Low molecular weight heparins may be associated with a higher incidence of bleeding than heparin due to their longer half-lives in renal failure and an inability to be predictably neutralized by protamine. Low molecular weight heparins should not be used in patients with HIT.

Prostacyclin (PGI_2, or epoprostenol) is an inhibitor of platelet aggregation and a vasodilator. It has been successfully employed both in combination with reduced doses of heparin, and alone in patients felt to be at risk of bleeding due to coagulopathy. Hypotension, an expected side effect, is generally not observed due to 30% to 40% clearance by filtration. Cost is the most commonly cited factor limiting its use.

Hirudin is a recombinant polypeptide which directly inhibits thrombin. It is 90% renally eliminated and has at least a 100-fold increase in its half-life in renal failure. Limited information is available regarding hirudin use in CRRT, and its use has been associated with hemorrhage. In addition, some patients develop antihirudin antibodies which further prolong the drug's elimination and complicate therapy. The aPTT does not correlate well with bleeding risk from hirudin.

Argatroban, an alternative direct thrombin inhibitor, may be the most promising option for patients on CRRT who have HIT. It is hepatically eliminated and a very effective option for HIT in critically ill patients with renal failure. Very little data is available regarding its clinical use in CRRT. Lower doses of 0.4-0.6 mcg/kg/min have been used for patients with combined liver and renal failure.

Another option for anticoagulation for patients with HIT or at high risk of bleeding is regional citrate. Citrate chelates calcium, which is necessary for activity of a number of factors in the clotting cascade. Numerous citrate anticoagulant procedures have been described to provide effective anticoagulation with filter durations ranging from 1-4 days with minimal bleeding rates. Anticoagulant citrate dextrose (ACD-A) solution or 4% trisodium citrate are generally administered prefilter at a rate to achieve a postfilter ionized Ca concentration of 0.25-0.35 mmol/L. Specialized dialysate solutions used in these procedures are low sodium, low or calcium-free, and low or bicarbonate-free. One potential complication of citrate anticoagulation is systemic alkalosis, since citrate is metabolized to bicarbonate. Citrate toxicity may also be observed when citrate is ineffectively removed in patients with liver failure, or hypoperfusion. High ratios of total calcium to ionized calcium occur when the citrate-calcium complex accumulates. Despite the need for specialized dialysate solutions, the additional need for intensive monitoring of ionized calcium concentrations, and the potential for metabolic alkalosis, citrate anticoagulation is growing in popularity due to its ability to provide longer filter life with a low incidence of bleeding.

CRRT in the absence of any anticoagulation is a final option. Saline flushes (100 mL/h) have provided filter patency for approximately 24 hours. This alternative may be an option for patients with bleeding risk, HIT, or liver failure.

DRUG DOSING IN CRRT

Many principles that apply to drug removal by traditional hemodialysis methods also apply to CRRT (refer to Chronic Renal Failure Chapter section on Dialysis Dosing). Similar drug (eg, molecular weight, protein binding, and volume of distribution) and procedure (eg, hemofilter) characteristics responsible for drug removal in intermittent dialysis are also important in CRRT. However, the large variety of procedures makes generalizations regarding removal of any individual drug difficult. In CRRT there is the possibility of more significant convection with or without diffusion, along with a variety of different dialysis membranes. In addition the dialysis/hemofiltration process is continual rather than for a limited time period. All of these factors make generalizations about the extent of drug removal by a specific type of CRRT procedure difficult to formulate. Nonrenal routes of elimination may become more important in renal failure. The amount of drug lost due to dialysis may be small compared to the amount cleared extrarenally. Some patients being treated with CRRT may have significant residual renal function, which may also contribute to drug clearance. Therefore, the patient's clinical status, liver and renal function, and the specific CRRT prescription should be closely evaluated when drug dosage recommendations are formulated.

During filtration processes such as CAVH and CVVH, the amount of drug removed is largely dependent on the filtration rate, the drug's protein binding characteristics, and the specific filter being utilized. Significant differences between filters have been documented with regard to the amount of drug removed by these procedures. The sieving coefficient is the ratio of drug found in ultrafiltrate to the prefilter plasma water concentration. The sieving coefficient often approximates the drug's free fraction in plasma. However, it can also vary with the specific filter used and as a result of altered plasma protein binding in renal disease or due to critical illness. Information regarding dosing alterations for filtration procedures is available for some drugs. When it is not available, the amount of drug removed during SCUF, CAVH, or CVVH can be estimated by the equation:

$$\text{Estimated amount removed}_{\text{(CVVH/CAVH)}} = \frac{(Q_f)\ (SC)\ (C_{pss})\ (\tau)}{(S)\ (F)}$$

where Q_f is the ultrafiltration rate, SC is the sieving coefficient, C_{pss} is the desired steady state plasma concentration, τ is the dosing interval, S is the salt form of the drug, and F is the fraction absorbed. When the sieving coefficient is unknown, f_{up} (free fraction in plasma) can be substituted. Once the amount of drug removed for a given interval can be estimated a clinical decision can be made with regard to the necessity of a supplemental dose or alteration in the dosage regimen. Typically dosage alterations are necessary when more than 25% to 30% of a dose is being removed over the specific interval.

For procedures that utilize diffusion (CVVHD and CAVHD), or both diffusion and convection (CVVHDF and CAVHDF), the amount of drug removed depends on the relative amounts of dialysis and filtration, along with the specific filter, and the drug's characteristics. The primary factor correlating with degree of drug removal is rate of dialysis, with ultrafiltration rate secondarily contributing. Drug dosage recommendations for these types of procedures are not widely available and uniform recommendations are difficult to formulate due to the large variety of potential combinations of dialysis rate, ultrafiltration rate and available filters. Case reports or studies are useful for assisting with development of dosing recommendations for individual patients undergoing these procedures. When dosing information is not available, the amount of drug removed during CVVHD/CAVHD, or CVVHDF/CAVHDF can be estimated by the following equations:

$$\text{Estimated amount removed}_{\text{(CVVHD/CAVHD)}} = \frac{(Q_{dial})\ (f_{up})\ (C_{pss})\ (\tau)}{(S)\ (F)}$$

$$\text{Estimated amount removed}_{\text{(CVVHDF/CAVHDF)}} = \frac{(Q_{dial} + Q_f)\ (f_{up})\ (C_{pss})\ (\tau)}{(S)\ (F)}$$

where Q_{dial} is the dialysate flow rate. As above, if the amount of drug removed is significant, an alteration in the dosage regimen to account for lost drug is necessary.

Close attention to a patient's CRRT therapy is needed for a number of reasons. The dialysis prescription should be evaluated to verify the presence of dialysis and or ultrafiltration, since terminologies for the procedures are often misused in the clinical setting. The dialysis prescription (dialysate rate, ultrafiltration rate) often changes frequently in order to adequately manage the patient's fluid, electrolyte,

CONTINUOUS RENAL REPLACEMENT THERAPY *(Continued)*

and hemodynamic status. Patency of the extracorporeal unit and the ability to continue dialysis is another challenge. Therefore, repeated alterations in drug dosing may be needed in order to best individualize the patient's pharmacotherapeutic regimen. Given the paucity of available information regarding drug dosing in CRRT, close monitoring of drug efficacy and safety is essential.

REFERENCES AND RECOMMENDED READING

Davenport A, "Anticoagulation for Continuous Renal Replacement Therapy," *Contrib Nephrol*, 2004, 144:228-38.

Joy MS, Matzke GR, Armstrong DK, et al, "A Primer on Continuous Renal Replacement Therapy for Critically Ill Patients," *Ann Pharamacother*, 1998, 32(3):362-75.

Matzke GR and Frye RF, "Drug Therapy Individualization for Patients With Renal Insufficiency," *Pharmacotherapy: A Pathophysiologic Approach*, DiPiro JT, Talbert RL, Yee GC, et al, eds, 5th ed, Stamford, CT: Appleton and Lange, 2002, 939-52.

Mueller BA, Pasko DA, and Sowinski KM, "Higher Renal Replacement Therapy Dose Delivery Influences on Drug Therapy," *Artif Organs*, 2003, 27(9):808-14.

Paganini EP, "Continuous Renal Replacement Therapy," *Critical Care Medicine: Principles of Diagnosis and Management in the Adult*, Parillo JE and Dellinger RP, eds, 2nd ed, St Louis, MO: Mosby, 2002, 270-94.

MANAGEMENT OF POSTOPERATIVE ARRHYTHMIAS

Arrhythmias commonly occur in the postoperative setting and can contribute to patient morbidity and mortality. Postoperative supraventricular arrhythmias have been reported to occur in a 3.2% to 13% incidence, depending on the surgical procedure. After cardiac surgery, atrial flutter and fibrillation occur in an even higher incidence (12% to 60%). The presence of serious ventricular arrhythmias (eg, sustained ventricular tachycardia, ventricular fibrillation) after cardiac surgery is becoming uncommon; it is even more so after noncardiac surgery. Patients with structural heart disease are most likely to experience arrhythmias in the postoperative setting. The duration of the arrhythmia, ventricular response rate, and the patient's underlying cardiac function are several of the factors that contribute to the physiologic consequences of an arrhythmia.

CLASSIFICATION OF ARRHYTHMIAS

Arrhythmias can be broadly grouped into tachyarrhythmias and bradyarrhythmias. Tachyarrhythmias are further divided by anatomical origin as either supraventricular or ventricular. Table 1 lists common supraventricular and ventricular arrhythmias. Further classifying tachyarrhythmias into those that do and do not traverse the atrioventricular (AV) node (Table 1) is useful when determining appropriate treatment. For example, pharmacologic agents that slow AV node conduction can be used to control the ventricular response if the arrhythmia traverses the AV node. Bradyarrhythmias include sinus bradycardia, sinoatrial (SA) block, sinus pause, and sinus arrest.

Table 1. Common Supraventricular and Ventricular Arrhythmias

Supraventricular Arrhythmias
Sinus tachycardia
Atrial flutter[1]
Atrial fibrillation[1]
Automatic (ectopic) atrial tachycardia[1]
Multifocal atrial tachycardia[1]
Junctional tachycardia
Atrioventricular nodal re-entrant tachycardias[1]
Atrioventricular reciprocating tachycardias[1]
Ventricular Arrhythmias
Premature ventricular beats
Ventricular tachycardia
Ventricular fibrillation

[1]Traverse the AV node.

PREDISPOSING FACTORS

Factors that predispose patients to postoperative arrhythmias can be found in Table 2. When specifically looking at atrial fibrillation after cardiac surgery, the following conditions may contribute to the development of this arrhythmia: Advanced age, male sex, history of preoperative atrial fibrillation, hypertension, history of congestive heart failure, need for postoperative intra-aortic balloon pump, postoperative pneumonia, ventilation for >24 hours, autonomic imbalance, electrolyte abnormalities, pericardial inflammation, inadequate atrial protection from cardioplegia during bypass, and atrial enlargement from volume overload and impaired hemodynamics encountered in the postoperative period. In the postoperative setting, factors that decrease sympathetic nervous system influence or increase parasympathetic nervous system activity can lead to sinus bradycardia (Table 3). Severe hypoxemia, SA nodal ischemia, and sick sinus syndrome

MANAGEMENT OF POSTOPERATIVE ARRHYTHMIAS *(Continued)*

can also reduce sinus rate. Postoperative ventricular tachycardia or fibrillation usually reflects severe myocardial ischemia, systemic acidemia, or hypoxemia. An important point to remember is that the genesis of arrhythmias can be multifactorial; caution should be taken not to attribute an arrhythmia to a single factor without fully considering the potential for multiple factors to be at play.

Table 2. Factors Predisposing Patients to Postoperative Arrhythmias

Myocardial ischemia	Acid-base imbalance
Endogenous or exogenous catecholamines	Electrolyte abnormalities
Hypoxemia	Mechanical factors
Hypercarbia	Administration of select medications

Table 3. Factors Predisposing Patients to Sinus Bradycardia

Decrease Sympathetic Activity
- High epidural or spinal anesthesia
- Severe acidemia/hypoxemia
- Withdrawal of stimulus
- Emptying bladder
- Sympatholytic medications (eg, beta-blockers, opioids, local anesthetics)

Increase Parasympathetic Activity
- Increased vagal tone
  - Carotid sinus massage
  - Valsalva maneuver
  - Gagging
  - Increased ocular pressure
  - Bladder distension
  - Pharyngeal stimulation
  - Anxiety/pain (centrally mediated response)
  - Surgery (eg, traction on peritoneum during vascular surgery)
- Parasympathomimetic medications (eg, acetylcholinesterase inhibitors, alpha-adrenergic drugs, opioids, succinylcholine)

PRINCIPLES / GOALS OF TREATMENT

Several principles must be kept in mind when managing patients with postoperative arrhythmias. The most important is to treat the patient and not the electrocardiogram (EKG). Questions one should ask include whether an arrhythmia is truly present (vs an artifact) and whether the rhythm seen on the EKG can account for the patient's condition. The urgency for treatment should then be decided. Items such as the patient's pulse, blood pressure, peripheral perfusion, and the presence of myocardial ischemia and congestive heart failure should be evaluated. For example, prompt electrical cardioversion is indicated in a patient who becomes unconscious or hemodynamically unstable in the presence of a tachyarrhythmia (excluding sinus tachycardia). Treatment should also be instituted if the arrhythmia is a precursor of a more severe arrhythmia. The type of arrhythmia will dictate the goals of therapy. Foremost is the need to establish hemodynamic stability. For tachyarrhythmias, attention is first given to slowing the ventricular response whereas with bradyarrhythmias, the ventricular rate must be increased. Once the patient is hemodynamically stable, restoration of sinus rhythm becomes the goal. If this is not possible, the focus should shift to preventing complications from occurring. In patients without overt cardiac disease, therapy of self-terminating arrhythmias is often not needed.

TREATMENT

Table 4. Common Drugs Used for Postoperative Arrhythmias

Drug	Dose	Indications	Adverse Reactions
Adenosine	6 mg rapid IVP (over 1-2 seconds); if no response within 1-2 minutes then 12 mg IVP; may repeat 12 mg dose if needed	PSVT	Transient heart block, facial flushing, chest pain, hypotension
Amiodarone	150 mg I.V. over 10 minutes, then 1 mg/minute over 6 hours, then 0.5 mg/minute; VF/ pulseless VT: 300 mg in 20-30 mL D_5W or NS IVP	VT or VF; rate control and conversion of AF	Hypotension, bradycardia, exacerbation of CHF, QT prolongation, AV nodal arrhythmias
Atropine	0.5-1 mg I.V. every 5 minutes, not to exceed a total of 3 mg or 0.04 mg/kg	Bradycardia or AV block	Excessive tachycardia, myocardial ischemia
Digoxin	10-15 mcg/kg IBW, divide into 2-3 doses over 6 hours (50% of dose initially, 25% of dose 3 hours later, 25% of dose 3 hours later)	Rate control	Arrhythmias, nausea, vomiting
Diltiazem	0.25 mg/kg I.V. over 2 minutes (20 mg average adult dose); if inadequate response after 15 minutes, 0.35 mg/kg I.V. over 2 minutes (25 mg average adult dose); maintenance infusion: 5-15 mg/hour	Rate control	Hypotension, bradycardia, dizziness, exacerbation of CHF, headache
Esmolol	500 mcg/kg I.V. over 1 minute, followed by infusion of 50 mcg/kg/minute; if inadequate response, repeat bolus after 5 minutes and increase infusion by 50 mcg/ kg/minute; infusion can be titrated to 300 mcg/kg/minute	Rapid rate control	Hypotension, nausea, dizziness, exacerbation of CHF, bronchospasm (dose >200 mcg/ kg/minute)
Ibutilide	1 mg (0.01 mg/kg if <60 kg) I.V. over 10 minutes, may repeat 10 minutes after end of initial infusion	Conversion of AF	QT prolongation, torsade de pointes, headache, hypotension
Lidocaine	1-1.5 mg/kg IVP over 1-1.5 minutes followed by infusion of 1-4 mg/minute (15-50 mcg/kg/ minute), repeat bolus of 0.5-1 mg/kg may be required 5-30 minutes after initial bolus	PVBs; VT; VF	CNS (eg, confusion, paresthesias, tremor, ataxia); seizures, sinus arrest
Metoprolol	5 mg IVP over 1 minute, repeat every 2 minutes for 3 doses	Rate control	Bronchospasm, hypotension, exacerbation of CHF
Procainamide	15-18 mg/kg I.V. over 25-30 minutes or 100-200 mg/dose every 5 minutes as needed to a total dose of 1 g; maintenance infusion of 1-6 mg/minute	VT or VF; ventricular premature beats; AF or A flutter	Hypotension, QT prolongation, torsade de pointes, headache

IVP = intravenous push; CHF = congestive heart failure; IBW = ideal body weight; AV = atrioventricular; PSVT = paroxysmal supraventricular tachycardia; AF = atrial fibrillation; A flutter = atrial flutter; VT = ventricular tachycardia; VF = ventricular fibrillation; PVB = premature ventricular beat.

MANAGEMENT OF POSTOPERATIVE ARRHYTHMIAS *(Continued)*

Bradycardia

Treatment of bradycardia centers on the elimination of factors causing autonomic nervous system imbalance. For example, if bradycardia is due to increased vagal tone, the provoking stimulus should be discontinued. No treatment is necessary if the bradycardia is transient and not associated with hemodynamic compromise. If hypotension occurs, atropine or beta-mimetic medications (eg, ephedrine) should be used to restore sinus rhythm. Cardiac pacing may be necessary in some patients.

Heart Block

Treatment for first-degree heart block is not necessary in the absence of hypotension or severe bradycardia. Treatment for Mobitz type I block is necessary only if bundle branch block, bradycardia, or congestive heart failure occurs. Transvenous pacing may be required. The use of a pacemaker is required for a Mobitz type II block as it may progress to complete heart block. Postoperative patients with high grade second- or third-degree atrioventricular block persisting for >7-14 days should be considered for permanent pacemaker implantation.

Sinus Tachycardia

Sinus tachycardia is common postoperatively, is nearly always associated with a physiologic increase in sympathetic nervous system influence, and is usually harmless. Common causes in the postoperative setting include pain, fever, anxiety, hypovolemia, hypoxemia, anemia, and medications. Treatment should be directed at the underlying cause and not the rhythm. For example, I.V. fluids can be administered for hypovolemia, sedatives for anxiety, and analgesics for pain. If the tachycardia constitutes a risk for myocardial ischemia, continuous use of a beta-blocker may be indicated.

Paroxysmal Supraventricular Tachycardia

AV nodal reentry is the most common paroxysmal supraventricular tachycardia. Sinus rhythm may be restored with carotid sinus massage or other vagal maneuvers. Adenosine is the initial drug of choice for this condition secondary to its short half-life (3-10 seconds) which minimizes its side effect potential. In the presence of circulatory insufficiency, cardioversion may be necessary. Beta-blockers or calcium channel blockers can also be used for this arrhythmia.

Atrial Premature Beats

Atrial premature beats occur when ectopic foci in the atria fire before the next expected impulse from the sinus node. The presence of these beats is common, benign (do not cause hemodynamic compromise), and usually requires no treatment.

Atrial Fibrillation

Prophylaxis. A beta-blocker should be administered preoperatively or early in the postoperative period for patients undergoing CABG surgery. Alternatively, amiodarone or sotalol may be considered for prophylaxis. Propafenone can be used as a prophylactic agent but the patient must be free of CAD. Evidence that these agents routinely reduce hospital length of stay and overall cost is currently lacking. Postoperative continuous atrial pacing in post-CABG patients has been demonstrated to reduce the incidence of atrial fibrillation and length of stay.

Treatment. In postsurgical patients who are hemodynamically unstable, direct current cardioversion (DCC) should be performed. In hemodynamically stable patients, the ventricular rate should be controlled with pharmacologic agents; digoxin is appropriate for mildly symptomatic patients. An intravenous beta-blocker or diltiazem should be used when faster ventricular rate control is needed (eg, symptomatic patient). Most patients with postoperative atrial fibrillation will spontaneously convert to sinus rhythm within 48 hours. Digoxin is the least effective and beta-blockers are the most effective for controlling ventricular response during atrial fibrillation. If this is not the case, anticoagulation with heparin should be considered. Ibutilide can be used to pharmacologically convert the patient to normal sinus rhythm. If pharmacologic conversion is not successful, DCC should be performed; it is not necessary to have the post-CABG patient anticoagulated for 3 weeks prior to attempting DCC.

Atrial Flutter

Atrial flutter is rare in postoperative patients. It is managed similar to atrial fibrillation, with some differences. Rapid atrial pacing may be effective in terminating the atrial flutter, especially when combined with a class IA antiarrhythmic agent. Care must be taken when using antiarrhythmic agents because sufficient slowing of the flutter rate may result in 1:1 conduction across the AV node.

Ventricular Premature Beats

Ventricular premature beats (VPBs) commonly occur in patients with or without cardiac disease. VPBs occurring in healthy individuals with no cardiac disease pose little, if any, risk and do not require treatment. The use of antiarrhythmic agents to suppress complex VPBs in patients with cardiac disease is controversial. Historically, lidocaine has been used for VPB suppression, specifically in the setting of acute myocardial infarction, as VPBs were felt to be a warning arrhythmia for ventricular fibrillation. However, warning arrhythmias are no more common in patients who experience ventricular fibrillation than in those who do not. Hence, treatment of the VPBs with an antiarrhythmic agent is not necessary beyond the routine use of beta-blockers. Although beta-blockers may be effective in suppressing VPBs, they are administered in the post-MI population for mortality reduction.

Nonsustained Ventricular Tachycardia

Nonsustained ventricular tachycardia is a common arrhythmia encountered in the ICU and has been extensively studied in cardiac surgery patients. Treatment is usually not necessary in patients with good ventricular function and the arrhythmia is not predictive of adverse outcomes. Monitoring, however, is required as it may be indicative of an underlying problem such as hypoxia, ischemia, or acidosis. In patients with poor postoperative cardiac output or those who have undergone valve replacement and have thick, hypertrophic hearts, there is an increased risk that nonsustained ventricular tachycardia may progress to sustained ventricular tachycardia or to ventricular fibrillation. It is not certain whether antiarrhythmic agents are beneficial in this situation. Antiarrhythmic agents may be useful in patients with nonsustained ventricular tachycardia who are at very high risk due to poor left ventricles or from hemodynamic instability. Amiodarone is most frequently used. Lidocaine and procainamide may be considered.

Sustained Monomorphic Ventricular Tachycardia

This reentrant arrhythmia is commonly seen >48 hours after myocardial infarction. Management depends on its rate, duration, and extent of underlying cardiac disease. In hemodynamically stable patients felt to be at risk for imminent circulatory collapse, amiodarone, lidocaine, or procainamide can be started. Direct current cardioversion is indicated in hemodynamically unstable patients or those with angina.

Sustained Polymorphic Ventricular Tachycardia

This arrhythmia is most commonly seen in patients with myocardial ischemia or infarction. Most episodes of polymorphic ventricular tachycardia terminate spontaneously. They can, however, lead to hemodynamic instability. Treatment is similar to that seen with monomorphic ventricular tachycardia. Direct current cardioversion should be used in unstable patients while antiarrhythmic agents that do not prolong the QT interval should be employed for sustained episodes. In addition to the treatment employed for the arrhythmia, beta-blockers and I.V. nitroglycerin should be used for the coronary disease present.

MANAGEMENT OF POSTOPERATIVE ARRHYTHMIAS
(Continued)

Torsade de Pointes

This is a rapid form of polymorphic ventricular tachycardia associated with QT prolongation. QT prolongation can be seen with various electrolyte abnormalities (eg, hypomagnesemia, hypokalemia), drugs (eg, type IA or type III antiarrhythmic agents, erythromycin, azole antifungal agents), and conditions such as cerebrovascular accident and hypothyroidism. For an acute episode of torsade de pointes, most patients will require DCC. All patients with suspected torsade de pointes should receive I.V. magnesium (2-6 g I.V. over several minutes followed by continuous infusion of 3-20 mg/minute for 5-48 hours), which suppresses triggered activity, as the benefits of doing so far outweigh the risk associated with it. Patients may also benefit from a short-term isoproterenol infusion until a temporary pacemaker can be inserted to increase ventricular rate.

Ventricular Fibrillation

The presence of postoperative ventricular fibrillation usually indicates severe myocardial ischemia, systemic academia, or hypoxemia. Please refer to the ACLS algorithm for the treatment of ventricular fibrillation *on page 1633*.

REFERENCES AND RECOMMENDED READING

Atlee JL, "Perioperative Cardiac Dysrhythmias: Diagnosis and Management," *Anesthesiology*, 1997, 86(6):1397-424.

Bauman JL and Schoen MD, "Arrhythmias", *Pharmacotherapy: A Pathophysiologic Approach*, DiPiro JT, et al, eds, Stamford CT: Appleton & Lange, 1999, 232-64.

Bigatello LM, "The Postanesthesia Care Unit," *Clinical Anesthesia Procedures of the Massachusetts General Hospital*, Hurford WE, et al, eds, Philadelphia PA: Lippincott Williams & Wilkins, 1998, 601-17.

Chow MSS and White CM, "Cardiac Arrhythmias," *Applied Therapeutics: The Clinical Use of Drugs*, Koda-Kimble MA, et al, eds, Philadelphia PA: Lippincott Williams & Wilkins, 2001, 18(1)-18(36).

Daoud EG, Strickberger SA, Man KC, et al, "Preoperative Amiodarone as Prophylaxis Against Atrial Fibrillation After Heart Surgery," *N Engl J Med*, 1997, 337(25):1785-91.

Eagle KA, Berger PB, Calkins H, et al, "ACC/AHA Guideline Update for Perioperative Cardiovascular Evaluation for Noncardiac Surgery - Executive Summary: A Report of the American College of Cardiology/American Heart Association Task Force on Practice Guidelines (Committee to Update the 1996 Guidelines on Perioperative Cardiovascular Evaluation for Noncardiac Surgery)," *J Am Coll Cardiol*, 2002, 39(3):542-53.

Forrest JB, Cahalan MK, Rehder K, et al, "Multicenter Study of General Anesthesia. II. Results," *Anesthesiology*, 1990, 72(2):262-8.

Gomes JA, Ip J, Santoni-Rugiu F, et al, "Oral d,l Sotalol Reduces the Incidence of Postoperative Atrial Fibrillation in Coronary Artery Bypass Surgery Patients: A Randomized, Double-Blind, Placebo-Controlled Study," *J Am Coll Cardiol*, 1999, 34(2):334-9.

Guarnieri T, Nolan S, Gottlieb SO, et al, "Intravenous Amiodarone for the Prevention of Atrial Fibrillation After Open-Heart Surgery: The Amiodarone Reduction in Coronary Heart (ARCH) Trial," *J Am Coll Cardiol*, 1999, 34(2):343-7.

"Guidelines 2000 for Cardiopulmonary Resuscitation and Emergency Cardiovascular Care: An International Consensus on Science," *Circulation*, 2000, 102:Supplement I.

Hillel Z and Thys DM, "Electrocardiography," *Anesthesia*, Miller RD, ed, Philadelphia PA: Churchill Livingstone, 2000, 1231-54.

Hollenberg SM and Dellinger RP, "Noncardiac Surgery: Postoperative Arrhythmias," *Crit Care Med*, 2000, 28(10 Suppl):N145-50.

Mahla E, Rotman B, Rehak P, et al, "Perioperative Ventricular Dysrhythmias in Patients With Structural Heart Disease Undergoing Noncardiac Surgery," *Anesth Analg*, 1998, 86(1):16-21.

Mecca RS, "Postoperative Recovery," *Clinical Anesthesia*, Barash PG, et al, eds, Philadelphia PA: Lippincott Williams & Wilkins, 1997, 1279-303.

Napolitano C, Priori SG, and Schwartz PJ, "Torsade de Pointes. Mechanisms and Management," *Drugs*, 1994, 47(1):51-65.

Ramsay JG, "Cardiac Management in the ICU," *Chest*, 1999, 115(5 Suppl):138S-144S.

Redle JD, Khurana S, Marzan R, et al, "Prophylactic Oral Amiodarone Compared With Placebo for Prevention of Atrial Fibrillation After Coronary Artery Bypass Surgery," *Am Heart J*, 1999, 138(1 Pt 1):144-50.

Rho RW, Bridges CR, and Kocovic D, "Management of Postoperative Arrhythmias," *Semin Thorac Cardiovasc Surg*, 2000, 12(4):349-61.

Tisdale JE, Padhi ID, Goldberg AD, et al, "A Randomized, Double-Blind Comparison of Intravenous Diltiazem and Digoxin for Atrial Fibrillation After Coronary Artery Bypass Surgery," *Am Heart J*, 1998, 135(5 Pt 1):739-47.

VanderLugt JT, Mattioni T, Denker S, et al, "Efficacy and Safety of Ibutilide Fumarate for the Conversion of Atrial Arrhythmias After Cardiac Surgery," *Circulation*, 1999, 100(4):369-75.

White CM, Caron MF, Kalus JS, et al, "Intravenous Plus Oral Amiodarone, Atrial Septal Pacing, or Both Strategies to Prevent Postcardiothoracic Surgery Atrial Fibrillation: The Atrial Fibrillation Suppression Trial II (AFIST II)," *Circulation*, 2003, 108 (Suppl 1):II200-6.

PERIOPERATIVE MANAGEMENT OF PATIENTS ON ANTISEIZURE MEDICATION

The pathophysiologic conditions that produce seizure activation and the drugs used to treat or prevent it will be discussed in addition to the recommended perioperative management for these situations.

ETIOLOGY OF SEIZURES

Brain injury:	Trauma, surgery, subarachnoid hemorrhage
Hypoxia/ischemia:	Stroke, cardiac arrest, shock, hypotension, hypoxemia, cerebral edema
Infection:	Meningitis, encephalitis, abscess
Metabolic:	Electrolyte abnormalities, hepatic or renal failure, hyperglycemia, hypoglycemia, genetic metabolic abnormalities
Drug toxicity:	Alcohol, cocaine, metrizamide
Pathologic states:	Drug withdrawal, eclampsia, cerebral tumor, AVM, cortical vein thrombosis
Idiopathic epilepsy:	Etiology unknown

TYPES OF SEIZURES

Seizures are recurrent, synchronous, rhythmic firings of cortical neurons. Seizures are classified into five major groups.

Classification of Seizures

1. Generalized seizures
   a. Excitatory (myoclonic, clonic/tonic)
   b. Inhibitors (absence, atonic)
2. Partial seizures
   a. Simple partial
   b. Complex partial
   c. Partial onset with generalization
3. Pseudoseizures
4. Status epilepticus
5. Unclassified seizures

Generalized Seizures

Excitatory seizures occur over the entire brain with no obvious focal onset. They may present with an aura followed by tonic-clonic motor activity. Loss of consciousness occurs along with loss of bladder and bowel sphincter tone. The patient becomes apneic with absence of respiratory effort. During the postictal period, the patient may be somnolent or confused. Seizure treatment is supportive, assuring ventilation/oxygenation and preventing the patient from becoming injured from the motor activity.

Inhibitory seizures include absence seizures (petit mal) and atonic seizures (person loses motor tone and falls down).

Partial Seizures

Partial seizure activity has a focal onset and is frequently asymptomatic (aura or simple seizure). Intracranial EEG recordings are often necessary to identify this type of seizure. Bilateral seizure activity must be sustained for at least 10-30 seconds before a physical manifestation occurs. The clinical response depends on the area of the brain containing the seizure focus (ie, uncontrollable hand moving = precentral gyrus; laughing, crying, fear = limbic; visual light flashes = occipital). These complex seizures are frequently termed psychomotor or temporal lobe seizures. When the seizure activity spreads throughout the entire brain it is called secondary generalization which presents as either tonic or clonic seizures.

Pseudoseizures

Pseudoseizures have no EEG abnormality and are usually attributed to malingering or the psychiatric condition of conversion disorder.

Status Epilepticus

Seizures are usually short-lived; however, when they are prolonged or recur without the patient regaining consciousness, the condition is called status epilepticus. Over 60,000 cases of status epilepticus occur per year in the United States. The longer the episode of untreated or inadequately treated status epilepticus, the more difficult it is to control and the greater the risk of permanent brain damage. Ventilation may need to be controlled since most of the drugs used to treat this condition can produce respiratory insufficiency.

Recommended Acute Intravenous Drug Therapy

1. Diazepam (0.2 mg/kg) or lorazepam (0.1-0.22 mg/kg) in adults. Watch for recurrence of seizures when the benzodiazepine redistributes from the brain, decreasing brain concentration.

   OR

2. Phenytoin (15-20 mg/kg in adults) and the prodrug fosphenytoin (15-20 mg/kg phenytoin equivalents [PE]) effectively treats 41% to 90% of patients. Phenytoin cannot be administered faster than 50 mg/minute without significant hypotension. Fosphenytoin can be administered up to a maximum rate of 150 mg PE/minute. It can be administered at a faster rate than phenytoin because it has fewer cardiovascular side effects.

   OR

3. Phenobarbital (20 mg/kg in adults) is also effective, however, this drug has a prolonged half-life and it is difficult to differentiate between drug-induced sedation vs postictal state vs other CNS concerns.

If these drug therapies are unsuccessful, general anesthesia using an inhalational agent (excluding enflurane, which has the potential to produce EEG seizure activity) can be used. This therapy is a temporizing measure, for upon withdrawal of the anesthetic gas the seizures may recommence.

Unclassified Seizures

Not all seizures are epileptic seizures, for example, alcohol withdrawal or toxic brain injury from liver failure. These seizures usually present with tonic/clonic activity.

PERIOPERATIVE MANAGEMENT OF PATIENTS ON ANTISEIZURE MEDICATION *(Continued)*

SEIZURE CLASSIFICATION AND SUGGESTED DRUG THERAPY

Type	Clinical Features	Drug Therapy
Generalized		
Myoclonic	Isolated clonic jerks	Valproic acid Phenobarbital Clonazepam Topiramate
Absence	Brief loss of consciousness; staring; little or no motor activity	Valproic acid Ethosuximide Clonazepam
Partial		
Simple partial	Focal motor or sensory disturbances	Valproic acid Carbamazepine Gabapentin Phenytoin Fosphenytoin Lamotrigine Topiramate Tiagabine Zonisamide
Complex partial	Aura; bizarre behavior with impaired consciousness	Valproic acid Carbamazepine Gabapentin Phenytoin Fosphenytoin Lamotrigine Topiramate Tiagabine Zonisamide
Status epilepticus	Continual seizure activity	Diazepam Phenytoin Fosphenytoin Phenobarbital

PATHOPHYSIOLOGY OF SEIZURES

As the mechanisms that produce seizure activity become evident, the use of specific antiseizure drugs becomes more logical. It is thought that partial seizures result from a reduction of inhibitory or an increase of excitatory synaptic activity. High frequency neuronal firing also produces seizures. Inactivation of the inner gate of the sodium channel prolongs the time the channels are inactive and inhibits rapid firing. This is probably the mechanism of action for carbamazepine, phenytoin, and valproate.

Another mechanism of seizure modulation involves GABA (gamma amino butyric acid) mediated synaptic inhibition, which reduces neuronal excitability and raises the seizure threshold. Activation of the GABAa receptor inhibits the postsynaptic neuron whereas a decrease in GABA receptor number or activity allows the unopposed excitatory activity to dominate. Benzodiazepines and barbiturates activate GABA receptors. Vigabatrin and valproate reduce the metabolism of GABA, and gabapentin enhances release of GABA from presynaptic cells.

Generalized seizures arise from reciprocal firing between the thalamus and cortex. Thalamic stimulation produces the 3/second spike and wave EEG pattern of absence seizures. These seizures are produced by voltage-regulated calcium currents. Drugs such as ethosuximide, trimethadione, and valproic acid inhibit this low threshold current.

PRINCIPLES OF SEIZURE THERAPY

Determine the cause of the seizure. Initiate therapy with a single drug. If this drug does not provide adequate control, another drug should be substituted. When discontinuing a drug, reduce the dosage gradually to prevent status epilepticus. Monitor for toxicity.

PERIOPERATIVE MANAGEMENT: THE PATIENT WITH EPILEPSY

For patients with epilepsy, it is important to maintain adequate antiseizure drug levels during the perioperative period. Since many seizure medications only exist as oral drugs, this needs to be taken into consideration, especially for long surgical procedures. Patients receiving antiseizure drug therapy are resistant to neuromuscular blocking agents, requiring both higher blood levels and more frequent dosing.

Anesthetic management includes continuation of the anticonvulsant therapy and avoidance of drugs that stimulate seizure activity (enflurane, methohexital). High-dose opioids and etomidate have been implicated in producing seizures; however, these drugs induce muscle hypertonus, producing a myoclonic action which can be mistaken for seizure activity. The only narcotic that has demonstrated seizure activity in humans is meperidine. Its metabolite normeperidine has a long half-life and is a known CNS stimulant. It has produced seizures in patients with renal failure and in cancer patients receiving large doses of meperidine over a prolonged time. It is a central sympathetic stimulant, but it also blocks neuronal NMDA receptor activation. (NMDA receptors are activated by glutamate, the major brain excitatory neurotransmitter.) These drug recommendations are not absolute.

PERIOPERATIVE MANAGEMENT: EXCISION OF SEIZURE FOCUS

When chronic medical therapy is unsuccessful in controlling epileptic seizures, patients may undergo craniotomy for resection of the epileptic foci. For these patients, their antiseizure medications are usually reduced or withdrawn prior to surgery to enhance identification of seizure prone tissue. Craniotomy may be performed under general anesthesia or local anesthesia with I.V. sedation, depending on the surgeon's preference, the patient's ability to cooperate, and the site of the seizure foci. The depth of anesthesia and/or sedation must be light enough not to mask seizure activity (ie, patients should not receive large doses of drugs that depress EEG activity or elevate the seizure threshold). Electrocorticography, or mapping the brain electrical activity using intraoperative cortical surface electrodes, identifies the target areas. Because anticonvulsant medications are discontinued preoperatively, there is a high possibility of stimulating generalized seizure activity, which needs to be treated so the sedated patient does not injure himself. For patients anesthetized with general anesthesia and muscle relaxants, the induced seizure activity may be less obvious. In either case, treatment is needed; however, large doses of long-acting anticonvulsants (eg, phenobarbital) may limit the sensitivity of additional electrocorticography.

PREGNANCY

Stillbirth and infant mortality are higher in epileptic mothers taking antiseizure medication during pregnancy. There is a significant correlation with multidrug therapy and higher blood drug levels. Teratogenicity is greatest for trimethadione. Valproate is associated with spinal bifida and neural tube defects. Carbamazepine is associated with craniofacial defects, fingernail hypoplasia, and developmental delays. The formation of epoxide intermediates from carbamazepine and phenytoin metabolism is associated with fetal malformation. However, this does not mean that every epileptic female should discontinue her antiseizure medications. Pregnant women should continue their antiseizure medication if needed for their safety. The effects of hypoxemia on the fetus from seizure-induced respiratory depression are more dangerous than seizure medication. The recommendations are to keep the dosage as small as possible, administer drugs in divided doses to avoid peak blood levels, and limit therapy to only one drug if at all possible.

PERIOPERATIVE MANAGEMENT OF PATIENTS ON ANTISEIZURE MEDICATION *(Continued)*

ECLAMPSIA

Pregnant women with preeclampsia routinely receive magnesium sulfate seizure prophylaxis treatment even though it is still debatable as to whether magnesium sulfate is an anticonvulsant. Because magnesium blocks calcium entry into myocytes, it causes smooth (vascular, uterine) muscle relaxation with a synergistic interaction with nondepolarizing muscle relaxants (ie, vecuronium, pancuronium). Magnesium is cleared via the kidney and must be given cautiously when renal function is decreased.

SUBARACHNOID HEMORRHAGE / HEAD TRAUMA

Seizures frequently occur with subarachnoid hemorrhage associated with rupture of a cerebral aneurysm or with head trauma. It is routine clinical practice to prophylactically treat these patients with antiseizure medication (primarily phenytoin). The benefit of seizure prophylaxis needs to be weighed against the side effects of the drug therapy.

FEBRILE SEIZURES

Although 2% to 4% of children experience a seizure during a febrile illness, only 2% to 3% of them will develop epilepsy later in life. This is a sixfold higher risk than in the general population. Febrile seizures do **not** have an infectious or metabolic origin within the CNS (eg, not produced by meningitis/encephalitis). Factors associated with this increased risk are pre-existing neurologic disorder, a family history of epilepsy, or a complicated febrile seizure (ie, lasting longer than 15 minutes or followed by another seizure within 24 hours). Fever is usually >102°F. The more rapid the rise in temperature, the greater the likelihood for seizure development. The most common age is between 3 months and 5 years. Adults can also experience febrile seizures. The use of chronic prophylactic antiseizure therapy is questionable because of the drug side effects, especially with regards to cognitive function. Temporary prophylaxis may be useful in subsequent febrile episodes (diazepam 0.33 mg/kg every 8 hours during the fever).

MAJOR ANTISEIZURE DRUGS AND SIDE EFFECTS

Name	Dose-Related Side Effect	Toxic Effect
Carbamazepine	Double vision, lethargy, leukopenia, photosensitivity	Skin rash, blood dyscrasia, hepatic/renal dysfunction, acute intermittent porphyria, Stevens-Johnson syndrome
Diazepam	Depression, lethargy, nystagmus, muscle weakness	Hypotension, respiratory depression
Lamotrigine	Somnolence, diplopia, ataxia	Rash, nausea
Phenobarbital	Irritability, lethargy, hallucinations	Rash, respiratory depression, hypotension
Phenytoin, Fosphenytoin	Ataxia, gingival hyperplasia, hirsutism, nystagmus	Neuropathy, rash, lupus (Stevens-Johnson), blood dyscrasia, hypotension, bradycardia
Tiagabine	Dizziness, CNS depression, tremor, ataxia, myalgia	Hepatic/renal dysfunction
Topiramate	Psychomotor slowing, speech problems, somnolence, weight loss, kidney stones	Metabolic acidosis
Valproic acid	Tremor, somnolence, anorexia, alopecia	Hepatic failure, thrombocytopenia
Zonisamide	Somnolence, dizziness, ataxia	Oligohydrosis, hepatic/renal dysfunction

PHARMACOKINETIC PRINCIPLES

1. Tight capillary endothelial junctions limit the passage of water soluble drugs (eg, phenytoin, carbamazepine) into the brain while permitting the rapid transit of lipid soluble drugs (benzodiazepines, barbiturates).
2. The therapeutic effect obtained from active drug concentration depends on drug absorption and bioavailability (ie, phenytoin binds to enteral feedings, which decrease drug absorption from the gastrointestinal tract).
3. Barbiturates enhance cytochrome P450 enzymes, which increase hepatic metabolism of antiseizure drugs.
4. Most antiseizure drugs are bound to plasma proteins. Therefore, a decrease in protein production in the severely ill patient can acutely increase the concentration of free active drug. Because alcohol and metoclopramide have greater plasma protein binding affinity, the benzodiazepine free fraction will increase with coadministration. It is recommended to assay for free drug rather than for total drug concentration for a better understanding of drug availability/activity.
5. Volume of distribution/redistribution. The first phase of distribution delivers antiseizure drugs directly to the brain for a rapid onset of action. During the second phase of distribution (called redistribution) the drug moves out of the brain and equilibrates with the total body's volume of distribution, thus decreasing brain concentration and diminishing the acute drug effect. During the third phase, the drug moves into adipose tissue and is slowly released into the circulation over time, thus slowly terminating drug concentration following discontinuation of the lipid soluble medication.
6. Metabolism of most antiepileptic drugs follows first order kinetics (ie, a constant rate is metabolized). Phenytoin demonstrates saturation kinetics. When the enzymes responsible for phenytoin become saturated, additional doses are not metabolized at the same rate and higher blood levels occur. This is important because the drug level increases exponentially after enzyme saturation occurs, which is at approximately 10 mcg/mL - the lower therapeutic level for phenytoin.
7. The therapeutic target drug level is the one at which the patient stops seizing. This is the level that provides the best protection from seizures; however, it may not be the best level regarding side effects.

REFERENCES AND RECOMMENDED READING

Litt B and Krauss GL, "Pharmacologic Approach to Acute Seizures and Antiepileptic Drugs P484-506," Chernow B, ed, *The Pharmacologic Approach to the Critically Ill Patient*, 3rd ed, Baltimore, MD: Williams & Wilkins, 1994, 484-506.

McNamara JO, "Drugs Effective in the Therapy of the Epilepsies," Gardman JG, Limbird LE, eds, *Goodman & Gilman's The Pharmacological Basis of Therapeutics*, 9th ed, New York, NY: McGraw Hill, 1996, 461-86.

Miller JW and Anderson HH, "The Effect of N-demethylation on Certain Pharmacologic Actions of Morphine, Codeine, and Meperidine in the Mouse," *J Pharmacol Exp Ther*, 1954, 112(2):191-6.

Rosman NP, Colton T, Labazzo J, et al, "A Controlled Trial of Diazepam Administered During Febrile Illnesses to Prevent Recurrence of Febrile Seizures," *N Engl J Med*, 1993, 329(2):79-84.

Runge JW and Allen FH, "Emergency Treatment of Status Epilepticus," *Neurology*, 1996, 46(6 Suppl 1):S20-3.

Szeto HH, "Accumulation of Normeperidine, An Active Metabolite of Meperidine in Patients With Renal Failure or Cancer," *Ann Int Med*, 1977, 86(6):738-41.

PERIOPERATIVE MANAGEMENT OF THE DIABETIC PATIENT

Diabetes is a disease that necessitates close consideration in the patient undergoing surgery due to the complexity of the disease and high risk of cardiovascular and/or renal complications. A review of the classification, associated diseases, risks and management of perioperative insulin, oral hypoglycemics, and glucose will be discussed.

CLASSIFICATION

Diabetes mellitus is classified as Type 1 (formerly, insulin-dependent diabetes mellitus) or Type 2 (formerly, noninsulin-dependent diabetes mellitus). The following table describes the general characteristics of the Type 1 and 2 diabetic patient.

	Type 1 (Insulin-Dependent)	**Type 2 (Noninsulin-Dependent)**
Age at onset	Juvenile	Adult
Insulin secretion	Very low	Normal or high
Physical characteristic	Lean	Obese
Response to insulin	Sensitive	Resistant
Ketosis likelihood	High	Low
Hereditary influence	Moderate	Great
Treatment	Insulin	Diet, oral agents, insulin

Characterizations are general; there may be overlap between the two types. Note that Type 2 diabetes may also be treated with insulin.

Modified from Morgan GE and Mikhail MS, "Anesthesia for Patients With Endocrine Disease," *Clinical Anesthesiology*, 2nd ed, Stamford, CT: Appleton and Lange, 1996, 637-49.

ASSOCIATED DISEASES AND PERIOPERATIVE RISKS

In the perioperative setting, mortality and morbidity is higher in both types of diabetes when compared to the nondiabetic patient. Diabetic patients undergoing major surgery will spend approximately 30% to 50% more time in the hospital, compared to a nondiabetic patient.

The perioperative mortality rate of the diabetic patient ranges between 3.7% to 13%. The major causes are secondary to cardiovascular complications and postoperative infections. Increased morbidity in the diabetic patient is secondary to their response to surgical procedures as well as underlying complications caused by the disease state.

ENDOCRINE AND METABOLIC RESPONSE TO SURGERY IN DIABETIC PATIENTS

Endocrine

- Increased secretion of counterregulatory hormones: Catecholamines, glucagon, cortisol (predominantly catabolic hormones), and growth hormone
- Decreased insulin secretion causes a loss of anticatabolic effects of insulin
- Decreased insulin action due to increased insulin resistance secondary to the counterregulatory hormones

Metabolic

- Increased hepatic glucose production leading to hyperglycemia
- Decreased glucose disposal (utilization)
- Increased glucose production secondary to glycogenolysis and gluconeogenesis
- Increased net protein catabolism
- Variable increase in lipolysis with ketone bodies formation
- General increase in metabolic rate and catabolism

Immediate and Long-Term Effects

- Dehydration and hemodynamic instability due to osmotic diuresis and volume loss during surgery
- Loss of lean body mass, negative nitrogen balance, impaired wound healing, decreased resistance to infection
- Loss of adipose tissue and energy reserve from fatty acids
- Deficiency of essential amino acids, vitamins, and minerals

In addition to the above, the diabetic patient is predisposed to disease-state complications. These complications include:

Dermopathy

Macrovascular disease – coronary atherosclerosis, peripheral vascular disease

Microvascular disease – nephropathy, retinopathy

Neuropathy – Distal polyneuropathies, neuromuscular disease, acute mononeuropathy, autonomic neuropathy (gastrointestinal, genitourinary, cardiovascular)

Because many diabetic patients have coronary artery disease, autonomic neuropathies and impaired renal function, their perioperative management must be vigilant in order to prevent significant complications. Furthermore, diabetics may present with asymptomatic cardiac ischemia. If undetected preoperatively, these patients are more likely to have an ischemic event during the perioperative time. If the patient suffers from cardiovascular autonomic neuropathy, he/she will be more likely to experience hypotension during induction of anesthesia, arrhythmias during the surgical procedure, and have an inadequate response to drugs such as atropine when used for treatment of bradycardia. In addition, many diabetic patients are predisposed to dehydration due to osmotic diuresis caused by glycosuria and electrolyte imbalance secondary to renal insufficiency, which can affect intraoperative and postoperative fluid management. It is for these reasons that comprehensive preoperative assessment of the diabetic patient by the physician and/or anesthesiologist is important.

PREOPERATIVE ASSESSMENT

A preoperative evaluation of the diabetic patient undergoing a surgical procedure should include the following:

Identification of Diabetes Type

- Type 1 – absolute need for continual insulin therapy
- Type 2 – associated with increased insulin needs

Determination of Level of Preceding Glycemic Control

- Self-monitoring of blood glucose levels – review blood glucose records
- Review glycosylated hemoglobin levels
- Frequency, timing, and severity of hypoglycemia

Determination of Presence of Diabetic Complications

- Nephropathy – fluid balance, hypotension, drug dosage
- Autonomic aeuropathy – cardiovascular response (arrhythmias, postural hypotension), gastrointestinal (gastroparesis, postoperative nausea or vomiting), bladder dysfunction (urinary retention)
- Retinopathy
- Peripheral vascular disease

Assessment of Operative Risk

- Cardiovascular disease, hypertension, congestive heart failure
- Pulmonary
- Renal
- Hematologic

PERIOPERATIVE MANAGEMENT OF THE DIABETIC PATIENT *(Continued)*

Pharmacological Regimen

- Medication type, dosage, and timing

Anticipated Surgery

- Type of procedure
- Type of anesthesia
- Duration of procedure

Complete blood count, electrolyte panel, renal function, and baseline electrocardiogram should be assessed. If the diabetic patient experiences cardiovascular, autonomic, or renal complications preoperatively, the patient should be optimized before undergoing the surgical procedure. In addition, control of these conditions must be maintained and closely evaluated throughout the surgical procedure to prevent increased morbidity and/or increased mortality.

PERIOPERATIVE INSULIN / GLUCOSE MANAGEMENT

Over the years, the management of perioperative glucose and insulin administration has changed. The one fact that remains consistent, however, is that the perioperative glucose and hypoglycemic agent of choice be diligently managed. The goal is to avoid hypoglycemia and prevent significant hyperglycemia. The usual desire is to maintain blood glucose between 120-180 mg/dL. Perioperative hyperglycemia increases morbidity for the diabetic patient and predisposes the patient to the following: infection, decreased wound healing, worsened neurologic outcome in the face of cerebral ischemia, and loss of metabolic control. Adequate management must start in the preoperative setting and follow through into the postoperative period.

Indications for Insulin Therapy During Major Surgery

Always	All insulin-taking diabetes (Type 1 and Type 2)
	Type 2 treated with diet and/or oral hypoglycemic agents, but with chronic hypoglycemia (fasting blood glucose [FBS] 100 mg/dL and glycosylated hemoglobin [HbA_{1c}] >10%)
Sometimes	Type 2 treated with diet or oral hypoglycemic agents and in acceptable control
	Average fasting blood glucose ≤140 mg/dL GHB >10% Surgery duration - 2 hours Body cavity not invaded Food intake anticipated after operation

INSULIN-TREATED / INSULIN-REQUIRING PATIENTS

Major Surgery

There are two methods for administering insulin in the perioperative setting. The first is administration of 33% to 50% of the patient's normal intermediate-acting insulin dose (ie, NPH) the morning of surgery. This method is sometimes referred to as the "split-dose method." The insulin dose should be administered after arrival at the hospital, after the morning blood glucose level is checked, and after the intravenous line is started for administration of a dextrose infusion. If the patient becomes hypoglycemic (<100 mg/dL) or hyperglycemic (>180 mg/dL) intraoperatively, intravenous dextrose or regular insulin, administered subcutaneously based on a sliding scale, should be given respectively. If insulin is administered as an intravenous bolus, its duration of action is only 20 minutes; therefore requiring frequent glucose evaluations and repeat boluses.

Regular Insulin Dosing Sliding Scale

Blood Glucose (mg/dL)	Regular Insulin (units)
<180	0
180-220	6
221-260	8
261-300	10
>300	12

Because of the potential for either hypoglycemia or hyperglycemia with this method, it is rarely the method of choice for perioperative insulin administration in the patient requiring a lengthy major surgical procedure. This method, however, is still commonly used in the insulin-requiring diabetic undergoing minor surgical procedures.

The second method for perioperative insulin administration is the continuous infusion method. This is a recommended method and is preferred because it allows for a more predictable and accurate way of administering insulin. For the brittle diabetic patient and patients that will have changing insulin requirements, it is advisable to use a separate insulin and dextrose infusion perioperatively.

Guidelines for Perioperative Diabetes Management With a Separate Insulin Infusion

- Insulin: Regular (human) 25 units in 250 mL of normal saline (1 unit/10 mL)
- Intravenous infusion of insulin: Flush 50 mL through line before connecting to patient; piggyback insulin line to perioperative maintenance fluid line
- Perioperative maintenance fluid: Fluids must contain 5% dextrose (rate: 100 mL/hour)
- Blood glucose: Monitor hourly intraoperatively; blood glucose value divided by 150 gives a reasonable estimate of infusion dosage (units/hour):

Blood Glucose	Insulin	
(mg/dL)	(units/h)	(mL/h)
<80	0.0	0.0
81-100	0.5	5.0
101-140	1.0	10
141-180	1.5	15
181-220	2.0	20
221-260	2.5	25
261-300	3.0	30
301-340	4.0	40
>341	5.0	50

- Blood glucose <80 mg/dL: Stop insulin and administer intravenous bolus of 50% dextrose in water (25 mL); once glucose >80 mg/dL, restart insulin infusion. It may be necessary to modify the algorithm.
- Decreased insulin needs: Patients treated with diet or oral agents, or <50 units insulin/day, endocrinologic deficiencies
- Increased insulin needs: Obesity, sepsis, steroid therapy, renal transplant, coronary artery bypass

PERIOPERATIVE MANAGEMENT OF THE DIABETIC PATIENT *(Continued)*

The approximate amount of regular insulin required by the patient can also be determined by the following formula:

units/hour = plasma glucose/150

The combination of insulin and glucose in a single I.V. bag is suitable treatment for those patients whose insulin requirements will remain steady throughout the surgical procedure.

The typical diabetic patient usually requires 0.5-3 units/hour of insulin. However, the following patients have a tendency toward insulin resistance and may require larger doses of insulin:

Obese: 2-3 units/hour of insulin
Sepsis: 3-4 units/hour of insulin
Corticosteroid therapy: 3-4 units/hour of insulin
CABG: 4-6 units/hour of insulin

For all patients receiving an insulin infusion for a major surgical procedure, blood glucose should be monitored every hour during and after the surgical procedure. Potassium levels should also be closely monitored because glucose/insulin will shift potassium intracellularly. For this reason, patients with normal potassium levels should have at least 20 mEq/L of potassium added to their perioperative maintenance fluids and adjust the amount according to the level.

Minor Surgery

For Type 1 diabetic patients undergoing minor surgical procedures or invasive diagnostic procedures, the administration of insulin is similar to that of the major surgical procedures. The "split-dose" insulin administration method is commonly used in this setting. The blood glucose monitoring is, however, less intense. These patients should have their blood glucose monitored every 1-4 hours, which is in contrast to every 1 hour for the patient undergoing a major surgical procedure.

ORAL HYPOGLYCEMIC TREATMENT

The diabetic patient taking an oral hypoglycemic agent for their disease state may be managed similar to the insulin requiring diabetic perioperatively or slightly different, depending on the length and type of surgical procedure. The oral hypoglycemic agent should be stopped before surgery. The following table is a list of the oral hypoglycemic agents currently available, their duration of action, and when they should be discontinued before surgery.

Agent	Duration (h)	Discontinue Prior to Surgery
Sulfonylureas, first-generation		
Chlorpropamide	24-72	24-72 h
Tolazamide	12-24	Day of surgery
Tolbutamide	6-24	Day of surgery
Sulfonylureas, second-generation		
Glimepiride	24	Day of surgery
Glipizide	12-24	Day of surgery
Glyburide	16-24	Day of surgery
Nonsulfonylureas		
Acarbose	?	?
Metformin	12	24-48 h
Pioglitazone	24	24 h
Repaglinide	24	?
Rosiglitazone	12-24	24 h
Troglitazone	24	?

Diabetic patients taking an oral hypoglycemic drug and undergoing a prolonged major surgical procedure should be managed like the insulin-requiring diabetic patient perioperatively. For the diabetic patient taking an oral hypoglycemic agent undergoing minor surgical procedures, the goal is "no glucose - no insulin." These patients should not receive dextrose-containing fluids or insulin, and must have their blood glucose checked before the surgical or invasive diagnostic procedure and again postoperatively. The patient should receive insulin, *if and only if*, the blood glucose is elevated. Regular insulin should be administered subcutaneously based on a sliding scale according to the blood glucose level.

POSTOPERATIVE MANAGEMENT

The immediate postoperative management of the diabetic patient is as critical as the intraoperative management. The following describes the postoperative management of the diabetic patient.

1. Continue perioperative insulin infusion until food is tolerated, then plan new regimen
2. Overlap (30-60 minutes) the initial subcutaneous dose of regular insulin before stopping insulin infusion
3. Type 2 previously treated with diet or oral hypoglycemic agent: Prescribe usual medication if BG is <180 mg/dL; elevated BG may administer regular insulin as per sliding scale; see *Regular Insulin Dosing Sliding Scale* table
4. Insulin-treated diabetics: Prescribe usual regimen or use prior 24- to 48-hour insulin dosage to develop a new basic dose regimen. Dose selected should be 80% to 100% of the previous day's total dose. Insulin requirements may be greater during persistent stress, infection, pain, steroid therapy, or high food intake (total parenteral nutrition); selected basic dose may be given premeal:

   Breakfast (25%) regular insulin
   Lunch (25%) regular insulin
   Dinner (25%) regular insulin
   Bedtime (25%) NPH insulin

   Aim to keep BG in a safe range (120-180 mg/dL)

Premeal Blood Glucose (mg/dL)	Basic Dose (regular insulin)
<80	4 units less
81-120	3 units less
121-180	Basic dose (no adjustment)
181-240	2 units more
241-300	3 units more
>300	4 units more

1. Modify the basic dose regularly (every 1-2 days) according to the sliding scale needs; additional doses of regular insulin may be needed at other times (eg, 10 PM, 2 AM)
2. Establish the most suitable insulin regimen or the patient's previous regimen before patient discharge

PERIOPERATIVE MANAGEMENT OF THE DIABETIC PATIENT *(Continued)*

CONCLUSION

The above recommendations are only guidelines. It is important to realize that the physician must individualize diabetic treatment based on the patient's coexisting diseases, type of diabetes, hypoglycemic agent, and surgical procedure. The health care professional must also remember that the disease-state complications of the diabetic patient (ie, cardiac, renal, fluid/electrolyte abnormalities) are major concerns in the perioperative setting. The associated diseases should always be optimized preoperatively and monitored closely in the intraoperative and postoperative period. Goal should be the prevention of complications as a result of hyperglycemia in the surgical patient.

REFERENCES AND RECOMMENDED READING

Boord JB, Graber AL, Christman JW, et al, "Practical Management of Diabetes in Critically Ill Patients," *Am J Respir Crit Care Med,* 2001, 164(10 Pt 1):1763-7.

Christoperson R, "Anesthesia for Endocrine Surgery," *Principles and Practice in Anesthesiology,* Rogers MC, Tinker JH, Covino BG, et al, St Louis, MO: CV Mosby Co, 1992, 2035-48.

Clement S, Braithwaite SS, Magee MF, et al, "Management of Diabetes and Hyperglycemia in Hospitals," *Diabetes Care,* 2004, 27(2):553-91.

Gavin LA, "Perioperative Management of the Diabetic Patient," *Endocrinol Metab Clin North Am,* 1992, 21(2):457-75.

Jacober SJ and Sowers JR, "An Update on Perioperative Management of Diabetes," *Arch Intern Med,* 1999, 159(20):2405-11.

Marks JB, "Perioperative Management of Diabetes," *Am Fam Physician,* 2003, 67(1):93-100.

Morgan GE and Mikhail MS, "Anesthesia for Patients With Endocrine Disease," *Clinical Anesthesiology,* 2nd ed, Stamford, CT: Appleton and Lange, 1996, 637-49.

Walts LF, Miller J, Davidson MB, et al, "Perioperative Management of Diabetes Mellitus," *Anesthesiology,* 1981, 55(2):104-9.

POSTOPERATIVE HYPERTENSION

It has been estimated that the overall incidence of postoperative hypertension (HTN) is approximately 3%. However, a higher incidence is seen with select surgical procedures (Table 1). It has been demonstrated that more than 50% of patients who develop postoperative HTN have pre-existing hypertension. Patients who do not take/receive their antihypertensive medications on the day of surgery are especially prone to present with hypertension postoperatively. Therefore, it is important to counsel patients to take their antihypertensive medications up until their surgical procedures.

Table 1. Incidence of Postoperative Hypertension

Surgery	Incidence
Abdominal aortic surgery	33% to 75%
Coronary artery bypass surgery	30% to 60%
Carotid endarterectomy	9% to 64%
Peripheral vascular surgery	29%
Neurosurgery	7% to 91%
Intraperitoneal or intrathoracic surgery	8%

Postoperative HTN has been defined in various manners (Table 2). A key point to keep in mind is that a diagnosis of postoperative hypertension should be made by considering the patient's preoperative blood pressure. A 20% increase over the baseline often defines treatment threshold; however, as always, each patient must be assessed on an individual basis. Most episodes of postoperative HTN are classified as hypertensive urgency (an increase in systemic arterial pressure without immediate risk of end-organ damage). It can result in various complications, some of them severe (Table 3), but there is no consensus among clinicians about when or how aggressively to treat postsurgical hypertension in the noncardiac surgery patient. Treatment is frequently made at the bedside taking into account the patient's underlying medical conditions. Cardiovascular surgery patients who develop postoperative hypertension are treated aggressively.

Table 2. Definitions of Postoperative Hypertension

- MAP >110 mm Hg
- SBP >160 mm Hg and DBP >90 mm Hg
- BP exceeding preoperative measurements with an increase ≥20% in systolic or diastolic blood pressure

MAP = mean arterial pressure.
SBP = systolic blood pressure.
DBP = diastolic blood pressure.
BP = blood pressure.

Table 3. Complications of Postoperative Hypertension

- Increased myocardial oxygen demand
- Myocardial ischemia
- Ventricular failure
- Rupture of grafts and suture lines
- Postoperative bleeding
- Neurologic defects and intracerebral hemorrhage
- Arrhythmias

POSTOPERATIVE HYPERTENSION *(Continued)*

Patients are most likely to develop blood pressure elevations and tachycardia during the induction of anesthesia. A significant increase in systolic blood pressure (up to 30 mm Hg in normotensive patients; up to 90 mm Hg in uncontrolled hypertensive patients) occurs during the intubation procedure. The recovery period is the next most likely segment where hypertension may occur. Blood pressure increases are usually less dramatic than with induction but occur because of enhanced sympathetic discharge and vascular tone of awakening. Postoperative blood pressure elevations usually begin 30 minutes after the surgery is completed and last for more than 3 hours in 20% of patients.

Other common contributing factors may include pain, anxiety, bladder distension, hypercarbia, hypoxia, fluid overload, hypothermia, antihypertensive withdrawal, and myocardial ischemia. Evaluation and treatment of causes of postoperative hypertension can frequently lower blood pressure. If after treatment, the hypertension has not resolved, antihypertensive drug therapy should be employed. Aggravation of postoperative bleeding, particularly at suture lines is often stated as being an indication for antihypertensive therapy. Systolic pressures ≥180 mm Hg have been associated with increased blood loss from wounds. Short-term injectable therapy in especially likely to be needed for patients who have pre-existing hypertension. Patients whose hypertension was controlled prior to surgery should have their antihypertensive medication reinstated as soon as possible postoperatively.

Patients with postoperative HTN should have their blood pressure frequently monitored. For patients undergoing major surgical procedures, an intra-arterial catheter may still be in place during the early postoperative period and can be used for continuous blood pressure monitoring.

A wide range of parenteral agents is now available for management of postoperative HTN when a patient is not yet tolerating the oral route of administration (Table 4). The drug of choice for a specific patient depends on that patient's circumstances. Table 5 presents some suggested uses for the parenteral agents commonly employed in the treatment of postoperative HTN. The dosages of antihypertensive agents are often titrated to attain a blood pressure value 10% above the patient's normal blood pressure to prevent overshooting the desired value. Unless the situation warrants an immediate reduction in blood pressure (eg, myocardial infarction, dissecting aortic aneurysm, malignant hypertension), the reduction can be achieved over a longer period of time.

Table 4. Select I.V. Agents Used in the Treatment of Postoperative Hypertension

Drug	Dose	Onset	Duration	Mechanism of Action	Potential Adverse Effects
Sodium nitroprusside (Nitropress®)	I.V. infusion: 0.25-0.5 mcg/kg/min initially, titrate every 1-2 min (maximum: 10 mcg/kg/min, limit to <10 min duration)	Immediate	1-2 min	Vasodilator	Nausea, vomiting, muscle twitching, hypotension, sweating, cyanide or thiocyanate toxicity, elevated ICP
Nitroglycerin (Tridil®, Nitro-Bid®)	I.V. infusion: 5 mcg/min initially, titrate every 3-5 min by 5-20 mcg/min increments	2-5 min	5-10 min	Vasodilator	Headache, tachycardia, hypotension (especially in volume-depleted patients), tolerance
Nicardipine (Cardene®)	I.V. infusion: 5 mg/h initially, titrate every 5-15 min by 2.5 mg/h increments; maintenance: 3 mg/h once blood pressure goals have been met (maximum: 15 mg/h)	5-10 min	15-30 min, up to ≥4 h	Vasodilator	Headache, tachycardia, flushing, phlebitis, hypotension
Enalaprilat (Vasotec®)	Intermittent I.V.: 0.625-1.25 mg every 6 h; use lower dose if hyponatremia, volume depletion, renal failure, or concurrent diuretic therapy in use (maximum: 20 mg/24 h period)	15-30 min	6-12 h	Vasodilator	Hypotension, renal dysfunction, hyperkalemia, angioedema
Hydralazine (Apresoline®)	Intermittent I.V.: 3-20 mg; use lower end of dosing range immediately postoperatively. Can dose every 20-60 min for desired response.	10-20 min	1-4 h	Vasodilator	Headache, flushing, tachycardia, vomiting, aggravation of angina
Fenoldopam (Corlopam®)	I.V. infusion: 0.1-0.3 mcg/kg/min initially, titrate every 15 min by 0.1 mcg/kg/min (maximum: 1.6 mcg/kg/min)	<5 min	30 min	Vasodilator	Headache, flushing, nausea, tachycardia, hypotension

POSTOPERATIVE HYPERTENSION *(Continued)*

Table 4. Select I.V. Agents Used in the Treatment of Postoperative Hypertension *(continued)*

Drug	Dose	Onset	Duration	Mechanism of Action	Potential Adverse Effects
Labetalol (Normodyne®, Trandate®)	Intermittent I.V.: 10-20 mg over 2 min initially; repeat every 10 min (maximum single dose: 80 mg; maximum cumulative dose: 300 mg/day); higher doses may be well tolerated. I.V. infusion: 0.5-4 mg/min initially; titrate every 10 min until desired effect, toxicity, or a cumulative dose of 300 mg in a 24 h period	5-10 min	3-6 h	Alpha and beta blocker	Bronchoconstriction, hypotension, bradycardia, conduction delays, left ventricular dysfunction
Esmolol (Brevibloc®)	I.V. infusion: 250-500 mcg/kg/min for 1 min initially, then 50-100 mcg/kg/min (maximum: 300 mcg/kg/min); can repeat bolus in 5 min and increase infusion by 50 mcg/kg/min	1-2 min	10-30 min	Beta blocker, $beta_1$ selective	Bronchoconstriction, hypotension, bradycardia, conduction delays, left ventricular dysfunction

Table 5. Suggested Uses for Select I.V. Antihypertensive Agents in Postoperative Hypertension

Drug	Use(s)
Sodium nitroprusside	Patients with CHF. Use caution with high intracranial pressure (in unanesthetized patients ICP can increase), renal dysfunction. Not for patients with acute myocardial ischemia or neurological emergencies
Nitroglycerin	Acute hypertension with concurrent CHF, coronary ischemia, postcoronary bypass surgery, or myocardial infarction; may decrease cerebral blood flow
Nicardipine	Postoperative HTN in cardiac and noncardiac procedures. Use caution with acute heart failure and cardiac ischemia.
Enalaprilat	Acute hypertension with concurrent CHF. Use caution with acute myocardial infarction.
Hydralazine	Not recommended for use in postoperative hypertension
Fenoldopam	Postoperative hypertension, where renal blood flow is compromised. Use caution with glaucoma.
Labetalol	Postoperative HTN after aortocoronary bypass surgery, neurosurgical patients with postoperative HTN; acute hypertension associated with MI. Use caution with acute heart failure; ejection fraction <40% or cardiac index <2.5 L/min/m^2; asthma; severe sinus bradycardia, or heart block.
Esmolol	Hypertension associated with tachycardia, acute aortic dissection. Avoid administration in patients with poor cardiac function or bronchospastic disease

The use of nifedipine capsules sublingually in the treatment of postoperative hypertension is discouraged. Nifedipine capsules have not been approved by the Food and Drug Administration (FDA) for the treatment of any form of hypertension. Further, there is no outcome data demonstrating its effectiveness for this indication. The Sixth Report of the Joint National Committee on Prevention. Detection, Evaluation, and Treatment of High Blood Pressure (JNC VI) states that the routine use of sublingual nifedipine, whenever blood pressure rises beyond a predetermined level in postoperative patients, is unacceptable. In addition, the literature is replete with many reports of serious adverse effects resulting from the sublingual administration of nifedipine (eg, severe hypotension, cerebrovascular ischemia, acute myocardial infarction, conduction disturbances, and death).

REFERENCES AND RECOMMENDED READING

Abdelwahab W, Frishman W, and Landau A, "Management of Hypertensive Urgencies and Emergencies," *J Clin Pharmacol,* 1995, 35(8):747-62.

Chobanian AV, Bakris GI, Black HR, et al, "Seventh Report of the Joint National Committee on Prevention, Detection, Evaluation, and Treatment of High Blood Pressure," *Hypertension,* 2003, 42(6):1206-52.

"Efficacy and Safety of Intravenous Nicardipine in the Control of Postoperative Hypertension," I.V. Nicardipine Study Group, *Chest,* 1991, 99(2):393-8.

Erstad BL and Barletta JF, "Treatment of Hypertension in the Perioperative Patient," *Ann Pharmacother,* 2000, 34(1):66-79.

"Fenoldopam - A New Drug for Parenteral Treatment of Severe Hypertension," *Med Lett Drugs Ther,* 1998, 40(1027):57-8.

Feeley TW and Macario A, "The Postanesthesia Care Unit," *Anesthesia,* 5th ed, Miller RD, ed, Philadelphia, PA: Churchill Livingstone, 2000, 2302-22.

Gal TJ and Cooperman LH, "Hypertension in the Immediate Postoperative Period," *Br J Anaesth,* 1975, 47(1):70-4.

Goldberg ME and Larijani GE, "Perioperative Hypertension," *Pharmacotherapy,* 1998, 18(5):911-4.

Graves JW, "Prolonged Continuous Infusion Labetalol: A New Alternative for Parenteral Antihypertensive Therapy," *Crit Care Med,* 1989, 17(8):759-61.

POSTOPERATIVE HYPERTENSION *(Continued)*

Grossman E, Messerli FH, Grodzicki T, et al, "Should a Moratorium Be Placed on Sublingual Nifedipine Capsules Given for Hypertensive Emergencies and Pseudoemergencies?" *JAMA,* 1996, 276(16):1328-31.

Haas CE and LeBlanc JM, "Acute Postoperative Hypertension: A Review of Therapeutic Options," *Am J Health-Syst Pharm,* 2004, 61:1661-75.

Halpern NA, Goldberg M, Neely C, et al, "Postoperative Hypertension: A Multicenter, Prospective, Randomized Comparison Between Intravenous Nicardipine and Sodium Nitroprusside," *Crit Care Med,* 1992, 20(12):1637-43.

Higgins TL, Yared JP, and Ryan T, "Immediate Postoperative Care of Cardiac Surgical Patients," *J Cardiothorac Vasc Anesth,* 1996, 10(5):643-58.

Laslett L, "Hypertension: Preoperative Assessment and Perioperative Management," *West J Med,* 1995, 162(3):215-9.

Murray MJ, "Perioperative Hypertension: Evaluation and Management," *ASA Refresher Courses in Anesthesiology,* 1998, 26:125-35.

Rose JC and Mayer SA, "Optimizing Blood Pressure in Neurological Emergencies," *Neurocrit Care,* 2004, 1(3):287-99.

Seltzer JL, Gerson JI, and Grogono AW, "Hypertension in Perioperative Period," *NY J State Med,* 1980, 80(1):29-31.

Shusterman NH, Elliott WJ, and White WB, "Fenoldopam, but not Nitroprusside, Improves Renal Function in Severely Hypertensive Patients With Impaired Renal Function," *Am J Med,* 1993, 95(2):161-8.

"The Sixth Report of the Joint National Committee on Prevention, Detection, Evaluation, and Treatment of High Blood Pressure," *Arch Intern Med,* 1997, 157(21):2413-46.

Udeh EC and Chow MSS, "Acute Hypertension: An Appraisal of New and Old Pharmacologic Agents," *Formulary,* 1996, 31:1178-98.

POSTOPERATIVE NAUSEA AND VOMITING

Postoperative nausea and vomiting (PONV) has been called the "biggest little problem" that affects surgical patients. The overall incidence is about 30%, with reports ranging from 0% to over 85%. It is a common postoperative problem and a leading cause of prolonged recovery room stay and unanticipated hospital admission.

The goals of this discussion are:

1. to explain the pathophysiology of PONV
2. to describe the patient risk factors associated with PONV
3. to discuss a rational approach to the prophylaxis and treatment of PONV; and
4. to discuss both commonly used drug treatments and less commonly used therapy

PATHOPHYSIOLOGY OF PONV

Figure 1 presents a simplified scheme of the neural circuits involved in nausea and vomiting. There are four major interconnected centers. Three are located in the medulla: chemoreceptor trigger zone (CTZ), area postrema, and nucleus tractus solitarius. They are jointly identified in this illustration as CTZ. The fourth center, located in the reticular formation, is the vomiting center, whose efferents produce the physical process of vomiting. The vomiting center is reflex activated through the CTZ. The major inputs into the CTZ are metabolic, including hypoglycemia, hypokalemia, and uremia; drugs such as opioid analgesics and chemotherapy agents; and hormones. The CTZ is rich in serotonin type 3 (5-HT_3), histamine type 1 (H_1), muscarinic cholinergic type 1 (M_1), dopamine type 2 (D_2), neurokinin type 1 (NK_1), and mu-opioid receptors. Stimulation of one or more of these receptors can cause nausea and vomiting. Another input to the CTZ is from the vestibular labyrinth via muscarinic (acetylcholine) and histamine receptor activation. If stimulation of the vestibular labyrinth is expected to cause nausea and vomiting following surgery, it makes sense to administer an anticholinergic (eg, transdermal scopolamine) or an antihistamine (eg, diphenhydramine) to prevent it.

Figure 1: Mechanisms of Nausea and Vomiting

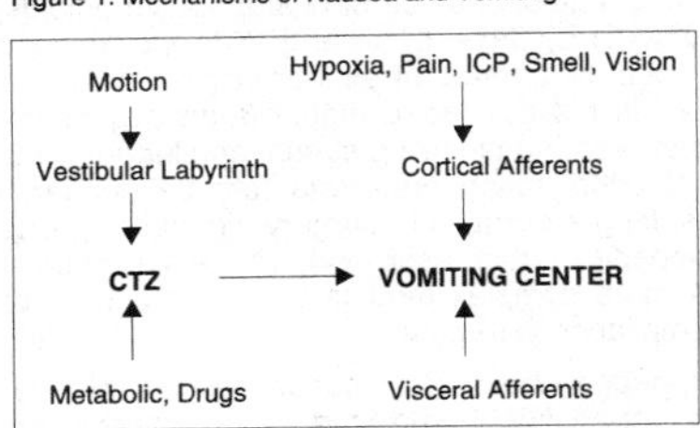

Anxiety, emotions, sights, and smells can activate the vomiting center by stimulating afferents from the cerebral cortex. It is well known that the sights and sounds of nausea and vomiting are quite effective in producing a similar response in a previously comfortable patient.

The last central input to the vomiting center originates in the periphery – the enterochromaffin cells located in the mucosa of the duodenum. They release serotonin, which stimulates vagal afferent nerves to the vomiting center. Therefore, antiserotonin drugs would be appropriate therapy for this vomiting stimulus.

A completely peripheral antinausea action (not presented in figure 1) is mediated via acetylcholine in the GI tract. Drugs such as metoclopramide enhance gastric sensitivity to acetylcholine and increase gastric peristalsis. It is prokinetic drug therapy for nausea and vomiting.

POSTOPERATIVE NAUSEA AND VOMITING *(Continued)*

RISK FACTORS

Risk factors for PONV in adults are listed below. These can be used to identify patients at a higher risk for PONV, which are those who would potentially benefit from prophylactic antiemetic administration.

Table 1. Risk Factors for PONV in Adults

Patient-Specific		
	Gender (female sex)	
	Nonsmoking status	
	Prior PONV	
	History of motion sickness	
Surgical		
	Duration of surgery	ENT surgery
	Breast surgery	Neurosurgery
	Laparoscopic surgery	Strabismus surgery
	Laparotomy	Plastic surgery
Anesthetic		
	Use of volatile anesthetics w/i 0-2 hours	
	Opioid use	
	Nitrous oxide use	
Postoperative		
	Inadequate analgesia	
	Postural hypotension	
	Patient movement	
	Oral fluid consumption	

ASSESSMENT OF RISK

Prophylaxis for PONV is not needed in every patient. Using the risk factors above, several simplified risk factor models have been developed that easily allow the level of risk (eg, low, moderate, high) for PONV to be estimated. Apfel et al used four risk factors in his model (female gender, history of PONV and/or motion sickness, nonsmoking status, and use of postoperative opioids), and was able to demonstrate a 10%, 21%, 39%, 61%, and 79% incidence of PONV with the presence of none, one, two, three, or all four of the risk factors. Koivuranta et al used five predictors in his risk factor model (female gender, history of PONV, history of motion sickness, nonsmoking status, and longer (>60 minutes) surgery) while Sinclair et al used seven predictors (female gender, history of PONV, nonsmoking status, longer duration of surgery, younger age, general anesthesia, and plastic or orthopedic shoulder surgery). These simplified risk models appear to be as good as more complex models but are much easier to use, thereby ensuring better compliance with them.

There does not appear to be a clear consensus on surgery type as an independent risk factor for PONV. Some studies have shown an increased risk of PONV in patients undergoing select surgical procedures while other studies have concluded that surgery type is not an independent risk factor.

REDUCING BASELINE RISK FACTORS

Whenever possible, baseline risk factors should be reduced to decrease the incidence of PONV.

Intraoperatively. Strategies to reduce baseline risk factors include use of *propofol for induction* and maintenance of anesthesia, use of regional anesthesia, use of hydration, use of supplemental oxygen, avoidance of volatile anesthetics, avoidance of nitrous oxide, minimization of neostigmine use, and minimization of intraoperative and postoperative opioids.

Postoperatively. Although opioids can cause nausea and vomiting, postoperative patients with pain experience nausea and vomiting, and treatment of the pain eliminates this. When these patients are challenged with naloxone, the pain returns and so does the nausea and vomiting. The key is to use the lowest opioid dose that will adequately treat the patient's pain. Inadequate hydration can lead to postural hypotension which can result in PONV. Rapid changes in patient position, or even rapid head movements, will produce PONV, probably via stimulation of the vestibular system. These types of movement in patients should be avoided.

Most recovery room criteria for discharge of ambulatory patients include the requirement for oral fluid consumption. The theory is that if patients can retain oral fluids, they will not become dehydrated due to vomiting when they go home. This practice has been questioned. Schreiner et al divided recovery room patients into two groups (mandatory drinkers and optional drinkers) with PONV significantly less in the latter group (23% vs 14%) and a longer recovery room stay for the mandatory group.

PONV PROPHYLAXIS

The patient's risk level for PONV will dictate whether prophylactic therapy is administered and, if so, how many agents are given to the patient. For example, patients at a low risk (eg, 0-1 risk factors in Apfel's model) for PONV should not receive a prophylactic antiemetic unless vomiting would lead to complications postoperatively. For patients at moderate risk (eg, 2-3 risk factors in Apfel's model) for PONV, a single antiemetic agent should be administered for prophylaxis. For patients at high risk (eg, all 4 risk factors in Apfel's model) for PONV, two or three antiemetic agents should be administered. It is important that these agents be from different classes (have different mechanisms of action).

A PONV Consensus Panel, after reviewing the literature and taking into consideration expert opinion, recommended that droperidol, dexamethasone, and the serotonin receptor antagonists be first-line agents for the prophylaxis of PONV. Droperidol's black box warning has made this agent a less attractive option. Dexamethasone has been shown to be as effective as the serotonin receptor antagonists and droperidol, and may have an advantage in postdischarge nausea and vomiting (PDNV) as its late efficacy seems to be more pronounced. In addition, dexamethasone may offer advantages over traditional antiemetics. When 8 mg of dexamethasone was administered I.V. 90 minutes before laparoscopic cholecystectomy, patients reported less pain, fatigue, nausea, vomiting, and duration of convalescence than patients who received placebo (Bisgaard). A specific serotonin receptor antagonist was not recommended as the panel concluded that there is no evidence of any difference in the safety and efficacy profiles of these agents. The panel stated that these agents can be used alone or in combination depending on PONV risk. It is important to keep in mind that these are general recommendations. One must always consider the specific patient when selecting a prophylactic antiemetic agent. For example, promethazine may be a more appropriate choice for PONV prophylaxis in a patient with motion sickness or who is undergoing surgery affecting the vestibular apparatus.

As a general rule, better efficacy is seen when the prophylactic antiemetic agents are administered at the end of surgery rather than prior to induction. The exception is dexamethasone; it appears to be most effective when administered before induction.

TREATMENT OF PONV

If a patient received no antiemetic prophylaxis and develops nausea and vomiting postoperatively, an appropriate agent (eg, 5-HT_3 receptor antagonist) should be administered. Dexamethasone is not recommended for the acute treatment of PONV secondary to its longer onset of action. It has been suggested that treatment doses of the serotonin receptor antagonists can be as low as a quarter of the prophylactic dose. If a patient received one or more prophylactic agents and still develops PONV, a drug from a different class (different mechanism of action) should be used. However, the Consensus Panel's recommendations allow repeat dosing of the serotonin receptor antagonists and droperidol when PONV occurs more than 6 hours after surgery (more than 8 hours for dexamethasone).

POSTOPERATIVE NAUSEA AND VOMITING *(Continued)*

Antiemetic Agents

Antiemetic Drug	Proposed Receptor Site of Action	Usual Dose[1]	Duration of Action	Adverse Effects	Comments and Recommendations for Use
Butyrophenones					
Droperidol (Inapsine®)	D_2	**Adults:** I.V.: 0.625-1.25 mg **Pediatrics:** I.V.: 20-50 mcg/kg	12-24 h	Sedation, hypotension (especially in hypovolemic patients), EPS	Monitor ECG for QT prolongation/ torsade de pointes; duration of action depends on size of dose; antinausea effect greater than antivomiting effect
Phenothiazines					
Prochlorperazine (Compazine®)	D_2	**Adults:** I.V./ I.M.: 5-10 mg P.R.: 25 mg **Pediatrics[2]:** P.O.: 0.1 mg/kg I.M.: 0.13 mg/kg P.R.: 2.5 mg	2-6 h (12 h when given P.R.)	Sedation, hypotension (especially in hypovolemic patients), EPS	Effective first-line agent; faster onset and less sedation vs promethazine
Antimuscarinics					
Dimenhydrinate (Dramamine®)	H_1, M_1	**Adults:** I.V./I.M.: 50-100 mg **Pediatrics:** I.V./I.M.: 1.25 mg/kg[4]	6-8 h	Sedation, dry mouth, blurred vision, urinary retention	Good for patients with motion sickness or undergoing surgery affecting the vestibular apparatus
Diphenhydramine (Benadryl®)	H_1, M_1	**Adults:** I.V./I.M.: 12.5-50 mg **Pediatrics:** P.O./I.V.: 1 mg/kg (max: 25 mg for <6 y old)	4-6 h	Sedation, dry mouth, blurred vision, urinary retention	Good for patients with motion sickness or undergoing surgery affecting the vestibular apparatus
Promethazine (Phenergan®)	D_2, H_1, M_1	**Adults:** I.V./I.M./P.R.: 6.25-25 mg **Pediatrics (>2 y):** I.V./I.M./P.R.: 0.25-0.5 mg/kg[3]	4 h	Sedation, hypotension (especially in hypovolemic patients), EPS	Good for patients with motion sickness or undergoing surgery affecting the vestibular apparatus

Antiemetic Agents *(continued)*

Antiemetic Drug	Proposed Receptor Site of Action	Usual Dose[1]	Duration of Action	Adverse Effects	Comments and Recommendations for Use
Scopolamine (Transderm Scōp®)	M_1	**Adults:** 1.5 mg transdermal patch **Pediatrics:** N/A	72 h[5]	Sedation, dry mouth, visual disturbances, dysphoria, confusion, disorientation, hallucinations	Good for patients with motion sickness or undergoing surgery affecting the vestibular apparatus; therapeutic plasma levels are obtained 4 hours after patch is placed; important for patch to be applied/removed correctly
Benzamides					
Metoclopramide (Reglan®)	D_2	**Adults:** I.V.: 20 mg **Pediatrics:** I.V.: 0.25 mg/kg	6-8 h	Sedation, hypotension, EPS	Good if N/V is due to gastric stasis; 10 mg dose not effective for preventing PONV; reduce dose to 5 mg in renal impairment; give slow I.V. push
Serotonin Antagonists					
Dolasetron (Anzemet®)	$5\text{-}HT_3$	**Adults:** I.V.: 12.5 mg **Pediatrics:** I.V.: 0.35 mg/kg	Up to 24 h	Headache, lightheadedness	Much more effective for vomiting than nausea
Granisetron (Kytril®)	$5\text{-}HT_3$	**Adults:** I.V.: 0.35-1 mg **Pediatrics:** Not known	Up to 24 h	Headache, lightheadedness	Much more effective for vomiting than nausea
Ondansetron (Zofran®)	$5\text{-}HT_3$	**Adults:** I.V.: 4 mg **Pediatrics:** I.V.: 0.05-0.1 mg/kg	Up to 24 h	Headache, lightheadedness	Much more effective for vomiting than nausea
Other					
Dexamethasone (Decadron®)	None	**Adults:** I.V.: 4-8 mg **Pediatrics:** I.V.: 0.5-1 mg/kg	Up to 24 h	Watch blood sugar in diabetics; watch for fluid retention in cardiac patients	Well tolerated in healthy patients
Ephedrine	None	**Adults:** I.M.: 0.5 mg/kg **Pediatrics:** N/A	Up to 24 h	Transient elevations in blood pressure	Consider for treatment of PONV when postural hypotension is present; may want to avoid use in patients with hypertension or organic heart disease

POSTOPERATIVE NAUSEA AND VOMITING *(Continued)*

Antiemetic Agents *(continued)*

Antiemetic Drug	Proposed Receptor Site of Action	Usual Dose[1]	Duration of Action	Adverse Effects	Comments and Recommendations for Use
Propofol (Diprivan®)	None	**Adults:** I.V.: 10-20 mg **Pediatrics:** N/A	<10 minutes	Sedation	Very short acting; excessive sedation may be a concern
Trimethobenzamide (Tigan®)	? (probably M_1, D_2)	**Adults:** I.M./P.R.: 200 mg **Pediatrics:** P.R.: 5 mg/kg	6-8 h	Sedation, hypotension, blurred vision	Probably less effective than traditional agents

D_2 = dopamine type 2 receptor; H_1 = histamine type 1 receptor; M_1 = muscarinic cholinergic type 1 receptor; 5-HT_3 = serotonin type 3 receptor; EPS = extrapyramidal symptoms such as motor restlessness or acute dystonia; N/A = not applicable; I.V. = intravenous; I.M. = intramuscular; P.R. = per rectum; P.O. = per os (by mouth); ECG = electrocardiogram; N/V = nausea and/or vomiting.

[1]Pediatric doses should not exceed the adult dose, unless otherwise indicated.

[2]Children >10 kg or 2 years of age only; change from I.M. to oral as soon as possible. When administering P.R., the dosing interval varies from 8-24 hours depending upon the child's weight.

[3]Maximum of 12.5 mg in children <12 years of age.

[4]Children >2 years of age only. Do not exceed 75 mg/dose or 300 mg/day.

[5]Remove after 24 hours. Instruct patients to wash the site where the patch was, as well as their hands, thoroughly.

LESS CONVENTIONAL THERAPY

Stimulation of the P-6 acupuncture point has been shown (Stein; Schlager) to be effective in the prevention of PONV. For both cesarean section and strabismus surgery, this technique decreases PONV when compared to placebo, with no associated drug-induced side effects.

Isopropyl alcohol, when sniffed from a cotton ball or alcohol swab, has been reported to have a significant antiemetic effect (Langevin). The nausea severity score did not change with saline treatment but decreased by 8 points (on a 10-point scale) with alcohol inhalation.

CONCLUSION

It is well known that specific risk factors predispose patients to PONV. These can be classified as patient-specific, surgical, anesthetic, and postoperative. Drug therapy, when tailored to the patient's risk factors, is effective in the prevention or treatment of PONV.

REFERENCES AND RECOMMENDED READING

Aasboe V, Raeder JC, and Groegaard B, "Betamethasone Reduces Postoperative Pain and Nausea After Ambulatory Surgery," *Anesth Analg,* 1998, 87(2):319-23.

Alon E and Himmelseher S, "Ondansetron in the Treatment of Postoperative Vomiting: A Randomized, Double-Blind Comparison With Droperidol and Metoclopramide," *Anesth Analg,* 1992, 75(4):561-5.

Andrews PL, "Physiology of Nausea and Vomiting," *Br J Anaesth,* 1992, 69(Suppl 1):2S-19S.

Aouad MT, Siddik SS, Rizk LB, et al, "The Effect of Dexamethasone on Postoperative Vomiting After Tonsillectomy," *Anesth Analg,* 2001, 92(3):636-40.

Apfel CC, Laara E, Koivuranta M, et al, "A Simplified Risk Score for Predicting Postoperative Nausea and Vomiting: Conclusions From Cross-Validations Between Two Centers," *Anesthesiology,* 1999, 91(3):693-700.

Beattie WS, Lindblad T, Buckley DN, et al, "Menstruation Increases the Risk of Nausea and Vomiting After Laparoscopy. A Prospective Randomized Study," *Anesthesiology,* 1993, 78(2):272-6.

Benedict CR, Arbogast R, Martin L, et al, "Single-Blind Study of the Effects of Intravenous Dolasetron Mesylate Versus Ondansetron on Electrocardiographic Parameters in Normal Volunteers," *J Cardiovasc Pharmacol,* 1996, 28(1):53-9.

Bisgaard T, Klarskov B, Kehlet H, et al, "Preoperative Dexamethasone Improves Surgical Outcome After Laparoscopic Cholecystectomy: A Randomized Double-Blind Placebo-Controlled Trial," *Ann Surg,* 2003, 238(5):651-60.

Borgeat A, Wilder-Smith OH, Saiah M, et al, "Subhypnotic Doses of Propofol Possess Direct Antiemetic Properties," *Anesth Analg,* 1992, 74(4):539-41.

Chen JJ, Frame DG, and White TJ, "Efficacy of Ondansetron and Prochlorperazine for the Prevention of Postoperative Nausea and Vomiting After Total Hip Replacement or Total Knee Replacement Procedures: A Randomized, Double-Blind, Comparative Trial," *Arch Intern Med,* 1998, 158(19):2124-8.

DeSilva PH, Darvish AH, McDonald SM, et al, "The Efficacy of Prophylactic Ondansetron, Droperidol, Perphenazine, and Metoclopramide in the Prevention of Nausea and Vomiting After Major Gynecologic Surgery," *Anesth Analg,* 1995, 81(1):139-43.

Elhakim M, el-Sebiae S, Kaschef N, et al, "Intravenous Fluid and Postoperative Nausea and Vomiting After Day-Case Termination of Pregnancy," *Acta Anaesthesiol Scand,* 1998, 42(2):216-9.

Fan CF, Tanhui E, Joshi S, et al, "Acupressure Treatment for Prevention of Postoperative Nausea and Vomiting," *Anesth Analg,* 1997, 84(4):821-5.

Fujii Y, Toyooka H, and Tanaka H, "Prophylactic Antiemetic Therapy With a Combination of Granisetron and Dexamethasone in Patients Undergoing Middle Ear Surgery," *Br J Anaesth,* 1998, 81(5):754-6.

Gan TJ, Glass PSA, Ginsberg B, et al, "Propofol Patient-Controlled Antiemesis Is a Safe and Effective Method for Treatment of Postoperative Nausea and Vomiting," *Anesthesiology,* 1997, 87:A49.

Gan TJ, Meyer T, Apfel CC, et al, "Consensus Guidelines for Managing Postoperative Nausea and Vomiting," *Anesth Analg,* 2003, 97(1):62-71.

Goll V, Akca O, Greif R, et al, "Ondansetron Is no More Effective Than Supplemental Intraoperative Oxygen for Prevention of Postoperative Nausea and Vomiting," *Anesth Analg,* 2001, 92(1):112-7.

Graczyk SG, McKenzie R, Kallar S, et al, "Intravenous Dolasetron for the Prevention of Postoperative Nausea and Vomiting After Outpatient Laparoscopic Gynecologic Surgery," *Anesth Analg,* 1997, 84(2):325-30.

Harper I, Della-Marta E, Owen H, et al, "Lack of Efficacy of Propofol in the Treatment of Early Postoperative Nausea and Vomiting," *Anaesth Intensive Care,* 1998, 26(4):366-70.

Henzi I, Walder B, and Tramer MR, "Dexamethasone for the Prevention of Postoperative Nausea and Vomiting: A Quantitative Systematic Review," *Anesth Analg,* 2000, 90(1):186-94.

Hovorka J, Korttila K, and Erkola O, "Nitrous Oxide Does Not Increase Nausea and Vomiting Following Gynaecological Laparoscopy," *Can J Anaesth,* 1989, 36(2):145-8.

POSTOPERATIVE NAUSEA AND VOMITING *(Continued)*

Joshi GP, Garg SA, Hailey A, et al, "The Effects of Antagonizing Residual Neuromuscular Blockade by Neostigmine and Glycopyrrolate on Nausea and Vomiting After Ambulatory Surgery," *Anesth Analg,* 1999, 89(3):628-31.

Koivuranta M, Laara E, Snare L, et al, "A Survey of Postoperative Nausea and Vomiting," *Anaesthesia,* 1997, 52(5):443-9.

Kovac AL, O'Connor TA, Pearman MH, et al, "Efficacy of Repeat Intravenous Dosing of Ondansetron in Controlling Postoperative Nausea and Vomiting: A Randomized, Double-Blind, Placebo-Controlled Multicenter Trial," *J Clin Anesth,* 1999, 11(6):453-9.

Langevin A, "Simple, Innocuous, and Inexpensive Treatment for Postoperative Nausea and Vomiting," *Anesth Analg,* 1998, 84:S15.

Lauder GR, McQuillan PJ, and Pickering RM, "Psychological Adjunct to Perioperative Antiemesis," *Br J Anaesth,* 1995, 74(3):266-70.

Liu K, Hsu CC, and Chia YY, "Effect of Dexamethasone on Postoperative Emesis and Pain," *Br J Anaesth,* 1998, 80(1):85-6.

Lonie DS and Harper NJ, "Nitrous Oxide Anaesthesia and Vomiting. The Effect of Nitrous Oxide Anaesthesia on the Incidence of Vomiting Following Gynaecological Laparoscopy," *Anaesthesia,* 1986, 41(7):703-7.

Lopez-Orlando L, Carrascosa F, Pueyo FJ, et al, "Combination of Ondansetron and Dexamethasone in the Prophylaxis of Postoperative Nausea and Vomiting," *Br J of Anaesth,* 1996, 76(6):835-40.

Lussos SA, Bader AM, Thornhill ML, et al, "The Antiemetic Efficacy and Safety of Prophylactic Metoclopramide for Elective Cesarean Delivery During Spinal Anesthesia," *Reg Anesth,* 1992, 17(3):126-30.

Maroof M, Ahmed SM, Khan RM, et al, "Intraoperative Suggestions Reduce Incidence of Posthysterectomy Emesis," *JPMA J Pak Med Assoc,* 1997, 47(8):202-4.

Nelskyla K, Yli-Hankala A, Soikkeli A, et al, "Neostigmine With Glycopyrrolate Does Not Increase the Incidence or Severity of Postoperative Nausea and Vomiting in Outpatients Undergoing Gynaecological Laparoscopy," *Br J Anaesth,* 1998, 81(5):757-60.

Pandit SK, Kothary SP, Pandit UA, et al, "Dose-Response Study of Droperidol and Metoclopramide as Antiemetics for Outpatient Anesthesia," *Anesth Analg,* 1989, 68(6):798-802.

Pueyo FJ, Carrascosa F, Lopez L, et al, "Combination of Ondansetron and Droperidol in the Prophylaxis of Postoperative Nausea and Vomiting," *Anesth Analg,* 1996, 83(1):117-22

Quaynor H and Raeder JC, "Incidence and Severity of Postoperative Nausea and Vomiting Are Similar After Metoclopramide 20 mg and Ondansetron 8 mg Given by the End of Laparoscopic Cholecystectomies," *Acta Anaesthesiol Scand,* 2002, 46(1):109-13.

Rothenberg DM, Parnass SM, Litwack K, et al, "Efficacy of Ephedrine in the Prevention of Postoperative Nausea and Vomiting," *Anesth Analg,* 1991, 72(1):58-61.

Schlager A, Offer T, and Baldissera I, "Laser Stimulation of Acupuncture Point P6 Reduces Postoperative Vomiting in Children Undergoing Strabismus Surgery," *Br J Anaesth,* 1998, 81(4):529-32.

Schreiner MS, Nicolson SC, Martin T, et al, "Should Children Drink Before Discharge From Day Surgery?" *Anesthesiology,* 1992, 76(4):528-33.

Schwartz RH and Beveridge RA, "Marijuana as an Antiemetic Drug: How Useful Is It Today? Opinions From Clinical Oncologists," *J Addict Dis,* 1994, 13(1):54-65.

Scuderi PE, D'Angelo R, Harris L, et al, "Small-Dose Propofol by Continuous Infusion Does Not Prevent Postoperative Vomiting in Females Undergoing Outpatient Laparoscopy," *Anesth Analg,* 1997, 84(1):71-5.

Sinclair DR, Chung F, and Mezei G, "Can Postoperative Nausea and Vomiting Be Predicted?" *Anesthesiology,* 1999, 91(1):109-18.

Stein DJ, Birnbach DJ, Danzer BI, et al, "Acupressure Versus Intravenous Metoclopramide to Prevent Nausea and Vomiting During Spinal Anesthesia for Cesarean Section," *Anesth Analg,* 1997, 84(2):342-5.

Tang J, Wang B, White PF, et al, "The Effect of Timing of Ondansetron Administration on Its Efficacy, Cost-Effectiveness, and Cost-Benefit as a Prophylactic Antiemetic in the Ambulatory Setting," *Anesth Analg,* 1998, 86:274-82.

Tang J, Watcha MF, and White PF, "A Comparison of Costs and Efficacy of Ondansetron and Droperidol as Prophylactic Antiemetic Therapy for Elective Outpatient Gynecologic Procedures," *Anesth Analg,* 1996, 83(2):304-13.

Tramer M, Moore RA, Reynolds DJ, et al, "A Quantitative Systemic Review of Ondansetron in Treatment of Established Postoperative Nausea and Vomiting," *BMJ,* 1997, 314(7087):1088-92.

Wang JJ, Ho ST, Lee SC, et al, "The Prophylactic Effect of Dexamethasone on Postoperative Nausea and Vomiting in Women Undergoing Thyroidectomy: A Comparison of Droperidol With Saline," *Anesth Analg,* 1999, 89(1):200-3.

Yogendran S, Asokumar B, Cheng DC, et al, "A Prospective Randomized Double-Blinded Study of the Effect of Intravenous Fluid Therapy on Adverse Outcomes on Outpatient Surgery," *Anesth Analg,* 1995, 80(4):682-6.

PREOPERATIVE EVALUATION OF THE CARDIAC PATIENT FOR NONCARDIAC SURGERY

As age increases, so does the prevalence of cardiac disease. Annually, 10% of the United States population has noncardiac surgery, with an overall cardiac morbidity/mortality rate of less than 6% for patients older than 40 years of age undergoing major operations.[1,2] This risk is increased in older patients and those with cardiac disease. The number of patients older than 65 years old presenting for surgery will increase substantially over the next several decades.

The purpose of this chapter is to identify those patients at high risk for postoperative cardiac complications. The preoperative evaluation should stratify patients with preexisting cardiac disease and recommend further workup for those at high risk, while avoiding additional testing for those patients with low potential for postoperative cardiac morbidity or mortality. Preoperative testing should be restricted to those patients in whom the results will affect patient treatment and outcome.

HISTORY OF CARDIAC RISK ASSESSMENTS

Coronary artery disease and congestive heart failure are two clinical conditions closely correlated with postoperative cardiac morbidity (see Table 1). Classic teaching based on the works by Tarhan[3] and Steen[4] in the 1970s reported approximately 30% reinfarction/mortality risk in patients who had surgery within 3 months of their myocardial infarction, decreasing to about 15% if their surgery was within 4-6 months of their MI, and 6% if the surgery was delayed more than 6 months. By 1983, Rao et al reported a reduction in the risk of recurrent MI/cardiac mortality to 6% if operated on within 3 months of a prior MI and 2% if surgery occurred between 4-6 months.[5] Shah confirmed Rao's data of improved cardiac risk in the 1990s.[6] The purposed reasons for this improvement in risk included the intensive postoperative care/monitoring and tight control of hemodynamic variables.

Table 1. Incidence of Perioperative Myocardial Reinfarction

Time Elapsed Since Prior Myocardial Infarction (mo)	Tarhan, et al[1] (%)	Steen, et al[2] (%)	Rao, et al[3] (%)	Shah, et al[4] (%)
0-3	37	27	5.7	4.3
4-6	16	11	2.3	0
>6	5	6		5.7

[1]Tarhan S, Moffitt EA, Taylor WF, et al, "Myocardial Infarction After General Anesthesia," *JAMA*, 1972, 220(11):1451-4.

[2]Steen PA, Tinker JH, and Tarhan S, "Myocardial Infarction After Anesthesia and Surgery," *JAMA*, 1978, 239(24):2566-70.

[3]Rao TL, Jacobs KH, and El-Etr AA, "Reinfarction Following Anesthesia in Patients With Myocardial Infarction," *Anesthesiology*, 1983, 59(6):499-505.

[4]Shah KB, Kleinman BS, Sami H, et al, "Reevaluation of Perioperative Myocardial Infarction in Patients With Prior Myocardial Infarction Undergoing Noncardiac Operations," *Anesth Analg*, 1990, 71(3):231-5.

CARDIAC RISK INDEXES

In the 1970s, Goldman[2] identified nine independent correlates of perioperative cardiac events and assigned them relative value points (see Table 2). The Goldman Cardiac Risk Index). This index stratified patients by cumulative points into four risk classes: Class 1 = 1-5 points (1% to 2% risk of death/major complications. Class II = 6-12 points (5% risk). Class III = 13-25 points (15% risk). Class IV = >25 points (56% risk).

PREOPERATIVE EVALUATION OF THE CARDIAC PATIENT FOR NONCARDIAC SURGERY *(Continued)*

Table 2. Goldman Cardiac Risk Index

Variable	Point Score
History	
Age >70 years	5
Preoperative MI within 6 months	10
Physical examination	
S3 gallop or increased JVP >12	11
Significant valvular aortic stenosis	3
EKG	
Rhythm other than sinus or atrial ectopy	7
PVCs >5/minute at any time	7
General medical status	3
PO_2 <60 or PCO_2 >59	
K^+ <3 or HCO_3 <20	
BUN >50 or creatinine >3	
Chronic liver disease or debilitation	
Operation	
Intraperitoneal, intrathoracic, or aortic	3
Emergency	4
Total possible points	53
Class I	0-5
Class II	6-12
Class III	13-25
Class IV	>25

Adapted from Goldman L, Caldera DL, Nussbaum SR, et al, "Multifactorial Index of Cardiac Risk in Noncardiac Surgical Procedures," *N Engl J Med*, 1977, 297(16):845-50.

In 1999, the Revised Goldman Cardiac Risk Index was developed to simplify risk assessment (using data from approximately 4500 patients) that identified six independent predictors of cardiac complications (see Table 3). Rates of major complications with 0, 1, 2, and 3+ of these factors were 0.4%, 0.9%, 7%, and 11% respectively.[7] Two other indexes focused primarily on high-risk patients. The Detsky risk index[8] added angina and pulmonary edema to Goldman's original criteria, and Eagle Criteria[9] looked at only patients undergoing major vascular surgery. These indexes were more specific to the high-risk population and not very sensitive to patients at the lower risk level.

Table 3. Revised Goldman Cardiac Risk Index

High risk type of surgery
History of ischemic heart disease
History of heart failure
History of cerebrovascular disease
Preoperative treatment with insulin
Preoperative serum creatinine >2 mg/dL

Adapted from Lee TH, Marcantonio ER, Mangione CM, et al, "Derivation and Prospective Validation of a Simple Index for Prediction of Cardiac Risk of Major Noncardiac Surgery," *Circulation*, 1999, 100(10):1043-9.

In 2002, the American College of Cardiology in association with the American Heart Association published practice guidelines to assist anesthesiologists and cardiologists in the preoperative evaluation of the cardiac patient for noncardiac surgery.[10] These guidelines originate from review/evaluation of the literature and provide the physician with a framework for evaluation and management of perioperative cardiac risk.

The perioperative anesthesiologist needs to assess the severity and stability of the patient's cardiac status and determine if additional workup will provide important information prior to the proposed surgery. Following a thorough history and physical examination, the anesthesiologist needs to risk stratify the patient. The predictors of increased perioperative cardiovascular risk, which can lead to myocardial infarction, heart failure, and death, are divided into three categories: **Clinical Predictors**, **Functional Capacity**, and **Risk of Surgical Procedure**. The need for further cardiac workup is based on the patient's classification in these three categories. Preoperative cardiac intervention is rarely indicated to solely decrease surgical risk, unless the intervention is needed regardless of the planned surgical procedure (see Table 4).

Table 4. ACC / AHA Predictors of Perioperative Cardiac Risk (MI, Heart Failure, Death)

Clinical Predictors

Major: Unstable coronary syndromes (including MI within 1 month, unstable or severe angina), decompensated heart failure, high grade AV block, symptomatic ventricular arrhythmias, supraventricular arrhythmias with uncontrolled ventricular rate, and severe valvular disease

Intermediate: Mild angina, previous MI by history or Q waves on ECG, prior heart failure, diabetes – especially insulin dependent, and renal insufficiency (creatinine >2 mg/dL)

Minor: Advanced age, abnormal ECG (LVH, LBBB, ST-T abnormalities), rhythm other than normal sinus, low functional capacity, stroke, uncontrolled HTN

Functional Capacity

1-4 Metabolic equivalents (METs): Able to do activities of daily living, walk 1-2 blocks on level ground, light housework (eg, dusting, washing dishes)

4-10 METs: Able to climb a flight of stairs, walk on level ground at 4 mph, do heavy housework, participate in physical activities like dancing, doubles tennis, golf

>10 METs: Strenuous sports (eg, swimming, football, basketball, skiing, singles tennis)

Risk of Surgical Procedure

High (cardiac risk >5%): Emergent surgery, vascular surgery including aortic and peripheral vascular (due to concurrent coronary artery disease), long procedures with large fluid shifts and/or blood loss

Intermediate (cardiac risk <5%): Carotid endarterectomy, head and neck, intraperitoneal, intrathoracic, orthopedic, and prostate surgery

Low (cardiac risk <1%): Endoscopic, superficial, cataract, and breast procedures

Adapted from Eagle KA, Berger PB, Calkins H, et al, "ACC/AHA Guideline Update for Perioperative Cardiovascular Evaluation for Noncardiac Surgery – Executive Summary: A Report of the American College of Cardiology/American Heart Association Task Force on Practice Guidelines (Committee to Update the 1996 Guidelines on Perioperative Cardiovascular Evaluation for Noncardiac Surgery)," *J Am Coll Cardiol*, 2002, 39(3):542-53.

PREOPERATIVE EVALUATION OF THE CARDIAC PATIENT FOR NONCARDIAC SURGERY *(Continued)*

SUMMARY OF ACA / AHA PREDICTORS OF CARDIAC RISK

A patient is considered at cardiac risk and needs additional cardiac evaluation if he/she has two of the following three conditions:

- Intermediate clinical risk predictor
- Low functional capacity (1-4 METs)
- High-risk surgery

Figure 1 is the complex approach to preoperative cardiac assessment developed by the ACC/AHA task force. It is provided here for completeness. Key points to remember include the following:

Step 1:	If the patient needs emergency surgery, there will be no time for a cardiac evaluation. Careful management of blood pressure, heart rate, and volume status is required intraoperatively. The patient should be risk stratified in the postoperative period and additional cardiac workup performed as indicated.
Step 2:	If the patient has had a coronary artery bypass operation within the past 5 years, or percutaneous coronary intervention between 6 months and 5 years ago, and the clinical status is stable with no ischemia, then additional workup is not needed because the risk of MI is very small.
Step 3:	If the patient has had cardiac evaluation within the last 2 years with good results, and the clinical condition has not changed, the patient does not need additional testing.
Step 4:	If the patient had a previous MI with ongoing evidence of ischemia (unstable angina, CHF, arrhythmias, significant valvular disease), then elective surgery should be postponed until the cardiac condition is treated.
Step 5:	If the patient has intermediate clinical predictors (see Table 1), then the functional capacity and surgery-specific risk are considered. Functional capacity is an excellent predictor of cardiac risk. A MET is equal to the oxygen consumption of a resting 40-year-old, 70 kg male. Perioperative MI and cardiovascular problems are high in patients with poor exercise tolerance (low functional capacity). The surgery specific-risk also contributes to perioperative cardiac morbidity, with very stressful surgical procedures increasing the incidence of cardiac complications. Patients undergoing low risk surgeries do not need additional work-up.
Step 6 and 7:	Patients with intermediate clinical predictors and moderate or excellent functional capacity can undergo intermediate risk surgical procedures without additional concern. Patients with poor functional capacity or with moderate functional capacity but high-risk surgery require additional noninvasive testing.
Step 7:	Patients with minor clinical predictors and moderate or excellent functional capacity can undergo any risk surgery.
Step 8:	Noninvasive testing can lead to invasive testing/therapy or change in medical therapy.

Figure 1. Stepwise Approach to Preoperative Cardiac Assessment

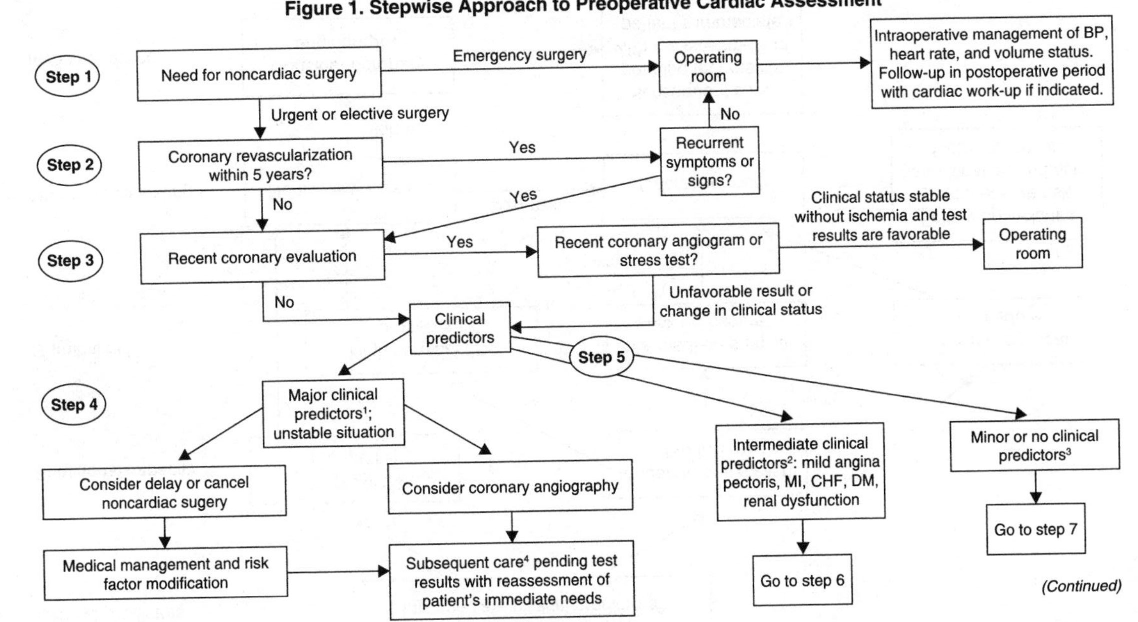

(Continued)

PREOPERATIVE EVALUATION OF THE CARDIAC PATIENT FOR NONCARDIAC SURGERY *(Continued)*

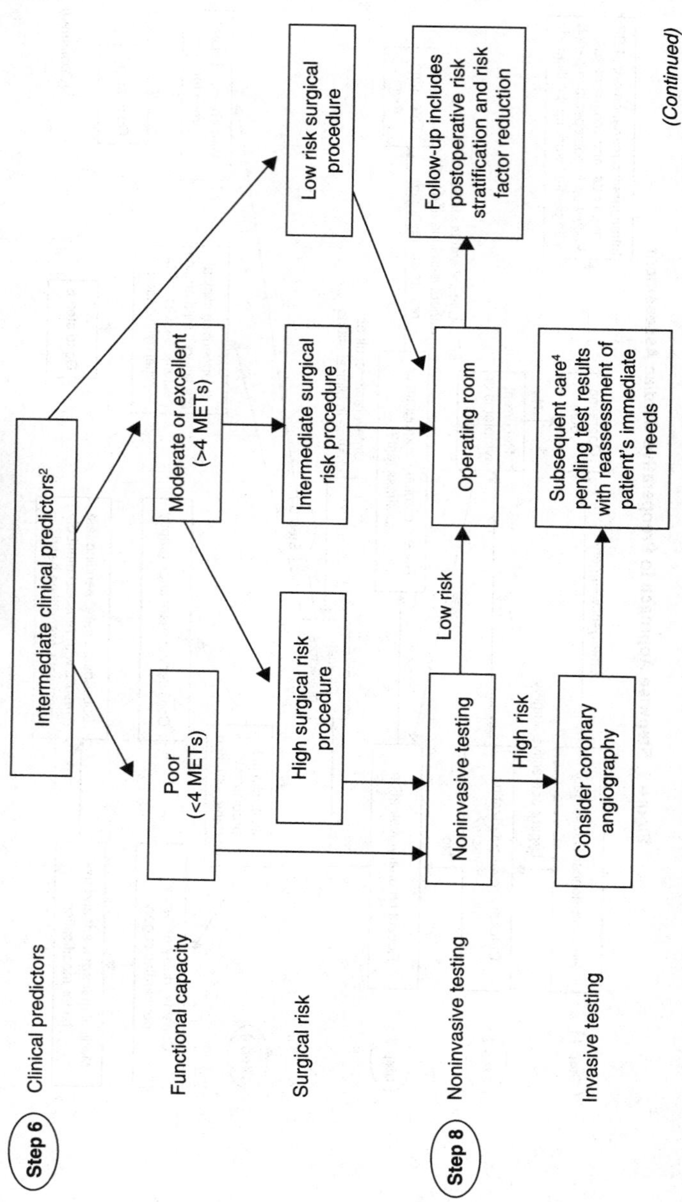

(Continued)

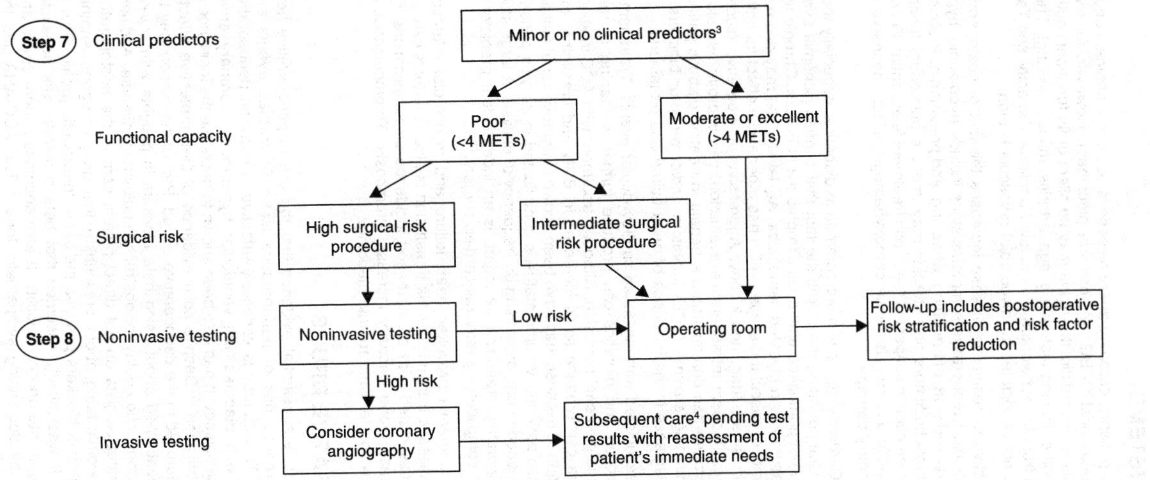

MET = metabolic equivalent.

[1]**Major clinical predictors:** Unstable coronary syndromes; decompensated congestive heart failure; significant arrhythmias; severe valvular disease.

[2]**Intermediate clinical predictors:** Mild angina pectoris; prior myocardial infarction; compensated or prior congestive heart failure; diabetes mellitus; renal insufficiency.

[3]**Minor clinical predictors:** Advanced age; abnormal ECG; rhythm other than sinus; low fuctional capacity; history of stroke; uncontrolled systemic hypertension.

[4]Subsequent care may include cancellation or delay of surgery, coronary revascularization followed by noncardiac surgery, or intensified care.

Adapted from Eagle KA, Berger PB, Calkins H, et al, "ACC/AHA Guideline Update for Perioperative Cardiovascular Evaluation for Noncardiac Surgery - Executive Summary: A Report of the American College of Cardiology/American Heart Association Task Force on Practice Guidelines (Committee to Update the 1996 Guidelines on Perioperative Cardiovascular Evaluation for Noncardiac Surgery)," *J Am Coll Cardiol*, 2002, 39(3):542-53.

PREOPERATIVE EVALUATION OF THE CARDIAC PATIENT FOR NONCARDIAC SURGERY *(Continued)*

REVIEW OF SYSTEMS

Cardiac: With some patients, coronary artery disease is obvious – angina, congestive heart failure, status post CABG, and/or stent placement. However, for many patients the diagnosis is more difficult. Angina may be silent or its functional activity level unclear due to other limiting factors (eg, age, arthritis, muscle wasting). These patients may benefit from further workup (due to low *Functional Capacity*, see Table 4) – unless they are not candidates for myocardial revascularization.

Pulmonary: Obstructive or restrictive disease increases the risk of postoperative respiratory complications. Preoperative symptoms/signs include hypoxemia, hypercapnia, acidosis, increased work of breathing, wheezing, and pneumonia. Preoperative treatment with bronchodilators and steroids may improve pulmonary function and gas exchange. If infection is suspected, antibiotic treatment is essential. Encouragement to stop tobacco use can decrease carboxyhemoglobin and decrease the progression of pulmonary damage.

Diabetes mellitus: Cardiac disease is more common in diabetics, especially those who require insulin. Compounding the risk is the fact that cardiac ischemia symptoms are silent, often not unmasked until a catastrophic event occurs. Chronic tight glucose control (measured by a glycated hemoglobin A_{1c} level <7%) may decrease the severity and rapidity of vascular disease, which has a beneficial effect for critical organs such as brain, heart, lung, and kidney. Aggressive perioperative glucose control, which requires frequent intraoperative evaluation, can improve neurologic outcome. Recent literature has demonstrated a benefit in treating diabetic patients with angiotensin converting enzyme (ACE) inhibitors and/or receptor blockers as demonstrated by a decrease in the incidence of heart failure and proteinuria.

Renal: Azotemia is associated with increased cardiovascular events. Treatment of CHF with fluid restriction and diuretics can produce further worsening of renal function by decrease in glomeruli perfusion. Although treatment with ACE inhibitors and receptor blockers can produce small increases in BUN and creatinine, they should not be discontinued because they have been shown to improve renal function and survival of diabetic patients. Volume status is complicated in dialysis patients, fluctuating from overloaded to dry, depending on frequency of dialysis. A large study has shown that preoperative creatinine >2 mg/dL is an independent predictor of postoperative cardiac complications after noncardiac surgery.[11]

Hematologic: Severe anemia provokes heart failure and myocardial infarction. Although concern for disease transmission via transfusion of blood products exists, a hematocrit <28% is associated with an increased incidence of complications.[12-14] Conditions that increase blood viscosity increase thrombosis. Thrombocytopenia and decreased coagulation factors promote bleeding.

NEW PERIOPERATIVE DRUGS

Beta Blockade: There is substantial evidence that the use of perioperative beta blocker therapy decreases risk of perioperative ischemic cardiac events and long-term mortality.[15] This therapy is especially effective in reducing perioperative mortality in patients with diabetes, left ventricular hypertrophy, coronary artery disease, and renal insufficiency. It has also been shown to decrease the incidence of postoperative atrial fibrillation.[16] Despite solid evidence of their protective effects, they are currently underused in the perioperative period. Part of the reason may be that physicians are concerned about using beta blockers in patients with severe cardiomyopathy, A-V conduction delay, or obstructive pulmonary disease. Additionally, since most anesthesiologists do not direct patient care in the postoperative period, many feel uncomfortable about prescribing this drug category. Another concern is whether all beta blockers possess the same therapeutic profile. This is not currently known. It was initially assumed that beta blockade was beneficial because it reduces heart rate and contractility. It also decreases shear stress and reduces inflammation by decreasing sympathetic tone.[17] The ACC/AHA and the American College of Physicians have recommended that beta blockers be prescribed perioperatively to all patients with a higher risk for perioperative cardiac morbidity.[10] They feel that a cardioselective beta blocker (eg, metoprolol, bisoprolol) should be started days to weeks before surgery with the goal of achieving a resting heart rate of 60 beats/minute. They also support the intraoperative and postoperative use of beta blockade.

Angiotensin converting enzyme (ACE) inhibitors/blockers: The perioperative use of these drugs is still debated. They have been shown to decrease the decline in renal function for patients with diabetes and to improve cardiac function in patients with congestive heart failure. There is some concern about reports of severe intraoperative hypotension with chronic drug administration[18] and several studies have reported increased cardiac and renal complications, although this has not been confirmed by additional studies.

SUMMARY

Preoperative evaluation of the cardiac patient involves careful analysis of the risk factors (clinical predictors, functional capacity, and risk of the surgical procedure). It also involves evaluation of the comorbid disease states that commonly coexist with cardiac dysfunction. The ACC/AHA Guidelines offer the preoperative physician a methodology for the evaluation of these patients.

FOOTNOTES

[1]Goldman L, "Assessment of Perioperative Cardiac Risk," *N Engl J Med*, 1994, 330(10):707-9.

[2]Goldman L, Caldera DL, Nussbaum SR, et al, "Multifactorial Index of Cardiac Risk in Noncardiac Surgical Procedures," *N Engl J Med*, 1977, 297(16):845-50.

[3]Tarhan S, Moffitt EA, Taylor WF, et al, "Myocardial Infarction After General Anesthesia," *JAMA*, 1972, 220(11):1451-4.

[4]Steen PA, Tinker JH, and Tarhan S, "Myocardial Infarction After Anesthesia and Surgery," *JAMA*, 1978, 239(24):2566-70.

[5]Rao TL, Jacobs KH, and El-Etr AA, "Reinfarction Following Anesthesia in Patients With Myocardial Infarction," *Anesthesiology*, 1983, 59(6):499-505.

[6]Shah KB, Kleinman BS, Sami H, et al, "Reevaluation of Perioperative Myocardial Infarction in Patients With Prior Myocardial Infarction Undergoing Noncardiac Operations," *Anesth Analg*, 1990, 71(3):231-5.

[7]Lee TH, Marcantonio ER, Mangione CM, et al, "Derivation and Prospective Validation of a Simple Index for Prediction of Cardiac Risk of Major Noncardiac Surgery," *Circulation*, 1999, 100(10):1043-9.

[8]Detsky AS, Abrams HB, Forbath N, et al, "Cardiac Assessment for Patients Undergoing Noncardiac Surgery. A Multifactorial Clinical Risk Index," *Arch Intern Med*, 1986, 146(11):2131-4.

[9]Eagle KA, Coley CM, Newell JB, et al, "Combining Clinical and Thallium Data Optimizes Preoperative Assessment of Cardiac Risk Before Major Vascular Surgery," *Ann Intern Med*, 1989, 110(11):859-66.

[10]Eagle KA, Berger PB, Calkins H, et al, "ACC/AHA Guideline Update for Perioperative Cardiovascular Evaluation for Noncardiac Surgery – Executive Summary: A Report of the American College of Cardiology/American Heart Association Task Force on Practice Guidelines (Committee to Update the 1996 Guidelines on Perioperative Cardiovascular Evaluation for Noncardiac Surgery)," *J Am Coll Cardiol*, 2002, 39(3):542-53.

[11]Plotkin JS, Benitez RM, Kuo PC, et al, "Dobutamine Stress Echocardiography for Preoperative Cardiac Risk Stratification in Patients Undergoing Orthotopic Liver Transplantation," *Liver Transpl Surg*, 1998, 4(4):253-7.

[12]Hogue CW Jr, Goodnough LT, and Monk TG, "Perioperative Myocardial Ischemic Episodes Are Related to Hematocrit Level in Patients Undergoing Radical Prostatectomy," *Transfusion*, 1998, 38(10):924-31.

[13]Hahn RG, Nilsson A, Farahmand BY, et al, "Blood Haemoglobin and the Long-Term Incidence of Acute Myocardial Infarction After Transurethral Resection of the Prostate," *Eur Urol*, 1997, 31(2):199-203.

[14]Nelson AH, Fleisher LA, and Rosenbaum SH, "Relationship Between Postoperative Anemia and Cardiac Morbidity in High-Risk Vascular Patients in the Intensive Care Unit," *Crit Care Med*, 1993, 21(6):860-6.

[15]Mangano DT, Layug EL, Wallace A, et al, "Effect of Atenolol on Mortality and Cardiovascular Morbidity After Noncardiac Surgery. Multicenter Study of Perioperative Ischemia Research Group," *N Engl J Med*, 1996, 335(23):1713-20.

[16]Jakobsen CJ, Bille S, Ahlburg P, et al, "Perioperative Metoprolol Reduces the Frequency of Atrial Fibrillation After Thoracotomy for Lung Resection," *J Cardiothorac Vasc Anesth*, 1997, 11(6):746-51.

[17]Ohtsuka T, Hamada M, Hiasa G, et al, "Effect of Beta-Blockers on Circulating Levels of Inflammatory and Anti-inflammatory Cytokines in Patients With Dilated Cardiomyopathy," *J Am Coll Cardiol*, 2001, 37(2):412-7.

[18]Brabant SM, Bertrand M, Eyraud D, et al, "The Hemodynamic Effects of Anesthetic Induction in Vascular Surgical Patients Chronically Treated With Angiotensin II Receptor Antagonists," *Anesth Analg*, 1999, 89(6):1388-92.

STRESS REPLACEMENT OF CORTICOSTEROIDS

Recommendations for stress replacement of corticosteroids vary due to the inconsistent data to predict adrenal suppression in patients receiving steroids. Because of the low risk involved with supplementation, some advocate administration of corticosteroids for any patient who has received steroids, including topical steroids, within a year. However, patients receiving 5 mg/day or less of prednisone maintain an intact HPA axis. Supplementation of corticosteroids during stress or acute illness may be required to prevent adrenal suppression. Furthermore in severe sepsis, supplementation of corticosteroids will reduce catecholamine vasopressor requirements and may lead to decreased mortality and morbidity in patients with relative adrenal insufficiency. Lastly, patients on concurrent medications (such as phenytoin, barbiturates, rifampin, etc) may require larger doses of steroids due to increased metabolism.

Corticosteroid Supplementation

Steroid Status	Prednisone Dose[1]	Severity of Surgery	Steroid Regimen
Taking steroids	<10 mg/d	Any surgery	Additional steroid coverage not required; assume normal HPA response
	>10 mg/d	Minor surgery	25 mg hydrocortisone at induction on day of induction only
		Moderate surgery	Hydrocortisone 25 mg at induction, **plus** 50-100 mg hydrocortisone per day for ~24 hours Taper quickly over 1-2 days to usual dose
		Major surgery	Hydrocortisone 25 mg at induction **plus** 100-150 mg hydrocortisone per day for 48-72 hours Taper quickly over 1-2 days to usual dose
	High-dose immunosuppression	Any surgery	Give usual immunosuppressive doses during perioperative period
Critically ill: Sepsis-induced hypotension or shock after confirmation of relative adrenal insufficiency[2]			Dexamethasone 4 mg every 12 hours[3] **OR** Hydrocortisone 50 mg every 6 hours, **plus** fludrocortisone 50 mcg every 24 hours for a total of 7 days

[1]If patient receiving a different corticosteroid, please use the table below to convert to an equivalent prednisone dose.

[2]Relative adrenal insufficiency defined as an increase of cortisol <9 mcg/dL from the baseline cortisol level, measured at 30 or 60 minutes after the administration of 250 mcg of adrenocorticotropin hormone (ACTH). Some authors define adrenal insufficiency at a baseline cortisol level ≤15 mcg/dL in the critically ill.

[3]Dexamethasone will not interfere with the rapid ACTH stimulation test and may be given while determining the adrenal status of the patient.

Patients receiving prednisone ≤5 mg/day should receive normal dose of corticosteroid and should not need additional coverage.

Patients receiving prednisone >5 mg/day should receive regimen listed above based on surgical severity or stress, in addition to patient's maintenance therapy.

Steroid Status	Time Off Steroid	Comments
Not currently taking steroids	<3 months	Treat as if receiving steroids
	>3 months	No perioperative steroids necessary

Corticosteroid Potency and Equivalent Dose Conversion

Steroid	Relative Potency		Equivalent Dose (mg)
	Anti-inflammatory	Mineralo-corticoid	
Short-Acting			
Cortisone	0.8	0.8	25
Hydrocortisone	1	1	20
Intermediate-Acting			
Prednisone	4	0.8	5
Prednisolone	4	0.8	5
Methylprednisolone	5	0.5	4
Triamcinolone	5	0	4
Long-Acting			
Dexamethasone	25	0	0.75
Betamethasone	25	0	0.6-0.75

REFERENCES AND RECOMMENDED READING

Annane D, Sebille V, Charpentier C, et al, "Effect of Treatment With Low Doses of Hydrocortisone and Fludrocortisone on Mortality in Patients with Septic Shock," *JAMA*, 2002, 288(7):862-71.

Cooper MS and Stewart PM, "Corticosteroid Insufficiency in Acutely Ill Patients," *N Engl J Med*, 2003, 348(8):727-34.

Coursin DB and Wood KE, "Corticosteroid Supplementation for Adrenal Insufficiency," *JAMA*, 2002, 287(2):236-40.

Gonzalez H, Nardi O, and Annane D, "Relative Adrenal Failure in the ICU: An Identifiable Problem Requiring Treatment," *Crit Care Clin*, 2006, 22(1):105-18.

Henriques HF III and Lebovic D, "Defining and Focusing Perioperative Steroid Supplementation," *Am Surg*, 1995, 61(9):809-13.

Marik PE and Zaloga GP, "Adrenal Insufficiency in the Critically Ill: A New Look at an Old Problem," *Chest*, 2002, 122(5):1784-96.

Nicholson G, Burrin JM, and Hall GM, "Perioperative Steroid Supplementation," *Anaesthesia*, 1998, 53(11):1091-104.

Salem M, Tainsh RE Jr, Bromberg J, et al, "Perioperative Glucocorticoid Coverage. A Reassessment 42 Years After Emergence of a Problem.," *Ann Surg*, 1994, 219(4):416-25.

SUBSTANCE ABUSE AND ANESTHESIA

Substance abuse is a problem that must be considered when evaluating a patient for general surgery under anesthesia. Many agents can potentially interfere with the anesthetics and other agents administered in the perioperative setting. Substances of abuse such as ethanol, central nervous system depressants (opioids, benzodiazepines, barbiturates), and cocaine can all influence the type and the amount of anesthetic administered. Below are brief discussions and tables referring to drugs of abuse and how to perioperatively manage those patients who are abusing the agents.

ETHANOL

Chronic Alcohol Abuse

Chronic ethanol abuse results in induction of the cytochrome P450 system which can affect many of the anesthetic and other medications used perioperatively. Because of this induction, certain agents may need to be dosed more frequently to achieve the desired effect. Larger doses of many of the anesthetic agents are needed in chronic alcohol abusers because of potential cross tolerance. It has been proven that the doses of certain opioids must be significantly increased in the chronic alcoholic to obtain the desired effect. Following is a list of anesthetic drugs that must be altered in the chronic alcoholic.

Agent	Dose
Volatile agents	Increased
Opioids	Increased
Benzodiazepines	Increased
Barbiturates	Increased

Acute Ethanol Abuse

Acute ethanol intoxication causes significant central nervous system (CNS) depression. For those individuals, including chronic alcoholics, undergoing anesthesia while intoxicated, the amount of anesthetic agent used should be decreased.

Agent	Dose
Volatile agents	Decreased
Opioids	Decreased
Benzodiazepines	Decreased
Barbiturates	Decreased

CENTRAL NERVOUS SYSTEM DEPRESSANTS

Patients taking CNS depressants on a chronic basis will frequently need increased doses of certain anesthetic agents. Patients who are taking barbiturates chronically will have enzyme induction and may have an increased requirement for some of the anesthetic agents. Patients on chronic opioids will have an increased requirement for opioids perioperatively. In fact, like chronic alcoholics, patients taking opioids and benzodiazepines chronically, may have a cross tolerance to other agents and the dose of many intravenous anesthetic agents may need to be increased. Following is a list of anesthetic drugs that may need to be altered.

Agent	Dose
Barbiturates	Increased barbiturates
Opioids	Increased - opioids, benzodiazepines (?)
Benzodiazepines	Increased - benzodiazepines, opioids, barbiturates

COCAINE

Cocaine addiction is a common problem in our society. The National Institute of Drug Abuse estimated that there was a fivefold increase in cocaine abuse from the mid 1970s to the mid 1980s. This increased prevalence of cocaine use makes it a significant consideration in the perioperative patient. Acute cocaine use places the surgical candidate in jeopardy of systemic adverse effects and drug interactions. Although the incidence of preoperative patients with a positive urine cocaine screen has not been determined, it is not uncommon for patients to arrive for surgery with a positive screen. It is frequently recommended that preoperative patients with a positive urine toxicology screen wait at least 48-72 hours before undergoing a surgical procedure. Although an increase in morbidity and mortality has occurred in the surgical patient following acute cocaine ingestion, many debates and questions remain as to the time delay for surgery and the potential risks of the surgical procedure in patients with a positive screen. Because a positive urine toxicology screen does not yield precise information on the chronicity or the amount of drug used, more emphasis should be focused on the management of the perioperative effects following acute cocaine administration.

The urine toxicology screen for cocaine detects not only the parent compound but also its metabolites. The metabolites of cocaine include ecgonine methyl ether (EME), benzoylecgonine, and norcocaine. A positive urine toxicology screen occurs up to 48-120 hours after cocaine use. This factor must be kept in mind when evaluating patients with a positive cocaine screen.

Perioperative management of the suspected cocaine intoxicated patient should be aimed at cardiovascular stability. It is very important to have an intravenous antihypertensive available or on board in order to blunt acute hyperdynamic responses. Arrhythmia agents must also be readily available.

For the cocaine intoxicated patient, the dose of many anesthetic agents will need to be increased. Following is a list of anesthetic drugs that must be altered in the cocaine intoxicated patient.

Agent	Dose
Volatile agents	Increased
Opioids	Increased
Benzodiazepines	Increased
Barbiturates	Increased

Management of induction of anesthesia for the cocaine-intoxicated patient should resemble that of the hypertensive patient and the same techniques should be used. The following measures can be taken to prevent the exaggerated increase in blood pressure during intubation from occurring.

Coadminister opioids during induction

- Fentanyl
- Alfentanil
- Remifentanil
- Sufentanil

Administer beta-antagonist during induction

- Esmolol
- Propranolol
- Labetalol
- Metoprolol

Administer topical local anesthetic prior to intubation

For maintenance anesthesia, it is important to avoid halothane in this patient population so as not to increase the risk of arrhythmia secondary to the myocardial sensitivity to catecholamines (epinephrine).

Anesthetic management of the cocaine-intoxicated patient remains an unresolved issue. The anesthesiologist and the surgeon should consider the risk/benefit

SUBSTANCE ABUSE AND ANESTHESIA *(Continued)*

analysis of delaying the procedure. If the surgery is elective, it should be delayed for 48-72 hours or until a negative urine toxicology is achieved. If the procedure is emergent, it need not be postponed and the above precautions and techniques should be considered. It is important to remember, however, that if the procedure occurs, events or medications which exacerbate the adrenergic state should be anticipated or avoided.

APPENDIX TABLE OF CONTENTS

APPENDIX TABLE OF CONTENTS *(Continued)*

BODY SURFACE AREA OF ADULTS AND CHILDREN

Calculating Body Surface Area in Children

In a child of average size, find weight and corresponding surface area on the boxed scale to the left; or, use the nomogram to the right. Lay a straightedge on the correct height and weight points for the child, then read the intersecting point on the surface area scale. (**Note:** 2.2 lb = 1 kg)

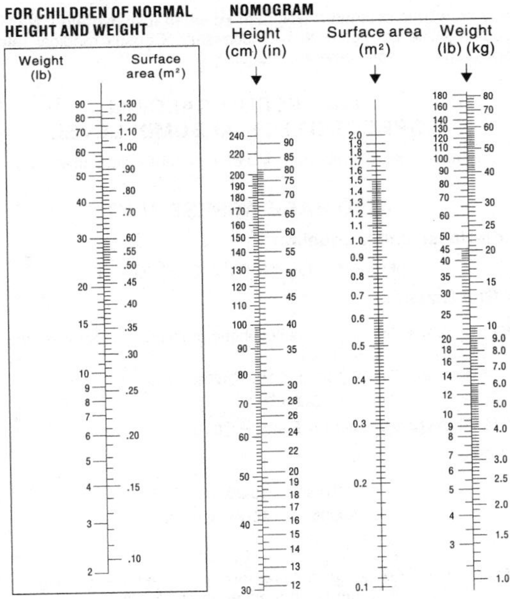

BODY SURFACE AREA FORMULA (Adult and Pediatric)

$$BSA\ (m^2) = \sqrt{\frac{Ht\ (in) \times Wt\ (lb)}{3131}}$$

or, in metric:

$$BSA\ (m^2) = \sqrt{\frac{Ht\ (cm) \times Wt\ (kg)}{3600}}$$

References

Lam TK and Leung DT, "More on Simplified Calculation of Body Surface Area," *N Engl J Med*, 1988, 318(17):1130 (Letter).

Mosteller RD, "Simplified Calculation of Body Surface Area", *N Engl J Med*, 1987, 317(17):1098 (Letter).

FORMULAS AND EQUATIONS

CORRECTED SODIUM

Corrected Na^+ = measured Na^+ + [1.5 x (glucose – 150 divided by 100)]

Note: Do not correct for glucose <150.

WATER DEFICIT

Water deficit = 0.6 x body weight [1 – (140 divided by Na^+)]

Note: Body weight is estimated weight in kg when fully hydrated; $\mathbf{Na^+}$ is serum or plasma sodium. Use corrected Na^+ if necessary. Consult medical references for recommendations for replacement of deficit.

TOTAL SERUM CALCIUM CORRECTED FOR ALBUMIN LEVEL

[(Normal albumin – patient's albumin) x 0.8] + patient's measured total calcium

ACID-BASE ASSESSMENT

Henderson-Hasselbalch Equation

$$pH = 6.1 + \log (HCO_3^- / (0.03)(pCO_2))$$

Alveolar Gas Equation

PIO_2 = FiO_2 x (total atmospheric pressure – vapor pressure of H_2O at 37°C)

= FiO_2 x (760 mm Hg – 47 mm Hg)

PAO_2 = $PIO_2 - PACO_2 / R$

Alveolar/arterial oxygen gradient = $PAO_2 - PaO_2$

Normal ranges:

Children	15-20 mm Hg
Adults	20-25 mm Hg

where:

PIO_2 = Oxygen partial pressure of inspired gas (mm Hg) (150 mm Hg in room air at sea level)

FiO_2 = Fractional pressure of oxygen in inspired gas (0.21 in room air)

PAO_2 = Alveolar oxygen partial pressure

$PACO_2$ = Alveolar carbon dioxide partial pressure

PaO_2 = Arterial oxygen partial pressure

R = Respiratory exchange quotient (typically 0.8, increases with high carbohydrate diet, decreases with high fat diet)

Acid-Base Disorders

Acute metabolic acidosis:

$PaCO_2$ expected = 1.5 (HCO_3^-) + 8 ± 2 **or**
Expected decrease in $PaCO_2$ = 1.3 (1-1.5) x decrease in HCO_3^-

Acute metabolic alkalosis:

Expected increase in $PaCO_2$ = 0.6 (0.5-1) x increase in HCO_3^-

Acute respiratory acidosis (<6 h duration):

For every $PaCO_2$ increase of 10 mm Hg, HCO_3 increases by 1 mEq/L

Chronic respiratory acidosis (>6 h duration):

For every $PaCO_2$ increase of 10 mm Hg, HCO_3 increases by 4 mEq/L

Acute respiratory alkalosis (<6 h duration):

For every $PaCO_2$ decrease of 10 mm Hg, HCO_3 decreases by 2 mEq/L

Chronic respiratory alkalosis (>6 h duration):
For every $PaCO_2$ decrease of 10 mm Hg, HCO_3 increases by 5 mEq/L

ACID-BASE EQUATION

H^+ (in mEq/L) = (24 x $PaCO_2$) divided by HCO_3^-

Aa GRADIENT

Aa gradient [(713)(FiO_2 – ($PaCO_2$ divided by 0.8))] – PaO_2

Aa gradient	=	alveolar-arterial oxygen gradient
FiO_2	=	inspired oxygen (expressed as a fraction)
$PaCO_2$	=	arterial partial pressure carbon dioxide (mm Hg)
PaO_2	=	arterial partial pressure oxygen (mm Hg)

OSMOLALITY

Definition: The summed concentrations of all osmotically active solute particles.

Predicted serum osmolality =
2 Na^+ + glucose (mg/dL) / 18 + BUN (mg/dL) / 2.8
The normal range of serum osmolality is 285-295 mOsm/L.

Differential diagnosis of increased serum osmolal gap (>10 mOsm/L)

Medications and toxins
- Alcohols (ethanol, methanol, isopropanol, glycerol, ethylene glycol)
- Mannitol

Calculated Osm

Osmolal gap = measured Osm – calculated Osm

0 to +10: Normal
>10: Abnormal
<0: Probable lab or calculation error

For drugs causing increased osmolar gap, see "Toxicology Information" section in this Appendix.

BICARBONATE DEFICIT

HCO_3^- deficit = (0.4 x wt in kg) x (HCO_3^- desired – HCO_3^- measured)

Note: In clinical practice, the calculated quantity may differ markedly from the actual amount of bicarbonate needed or that which may be safely administered.

ANION GAP

Definition: The difference in concentration between unmeasured cation and anion equivalents in serum.

Anion gap = Na^+ – (Cl^- + HCO_3^-)
(The normal anion gap is 10-14 mEq/L)

Differential Diagnosis of Increased Anion Gap Acidosis

Organic anions
- Lactate (sepsis, hypovolemia, seizures, large tumor burden)
- Pyruvate
- Uremia
- Ketoacidosis (β-hydroxybutyrate and acetoacetate)
- Amino acids and their metabolites
- Other organic acids

Inorganic anions
- Hyperphosphatemia
- Sulfates
- Nitrates

FORMULAS AND EQUATIONS *(Continued)*

Differential Diagnosis of Decreased Anion Gap

Organic cations

- Hypergammaglobulinemia

Inorganic cations

- Hyperkalemia
- Hypercalcemia
- Hypermagnesemia

Medications and toxins

- Lithium

Hypoalbuminemia

RETICULOCYTE INDEX

(% retic divided by 2) x (patient's Hct divided by normal Hct) **or**
(% retic divided by 2) x (patient's Hgb divided by normal Hgb)

Normal index: 1.0
Good marrow response: 2.0-6.0

IDEAL BODY WEIGHT CALCULATION

Adults (18 years and older)

IBW (male) = 50 + (2.3 x height in inches over 5 feet)
IBW (female) = 45.5 + (2.3 x height in inches over 5 feet)

IBW is in kg.

Children

a. 1-18 years

$$IBW = \frac{(height^2 \times 1.65)}{1000}$$

IBW is in kg.
Height is in cm.

b. 5 feet and taller

IBW (male) = 39 + (2.27 x height in inches over 5 feet)
IBW (female) = 42.2 + (2.27 x height in inches over 5 feet)

IBW is in kg.

ADJUSTED BODY WEIGHT CALCULATION

Adults (18 years and older)

ABW = IBW + 0.4 (actual body weight – IBW)

Note: This calculation is used in dosing certain medications when patient weighs >20% of his/her IBW. ABW is in kg.

MILLIEQUIVALENT AND MILLIMOLE CALCULATIONS

Definitions

mole	=	gram molecular weight of a substance (aka molar weight)
millimole (mM)	=	milligram molecular weight of a substance (a millimole is 1/1000 of a mole)
equivalent weight	=	gram weight of a substance which will combine with or replace one gram (one mole) of hydrogen; an equivalent weight can be determined by dividing the molar weight of a substance by its ionic valence
milliequivalent (mEq)	=	milligram weight of a substance which will combine with or replace one milligram (one millimole) of hydrogen (a milliequivalent is 1/1000 of an equivalent)

Calculations

$$\text{moles} = \frac{\text{weight of a substance (grams)}}{\text{molecular weight of that substance (grams)}}$$

$$\text{millimoles} = \frac{\text{weight of a substance (milligrams)}}{\text{molecular weight of that substance (milligrams)}}$$

equivalents = moles x valence of ion

milliequivalents = millimoles x valence of ion

$$\text{moles} = \frac{\text{equivalents}}{\text{valence of ion}}$$

$$\text{millimoles} = \frac{\text{milliequivalents}}{\text{valence of ion}}$$

millimoles = moles x 1000

milliequivalents = equivalents x 1000

Note: Use of equivalents and milliequivalents is valid only for those substances which have fixed ionic valences (eg, sodium, potassium, calcium, chlorine, magnesium bromine, etc). For substances with variable ionic valences (eg, phosphorous), a reliable equivalent value cannot be determined. In these instances, one should calculate millimoles (which are fixed and reliable) rather than milliequivalents.

MILLIEQUIVALENT CONVERSIONS

To convert mg/100 mL to mEq/L the following formula may be used:

$$\frac{(\text{mg}/100\text{ mL}) \times 10 \times \text{valence}}{\text{atomic weight}} = \text{mEq/L}$$

To convert mEq/L to mg/100 mL the following formula may be used:

$$\frac{(\text{mEq/L}) \times \text{atomic weight}}{10 \times \text{valence}} = \text{mg}/100\text{ mL}$$

To convert mEq/L to volume of percent of a gas the following formula may be used:

$$\frac{(\text{mEq/L}) \times 22.4}{10} = \text{volume percent}$$

Valences and Atomic Weights of Selected Ions

Substance	Electrolyte	Valence	Molecular Wt
Calcium	Ca^{++}	2	40
Chloride	Cl^{-}	1	35.5
Magnesium	Mg^{++}	2	24
Phosphate	HPO_4^{--} (80%)	1.8	96*
pH = 7.4	$H_2PO_4^{-}$ (20%)	1.8	96*
Potassium	K^{+}	1	39
Sodium	Na^{+}	1	23
Sulfate	SO_4^{--}	2	96*

*The molecular weight of phosphorus only is 31, and sulfur only is 32.

Approximate Milliequivalents — Weights of Selected Ions

Salt	mEq/g Salt	Mg Salt/mEq
Calcium carbonate [$CaCO_3$]	20	50
Calcium chloride [$CaCl_2 \bullet 2H_2O$]	14	74
Calcium gluceptate [$Ca(C_7H_{13}O_8)_2$]	4	245
Calcium gluconate [$Ca(C_6H_{11}O_7)_2 \bullet H_2O$]	5	224
Calcium lactate [$Ca(C_3H_5O_3)_2 \bullet 5H_2O$]	7	154
Magnesium gluconate [$Mg(C_6H_{11}O_7)_2 \bullet H_2O$]	5	216
Magnesium oxide [MgO]	50	20
Magnesium sulfate [$MgSO_4$]	17	60
Magnesium sulfate [$MgSO_4 \bullet 7H_2O$]	8	123
Potassium acetate [$K(C_2H_3O_2)$]	10	98
Potassium chloride [KCl]	13	75
Potassium citrate [$K_3(C_6H_5O_7) \bullet H_2O$]	9	108
Potassium iodide [KI]	6	166
Sodium acetate [$Na(C_2H_3O_2)$]	12	82
Sodium acetate [$Na(C_2H_3O_2) \bullet 3H_2O$]	7	136
Sodium bicarbonate [$NaHCO_3$]	12	84
Sodium chloride [$NaCl$]	17	58
Sodium citrate [$Na_3(C_6H_5O_7) \bullet 2H_2O$]	10	98
Sodium iodine [NaI]	7	150
Sodium lactate [$Na(C_3H_5O_3)$]	9	112
Zinc sulfate [$ZnSO_4 \bullet 7H_2O$]	7	144

POUNDS / KILOGRAMS CONVERSION

1 pound = 0.45359 kilograms
1 kilogram = 2.2 pounds

lb	= kg	lb	= kg	lb	= kg
1	0.45	70	31.75	140	63.50
5	2.27	75	34.02	145	65.77
10	4.54	80	36.29	150	68.04
15	6.80	85	38.56	155	70.31
20	9.07	90	40.82	160	72.58
25	11.34	95	43.09	165	74.84
30	13.61	100	45.36	170	77.11
35	15.88	105	47.63	175	79.38
40	18.14	110	49.90	180	81.65
45	20.41	115	52.16	185	83.92
50	22.68	120	54.43	190	86.18
55	24.95	125	56.70	195	88.45
60	27.22	130	58.91	200	90.72
65	29.48	135	61.24		

TEMPERATURE CONVERSION

Celsius to Fahrenheit = (°C x 9/5) + 32 = °F
Fahrenheit to Celsius = (°F – 32) x 5/9 = °C

°C	= °F	°C	= °F	°C	= °F
100.0	212.0	39.0	102.2	36.8	98.2
50.0	122.0	38.8	101.8	36.6	97.9
41.0	105.8	38.6	101.5	36.4	97.5
40.8	105.4	38.4	101.1	36.2	97.2
40.6	105.1	38.2	100.8	36.0	96.8
40.4	104.7	38.0	100.4	35.8	96.4
40.2	104.4	37.8	100.1	35.6	96.1
40.0	104.0	37.6	99.7	35.4	95.7
39.8	103.6	37.4	99.3	35.2	95.4
39.6	103.3	37.2	99.0	35.0	95.0
39.4	102.9	37.0	98.6	0	32.0
39.2	102.6				

ALDRETE SCORING SYSTEM

Activity	
Able to move 4 extremities voluntarily or on command	2
Able to move 2 extremities voluntarily or on command	1
Not able to move extremities voluntarily or on command	0
Respiration	
Able to deep breathe and cough freely	2
Dyspnea, shallow or limited breathing	1
Apneic	0
Circulation	
Blood pressure ± 20 mm of preanesthesia level	2
Blood pressure ± 20 to 50 mm of preanesthesia level	1
Blood pressure ± 50 mm of preanesthesia level	0
Consciousness	
Fully awake	2
Arousable on calling	1
Not responding	0
Color	
Normal	2
Pale, dusky, blotchy	1
Cyanotic	0

Note: This scoring system is used to determine readiness of patient to be discharged to unit (if inpatient) or to phase II recovery (if outpatient); patients with a score of 9 or above are considered fit for discharge.

Adapted from Aldrete JA and Kroulik D, "A Postanesthetic Recovery Score," *Anes Analg*, 1970, 49:924-34.

AMERICAN SOCIETY OF ANESTHESIOLOGISTS (ASA) PHYSICAL STATUS CLASSIFICATION

Category	Description
ASA 1	Normal, healthy patient
ASA 2	Mild systemic disease — no functional limitation (eg, anemia, chronic bronchitis, controlled hypertension, extremes of age, mild diabetes mellitus, morbid obesity)
ASA 3	Severe systemic disease — definite functional limitation (eg, angina pectoris, diabetes mellitus with vascular complications, history of prior myocardial infarction, obstructive pulmonary disease, poorly controlled hypertension)
ASA 4	Severe systemic disease that is a constant threat to life (eg, advanced pulmonary or hepatic dysfunction, congestive heart failure, heart failure, renal failure)
ASA 5	Moribund patient unlikely to survive 24 hours with or without operation

For procedures performed on an emergency basis, the letter "**E**" should be added to the ASA status.

ASA DIFFICULT AIRWAY ALGORITHM

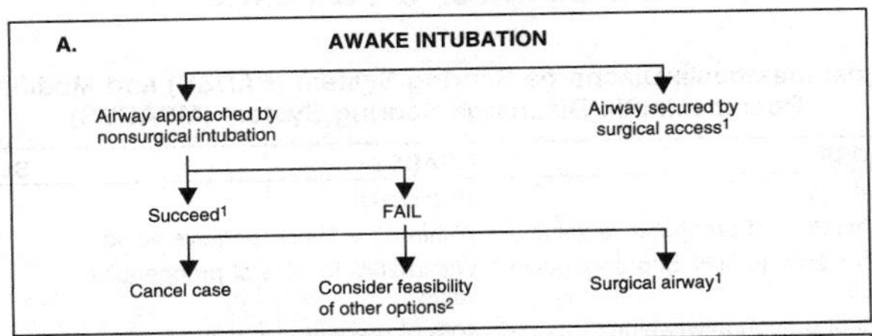

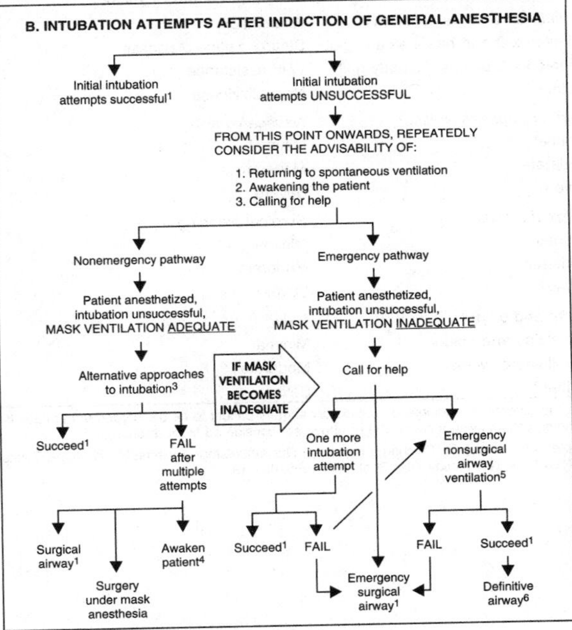

1 Confirm intubation with exhaled CO_2.

2 Other options include (but are not limited to): surgery under mask anesthesia, surgery under local anesthesia infiltration or regional nerve blockade, or intubation attempts after induction of general anesthesia.

3 Alternative approaches to difficult intubation include (but are not limited to): use of different laryngoscope blades, awake intubation, blind oral or nasal intubation, fiberoptic intubation, intubating stylet or tube changer, light wand, retrograde intubation, and surgical airway access.

4 See awake intubation.

5 Options for emergency nonsurgical airway ventilation include (but are not limited to): transtracheal jet ventilation, laryngeal mask ventilation, or esophageal-tracheal combitube ventilation.

6 Options for establishing a definitive airway include (but are not limited to): returning to awake state with spontaneous ventilation, tracheotomy, or endotracheal intubation.

Modified with permission from "Practice Guidelines for Management of the Difficult Airway. A Report by the ASA Task Force on Management in the Difficult Airway," *Anesthesiology*, 1993, 78:597-602.

AMBULATORY SURGERY DISCHARGE SCORING SYSTEMS

Postanesthesia Discharge Scoring System (PADSS) and Modified Postanesthetic Discharge Scoring System (MPADSS)[1]

PADSS	MPADSS	Score
Vital signs	*Vital signs*	
Within 20% of preoperative value	Within 20% of preoperative value	2
Within 20% to 40% of preoperative value	Within 20% to 40% of preoperative value	1
40% of preoperative value	40% of preoperative value	0
Ambulation and mental status	*Ambulation*	
Oriented x 3 **and** has a steady gait	Steady gait/no dizziness	2
Oriented x 3 **or** has a steady gait	With assistance	1
Neither	None/dizziness	0
Pain, or nausea/vomiting	*Nausea/vomiting*	
Minimal	Minimal	2
Moderate	Moderate	1
Severe	Severe	0
Surgical bleeding	*Surgical bleeding*	
Minimal	Minimal	2
Moderate	Moderate	1
Severe	Severe	0
Intake and output	*Pain*	
P.O. fluids **and** voided	Minimal	2
P.O. fluids **or** voided	Moderate	1
Neither	Severe	0

[1]Used to determine readiness of ambulatory surgery patient to be discharged from phase II recovery; patients with a score of 9 or above are considered fit for discharge.

Adapted from Chung F, "Discharge Process," *The Ambulatory Anesthesia Handbook*, Twersky RS, ed, New York, NY: Mosby-Year Book, Inc, 1995, 431-49.

CRITERIA FOR ASSESSING FAST-TRACK ELIGIBILITY IN OUTPATIENTS[1] [ABILITY TO SKIP PHASE I (PACU) RECOVERY]

The patient must meet all the criteria below to be eligible to bypass phase I (PACU) recovery and in the judgment of the anesthesia provider, be capable of transfer to the step-down unit.

- Awake, alert, oriented, responsive (or return to baseline)
- Minimal pain
- Minimal nausea
- No vomiting
- No active bleeding
- Vital signs stable (not likely to require pharmacologic intervention)
- Patient can perform a 5-second head lift if a nondepolarizing neuromuscular blocking agent used
- Oxygen saturation of 94% on room air (3 minutes or longer) **or** return of oxygen saturation to baseline or higher

A minimal score of 12 (with no score <1 in any individual category) is required to bypass phase I (PACU) recovery

	Score
Level of consciousness	
Awake and oriented	2
Arousable with minimal stimulation	1
Responsive only to tactile stimulation	0
Physical activity	
Able to move all extremities on command	2
Some weakness in movement of extremities	1
Unable to voluntarily move extremities	0
Hemodynamic stability	
Blood pressure <15% of baseline mean arterial pressure (MAP)	2
Blood pressure 15% to 30% of baseline MAP	1
Blood pressure >30% below baseline MAP value	0
Respiratory stability	
Able to breathe deeply	2
Tachypnea with good cough	1
Dyspneic with weak cough	0
Oxygen saturation status	
Maintains value >90% on room air	2
Requires supplemental oxygen (nasal prongs)	1
Saturation <90% with supplemental oxygen	0
Postoperative pain assessment	
None or mild discomfort	2
Moderate to severe pain controlled with I.V. analgesics	1
Persistent severe pain	0
Postoperative emetic symptoms	
None or mild nausea with no active vomiting	2
Transient vomiting or retching	1
Persistent moderate to severe nausea and vomiting	0
Total score	**14**

[1]Patients evaluated in the operating room suite using the criteria.

References

Apfelbaum JL, "Current Controversies in Adult Outpatient Anesthesia," ASA Annual Refresher Course Lecture, Dallas, TX, 1999.

White PF and Song D, "New Criteria for Fast-Tracking After Outpatient Anesthesia: A Comparison With the Modified Aldrete's Scoring System," *Anesth Analg*, 1999, 88(5):1069-72.

CRITICAL CARE INFUSION ADMINISTRATION CHARTS

DILTIAZEM 1 mcg/mL

125 mg in 125 mL D_5W or NS			
mg/h	mL/h	mg/h	mL/h
1	1	11	11
2	2	12	12
3	3	13	13
4	4	14	14
5	5	15	15
6	6	16	16
7	7	17	17
8	8	18	18
9	9	19	19
10	10	20	20

Initial dose is 0.25 mg/kg (~20 mg for the average adult) as a bolus administered over 2 minutes.

A second bolus dose may be administered after 15 minutes if the response is adequate. The second bolus dose should be 0.35 mg/kg (~25 mg for the average patient) administered over 2 minutes.

Begin I.V. infusion after bolus dose. Recommended initial infusion rate is 10 mg/hour but some patients may respond to a rate of 5 mg/hour.

The infusion rate may be increased in 5 mg/hour increments, up to 15 mg/hour as needed.

Infusion duration >24 hours and infusion rates >15 mg/hour are not recommended (due to potential accumulation of metabolites and increased toxicity) but have been used.

DOBUTAMINE

	2 mg/mL (500 mg/250 mL of D_5W or NS)																
	WEIGHT (kg)																
	40	**45**	**50**	**55**	**60**	**65**	**70**	**75**	**80**	**85**	**90**	**95**	**100**	**105**	**110**	**115**	**120**
mL/h	*(mcg/kg/minute)*																
3	2.5	2.2	2.0														
4	3.3	3.0	2.7	2.4	2.2	2.1											
5	4.2	3.7	3.3	3.0	2.8	2.6	2.4	2.2									
6	5.0	4.4	4.0	3.6	3.3	3.1	2.9	2.7	2.5	2.4	2.2						
7	5.8	5.2	4.7	4.2	3.9	3.6	3.3	3.1	2.9	2.7	2.6	2.5	2.3				
8	6.7	5.9	5.3	4.8	4.4	4.1	3.8	3.6	3.3	3.1	3.0	2.8	2.7	2.5	2.4	2.3	
9	7.5	6.7	6.0	5.5	5.0	4.6	4.3	4.0	3.8	3.5	3.3	3.2	3.0	2.9	2.7	2.6	2.5
10	8.3	7.4	6.7	6.1	5.6	5.1	4.8	4.4	4.2	3.9	3.7	3.5	3.3	3.2	3.0	2.9	2.8
11	9.2	8.1	7.3	6.7	6.1	5.6	5.2	4.9	4.6	4.3	4.1	3.9	3.7	3.5	3.3	3.2	3.1
12	10.0	8.9	8.0	7.3	6.7	6.2	5.7	5.3	5.0	4.7	4.4	4.2	4.0	3.8	3.6	3.5	3.3
13	10.8	9.6	8.7	7.9	7.2	6.7	6.2	5.8	5.4	5.1	4.8	4.6	4.3	4.1	3.9	3.8	3.6
14	11.7	10.4	9.3	8.5	7.8	7.2	6.7	6.2	5.8	5.5	5.2	4.9	4.7	4.4	4.2	4.1	3.9
15	12.5	11.1	10.0	9.1	8.3	7.7	7.1	6.7	6.3	5.9	5.6	5.3	5.0	4.8	4.5	4.3	4.2
16	13.3	11.9	10.7	9.7	8.9	8.2	7.6	7.1	6.7	6.3	5.9	5.6	5.3	5.1	4.8	4.6	4.4
17	14.2	12.6	11.3	10.3	9.4	8.7	8.1	7.6	7.1	6.7	6.3	6.0	5.7	5.4	5.2	4.9	4.7
18	15.0	13.3	12.0	10.9	10.0	9.2	8.6	8.0	7.5	7.1	6.7	6.3	6.0	5.7	5.5	5.2	5.0
19	15.8	14.1	12.7	11.5	10.6	9.7	9.0	8.4	7.9	7.5	7.0	6.7	6.3	6.0	5.8	5.5	5.3
20	16.7	14.8	13.3	12.1	11.1	10.3	9.5	8.9	8.3	7.8	7.4	7.0	6.7	6.3	6.1	5.8	5.6
21	17.5	15.6	14.0	12.7	11.7	10.8	10.0	9.3	8.8	8.2	7.8	7.4	7.0	6.7	6.4	6.1	5.8
22	18.3	16.3	14.7	13.3	12.2	11.3	10.5	9.8	9.2	8.6	8.1	7.7	7.3	7.0	6.7	6.4	6.1
23	19.2	17.0	15.3	13.9	12.8	11.8	11.0	10.2	9.6	9.0	8.5	8.1	7.7	7.3	7.0	6.7	6.4
24	20.0	17.8	16.0	14.5	13.3	12.3	11.4	10.7	10.0	9.4	8.9	8,4	8.0	7.6	7.3	7.0	6.7
25	20.8	18.5	16.7	15.2	13.9	12.8	11.9	11.1	10.4	9.8	9.3	8.8	8.3	7.9	7.6	7.2	6.9
26	21.7	19.3	17.3	15.8	14.4	13.3	12.4	11.6	10.8	10.2	9.6	9.1	8.7	8.3	7.9	7.5	7.2
27	22.5	20.0	18.0	16.4	15.0	13.8	12.9	12.0	11.3	10.6	10.0	9.5	9.0	8.6	8.2	7.8	7.5
28	23.3	20.7	18.7	17.0	15.6	14.4	13.3	12.4	11.7	11.0	10.4	9.8	9.3	8.9	8.5	8.1	7.8
29	24.2	21.5	19.3	17.6	16.1	14.9	13.8	12.9	12.1	11.4	10.7	10.2	9.7	9.2	8.8	8.4	8.1
30	25.0	22.2	20.0	18.2	16.7	15.4	14.3	13.3	12.5	11.8	11.1	10.5	10.0	9.5	9.1	8.7	8.3
31	25.8	23.0	20.7	18.8	17.2	15.9	14.8	13.8	12.9	12.2	11.5	10.9	10.3	9.8	9.4	9.0	8.6
32	26.7	23.7	21.3	19.4	17.8	16.4	15.2	14.2	13.3	12.5	11.9	11.2	10.7	10.2	9.7	9.3	8.9
33	27.5	24.4	22.0	20.0	18.3	16.9	15.7	14.7	13.8	12.9	12.2	11.6	11.0	10.5	10.0	9.6	9.2
34	28.3	25.2	22.7	20.6	18.9	17.4	16.2	15.1	14.2	13.3	12.6	11.9	11.3	10.8	10.3	9.9	9.4
35	29.2	25.9	23.3	21.2	19.4	17.9	16.7	15.6	14.6	13.7	13.0	12.3	11.7	11.1	10.6	10.1	9.7
36	30.0	26.7	24.0	21.8	20.0	18.5	17.1	16.0	15.0	14.1	13.3	12.6	12.0	11.4	10.9	10.4	10.0
37	30.8	27.4	24.7	22.4	20.6	19.0	17.6	16.4	15.4	14.5	13.7	13.0	12.3	11.7	11.2	10.7	10.3
38	31.7	28.1	25.3	23.0	21.1	19.5	18.1	16.9	15.8	14.9	14.1	13.3	12.7	12.1	11.5	11.0	10.6
39	32.5	28.9	26.0	23.6	21.7	20.0	18.6	17.3	16.3	15.3	14.4	13.7	13.0	12.4	11.8	11.3	10.8
40	33.3	29.6	26.7	24.2	22.2	20.5	19.0	17.8	16.7	15.7	14.8	14.0	13.3	12.7	12.1	11.6	11.1
41	34.2	30.4	27.3	24.8	22.8	21.0	19.5	18.2	17.1	16.1	15.2	14.4	13.7	13.0	12.4	11.9	11.4
42	35.0	31.1	28.0	25.5	23.3	21.5	20.0	18.7	17.5	16.5	15.6	14.7	14.0	13.3	12.7	12.2	11.7
43	35.8	31.9	28.7	26.1	23.9	22.1	20.5	19.1	17.9	16.9	15.9	15.1	14.3	13.7	13.0	12.5	11.9
44	36.7	32.6	29.3	26.7	24.4	22.6	21.0	19.6	18.3	17.3	16.3	15.4	14.7	14.0	13.3	12.8	12.2
45	37.5	33.3	30.0	27.3	25.0	23.1	21.4	20.0	18.8	17.6	16.7	15.8	15.0	14.3	13.6	13.0	12.5

Usual dobutamine starting dose: 5 mcg/kg/minute.

Usual dosing range: 2.5-20 mcg/kg/minute.

CRITICAL CARE INFUSION ADMINISTRATION CHARTS
(Continued)

DOPAMINE

	3.2 mg/mL (800 mg/250 mL of D_5W or NS)																
	WEIGHT (kg)																
	40	**45**	**50**	**55**	**60**	**65**	**70**	**75**	**80**	**85**	**90**	**95**	**100**	**105**	**110**	**115**	**120**
mL/h	*(mcg/kg/minute)*																
1	1.3	1.2	1.1	1.0	0.9	0.8	0.8	0.7	0.7	0.6	0.6	0.6	0.5	0.5	0.5	0.5	0.4
2	2.7	2.4	2.1	1.9	1.8	1.6	1.5	1.4	1.3	1.3	1.2	1.1	1.1	1.0	1.0	0.9	0.9
3	4.0	3.6	3.2	2.9	2.7	2.5	2.3	2.1	2.0	1.9	1.8	1.7	1.6	1.5	1.5	1.4	1.3
4	5.3	4.7	4.3	3.9	3.6	3.3	3.0	2.8	2.7	2.5	2.4	2.2	2.1	2.0	1.9	1.9	1.8
5	6.7	5.9	5.3	4.8	4.4	4.1	3.8	3.6	3.3	3.1	3.0	2.8	2.7	2.5	2.4	2.3	2.2
6	8.0	7.1	6.4	5.8	5.3	4.9	4.6	4.3	4.0	3.8	3.6	3.4	3.2	3.0	2.9	2.8	2.7
7	9.3	8.3	7.5	6.8	6.2	5.7	5.3	5.0	4.7	4.4	4.1	3.9	3.7	3.6	3.4	3.2	3.1
8	10.7	9.5	8.5	7.8	7.1	6.6	6.1	5.7	5.3	5.0	4.7	4.5	4.3	4.1	3.9	3.7	3.6
9	12.0	10.7	9.6	8.7	8.0	7.4	6.9	6.4	6.0	5.6	5.3	5.1	4.8	4.6	4.4	4.2	4.0
10	13.3	11.9	10.7	9.7	8.9	8.2	7.6	7.1	6.7	6.3	5.9	5.6	5.3	5.1	4.8	4.6	4.4
11	14.7	13.0	11.7	10.7	9.8	9.0	8.4	7.8	7.3	6.9	6.5	6.2	5.9	5.6	5.3	5.1	4.9
12	16.0	14.2	12.8	11.6	10.7	9.8	9.1	8.5	8.0	7.5	7.1	6.7	6.4	6.1	5.8	5.6	5.3
13	17.3	15.4	13.9	12.6	11.6	10.7	9.9	9.2	8.7	8.2	7.7	7.3	6.9	6.6	6.3	6.0	5.8
14	18.7	16.6	14.9	13.6	12.4	11.5	10.7	10.0	9.3	8.8	8.3	7.9	7.5	7.1	6.8	6.5	6.2
15	20.0	17.8	16.0	14.5	13.3	12.3	11.4	10.7	10.0	9.4	8.9	8.4	8.0	7.6	7.3	7.0	6.7
16	21.3	19.0	17.1	15.5	14.2	13.1	12.2	11.4	10.7	10.0	9.5	9.0	8.5	8.1	7.8	7.4	7.1
17	22.7	20.1	18.1	16.5	15.1	13.9	13.0	12.1	11.3	10.7	10.1	9.5	9.1	8.6	8.2	7.9	7.6
18	24.0	21.3	19.2	17.5	16.0	14.8	13.7	12.8	12.0	11.3	10.7	10.1	9.6	9.1	8.7	8.3	8.0
19	25.3	22.5	20.3	18.4	16.9	15.6	14.5	13.5	12.7	11.9	11.3	10.7	10.1	9.7	9.2	8.8	8.4
20	26.7	23.7	21.3	19.4	17.8	16.4	15.2	14.2	13.3	12.5	11.9	11.2	10.7	10.2	9.7	9.3	8.9
21	28.0	24.9	22.4	20.4	18.7	17.2	16.0	14.9	14.0	13.2	12.4	11.8	11.2	10.7	10.2	9.7	9.3
22	29.3	26.1	23.5	21.3	19.6	18.1	16.8	15.6	14.7	13.8	13.0	12.4	11.7	11.2	10.7	10.2	9.8
23	30.7	27.3	24.5	22.3	20.4	18.9	17.5	16.4	15.3	14.4	13.6	12.9	12.3	11.7	11.2	10.7	10.2
24	32.0	28.4	25.6	23.3	21.3	19.7	18.3	17.1	16.0	15.1	14.2	13.5	12.8	12.2	11.6	11.1	10.7
25	33.3	29.6	26.7	24.2	22.2	20.5	19.0	17.8	16.7	15.7	14.8	14.0	13.3	12.7	12.1	11.6	11.1
26	34.7	30.8	27.7	25.2	23.1	21.3	19.8	18.5	17.3	16.3	15.4	14.6	13.9	13.2	12.6	12.1	11.6
27	36.0	32.0	28.8	26.2	24.0	22.2	20.6	19.2	18.0	16.9	16.0	15.2	14.4	13.7	13.1	12.5	12.0
28	37.3	33.2	29.9	27.2	24.9	23.0	21.3	19.9	18.7	17.6	16.6	15.7	14.9	14.2	13.6	13.0	12.4
29	38.7	34.4	30.9	28.1	25.8	23.8	22.1	20.6	19.3	18.2	17.2	16.3	15.5	14.7	14.1	13.4	12.9
30	40.0	35.6	32.0	29.1	26.7	24.6	22.9	21.3	20.0	18.8	17.8	16.8	16.0	15.2	14.5	13.9	13.3
31	41.3	36.7	33.1	30.1	27.6	25.4	23.6	22.0	20.7	19.5	18.4	17.4	16.5	15.7	15.0	14.4	13.8
32	42.7	37.9	34.1	31.0	28.4	26.3	24.4	22.8	21.3	20.1	19.0	18.0	17.1	16.3	15.5	14.8	14.2
33	44.0	39.1	35.2	32.0	29.3	27.1	25.1	23.5	22.0	20.7	19.6	18.5	17.6	16.8	16.0	15.3	14.7
34	45.3	40.3	36.3	33.0	30.2	27.9	25.9	24.2	22.7	21.3	20.1	19.1	18.1	17.3	16.5	15.8	15.1
35	46.7	41.5	37.3	33.9	31.1	28.7	26.7	24.9	23.3	22.0	20.7	19.6	18.7	17.8	17.0	16.2	15.6
36	48.0	42.7	38.4	34.9	32.0	29.5	27.4	25.6	24.0	22.6	21.3	20.2	19.2	18.3	17.5	16.7	16.0
37	49.3	43.9	39.5	35.9	32.9	30.4	28.2	26.3	24.7	23.2	21.9	20.8	19.7	18.8	17.9	17.2	16.4
38	50.7	45.0	40.5	36.8	33.8	31.2	29.0	27.0	25.3	23.8	22.5	21.3	20.3	19.3	18.4	17.6	16.9
39		46.2	41.6	37.8	34.7	32.0	29.7	27.7	26.0	24.5	23.1	21.9	20.8	19.8	18.9	18.1	17.3
40		47.4	42.7	38.8	35.6	32.8	30.5	28.4	26.7	25.1	23.7	22.5	21.3	20.3	19.4	18.6	17.8
41		48.6	43.7	39.8	36.4	33.6	31.2	29.2	27.3	25.7	24.3	23.0	21.9	20.8	19.9	19.0	18.2
42		49.8	44.8	40.7	37.3	34.5	32.0	29.9	28.0	26.4	24.9	23.6	22.4	21.3	20.4	19.5	18.7
43			45.9	41.7	38.2	35.3	32.8	30.6	28.7	27.0	25.5	24.1	22.9	21.8	20.8	19.9	19.1
44			46.9	42.7	39.1	36.1	33.5	31.3	29.3	27.6	26.1	24.7	23.5	22.3	21.3	20.4	19.6
45			48.0	43.6	40.0	36.9	34.3	32.0	30.0	28.2	26.7	25.3	24.0	22.9	21.8	20.9	20.0

Dosing: 0.5-3 mcg/kg/minute. **Receptor:** DA-1 and DA-2. **Effects:** Enhances renal blood flow.

Dosing: 3-10 mcg/kg/minute. **Receptor:** Beta-adrenergic. **Effects:** ↑HR and contract, maintains renal blood flow.

Dosing: 10-50 mcg/kg/minute. **Receptor:** Alpha-adrenergic. **Effects:** Vasoconstriction.

EPINEPHRINE 32 mcg/mL

8 mg in 250 mL D_5W or NS							
mL/h	mcg/min	mL/h	mcg/min	mL/h	mcg/min	mL/h	mcg/min
1	0.53	21	11.20	41	21.87	61	32.53
2	1.07	22	11.73	42	22.40	62	33.07
3	1.60	23	12.27	43	22.93	63	33.60
4	2.13	24	12.80	44	23.47	64	34.13
5	2.67	25	13.33	45	24.00	65	34.67
6	3.20	26	13.87	46	24.53	66	35.20
7	3.73	27	14.40	47	25.07	67	35.73
8	4.27	28	14.93	48	25.60	68	36.27
9	4.80	29	15.47	49	26.13	69	36.80
10	5.33	30	16.00	50	26.67	70	37.33
11	5.87	31	16.53	51	27.20	71	37.87
12	6.40	32	17.07	52	27.73	72	38.40
13	6.93	33	17.60	53	28.27	73	38.93
14	7.47	34	18.13	54	28.80	74	39.47
15	8.00	35	18.67	55	29.33	75	40.00
16	8.53	36	19.20	56	29.87	76	40.53
17	9.07	37	19.73	57	30.40	77	41.07
18	9.60	38	20.27	58	30.93	78	41.60
19	10.13	39	20.80	59	31.47	79	42.13
20	10.67	40	21.33	60	32.00	80	42.67

Usual dosing range: 1-20 mcg/minute.

EPINEPHRINE 64 mcg/mL

16 mg in 250 mL D_5W or NS							
mL/h	mcg/min	mL/h	mcg/min	mL/h	mcg/min	mL/h	mcg/min
1	1.07	21	22.40	41	43.73	61	65.07
2	2.13	22	23.47	42	44.80	62	66.13
3	3.20	23	24.53	43	45.87	63	67.20
4	4.27	24	25.60	44	46.93	64	68.27
5	5.33	25	26.67	45	48.00	65	69.33
6	6.40	26	27.73	46	49.07	66	70.40
7	7.47	27	28.80	47	50.13	67	71.47
8	8.53	28	29.87	48	51.20	68	72.53
9	9.60	29	30.93	49	52.27	69	73.60
10	10.67	30	32.00	50	53.33	70	74.67
11	11.73	31	33.07	51	54.40	71	75.73
12	12.80	32	34.13	52	55.47	72	76.80
13	13.87	33	35.20	53	56.53	73	77.87
14	14.93	34	36.27	54	57.60	74	78.93
15	16.00	35	37.33	55	58.67	75	80.00
16	17.07	36	38.40	56	59.73	76	81.07
17	18.13	37	39.47	57	60.80	77	82.13
18	19.20	38	40.53	58	61.87	78	83.20
19	20.27	39	41.60	59	62.93	79	84.27
20	21.33	40	42.67	60	64.00	80	85.33

Usual dosing range: 1-20 mcg/minute.

CRITICAL CARE INFUSION ADMINISTRATION CHARTS
(Continued)

MILRINONE 200 mcg/mL

	20 mg/100 mL of D_5W or NS																
	WEIGHT (kg)																
	40	**45**	**50**	**55**	**60**	**65**	**70**	**75**	**80**	**85**	**90**	**95**	**100**	**105**	**110**	**115**	**120**
mL/h	*(mcg/kg/minute)*																
1	0.08	0.07	0.07	0.06	0.06	0.05	0.05	0.04	0.04	0.04	0.04	0.04	0.03	0.03	0.03	0.03	0.03
2	0.17	0.15	0.13	0.12	0.11	0.10	0.10	0.09	0.08	0.08	0.07	0.07	0.07	0.06	0.06	0.06	0.06
3	0.25	0.22	0.20	0.18	0.17	0.15	0.14	0.13	0.13	0.12	0.11	0.11	0.10	0.10	0.09	0.09	0.08
4	0.33	0.30	0.27	0.24	0.22	0.21	0.19	0.18	0.17	0.16	0.15	0.14	0.13	0.13	0.12	0.12	0.11
5	0.42	0.37	0.33	0.30	0.28	0.26	0.24	0.22	0.21	0.20	0.19	0.18	0.17	0.16	0.15	0.14	0.14
6	0.50	0.44	0.40	0.36	0.33	0.31	0.29	0.27	0.25	0.24	0.22	0.21	0.20	0.19	0.18	0.17	0.17
7	0.58	0.52	0.47	0.42	0.39	0.36	0.33	0.31	0.29	0.27	0.26	0.25	0.23	0.22	0.21	0.20	0.19
8	0.67	0.59	0.53	0.48	0.44	0.41	0.38	0.36	0.33	0.31	0.30	0.28	0.27	0.25	0.24	0.23	0.22
9	0.75	0.67	0.60	0.55	0.50	0.46	0.43	0.40	0.38	0.35	0.33	0.32	0.30	0.29	0.27	0.26	0.25
10		0.74	0.67	0.61	0.56	0.51	0.48	0.44	0.42	0.39	0.37	0.35	0.33	0.32	0.30	0.29	0.28
11			0.73	0.67	0.61	0.56	0.52	0.49	0.46	0.43	0.41	0.39	0.37	0.35	0.33	0.32	0.31
12				0.73	0.67	0.62	0.57	0.53	0.50	0.47	0.44	0.42	0.40	0.38	0.36	0.35	0.33
13					0.72	0.67	0.62	0.58	0.54	0.51	0.48	0.46	0.43	0.41	0.39	0.38	0.36
14						0.72	0.67	0.62	0.58	0.55	0.52	0.49	0.47	0.44	0.42	0.41	0.39
15							0.71	0.67	0.63	0.59	0.56	0.53	0.50	0.48	0.45	0.43	0.42
16								0.71	0.67	0.63	0.59	0.56	0.53	0.51	0.48	0.46	0.44
17									0.71	0.67	0.63	0.60	0.57	0.54	0.52	0.49	0.47
18									0.75	0.71	0.67	0.63	0.60	0.57	0.55	0.52	0.50
19										0.75	0.70	0.67	0.63	0.60	0.58	0.55	0.53
20											0.74	0.70	0.67	0.63	0.61	0.58	0.56
21												0.74	0.70	0.67	0.64	0.61	0.58
22													0.73	0.70	0.67	0.64	0.61
23														0.73	0.70	0.67	0.64
24															0.73	0.70	0.67
25																0.72	0.69
26																0.75	0.72
27																	0.75

Loading dose: 50 mcg/kg I.V. slowly over 10 minutes.

Maintenance dose: 0.375-0.75 mcg/kg/minute.

DOSING IN RENAL FAILURE

Creatinine Clearance (mL/min/1.73 m^2)	Infusion Rate (mcg/kg/min)	Rated Delivery[1] (mL/kg/h)
5	0.20	0.060
10	0.23	0.069
20	0.28	0.084
30	0.33	0.099
40	0.38	0.114
50	0.43	0.129

[1]200 mcg/mL concentration.

NICARDIPINE

0.1 mg/mL (25 mg in 250 mL D_5W or NS)				0.2 mg/mL (50 mg in 250 mL D_5W or NS)			
mg/h	**mL/h**	**mg/h**	**mL/h**	**mg/h**	**mL/h**	**mg/h**	**mL/h**
0.5	5	8	80	0.5	2.5	8	40
1	10	8.5	85	1	5	8.5	42.5
1.5	15	9	90	1.5	7.5	9	45
2	20	9.5	95	2	10	9.5	47.5
2.5	25	10	100	2.5	12.5	10	50
3	30	10.5	105	3	15	10.5	52.5
3.5	35	11	110	3.5	17.5	11	55
4	40	11.5	115	4	20	11.5	57.5
4.5	45	12	120	4.5	22.5	12	60
5	50	12.5	125	5	25	12.5	62.5
5.5	55	13	130	5.5	27.5	13	65
6	60	13.5	135	6	30	13.5	67.5
6.5	65	14	140	6.5	32.5	14	70
7	70	14.5	145	7	35	14.5	72.5
7.5	75	15	150	7.5	37.5	15	75

Maintenance dose: Begin at 5 mg/hour and increase by 2.5 mg/hour every 5-15 minutes. Decrease to 3 mg/hour once blood pressure goal is achieved.

Maximum rate: 15 mg/hour.

NICARDIPINE

0.5 mg/mL (25 mg in 250 mL D_5W or NS)				1 mg/mL (250 mg in 250 mL D_5W or NS)			
mg/h	**mL/h**	**mg/h**	**mL/h**	**mg/h**	**mL/h**	**mg/h**	**mL/h**
0.5	1	8	16	0.5	0.5	8	8
1	2	8.5	17	1	1	8.5	8.5
1.5	3	9	18	1.5	1.5	9	9
2	4	9.5	19	2	2	9.5	9.5
2.5	5	10	20	2.5	2.5	10	10
3	6	10.5	21	3	3	10.5	10.5
3.5	7	11	22	3.5	3.5	11	11
4	8	11.5	23	4	4	11.5	11.5
4.5	9	12	24	4.5	4.5	12	12
5	10	12.5	25	5	5	12.5	12.5
5.5	11	13	26	5.5	5.5	13	13
6	12	13.5	27	6	6	13.5	13.5
6.5	13	14	28	6.5	6.5	14	14
7	14	14.5	29	7	7	14.5	14.5
7.5	15	15	30	7.5	7.5	15	15

Maintenance dose: Begin at 5 mg/hour and increase by 2.5 mg/hour every 5-15 minutes. Decrease to 3 mg/hour once blood pressure goal is achieved.

Maximum rate: 15 mg/hour.

CRITICAL CARE INFUSION ADMINISTRATION CHARTS
(Continued)

NITROGLYCERIN

200 mcg/mL (50 mg in 250 mL D_5W or NS)					
mL/h	mcg/min	mL/h	mcg/min	mL/h	mcg/min
1	3.33	21	70.00	41	136.67
2	6.67	22	73.33	42	140.00
3	10.00	23	76.67	43	143.33
4	13.33	24	80.00	44	146.67
5	16.67	25	83.33	45	150.00
6	20.00	26	86.67	46	153.33
7	23.33	27	90.00	47	156.67
8	26.67	28	93.33	48	160.00
9	30.00	29	96.67	49	163.33
10	33.33	30	100.00	50	166.67
11	36.67	31	103.33	51	170.00
12	40.00	32	106.67	52	173.33
13	43.33	33	110.00	53	176.67
14	46.67	34	113.33	54	180.00
15	50.00	35	116.67	55	183.33
16	53.33	36	120.00	56	186.67
17	56.67	37	123.33	57	190.00
18	60.00	38	126.67	58	193.33
19	63.33	39	130.00	59	196.67
20	66.67	40	133.33	60	200.00

Initial rate: 5 mcg/minute, increase by 5 mcg/minute every 3-5 minutes to 20 mcg/minute; if no response at 20 mcg/minute, increase by 10 mcg/minute every 3-5 minutes, up to 200 mcg/minute.

Maximum rate: 200 mcg/minute.

NITROGLYCERIN

400 mcg/mL (100 mg in 250 mL D_5W or NS)					
mL/h	mcg/min	mL/h	mcg/min	mL/h	mcg/min
1	6.67	11	73.33	21	140.00
1.5	10.00	11.5	76.67	21.5	143.33
2	13.33	12	80.00	22	146.67
2.5	16.67	12.5	83.33	22.5	150.00
3	20.00	13	86.67	23	153.33
3.5	23.33	13.5	90.00	23.5	156.67
4	26.67	14	93.33	24	160.00
4.5	30.00	14.5	96.67	24.5	163.33
5	33.33	15	100.00	25	166.67
5.5	36.67	15.5	103.33	25.5	170.00
6	40.00	16	106.67	26	173.33
6.5	43.33	16.5	110.00	26.5	176.67
7	46.67	17	113.33	27	180.00
7.5	50.00	17.5	116.67	27.5	183.33
8	53.33	18	120.00	28	186.67
8.5	56.67	18.5	123.33	28.5	190.00
9	60.00	19	126.67	29	193.33
9.5	63.33	19.5	130.00	29.5	196.67
10	66.67	20	133.33	30	200.00
10.5	70.00	20.5	136.67		

Initial rate: 5 mcg/minute, increase by 5 mcg/minute every 3-5 minutes to 20 mcg/minute; if no response at 20 mcg/minute, increase by 10 mcg/minute every 3-5 minutes, up to 200 mcg/minute.

Maximum rate: 200 mcg/minute.

NITROPRUSSIDE (Nipride®)

	200 mcg/mL (50 mg/250 mL of D_5W) WEIGHT (kg)																
	40	45	50	55	60	65	70	75	80	85	90	95	100	105	110	115	120
mL/h	*(mcg/kg/minute)*																
3	0.25	0.22	0.20	0.18	0.17												
5	0.42	0.37	0.33	0.30	0.28	0.26	0.24										
7	0.58	0.52	0.47	0.42	0.39	0.36	0.33	0.31	0.29	0.27	0.26	0.25					
9	0.75	0.67	0.60	0.55	0.50	0.46	0.43	0.40	0.38	0.35	0.33	0.32	0.30	0.29	0.27	0.26	0.25
11	0.92	0.81	0.73	0.67	0.61	0.56	0.52	0.49	0.46	0.43	0.41	0.39	0.37	0.35	0.33	0.32	0.31
13	1.08	0.96	0.87	0.79	0.72	0.67	0.62	0.58	0.54	0.51	0.48	0.46	0.43	0.41	0.39	0.38	0.36
15	1.25	1.11	1.00	0.91	0.83	0.77	0.71	0.67	0.63	0.59	0.56	0.53	0.50	0.48	0.45	0.43	0.42
17	1.42	1.26	1.13	1.03	0.94	0.87	0.81	0.76	0.71	0.67	0.63	0.60	0.57	0.54	0.52	0.49	0.47
19	1.58	1.41	1.27	1.15	1.06	0.97	0.90	0.84	0.79	0.75	0.70	0.67	0.63	0.60	0.58	0.55	0.53
21	1.75	1.56	1.40	1.27	1.17	1.08	1.00	0.93	0.88	0.82	0.78	0.74	0.70	0.67	0.64	0.61	0.58
23	1.92	1.70	1.53	1.39	1.28	1.18	1.10	1.02	0.96	0.90	0.85	0.81	0.77	0.73	0.70	0.67	0.64
25	2.08	1.85	1.67	1.52	1.39	1.28	1.19	1.11	1.04	0.98	0.93	0.88	0.83	0.79	0.76	0.72	0.69
27	2.25	2.00	1.80	1.64	1.50	1.38	1.29	1.20	1.13	1.06	1.00	0.95	0.90	0.86	0.82	0.78	0.75
29	2.42	2.15	1.93	1.76	1.61	1.49	1.38	1.29	1.21	1.14	1.07	1.02	0.97	0.92	0.88	0.84	0.81
31	2.58	2.30	2.07	1.88	1.72	1.59	1.48	1.38	1.29	1.22	1.15	1.09	1.03	0.98	0.94	0.90	0.86
33	2.75	2.44	2.20	2.00	1.83	1.69	1.57	1.47	1.38	1.29	1.22	1.16	1.10	1.05	1.00	0.96	0.92
35	2.92	2.59	2.33	2.12	1.94	1.79	1.67	1.56	1.46	1.37	1.30	1.23	1.17	1.11	1.06	1.01	0.97
37	3.08	2.74	2.47	2.24	2.06	1.90	1.76	1.64	1.54	1.45	1.37	1.30	1.23	1.17	1.12	1.07	1.03
39	3.25	2.89	2.60	2.36	2.17	2.00	1.86	1.73	1.63	1.53	1.44	1.37	1.30	1.24	1.18	1.13	1.08
41	3.42	3.04	2.73	2.48	2.28	2.10	1.95	1.82	1.71	1.61	1.52	1.44	1.37	1.30	1.24	1.19	1.14
43	3.58	3.19	2.87	2.61	2.39	2.21	2.05	1.91	1.79	1.69	1.59	1.51	1.43	1.37	1.30	1.25	1.19
45	3.75	3.33	3.00	2.73	2.50	2.31	2.14	2.00	1.88	1.76	1.67	1.58	1.50	1.43	1.36	1.30	1.25
47	3.92	3.48	3.13	2.85	2.61	2.41	2.24	2.09	1.96	1.84	1.74	1.65	1.57	1.49	1.42	1.36	1.31
49	4.08	3.63	3.27	2.97	2.72	2.51	2.33	2.18	2.04	1.92	1.81	1.72	1.63	1.56	1.48	1.42	1.36
51	4.25	3.78	3.40	3.09	2.83	2.62	2.43	2.27	2.13	2.00	1.89	1.79	1.70	1.62	1.55	1.48	1.42
53	4.42	3.93	3.53	3.21	2.94	2.72	2.52	2.36	2.21	2.08	1.96	1.86	1.77	1.68	1.61	1.54	1.47
55	4.58	4.07	3.67	3.33	3.06	2.82	2.62	2.44	2.29	2.16	2.04	1.93	1.83	1.75	1.67	1.59	1.53
57	4.75	4.22	3.80	3.45	3.17	2.92	2.71	2.53	2.38	2.24	2.11	2.00	1.90	1.81	1.73	1.65	1.58
59	4.92	4.37	3.93	3.58	3.28	3.03	2.81	2.62	2.46	2.31	2.19	2.07	1.97	1.87	1.79	1.71	1.64
61	5.08	4.52	4.07	3.70	3.39	3.13	2.90	2.71	2.54	2.39	2.26	2.14	2.03	1.94	1.85	1.77	1.69
63	5.25	4.67	4.20	3.82	3.50	3.23	3.00	2.80	2.63	2.47	2.33	2.21	2.10	2.00	1.91	1.83	1.75
65	5.42	4.81	4.33	3.94	3.61	3.33	3.10	2.89	2.71	2.55	2.41	2.28	2.17	2.06	1.97	1.88	1.81
67	5.58	4.96	4.47	4.06	3.72	3.44	3.19	2.98	2.79	2.63	2.48	2.35	2.23	2.13	2.03	1.94	1.86
69	5.75	5.11	4.60	4.18	3.83	3.54	3.29	3.07	2.88	2.71	2.56	2.42	2.30	2.19	2.09	2.00	1.92
71	5.92	5.26	4.73	4.30	3.94	3.64	3.38	3.16	2.96	2.78	2.63	2.49	2.37	2.25	2.15	2.06	1.97
73	6.08	5.41	4.87	4.42	4.06	3.74	3.48	3.24	3.04	2.86	2.70	2.56	2.43	2.32	2.21	2.12	2.03
75	6.25	5.56	5.00	4.55	4.17	3.85	3.57	3.33	3.13	2.94	2.78	2.63	2.50	2.38	2.27	2.17	2.08
77	6.42	5.70	5.13	4.67	4.28	3.95	3.67	3.42	3.21	3.02	2.85	2.70	2.57	2.44	2.33	2.23	2.14
79	6.58	5.85	5.27	4.79	4.39	4.05	3.76	3.51	3.29	3.10	2.93	2.77	2.63	2.51	2.39	2.29	2.19
81	6.75	6.00	5.40	4.91	4.50	4.15	3.86	3.60	3.38	3.18	3.00	2.84	2.70	2.57	2.45	2.35	2.25
83	6.92	6.15	5.53	5.03	4.61	4.26	3.95	3.69	3.46	3.25	3.07	2.91	2.77	2.63	2.52	2.41	2.31
85	7.08	6.30	5.67	5.15	4.72	4.36	4.05	3.78	3.54	3.33	3.15	2.98	2.83	2.70	2.58	2.46	2.36
87	7.25	6.44	5.80	5.27	4.83	4.46	4.14	3.87	3.63	3.41	3.22	3.05	2.90	2.76	2.64	2.52	2.42

Initial rate: 0.25 mcg/kg/minute; increase rate every 5 minutes by 0.25 mcg/kg/minute until desired mean systolic blood pressure is achieved.

Maximum rate: 10 mcg/kg/minute.

CRITICAL CARE INFUSION ADMINISTRATION CHARTS

(Continued)

NITROPRUSSIDE (Nipride®)

	400 mcg/mL (100 mg/250 mL of D_5W)																
	WEIGHT (kg)																
	40	**45**	**50**	**55**	**60**	**65**	**70**	**75**	**80**	**85**	**90**	**95**	**100**	**105**	**110**	**115**	**120**
mL/h	*(mcg/kg/minute)*																
1	0.17	0.15	0.13	0.12	0.11	0.10											
3	0.50	0.44	0.40	0.36	0.33	0.31	0.29	0.27	0.25	0.24	0.22	0.21	0.20	0.19	0.18	0.17	0.17
5	0.83	0.74	0.67	0.61	0.56	0.51	0.48	0.44	0.42	0.39	0.37	0.35	0.33	0.32	0.30	0.29	0.28
7	1.17	1.04	0.93	0.85	0.78	0.72	0.67	0.62	0.58	0.55	0.52	0.49	0.47	0.44	0.42	0.41	0.39
9	1.50	1.33	1.20	1.09	1.00	0.92	0.86	0.80	0.75	0.71	0.67	0.63	0.60	0.57	0.55	0.52	0.50
11	1.83	1.63	1.47	1.33	1.22	1.13	1.05	0.98	0.92	0.86	0.81	0.77	0.73	0.70	0.67	0.64	0.61
13	2.17	1.93	1.73	1.58	1.44	1.33	1.24	1.16	1.08	1.02	0.96	0.91	0.87	0.83	0.79	0.75	0.72
15	2.50	2.22	2.00	1.82	1.67	1.54	1.43	1.33	1.25	1.18	1.11	1.05	1.00	0.95	0.91	0.87	0.83
17	2.83	2.52	2.27	2.06	1.89	1.74	1.62	1.51	1.42	1.33	1.26	1.19	1.13	1.08	1.03	0.99	0.94
19	3.17	2.81	2.53	2.30	2.11	1.95	1.81	1.69	1.58	1.49	1.41	1.33	1.27	1.21	1.15	1.10	1.06
21	3.50	3.11	2.80	2.55	2.33	2.15	2.00	1.87	1.75	1.65	1.56	1.47	1.40	1.33	1.27	1.22	1.17
23	3.83	3.41	3.07	2.79	2.56	2.36	2.19	2.04	1.92	1.80	1.70	1.61	1.53	1.46	1.39	1.33	1.28
25	4.17	3.70	3.33	3.03	2.78	2.56	2.38	2.22	2.08	1.96	1.85	1.75	1.67	1.59	1.52	1.45	1.39
27	4.50	4.00	3.60	3.27	3.00	2.77	2.57	2.40	2.25	2.12	2.00	1.89	1.80	1.71	1.64	1.57	1.50
29	4.83	4.30	3.87	3.52	3.22	2.97	2.76	2.58	2.42	2.27	2.15	2.04	1.93	1.84	1.76	1.68	1.61
31	5.17	4.59	4.13	3.76	3.44	3.18	2.95	2.76	2.58	2.43	2.30	2.18	2.07	1.97	1.88	1.80	1.72
33	5.50	4.89	4.40	4.00	3.67	3.38	3.14	2.93	2.75	2.59	2.44	2.32	2.20	2.10	2.00	1.91	1.83
35	5.83	5.19	4.67	4.24	3.89	3.59	3.33	3.11	2.92	2.75	2.59	2.46	2.33	2.22	2.12	2.03	1.94
37	6.17	5.48	4.93	4.48	4.11	3.79	3.52	3.29	3.08	2.90	2.74	2.60	2.47	2.35	2.24	2.14	2.06
39	6.50	5.78	5.20	4.73	4.33	4.00	3.71	3.47	3.25	3.06	2.89	2.74	2.60	2.48	2.36	2.26	2.17
41	6.83	6.07	5.47	4.97	4.56	4.21	3.90	3.64	3.42	3.22	3.04	2.88	2.73	2.60	2.48	2.38	2.28
43	7.17	6.37	5.73	5.21	4.78	4.41	4.10	3.82	3.58	3.37	3.19	3.02	2.87	2.73	2.61	2.49	2.39
45	7.50	6.67	6.00	5.45	5.00	4.62	4.29	4.00	3.75	3.53	3.33	3.16	3.00	2.86	2.73	2.61	2.50
47	7.83	6.96	6.27	5.70	5.22	4.82	4.48	4.18	3.92	3.69	3.48	3.30	3.13	2.98	2.85	2.72	2.61
49	8.17	7.26	6.53	5.94	5.44	5.03	4.67	4.36	4.08	3.84	3.63	3.44	3.27	3.11	2.97	2.84	2.72
51	8.50	7.56	6.80	6.18	5.67	5.23	4.86	4.53	4.25	4.00	3.78	3.58	3.40	3.24	3.09	2.96	2.83
53	8.83	7.85	7.07	6.42	5.89	5.44	5.05	4.71	4.42	4.16	3.93	3.72	3.53	3.37	3.21	3.07	2.94
55	9.17	8.15	7.33	6.67	6.11	5.64	5.24	4.89	4.58	4.31	4.07	3.86	3.67	3.49	3.33	3.19	3.06
57	9.50	8.44	7.60	6.91	6.33	5.85	5.43	5.07	4.75	4.47	4.22	4.00	3.80	3.62	3.45	3.30	3.17
59	9.83	8.74	7.87	7.15	6.56	6.05	5.62	5.24	4.92	4.63	4.37	4.14	3.93	3.75	3.58	3.42	3.28
61	10.17	9.04	8.13	7.39	6.78	6.26	5.81	5.42	5.08	4.78	4.52	4.28	4.07	3.87	3.70	3.54	3.39
63		9.33	8.40	7.64	7.00	6.46	6.00	5.60	5.25	4.94	4.67	4.42	4.20	4.00	3.82	3.65	3.50
65		9.63	8.67	7.88	7.22	6.67	6.19	5.78	5.42	5.10	4.81	4.56	4.33	4.13	3.94	3.77	3.61
67		9.93	8.93	8.12	7.44	6.87	6.38	5.96	5.58	5.25	4.96	4.70	4.47	4.25	4.06	3.88	3.72
69		10.22	9.20	8.36	7.67	7.08	6.57	6.13	5.75	5.41	5.11	4.84	4.60	4.38	4.18	4.00	3.83
71			9.47	8.61	7.89	7.28	6.76	6.31	5.92	5.57	5.26	4.98	4.73	4.51	4.30	4.12	3.94
73			9.73	8.85	8.11	7.49	6.95	6.49	6.08	5.73	5.41	5.12	4.87	4.63	4.42	4.23	4.06
75			10.00	9.09	8.33	7.69	7.14	6.67	6.25	5.88	5.56	5.26	5.00	4.76	4.55	4.35	4.17
77				9.33	8.56	7.90	7.33	6.84	6.42	6.04	5.70	5.40	5.13	4.89	4.67	4.46	4.28
79				9.58	8.78	8.10	7.52	7.02	6.58	6.20	5.85	5.54	5.27	5.02	4.79	4.58	4.39
81				9.82	9.00	8.31	7.71	7.20	6.75	6.35	6.00	5.68	5.40	5.14	4.91	4.70	4.50
83				10.06	9.22	8.51	7.90	7.38	6.92	6.51	6.15	5.82	5.53	5.27	5.03	4.81	4.61
85					9.44	8.72	8.10	7.56	7.08	6.67	6.30	5.96	5.67	5.40	5.15	4.93	4.72
87					9.67	8.92	8.29	7.73	7.25	6.82	6.44	6.11	5.80	5.52	5.27	5.04	4.83

Initial rate: 0.25 mcg/kg/minute; increase rate every 5 minutes by 0.25 mcg/kg/minute until desired mean systolic blood pressure is achieved.

Maximum rate: 10 mcg/kg/minute.

NOREPINEPHRINE (Levophed®) 32 mcg/mL

8 mg in 250 mL D_5W or NS							
mL/h	mcg/min	mL/h	mcg/min	mL/h	mcg/min	mL/h	mcg/min
1	0.53	21	11.20	41	21.87	61	32.53
2	1.07	22	11.73	42	22.40	62	33.07
3	1.60	23	12.27	43	22.93	63	33.60
4	2.13	24	12.80	44	23.47	64	34.13
5	2.67	25	13.33	45	24.00	65	34.67
6	3.20	26	13.87	46	24.53	66	35.20
7	3.73	27	14.40	47	25.07	67	35.73
8	4.27	28	14.93	48	25.60	68	36.27
9	4.80	29	15.47	49	26.13	69	36.80
10	5.33	30	16.00	50	26.67	70	37.33
11	5.87	31	16.53	51	27.20	71	37.87
12	6.40	32	17.07	52	27.73	72	38.40
13	6.93	33	17.60	53	28.27	73	38.93
14	7.47	34	18.13	54	28.80	74	39.47
15	8.00	35	18.67	55	29.33	75	40.00
16	8.53	36	19.20	56	29.87	76	40.53
17	9.07	37	19.73	57	30.40	77	41.07
18	9.60	38	20.27	58	30.93	78	41.60
19	10.13	39	20.80	59	31.47	79	42.13
20	10.67	40	21.33	60	32.00	80	42.67

Usual dosing range: 2-30 mcg/minute.

NOREPINEPHRINE (Levophed®) 64 mcg/mL

16 mg in 250 mL D_5W or NS							
mL/h	mcg/min	mL/h	mcg/min	mL/h	mcg/min	mL/h	mcg/min
1	1.07	21	22.40	41	43.73	61	65.07
2	2.13	22	23.47	42	44.80	62	66.13
3	3.20	23	24.53	43	45.87	63	67.20
4	4.27	24	25.60	44	46.93	64	68.27
5	5.33	25	26.67	45	48.00	65	69.33
6	6.40	26	27.73	46	49.07	66	70.40
7	7.47	27	28.80	47	50.13	67	71.47
8	8.53	28	29.87	48	51.20	68	72.53
9	9.60	29	30.93	49	52.27	69	73.60
10	10.67	30	32.00	50	53.33	70	74.67
11	11.73	31	33.07	51	54.40	71	75.73
12	12.80	32	34.13	52	55.47	72	76.80
13	13.87	33	35.20	53	56.53	73	77.87
14	14.93	34	36.27	54	57.60	74	78.93
15	16.00	35	37.33	55	58.67	75	80.00
16	17.07	36	38.40	56	59.73	76	81.07
17	18.13	37	39.47	57	60.80	77	82.13
18	19.20	38	40.53	58	61.87	78	83.20
19	20.27	39	41.60	59	62.93	79	84.27
20	21.33	40	42.67	60	64.00	80	85.33

Usual dosing range: 2-30 mcg/minute.

CRITICAL CARE INFUSION ADMINISTRATION CHARTS
(Continued)

PHENYLEPHRINE 500 mcg/mL

50 mg in 100 mL D_5W or NS			
mL/h	**mcg/min**	**mL/h**	**mcg/min**
0.5	4.17	15.5	129.17
1	8.33	16	133.33
1.5	12.50	16.5	137.50
2	16.67	17	141.67
2.5	20.83	17.5	145.83
3	25.00	18	150.00
3.5	29.17	18.5	154.17
4	33.33	19	158.33
4.5	37.50	19.5	162.50
5	41.67	20	166.67
5.5	45.83	20.5	170.83
6	50.00	21	175.00
6.5	54.17	21.5	179.17
7	58.33	22	183.33
7.5	62.50	22.5	187.50
8	66.67	23	191.67
8.5	70.83	23.5	195.83
9	75.00	24	200.00
9.5	79.17	24.5	204.17
10	83.33	25	208.33
10.5	87.50	25.5	212.50
11	91.67	26	216.67
11.5	95.83	26.5	220.83
12	100.00	27	225.00
12.5	104.17	27.5	229.17
13	108.33	28	233.33
13.5	112.50	28.5	237.50
14	116.67	29	241.67
14.5	120.83	29.5	245.83
15	125.00	30	250.00

Usual maintenance dose: 20-200 mcg/minute.

PROPOFOL (Diprivan®) 10 mg/mL

	CONTINUOUS INFUSION FOR ICU SEDATION																
	WEIGHT (kg)																
	40	45	50	55	60	65	70	75	80	85	90	95	100	105	110	115	120
mL/h	*(mcg/kg/minute)*																
1	4.2	3.7	3.3	3.0	2.8	2.6	2.4	2.2	2.1	2.0	1.9	1.8	1.7	1.6	1.5	1.4	1.4
2	8.3	7.4	6.7	6.1	5.6	5.1	4.8	4.4	4.2	3.9	3.7	3.5	3.3	3.2	3.0	2.9	2.8
3	12.5	11.1	10.0	9.1	8.3	7.7	7.1	6.7	6.3	5.9	5.6	5.3	5.0	4.8	4.5	4.3	4.2
4	16.7	14.8	13.3	12.1	11.1	10.3	9.5	8.9	8.3	7.6	7.4	7.0	6.7	6.3	6.1	5.8	5.6
5	20.8	18.5	16.7	15.2	13.9	12.8	11.9	11.1	10.4	9.8	9.3	8.8	8.3	7.9	7.6	7.2	6.9
6	25.0	22.2	20.0	18.2	16.7	15.4	14.3	13.3	12.5	11.8	11.1	10.5	10.0	9.5	9.1	8.7	8.3
7	29.2	25.9	23.3	21.2	19.4	17.9	16.7	15.6	14.6	13.7	13.0	12.3	11.7	11.1	10.6	10.1	9.7
8	33.3	29.6	26.7	24.2	22.2	20.5	19.0	17.8	16.7	15.7	14.8	14.0	13.3	12.7	12.1	11.6	11.1
9	37.5	33.3	30.0	27.3	25.0	23.1	21.4	20.0	18.8	17.6	16.7	15.8	15.0	14.3	13.6	13.0	12.5
10	41.7	37.0	33.3	30.3	27.8	25.6	23.8	22.2	20.8	19.6	18.5	17.5	16.7	15.9	15.2	14.5	13.9
11	45.8	40.7	36.7	33.3	30.6	28.2	26.2	24.4	22.9	21.6	20.4	19.3	18.3	17.5	16.7	15.9	15.3
12	50.0	44.4	40.0	36.4	33.3	30.8	28.6	26.7	25.0	23.5	22.2	21.1	20.0	19.0	18.2	17.4	16.7
13	54.2	48.1	43.3	39.4	36.1	33.3	31.0	28.9	27.1	25.5	24.1	22.8	21.7	20.6	19.7	18.8	18.1
14	56.3	51.9	46.7	42.4	38.9	35.9	33.3	31.1	29.2	27.5	25.9	24.6	23.3	22.2	21.2	20.3	19.4
15	62.5	55.6	50.0	45.5	41.7	38.5	35.7	33.3	31.3	29.4	27.8	26.3	25.0	23.8	22.7	21.7	20.8
16	66.7	59.3	53.3	48.5	44.4	41.0	38.1	35.6	33.3	31.4	29.6	28.1	26.7	25.4	24.2	23.2	22.2
17	70.8	63.0	56.7	51.5	47.2	43.6	40.5	37.8	35.4	33.3	31.5	29.8	28.3	27.0	25.8	24.6	23.6
18	75.0	66.7	60.0	54.5	50.0	46.2	42.9	40.0	37.5	35.3	33.3	31.6	30.0	28.6	27.3	26.1	25.0
19		70.4	63.3	57.6	52.8	48.7	45.2	42.2	39.6	37.3	35.2	33.3	31.7	30.2	28.8	27.5	26.4
20		74.1	66.7	60.6	55.6	51.3	47.6	44.4	41.7	39.2	37.0	35.1	33.3	31.7	30.3	29.0	27.8
21			70.0	63.6	58.3	53.8	50.0	46.7	43.8	41.2	38.9	36.8	35.0	33.3	31.8	30.4	29.3
22			73.3	66.7	61.1	56.4	52.4	48.9	45.6	43.1	40.7	38.6	36.7	34.9	33.3	31.9	30.6
23			76.7	69.7	63.9	59.0	54.8	51.1	47.9	45.1	42.6	40.4	38.3	36.5	34.8	33.3	31.9
24				72.7	66.7	61.5	57.1	53.3	50.0	47.1	44.4	42.1	40.0	38.1	36.4	34.8	33.3
25				75.8	69.4	64.1	59.5	55.6	52.1	49.0	46.3	43.9	41.7	39.7	37.9	36.2	34.7
26					72.2	66.7	61.9	57.8	54.2	51.0	48.1	45.6	43.3	41.3	39.4	37.7	36.1
27					75.0	69.2	64.3	60.0	56.3	52.9	50.0	47.4	45.0	42.9	40.9	39.1	37.5
28						71.8	66.7	62.2	58.3	54.9	51.9	49.1	46.7	44.4	42.4	40.6	38.9
29						74.4	69.0	64.4	60.4	56.9	53.7	50.9	48.3	46.0	43.9	42.0	40.3
30						76.9	71.4	66.7	62.5	58.8	55.6	52.6	50.0	47.6	45.5	43.5	41.7
31							73.8	68.9	64.6	60.8	57.4	54.4	51.7	49.2	47.0	44.9	43.1
32							76.2	71.1	66.7	62.7	59.3	56.1	53.3	50.8	48.5	46.4	44.4
33								73.3	68.8	64.7	61.1	57.9	55.0	52.4	50.0	47.8	45.8
34								75.6	70.8	66.7	63.0	59.6	56.7	54.0	51.5	49.3	47.2
35									72.9	68.6	64.8	61.4	58.3	55.6	53.0	50.7	48.6
36									75.0	70.6	66.7	63.2	60.0	57.1	54.5	52.2	50.0
37										72.5	68.5	64.9	61.7	58.7	56.1	53.6	51.4
38										74.5	70.4	66.7	63.3	60.3	57.6	55.1	52.8
39										76.5	72.2	68.4	65.0	61.9	59.1	56.5	54.2
40											74.1	70.2	66.7	63.5	60.6	58.0	55.6
41											75.9	71.9	68.3	65.1	62.1	59.4	56.9
42												73.7	70.0	66.7	63.6	60.9	58.3
43												75.4	71.7	68.3	65.2	62.3	59.7
44													73.3	69.8	66.7	63.8	61.1
45													75.0	71.4	68.2	65.2	62.5

Recommended starting dose: 17-50 mcg/kg/minute with adjustments in dose made at 3- to 5-minute intervals; once sedation is established, dose should be decreased for the maintenance infusion period and adjusted to response.

Usual maintenance dose: 25-75 mcg/kg/minute.

FACTORS ASSOCIATED WITH POSTOPERATIVE NAUSEA AND VOMITING (PONV)

Patient-Related

- Female gender
- Obesity
- Infants and small children
- Surgery during days of menstruation and ovulation
- History of previous PONV
- History of motion sickness
- Gastroparesis
- Preoperative anxiety

Surgical Procedure

- Children
  - Middle ear surgery, eye surgery (especially strabismus surgery), hernia surgery, tonsillectomy/adenoidectomy, otoplasty, orchiopexy
- Adults
  - Laparoscopic gynecological surgery, extracorporeal shock-wave lithotripsy, abortion, head and neck surgery, gastrointestinal (GI) surgery, ear surgery
- Increased incidence with increased duration of surgery

Anesthetic

- Premedication with opioids
- Inappropriate mask and bag ventilation
- Inhalation anesthesia (vs total I.V. anesthesia)
- Nitrous oxide-opioid-relaxant technique
- Ketamine induction/maintenance
- Etomidate induction
- Use of anticholinesterase (eg, neostigmine) agents

Postoperative

- Pain
- Dizziness
- Ambulation attempted too early
- Changes in position
- Hypotension
- Oral intake attempted too early
- Opioid administration

HEPARIN AND LOW MOLECULAR WEIGHT HEPARIN (LMWH)

Guidelines for Use in Regional Anesthesia

Drug	Guidelines
Heparin I.V.	Therapeutic heparinization performed at least 60 minutes after needle placement for spinal or epidural anesthesia
	Heparin effect appropriately monitored; APTT maintained in therapeutic range
	Indwelling catheter removed when heparin activity is low or completely reversed
Heparin S.C.	Needle placement or catheter removal avoided within 4 hours of heparin administration
	Anticoagulant effect monitored in patients with liver disease or long-term thromboprophylaxis
LMWH	***Patients receiving LMWH preoperatively***[1]
	Needle placement at least 10-12 hours after the last dose of LMWH
	Further dosing of LMWH at least 2 hours after needle placement
	Postoperative initiation of LMWH[2]
	With continuous catheter techniques, the first dose of LMWH should be administered 2 hours after catheter removal, ideally with the catheter having been left indwelling overnight
	Catheter removal should not be performed for 10-12 hours after a dose of LMWH
	Beginning LMWH in presence of indwelling catheter must be done with caution and patient's neurologic status monitored closely

[1]Single-dose spinal anesthetic may be safest technique in this patient population.

[2]Single-dose or continuous catheter techniques can be used.

Monitor for early signs of cord compression in the perioperative period:

- progression of numbness/weakness
- bowel/bladder dysfunction
- severe back pain may or may not be present

Reference

Horlocker TT and Heit JA, "Low Molecular Weight Heparin: Biochemistry, Pharmacology, Perioperative Prophylaxis Regimens, and Guidelines for Regional Anesthetic Management," *Anesth Analg,* 1997, 85(4):874-85.

INHALATIONAL ANESTHETICS

Factors Affecting Minimum Alveolar Concentration (MAC)

Variable	Effect on MAC
Age	
Young	↑
Elderly	↓
Alcohol	
Acute intoxication	↓
Chronic abuse	↑
Anemia	
Hematocrit <10%	↓
Blood pressure	
MAP <40 mm Hg	↓
Drugs	
Anesthetics, local	↓
Barbiturates	↓
Benzodiazepines	↓
Ketamine	↓
Lithium	↓
Opioids	↓
Sympatholytics	
Clonidine	↓
Dexmedetomidine	↓
Sympathomimetics	
Amphetamine	
Acute	↑
Chronic	↓
Cocaine	↑
Ephedrine	↑
MAOI	↑
Verapamil	↓
Electrolytes	
Hypercalcemia	↓
Hypernatremia	↑
Hyponatremia	↓
PaO_2 <40 mm Hg	↓
$PaCO_2$ >95 mm Hg	↓
Pregnancy	↓
Temperature	
Hyperthermia (>42°C)	↑
Hypothermia	↓
Thyroid	
Hyperthyroid	No change
Hypothyroid	No change

Modified from Morgan GE and Mikhail MS, eds, *Clinical Anesthesiology*, East Norwalk, CT: Appleton & Lange, 1992.

Modified from Stoelting RK and Miller RD, eds, *Basics of Anesthesia*, 3rd ed, New York, NY: Churchill Livingstone, 2000.

Effects of Inhalational Anesthetics on Organ Systems

	Desflurane	Enflurane	Halothane	Isoflurane	Nitrous Oxide	Sevoflurane
MAC (%)[1]	6.0	1.68	0.74	1.2	105	2.6
Blood/Gas Partition Coefficient[2]	0.42	1.9	2.4	1.4	0.47	0.63
Cardiovascular						
Blood pressure	↓↓	↓↓	↓↓	↓↓	No change	↓↓
Cardiac output[3]	No change	↓↓	↓	No change	No change	No change
Heart rate	↑	↑	↓	↑	No change	No change
Systemic vascular resistance	↓↓	↓	No change	↓↓	No change	↓
Cerebral						
Blood flow	↑	↑	↑↑	↑	↑↑	↑
Intracranial pressure	↑	↑↑	↑↑	↑	↑	↑
Seizures	↓	↑	↓	↓	↓	↓
Hepatic						
Blood flow	↓	↓↓	↓↓	↓	↓	↓
Metabolism[4]	0.02%	2% to 5%	15% to 50%	0.2%	0.004%	3% to 5%
Neuromuscular						
Nondepolarizing blockade	↑↑↑	↑↑↑	↑↑	↑↑↑	↑	↑↑↑
Renal						
Glomerular filtration rate	?	↓↓	↓↓	↓↓	↓↓	?
Renal blood flow	↓	↓↓	↓↓	↓↓	↓↓	↓
Urinary output	?	↓↓	↓↓	↓↓	↓↓	?

INHALATIONAL ANESTHETICS *(Continued)*

Effects of Inhalational Anesthetics on Organ Systems *(continued)*

	Desflurane	Enflurane	Halothane	Isoflurane	Nitrous Oxide	Sevoflurane
Respiratory						
$PaCO_2$						
Resting	↑	↑↑	↑	↑	No change	↑
Challenge	↑	↑↑	↑	↑	↑	↑
Respiratory rate	↑	↑↑	↑↑	↑	↑	↑
Tidal volume	↓	↓	↓	↓	↓	↓

[1]Minimum alveolar concentration (MAC) = percentage of inspired concentration to prevent 50% of patients from moving to surgical stimulus (ED_{50}).

[2]Solubility of gas in blood at 37°C; less soluble gases have faster onset of action.

[3]Controlled ventilation.

[4]Metabolism = percentage of absorbed anesthetic undergoing metabolism.

Modified from Morgan GE and Mikhail MS, "Clinical Anesthesiology," New York, NY: Lange Medical Books/McGraw-Hill, 1996:138.

INTRAVENOUS ANESTHETIC AGENTS

Agent	Anesthesia Bolus	Anesthesia Maintenance	Sedation Bolus	Sedation Maintenance
Diazepam	0.3-0.6 mg/kg	—	0.04-0.2 mg/kg	—
Etomidate	0.2-0.5 mg/kg	10-20 mcg/kg/min	—	—
Ketamine	1-2 mg/kg	15-75 mcg/kg/min	0.5-1 mg/kg	—
Lorazepam	0.02-0.05 mg/kg	—	0.03-0.05 mg/kg	—
Methohexital	1-2 mg/kg	50-150mcg/kg/min	0.25-1 mcg/kg	10-50 mcg/kg/min
Midazolam	0.2-0.6 mg/kg	0.25-2 mcg/kg/min	0.01-0.1 mg/kg	
Propofol	1.5-2.5 mg/kg	100-200 mcg/kg/min	0.25-1 mcg/kg	25-100 mcg/kg/min
Thiopental	3-5 mg/kg	30-200 mcg/kg/min	0.5-1.5 mg/kg	—

LOCAL ANESTHETICS

Amides – Use / Concentration

Agent	Use	Concentration
Bupivacaine	Infil, PNB, epid, spin	0.25% (infil); 0.25%, 0.5% (PNB); 0.25%, 0.5%, 0.75% (epid); 0.5%, 0.75% (spin)
Etidocaine	Infil, PNB, epid	0.25%, 0.5% (infil); 0.5%, 1% (PNB, epid)
Lidocaine	PNB, epid, infil, spin, topical, bier	1%, 1.5%, 2% (PNB, epid); 5% (spin); 2%, 2.5%, 5% (topical); 0.5%, 1% (infil); 0.5% (bier)
Mepivacaine	Infil, PNB, epid	1% (infil); 1%, 2% (PNB), 1%, 1.5%, 2% (epid)
Prilocaine	Infil, PNB. epid	1%, 2% (infil); 1%, 2%, 3% (PNB, epid)
Ropivacaine	Infil, PNB, epid, spin	0.5% (infil); 0.5% (PNB), 0.5%, 0.75% (epid)

epid = epidural; infil = infiltration; PNB = peripheral nerve block; spin = spinal.

Esters – Use / Concentration

Agent	Use	Concentration
Chloroprocaine	Epid, infil, PNB	1% (infil); 1%, 2% (PNB); 2%, 3% (epid, spin)
Cocaine	Anesthetize and constrict nasal mucosa prior to nasal intubation; nasal surgery; vasoconstriction properties	4% (topical)
Procaine	Infil, PNB, spin	1%, 2% (infil); 5% (spinal)
Tetracaine	Spinal, topical	0.1%, 0.5% (spinal); 2% (topical)

epid = epidural; infil = infiltration; PNB = peripheral nerve block; spin = spinal.

Pharmacodynamics / Kinetics, Maximum Dose, and Toxic Threshold Concentration

Agent	pKa	Protein Binding (%)	Onset	Duration[1] (h)	Maximum Dose (mg/kg)	Toxic Threshold Concentration (mcg/mL)
Bupivacaine	8.1	95	Intermediate	1.5-8.5	2.5	1.6
Chloroprocaine	9.2	<10	Rapid	0.5-1	12	—
Etidocaine	7.7	90-94	Rapid	4-10	4	2.0
Lidocaine	7.8	70-75	Rapid	1-4	5 w/o epi; 7 w/epi	5-6
Mepivacaine	7.6	75	Rapid	2-3	5 w/o epi; 7 w/epi	5-6
Prilocaine	7.8	50	Rapid	2-6	8	5-6
Procaine	8.9	<10	Slow	0.5-1	12	—
Ropivacaine	8.1	95	Intermediate	1.5-9	3	ND
Tetracaine	8.2	75-80	Slow	1-3 (topical)	3	—

[1]Duration of action depends on site of local anesthetic administration.

MALIGNANT HYPERTHERMIA

SIGNS AND SYMPTOMS

Tachycardia (unexplained)
Increased end-tidal carbon dioxide
Arrhythmias (ventricular)
Acidosis (respiratory, metabolic)
Muscle rigidity
Tachypnea
Fever
Cyanosis
Hypoxemia
Hyperkalemia
Coagulopathy (eg, DIC)
Myoglobinuria

THERAPY FOR MALIGNANT HYPERTHERMIA EMERGENCY

CAUTION: This protocol may not apply to every patient and must of necessity be altered according to specific patient needs.

1. Immediately discontinue all inhalation anesthetics and succinylcholine. Hyperventilate with 100% oxygen at high gas flows (≥10 L/minute).
2. In the absence of blood gas analysis, bicarbonate 1-2 mEq/kg should be administered.
3. Dantrolene sodium should be obtained, mixed with 60 mL of sterile water for injection USP (without a bacteriostatic agent), and 2.5 mg/kg administered intravenously. At present, dantrolene is packaged as a lyophilized preparation that contains 20 mg of dantrolene and 3 g mannitol per vial.
4. Simultaneously, cooling should be started by all routes: surface, nasogastric lavage, intravenous cold solutions, wound, and rectally.
5. Arrhythmias will usually respond to treatment of acidosis and hyperkalemia. If they persist or are life-threatening, standard antiarrhythmic agents may be used, with the exception of calcium channel blockers.
6. Administer further doses of dantrolene as necessary titrated to heart rate, muscle rigidity, and temperature. Response to dantrolene should begin to occur in minutes; if not, more drug should be administered. Although the average successful dose of dantrolene is about 2.5 mg/kg, much higher doses may be needed (≥10 mg/kg). Fortunately, dantrolene does not produce significant myocardial depression at these doses.
7. Change anesthetic tubing.
8. Determine and monitor closely urine output, serum potassium, calcium, arterial blood gases, end tidal CO_2, and clotting studies. Hyperkalemia is common in the acute phase of MH and should be treated with intravenous glucose and insulin.
9. Observe the patient in an ICU setting for at least 24 hours since recrudescence of MH may occur, particularly following a case that was difficult to treat.
10. Follow CK, calcium, potassium, and clotting studies until such time as they return.
11. ECG should also be obtained and followed postoperatively.
12. Monitor body temperature closely since overvigorous treatment of MH may lead to hypothermia. Temperature instability may persist for several days after the acute episode. Body temperatures of 41°C to 42°C are compatible with survival and normal brain function if treated promptly.
13. Ensure urine output >1 mL/kg/hour. Consider CVP monitoring because of fluid shifts that may occur.
14. When the patient's condition has stabilized, convert from intravenous to oral dantrolene. Although data are not available regarding optimal doses and duration of treatment with dantrolene after an episode, the patient should probably receive a total dose of 4 mg/kg/day in divided doses for 48 hours postoperatively.
15. Counsel the patient and family regarding MH and further precautions. Refer patient to the Malignant Hyperthermia Association of the United States (MHAUS).

Malignant Hyperthermia Hotline (209) 634-4917

OPIOIDS

Opioid Agonist-Antagonists

Agent	I.V.	I.M.	Oral	Epidural	Nasal
Buprenorphine	0.3 mg; 4-6 h	0.3 mg; 4-6 h	—	—	—
Butorphanol	0.5-2 mg; 3-4 h	1-4 mg; 3-4 h	—	2 mg	1 spray/nostril
Dezocine	2.5-10 mg; 2-4 h	5-20 mg; 3-6 h	—	—	—
Pentazocine	30 mg; 3-4 h	30-60 mg; 3-4 h	50 mg; 3-4 h	50 mg; 3-4 h	—

Analgesic Doses

Agent	PCA Load Dose	PCA Bolus Dose	PCA Lockout	Epidural Bolus Dose
Alfentanil	50-100 mcg	10-100 mcg	3-10 min	500-1000 mcg
Fentanyl	25-75 mcg	10-20 mcg	2-10 min	25-100 mcg
Hydromorphone	0.25 mg	0.05-0.25 mg	5-10 min	1-2 mg
Meperidine	50-100 mg	5-30 mg	10-20 min	20-50 mg
Morphine	5-10 mg	0.5-3 mg	5-12 min	2-6 mg
Nalbuphine	2-5 mg	1-5 mg	5-15 min	1-10 mg
Sufentanil	2-5 mcg	2-10 mcg	2-10 min	10-60 mcg

Agent	Epidural Continuous Infusion	Intrathecal Bolus Dose	Intermittent I.M.	Intermittent I.V.
Alfentanil	200 mcg/h	—	—	—
Fentanyl	25-100 mcg/h	5-25 mcg	—	1-2 mcg/kg
Hydromorphone	0.1-0.2 mg/h	—	1.5 mg	1-2 mg
Meperidine	10-50 mg/h	10-30 mg	75-100 mg	75-100 mg
Morphine	0.2-1 mg/h	0.1-0.5 mg	2-10 mg	2-10 mg
Nalbuphine	0.5 mg/h	—	10 mg	5-10 mg
Sufentanil	5-30 mcg/h	0.02-0.05 mcg/kg	—	0.2-0.5 mcg/kg

PATIENTS WITH GREATER RISK FOR PULMONARY ASPIRATION

- Pregnant patients
- Diabetic patients
- Obese patients
- Patients with history of gastroesophageal reflux (GER)
- Trauma patients
- Patients with an anticipated difficult airway
- Patients at the extremes of age
- Patients undergoing emergency surgery

Note: Recommended that these patients and any other patients felt to be at risk should be premedicated with a H_2-antagonist, metoclopramide, and/or nonparticulate antacid.

Mallampati Airway Classification[1,2]

Class	Description
1	Faucial pillars, soft palate, and uvula are visible
2	Faucial pillars and soft palate are visible, but uvula is masked by the base of the tongue
3	Only soft palate is visible

[1]Evaluation made with patient sitting upright, the mouth open, and the tongue protruded maximally.

[2]Intubation is predicted to be difficult in patients with class 3 airways.

SKIN DERMATOMES

A dermatome is defined as that area of the skin supplied by a single spinal nerve. The body, with the exception of the face, is supplied in sequence by dermatomes C2 through S5. Knowledge of the distribution of spinal nerves is helpful in interpreting the effects of epidural and spinal anesthesia.

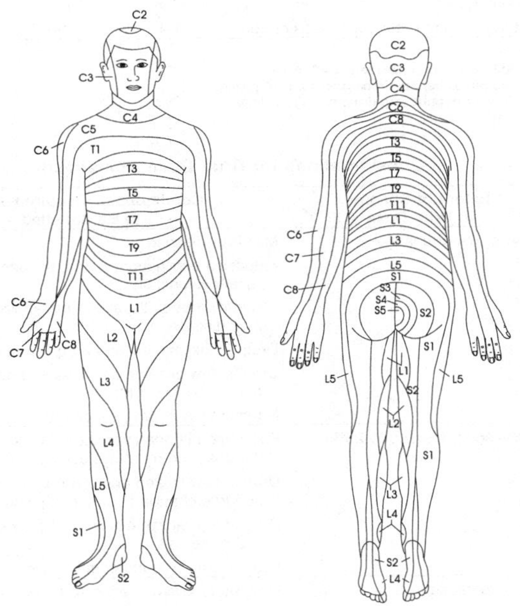

Skin dermatomes corresponding to respective sensory innervation by spinal nerves.

LIVER DISEASE

Pugh's Modification of Child's Classification for Severity

Parameter	Points for Increasing Abnormality 1	2	3
Encephalopathy	None	1 or 2	3 or 4
Ascites	Absent	Slight	Moderate
Bilirubin (mg/dL)	<2.9	2.9-5.8	>5.8
Albumin (g/dL)	>3.5	2.8-3.5	<2.8
Prothrombin time (seconds over control)	1-4	4-6	>6

Scores:

Mild hepatic impairment = <6 points.
Moderate hepatic impairment = 6-10 points.
Severe hepatic impairment = >10 points.

Considerations for Drug Dose Adjustment

Extent of Change in Drug Dose	Conditions or Requirements to Be Satisfied
None or minor change	Mild liver disease
	Extensive elimination of drug by kidneys and no renal dysfunction
	Elimination by pathways of metabolism spared by liver disease
	Drug is enzyme-limited and given acutely
	Drug is flow/enzyme-sensitive and only given acutely by I.V. route
	No alteration in drug sensitivity
Decrease in dose up to 25%	Elimination by the liver does not exceed 40% of the dose; no renal dysfunction
	Drug is flow-limited and given by I.V. route, with no large change in protein binding
	Drug is flow/enzyme-limited and given acutely by oral route
	Drug has a large therapeutic ratio
>25% decrease in dose	Drug metabolism is affected by liver disease; drug administered chronically
	Drug has a narrow therapeutic range; protein binding altered significantly
	Drug is flow-limited and given orally
	Drug is eliminated by kidneys and renal function severely affected
	Altered sensitivity to drug due to liver disease

Reference

Arns PA, Wedlund PJ, and Branch RA, "Adjustment of Medications in Liver Failure," *The Pharmacologic Approach to the Critically Ill Patient*, 2nd ed, Chernow B, ed, Baltimore, MD: Williams & Wilkins, 1988, 85-111.

CREATININE CLEARANCE ESTIMATING METHODS IN PATIENTS WITH STABLE RENAL FUNCTION

These formulas provide an acceptable estimate of the patient's creatinine clearance **except** in the following instances.

- Patient's serum creatinine is changing rapidly (either up or down).
- Patients are markedly emaciated.

In above situations, certain assumptions have to be made.

- In patients with rapidly rising serum creatinine (ie, >0.5-0.7 mg/dL/day), it is best to assume that the patient's creatinine clearance is probably <10 mL/minute.
- In emaciated patients, although their actual creatinine clearance is less than their calculated creatinine clearance (because of decreased creatinine production), it is not possible to easily predict how much less.

Infants

Estimation of creatinine clearance using serum creatinine and body length (to be used when an adequate timed specimen cannot be obtained). **Note:** This formula may not provide an accurate estimation of creatinine clearance for infants younger than 6 months of age and for patients with severe starvation or muscle wasting.

$$Cl_{cr} = K \times L/S_{cr}$$

where:

Cl_{cr} = creatinine clearance in mL/minute/1.73 m^2
K = constant of proportionality that is age specific

Age	K
Low birth weight ≤1 y	0.33
Full-term ≤1 y	0.45
2-12 y	0.55
13-21 y female	0.55
13-21 y male	0.70

L = length in cm
S_{cr} = serum creatinine concentration in mg/dL

Reference

Schwartz GJ, Brion LP, and Spitzer A, "The Use of Plasma Creatinine Concentration for Estimating Glomerular Filtration Rate in Infants, Children and Adolescents," *Pediatr Clin North Am*, 1987, 34(3):571-90.

Children (1-18 years)

Method 1: (Traub SL and Johnson CE, *Am J Hosp Pharm*, 1980, 37(2):195-201)

$$Cl_{cr} = \frac{0.48 \times (\text{height})}{S_{cr}}$$

where:

Cl_{cr} = creatinine clearance in mL/min/1.73 m^2
S_{cr} = serum creatinine in mg/dL
Height = height in cm

CREATININE CLEARANCE ESTIMATING METHODS IN PATIENTS WITH STABLE RENAL FUNCTION *(Continued)*

Method 2: Nomogram (Traub SL and Johnson CE, *Am J Hosp Pharm*, 1980, 37(2):195-201)

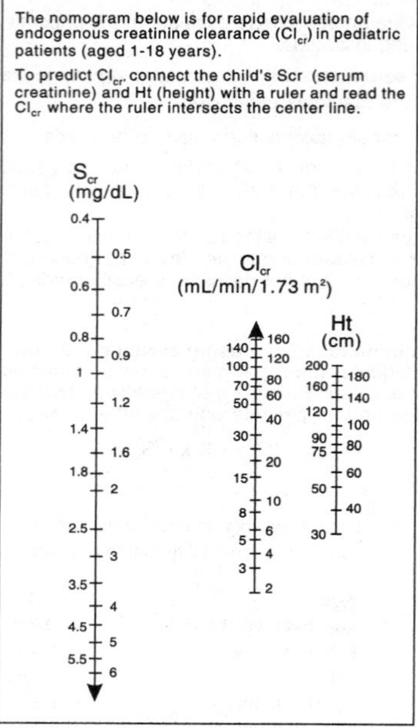

Adults (18 years and older)

Method 1: (Cockroft DW and Gault MH, *Nephron*, 1976, 16:31-41)

Estimated creatinine clearance (Cl_{cr}) (mL/min):

$$\text{Male} = \frac{(140 - \text{age})\ \text{IBW (kg)}}{72 \times S_{cr}}$$

$$\text{Female} = \text{estimated } Cl_{cr} \text{ male} \times 0.85$$

Note: Use of actual body weight (BW) in obese patients (and possibly patients with ascites) may significantly overestimate creatinine clearance. Some clinicians prefer to use an adjusted ideal body weight (IBW) in such cases [eg, IBW + 0.4(ABW-IBW)], especially when calculating dosages for aminoglycoside antibiotics.

Method 2: (Jelliffe RW, *Ann Intern Med*, 1973, 79:604)

Estimated creatinine clearance (Cl_{cr}) (mL/min/1.73 m^2):

$$\text{Male} = \frac{98-0.8\ (\text{age} - 20)}{\text{serum creatinine}}$$

$$\text{Female} = \text{estimated } Cl_{cr} \text{ male} \times 0.90$$

RENAL FUNCTION TESTS

Endogenous Creatinine Clearance vs Age (timed collection)

Creatinine clearance (mL/min/1.73 m^2) = (Cr_uV/Cr_sT) (1.73/A)

where:

Cr_u	=	urine creatinine concentration (mg/dL)
V	=	total urine collected during sampling period (mL)
Cr_s	=	serum creatinine concentration (mg/dL)
T	=	duration of sampling period (min) (24 h = 1440 min)
A	=	body surface area (m^2)

Age-specific normal values

5-7 d	50.6 ± 5.8 mL/min/1.73 m^2
1-2 mo	64.6 ± 5.8 mL/min/1.73 m^2
5-8 mo	87.7 ± 11.9 mL/min/1.73 m^2
9-12 mo	86.9 ± 8.4 mL/min/1.73 m^2
≥18 mo	
male	124 ± 26 mL/min/1.73 m^2
female	109 ± 13.5 mL/min/1.73 m^2
Adults	
male	105 ± 14 mL/min/1.73 m^2
female	95 ± 18 mL/min/1.73 m^2

Note: In patients with renal failure (creatinine clearance <25 mL/min), creatinine clearance may be elevated over GFR because of tubular secretion of creatinine.

Calculation of Creatinine Clearance From a 24-Hour Urine Collection

Equation 1:

$$Cl_{cr} = \frac{U \times V}{P}$$

where:

Cl_{cr}	=	creatinine clearance
U	=	urine concentration of creatinine
V	=	total urine volume in the collection
P	=	plasma creatinine concentration

Equation 2:

$$Cl_{cr} = \frac{\text{(total urine volume [mL]) x (urine Cr concentration [mg/dL])}}{\text{(serum creatinine [mg/dL]) x (time of urine collection [minutes])}}$$

Occasionally, a patient will have a 12- or 24-hour urine collection done for direct calculation of creatinine clearance. Although a urine collection for 24 hours is best, it is difficult to do since many urine collections occur for a much shorter period. A 24-hour urine collection is the desired duration of urine collection because the urine excretion of creatinine is diurnal and thus the measured creatinine clearance will vary throughout the day as the creatinine in the urine varies. When the urine collection is less than 24 hours, the total excreted creatinine will be affected by the time of the day during which the collection is performed. A 24-hour urine collection is sufficient to be able to accurately average the diurnal creatinine excretion variations. If a patient has 24 hours of urine collected for creatinine clearance, equation 1 can be used for calculating the creatinine clearance. To use equation 1 to calculate the creatinine clearance, it will be necessary to know the duration of urine collection, the urine collection volume, the urine creatinine concentration, and the serum creatinine value that reflects the urine collection period. In most cases, a serum creatinine concentration is drawn anytime during the day, but it is best to have the value drawn halfway through the collection period.

RENAL FUNCTION TESTS *(Continued)*

Amylase:Creatinine Clearance Ratio

$$\frac{\text{Amylase}_u \times \text{creatinine}_p}{\text{Amylase}_p \times \text{creatinine}_u} \times 100$$

u = urine; p = plasma

Serum BUN:Serum Creatinine Ratio

Serum BUN (mg/dL:serum creatinine (mg/dL))

Normal BUN:creatinine ratio is 10-15

BUN:creatinine ratio >20 suggests prerenal azotemia (also seen with high urea-generation states such as GI bleeding)

BUN:creatinine ratio <5 may be seen with disorders affecting urea biosynthesis such as urea cycle enzyme deficiencies and with hepatitis.

Fractional Sodium Excretion

Fractional sodium secretion (FENa) = Na_uCr_s/Na_sCr_u x 100%

where:

Na_u = urine sodium (mEq/L)
Na_s = serum sodium (mEq/L)
Cr_u = urine creatinine (mg/dL)
Cr_s = serum creatinine (mg/dL)

FENa <1% suggests prerenal failure
FENa >2% suggest intrinsic renal failure
(for newborns, normal FENa is approximately 2.5%)

Note: Disease states associated with a falsely elevated FENa include severe volume depletion (>10%), early acute tubular necrosis, and volume depletion in chronic renal disease. Disorders associated with a lowered FENa include acute glomerulonephritis, hemoglobinuric or myoglobinuric renal failure, nonoliguric acute tubular necrosis, and acute urinary tract obstruction. In addition, FENa may be <1% in patients with acute renal failure **and** a second condition predisposing to sodium retention (eg, burns, congestive heart failure, nephrotic syndrome).

Urine Calcium:Urine Creatinine Ratio (spot sample)

Urine calcium (mg/dL): urine creatinine (mg/dL)

Normal values <0.21 (mean values 0.08 males, 0.06 females)

Premature infants show wide variability of calcium:creatinine ratio, and tend to have lower thresholds for calcium loss than older children. Prematures without nephrolithiasis had mean Ca:Cr ratio of 0.75 ± 0.76. Infants with nephrolithiasis had mean Ca:Cr ratio of 1.32 ± 1.03 (Jacinto JS, Modanlou HD, Crade M, et al, "Renal Calcification Incidence in Very Low Birth Weight Infants," *Pediatrics*, 1988, 81:31.)

Urine Protein:Urine Creatinine Ratio (spot sample)

P_u/Cr_u	Total Protein Excretion ($mg/m^2/d$)
0.1	80
1	800
10	8000

where:

P_u = urine protein concentration (mg/dL)
Cr_u = urine creatinine concentration (mg/dL)

ACETAMINOPHEN AND NSAIDs, DOSING DATA

Drug	Usual Dose for Adults >50 kg Body Weight	Usual Dose for Adults[1] <50 kg Body Weight
Acetaminophen and Over-the-Counter NSAIDs		
Acetaminophen[2]	650 mg q4h	10-15 mg/kg q4h
	975 mg q6h	15-20 mg/kg q4h (rectal)
Aspirin[3]	650 mg q4h	10-15 mg/kg q4h
	975 mg q6h	15-20 mg/kg q4h (rectal)
Ibuprofen (Motrin®, others)	400-600 mg q6h	10 mg/kg q6-8h
Magnesium salicylate (Doan's®)	304 mg q4h	
Prescription NSAIDs		
Celecoxib (Celebrex)[4]	200 mg q12h	
Choline magnesium trisalicylate (Trilisate®)[4]	1000-1500 mg tid	25 mg/kg tid
Choline salicylate (Arthropan®)[4]	870 mg q3-4h	
Diflunisal (Dolobid®)[5]	500 mg q12h	
Etodolac (Lodine®)	200-400 mg q6-8h	≤20 mg/kg/day
Fenoprofen calcium (Nalfon®)	300-600 mg q6h	
Ketoprofen (Oruvail®)	100-300 mg q24h	
Ketorolac tromethamine (Toradol)[6]	10 mg q4-6h to a maximum of 40 mg/d	
Meclofenamate sodium (Meclomen®)[7]	50-100 mg q6h	
Mefenamic acid (Ponstel®)	250 mg q6h	
Naproxen (Naprosyn®)	250-275 mg q6-8h	5 mg/kg q8h
Naproxen sodium (Anaprox®)	275 mg q6-8h	
Rofecoxib (Vioxx)[4]	50 mg q24h	
Sodium salicylate	325-650 mg q3-4h	
Parenteral NSAIDs		
Ketorolac tromethamine[7,8] (Toradol®)	60 mg I.M. or 30 mg I.V. initially, then 30 mg q6h, dose not to exceed 5 days	30 mg I.M. or 15 mg I.V. initially, then 15 mg q6h, dose not to exceed 5 days

[1]Acetaminophen and NSAID dosages for adults weighing <50 kg should be adjusted for weight.

[2]Acetaminophen lacks the peripheral anti-inflammatory and antiplatelet activities of the other NSAIDs

[3]The standard against which other NSAIDs are compared. May inhibit platelet aggregation for ≥1 week and may cause bleeding.

[4]May have minimal antiplatelet activity.

[5]Administration with antacids may decrease absorption

[6]For short-term use only.

[7]Coombs'-positive autoimmune hemolytic anemia has been associated with prolonged use.

[8]Has the same GI toxicities as oral NSAIDs, dosing for patients with normal renal function.

Note: Only the above NSAIDs have FDA approval for use as simple analgesics, but clinical experience has been gained with other drugs as well.

ANGIOTENSIN AGENTS

ACE Inhibitors: Comparison of Indications and Adult Dosages

Drug	Hypertension	CHF	Renal Dysfunction	Dialyzable	Strengths (mg)
Benazepril (Lotensin®)	10-40 mg/day	Not FDA approved	Cl_{cr} <30 mL/min: 5 mg/day initially Maximum: 40 mg/day	Yes	Tablets 5, 10, 20, 40
Captopril (Capoten®)	25-100 mg/day bid-tid	6.25-100 mg tid Maximum: 450 mg/day	Cl_{cr} 10-50 mL/min: 75% of usual dose Cl_{cr} <10 mL/min: 50% of usual dose	Yes	Tablets 12.5, 25, 50, 100
Enalapril (Vasotec®)	2.5-40 mg/day qd-bid	2.5-20 mg bid Maximum: 20 mg bid	Cl_{cr} 30-80 mL/min: 5 mg/day initially Cl_{cr} <30 mL/min: 2.5 mg/day initially	Yes	Tablets 2.5, 5, 10, 20
Enalaprilat[1]	0.625 mg, 1.25 mg, 2.5 mg q6h Maximum: 5 mg q6h	Not FDA approved	Cl_{cr} <30 mL/min: 0.625 mg q6h	Yes	2.5 mg/2 mL vial
Fosinopril (Monopril®)	10-40 mg/day	10-40 mg/day	No dosage reduction necessary	Not well dialyzed	Tablets 10, 20, 40
Lisinopril (Prinivil®, Zestril®)	10-40 mg/day Maximum: 40 mg/day	5-40 mg/day	Cl_{cr} 10-30 mL/min: 5 mg/day initially Cl_{cr} <10 mL/min: 2.5 mg/day initially	Yes	Tablets 2.5, 5, 10, 20, 30, 40
Moexipril (Univasc®)	7.5-30 mg/day qd-bid Maximum: 30 mg/day	LV dysfunction (post-MI): 7.5-30 mg/day	Cl_{cr} <40 mL/min: 3.75 mg/day initially Maximum: 15 mg/day	Unknown	Tablets 7.5, 15
Perindopril (Aceon®)	4-8 mg/day	4-8 mg/day Maximum: 16 mg/day	Cl_{cr} 30-60 mL/min: 2 mg/day Cl_{cr} 15-29 mL/min: 2 mg qod Cl_{cr} <15 mL/min: 2 mg on dialysis days	Yes	Tablets 2, 4, 8
Quinapril (Accupril®)	10-40 mg/day qd-bid	5-20 mg bid	Cl_{cr} 30-60 mL/min: 5 mg/day initially Cl_{cr} <10-30 mL/min: 2.5 mg/day initially	Not well dialyzed	Tablets 5, 10, 20, 40
Ramipril (Altace®)	2.5-20 mg/day qd-bid	2.5-10 mg/day	Cl_{cr} <40 mL/min: 25% of normal dose	Unknown	Capsules 1.25, 2.5, 5, 10
Trandolapril (Mavik®)	1-4 mg/day Maximum: 8 mg/day qd-bid	LV dysfunction (post-MI): 1-4 mg/day	Cl_{cr} <30 mL/min: 0.5 mg/day initially	No	Tablets 1, 2, 4

Dosage is based on 70 kg adult with normal hepatic and renal function.

[1]Enalaprilat is the only available ACE inhibitor in a parenteral formulation.

Angiotensin II Receptor Blockers: Comparison of Indications and Adult Dosages

Drug	Hypertension	CHF	Renal Dysfunction	Dialyzable	Strengths (mg)
Candesartan (Atacand®)	8-32 mg/day	Target: 32 mg once daily	No dosage adjustment necessary	No	Tablets 4, 8, 16, 32
Eprosartan (Teveten®)	400-800 mg/day qd-bid	Not FDA approved	No dosage adjustment necessary	Unknown	Tablets 400, 600
Irbesartan (Avapro®)	150-300 mg/day	Not FDA approved	No dosage reduction necessary	No	Tablets 75, 150, 300
Losartan (Cozaar®)	25-100 mg qd or bid	Not FDA approved	No dosage adjustment necessary	No	Tablets 25, 50, 100
Olmesartan (Benicar®)	20-40 mg/day	Not FDA approved	No dosage adjustment necessary	Unknown	Tablets 5, 20, 40
Telmisartan (Micardis®)	20-80 mg/day	Not FDA approved	No dosage reduction necessary	No	Tablets 20, 40, 80
Valsartan (Diovan®)	80-320 mg/day	Target: 160 mg bid	Decrease dose only if Cl_{cr} <10 mL/minute	No	Tablets 40, 80, 160, 320

Dosage is based on 70 kg adult with normal hepatic and renal function.

ANGIOTENSIN AGENTS *(Continued)*

ACE Inhibitors: Comparative Pharmacokinetics

Drug	Prodrug	Absorption (%)	Serum $t_{1/2}$ (h) Normal Renal Function	Serum Protein Binding (%)	Elimination	Onset of BP Lowering Action (h)	Peak BP Lowering Effects (h)	Duration of BP Lowering Effects (h)
Benazepril	Yes	37		~97	Renal (32%), biliary (~12%)	1	2-4	24
Benazeprilat			10-11 (effective)	~95%				
Captopril	No	60-75 (fasting)	1.9 (elimination)	25-30	Renal	0.25-0.5	1-1.5	~6
Enalapril	Yes	55-75	2	50-60	Renal (60%-80%), fecal	1	4-6	12-24
Enalaprilat			11 (effective)					
Fosinopril		36			Renal (~50%), biliary (~50%)	1		24
Fosinoprilat			12 (effective)	>99				
Moexipril	Yes		1	90	Fecal (53%), renal (8%)		1-2	>24
Moexiprilat			2-10	50				
Perindopril	Yes		1.5-3	60	Renal		3-7	
Perindoprilat			3-10 (effective)	10-20				
Quinapril	Yes	>60	0.8	97	Renal (~60%) as metabolite, fecal	1	2-4	24
Quinaprilat			2					
Ramipril	Yes	50-60	1-2	73	Renal (60%), fecal (40%)	1-2	3-6	24
Ramiprilat			13-17 (effective)	56				
Trandolapril	Yes		6	80	Renal (33%), fecal (66%)	1-2	6	≥24
Trandolaprilat			10	65-94				

Angiotensin II Receptor Blockers: Comparative Pharmacokinetics

	Candesartan (Atacand®)	Eprosartan (Teveten®)	Irbesartan (Avapro®)	Losartan (Cozaar®)	Olmesartan (Benicar®)	Telmisartan (Micardis®)	Valsartan (Diovan®)
Prodrug	Yes[1]	No	No	Yes[2]	Yes	No	No
Time to peak	3-4 h	1-2 h	1.5-2	1 h / 3-4 h[2]	1-2 h	0.5-1 h	2-4 h
Bioavailability	15%	13%	60%-80%	33%	26%	42%-58%	25%
Food – area-under-the-curve	No effect	No effect	No effect	9%-10%	No effect	9.6%-20%	9%-40%
Elimination half-life	9 h	5-9 h	11-15 h	1.5-2 h / 6-9 h[2]	13 h	24 h	6 h
Elimination altered in renal dysfunction	Yes[3]	No	No	No	Yes	No	No
Precautions in severe renal dysfunction	Yes	Yes	Yes	Yes	Yes	Yes	Yes
Elimination altered in hepatic dysfunction	No	No	No	Yes	Yes	Yes	Yes
Precautions in hepatic dysfunction	No	Yes	No	No	No	Yes	No
Protein binding	>99%	98%	90%	~99%	99%	>99.5%	95%

[1]Candesartan cilexetil: Active metabolite candesartan.

[2]Losartan: Active metabolite E-3174.

[3]Dosage adjustments are not necessary.

ANTIARRHYTHMIC DRUGS

Vaughan Williams Classification of Antiarrhythmic Drugs Based on Cardiac Effects

Class	Drug(s)	Conduction Velocity[1]	Refractory Period	Automaticity
I	Moricizine	↓	↓	↓ (0 on SA node)
Ia	Disopyramide Procainamide Quinidine	↓	↑	↓
Ib	Lidocaine Mexiletine	0/↓	↓	↓
Ic	Flecainide Propafenone[2]	↓↓	0	↓
II	Beta-blockers	0	0	↓
III	Amiodarone Bretylium Dofetilide Ibutilide Sotalol[2]	0	↑↑	0
IV	Diltiazem Verapamil[3]	↓	↑	↓

[1]Variables for normal tissue models in ventricular tissue.

[2]Also has type II, beta-blocking action.

[3]Variables for SA and AV nodal tissue only.

Vaughan Williams Classification of Antiarrhythmic Agents and Their Indications / Adverse Effects

Class	Drug(s)	Indication	Route of Administration	Adverse Effects
I	Moricizine	VT	P.O.	Dizziness, nausea, rash, seizures
Ia	Disopyramide	AF, VT	P.O.	Anticholinergic effects, CHF
	Procainamide	AF, VT, WPW	P.O./I.V.	GI, CNS, lupus, fever, hematological, anticholinergic effects
	Quinidine	AF, PSVT, VT, WPW	P.O./I.V.	Hypotension, GI, thrombocytopenia, cinchonism
Ib	Lidocaine	VT, VF, PVC	I.V.	CNS, GI
	Mexiletine	VT	P.O.	GI, CNS
Ic	Flecainide	VT	P.O.	CHF, GI, CNS, blurred vision
	Propafenone	VT	P.O.	GI, blurred vision, dizziness
II	Esmolol	VT, SVT	I.V.	CHF, CNS, lupus-like syndrome, hypotension, bradycardia, bronchospasm
	Propranolol	SVT, VT, PVC, digoxin toxicity	P.O./I.V.	CHF, bradycardia, hypotension, CNS, fatigue
III	Amiodarone	VT	P.O.	CNS, GI, thyroid, pulmonary fibrosis, liver, corneal deposits
	Bretylium	VT, VF	I.V.	GI, orthostatic hypotension, CNS
	Dofetilide	AF	P.O.	Headache, dizziness, VT, torsade de pointes
	Ibutilide	AF	I.V.	Torsade de pointes, hypotension, branch bundle block, AV block, nausea, headache
	Sotalol	AF, VT	P.O.	Bradycardia, hypotension, CHF, CNS, fatigue
IV	Diltiazem	AF, PSVT	P.O./I.V.	Hypotension, GI, liver
	Verapamil	AF, PSVT	P.O./I.V.	Hypotension, CHF, bradycardia, vertigo, constipation
Miscellaneous	Adenosine	SVT, PSVT	I.V.	Flushing, dizziness, bradycardia, syncope
	Digoxin	AF, PSVT	P.O./I.V.	GI, CNS, arrhythmias
	Magnesium	VT, VF	I.V.	Hypotension, CNS, hypothermia, myocardial depression

AF = atrial fibrillation; PSVT = paroxysmal supraventricular tachycardia; VT = ventricular tachycardia; WPW = Wolf-Parkinson-White arrhythmias; VF = ventricular fibrillation; SVT = supraventricular tachycardia.

ANTIARRHYTHMIC DRUGS *(Continued)*

Comparative Pharmacokinetic Properties of Antiarrhythmic Agents

Class	Drug(s)	Bioavailability (%)	Primary Route of Elimination	Volume of Distribution (L/kg)	Protein Binding (%)	Half-Life	Therapeutic Range (mcg/mL)
I	Moricizine	34-38	Hepatic	6-11	92-95	1-6 h	—
Ia	Disopyramide	70-95	Hepatic/renal	0.8-2	50-80	4-8 h	2-6
	Procainamide	75-95	Hepatic/renal	1.5-3	10-20	2.5-5 h	4-15
	Quinidine	70-80	Hepatic	2-3.5	80-90	5-9 h	2-6
Ib	Lidocaine	20-40	Hepatic	1-2	65-75	60-180 min	1.5-5
	Mexiletine	80-95	Hepatic	5-12	60-75	6-12 h	0.75-2
Ic	Flecainide	90-95	Hepatic/renal	8-10	35-45	12-30 h	0.3-2.5
	Propafenone[1]	11-39	Hepatic	2.5-4	85-95	12-32 h 2-10 h	—
II	Esmolol	Refer to Beta-Blocker Comparison Chart					
	Propranolol	Refer to Beta-Blocker Comparison Chart					
III	Amiodarone	22-28	Hepatic	70-150	95-97	15-100 d	1-2.5
	Bretylium	15-20	Renal	4-8	Negligible	5-10 h	0.5-2
	Dofetilide	>90%	Renal	3 L/kg	60-70	10 h	—
	Ibutilide	NA	Hepatic	11	40	2-12 h	—
	Sotalol	90-95	Renal	1.6-2.4	Negligible	12-15 h	—
IV	Diltiazem	80-90	Hepatic/renal	1.7	77-85	4-6 h	0.05-0.2
	Verapamil	20-40	Hepatic	1.5-5	95-99	4-12 h	>50 ng/mL

[1]**Top** numbers reflect **poor** metabolizers and **bottom** numbers reflect **extensive** metabolizers.

ANTIDEPRESSANT AGENTS

Comparison of Usual Dosage, Mechanism of Action, and Adverse Effects

Drug	Initial Dose	Usual Dosage (mg/d)	Dosage Forms	Adverse Effects						Comments
				ACH	Drowsiness	Orthostatic Hypotension	Conduction Abnormalities	GI Distress	Weight Gain	
Tricyclic Antidepressants and Related Compounds[1]										
Amitriptyline	25-75 mg qhs	100-300	T, I	4+	4+	3+	3+	1	4+	Also used in chronic pain, migraine, and as a hypnotic; contraindicated with cisapride
Amoxapine	50 mg bid	100-400	T	2+	2+	2+	2+	0	2+	May cause extrapyramidal symptom (EPS)
Clomipramine[2] (Anafranil®)	25-75 mg qhs	100-250	C	4+	4+	2+	3+	1+	4+	Approved for OCD
Desipramine (Norpramin®)	25-75 mg qhs	100-300	T	1+	2+	2+	2+	0	1+	Blood levels useful for therapeutic monitoring
Doxepin (Sinequan®, Zonalon®)	25-75 mg qhs	100-300	C, L	3+	4+	2+	2+	0	4+	
Imipramine (Tofranil®, Tofranil-PM®)	25-75 mg qhs	100-300	T, C	3+	3+	4+	3+	1+	4+	Blood levels useful for therapeutic monitoring
Maprotiline	25-75 mg qhs	100-225	T	2+	3+	2+	2+	0	2+	
Nortriptyline (Pamelor®)	25-50 mg qhs	50-150	C, L	2+	2+	1+	2+	0	1+	Blood levels useful for therapeutic monitoring
Protriptyline (Vivactil®)	15 mg qAM	15-60	T	2+	1+	2+	3+	1+	1+	
Trimipramine (Surmontil®)	25-75 mg qhs	100-300	C	4+	4+	3+	3+	0	4+	

ANTIDEPRESSANT AGENTS *(Continued)*

Comparison of Usual Dosage, Mechanism of Action, and Adverse Effects *(continued)*

Drug	Initial Dose	Usual Dosage (mg/d)	Dosage Forms	Adverse Effects						Comments
				ACH	Drowsiness	Orthostatic Hypotension	Conduction Abnormalities	GI Distress	Weight Gain	
Selective Serotonin Reuptake Inhibitors[3]										
Citalopram (Celexa™)	20 mg qAM	20-60	T	0	0	0	0	3+[4]	1+	
Escitalopram (Lexapro™)	10 mg qAM	10-20	T	0	0	0	0	3+	1+	S-enantiomer of citalopram
Fluoxetine (Prozac®, Prozac® Weekly™, Sarafem™)	10-20 mg qAM	20-80	C, L, T	0	0	0	0	3+[4]	1+	CYP2B6 and 2D6 inhibitor
Fluvoxamine[2]	50 mg qhs	100-300	T	0	0	0	0	3+[4]	1+	Contraindicated with pimozide, thioridazine, mesoridazine, CYP1A2, 2B6, 2C19, and 3A4 inhibitors
Paroxetine (Paxil®, Paxil® CR™)	10-20 mg qAM	20-50	T, L	1+	1+	0	0	3+[4]	2+	CYP2B6 and 2D6 inhibitor
Sertraline (Zoloft®)	25-50 mg qAM	50-200	T	0	0	0	0	3+[4]	1+	CYP2B6 and 2C19 inhibitor
Dopamine-Reuptake Blocking Compounds										
Bupropion (Wellbutrin®, Wellbutrin SR®, Wellbutrin XL™, Zyban®)	100 mg bid-tid IR[5] 150 mg qAM-bid SR[6]	300-450[7]	T	0	0	0	1+/0	1+	0	Contraindicated with seizures, bulimia, and anorexia; low incidence of sexual dysfunction IR: A 6-h interval between doses preferred SR: An 8-h interval between doses preferred
Serotonin / Norepinephrine Reuptake Inhibitors[8]										
Duloxetine (Cymbalta®)	40-60 mg qd	40-60	C	1+	1+	0	1+	3+[4]	0	
Venlafaxine (Effexor®, Effexor® XR)	25 mg bid-tid IR 37.5 mg qd XR	75-375	T	1+	1+	0	1+	3+[4]	0	High-dose is useful to treat refractory depression; frequency of hypertension increases with dosage >225 mg/d

Comparison of Usual Dosage, Mechanism of Action, and Adverse Effects *(continued)*

Drug	Initial Dose	Usual Dosage (mg/d)	Dosage Forms	Adverse Effects						Comments
				ACH	Drowsiness	Orthostatic Hypotension	Conduction Abnormalities	GI Distress	Weight Gain	
5-HT$_2$ Receptor Antagonist Properties										
Nefazodone	100 mg bid	300-600	T	1+	1+	2+	1+	1+	0	Contraindicated with carbamazepine, pimozide, astemizole, cisapride, and terfenadine; caution with triazolam and alprazolam; low incidence of sexual dysfunction
Trazodone (Desyrel®)	50 mg tid	150-600	T	0	4+	3+	1+	1+	2+	
Noradrenergic Antagonist										
Mirtazapine (Remeron®, Remeron® SolTab®)	15 mg qhs	15-45	T	1+	3+	1+	1+	0	3+	Dose >15 mg/d less sedating, low incidence of sexual dysfunction
Monoamine Oxidase Inhibitors										
Isocarboxazid (Marplan®)	10 mg tid	10-30	T	2+	2+	2+	1+	1+	2+	Diet must be low in tyramine; contraindicated with sympathomimetics and other antidepressants
Phenelzine (Nardil®)	15 mg tid	15-90	T	2+	2+	2+	0	1+	3+	
Tranylcypromine (Parnate®)	10 mg bid	10-60	T	2+	1+	2+	1+	1+	2+	

ACH = anticholinergic effects (dry mouth, blurred vision, urinary retention, constipation); 0 - 4+ = absent or rare - relatively common. T = tablet, L = liquid, I = injectable, C = capsule; IR = immediate release, SR = sustained release.

[1]**Important note:** A 1-week supply taken all at once in a patient receiving the maximum dose can be fatal.

[2]Not approved by FDA for depression. Approved for OCD.

[3]Flat dose response curve, headache, nausea, and sexual dysfunction are common side effects for SSRIs.

[4]Nausea is usually mild and transient.

[5]IR: 100 mg bid, may be increased to 100 mg tid no sooner than 3 days after beginning therapy.

[6]SR: 150 mg qAM, may be increased to 150 mg bid as early as day 4 of dosing.

[7]To minimize seizure risk, do not exceed IR 150 mg/dose or SR 200 mg/dose.

[8]Do not use with sibutramine; relatively safe in overdose.

ANTIFUNGAL AGENTS

Activities of Various Agents Against Specific Fungi

Fungus	Amphotericin B[1]	Caspofungin	Fluconazole	Flucytosine
Aspergillus	FA	FA	N	?
Blastomyces dermatitidis	FA	?	A	N
Candida albicans	FA	FA	FA	FA
Candida glabrata	A	A	?	A
Candida krusei	FA	A	?	A
Candida tropicalis	FA	A	?	A
Coccidioides immitis	FA	?	A	N
Cryptococcus sp	FA	N	FA	FA
Dermatophytes	A	?	A	?
Fusarium	A	N	N	N
Histoplasma capsulatum	FA	A?	A	N
Penicillium	A	?	?	A
Pseudoallescheria boydii	?	A	N	N
Sporothrix schenckii	A	?	?	?
Zygomycetes (Mucor, Rhizopus)	A	N	N	N

Fungus	Griseofulvin	Itraconazole	Ketoconazole	Micafungin
Aspergillus	N	FA	N	A
Blastomyces dermatitidis	N	FA	FA	?
Candida albicans	N	FA	FA	FA
Candida glabrata	N	?	?	FA
Candida krusei	N	A	?	A
Candida tropicalis	N	?	?	A
Coccidioides immitis	N	A	FA	?
Cryptococcus sp	N	A	A	N
Dermatophytes	FA	A	A	?
Fusarium	N	N	N	?
Histoplasma capsulatum	N	FA	FA	?
Penicillium	N	?	N	?
Pseudoallescheria boydii	N	N	N	?
Sporothrix schenckii	N	?	N	?
Zygomycetes (Mucor, Rhizopus)	N	N	N	N

Fungus	Miconazole	Nystatin	Terbinafine	Voriconazole
Aspergillus	N	A	N	FA
Blastomyces dermatitidis	N	A	N	A
Candida albicans	FA	FA	A	A
Candida glabrata	?	A	?	A
Candida krusei	?	A	?	A
Candida tropicalis	?	A	?	A
Coccidioides immitis	A	N	N	A
Cryptococcus sp	A	N	N	A
Dermatophytes	N	N	FA	?
Fusarium	N	N	N	FA
Histoplasma capsulatum	N	N	N	A
Penicillium	N	N	N	?
Pseudoallescheria boydii	N	N	N	FA
Sporothrix schenckii	?	N	N	?
Zygomycetes (Mucor, Rhizopus)	N	N	N	N?

FA = FDA approved indication. A = active. ? = unknown or questionable. N = not active.

[1]Various lipid products have differing indications, but all have activity against the same organisms.

BENZODIAZEPINES

Agent	Dosage Forms	Approximate Equivalent Dose (mg)	Peak Blood Levels (oral) (h)	Protein Binding (%)	Volume of Distribution (L/kg)	Major Active Metabolite	Half-Life (parent) (h)	Half-Life[1] (metabolite) (h)	Usual Initial Dose	Adult Oral Dosage Range
Anxiolytic										
Alprazolam (Alprazolam Intensol®, Xanax®)	Sol, tab	0.5	1-2	80	0.9-1.2	No	12-15	—	0.25-0.5 mg tid	0.75-4 mg/d
Chlordiazepoxide (Librium®)	Cap, powder for inj	10	2-4	90-98	0.3	Yes	5-30	24-96	5-25 mg tid-qid	15-100 mg/d
Diazepam (Diastat® Rectal Delivery System, Diazepam Intensol®, Valium®)	Gel, inj, sol, tab	5	0.5-2	98	1.1	Yes	20-80	50-100	2-10 mg bid-qid	4-40 mg/d
Lorazepam (Ativan®)[2]	Inj, sol, tab	1	1-6	88-92	1.3	No	10-20	—	0.5-2 mg tid-qid	2-4 mg/d
Oxazepam (Serax®)	Cap, tab	15-30	2-4	86-99	0.6-2	No	5-20	—	10-30 mg tid-qid	30-120 mg/d
Sedative / Hypnotic										
Estazolam (ProSom®)	Tab	0.3	2	93	—	No	10-24	—	1 mg qhs	1-2 mg
Flurazepam (Dalmane®)	Cap	5	0.5-2	97	—	Yes	Not significant	40-114	15 mg qhs	15-60 mg
Quazepam (Doral®)	Tab	5	2	95	5	Yes	25-41	28-114	15 mg qhs	7.5-15 mg
Temazepam (Restoril®)	Cap	5	2-3	96	1.4	No	10-40	—	15-30 mg qhs	15-30 mg
Triazolam (Halcion®)	Tab	0.1	1	89-94	0.8-1.3	No	2.3	—	0.125-0.25 mg qhs	0.125-0.25 mg

BENZODIAZEPINES *(Continued)*

Agent	Dosage Forms	Approximate Equivalent Dose (mg)	Peak Blood Levels (oral) (h)	Protein Binding (%)	Volume of Distribution (L/kg)	Major Active Metabolite	Half-Life (parent) (h)	Half-Life[1] (metabolite) (h)	Usual Initial Dose	Adult Oral Dosage Range
Miscellaneous										
Clonazepam (Klonopin®)	Tab	0.25-0.5	1-2	86	1.8-4	No	18-50 h	—	0.5 mg tid	1.5-20 mg/d
Clorazepate (Tranxene®)	Cap, tab	7.5	1-2	80-95	—	Yes	Not significant	50-100 h	7.5-15 mg bid-qid	15-60 mg
Midazolam	Inj	NA	0.4-0.7[3]	95	0.8-6.6	No	2-5 h	—	NA	NA

[1]Significant metabolite.

[2]Reliable bioavailability when given I.M.

[3]I.V. only.

NA = not available.

BETA-BLOCKERS

Agent	Adrenergic Receptor Blocking Activity	Lipid Solubility	Protein Bound (%)	Half-Life (h)	Bioavailability (%)	Primary (Secondary) Route of Elimination	Indications	Usual Dosage
Acebutolol (Sectral®)	beta$_1$	Low	15-25	3-4	40 7-fold[1]	Hepatic (renal)	Hypertension, arrhythmias	P.O.: 400-1200 mg/d
Atenolol (Tenormin®)	beta$_1$	Low	<5-10	6-9[2]	50-60 4-fold[1]	Renal (hepatic)	Hypertension, angina pectoris, acute MI	P.O.: 50-200 mg/d I.V.: 5 mg x 2 doses
Betaxolol (Kerlone®)	beta$_1$	Low	50-55	14-22	84-94	Hepatic (renal)	Hypertension	P.O.: 10-20 mg/d
Bisoprolol (Zebeta®)	beta$_1$	Low	26-33	9-12	80	Renal (hepatic)	Hypertension, heart failure	P.O.: 2.5-5 mg
Carteolol (Cartrol®)	beta$_1$ beta$_2$	Low	20-30	6	80-85	Renal	Hypertension	P.O.: 2.5-10 mg/d
Carvedilol (Coreg®)	beta$_1$ beta$_2$ alpha$_1$	ND	98	7-10	25-35	Bile into feces	Hypertension, heart failure (mild to severe)	P.O.: 6.25 mg twice daily
Esmolol (Brevibloc®)	beta$_1$	Low	55	0.15	NA 5-fold[1]	Red blood cell	Supraventricular tachycardia, sinus tachycardia	I.V. infusion: 25-300 mcg/kg/min
Labetalol (Trandate®)	alpha$_1$ beta$_1$ beta$_2$	Moderate	50	5.5-8	18-30 10-fold[1]	Renal (hepatic)	Hypertension	P.O.: 200-2400 mg/d I.V.: 20-80 mg at 10-min intervals up to a maximum of 300 mg **or** continuous infusion of 2 mg/min
Metoprolol (Lopressor®, Toprol-XL®)	beta$_1$	Moderate	10-12	3-7	50 10-fold[1] (Toprol XL®: 77)	Hepatic/renal	Hypertension, angina pectoris, acute MI, heart failure (mild to moderate; XL formulation only)	P.O.: 100-450 mg/d I.V.: Post-MI 15 mg Angina: 15 mg then 2-5 mg/hour Arrhythmias: 0.2 mg/kg
Nadolol (Corgard®)	beta$_1$ beta$_2$	Low	25-30	20-24	30 5- to 8-fold[1]	Renal	Hypertension, angina pectoris	P.O.: 40-320 mg/d
Penbutolol (Levatol®)	beta$_1$ beta$_2$	High	80-98	5	≅100	Hepatic (renal)	Hypertension	P.O.: 20-80 mg/d
Pindolol	beta$_1$ beta$_2$	Moderate	57	3-4[2]	90 4-fold[1]	Hepatic (renal)	Hypertension	P.O.: 20-60 mg/d

BETA-BLOCKERS *(Continued)*

Agent	Adrenergic Receptor Blocking Activity	Lipid Solubility	Protein Bound (%)	Half-Life (h)	Bioavail-ability (%)	Primary (Secondary) Route of Elimination	Indications	Usual Dosage
Propranolol (Inderal®, various)	$beta_1$ $beta_2$	High	90	3-5[2]	30 20-fold[1]	Hepatic	Hypertension, angina pectoris, arrhythmias	P.O.: 40-480 mg/d I.V.: Reflex tachycardia 1-10 mg
Propranolol long-acting (Inderal-LA®)	$beta_1$ $beta_2$	High	90	9-18	20- to 30-fold[1]	Hepatic	Hypertrophic subaortic stenosis, prophylaxis (post-MI)	P.O.: 180-240 mg/d
Sotalol (Betapace®, Betapace AF®, Sorine®)	$beta_1$ $beta_2$	Low	0	12	90-100	Renal	Ventricular arrhythmias/ tachyarrhythmias	P.O. 160-320 mg/d
Timolol (Blocadren®)	$beta_1$ $beta_2$	Low to moderate	<10	4	75 7-fold[1]	Hepatic (renal)	Hypertension, prophylaxis (post-MI)	P.O.: 20-60 mg/d P.O.: 20 mg/d

Dosage is based on 70 kg adult with normal hepatic and renal function.

Note: All $beta_1$-selective agents will inhibit $beta_2$ receptors at higher doses.

[1]Interpatient variations in plasma levels.

[2]Half-life increased to 16-27 hours in creatinine clearance of 15-35 mL/minute and >27 hours in creatinine clearance <15 mL/minute.

CALCIUM CHANNEL BLOCKERS

Comparative Pharmacokinetics

Agent	Bioavailability (%)	Protein Binding (%)	Onset of BP Effect (min)	Duration of BP Effect (h)	Half-Life (h)	Volume of Distribution	Route of Metabolism	Route of Excretion
Dihydropyridines								
Amlodipine (Norvasc®)	64-90	93-98	30-50	24	30-50	21 L/kg	Hepatic; inactive metabolites	Urine; 10% as parent
Felodipine (Plendil®)	20	>99	2-5 h	24	11-16	10 L/kg	Hepatic; CYP3A4 substrate (major); inactive metabolites; extensive first pass	Urine (70%; as metabolites); feces 10%
Isradipine (DynaCirc® [DSC]) (immediate release)	15-24	95	20	>12	8	3 L/kg	Hepatic; CYP3A4 substrate (major); inactive metabolites; extensive first pass	Urine as metabolites
Nicardipine (Cardene®) (immediate release)	35	>95	30	≤8	2-4		Hepatic; CYP3A4 substrate (major); saturable first pass	Urine (60%; as metabolites); feces 35%
Nifedipine (Procardia®) (immediate release)	40-77	92-98	Within 20		2-5		Hepatic; CYP3A4 substrate (major); inactive metabolites	Urine as metabolites
Nimodipine (Nimotop®)	13	>95	ND	4-6	1-2		Hepatic; CYP3A4 substrate (major); metabolites inactive or less active than parent; extensive first pass	Urine (50%; as metabolites); feces 32%
Nisoldipine (Sular®)	5	>99	ND	6-12	7-12		Hepatic; CYP3A4 substrate (major); 1 active metabolite (10% of parent); extensive first pass	Urine as metabolites

CALCIUM CHANNEL BLOCKERS *(Continued)*

Comparative Pharmacokinetics *(continued)*

Agent	Bioavailability (%)	Protein Binding (%)	Onset of BP Effect (min)	Duration of BP Effect (h)	Half-Life (h)	Volume of Distribution	Route of Metabolism	Route of Excretion
Phenylalkylamines								
Verapamil (Calan®) (immediate release)	20-35	90	30	6-8	4.5-12		Hepatic; CYP3A4 substrate (major); 1 active metabolite (20% of parent); extensive first pass	Urine (70%; 3%-4% as unchanged drug); feces 16%
Benzothiazepines								
Diltiazem (Cardizem®) (immediate release)	~40	70-80	30-60	6-8	3-4.5	3-13 L/kg	Hepatic; CYP3A4 substrate (major); 1 major metabolite (20%-50% of parent); extensive first pass	Urine as metabolites

CORTICOSTEROIDS

Corticosteroids, Systemic Equivalencies

Glucocorticoid	Pregnancy Category	Approximate Equivalent Dose (mg)	Routes of Administration	Relative Anti-inflammatory Potency	Relative Mineralocorticoid Potency	Protein Binding (%)	Half-life	
							Plasma (min)	Biologic (h)
Short-Acting								
Cortisone	D	25	P.O., I.M.	0.8	2	90	30	8-12
Hydrocortisone	C	20	I.M., I.V.	1	2	90	80-118	8-12
Intermediate-Acting								
Methylprednisolone[1]	—	4	P.O., I.M., I.V.	5	0	—	78-188	18-36
Prednisolone	B	5	P.O., I.M., I.V., intra-articular, intradermal, soft tissue injection	4	1	90-95	115-212	18-36
Prednisone	B	5	P.O.	4	1	70	60	18-36
Triamcinolone[1]	C	4	P.O., I.M., intra-articular, intradermal, intrasynovial, soft tissue injection	5	0	—	200+	18-36
Long-Acting								
Betamethasone	C	0.6-0.75	P.O., I.M., intra-articular, intradermal, intrasynovial, soft tissue injection	25	0	64	300+	36-54
Dexamethasone	C	0.75	P.O., I.M., I.V., intra-articular, intradermal, soft tissue injection	25-30	0	—	110-210	36-54
Mineralocorticoids								
Fludrocortisone	C	—	P.O.	10	125	42	210+	18-36

[1]May contain propylene glycol as an excipient in injectable forms.

CORTICOSTEROIDS *(Continued)*

GUIDELINES FOR SELECTION AND USE OF TOPICAL CORTICOSTEROIDS

The quantity prescribed and the frequency of refills should be monitored to reduce the risk of adrenal suppression. In general, short courses of high-potency agents are preferable to prolonged use of low potency. After control is achieved, control should be maintained with a low potency preparation.

1. Low-to-medium potency agents are usually effective for treating thin, acute, inflammatory skin lesions; whereas, high or super-potent agents are often required for treating chronic, hyperkeratotic, or lichenified lesions.
2. Since the stratum corneum is thin on the face and intertriginous areas, low-potency agents are preferred but a higher potency agent may be used for 2 weeks.
3. Because the palms and soles shave a thick stratum corneum, high or super-potent agents are frequently required.
4. Low potency agents are preferred for infants and the elderly. Infants have a high body surface area to weight ratio; elderly patients have thin, fragile skin.
5. The vehicle in which the topical corticosteroid is formulated influences the absorption and potency of the drug. Ointment bases are preferred for thick, lichenified lesions; they enhance penetration of the drug. Creams are preferred for acute and subacute dermatoses; they may be used on moist skin areas or intertriginous areas. Solutions, gels, and sprays are preferred for the scalp or for areas where a nonoil-based vehicle is needed.
6. In general, super-potent agents should not be used for longer than 2-3 weeks unless the lesion is limited to a small body area. Medium-to-high potency agents usually cause only rare adverse effects when treatment is limited to 3 months or less, and use on the face and intertriginous areas are avoided. If long-term treatment is needed, intermittent vs continued treatment is recommended.
7. Most preparations are applied once or twice daily. More frequent application may be necessary for the palms or soles because the preparation is easily removed by normal activity and penetration is poor due to a thick stratum corneum. Every-other-day or weekend-only application may be effective for treating some chronic conditions.

Corticosteroids, Topical

	Steroid	Vehicle
Very High Potency		
0.05%	Betamethasone dipropionate, augmented	Ointment, lotion
0.05%	Clobetasol propionate	Cream, foam, gel, lotion, ointment, shampoo, spray
0.05%	Diflorasone diacetate	Ointment
0.05%	Halobetasol propionate	Cream, ointment
High Potency		
0.1%	Amcinonide	Cream, ointment, lotion
0.05%	Betamethasone dipropionate, augmented	Cream
0.05%	Betamethasone dipropionate	Cream, ointment
0.1%	Betamethasone valerate	Ointment
0.05%	Desoximetasone	Gel
0.25%	Desoximetasone	Cream, ointment
0.05%	Diflorasone diacetate	Cream, ointment
0.05%	Fluocinonide	Cream, ointment, gel
0.1%	Halcinonide	Cream, ointment
0.5%	Triamcinolone acetonide	Cream

Corticosteroids, Topical *(continued)*

	Steroid	Vehicle
Intermediate Potency		
0.05%	Betamethasone dipropionate	Lotion
0.1%	Betamethasone valerate	Cream
0.1%	Clocortolone pivalate	Cream
0.05%	Desoximetasone	Cream
0.025%	Fluocinolone acetonide	Cream, ointment
0.05%	Flurandrenolide	Cream, ointment, lotion, tape
0.005%	Fluticasone propionate	Ointment
0.05%	Fluticasone propionate	Cream
0.1%	Hydrocortisone butyrate[1]	Ointment, solution
0.2%	Hydrocortisone valerate[1]	Cream, ointment
0.1%	Mometasone furoate[1]	Cream, ointment, lotion
0.1%	Prednicarbate	Cream, ointment
0.025%	Triamcinolone acetonide	Cream, ointment, lotion
0.1%	Triamcinolone acetonide	Cream, ointment, lotion
Low Potency		
0.05%	Alclometasone dipropionate[1]	Cream, ointment
0.05%	Desonide	Cream
0.01%	Fluocinolone acetonide	Cream, solution
0.5%	Hydrocortisone[1]	Cream, ointment, lotion
0.5%	Hydrocortisone acetate[1]	Cream, ointment
1%	Hydrocortisone acetate[1]	Cream, ointment
1%	Hydrocortisone	Cream, ointment, lotion, solution
2.5%	Hydrocortisone	Cream, ointment, lotion

[1]Not fluorinated.

CYCLOPLEGIC MYDRIATICS

Agent	Peak Mydriasis	Peak Cycloplegia	Time to Recovery
Atropine	30-40 min	1-3 h	>14 d
Cyclopentolate	25-75 min	25-75 min	24 h
Homatropine	30-90 min	30-90 min	6 h - 4 d
Scopolamine	20-30 min	30 min - 1 h	5-7 d
Tropicamide	20-40 min	20-35 min	1-6 h

DIURETICS, LOOP

Agent	Equivalent Potency	Usual Dose	Oral Bioavailability (%)	Duration of Action (h)
Bumetanide				
oral	1	0.5-2 mg qd	72-95	4
I.V. injection	1	0.5-1 mg qd	—	2-3
Ethacrynic acid				
oral	100	50-100 mg qd-bid	90-100	6-12
I.V. injection	100	50 mg IVPB[1]	—	2
Furosemide				
oral	40	20-80 mg bid	60-70	6-8
I.V. injection	40	1-5 mg q6h	—	2
Torsemide				
oral	10-20	5-10 mg qd	80-90	6
I.V. injection	10-20	10-20 mg qd	—	6

[1]Repeat doses may be required based upon response to initial doses.

Dosage is based on 70 kg adult with normal hepatic and renal function.

HEMODYNAMIC SUPPORT, INTRAVENOUS

Drug	Dose	Hemodynamic Effects				
		HR	MAP	PAOP	CI	SVR
Dopamine	1-3 mcg/kg/min 3-10 mcg/kg/min >10-20 mcg/kg/min	↑ ↑ ↑↑	0 ↑ ↑↑	↓ 0 0	0/↑ ↑ ↑	0/↓ 0 ↑
Epinephrine	0.01-0.05 mcg/kg/min >0.05 mcg/kg/min	↑ ↑↑	↑ ↑↑	0/↓ ↑	↑↑ ↑↑	0/↓ ↑↑
Norepinephrine	0.02-3 mcg/kg/min	0/↑	↑↑↑	↑↑	0/↓/↑	↑↑↑
Phenylephrine	0.5-9 mcg/kg/min	0/↓	↑	↑	0/↓/↑	↑↑↑
Vasopressin	0.04 units/min	0/↓	↑↑	↑	0/↓	↑↑
Dobutamine	2-10 mcg/kg/min >10-20 mcg/kg/min	0/↑ ↑↑	↑ ↓/↑	↓ ↓	↑ ↑	0/↓ ↓
Milrinone	0.375-0.75 mcg/kg/min	↑↑	0/↓/↑	↓	↑	↓↓
Nesiritide	2 mcg/kg bolus; 0.01-0.03 mcg/kg/min	0	↓	↓	0/↑	↓
Nitroglycerin	0.1-2 mcg/kg/min	0/↑	0/↓	↓	0/↑	↓
Nitroprusside	0.25-3 mcg/kg/min	0/↑	0/↓	↓	↑	↓

HR = heart rate; MAP = mean arterial pressure; PAOP = pulmonary artery occlusion pressure; CI = cardiac index; SVR = systemic vascular resistance

↑ = increase; ↓ = decrease; 0 = no change.

Drug	Dose	Receptor Activity				
		α_1	α_2	β_1	β_2	DA_1
Dobutamine	2-10 mcg/kg/min >10-20 mcg/kg/min	+ ++	0 0	+++ ++++	++ +++	0 0
Dopamine	1-3 mcg/kg/min 3-10 mcg/kg/min >10-20 mcg/kg/min	0 0/+ +++	0 0 0	+ ++++ ++++	0 ++ +	++++ ++++ 0
Epinephrine	0.01-0.05 mcg/kg/min >0.05 mcg/kg/min	++ ++++	++ ++++	++++ +++	+++ +	0 0
Norepinephrine	0.02-3 mcg/kg/min	++++	++	++	0	0
Phenylephrine	0.5-9 mcg/kg/min	++++	+	0	0	0
Vasopressin	0.04 units/min	0	0	0	0	0

Activity ranges from no activity (0) or maximal activity (++++).

DA = dopaminergic.

Reference

Sypniewski ES, "Hypovolemic and Cardigenic Shock," *Pharmacotherapy: A Pathophysiologic Approach*, 3rd ed, Dipiro JT, Talbert RL, Hayes PE, et al, eds, Stamford, CT: McGraw-Hill, 1997, 522-3.

LAXATIVES, CLASSIFICATION AND PROPERTIES

Laxative	Onset of Action	Site of Action	Mechanism of Action
Saline			
Magnesium citrate Magnesium hydroxide (Phillips'® Milk of Magnesia)	30 min to 3 h	Small and large intestine	Attract/retain water in intestinal lumen increasing intraluminal pressure; cholecystokinin release
Sodium phosphates (Fleet® Enema)	2-15 min	Colon	
Irritant / Stimulant			
Senna (Senokot®)	6-10 h	Colon	Direct action on intestinal mucosa; stimulate myenteric plexus; alter water and electrolyte secretion
Bisacodyl (Dulcolax®) tablets, suppositories	15 min to 1 h	Colon	
Castor oil	2-6 h	Small intestine	
Bulk-Producing			
Methylcellulose (Citrucel®) Psyllium (Metamucil®)	12-24 h (up to 72 h)	Small and large intestine	Holds water in stool; mechanical distention; malt soup extract reduces fecal pH
Lubricant			
Mineral oil	6-8 h	Colon	Lubricates intestine; retards colonic absorption of fecal water; softens stool
Surfactants / Stool Softener			
Docusate sodium (Colace®) Docusate calcium (Surfak®)	24-72 h	Small and large intestine	Detergent activity; facilitates admixture of fat and water to soften stool
Miscellaneous and Combination Laxatives			
Glycerin suppository	15-30 min	Colon	Local irritation; hyperosmotic action
Lactulose	24-48 h	Colon	Delivers osmotically active molecules to colon
Docusate/senna (Peri-Colace®)	8-12 h	Small and large intestine	Senna – mild irritant; docusate – stool softener
Polyethylene glycol 3350 (GlycoLax™, MiraLax™)	48 h	Small and large intestine	Nonabsorbable solution which acts as an osmotic agent
Sorbitol 70%	24-48 h	Colon	Delivers osmotically active molecules to colon

NARCOTIC / OPIOID ANALGESICS

Dose Equivalents for Opioid Analgesics

Drug	Approximate Equianalgesic Dose	
	Oral	Parenteral
Morphine-Like Agonists (mu agonists)		
Morphine	30 mg	10 mg
Oxycodone	20 mg	NA
Hydromorphone (Dilaudid®)	7.5 mg	1.5 mg
Levorphanol (Levo-Dromoran®)	Acute: 4 mg Chronic: 1 mg	Acute: 2 mg Chronic: 1 mg
Meperidine (Demerol®)	300 mg	75 mg
Methadone (Dolophine®, others)	10 mg	5 mg
Oxymorphone (Numorphan®)	NA	1 mg
Mixed Agonist-Antagonists (kappa agonists)		
Butorphanol (Stadol®)	NA	2 mg
Nalbuphine (Nubain®)	NA	10 mg
Pentazocine (Talwin®, others)	50 mg	30 mg
Partial Agonist		
Buprenorphine (Buprenex®)	NA	0.4 mg

Adapted from *Principles of Analgesic Use in the Treatment of Acute Pain and Cancer Pain*, 5th ed, Glenview, IL: American Pain Society, 2003, 16.

AHCPR Usual Starting Dosage for Opioid Analgesics for Moderate to Severe Pain in Opioid-Naive Adults*

Drug	Usual Starting Dose Adults <50 kg		Usual Starting Dose Adults ≥50 kg	
	Oral	Parenteral	Oral	Parenteral
Opioid Agonist				
Morphine[1]	0.3 mg/kg q3-4h	0.1 mg/kg q3-4h	30 mg q3-4h	10 mg q3-4h
Codeine[2] (also in combination with aspirin or acetaminophen)	0.5-1 mg/kg q3-4h	NR	60 mg q3-4h	60 mg q2h (I.M./SubQ)
Hydromorphone[1] (Dilaudid®)	0.06 mg/kg q3-4h	0.015 mg/kg q3-4h	6 mg q3-4h	1.5 mg q3-4h
Levorphanol (Levo-Dromoran®)	0.04 mg/kg q6-8h	0.02 mg/kg q6-8h	4 mg q6-8h	2 mg q6-8h (SubQ)
Meperidine[3] (Demerol®; Meperitab®)	NR	0.74 mg/kg q2-3h	NR	100 mg q3h
Methadone (Dolophine®, others)	0.2 mg/kg q6-8h	0.1 mg/kg q6-8h	20 mg q6-8h	10 mg q6-8h
Oxycodone (Roxicodone®, also in Percocet®, Percodan®, Tylox®, others)	0.2 mg/kg q3-4h	NA	10 mg q3-4h	NA
Oxymorphone[1] (Numorphan®)	NA	NR	NA	1 mg q3-4h
Combination Opioid / NSAID Preparations[4]				
Hydrocodone (in Lorcet®, Lortab®, Vicodin®, others)	0.2 mg/kg q3-4h	NA	10 mg q3-4h	NA
Oxycodone (in Percocet®, Percodan®, Tylox®, others)	0.2 mg/kg q3-4h	NA	10 mg q3-4h	NA
Opioid Agonist-Antagonist and Partial Agonist				
Buprenorphine (Buprenex®)	NA	0.0004 mg/kg q6-8h	NA	0.4 mg q6-8h
Butorphanol (Stadol®)	NA	NR	NA	2 mg q3-4h
Nalbuphine (Nubain®)	NA	0.1 mg/kg q3-4h	NA	10 mg q3-4h
Pentazocine (Talwin®, others)	NR	NR	50 mg q4-6h	NR

Note: Dosage of opiates must be individualized. Lower initial doses may be appropriate in selected patients (consult individual drug monographs).

Caution: Recommended doses do not apply to patients with renal or hepatic insufficiency or other conditions affecting drug metabolism and kinetics.

[1]**Caution:** For morphine, hydromorphone, and oxymorphone, rectal administration is an alternate route for patients unable to take oral medications. Equianalgesic doses may differ from oral and parenteral doses because of pharmacokinetic differences. **Note:** A short-acting opioid should normally be used for initial therapy of moderate to severe pain.

[2]**Caution:** Doses >1.5 mg/kg not recommended. 60 mg oral codeine = 650 mg aspirin or acetaminophen.

[3]For short-term treatment of acute pain only.

[4]**Caution:** Doses of aspirin and acetaminophen in combination opioid/NSAID preparations must also be adjusted to the patient's body weight.

NA = not available; NR = not recommended.

Adapted from Acute Pain Management Guideline Panel, "Acute Pain Management: Operative or Medical Procedures and Trauma," Clinical Practice Guideline, AHCPR Publication No. 92-0032, Rockville, MD: Agency for Health Care Policy and Research, Public Health Service, U.S. Department of Health and Human Services, February 1992.
Available at http://www.ncbi.nlm.nih.gov/books/bv.fcgi?rid=hstat6.chapter.8991, Appendix C.

NARCOTIC / OPIOID ANALGESICS *(Continued)*

Comparative Pharmacokinetics

Drug	Onset (min)	Peak (h)	Duration (h)	Half-Life (h)	Average Dosing Interval (h)		Equianalgesic Doses[1] (mg)	
							I.M.	Oral
Alfentanil	Immediate	ND	ND	1-2	—	—	ND	NA
Buprenorphine	15	1	4-8	2-3			0.4	—
Butorphanol	I.M.: 30-60; I.V.: 4-5	0.5-1	3-5	2.5-3.5	3	(3-6)	2	—
Codeine	P.O.: 30-60; I.M.: 10-30	0.5-1	4-6	3-4	3	(3-6)	120	200
Fentanyl	I.M.: 7-15 I.V.: Immediate	ND	1-2	1.5-6	1	(0.5-2)	0.1	NA
Hydrocodone	ND	ND	4-8	3.3-4.4	6	(4-8)	ND	ND
Hydromorphone	P.O.: 15-30	0.5-1	4-6	2-4	4	(3-6)	1.5	7.5
Levorphanol	P.O.: 10-60	0.5-1	4-8	12-16	6	(6-24)	2 (A) 1 (C)	4 (A) 1 (C)
Meperidine	P.O./I.M./Sub-Q: 10-15 I.V.: ≤5	0.5-1	2-4	3-4	3	(2-4)	75	300
Methadone	P.O.: 30-60; I.V.: 10-20	0.5-1	4-6 (acute); >8 (chronic)	15-30	8	(6-12)	10 (A) 2-4 (C)	20 (A) 2-4 (C)
Morphine	P.O.: 15-60 I.V.: ≤5	P.O./I.M./Sub-Q: 0.5-1; I.V.: 0.3	3-6	2-4	4	(3-6)	10	60[2] (A) 30 (C)
Nalbuphine	I.M.: 30; I.V.: 1-3	1	3-6	5		—	10	—
Oxycodone	P.O.: 10-15	0.5-1	4-6	3-4	4	(3-6)	NA	20
Oxymorphone	5-15	0.5-1	3-6				1	10[3]
Pentazocine	15-20	0.25-1	3-4	2-3	3	(3-6)		
Propoxyphene	P.O.: 30-60	2-2.5	4-6	3.5-15	6	(4-8)	ND	130[4]-200[5]
Remifentanil	1-3	<0.3	0.1-0.2	0.15-0.3	—	—	ND	ND
Sufentanil	1.3-3	ND	ND	2.5-3	—	—	0.02	NA

ND = no data available. NA = not applicable. (A) = acute, (C) = chronic.

[1]Based on acute, short-term use. Chronic administration may alter pharmacokinetics and decrease the oral parenteral dose ratio. The morphine oral-parenteral ratio decreases to ~1.5-2.5:1 upon chronic dosing.

[2]Extensive survey data suggest that the relative potency of I.M.:P.O. morphine of 1:6 changes to 1:2-3 with chronic dosing.

[3]Rectal

[4]HCl salt

[5]Napsylate salt

Adapted from *Principles of Analgesic Use in the Treatment of Acute Pain and Cancer Pain*, 4th ed, Skokie, IL: The American Pain Society, 1999.

Comparative Pharmacology

Drug	Analgesic	Antitussive	Constipation	Respiratory Depression	Sedation	Emesis
Phenanthrenes						
Codeine	+	+++	+	+	+	+
Hydrocodone	+	+++		+		
Hydromorphone	++	+++	+	++	+	+
Levorphanol	++	++	++	++	++	+
Morphine	++	+++	++	++	++	++
Oxycodone	++	+++	++	++	++	++
Oxymorphone	++	+	++	+++		+++
Phenylpiperidines						
Alfentanil	++					
Fentanyl	++			+		+
Meperidine	++	+	+	++	+	
Remifentanil	++			++	+++	++
Sufentanil	+++					
Diphenylheptanes						
Methadone	++	++	++	++	+	+
Propoxyphene	+			+	+	+
Agonist / Antagonist						
Buprenorphine	++	N/A	+++	+++	++	++
Butorphanol	++	N/A	+++	+++	++	+
Nalbuphine	++	N/A	+++	+++	++	++
Pentazocine	++	N/A	+	++	++ or stimulation	++

NEUROMUSCULAR BLOCKING AGENTS

Suggested Dosing Guidelines for the Use of Neuromuscular Blocking Agents in the Intensive Care Unit

Agent	Intermittent Injection	Continuous Infusion
	Short Duration	
Mivacurium (Mivacron®)	0.15-0.25 mg/kg followed by 0.1 mg/kg every 15 minutes	1-15 mcg/kg/min
	Intermediate Duration	
Atracurium (Tracrium®)	0.4-0.5 mg/kg every 25-35 minutes	0.4-1 mg/kg/h
Cisatracurium (Nimbex®)	0.15-0.2 mg/kg every 40-60 minutes	0.03-0.6 mg/kg/h
Rocuronium (Zemuron®)	0.6 mg/kg every 30 minutes	0.6 mg/kg/h
Vecuronium	0.1 mg/kg every 35-45 minutes	0.05-0.1 mg/kg/h
	Long Duration	
Doxacurium (Nuromax®)	0.025 mg/kg every 2-3 hours	0.015-0.045 mg/kg/h
Pancuronium	0.1 mg/kg every 90-100 minutes	0.05-0.1 mg/kg/h

Pharmacokinetic and Pharmacodynamic Properties of Neuromuscular Blocking Agents

Agent	Clearance (mL/kg/min)	V_{dss} (L/kg)	Half-life (min)	ED95[1] (mg/kg)	Initial Adult Dose[2,3] (mg/kg)	Onset (min)	Clinical Duration of Action of Initial Dose (min)	Administration as an Intraoperative Infusion (mcg/kg/min)
Ultra-Short Duration								
Succinylcholine	Unknown	Unknown	Unknown	0.2	1-1.5	0.5-1	4-8	10-100
Short Duration								
Mivacurium	50-100[2]	0.2	2[4]	0.07	0.15-0.25	1.5-3	12-20	1-15
Intermediate Duration								
Atracurium	5-7	0.2	20	0.2	0.4-0.5	2-3	20-45	4-12
Cisatracurium	4.6	0.15	22-29	0.05	0.15-0.2	2-3	40-60	1-3
Rocuronium	4	0.17-0.29	60-70	0.3	0.6-1.2	1-1.5	31-67	4-16
Vecuronium	4.5	0.16-0.27	51-80	0.05	0.08-0.1	2-3	20-40	0.8-2
Long Duration								
Doxacurium	1-2.5	0.2	100-200	0.025	0.05-0.08	4-6	100-160	n/a
Pancuronium	1-2	0.18-0.26	107-169	0.07	0.08-0.1	3-5	60-100	n/a

[1]ED95: Effective dose causing 95% blockade.

[2]Initial dose (intubation dose) is usually 2 x ED95 with the exception of cisatracurium where the recommended initial dose is 3-4 x ED95.

[3]Prior administration of succinylcholine generally enhances the magnitude and duration of nondepolarizing NMB agents; initial doses should be lower.

[4]Values reflect contribution of cis-trans and trans-trans isomers only.

NITRATES

Nitrates[1]	Dosage Form	Onset (min)	Duration
Nitroglycerin	I.V.	1-2	3-5 min
	Sublingual	1-3	30-60 min
	Translingual spray	2	30-60 min
	Oral, sustained release	40	4-8 h
	Topical ointment	20-60	2-12 h
	Transdermal	40-60	18-24 h
Isosorbide dinitrate	Sublingual and chewable	2-5	1-2 h
	Oral	20-40	4-6 h
	Oral, sustained release	Slow	8-12 h
Isosorbide mononitrate	Oral	60-120	5-12 h

[1]Hemodynamic and antianginal tolerance often develops within 24-48 hours of continuous nitrate administration.

Adapted from Corwin S and Reiffel JA, "Nitrate Therapy for Angina Pectoris," *Arch Intern Med*, 1985, 145:538-43 and Franciosa JA, "Nitroglycerin and Nitrates in Congestive Heart Failure," *Heart and Lung*, 1980, 9(5):873-82.

NONSTEROIDAL ANTI-INFLAMMATORY AGENTS

Comparative Dosages and Pharmacokinetics

Drug	Maximum Recommended Daily Dose (mg)	Time to Peak Levels (h)[1]	Half-life (h)
Acetic Acids			
Diclofenac potassium immediate release (Cataflam®)	200	1	1-2
Diclofenac sodium delayed release (Voltaren®)	225	2-3	1-2
Etodolac (Lodine®)	1200	1-2	7.3
Indomethacin (Indocin®)	200	1-2	4.5
Indomethacin sustained release (Indocin® SR)	150	2-4	4.5-6
Ketorolac (Toradol®)	I.M.: 120[2] P.O.: 40	0.5-1	3.8-8.6
Sulindac (Clinoril®)	400	2-4	7.8 (16.4)[3]
Tolmetin (Tolectin®)	2000	0.5-1	1-1.5
Fenamates (Anthranilic Acids)			
Meclofenamate	400	0.5-1	2 (3.3)[4]
Mefenamic acid (Ponstel®)	1000	2-4	2-4
Propionic Acids			
Fenoprofen (Nalfon®)	3200	1-2	2-3
Flurbiprofen (Ansaid®)	300	1.5	5.7
Ibuprofen (various)	3200	1-2	1.8-2.5
Ketoprofen (Orudis®, others)	300	0.5-2	2-4
Naproxen (Naprosyn®)	1500	2-4	12-15
Naproxen sodium (Anaprox®, others)	1375	1-2	12-13
Oxaprozin (Daypro®)	1800	3-5	42-50
Nonacidic Agent			
Nabumetone (Relafen®)	2000	3-6	24
Salicylic Acid Derivative			
Diflunisal (Dolobid®)	1500	2-3	8-12
Salsalate	3000	2-3	7-8
COX-2 Inhibitors			
Celecoxib (Celebrex®)	400	3	11
Valdecoxib (Bextra®) [withdrawn from market]	40	2.25-3	8-11
Oxicam			
Meloxicam (Mobic®)	15	4-5	15-20
Piroxicam (Feldene®)	20	3-5	30-86

Dosage is based on 70 kg adult with normal hepatic and renal function.

[1]Food decreases the rate of absorption and may delay the time to peak levels.

[2]150 mg on the first day.

[3]Half-life of active sulfide metabolite.

[4]Half-life with multiple doses.

SEDATIVE AGENTS IN THE INTENSIVE CARE UNIT

Comparative Dosages of Sedative Agents

Drug	Recommended Pediatric Dosage	Recommended Adult Dosage	Continuous Infusion Dosage
Benzodiazepines			
Diazepam	P.O.: 0.12-0.8 mg/kg/d in divided doses q6-8h I.M./I.V.: 0.04-0.3 mg/kg/dose q2-4h to a maximum of 0.6 mg/kg/8 h period	I.V.: 0.03-0.1 mg/kg q0.5-6h	**Not recommended** due to poor stability
Lorazepam	I.M./P.O.: 0.05 mg/kg/dose (maximum: 2 mg/dose) q4-8h prn	Intermittent I.V. dose: 0.02-0.06 mg/kg q2-6h	May precipitate; 0.01-0.1 mg/kg/h
Midazolam	P.O.: <5 y: 0.5 mg/kg/dose >5 y: 0.4-0.5 mg/kg/dose Usual duration: 2 h I.M.: 0.1-0.15 mg/kg/dose I.V.: 0.025-0.1 mg/kg/dose which may be repeated up to a total dose of 0.6 mg/kg (6 mg) for children 6 months to 5 years and 0.4 mg/kg (10 mg) for children 6-12 years **Intranasal:** 0.2 mg/kg by needleless syringe to nares over 15 sec and may be repeated in 5-15 min	Acute agitation: I.V.: 2-5 mg q5-15min until controlled Intermittent I.V. dose: 0.02-0.08 mg/kg q0.5-2h	100 mg in 250 mL D_5W or NS: Children: 0.05-0.2 mg/kg loading dose followed by 1-2 mcg/kg/min titrated to desired effect (usual range: 0.4-6 mcg/kg/min) Adults: 0.04-0.2 mg/kg/h
Other Agents			
Haloperidol	Limited Data	I.M./I.V.: Mild agitation: 0.5-2 mg Moderate agitation: 2-5 mg Severe agitation: 10-20 mg Repeat dose after 30 minutes; double dose and administer after another 30 minutes and continue until calm achieved; may repeat additional doses at 6- to 12-hour intervals Acute delirium: I.V.: 2-10 mg q20-30min until controlled, then 25% loading dose every 4-6 h Intermittent I.V. dose: 0.03-0.15 mg/kg q0.5-6h	Adults: Dilutions of up to 3 mg/mL in D_5W and up to 0.75 mg/mL in 0.9% NaCl Infusion rates of 3-25 mg/h for treatment durations of 2-12 days have been reported
Propofol	Limited Data	–	Adults: 5-80 mcg/kg/min (0.3-4.8 mg/kg/h)

American College of Critical Care Medicine of the Society of Critical Care Medicine, American Society of Health-System Pharmacists, American College of Chest Physicians, "Clinical Practice Guidelines for the Sustained Use of Sedatives and Analgesics in the Critically Ill Adult," *Am J Health Syst Pharm*, 2002, 59(2):150-78.

THIAZOLIDINEDIONES

Lipid Effects

Parameter	Pioglitazone (Actos®)	Rosiglitazone (Avandia®)
LDL	No significant change	↑ up to 12.1%
HDL	↑ up to 13%	↑ up to 18.5%
Total cholesterol	No significant change	↑
Total cholesterol/HDL ratio	–	–
LDL/HDL ratio	–	No change
Triglycerides	↓ up to 28%	Variable effects

Thiazolidinedione Pharmacokinetics

Parameter	Pioglitazone (Actos®)	Rosiglitazone (Avandia®)
Absorption	Food slightly delays but does not alter the extent of absorption	Absolute bioavailability is 99% Food ↓ C_{max} and delays T_{max}, but not change in AUC
C_{max}	156-342 ng/mL	–
T_{max}	2 hours	1 hour
Distribution	0.63 ± 0.41 L/kg	17.6 L
Plasma protein binding	>99% to serum albumin	99.8% to serum albumin
Metabolism	Extensive liver metabolism by hydroxylation and oxidation. Some metabolites are pharmacologically active. CYP2C8 and CYP3A4 metabolism	Extensive metabolism via N-demethylation and hydroxylation with no unchanged drug excreted in the urine CYP2C8 and some CYP2C9 metabolism
Excretion	Urine (15% to 30%) and bile	Urine (64%) and feces (23%)
Half-life	3-6 hours (pioglitazone) 16-24 hours (pioglitazone and metabolites)	3.15-3.59 hours
Effect of hemodialysis	Not removed	Not removed

Thiazolidinedione Derivatives Approved Indications

Indication	Pioglitazone (Actos®)	Rosiglitazone (Avandia®)
Monotherapy	x	x
Combination Therapy – Dual Therapy		
Combination with sulfonylureas	x	x
Combination therapy with metformin (Glucophage®)	x	x
Combination therapy with insulin	x	x
Combination Therapy – Triple Therapy		
Combination therapy with sulfonylureas and metformin (Glucophage®)	–	x

COMMONLY USED HERBAL MEDICINES

The use of herbal medicines by the general population continues to increase. In 1988, retail sales of herbal products was approximately $200 million with this number increasing to $5.1 billion in 1997. If the current trend in herbal medicine use continues, annual sales of $25 billion are expected by the year 2010. A survey of surgical patients performed in 1999 revealed that 17.4% reported taking herbals or nutrachemicals. In this survey, the most common herbs taken were gingko (32.4%), garlic (26.5%), ginger (26.5%), ginseng (14%), and St John's wort (14%). A major problem with herbal medicine use is that patients frequently do not report this use to their healthcare providers. This results in the potential for adverse interactions between the patient's prescription medications and herbal products. Further, the use of herbal medicine may cause problems not anticipated by the healthcare provider (eg, increased bleeding potential) if its use is not communicated. Hence, it is critical that all healthcare providers question patients about herbal use as part of their routine medication history. One may also want to consider having the patient stop taking select herbal medicines up to 2 weeks prior to surgery, if possible, secondary to their potential effects on coagulation (eg, feverfew, garlic, ginger, ginkgo, horse chestnut seed, kava-kava). Although there are hundreds of herbal products available on the market, a relatively small number (10-20) account for the majority of sales. The table that follows lists some of the most commonly used herbal medicines, their traditional uses, and cautions and contraindications with regard to their use. Keep in mind that there are few well-designed studies assessing these products, as they are considered dietary supplements, and as such, are not held to the rigid FDA testing standards for drugs.

Herb	Use(s)	Cautions and Contraindications
Cat's claw *(Unacaria tomentosa)*	– Treatment of allergies, arthritis – Adjunct therapy for AIDS – Adjunct agent for cancer therapy – Immune stimulant – Postradiation therapy – Antiparasitic	– Should not be taken when pregnant, nursing, or by transplant recipients – May see diarrhea or changes in bowel movement – Use with caution in conjunction with anticoagulants (may increase risk of bleeding due to platelet activating factor inhibition) – Use with caution with NSAIDs (may increase risk of GI bleeding)
Cayenne *(Capsicum annuum)*	– **External:** Muscle spasm or soreness, shingles, diabetic neuropathy, cluster headache, osteoarthritis, rheumatoid arthritis – **Internal:** GI tract disorders	– **External:** Potential for skin ulceration and blistering with >2 days' use – **Internal:** Overdose may cause severe hypothermia
Echinacea *(Echinacea purpurea)*	– Prevention and treatment of colds and flu, allergies, infections, tonsillitis, sore throat – Chronic skin complaints	– Should not be administered with immunosuppressants – People with chronic suppressed immunity should not take for extended periods of time (>10-14 days)

Herb	Use(s)	Cautions and Contraindications
Ephedra *(Ephedra sinica)*	– Over-the-counter diet aids – Antitussive – Enhance athletic performance (CNS stimulant)	– Active constituent is ephedrine – Intraoperative hemodymanic instability – Palpitations and increased blood pressure can be seen with its use – Potential for increased blood pressure when combined with caffeine-containing botanicals (eg, Metabolife™, Formula One™) – Enhanced sympathomimetic effects with guanethedine and MAOIs – Hypertension when given with oxytocin – Arrhythmias with halothane or cardiac glycosides – Higher doses produce euphoria – Misuse has resulted in death
Evening primrose oil *(Oenothera biennis)*	– Reduce cholesterol – Allergic/inflammatory conditions – Treatment of PMS	– Reduces platelet aggregation (monitor bleeding times and PT in patients on antiplatelet drugs, warfarin, or other anticoagulant drugs)
Feverfew *(Tanacetum parthenium)*	– Treatment of arthritis – Migraine prophylaxis/ treatment – Antipyretic	– Can inhibit platelet activity and increase bleeding; avoid use in patients on warfarin or other anticoagulants or antiplatelet drugs – Rebound headache with sudden cessation – Avoid in pregnant women (uterine stimulant) – Users may develop aphthous ulcers or GI tract irritation (5% to 15%) – Use with caution when administering with drugs that increase serotonin (eg, fluoxetine, sumatriptan) secondary to increased risk of serotonin syndrome
Garlic *(Allium sativum)*	– Lower cholesterol and blood pressure – Has antiplatelet, antioxidant, and antithrombotic qualities – Prevent infections	– Reduces platelet aggregation and increases fibrinolytic activity; monitor bleeding times and PT in patients on antiplatelet drugs and warfarin – Monitor blood glucose (decreased blood glucose secondary to increased serum insulin levels) – May potentiate antihypertensives – Vasodilator properties
Ginger *(Zingiber officinale)*	– Antinauseant – Antispasmodic	– Potent inhibitor of thromboxane synthetase; may increase bleeding time – May interact with anticoagulant and antiplatelet drugs to increase risk of bleeding – May alter effects of calcium channel blockers (ginger increases calcium uptake by the heart)

COMMONLY USED HERBAL MEDICINES *(Continued)*

Herb	Use(s)	Cautions and Contraindications
Ginkgo *(Ginkgo biloba)*	– Treatment of dementia associated with Alzheimer's disease or other conditions associated with cerebral vascular insufficiency – Treatment of vertigo, headache, tinnitus, depression, peripheral vascular disease, Raynaud's disease	– Ginkgolides inhibit platelet activating factor and antagonize thrombus formation; may enhance bleeding in patients on anticoagulant or antithrombotic therapy
Ginseng *(Panax schinseng)*	– Enhance mental and physical performance – Increase energy, decrease stress – Improve immune function – Adaptogen – Antioxidant	– Use caution in patients on digoxin therapy – Hypoglycemic effect – Ginsenosides inhibit platelet aggregation and enhance fibrinolysis; may interact with warfarin or antiplatelet drugs to increase risk of bleeding – Should not be used in pregnancy or acute infection – May potentiate action of MAOIs
Goldenseal *(Hydrastis canadensis)*	– Diuretic – Hemostatic – Anti-inflammatory – Laxative	– High doses may induce paralysis – Should not be taken during pregnancy or while nursing – Functions as an aquaretic – Functions as an oxytocic
Grape seed extract *(Vitis vinifera)*	– Treatment of allergies, asthma – Improve peripheral circulation – Decrease platelet aggregation, capillary fragility – Improve general circulation – Antioxidant	– Monitor bleeding times and PT in patients on antiplatelet drugs and warfarin
Green tea leaf *(Camellia sinensis)*	– Antioxidant/free radical scavenger – Preventative for cancer and cardiovascular disease – Preventative for atherosclerosis and hypertension – Antibacterial – Lower cholesterol – Platelet inhibition actions	– Use with caution in patients on anticoagulant therapy
Hawthorn *(Crataegus oxyacantha)*	– Treatment for angina, arrhythmias, tachycardia, hypo-/hypertension, irregular heartbeat, peripheral vascular disorders, vascular spasms – Lower cholesterol	– May potentiate digoxin and ACE inhibitors
Horse chestnut seed *(Aesculus hippocastanum)*	– Treatment of varicose veins, hemorrhoids, venous insufficiencies	– Contains coumarin and aescin constituents; use with caution in patients on anticoagulant or antiplatelet therapy (can cause severe bleeding or bruising)

Herb	Use(s)	Cautions and Contraindications
Kava-kava *(Piper methysticum)*	– Anxiolytic – Analgesic – Antidepressant – Insomnia	– Kava lactones (active constituents of kava-kava) potentiate the effects of other CNS depressants such as barbiturates, benzodiazepines, opioids, and anesthetics – Can potentiate ethanol effects – Avoid in endogenous depression – May worsen symptoms of Parkinson's disease (kava-kava antagonizes dopamine)
Licorice root *(Glycyrrhiza glabra)*	– Gastric and duodenal ulcers – Adrenal insufficiency – Expectorant and antitussive	– Contraindicated in many chronic liver conditions, severe kidney insufficiency, hypertension, cardiac disease, hypokalemia – Contraindicated in pregnancy and diabetes – Glycyrrhizic acid in licorice may cause high blood pressure, hypokalemia, and edema
Passionflower vine *(Passiflora incarnata)*	– Sedative and hypnotic – In combination with valerian to produce restful sleep	– May potentiate sedative actions of pharmaceuticals – Use with caution in patients on MAOI therapy – Use with caution with consumption of alcohol
Saw palmetto *(Serenoa repens)*	– Benign prostatic hypertrophy	– Antiestrogen effect (avoid during pregnancy and in patients with breast cancer) – Can cause hypertension and GI disturbances
St John's wort *(Hypericum perforatum)*	– **External:** Herpes simplex 1, minor wounds and burns – **Internal:** Treatment for depression, nervousness, anxiety	– May prolong effects of anesthesia – Photosensitivity in large doses in light-skinned people – Serotonin syndrome that is reversed by decreasing dose – May be prudent to avoid SSRIs, MAOIs, and meperidine – Increases metabolism of many perioperative drugs
Turmeric *(Curcuma longa)*	– Antioxidant – Anti-inflammatory – Antirheumatic – Lower blood lipid levels	– Use with caution if currently taking anticoagulant medications – Use with caution if peptic ulceration is present – Do not use if biliary obstruction is present
Valerian *(Valeriana officinalis)*	– Mild sedative and anxiolytic	– May potentiate the effects of CNS depressants (eg, barbiturates, anesthetics) and anxiolytics – May decrease symptoms of benzodiazepine withdrawal – Many extracts contain alcohol; potential to interact with disulfiram

COMMONLY USED HERBAL MEDICINES *(Continued)*

References

American Society of Anesthesiologists, "Considerations for Anesthesiologists: What You Should Know About Your Patients' Use of Herbal Medicines," 1999 (brochure).

Ang-Lee MK, Moss J, and Yuan CS, "Herbal Medicines and Perioperative Care," *JAMA*, 2001, 286(2):208-16.

Blumenthal M, *The Complete German Commission E Monographs. Therapeutic Guide to Herbal Medicines,* Austin, Texas: American Botanical Council, 1998.

DerMarderosian A, *The Review of Natural Products,* St Louis, MO: Facts and Comparisons, 1999.

Eisenberg DM, Davis RB, Ettner SL, et al, "Trends in Alternative Medicine Use in the United States, 1990-1997: Results of a Follow-up National Survey," *JAMA,* 1998, 280(18):1569-75.

Klepser TB and Klepser ME, "Unsafe and Potentially Safe Herbal Therapies," *Am J Health Syst Pharm,* 1999, 56(2):125-38.

LaValle JB, "Phytotherapy: A Guide to the Safe and Effective Use of Medicinal Herbs," *Pharmacy Practice News,* 1999, 26(11):57-61.

Mahady GB, "Herbal Medicine and Pharmacy Education," *J Amer Pharm Assoc,* 1998, 38:274.

McDermott JH, "Herbal Chart for Healthcare Professionals," *Pharmacy Today,* 1999, 5(8) (centerfold poster).

McLeskey CH, Meyer TA, Baisden CE, et al, "The Incidence of Herbal and Selected Nutrachemical Use in Surgical Patients," *Anesthesiology,* 1999, 91:A1168.

Miller LG, "Herbal Medicinals: Selected Clinical Considerations Focusing on Known or Potential Drug-Herb Interactions," *Arch Intern Med,* 1998, 158(20):2200-11.

Murphy JM, "Preoperative Considerations With Herbal Medicines," *AORN J,* 1999, 69(1):173-5, 177-8, 180-3.

Murray M, *The Healing Power of Herbs: The Enlightened Person's Guide to the Wonders of Medicinal Plants,* Rocklin, CA: Prima Publishing, 1995.

Newall CA, Anderson LA, and Phillipson JD, *Herbal Medicines: A Guide for Health Care Professionals,* London, England: The Pharmaceutical Press, 1996.

Schulz V, Hansel R, and Tyler VE, *Rational Phytotherapy, A Physician's Guide to Herbal Medicine,* New York, NY: Springer, 1998.

Zaglaniczny KL, "An Introduction to Herbal Medicine and Anesthetic Considerations," *Nurse Anesthetist, Forum,* 1999, 2(3):4-5,11.

PREVENTION OF BACTERIAL ENDOCARDITIS

Recommendations by the American Heart Association (*JAMA*, 1997, 277:1794-801)

Consensus Process – The recommendations were formulated by the writing group after specific therapeutic regimens were discussed. The consensus statement was subsequently reviewed by outside experts not affiliated with the writing group and by the Science Advisory and Coordinating Committee of the American Heart Association. These guidelines are meant to aid practitioners but are not intended as the standard of care or as a substitute for clinical judgment.

Table 1. Cardiac Conditions[1]

Endocarditis Prophylaxis Recommended

High-Risk Category
- Prosthetic cardiac valves, including bioprosthetic and homograft valves
- Previous bacterial endocarditis
- Complex cyanotic congenital heart disease (eg, single ventricle states, transposition of the great arteries, tetralogy of Fallot)
- Surgically constructed systemic pulmonary shunts or conduits

Moderate-Risk Category
- Most other congenital cardiac malformations (other than above and below)
- Acquired valvar dysfunction (eg, rheumatic heart disease)
- Hypertrophic cardiomyopathy
- Mitral valve prolapse with valvar regurgitation and/or thickened leaflets

Endocarditis Prophylaxis Not Recommended

Negligible-Risk Category (no greater risk than the general population)
- Isolated secundum atrial septal defect
- Surgical repair of atrial septal defect, ventricular septal defect, or patent ductus arteriosus (without residua beyond 6 months)
- Previous coronary artery bypass graft surgery
- Mitral valve prolapse without valvar regurgitation
- Physiologic, functional, or innocent heart murmurs
- Previous Kawasaki disease without valvar dysfunction
- Previous rheumatic fever without valvar dysfunction
- Cardiac pacemakers (intravascular and epicardial) and implanted defibrillators

[1]This table lists selected conditions but is not meant to be all-inclusive.

PREVENTION OF BACTERIAL ENDOCARDITIS *(Continued)*

Patient With Suspected Mitral Valve Prolapse

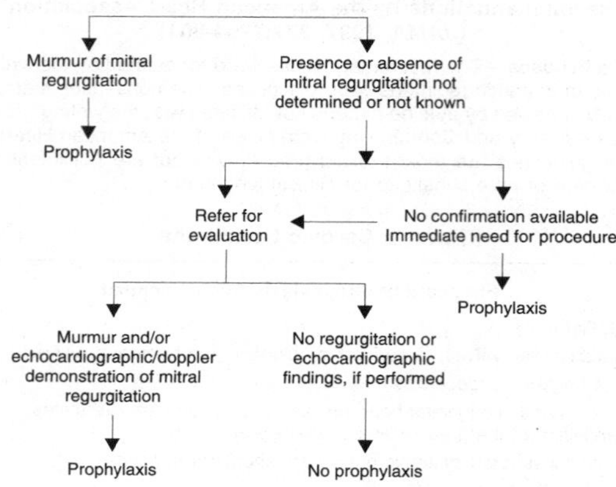

Table 2. Dental Procedures and Endocarditis Prophylaxis

Endocarditis Prophylaxis Recommended[1]
Dental extractions
Periodontal procedures including surgery, scaling and root planing, probing, and recall maintenance
Dental implant placement and reimplantation of avulsed teeth
Endodontic (root canal) instrumentation or surgery only beyond the apex
Subgingival placement of antibiotic fibers or strips
Initial placement of orthodontic bands but not brackets
Intraligamentary local anesthetic injections
Prophylactic cleaning of teeth or implants where bleeding is anticipated
Endocarditis Prophylaxis Not Recommended
Restorative dentistry[2] (operative and prosthodontic) with or without retraction cord[3]
Local anesthetic injections (nonintraligamentary)
Intracanal endodontic treatment; post placement and buildup[3]
Placement of rubber dams[3]
Postoperative suture removal
Placement of removable prosthodontic or orthodontic appliances
Taking of oral impressions[3]
Fluoride treatments
Taking of oral radiographs
Orthodontic appliance adjustment
Shedding of primary teeth

[1]Prophylaxis is recommended for patients with high- and moderate-risk cardiac conditions.

[2]This includes restoration of decayed teeth (filling cavities) and replacement of missing teeth.

[3]Clinical judgment may indicate antibiotic use in selected circumstances that may create significant bleeding.

Table 3. Recommended Standard Prophylactic Regimen for Dental, Oral, or Upper Respiratory Tract Procedures in Patients Who Are at Risk

Endocarditis Prophylaxis Recommended

Respiratory Tract
- Tonsillectomy and/or adenoidectomy
- Surgical operations that involve respiratory mucosa
- Bronchoscopy with a rigid bronchoscope

Gastrointestinal Tract[1]
- Sclerotherapy for esophageal varices
- Esophageal stricture dilation
- Endoscopic retrograde cholangiography with biliary obstruction
- Biliary tract surgery
- Surgical operations that involve intestinal mucosa

Genitourinary Tract
- Prostatic surgery
- Cystoscopy
- Urethral dilation

Endocarditis Prophylaxis Not Recommended

Respiratory Tract
- Endotracheal intubation
- Bronchoscopy with a flexible bronchoscope, with or without biopsy[2]
- Tympanostomy tube insertion

Gastrointestinal Tract
- Transesophageal echocardiography[2]
- Endoscopy with or without gastrointestinal biopsy[2]

Genitourinary Tract
- Vaginal hysterectomy[2]
- Vaginal delivery[2]
- Cesarean section
- In uninfected tissues:
  - Urethral catheterization
  - Uterine dilatation and curettage
  - Therapeutic abortion
  - Sterilization procedures
  - Insertion or removal of intrauterine devices

Other
- Cardiac catheterization, including balloon angioplasty
- Implanted cardiac pacemakers, implanted defibrillators, and coronary stents
- Incision or biopsy or surgically scrubbed skin
- Circumcision

[1]Prophylaxis is recommended for high-risk patients, optional for medium-risk patients.
[2]Prophylaxis is optional for high-risk patients.

PREVENTION OF BACTERIAL ENDOCARDITIS *(Continued)*

Table 4. Prophylactic Regimens for Dental, Oral, Respiratory Tract, or Esophageal Procedures

Situation	Agent	Regimen[1]	
		Adults	Children
Standard general prophylaxis	Amoxicillin	2 g P.O. 1 h before procedure	50 mg/kg P.O. 1 h before procedure
Unable to take oral medications	Ampicillin	2 g I.M./I.V. within 30 min before procedure	50 mg/kg I.M./I.V. within 30 min before procedure
Allergic to penicillin	Clindamycin or	600 mg P.O. 1 h before procedure	20 mg/kg P.O. 1 h before procedure
	Cephalexin[2] or cefadroxil[2] or	2 g P.O 1 h before procedure	50 mg/kg P.O. 1 h before procedure
	Azithromycin or clarithromycin	500 mg P.O. 1 h before procedure	15 mg/kg P.O. 1 h before procedure
Allergic to penicillin and unable to take oral medications	Clindamycin or	600 mg I.V. within 30 min before procedure	20 mg/kg I.V. within 30 min before procedure
	Cefazolin[2]	1 g I.M./I.V. within 30 min before procedure	25 mg/kg I.M./I.V. within 30 min before procedure

[1]Total children's dose should not exceed adult dose.

[2]Cephalosporins should not be used in individuals with immediate-type hypersensitivity reaction (urticaria, angioedema, or anaphylaxis) to penicillins.

Table 5. Prophylactic Regimens for Genitourinary / Gastrointestinal (Excluding Esophageal) Procedures

Situation	Agents	Regimen[1,2] Adults	Children
High-risk[3] patients	Ampicillin plus gentamicin	Ampicillin 2 g I.M. or I.V. plus gentamicin 1.5 mg/kg (not to exceed 120 mg) within 30 min of starting the procedure; 6 h later, ampicillin 1 g I.M./I.V. or amoxicillin 1 g orally	Ampicillin 50 mg/kg I.M./I.V. (not to exceed 2 g) plus gentamicin 1.5 mg/kg within 30 min of starting the procedure; 6 h later, ampicillin 25 mg/kg I.M./I.V. or amoxicillin 25 mg/kg orally
High-risk[3] patients allergic to ampicillin/amoxicillin	Vancomycin plus gentamicin	Vancomycin 1 g I.V. over 1-2 h plus gentamicin 1.5 mg/kg I.M./I.V. (not to exceed 120 mg); complete injection/infusion within 30 min of starting the procedure	Vancomycin 20 mg/kg I.V. over 1-2 h plus gentamicin 1.5 mg/kg I.M./I.V.; complete injection/infusion within 30 min of starting the procedure
Moderate-risk[4] patients	Amoxicillin or ampicillin	Amoxicillin 2 g orally 1 h before procedure, or ampicillin 2 g I.M./I.V within 30 min of starting the procedure	Amoxicillin 50 mg/kg orally 1 h before procedure, or ampicillin 50 mg/kg I.M./I.V. within 30 min of starting the procedure
Moderate-risk[4] patients allergic to ampicillin/amoxicillin	Vancomycin	Vancomycin 1 g I.V. over 1-2 h; complete infusion within 30 min of starting the procedure	Vancomycin 20 mg/kg I.V. over 1-2 h; complete infusion within 30 min of starting the procedure

[1]Total children's dose should not exceed adult dose.

[2]No second dose of vancomycin or gentamicin is recommended.

[3]High-risk: Patients are those who have prosthetic valves, a previous history of endocarditis (even in the absence of other heart disease, complex cyanotic congenital heart disease, or surgically constructed systemic pulmonary shunts or conduits).

[4]Moderate-risk: Individuals with certain other underlying cardiac defects. Congenital cardiac conditions include the following uncorrected conditions: Patent ductus arteriosus, ventricular septal defect, ostium primum atrial septal defect, coarctation of the aorta, and bicuspid aortic valve. Acquired valvar dysfunction and hypertrophic cardiomyopathy are also moderate risk conditions.

PREVENTION OF WOUND INFECTION AND SEPSIS IN SURGICAL PATIENTS

Nature of Operation	Likely Pathogens	Recommended Drugs	Adult Dosage Before Surgery[1]
Cardiac	*S. aureus*, *S. epidermidis*	Cefazolin or cefuroxime or vancomycin[3] or clindamycin	1-2 g I.V.[2] 1.5 g I.V.[2] 1 g I.V. 600-900 mg I.V.
Gastrointestinal			
Esophageal, gastroduodenal	Enteric gram-negative bacilli, gram-positive cocci	*High risk[4] only:* Cefazolin[5]	1-2 g I.V.
Biliary tract	Enteric gram-negative bacilli, enterococci, clostridia	*High risk[6] only:* Cefazolin[5]	1-2 g I.V.
Colorectal	Enteric gram-negative bacilli, anaerobes, enterococci	*Oral:* Neomycin + erythromycin base[7] or neomycin + metronidazole[7]	
		Parenteral:	
		Cefotetan[8] or cefoxitin or cefazolin + metronidazole[5]	1-2 g I.V. 1-2 g I.V. 1-2 g I.V. 0.5-1 g I.V.
Appendectomy, nonperforated	Enteric gram-negative bacilli, anaerobes, enterococci	Cefoxitin or cefotetan[8] or cefazolin + metronidazole[5]	1-2 g I.V. 1-2 g I.V. 1-2 g I.V. 0.5-1 g I.V.
Ruptured viscus	Enteric gram-negative bacilli, anaerobes, enterococci	Cefoxitin or cefotetan[8] ± gentamicin[5,9]	1-2 g I.V. q6h 1-2 g I.V. q12h 1.5 mg/kg I.V. q8h
Genitourinary	Enteric gram-negative bacilli, enterococci	*High risk[10] only:* Ciprofloxacin	500 mg P.O. or 400 mg I.V.
Gynecologic and Obstetric			
Vaginal, abdominal, or laparoscopic hysterectomy	Enteric gram-negative bacilli, anaerobes, group B streptococci, enterococci	Cefotetan[8] or cefoxitin or cefazolin[5] or cefuroxime	1-2 g I.V. 1-2 g I.V 1-2 g I.V 1.5 g I.V.
Cesarean section	Same as for hysterectomy	Cefazolin	1-2 g I.V. after cord clamping
Abortion	Same as for hysterectomy	*First trimester, high-risk[11]:*	
		Aqueous penicillin G or doxycycline	2 mill units I.V. 300 mg P.O.[12]
		Second trimester:	
		Cefazolin	1-2 g I.V.
Head and Neck			
Incisions through oral or pharyngeal mucosa	Anaerobes, enteric gram-negative bacilli, *S. aureus*	Clindamycin + gentamicin or cefazolin	600-900 mg I.V. 1.5 mg/kg I.V. 1-2 g I.V.
Neurosurgery	*S. aureus*, *S. epidermidis*	Cefazolin or vancomycin[3]	1-2 g I.V. 1 g I.V.
Ophthalmic	*S. epidermidis*, *S. aureus*, streptococci, enteric gram-negative bacilli, *Pseudomonas*	Gentamicin, tobramycin, ciprofloxacin, gatifloxacin, levofloxacin, moxifloxacin, ofloxacin, or neomycin-gramicidin-polymyxin B	Multiple drops topically over 2-24 hours
		Cefazolin	100 mg subconjunctivally

Nature of Operation	Likely Pathogens	Recommended Drugs	Adult Dosage Before Surgery[1]
Orthopedic			
Total joint replacement, internal fixation of fractures	*S. aureus*, *S. epidermidis*	Cefazolin[13] or vancomycin[3,13]	1-2 g I.V. 1 g I.V.
Hip or knee arthroplasty	*S. aureus*, *S. epidermidis*	Cefazolin or cefuroxime[14] or vancomycin or clindamycin	1-2 g I.V. 1.5 g I.V. 1 g I.V. 600-900 mg I.V.
Thoracic (Noncardiac)	*S. aureus*, *S. epidermidis*, streptococci, enteric gram-negative bacilli	Cefazolin or cefuroxime or vancomycin[3]	1-2 g I.V. 1.5 g I.V. 1 g I.V.
Vascular			
Arterial surgery involving a prosthesis, the abdominal aorta, or a groin incision	*S. aureus*, *S. epidermidis*, enteric gram-negative bacilli	Cefazolin or cefuroxime or vancomycin[3] ± gentamicin or clindamycin	1-2 g I.V. 1.5 g I.V. 1 g I.V. 1.5 mg/kg I.V. 600-900 mg I.V.
Lower extremity amputation for ischemia	*S. aureus*, *S. epidermidis*, enteric gram-negative bacilli, clostridia	Cefazolin OR vancomycin[3]	1-2 g I.V. 1 g I.V.

[1]Parenteral prophylactic antimicrobials can be given as a single I.V. dose begun 60 minutes or less before the operation. For prolonged operations, additional intraoperative doses should be given at intervals 1-2 times the half-life of the drug for the duration of the procedure. If vancomycin or a fluoroquinolone is used, the infusion should be started 60-120 minutes before incision in order to minimize the possibility of an infusion reaction close to the time of induction of anesthesia and to have adequate tissue levels at the time of incision.

[2]Some consultants recommend an additional dose when patients are removed from bypass during open-heart surgery.

[3]For hospitals in which methicillin-resistant *S. aureus* and *S. epidermidis* are a frequent cause of postoperative wound infection, for patients previously colonized with MRSA, or for patients allergic to penicillins or cephalosporin. Rapid I.V. administration may cause hypotension, which could be especially dangerous during induction of anesthesia. Even if the drug is given over 60 minutes, hypotension may occur; treatment with diphenhydramine (Benadryl® and others) and further slowing of the infusion rate may be helpful. For procedures in which enteric gram-negative bacilli are likely pathogens, such as vascular surgery involving a groin incision, cefazolin or cefuroxime should be included in the prophylaxis regimen for patients not allergic to cephalosporins; ciprofloxacin, levofloxacin (750 mg), gentamicin, or aztreonam, each one in combination with vancomycin, can be used in patients who cannot tolerate a cephalosporin.

[4]Morbid obesity, esophageal obstruction, decreased gastric acidity, or gastrointestinal motility.

[5]For patients allergic to cephalosporins, clindamycin with either gentamicin, ciprofloxacin, levofloxacin (750 mg), or aztreonam is a reasonable alternative.

[6]Age >70 years, acute cholecystitis, nonfunctioning gallbladder, obstructive jaundice, or common duct stones.

[7]After appropriate diet and catharsis, 1 g of neomycin plus 1 g of erythromycin at 1 PM, 2 PM, and 11 PM or 2 g of neomycin plus 2 g of metronidazole at 7 PM and 11 PM the day before an 8 AM operation.

[8]Cefotetan is no longer manufactured in the U.S. although some hospitals may still have it available.

[9]Therapy is often continued for about 5 days. Ruptured viscus in postoperative setting (dehiscence) requires antibacterials to include coverage of nosocomial pathogens.

[10]Urine culture positive or unavailable, preoperative catheter, transrectal prostatic biopsy, placement of prosthetic material.

[11]Patients with previous pelvic inflammatory disease, previous gonorrhea, or multiple sex partners.

[12]Divided into 100 mg 1 hour before the abortion and 200 mg 30 minutes after.

[13]If a tourniquet is to be used in the procedure, the entire dose of antibiotic must be infused prior to its inflation.

[14]For total hip arthroplasty.

References

"Antimicrobial Prophylaxis for Surgery," *Treatment Guidelines*, 2004, 2(20):28-9.

Bratzler DW, Houck PM, Surgical Infection Prevention Guideline Writers Workgroup, et al, "Antimicrobial Prophylaxis for Surgery: An Advisory Statement From the National Surgical Infection Prevention Project," *Clin Infect Dis*, 2004, 38(12):1706-15.

REFERENCE VALUES FOR ADULTS

Automated Chemistry (CHEMISTRY A)

Test	Values	Remarks
SERUM / PLASMA		
Acetone	Negative	
Albumin	3.2-5 g/dL	
Alcohol, ethyl	Negative	
Aldolase	1.2-7.6 IU/L	
Ammonia	20-70 mcg/dL	Specimen to be placed on ice as soon as collected.
Amylase	30-110 units/L	
Bilirubin, direct	0-0.3 mg/dL	
Bilirubin, total	0.1-1.2 mg/dL	
Calcium	8.6-10.3 mg/dL	
Calcium, ionized	2.24-2.46 mEq/L	
Chloride	95-108 mEq/L	
Cholesterol, total	≤200 mg/dL	Fasted blood required – normal value affected by dietary habits. This reference range is for a general adult population.
HDL cholesterol	40-60 mg/dL	Fasted blood required – normal value affected by dietary habits.
LDL cholesterol	<160 mg/dL	If triglyceride is >400 mg/dL, LDL cannot be calculated accurately (Friedewald equation). Target LDL-C depends on patient's risk factors.
CO_2	23-30 mEq/L	
Creatine kinase (CK) isoenzymes		
CK-BB	0%	
CK-MB (cardiac)	0%-3.9%	
CK-MM (muscle)	96%-100%	
CK-MB levels must be both ≥4% and 10 IU/L to meet diagnostic criteria for CK-MB positive result consistent with myocardial injury.		
Creatine phosphokinase (CPK)	8-150 IU/L	
Creatinine	0.5-1.4 mg/dL	
Ferritin	13-300 ng/mL	
Folate	3.6-20 ng/dL	
GGT (gamma-glutamyltranspeptidase)		
male	11-63 IU/L	
female	8-35 IU/L	
GLDH	To be determined	
Glucose (preprandial)	<115 mg/dL	Goals different for diabetics.
Glucose, fasting	60-110 mg/dL	Goals different for diabetics.
Glucose, nonfasting (2-h postprandial)	<120 mg/dL	Goals different for diabetics.
Hemoglobin A_{1c}	<8	
Hemoglobin, plasma free	<2.5 mg/100 mL	
Hemoglobin, total glycosolated (Hb A_1)	4%-8%	
Iron	65-150 mcg/dL	
Iron binding capacity, total (TIBC)	250-420 mcg/dL	
Lactic acid	0.7-2.1 mEq/L	Specimen to be kept on ice and sent to lab as soon as possible.
Lactate dehydrogenase (LDH)	56-194 IU/L	

Automated Chemistry (CHEMISTRY A) *(continued)*

Test	Values	Remarks
Lactate dehydrogenase (LDH) isoenzymes		
LD_1	20%-34%	
LD_2	29%-41%	
LD_3	15%-25%	
LD_4	1%-12%	
LD_5	1%-15%	
Flipped LD_1/LD_2 ratios (>1 may be consistent with myocardial injury) particularly when considered in combination with a recent CK-MB positive result.		
Lipase	23-208 units/L	
Magnesium	1.6-2.5 mg/dL	Increased by slight hemolysis.
Osmolality	289-308 mOsm/kg	
Phosphatase, alkaline		
adults 25-60 y	33-131 IU/L	
adults 61 y or older	51-153 IU/L	
infancy-adolescence	Values range up to 3-5 times higher than adults	
Phosphate, inorganic	2.8-4.2 mg/dL	
Potassium	3.5-5.2 mEq/L	Increased by slight hemolysis.
Prealbumin	>15 mg/dL	
Protein, total	6.5-7.9 g/dL	
SGOT (AST)	<35 IU/L (20-48)	
SGPT (ALT) (10-35)	<35 IU/L	
Sodium	134-149 mEq/L	
Transferrin	>200 mg/dL	
Triglycerides	45-155 mg/dL	Fasted blood required.
Troponin I	<1.5 ng/mL	
Urea nitrogen (BUN)	7-20 mg/dL	
Uric acid		
male	2-8 mg/dL	
female	2-7.5 mg/dL	
CEREBROSPINAL FLUID		
Glucose	50-70 mg/dL	
Protein		
adults and children	15-45 mg/dL	CSF obtained by lumbar puncture.
newborn infants	60-90 mg/dL	

On CSF obtained by cisternal puncture: About 25 mg/dL

On CSF obtained by ventricular puncture: About 10 mg/dL

Note: Bloody specimen gives erroneously high value due to contamination with blood proteins

URINE **(24-hour specimen is required for all these tests unless specified)**		
Amylase	32-641 units/L	The value is in units/L and **not** calculated for total volume.
Amylase, fluid (random samples)		Interpretation of value left for physician, depends on the nature of fluid.
Calcium	Depends upon dietary intake	
Creatine		
male	150 mg/24 h	Higher value on children and during pregnancy.
female	250 mg/24 h	
Creatinine	1000-2000 mg/24 h	

REFERENCE VALUES FOR ADULTS *(Continued)*

Automated Chemistry (CHEMISTRY A) *(continued)*

Test	Values	Remarks
Creatinine clearance (endogenous)		
male	85-125 mL/min	A blood sample must accompany urine specimen.
female	75-115 mL/min	
Glucose	1 g/24 h	
5-hydroxyindoleacetic acid	2-8 mg/24 h	
Iron	0.15 mg/24 h	Acid washed container required.
Magnesium	146-209 mg/24 h	
Osmolality	500-800 mOsm/kg	With normal fluid intake.
Oxalate	10-40 mg/24 h	
Phosphate	400-1300 mg/24 h	
Potassium	25-120 mEq/24 h	Varies with diet; the interpretation of urine electrolytes and osmolality should be left for the physician.
Sodium	40-220 mEq/24 h	
Porphobilinogen, qualitative	Negative	
Porphyrins, qualitative	Negative	
Proteins	0.05-0.1 g/24 h	
Salicylate	Negative	
Urea clearance	60-95 mL/min	A blood sample must accompany specimen.
Urea N	10-40 g/24 h	Dependent on protein intake.
Uric acid	250-750 mg/24 h	Dependent on diet and therapy.
Urobilinogen	0.5-3.5 mg/24 h	For qualitative determination on random urine, send sample to urinalysis section in Hematology Lab.
Xylose absorption test		
children	16%-33% of ingested xylose	
FECES		
Fat, 3-day collection	<5 g/d	Value depends on fat intake of 100 g/d for 3 days preceding and during collection.
GASTRIC ACIDITY		
Acidity, total, 12 h	10-60 mEq/L	Titrated at pH 7.

Blood Gases

	Arterial	Capillary	Venous
pH	7.35-7.45	7.35-7.45	7.32-7.42
pCO_2 (mm Hg)	35-45	35-45	38-52
pO_2 (mm Hg)	70-100	60-80	24-48
HCO_3 (mEq/L)	19-25	19-25	19-25
TCO_2 (mEq/L)	19-29	19-29	23-33
O_2 saturation (%)	90-95	90-95	40-70
Base excess (mEq/L)	-5 to +5	-5 to +5	-5 to +5

HEMATOLOGY VALUES

Complete Blood Count

Age	Hgb (g/dL)	Hct (%)	RBC (mill/mm^3)	RDW
0-3 d	15.0-20.0	45-61	4.0-5.9	<18
1-2 wk	12.5-18.5	39-57	3.6-5.5	<17
1-6 mo	10.0-13.0	29-42	3.1-4.3	<16.5
7 mo to 2 y	10.5-13.0	33-38	3.7-4.9	<16
2-5 y	11.5-13.0	34-39	3.9-5.0	<15
5-8 y	11.5-14.5	35-42	4.0-4.9	<15
13-18 y	12.0-15.2	36-47	4.5-5.1	<14.5
Adult male	13.5-16.5	41-50	4.5-5.5	<14.5
Adult female	12.0-15.0	36-44	4.0-4.9	<14.5

Age	MCV (fL)	MCH (pg)	MCHC (%)	PLTS (x 10^3/mm^3)
0-3 d	95-115	31-37	29-37	250-450
1-2 wk	86-110	28-36	28-38	250-450
1-6 mo	74-96	25-35	30-36	300-700
7 mo to 2 y	70-84	23-30	31-37	250-600
2-5 y	75-87	24-30	31-37	250-550
5-8 y	77-95	25-33	31-37	250-550
13-18 y	78-96	25-35	31-37	150-450
Adult male	80-100	26-34	31-37	150-450
Adult female	80-100	26-34	31-37	150-450

WBC and Differential

Age	WBC (x 10^3/mm^3)	Segs	Bands	Lymphs	Monos
0-3 d	9.0-35.0	32-62	10-18	19-29	5-7
1-2 wk	5.0-20.0	14-34	6-14	36-45	6-10
1-6 mo	6.0-17.5	13-33	4-12	41-71	4-7
7 mo to 2 y	6.0-17.0	15-35	5-11	45-76	3-6
2-5 y	5.5-15.5	23-45	5-11	35-65	3-6
5-8 y	5.0-14.5	32-54	5-11	28-48	3-6
13-18 y	4.5-13.0	34-64	5-11	25-45	3-6
Adults	4.5-11.0	35-66	5-11	24-44	3-6

Age	Eosinophils	Basophils	Atypical Lymphs	No. of NRBCs
0-3 d	0-2	0-1	0-8	0-2
1-2 wk	0-2	0-1	0-8	0
1-6 mo	0-3	0-1	0-8	0
7 mo to 2 y	0-3	0-1	0-8	0
2-5 y	0-3	0-1	0-8	0
5-8 y	0-3	0-1	0-8	0
13-18 y	0-3	0-1	0-8	0
Adults	0-3	0-1	0-8	0

Segs = segmented neutrophils.

Bands = band neutrophils.

Lymphs = lymphocytes.

Monos = monocytes.

ASTHMA

MANAGEMENT OF ASTHMA IN ADULTS AND CHILDREN >5 YEARS OF AGE

Goals of Asthma Treatment

- Minimal or no chronic symptoms day or night
- Minimal or no exacerbations
- No limitations on activities; no school/work missed
- Minimal use of inhaled short-acting beta$_2$-agonist (<1 time/day, <1 canister/month)
- Minimal or no adverse effects from medications
- Children >5 years of age and adults only: PEF >80% of personal best

All Patients

- Short-acting bronchodilator: **Inhaled beta$_2$-agonists** as needed for symptoms.
- Intensity of treatment will depend on severity of exacerbation; see "Management of Asthma Exacerbations".
- Use of short-acting inhaled beta$_2$-agonists on a daily basis, or increasing use, indicates the need to initiate or titrate long-term control therapy.

Education

- Teach self-management.
- Teach about controlling environmental factors (avoidance of allergens or other factors that contribute to asthma severity).
- Review administration technique and compliance with patient.
- May use a written action plan to help educate.

Stepwise Approach for Managing Asthma in Adults and Children >5 Years of Age: Treatment[1]

Symptoms[2]	Lung Function[3]	Long-Term Control (Daily Medications)
STEP 4: Severe Persistent		
Day: Continual Night: Frequent	PEF/FEV$_1$ ≤60% PEF variability >30%	**• Preferred treatment:** **– High dose inhaled corticosteroid** **AND** **– Long-acting inhaled beta$_2$-agonist** AND, if needed – Long-term oral corticosteroids (2 mg/kg/day, generally do not exceed 60 mg/day). (Make repeated attempts to reduce systemic corticosteroids and maintain control with high-dose inhaled corticosteroids.)

Symptoms[2]	Lung Function[3]	Long-Term Control (Daily Medications)
STEP 3: Moderate Persistent		
Day: Every day Night: >1 night/week	PEF/FEV_1 >60% - <80% PEF variability >30%	• **Preferred treatment:** **– Low-medium dose inhaled corticosteroid** **AND** **– Long-acting inhaled beta$_2$-agonist** • Alternatives: – Increase inhaled corticosteroids within medium-dose range **OR** – Low-medium dose inhaled corticosteroids and either leukotriene receptor antagonist or theophylline
		If needed (especially with recurring severe exacerbations): • **Preferred treatment:** – Increase inhaled corticosteroids within medium-dose range, and add long-acting inhaled beta$_2$-agonist • Alternatives: – Increase inhaled corticosteroids in medium-dose range, and add either leukotriene receptor antagonist or theophylline
STEP 2: Mild Persistent		
Day: >2 days/week but <1 time/day Night: >2 nights/month	PEF/FEV_1 ≥80% PEF variability 20%-30%	• **Preferred treatment:** **– Low-dose inhaled corticosteroid** • Alternatives: Cromolyn, leukotriene receptor antagonist, nedocromil, or sustained release theophylline (serum concentration 5-15 mcg/mL)
STEP 1: Mild Intermittent		
Day: ≤2 days/week Night: ≤2 nights/month	PEF/FEV_1 ≥80% PEF variability <20%	No daily medication needed. A course of systemic corticosteroids is recommended for severe exacerbations.

[1]Classify severity. The presence of one of the features of severity is sufficient to place a patient in that category. An individual should be assigned to the most severe grade in which any feature occurs. The characteristics noted are general and may overlap because asthma is highly variable. Furthermore, an individual's classification may change over time.

[2]Patients at any level of severity can have mild, moderate, or severe exacerbations. Some patients with intermittent asthma experience severe and life-threatening exacerbations separated by long periods of normal lung function and no symptoms.

[3]PEF is % of personal best and FEV_1 is % predicted.

↓ Step down
Review treatment every 1-6 months; a gradual stepwise reduction in treatment may be possible.

↑Step up
If control is not maintained, consider step up. First, review patient medication technique, adherence, and environmental control.

ASTHMA *(Continued)*

Notes:

- **The stepwise approach presents general guidelines to assist clinical decision making; it is not intended to be a specific prescription. Asthma is highly variable; clinicians should tailor specific medication plans to the needs and circumstances of individual patients.**
- Gain control as quickly as possible; then decrease treatment to the least medication necessary to maintain control.
- A rescue course of systemic corticosteroids may be needed at any time and at any step.
- Some patients with intermittent asthma experience severe and life-threatening exacerbations separated by long periods of normal lung function and no symptoms. This may be especially common with exacerbations provoked by respiratory infections. A short course of systemic corticosteroids is recommended.
- At each step, patients should control their environment to avoid or control factors that make their asthma worse.
- Antibiotics are not recommended for treatment of acute asthma exacerbations except where there is evidence or suspicion of bacterial infection.
- Consultation with an asthma specialist is recommended for moderate or severe persistent asthma.
- Peak flow monitoring for patients with moderate-severe asthma should be considered.

MANAGEMENT OF ASTHMA IN INFANTS AND YOUNG CHILDREN

All Patients

- Bronchodilator as needed for symptoms ≤2 times/week. Intensity of treatment will depend upon severity of exacerbation (see "Management of Asthma Exacerbations"). Either:
  - Preferred treatment: Inhaled short-acting beta$_2$-agonist by nebulizer or face mask and spacer/holding chamber

    or
  - Alternative treatment: Oral beta$_2$-agonist
- With viral respiratory infection:
  - Bronchodilator q4-6h up to 24 hours (longer with physician consult) but, in general, repeat no more than once every 6 weeks.
  - Consider systemic corticosteroid if current exacerbation is severe or patient has history of severe exacerbations.
- Use of short-acting inhaled beta$_2$-agonist on a daily basis, or increasing use, indicates the need to initiate or titrate long-term control therapy.

Education

- Teach self-management or caregiver management.
- Teach about controlling environmental factors.
- Review administration technique and compliance with patient.
- May use a written action plan to help educate.

Stepwise Approach for Managing Infants and Young Children (≤5 Years of Age) With Acute or Chronic Asthma[1]

Symptoms[2]	Long-Term Control (Daily Medications)
STEP 4: Severe Persistent	
Day: Continual Night: Frequent	• **Preferred treatment:** **– High dose inhaled corticosteroid** **AND** **– Long-acting inhaled beta$_2$-agonist** AND, if needed – Long-term oral corticosteroids (2 mg/kg/day, generally do not exceed 60 mg/day). (Make repeated attempts to reduce systemic corticosteroids and maintain control with high-dose inhaled corticosteroids.)
STEP 3: Moderate Persistent	
Day: Every day Night: >1 night/week	• **Preferred treatment:** **– Low-dose inhaled corticosteroid** **AND** **Long-acting inhaled beta$_2$-agonist** **OR** **Medium-dose inhaled corticosteroid** • Alternatives: – Low-dose inhaled corticosteroid and either leukotriene receptor antagonist or theophylline
	If needed (especially with recurring severe exacerbations): • **Preferred treatment:** **– Medium-dose inhaled corticosteroid and long-acting inhaled beta$_2$-agonist** • Alternatives: – Medium-dose inhaled corticosteroid and either leukotriene receptor antagonist or theophylline
STEP 2: Mild Persistent	
Day: >2 days/week but <1 time/day Night: >2 nights/month	• **Preferred treatment:** **– Low-dose inhaled corticosteroid (with nebulizer or MDI with holding chamber with or without face mask or DPI)** • Alternatives: Cromolyn (nebulizer is preferred or MDI with holding chamber) **OR** Leukotriene receptor antagonist

ASTHMA *(Continued)*

Stepwise Approach for Managing Infants and Young Children (≤5 Years of Age) With Acute or Chronic Asthma[1]

Symptoms[2]	Long-Term Control (Daily Medications)
STEP 1: Mild Intermittent	
Day: ≤2 days/week Night: ≤2 nights/month	No daily medication needed

[1]Classify severity. The presence of one of the features of severity is sufficient to place a patient in that category. An individual should be assigned to the most severe grade in which any feature occurs. The characteristics noted in this figure are general and may overlap because asthma is highly variable. Furthermore, an individual's classification may change over time.

[2]Patients at any level of severity can have mild, moderate, or severe exacerbations. Some patients with intermittent asthma experience severe and life-threatening exacerbations separated by long periods of normal lung function and no symptoms.

↓ Step Down
Review treatment every 1-6 month; a gradual stepwise reduction in treatment may be possible.

↑ Step Up
If control is not achieved, consider step up. But first: review patient medication technique, adherence, and environmental control (avoidance of allergens or other precipitant factors)

Notes:

- **The stepwise approach presents guidelines to assist clinical decision making. Asthma is highly variable; clinicians should tailor specific medication plans to the needs and circumstances of individual patients.**
- Gain control as quickly as possible; then decrease treatment to the least medication necessary to maintain control.
- A rescue course of systemic corticosteroid may be needed at any time and step.
- In general, use of a short-acting beta$_2$-agonist on a daily basis indicates the need for additional long-term control therapy.
- There are very few studies on asthma therapy for infants.
- Studies comparing medications in children <5 years of age are not available.
- Consultation with an asthma specialist is recommended for moderate or severe persistent asthma. Consider consultation for patient with mild persistent asthma.
- Initiation of long-term control therapy should be considered in infants and young children who have had >3 episodes of wheezing in the past year that lasted >1 day and affected sleep and who have risk factors for asthma.
- Inhaled corticosteroids improve health outcomes for children with mild-moderate persistent asthma. Monitor growth of children taking corticosteroids by any route. If growth appears slowed, weigh the benefits against the risks.
- Antibiotics are not recommended for treatment of acute asthma exacerbations except where there is evidence or suspicion of bacterial infection.

Management of Asthma Exacerbations: Home Treatment[1]

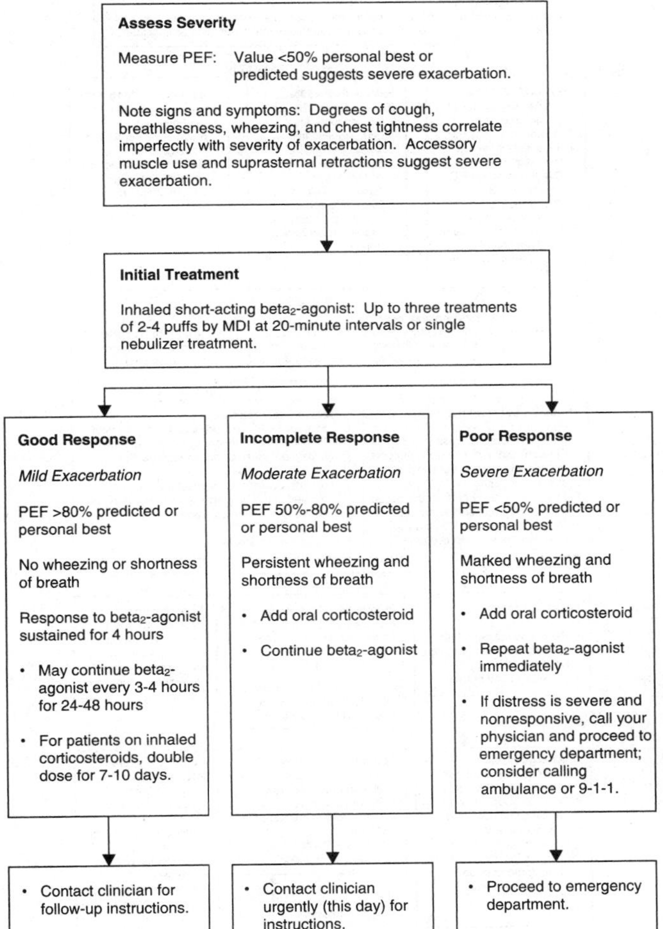

[1]Patients at high risk of asthma-related death should receive immediate clinical attention after initial treatment. Additional therapy may be required.

ASTHMA *(Continued)*

Management of Asthma Exacerbations: Emergency Department and Hospital-Based Care

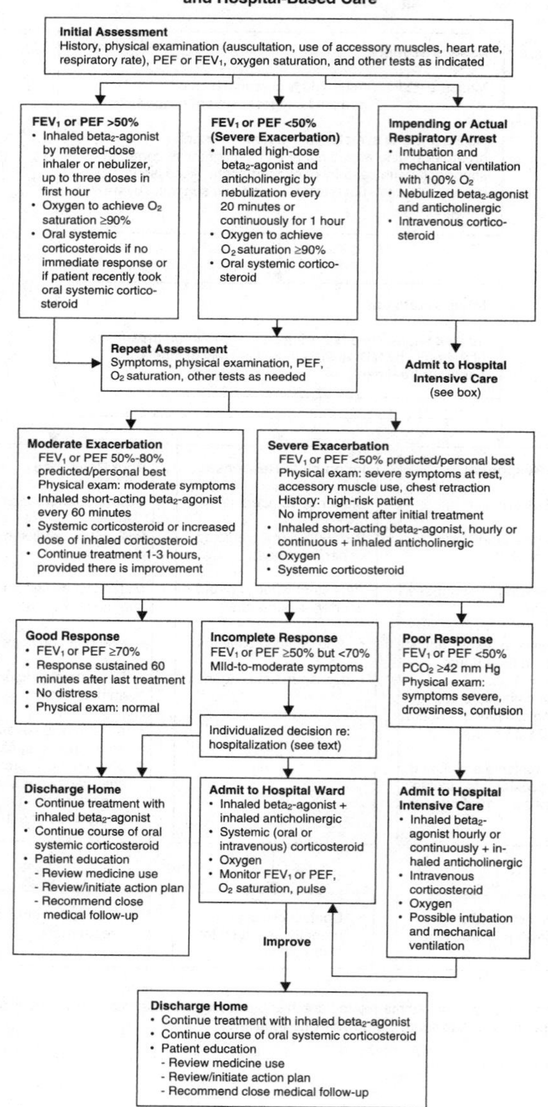

ESTIMATED COMPARATIVE DAILY DOSAGES FOR INHALED CORTICOSTEROIDS

Adults

Drug	Low Dose	Medium Dose	High Dose
Beclomethasone dipropionate	168-504 mcg	504-840 mcg	>840 mcg
42 mcg/puff	4-12 puffs	12-20 puffs	>20 puffs
84 mcg/puff	2-6 puffs	6-10 puffs	>10 puffs
Beclomethasone dipropionate HFA	80-240 mcg	240-480 mcg	>480 mcg
40 mcg/puff	2-6 puffs	12 puffs	>12 puffs
80 mcg/puff	1-3 puffs	6 puffs	>6 puffs
Budesonide Turbuhaler®	200-600 mcg	600-1200 mcg	>1200 mcg
200 mcg/inhalation	1-3 inhalations	3-6 inhalations	>6 inhalations
Flunisolide	500-1000 mcg	1000-2000 mcg	>2000 mcg
250 mcg/puff	2-4 puffs	4-8 puffs	>8 puffs
Fluticasone MDI 44, 110, 220 mcg/puff	88-264 mcg	264-660 mcg	>660 mcg
Fluticasone DPI 50, 100, 250 mcg/dose	100-300 mcg	300-600 mcg	>600 mcg
Triamcinolone acetonide	400-1000 mcg	1000-2000 mcg	>2000 mcg
100 mcg/puff	4-10 puffs	10-20 puffs	>20 puffs

Children

Drug	Low Dose	Medium Dose	High Dose
Beclomethasone dipropionate	84-336 mcg	336-672 mcg	>672 mcg
42 mcg/puff	2-8 puffs	8-16 puffs	>16 puffs
84 mcg/puff	1-4 puffs	4-8 puffs	>8 puffs
Beclomethasone dipropionate HFA	80-160 mcg	160-320 mcg	>320 mcg
40 mcg/puff	2-4 puffs	4-8 puffs	>8 puffs
80 mcg/puff	1-2 puffs	2-4 puffs	>4 puffs
Budesonide Turbuhaler®	200-400 mcg	400-800 mcg	>800 mcg
200 mcg/inhalation	1-2 inhalations	2-4 inhalations	>4 inhalations
Budesonide inhalation suspension for nebulization	0.5 mg	1 mg	2 mg
Flunisolide	500-750 mcg	1000-1250 mcg	>1250 mcg
250 mcg/puff	2-3 puffs	4-5 puffs	>5 puffs
Fluticasone MDI 44, 110, 220 mcg/puff	88-176 mcg	176-440 mcg	>440 mcg
Fluticasone DPI 50, 100, 250 mcg/dose	100-200 mcg	200-400 mcg	>400 mcg
Triamcinolone acetonide	400-800 mcg	800-1200 mcg	>1200 mcg
100 mcg/puff	4-8 puffs	8-12 puffs	>12 puffs

References

National Asthma Education and Prevention Program (NAEPP), Clinical Practice Guidelines, Expert Panel Report 2, "Guidelines for the Diagnosis and Management of Asthma," NIH Publication No. 97-4051, July 1997.

National Asthma Education and Prevention Program (NAEPP) Expert Panel Report, "Guidelines for the Diagnosis and Management of Asthma – Update on Selected Topics 2002," NIH Publication No. 02-5075 (www.nhlbi.nih.gov/guidelines/asthma/index.html)

CONTRAST MEDIA REACTIONS, PREMEDICATION FOR PROPHYLAXIS

American College of Radiology Guidelines for Use of Nonionic Contrast Media

It is estimated that approximately 5% to 10% of patients will experience adverse reactions to administration of contrast dye (less for nonionic contrast). In approximately 1000-2000 administrations, a life-threatening reaction will occur.

A variety of premedication regimens have been proposed, both for pretreatment of "at risk" patients who require contrast media and before the routine administration of the intravenous high osmolar contrast media. Such regimens have been shown in clinical trials to decrease the frequency of all forms of contrast medium reactions. Pretreatment with a 2-dose regimen of methylprednisolone 32 mg, 12 and 2 hours prior to intravenous administration of HOCM (ionic), has been shown to decrease mild, moderate, and severe reactions in patients at increased risk and perhaps in patients without risk factors. Logistical and feasibility problems may preclude adequate premedication with this or any regimen for all patients. It is unclear at this time that steroid pretreatment prior to administration of ionic contrast media reduces the incidence of reactions to the same extent or less than that achieved with the use of nonionic contrast media alone. Information about the efficacy of nonionic contrast media combined with a premedication strategy, including steroids, is preliminary or not yet currently available. For high-risk patients (ie, previous contrast reactors), the combination of a pretreatment regimen with nonionic contrast media has empirical merit and may warrant consideration. Oral administration of steroids appears preferable to intravascular routes, and the drug may be prednisone or methylprednisolone. Supplemental administration of H_1 and H_2 antihistamine therapies, orally or intravenously, may reduce the frequency of urticaria, angioedema, and respiratory symptoms. Additionally, ephedrine administration has been suggested to decrease the frequency of contrast reactions, but caution is advised in patients with cardiac disease, hypertension, or hyperthyroidism. No premedication strategy should be a substitute for the ABC approach to preadministration preparedness listed above. Contrast reactions do occur despite any and all premedication prophylaxis. The incidence can be decreased, however, in some categories of "at risk" patients receiving high osmolar contrast media plus a medication regimen. For patients with previous contrast medium reactions, there is a slight chance that recurrence may be more severe or the same as the prior reaction, however, it is more likely that there will be no recurrence.

General Premedication Regimen

Methylprednisolone	32 mg orally 12 and 2 hours prior to procedure
Diphenhydramine	50 mg orally 1 hour prior to the procedure

Alternative Premedication Regimen

Prednisone	50 mg orally 13, 7, and 1 hour before the procedure
Diphenhydramine	50 mg orally 1 hour before the procedure
Ephedrine	25 mg orally 1 hour before the procedure (except when contraindicated)

Unlabeled Use (Nephroprotective)

N-acetylcysteine, P.O.	600 mg orally twice daily on the day before and the day of the scan in addition to hydration with 0.45% saline intravenously

Indications for Nonionic Contrast

- Previous reaction to contrast – premedicate[1]
- Known allergy to iodine or shellfish
- Asthma, especially if on medication
- Myocardial instability or CHF
- Risk for aspiration or severe nausea and vomiting
- Difficulty communicating or inability to give history
- Patients taking beta-blockers
- Small children at risk for electrolyte imbalance or extravasation
- Renal failure with diabetes, sickle cell disease, or myeloma
- At physician or patient request

[1]Life-threatening reactions (throat swelling, laryngeal edema, etc), consider omitting the intravenous contrast.

EPILEPSY

CONVULSIVE STATUS EPILEPTICUS

Recommendations of the Epilepsy Foundation of America's Working Group on Status Epilepticus

(*JAMA*, 1993, 270:854-9)

Convulsive status epilepticus is an emergency that is associated with high morbidity and mortality. The outcome largely depends on etiology, but prompt and appropriate pharmacological therapy can reduce morbidity and mortality. Etiology varies in children and adults and reflects the distribution of disease in these age groups. Antiepileptic drug administration should be initiated whenever a seizure has lasted 10 minutes. Immediate concerns include supporting respiration, maintaining blood pressure, gaining intravenous access, and identifying and treating the underlying cause. Initial therapeutic and diagnostic measures are conducted simultaneously. The goal of therapy is rapid termination of clinical and electrical seizure activity; the longer a seizure continues, the greater the likelihood of an adverse outcome. Several drug protocols now in use will terminate status epilepticus. Common to all patients is the need for a clear plan, prompt administration of appropriate drugs in adequate doses, and attention to the possibility of apnea, hypoventilation, or other metabolic abnormalities.

Figure 1. Algorithm for the Initial Management of Status Epilepticus

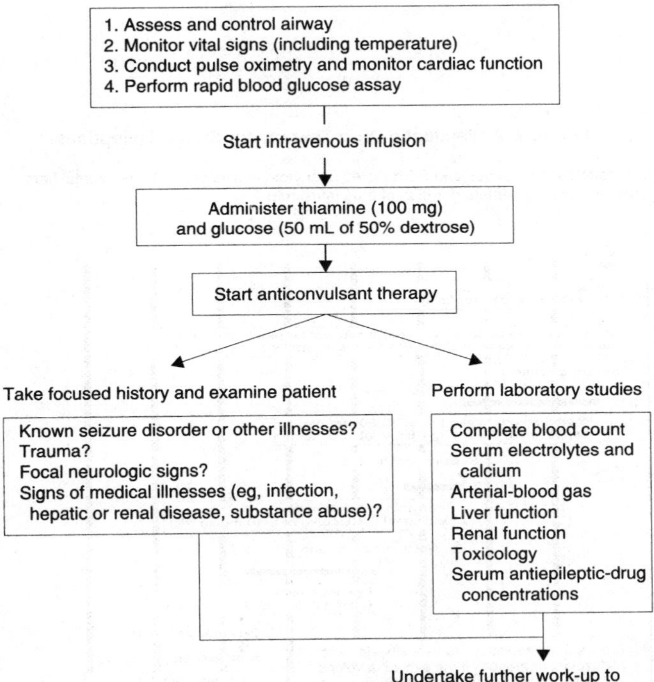

Adapted from Lowenstein A, "Current Concepts: Status Epilepticus," *N Engl J Med*, 1998, 338:970-6 with permission.

EPILEPSY *(Continued)*

Figure 2. Antiepileptic Drug Therapy for Status Epilepticus

I.V. denotes intravenous and PE denotes phenytoin equivalents. The horizontal bars indicate the approximate duration of drug infusions.

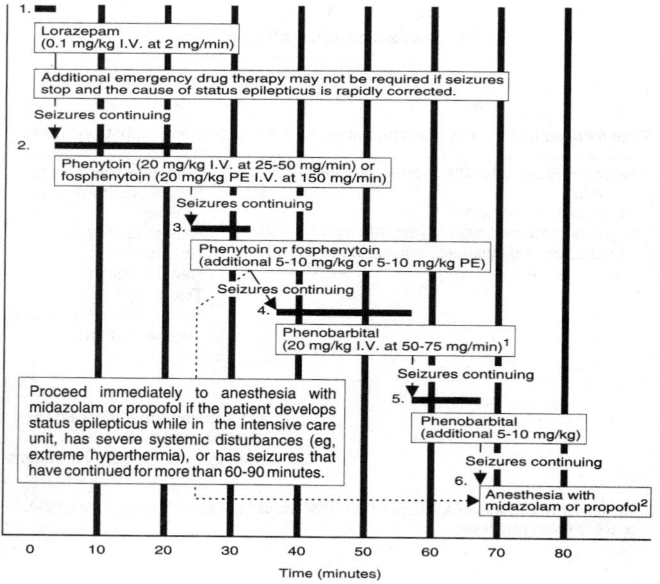

[1]Or pentobarbital (10-20 mg/kg over 1-2 hours).
[2]Or valproate sodium (15-25 mg/kg administered at 3 mg/kg/minute).

Adapted from Lowenstein A, "Current Concepts: Status Epilepticus," *N Engl J Med*, 1998, 338:970-6 with permission.

HEART FAILURE (SYSTOLIC)

INTRODUCTORY COMMENTS

This chapter summarizes the pharmacotherapy of patients with systolic heart failure with respect to treating mild-moderate exacerbations and chronic therapy. A more detailed discussion is available at: www.acc.org/clinical/guidelines/failure;index.pdf.

It should be recognized that the most common cause for exacerbations of patents' heart failure is poor adherence to therapy (medications and diet restriction). Health-care providers need to educate patients about the importance of adherence to medical regimens.

For many years, therapy of heart failure focused on correcting the hemodynamic imbalances that occurred in heart failure. It is now recognized that heart failure triggers the release of several neurohormones that, in the short-run, help the patient; but, in the long-run, are detrimental. Newer pharmacotherapeutic approaches address counteracting the actions of these harmful neurohormones as well as address hemodynamic issues.

Diuretics

Although data have yet to demonstrate that diuretics reduce the mortality associated with heart failure, they relieve symptoms seen in heart failure. Diuretics should only be used in patients experiencing congestion with their heart failure. Although not usually the case, some patients do have heart failure without any congestion. In such rare instances, diuretic therapy is not indicated since they further stimulate the deleterious neurohormonal responses seen.

Although some heart failure patients with congestion can be controlled with thiazide diuretics, most will require the more potent loop diuretics, either because a strong diuretic effect is needed or the renal function of the patients is compromised (thus limiting the effectiveness of the thiazide diuretic). When patients with heart failure are discovered to have mild-moderate worsening congestion, they often can be controlled by adjusting their oral loop diuretic dose or, if applicable, initiating a loop diuretic regimen. If a more aggressive diuresis is indicated, especially if the patient is suffering from pulmonary congestion, intravenous loop diuretics would be indicated. When loop diuretics are given intravenously, before any diuretic effect occurs, they benefit the patient by dilating veins and reducing preload, thus relieving pulmonary congestion. Intravenous loop diuresis may also be considered in a patient where concerns exist about the ability of the patient to absorb the orally administered medication.

If already on an oral loop diuretic, the dosage should be increased (generally, 1.5-2 times their current regimen) in an effort for the patient to lose about 1-1.5 liters of fluid per day (about equivalent to 1-1.5 kg of weight per day). If the patient had yet to be started on a diuretic or was previously receiving a thiazide diuretic, initiating furosemide at 20-40 mg once or twice daily is a reasonable consideration. If the initial increase (or initiation) in dosage fails to induce a diuretic response, the dosage may be increased. If the initial increase (or initiation) does induce a diuretic response but the patient fails to lose weight or is not losing more fluids than taking in, the frequency of giving the loop diuretic can be increased. When an effective regimen is achieved, this regimen should be continued until the patient achieves a goal "dry" weight. Once this weight is attained, a decision needs to be made on how to continue the patient on diuretic therapy. If the patient had not been on a diuretic at home, continuation of the loop diuretic at a reduced dose is a worthy consideration. If the exacerbation was related to noncompliance with the diuretic or diet, the previous home dose might be continued with education on compliance. If the exacerbation was caused by an inadequate pharmacotherapeutic regimen (such as vasodilator was not being use), the previous home dose might be continued in conjunction with a more complete pharmacotherapeutic regimen. If the patient was compliant and on an acceptable pharmacotherapeutic regimen, the patient's original diuretic dose would be increased to some dosage greater than their home regimen, yet generally less than what was just used to achieve their dry weight.

The use of loop diuretics can lead to hypokalemia and/or hypomagnesemia. Electrolyte disturbances can predispose a patient to serious cardiac arrhythmias particularly if the patient is concurrently receiving digoxin. Fluid depletion, hypotension, and azotemia can also result from excessive use of diuretics. In contrast to thiazide

HEART FAILURE (SYSTOLIC) *(Continued)*

diuretics, a loop diuretic can also lower serum calcium concentrations. For some patients, despite higher doses of loop diuretic treatment, an adequate diuretic response cannot be attained. Diuretic resistance can usually be overcome by intravenous administration (including continuous infusion), the use of 2 diuretics together (eg, furosemide and metolazone), or the use of a diuretic with a positive inotropic agent. When such combinations are used, serum electrolytes need to be monitored even more closely.

When loop diuretics are used in patients with renal dysfunction, to achieve the desired diuretic response, dosages typically will need to be greater than what is used in patients with normal renal function.

Due to its long existence and inexpensive price, furosemide tends to be the loop diuretic most commonly used. Bumetanide is now available as a generic and its use has been increasing consequently. The oral bioavailability of bumetanide and torsemide are nearly 100%; whereas, furosemide's oral bioavailability averages about 50%. A useful rule of thumb for conversion of intravenous loop diuretics is 40 mg of furosemide is equal to 1 mg bumetanide is equal to 15 mg torsemide. A few patients have allergies to diuretics because many contain a sulfur element. The only loop diuretic that lacks a sulfur element is ethacrynic acid.

Vasodilators

Vasodilator therapy, specifically the combination of hydralazine and isosorbide dinitrate, was the first pharmacotherapeutic treatment demonstrated to enhance survival of heart failure patients. The use of hydralazine 75 mg (which reduces afterload) and isosorbide dinitrate 40 mg four times a day (which reduces preload) demonstrated enhanced survival compared to placebo and prazosin. Unfortunately, many patients were unable to tolerate this regimen (primarily due to headaches and gastrointestinal disturbances) and the magnitude of benefit in survival dissipated with time.

Later, a series of investigations demonstrated that enalapril (which reduces both afterload and preload) enhances the survival of heart failure patients. Dosages used in these trials averaged about 10 mg twice daily. Since these trials, other ACE inhibitors were proven to benefit heart failure patients.

ACE Inhibitors

This led to the question, which is superior, ACE inhibitor or the combination of hydralazine and isosorbide dinitrate? In a comparative trial, using doses described above, enalapril was superior to the combination of hydralazine and isosorbide dinitrate, making an ACE inhibitor the vasodilator of choice in heart failure patients. An ACE inhibitor can alleviate symptoms, improve clinical status, and enhance a patient's quality of life. In addition an ACE inhibitor can reduce the risk of death and the combined risk of death or hospitalization.

Adverse effects associated with ACE inhibitors include hyperkalemia, rash, dysgeusia, dry cough, and (rarely) angioedema. Patients sometime develop renal dysfunction with the initiation of ACE inhibitors. This is not due to direct nephrotoxicity of the kidney but related to the ACE inhibitor dilating the efferent renal artery of the kidney, thus shunting blood away from being filtered in the glomerulus. The risk for renal dysfunction is increased when the ACE inhibitor is introduced to a patient who is hypovolemic, is being aggressively diuresed, is on an NSAID, or has bilateral renal artery stenosis (unilateral if only one kidney is present). Avoid NSAIDs in heart failure patients. ACE inhibitors should be avoided in patients with known renal artery stenosis. Monitor renal function and serum potassium within 1 to 2 weeks of initiation of therapy and routinely thereafter especially in patients with pre-existing hypotension, hyponatremia, diabetes, azotemia, or in those taking potassium supplements. Some patients will have an exaggerated hypotensive response following the initial doses (especially the first dose) of an ACE inhibitor.

A major limitation to using ACE inhibitors treatment in heart failure can be the dry cough that some patients develop. Lowering the ACE inhibitor dose sometimes can control it, but this may limit the effectiveness of the ACE inhibitor treatment. The development of angiotensin receptor blockers (ARBs) has helped address this issue. ARBs were demonstrated to enhance survival of heart failure patients. Although they are not the vasodilator of first choice in heart failure, they are a reasonable alternative in patients who cannot tolerate an ACE inhibitor due to the cough or some other adverse effect (with the exception of hyperkalemia and renal dysfunction; ARBs can induce as well). ARBs do not cause an accumulation of kinins as ACE inhibitors do.

Can ARBs can be used in patients who suffer angioedema with ACE inhibitors. Reports are available in the literature describing patients who experienced angioedema with both ACE inhibitors and ARBs. These cases do not indicate how safe an ARB is in a patient who has experienced ACE inhibitor-induced angioedema. The CHARM-Alternative trial confirmed that only one of 39 patients (~2.6%) who experienced angioedema with an ACE inhibitors also experienced it with an ARB.

Concurrent Use of an ACE Inhibitor and an ARB

In Val-HeFT, valsartan added to conventional treatment (included ACE inhibitor treatment) did not impact survival but did reduce morbidity. Of note, a subgroup analysis of this trial suggested the combination of valsartan and an ACE inhibitor may be detrimental to patients also receiving a beta-blocker. In CHARM-Added, candesartan added to ACE inhibitor therapy was of benefit to heart failure patients (modest reduction in hospitalization; increased risk of hyperkalemia and renal dysfunction), even for those receiving a beta-blocker. As a result, the recently released ACC/AHA Practice Guidelines do not speak against using the combination of ACE inhibitors and ARBs. However, few patients in these trials were receiving an aldosterone blocker (such as spironolactone), which is now known to be of benefit to heart failure patients. Since there is enhanced risk for hyperkalemia and outcome data are currently unknown, the ACC/AHA Practice Guidelines for heart failure do not advocate the combined use of ACE inhibitors, ARBs, and an aldosterone inhibitor.

In summary, vasodilator therapy should initially consist of an ACE inhibitor. If such therapy cannot be tolerated due to renal failure or hyperkalemia, the combination of hydralazine and isosorbide dinitrate may be considered as ARBs can also cause renal failure and hyperkalemia. If the ACE inhibitor cannot be tolerated due to adverse effects such as dry cough, an ARB may be considered. If an ACE inhibitor and beta blocker have been maximized yet heart failure symptoms persist, consider adding hydralazine and isosorbide dinitrate. This approach, in fact, has been demonstrated to enhance the survival of African-American patients with heart failure. Another approach may be to add an ARB to the ACE inhibitor; but caution should occur, due to the risk of hyperkalemia.

Beta-Blockers

Despite being negative inotropes, beta-blockers have been demonstrated to enhance the survival of systolic heart failure patients. Their benefit is attributed to their ability to protect the myocardium from the "bombardment" of catecholamines present in heart failure that can lead to ventricular remodeling. Bisoprolol, metoprolol succinate (extended release), and carvedilol have been demonstrated in trials to improve survival. At present, superiority of one agent over another has not been definitively demonstrated. For patients to be able to tolerate this therapy, beta-blocker treatment needs to be initiated at low doses and titrated slowly (generally, the dose is double every two weeks). Following the initiation of treatment and the increase in dosage, patients may feel that their disease is worsening but this should dissipate after a few days. If this ill feeling continues beyond a few days, consideration should be given to regimen adjustments. If the patient is congested, increase the diuretic dosage. If the patient's discomfort is related to hypotension, staggering the beta-blocker dose with the vasodilator dose and/or lowering the vasodilator dosage may be helpful. If these approaches are ineffective or cannot explain the patient's ill feeling, consideration should be given to lowering the beta-blocker dosage and attempt a titration later on. Sometimes, a patient may not be able to tolerate "goal" doses of both beta-blockers and concurrent vasodilator treatment due to hypotension. It is the consensus opinion that a reduced dose of each agent is better than a goal dose of just one agent. Beta-blockers are not necessarily contraindicated but need to be used cautiously in patients with bronchospastic disease, peripheral artery disease, or diabetes mellitus.

Aldosterone Blockers

Of the pharmacotherapeutic treatments of heart failure demonstrated to benefit patients, the use of aldosterone blockers is the newest. It has been demonstrated, especially in the more severe forms of heart failure, that spironolactone, at an average dose of 25 mg daily, enhances the survival of heart failure patients. In patients who suffer hyperkalemia at this relatively low dosage, lowering the dose to

HEART FAILURE (SYSTOLIC) *(Continued)*

25 mg every other day may be attempted. In patients who are still symptomatic with their heart failure and have maximized the other proven treatments of heart failure and whose potassium concentrations can tolerate it, the spironolactone dose may be increased to 50 mg daily.

Obviously, hyperkalemia is a concern with this treatment, especially since patients generally will also be on an ACE inhibitor or ARB. It has been demonstrated that the number of emergency visits related to hyperkalemia in heart failure has increased with the introduction of aldosterone blocking therapy in treating heart failure. About 10% of patients will experience endocrinological effects with spironolactone. In men, breast tenderness and gynecomastic can occur. In women, menstrual irregularities may occur. In such instances, the use of eplerenone may be considered. Eplerenone is less apt to induce endocrinological effects but it is more expensive. A typical dose is 25-50 mg daily. Eplerenone has been demonstrated to enhance survival of post-MI patients with reduced ejection fractions. Spironolactone has not been studied in this patient group.

These medications should not be started in patients with renal insufficiency. These medications should be avoided if the serum creatinine exceeds 2.5 mg/dL in men (2 mg/dL in women) or if baseline potassium ≥5 mEq/L.

Digoxin

The value of digoxin in heart failure has crossed the spectrum. In the late 1980s further investigation with digoxin suggested that indeed it may have a role in heart failure treatment, but the methods of these trials were not ideal (digoxin was taken away from stabilized patients to see if the condition of patients worsened – it did). Finally, digoxin was studied in a prospective manner where patients were on known optimal heart failure treatment at the time and randomized to placebo or digoxin. The digoxin dosage used resulted in digoxin steady-state concentrations of 1 mcg/L. This trial revealed that digoxin did not impact survival but reduced the number of patient hospitalizations, suggesting digoxin has a morbidity benefit. Many are of the opinion that digoxin's benefit is unrelated to its positive inotropic activity but related to inhibiting neurohormal activity. Healthcare providers may consider adding digoxin in patients with persistent heart failure symptoms as a fourth line agent.

Digoxin is primarily renally eliminated; therefore, renal function of patients should be closely monitored and the dose adjusted. Digoxin does become difficult to use in patients whose renal function is unstable. In the DIG trial, effective digoxin steady-state concentrations were around 0.7-1 mcg/L. Levels much beyond 1 mcg/L were associated with worsened outcomes, especially in women. Since digoxin's benefit is long-term, a loading dose is not necessary. When checking a digoxin serum concentration, the sample should not be obtained until 12 hours after a dose, especially if it was oral, since digoxin has a relatively long distribution phase. It should also be assured that the patient is at steady-state (recall that the half-life of digoxin in a patient with normal renal function is 36 hours and that patients with heart failure generally have worsened renal function).

Hypokalemia, hypomagnesia, and hypercalcemia can precipitate digoxin toxicity in the presence of a therapeutic digoxin concentration. This toxicity can be alleviated by correcting the electrolyte abnormality. In acute digoxin overdoses, hyperkalemia can occur since digoxin inhibits the sodium-potassium ATPase pump. For this reason, one should not assume potassium is given to just **any** patient with digoxin toxicity. Digoxin toxicity can present as bradyarrhythmias, heart blocks, ventricular tachyarrhythmias, and atrial tachyarrhythmias (PAT with block is pathognomic). Other toxic manifestations include visual disturbances (including greenish-yellowish vision and halos around lights), gastrointestinal disturbances, anorexia, and altered mental status. Many medications elevate digoxin concentrations and a patient's regimen should be assessed for potential interactions.

Other Heart Failure Therapeutic Considerations

- If a calcium channel blocker is desired, amlodipine and felodipine are preferred choices.
- To treat arrhythmias, amiodarone and dofetilide are best documented to lack much proarrhythmic propensity in heart failure patients.

- In heart failure patients with diabetes mellitus, metformin should not be used and "glitazones" should not be used in severe heart failure (NYHA III and IV) and used cautiously, if at all, in mild-moderate heart failure.
- The use of cilostazol, because it has type III phosphodiesterase-inhibiting properties, is contraindicated in heart failure. This is because the chronic use of oral milrinone and inamrinone, also type III phosphodiesterase inhibitors, resulted in enhanced mortality in heart failure patients (and therefore, these two agents were never FDA-approved for oral use).
- NSAID use should be avoided or used minimally as these agents antagonize the effects of diuretics and ACE inhibitors.
- Retrospective data suggests that daily aspirin may also negate the effects of ACE inhibitors but this has yet to be definitively proven in prospective trials. Using the lowest possible aspirin dose with the highest possible ACE inhibitor dose has been suggested as a way to best circumvent this issue.
- Routine intermittent infusions of positive inotropes are not recommended. Can be used as palliation in end-stage disease.

Dosing of ACE Inhibitors in Heart Failure[1]

ACEI	Initial Dose	Maximum Dose
Captopril	6.25 mg tid	50 mg tid
Enalapril	2.5 mg bid	10-20 mg bid
Fosinopril	5-10 mg daily	40 mg daily
Lisinopril	2.5-5 mg daily	20-40 mg daily
Perindopril	2 mg daily	8-16 mg daily
Quinapril	5 mg bid	20 mg bid
Ramipril	1.25-2.5 mg daily	10 mg daily
Trandolapril	1 mg daily	4 mg daily

[1]From ACC/AHA Guidelines.

Dosing of ARBs in Heart Failure[1]

ARB	Initial Dose	Maximum Dose
Candesartan	4-8 mg daily	32 mg daily
Losartan	25-50 mg daily	50-100 mg daily
Valsartan	20-40 mg bid	160 mg bid

[1]From ACC/AHA Guidelines.

Initial and Target Doses for Beta-Blocker Therapy in Heart Failure[1]

Beta-Blocker	Starting Dose	Target Dose	Comment
Bisoprolol	1.25 mg daily	10 mg daily	β_1-Selective blocker Inconvenient dosage forms for initial dose titration
Carvedilol	3.125 mg bid	25 mg bid (≤85 kg) 50 mg bid >85 kg)	β-Nonselective blocker α-Blocking properties
Metoprolol succinate, extended release	12.5-25 mg daily	200 mg daily	β_1-Selective blocker

[1]From ACC/AHA Guidelines.

References

Brater DC, "Diuretic Therapy," *N Engl J Med*, 1998, 339(6):387-95.

Granger CB, McMurray JJ, Yusuf S, et al, "Effects of Candesartan in Patients With Chronic Heart Failure and Reduced Left-Ventricular Systolic Function Intolerant to Angiotensin-Converting-Enzyme Inhibitors: The CHARM-Alternative Trial," *Lancet*, 2003, 362(9386):772-6.

HEART FAILURE (SYSTOLIC) *(Continued)*

Hunt SA, Abraham WT, Chin MH, et al, "ACC/AHA 2005 Guideline Update for the Diagnosis and Management of Chronic Heart Failure in the Adult. A Report of the American College of Cardiology/American Heart Association Task Force on Practice Guidelines (Writing Committee to Update the 2001 Guidelines for the Evaluation and Management of Heart Failure), *J Am Coll Cardiol*, 2005, 46(6):1116-43. Available online at www.acc.org.

McMurray JJ, Ostergren J, Swedberg K, et al, "Effects of Candesartan in Patients With Chronic Heart Failure and Reduced Left-Ventricular Systolic Function Taking Angiotensin-Converting-Enzyme Inhibitors: The CHARM-Added Trial," *Lancet*, 2003, 362(9386):767-71.

Taylor AL, Ziesche S, Yancy C, et al, "Combination of Isosorbide Dinitrate and Hydralazine in Blacks With Heart Failure," *N Engl J Med*, 2004, 351(20):2049-57.

HELICOBACTER PYLORI TREATMENT

Multiple Drug Regimens for the Treatment of *H. pylori* Infection

Drug	Dosages	Duration of Therapy
H_2-receptor antagonist[1]	Any one given at appropriate dose	4 weeks
plus Bismuth subsalicylate	525 mg 4 times/day	2 weeks
plus Metronidazole	250 mg 4 times/day	2 weeks
plus Tetracycline	500 mg 4 times/day	2 weeks
Proton pump inhibitor[1]	Esomeprazole 40 mg once daily	10 days
plus Clarithromycin	500 mg twice daily	10 days
plus Amoxicillin	1000 mg twice daily	10 days
Proton pump inhibitor[1]	Lansoprazole 30 mg twice daily or Omeprazole 20 mg twice daily	10-14 days
plus Clarithromycin	500 mg twice daily	10-14 days
plus Amoxicillin	1000 mg twice daily	10-14 days
Proton pump inhibitor[1]	Rabeprazole 20 mg twice daily	7 days
plus Clarithromycin	500 mg twice daily	7 days
plus Amoxicillin	1000 mg twice daily	7 days
Proton pump inhibitor	Lansoprazole 30 mg twice daily or Omeprazole 20 mg twice daily	2 weeks
plus Clarithromycin	500 mg twice daily	2 weeks
plus Metronidazole	500 mg twice daily	2 weeks
Proton pump inhibitor	Lansoprazole 30 mg once daily or Omeprazole 20 mg once daily	2 weeks
plus Bismuth	525 mg 4 times/day	2 weeks
plus Metronidazole	500 mg 3 times/day	2 weeks
plus Tetracycline	500 mg 4 times/day	2 weeks

[1]FDA-approved regimen.

Modified from Howden CS and Hunt RH, "Guidelines for the Management of *Helicobacter pylori* Infection," *AJG*, 1998, 93:2336.

HYPERLIPIDEMIA MANAGEMENT

MORTALITY

There is a strong link between serum cholesterol and cardiovascular mortality. This association becomes stronger in patients with established coronary artery disease. Lipid-lowering trials show that reductions in LDL cholesterol are followed by reductions in mortality. In general, each 1% fall in LDL cholesterol confers a 2% reduction in cardiovascular events. The aim of therapy for hyperlipidemia is to decrease cardiovascular morbidity and mortality by lowering cholesterol to a target level using safe and cost-effective treatment modalities. The target LDL cholesterol is determined by the number of patient risk factors (see the following Risk Factors and Goal LDL Cholesterol tables). The goal is achieved through diet, lifestyle modification, and drug therapy. The basis for these recommendations is provided by longitudinal interventional studies, demonstrating that lipid-lowering in patients with prior cardiovascular events (secondary prevention) and in patients with hyperlipidemia but no prior cardiac event (primary prevention) lowers the occurrence of future cardiovascular events, including stroke.

Major Risk Factors That Modify LDL Goals

Positive risk factors	Male ≥45 years
	Female ≥55 years
	Family history of premature coronary heart disease, defined as CHD in male first-degree relative <55 years; CHD in female first-degree relative <65 years
	Cigarette smoking
	Hypertension (blood pressure ≥140/90 mm Hg) or taking antihypertensive medication
	Low HDL (<40 mg/dL [1.03 mmol/L])
Negative risk factors	High HDL (≥60 mg/dL [1.6 mmol/L])[1]

[1]If HDL is ≥60 mg/dL, may subtract one positive risk factor.

Adult Treatment Panel (ATP) III LDL-C Goals and Cutpoints for Therapeutic Lifestyle Changes (TLC) and Drug Therapy in Different Risk Categories

Risk Category	LDL-C Goal	Initiate TLC	Consider Drug Therapy[1]
High risk: CHD[2] or CHD risk equivalents[3] (10-year risk >20%)	<100 mg/dL (optional goal: <70 mg/dL)[4]	≥100 mg/dL[5]	≥100 mg/dL[6] (<100 mg/dL: Consider drug options)[1]
Moderately high risk: 2+ risk factors[7] (10-year risk 10% to 20%)[8]	<130 mg/dL[9]	≥130 mg/dL[5]	≥130 mg/dL (100-120 mg/dL: Consider drug options)[10]
Moderate risk: 2+ risk factors[7] (10-year risk <10%)[8]	<130 mg/dL	≥130 mg/dL	≥160 mg/dL
Lower risk: 0-1 risk factor[11]	<160 mg/dL	≥160 mg/dL	≥190 mg/dL (160-189 mg/dL: LDL-lowering drug optional)

[1]When LDL-lowering drug therapy is employed, it is advised that intensity of therapy be sufficient to achieve at least a 30% to 40% reduction in LDL-C levels.

[2]CHD includes history of myocardial infarction, unstable angina, stable angina, coronary artery procedures (angioplasty or bypass surgery), or evidence of clinically significant myocardial ischemia.

[3]CHD risk equivalents include clinical manifestations of noncoronary forms of atherosclerotic disease (peripheral arterial disease, abdominal aortic aneurysm, and carotid artery disease [transient ischemic attacks or stroke of carotid origin or >50% obstruction of a carotid artery]), diabetes, and 2+ risk factors with 10-year risk for hard CHD >20%.

[4]Very high risk favors the optional LDL-C goal of <70 mg/dL, and in patients with high triglycerides, non-HDL-C <100 mg/dL.

[5]Any person at high risk or moderately high risk who has lifestyle-related risk factors (eg, obesity, physical inactivity, elevated triglyceride, low HDL-C, or metabolic syndrome) is a candidate for therapeutic lifestyle changes to modify these risk factors regardless of LDL-C level.

[6]If baseline LDL-C is <100 mg/dL, institution of an LDL-lowering drug is a therapeutic option on the basis of available clinical trial results. If a high-risk person has high triglycerides or low HDL-C, combining a fibrate or nicotinic acid with an LDL-lowering drug can be considered.

[7]Risk factors include cigarette smoking, hypertension (BP ≥140/90 mm Hg or on antihypertensive medication), low HDL cholesterol (<40 mg/dL), family history of premature CHD (CHD in male first-degree relative <55 years of age; CHD in female first-degree relative <65 years of age), and age (men ≥45 years; women ≥55 years).

[8]Electronic 10-year risk calculators are available at www.nhlbi.nih.gov/guidelines/cholesterol.

[9]Optional LDL-C goal <100 mg/dL.

[10]For moderately high-risk persons, when LDL-C level is 100-129 mg/dL, at baseline or on lifestyle therapy, initiation of an LDL-lowering drug to achieve an LDL-C level <100 mg/dL is a therapeutic option on the basis of available clinical trial results.

[11]Almost all people with zero or 1 risk factor have a 10-year risk <10%, and 10-year risk assessment in people with zero or 1 risk factor thus not necessary.

Any person with elevated LDL cholesterol or other form of hyperlipidemia should undergo evaluation to rule out secondary dyslipidemia. Causes of secondary dyslipidemia include diabetes, hypothyroidism, obstructive liver disease, chronic renal failure, and drugs that increase LDL and decrease HDL (progestins, anabolic steroids, corticosteroids).

Elevated Serum Triglyceride Levels

Elevated serum triglyceride levels may be an independent risk factor for coronary heart disease. Factors that contribute to hypertriglyceridemia include obesity, inactivity, cigarette smoking, excess alcohol intake, high carbohydrate diets (>60% of energy intake), type 2 diabetes, chronic renal failure, nephrotic syndrome, certain medications (corticosteroids, estrogens, retinoids, higher doses of beta-blockers), and genetic disorders. Non-HDL cholesterol (total cholesterol minus HDL cholesterol) is a secondary focus for clinicians treating patients with high serum triglyceride levels (≥200 mg/dL). The goal for non-HDL cholesterol in patients with high serum triglyceride levels can be set 30 mg/dL higher than usual LDL cholesterol goals. Patients with serum triglyceride levels <200 mg/dL should aim for the target LDL cholesterol goal.

ATP classification of serum triglyceride levels:

- Normal triglycerides: <150 mg/dL
- Borderline-high: 150-199 mg/dL
- High: 200-499 mg/dL
- Very high: ≥500 mg/dL

NONDRUG THERAPY

Dietary therapy and lifestyle modifications should be individualized for each patient. A total lifestyle change is recommended for all patients. Dietary and lifestyle modifications should be tried for 3 months, if deemed appropriate. Nondrug and drug therapy should be initiated simultaneously in patients with highly elevated cholesterol (see LDL Cholesterol Goals and Cutpoints for Therapeutic Lifestyle Changes and Drug Therapy in Different Risk Categories table). Increasing physical activity and smoking cessation will aid in the treatment of hyperlipidemia and improve cardiovascular health.

Note: Refer to the National Cholesterol Education Program reference for details concerning the calculation of 10-year risk of CHD using Framingham risk scoring. Risk assessment tool is available on-line at http://hin.nhlbi.nih.gov/atpiii/calculator.asp?usertype=prof, last accessed March 14, 2002.

Total Lifestyle Change (TLC) Diet

	Recommended Intake
Total fat	25%-35% of total calories
Saturated fat[1]	<7% of total calories
Polyunsaturated fat	≤10% of total calories
Monounsaturated fat	≤20% of total calories
Carbohydrates[2]	50%-60% of total calories
Fiber	20-30 g/day
Protein	~15% of total calories
Cholesterol	<200 mg/day

HYPERLIPIDEMIA MANAGEMENT *(Continued)*

Total Lifestyle Change (TLC) Diet *(continued)*

	Recommended Intake
Total calories[3]	Balance energy intake and expenditure to maintain desirable body weight/prevent weight gain

[1]*Trans* fatty acids (partially hydrogenated oils) intake should be kept low. These are found in potato chips, other snack foods, margarines and shortenings, and fast-foods.

[2]Complex carbohydrates including grains (especially whole grains, fruits, and vegetables).

[3]Daily energy expenditure should include at least moderate physical activity.

DRUG THERAPY

Drug therapy should be selected based on the patient's lipid profile, concomitant disease states, and the cost of therapy. The following table lists specific advantages and disadvantages for various classes of lipid-lowering medications. The expected reduction in lipids with therapy is listed in the Lipid-Lowering Agents table. Refer to individual drug monographs for detailed information.

Advantages and Disadvantages of Specific Lipid-Lowering Therapies

	Advantages	Disadvantages
Bile acid sequestrants	Good choice for ↑ LDL, especially when combined with a statin (↓ LDL ≤50%); low potential for systemic side effects; good choice for younger patients	May increase triglycerides; higher incidence of adverse effects; moderately expensive; drug interactions; inconvenient dosing
Niacin	Good choice for almost any lipid abnormality; inexpensive; greatest increase in HDL	High incidence of adverse effects; may adversely affect NIDDM and gout; sustained release niacin may decrease the incidence of flushing and circumvent the need for multiple daily dosing; sustained release niacin may not increase HDL cholesterol or decrease triglycerides as well as immediate release niacin
HMG-CoA reductase inhibitors	Produces greatest ↓ in LDL; generally well-tolerated; convenient once-daily dosing; proven decrease in mortality	Expensive
Gemfibrozil	Good choice in patients with ↑ triglycerides where niacin is contraindicated or not well-tolerated; gemfibrozil is well tolerated	Variable effects on LDL
Ezetimibe	Additional cholesterol-lowering effects when combined with HMG-CoA reductase inhibitors	Effects similar to bile acid sequestrants

Lipid-Lowering Agents

Drug	Dose / Day	Effect on LDL (%)	Effect on HDL (%)	Effect on TG (%)
HMG-CoA Reductase Inhibitors				
Atorvastatin	10 mg	-39	+6	-19
	20 mg	-43	+9	-26
	40 mg	-50	+6	-29
	80 mg	-60	+5	-37
Fluvastatin	20 mg	-22	+3	-12
	40 mg	-25	+4	-14
	80 mg	-36	+6	-18
Lovastatin	10 mg	-21	+5	-10
	20 mg	-27	+6	-8
	40 mg	-31	+5	-8
	80 mg	-40	+9.5	-19

Lipid-Lowering Agents *(continued)*

Drug	Dose / Day	Effect on LDL (%)	Effect on HDL (%)	Effect on TG (%)
Pravastatin	10 mg 20 mg 40 mg 80 mg	-22 -32 -34 -37	+7 +2 +12 +3	-15 -11 -24 -19
Rosuvastatin	5 mg 10 mg 20 mg 40 mg	-45 -52 -55 -63	+13 +14 +8 +10	-35 -10 -23 -28
Simvastatin	5 mg 10 mg 20 mg 40 mg 80 mg	-26 -30 -38 -41 -47	+10 +12 +8 +13 +16	-12 -15 -19 -28 -33
Bile Acid Sequestrants				
Cholestyramine	4-24 g	-15 to -30	+3 to +5	+0 to +20
Colestipol	7-30 g	-15 to -30	+3 to +5	+0 to +20
Colesevelam	6 tablets 7 tablets	-15 -18	+3 +3	+10 +9
Fibric Acid Derivatives				
Fenofibrate	67-200 mg	-20 to -25	+1 to -34	-30 to -50
Gemfibrozil	600 mg twice daily	-5 to -10[1]	+10 to +20	-40 to -60
Niacin	1.5-6 g	-21 to -27	+10 to +35	-10 to -50
2-Azetidinone				
Ezetimibe	10 mg	-18	+1	-8
Omega-3-Acid Ethyl Esters	4 g	+44.5	+9.1	-44.9
Combination Products				
Ezetimibe and simvastatin	10/10 mg 10/20 mg 10/40 mg 10/80 mg	-45 -52 -55 -60	+8 +10 +6 +6	-23 -24 -23 -31
Niacin and lovastatin	1000/20 mg 1000/40 mg 1500/40 mg 2000/40 mg	-30 -36 -37 -42	+20 +20 +27 +30	-32 -39 -44 -44

[1]May increase LDL in some patients.

Recommended Liver Function Monitoring for HMG-CoA Reductase Inhibitors

Agent	Initial and After Elevation in Dose	6 Weeks[1]	12 Weeks[1]	Periodically
Atorvastatin (Lipitor®)	x		x	x
Fluvastatin (Lescol®)	x		x	x
Lovastatin (Mevacor®)	x	x	x	x
Pravastatin (Pravachol®)	x			x
Simvastatin (Zocor®)	x			x

[1]After initiation of therapy or any elevation in dose.

DRUG SELECTION

Lipid Profile	Monotherapy	Combination Therapies
Increased LDL with normal HDL and triglycerides (TG)	Resin Niacin[1] Statin	Resin plus niacin[1] or statin Statin plus niacin[1,2]
Increased LDL and increased TG (200-499 mg/dL)[2]	Intensify LDL-lowering therapy	Statin plus niacin[1,3] Statin plus fibrate[3]
Increased LDL and increased TG (≥500 mg/dL)[2]	Consider combination therapy (niacin,[1] fibrates, statin)	
Increased TG	Niacin[1] Fibrates	Niacin[1] plus fibrates

HYPERLIPIDEMIA MANAGEMENT *(Continued)*

(continued)

Lipid Profile	Monotherapy	Combination Therapies
Increased LDL and low HDL	Niacin[1] Statin	Statin plus niacin[1,2]

[1]Avoid in diabetics.

[2]Emphasize weight reduction and increased physical activity.

[3]Risk of myopathy with combination.

Resins = bile acid sequestrants; statins = HMG-CoA reductase inhibitors; fibrates = fibric acid derivatives (eg, gemfibrozil, fenofibrate).

Progression of Drug Therapy in Primary Prevention

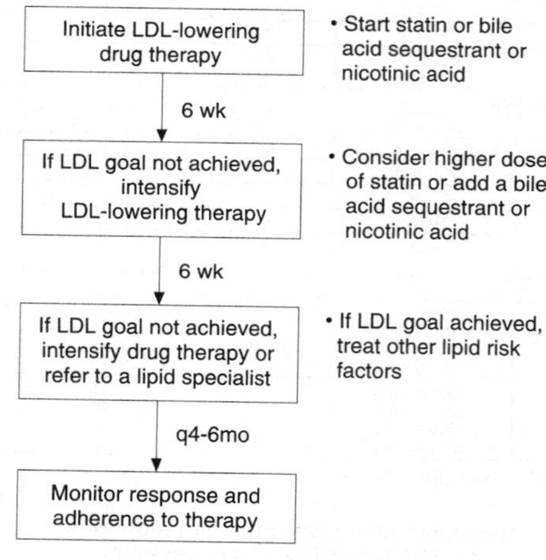

COMBINATION DRUG THERAPY

If after at least 6 weeks of therapy at the maximum recommended or tolerated dose, the patient's LDL cholesterol is not at target, consider optimizing nondrug measures, prescribing a higher dose of current lipid-lowering drug, or adding another lipid-lowering medication to the current therapy. Successful drug combinations include statin and niacin, statin and bile acid sequestrant, or niacin and bile acid sequestrant. At maximum recommended doses, LDL cholesterol may be decreased by 50% to 60% with combination therapy. This is the same reduction achieved by atorvastatin 40 mg twice daily. If a bile acid sequestrant is used with other lipid-lowering agents, space doses 1 hour before or 4 hours after the bile acid sequestrant administration. Statins combined with either fenofibrate, clofibrate, gemfibrozil, or niacin increase the risk of rhabdomyolysis. In this situation, patient education (muscle pain/weakness) and careful follow-up are warranted.

References

Guidelines

Gavin JR, Alberti KGMM, Davidson MB, et al, for the Members of the Expert Committee on the Diagnosis and Classification of Diabetes Mellitus, "American Diabetes Association: Clinical Practice Recommendations," *Diabetes Care*, 1999, 22(Suppl 1):S1-S114.

National Cholesterol Education Program, "Third Report of the Expert Panel on Detection, Evaluation, and Treatment of High Blood Cholesterol in Adults (Adult Treatment Panel III)," *JAMA*, 2001, 285:2486-97.

Grundy SM, Cleeman JI, Merz CN, et al, "Implications of Recent Clinical Trials for the National Cholesterol Education Program Adult Treatment Panel III Guidelines," *JACC*, 2004, 44(3):729.

Mosca L, Appel LJ, Benjamin EJ, et al, "Evidence-Based Guidelines for Cardiovascular Disease Prevention in Women," *J Am Coll Cardiol*, 2004, 43(5):900-21.

Others

Berthold HK, Sudhop T, and von Bergmann K, "Effect of a Garlic Oil Preparation on Serum Lipoproteins and Cholesterol Metabolism: A Randomized Controlled Trial," *JAMA*, 1998, 279:1900-2.

Bertolini S, Bon GB, Campbell LM, et al, "Efficacy and Safety of Atorvastatin Compared to Pravastatin in Patients With Hypercholesterolemia," *Atherosclerosis*, 1997, 130:191-7.

Blankenhorn DH, Nessim SA, Johnson RL, et al, "Beneficial Effects of Combined Colestipol-Niacin Therapy on Coronary Atherosclerosis and Venous Bypass Grafts," *JAMA*, 1987, 257:3233-40.

Brown G, Albers JJ, Fisher LD, et al, "Regression of Coronary Artery Disease as a Result of Intensive Lipid-Lowering Therapy in Men With High Levels of Apolipoprotein B," *N Engl J Med*, 1990, 323:1289-98.

Capuzzi DM, Guyton JR, Morgan JM, et al, "Efficacy and Safety of an Extended-Release Niacin (Niaspan®): A Long-Term Study," *Am J Cardiol*, 1998, 82:74U-81U.

Coronary Drug Project Research Program, "Clofibrate and Niacin in Coronary Heart Disease," *JAMA*, 1975, 231:360-81.

Dart A, Jerums G, Nicholson G, et al, "A Multicenter, Double-Blind, One-Year Study Comparing Safety and Efficacy of Atorvastatin Versus Simvastatin in Patients With Hypercholesterolemia," *Am J Cardiol*, 1997, 80:39-44.

Davidson MH, Dillon MA, Gordon B, et al, "Colesevelam Hydrochloride (Cholestagel): A New Potent Bile Acid Sequestrant Associated With a Low Incidence of Gastrointestinal Side Effects," *Arch Intern Med*, 1999, 159(16):1893-900.

Davidson M, McKenney J, Stein E, et al, "Comparison of One-Year Efficacy and Safety of Atorvastatin Versus Lovastatin in Primary Hypercholesterolemia," *Am J Cardiol*, 1997, 79:1475-81.

Frick MH, Heinonen OP, Huttunen JK, et al, "Helsinki Heart Study: Primary-Prevention Trial With Gemfibrozil in Middle-Aged Men With Dyslipidemia," *N Engl J Med*, 1987, 317:1237-45.

Garber AM, Browner WS, and Hulley SB, "Clinical Guideline, Part 2: Cholesterol Screening in Asymptomatic Adults, Revisited," *Ann Intern Med*, 1995, 124:518-31.

Johannesson M, Jonsson B, Kjekshus J, et al, "Cost-Effectiveness of Simvastatin Treatment to Lower Cholesterol Levels in Patients With Coronary Heart Disease. Scandinavian Simvastatin Survival Study Group," *N Engl N Med*, 1997, 336:332-6.

Jones P, Kafonek S, Laurora I, et al, "Comparative Dose Efficacy Study of Atorvastatin Versus Simvastatin, Pravastatin, Lovastatin, and Fluvastatin in Patients With Hypercholesterolemia," *Am J Cardiol*, 1998, 81:582-7.

Kasiske BL, Ma JZ, Kalil RS, et al, "Effects of Antihypertensive Therapy on Serum Lipids," *Ann Intern Med*, 1995, 133-41.

Lipid Research Clinics Program, "The Lipid Research Clinics Coronary Primary Prevention Trial Results: I. Reduction in Incidence of Coronary Heart Disease," *JAMA*, 1984, 251:351-64.

Mauro VF and Tuckerman CE, "Ezetimibe for Management of Hypercholesterolemia," *Ann Pharmacother*, 2003, 37(6):839-48.

Multiple Risk Factor Intervention Trial Research Group, "Multiple Risk Factor Intervention Trial: Risk Factor Changes and Mortality Results," *JAMA*, 1982, 248:1465-77.

Pitt B, Waters D, Brown WV, et al, "Aggressive Lipid-Lowering Therapy Compared With Angioplasty in Stable Coronary Artery Disease. Atorvastatin Versus Revascularization Treatment Investigators," *N Engl J Med*, 1999, 341(2):70-6.

Ross SD, Allen IE, Connelly JE, et al, "Clinical Outcomes in Statin Treatment Trials: A Meta-Analysis," *Arch Intern Med*, 1999, 159:1793-802.

Sacks FM, Pfeffer MA, Moye LA, et al, "The Effect of Pravastatin on Coronary Events After Myocardial Infarction in Patients With Average Cholesterol Levels," *N Engl J Med*, 1996, 335:1001-9.

Scandinavian Simvastatin Survival Study, "Randomized Trial of Cholesterol Lowering in 4444 Patients With Coronary Heart Disease: The Scandinavian Simvastatin Survival Study (4S)," *Lancet*, 1994, 344:1383-9.

Schrott HG, Bittner V, Vittinghoff E, et al, "Adherence to National Cholesterol Education Program Treatment Goals in Postmenopausal Women With Heart Disease. The Heart and Estrogen/Progestin Replacement Study (HERS)," *JAMA*, 1997, 277:1281-6.

Shepherd J, Cobbe SM, Ford I, et al, "Prevention of Coronary Heart Disease With Pravastatin in Men With Hypercholesterolemia, The West of Scotland Coronary Prevention Study Group," *N Engl J Med*, 1995, 333:1301-7.

Stein EA, Davidson MH, Dobs AS, et al, "Efficacy and Safety of Simvastatin 80 mg/day in Hypercholesterolemic Patients. The Expanded Dose Simvastatin U.S. Study Group," *Am J Cardiol*, 1998, 82:311-6.

HYPERTENSION

The optimal blood pressure for adults is <120/80 mm Hg. Consistent systolic pressure ≥140 mm Hg or a diastolic pressure ≥90 mm Hg, in the absence of a secondary cause, defines hypertension. Hypertension affects approximately 25% (50 million people) in the United States. Of those patients on antihypertensive medication, only one in three have their blood pressure controlled (<140/90 mm Hg).

Controlling systolic hypertension has been much more difficult than controlling diastolic hypertension. Educating patients in lifestyle management, cardiovascular risk reduction, and drug therapy aids in improving the morbidity and mortality of patients with hypertension.

The Seventh Report of the Joint National Committee (JNC VII) is an excellent reference and guide for the treatment of hypertension (Chobanian AV, Bakris GL, Black HR, et al, "The Seventh Report of the Joint National Committee on Prevention, Detection, Evaluation, and Treatment of High Blood Pressure: The JNC 7 Report," *JAMA*, 2003, 289(19):2560-71). For adults, hypertension is classified in stages (see following table).

Adult Classification of Blood Pressure

Category	Systolic (mm Hg)		Diastolic (mm Hg)
Normal	<120	and	<80
Prehypertension	120-139	or	80-89
Hypertension			
Stage 1	140-159	or	90-99
Stage 2	≥160	or	≥100

Adapted from Chobanian AV, Bakris GL, Black HR, et al, "The Seventh Report of the Joint National Committee on Prevention, Detection, Evaluation, and Treatment of High Blood Pressure: The JNC 7 Report," *JAMA*, 2003, 289(19):2560-71.

Normal Blood Pressure in Children

Age (y)	Girls' SBP / DBP (mm Hg)		Boys' SBP / DBP (mm Hg)	
	50th Percentile for Height	75th Percentile for Height	50th Percentile for Height	75th Percentile for Height
1	104/58	105/59	102/57	104/58
6	111/73	112/73	114/74	115/75
12	123/80	124/81	123/81	125/82
17	129/84	130/85	136/87	138/88

SBP = systolic blood pressure.

DBP = diastolic blood pressure.

Adapted from the report by the NHBPEP Working Group on Hypertension Control in Children and Adolescents, *Pediatrics*, 1996, 98(4 Pt 1):649-58.

PATIENT ASSESSMENT

- **Cardiovascular Risk Factors:** Hypertension, cigarette smoking, obesity (BMI ≥30), inactive lifestyle, dyslipidemia, diabetes mellitus, microalbuminuria or estimated GFR <60 mL/minute, age (>55 years for men, >65 years for women), family history of premature cardiovascular disease (men <55 years or women >65 years).

  Components of metabolic syndrome include hypertension, obesity, dyslipidemia, diabetes mellitus.

- Identify causes of high BP.
- Assess target-organ damage and CVD.

Target-Organ Disease

Organ System	Manifestation
Cardiac	Clinical, ECG, or radiologic evidence of coronary artery disease; prior MI, angina, post-CABG; left ventricular hypertrophy (LVH); left ventricular dysfunction or cardiac failure, prior coronary revascularization
Cerebrovascular	Transient ischemic attack or stroke
Peripheral vascular	Absence of pulses in extremities (except dorsalis pedis), claudication, aneurysm, peripheral arterial disease
Renal	Serum creatinine ≥130 μmol/L (1.5 mg/dL); proteinuria (≥1+); microalbuminuria, chronic kidney disease
Eye	Hemorrhages or exudates, with or without papilledema; retinopathy

Adapted from Chobanian AV, Bakris GL, Black HR, et al, "The Seventh Report of the Joint National Committee on Prevention, Detection, Evaluation, and Treatment of High Blood Pressure: The JNC 7 Report," *JAMA*, 2003, 289(19):2560-71.

BLOOD PRESSURE MEASUREMENT

At an office visit, patients should be seated quietly for ≥5 minutes in a chair with feet on the floor and arm supported at heart level. At least two measurements should be made. Patients should be given their results and their goal BP.

Ambulatory BP monitoring is useful in evaluating "white coat hypertension" (no end-organ damage), drug resistance, hypotensive symptoms, episodic hypertension, and autonomic dysfunction. Ambulatory BP monitoring correlates better with end-organ damage than office measurements.

Having patients monitor their own BP helps to improve compliance and provides information on response to therapeutic interventions.

Based on these initial assessments, treatment strategies for patients with hypertension are stratified based on their blood pressure and comorbidities (compelling indications).

Management of Blood Pressure

	Management: Based upon highest BP category		
BP Classification	**Lifestyle Modification**	**Initial Therapy Without Compelling Indication**	**Initial Therapy With Compelling Indication[1]**
Normal	Encourage	None	None
Prehypertensive	Yes	None	Treat patients with chronic kidney disease or diabetes to BP goal of <130/80 mm Hg
Hypertension Stage 1	Yes	Thiazide-type diuretic for most; consider ACEI, ARB, β-blocker, CCB, or combination	Drugs for the compelling indications; other antihypertensives as needed
Hypertension Stage 2	Yes	Two drug combos (typically a thiazide-type diuretic and ACEI or ARB or β-blocker or CCB). Use combo cautiously in patients at risk for orthostasis.	Drugs for the compelling indications; other antihypertensives as needed

[1]Compelling Indication: Conditions for which specific classes of antihypertensive drugs have proven beneficial.

Adapted from Chobanian AV, Bakris GL, Black HR, et al, "The Seventh Report of the Joint National Committee on Prevention, Detection, Evaluation, and Treatment of High Blood Pressure: The JNC 7 Report," *JAMA*, 2003, 289(19):2560-71.

HYPERTENSION *(Continued)*

ACHIEVING BLOOD PRESSURE CONTROL

Treatment of hypertension should be individualized. Lower blood pressure (goal <130/80 mm Hg) should be achieved in patients with diabetes or chronic renal disease. The following Hypertension Treatment Algorithm may be used to select specific antihypertensives based on compelling indications.

Special consideration for starting combination therapy should be made in each patient.

Starting drug therapy at a low dose and titrating upward if blood pressure is not controlled is recommended.

Most patients with hypertension will require two or more drugs to achieve their BP goals.

Adding a second drug from a different class will help when a single drug at reasonable doses has failed to achieve the goal.

If the untreated BP is >20/10 mm Hg away from the goal, consider initiating therapy with two drugs. Use caution in those at risk for orthostasis (eg, diabetics, geriatrics, and those with autonomic dysfunction).

Low-dose aspirin therapy should be considered when BP is controlled; use in uncontrolled hypertension can increase the risk of hemorrhagic stroke.

Lifestyle modification and risk reduction should always be reviewed and reinforced.

MONITORING THERAPY

Generally, monthly follow-up is recommended until BP control is reached.

More frequent monitoring is required for those patients with Stage 2 hypertension or those with complications.

Serum potassium and serum creatinine should be monitored at least twice yearly.

When BP is at goal and stable, follow-up can be maintained every 3-6 months. Treat other cardiovascular risk factors if present.

Hypertension Treatment Algorithm

Begin or continue lifestyle modifications

↓

Not at goal blood pressure (<140/90 mm Hg or <130/80 mm Hg for patients with diabetes or chronic renal disease)

↓

Initial Drug Choice

Hypertension

Stage I
Thiazide-type diuretic for most. Consider ACEI, ARB, β-blocker, CCB, or combo.

Stage 2
Two-drug combo for most (typically thiazide-type diuretic + ACEI or ARB or β-blocker or CCB)

Compelling Indications

Chronic kidney disease
- ACEI
- ARB

Diabetes mellitus
- ACEI
- ARB
- β-blocker
- CCB
- Diuretic

Heart failure
- ACEI
- Aldosterone blocker
- ARB
- β-blocker
- Diuretic

High coronary risk
- ACEI
- β-blocker
- CCB
- Diuretic

Myocardial infarction
- ACEI
- Aldosterone blocker
- β-blocker

Recurrent stroke prevention
- ACEI
- Diuretic

↓

Not at goal blood pressure

↓ Optimize dosages or add additional drugs until goal BP achieved.

↓ Consider consultation with hypertension specialist.

HYPERTENSION *(Continued)*

Additional Considerations for Specific Therapies

Indication	Drug Therapy
Atrial tachyarrhythmias	β-blocker, CCB (non-DHP)
Chronic kidney disease	
Cl_{cr} <60 mL/min or albuminuria	ACEI or ARB
Cl_{cr} <30 mL/min	Increase loop diuretic
Diabetes	Thiazide diuretic, β-blocker, ACEI, ARB, CCB
Nephropathy	ACEI, ARB
Essential tremor	β-blocker (noncardioselective)
Heart failure	
Ventricular dysfunction (asymptomatic)	ACEI, β-blocker
Ventricular dysfunction (symptomatic)	ACEI, β-blocker, ARB, aldosterone blocker, loop diuretic
Hypertensive women who are pregnant	Methyldopa, β-blocker, vasodilator
Ischemic heart disease	
Angina	β-blocker, CCB (long-acting)
Acute coronary syndromes	β-blocker, ACEI
Migraine	β-blocker (noncardioselective), CCB (long-acting, non-DHP)
Osteoporosis	Thiazide diuretic
Perioperative hypertension	β-blocker
Prostatism (BPH)	Alpha-adrenergic blocking agent
Raynaud syndrome	CCB
Thyrotoxicosis	β-blocker

Note: ACEI = angiotensin-converting enzyme inhibitor; ARB = angiotensin receptor blocker; CCB = calcium channel blocker; DHP = dihydropyridine.

May Have Unfavorable Effects on Comorbid Conditions

Condition	Drug Therapy to Avoid
Angioedema	ACEI
Bronchospastic disease	β-blocker
Gout	Thiazide diuretic
Heart block (second or third degree)	β-blocker, CCB (non-DHP)
Hyponatremia	Thiazide diuretic
Potassium >5 mEq/L before treatment	Potassium-sparing diuretic, aldosterone antagonist
Pregnancy or those likely to become pregnant	ACEI, ARB

Note: ACEI = angiotensin-converting enzyme inhibitor; ARB = angiotensin receptor blocker; CCB = calcium channel blocker; DHP = dihydropyridine.

HYPERTENSIVE EMERGENCIES AND URGENCIES

General Treatment Principles in the Treatment of Hypertensive Emergencies

Principle	Considerations
Admit the patient to the hospital, preferably in the ICU. Monitor vital signs appropriately.	Establish I.V. access and place patient on a cardiac monitor. Place a femoral intra-arterial line and pulmonary arterial catheter, if indicated, to assess cardiopulmonary function and intravascular volume status.
Perform rapid but thorough history and physical examination.	Determine cause of, or precipitating factors to, hypertensive crisis if possible (remember to obtain a medication history including Rx, OTC, and illicit drugs). Obtain details regarding any prior history of hypertension (severity, duration, treatment), as well as other coexisting illnesses. Assess the extent of hypertensive end organ damage. Determine if a hypertensive urgency or emergency exists.
Determine goal blood pressure based on premorbid level, duration, severity and rapidity of increase of blood pressure, concomitant medical conditions, race, and age.	Acute decreases in blood pressure to normal or subnormal levels during the initial treatment period may reduce perfusion to the brain, heart, and kidneys, and must be avoided except in specific instances (ie, dissecting aortic aneurysm). Gradually establish a normal (or reasonable) blood pressure over the next 1-2 weeks.
Select an appropriate antihypertensive regimen depending on the individual patient and clinical setting.	Initiate a controlled decrease in blood pressure. Avoid concomitant administration of multiple agents that may cause precipitous falls in blood pressure. Select the agent with the best hemodynamic profile based on the primary treatment goal. Avoid diuretics and sodium restriction during the initial treatment period unless there is a clear clinical indication (ie, CHF, pulmonary edema). Avoid sedating antihypertensives in patients with hypertensive encephalopathy, CVA, or other CNS disorders in whom mental status must be monitored. Use caution with direct vasodilating agents that induce reflex tachycardia or increase cardiac output in patients with coronary heart disease, history of angina or myocardial infarction, or dissecting aortic aneurysm. Preferably choose an agent that does not adversely affect glomerular filtration rate or renal blood flow and also agents that have favorable effects on cerebral blood flow and its autoregulation, especially for patients with hypertensive encephalopathy or CVAs. Select the most efficacious agent with the fewest adverse effects based on the underlying cause of the hypertensive crisis and other individual patient factors.
Initiate a chronic antihypertensive regimen after the patient's blood pressure is stabilized	Begin oral antihypertensive therapy once goal blood pressure is achieved before gradually tapering parenteral medications. Select the best oral regimen based on cost, ease of administration, adverse effect profile, and concomitant medical conditions.

Oral Agents Used in the Treatment of Hypertensive Urgencies

Drug	Dose	Onset	Cautions
Captopril[1]	P.O.: 25 mg, repeat as required	15-30 min	Hypotension, renal failure in bilateral renal artery stenosis
Clonidine	P.O.: 0.1-0.2 mg, repeated every hour as needed to a total dose of 0.6 mg	30-60 min	Hypotension, drowsiness, dry mouth
Labetalol	P.O.: 200-400 mg, repeat every 2-3 h	30 min to 2 h	Bronchoconstriction, heart block, orthostatic hypotension

[1]There is no clearly defined clinical advantage in the use of sublingual over oral routes of administration with these agents.

HYPERTENSION *(Continued)*

Recommendations for the Use of Intravenous Antihypertensive Drugs in Selected Hypertensive Emergencies

Condition	Agent(s) of Choice	Agent(s) to Avoid or Use With Caution	General Treatment Principles
Hypertensive encephalopathy	Nitroprusside, labetalol, diazoxide	Methyldopa, reserpine	Avoid drugs with CNS-sedating effects.
Acute intracranial or subarachnoid hemorrhage	Nicardipine,[1] nitroprusside	β-blocker	Careful titration with a short-acting agent.
Cerebral infarction	Nicardipine,[1] nitroprusside, labetalol	β-blocker, minoxidil, diazoxide	Careful titration with a short-acting agent. Avoid agents that may decrease cerebral blood flow.
Head trauma	Esmolol, labetalol	Methyldopa, reserpine, nitroprusside, nitroglycerin, hydralazine	Avoid drugs with CNS-sedating effects, or those that may increase intracranial pressure.
Acute myocardial infarction, myocardial ischemia	Nitroglycerin, nicardipine[1] (calcium channel blocker), labetalol	Hydralazine, diazoxide, minoxidil	Avoid drugs which cause reflex tachycardia and increased myocardial oxygen consumption.
Acute pulmonary edema	Nitroprusside, nitroglycerin, loop diuretics	β-blocker (labetalol), minoxidil, methyldopa	Avoid drugs which may cause sodium and water retention and edema exacerbation.
Renal dysfunction	Hydralazine, calcium channel blocker	Nitroprusside, ACE inhibitors, β-blocker (labetalol)	Avoid drugs with increased toxicity in renal failure and those that may cause decreased renal blood flow.
Eclampsia	Hydralazine, labetalol, nitroprusside[2]	Diuretics, diazoxide (diazoxide may cause cessation of labor)	Avoid drugs that may cause adverse fetal effects, compromise placental circulation, or decrease cardiac output.
Pheochromocytoma	Phentolamine, nitroprusside, β-blocker (eg, esmolol) only after alpha blockade (phentolamine)	β-blocker in the absence of alpha blockade, methyldopa, minoxidil	Use drugs of proven efficacy and specificity. Unopposed beta blockade may exacerbate hypertension.
Dissecting aortic aneurysm	Nitroprusside and beta blockade	Hydralazine, diazoxide, minoxidil	Avoid drugs which may increase cardiac output.
Postoperative hypertension	Nitroprusside, nicardipine,[1] labetalol		Avoid drugs which may exacerbate postoperative ileus.

[1]The use of nicardipine in these situations is by the recommendation of the author based on a review of the literature.

[2]Reserve nitroprusside for eclamptic patients with life-threatening hypertension unresponsive to other agents due to the potential risk to the fetus (cyanide and thiocyanate metabolites may cross the placenta).

Selected Intravenous Agents for Hypertensive Emergencies

Drug	Dose[1]	Onset of Action	Duration of Action	Adverse Effects[2]	Special Indications
Vasodilators					
Sodium nitroprusside	0.25-10 mcg/kg/min as I.V. infusion[3] (max: 10 min only)	Immediate	1-2 min	Nausea, vomiting, muscle twitching, sweating, thiocyanate and cyanide intoxication	Most hypertensive emergencies; caution with high intracranial pressure or azotemia
Nicardipine hydrochloride	5-15 mg/h I.V.	5-10 min	1-4 h	Tachycardia, headache, flushing, local phlebitis	Most hypertensive emergencies except acute heart failure; caution with coronary ischemia
Fenoldopam mesylate	0.1-0.3 mcg/kg/min as I.V. infusion	<5 min	30 min	Tachycardia, headache, nausea, flushing	Most hypertensive emergencies; caution with glaucoma
Nitroglycerin	5-100 mcg/min as I.V. infusion[3]	2-5 min	3-5 min	Headache, vomiting, methemoglobinemia, tolerance with prolonged use	Coronary ischemia
Enalaprilat	1.25-5 mg every 6 hours I.V.	15-30 min	6 h	Precipitous fall in pressure in high-renin states; response variable	Acute left ventricular failure; avoid in acute myocardial infarction
Hydralazine hydrochloride	10-20 mg I.V. 10-50 mg I.M.	10-20 min 20-30 min	3-8 h	Tachycardia, flushing, headache, vomiting, aggravation of angina	Eclampsia
Diazoxide	50-100 mg I.V. bolus repeated, or 15-30 mg/min infusion	2-4 min	6-12 h	Nausea, flushing, tachycardia, chest pain	Now obsolete; when no intensive monitoring available
Adrenergic Inhibitors					
Labetalol hydrochloride	20-80 mg I.V. bolus every 10 min; 0.5-2 mg/min as I.V. infusion	5-10 min	3-6 h	Vomiting, scalp tingling, burning in throat, dizziness, nausea, heart block, orthostatic hypotension	Most hypertensive emergencies except acute heart failure
Esmolol hydrochloride	250-500 mcg/kg/min for 1 min, then 50-100 mcg/kg/min for 4 min; may repeat	1-2 min	10-20 min	Hypotension, nausea	Aortic dissection, perioperative
Phentolamine	5-15 mg I.V.	1-2 min	3-10 min	Tachycardia, flushing, headache	Catecholamine excess

[1]These doses may vary from those in the *Physicians' Desk Reference* (51st edition).

[2]Hypotension may occur with all agents.

[3]Require special delivery system.

HYPERTENSION *(Continued)*

References

Guidelines

1999 World Health Organization-International Society of Hypertension Guidelines for the Management of Hypertension. Guidelines Subcommittee, *J Hypertens*, 1999, 17:151-83.

Chobanian AV, Bakris GL, Black HR, et al, "The Seventh Report of the Joint National Committee on Prevention, Detection, Evaluation, and Treatment of High Blood Pressure: The JNC 7 Report," *JAMA*, 2003, 289(19):2560-71.

National High Blood Pressure Education Program Working Group on Hypertension Control in Children and Adolescents. Update on the 1987 Task Force Report on High Blood Pressure in Children and Adolescents: A Working Group Report From the National High Blood Pressure Education Program, *Pediatrics*, 1996, 98(4 Pt 1):649-58.

National High Blood Pressure Education Program Working Group. 1995 Update of the Working Group Reports on Chronic Renal Failure and Renovascular Hypertension, *Arch Intern Med*, 1996, 156:1938-47.

"The Sixth Report of the National Committee on Detection, Evaluation, and Treatment of High Blood Pressure (JNC-VI)," *Arch Intern Med*, 1997, 157:2413-46.

Others

Appel LJ, Moore TJ, Obarzanek E, et al, "A Clinical Trial of the Effect of Dietary Patterns on Blood Pressure. The DASH Collaborative Research Group," *N Engl J Med*, 1997, 336:1117-24.

Epstein M and Bakris G, "Newer Approaches to Antihypertensive Therapy: Use of Fixed-Dose Combination Therapy," *Arch Intern Med*, 1996, 156:1969-78.

Estacio RO and Schrier RW, "Antihypertensive Therapy in Type II Diabetes: Implications of the Appropriate Blood Pressure Control in Diabetes (ABCD) Trial," *Am J Cardiol*, 1998, 82:9R-14R.

Flack JM, Neaton J, Grimm RJ, et al, "Blood Pressure and Mortality Among Men With Prior Myocardial Infarction. The Multiple Risk Factor Intervention Trial Research Group," *Circulation*, 1995, 92:2437-45.

Frishman WH, Bryzinski BS, Coulson LR, et al, "A Multifactorial Trial Design to Assess Combination Therapy in Hypertension: Treatment With Bisoprolol and Hydrochlorothiazide," *Arch Intern Med*, 1994, 154:1461-8.

Furberg CD, Psaty BM, and Meyer JV, "Nifedipine: Dose-Related Increase in Mortality in Patients With Coronary Heart Disease," *Circulation*, 1995, 92:1326-31.

Glynn RJ, Brock DB, Harris T, et al, "Use of Antihypertensive Drugs and Trends in Blood Pressure in the Elderly," *Arch Intern Med*, 1995, 155:1855-60.

Gradman AH, Cutler NR, Davis PJ, et al, "Combined Enalapril and Felodipine Extended Release (ER) for Systemic Hypertension. The Enalapril-Felodipine ER Factorial Study Group," *Am J Cardiol*, 1997, 79:431-5.

Grim RH Jr, Flack JM, Grandits GA, et al, "Long-Term Effects on Plasma Lipids of Diet and Drugs to Treat Hypertension. The Treatment of Mild Hypertension Study (TOMHS) Research Group," *JAMA*, 1996, 275:1549-56.

Grim RH Jr, Grandits GA, Cutler JA, et al, "Relationships of Quality-of-Life Measures to Long-Term Lifestyle and Drug Treatment in the Treatment of Mild Hypertension Study. The TOMHS Research Group," *Arch Intern Med*, 1997, 157:638-48.

Grossman E, Messerli FH, Grodzicki T, et al, "Should a Moratorium Be Placed on Sublingual Nifedipine Capsules Given for Hypertensive Emergencies and Pseudoemergencies?" *JAMA*, 1996, 276:1328-31.

Hansson L, Zanchetti A, Carruthers SG, et al, "Effects of Intensive Blood Pressure Lowering and Low-Dose Aspirin in Patients With Hypertension: Principal Results of the Hypertension Optimal Treatment (HOT) Randomized Trial. HOT Study Group," *Lancet*, 1998, 351:1755-62.

Kaplan NM and Gifford RW Jr, "Choice of Initial Therapy for Hypertension," *JAMA*, 1996, 275:1577-80.

Kasiske BL, Ma JZ, Kalil RSN, et al, "Effects of Antihypertensive Therapy in Serum Lipids," *Ann Intern Med*, 1995, 122:133-41.

Kostis JB, Davis BR, Cutler J, et al, "Prevention of Heart Failure by Antihypertensive Drug Treatment in Older Persons With Isolated Systolic Hypertension. SHEP Cooperative Research Group," *JAMA*, 1997, 278:212-6.

Lazarus JM, Bourgoignie JJ, Buckalew VM, et al, "Achievement and Safety of a Low Blood Pressure Goal in Chronic Renal Disease: The Modification of Diet in Renal Disease Study Group," *Hypertension*, 1997, 29:641-50.

Lindheimer MD, "Hypertension in Pregnancy," *Hypertension*, 1993, 22:127-37.

Materson BJ, Reda DJ, Cushman WC, et al, "Single-Drug Therapy for Hypertension in Men: A Comparison of Six Antihypertensive Agents With Placebo. The Department of Veterans Affairs Cooperative Study Group on Antihypertensive Agents," *N Engl J Med*, 1993, 328:914-21.

Miller NH, Hill M, Kottke T, et al, "The Multi-Level Compliance Challenge: Recommendations for a Call to Action; A Statement for Healthcare Professionals," *Circulation*, 1997, 95:1085-90.

Neaton JD and Wentworth D, "Serum Cholesterol, Blood Pressure, Cigarette Smoking, and Death From Coronary Heart Disease: Overall Findings and Differences by Age for 316,099 White Men. The Multiple Risk Factor Intervention Trial Research Group," *Arch Intern Med*, 1992, 152:56-64.

Neaton JD, Grim RH, Prineas RJ, et al, "Treatment of Mild Hypertension Study (TOHMS). Final Results," *JAMA*, 1993, 270:721-31.

Oparil S, Levine JH, Zuschke CA, et al, "Effects of Candesartan Cilexetil in Patients With Severe Systemic Hypertension," *Am J Cardiol*, 1999, 84:289-93.

Perloff D, Grim C, Flack J, et al, "Human Blood Pressure Determination by Sphygmomanometry," *Circulation*, 1993, 88:2460-7.

Perry HM Jr, Bingham S, Horney A, et al, "Antihypertensive Efficacy of Treatment Regimens Used in Veterans Administration Hypertension Clinics. Department of Veterans Affairs Cooperative Study Group on Antihypertensive Agents," *Hypertension*, 1998, 31:771-9.

Preston RA, Materson BJ, Reda DJ, et al, "Age-Race Subgroup Compared With Renin Profile as Predictors of Blood Pressure Response to Antihypertensive Therapy," *JAMA*, 1998, 280:1168-72.

Psaty BM, Smith NL, Siscovick DS, et al, "Health Outcomes Associated With Antihypertensive Therapies Used as First-Line Agents. A Systemic Review and Meta-analysis," *JAMA*, 1997, 277:739-45.

Radevski IV, Valtchanova SP, Candy GP, et al, "Comparison of Acebutolol With and Without Hydrochlorothiazide Versus Carvedilol With and Without Hydrochlorothiazide in Black Patients With Mild to Moderate Systemic Hypertension," *Am J Cardiol*, 1999, 84(1):70-5.

Setaro JF and Black HR, "Refractory Hypertension," *N Engl J Med*, 1992, 327:543-7.

SHEP Cooperative Research Group, "Prevention of Stroke by Antihypertensive Drug Treatment in Older Persons With Isolated Systolic Hypertension: Final Results of the Systolic Hypertension in the Elderly Program (SHEP)," *JAMA*, 1991, 265:3255-64.

Sibai BM, "Treatment of Hypertension in Pregnant Women," *N Engl J Med*, 1996, 335:257-65.

Sowers JR, "Comorbidity of Hypertension and Diabetes: The Fosinopril Versus Amlodipine Cardiovascular Events Trial," *Am J Cardiol*, 1998, 82:15R-19R.

Sternberg H, Rosenthal T, Shamiss A, et al, "Altered Circadian Rhythm of Blood Pressure in Shift Workers," *J Hum Hypertens*, 1995, 9:349-53.

"The Hypertension Prevention Trial: Three-Year Effects of Dietary Changes on Blood Pressure. Hypertension Prevention Trial Research Group," *Arch Intern Med*, 1990, 150:153-62.

Trials of Hypertension Prevention Collaborative Research Group, "Effects of Weight Loss and Sodium Reduction Intervention on Blood Pressure and Hypertension Incidence in Overweight People With High-Normal Blood Pressure: The Trials of Hypertension Prevention, Phase II," *Arch Intern Med*, 1997, 157:657-67.

Tuomilehto J, Rastenyte D, Birkenhager WH, et al, "Effects of Calcium Channel Blockade in Older Patients With Diabetes and Systolic Hypertension," *N Engl J Med*, 1999, 340:677-84.

Veelken R and Schmieder RE, "Overview of Alpha-1 Adrenoceptor Antagonism and Recent Advances in Hypertensive Therapy," *Am J Hypertens*, 1996, 9:139S-49S.

White WB, Black HR, Weber MA, et al, "Comparison of Effects of Controlled Onset Extended Release Verapamil at Bedtime and Nifedipine Gastrointestinal Therapeutic System on Arising on Early Morning Blood Pressure, Heart Rate, and the Heart Rate-Blood Pressure Product," *Am J Cardiol*, 1998, 81:424-31.

PEDIATRIC ALS ALGORITHMS

PALS Bradycardia Algorithm

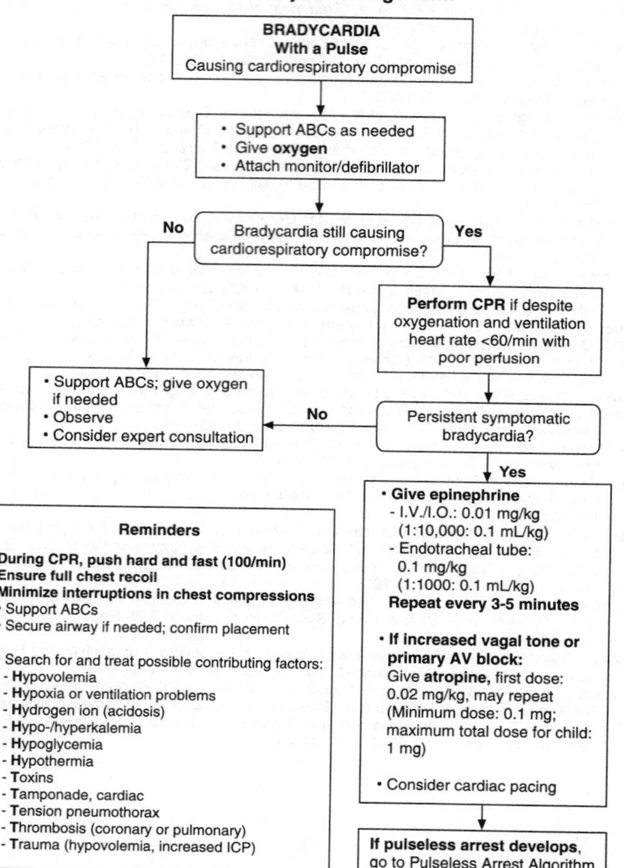

Adapted from American Heart Association Emergency Cardiovascular Care Committee, "2005 American Heart Association (AHA) Guidelines for Cardiopulmonary Resuscitation (CPR) and Emergency Cardiovascular Care (ECC)," *Circulation*, 2005, 112(24 Suppl):IV-176.

PALS Pulseless Arrest Algorithm

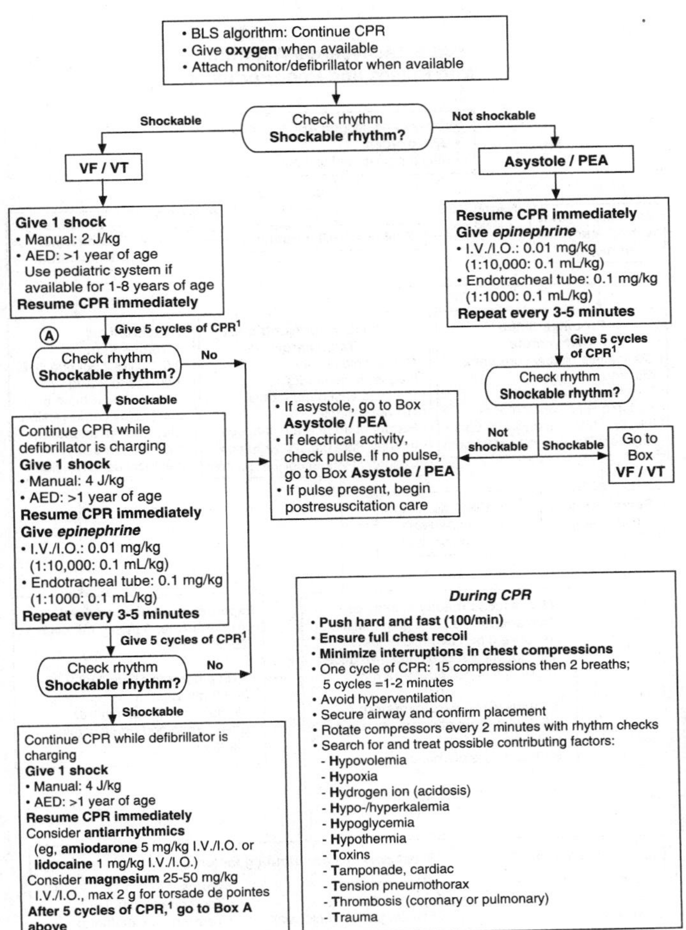

VF = ventricular fibrillation; VT = ventricular tachycardia; PEA = pulseless electrical activity; AED = automated external defibrillator.

[1]After an advanced airway is placed, rescuers no longer deliver "cycles" of CPR. Give continuous chest compressions without pauses for breaths. Give 8-10 breaths/min. Check rhythm every 2 minutes.

Adapted from American Heart Association Emergency Cardiovascular Care Committee, "2005 American Heart Association (AHA) Guidelines for Cardiopulmonary Resuscitation (CPR) and Emergency Cardiovascular Care (ECC)," *Circulation*, 2005, 112(24 Suppl):IV-173.

PEDIATRIC ALS ALGORITHMS *(Continued)*

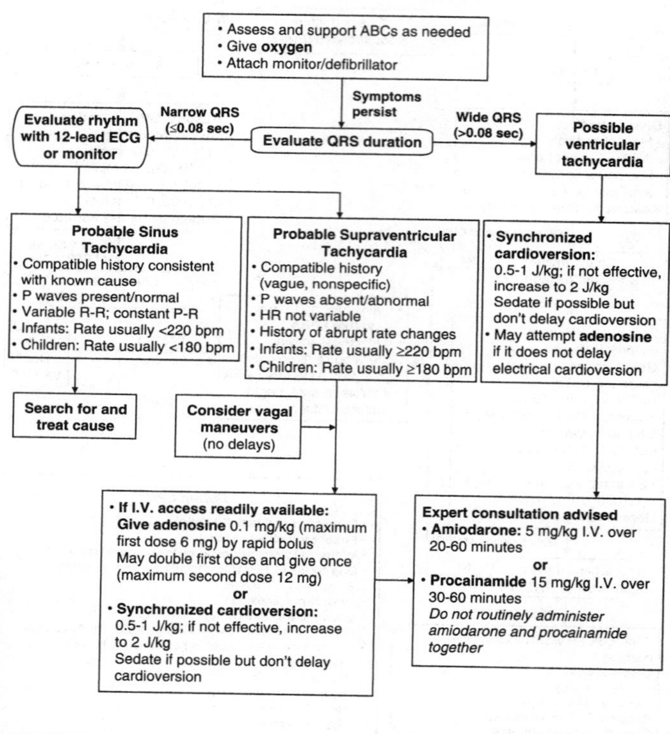

During Evaluation

- Secure, verify airway and vascular access when possible
- Consider expert consultation
- Prepare for cardioversion

Treat possible contributing factors:

- **Hyp**ovolemia
- **Hyp**oxia
- **H**ydrogen ion (acidosis)
- **Hyp**o-/hyperkalemia
- **Hyp**oglycemia
- **Hyp**othermia
- **T**oxins
- **T**amponade, cardiac
- **T**ension pneumothorax
- **T**hrombosis (coronary or pulmonary)
- **T**rauma (hypovolemia)

Adapted from American Heart Association Emergency Cardiovascular Care Committee, "2005 American Heart Association (AHA) Guidelines for Cardiopulmonary Resuscitation (CPR) and Emergency Cardiovascular Care (ECC)," *Circulation*, 2005, 112(24 Suppl):IV-177.

ADULT ACLS ALGORITHMS

Bradycardia Algorithm

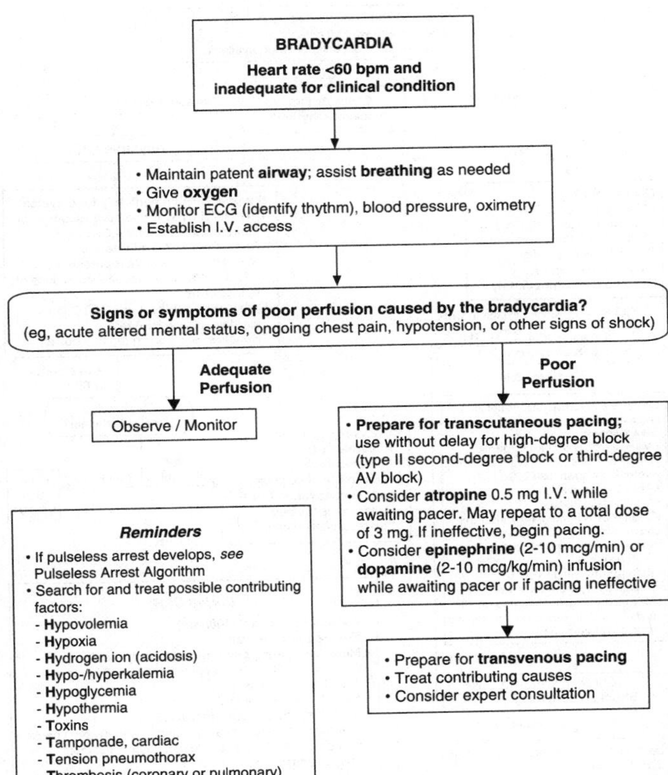

Adapted from American Heart Association Emergency Cardiovascular Care Committee, "2005 American Heart Association (AHA) Guidelines for Cardiopulmonary Resuscitation (CPR) and Emergency Cardiovascular Care (ECC)," *Circulation*, 2005, 112(24 Suppl):IV-68.

ADULT ACLS ALGORITHMS *(Continued)*

ACLS Pulseless Arrest Algorithm

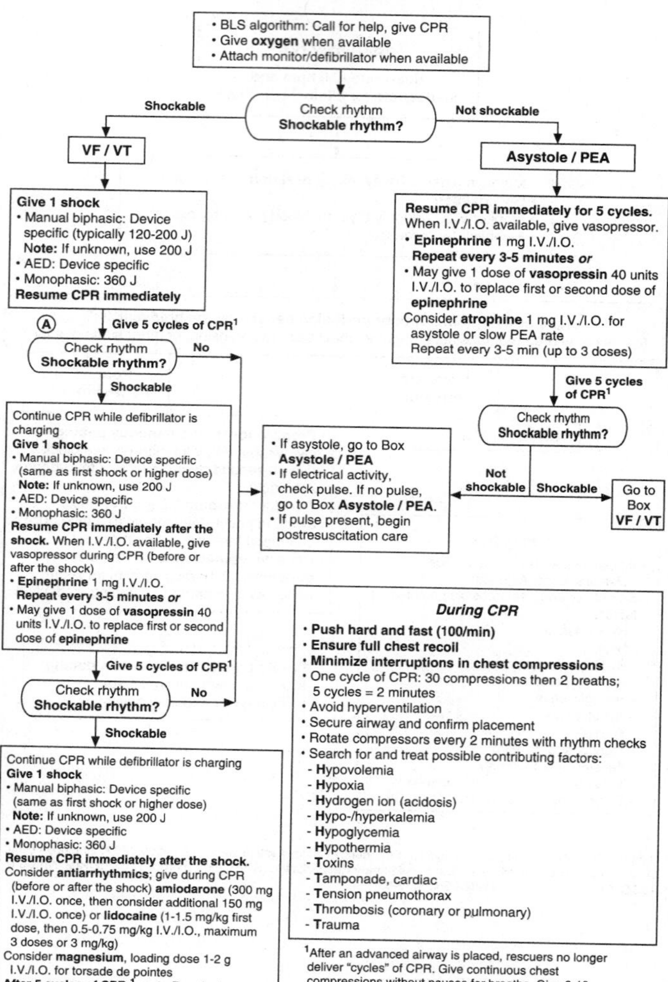

[1]After an advanced airway is placed, rescuers no longer deliver "cycles" of CPR. Give continuous chest compressions without pauses for breaths. Give 8-10 breaths/min. Check rhythm every 2 minutes.

VF = ventricular fibrillation; VT = ventricular tachycardia; PEA = pulseless electrical activity; AED = automated external defibrillator.

Adapted from American Heart Association Emergency Cardiovascular Care Committee, "2005 American Heart Association (AHA) Guidelines for Cardiopulmonary Resuscitation (CPR) and Emergency Cardiovascular Care (ECC)," *Circulation*, 2005, 112(24 Suppl):IV-59.

ACLS Tachycardia Algorithm With Pulses

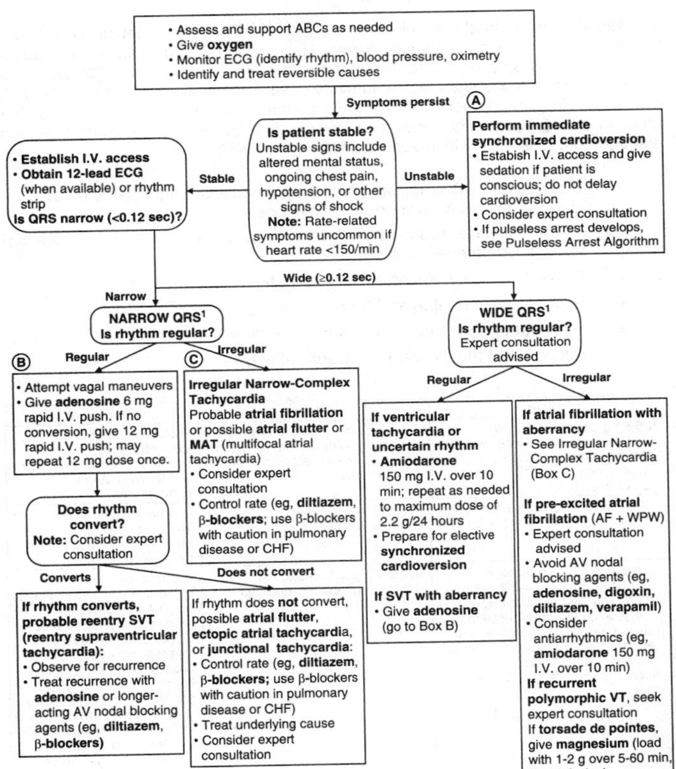

During Evaluation	***Treat possible contributing factors:***	
• Secure, verify airway and vascular access when possible • Consider expert consultation • Prepare for cardioversion	• **H**ypovolemia • **H**ypoxia • **H**ydrogen ion (acidosis) • **H**ypo-/hyperkalemia • **H**ypoglycemia • **H**ypothermia	• **T**oxins • **T**amponade, cardiac • **T**ension pneumothorax • **T**hrombosis (coronary or pulmonary) • **T**rauma (hypovolemia)

SVT = supraventricular tachycardia; VT = ventricular tachycardia.

[1]If patient becomes unstable, go to Box A.

Adapted from American Heart Association Emergency Cardiovascular Care Committee, "2005 American Heart Association (AHA) Guidelines for Cardiopulmonary Resuscitation (CPR) and Emergency Cardiovascular Care (ECC)," *Circulation*, 2005, 112(24 Suppl):IV-70.

TOXICOLOGY INFORMATION

Initial Stabilization of the Patients

The recommended treatment plan for the poisoned patient is not unlike general treatment plans taught in advanced cardiac life support (ACLS) or advanced trauma life support (ATLS) courses. In this manner, the initial approach to the poisoned patient should be essentially similar in every case, irrespective of the toxin ingested, just as the initial approach to the trauma patient is the same irrespective of the mechanism of injury. This approach, which can be termed as routine poison management, essentially includes the following aspects.

- Stabilization: ABCs (airway, breathing, circulation; administration of glucose, thiamine, oxygen, and naloxone
- History, physical examination leading toward the identification of class of toxin (toxidrome recognition)
- Prevention of absorption (decontamination)
- Specific antidote, if available
- Removal of absorbed toxin (enhancing excretion)
- Support and monitoring for adverse effects

Drug	Effect	Comment
25-50 g **dextrose** ($D_{50}W$) intravenously to reverse the effects of drug-induced hypoglycemia (adult) 1 mL/kg $D_{50}W$ diluted 1:1 (child)	This can be especially effective in patients with limited glycogen stores (ie, neonates and patients with cirrhosis)	Extravasation into the extremity of this hyperosmolar solution can cause Volkmann's contractures
50-100 mg intravenous **thiamine**	Prevent Wernicke's encephalopathy	A water-soluble vitamin with low toxicity; rare anaphylactoid reactions have been reported
Initial dosage of **naloxone** should be 2 mg in adult patients preferably by the intravenous route, although intramuscular, subcutaneous, intralingual, and endotracheal routes may also be utilized. Pediatric dose is 0.1 mg/kg from birth until 5 years of age	Specific opioid antagonist without any agent properties	It should be noted that some semisynthetic opiates (such as meperidine or propoxyphene) may require higher initial doses for reversal, so that a total dose of 6-10 mg is not unusual for the adults. If the patient responds to a bolus dose and then relapses to a lethargic or comatose state, a naloxone drip can be considered. This can be accomplished by administering two-thirds of the bolus dose that revives the patient per hour or injecting 4 mg naloxone in 1 L crystalloid solution and administering at a rate of 100 mL/hour 0.4 mg/hour)
Oxygen, utilized in 100% concentration	Useful for carbon monoxide, hydrogen, sulfide, and asphyxiants	While oxygen is antidotal for carbon monoxide intoxication, the only relative toxic contraindication is in paraquat intoxication (in that it can promote pulmonary fibrosis)
Flumazenil	Benzodiazepine antagonist	Not routinely recommended due to increased risk of seizures

Laboratory Evaluation of Overdose

Unknown ingestion: Electrolytes, anion gap, serum osmolality, arterial blood gases, serum drug concentration

Known ingestion: Labs tailored to agent

Toxins Affecting the Anion Gap

Drugs Causing Increased Anion Gap (>12 mEq/L)

Nonacidotic

- Carbenicillin
- Sodium salts

Metabolic Acidosis

- Acetaminophen (ingestion >75-100 g)
- Acetazolamide
- Amiloride
- Ascorbic acid
- Benzalkonium chloride
- Benzyl alcohol
- Beta-adrenergic drugs
- Bialaphos
- 2-Butanone
- Carbon monoxide
- Centrimonium bromide
- Chloramphenicol
- Colchicine
- Cyanide
- Dapsone
- Dimethyl sulfate
- Dinitrophenol
- Endosulfan
- Epinephrine (I.V. overdose)
- Ethanol
- Ethylene dibromide
- Ethylene glycol
- Fenoprofen
- Fluoroacetate
- Formaldehyde
- Fructose (I.V.)
- Glycol ethers
- Hydrogen sulfide
- Ibuprofen (ingestion >300 mg/kg)
- Inorganic acid
- Iodine
- Iron
- Isoniazid
- Ketamine
- Ketoprofen
- Metaldehyde
- Metformin
- Methanol
- Methenamine mandelate
- Monochloracetic acid
- Nalidixic acid
- Naproxen
- Niacin
- Papaverine
- Pennyroyal oil
- Pentachlorophenol
- Phenelzine
- Phenformin (off the market)
- Phenol
- Phenylbutazone
- Phosphoric acid
- Potassium chloroplatinite
- Propylene glycol
- Salicylates
- Sorbitol (I.V.)
- Strychnine
- Surfactant herbicide
- Tetracycline (outdated)
- Theophylline
- Tienilic acid
- Toluene
- Tranylcypromine
- Vacor
- Verapamil

Drugs Causing Decreased Anion Gap (<6 mEq/L)

Acidosis

- Ammonium chloride
- Bromide
- Iodide
- Lithium
- Polymyxin B
- Tromethamine

TOXICOLOGY INFORMATION *(Continued)*

Drugs Causing Increased Osmolar Gap

(by freezing-point depression, gap is >10 mOsm)

- Ethanol[1]
- Ethylene glycol[1]
- Glycerol
- Hypermagnesemia (>9.5 mEq/L)
- Isopropanol[1] (acetone)
- Iodine (questionable)
- Mannitol
- Methanol[1]
- Propylene glycol
- Severe alcoholic ketoacidosis or lactic acidosis
- Sorbitol[1]

[1]Toxins increasing both anion and osmolar gap.

Toxins Associated With Oxygen Saturation Gap

(>5% difference between measured and calculated value)

- Carbon monoxide
- Cyanide (questionable)
- Hydrogen sulfide (possible)
- Methemoglobin

Acetaminophen Toxicity

The Toxicology Laboratory is also very useful for determining levels of toxin in body fluids. Often these drug levels will guide therapy. For example, use of the Rumack-Matthew nomogram for acute acetaminophen poisoning can direct N-acetylcysteine therapy if the serum acetaminophen level falls above the treatment line.

Acetaminophen Toxicity Nomogram

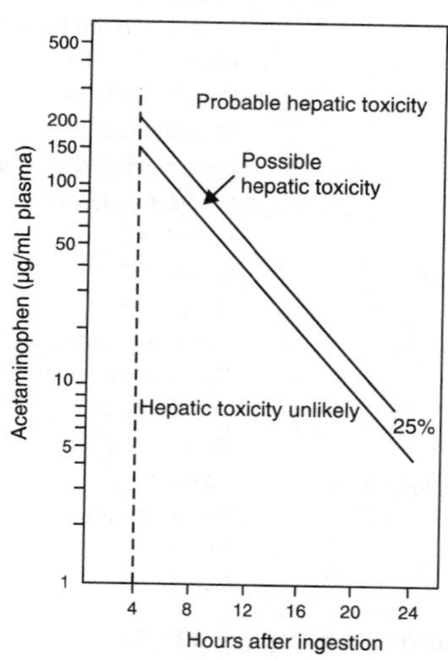

The Rumack-Matthew nomogram, relating expected severity of liver toxicity to serum acetaminophen concentrations.

From Smilkstein MJ, Bronstein AC, Linden C, et al, "Acetaminophen Overdose: A 48-Hour Intravenous N-Acetylcysteine Treatment Protocol," *Ann Emerg Med*, 1991, 20(10):1058, with permission.

Ibuprofen Toxicity Nomogram

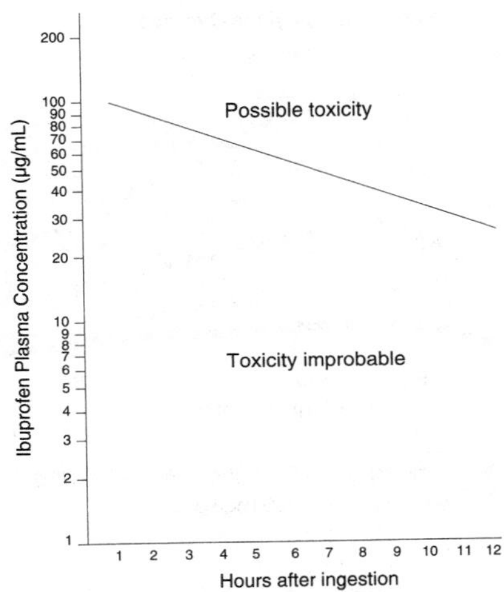

Adapted from Hall AH, Smolinske SC, Stover B, et al, "Ibuprofen Overdose in Adults," *J Toxicol Clin Toxicol*, 1992, 30:34.

Serum Salicylate Intoxication

Similarly, the Done nomogram is somewhat useful in predicting salicylate toxicity in pediatric patients. Neither nomogram should be utilized with chronic ingestions. Recently, a nomogram has been devised for theophylline ingestion; see the following nomogram.

Serum Salicylate Level and Severity of Intoxication Single Dose Acute Ingestion Nomogram

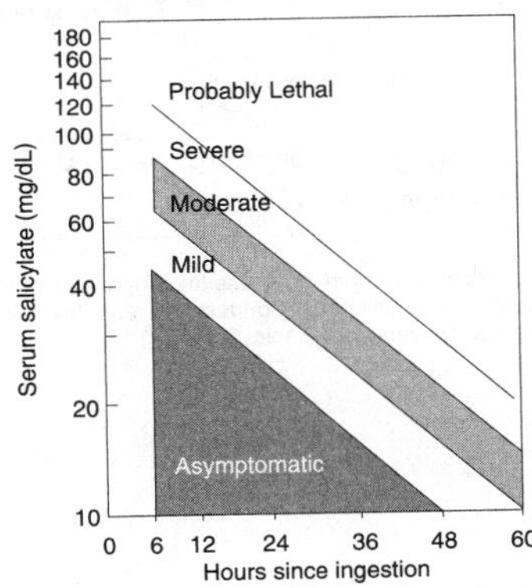

Done nomogram for salicylate poisoning. Note that this nomogram is not accurate for chronic ingestions nor for acute ingestions with enteric coated tabs. Clinical laboratory signs and symptoms are best indicators for assessments. (From Done AK, "Salicylate Intoxication: Significance of Measurements of Salicylate in Blood in Cases of Acute Ingestions," *Pediatrics*, 1960, 26:800; copyright American Academy of Pediatrics, 1960.)

TOXICOLOGY INFORMATION *(Continued)*

Serum Theophylline Overdose

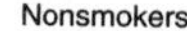

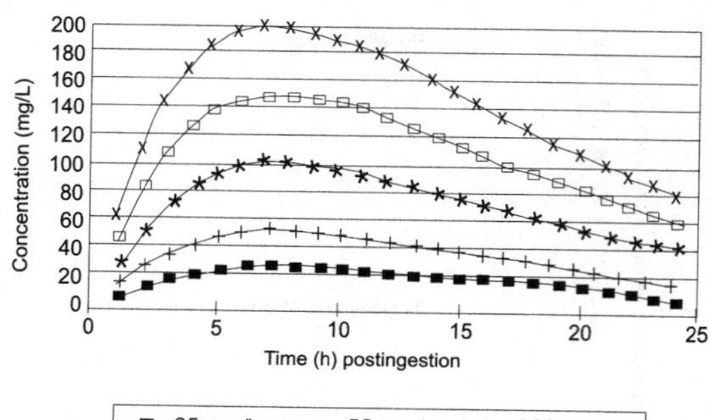

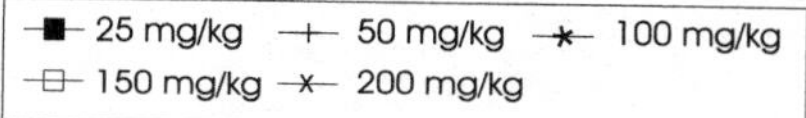

Serum Theophylline Overdose

Smokers and Children

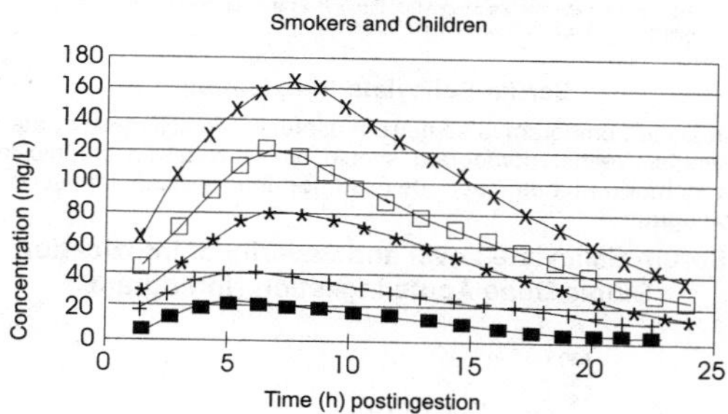

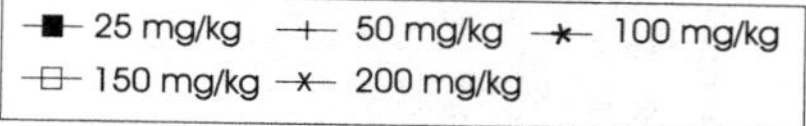

Nomogram for overdose of sustained-release theophylline in 1) nonsmoking adults, and 2) smokers and children. (Courtesy of Frank Paloucek, PharmD, College of Pharmacy, University of Illinois, Chicago.)

History and Physical Examination

While the history and physical examination is the cornerstone of clinical patient management, it takes on special meaning with regard to the toxic patient. While taking a history may be a more direct method of the determination of the toxin, quite often is is not reliable. Information obtained may prove minimal in some cases and could be considered partial or inaccurate in suicide gestures and addicts. A quick physical examination often leads to important clues about the nature of the toxin. These clues can be specific symptom complexes associated with certain toxins and can be referred to as "toxidromes".

Prevention of Absorption

Toxic substances can enter the body through the dermal, ocular, pulmonary, parenteral, and gastrointestinal routes. The basic principle of decontamination involves appropriate copious irrigation of the toxic substances relatable to the route of exposure. For example, with ocular exposure, this can be done with normal saline for 30-40 minutes through a Morgan therapeutic lens. With alkali exposures, the pH should be checked until the runoff of the solution is either neutral or slightly acidic. Skin decontamination involves removal of the toxin with nonabrasive soap. This should especially be considered for organophosphates, methylene chloride, dioxin, radiation, hydrocarbons, and herbicide exposure. Separate drainage areas should be obtained for the contaminated runoff.

Since >80% of incidents of accidental poisoning in children occur through the gastrointestinal tract, a thorough knowledge of gastric decontamination is essential. There are essentially four modes of gastric decontamination, of which three are physical removal (emesis, gastric lavage, and whole bowel irrigation). Activated charcoal associated with a cathartic is the fourth mode for preventing absorption.

Methods of Enhanced Elimination of Toxic Substances/Drugs

Emesis with Syrup of Ipecac

Indications

- Use within 1 hour of ingestion
- Hydrocarbons with "dangerous additives"
- Heavy metals
- Toxic insecticides

Contraindications

- Children <6 months of age
- Nontoxic ingestion
- Lack of gag reflex
- Caustic/corrosive ingestions
- Hemorrhagic diathesis
- Sharp object ingestion
- Prior vomiting
- Ingestion of pure petroleum distillate

Dose: + 15 mL H_2O

Children:	6-12 months: 10 mL
	1-5 years: 15 mL
	>5 years: 30 mL
Adults:	30 mL

Note: Ipecac use is becoming less frequently recommended since <30% of the stomach is usually emptied and its use may delay the use of activated charcoal.

Gastric Lavage

Indications

- Use within 1 hour of ingestion
- Comatose patient with significant ingestion without contraindications
- Failure to respond to ipecac
- Large quantities of toxins

Contraindications

- Seizures
- Nontoxic ingestion
- Significant hemorrhagic diathesis
- Caustic ingestions, hydrocarbons
- Usually unable to use large enough tube in children <12 years of age

TOXICOLOGY INFORMATION *(Continued)*

Note: Lavage is not routinely recommended except for recent and very large ingestions of noncontraindicated toxins since it is believed to actually push a significant portion of drug into the intestine and may delay administration of activated charcoal.

Enhancement of Elimination

Only recently has this aspect of poison management received more than cursory attention in practice and in the literature. The standard practice for enhancement of elimination consisted primarily of forced diuresis in order to excrete the toxin. However, the past 10 years experience has produced a radical change in the approach to this and therefore, a more focused methodology to eliminating absorbed toxins. Essentially, there are three methods by which absorbed toxins may be eliminated: recurrent adsorption with multiple dosings of activated charcoal, use of forced diuresis in combination with possible alkalinization of the urine, and use of dialysis or charcoal hemoperfusion.

Activated Charcoal Indications

Indications

- Single dose for agents known to be bound
- Multiple dose for drugs with favorable characteristics: Small volume of distribution (<1 L/kg), low plasma protein binding, biliary or gastric secretion, active metabolites that recirculate, drugs that exhibit a large free fraction (eg, dapsone, carbamazepine, digitalis, methotrexate, phenobarbital, salicylates, theophylline, tricyclic antidepressants), unchanged, lipophilic, long half-life

Recently, multiple dosing of activated charcoal ("pulse dosing") has been advocated as a method for removal of absorbed drug. This procedure has been demonstrated to be efficacious in drugs that re-enter the gastrointestinal tract through enterohepatic circulation (ie, digitoxin, carbamazepine, glutethimide) and with drugs that diffuse from the systemic circulation into the gastrointestinal tract due to formation of a concentration gradient ("the infinite sink" hypothesis).

Toxins Eliminated by Multiple Dosing of Activated Charcoal (MDAC)

Acetaminophen	Meprobamate
Amitriptyline	Methotrexate
Amoxapine	Methyprylon
Baclofen (?)	Nadolol
Benzodiazepines (?)	Nortriptyline
Bupropion (?)	Phencyclidine
Carbamazepine[1]	Phenobarbital[1]
Chlordecone	Phenylbutazone
Cyclosporine	Phenytoin (?)
Dapsone	Piroxicam
Diazepam	Propoxyphene
Digoxin	Propranolol
Disopyramide	Salicylates (?)[1]
Glutethimide	Theophylline[1]
Maprotiline	Valproic acid[1]

[1]Only agents routinely recommended for removal with MDAC.

Contraindications

- Absence of hypoactive bowel sounds
- Caustic ingestions
- Drugs without effect: Acids, alkalis, alcohols, cyanide, iron, heavy metals, lithium, insecticides

Dose

Children and Adults: 50-100 g initially or 1 g/kg weight; repeat doses of 25 g or 0.5 g/kg every 2-4 hours

Most effective at 1-hour postingestion but can remove at >1-hour postingestion

Doses subsequent to first may be admixed with water rather than a cathartic such as sorbitol to avoid diarrhea and consequent electrolyte disturbances.

Whole Bowel Irrigation – propylene glycol based solutions

Initial dose of charcoal is necessary prior to use. Avoid pretreatment with ipecac.

Indications

- Iron, lead, lithium
- Agents not bound by charcoal
- Modified or sustained release dosage forms
- Body packers

Contraindications

- Bowel perforation
- Obstruction
- Ileus
- Gastrointestinal bleed

Dose

Maximum: 5-10 L
Toddlers/preschool: 250-500 mL/hour or 35 mL/kg
Adults: 1-2 L/hour
Terminate when rectal effluent = infusate = clear

Urinary Ion Trapping – to alkalinize the urine

Indications

- Salicylates
- Phenobarbital

Toxins Eliminated by Forced Saline Diuretics	Toxins Eliminated by Alkaline Diuresis
Bromidex	2,4-D chlorphenoxyacetic acid
Chromium	Fluoride
Cimetidine (?)	Isoniazid (?)
Cis-platinum	Mephobarbital
Cyclophosphamide	Methotrexate
Hydrazine	Phenobarbital
Iodide	Primidone
Iodine	Quinolones antibiotic
Isoniazid (?)	Salicylates
Lithium	Uranium
Methyl iodide	
Potassium chloroplatinite	
Thallium	

Dose

Sodium bicarbonate 1-2 mEq/kg every 3-4 hours or 100 mEq $NaHCO_3$ in 1 L $D_5{}^1/_4NS$ at 200 mL/hour (desired urine pH: 7.6-7.8)

A urine flow of 3-5 mL/kg/hour should be achieved with a combination of isotonic fluids or diuretics. Although several drugs can exhibit enhanced elimination through an acidic urine (quinine, amphetamines, PCP, nicotine, bismuth, ephedrine, flecainide), the practice of acidifying the urine should be discouraged in that it can produce metabolic acidosis and promote renal failure in the presence of rhabdomyolysis. **Note:** Use caution in alkalinizing urine of children to avoid fluid overdose.

Hemodialysis

Indications

Drugs with favorable characteristics

- Low molecular weight (<500 daltons)
- Ionically charged
- H_2O soluble
- Low plasma protein binding (<70%-80%)
- Small volume of distribution (<1 L/kg)
- Low tissue binding
- Methanol, ethylene glycol

TOXICOLOGY INFORMATION *(Continued)*

Drugs and Toxins Removed by Hemodialysis

Acetaminophen
Acyclovir
Amanita phalloides (?)
Amantadine (?)
Ammonium chloride
Amphetamine
Anilines
Atenolol
Bromides
Bromisoval
Calcium
Captopril (?)
Carbromal
Carisoprodol
Chloral hydrate
Chlorpropamide
Chromium
Cimetidine (?)
Cyclophosphamide
Dapsone
Disopyramide
Enalapril (?)
Ethanol
Ethylene glycol
Famotidine (?)
Fluoride
Folic acid
Formaldehyde
Foscarnet sodium
Gabapentin
Glycol ethers
Hydrazine (?)
Hydrochlorothiazide
Iodides
Isoniazid
Isopropanol
Ketoprofen
Lithium
Magnesium
Meprobamate
Metal-chelate compounds
Metformin (?)
Methanol
Methaqualone
Methotrexate
Methyldopa
Methylprylone
Monochloroacetic acid
Nadolol
Oxalic acid
Phenelzine (?)
Phenobarbital
Phosphoric acid
Potassium
Procainamide
Quinidine
Ranitidine (?)
Rifabutin
Salicylates
Sotalol
Strychnine
Thallium
Theophylline
Thiocyanates
Tranylcypromine sulfate (?)
Verapamil (?)

Hemoperfusion

Indications

Drugs with favorable characteristics:

- Affinity for activated charcoal
- Tissue binding
- High rate of equilibration from peripheral tissues to blood

Examples: Barbiturates, carbamazepine, ethchlorvynol, methotrexate, phenytoin, theophylline

Drugs and Toxins Removed by Hemoperfusion (Charcoal)

Aconitine
Amanita phalloides (?)
Atenolol (?)
Bromisoval
Bromoethylbutyramide
Caffeine
Carbamazepine
Carbon tetrachloride (?)
Carbromal
Chloral hydrate (trichloroethanol)
Chloramphenicol
Chlorpropamide
Colchicine (?)
Creosote (?)
Dapsone
Diltiazem (?)
Disopyramide
Ethchlorvynol
Ethylene oxide
Glutethimide
Lindane
Meprobamate
Methaqualone
Methotrexate
Methsuximide
Methyprylon (?)
Metoprolol (?)
Nadolol (?)
Oxalic acid (?)
Paraquat
Phenelzine (?)
Phenobarbital
Phenytoin
Podophyllin (?)
Procainamide (?)
Quinidine (?)
Rifabutin (?)
Sotalol (?)
Thallium
Theophylline
Verapamil (?)

Exchange transfusion is another mode of extracorporeal removal of toxins that can be utilized in neonatal infant drug toxicity. It may be especially useful for barbiturate, iron, caffeine, sodium nitrite, or theophylline overdose.

CYTOCHROME P450 ENZYMES: SUBSTRATES, INHIBITORS, AND INDUCERS

INTRODUCTION

Most drugs are eliminated from the body, at least in part, by being chemically altered to less lipid-soluble products (ie, metabolized), and thus are more likely to be excreted via the kidneys or the bile. Phase I metabolism includes drug hydrolysis, oxidation, and reduction, and results in drugs that are more polar in their chemical structure, while Phase II metabolism involves the attachment of an additional molecule onto the drug (or partially metabolized drug) in order to create an inactive and/or more water soluble compound. Phase II processes include (primarily) glucuronidation, sulfation, glutathione conjugation, acetylation, and methylation.

Virtually any of the Phase I and II enzymes can be inhibited by some xenobiotic or drug. Some of the Phase I and II enzymes can be induced. Inhibition of the activity of metabolic enzymes will result in increased concentrations of the substrate (drug), whereas induction of the activity of metabolic enzymes will result in decreased concentrations of the substrate. For example, the well-documented enzyme-inducing effects of phenobarbital may include a combination of Phase I and II enzymes. Phase II glucuronidation may be increased via induced UDP-glucuronosyltransferase (UGT) activity, whereas Phase I oxidation may be increased via induced cytochrome P450 (CYP) activity. However, for most drugs, the primary route of metabolism (and the primary focus of drug-drug interaction) is Phase I oxidation, and specifically, metabolism.

CYP enzymes may be responsible for the metabolism (at least partial metabolism) of approximately 75% of all drugs, with the CYP3A subfamily responsible for nearly half of this activity. Found throughout plant, animal, and bacterial species, CYP enzymes represent a superfamily of xenobiotic metabolizing proteins. There have been several hundred CYP enzymes identified in nature, each of which has been assigned to a family (1, 2, 3, etc), subfamily (A, B, C, etc), and given a specific enzyme number (1, 2, 3, etc) according to the similarity in amino acid sequence that it shares with other enzymes. Of these many enzymes, only a few are found in humans, and even fewer appear to be involved in the metabolism of xenobiotics (eg, drugs). The key human enzyme subfamilies include CYP1A, CYP2A, CYP2B, CYP2C, CYP2D, CYP2E, and CYP3A.

CYP enzymes are found in the endoplasmic reticulum of cells in a variety of human tissues (eg, skin, kidneys, brain, lungs), but their predominant sites of concentration and activity are the liver and intestine. Though the abundance of CYP enzymes throughout the body is relatively equally distributed among the various subfamilies, the relative contribution to drug metabolism is (in decreasing order of magnitude) CYP3A4 (nearly 50%), CYP2D6 (nearly 25%), CYP2C8/9 (nearly 15%), then CYP1A2, CYP2C19, CYP2A6, and CYP2E1. Owing to their potential for numerous drug-drug interactions, those drugs that are identified in preclinical studies as substrates of CYP3A enzymes are often given a lower priority for continued research and development in favor of drugs that appear to be less affected by (or less likely to affect) this enzyme subfamily.

Each enzyme subfamily possesses unique selectivity toward potential substrates. For example, CYP1A2 preferentially binds medium-sized, planar, lipophilic molecules, while CYP2D6 preferentially binds molecules that possess a basic nitrogen atom. Some CYP subfamilies exhibit polymorphism (ie, multiple allelic variants that manifest differing catalytic properties). The best described polymorphisms involve CYP2C9, CYP2C19, and CYP2D6. Individuals possessing "wild type" gene alleles exhibit normal functioning CYP capacity. Others, however, possess allelic variants that leave the person with a subnormal level of catalytic potential (so called "poor metabolizers"). Poor metabolizers would be more likely to experience toxicity from drugs metabolized by the affected enzymes (or less effects if the enzyme is responsible for converting a prodrug to it's active form as in the case of codeine). The percentage of people classified as poor metabolizers varies by enzyme and population group. As an example, approximately 7% of Caucasians and only about 1% of Orientals appear to be CYP2D6 poor metabolizers.

CYP enzymes can be both inhibited and induced by other drugs, leading to increased or decreased serum concentrations (along with the associated effects), respectively. Induction occurs when a drug causes an increase in the amount of

CYTOCHROME P450 ENZYMES: SUBSTRATES, INHIBITORS, AND INDUCERS *(Continued)*

smooth endoplasmic reticulum, secondary to increasing the amount of the affected CYP enzymes in the tissues. This "revving up" of the CYP enzyme system may take several days to reach peak activity, and likewise, may take several days, even months, to return to normal following discontinuation of the inducing agent.

CYP inhibition occurs via several potential mechanisms. Most commonly, a CYP inhibitor competitively (and reversibly) binds to the active site on the enzyme, thus preventing the substrate from binding to the same site, and preventing the substrate from being metabolized. The affinity of an inhibitor for an enzyme may be expressed by an inhibition constant (Ki) or IC50 (defined as the concentration of the inhibitor required to cause 50% inhibition under a given set of conditions). In addition to reversible competition for an enzyme site, drugs may inhibit enzyme activity by binding to sites on the enzyme other than that to which the substrate would bind, and thereby cause a change in the functionality or physical structure of the enzyme. A drug may also bind to the enzyme in an irreversible (ie, "suicide") fashion. In such a case, it is not the concentration of drug at the enzyme site that is important (constantly binding and releasing), but the number of molecules available for binding (once bound, always bound).

Although an inhibitor or inducer may be known to affect a variety of CYP subfamilies, it may only inhibit one or two in a clinically important fashion. Likewise, although a substrate is known to be at least partially metabolized by a variety of CYP enzymes, only one or two enzymes may contribute significantly enough to its overall metabolism to warrant concern when used with potential inducers or inhibitors. Therefore, when attempting to predict the level of risk of using two drugs that may affect each other via altered CYP function, it is important to identify the relative effectiveness of the inhibiting/inducing drug on the CYP subfamilies that significantly contribute to the metabolism of the substrate. The contribution of a specific CYP pathway to substrate metabolism should be considered not only in light of other known CYP pathways, but also other nonoxidative pathways for substrate metabolism (eg, glucuronidation) and transporter proteins (eg, P-glycoprotein) that may affect the presentation of a substrate to a metabolic pathway.

HOW TO USE THE TABLES

The following CYP SUBSTRATES, INHIBITORS, and INDUCERS tables provide a clinically relevant perspective on drugs that are affected by, or affect, cytochrome P450 (CYP) enzymes. Not all human, drug-metabolizing CYP enzymes are specifically (or separately) included in the tables. Some enzymes have been excluded because they do not appear to significantly contribute to the metabolism of marketed drugs (eg, CYP2C18). In the case of CYP3A4, the industry routinely uses this single enzyme designation to represent all enzymes in the CYP3A subfamily. CYP3A7 is present in fetal livers. It is effectively absent from adult livers. CYP3A4 (adult) and CYP3A7 (fetal) appear to share similar properties in their respective hosts. The impact of CYP3A7 in fetal and neonatal drug interactions has not been investigated.

The **CYP Substrates table** contains a list of drugs reported to be metabolized, at least in part, by one or more CYP enzymes. An enzyme that appears to play a clinically significant (major) role in a drug's metabolism is indicated by "●", and an enzyme whose role appears to be clinically insignificant (minor) is indicated by "○". A clinically significant designation is the result of a two-phase review. The first phase considered the contribution of each CYP enzyme to the overall metabolism of the drug. The enzyme pathway was considered potentially clinically relevant if it was responsible for at least 30% of the metabolism of the drug. If so, the drug was subjected to a second phase. The second phase considered the clinical relevance of a substrate's concentration being increased twofold, or decreased by one-half (such as might be observed if combined with an effective CYP inhibitor or inducer, respectively). If either of these changes was considered to present a clinically significant concern, the CYP pathway for the drug was designated "major." If neither change would appear to present a clinically significant concern, or if the CYP enzyme was responsible for a smaller portion of the overall metabolism (ie, <30%), the pathway was designated "minor."

The **CYP Inhibitors table** contains a list of drugs that are reported to inhibit one or more CYP enzymes. Enzymes that are strongly inhibited by a drug are indicated by "●". Enzymes that are moderately inhibited are indicated by "◑". Enzymes that are weakly inhibited are indicated by "○". The designations are the result of a review of published clinical reports, available Ki data, and assessments published by other experts in the field. As it pertains to Ki values set in a ratio with achievable serum drug concentrations ([I]) under normal dosing conditions, the following parameters were employed: [I]/Ki ≥1 = strong; [I]/Ki 0.1-1 = moderate; [I]/Ki <0.1 = weak.

The **CYP Inducers table** contains a list of drugs that are reported to induce one or more CYP enzymes. Enzymes that appear to be effectively induced by a drug are indicated by "●", and enzymes that do not appear to be effectively induced are indicated by "○". The designations are the result of a review of published clinical reports and assessments published by experts in the field.

In general, clinically significant interactions are more likely to occur between substrates and either inhibitors or inducers of the same enzyme(s), all of which have been indicated by "●". However, these assessments possess a degree of subjectivity, at times based on limited indications regarding the significance of CYP effects of particular agents. An attempt has been made to balance a conservative, clinically-sensitive presentation of the data with a desire to avoid the numbing effect of a "beware of everything" approach. Even so, other potential interactions (ie, those involving enzymes indicated by "○") may warrant consideration in some cases. It is important to note that information related to CYP metabolism of drugs is expanding at a rapid pace, and thus, the contents of this table should only be considered to represent a "snapshot" of the information available at the time of publication.

Selected Readings

Bjornsson TD, Callaghan JT, Einolf HJ, et al, "The Conduct of *in vitro* and *in vivo* Drug-Drug Interaction Studies: A PhRMA Perspective," *J Clin Pharmacol*, 2003, 43(5):443-69.

Drug-Drug Interactions, Rodrigues AD, ed, New York, NY: Marcel Dekker, Inc, 2002.

Levy RH, Thummel KE, Trager WF, et al, eds, *Metabolic Drug Interactions*, Philadelphia, PA: Lippincott Williams & Wilkins, 2000.

Michalets EL, "Update: Clinically Significant Cytochrome P-450 Drug Interactions," *Pharmacotherapy*, 1998, 18(1):84-112.

Thummel KE and Wilkinson GR, "*In vitro* and *in vivo* Drug Interactions Involving Human CYP3A," *Annu Rev Pharmacol Toxicol*, 1998, 38:389-430.

Zhang Y and Benet LZ, "The Gut as a Barrier to Drug Absorption: Combined Role of Cytochrome P450 3A and P-Glycoprotein," *Clin Pharmacokinet*, 2001, 40(3):159-68.

Selected Websites

http://www.gentest.com
http://www.imm.ki.se/CYPalleles
http://medicine.iupui.edu/flockhart
http://www.mhc.com/Cytochromes

CYP Substrates

● = major substrate
○ = minor substrate

Drug	1A2	2A6	2B6	2C8	2C9	2C19	2D6	2E1	3A4
Acenocoumarol	●				●	○			
Acetaminophen	○	○			○		○	○	○
Albendazole	○								○
Albuterol									●
Alfentanil									●
Almotriptan							○		○
Alosetron	○				●				○
Alprazolam									●
Aminophylline	●							○	○
Amiodarone	○			●		○	○		●
Amitriptyline	○		○		○	○	●		○
Amlodipine									●
Amoxapine							●		
Amphetamine							○		
Amprenavir					○				●
Aprepitant	○					○			●
Argatroban									○
Aripiprazole							●		●
Aspirin					○				
Atazanavir									●
Atomoxetine						○	●		
Atorvastatin									●
Azelastine	○					○	○		○
Azithromycin									○

CYTOCHROME P450 ENZYMES: SUBSTRATES, INHIBITORS, AND INDUCERS *(Continued)*

CYP Substrates *(continued)*

Drug	1A2	2A6	2B6	2C8	2C9	2C19	2D6	2E1	3A4
Benzphetamine			○						●
Benztropine							○		
Betaxolol	●						●		
Bexarotene									○
Bezafibrate									○
Bisoprolol							○		●
Bortezomib	○				○	○	○		●
Bosentan					●				●
Brinzolamide									○
Bromazepam									●
Bromocriptine									●
Budesonide									●
Bupivacaine	○					○	○		○
Buprenorphine									●
BuPROPion	○	○	●		○		○	○	○
BusPIRone							○		●
Busulfan									●
Caffeine	●				○		○	○	○
Candesartan					○				
Capsaicin								○	
Captopril							●		
Carbamazepine				○					●
Carisoprodol						●			
Carteolol							○		
Carvedilol	○				●		●	○	○
Celecoxib					●				○
Cerivastatin									●
Cetirizine									○
Cevimeline							○		○
Chlordiazepoxide									●
Chloroquine							●		●
Chlorpheniramine							○		●
ChlorproMAZINE	○						●		○
ChlorproPAMIDE					○				
Chlorzoxazone	○	○					○	●	○
Cilostazol	○					●	○		●
Cinacalcet	○						○		○
Cisapride	○	○	○		○	○			●
Citalopram						●	○		●
Clarithromycin									●
Clobazam						●			●
Clofibrate									○
ClomiPRAMINE	●					●	●		○
Clonazepam									●
Clopidogrel	○								○
Clorazepate									●
Clozapine	●	○			○	○	○		○
Cocaine									●
Codeine[1]							●		○
Colchicine									●
Conivaptan									●
Cyclobenzaprine	●						○		○
Cyclophosphamide[2]		○	●		○	○			●
CycloSPORINE									●
Dacarbazine	●							●	
Dantrolene									●
Dapsone				○	●	○		○	●
Delavirdine							○		●
Desipramine	○						●		
Desogestrel						●			

CYP Substrates *(continued)*

Drug	1A2	2A6	2B6	2C8	2C9	2C19	2D6	2E1	3A4
Dexamethasone									○
Dexmedetomidine		●							
Dextroamphetamine							●		
Dextromethorphan		○			○	○	●	○	○
Diazepam	○		○		○	●			●
Diclofenac	○		○	○	○	○	○		○
Digitoxin									●
Digoxin									○
Dihydrocodeine[1]							●		
Dihydroergotamine									●
Diltiazem					○		○		●
Dirithromycin									○
Disopyramide									●
Disulfiram	○	○	○				○	○	○
Docetaxel									●
Dofetilide									○
Dolasetron					○				○
Domperidone									○
Donepezil							○		○
Dorzolamide					○				○
Doxepin	●						●		●
DOXOrubicin							●		●
Doxycycline									●
Drospirenone									○
Duloxetine	●						●		
Dutasteride									○
Efavirenz			●						●
Eletriptan									●
Enalapril									●
Enflurane								●	
Eplerenone									●
Ergoloid mesylates									●
Ergonovine									●
Ergotamine									●
Erythromycin			○						●
Escitalopram						●			●
Esomeprazole						●			○
Estazolam									○
Estradiol	●	○	○		○	○	○	○	●
Estrogens, conjugated A/synthetic	●	○	○		○	○	○	○	●
Estrogens, conjugated equine	●	○	○		○	○	○	○	●
Estrogens, conjugated esterified	●		○		○			○	●
Estrone	●		○		○			○	●
Estropipate	●		○		○			○	●
Ethinyl estradiol					○				●
Ethosuximide									●
Etonogestrel									○
Etoposide	○							○	●
Exemestane									●
Felbamate								○	●
Felodipine									●
Fenofibrate									○
Fentanyl									●
Fexofenadine									○
Finasteride									○
Flecainide	○						●		
Fluoxetine	○		○		●	○	●	○	○
Fluphenazine							●		
Flurazepam									●
Flurbiprofen					○				
Flutamide	●								●

CYTOCHROME P450 ENZYMES: SUBSTRATES, INHIBITORS, AND INDUCERS *(Continued)*

CYP Substrates *(continued)*

Drug	1A2	2A6	2B6	2C8	2C9	2C19	2D6	2E1	3A4
Fluticasone									●
Fluvastatin					○		○		○
Fluvoxamine	●						●		
Formoterol		○			○	○	○		
Fosamprenavir (as amprenavir)					○				●
Fosphenytoin (as phenytoin)					●	●			○
Frovatriptan	○								
Fulvestrant									○
Galantamine							○		○
Gefitinib									●
Gemfibrozil									○
Glimepiride					●				
GlipiZIDE					●				
Granisetron									○
Guanabenz	●								
Halazepam									○
Halofantrine					○		○		●
Haloperidol	○						●		●
Halothane		○	○		○		○	●	○
Hydrocodone[1]							●		
Hydrocortisone									○
Ibuprofen					○	○			
Ifosfamide[3]		○	○	○	○	○			●
Imatinib	○				○	○	○		●
Imipramine	○		○			●	●		○
Imiquimod	○								○
Indinavir							○		●
Indomethacin					○	○			
Irbesartan					○				
Irinotecan			●						●
Isoflurane								●	
Isoniazid								●	
Isosorbide									●
Isosorbide dinitrate									●
Isosorbide mononitrate									●
Isradipine									●
Itraconazole									●
Ivermectin									○
Ketamine			●		●				●
Ketoconazole									●
Labetalol							●		
Lansoprazole					○	●			●
Letrozole		○							●
Levobupivacaine	○								○
Levonorgestrel									●
Lidocaine	○	○	○		○		●		●
Lomustine							●		
Lopinavir									○
Loratadine							○		○
Losartan					●				●
Lovastatin									●
Maprotiline							●		
MedroxyPROGESTERone									●
Mefenamic acid					○				
Mefloquine									●
Meloxicam					○				○
Mephobarbital			○		○	●			
Mestranol[4]					●				●
Methadone					○	○	○		●

CYP Substrates *(continued)*

Drug	1A2	2A6	2B6	2C8	2C9	2C19	2D6	2E1	3A4
Methamphetamine							●		
Methoxsalen		○							
Methsuximide						●			
Methylergonovine									●
Methylphenidate							●		
MethylPREDNISolone									○
Metoclopramide	○						○		
Metoprolol						○	●		
Mexiletine	●						●		
Miconazole									●
Midazolam			○						●
Mifepristone									○
Miglustat									●
Mirtazapine	●				○		●		●
Moclobemide						●	●		
Modafinil									●
Mometasone furoate									○
Montelukast					●				●
Moricizine									●
Morphine sulfate							○		
Naproxen	○				○				
Nateglinide					●				●
Nefazodone							●		●
Nelfinavir					○	●	○		●
Nevirapine			○				○		●
NiCARdipine	○				○		○	○	●
Nicotine	○	○	○		○	○	○	○	○
NIFEdipine							○		●
Nilutamide						●			
Nimodipine									●
Nisoldipine									●
Nitrendipine									●
Norelgestromin									○
Norethindrone									●
Norgestrel									●
Nortriptyline	○					○	●		○
Olanzapine	○						○		
Omeprazole		○			○	●	○		○
Ondansetron	○				○		○	○	●
Orphenadrine	○		○				○		○
Oxybutynin									○
Oxycodone[1]							●		
Paclitaxel				●	●				●
Palonosetron	○						○		○
Pantoprazole						●			○
Paroxetine							●		
Pentamidine						●			
Pergolide									●
Perphenazine	○				○	○	●		○
Phencyclidine									●
Phenobarbital					○	●		○	
Phenytoin					●	●			○
Pimecrolimus									○
Pimozide	●								●
Pindolol							●		
Pioglitazone				●					○
Pipotiazine							●		●
Piroxicam					○				
Pravastatin									○
Prazepam									○
PrednisoLONE									○
PredniSONE									○
Primaquine									●

CYTOCHROME P450 ENZYMES: SUBSTRATES, INHIBITORS, AND INDUCERS *(Continued)*

CYP Substrates *(continued)*

Drug	1A2	2A6	2B6	2C8	2C9	2C19	2D6	2E1	3A4
Procainamide							●		
Progesterone	○	○			○	●	○		●
Proguanil	○					○			○
Promethazine			●				●		
Propafenone	○						●		○
Propofol	○	○	●		●	○	○	○	○
Propranolol	●					○	●		○
Protriptyline							●		
Quazepam									○
Quetiapine							○		●
Quinidine					○			○	●
Quinine	○					○			○
Rabeprazole						●			●
Ranitidine	○					○	○		
Ranolazine							○		●
Repaglinide				●					●
Rifabutin									●
Riluzole	●								
Risperidone							●		○
Ritonavir	○		○				○		●
Rofecoxib					○				
Ropinirole	●								○
Ropivacaine	○		○				○		○
Rosiglitazone				●	○				
Rosuvastatin					○				○
Salmeterol									●
Saquinavir							○		●
Selegiline	○	○	●	○		○	○		○
Sertraline			○		○	●	●		○
Sevoflurane		○	○					●	○
Sibutramine									●
Sildenafil					○				●
Simvastatin									●
Sirolimus									●
Sorafenib									○
Spiramycin									●
Sufentanil									●
SulfaDIAZINE					●			○	○
Sulfamethoxazole					●				○
Sulfinpyrazone					●				○
SulfiSOXAZOLE					●				
Sunitinib									●
Tacrine	●								
Tacrolimus									●
Tamoxifen		○	○		●		●	○	●
Tamsulosin							●		●
Telithromycin	○								●
Temazepam			○		○	○			○
Teniposide									●
Terbinafine	○				○	○			○
Testosterone			○		○	○			○
Tetracycline									●
Theophylline	●				○		○	●	●
Thiabendazole	○								
Thioridazine						○	●		
Thiothixene	●								
Tiagabine									●
Ticlopidine									●
Timolol							●		
Tinidazole									○

CYP Substrates *(continued)*

Drug	1A2	2A6	2B6	2C8	2C9	2C19	2D6	2E1	3A4
Tiotropium							○		○
Tipranavir									●
TOLBUTamide					●	○			
Tolcapone		○							○
Tolterodine					○	○	●		●
Toremifene	○								●
Torsemide				○	●				
Tramadol[1]			○				●		○
Trazodone							○		●
Tretinoin		○	○	●	○				
Triazolam									●
Trifluoperazine	●								
Trimethadione					○	○		●	○
Trimethoprim					●				●
Trimipramine						●	●		●
Troleandomycin									●
Valdecoxib					○				○
Valproic acid		○	○		○	○		○	
Vardenafil									●
Venlafaxine					○	○	●		●
Verapamil	○		○		○			○	●
VinBLAStine							○		●
VinCRIStine									●
Vinorelbine							○		●
Voriconazole					●	●			○
Warfarin	○				●	○			○
Yohimbine							○		
Zafirlukast					●				
Zaleplon									○
Zidovudine		○			○	○			○
Zileuton	○				○				○
Ziprasidone	○								○
Zolmitriptan	○								
Zolpidem	○				○	○	○		●
Zonisamide						○			●
Zopiclone					●				●
Zuclopenthixol							●		

[1]This opioid analgesic is bioactivated *in vivo* via CYP2D6. Inhibiting this enzyme would decrease the effects of the analgesic. The active metabolite might also affect, or be affected by, CYP enzymes.
[2]Cyclophosphamide is bioactivated *in vivo* to acrolein via CYP2B6 and 3A4. Inhibiting these enzymes would decrease the effects of cyclophosphamide.
[3]Ifosfamide is bioactivated *in vivo* to acrolein via CYP3A4. Inhibiting this enzyme would decrease the effects of ifosfamide.
[4]Mestranol is bioactivated *in vivo* to ethinyl estradiol via CYP2C8/9. See Ethinyl Estradiol for additional CYP information.

CYTOCHROME P450 ENZYMES: SUBSTRATES, INHIBITORS, AND INDUCERS *(Continued)*

CYP Inhibitors

● = strong inhibitor
◑ = moderate inhibitor
○ = weak inhibitor

Drug	1A2	2A6	2B6	2C8	2C9	2C19	2D6	2E1	3A4
Acebutolol							○		
Acetaminophen									○
AcetaZOLAMIDE									○
Albendazole	○								
Alosetron	○							○	
Amiodarone	○	◑	○		◑	○	◑		◑
Amitriptyline	○				○	○	○	○	
Amlodipine	◑	○	○	○	○		○		○
Amphetamine							○		
Amprenavir						○			●
Anastrozole	○			○	○				○
Aprepitant					○	○			◑
Atazanavir	○			●	○				●
Atorvastatin									○
Azelastine			○		○	○	○		○
Azithromycin									○
Bepridil							○		
Betamethasone									○
Betaxolol							○		
Biperiden							○		
Bortezomib	○				○	◑	○		○
Bromazepam								○	
Bromocriptine	○								○
Buprenorphine	○	○				○	○		
BuPROPion							○		
Caffeine	●								◑
Candesartan				○	○				
Celecoxib				◑			○		
Cerivastatin									○
Chloramphenicol					○				○
Chloroquine							◑		
Chlorpheniramine							○		
ChlorproMAZINE							●	○	
Chlorzoxazone								○	○
Cholecalciferol					○	○	○		
Cimetidine	◑				○	◑	◑	○	◑
Cinacalcet							○		
Ciprofloxacin	●								○
Cisapride							○		○
Citalopram	○		○			○	○		
Clarithromycin	○								●
Clemastine							○		○
Clofazimine									○
Clofibrate		○							
ClomiPRAMINE							◑		
Clopidogrel					○				
Clotrimazole	○	○	○	○	○	○	○	○	◑
Clozapine	○				○	○	◑	○	○
Cocaine							●		○
Codeine							○		
Conivaptan									●
Cyclophosphamide									○

CYP Inhibitors *(continued)*

Drug	1A2	2A6	2B6	2C8	2C9	2C19	2D6	2E1	3A4
CycloSPORINE					○				◑
Danazol									○
Delavirdine	○				●	●	●		●
Desipramine		◑	◑				◑	○	◑
Dexmedetomidine	○				○		●		○
Dextromethorphan							○		
Diazepam						○			○
Diclofenac	◑				○			○	●
Dihydroergotamine									○
Diltiazem					○		○		◑
Dimethyl sulfoxide					○	○			
DiphenhydrAMINE							◑		
Disulfiram	○	○	○		○		○	●	○
Docetaxel									○
Dolasetron							○		
DOXOrubicin			◑				○		○
Doxycycline									◑
Drospirenone	○				○	○			○
Duloxetine							◑		
Econazole								○	
Efavirenz					○	○			○
Enoxacin	●								●
Entacapone	○	○			○	○	○	○	○
Eprosartan					○				
Ergotamine									○
Erythromycin	○								◑
Escitalopram							○		
Estradiol	○			○					
Estrogens, conjugated A/synthetic	○								
Estrogens, conjugated equine	○								
Ethinyl estradiol	○		○	○		○			○
Ethotoin						○			
Etoposide					○				○
Felbamate						○			
Felodipine				◑	○		○		○
Fenofibrate		○		◑	◑	○			
Fentanyl									○
Fexofenadine							○		
Flecainide							○		
Fluconazole	○				●	●			◑
Fluoxetine	◑		○		○	◑	●		○
Fluphenazine	○				○		○	○	
Flurazepam								○	
Flurbiprofen					●				
Flutamide	○								
Fluvastatin	○			○	◑		○		○
Fluvoxamine	●		○		○	●	○		○
Fosamprenavir (as amprenavir)						○			●
Gefitinib						○	○		
Gemfibrozil	◑			●	●	●			
Glyburide				○					○
Grapefruit juice									◑
Halofantrine							○		
Haloperidol							◑		◑
HydrALAZINE									○
HydrOXYzine							○		
Ibuprofen					●				
Ifosfamide									○

CYTOCHROME P450 ENZYMES: SUBSTRATES, INHIBITORS, AND INDUCERS *(Continued)*

CYP Inhibitors *(continued)*

Drug	1A2	2A6	2B6	2C8	2C9	2C19	2D6	2E1	3A4
Imatinib					○		○		●
Imipramine	○					○	◑	○	
Indinavir					○	○	○		●
Indomethacin					●	○			
Interferon alfa-2a	○								
Interferon alfa-2b	○								
Interferon gamma-1b	○							○	
Irbesartan				◑	◑		○		○
Isoflurane			○						
Isoniazid	○	◑			○	●	◑	◑	●
Isradipine									○
Itraconazole									●
Ketoconazole	●	◑	○	○	●	◑	◑		●
Ketoprofen					○				
Labetalol							○		
Lansoprazole					○	◑	○		○
Leflunomide					○				
Letrozole		●				○			
Lidocaine	●						◑		◑
Lomefloxacin	○								
Lomustine							○		○
Loratadine				○		◑	○		
Losartan	○			◑	◑	○			○
Lovastatin					○		○		○
Mefenamic acid					●				
Mefloquine							○		○
Meloxicam					○				
Mephobarbital						○			
Mestranol	○		○			○			○
Methadone							◑		○
Methimazole	○	○	○		○	○	◑	○	○
Methotrimeprazine							○		
Methoxsalen	●	●			○	○	○	○	○
Methsuximide						○			
Methylphenidate							○		
MethylPREDNISolone				○					○
Metoclopramide							○		
Metoprolol							○		
Metronidazole					○				◑
Metyrapone		○							
Mexiletine	●								
Miconazole	◑	●	○		●	●	●	◑	●
Midazolam				○	○				○
Mifepristone							○		○
Mirtazapine	○								○
Mitoxantrone									○
Moclobemide	○					○	○		
Modafinil	○	○			○	●		○	○
Montelukast				○	○				
Nalidixic acid	○								
Nateglinide					○				
Nefazodone	○		○	○			○		●
Nelfinavir	○		○		○	○	○		●
Nevirapine	○						○		○
NiCARdipine					●	◑	◑		●
Nicotine		○						○	
NIFEdipine	◑				○		○		○

CYP Inhibitors *(continued)*

Drug	1A2	2A6	2B6	2C8	2C9	2C19	2D6	2E1	3A4
Nilutamide						○			
Nisoldipine	○								○
Nitrendipine									○
Nizatidine									○
Norfloxacin	●								◑
Nortriptyline							○	○	
Ofloxacin	●								
Olanzapine	○				○	○	○		○
Omeprazole	○				◑	●	○		○
Ondansetron	○				○		○		
Orphenadrine	○	○	○		○	○	○	○	○
Oxcarbazepine						○			
Oxprenolol							○		
Oxybutynin				○			○		○
Pantoprazole					◑				
Paroxetine	○		◑		○	○	●		○
Peginterferon alfa-2a	○								
Peginterferon alfa-2b	○								
Pentamidine					○	○	○		○
Pentoxifylline	○								
Pergolide							●		○
Perphenazine	○						○		
Phencyclidine									○
Pilocarpine		○						○	○
Pimozide						○	○	○	○
Pindolol							○		
Pioglitazone				◑	○	○	◑		
Piroxicam					●				
Pravastatin					○		○		○
Praziquantel							○		
PrednisoLONE									○
Primaquine	●						○		○
Probenecid						○			
Progesterone					○	○			○
Promethazine							○		
Propafenone	○						○		
Propofol	◑				○	◑	○	○	●
Propoxyphene					○		○		○
Propranolol	○						○		
Pyrimethamine					◑		◑		
Quinidine					○		●		●
Quinine				◑	◑		●		○
Quinupristin									○
Rabeprazole				◑		◑	○		○
Ranitidine	○						○		
Ranolazine							○		○
Risperidone							○		○
Ritonavir				●	○	○	●	○	●
Rofecoxib	○								
Ropinirole	○						●		
Rosiglitazone				◑	○	○	○		
Saquinavir					○	○	○		◑
Selegiline	○	○			○	○	○	○	○
Sertraline	○		◑	○	○	◑	◑		◑
Sildenafil	○				○	○	○	○	○
Simvastatin				○	○		○		
Sirolimus									○
Sorafenib			○	○					
Sulconazole	○	○			○	○	○	○	○
SulfaDIAZINE					●				

CYTOCHROME P450 ENZYMES: SUBSTRATES, INHIBITORS, AND INDUCERS *(Continued)*

CYP Inhibitors *(continued)*

Drug	1A2	2A6	2B6	2C8	2C9	2C19	2D6	2E1	3A4
Sulfamethoxazole					◑				
Sulfinpyrazone					◑				
SulfiSOXAZOLE					●				
Tacrine	○								
Tacrolimus									○
Tamoxifen			○	◑	○				○
Telithromycin							○		●
Telmisartan						○			
Teniposide					○				○
Tenofovir	○								
Terbinafine							●		
Testosterone									○
Tetracycline									◑
Theophylline	○								
Thiabendazole	●								
Thioridazine	○				○		◑	○	
Thiotepa			○						
Thiothixene							○		
Ticlopidine	○				○	●	◑	○	○
Timolol							○		
Tioconazole	○	○			○	○	○	○	
Tocainide	○								
TOLBUTamide				○	●				
Tolcapone					○				
Topiramate						○			
Torsemide						○			
Tranylcypromine	◑	●		○	○	◑	◑	○	○
Trazodone							◑		○
Tretinoin					○				
Triazolam				○	○				
Trimethoprim				◑	◑				
Tripelennamine							◑		
Triprolidine							○		
Troleandomycin									◑
Valdecoxib				○	○	○			
Valproic acid					○	○	○		○
Valsartan					○				
Venlafaxine			○				○		○
Verapamil	○				○		○		◑
VinBLAStine							○		○
VinCRIStine									○
Vinorelbine							○		○
Voriconazole					○	○			◑
Warfarin					◑	○			
Yohimbine							○		
Zafirlukast	○			○	◑	○	○		○
Zileuton	◑								
Ziprasidone							○		○

CYP Inducers

● = effectively induced
○ = not effectively induced

Drug	1A2	2A6	2B6	2C8	2C9	2C19	2D6	2E1	3A4
Aminoglutethimide	●					●			●
Amobarbital		●							
Aprepitant					○				○
Bexarotene									○
Bosentan					○				○
Calcitriol									○
Carbamazepine	●		●	●	●	●			●
Clofibrate			○					○	○
Colchicine				○	○			○	○
Cyclophosphamide			○	○	○				
Dexamethasone		○	○	○	○				○
Dicloxacillin									○
Efavirenz (in liver only)			○						○
Estradiol									○
Estrogens, conjugated A/synthetic									○
Estrogens, conjugated equine									○
Exemestane									○
Felbamate									○
Fosphenytoin (as phenytoin)			●	●	●	●			●
Griseofulvin	○			○	○				○
Hydrocortisone									○
Ifosfamide				○	○				
Insulin preparations	○								
Isoniazid (after D/C)								○	
Lansoprazole	○								
MedroxyPROGESTERone									○
Mephobarbital		○							
Metyrapone									○
Modafinil	○		○						○
Moricizine	○								○
Nafcillin									●
Nevirapine			●						●
Norethindrone						○			
Omeprazole	○								
Oxcarbazepine									●
Paclitaxel									○
Pantoprazole	○								○
Pentobarbital		●							●
Phenobarbital	●	●	●	●	●				●
Phenytoin			●	●	●	●			●
Pioglitazone									○
PredniSONE						○			○
Primaquine	○								
Primidone[1]	●		●	●	●				●
Rifabutin									●
Rifampin	●	●	●	●	●	●			●
Rifapentine				●	●				●
Ritonavir (long-term)	○			○	○				○
Rofecoxib									○
Secobarbital		●		●	●				
Sulfinpyrazone									○
Terbinafine									○
Topiramate									○
Tretinoin								○	
Troglitazone									○
Valproic acid		○							

[1]Primidone is partially metabolized to phenobarbital. See Phenobarbital for additional CYP information.

EXTRAVASATION TREATMENT OF DRUGS

Medication Extravasated	Cold / Warm Pack	Antidote
Vasopressors		
Dobutamine Dopamine Epinephrine Norepinephrine Phenylephrine	None	Phentolamine (Regitine®) Mix 5 mg with 9 mL of NS Inject a small amount of this dilution into extravasated area. Blanching should reverse immediately. Monitor site. If blanching should recur, additional injections of phentolamine may be needed.
I.V. Fluids and Other Medications		
Aminophylline Calcium Dextrose, 10% Electrolyte solutions Esmolol Magnesium sulfate Metoprolol Nafcillin Parenteral nutrition preparations Phenytoin Potassium Radiocontrast media Sodium solutions	Cold	

FEVER DUE TO DRUGS

Most Common

Atropine	Cephalosporins	Procainamide
Amphotericin B	Interferon	Quinidine
Asparaginase	Methyldopa	Salicylates (high doses)
Barbiturates	Penicillins	Streptomycin
Bleomycin	Phenytoin	Sulfonamides

Less Common

Allopurinol	Hydralazine	Nitrofurantoin
Antihistamines	Hydroxyurea	Pentazocine
Azathioprine	Imipenem	Procarbazine
Carbamazepine	Iodides	Propylthiouracil
Cimetidine	Isoniazid	Rifampin
Cisplatin	Mercaptopurine	Streptokinase
Colistimethate	Metoclopramide	Triamterene
Diazoxide	Nifedipine	Vancomycin
Folic acid	NSAIDs	

References

Cunha BA, "Antibiotic Side Effects," *Med Clin North Am*, 2001, 85(1):149-85.

Mackowiak PA and LeMaistre CF, "Drug Fever: A Critical Appraisal of Conventional Concepts. An Analysis of 51 Episodes in Two Dallas Hospitals and 97 Episodes Reported in the English Literature," *Ann Intern Med*, 1987, 106(5):728-33.

Tabor PA, "Drug-Induced Fever," Table 2, "Drugs Implicated in Causing a Fever," *Drug Intell Clin Pharm*, 1986, 20(6):416.

PORPHYRIA: SAFE AND UNSAFE DRUGS

Categories of Safe and Unsafe Drugs in Acute Intermittent Porphyria, Hereditary Coproporphyria, and Variegate Porphyria

Unsafe	Safe
Alcohol	Acetaminophen
Aminolevulinic acid	Aspirin
Barbiturates	Atropine
Carbamazepine	Bromides
Carisoprodol	Glucocorticoids
Danazol	Insulin
Ergots	Narcotic analgesics
Ethchlorvynol	Penicillin and derivatives
Glutethimide	Phenothiazines
Griseofulvin	Streptomycin
Mephenytoin	
Meprobamate	
Methyprylon	
Mifepristone	
Phenytoin	
Porfimer	
Pyrazolones	
Succinimides	
Sulfonamide antibiotics	
Synthetic estrogens and progestins	
Valproic acid	
Verteporfin	

INTERNATIONAL BRAND NAME INDEX

The following countries are included in this index and are abbreviated as follows:

Argentina (AR)
Australia (AU)
Austria (AT)
Bangladesh (BD)
Belgium (BE)
Brazil (BR)
Bulgaria (BG)
Canada (CA)
Chile (CL)
China (CN)
Colombia (CO)
Costa Rica (CR)
Croatia / Hrvatska (HR)
Cypress (CY)
Czech Republic (CZ)
Denmark (DK)
Dominican Republic (DO)
Ecuador (EC)
Egypt (EG)
El Salvador (SV)
Finland (FI)
France (FR)
Germany (DE)
Great Britain [UK] (GB)
Greece (GR)
Guatemala (GT)
Honduras (HN)
Hong Kong (HK)
Hungary (HU)
Iceland (IS)
India (IN)
Indonesia (ID)
Ireland (IE)
Israel (IL)
Italy (IT)
Japan (JP)
Jordan (JO)
Korea [South] (KR)
Kuwait (KW)
Lebanon (LB)
Lithuania (LT)
Luxemborg (LU)
Malta (MT)
Malaysia (MY)
Mexico (MX)
Monaco (MC)
Morocco (MA)
Netherlands (NL)
New Zealand (NZ)
Norway (NO)
Panama (PA)
Peru (PE)
Phillipines (PH)
Poland (PL)
Portugal (PT)
Puerto Rico (PR)
Romania (RO)
Russian Federation (RU)
Singapore (SG)
Slovak Republic (SK)
Slovenia (SI)
South Africa (ZA)
Spain (ES)
Sri Lanka (LK)
Sweden (SE)
Switzerland (CH)
Syria (SY)
Taiwan (TW)
Thailand (TH)
Turkey (TR)
Ukraine (UA)
Uruguay (UY)
Venezuela (VE)
Viet Nam (VN)
Yugoslavia (YU)

Other Products Offered by Lexi-Comp®

Drug Information Handbook

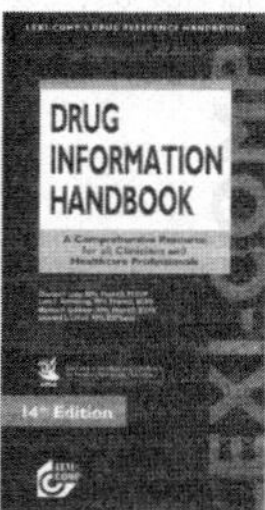

This easy-to-use reference is compiled especially for the pharmacist, physician, or other healthcare professional needing quick access to drug information. The book is organized in four sections for easy retrieval of critical information. Includes drug monographs, listed alphabetically, with extensive cross-referencing.

Includes: Over 1300 drug monographs; Drug Interaction information; Labeled and Investigational indications; Up to 33 key fields per monograph including Medication Safety Issues; Pharmacodynamics/Kinetics; Dosing for renal/hepatic impairment; and a Pharmacologic Category Index

The valuable Appendix information includes hundreds of charts and reviews of special topics such as guidelines for treatment and therapy recommendations.

Published in cooperation with APhA.

Drug Interactions Handbook

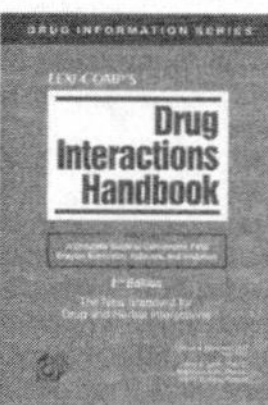

The new standard for evaluating drug and herbal interactions, this comprehensive handbook was designed to allow convenient access to interaction data. More than 150,000 interactions are documented in a user-friendly structure that is extensively indexed and fully cross referenced by page number.

Includes: The most comprehensive and clinically-relevant table of Cytochrome P450 enzyme substrates, inducers, and inhibitors in the industry;the greatest number of potential interactions compared to any other interactions references; Drug, food, herbal, and alcohol interactions; Reliability Rating - Indicating the quality and nature of documentation for an interaction; Risk Rating - A: No Known Interaction, B: No Action Needed, C: Monitor Therapy, D: Consider Therapy Modification, X: Avoid; and Severity Rating - Indicating the reported or possible magnitude of an interaction

Geriatric Dosage Handbook

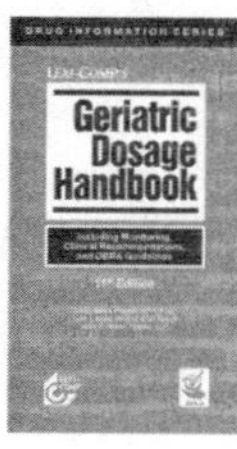

Designed for any healthcare professional managing geriatric patients.

Includes: Complete adult and geriatric dosing; Special geriatric considerations; Up to 36 key fields of information in each monograph including Medication Safety Issues; and Extensive information on drug interactions as well as dosing for patients with renal/hepatic impairment

To order call Customer Service at 1-866-397-3433 or go to www.lexi.com.
Outside of the U.S. call: 330-650-6506 or www.lexi.com

Other Products Offered by Lexi-Comp®

Pediatric Dosage Handbook

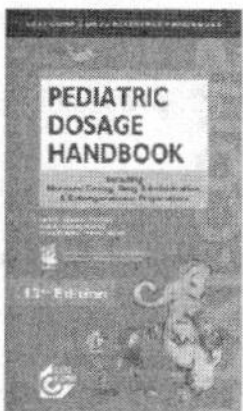

Designed for any healthcare professional requiring quick access to comprehensive, pediatric drug information.

Includes: Over 745 drug monographs, including vaccines; Extemporaneous preparation formulas; Up to 35 key fields of information per monograph including Medication Safety Issues, Neonatal and Pediatric Dosing

Pharmacology Companion Guide

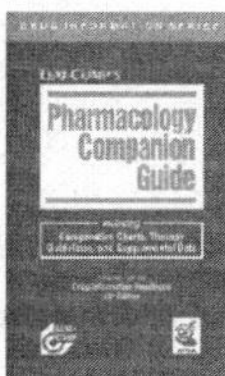

This guide supplies the best of Lexi-Comp's comparative charts, therapy guidelines, and supplemental data. Ideal for healthcare providers who require a quick reference to all the key appendix information found in our popular *Drug Information Handbook* or as a companion to our PDA software.

Includes: Abbreviations and measurements; ACLS Algorithms; Cytochrome P450 and Drug Interactions; and Laboratory Values

Pediatric Pharmacology Companion Guide

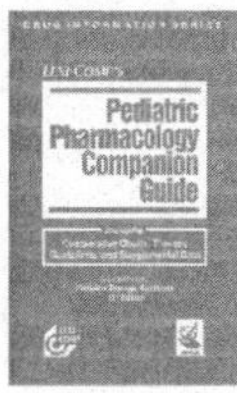

This guide supplies the best of Lexi-Comp's comparative charts, therapy guidelines, and supplemental data. Ideal as a quick reference to all the key appendix information found in our popular *Pediatric Dosage Handbook* or as a companion to our PDA software.

Includes: Apgar Scoring System; CPR Pediatric Drug Dosages; Immunization Guidelines; and Pediatric ALS Algorithms

Drug-Induced Nutrient Depletion Handbook

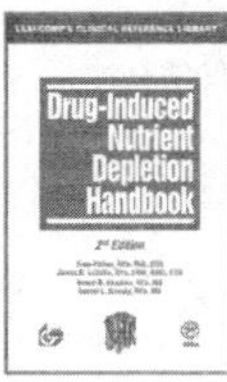

Provides a complete listing of drugs known to deplete the body of nutritional compounds.

Includes: Alphabetical listing of drugs most commonly prescribed (by Brand and Generic name) cross-referenced by page number to nutrients depleted; Key points of information include Abstract & Studies section; and Nutrient monographs with concise descriptions of the effects of depletion, biological function and effect, sources of repletion, RDA, dosage range, and dietary sources for nutrients

To order call Customer Service at 1-866-397-3433 or go to www.lexi.com.
Outside of the U.S. call: 330-650-6506 or www.lexi.com

Other Products Offered by Lexi-Comp®

Drug Information Handbook for Perioperative Nursing

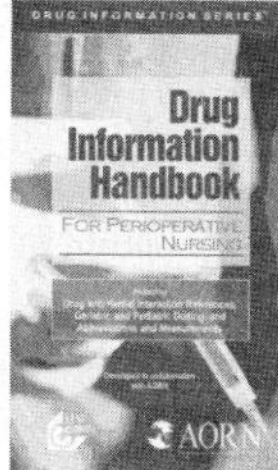

Designed especially for perioperative nurses, Registered Nurses practicing in operative and interventional procedure settings, and upper-division nursing students seeking a distinctive reference for dosing, administration, monitoring, and patient education criteria for perioperative patient care environments

Includes: Up to 40 fields per monograph including Medication Safety data; Adult, Pediatric, and Geriatric Dosing guidelines; and information on each phase of the perioperative encounter and how it is addressed, with emphasis on special situations central to perioperative patient care

Pharmacogenomics Handbook

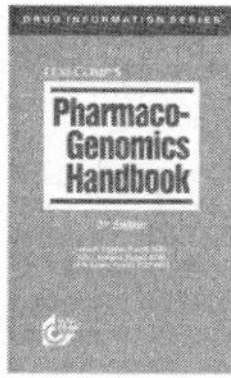

Ideal for any healthcare professional or student wishing to gain insight into the emerging field of pharmacogenomics.

Includes: Information concerning key genetic variations that may influence drug disposition and/or sensitivity; brief introductions to fundamental concepts in genetics and genomics. A foundation for all clinicians who will be called on to integrate rapidly-expanding genomic knowledge into the management of drug therapy,

Laboratory Test Handbook

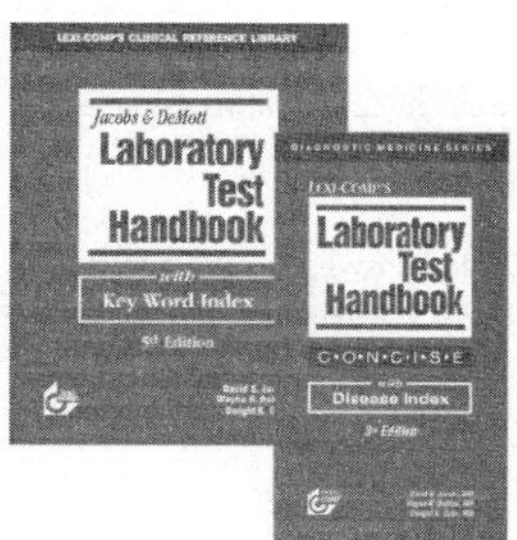

An invaluable source of information for anyone interested in diagnostic laboratory testing.

Includes: 960 tests; Up to 25 fields per test; Extensive cross-referencing; Over 12,000 references; and Key Word Index: test result, disease, organ system and syndrome

Clinicians, nurse practitioners, residents, nurses, and students will appreciate the Concise version of the *Laboratory Test Handbook* for its convenience as a quick reference. This abridged version includes 876 tests.

To order call Customer Service at 1-866-397-3433 or go to www.lexi.com.
Outside of the U.S. call: 330-650-6506 or www.lexi.com

Other Products Offered by Lexi-Comp®

Drug Information Handbook for Oncology

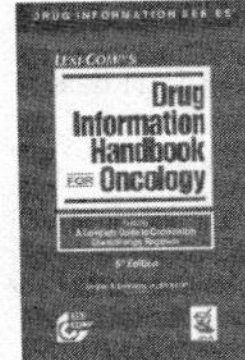

Designed for oncology professionals requiring information on combination chemotherapy regimens and dosing protocols.

Includes: Monographs containing warnings, adverse reaction profiles, drug interactions, dosing for specific indications, vesicant, emetic potential, combination regimens, and more; Where applicable, a special Combination Chemotherapy field that will link you to specific oncology monographs; Special Topics such as Cancer Treatment Related Complications, Bone Marrow Transplantation, and Drug Development

Diagnostic Procedures Handbook

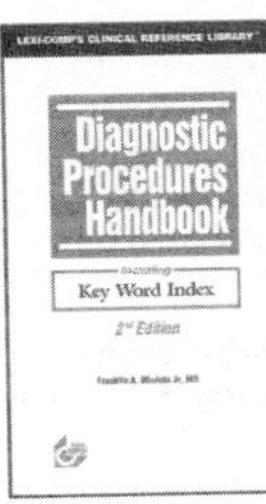

A concise resource for physicians, nurses, students, medical records personnel, or anyone needing quick access to diagnostic procedure information. An excellent source of information in areas such as allergy, infectious diseases, cardiology, urology, and many more.

Includes: 309 common (and less common) procedures; and up to 28 fields of information per monograph

Drug Information Handbook for the Allied Health Professional

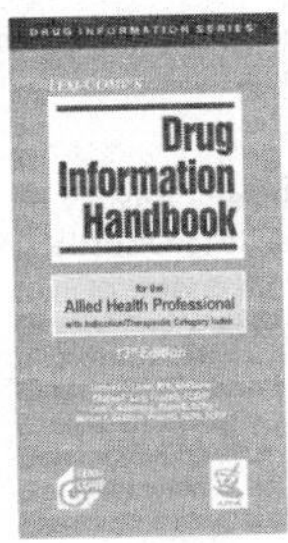

Designed for medical secretaries, transcriptionists, pharmacy technicians, and other allied health professionals requiring quick access to basic information regarding medications.

Includes: Over 1600 monographs offering up to 13 key fields of information and 125 pages of updated, valuable charts and tables

To order call Customer Service at 1-866-397-3433 or go to www.lexi.com.
Outside of the U.S. call: 330-650-6506 or www.lexi.com

Other Products Offered by Lexi-Comp®

Drug Information Handbook for Psychiatry

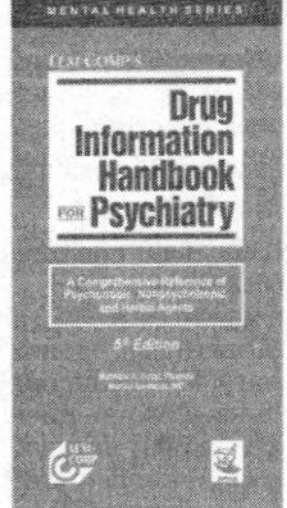

Designed for any healthcare professional requiring quick access to comprehensive drug information as it relates to mental health issues.

Includes: Detailed drug monographs for psychotropic, nonpsychotropic, and herbal medications; Special fields such as Mental Health Comment (useful clinical pearls), Medication Safety Issues, Effects on Mental Status, and Effects on Psychiatric Treatment

Psychotropic Drug Information Handbook

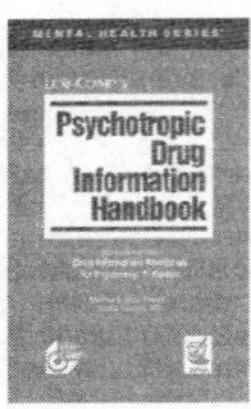

Designed for any healthcare professional requiring a small, portable, quick reference to psychotropic drug information. This is a pocket-sized companion to the *Drug Information Handbook for Psychiatry*.

Includes: All psychotropic agents; Adult and pediatric dosing; FDA-approved and unlabeled uses; Medication safety issues; and Useful clinical pearls

Rating Scales for Mental Health

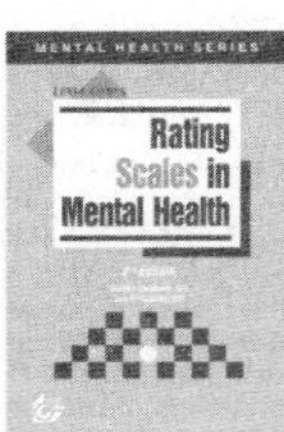

Ideal for clinicians as well as administrators, this book provides an overview of over 100 recommended rating scales for mental assessment.

Includes: Rating scales for conditions such as General Anxiety, Social/Family Functioning, Eating Disorders, and Sleep Disorders; and Monograph format covering such topics as Overview of Scale, General Applications, Psychometric Properties, and References